BSAVA Textbook of
Veterinary Nursing
6th edition

Editors

Barbara Cooper CertEd LicIPD DTM HonAssocRCVS RVN
The College of Animal Welfare,
Headland House, Chord Business Park, London Road, Godmanchester,
Huntingdon, Cambridgeshire PE29 2BQ

Elizabeth Mullineaux BVM&S CertSHP DVM&S MRCVS
Capital Veterinary Services Ltd,
Haddington, East Lothian EH41 4JN

Lynn Turner MA VetMB MRCVS
St David's Farm and Equine Practice,
Nutwell Estate, Lympstone, Exeter EX8 5AN

NEW – 3D models added to this edition – see page xiv for details
BSAVA has partnered with Ludenso to add augmented reality (AR) to this book.
See page xiv for details of how to download the **Ludenso Explore app** and
access these enrichments.

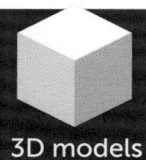

3D models

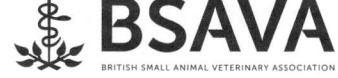

BRITISH SMALL ANIMAL VETERINARY ASSOCIATION

19470PUBS24

Published by:

British Small Animal Veterinary Association
Woodrow House, 1 Telford Way,
Waterwells Business Park, Quedgeley,
Gloucester GL2 2AB

A Company Limited by Guarantee in England
Registered Company No. 2837793
Registered as a Charity

The publishers, editors and contributors cannot take responsibility for information
provided on dosages and methods of application of drugs mentioned or referred to in
this publication. Details of this kind must be verified in each case by individual users
from up to date literature published by the manufacturers or suppliers of those
drugs. Veterinary nurses are reminded that in each case they must follow all
appropriate national legislation and regulations from time to time in force.

Printed in the UK by Zenith Media, Pontypool NP4 0DG
Printed on FSC® certified timber supporting sustainable forestry/forest management.

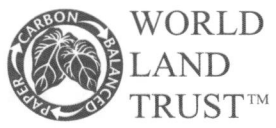

WORLD
LAND
TRUST™

www.carbonbalancedpaper.com
CBP023712

Carbon Balancing is delivered by World Land
Trust, an international conservation charity, who
protects the world's most biologically important
and threatened habitats acre by acre. Their
Carbon Balanced Programme offsets emissions
through the purchase and preservation of high
conservation value forests.

MIX
Paper | Supporting
responsible forestry
FSC® C019670

Contents

Contributors

Nicola Ackerman PGDip RVN CertSAN CertVNECC VTS(Nutrition) HonMBVNA
Plymouth Veterinary Group
Plymouth
Devon PL6 8RP

Wendy Adams RVN
Guide Dogs National Breeding Centre
Banbury Road
Bishop's Tachbrook
Leamington Spa
Warwickshire CV33 9WF

Davina Anderson MA VetMB PhD DipSAS(ST) DipECVS MRCVS
Anderson Moores Veterinary Specialists Ltd
The Granary
Bunstead Barns
Poles Lane
Hursley
Winchester SO21 2LL

Amanda Boag MA VetMB DipACVIM DipACVECC DipECVECC FHEA MRCVS
IVC Evidensia UK
The Chocolate Factory
Keynsham
Bristol BS31 2AU

Victoria Bowes DipHE DipRSA RVN
Moreton Morrell College
Moreton Morrell
Warwickshire CV35 9BL

Abby Caine MA VetMB DipECVDI CertVDI MRCVS
Dick White Referrals
Station Farm
London Road
Six Mile Bottom
Cambridgeshire CB8 0UH

Barbara Cooper CertEd LicIPD DTM HonAssocRCVS RVN
The College of Animal Welfare
Headland House
Chord Business Park
London Road
Godmanchester
Huntingdon
Cambridgeshire PE29 2BQ

Susan Dawson BVMS PhD MRCVS
Institute of Veterinary Science
University of Liverpool
Chester High Road
Neston CH64 7TE

Claire Defries PGDip DipAVN(Medical) RVN
The College of Animal Welfare
Headland House
Chord Business Park
London Road
Godmanchester
Huntingdon
Cambridgeshire PE29 2BQ

Ruth Dennis MA VetMB DVR DipECVDI FRCVS
Animal Health Trust
Lanwades Park
Kentford
Newmarket
Suffolk CB8 7UU

Gary England BVetMed PhD DVetMed DVR CertVA DVRep DipACT DipECAR PFHEA FRCVS
School of Veterinary Medicine and Science
University of Nottingham
Sutton Bonington
Loughborough
Leicestershire LE12 5RD

Maggie Fisher BVetMed CBiol FRSB DipEVPC MRCVS
Veterinary Research Management
The Mews Studio
Portland Road
Malvern
Worcestershire WR14 2TA

Stuart Ford-Fennah BSc(Hons) RVN PGDipBusAdmin AIOSH MCMI MInstLM
Cave Veterinary Specialists
West Buckland
Wellington
Somerset TA21 9LE

Vicky Ford-Fennah BSc(Hons) RVN VTS(Anesthesia/Analgesia) A1 VPAC
Linnaeus, Friars Gate
1011 Stratford Road
Shirley
Solihull B90 4NH

Mary Fraser BVMS PhD CertVD MAcadMEd PGCHE FHEA CBiol FRSB FRSPH FRCVS
G&F Academy
Glenfarg
Perth PH2 9QD

Isuru Gajanayake BVSc CertSAM DipACVIM DipECVIM-CA DipACVN MRCVS
Willows Veterinary Centre & Referral Service
Highlands Road
Shirley
Solihull
West Midlands B90 4NH

Robyn Gear BVSc DipSAM DipECVIM-CA
School of Environmental and Animal Sciences
Unitec Institute of Technology
Private Bag 92025
Victoria Street West
Auckland 1142
New Zealand

Julie Gerrish VTS(Surgery) DipAVN(Surg) RVN
North Downs Specialist Referrals
Friesian Buildings 3&4
The Brewerstreet Dairy Business Park
Brewer Street
Bletchingley RH1 4QP

Simon Girling BVMS(Hons) DipZooMed DipECZM(ZHM) CBiol FRSB EurProBiol FRCVS
Royal Zoological Society of Scotland
134 Corstorphine Road
Edinburgh EH12 6TS

Andrea Jeffery MSc FHEA DipAVN CertEd RVN
University of Bristol
Langford House
Bristol BS40 5HB

Anne Lawson BVMS TechIOSH MRCVS
Ashgrove Veterinary Centre
10 Belmont Road
Aberdeen AB25 3SR

Philip Lhermette BSc(Hons) CBiol FRSB BVetMed FRCVS
Elands Veterinary Clinic
St John's Church
London Road
Dunton Green
Sevenoaks TN13 2TE

Jill Macdonald DipAVN(Surgical) RVN FHEA
ONCORE ePD
Walnut Lodge
Farm Lane
South Littleton
Evesham WR11 8TL

Racheal Marshall RVN CertVNECC
Vets Now, Penguin House
Castle Riggs
Dunfermline
Fife KY11 8SG

Helen Mathie Chartered Physiotherapist MSc(Vet Phys) MCSP HCPC Veterinary Physiotherapist ACPAT Cat A RAMP
SyncThermology
Crewe Farm
Crewe Hill Lane
Crewe by Farndon
Cheshire CH3 6PD

John McGarry MSc PhD
Institute of Veterinary Science
University of Liverpool
Chester High Road
Neston CH64 7TE

Cathryn S. Mellersh BSc PhD
Animal Health Trust
Lanwades Park
Kentford
Newmarket
Suffolk CB8 7UU

Elizabeth Mullineaux BVM&S CertSHP DVM&S MRCVS
Capital Veterinary Services Ltd
Haddington
East Lothian EH41 4JN

Jo Murrell BVSc(Hons) PhD DipECVAA MRCVS
Highcroft Veterinary Referrals
Whitchurch
Bristol BS14 9BE

Louise O'Dwyer † MBA BSc(Hons) VTS(Anesthesia/Analgesia, & ECC) DipAVN(Medical & Surgical) RVN
Vets Now
Penguin House
Castle Riggs
Dunfermline
Fife KY11 8SG

James A.C. Oliver BVSc PhD CertVOphthal DipECVO MRCVS
Dick White Referrals
Station Farm
London Road
Six Mile Bottom
Cambridgeshire CB8 0UH

Ursula van der Riet DipVetNur
Cape Animal Dentistry Service
78 Rosmead Avenue
Kenilworth
Cape Town
Western Cape 7708
South Africa

Julie Sales DCR
Davies Veterinary Specialists
Manor Farm Business Park
Higham Gobion
Hitchin SG5 3HR

Jenny Smith BSc(Hons) DipAVN(Surgical) RVN
School of Veterinary Medicine and Science
University of Nottingham
Sutton Bonington
Loughborough
Leicestershire LE12 5RD

Lynn Turner MA VetMB MRCVS
St David's Farm and Equine Practice
Nutwell Estate
Lympstone
Exeter EX8 5AN

Cedric Tutt BVSc MMedVet(Med) DipEVDC MRCVS
Cape Animal Dentistry Service
78 Rosmead Avenue
Kenilworth
Cape Town
Western Cape 7708
South Africa

Clare Wilson MA VetMB CCAB PGDipCABC MRCVS
Behaviour Veterinary Practice
Bramley House
Coventry Road
Church Lawford
Rugby CV23 9HB

Elizabeth Wright MPharm PgDip
The Royal (Dick) School of Veterinary Studies
and The Roslin Institute
Easter Bush Campus
Midlothian EH25 9RG

Alison Young DipAVN(Surgery) VTS(Surgery) RVN
Queen Mother Hospital for Animals
The Royal Veterinary College
Hawkshead Lane
North Mymms
Hatfield
Hertfordshire AL9 7TA

Foreword

I am delighted to be able to write the foreword to this sixth edition of the *BSAVA Textbook of Veterinary Nursing*. The evolution of this text, since the first edition was published in 1966, has closely followed the path of the veterinary nursing profession as it has grown and developed. The range of skills expected from the registered veterinary nurse (RVN) is highlighted by the length and breadth of this completely updated text book.

The addition of new chapters on Nurse-led clinics, Managing the hospital ward and basic patient care and Nursing interventions in hospitalized animals, clearly illustrates that the RVN is an essential and integral part of the veterinary team and that they play vital parts in so many different aspects of both primary care and referral practice. As recognition of the pressures all veterinary professionals, including RVNs, face in practice, there is information on mental health and wellbeing in several chapters. Chapter 9 particularly considers staff wellbeing in the context of communicating with colleagues, and acknowledges the emotional impact of client relationships and quality of life discussions.

Each chapter is clearly laid out with specific learning objectives and illustrated with a myriad of high-quality colour photographs, together with numerous tables and diagrams that make this an easy text to use. The references and further reading list, together with useful websites, allows the interested nurse to read around the subject if needed. The provision of self-assessment questions at the end of each chapter allows the reader to ensure they have a good understanding of each section and provides a basis for reflection on their learning.

This sixth edition, which focuses on dogs, cats and exotic pets, has been written with the input and expertise of numerous subject specialists. The authors, editors and publication team at Woodrow House must be congratulated on producing this superb new edition that will be an invaluable resource for both trainee and qualified veterinary nurses.

Sue Paterson MA VetMB DVD DipECVD FRCVS
BSAVA President 2019–2020

Preface

This is the sixth edition of the *BSAVA Textbook of Veterinary Nursing*. It is the perfect resource for veterinary nurse students undertaking or that have recently completed their Level 3 Diploma or Degree in Veterinary Nursing. The book introduces the full range of veterinary nursing skills, theory and knowledge that students will need to succeed; the biological science underpinning veterinary nursing and the core clinical skills for effective practice.

The book has put the theory into context, bringing the subject to life. Whether preparing for the first practice placement, completing an assignment, revising for an examination or starting a first veterinary nursing job, this edition will provide support to the reader.

In addition to covering the many veterinary procedures that a student veterinary nurse will come across, the book provides a quickly accessible and thorough guide to patient assessment techniques, patient care, preoperative and postoperative routines, pain management, disease prevention, the administration of drugs, diagnostic aids and current approaches to wound management.

The thoughtfully organized index makes finding relevant information convenient. This sixth edition also includes a range of new learning features throughout each chapter. Each chapter is designed to assist the reader as they use the book to support their learning in clinical practice. The chapters have been organized as far as possible to enable the reader to extend their knowledge further, starting with identifying what the reader can expect to know after working through the chapter and completing the self-assessment at the end. Definitions are explained and technical concepts expanded upon. Professional and legal issues are identified where relevant and, where appropriate, evidence-based principles are applied. Each chapter finishes with a combined reference and reading list along with details of useful websites.

The work of 39 contributors, in addition to the expertise of the publishing team, has resulted in the production of a contemporary textbook that satisfies the requirement upon us all to delivery high-quality care for both the patient and the client.

Barbara Cooper
Elizabeth Mullineaux
Lynn Turner
February 2020

NEW – 3D models added to this edition

Powered by 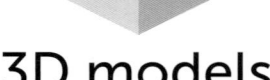 **LUDENSO**

What enrichment is in this book?...

3D models

Where to find them...

Look for visual AR markings next to the image in your book. These symbols indicate digital enhancements.

Open the app and find a list of enriched resources linked to your book.

How to use...

SCAN ME

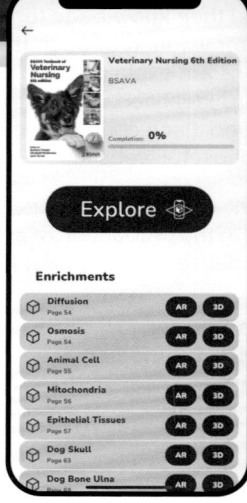
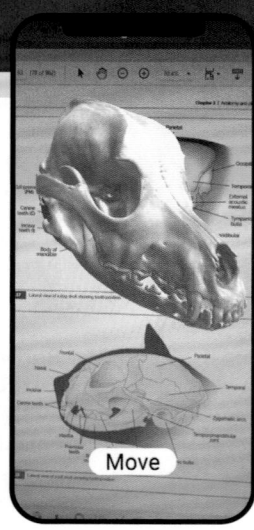

1. Scan the QR code with your phone or tablet and download the Ludenso Explore app. You will automatically be directed to the ***BSAVA Textbook of Veterinary Nursing 6th edition***.

2. Click on the 'AR' button next to your chosen enrichment and hover your phone over the relevant page of the book or ebook.

Send us your feedback

If you have any questions or comments on these new features, or ideas for new enrichment that could be added, we'd love to hear from you – please contact us at **publications@bsava.com**.

Let your colleagues and friends know

Anyone who already owns a copy of the 6th edition of the Textbook, or has access to the ebook version, should also be able to see the 3D models – but they won't know about it! If you enjoy these additions please help to spread the word to the thousands of people who already have this book.

Android & iOS

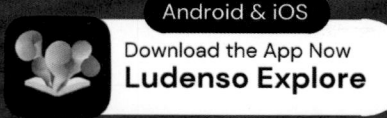
Download the App Now
Ludenso Explore

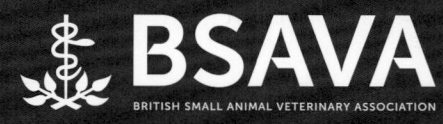
BSAVA
BRITISH SMALL ANIMAL VETERINARY ASSOCIATION

Chapter 1

Professional veterinary nursing

Claire Defries

Learning objectives

After studying this chapter, readers will have the knowledge to:

- Interpret the Royal College of Veterinary Surgeons (RCVS) Code of Professional Conduct for Veterinary Nurses
- Identify the legal and ethical aspects of veterinary nursing
- Demonstrate knowledge of the organization and legislation related to a veterinary business
- Critically review and evaluate literature and presentations
- Discuss the nature of evidence-based veterinary nursing
- Identify personal and professional limits, and know how to seek professional advice, assistance and support when necessary
- Demonstrate a commitment to learning and professional development, both personally and as a member of a profession actively engaged in work-based learning

Introduction

In recent years, veterinary nurses in the United Kingdom (UK) have embraced changes in regulations that make Registered Veterinary Nurses (RVNs) accountable and responsible for their actions. Veterinary nursing is now recognized as a profession in its own right, which means that veterinary nurses must be professional, responsible and accountable; these terms are defined in Figure 1.1.

In this chapter various frameworks are discussed that can be applied by veterinary nurses to work through every day scenarios and more difficult or complicated situations.

Term	Definition
Responsibility	Something that is your job or duty to deal with
Accountability	An obligation or willingness to be answerable or culpable for something
Professionalism	The combination of all the qualities that are connected with trained and skilled people (e.g. character, status, high standards, integrity and trust)

1.1 Definition of terms encountered in professional veterinary nursing.

When making decisions on a course of action veterinary nurses should be clear about their role within the practice and the profession, and be mindful of any possible consequences. As a result of being accountable for their actions temperance, prudence and patience should be exercised to ensure that actions taken are responsible and can be justified. Resilience is also a key quality for veterinary nurses to develop, particularly when dealing with difficult and challenging circumstances. When making decisions or reflecting on decisions made the following questions can be considered:

- Has good animal welfare been promoted?
- Has the animal's welfare been compromised?
- Have legal and professional frameworks been adhered to?
- Was the decision made ethical?

The overarching issue for veterinary nurses is always the welfare of the patient; however, there are other factors to take into account such as ethics, professional conduct and, perhaps most importantly, working within the law. Some examples of how all these things can be considered together in practice are given at the end of the chapter.

The RCVS Code of Professional Conduct for Veterinary Nurses

In 2012 the Royal College of Veterinary Surgeons (RCVS) published The Code of Professional Conduct for Veterinary Nurses, which superseded The Guide to Professional Conduct of 2010. The Code of Professional Conduct provides guidance for RVNs and outlines the responsibilities of veterinary nurses in relation to animals, clients, the profession, the veterinary team, the RCVS and the public (RCVS, 2012). When deciding whether or not there has been professional misconduct the RCVS will take into account The Code of Professional Conduct, but regulate veterinary nurses through The Veterinary Surgeons Act 1966, the Royal Charter and the Veterinary Nurse Conduct and Discipline Rules 2014. The primary purpose of professional regulation being to protect the public interest and to safeguard the health and welfare of animals.

From 1st April 2012, veterinary nurses entering the RCVS VN register make the following declaration:

'I promise and solemnly declare that I will pursue the work of my profession with integrity and accept my responsibilities to the public, my clients, the profession and the Royal College of Veterinary Surgeons, and that, **above all**, my constant endeavour will be to ensure the health and welfare of animals committed to my care' (RCVS, 2012)

In relation to these professional responsibilities The Code of Professional Conduct outlines the five principles of practice, which are:

1. Professional competence.
2. Honesty and integrity.
3. Independence and impartiality.
4. Client confidentiality and trust.
5. Professional accountability.

In conjunction with The Code of Professional Conduct, the supporting guidance can be accessed online (www.rcvs.org.uk) to provide further guidance in specific situations. The key professional responsibilities to animals, clients, the profession, the veterinary team, the RCVS and the public, as set out in The Code of Professional Conduct (www.rcvs.org.uk/setting-standards/advice-and-guidance/code-of-professional-conduct-for-veterinary-nurses/) are illustrated in Figure 1.2.

In a situation where a veterinary nurse finds themselves facing an ethical dilemma, perhaps pertaining to principles of patient care, or conduct of a colleague or client, The Code of Professional Conduct and supporting guidance pages can provide detailed guidance. However, the decision regarding the action taken remains the responsibility of the RVN, who must ensure that animal welfare is balanced with professional responsibilities. There are various ethical frameworks that can be applied when making these decisions, as well as organizations that can provide confidential information, advice and guidance. Some of these organizations include The British Veterinary Nursing Association (BVNA), Royal Society for the Prevention of Cruelty to Animals (RSPCA), Citizens Advice Bureau and Public Concern at Work (PCAW). A full list of organizations can be found in Section 20 of the supporting guidance.

Professional regulation

In addition to The Code of Professional Conduct, there have been other recent advances towards statutory regulation of the profession. In 2011 a disciplinary system was introduced for RVNs which meant that concerns could be raised about veterinary nurses and investigated by the RCVS, in a similar way to veterinary surgeons. This involves a three-stage process (Figure 1.3), with around 20% of concerns progressed beyond Stage 1. Concerns remain confidential at Stages 1 and 2, but disciplinary hearings (Stage 3) are usually public; these hearings are also listed on the RCVS website for 3 years.

At Stages 1 and 2, if a concern is not progressed, the respondent is informed in writing that the case has been closed; there may also be formal advice issued. The Preliminary

Veterinary nurses and animals

- Veterinary nurses must make animal health and welfare their first consideration when attending to animals
- Veterinary nurses must keep within their own area of competence and refer cases responsibly
- Veterinary nurses must provide veterinary nursing care that is appropriate and adequate
- Veterinary nurses in practice must take steps to provide emergency first aid and pain relief to animals according to their skills and the specific situation
- Veterinary nurses who supply and administer medicines must do so responsibly
- Veterinary nurses must communicate with veterinary surgeons and each other to ensure the health and welfare of the animal or group of animals
- Veterinary nurses must ensure that clinical governance forms part of their professional activities

Veterinary nurses and clients

- Veterinary nurses must be open and honest with clients and respect their needs and requirements
- Veterinary nurses must provide independent and impartial advice and inform a client of any conflict of interest
- Veterinary nurses must provide appropriate information to clients about the practice, including the costs of services and medicines
- Veterinary nurses must communicate effectively, including in written and spoken English, with clients and ensure informed consent is obtained before treatments or procedures are carried out
- Veterinary nurses must keep clear, accurate and detailed clinical nursing and client records
- Veterinary nurses must not disclose information about a client or the client's animals to a third party, unless the client gives permission or animal welfare or the public interest may be compromised
- Veterinary nurses must respond promptly, fully and courteously to clients' complaints and criticism

1.2 Key professional responsibilities of veterinary nurses set out by RCVS Code of Professional Conduct. *continues* ▶

Veterinary nurses and the profession

- Veterinary nurses must take reasonable steps to address adverse physical or mental health or performance that could impair fitness to practise; or, that results in harm, or a risk of harm, to animal health or welfare, public health or the public interest
- Veterinary nurses who are concerned about a professional colleague's fitness to practise must take steps to ensure that animals are not put at risk and that the interests of the public are protected
- Veterinary nurses must maintain and develop the knowledge and skills relevant to their professional practice and competence and comply with RCVS requirements on the Period of Supervised Practice (PSP) and continuing professional development (CPD)
- Veterinary nurses must ensure that all their professional activities are covered by professional indemnity insurance or equivalent arrangements
- Veterinary nurses must not: hold out themselves or others as having expertise they cannot substantiate; hold out others as specialists or advanced practitioners unless appropriately listed with the RCVS; or, hold out others as veterinary nurses unless appropriately registered with the RCVS

Veterinary nurses and the veterinary team

- Veterinary nurses must work together and with others in the veterinary team and business, to co-ordinate the care of animals and the delivery of services
- Veterinary nurses must ensure that tasks are delegated only to those who have the appropriate competence and registration
- Veterinary nurses must maintain minimum practice standards equivalent to the Core Standards of the RCVS Practice Standards Scheme
- Veterinary nurses must not impede professional colleagues seeking to comply with legislation and these standards or with the RCVS Code of Professional Conduct for Veterinary Surgeons
- Veterinary nurses must communicate effectively, including in written and spoken English, with the veterinary team and other veterinary professionals in the UK

Veterinary nurses and the RCVS

- Veterinary nurses other than student veterinary nurses must be entered in the Register of Veterinary Nurses
- Veterinary nurses must provide the RCVS with their PSP and CPD records when requested to do so
- Veterinary nurses and those applying to be registered as veterinary nurses must disclose to the RCVS any caution or conviction, including absolute and conditional discharges, or adverse finding which may affect registration, whether in the UK or overseas (except for spent convictions and minor offences excluded from disclosure by the RCVS)
- Veterinary nurses and those applying to be registered as veterinary nurses must comply with reasonable requests from the RCVS as part of the regulation of the profession, and comply with any undertakings they give to the RCVS
- Veterinary nurses must report to the RCVS those veterinary nurses removed from the RCVS register at the direction of the VN Disciplinary Committee who nevertheless continue to give medical treatment or carry out minor surgery unlawfully

Veterinary nurses and the public

- Veterinary nurses must seek to ensure the protection of public health and animal health and welfare, and must consider the impact of their actions on the environment
- Veterinary nurses must report facts and opinions honestly and with due care, taking into account the 10 Principles of Certification
- Veterinary nurses promoting and advertising products and services must do so in a professional manner
- Veterinary nurses must comply with legislation relevant to the provision of veterinary services
- Veterinary nurses must not engage in any activity or behaviour that would be likely to bring the profession into disrepute or undermine public confidence in the profession

1.2 *continued* Key professional responsibilities of veterinary nurses set out by RCVS Code of Professional Conduct.

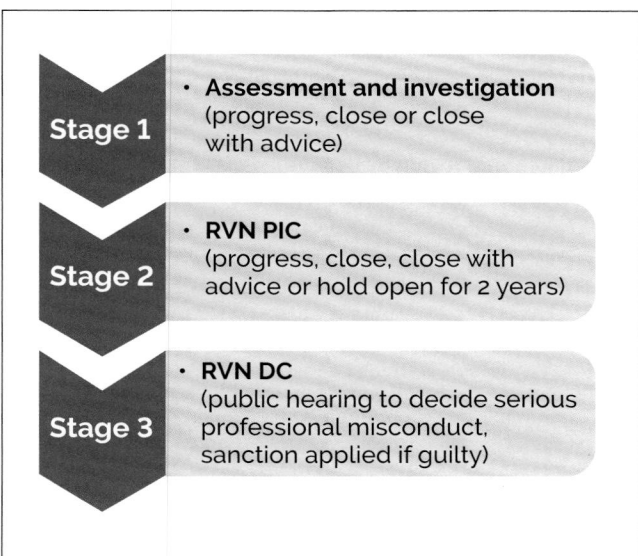

1.3 Disciplinary system structure for RVNs introduced in 2011. DC = Disciplinary Committee; PIC = Preliminary Investigation Committee.

Investigation Committee (PIC) may also direct that a case is held open for up to 2 years (for example, where a follow up visit from a veterinary investigator may be required). At each stage the committees comprise veterinary and non-veterinary members; the chair is a non-veterinary member. For a disciplinary hearing five members may sit; however, the quorum is three; an RVN, a veterinary surgeon and a non-veterinary member. If a respondent is found guilty of disgraceful conduct in a professional respect, or considered unfit to practise, a sanction will be applied taking into account mitigating and aggravating circumstances. The standard of proof required for the Disciplinary Committee (DC) is tantamount to the criminal standard (i.e. 'so that it is sure') and there are three possible sanctions that can be applied.

- Reprimand or warning as to future conduct.
- Suspension (no more than 2 years).
- Removal from the register.

Removal from the register means that a veterinary nurse can no longer practise under Schedule 3 of the Veterinary Surgeons Act 1966 and, therefore, can carry serious consequences for the respondent. The Disciplinary Procedure Guidance recommends that removal is not imposed as a punitive measure, rather as a means of protecting animal welfare and the public interest. A respondent may apply to the committee for restoration after a period of 10 months.

The Veterinary Client Mediation Service (VCMS) is a voluntary, independent and free mediation service for clients whose animals have received veterinary care and for the veterinary professionals providing that care. Using the process of mediation, VCMS offer help and guidance to resolve complaints that is unbiased and non-judgmental. The service is funded by the RCVS. All veterinary practices have their own complaints procedures to deal with concerns raised by clients. However, where a complaint cannot be resolved within the practice, either party can refer the complaint to the VCMS.

The Royal Charter

On 17th February 2015 the new Royal Charter came into effect, meaning that the 'list' and 'register' of veterinary nurses that had existed prior to that date, were merged into a single register. The Charter is a step towards statutory protection of the title 'veterinary nurse', but at the time of writing does not yet protect the title. It does, however, strengthen the argument for statutory protection and underpin the regulation of veterinary nurses. Thus, RVNs must ensure that their professional activities are covered by professional indemnity insurance. The Veterinary Defence Society (VDS), for example, now covers both veterinary surgeons and veterinary nurses within the practice policy. If a veterinary nurse is working as a locum, it is recommended they seek to ensure they have a personal policy in place, as they are unlikely to be on the practice list of RVNs.

Schedule 3 procedures

In light of recent regulatory developments within the profession, it is imperative that RVNs are familiar with the provisions of Schedule 3 (amended 2002) of the Veterinary Surgeons Act 1966. The Act defines veterinary surgery and who may practise veterinary surgery in the UK. Schedule 3 sets out exemptions to this rule, which includes amongst others veterinary nurses and student veterinary nurses.

The Veterinary Surgeons Act defines veterinary surgery as the art and science of veterinary surgery and medicine to include:

- Diagnosis of diseases in, and injuries to, animals including tests performed on animals for diagnostic purposes
- Giving of advice based upon such diagnosis
- Medical or surgical treatment of animals
- Performance of surgical operations on animals.

Schedule 3 of the Act permits in Part I certain exemptions:

- Minor medical treatment to be given to an animal by the owner, another member of the household or an employee of the owner
- Medical treatment or minor surgery (not involving entry into a body cavity) given to an animal used in agriculture by the owner or an employee of the owner

- First aid for the purpose of saving life or relieving pain or suffering (by anyone).

Other notable exemptions to be carried out by *anyone over the age of eighteen* include:

- The castration of a male animal or the caponizing of an animal, whether by chemical means or otherwise
- The docking of the tail of a lamb
- The amputation of the dew claws of a dog before its eyes are open.

Paragraphs six and seven of Schedule 3 set out exemptions in relation to veterinary nurses and student veterinary nurses. A veterinary nurse is defined as a nurse whose name is entered on the 'list' (now the register) of veterinary nurses maintained by the RCVS. A student veterinary nurse is defined as a person enrolled for the purpose of undergoing training as a veterinary nurse at an approved training centre or veterinary practice. Both may carry out the same procedures, but with differing levels of supervision and under different circumstances (Figure 1.4). Part II of Schedule 3 covers a number of exclusions from Part I, most of which relate to farm animals, but makes it clear that spaying and castrating dogs and cats is an act of veterinary surgery.

In terms of 'minor medical and surgical treatments', Schedule 3 does not provide a definitive list of what these might be. Therefore, veterinary nurses must consider their own scope of competence, experience, qualifications and the risks and benefits of a procedure, before undertaking any delegation. Similarly, veterinary surgeons should be mindful of the same considerations before delegating to veterinary nurses. This part of veterinary nursing practice is considered to be a grey area, and at the time of writing Schedule 3 is

Veterinary nurses
Any medical treatment or minor surgery (not involving entry into a body cavity) to any animal providing:
<ul><li>The animal is, for the time being, under the care of a registered veterinary surgeon or veterinary practitioner and the medical treatment or minor surgery is carried out by the veterinary nurse at their direction</li><li>The registered veterinary surgeon or veterinary practitioner is the employer or is acting on behalf of the employer of the veterinary nurse</li><li>The registered veterinary surgeon or veterinary practitioner directing the medical treatment or minor surgery is satisfied that the veterinary nurse is qualified to carry out the treatment or surgery</li></ul>
Student veterinary nurses
Any medical treatment or minor surgery (not involving entry into a body cavity) to any animal by a student veterinary nurse if the following conditions are complied with:
<ul><li>The animal is, for the time being, under the care of a registered veterinary surgeon or veterinary practitioner and the medical treatment or minor surgery is carried out by the student veterinary nurse at his direction *and in the course of the student veterinary nurse's training*</li><li>The registered veterinary surgeon or veterinary practitioner is the employer or is acting on behalf of the employer of the veterinary nurse</li><li>The treatment or surgery is supervised by a registered veterinary surgeon, veterinary practitioner or veterinary nurse and, *in the case of surgery, the supervision is direct, continuous and personal*</li></ul>

1.4 Schedule 3 exemptions in relation to veterinary nurses and student veterinary nurses.

under review. There is, however, some detailed information within the supporting guidance of The Code of Professional Conduct in relation to some of the areas of practice commonly delegated to veterinary nurses.

Maintenance and monitoring of anaesthesia

In the supporting guidance pertaining to delegation to veterinary nurses, inducing anaesthesia using a specific quantity of medicine (e.g. medetomidine and ketamine) may be carried out by a veterinary nurse, or student veterinary nurse under supervision, providing the task has been delegated by a veterinary surgeon. Administering medicine incrementally to induce and maintain anaesthesia (e.g. propofol) should only be carried out by a veterinary surgeon.

It is recognized that the most suitable person to assist a veterinary surgeon to monitor and maintain anaesthesia is a veterinary nurse, or a student veterinary nurse under supervision. However, in practice this is not always possible and aspects of anaesthesia that do not involve acts of veterinary surgery may instead be carried out by a 'suitably trained person', but remain the overall responsibility of the veterinary surgeon. Examples of this include:

- Acting as the veterinary surgeon's hands by moving dials
- Monitoring the patient during the anaesthesia and recovery period.

A Level 2 Certificate in Assisting Veterinary Surgeons in the Monitoring of Animal Patients Under Anaesthesia and Sedation is available, which was developed in partnership with LANTRA and with support from the Society of Practising Veterinary Surgeons (SPVS). The aim of the qualification being to support lay staff and veterinary care assistants who are assisting veterinary surgeons in this way, to develop their skills whilst working safely and professionally.

Vaccination of companion animals

Any patient receiving a first vaccination (POM-V; see Chapter 8) or booster vaccination must be under the care of the prescribing veterinary surgeon and must also have undergone a clinical assessment. Following this the veterinary surgeon may administer the vaccination, or direct a veterinary nurse or student veterinary nurse to do so. For a second vaccination given close in time to the first, a veterinary nurse or student veterinary nurse may administer the vaccine, which is usually prescribed by the veterinary surgeon at the time of the clinical assessment and first vaccination. The Code of Professional Conduct advises, however, that it is helpful for a veterinary surgeon to be on the premises in case of adverse reaction.

If certification is required then it is recommended that the veterinary surgeon vaccinates the animal themselves or witnesses it done, therefore, this should be taken into consideration when delegating or accepting delegation of a vaccination. It is recommended that for clarity the phrase 'under the direction of...' is added to the clinical record if an RVN is signing. Official certification, such as that for rabies vaccinations, should be signed only by the veterinary surgeon administering the vaccination. In addition, the veterinary nurse must also consider their own scope of competence in relation to the task.

Dentistry

The guidance within The Code of Professional Conduct regarding dental procedures clearly states, that the RCVS considers the extraction of teeth using instruments to be outside the meaning of 'minor surgery'. Therefore, veterinary nurses and student veterinary nurses may carry out routine dental hygiene work only, under the direction of a veterinary surgeon.

Professional competence

Professional competence and due care imposes the following obligations on all professional staff:

- Veterinary nurses must maintain professional knowledge and skill at the level required to ensure that their employers, clients and patients receive competent professional care
- Veterinary nurses must act diligently in accordance with applicable technical and professional standards when performing their duties
- Veterinary nurses must take reasonable steps to address adverse physical or mental health or performance that could impair their fitness to practise; or that results in harm, or the risk of harm, to animal health or welfare, public health or the public interest
- Veterinary nurses, and those applying to be registered as veterinary nurses, are required to disclose to the RCVS any caution or conviction, including absolute and conditional discharges and spent convictions, or adverse finding which may affect registration, whether in the UK or overseas (except for minor offences excluded from disclosure by the RCVS).

Fitness to practise

In March 2016, the RCVS published a new guide entitled *Fitness to Practise – A Guide for UK Providers of Veterinary Nursing Education and Student Veterinary Nurses*. The guide assists training providers in identifying and addressing fitness to practise concerns, and sets out principles that student veterinary nurses are expected to follow. The guide sets out principles and behaviours relating to people, practice and private and student life; it also gives examples of particular concerns that may affect a student's fitness to practise

Personal and professional development: reflective insight

As regulated professionals it is important that veterinary nurses develop reflective insight to explain why we react and think in certain ways. This gives us an opportunity to change and develop, as well as allows us to identify resources available to aid us. This might be evidence-based literature, or colleagues, family and friends. The RCVS Code of Professional Conduct supporting guidance makes several recommendations in relation to clinical governance:

- Keeping up-to-date with continuing professional development (CPD) and new developments relevant to the area of work
- Reflecting upon performance, preferably in the form of a learning diary, and making appropriate changes to practice
- Reflecting upon any unexpected critical events and learning from the outcome and making appropriate changes to practice
- Critically analysing the evidence base for procedures used and making appropriate changes to practice
- Reflecting upon communication with other members of the work team and making appropriate changes to practice
- Reflecting upon communication with clients and making appropriate changes to practice
- Assessing professional competence in consultation with more experienced or better qualified colleagues and limiting your practice appropriately.

Continuing professional development

Veterinary nurses must maintain and develop the knowledge and skills relevant to their professional practice and competence, and comply with the RCVS requirements on the Period of Supervised Practice (PSP) and CPD. They must ensure that all their professional activities are covered by professional indemnity insurance, or equivalent arrangements, and must not hold themselves or others as having expertise they cannot substantiate or call themselves a 'specialist' or similar where to do so it might mislead or misrepresent.

From 2020, veterinary nurses are required to complete a minimum of 15 hours of CPD in a calendar year. This is a change from the previous requirement of 45 hours over a 3-year period.

This can be part of a planned development programme or through attending organized courses, lectures or seminars, shadowing someone, discussing case reports, in-house training, secondment to another practice, reading veterinary journals and other relevant publications (and keeping a reading diary or notes) or completing research. It can also include research in preparation for giving lectures, seminars or presentations. Veterinary nurses are encouraged to use reflection to deepen their understanding and review the effectiveness of the skills learnt.

Integrating personal and professional experience

Personal experience is a rich resource that may not always be seen as relevant to professional life or experience. However, personal experience in terms of skills and knowledge can be used as a foundation to build professional identity and skills. Personal experiences such as parenting, animal ownership, coaching, volunteering or membership of social groups bring valuable experiences that can be integrated with professional experience, to advance knowledge and practice in different ways. For example, volunteering for a charity or coaching a sports team may have developed your leadership skills, or having children and/or animals that are dependent on you may have enhanced your organization skills. Integrating personal and professional experiences involves reflecting upon what your personal experience has taught you and identifying how this relates to your professional experience.

Self-evaluation

There are many reflective models that can be used as frameworks to reflect on and evaluate your own performance.

The Gibbs reflective cycle (Gibbs, 1988) and Kolb's experiential learning model (Kolb, 1984) are popular and often used by students to assist with reflective writing (Figure 1.5). Schön (1983) describes two approaches to reflection: reflection-in-action and reflection-on-action.

- Reflection-in-action – during the experience.
- Reflection-on-action – after the experience.

Reflection-on-action comes more naturally; reflection-in-action is something we can build on with more experience. Keeping a reflective diary can be helpful and is a useful place to start.

Some training providers ask student veterinary nurses to keep a *reflective diary*, so that they can begin to develop these skills in preparation for professional practice. In 2016, the new Nursing Progress Log (NPL) was introduced which includes a *professional behaviour assessment*. As part of this assessment the student is asked to reflect on their own performance in a range of professional and developmental areas and score themselves between 1 and 5, where 1 is the lowest score and 5 the highest. The student then asks a peer to complete the assessment, then their clinical coach, and finally the assessment is reviewed by the student's tutor. This provides an opportunity for self-reflection, evaluation and action planning. The behaviours and attitudes assessed are:

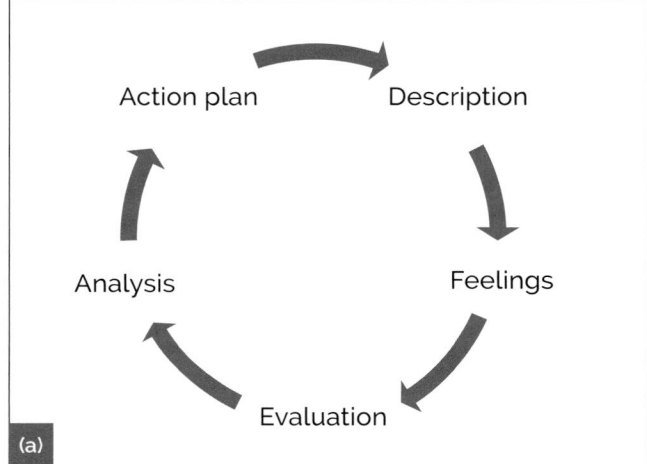

(a)

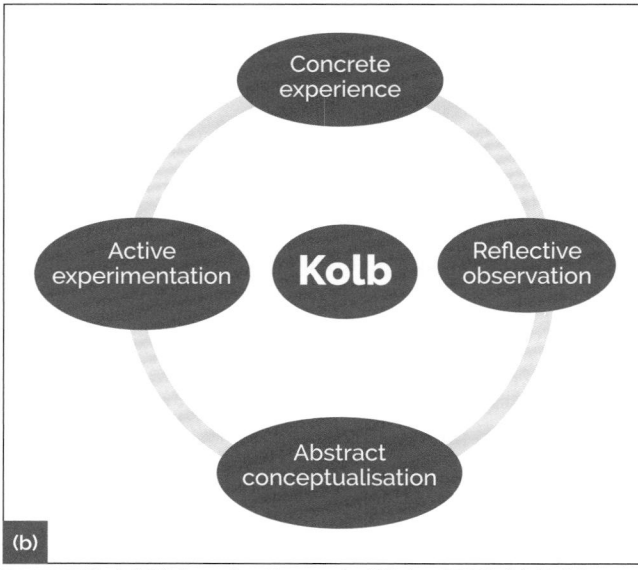

(b)

1.5 **(a)** Gibbs reflective cycle (Gibbs, 1988). **(b)** Kolb's experiential learning model (Kolb, 1984).

- Knowledge and skills
- Reliability and adaptability
- Works within legal and ethical limits
- Initiative and confidence
- Time management and ability to organize own work
- Communication skills
- Attitude to feedback and guidance
- Professional accountability
- Professional development
- Professional and clinical appearance.

Later on as the veterinary nurse develops their professional career, the RCVS requires a record of professional development in the form of an online log called a *professional development record* (PDR) or similar to be kept. This online log can be audited by the RCVS upon request and can also be shared with others, for example your employer. The record should be reflective, relevant to your area of practice and include a development plan and a diary.

Those who struggle with reflective models may find reflective questions useful, or a combination of both. It is important to evaluate your performance as soon as possible after the event, identifying areas of strength and development. Below are questions some may find helpful for self-evaluation upon completion of an assessment activity.

- What were you aiming to achieve when starting out?
- Did your aims change? Why?
- What did you want to get out of the assessment? How do you know this?
- Did you notice anything about a person's body language? How did you tackle this?
- Who did you liaise with before the assessment? Was this helpful? Why/why not?
- Do you think you managed to collect all the information you needed to carry out a particular task? If yes, what strategies helped you in this case?
- What, if any, were the barriers to change? How do you know this? How did you tackle them? Was your strategy successful? How do you know this?
- Did you give any advice? Do you think it helped? How do you know this?
- Do you think your knowledge was adequate in this case? Do you have evidence to back up your advice (e.g. books or journals)? Was there anything you were unsure about? If yes, what could you do about this?
- What actions do you need to take after the assessment? Do you feel competent to tackle these?
- What pleased you most about this assessment and why? What troubled you most about this assessment and why?
- What would you do differently next time and why?

Evidence-based veterinary nursing

Evidence-based veterinary medicine (EBVM) is a growing influence that is not only relevant to veterinary surgeons, but also RVNs. Veterinary nurses are now accountable for their practise and therefore should be able to *question and appraise current practice and literature*. A simple five-step process can be used to form the basis of EBVM, as recommended by the EVBM network (Macdonald *et al.*, 2017). This will be of benefit when training staff and drawing up systems of work/updating practice protocols.

- **Ask** – formulation of a clinical question.
- **Acquire** – conducting a search for the current evidence according to the clinical question.

- **Appraise** – evaluating the validity and strength of the evidence that has been found. The hierarchy of evidence may help with this.
- **Apply** – applying your newly found answer into day-to-day practice.
- **Assess** – assessing how the application of the evidence in your practice has impacted on yourself, your patients, their owners and even your colleagues.

Like any new concept there may be scepticism in terms of having the time to apply this process, as well as its relevance to veterinary nursing. Currently we know that there are gaps in the evidence base for veterinary nursing, and a search for current evidence may be unsuccessful. This highlights an area for future veterinary nursing research and may inspire RVNs to become involved in this area; for example, there are now several peer-reviewed journals for veterinary nursing. RCVS knowledge groups are also available for veterinary nursing and other related areas (e.g. client education and support, and trauma, wounds and bites).

Knowledge summaries (KS) are developed to answer a relevant question based on the current evidence. This is achieved by creating a 'PICO question' (patient, intervention, comparison, outcome), conducting a literature search, evaluating the current evidence available and formulating a conclusion to the question based upon the evidence. Guidance and support is provided by RCVS Knowledge, providing opportunities for learning and CPD as well as potential publication. There is a variety of knowledge groups available through RCVS Knowledge that RVNs are encouraged to join. As the evidence-based approach grows in the veterinary profession, it is hoped the same will happen for veterinary nursing.

Reviewing the literature

A literature review is a search and evaluation of the available literature in a particular subject or topic. The purpose of completing a review of the literature is to:

- Establish what is available on the topic
- Synthesize the information in the literature into a summary
- Critically analyse the information gathered by identifying gaps in current knowledge
- Present the literature in an organized way.

Completing a comprehensive review of the literature allows an in-depth grasp of a subject. It also enables the identification of gaps in the available information and what research needs to be undertaken to add to an existing body of agreed knowledge.

Health and wellbeing

The World Health Organization (WHO) defines **health** as 'a state of complete physical, mental and social **wellbeing** and not merely the absence of disease or infirmity' (WHO, 1948). Mental health and physical health are inextricably linked, with evidence for a strong relationship between the two. The nature of this relationship is two-way, with mental health influencing physical health and *vice versa*. With this in mind, veterinary nurses should seek to look after themselves as well as others, particularly if they are responsible for managing staff.

An appreciation of the factors that influence wellbeing, along with the strategies to support wellbeing include:

- Relationship with a partner
- Network of friends
- Enjoyable and fulfilling career
- Sufficient money
- Regular exercise
- Suitable diet
- Sufficient sleep
- Spiritual or religious beliefs.

The NHS has developed a range of resources that can be accessed to support wellbeing (www.nhs.uk/oneyou/every-mind-matters/top-tips-to-improve-your-mental-wellbeing/), including how to:

- Reframe unhelpful thoughts
- Be in the present. Be mindful and meditate
- Get good quality sleep
- Spend quality time with friends or family
- Live a healthy life by being active, having a balanced diet and removing bad habits (e.g. smoking, alcohol, caffeine)
- Take up a hobby and do something for yourself.

If you are concerned about yourself or a colleague, the following helplines and support groups can offer expert advice:

- Anxiety UK – a charity providing support if you have been diagnosed with an anxiety condition (www.anxietyuk.org.uk)
- The Mental Health Foundation – providing information and support for anyone with mental health problems or learning disabilities (www.mentalhealth.org.uk)
- Mind Matters Initiative (MMI) – aims to improve the mental health and wellbeing of those in the veterinary team, including students, veterinary nurses, veterinary surgeons and practice managers. MMI was launched in 2015 and is funded and run by RCVS (www.vetmindmatters.org/)
- NHS A-Z (www.nhs.uk/conditions/stress-anxiety-depression/improve-mental-wellbeing/)
- No Panic – voluntary charity offering support for sufferers of panic attacks and obsessive compulsive disorder (OCD), offering a course to help overcome your phobia or OCD (www.nopanic.org.uk)
- Papyrus – young suicide prevention society (www.papyrus-uk.org; telephone: 0800 068 4141)
- Vetlife – independent, confidential and free help for everyone in the veterinary community, including nurses and students (www.vetlife.org.uk).

Use of social media

Within the Fitness to Practise Guide and the supporting guidance of The Code of Professional Conduct, advice has been issued on the use of social media (see also Chapter 9). The term social media pertains to websites and other online applications that involve some sort of interaction between users and content developers. It includes sharing of opinions, insights, information, knowledge, ideas and interests, and involves the building of public networks. Examples include:

- Twitter
- Facebook
- YouTube
- Instagram
- LinkedIn
- Snapchat.

There may be some overlap of personal and professional networks with some of these applications (e.g. private groups for a specific interest, such as student nurse groups on Facebook). It is important to remember that these groups may have a large number of members and are unlikely to be truly 'private'. Other users may comment on, circulate or copy information posted online and, generally, once something is posted it is difficult or even impossible to remove. Examples of inappropriate social media conduct are:

- Posts that contravene internet/social media policies set out by a training provider
- Posts that cause undue stress or provoke antisocial behaviour
- Offensive/false/inaccurate/unjustified posts
- Posts that involve abuse, bullying, victimization, harassment, threats or intimidation to fellow students, colleagues, staff or others
- Posts that discriminate against an individual based on their race, gender, disability, sexual orientation, age, religion or beliefs, or national origin
- Posts that breach client confidentiality.

Example 1

A student veterinary nurse posts on a social media site a discussion about a recent assessment; several other students reply to the post, one of whom makes personal and disparaging remarks about a fellow student. Although the student who the remarks are about has no direct link with the person who made them, they see the post through a mutual connection. They are understandably upset and distressed by this and inform their training provider

Example 2

A private page within a social media networking site is set up by a student representative for a particular cohort of students. A discussion thread is started about one of the class tutors; within this discussion, two students comment describing how they would inflict physical violence on the tutor and a third student reacts to this. A fellow student raises a concern with the training provider about these comments, providing a screen shot of the discussion

In the examples above, it is clear that the posts have caused undue stress to the person the remarks were made about and others. These concerns relate to students' conduct and can be investigated by the training provider, using their own fitness to practise policies. A subsequent adverse finding may incur a sanction and must also be disclosed to the RCVS at the point of registration. In other words, this misconduct may affect the student's registration status and their ability to practise as a veterinary nurse.

It is important to ensure that as a user of social media, professionals (and students) protect their privacy (by using appropriate privacy/security settings); however, there is also a responsibility to behave appropriately as one would in the real world and be mindful that information posted online could be viewed by anybody, including clients, fellow students and training providers.

Whistleblowing

Veterinary nurses may feel they have witnessed poor standards of care or inappropriate conduct in the workplace. Addressing these concerns can be difficult; however, there is a duty of care for professional staff to uphold ethical standards of practice. The term whistleblowing is used when an employee raises concerns over an act, or acts of wrongdoing they believe to be going on in their workplace.

As a regulated profession, it is expected by the general public that veterinary nurses will demonstrate qualities such as professional integrity, transparency and trust. Hand in hand with this is the expectation that they have a moral obligation to report any acts of misconduct or malpractice that they may witness, if it is in the public's interest to do so. The RCVS provides some assistance within the supporting guidance of The Code of Professional Conduct, but there are perhaps wider issues to consider alongside this, including the Public Interest Disclosure Act 1998.

The guidance from the RCVS is to first try and resolve the matter within the practice, with your line manager or a senior veterinary surgeon for example. Internal practice policies may be used to reach a solution. Most problems can be successfully managed in this way (further information on communicating with colleagues can be found in Chapter 9). If the matter cannot be resolved using this approach, concerns should be brought to the attention of the RCVS Professional Conduct Department. It is likely at this stage that the person will be asked to submit a formal complaint. In some cases, it may not be appropriate to follow this course of action, for example if the misconduct involves senior members of the practice. In this situation, various organizations, including the Veterinary Defence Society (VDS) and the British Veterinary Nursing Association (BVNA), can be approached for advice and guidance, or the veterinary nurse may consider taking the matter straight to the RCVS, bypassing any practice policy that may be in place.

The RCVS may not be able to investigate anonymous claims fully, which brings about other considerations for the whistle-blower in terms of personal and professional relationships. On the one hand those that choose to blow the whistle may be considered 'moral heroes' and 'admirable exemplars of integrity'; however, there may also be fears of retribution and reprisal, professional suicide and risk of damaging the functioning of the profession if all other avenues have not been fully explored. That said, it is important for veterinary nurses to be able to distinguish between genuine errors and acts of wrongdoing; conducting regular clinical audits and keeping a record of incidents that occur can be useful in this respect and help identify areas of professional development for employees. The RCVS may also inform other agencies such as the police, depending on the nature of the complaint.

Where an RVN is concerned about the health of a colleague in relation to their conduct or fitness to practise, this should be reported to the RCVS as soon as is reasonably practicable. Further investigation and/or undertakings may be carried out (under the health protocol), which may not necessarily involve disciplinary action.

Any situation involving whistleblowing can be fraught with worry and emotion, both on a personal and professional level. There is legislation in place to protect whistleblowing in the form of the Public Interest Disclosure Act 1998, but the whistler-blower should be aware that if the complaint involves disclosure of client information, this should only be for public interest or animal welfare reasons.

Veterinary nurses may also seek further advice and support from the various organizations listed at the end of this chapter and within the RCVS Code of Professional Conduct supporting guidance. Membership of trade unions or similar organizations, such as the BVNA, may be of benefit. Veterinary surgeons and veterinary nurses will have indemnity insurance cover through the practice policy. RVNs working as locums can also take out personal insurance cover.

Consent to treatment

The RCVS Code of Professional Conduct states that veterinary nurses must communicate effectively, including in written and spoken English, with clients and ensure informed consent is obtained before treatments or procedures are carried out. Consent is a contractual relationship between the client and the veterinary practice and further information is provided in the supporting guidance to define what consent is, who can give consent and perhaps most importantly what constitutes informed consent. It is worth noting that around 80% of complaints received by the RCVS involve communication and consent in some way.

What is consent?

- Consent is a formal agreement whereby the owner agrees to a medical or surgical course of action proposed, usually including some sort of acknowledgment of estimate of the associated fees. The word consent is derived from the Latin term consentire, meaning 'agree', the legal definition of consent being 'deliberate or implied affirmation: compliance with a course of proposed action'.
- Consent is usually given in written form, but does not have to be; other forms of consent (verbal or by implication) are equally valid in law. Written evidence of consent may be useful in the event of a complaint or dispute.
- Written consent is usually obtained for medical treatment/surgery/euthanasia and use of 'off label' drugs.
- Consent should be obtained from the owner of the animal. If this is not possible, a friend or relative of the owner may consent on their behalf; they should do so by signing as 'Owners agent' stating their relationship to the owner.
- Owners must understand what they are signing for (i.e. consent must be 'informed', see below); therefore, procedures should be clearly outlined on a consent form without the use of jargon or abbreviations. Phrases such as 'any other treatment as required' should also be avoided.
- *Informed consent*, which is an essential part of any contract, can only be given by a client who has had the opportunity to consider a range of reasonable treatment options, with associated fee estimates, and had the significance and main risks explained to them (RCVS, 2016).

Who can give consent?

Obtaining consent is a task often delegated to veterinary nurses, who should assume the same level of responsibility as a veterinary surgeon when dealing with clients in this regard. Therefore, there may be occasions where a veterinary nurse considers it appropriate to refer to a veterinary surgeon or more experienced colleague. It is important to treat clients fairly and without discrimination whilst providing clear and accurate information about treatment options, staff involved and a range of options. Consent can be expressed verbally, in writing or by implication; however, in most circumstances written evidence is recommended. This may not be possible in some circumstances, for example where the owner is absent or in an emergency situation. The RCVS recommends that written consent is obtained as soon as possible in these circumstances. Where consent is given over the telephone verbally, it is common practice for two separate members of the veterinary team to confirm this with the owner to ensure their wishes are fully understood.

- Firstly, a veterinary nurse should take reasonable steps to ensure they are satisfied that the person giving consent is authorized to do so, for example by checking practice records (including ID chip information).
- When dealing with somebody who is not the owner, veterinary nurses should be satisfied that the person is authorized to give consent.
- If an animal is jointly owned, veterinary nurses should be sure that the wishes of the absent partner are the same as the person presenting the animal.
- In the event that a boarding establishment presents an animal on the owner's behalf, it should be confirmed that authority has been delegated to the owner of that establishment.
- Where an animal is presented by a carer on behalf of the owner, it should be established that the carer does, in fact, have the authorization of the owner.
- If an animal is presented by someone over the age of 16 but under 18 years of age, they are not considered a minor, but also are not legally considered an adult in terms of entering into a financial agreement. This is somewhat of a grey area and the veterinary nurse or veterinary surgeon must use their judgment, to consider whether the young person has the capacity to understand what they are consenting to and what the possible consequences might be. A note should be made in the clinical record that the animal was presented by a 16–18 year old.

Informed consent

Informed consent, which is an essential part of any contract, can only be given by a client who has had the opportunity to consider a range of reasonable treatment options, with associated fee estimates, and had the significance and main risks explained to them. It is important that the person gaining consent seeks to ensure that what is said is understood on both sides. This can be achieved by asking questions and summarizing the key points of the discussion. Contemporaneous clinical records will also be of benefit if an owner's understanding is called into question later on.

Clients should be encouraged to ask questions and take part in the discussions; however, where a client's ability to understand is called into question steps should be taken to assist their understanding. This can be achieved in a number of ways, including providing written and diagrammatic information, extra time to consider the information and ask questions, or asking a family member or friend to be present during discussions.

Provision for unexpected outcomes should be made, for example, by obtaining contact details for use during an emergency or contingency planning for the veterinary surgeon to act without the owner's consent in the best interest for the animal. It is important to remember, however, that the wishes of the veterinary surgeon or veterinary nurse cannot override those of the owners, other than under exceptional circumstances (e.g. welfare grounds).

The RCVS Practice Standards Scheme Manual recommends signed consent forms are obtained for all procedures and for admittance to the practice. It is also recommended that the person signing the form receives a copy. The form should be completed in indelible ink, signed, initialled and dated if amended and safely stored. There are no recommendations for how long practice records should be kept (with the exception of prescription-only medicines), but presently the majority of records are held in digital format and therefore become a permanent record linked to the animal's digital clinical records.

Mental incapacity

The Mental Capacity Act 2005 (applicable in England and Wales) states: 'A person lacks capacity in relation to a matter if at the material time he is unable to make a decision for himself in relation to the matter because of an impairment of, or a disturbance in the functioning of, the mind or brain. It does not matter whether the impairment or disturbance is permanent or temporary.' Similar legislation exists in Scotland and Northern Ireland in the form of The Adults with Incapacity (Scotland) Act 2000 and the Mental Capacity Act (Northern Ireland) 2016, respectively.

Veterinary surgeons and veterinary nurses may find themselves in a situation where they are judging a client's capacity or ability to make a decision. In this situation, The Code of Practice on using the Mental Capacity Act 2005 suggests using the following guidelines:

- Does the client have a general understanding of what decision they need to make and why they need to make it?
- Does the client have a general understanding of the likely consequences of making, or not making this decision?
- Is the client able to understand, retain, use and weigh up the information relevant to this decision?
- Can the client communicate their decision (by talking, using sign language or by any other means)?

It is the veterinary professional's responsibility to ensure that the client has been given every opportunity to understand the information provided, thereby placing the onus on the professional to ensure their communication skills are well developed.

Animal welfare

On entering the register of veterinary nurses held by the RCVS, veterinary nurses declare that they will ensure the health and welfare of animals in their care. The concept of animal welfare links closely with other ethical principles and can have different meanings for different people. For example, some welfare organizations may campaign for a reduction in the use of animals in experiments and some may campaign for a total ban. There are many different definitions of animal welfare and, since 2007, modern legislation has been in place to protect animals in the form of the Animal Welfare Act 2006 in England and Wales, the Animal Health and Welfare (Scotland) Act 2006, and the Welfare of Animals Act (Northern Ireland) 2011.

Broom (1991) defines the term 'welfare' as referring to the state of an individual in relation to its environment. This can be measured in terms of failure to cope with the environment and difficulty in coping, which can both be indicators of poor welfare. Often poor welfare is associated with suffering; however, welfare can be poor without suffering, which is reflected in the Animal Welfare Acts. Indicators of poor welfare can include: reduced life expectancy; impaired growth; impaired reproduction; body damage; disease; immunosuppression; and behaviour anomalies. Broom (1991) also recognizes that animals have a range of needs and that suffering occurs when unpleasant subjective feelings are acute or continue for a long time.

Dawkins (2004) identified two key questions to answer when considering animal welfare:

- Are the animals healthy?
- Do they have what they want?

Within the context of veterinary practice, the first question is perhaps the easiest to answer, in terms of assessing an animal's health status and diagnosing disease. The second question involves considering the mental state of the animal and calls into question whether it is more important to consider an individual's wants or their needs. Historically, it was thought that animals were without reason (i.e. they were not considered to be sentient beings) (Legood, 2000). However, over the last 150 years, developments in animal welfare legislation have meant that animal needs have been recognized and can be used to measure welfare standards. Both in academic and legal circles a single clear and precise meaning of 'welfare' is yet to be agreed, therefore many methods of assessment involve both subjective and objective observations. It is generally considered that unnecessary suffering amounts to cruelty and constitutes a criminal offence. It is important that when we conclude an animal is suffering, that we have been consistent and logical, considering what matters to the animal and not just to us.

When evaluating the welfare status of animals, it is common for humans to apply their own values, perceptions and experiences perhaps without regard of how animals perceive the world. This is known as *anthropocentrism*. For example, many animals use a variety of senses to interpret their environment such as their sense of smell or hearing, whereas humans primarily rely on vision. Some animal behaviours can be misinterpreted by humans, such as a cat bringing home prey or a dog chewing their favourite shoes. Often these actions are considered to be undesirable or even malicious by owners, attributing human characteristics to the animal otherwise known as *anthropomorphism*.

Animal welfare legislation

Although modern day British society regards itself as 'a nation of animal lovers', historically animal cruelty was rife and legislative provision for animal cruelty was not introduced until 1822 in the form of 'Martins Act'. This Act made it an offence for any person to wantonly and cruelly beat, abuse or ill-treat any horse, mare, gelding, mule, ass, ox, cow, heifer, steer, sheep or other cattle. Following the introduction of this statute unsuccessful attempts were made to extend

protection to domestic animals, and to ban cruel sports; a debate that extends to the present day. From this approach the beginnings of the RSPCA were formed, who campaigned for the mitigation of animal suffering. In the years following this, legislation was amended and added to, eventually being consolidated into the Protection of Animals Act 1911. In modern day society this Act was considered to be cumbersome and old-fashioned, in terms of the language and terminology used in relation to the current status of animals in society. Under this Act enforcement bodies could not intervene until cruelty had first taken place, even if they could see an animal was about to suffer.

The Animal Welfare Act 2006 (AWA) came into force in April 2007 in England and Wales (similar legislation came into force in Scotland and Northern Ireland in 2006 and 2011, respectively). Section 9 of the Act places a duty of care on owners and keepers of animals to ensure they take reasonable steps in all circumstances to meet the welfare needs of animals in their care. This means that enforcement agencies can now act by advising and educating owners, before an animal suffers. If this advice is not met then action can be taken, which in some cases may involve prosecution. The five welfare 'needs' as set out by the Act are:

- Need for a suitable environment
- Need for a suitable diet
- Need to be able to exhibit normal behaviour patterns
- Need to be housed with, or apart, from other animals
- Need to be protected from pain, suffering, injury and disease.

These needs were first set out as the Five Freedoms proposed by the Farm Animal Welfare Council in 1979 (https://webarchive.nationalarchives.gov.uk/20121010012427/http://www.fawc.org.uk/freedoms.htm), setting out guidelines for an acceptable level of welfare in farmed animals.

- Freedom from hunger and thirst – by ready access to food and fresh water in order to maintain full health and vigour.
- Freedom from discomfort – by providing an appropriate environment, including shelter and a comfortable resting area.
- Freedom from pain, injury or disease – by prevention and/or rapid diagnosis and treatment.
- Freedom to express normal behaviour – by providing sufficient space, proper facilities and, where necessary, company of the animal's own kind.
- Freedom from fear and distress – by ensuring conditions and treatment that avoid mental suffering.

The Five Freedoms provide guidance and are aspirational, as opposed to the five welfare 'needs' which are now enshrined in law.

Codes of Practice for the welfare of dogs, cats, horses, ponies and donkeys, and non-human primates have been developed by the Department for Environment, Food and Rural Affairs (Defra) and can be used as a reference guide by the general public and professionals caring for any of these species. These codes are crucial for keepers in order to know what needs to be done to meet welfare needs in relation to the Animal Welfare Acts. Veterinary nurses may find these codes useful when advising clients on best practice for meeting their animal's needs, and indeed when caring for animals committed to their care. The RSPCA and other enforcement agencies also use these codes to demonstrate best practice.

Quality of life

Quality of Life (QoL) is a concept derived from human medicine which balances longevity with suffering (Rollin, 2006). Three overlapping areas of concern were previously identified by Benson and Rollin (2004) in terms of QoL: biological function, affective states and nature (Figure 1.6). Biological function considers normal health, growth, behaviour and development (i.e. is the animal healthy? (Dawkins, 2004) and can it cope with its environment? (Broom, 1991)). Affective states refer to an animal's emotions or feelings, in particular unpleasant states such as fear, pain, hunger and distress. This theory assumes that subjective states of animals can be scientifically assessed by examining preferences and motivations. Lastly is the ability to lead a natural life. It has been identified that it is important for animals to be able to exhibit normal behaviour for the species, fulfilling a full behavioural repertoire. An inability to meet this need can be viewed as detrimental to an animal's welfare.

Owners who have become emotionally dependant on their animals may wish to pursue treatment, regardless of the level of suffering it may incur for the animal. This can lead to conflict with the veterinary team in terms of how to balance length of life with levels of suffering. With this in mind it is important to advocate for the patient by communicating carefully with owners early on regarding end of life care. The major difference between human and veterinary care being, that we have the option of euthanasia to end the suffering of an animal.

Villalobos and Kaplan (2008) developed the Quality of Life Scale to support owners in coming to a decision about QoL. This model uses a scoring system where a total score of over 35 points indicates an acceptable QoL. For each criterion a score of 10 represents the ideal and a score of 5 is acceptable (Figure 1.7). The criteria used in the model are: Hurt, Hunger, Hydration, Hygiene, Happiness, Mobility, and More good days than bad; enabling a more objective and perhaps less emotional evaluation of QoL.

The World Health Organization (WHO) has developed a holistic QoL assessment, encompassing six domains subdivided into 24 facets, each containing four items that are scored on a five-point scale (100 items in total). This cross-cultural assessment (WHOQOL) (www.who.int/mental_health/publications/whoqol/en/) may be relevant to animals in some of the facets, for example energy and fatigue, pain and discomfort, sleep and rest. Some facets, however, are less relevant, such as body image and appearance.

Further information on client communication, including dealing with bereavement, is given in Chapter 9.

1.6 The three overlapping areas of concern identified in the Quality of Life concept. (Benson and Rollin, 2004)

Accountability and the law

As professionals, veterinary nurses hold a position of responsibility. They are professionally accountable to the RCVS, contractually accountable to their employer and, of course, accountable to the law for their actions. When deciding on whether a particular course of action should be taken, it is important to take into account whether such an action would break the law. There are multiple pieces of legislation that affect veterinary nurses (Figure 1.8), including those relating

Score	Criterion	Comments
0–10	Hurt	Adequate pain control, including breathing ability, is first and foremost on the scale. Is the pet's pain successfully managed? Is oxygen necessary?
0–10	Hunger	Is the pet eating enough? Does hand-feeding help? Does the patient require a feeding tube?
0–10	Hydration	Is the patient dehydrated? For patients not drinking enough, use subcutaneous fluids once or twice daily to supplement fluid intake
0–10	Hygiene	The patient should be kept brushed and cleaned, particularly after elimination, avoid pressure sores and keep all wounds clean
0–10	Happiness	Does the pet express joy and interest? Is he responsive to things around him (e.g. family, toys)? Is the pet depressed, anxious, bored or afraid? Can the pet's bed be placed close to the family activities and not be isolated?
0–10	Mobility	Can the patient get up without assistance? Does the pet need human or mechanical help (e.g. a cart)? Does he feel like going for a walk? Is he having seizures or stumbling? Note: Some caregivers feel euthanasia is preferable to amputation, yet an animal who has limited mobility but is still alert and responsive can have a good quality of life as long as his caregivers are committed to helping him
0–10	More good days than bad	When there are too many bad days in a row, quality of life is too compromised. When a healthy human–animal bond is no longer possible, the caretaker must be made aware the end is near. The decision needs to be made if the pet is suffering. If death comes peacefully and painlessly, that is okay

1.7 Quality of Life Scale developed to help support owners in coming to a decision about quality of life. 0 = unacceptable; 10 = excellent. A total score of >35 is an acceptable quality of life for pets. (Villalobos and Kaplan, 2008)

Legislation relevant to veterinary practice includes:

- Veterinary Surgeons Act 1966
- Animal Welfare Act 2006 in England and Wales
- Animal Health and Welfare (Scotland) Act 2006
- Welfare of Animals Act (Northern Ireland) 2011
- Veterinary Medicines Regulations 2006
- Health and Safety at Work Act 1974
- Ionising Radiations Regulations 2017
- Control of Substances Hazardous to Health Regulations 2002
- Data Protection Act 2018
- Public Interest Disclosure Act 1998
- Animals (Scientific Procedures Act) 1986
- Equality Act 2010

Other legislation exists pertaining to employment, Inland Revenue, VAT and social security, disease control, animal breeding, public health and zoonoses

1.8 Legislation relevant to veterinary nurses in practice.

to health and safety and employment. Veterinary nurses may also be called upon as professional or expert witnesses in criminal or civil proceedings or as witnesses to fact in a professional hearing.

Types of law

A veterinary nurse needs to be aware of the two main branches of the UK legal system: *criminal* and *civil*. Each serves a different purpose and requires a different standard of proof. Veterinary surgeons or veterinary nurses could be involved in either. They may be called as an expert witness under criminal law (e.g. in a welfare case) or prosecuted themselves for not obeying the law. In the case of the latter, it is a requirement to notify the RCVS. If a negligence case is brought by an owner against a veterinary practice, this occurs under civil law. The structure of the court system is complicated; different types of cases are dealt with in different courts. The system in England and Wales is illustrated in Figure 1.9.

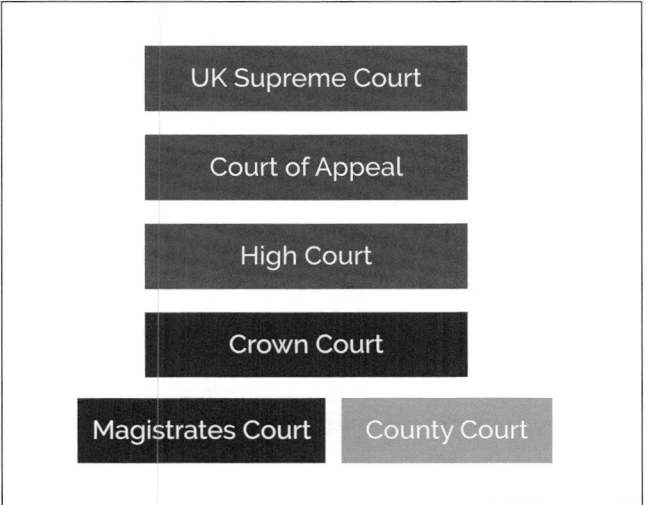

1.9 The structure of the court system in England and Wales. Blue = courts that deal with both criminal (e.g. an animal welfare case brought by RSPCA) and civil (e.g. a negligence case brought by an owner against a veterinary practice) cases. Red = courts that deal with criminal cases. Green = courts that deal with civil cases.

Criminal law

The purpose of this type of legislation is to *maintain law and order and protect the public* (e.g. the state *versus* a person). In cases of a breach of the Animal Welfare Act, the prosecutor can be an organization such as the RSPCA, but otherwise would be the police or the Crown Prosecution Service. In England, Wales and Northern Ireland the case is held in either the Magistrates (District Court in Scotland) or Crown Court (Sheriff Court in Scotland) and the standard of proof is 'beyond reasonable doubt'. The defendant may be found 'guilty' or 'not guilty'. If found guilty, the possible sanctions are:

- Conditional discharge
- Fine
- Community order
- Custodial sentence.

In the case of a breach of the Animal Welfare Act, a ban from keeping animals may be applied. Any of these outcomes will result in a criminal record for the individual, which may have a serious impact on their future.

Civil law

The purpose of this type of law is to *uphold the rights of an individual*. The individual bringing the case is referred to as the plaintiff and instigates a case against the defendant if they feel they have suffered loss or their rights have been affected (e.g. breach of a contract). In England, Wales and Northern Ireland the case is heard in a County Court (Sheriff Court in Scotland) or High Court (Court of Session in Scotland) with a judge hearing the case. The branch of civil law that deals specifically with negligence is known as 'Tort' or 'Delict' in Scotland. The standard of proof is on the 'balance of probability'. The defendant is found 'liable' or 'not liable'. If the defendant is found 'liable', they may have to pay compensation or damages plus costs to the plaintiff. Injunctions may also be imposed.

Negligence

The theory of negligence is based around the concept of *duty of care*. Veterinary nurses have a duty of care in law not to cause harm or loss to clients. Animals count as property or chattel and any harm must result in loss to the owner for the case to be considered as negligence (for example, accidental spaying of a pedigree cat which prevents the owner from breeding from it). Thus, negligence cases are civil cases, unless legislation such as the Veterinary Surgeons Act or Animal Welfare Act is found to have been breached.

There are three stages to proving negligence:

1. Is there a duty of care?
2. Has there been a breach of that duty of care?
3. Has this resulted in damage which would have been reasonably foreseeable?

The case precedent for Stage 1 is *Donoghue versus Stevenson* (1932). Mrs Donoghue, whilst drinking ginger beer from an opaque bottle in a café in Paisley, discovered a decomposed snail in the bottle and subsequently suffered personal injury. Her claim against the manufacturer of the ginger beer, Mr Stevenson was successful. Lord Atkin in his decision applied the 'neighbour test', i.e. you must take reasonable care to avoid acts or omissions which you can reasonably foresee would be likely to injure your neighbour. This case is sometimes referred to as 'The Paisley Snail'.

The case precedent for Stage 2 is *Bolam versus Friern Hospital Management Committee (1957)*. A patient was admitted to the hospital for electroconvulsive therapy (ECT) for depression, which involves applying an electrical current to the brain via skull electrodes. The patient was restrained by two nurses, but sustained bilateral hip fractures when he flew from the couch. The patient argued that the doctor was negligent for not giving a muscle relaxant or providing adequate restraint. The ruling in this case was that a 'medical professional is not guilty of negligence if he has acted in accordance with a practice accepted as proper by a responsible body of medical men skilled in that particular art'. In other words, to fulfil the Bolam test professionals are judged against the standards of others undertaking similar work. At this time risks were associated both with and without the use of muscle relaxants and the expert witness testimony supported the hospital in their policy not to warn patients of small risks, unless they were asked.

In relation to Stage 3, the courts must decide how likely it would be that a specific action would cause harm. The consequences of a tortious act must be foreseeable by a reasonable person, in the given circumstances.

Inexperience is never a valid excuse for negligence. Before accepting professional responsibility, the individual must judge what they have been trained to do and what they are capable of doing. Those with further training or qualifications may be judged against higher standards.

Animal abuse

There is increasing research and clinical evidence suggesting that sometimes there are links between the abuse of children, vulnerable adults and animals (Munro and Munro, 2008). As veterinary nurses often deal with the families of animals under their care, they may come across situations where they have concerns about the welfare of children and/or animals. The four categories of abuse are:

- Physical (children and animals)
- Emotional (children)
- Sexual (children and animals)
- Neglect (children and animals).

The links under these categories have been made in both the UK and the United States of America (USA) and include the following key indicators:

- If a child inflicts cruelty on an animal, in a minority of cases, it may be associated with abuse of that child
- Where serious animal abuse has taken place in a household there is increased risk of other types of abuse taking place
- Animal abuse may be used to coerce, control and intimidate vulnerable people by their abusers
- Where an animal has been abused, there is an increased likelihood that the animal has bitten/attacked adults and children within the household.

Professionals working with animals, such as veterinary nurses, are advised to discuss their concerns with a line manager or senior colleague and report concerns about animal abuse to the appropriate authority according to professional body guidance. Concerns about child abuse can be discussed with agencies such as the National Society for the Prevention of Cruelty to Children (NSPCC) or children's social services. Several agencies, including the NSPCC and RSPCA, have come together to produce guidelines for dealing with these types of concerns titled *Understanding the links* (www.nspcc.org.uk/globalassets/documents/research-reports/understanding-links-child-abuse-animal-abuse-domestic-violence.pdf).

This literature provides information, advice and guidance for raising concerns with the appropriate agencies. In addition, the Animal Welfare Foundation (www.animalwelfarefoundation.org.uk) and the Links Group (thelinksgroup.org.uk) have produce a booklet entitled *Recognizing abuse in animals and humans: comprehensive guidance for the veterinary team*, which can be downloaded from their websites (www.animalwelfarefoundation.org.uk/wp-content/uploads/2017/12/20160415-AWF-Recognising-abuse-in-animals-and-humans-v10-web.pdf or thelinksgroup.org.uk/wp-content/uploads/2019/04/Links-Group-Recognising-abuse-in-animals-and-humans-1.pdf); this provides useful information on the subject.

Ethics

The term ethics is derived from the Greek word 'ethos', meaning custom, characteristic or habit and relates to making decisions based on our moral values. It concerns the reasons behind our opinions on morally challenging decisions and goes beyond what is 'common practice'. It comprises notions such as 'good', 'bad', 'right' and 'wrong'. Many of us will have had to make challenging decisions in our life, but not necessarily have thought about the theory of the type of reasoning behind our decisions. Student veterinary nurses are now required as part of their syllabus to study ethics and morality in relation to veterinary nursing practice by utilizing ethical schools of thought and principles. These frameworks ensure that a consistent and logical approach is taken when making decisions in challenging situations.

Ethics and morality

In simple terms:

- *Morality* tells us if a decision is 'good', 'bad, 'right' or 'wrong'
- *Ethics* explores the rationale behind the decision.

Example

The neutering of stray pregnant cats, which is commonplace in some welfare organizations and veterinary practices.

- Some would argue that this is a 'good' and 'right' action as it prevents this cat and her offspring from adding to the stray cat population. There are already a large number of stray cats in need of homes.
- Others may believe that this is 'wrong' or 'bad' as this will cause the death of the unborn kittens, which is not acceptable, as well as increase the risks to the queen of neutering whilst pregnant.
- Some would consider routine neutering to be an essential part of responsible ownership.

> ### Example *continued*
> - Others may even believe that it is wrong to neuter altogether because they feel it causes unnecessary suffering.
>
> From this example it is clear that what one person believes to be 'right' or 'good' may seem 'wrong' or 'bad' to someone else.

Ethical dilemmas

In most situations, decisions and actions can be undertaken without much thought (for example, telling a colleague that a medication has been missed). However, there may be certain situations where an individual finds it difficult to make a decision about whether a course of action is 'good' or 'right'.

> ### Example
> A 16-year-old Shih Tzu, hospitalized to treat chronic end-stage renal failure, is recumbent, anorexic and on intravenous fluid therapy receiving palliative nursing care. The veterinary team feels that the 'right' course of action is euthanasia; however, due to the owner's religious beliefs the owner does not want to consent to this. As a result of being recumbent the patient develops a melting corneal ulcer and following discussions with the veterinary surgeon the owner consents to anaesthesia and eye enucleation. The nursing team feel strongly that this course of action is 'wrong' but are asked by the veterinary surgeon to participate in the patient's care

There are many factors that affect the way we think and feel about a situation and philosophers have attempted to answer the question about how decisions about 'right' and 'wrong' are made. Various frameworks have been written, providing useful tools to help with the decision-making process.

Ethical schools of thought

There are many theories; however, the majority can be grouped under two main headings.

- *Non-consequentialism:* this theory involves deciding on whether an action is 'right' or 'wrong' by examining obligations. Non-consequentialists claim that the right thing should be done, whatever the consequences might be. These are known as *deontological theories*. For example, the owner of a brachycephalic dog who is a long-standing client asks the veterinary nurse on duty if she thinks it is a good idea to breed from her dog. The client has asked for an opinion; the veterinary nurse must tell the client the truth because it is 'wrong' to lie.
- *Consequentialism:* this theory involves examining the outcome of an action to decide whether it is 'good' or 'bad'. The most popular of these outcome-based theories is *utilitarianism*. Using the example above, the veterinary nurse believes that it is unethical to breed from this brachycephalic dog with severe conformational abnormalities due to the complications that may arise. However, the nurse would decide that it is better to tell

the client that breeding is a possibility if the consequence of what they actually believe would not produce a good outcome. For example, the client becoming disengaged from the practice and not seeking veterinary advice.

Deontology

As non-consequentialists, deontologists believe that rules must be followed, no matter what the consequences may be. Therefore, it is the 'actions' that are 'right' or 'wrong' not the consequences. This is termed the *categorical imperative* (meaning unconditional and vital). Immanuel Kant (1724–1804) was an influential deontologist who held a firm belief in this theory. Kant believed that it is our duty not to lie, even if a lie would be directing a murderer away from their intended victim. Deontological theories encompass 'individual rights', which are often linked to laws or professional codes. It is accepted that choosing a rule that is applicable in every situation can be difficult and that duties or rights may conflict with each other. With this in mind it is recognized that exceptions may need to be made for certain circumstances and that sometimes, where there is conflict, avoiding the worst harm would be the right course of action to take.

> ### Example
> The practice manager has introduced a number of protocols to reduce costs as the wholesaler bill for consumables has become too large. They have said that animals undergoing a general anaesthetic are not to routinely have an intravenous catheter placed. The veterinary nursing team argues that there will be an increased risk of complications that could result in loss of life, but the practice manager states the financial benefits outweigh the risks.
>
> Using the *categorical imperative*, it could be questioned whether it would be acceptable for all veterinary practices to adopt this policy. If it was believed that this would be acceptable, the policy should be implemented. If not, then a refusal could be given, supported by this rationale

Utilitarianism

Early utilitarian Jeremy Bentham (1748–1832) considered 'happiness' to be linked to pleasurable experiences and the absence of pain (Mullan, 2006). This theory has been adapted slightly over time to include other forms of happiness (for example, when considering animals and their capabilities). Utilitarians believe that decisions should be taken to ensure that the consequences are the best possible for all involved. In other words, '*the greatest good for the greatest number*'.

Other ethical frameworks

'*Virtue ethics*' maintains that it is how we are that is important and that if we are a 'virtuous' or 'morally good' person then we will naturally act correctly in accordance with our character' (Mullan, 2006). This should perhaps be considered in relation to how we should act as professionals, and what the public perception of a veterinary nurse is both in and out of the workplace (Opperman, 2014).

'*Medical ethics*', the development of four principles to assist with decision making in healthcare, was proposed by Beauchamp and Childress (2013):

- **Non-maleficence** – the principle of doing no harm. This is often seen as the first, most important principle to follow. However, it is recognized that in veterinary practice sometimes short-term harm is inflicted on animals that is weighed up against the long-term good (e.g. orthopaedic surgery)
- **Beneficence** – the principle of promoting good and doing no harm. This is often taken into consideration on balance with non-maleficence in order to determine what course of action is in the best interest of the patient
- **Autonomy** – relates to the ability of an individual to be self-governing. This can be challenging to apply to animal patients as very often decision making is the responsibility of the client, guided by the veterinary surgeon
- **Justice** – treating all animals and people fairly and equally (i.e. as individuals).

Making ethical decisions

Consideration of these frameworks can be challenging and complicated. Mullan (2006) suggested the following practical framework for decision making in practice:

1. Identify all the possible courses of action.
2. Establish the interests of affected parties, including legal and professional guidance.
3. Formulate an ethical decision.
4. Minimize the impact of the decision.

Example

The stray pregnant cat neuter scenario from above: imagine there is conflict within the team about whether or not to neuter an individual.

Step one: List all the parties that will be affected by the decision.

- The cat – will awake from general anaesthesia no longer pregnant; there is also an increased risk from the general anaesthetic associated with neutering pregnant animals.
- The kittens – have no autonomy; others are making a decision about whether they live or die.
- The charity – will accept financial liability for either the neutering cost, or the cost of raising and re-homing a litter of kittens. They will also need to provide for the needs of, and re-home, the cat.
- The veterinary surgeon – will perform the surgery.
- The veterinary nurses – will provide care for the cat and kittens.
- Society as a whole – there is a large stray cat population already, what will the public think? Will they think spay and termination of the pregnancy is the most cost efficient approach? Or, will they think that preserving the life of the kittens should be the priority?
- The practice – would the decision to go ahead with the spay have an effect on the staff and/or the reputation of the practice?
- The profession – would this procedure be a positive or negative step?

Step two: Consider the potential *costs* and *benefits* of the procedure to each of the parties involved. →

Example *continued*

Costs:
- The cat will have to adapt to no longer being pregnant
- The kittens will be dead
- The charity will provide more assistance to the cat in terms of finances and resources if it is not neutered
- The veterinary surgeon and veterinary nurses may be acting against their own moral code if the pregnancy is terminated.

Benefits:
- The cat will spend less time in the care of the charity and will be re-homed much more quickly
- The charity will be able to use their resources to help more animals in need if there are no kittens to support
- The cat can be re-homed and will not contribute further to the stray cat population. As a result of this procedure, the potential offspring of the cat will also not contribute to the growing stray cat population
- Society as a whole will benefit from this reduction in the stray cat population.

Step three: Consideration of the costs and benefits for all parties.

Animal welfare should be the primary concern and it is clear from this approach that it is not an easy decision to make. It can be difficult to weigh up the costs and benefits, as different people will place differing importance on certain aspects of the situation. On the one hand, it could be argued that more animals will benefit from the neutering; however, the counter argument is that preserving the life of the kittens is more important.

Step four: Make a decision.
There are two options in this scenario:

- Spay the cat, resulting in termination of the pregnancy, but providing other benefits elsewhere
- Do not spay the cat, allow the pregnancy to continue, spay the cat at a later date, re-home the cat and kittens. This will incur extra costs for the charity but preserve the life of the kittens. There will be a risk that not all of the animals will find homes.

This example illustrates the difficulties that can be faced in making a decision as a team that is in the patient's best interest. The process above is useful as it ensures that everyone considers all alternatives, rather than making decisions based on emotion alone. Ultimately, the decision would be the owner's (in this case the charity), guided by the veterinary surgeon.

Applying regulatory, legal and welfare considerations to veterinary practice

Veterinary nurses should ensure that they are familiar with and take into account the relevant regulations, legislation and welfare considerations when working within veterinary practice. Examples of scenarios that may be encountered in practice are given below.

Scenario 1: Owners wishes

Cara, an RVN, has been qualified for a number of years in the practice she initially trained in, and has recently been involved in the care of an elderly feline patient named 'Orlando'. The patient is 14 years old and has been treated for several age-related conditions, including an abdominal mass. More recently, his condition has deteriorated and his owners have decided they would like for him to be euthanased, rather than undergo any more invasive therapies. Petra, the veterinary surgeon, confirms with both owners of 'Orlando' that they wish to go ahead with euthanasia and prepares the drugs. The owners of 'Orlando' do not wish to be present and do not want his ashes back following the cremation.

Cara expresses sadness at this decision and offers to take 'Orlando' home for some intensive nursing to see whether he will improve. Petra agrees to this course of action on the condition that 'Orlando' is euthanased if no improvement is seen. 'Orlando's' owners are not contacted to discuss this option and as far as they are concerned he has been euthanased. Unfortunately, 10 days later 'Orlando' escapes from Cara's home via an open window. 'Orlando' is microchipped and Cara begins to worry about what may happen if he is found and his owners are contacted.

Regulatory considerations	Legal considerations	Ethical and welfare considerations
Consent		
As an RVN Cara is accountable to the RCVS. She has responsibilities to animals, clients, colleagues, the profession and the general public The owners of 'Orlando' have not consented to this course of action. The Code of Professional Conduct gives clear guidance that the wishes of the RVN cannot override those of the owner except in exceptional circumstances. If a concern was raised it would be fully investigated by the practice and it is likely it would also be referred to the RCVS	It is likely that 'Orlando's' owners would not have consented to this course of action. However, this cannot be fully determined as they were never given the opportunity to consider this as part of the consent process	The patient's welfare is at risk
Dishonesty		
In terms of the five principles of practice, honesty and integrity, client confidentiality and trust and professional accountability should be taken into consideration. Dishonesty is seen by the RCVS as grounds for disgraceful conduct in a professional respect, although the procedure for investigating complaints would have to be followed before any formal decision was made. In a disciplinary hearing, if charges were proved a sanction would be applied. Cara's actions have also put the veterinary surgeon's professional registration at risk as she agreed to Cara taking 'Orlando' home	In law, 'Orlando' is regarded as the property of the owner. Therefore, the theft of a cat is treated as the theft of any other property under The Theft Act (1968). The owners of 'Orlando' could launch civil proceedings against the practice/Cara/Petra in relation to negligence. The three stages of negligence would be applied: 1. Is there a duty of care? 2. Has the duty of care been breached? 3. Has this resulted in damage, which would have been reasonably foreseeable?	'Orlando's' welfare has been put at significant risk because at the time he escaped he was terminally ill. The five animal needs as detailed in The Animal Welfare Act (2006) may be taken into consideration; for example, in this case the need to be protected from pain, suffering, injury and disease is likely to have been breached

Scenario 2: Professional conduct

Oliver is working at a veterinary practice as a locum RVN; the booking involves working long shifts from 8am until 7pm for 1 week. Accommodation is provided in a flat above the practice. During the course of the day, it is noticed by other members of staff that Oliver is making frequent visits to the flat, approximately every half an hour to an hour. When he returns he is usually eating something, drinking a glass of squash or chewing gum. Other members of staff think this is unusual as there are toilet and rest facilities within the practice building.

Daisy, a veterinary surgeon at the practice, and Maria, an RVN, also notice that Oliver is unsteady on his feet, slurring his words and his face is flushed. Daisy also notices an open bottle of wine in Oliver's bag and confronts him. Oliver says that he does like a drink but that it does not affect his work. When asked about his frequent visits to the flat, Oliver says that he is diabetic and needs to eat regularly, but that his diabetes is under control. Daisy also has some concerns about Oliver's ability to interpret instructions given to him relating to patient care; for example, she has told him several times which patient monitors to attach to anaesthetized patients but he fails to do this.

Several weeks later, the practice is contacted by the RCVS who inform them that another practice has raised concerns about Oliver being under the influence of alcohol whilst working as a locum RVN. Daisy and Maria are asked to provide witness statements; it also transpires that 3 years earlier Oliver was convicted of driving under the influence of alcohol.

continues ▶

Scenario 2: Professional conduct *continued*

Regulatory considerations	Legal considerations	Ethical and welfare considerations
Whistleblowing		
It is considered by both the RCVS and the general public that veterinary surgeons and veterinary nurses will report any acts of misconduct. This is part of being a regulated professional. Daisy and Maria should engage with the investigation fully, providing written statements when asked and possibly attending a disciplinary hearing as witnesses if requested. Oliver should engage with the RCVS investigation fully. The three-stage process will be followed. There is support available from various organizations, including Vetlife and Oliver's indemnity insurer	The Public Interest Disclosure Act 1998 covers employees, contractors, students, locum staff and staff working at home. The usual employment law restrictions on minimum qualification period and age do not apply to this Act	Oliver's conduct may have had an impact on the welfare of patients, either directly or indirectly. There is also the potential for the welfare of patients under his care to be compromised in the future
Fitness to practise		
Under the health protocol, Oliver may be medically assessed and asked to agree to undertakings relating to his fitness to practise. If a breach of these undertakings occurs, it is likely Oliver will be referred to the RVN DC by the RVN PIC. Alternatively, the PIC may make a decision to refer straight to the RVN DC (e.g. if Oliver refuses to respond to the RCVS during the investigation)	Although Oliver's previous conviction alone is unlikely to render him unfit for practise, it is likely to be taken into consideration in relation to this concern and subsequent investigation	The RCVS will consider whether there was any danger to animals under Oliver's care during their investigation
Insight		
A disciplinary committee would consider whether there is any insight in relation to the misconduct. If a respondent shows insight and engages with support, for example via the health protocol, a disciplinary hearing may be postponed. A lack of insight may contribute to a harsher sanction in a disciplinary hearing, for example removal from the register		Under the health protocol Oliver may still be permitted to practice with undertakings (e.g. a workplace supervisor and/or blood/urine/medical tests)
Public protection		
This is the primary purpose of professional regulation. The disciplinary committee will consider public protection when considering professional misconduct and sanctions		If there was harm to animals directly or indirectly as a result of Oliver's conduct, this would be taken into consideration, as well as the possibility of any future harm

Scenario 3: Delegation

Pauline, a student veterinary nurse, is asked to admit an elderly Bichon Frise for a dental scale and polish on behalf of the veterinary surgeon who is busy with another patient. Pauline has never carried out an admission on her own before; however, she has watched RVNs and the practice has a checklist so she goes ahead and admits the patient. Afterwards she is pleased with how it went but realizes she forgot to ask the owner if they wanted pre-anaesthetic blood tests, something that the practice routinely recommend. The veterinary surgeon has a reputation for being a little short-tempered and abrupt and Pauline is a little intimidated by them, so she decides not to tell them about this oversight. The procedure goes ahead but the patient is very unstable under the anaesthetic; the veterinary surgeon realizes the blood tests were not done and runs them immediately. The results show that the patient is in chronic renal failure and the veterinary surgeon is displeased with Pauline, as they would have taken a different course of action had they seen the results prior to the procedure.

Regulatory considerations	Legal considerations	Ethical and welfare considerations
Personal scope of competence		
It was not inappropriate to delegate this task to a student veterinary nurse; however, it should have been taken into account whether or not Pauline understood the procedure and had the experience and good sense to react appropriately if problems arose. There should have also been an appropriate level of supervision and/or someone to call upon for assistance. In light of the fact that Pauline had never completed an admission by herself, it may have been appropriate to delegate the task to someone else, or have an observer in the room to step in and assist if necessary		The welfare of the patient could be compromised by the omission

continues ▶

Scenario 3: Delegation *continued*

Communication and consent		
In order for informed consent to have taken place, the client should have been given a range of options and had all of the risks and benefits explained to them. If the client was not aware of the option of a pre-anaesthetic blood test, they may not have been able to make a fully informed decision. Pauline had a responsibility to communicate to the veterinary surgeon that she had overlooked the option of the blood test, however difficult that may be. The veterinary surgeon also had a responsibility to check the patient record prior to starting the procedure and to follow up on the delegation appropriately. The student should have their work directly supervised at all times	There is the potential for a negligence case to brought against the practice/veterinary surgeon	The welfare of the patient could be compromised due to the breakdown in communication
Risk to the patient		
The patient was at risk and the client could raise a concern with the practice. If they felt that there was no resolution following this they could also raise a concern with the RCVS		The procedure was potentially unnecessary in light of the findings from the blood test. It is possible that the patient would have been stabilized in terms of renal function first, before undertaking the dental procedure at a later date. It is likely that suffering did not occur as the patient survived the anaesthetic and then would have been treated for the renal failure

References and further reading

Beauchamp TL and Childress JE (2013) *Principles of Biomedical Ethics, 7th edn.* Oxford University Press, Oxford

Benson GJ and Rollin BE (2004) *The Well-Being of Farm Animals: Challenges and Solution.* Blackwell Publishing, Oxford

Boud D, Keogh R and Walker D (1985) *Reflection: Turning Experience into Learning.* Kogan Page, London

Broom DM (1991) Animal welfare: concepts and measurement. *Journal of Animal Science* **69**, 4167–4175

Dawkins MS (2004) Using behaviour to assess animal welfare. *Animal Welfare* **13**, 3–7

Earl E (2006) Negligence and whistle-blowing. In: *Ethics, Law and the Veterinary Nurse,* ed. S Pullen and C Gray, pp. 29–33. Elsevier

Fraser D (2008) *Understanding Animal Welfare: The Science in its Cultural Context (UFAW Animal Welfare).* Wiley-Blackwell, Oxford

Fraser D (2012) A 'practical' ethic for animals. *Journal of Agricultural and Environmental Ethics* **25(5)**, 721–746

Gibbs G (1988) *Learning by doing: a guide to teaching and learning methods.* Further Education Unit. Oxford Polytechnic, Oxford

Kolb DA (1984) *Experimental Learning: Experience as the Source of Learning and Development.* Prentice Hall, New Jersey

Legood G (2000) *Veterinary Ethics.* Continuum, UK

Macdonald J, Buckley L and Mann A (2017) Evidence-based veterinary nursing – it's more sexy than you might think! *Veterinary Nursing Journal* **32**, 78–81

Macdonald J and Gray C (2014) Informed consent – how do we get it right? *Veterinary Nursing Journal* **29**, 101–103

Merry A and McCall Smith A (2004) *Errors, Medicine and the Law.* Cambridge University Press, UK

Mullan S (2006) Introduction to ethical principles. In: *Ethics, Law and the Veterinary Nurse,* ed. S Pullen and C Gray, pp. 11–22. Elsevier, UK

Munro R and Munro HMC (2008) *Animal Abuse and Unlawful Killing: Veterinary Forensic Pathology.* Saunders Elsevier, Oxford

Opperman E (2014) What it means to be professional – a personal viewpoint. *Veterinary Nursing Journal* **29**, 99–100

Pullen S and Gray C (2006) *Ethics, Law and the Veterinary Nurse.* Elsevier, UK

Pullen S, Wright A and Cooper C (2011) Professional responsibilities, regulation and the ethics of veterinary nursing. In: *BSAVA Textbook of Veterinary Nursing, 5th edn,* ed. B Cooper et al., pp. 1–15. BSAVA Publications, Gloucester

Rollin BE (2006) Euthanasia and quality of life. *Journal of American Veterinary Medical Association* **228(7)**, 1014–1016

Schön DA (1983) *The Reflective Practitioner: How Professionals Think in Action.* Basic Books Inc., USA

Villalobos A and Kaplan L (2008) *Canine and Feline Geriatric Oncology: Honoring the Human–Animal Bond.* Blackwell, USA

Welsh P and Bayliss S (2012) Whistle-blowing explained: to be or not to be a whistle-blower, that is the question. *The Veterinary Nurse* **3**, 122–126

Yeates J (2013) *Animal Welfare in Veterinary Practice (UFAW Animal Welfare).* Wiley-Blackwell, Oxford

Useful websites

Advisory, Conciliation and Arbitration Service (ACAS): www.acas.org.uk

Animal Welfare Foundation: www.animalwelfarefoundation.org.uk
- Recognizing abuse in animals and humans: comprehensive guidance for the veterinary team: www.animalwelfarefoundation.org.uk/wp-content/uploads/2017/12/20160415-AWF-Recognising-abuse-in-animals-and-humans-v10-web.pdf

British Small Animal Veterinary Association (BSAVA): www.bsava.com

British Veterinary Association (BVA): www.bva.co.uk

British Veterinary Nursing Association (BVNA): www.bvna.org.uk

Citizens Advice Bureau: www.citizensadvice.org.uk

Department for Environment, Food and Rural Affairs (Defra): www.defra.gov.uk

Health and Safety Executive (HSE): www.hse.gov.uk

The Kennel Club:
www.thekennelclub.org.uk

Law Society:
www.lawsociety.org.uk

Links Group:
thelinksgroup.org.uk
- Recognizing abuse in animals and humans: comprehensive guidance for the veterinary team: thelinksgroup.org.uk/wp-content/uploads/2019/04/Links-Group-Recognising-abuse-in-animals-and-humans-1.pdf

Mental Health Act 1983 – Code of Practice:
www.gov.uk/government/publications/code-of-practice-mental-health-act-1983

National Society for the Prevention of Cruelty to Children (NSPCC):
www.nspcc.org.uk
- Understanding the links – child abuse, animal abuse and domestic violence: www.nspcc.org.uk/globalassets/documents/research-reports/understanding-links-child-abuse-animal-abuse-domestic-violence.pdf

Public Concern at Work (PCAW):
www.pcaw.co.uk

The Ralph Site:
www.theralphsite.com

Refuge:
www.refuge.org.uk

Royal College of Veterinary Surgeons (RCVS):
www.rcvs.org.uk
- Code of Professional Conduct for Veterinary Nurses: www.rcvs.org.uk/advice-and-guidance/code-of-professional-conduct-for-veterinary-nurses/
- Communication and Consent: www.rcvs.org.uk/setting-standards/advice-and-guidance/code-of-professional-conduct-for-veterinary-surgeons/supporting-guidance/communication-and-consent/
- Fitness to Practise – A Guide for UK Providers of Veterinary Nursing Education and Student Veterinary Nurses: www.rcvs.org.uk/news-and-views/news/new-fitness-to-practise-guidance-for-student-veterinary-nurses/
- Knowledge: https://knowledge.rcvs.org.uk

Royal Society for the Protection of Cruelty to Animals (RSPCA):
www.rspca.org.uk

Society for Companion Animal Studies (SCAS):
www.scas.org.uk

Veterinary Defence Society (VDS):
www.thevds.co.uk

Veterinary Client Mediation Service (VCMS):
www.vetmediation.co.uk

Vetlife:
www.vetlife.org.uk/how-we-help/vetlife-health-support/

VN Futures:
www.vetfutures.org.uk/vnfutures/

Self-assessment questions

1. What is the definition of accountability?
2. State at least three of the five principles of practice.
3. In relation to The Code of Professional Conduct for Veterinary Nurses, identify the key areas of responsibility the RVN has.
4. What is the definition of informed consent?
5. Who can give legal consent?
6. What is the standard of proof for a) criminal cases and b) civil cases?
7. Which ethical school of thought considers the consequences of decisions made?
8. What is the meaning of non-maleficence?
9. What is the definition of evidence-based veterinary medicine?
10. With whom should concerns about standards of care or professional conduct be raised?

Chapter 2

Principles of health and safety

Anne Lawson

Learning objectives

After studying this chapter, readers will have the knowledge to:

- Describe the aims of effective health and safety in the workplace
- Summarize the requirements of effective risk management and be able to conduct a workplace risk assessment
- Identify the principle risks associated with health and safety in a veterinary practice
- Describe and apply safe principles of health and safety practice in relation to a range of situations in the veterinary practice
- Implement good health and safety systems into practice management
- Identify where to find further information on health and safety topics

The aims of effective health and safety management

The veterinary nurse has a crucial role in the effective implementation of health and safety in the workplace.

Health and safety management is not a standalone item in veterinary practice, it is an integral part of how all veterinary practices, regardless of size, have to be run on a daily basis.

The existence of a health and safety management system alone is not sufficient to ensure that health and safety is effectively implemented in practice. The success of the system is dependent on the attitude and behaviour of the team, often referred to as the 'safety culture'. The veterinary nurse is instrumental in the development of a positive safety culture.

Keys to effective health and safety management

- Members of staff in leadership and management positions who are committed to health and safety in the practice
- A competent workforce who are trained in the requirements of effective health and safety

→

Keys to effective health and safety management *continued*

- Clear health and safety policies, procedures, standard operating procedures (SOPs) and guidelines
- A comprehensive understanding of the health and safety risks associated with the veterinary practice, how to manage these risks, and their regular review
- Creating a culture and environment where the whole team is engaged and actively involved in health and safety management

The role of clinical audit

Clinical audit is a rapidly developing area in veterinary practice. It is a process for monitoring standards of clinical care to determine how it is being carried out compared with best practice and evidence-based veterinary medicine (EBVM). The Royal College of Veterinary Surgeons (RCVS) Knowledge website (https://knowledge.rcvs.org.uk/home/) has simple to use audit tools available. These tools are ideal to integrate with good safety management, and there are numerous safety subjects to audit, including Controlled Drugs recording, fire safety checks and waste management.

The legal framework

Health and safety law is enforced in the United Kingdom by the Health and Safety Executive (HSE). They are a government appointed regulator and have a number of powers, including requesting entry into a business, questioning employees, examining the workplace and looking at documentation. The HSE can issue sanctions such as letters of contravention, improvement notices, prohibition notices and prosecutions.

The key pieces of legislation underpinning Health and safety law for veterinary practice are:

- The Health and Safety at Work Act 1974
- The Management of Health and Safety at Work Regulations (MHSWR) 1999.

The basis of health and safety law in Great Britain is the Health and Safety at Work Act 1974 and in Northern Ireland is the Health and Safety at Work (Northern Ireland) Order 1978. These set out the general duties which employers have to employees and members of the public, and employees have to themselves and to each other. The MHSWR (Management Regulations) require employers to put in place arrangements to control health and safety risks (Figure 2.1).

- A health and safety policy (written if you employ five or more people)
- Assessment of the risks to employees, contractors, clients, partners and any other people who could be affected by your activities
- Arrangements for preventive and protective measures arising from your risk assessment
- Access to competent health and safety advice
- Provision of information to employees about workplace risks and how they are protected
- Instruction and training for employees in how to deal with the risks
- Ensure adequate and appropriate supervision is in place
- Consultation with employees about their risks at work and current preventive and protective measures

2.1 Key requirements of the Management of Health and Safety at Work Regulations 1999.

The HSE enforce legislation, publish the Approved Codes of Practice (ACOPs) and produce guidance to help interpret legislation and the ACOPs.

- Legislation are laws approved by the government.
- ACOPs offer practical examples of good practice and have a special legal status. If employers are prosecuted for a breach of health and safety law, and it is proved that they have not followed the relevant provisions of the ACOPs, a court can find them at fault unless they can show that they have complied with the law in some other way.
- Guidance documents – compliance with these is not compulsory and employers are free to take other action. However, it should be noted that if the guidance is followed, then the legal requirements are likely to have been met.

All this information is available free of charge on the HSE website (www.hse.gov.uk/). Other pieces of relevant legislation are referenced throughout the chapter.

RCVS Practice Standard Scheme

The RCVS Practice Standards Scheme (PSS) is an accreditation scheme, which quality assures veterinary practices. If the practice is part of the scheme, health and safety standards and implementation will be checked by the PSS Assessor during their visit

Health and safety policy

Legislation

- The Health and Safety at Work Act 1974
- The Health and Safety Information for Employees Regulations 1989
- Employers Liability (Compulsory Insurance) Act 1969

A health and safety policy should state the aims of the veterinary practice with regard to health and safety. It should detail who has overall responsibility for health and safety in the practice and who is responsible for the day-to-day implementation of the policy. Individuals need to be appointed for specific roles regarding health and safety, such as fire officer and appointed first aider. The health and safety policy should reference the practice arrangements and what measures are in place for implementing the policy. If there are fewer than five employees, the policy does not need to be written down; however it is recommended that it is. The HSE provide a health and safety policy template. Figure 2.2 shows a completed example for a general veterinary practice.

By law, an official health and safety law poster must be completed and displayed, or an equivalent leaflet provided to each worker. It is sensible to display the poster in an area where all team members will have access to it, such as the refreshments area or a team notice board. The practice is also obliged by law to have employers' liability insurance against accidents and ill health of their employees and to display a copy of the up to date certificate.

Risk assessment

Legislation

- The Management of Health and Safety at Work Regulations (MHSWR) 1999 (Management Regulations)

The MHSWR require employers to carry out a risk assessment. Understanding risk assessment principles is crucial to good health and safety management.

Risk is assessed by identifying common hazards (things that may cause harm) in the workplace, evaluating the likelihood of harm occurring and the severity of harm should it occur. Put simply, a risk assessment involves thinking about the things that could cause harm in the veterinary environment and considering whether there are sufficient controls in place to prevent this harm occurring.

Health and safety policy

This is the statement of general policy and arrangements for: A N Other Vets Ltd

Name. For example, Practice Owner, Clinical Director — **has overall and final responsibility for health and safety**

Name. For example, Head Veterinary Nurse — **has day-to-day responsibility for ensuring this policy is put into practice**

Statement of general policy	Responsibility: name/title	Action/arrangements (what are we going to do?)
Prevent accidents and cases of work-related ill health (physical and mental) by managing the health and safety risks in the workplace	**Name** Practice Owner	Implement a risk assessment programme with regular reviews; Ensure any accident or incident is investigated and reported; Provide information on Health and Safety on the noticeboard
Provide clear instructions and information, and adequate training, to ensure employees are competent to do their work	**Name** Practice Manager	Maintain an up to date employee handbook; Ensure induction training, task-specific and refresher training is given to all personnel; Develop and maintain SOPs for all activities that pose a risk to employee health and safety; Provide regular health and safety updates at team meetings
Engage and consult with employees on day-to-day health and safety conditions	**Name** Practice Owner	Appoint a Safety Representative to aid employee consultation; Conduct regular team meetings and address any matters arising
Maintain safe and healthy working conditions, provide and maintain plant, equipment and machinery, and ensure safe storage/use of substances	**Name** Practice Manager	Establish and keep up to date equipment maintenance records and contracts; Implement a reporting system for faulty equipment and workplace health and safety concerns; Provide hazardous substance training and suitable facilities and controls for storage and use
Implement emergency procedures – evacuation in case of fire or other significant incident	**Name** Practice Manager	Conduct and maintain an up to date fire risk assessment; Ensure effective fire prevention and detection by regular checks and maintenance of fire alarm, detection systems, and extinguishers; Conduct fire training and evacuation drills at regular intervals; Complete and record weekly housekeeping checks and address any shortfalls; Display appropriate signs and notices to ensure escape routes and fire safety information is communicated effectively

Health and safety law poster displayed at	Kitchen
First-aid box(es) located at	Staff room/reception
Accident book is located at	Reception desk

All employees must:

- Cooperate with the Practice Owner, Manager and Supervisors on health and safety matters
- Take reasonable care of their own health and safety
- Report all health and safety concerns to an appropriate person (as detailed above).

Signed: Practice Owner	Date	Signed: Practice Manager	Date

2.2 Example of a general health and safety policy for a veterinary practice.

Risk assessments do not need to be complicated, generally do not require external expertise, and the individual does not have to be a health and safety expert to carry them out. The veterinary nurse may be involved in carrying out risk assessments or in reviewing assessments completed by others.

Hazards and risks are often misunderstood (Figure 2.3).

- A **hazard** is anything that may cause harm. Hazards can result in injury or ill health (either physical or mental ill health).
- **Risk** is the combination of the **likelihood** of the hazard causing harm occurring (high or low), together with the **severity** (how serious) the harm could be.

Risk assessments are carried out for a number of reasons: to assess an area (e.g. waiting room), a task (e.g. use of the autoclave) or a specific legislative requirement (e.g. Control of Substances Hazardous to Health (COSHH), ionizing radiation, fire safety). Some areas of risk assessment overlap; for example, a laboratory area assessment may identify spillage of stains as a hazard, with skin or eye irritation as the consequence. This would also be identified in a COSHH risk assessment as a hazardous chemical with associated handling risks. The controls would be the same – spill kit, information for users readily available, training for team members, clear

labelling of products, storage of stains within a spill tray and use of personal protective equipment (PPE).

Figure 2.4 summarizes the steps required to carry out a risk assessment and keep it up to date. When preparing or reviewing a risk assessment, working through the five steps discussed below will help the veterinary professional to establish whether all the necessary steps have been completed. A copy of these rules affixed to the front of the risk assessment folder provides an easy aide memoire.

- **Step one** – identify the hazards
- **Step two** – decide who might be harmed and how
- **Step three** – evaluate the risks and decide on precautions
- **Step four** – record your significant findings
- **Step five** – review your assessment and update if necessary

2.4 The five steps of risk assessment.

Step one – identify the hazards

- The best advice for identifying hazards is to print a blank risk assessment form, walk around a work area or where a task is taking place, look for potential hazards and record the findings.
- Look at equipment, servicing and maintenance (routine and emergency).
- Look at the layout of the premises.
- Look at accident and ill health records.
- Remember to take into consideration long-term health effects that may not be visible (e.g. exposure to anaesthetics, effects of ionizing radiation).
- Consider human factors (e.g. why PPE is available for some tasks but not used).
- It is a common misbelief that every single possibility must be considered and recorded. Events need to be considered only if they are plausible.

Step two – decide who might be harmed and how

Who

- In the veterinary practice, consideration should be given to a wide range of people:
  - Team members
  - Third parties – clients or members of the public, people undertaking work experience, contractors.
- Special situations – new and young workers, new or expectant mothers, people with disabilities, locums, lone workers (Figure 2.5).
- Practices in shared premises like pet shops or emergency clinics – each party must consider how their work affects the other and cooperate to ensure health and safety obligations are met.

How

- Think of the likely consequence in terms of severity; what is the worst that could realistically happen? It is important to get this right for the assessment to be taken seriously.
- Once the worst credible scenario has been determined, suitable risk precautions can be applied.

Sensible risk management

Remember that HAZARD (anything that can cause harm)

is not the same as RISK (likelihood harm will occur and its severity)

High risk

Low risk

2.3 Understanding risk. The lion represents the hazard and the two examples of risk are represented by the person photographing the lion in the wild (high risk) and the person photographing the lion in a cage (low risk).

CASE EXAMPLE – Paris *versus* Stepney Borough Council (1951)

This is a pivotal case in health and safety law

- Paris had sight in one eye. During the course of his Council employment, a splinter of metal went into his sighted eye causing him to become completely blind
- The employer did not provide safety goggles to workers engaged in the type of work Paris was undertaking
- The Council argued there was no breach of duty as they did not provide goggles to workers with vision in both eyes and it was not standard practice to do so. They said there was therefore no obligation to provide Paris with goggles

The House of Lords found there was a breach of duty by the Council. The employer should have provided goggles to Paris because the seriousness of harm to him would have been greater than that experienced by workers with sight in both eyes. The duty is owed to the particular claimant, not to a class of persons of reasonable workers

Why is this case relevant?

- The concept of **negligence** is that people should exercise reasonable care in their actions, by taking account of the **harm that they might foreseeably cause to other people or property**
- This case demonstrates the **increased duty of care** to persons affected by work activities with special requirements (e.g. persons with disabilities, new and expectant mothers, young people)

2.5 Case law (Paris *versus* Stepney Borough Council, 1951) demonstrating the importance of effective risk management. In this case, the Council were found to be negligent because they failed to identify that Paris was at increased risk and to take additional precautions.

Step three – evaluate the risks and decide on precautions (also known as controls)

- Evaluating the risks can be done either by assigning a score or by objectively assessing the likelihood and severity of harm.
- An important question is: can the hazard be removed altogether? For example, do not do the task or do it a different way. A simple example of this is examining a large dog on the floor rather than lifting it on to a table, reducing the risk of injury from manual handling.
- Think about what is already in place and make a list of these items.
- Think about what other precautions or controls are needed so that the risk is as low as is reasonably practicable (Figures 2.6 and 2.7).
- A good general rule for risk assessment is that the higher the likelihood of harm and/or the severity of harm, the more controls should be in place to prevent the harm occurring.

CASE EXAMPLE – Edwards *versus* National Coal Board (NCB) (1949)

The reasonably practicable test

Mr Edwards was killed when a section of underground roadway in a mine collapsed. The NCB stated that the cost of shoring up the roadway would have been prohibitive and therefore was not justified. The Court of Appeal found for the widow of Mr Edwards, considering that the NCB had failed to establish an adequate defence, determining that the risk far outweighted any sacrifice in shoring up the road.

The reasonably practicable risk test is a balancing act, with the degree of risk being placed on one side of the scales and the sacrifice involved in the control measures needed to avert the risk – that is, time, money and trouble – placed on the other side.

Extreme examples of this are:

- To spend £1 million to prevent a member of staff suffering bruised knees is obviously grossly disproportionate
- But, to spend £1 million to prevent a major explosion capable of killing 150 people is obviously proportionate

2.7 The reasonably practicable test – Edwards *versus* National Coal Board (NCB), 1949.

As low as is reasonably practicable (ALARP)

- This is a term that frequently occurs in safety legislation
- It means that you need to weigh a risk against the cost needed to control it

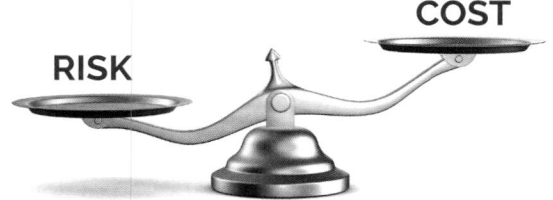

Cost of additional precautions should be considered

- Trouble
- Time/effort

2.6 As low as reasonably practicable – an explanation of the terminology.

Step four – record your significant findings

Where five or more persons are employed, the significant findings of risk assessments must be recorded. Where fewer than five persons are employed, it is not required for them to be in writing; however, it is considered best practice to record all risk assessments. There are many formats for risk assessment recording but as a general rule, a simple format is most effective.

The HSE have produced a template risk assessment that is simple to understand and easy to use. Figure 2.8 is an example of a veterinary risk assessment completed using this template.

Risk assessments can incorporate a risk rating score. This can be useful to help prioritise actions. High score items necessitate immediate action, whilst lower score items may have sufficient controls. Figure 2.9 is an example of a simple scored rating system, using guide words to help with accurate and consistent scoring. The matrix provides guidance on the appropriate response required for each risk rating

Risk assessment – consulting room

Company name: A N Other Vets Ltd

Date of risk assessment: 21 May 2019

What are the hazards?	Who might be harmed and how?	What are you already doing?	Do you need to do anything else to control this risk?	Action by who?	Action by when?	Done
Slips and trips	■ Vet, nurse or client ■ Slips and trips resulting in injury • Mid-day cleaning and spot cleaning animal urine/faeces • Trailing vacuum cables • Small step outside consulting room door	■ Non-slip flooring ■ Cleaning with non-slip floor cleaner ■ Non-slip footwear for team ■ Trailing leads or cables used only when no clients are in practice ■ Move plug points regularly to decrease trip risk ■ Well-lit area	Provide training regarding slips and trips Dry floor after spot cleaning Highlight small step to make more visible (short term) Remove step at next planned refurbishment	Practice Manager Vet or nurse Practice Manager Practice Manager	29/5/2019 At time 29/5/2019 21/11/2019	Complete 28/5/2019 Complete 28/5/2019
Manual handling of animals	■ Vet, nurse or client ■ Back injury from incorrect handling	■ Manual handling training completed ■ Large dogs examined on floor ■ Table is height adjustable ■ Additional help available if needed	Advise clients not to lift large dogs on to table	Practice Manager	31/5/2019 Practice Meeting agenda item	Complete 3/6/2019
Animal bites	■ Vet, nurse or client ■ Bite injury to hands, arm or face	■ Muzzles, towels and other restraints available ■ Additional team members available to help ■ Trained team only handle animals ■ System provides details of animals known to bite	Engage clients with positive reinforcement methods for dogs – produce information sheets to help	Nurse team	21/8/2019	
Handling reptiles	■ Vet, nurse or client ■ Salmonellosis from contact	■ PPE (gloves) ■ Good hygiene practice ■ Sinks and soap in consulting room ■ Refer to the BSAVA Manual of Reptiles for information on correct handling ■ Zoonoses SOP	Public Health England information sheet for clients not on server – to be added Ensure soap is regularly replaced as sometimes not replaced when empty. Add to daily consulting room checklist	Reception Head Nurse	Immediately 28/5/2019	Complete 21/5/2019 Complete 22/5/2019
Handling birds	■ Vet or nurse ■ Injury from beak or claws ■ Zoonotic disease from direct contact or inhalation ■ Escape of pet leading to harm or loss	■ Zoonoses SOP ■ Specific team members designated for all avian work ■ PPE (gloves) ■ Good hygiene practice ■ Sinks and soap in consulting room ■ Secure room available with lock on door to prevent escape	Ensure soap is regularly replaced Add to daily consulting room checklist Ensure new team members made aware of SOP Add SOPs to induction file	Head Nurse Practice Manager Practice Manager	28/5/2019 Ongoing 28/5/2019	Complete 22/5/19 Complete 27/5/2019
Hazardous substances	■ Vet or nurse ■ Range of acute and chronic health effects from harmful substances ■ Examples in consulting room: • Cleaning products – irritation • Surgical spirit – flammable/harmful by inhalation or skin contact • Chlorhexidine – dermatitis	■ Specific COSHH risk assessment for hazardous substances to be followed ■ High risk products identified with red stickers ■ Datasheets available online and links on all computer terminals ■ PPE readily available and used ■ Refer to COSHH assessment for full assessment	See COSHH risk assessment for full information on products stocked	N/A	N/A	

2.8 HSE template used to complete a risk assessment for a consulting room.

continues ▲

Risk assessment – consulting room

What are the hazards?	Who might be harmed and how?	What are you already doing?	Do you need to do anything else to control this risk?	Action by who?	Action by when?	Done
Contact with zoonoses	▪ Vet or nurse ▪ Infectious diseases	▪ Sink in consulting room for handwashing ▪ Trained team members ▪ Zoonoses SOP ▪ Cleaning with approved materials ▪ Cleaning SOP ▪ Cleaning records and regular audit	Ensure soap is regularly replaced	Head Nurse	28/5/19	Complete 22/5/19
			Ensure new team members made aware of SOP on zoonoses	Practice Manager	Ongoing	
			Display Bella Moss guidelines on handwashing in consulting rooms	Head Nurse	28/5/2109	Complete 27/5/19
Standing for long periods	▪ Vet or nurse ▪ Back pain, musculoskeletal injury, varicose veins	▪ Rest breaks built into consulting time ▪ Vet/nurse leaves consulting room to call through next client ▪ Comfortable footwear	Provide suitable seating	Practice Manager	29/6/2019	
			Workstation assessment for computer to be completed	Practice Manager	28/5/2019	Complete 27/5/19

2.8 *continued* HSE template used to complete a risk assessment for a consulting room.

		Medium risk **3**	High risk **6**	High risk **9**
Likelihood (L)	3. Very likely (known to happen regularly)			
	2. Likely (known to happen infrequently)	Low risk **2**	Medium risk **4**	High risk **6**
	1. Unlikely (unknown to happen)	Low risk **1**	Low risk **2**	Medium risk **3**
		1. Minor (cut or bruise)	2. Moderate (serious injury or illness resulting in time off work)	3. Major (life-changing injury, illness or fatality)
		Severity (S)		

1 or 2 = Low risk	Proceed with existing controls in place
3 or 4 = Medium risk	Consider additional controls. Proceed when all reasonably practicable controls have been applied
6 or 9 = High risk	Do not continue until additional controls have been applied and the risk is reduced to low or medium

2.9 Risk assessment rating score matrix and guidance.

(high, medium or low risk). Scoring is not a legal requirement and it can cause confusion for some users; it is important to establish a method that works well for the practice. An example of a scored risk assessment is given in Figure 2.10.

Step five – review your assessment and update if necessary

A risk assessment should be reviewed periodically. There is no set time frame for this and it is the assessor's responsibility to make sure it stays up to date. A risk assessment should be reviewed:

- If it is no longer valid
- If there has been a significant change
- If the workplace changes (e.g. new equipment, procedures, facilities alteration, job description changes).

It is common practice in many businesses to review risk assessments annually, but some may require more frequent review; for example, risk assessments where there are many controls that require implementation and risk assessments relating to highly hazardous occurrences such as fire.

By law, any risk assessment must be 'suitable and sufficient'. It should show that a proper check for hazards was made and that thought was given to who might be affected and how. It should record which controls are in place and which are needed, so that precautions are reasonable and the remaining risk is low. If the five steps to risk assessment are followed in this way, and management and team members are also involved in developing the risk assessment and implementing solutions, the risk assessment should be suitable and sufficient.

Each veterinary practice is different with variations in facilities, team members, case load and location. Figure 2.11 shows the typical subjects that may be covered in a risk assessment; it is up to each individual practice to ensure that the type and number of assessments carried out meet the needs of the practice. In addition to these planned risk assessments, some circumstances will require a risk assessment at the time of the activity (dynamic), for example, unplanned events. New and expectant mothers and persons with disabilities or health problems such as dermatitis also require specific individual risk assessments.

Young persons

Young persons (defined in law as a person under 18) may be employed by a veterinary practice or be present in a training capacity either to gain work experience before commencing training or to gain practical experience during their veterinary nurse training. There are significant hazards in the veterinary environment and it is recommended that a separate young person risk assessment is drawn up and/or young persons are considered in each individual risk assessment.

The specific hazards relating to a young person include lack of workplace experience, maturity (physical and psychological) and lack of awareness of potential risks. Young people may be less likely to ask for help or advice than more experienced team members. Young people also require additional supervision and regular breaks. Induction training should take place for all young persons and should include items such as: checking contact information, allergy status, fire and first aid safety, details of supervising team member, and general rules such as footwear, appearance and taking breaks. Training should also include a list of tasks they should not do as a young person within the practice. It should be clear to the young worker and to the team that they must be supervised at all times.

Date	02/09/2019	Risk assessment title	New and expectant mother	Name of Mother	Name
Assessed by	Practice Manager Name	Risk assessment type	Special	Job role	Veterinary nurse
Approved by	Practice Owner Name	Next planned review date	Weekly during pregnancy	Baby due date/ date born	16/03/2020

No.	Activity/plant/ materials, etc.	Hazard	Risks to the new or expectant mother/child	Severity (S)	Likelihood (L)	Risk rating (SxL)	Risk controls/actions required	Acceptable yes/no
1	Moving sedated/ anaesthetized dogs to and from kennels	Strenuous manual handling	Risk to mother – hormone changes can affect ligaments causing susceptibility to injury or postural problems	2	2	4	Reduce amount of physical lifting/ carrying Job rotation Use trolleys or stretchers where necessary	Yes
2	Monitoring anaesthesia	Exposure to anaesthetic gases	Anaesthetic gases can affect unborn child and increase risk of miscarriage	2	3	6	Avoid by job rotation Active scavenging in place Anaesthetic machine serviced regularly Anaesthetic badge monitoring Minimize exposure in recovery wards/ kennels	Yes
3	Assisting with radiography	Exposure to ionizing radiation	Damage to unborn child	2	3	6	Do not include pregnant women in work involving exposure to ionizing radiation Amend shifts/duties etc. or find alternative work	Yes
4	Cleaning kennels	Handling cat/dog faeces	*Toxoplasma* in cat faeces. Risk of miscarriage in early pregnancy and infection in unborn child in later pregnancy	1	3	3	Nurse not to handle cat litter trays Cleaning kennels – wear PPE (mask, apron and gloves)	Yes
5	Dispensing medication	Active substances in some drugs	Some drugs are teratogenic – can damage unborn child Some drugs can cause miscarriage	2	3	6	Avoid dispensing drugs classified as teratogenic or causing miscarriages Wear gloves for all dispensing Good dispensary practice Check COSHH assessment and SPCs for drugs used	Yes
6	Standing for long periods	Tiredness Dizziness/ fainting	Affects mother	1	2	2	Regular rest breaks with somewhere to sit or lie down provided	Yes
7	Working long hours, overtime, night shifts	Tiredness	Affects mother	1	2	2	Regular rest breaks Review in a month	Yes
8	Any specific advice from GP, midwife or health visitor							

Risk rating: 1–2 = low risk; 3–4 = medium risk; 6–9 = high risk
Evaluate risk rating and controls/actions to determine whether they are sufficient and if the risk is acceptable for work to continue

2.10 An example of a completed risk assessment for a new and expectant mother, using a risk rating score.

Area
■ Access (car park, surrounding areas)
■ Waiting area
■ Consulting rooms
■ Team rest facilities
■ Preparation area
■ Radiography
■ Isolation
■ Kennels and cattery
■ Exotic pets
■ Storage areas
■ Sterile theatre
■ Laboratory
■ Medical gas store
■ Dispensary
■ Office

Task or hazard
■ Lone working
■ Driving
■ Use of autoclave
■ Cleaning
■ Use of laboratory
■ Dentistry
■ Handling reptiles
■ Handling birds
■ Laser
■ Waste and cadavers
■ Post-mortem examinations
■ Sharps
■ Handling animals
■ Zoonoses
■ Office work

Legislative
■ Fire
■ First aid
■ Manual handling
■ Display screen equipment
■ Control of Substances Hazardous to Health
■ New and expectant mothers
■ Young persons
■ Mental health/stress
■ Asbestos
■ *Legionella*
■ Ionizing radiation

2.11 List of typical subjects for risk assessment.

New and expectant mothers

When an employee is pregnant, has given birth in the last six months or is breastfeeding, the general risk assessment for new and expectant mothers should be revisited and completed for the individual involved. The aim of this risk assessment is to prevent harm to the mother, unborn and newborn child (see Figure 2.10). When carrying out the risk assessment for the individual, ask whether the risks can be removed or reduced, then whether conditions and hours can be adjusted, or whether suitable alternative work can be found if there are no other adaptations possible. Good communication is key to this process and regular discussions should be held with the new or expectant mother, and the risk assessment reviewed and updated as required.

People with disabilities

The veterinary employer is responsible for the health, safety and welfare of all employees, including those with a disability.

Health and safety legislation should not be used as an excuse to justify discriminating against disabled workers and should not prevent disabled people finding employment.

The practice has a duty to make reasonable adjustments for disabled workers to ensure the worker has the same access to everything involved with attaining, doing and keeping a job as a non-disabled person. Many adjustments may be simple and low cost, such as relocating equipment or altering work rotas. It may be helpful to enlist the help of a disability employment advisor for more complex situations. Consent of the disabled person must be obtained before approaching any third parties to help. People with unapparent disabilities, for example mental health conditions, may also require adjustments in the workplace to help them carry out their work.

Fire safety

Legislation
■ The Regulatory Reform (Fire Safety) Order 2005 (England and Wales)
■ Fire Safety (Scotland) Regulations 2006
■ Fire Safety Regulations (Northern Ireland) 2010
■ Health and Safety (Safety Signs and Signals) Regulations 1996

In the majority of UK premises, local fire and rescue authorities are responsible for enforcing fire safety legislation. Fire prevention is a significant moral, legal and economic responsibility for veterinary practices. The consequences of a fire can be devastating, ranging from injury to team members and animals, to loss of livelihood and loss of life. The average cost of a fire in commercial premises is around £70,000 and it is estimated that 60% of businesses do not re-open after a fire (Gov.uk, 2011).

For a fire to occur three things are needed: a source of ignition (heat), a source of fuel (something that burns) and oxygen (Figure 2.12). If one of these elements is removed, a fire will not occur or will go out rather than continue to burn.

Fire safety can be divided into three main areas:

■ Fire risk assessment
■ Fire prevention and detection
■ Emergency response.

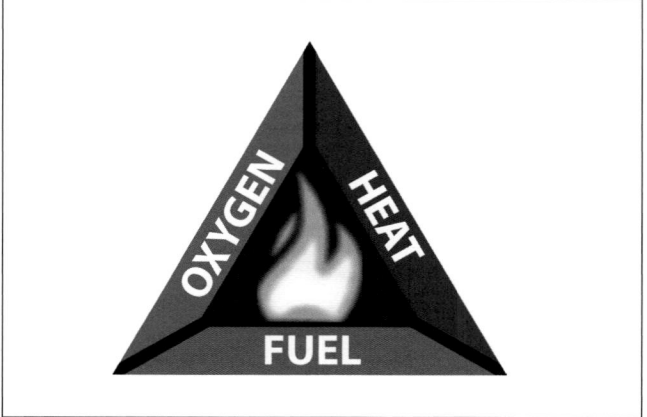

2.12 Fire triangle.

There are many sources of information available to help with fire safety. The gov.uk website provides a useful starting point and has a link to a fire risk assessment for premises with animals (www.gov.uk/workplace-fire-safety-your-responsibilities). However, many practices may choose to seek external assistance with some aspects of fire safety management.

Figure 2.13 summarizes the main fire safety requirements for veterinary practices.

Fire risk assessment

A fire risk assessment should be completed following the five steps described previously (see 'Risk assessment', above). Figure 2.14 is a checklist that can be used to help formulate the risk assessment.

Fire prevention and detection

Prevention

Good housekeeping is essential. This involves avoiding the build-up of rubbish, keeping fire exits unobstructed at all times and ensuring locks and door openings are used as intended. It is useful to carry out a weekly housekeeping inspection. Suitable storage areas within the practice should be created to ensure possible sources of ignition, fuel and oxygen are kept apart and securely stored.

Detection and warning equipment

Fire detection and warning equipment should ensure people are alerted promptly, so that they can escape to a

place of safety. Equipment can range from a simple manually operated device, like an air horn, that can be heard by everyone when operated from a single point, to an electrical fire detection and alarm system. In larger premises, and premises where fire may start and spread without being noticed, automatic fire detection is likely to be required. Consideration should be given to people working alone; for example, veterinary nurses checking inpatients during the night.

Emergency response

Firefighting equipment

Correct use of the appropriate fire extinguisher to control a fire in its early stages can significantly reduce the risk to people (and animals) in the veterinary premises and reduce the likelihood of a small fire (e.g. in a wastepaper bin) developing into a larger one. Only persons trained in the use of the firefighting equipment should attempt to extinguish a fire. Extinguishers must be suitable for the type of fire likely to be encountered and may need to be different for each area of the practice (Figure 2.15).

Escape routes and emergency lighting

Fire escape routes should ensure, as far as possible, that any person confronted by a fire should be able to turn away from the fire and escape to a place of relative safety, either directly outside or to a protected staircase. From there, they should be able to proceed to an assembly point, away from the affected building(s). Escape should be possible unaided and without the assistance of the fire and rescue

Requirement	Comments
Risk assessment	
Carry out a fire safety risk assessment	■ If required, seek external competent advice ■ Review and update when necessary ■ Train team on contents of risk assessment
Fire prevention	
Keep sources of ignition and flammable substances apart	■ Keep naked flames or sparks away from flammable gas ■ Ensure smoking shelter is not near the waste collection point
Avoid accidental fires	■ Make sure heaters are kept away from flammable surfaces ■ Keep electrical equipment in good condition
Ensure good housekeeping at all times	■ Avoid build-up of flammable waste ■ Carefully store flammable chemicals ■ Conduct regular workplace inspections and keep records (a fire logbook is a useful place to record this information)
Fire detection	
Establish a method to detect fires and warn people promptly if they start	■ Install heat and/or smoke alarms, fire alarms and sounders ■ Test and maintain the system
Have the correct firefighting equipment for a possible fire	■ Match fire extinguisher type to the area and likely class of fire ■ Ensure they are installed and maintained by competent person ■ Ensure team members are trained in their use
Emergency response	
Keep fire exits and escape routes clearly marked and unobstructed at all times	■ A premises fire safety drawing is useful to show escape routes, muster points, medical gas storage area and fire extinguisher locations
Train workers	■ Training to cover sources of fire, fire prevention and actions required to respond to a fire. Includes training in the use of firefighting equipment, sounding the alarm and evacuation (fire drills)

2.13 Fire safety requirements.

FIRE SAFETY RISK ASSESSMENT

▶ Follow the 5 key steps ▶ Fill in the checklist ▶ Assess your fire risk and plan fire safety

1 Fire hazards

Fire starts when heat (source of ignition) comes into contact with fuel (anything that burns), and oxygen (air).

You need to keep sources of ignition and fuel **apart**.

How could a fire start?
Think about heaters, lighting, naked flames, electrical equipment, hot processes such as welding or grinding, cigarettes, matches and anything else that gets very hot or causes sparks.

What could burn?
Packaging, rubbish and furniture could all burn, just like the more obvious fuels such as petrol, paint, varnish and white spirit. Also think about wood, paper, plastic, rubber and foam. Do the walls or ceilings have hardboard, chipboard, or polystyrene? Check outside, too.

☐ Have you found anything that could start a fire?
   Make a note of it.

☐ Have you found anything that could burn?
   Make a note of it.

2 People at risk

People at risk
Everyone is at risk if there is a fire. Think whether the risk is greater for some because of when or where they work, such as night staff, or because they're not familiar with the premises, such as visitors or customers. Children, the elderly or disabled people are especially vulnerable.

Have you identified?
☐ Who could be at risk?
☐ Who could be especially at risk?
   Make a note of what you have found.

3 Evaluate, and act

Evaluate
First, think about what you have found in steps 1 and 2: what are the risks of a fire starting, and what are the risks to people in the building and nearby?

Remove and reduce risk
How can you avoid accidental fires? Could a source of heat or sparks fall, be knocked or pushed into something that would burn? Could that happen the other way round?

Protect
Take action to protect your premises and people from fire.

☐ Have you assessed the risks of fire in your workplace?
☐ Have you assessed the risk to staff and visitors?

☐ Have you kept any source of fuel and heat/sparks apart?
☐ If someone wanted to start a fire deliberately, is there anything around they could use?
☐ Have you removed or secured any fuel an arsonist could use?
☐ Have you protected your premises from accidental fire or arson?

How can you make sure everyone is safe in case of fire?
☐ Will you know there is a fire?
☐ Do you have a plan to warn others?
☐ Who will make sure everyone gets out?
☐ Who will call the fire service?
☐ Could you put out a small fire quickly and stop it spreading?

How will everyone escape?
☐ Have you planned escape routes?
☐ Have you made sure people will be able to safely find their way out, even at night if necessary?
☐ Does all your safety equipment work?
☐ Will people know what to do and how to use equipment?
   Make a note of what you have found.

4 Record, plan and train

Record
Keep a record of any fire hazards and what you have done to reduce or remove them. If your premises are small, a record is a good idea. If you have five or more staff or have a licence then you must keep a record of what you have found and what you have done.

Plan
You must have a clear plan of how to prevent fire and how you will keep people safe in case of fire. If you share a building with others, you need to coordinate your plan with them.

Train
You need to make sure your staff know what to do in case of fire, and if necessary, are trained for their roles.

☐ Have you made a record of what you have found, and action you have taken?

☐ Have you planned what everyone will do if there is a fire?
☐ Have you discussed the plan with all staff?

Have you?
☐ Informed and trained people (practised a fire drill and recorded how it went)?
☐ Nominated staff to put in place your fire prevention measures, and trained them?
☐ Made sure everyone can fulfil their role?
☐ Informed temporary staff?
☐ Consulted others who share a building with you, and included them in your plan?

5 Review

Keep your risk assessment under regular review. Over time, the risks may change.

If you identify significant changes in risk or make any significant changes to your plan, you must tell others who share the premises and where appropriate re-train staff.

Have you?
☐ Made any changes to the building inside or out?
☐ Had a fire or near miss?
☐ Changed work practices?
☐ Begun to store chemicals or dangerous substances?
☐ Significantly changed your stock, or stock levels?
☐ Have you planned your next fire drill?

Completed the checklist?
Do you need more information?

The checklist above can help you with the Fire Risk Assessment but you may need additional information especially if you have large or complex premises.

We have produced a series of guides for different business sectors. These guides will give you more information about how to carry out a Fire Risk Assessment, with specific advice for your type of premises. These guides are free to download at www.communities.gov.uk/fire

2.14 Fire safety risk assessment checklist. (Contains public sector information licensed under the Open Government Licence v3.0)

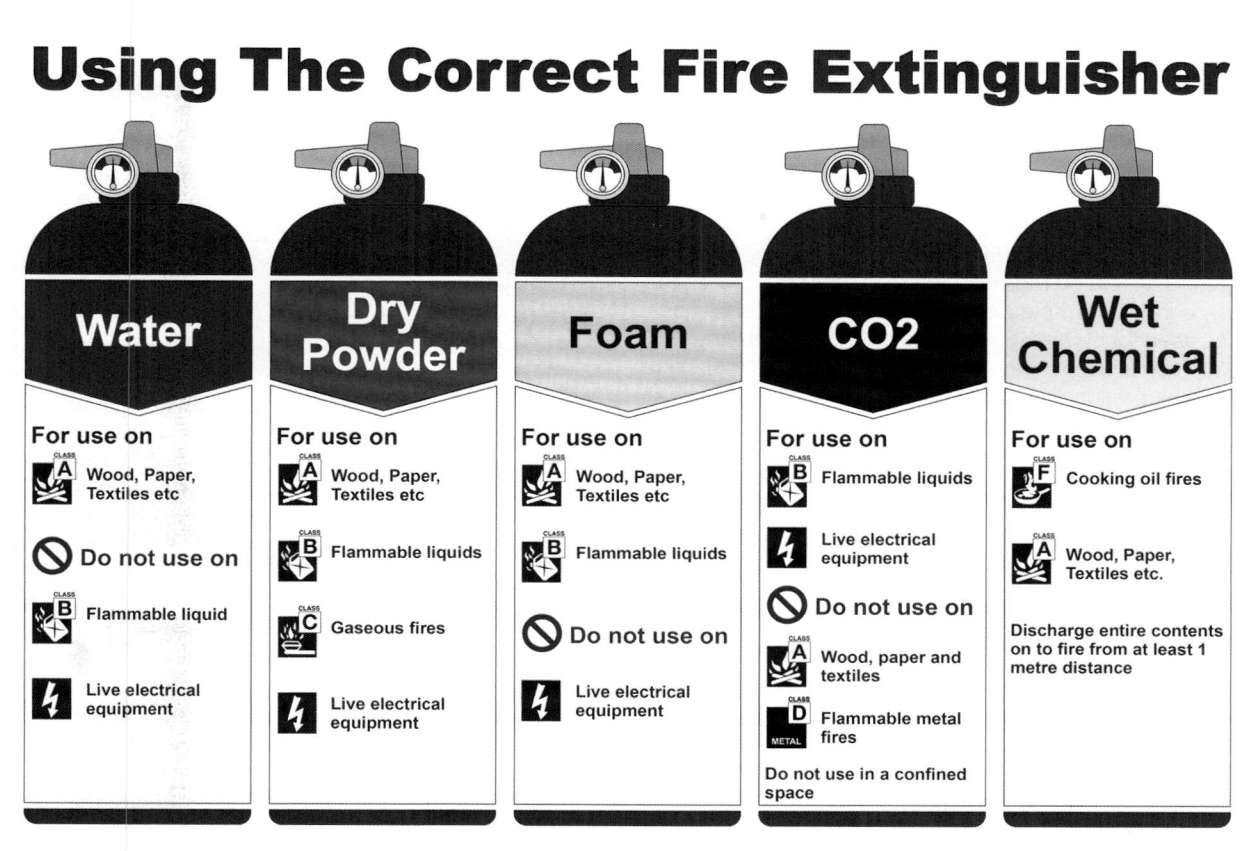

Using The Correct Fire Extinguisher

Water

For use on

- Wood, Paper, Textiles etc

Do not use on

- Flammable liquid
- Live electrical equipment

Dry Powder

For use on

- Wood, Paper, Textiles etc
- Flammable liquids
- Gaseous fires
- Live electrical equipment

Foam

For use on

- Wood, Paper, Textiles etc
- Flammable liquids

Do not use on

- Live electrical equipment

CO2

For use on

- Flammable liquids
- Live electrical equipment

Do not use on

- Wood, paper and textiles
- Flammable metal fires

Do not use in a confined space

Wet Chemical

For use on

- Cooking oil fires
- Wood, Paper, Textiles etc.

Discharge entire contents on to fire from at least 1 metre distance

2.15   Types of fire extinguisher. (© Safety First Aid Group)

service. However, some people with disabilities or special requirements may need help from other people and the use of specialized equipment. Escape routes should have sufficient levels of lighting, and emergency lighting is likely to be needed to allow safe escape from routes without windows and from premises that are used during periods of darkness (Figure 2.16). Emergency lighting should be tested periodically and maintained as required.

Signs

Signs must be used to help people identify escape routes, find firefighting equipment and to identify fire warning devices. They must be in pictogram form (see Figure 2.16). The pictogram can be supplemented by text if this is considered necessary to make the sign more easily understood.

2.16   Fire exit sign and emergency lighting. (Courtesy of Ashgrove Vets, Aberdeen)

Team training

All team members and visitors, including work experience students and contractors, should be given fire safety information and instruction, in an easily understood format, as soon as possible after they start work. Regular updates should also take place and records should be kept. Training should cover the items detailed in Figure 2.17.

Fire action training

- Procedures for alerting other team members that there is a fire
- Procedure for evacuating the team and members of the public, visitors and contractors to an assembly point at a safe location
- Procedure for animal inpatients
- Arrangements and responsibility for calling the fire and rescue service
- Appointment of fire wardens with responsibility for securing the building, doors, roll call and preventing re-entry until all clear
- Location and, when appropriate, use of the provided firefighting equipment
- The location of escape routes, especially those not in regular use
- The importance of closing fire-resisting doors to prevent the spread of fire, heat and smoke
- How to isolate supply sources, such as piped gases, if it is safe to do so

2.17   Fire action training requirement.

Medical gases

Medical gases are commonly used in veterinary practice.

- Oxidizing agents – examples include oxygen (see *Oxygen use in the workplace*; www.hse.gov.uk) and nitrous oxide. These agents support and can increase the intensity of burning. Oxygen enrichment occurs when there is an increased level of oxygen in the air (e.g. from a leaking cylinder), which means a fire will start more easily, burn aggressively and be more difficult to extinguish.
- Asphyxiants – examples include nitrous oxide and some gases used for cryosurgery. These agents deplete the oxygen in the surrounding air. These gases are odourless and if their presence is not detected this depletion can cause giddiness, mental confusion, loss of judgment, loss of coordination, weakness, nausea, fainting, loss of consciousness and eventually death.

Gas cylinders also present explosion hazards. They should be stored in a secure, well ventilated area, and different products may need to be stored in different areas. Smaller cylinders are stored horizontally and larger ones vertically and secured to prevent falling or damage to the cylinders. It is recommended that a purpose-built trolley be used when moving cylinders. Cylinders should be kept clean and team members should be trained in their safe use. There should be clear signage wherever medical gases are used or stored and the fire service informed.

Practice equipment

Legislation

- Provision and Use of Work Equipment Regulations (PUWER) 1998
- Pressure Systems Safety Regulations (PSSR) 2000
- Personal Protective Equipment at Work Regulations 1992
- Electricity at Work Regulations 1989
- Ionising Radiation Regulations 2017
- Control of Artificial Optical Radiation at Work Regulations 2010

Work equipment

The practice has a duty to ensure work equipment is:

- Suitable for purpose (e.g. fire extinguishers specific for the hazard)
- Safe, maintained and inspected to ensure it has not deteriorated (e.g. anaesthetic equipment annual service and maintenance)
- Only used or maintained by suitably trained persons
- Fitted with suitable health and safety measures (e.g. isolation switch distant from X-ray head, signage, warning lights).

Work equipment may require internal and/or external maintenance. Maintenance logs can be a helpful way of ensuring equipment maintenance occurs, for recording maintenance problems and history. SOPs detailing correct use of the equipment are useful for reminding team members how to carry out tasks, although they are not a substitute for training.

Autoclaves

Autoclaves are commonly used in veterinary practice for sterilizing equipment. They are classed as high risk equipment because failure can lead to the high pressure ejection of parts, fluid or contents. Veterinary practices need to ensure that a suitable written scheme of examination is in place before the system is operated and should be available for inspection and update, if necessary, throughout the life of the machine. The written scheme should cover all items within the self-contained pressurized system that may give rise to danger.

Veterinary practices also need to maintain pressurized equipment; this should be undertaken by a competent person and records of the maintenance retained. The competent person should refer to the written scheme and over the lifetime of the equipment may alter the written scheme to reflect changes to the equipment. It is important to note that these are two separate requirements and not to assume that a service certificate is the same as a written scheme of examination.

Team members should be trained in use of the autoclave; for example, checking the pressure indicator to verify nil pressure before opening, identifying and reporting any damaged parts (such as door seals) and knowledge of emergency procedures.

Gas cylinders and distribution systems

The PSSR are also relevant to piped medical gases. Equipment for use with medical gas cylinders and gas distribution systems (i.e. pipework and hoses) should be routinely inspected and maintained in accordance with the manufacturers' recommendations.

Personal protective equipment

Personal protective equipment (PPE) is equipment that protects the user against health or safety risks at work and has specific requirements (Figure 2.18). PPE should be used as a last resort; other control measures should be chosen first. For example, if a medicinal product is available in a blister pack or as loose tablets, and the loose tablets require the handler to wear gloves, the blister pack should be chosen first as it reduces the employee's exposure to hazards. This is an example of substitution in COSHH assessments.

Where the use of PPE is deemed necessary, it should be properly selected and CE marked to ensure that it is appropriate for the task. It should be cleaned and carefully stored if it is reusable. If PPE is required for a task, it is not acceptable to avoid wearing it because 'it will only take a few minutes' or because 'it is an emergency situation'.

The employer has a duty concerning the provision and use of PPE at work. PPE must be provided to protect the user against health and safety risks at work. This can include items such as gloves, aprons, eye protection, lead aprons, safety footwear and masks. PPE should always be provided free of charge by an employer. Different PPE may be required for

Requirement	Comments
CE[a] marked	Should show a CE mark of at least 5 mm, as well as the standard of protection provided
Fit for purpose	Confirmed as suitable for the task or product it is protecting the user from. For example, standard safety eyewear may not be suitable for handling chemotherapy drugs
Maintained and stored properly	For example, eye protection should be clean, not scratched and easily accessible
Used correctly by employees	It is only protective if it is being used in the correct way for the appropriate tasks. Note: regular prescription eyewear is not a substitute for eye protection
Training	How, when and why it is used?
Compatible with other PPE	For example, masks may make some safety spectacles fog up, therefore, different safety eyewear should be considered, such as visors or non-fogging goggles

2.18 PPE requirements. [a] The CE mark is a certification mark that indicates that a product conforms with relevant EU directives regarding health and safety or environmental protection.

team members to ensure correct comfort and fit. Team members should be trained in the correct use and storage of PPE.

Common examples of PPE for dentistry are shown in Figure 2.19 and for radiography are shown in Figure 2.20.

Eye protection

This is required for tasks such as dentistry (see Figure 2.19) and for handling certain chemicals such as some chemotherapy agents. Safety datasheets and suppliers can advise the practice about the correct type of eye protection.

Hearing protection

Occasionally, veterinary nurses may be exposed to noise hazards (e.g. working in large kennels or for prolonged periods of time). The combination of sound level and

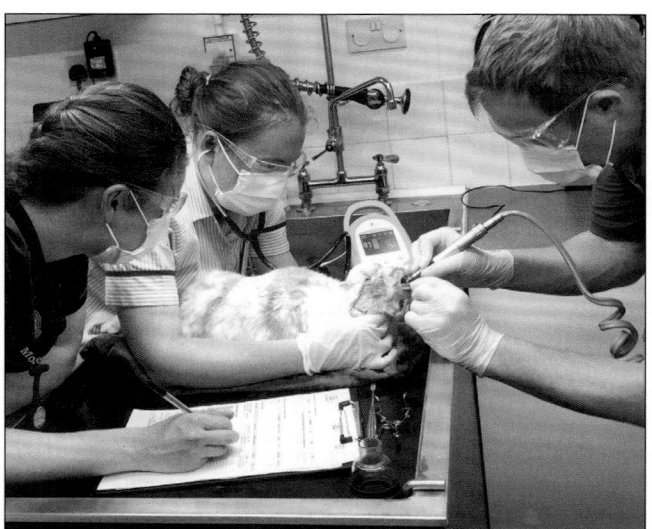

2.19 PPE required for dental procedures may include masks, goggles and gloves. (Courtesy of Ashgrove Vets, Aberdeen)

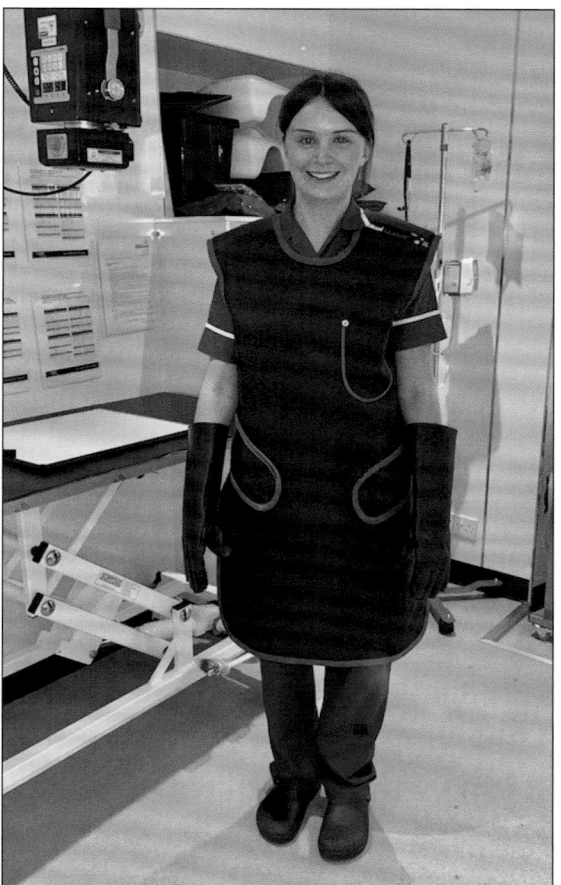

2.20 PPE required for radiographic procedures may include gowns and gloves, as well as sleeves and a thyroid collar (not shown here). (Courtesy of Ashgrove Vets, Aberdeen)

duration of exposure should be considered. If this hazard is identified, hearing protection should be provided. It should be ensured that ear plugs are designed for hearing protection and remembered that cotton wool is not suitable for this purpose. Training should be provided on how to fit and use hearing protection. (A good rule of thumb is that if you need to shout to make yourself heard at a distance of 2 m, you are likely to need to address the noise hazard, either by reducing exposure (moving out of the area) or providing hearing protection.)

Hand protection

There are currently an estimated 17,000 people in work with skin problems they regard as caused or made worse by work. Contact dermatitis often occurs at a young age (<35 years old), particularly amongst female workers (HSE, 2018). The most effective and reliable way to prevent skin problems is to design and operate processes to avoid contact with harmful substances, before resorting to the use of protective gloves.

A variety of gloves are available for use in veterinary practice and the type selected will depend on the task being undertaken. Latex and nitrile gloves are commonly used in veterinary practice. The proteins in latex can trigger allergic responses in a small number of individuals and for this reason the HSE recommends using non-latex gloves unless there are no alternatives that provide the protection needed. If latex gloves are used, low-protein, powder-free gloves are preferable to powdered gloves, as the use of powder increases the risk of allergic response.

Wearing gloves for long periods of time can make the skin hot and sweaty, leading to skin problems. The use of separate cotton inner gloves can help prevent this from occurring.

Respiratory protection

Handling or preparing certain chemicals requires the use of respiratory protection to prevent the breathing in of harmful substances. The fitting and use of respiratory protective equipment is a specialist subject for which competent help should be sought and individuals should be trained in its use.

Bioaerosols generated during dental treatment are a potential hazard for team members. The use of a simple facemask during these procedures provides sufficient protection from these organisms. In addition, adequate cleaning and sterilization of dental equipment and instruments is an important factor in decreasing pathogen contamination.

Footwear

Veterinary footwear should primarily protect the wearer from slipping, cuts, falling objects and splashes from medicines. They should be capable of being cleaned to prevent the spread of infectious disease. Open-toed or heeled footwear should not be worn.

Electricity and electrical appliances

Electrical installation checks (also known as fixed wiring or electrical integrity testing) should be carried out to ensure there is no deterioration of electrical systems. These checks should be carried out by a competent person, commonly every 5 years or on a rolling programme over 5 years.

A portable appliance is defined as any item that can be moved, either connected or disconnected, from an electrical supply. They usually have a plug and cable and the law requires that such equipment is maintained. It is common practice to carry out portable appliance tests (PAT) annually (Figure 2.21); however, this interval is not mandatory and low risk environments and equipment may require only inspection. Team members should be trained to note if electrical appliances are damaged or in poor condition, and how to mark them out of use and segregate them. Further information with specific examples is available on the HSE website (www.hse.gov.uk).

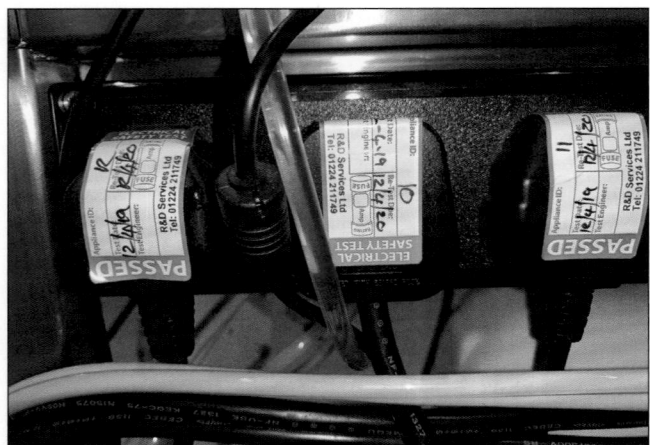

2.21 PAT testing. (Courtesy of Ashgrove Vets, Aberdeen)

Radiography

There is an ACOP available on the HSE website to help with interpretation of the legislation. In addition, the BVA have published guidance notes on the use of ionizing radiation in veterinary practice (see *Ionising radiation – myth busting guide*; www.bva.co.uk/resources-support/practice-management/ionising-radiation-irr17-myth-busting-guide/). For further information on radiation safety, see Chapter 16.

When ionizing radiation passes through tissue, the energy creates ions. This action can cause harmful effects in human tissue. High doses of ionizing radiation can cause severe harm, but even low doses can cause DNA damage in cells, which makes them more likely to develop tumours in the future. Harm may also be caused to the fetus during pregnancy, it is therefore in the best interests of a pregnant employee to inform their employer in writing as soon as possible so that any required changes can be implemented. Radiation exposure can be controlled by three factors:

- Shielding
- Time
- Distance.

The system of work for ionizing radiation in the veterinary practice should include all three factors, to reduce exposure to as low a level as reasonably practicable.

Radiation safety roles

- A Radiation Protection Adviser (RPA) must be appointed to help the practice comply with the regulations. The RPA must meet specified criteria of competence and have the relevant experience for veterinary practice.
- The Radiation Protection Supervisor (RPS) is an appointed member of the practice team and should be a veterinary surgeon or veterinary nurse with sufficient supervisory authority in the premises. They should be trained in the legislative requirements and know where to seek further information. They should also know what to do in an emergency. In addition, they should also undertake periodic refresher training to maintain competency levels.

All employees working with ionizing radiation should receive training so they understand the key health risks related to exposure, the control measures in place and what to do if things go wrong.

A practice must apply to notify, register or get consent to use ionizing radiation from the HSE and this can be done online. A risk assessment for ionizing radiation must also be carried out and this should include dental radiography where applicable. The RPA may advise on the completion of the risk assessment for ionizing radiation. The RPA will also write the local rules, which are a set of key working instructions that set out the arrangements for restricting exposure to ionizing radiation. Local rules should be displayed in the X-ray room. Digital radiography systems are almost exclusively used in veterinary practices now; however, if X-ray film and wet processing are still used, factors relating to chemical handling, ventilation and the disposal of chemicals should also be taken into account.

Local rules

HSE Working with Ionising Radiation – Ionising Radiation Regulations 2017
Approved Code of Practice (ACOP) 18(1)-(2)340 – Making local rules effective

"Local rules are effective if they:
a. Are brief and concentrate on the activities which give the greatest risks;
b. Focus on the key working instructions to be followed by everyone to keep radiation doses as low as reasonably practicable;
c. Are 'local' by referring directly to work at a particular location and by taking account of the environment in and around the working area;
d. Contain clear instructions which reflect actual work practice rather than an ideal which is not attainable;
e. Are reviewed periodically to check that they remain relevant."

A controlled area should be designated for radiography. This should be clearly demarcated and signed, with access restricted to authorized personnel only (Figures 2.22 and 2.23). An exposure log should be completed for each radiographic exposure. This should detail the views taken, the exposures used, the quality of the images and the personnel involved. It can be useful to audit the X-ray exposure, for example, image quality and collimation may be checked.

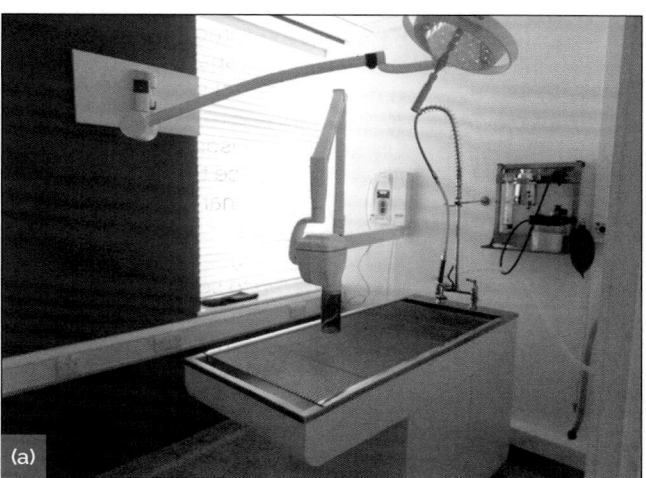

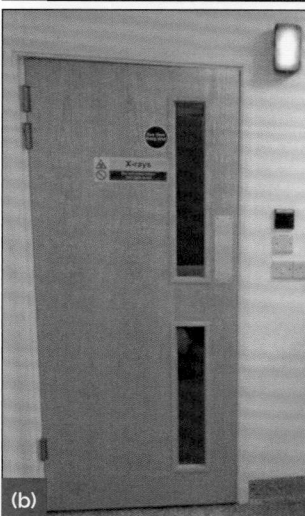

2.22 (a) Dental X-ray machine in a designated dental treatment room. (b) Entrance to the dental treatment room showing controlled area warning light and signage. (Courtesy of Peter Cockett)

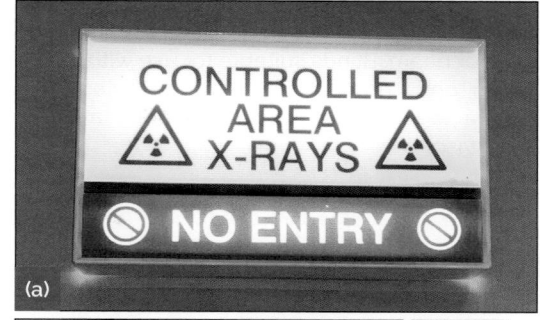

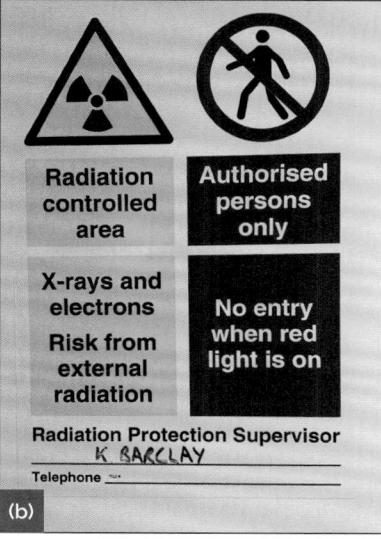

2.23

(a) Two-stage illuminated warning sign outside an X-ray room. (b) Controlled area signage. (Courtesy of Ashgrove Vets, Aberdeen).

PPE for radiography may include gowns, gloves, sleeves and a thyroid collar (see Figure 2.20). PPE should be inspected regularly for damage and stored without creasing or folding. Gowns should be hung over a large diameter bar to prevent damage.

Manual restraint of animals should be avoided wherever possible. Judicious use of modern sedative techniques, along with the use of a range of positioning aids such as foam wedges and sandbags, means that many animals can be safely imaged without the need for manual restraint. A good safety culture helps discourage manual restraint.

The equipment used for radiography should be regularly serviced and records maintained.

Lasers

Light Amplification by the Stimulated Emission of Radiation (laser) is a form of artificial optical radiation. Lasers are used in practice for a variety of purposes, including rehabilitation and amelioration of wound healing. Lasers can cause injury to the user, primarily to the tissues of the eye and, in some cases, to the skin. Thus, measures must be put in place to reduce worker exposure to as low as is reasonably practicable.

A risk assessment should be carried out. The risk assessment should include an exposure limit value (specialist help may be required to determine this value). The key risk to workers is eye damage. Protective eyewear protects the user from the damaging effects of the laser on the eye. The eyewear is specific to the type of beam emitted by the laser. Other PPE may be required, including skin protection, depending on the function of the laser.

A designated area with restricted access should be used for laser treatment. This are should be clearly marked with appropriate signage. In addition, care must be taken to prevent exposure of third parties (e.g. clients in adjoining rooms) to the laser beam. Blinds suitable for use with lasers must be placed on windows and door portholes. It is useful to keep a log of usage and to appoint a Laser Protection Supervisor.

Hazardous substances

Legislation
- Control of Substances Hazardous to Health (COSHH) Regulations 2002

COSHH regulations aim to prevent or control exposure of substances hazardous to health. In veterinary practice, there are a variety of such substances encountered, including:

- Drugs and medical gases
- Cleaning products
- Biological agents – bacteria, viruses, fungi, protozoa and parasites.

In addition, some substances can be hazardous to some people but not everyone. This may be due to individual susceptibilities (e.g. allergic reaction to penicillin or latex) or individuals being at increased risk, including young, old, pregnant and immunocompromised (YOPI).

COSHH requires a risk assessment to be conducted where workers may be exposed to hazardous substances. The risk assessment will follow the general principles covered previously (see 'Risk assessment', above), along with some additional requirements. It is a common misconception that to satisfy COSHH you simply have to keep a product safety datasheet (SDS). In practice, the SDS is an input to the overall hazardous substance management process. Figure 2.24 shows the key factors to be considered to fulfil the requirements of COSHH.

Sources of information

Datasheets are provided for veterinary drugs; these give information on prescribing and any warnings regarding use, handling and disposal of the product. A large number of companies use the NOAH compendium (www.noahcompendium.co.uk/), which collates datasheets in an easily accessible online and paper format. All authorized veterinary products have a summary of product characteristics (SPC) available via the Veterinary Medicines Directorate (VMD) website (www.vmd.defra.gov.uk/ProductInformationDatabase). Products are arranged alphabetically by their tradename. For human prescription-only medicines, used under the Prescribing Cascade (see Chapter 8), information can be obtained via the Electronic Medicines Compendium (eMc) (www.medicines.org.uk/emc/). BSAVA also produces medicines information for clients on drugs prescribed under the Cascade, as well as for other products such as steroids. These are available to members via the BSAVA library (www.bsavalibrary.com). These leaflets are an excellent way of providing clients with information about the products being dispensed. Chemicals and cleaning products must have a safety datasheet provided by the manufacturer and information can be accessed online.

Risk assessment
Step one – identify the hazards

Assessment must cover all harmful substances, including those brought into the workplace (e.g. chemicals and medication), biological agents and those created by work processes (e.g. anaesthetic gases). The information from the SDS and suppliers should be used to form the basis of the risk assessment. These documents will detail all the key information, including the hazardous properties (e.g. irritant, corrosive, toxic), the health effects, route of entry into the body and the harm that could result, and a work exposure limit (WEL), if applicable. They also have key information for storage and disposal, first aid and emergency requirements. For assessment purposes, low risk drugs may be assessed collectively. Medium and high risk drugs or processes (e.g. chemotherapeutics) should be assessed individually (Figure 2.25).

Factor	Comments
Establish what the health hazards are	Identify harmful substances and processes that may cause harm
Conduct a risk assessment	Assess how these substances may cause harm
Establish control measures to reduce harm to health	Follow the hierarchy of control: - Eliminate - Substitute - Apply engineering controls - Minimize exposure - Train workers - Personal protective equipment (PPE)
Make sure controls are used	Supervision, inspections and audits
Maintain control measures in good working order	Equipment maintenance and cleaning
Provide information, instruction and training for employees and others	Nature of the hazards and potential health effects, the importance of controls and how to apply them
Conduct monitoring and health surveillance in appropriate cases	Monitoring and health surveillance as required for individual exposure to certain products
Plan for emergencies	Plan for likely incidents (e.g. spillage, overexposure or contamination from substance)

2.24 Factors to be considered to satisfy COSHH.

Low risk substances
■ Topical shampoos
■ Most antibiotics
■ Anti-inflammatory drugs
■ Nutraceuticals
■ Ectoparasiticides

Medium and high risk substances
■ Chemotherapeutic agents
■ Latex
■ Hormones
■ Steroids
■ Laboratory substances

2.25 Examples of low, medium and high risk substances.

Step two – decide who might be harmed and how

Consider who might be exposed, including team members, clients, contractors, groups including young, pregnant or disabled workers and susceptible persons, and the extent of the exposure against the WEL, if applicable. Determine how they can be harmed by the substance. This may include inhalation, ingestion of either directly contaminated food or via fingers, absorption through the skin or eyes, or injection into the body by high-pressure equipment or contaminated sharp objects. Carcinogens are chemicals that can cause cancer or increase its incidence. Mutagens are chemicals that induce heritable genetic diseases or increase its incidence. Products identified with these descriptors (found in the SDS) must have additional controls, such as enclosure of the process, signage, labelling and specific cleaning protocols.

Step three – evaluate the risks and decide on precautions

As a general rule, the higher the potential harm, the more controls should be in place to prevent that harm. For health effects that are more serious, such as cancer or allergic dermatitis, control measures might be extensive and need to control risk of both acute and chronic health effects. COSHH legislation specifies a hierarchy of controls (Figure 2.26); this is

Control	Example
Eliminate the use of a harmful substance and use a safer one	Change existing disinfectant for one that is less harmful
Use a safer form of the product	Use a paste rather than powder to decrease inhalation risk
Change the process to emit less of the substance at source	Purchase of preconstituted chemotherapy drugs
Enclose the process so that the product does not escape	Constituting chemotherapy drugs in a fume cupboard
Extract emissions of the substance near the source	Local exhaust ventilation for chemotherapy products
Have as few workers in harm's way as possible	Have rules to restrict access: authorized persons only; pregnant persons not permitted
Provide personal protective equipment (PPE) such as gloves, coveralls and a respirator	PPE must fit the wearer. It should be readily available and used. It should not be the only control in place

2.26 COSHH hierarchy of control.

a logical way of considering hazardous substances and reducing exposure to them. Once this has been evaluated, consideration should be given as to whether additional controls are needed and within what time scale.

Steps four and five – record significant findings, review the assessment and update if necessary

There is no set format for recording a COSHH risk assessment and the HSE state that any format for COSHH risk assessment is acceptable as long as the steps detailed here are followed. Written records are required for five or more employees; however, it is strongly recommended that any risk assessment is recorded in writing.

Review of risk assessments should take place periodically and after any significant ill health or incident, when the workplace or work processes have changed or when new substances are introduced. Review does not involve revisiting the entire process, simply checking that the controls are still valid and whether any additional controls are needed.

Information and training

Team members should be able to identify hazardous substances to which they are likely to be exposed, know about the health risks of these exposures, understand WELs, recognize zoonotic disease and know where to access SDS information on products. Information on COSHH should be provided in a form that is easily accessible and understood.

Veterinary nurses must be capable of evaluating and reacting correctly to exposure to hazardous substances on their own initiative. Veterinary nurses are also a vital link to clients, to provide them with sufficient and easily understood information on how to use and handle products dispensed from veterinary practices.

Monitoring and health surveillance

Monitoring is only required for a small number of products found in veterinary practice. These substances have set WELs. WELs relate to the concentrations of hazardous substances in the air, averaged over a specified period of time, referred to as a time-weighted average (TWA). Two time periods are used: long-term exposure limit (8 hours) and short-term exposure limit (15 minutes).

Monitoring exposure is a way of actively checking that the controls in place are effective in ensuring that there is no overexposure to hazardous substances. The most well-known substances with a WEL in veterinary practice are anaesthetic gases (e.g. isoflurane, sevoflurane, nitrous oxide; see Chapter 21) and ethylene oxide, which is used for sterilizing instruments (see Chapter 22).

Health surveillance is a selective COSHH requirement (i.e. not required in all cases). Individuals that are at increased risk or affected by work-related illness (e.g. dermatitis) may need to be part of a health surveillance programme to monitor their health. Occupational health advice may be required in these circumstances, as failure to appropriately manage these conditions (e.g. latex allergy) can lead to debilitating illness. It is often beneficial to consult a competent occupational health adviser for advice on health surveillance.

Planning for emergencies

Written guidelines for emergencies are one of the controls for COSHH. It is important that team members are aware of these and trained in them. The simplest way to teach and test COSHH emergency preparedness is to use SOPs for teaching and reference and use example scenarios for testing emergency planning.

Examples of training scenarios may include:

- Chemotherapy
  - In the event of a spill, are team members trained and know what to do (Figure 2.27)?
  - Is information on the product readily available?
  - Is there a spill kit (Figure 2.28)?
  - Does the area need to be evacuated?
  - How is the contaminated spill kit disposed of?
  - Why has the spill occurred?
  - Is the correct equipment being used?
  - Is the equipment in date?
- Use of an oil-based vaccine
  - The veterinary surgeon has injected their finger. What should be done?
  - Where is the product SPC?
  - Where do they go for help – first aid in-house or hospital?
  - Where is the accident recorded?
  - Was the product clearly marked?
  - Were team members aware of the increased risk associated with oil-based product handling?

Event	Procedure
Spillage of cytotoxic drugs	1. Call for assistance and warn others 2. Full personal protective clothing should be worn (including full face respirator and protective shoe coverings) 3. Use dry absorbent towels to absorb any fluid 4. Clean contaminated area with 70% alcohol and dry tissue three times 5. Dispose of all contaminated material as cytotoxic waste
Contamination of skin	Rinse with large amounts of water and wash with soap
Contamination of eyes	1. Seek help 2. Remove contact lenses (if worn) 3. Rinse eye(s) with large amounts of water; use eye wash facility if available for at least 20 minutes 4. Consult a doctor
All accidents should be reported according to local Health and Safety regulations	

2.27 Procedures in the event of accidental spillage or contamination. (Reproduced from the *BSAVA Manual of Canine and Feline Oncology*, 3rd edn)

- Disposable protective gown x 2
- Disposable chemotherapy gloves x 2 pairs
- Disposable shoe covers x 2 pairs
- Full face respirator and filters
- pH 5 soap tablet
- Sealable plastic bags
- Chemosorb™ pads
- Absorbent disposable towels

2.28 Contents of a spill kit for cytotoxic drugs (Reproduced from the *BSAVA Manual of Canine and Feline Oncology, 3rd edn*)

Zoonotic diseases

A zoonotic disease is defined as an infectious disease transmissible (under natural conditions) between animals and humans. There are approximately 40 potential zoonoses in the UK. The diseases they can cause range from mild, self-limiting disease to life-threatening conditions.

The assessment of risk for zoonoses should form part of the COSHH assessment. When assessing zoonotic diseases, consideration should be given to how the microorganism is transmitted, how easily the disease is spread, how severe and how easily treated the disease is, and how well the microorganism survives in the environment. Workers, persons not on the premises at all times, such as cleaners and clients, and persons that are at increased risk of zoonotic disease, such as the young, old, pregnant and immunocompromised (YOPI), should all be considered.

Zoonotic diseases may emerge and change over time and it is important to keep up to date with the relevant websites and literature.

Sources of information

There are various different sources of information available:

- A full list of zoonotic diseases found in the UK is available on the government website (www.gov.uk/government/publications/list-of-zoonotic-diseases/list-of-zoonotic-diseases#zoonotic-diseases-found-in-the-uk)
- Public Health England has produced an advice sheet for reptile owners, as reptiles may be asymptomatic carriers of *Salmonella* species (https://assets.publishing.service.gov.uk/government/uploads/system/uploads/attachment_data/file/377731/*Salmonella*_in_reptiles_factsheet_2_.pdf)
- In 2003, the HSE published *Infection at work: controlling the risks. A guide for employers and the self-employed on identifying, assessing and controlling the risks of infection in the workplace* (www.hse.gov.uk/pubns/infection.pdf)
- The Centre for Public Health and Zoonoses has produced a resource on worms and germs, with information for veterinary surgeons, pet owners and children (www.wormsandgermsblog.com/resources-pets/).

Infection control

The use of precautionary principles allows a basic level of infection control in the absence of information about the infection status of an animal. Precautionary principles include good hand hygiene, use of PPE, sharps management, spillage procedures, laundry protocols and management of hazardous waste. Where an animal suspected of carrying a zoonotic disease, additional controls will be required.

Good occupational hygiene is vital and the following should be in place:

- Wash hands and arms, if necessary, before eating, drinking, smoking, using the phone, applying make-up or contact lenses or taking medication – the approved World Health Organization (WHO) handwashing techniques should be followed (see Chapter 7)
- Cover all new and existing cuts with waterproof dressings and replace as often as needed
- Keep nails short and clean; no artificial nails or nail polish
- Take rest breaks away from clinical areas

- Wear appropriate PPE and dispose and/or clean regularly
- Dispose of waste appropriately (see 'Waste management', below)
- Use equipment that is easy to clean and decontaminate
- Clean work areas regularly (see Chapter 14).

The Bella Moss Foundation produces resources specific for veterinary practices on infection control. These guidelines should be used as the starting point for developing practice specific guidelines (www.thebellamossfoundation.com/practice-guidelines/).

Asbestos

> ### Legislation
> - Control of Asbestos Regulations 2012

Asbestos may be present in any premises built or refurbished up until the year 2000. If materials that contain asbestos are disturbed or damaged, fibres are released into the air. If these fibres are inhaled they can cause serious diseases, which take time to develop but are often fatal. Past exposure to asbestos currently kills around 4500 people a year in Great Britain, with those who carry out building maintenance and repair being at particular risk.

In veterinary practice, the owner or the person responsible for the maintenance or repair of the premises has a duty to manage any asbestos in that building. Asbestos is usually only dangerous when disturbed. If it is safely managed and contained, it does not present an immediate health hazard and removing it can sometimes be more hazardous than leaving it in place.

To manage asbestos effectively, the following steps need to be taken:

- Find out whether asbestos is present (many businesses make use of specialist advice for this aspect)
- If asbestos is identified, a record of location, type and condition of the asbestos should be made
- Conduct a risk assessment regarding who could be exposed to asbestos and how
- Prepare a plan detailing how to manage these risks
- Put the plan into action
- Review and monitor the plan and arrangements to ensure they are effective
- Establish a system to provide information relating to the location and condition of the material to anyone who is liable to work on or disturb the asbestos. This is usually when repairs, maintenance or building work are taking place, but may also be needed for practice employees when working in certain areas.

The HSE provide a guidance leaflet and checklist to help manage asbestos effectively (see 'References and further reading').

Legionella

The bacterium *Legionella pneumophila* and related bacteria are found in low numbers in natural water sources. Certain specific conditions in purpose built water systems (e.g. shower hoses for washing dogs), hot and cold water systems and spa pools (as used for canine and feline rehabilitation) can allow bacteria to grow. Inhalation of droplets can lead to pneumonia and other lung diseases, particularly in certain vulnerable groups.

A risk assessment should be carried out and a competent person appointed to be responsible for the risk assessment. Those with complex water systems may require external help with the risk assessment. The risk assessment should encompass management responsibilities, a description of the system, any potential risk sources, measures currently in place to control risks, monitoring, inspection and maintenance procedures, the monitoring of results and the inspection and checks carried out. The risk assessment should have a review date. If the risks are deemed insignificant, properly managed and legally compliant, no further action except periodic review is required.

Controls in place should include:

- Ensuring that the release of water spray is properly controlled
- Avoiding water temperatures between 20°C and 50°C and conditions (stagnation, biofilm and scale or sediment) in the water system that favour the growth of *Legionella*
- Ensuring water cannot stagnate by keeping pipe lengths as short as possible, removing redundant pipework or running taps regularly
- Avoiding materials that encourage the growth of *Legionella*
- Keeping the system and the water in it clean
- Treating water to either kill *Legionella* (and other microorganisms) or limit their ability to grow.

In veterinary practices, the most common situations in which *Legionella* may occur are with taps and showers that are infrequently used, and with any water system where deposits (such as sludge and organic matter) may exist that support bacterial growth. The key point is to design, maintain and operate the water services under conditions that prevent or adequately control the growth of *Legionella* bacteria.

Waste management

> ### Legislation
> - The Hazardous Waste Directive
> - Environmental Protection Act 1990

The modern veterinary practice produces various types of waste and it is important that all waste is handled, stored and disposed of in line with current legislation. Waste disposal is regulated by the Environment Agency (EA) in England and Wales (www.gov.uk/government/organisations/environment-agency), the Scottish Environment Protection Agency (SEPA) (www.sepa.org.uk) and the Northern Ireland Environment Agency (NIEA) (www.daera-ni.gov.uk/northern-ireland-environment-agency), respectively. In Scotland, the term 'special waste' is used to refer to the equivalent of hazardous waste. Non-special waste refers to non-hazardous waste in Scotland.

The British Veterinary Association (BVA) has produced a *Guide to Handling Veterinary Waste* and a range of reference posters that summarize the guidance in England and Wales, Scotland and Northern Ireland.

- BVA Good practice guide to handling veterinary waste in England and Wales (Figure 2.29) (www.bva.co.uk/resources-support/practice-management/handling-veterinary-waste-guidance-posters/).

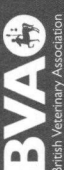

BVA British Veterinary Association

Good practice guide to handling veterinary waste in England and Wales

Veterinary assessment

All general waste must be subject to a veterinary risk assessment which must ask:

- Does the material arise from an animal that has any disease caused by a micro-organism, such that the material is contaminated with that micro-organism?
- Is there any other potential risk of infection?
- If the answer to either is **yes**, the waste is infectious, clinical waste ▼

Hazardous waste

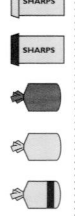
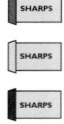
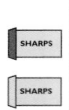

Register your premises, keep a Waste Register; use Consignment Notes, keep all records for at least three years.

Cytotoxic and cytostatic pharmaceuticals

Waste contaminated with cytotoxic and cytostatic pharmaceuticals, which are medicinal products that are toxic, carcinogenic, toxic for reproduction or mutagenic.

This includes:
- Glass bottles and vials
- Clinical items (for example, swabs, masks and gloves)
- Syringes and sharps
- Animal bedding.

DISPOSAL
- Segregate into appropriate purple and yellow containers — sharps, glass bottles and vials into purple-lidded sharps containers — for high-temperature incineration only
- EWC = 18 02 07*.

Contaminated sharps

Sharps must be subject to a risk assessment. Sharps contaminated with material (other than cytotoxic or cytostatic) that is deemed to present a risk of infection to any animal or person that may come into contact with it may include:

- Partially and fully discharged sharps, hypodermic needles and other sharp instruments and objects.

DISPOSAL
- EWC = 18 02 02* and 18 02 08
- Segregate into yellow sharps containers for high-temperature incineration only.

FOR BEST PRACTICE
- EWC = 18 02 02*
- Non-pharmaceutically contaminated sharps can be further segregated into orange-lidded bins for suitable alternative treatment (for example, autoclaving).

Infectious, clinical waste

Infectious, clinical waste is:

Waste containing viable micro-organisms or their toxins which are known or reliably believed to cause disease in humans or other living organisms; or waste which, following a veterinary assessment, is deemed to present a risk of infection to any animal or person that may come into contact with it.

This may include:
- Items used in treatment (for example, swabs, masks and gloves, which may include blood-contaminated items
- Animal bedding
- Blood and body parts.

DISPOSAL
- Segregate into appropriate yellow containers for high-temperature incineration only
- EWC = 18 02 02*.

FOR BEST PRACTICE
- Infectious waste, other than body parts and cadavers, can be further segregated into orange containers for suitable alternative treatment (for example, autoclaving) as best practice
- EWC = 18 02 02*.

Photographic chemicals

This may include:
- Waste fixer and developer solutions.

DISPOSAL
- Segregate into separate fixer and developer leak-proof containers for treatment at an appropriately permitted facility
- There is no standard packaging to accept specific requirements should be discussed with your waste contractor
- EWC = 09 01 01* (developer) and 09 01 04* (fixer).

Non-hazardous waste

Use transfer notes and keep all records for three years.

Offensive waste

Offensive waste is veterinary waste other than sharps that is not hazardous or clinical but which is unpleasant and may cause offence to the senses.

This waste must have been subjected to a detailed item and patient-specific assessment that clearly demonstrates it does not present a risk of infection or other potential hazard to any animal or person that may come into contact with it, even if mismanaged.

This is particularly important in the case of material contaminated with body fluids (for example, blood), where a veterinary surgeon must be able to demonstrate that they implemented procedures that meet the requirements set out in the accompanying web guidance (see www.bva.co.uk).

As a result of this assessment the veterinary surgeon is declaring that the waste is not hazardous, and is not clinical waste that requires incineration or other treatment prior to landfill.

Offensive waste may include:
- Items used in treatment (for example swabs, masks and gloves, which may include blood-contaminated items)
- Animal bedding
- Animal faeces.

These **must not** contain body parts or body tissues.

DISPOSAL
- Landfill or other suitable permitted facility
- EWC = 18 02 03.

Sharps

Sharps must be subject to a risk assessment that demonstrates they do not present a risk of infection to any animal or person that may come into contact with them.

This may include:
- An unused sharp that has been dropped on the floor prior to use.

If there is deemed to be a risk, however small, the sharp should be assumed to be hazardous and handled accordingly (see Contaminated sharps).

DISPOSAL
- EWC = 18 02 01
- If the sharps are classified as 18 02 01 the vet is indicating that they are not clinical waste and do not need to be rendered safe. In such circumstances disposal outlets may be more limited and less predictable, potentially including landfill without treatment. It is unlikely that a veterinary practice would produce a sharps waste stream which could be coded 18 02 01.

Pharmaceuticals (not cytotoxic or cytostatic)

Waste contaminated with pharmaceuticals (not cytotoxic or cytostatic).

This may include:
- Denatured controlled drugs
- Prescription-only medicines
- Out-of-date drugs
- Contaminated bottles, syringe bodies and packaging.

DISPOSAL OF CONTROLLED DRUGS
- All controlled drugs must be denatured or made not readily recoverable and then be disposed of with other pharmaceuticals (not cytotoxic or cytostatic)
- For Schedule 2 controlled drugs this should be done in the presence of an authorised person (for example, a veterinary surgeon from another practice).

DISPOSAL OF OTHER PHARMACEUTICALS
- Segregate into blue leak-proof containers
- Avoid mixing
- Incineration at an appropriately permitted facility
- EWC = 18 02 08.

Pet cadavers

Pet cadavers are now transferred and disposed of under animal by-product controls, except where the cadaver is suspected of harbouring a notifiable disease, in which case collection and disposal will be arranged by Defra.

DISPOSAL
- Burial at home
- Burial in a pet cemetery
- Cremation.

Domestic waste

Waste that only contains domestic rubbish. This includes separate recyclable and mixed non-recyclable materials. Batteries and hazardous items should not be placed in the mixed municipal waste.

Recyclables may include:
- Paper, card, unsoiled newspapers and magazines
- Plastic food containers
- Drink cans
- Batteries.

DISPOSAL
- Recycling or disposal at a suitably permitted or licensed site
- EWC = 20 03 01 (mixed).

Further information

It is the right and responsibility of the waste producer, that is, the practice, to classify and segregate their waste. Waste should be subjected to a detailed item and patient specific assessment to determine if it presents a risk of infection or other potential hazard to any animal or person that may come into contact with it.

All businesses have a duty of care to ensure that:
- All waste is stored and disposed of responsibly
- Waste is only handled or dealt with by those authorised to do so
- Appropriate records are kept of all waste that is transferred or received

This is a practical good practice guide to assist veterinary surgeons to comply with waste regulations in England and Wales

Supported by the

ENVIRONMENT AGENCY

The **Environment Agency** supports this *Good practice guide to handling veterinary waste in England and Wales* written and published by the British Veterinary Association.

Further information on handling veterinary waste is available at **www.bva.co.uk** and **www.environment-agency.gov.uk**

Published **December 2011** Copyright © British Veterinary Association. All rights reserved. No part of this publication may be reproduced by any process without written permission from the publisher. Requests and enquiries concerning reproduction and rights should be made to: BVA, 7 Mansfield Street, London W1G 9NQ. Email: bvahq@bva.co.uk

2.29 BVA Good practice guide to handling veterinary waste in England and Wales. (Reproduced with permission from the BVA).

- BVA Good practice guide to handling veterinary waste in Scotland (www.bva.co.uk/resources-support/practice-management/handling-veterinary-waste-guidance-posters/).
- BVA Good practice guide to handling veterinary waste in Northern Ireland (www.bva.co.uk/resources-support/practice-management/handling-veterinary-waste-guidance-posters/).

The veterinary practice has a legal 'duty of care' to ensure that waste is handled, stored and disposed of responsibly. The practice must also ensure that the company removing the waste is authorized to deal with the waste type and that the waste goes to an appropriate site for processing. The practice duty therefore does not end when the waste is passed on to the waste disposal company.

Each movement of waste must be accompanied by a waste transfer note for non-hazardous waste (retained for 2 years) or a consignment note for hazardous waste (retained for 3 years), which should be signed by both the practice and the waste collector. Waste transfer notes and consignment notes should contain a written description of the waste and the appropriate European Waste Catalogue (EWC) code(s). The use of EWC codes to describe waste is a legal requirement. Veterinary waste is coded 18-02–XX, with the final two digits dependant on the type of waste (e.g. cytotoxic/cytostatic medicines are 18-02-07). Information on EWC codes is available in the *BSAVA Guide to the Use of Veterinary Medicines*. All waste leaving the practice must carry the appropriate coding on each item.

A pre-acceptance waste audit should be completed before waste collection commences. This document identifies the waste a practice produces, the quantity produced and helps to ensure the waste is processed via the correct waste stream. A summary of waste classification is shown in Figure 2.30.

RCVS PSS assessors may check that appropriate bags and bins are used, and that paperwork such as pre-assessment audits, contracts, waste transfer and consignment notes are available and retained.

Type of waste	Description
Hazardous waste	
Infectious waste	Waste containing viable microorganisms or their toxins, which are known or reliably believed to cause disease in humans or other living organisms Waste which, following a veterinary assessment, is deemed to present a risk of infection to any animal or person that may come into contact with it Examples of this include waste from animals with infectious diseases
Cytotoxic and cytostatic pharmaceuticals	Waste contaminated with cytotoxic and cytostatic pharmaceuticals, which are medicinal products that are toxic, carcinogenic, toxic for reproduction or mutagenic Refer to the *BSAVA Guide to the Use of Veterinary Medicines* for full details of relevant medication for disposal. This includes: - Glass bottles - Syringes and sharps - Clinical items (e.g. PPE, swabs)
Sharps	Scalpel blades Needles Glass
Photographic chemicals	Used for wet developing Liaise with waste carrier Refer to datasheets
Non-hazardous waste	
Offensive waste	Offensive waste is veterinary waste other than sharps that is not hazardous or clinical but which is unpleasant and may cause offence to the senses Bedding Swabs Masks (depending on practice risk assessment)
Pharmaceutical waste	Waste contaminated with pharmaceuticals (not cytotoxic or cytostatic): - Denatured Controlled Drugs - Prescription-only medicines - Out-of-date drugs - Contaminated bottles, syringes and packaging Do not mix solids and liquids – the chemical reaction can lead to fire
Sanitary waste	Female sanitary items All toilets used by women should be provided with a suitable method for disposing of sanitary waste
Animal byproducts	
Cadavers	Options for owners are cremation at a licensed pet crematorium, burial at home or burial at a registered pet burial site Rarely, Defra may classify as hazardous if notifiable disease is present
Body parts	These should not be placed with hazardous waste; they should be separated and stored for cremation at a licensed facility

2.30 Examples of types of veterinary waste.

continues ▶

Type of waste	Description
Domestic waste	
Recycling	■ Paper, card, unsoiled newspapers and magazines ■ Plastic food containers ■ Glass ■ Metals and drink cans ■ Batteries Local authority requirements may vary
Mixed non-cycling	Domestic waste Black bag items In a veterinary practice this is mainly office waste
Electrical equipment	Electrical appliance disposal Waste electrical and electronic equipment includes most products that have a plug or need a battery Refer to the Waste Electrical and Electronic Equipment (WEEE) Regulations 2013 for specific disposal requirements

2.30 *continued* Examples of types of veterinary waste.

Definitions

Clinical waste

Clinical waste is defined as waste containing viable micro-organisms or their toxins which are known or reliably believed to cause disease in humans or other living organisms, or waste which, following a veterinary assessment, is deemed to present a risk of infection to any animal or person that may come into contact with it. This may include items used in treatment (e.g. swabs, masks, gloves) that become contaminated with blood, animal bedding or bodily fluids from patients with infectious disease.

The reader should note that the term 'clinical waste' may be more applicable to human healthcare rather than the veterinary environment. The use of the term 'hazardous' with subcategories of infectious, sharps, cytotoxic/cytostatic pharmaceuticals and photographic chemicals may be more accurate in the veterinary environment.

Hazardous waste

Hazardous wastes are those that are harmful to people, the environment or animals, either immediately or over an extended period of time. Key veterinary hazardous wastes include:

■ Cytotoxic and cytostatic pharmaceuticals
■ Infectious waste – any veterinary waste containing viable microorganisms or their toxins, which are known or reliably believed to cause disease in humans or other living organisms
■ Sharps contaminated with animal blood or pharmaceuticals that are deemed to present a risk of infection
■ Photographic chemicals such as fixer or developer solution.

Non-hazardous waste

This is veterinary waste that is not hazardous or clinical but which is unpleasant and may cause offence to the senses. Non-hazardous waste may include items used in the treatment of non-infectious cases (e.g. swabs, masks and gloves), and may include blood-contaminated items, bedding and animal faeces.

Medicines

Detailed information on all aspects of medicines handling, storage and disposal can be found in Chapter 8 and the *BSAVA Guide to the Use of Veterinary Medicines*, which is available on the BSAVA website (www.bsavalibrary.com/).

Pharmaceutical waste bin

The pharmaceutical waste disposal bin, also known as the 'pharmy bin', is the main disposal bin for pharmaceutical waste. This bin was previously referred to as the 'DOOP' bin; however, this term is now obsolete. The bin should be made of leak-proof plastic and the contents should not be hazardous. Examples of items commonly placed in the pharmaceutical waste include vaccination bottles, empty injection bottles, syringes, whole medicines and denatured Controlled Drugs. The contents of the bin should be recorded and the record made available to the disposal contractor. This also forms part of the practice medicine audit.

All syringes placed in the bin should have been fully discharged of content. Snap-top glass vials should not be placed in these bins; they should be placed in the sharps bin. Any unused content in syringes (e.g. induction anaesthetic agents) should be discharged into an absorbable material (such as cat litter) and this should be placed into the pharmaceutical waste bin. These products should not be disposed of down the sink. Cytotoxic and cytostatic medicines (e.g. injection bottles, whole medicines and used syringes) should be placed in the purple lidded bin (see 'Cytotoxic and cytostatic products', below).

Controlled Drugs

Controlled Drugs (CDs) are commonly used in veterinary practices, usually as analgesics and for seizure management. Their regulation is enforced by the Home Office. Practices will be visited by either RCVS PSS assessors or VMD representatives to review their medicine practices, with particular focus on the governance of CDs.

There are extensive rules relating to the requisition, storage, recording and disposal of CDs (see Chapter 8). The *BSAVA Guide to the Use of Veterinary Medicines* and the RCVS both offer practical guidance on the subject. These should be read and referred to as needed, so it can be ensured that CDs are adequately managed in practice. Writing easy-to-follow

SOPs will help manage CDs within the practice. SOPs should cover supply, use, recording and disposal, as well as procedures for the investigation of any discrepancies.

Out-of-date CDs must be denatured in a kit that renders the drug irretrievable, before disposal. The kit is then placed in the pharmaceutical bin. Denaturing of Schedule 2 CDs, such as ketamine, methadone and fentanyl, must be witnessed by a Controlled Drugs Liaison Officer (CDLO), an independent veterinary surgeon or a RCVS PSS assessor. Practices must apply for an exemption to allow denaturing of CDs on site. This is waste exemption T28 in England (www.gov.uk/guidance/register-your-waste-exemptions-environmental-permits). There is a link on the government webpage for practices in Northern Ireland, Wales and Scotland to complete the equivalent form for their area.

Sharps handling and disposal

The use of sharps such as injection needles, capillary tubes and scalpel blades should be risk assessed. The correct type of sharps bin should be used for different types of hazardous waste.

- A purple lidded bin is used for cytotoxic and cytostatic products (see below).
- Yellow or orange lidded bins (colour dependant on waste handling and company) are used for disposal of used needles, glass vials, scalpel blades and any other products that could cause a penetrating injury to the user.

Sharps bins (Figure 2.31) are commonly filled above the indicated fill line, which creates a risk of injury to team members. Once filled the bins should be sealed and stored securely awaiting collection. Clients with diabetic pets should be provided with a sharps bin for safe sharps disposal, and this should be returned to the practice for disposal when full.

Cytotoxic and cytostatic products

Cytotoxic and cytostatic drugs and cytotoxic waste should be disposed of in a purple lidded bin. This includes cancer chemotherapeutic drugs such as vincristine, ciclosporin, antivirals such as interferon, and hormonal drugs such as androgens and aglepristone. Chemotherapeutic equipment, including needles, syringes and giving sets, as well as out-of-date medicines, should be disposed of in this bin. For practices producing large volumes of such waste (e.g. oncology centres), larger volume bins will be needed. Carriage of cytotoxic and cytostatic waste in unlicensed vehicles is illegal, so transfer between practices is not acceptable.

Body parts and cadavers

Pet cadavers are collected and disposed of under animal by-products legislation. Body parts (e.g. tissue removed during surgery) should be disposed of in the same manner as pet cadavers.

Other waste

Practices should separate their domestic waste into products suitable for recycling and those which are not. Domestic waste is commonly placed in black refuse bags. The contents of these bags should essentially be office products.

Location of bins

Within a veterinary practice, it is common for each consultation room, preparatory room and kennel area to contain a bin for hazardous and non-hazardous waste. All team members in the practice should be familiar with items that should be placed in each bin; a detailed SOP may be useful in this regard. Laminated lists stuck near to or on bins can be helpful to remind team members which bin to use in each circumstance. Waste disposal should be carefully monitored and training on segregation and identification of appropriate waste streams should be carried out by the practice.

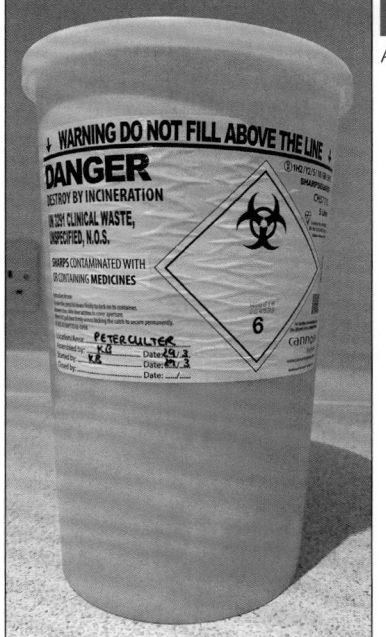

2.31 Sharps bin. (Courtesy of Ashgrove Vets, Aberdeen)

Lone working, house visits and practice security

Legislation

- Health and Safety at Work etc. Act 1974
- Management of Health and Safety at Work Regulations 1999

There are no specific regulations for lone working, but duties under the principle regulations require the employer to identify those who work alone and manage any health and safety risks when doing so. Lone workers are those who work by themselves, either away from the practice (e.g. house visits, attending emergencies for charitable organizations) or within the practice without supervision for long periods of time (lone veterinary surgeon in small or branch practice) or out of normal working hours (veterinary surgeons and veterinary nurses). The risks encountered vary greatly between practices and areas of the UK and it is vital that practice-specific (and branch-specific) risk assessments are carried out. The risk assessment should address all aspects of lone working, away from and within the practice.

Risk assessment

The risk assessment for lone working can be built into other risk assessments, but is often easier as a standalone assessment. The same format as other practice risk assessments should be used and may make reference to other risk assessments for generic risks. However, they should address specific lone worker risks, including:

- Increased risks of accidents, injury or ill health
- Increased vulnerability (e.g. in the event of violence, sudden illness, fire or other emergency)
- Special circumstances (e.g. a pregnant worker will require special consideration and the risk assessment may need to be updated throughout pregnancy).

Other considerations should include:

- Can one person complete the job safely? Is the animal too large or aggressive for one person to handle, or is the area of the visit too dangerous for a lone worker?
- Is the employee fit to work alone?
- What training is required to work alone (competent for all likely treatment) and also to deal with any unexpected situation such as violence or aggression?
- The boundaries for lone work – what is permitted and when help should be sought
- How will supervision be provided for those new to lone working?
- How are lone workers monitored? A pre-agreed contact routine can be good for veterinary practice. In addition, checking systems to ensure that the worker has returned safely when the visit is complete may be useful
- Arrangements for illness, accident or emergency – training and provision of first aid equipment and emergency contact arrangements
- Any previous accidents, incidents or near misses and what has been learnt from them.

The risk assessment should be developed with input from those who will be working alone. Once developed the team should be fully briefed on the risk assessment and trained with regard to the in-house protocols for lone working. The nature of lone working requires the ability of the employee to be able to assess each individual situation to ensure adequate controls are in place to carry out the required task professionally and safely. Contractors working alone in the practice should be fully briefed on the actions to take to ensure they can work safely in the event of any accident or emergency.

House visits

House visits may be necessary in small animal veterinary practice. They require preparation and planning, so that visits can be facilitated at short notice when required. A risk assessment must be carried out and an SOP is also helpful to ensure there is a standard approach for visits. It is common

practice for two persons to attend visits away from the practice. A mobile phone should be carried by the team members. A visit box should be prepared and ready to use with a list of contents available. The box should be replenished at the end of each visit.

A driving for work risk assessment should be completed, and should consider vehicle insurance, driver eligibility to drive in the UK, condition of the vehicle (practice or employees' own vehicle), vehicle breakdown and repair strategy, what to do in the event of an accident, vehicle and driver/passenger security and safe/secure storage of equipment. Where animals are transported, they should be placed in a secured crate or carrier to prevent escape, injury to pet or passengers, or any interference with driver concentration. The assessment of the risks from work-related road safety should include organizing journeys, driver training and vehicle maintenance. It should clearly set out everyone's roles and responsibilities for work-related road safety.

Practice security

A risk assessment should form the basis of decision making regarding practice security. Previous incidents, practice workload, location and demographics may influence the level of security required. Dispensary areas should not be accessible to the public and areas for authorized persons only are often protected by key pad entry. In larger practices, identification badges and area passes should be considered. All client-facing reception team members should be provided with an SOP for dealing with aggressive clients and should be trained in the procedures and action to take in these circumstances. Team training for these circumstances, including role play, can be helpful.

Manual handling

Legislation

- The Manual Handling Operations Regulations 2002
- Health and Safety (Display Screen Equipment) Regulations 1992

Work-related musculoskeletal disorders (WRMSDs) affect muscles, joints and tendons in all parts of the body, with most developing over time. An estimated 8.9 million working days in 2017 were lost due to WRMSDs, with an average of 14 days lost for each case. This represents 35% of all days lost due to work-related ill health in Great Britain (HSE, 2017). Figure 2.32 shows how WRMSDs can affect different areas of the body and their possible causes.

Type of injury	Area affected	Possibly veterinary workplace causes
Upper limb disorder (repetitive strain injuries)	Arm, shoulder and neck	Prolonged keyboard use, poor workstation design, incorrect use of equipment
Lower limb disorder	Hips to toes	Prolonged standing
Back pain	Neck to hips	Inappropriate manual handling tasks without adequate controls

2.32 Possible causes of work-related musculoskeletal disorders.

Manual handling is moving or supporting a load (object or animal), including pushing, pulling, carrying, lifting or placing down. Examples of tasks that may be hazardous in veterinary practice are:

■ Handling live animals (weight range in small animal practice can be 20 g to 100 kg!)
■ Moving cadavers
■ Handling medical gas cylinders
■ Lifting/carrying boxed goods, bags of food, laboratory equipment
■ Moving equipment
■ Computer work
■ Prolonged standing or kneeling.

Practices are required to:

■ Avoid the need for hazardous manual handling
■ Assess the risk of injury from any hazardous manual handling that cannot be avoided
■ Reduce the risk of injury.

A manual handling risk assessment should be carried out for all tasks that are likely to occur in the practice that involve hazardous manual handling. It should be remembered to consider and plan for emergency situations, such as movement of giant breed inpatients or transfer of emergency patients from the car park or house visit to the clinic.

For every manual handling task taking place, a dynamic risk assessment should be carried out. Many people will do this almost without thinking, and it does not have to be recorded. However, it is beneficial to pause, plan and discuss more complex manual handling tasks, involving more than one person, before proceeding. When following the general rules of manual handling, consideration should be given to:

■ Can handling be avoided? For example:
  • Can the dog walk to the area where it will be anaesthetized, rather than carrying it?
  • Can the oxygen cylinders be delivered directly to the storage area, rather than being left for team members to move?
  • The HSE has developed a 'Variable Manual Handling Assessment Chart (V-MAC) tool' for manual handling (www.hse.gov.uk/msd/mac/vmac/index.htm). However, this tool is limited in most veterinary situations (www.hse.gov.uk/msd/mac/vmac/1-advantages-limitations.htm), although it may be useful when moving and unpacking deliveries.
■ Assessing hazardous manual handling operations that cannot be avoided. The LITE risk assessment model is easy to use and remember (Figure 2.33). The HSE provide a useful manual handling assessment template that can be utilized for hazardous handling assessments (www.hse.gov.uk/pubns/ck5.pdf)
■ Reducing the risk of injury so far as is reasonably practicable. Training is a vital part of injury prevention and adopting good manual handling techniques will prevent team members from becoming injured or exacerbating existing injuries (see Chapter 11). Other practical solutions to reduce the risk of injury may include:
  • Using a lifting aid or equipment (Figure 2.34)
  • Improving workplace layout and lighting
  • Reducing carrying distances
  • Avoiding repetitive handling and vary the work, allowing one set of muscles to rest while another is used

Load	Individual
■ Size	■ Capability
■ Shape	■ Size
■ Weight	■ Training
■ Temperature	■ Strength
■ Stability	■ Pre-existing injury
■ Awkward	■ Pregnant
Task	**Environment**
■ Type of handling	■ Indoors
■ Pushing	■ Outdoors
■ Pulling	■ Hot/cold
■ Lifting	■ Slippery
■ Carrying	■ Uneven
■ Bending	■ Lighting
■ Stooping	■ Route to be taken
■ Twisting	

2.33 LITE manual handling assessment model.

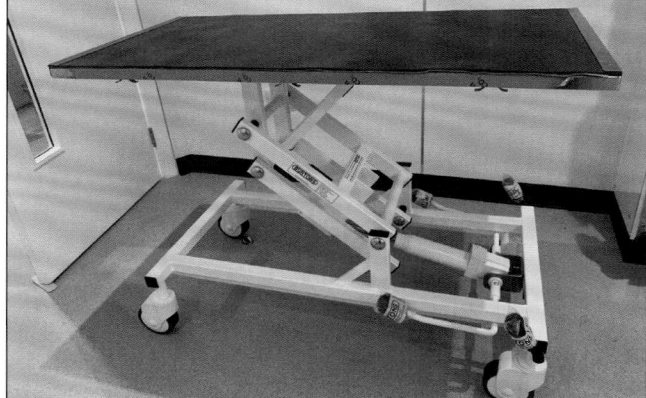

2.34 A height adjustable examination table. The table can be raised or lowered to avoid lifting large dogs and can be used to move patients within the practice. (Courtesy of Ashgrove Vets, Aberdeen)

• Pushing rather than pulling
• Paying particular attention to those who have a physical weakness
• Taking extra care of pregnant and young workers

Individual capabilities vary greatly. This is especially true with regard to new and expectant mothers, who are more vulnerable to injury. Those with pre-existing injuries require a special duty of care (as outlined in the section on 'Risk assessment', above). Handling aids, such as towels, hoists, harnesses and stretchers, as well as height adjustable tables, are available and minimize risk of injury when used correctly.

The work environment should be kept free from obstructions and problems such as uneven flooring, slip and trip hazards and poor housekeeping should be identified and rectified. A good safety culture will help prevent injuries, by encouraging team members to plan lifting operations and not to rush, nor to adopt an overly ambitious or self-reliant attitude to lifting. It should be remembered that most WRMSDs develop over time, so it is critical to prevent any injury early on in a veterinary nurse's career.

Workstation assessment

There are potential health risks associated with the use of display screen equipment (DSE) such as desktop computers, tablets and laptops. These risks relate to the development of upper limb disorders if work activities are not effectively managed.

The Health and Safety (Display Screen Equipment) Regulations 1992 apply to 'DSE users', usually defined as workers who use DSE daily, for an hour or more at a time. They do not apply to workers who use DSE infrequently or only use it for a short time. However, practices may choose to carry out general workstation assessments (Figure 2.35), to ensure work areas suit the ergonomics of the task, and this is to be recommended.

Changes may not need to be complex or expensive to be effective; for example, job rotation can reduce time spent in one position. Liaison with team members who actually do the job is important to ensure improvements do not create additional unforeseen risks.

If you have DSE users, you must:
- Analyse workstations to assess and reduce risks
- Make sure controls are in place
- Provide information and training
- Provide eyesight tests on request and special spectacles if needed
- Review the assessment when the user or the DSE changes

2.35 DSE user requirements.

Handling animals

Risk assessments should address the risks involved in handling small animal patients. Veterinary personnel need to be properly trained and know how to use appropriate handling equipment and PPE (see Chapter 11). Risk assessment controls should be aimed primarily at prevention of injury, with consideration given to first aid measures required in the event of injury. Animals in the practice should be restrained in suitable carriers or on leads. The reception team should be trained to ask clients to restrain their pets whilst in the waiting room. The use of aids such as muzzles, towels and buster collars can help with handling. Appropriate chemical restraint may be needed if the animal cannot otherwise be safely handled.

Dogs can be positively conditioned to veterinary visits and to wearing a muzzle. The use of correct handling techniques and equipment minimizes stress for the animal and reduces the risk to the handlers (see Chapter 11). (It should be remembered that the veterinary practice is also responsible for the safe handling of pets by their owners whilst they are in the practice.)

Feline handling safety can be improved by using separate cat areas in the practice, pheromone therapy and cat friendly handling techniques (see Chapter 11). Most clinically normal cats carry a variety of aerobic and anaerobic pathogenic bacteria in their oral cavities, including *Pasteurella multocida*, *Streptococcus* spp. and *Fusobacterium* organisms. Pathogenic bacteria can also be harboured in the nails and introduced through cat scratches. Kheiran *et al.* (2019) reported that cat bites lead to an infection rate of 30–60%, which is more than double the rate of infection caused by dog bites. Symptomatic cat bites to the upper limb must be treated promptly (i.e. within 48 hours). Failure to do so may lead to septic arthritis, osteomyelitis and the need for digital amputation. These negative outcomes are more likely in immunocompromised people (e.g. those with diabetes).

Appropriate techniques for handling rabbits, rodents, ferrets, birds and reptiles are detailed in Chapter 11 and the relevant BSAVA Manuals and should be referred to before handling these species.

Welfare and mental health

Legislation
- Workplace (Health, Safety and Welfare) Regulations 1992

Workplace welfare

Welfare facilities relate to those facilities that are necessary for the wellbeing of employees, such as toilets, washing, rest and changing facilities, and somewhere clean to eat and drink during breaks. In veterinary practice, food and drink should not be prepared or consumed in any clinical areas, for health and hygiene reasons. Legislation prohibits smoking in the workplace in the UK.

Changing facilities should ensure the privacy of the user and be provided with seating. Secure storage space should be provided to store workers' own clothing and uniforms. Pregnant and breastfeeding employees must be provided with somewhere to rest and, where necessary, this should include somewhere for them to lie down. It is not suitable for new mothers to use toilets for expressing milk. An employer may provide a private, healthy and safe environment for employees to express and store milk, although there is no legal requirement for this.

Welfare provision should ensure that disabled workers are not discriminated against, and the employer is required to make sure that arrangements include provision of suitable access to facilities, which are adequate for the number of people at work with a disability.

In an average week, employees should not work more than 48 hours, averaged over a 17-week period. There are notable exceptions to this general rule and employees can choose to opt out of this directive. Any opt-outs should be recorded in writing. Detailed information is available on the government website (www.gov.uk/maximum-weekly-working-hours).

Workplace stress

Veterinary nurses are part of a caring profession. The very traits of empathy and caring that make an individual an excellent veterinary nurse, can also expose veterinary nurses to the risk of occupational stress. The veterinary nurse may experience this on a personal level or may recognize signs of occupational stress in team members.

An RCVS study of veterinary staff in 2014 found stress to be second on the list of the main challenges facing the profession. The HSE (2017) states that workplace stress is a major cause of sickness absence in the workplace and costs over £5 billion a year in Great Britain.

The HSE recognizes that a degree of stimulation or pressure in the workplace is beneficial, but that excessive pressure can result in stress-related ill-health, describing stress as 'the adverse reaction people have to excessive pressures or other types of demand placed on them'.

- **Burnout** is considered an 'unintentional end point' for certain individuals who are exposed to chronic stress within their working environment. When suffering burnout, a person may experience emotional exhaustion, may become more cynical or they may have a reduced sense of personal accomplishment in regard to their own work. Signs of burnout can include increased levels of absence or decreased working standards. This could directly impact on patient care and safety (Lloyd and Campion, 2019).

■ **Compassion fatigue** may occur when there is a need to show compassion and empathy towards clients who are emotionally distressed. Workplace support may include appropriate debriefing sessions among willing participants, particularly after an emotionally stressful encounter. This is important for both experienced and inexperienced team members (Lloyd and Campion, 2019).

There are excellent sources of information and support available to the profession. Vetlife has an extensive range of resources available free of charge and provide a confidential contact service (email or phone). Details of Vetlife, or other support organizations, should be displayed so team members are aware of how to access these services.

There is a legal requirement to carry out a risk assessment relating to stress at work. The HSE Management Standards can be helpful when putting together a stress risk assessment (Figure 2.36). They cover six key areas of work design that, if not properly managed, are associated with poor health, lower productivity and increased accident and sickness absence rates.

Management Standard	Comments
Demands	Issues related to workload, work patterns and the work environment
Control	How much say the person has in the way they do their work
Support	Levels of encouragement, sponsorship and resources provided by the organization, line management and colleagues
Relationships	Promoting positive working to avoid conflict and dealing with unacceptable behaviour
Role	Whether people understand their role within the organization and whether the organization ensures they do not have conflicting roles
Change	How organizational change is managed and communicated in the organization

2.36 HSE Management Standards relating to stress in the workplace.

Practical guidance on how to implement these strategies in a veterinary practice is detailed by Mamo (2016), who describes how to tackle work-related stress, promote wellbeing and support those experiencing mental health problems. RCVS Mind Matters offer training courses, have conducted research and have produced a guide to managing stress in veterinary workplaces. Implementing one or two simple initiatives can make a difference to psychological health and team moral.

Substance abuse

Substance abuse is associated with increased accident rates and increased days lost to absence. It can be a significant cause of stress to colleagues.

The RCVS Code of Professional Conduct for Veterinary Nurses requires that veterinary nurses take reasonable steps to address adverse physical or mental health or performance that could impair fitness to practise. It also requires that veterinary nurses who are concerned about a professional colleague's fitness to practise must take steps to ensure that animals are not put at risk and that the interests of the public are protected (see Chapter 1). Training providers have a responsibility to address any potential fitness to practise concerns with their students.

Vetlife Health Support offers help to anyone in the veterinary community who is experiencing mental health difficulties, including alcohol and drug misuse, eating disorders and anxiety and depression.

First aid, accident and incident reporting

> ### Legislation
> ■ The Health and Safety (First-Aid) Regulations 1981
> ■ Reporting of Injuries, Diseases and Dangerous Occurrences Regulations (RIDDOR) 2013

Employers are required to provide appropriate equipment, facilities and personnel to ensure their employees receive immediate attention if they are injured or taken ill at work. These Regulations apply to all workplaces and to the self-employed. Notably, there is no legal requirement to provide first aid for non-employees, such as clients and contractors; however, there is a moral obligation to care for them and it is strongly recommended they are included in the assessment of first aid requirements.

Accidents and ill health can occur at any time, and it is important that suitable provision is made for all team work periods and locations. In the veterinary industry, this includes provision for those working at nights, weekends and those working away from the practice site.

First aid needs assessment

Employers are required to carry out an assessment of first aid needs. In simple terms, this is a first aid risk assessment and the factors to consider are shown in Figure 2.37. The findings of the first aid needs assessment should take into account

Factor	Comments
Work environment and location	Mobile service, single/multiple branches, rural location
Typical work undertaken	Laboratory work, feral cats, specific hazards related to niche workload (e.g. exotic pets)
Type and severity of potential injuries	Contents of first aid kit should be suitable for workload and maintained
Location of nearest emergency services	Contact details, arrangements and determination of suitability (e.g. if the support is an hour away, this should not be the primary care provision)
Training needs assessment	Number of persons and training required

2.37 Factors to be considered in a first aid needs assessment.

the circumstances particular to the workplace, as this will determine what first aid equipment, facilities and first aid training should be provided. It will also provide an indication of how many first aiders may be required (Figure 2.38). Team members may be trained as appointed persons or first aiders. The roles and requirements are detailed in Figure 2.39.

The minimum first aid provision on any work site is:
- A suitably stocked first aid kit
- An appointed person to take charge of first aid arrangements
- Information for employees about first aid arrangements

2.38 Minimum first aid provision.

Appointed person
- This is the minimum requirement
- The minimum role of this appointed person is to look after first aid equipment and facilities and call the emergency services when required
- An appointed person does not need first aid training. However, 1-day courses for appointed persons are available
- An appointed person is not necessary where there are an adequate number of appropriately trained first aiders

First aider
- A first aider is someone who has done training appropriate to the level identified in the first aids needs assessment
- Training can be provided by a variety of suppliers. It is important that the training is specific for the workplace needs and the hazards encountered in veterinary practice
- Options are:
  - First aid at work (FAW)
  - Emergency first aid at work (EFAW)
  - Other first aid training appropriate to the veterinary practice
- If the veterinary practice has sufficient first aiders, there is no need for additional appointed persons

2.39 First aid roles.

The first aid box contents should be determined from the first aid needs assessment. It should be suitably stocked at all times. A list of required contents should be kept with the box and the contents should be checked regularly by a designated person(s) and records kept. The location of first aid equipment is important, so it can be readily accessed. It is useful to provide eyewash facilities near laboratory equipment and dispensary areas. It is recommended that tablets and other medicines are not kept in the first aid box.

First aid box contents

The decision about what should be provided in a workplace first aid box is determined by the findings of the first aid needs assessment. As a general guide, where work activities involve low risk hazards, the minimum that should be stocked in the first aid box includes:
- A leaflet giving general guidance on first aid (e.g. the HSE booklet on Basic advice of first aid at work; www.hse.gov.uk/pubns/firindex.htm)
- Individually wrapped sterile plasters (assorted sizes), appropriate to the type of work (hypoallergenic plasters can be provided, if necessary) ➔

First aid box contents *continued*
- Sterile eye pads
- Individually wrapped triangular bandages, preferably sterile
- Safety pins
- Large sterile, individually wrapped, non-medicated wound dressings
- Medium-sized sterile, individually wrapped, non-medicated wound dressings
- Disposable gloves (see 'Hand protection', above for information about glove selection).
  A suggested list of contents for a basic first aid box can be found on the HSE website (www.hse.gov.uk/firstaid/faqs.htm).

A useful way of informing the team about first aid provision is to cover this during induction training. Thereafter, a simple method of keeping team members informed is use of first aid notices. These can be displayed in prominent locations within the practice.

Recording and reporting accidents

An accident book is required by law to record and report details of specified work-related injuries and incidents. However, it is good practice to record all accidents and injuries in order to prevent recurrence where possible, and to minimize harm if recurrence occurs. Once completed, most books have a tear out system to ensure sensitive personal information is securely stored. Practices may choose to record accidents, incidents and near misses on their own recording systems. It is good practice to review records of accidents to identify trends. In addition, recording near miss events provides an excellent learning and training opportunity for the practice and team members to prevent future accidents.

RIDDOR requires employers, the self-employed and people in control of work premises to report serious workplace accidents, occupational diseases and specified dangerous occurrences. Reporting can be undertaken using an online form (www.hse.gov.uk/riddor/report.htm). Typical examples of reportable injuries in veterinary practice are most fractures, over 7-day injuries to workers (i.e. where a worker is not able to carry out their work for 7 days, not counting the day of the accident), occupational diseases such as occupational dermatitis or carpal tunnel syndrome, and injuries to non-workers (e.g. clients) that involve the person being taken from the scene of the accident to the hospital. The criteria for reporting is very specific and the information should be reviewed before deciding to report an injury or incident.

References and further reading

BSAVA (2018) *BSAVA Guide to the Use of Veterinary Medicines*. Available at: www.bsavalibrary.com/content/book/10.22233/9781905319862
Dobson J and Lascelles DX (2011) *BSAVA Manual of Canine and Feline Oncology, 3rd edn*. BSAVA Publications, Gloucester
Girling S and Raiti P (2019) *BSAVA Manual of Reptiles, 3rd edn*. BSAVA Publications, Gloucester

Gov.uk (2006) *Fire safety risk assessment: 5-step checklist.* Available at: https://assets.publishing.service.gov.uk/government/uploads/system/uploads/attachment_data/file/14899/fsra-5-step-checklist.pdf

Gov.uk (2007) *Fire safety risk assessment for animal premises and stables.* Available at: https://assets.publishing.service.gov.uk/government/uploads/system/uploads/attachment_data/file/14895/fsra-animals.pdf

Gov.uk (2011) The economic cost of fire: estimates for 2008. *Fire Research Report 3/2011.* Available at https://webarchive.nationalarchives.gov.uk/20121105004836/http://www.communities.gov.uk/documents/corporate/pdf/1838338.pdf

Gov.uk (2014) *Waste exemption: T28 sort and denature controlled drugs for disposal.* Available at: www.gov.uk/guidance/waste-exemption-t28-sort-and-denature-controlled-drugs-for-disposal

HSE (2003) *Health and safety regulation: a short guide.* Available at: www.hse.gov.uk/pubns/hsc13.pdf

HSE (2005) *EH40/2005 Workplace exposure limits.* Available at: www.hse.gov.uk/pUbns/priced/eh40.pdf

HSE (2010) *Guidance for employers on the control of artificial optical radiation at work regulations (AOR) 2010.* Available at: www.hse.gov.uk/radiation/nonionising/employers-aor.pdf

HSE (2012) *Legionnaires' disease: a brief guide for dutyholders.* Available at: www.hse.gov.uk/pubns/indg458.pdf.

HSE (2012) *Maintaining portable electric equipment in low-risk environments.* Available at: www.hse.gov.uk/pubns/indg236.htm

HSE (2012) *Managing asbestos in buildings: a brief guide.* Available at: www.hse.gov.uk/pubns/indg223.pdf

HSE (2012) *Safety requirements for autoclaves: Guidance Note PM73 (rev3).* Available at: www.hse.gov.uk/pubns/guidance/pm73.pdf

HSE (2012) *Written schemes of examination: pressure systems safety regulations 2000.* Available at: www.hse.gov.uk/pubns/indg178.pdf

HSE (2013) *Managing for health and safety HSG 65.* Available at: www.hse.gov.uk/pibns/books/hsg65.htm

HSE (2013) *Oxygen use in the workplace: fire and explosion hazards.* Available at: www.hse.gov.uk/pubns/indg459.pdf

HSE (2013) *Personal protective equipment at work: a brief guide.* Available at: www.hse.gov.uk/pubns/indg174.pdf

HSE (2013) *Reporting accidents and incidents at work.* Available at: www.hse.gov.uk/pubns/indg453.pdf

HSE (2014) *A brief guide to controlling risks in the workplace.* Available at: www.hse.gov.uk/pubns/indg163.htm

HSE (2017) *Health and safety at work: summary statistics for Great Britain 2017.* Available at: www.hse.gov.uk/statistics/overall/hssh1617.pdf

HSE (2017) *Tackling work-related stress using the Management Standards approach: a step-by-step workbook.* Available at: www.hse.gov.uk/pubns/wbk01.pdf

HSE (2018) *First aid at work: your questions answered.* Available at: www.hse.gov.uk/pubns/indg214.pdf

HSE (2018) *Work-related skin disease in Great Britain (2018).* Available at: www.hse.gov.uk/statistics/causdis/dermatitis/skin.pdf

Kheiran A, Palial V, Rollett R, Wildin CJ, Chatterji U and Singh HP (2019) Cat bite: an injury not to underestimate. *Journal of Plastic Surgery and Hand Surgery* **9**, 1–6

Lloyd C and Campion DP (2019) Occupational stress and the importance of self-care and resilience. *Veterinary Ireland Journal* **9(4)**, 1–7

Mamo E (2016) Why creating a mentally healthy workplace is so important in veterinary practice. *In Practice* **38**, 355–357

Mindmatters (2018) *A guide to enhancing wellbeing and managing work stress in the veterinary workplace.* Available at: www.vetmind-matters.org/wp-content/uploads/20101/MMI-12pp-web.pdf

RCVS (2014) *RCVS survey of the veterinary profession.* Available at: www.rcvs.org.uk/news-and-views/publications/rcvs-survey-of-the-veterinary-profession-2014

RCVS (2015) *Controlled drugs guidance.* Available at: www.rcvs.org.uk/news-and-views/publications/controlled-drugs-guidance/

RCVS Knowledge (2019) *Clinical Audit.* Available at: knowledge.rcvs.org.uk/quality-improvement/tools-and-resources/clinical-audit/

Useful websites

HSE:
- Control of Substances Hazardous to Health (COSHH) – www.hse.gov.uk/coshh/index.htm
- New and expectant mothers – www.hse.gov.uk/mothers
- Young people at work – www.hse.gov.uk/youngpeople/index.htm

Mind matters:
www.vetmindmatters.org

RCVS:
- Fitness to practise – www.rcvs.org.uk/news-and-views/publication/fitness-to-practise-a-guide-for-uk-providers-of-veterinary-nursing-education-and-student-veterinary-nurses-web.pdf
- Practice Standards Scheme – www.rcvs.org.uk/setting-standards/practice-standards-scheme/

Vetlife:
www.vetlife.org.uk

Self-assessment questions

1. What are the key principles of effective health and safety in the workplace?
2. What are the five steps of risk assessment?
3. Define hazard and risk.
4. What is a safety datasheet used for?
5. What does the acronym LITE mean with regard to manual handling?
6. What are the duties of an appointed person?
7. What are the three elements of fire safety?
8. What regulations apply to radiography in the veterinary workplace?
9. What is the purpose of health and safety consultation with employees?
10. Where can information on supporting mental health in the workplace be found?

Chapter 3

Anatomy and physiology

Mary Fraser and Simon Girling

Learning objectives

After studying this chapter, readers will have the knowledge to:

- **Recognize the terminology relating to anatomy and physiology**
- **Identify anatomical landmarks of the skeleton and soft tissues of dogs, cats and exotic animal species**
- **Identify the normal form and function of body systems in a range of mammalian species**
- **Describe the key anatomical features and body functions of birds and reptiles**
- **Describe the body systems and how they relate to each other**
- **Compare normal form and function with that seen in disease processes**
- **Relate anatomical and physiological features to radiography, ultrasonography, surgical and medical nursing**

Introduction

This chapter describes the anatomy and physiology of a wide range of species commonly encountered in veterinary practice: dogs, cats, small mammals, birds and reptiles. In each section basic generic anatomy is described, usually with the dog as a reference model; this is followed by consideration of the major anatomical differences between species or groups.

Terminology

- Anatomy – the physical structure of the body.
- Physiology – the way in which body systems work.

When describing the anatomy of animals, directional terms are used to provide more information about the structure and position of organs and tissues (Figure 3.1). Sectional planes are also used to describe the location of parts of the animal (Figure 3.2). Examples include:

- Median/mid-sagittal plane – a line that divides the body into right and left halves
- Sagittal/paramedian plane – any line parallel to the median plane
- Dorsal plane – parallel to the back of the animal
- Transverse plane – perpendicular to the long axis of the animal.

Other useful veterinary terminology, some of which can be applied to anatomical structures is given in Appendix 4.

Term	Description
Cranial (anterior)	Towards the head
Caudal (posterior)	Towards the tail
Lateral	Towards the side of the animal
Medial	Towards the middle of the animal
Ipsilateral	On the same side
Contralateral	On the opposite side
Dorsal	Near the back of the animal
Ventral	Near the underside of the animal
Palmar	The back or under surface of the front foot
Plantar	The back or under surface of the back foot
Rostral	Towards the nose
Proximal	Applies to limbs near the body
Distal	Applies to limbs near the toes
Superficial	Near the outside of the animal
Deep	Near the centre of the animal

3.1 Directional terminology.

BSAVA Textbook of Veterinary Nursing, sixth edition. Edited by Barbara Cooper, Elizabeth Mullineaux and Lynn Turner. ©BSAVA 2020

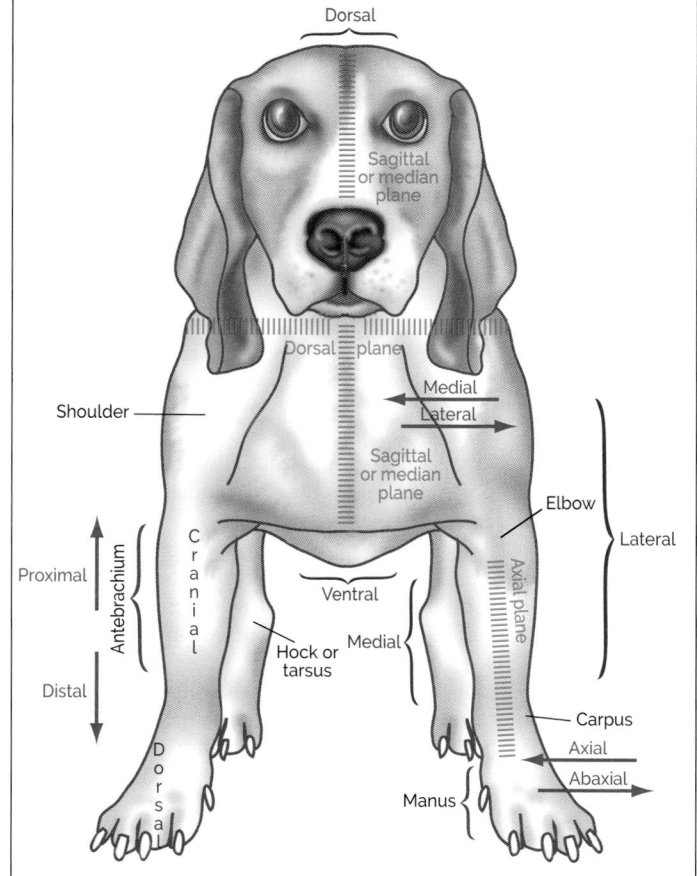
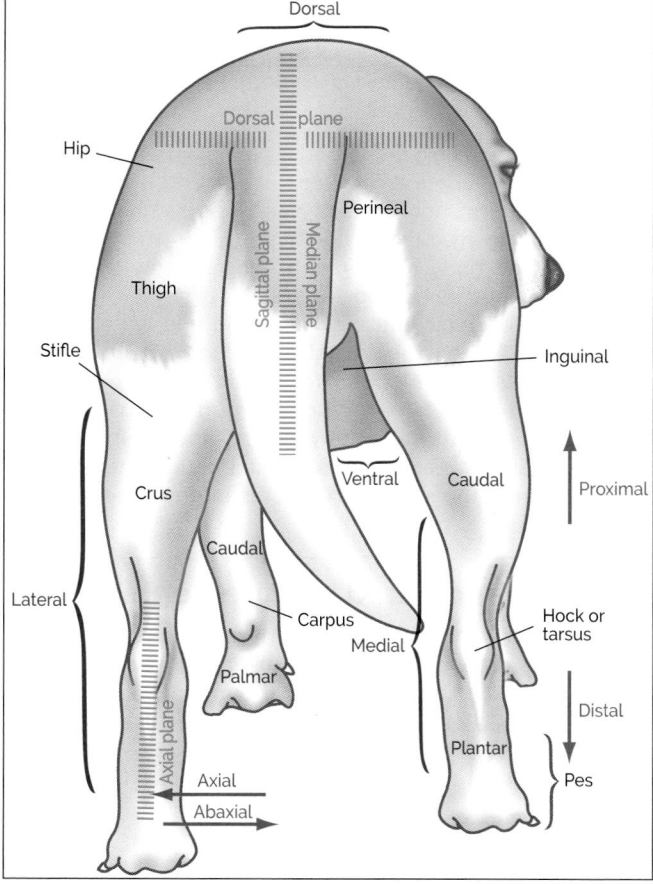

3.2 Anatomical planes and directions.

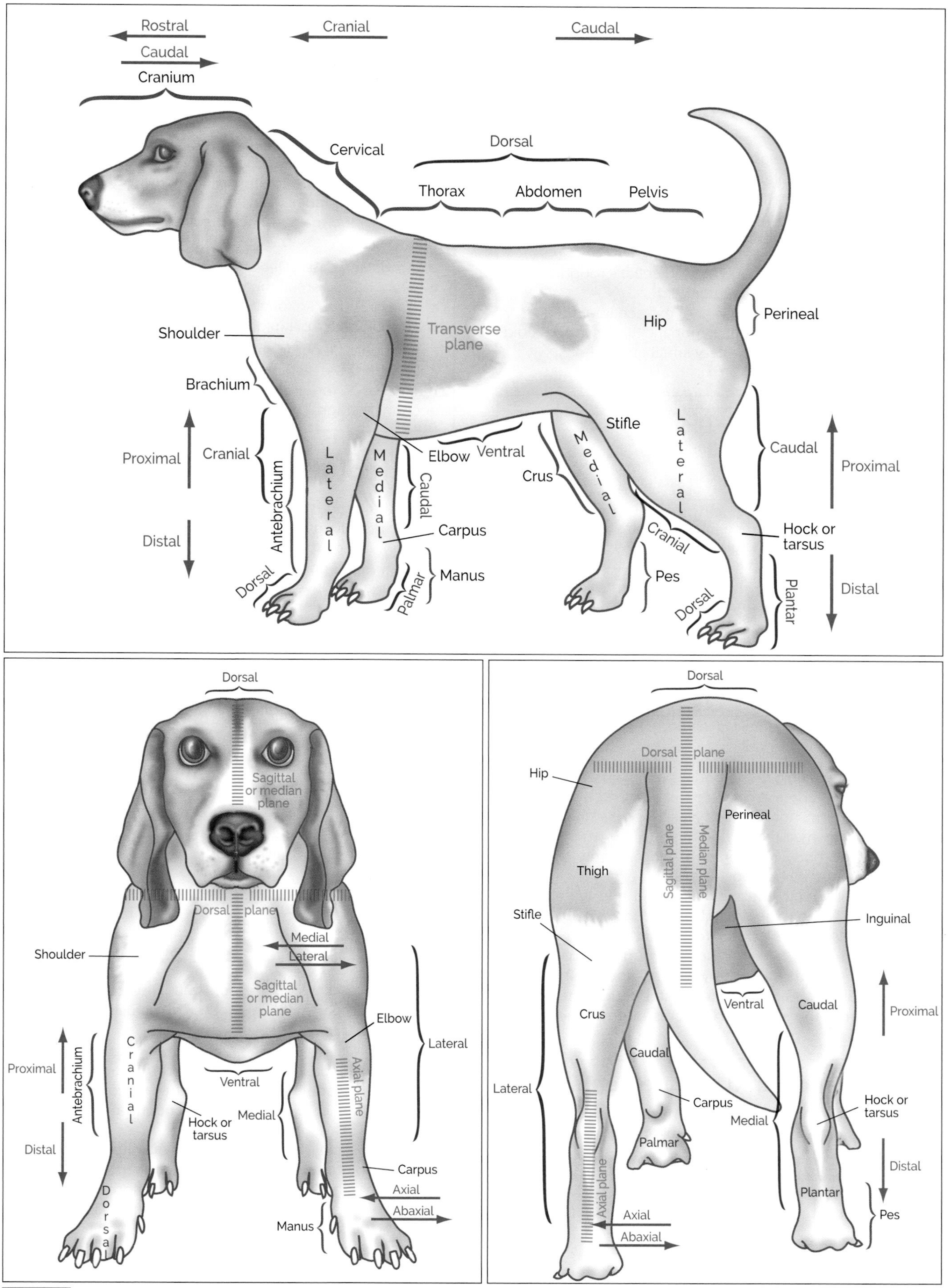

Body fluid

Approximately two-thirds of the body is made up of water. This varies between different species and is affected by both the age of animal and how fat or thin it is. Younger animals have a greater percentage of water than older animals. Thinner animals have a higher percentage of water than fatter animals.

Of the 60% bodyweight made up of water, approximately two-thirds is intracellular fluid and one-third is extracellular fluid (Figure 3.3). Intracellular fluid is the fluid found inside the individual cells of the body. Extracellular fluid is the fluid found outside the cells and comprises:

- Interstitial fluid (fluid found around cells) – roughly three-quarters of extracellular fluid
- Plasma – roughly one-quarter of extracellular fluid
- Transcellular fluid (such as lymphatic fluid, synovial fluid and cerebrospinal fluid) – very small amount of extracellular fluid.

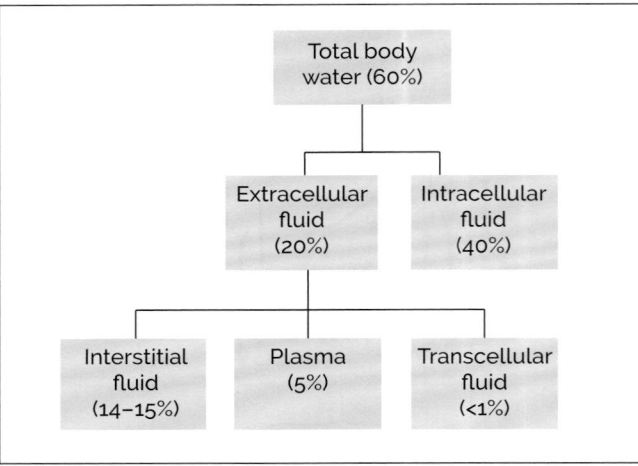

| 3.3 | Distribution of fluid in the body. Percentages are of bodyweight. |

The volume of fluid in the body is maintained within constant limits by controlling fluid intake and the amount excreted. The term 'homeostasis' describes the method used by the body to maintain parameters within narrow limits. Water content, body temperature and electrolyte balance are all maintained by homeostasis.

Fluid is taken into the body via food and water. Water is also produced from the breakdown of food products; this is an important source of water for many arid area-dwelling species. Fluid is lost from the body through normal physiological processes via the urinary tract, gastrointestinal tract, respiration and sweating. Water lost through the skin as sweat and from the respiratory tract is often termed insensible fluid loss.

Maintenance fluid requirements

Daily fluid loss in dogs and cats. These values can be used to determine maintenance fluid requirements.

Method of fluid loss	Volume of fluid lost
Urine	20 ml/kg/day
Faeces	10–20 ml/kg/day
Respiration and sweating (insensible losses)	20 ml/kg/day

→

Maintenance fluid requirements *continued*

Fluid requirements are influenced by both metabolic rate and physiological adaptations to the environment in which the animal lives. For example, reptiles often live in environments where water is scarce and have evolved to conserve water, with particular reference to the structure and function of the kidneys (see 'Kidneys' below).

Suggested maintenance fluid requirements are as follows:

- Dogs and cats: 50–60 ml/kg/day
- Rabbits and small mammals: 100 ml/kg/day
- Birds: 50 ml/kg/day
- Reptiles: 25 ml/kg/day.

It should be noted that metabolic scaling calculations are also often used to determine fluid maintenance requirements as these can take into account the age, size and species more accurately.

Electrolytes

Fluid in the body is not just made up of water; it consists of minerals dissolved in water (solution). Electrolytes are solutions containing free ions (such as sodium, potassium and chloride), which conduct electricity, and can have either a positive or a negative charge. Ions with a positive charge are known as cations; ions with a negative charge are known as anions (Figure 3.4). The number of electrolytes present determines the concentration of the solution (the higher the level of electrolytes, the greater the concentration).

Type of fluid	Cations (+)	Anions (−)
Intracellular	Potassium Magnesium Sodium	Phosphate Bicarbonate Chloride
Extracellular	Sodium Potassium Magnesium Calcium	Chloride Bicarbonate Phosphate

| 3.4 | Distribution of electrolytes in body fluid. |

Diffusion and osmosis

Electrolytes and water are not static but can move from one body compartment to another by diffusion, osmosis or active transport.

- Diffusion – a passive process whereby electrolytes pass from a solution of high electrolyte concentration to a solution of low electrolyte concentration (Figure 3.5).
- Osmosis – the passive movement of water molecules from a solution of low electrolyte concentration to a solution of high electrolyte concentration across a semi-permeable membrane (SPM) (Figure 3.5).
- Active transport – the movement of electrolytes against an osmotic gradient. Cells use energy to transport electrolytes across a cell membrane, enabling them to move from a solution of low concentration to a solution of high concentration.

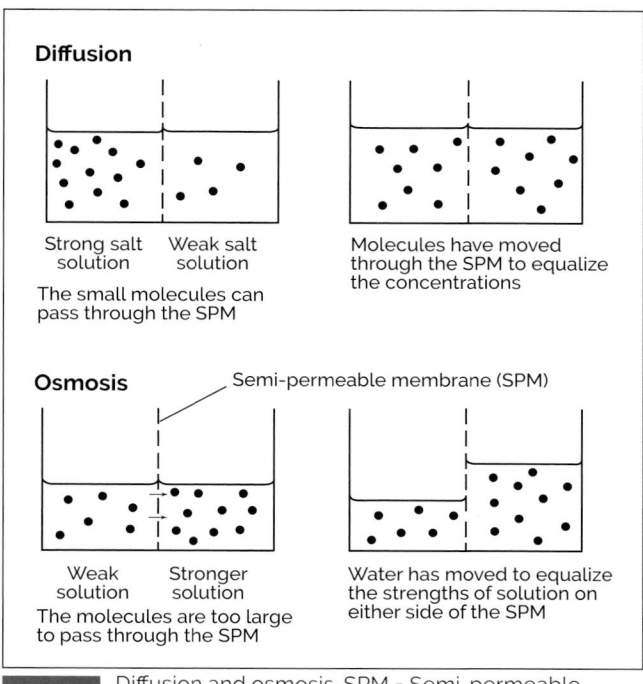

Diffusion

Strong salt solution | Weak salt solution

The small molecules can pass through the SPM

Molecules have moved through the SPM to equalize the concentrations

Osmosis

Semi-permeable membrane (SPM)

Weak solution | Stronger solution

The molecules are too large to pass through the SPM

Water has moved to equalize the strengths of solution on either side of the SPM

3.5 Diffusion and osmosis. SPM = Semi-permeable membrane.

In the body, different fluids can be separated by a semi-permeable membrane. This means that water, but not all electrolytes, can move passively across the membrane. If a solution has a high concentration of electrolytes, then it has a low concentration of water. Conversely, if a solution has a low concentration of electrolytes, then it has a high concentration of water. Water molecules move across a semi-permeable membrane from a solution of low electrolyte concentration, to a solution of high electrolyte concentration, until the solutions on either side of the semi-permeable membrane have the same equilibrated concentration. This process is called osmosis (Figure 3.5).

The pressure with which water molecules are drawn across the semi-permeable membrane is known as the osmotic pressure. Where fluids on either side of a semi-permeable membrane have the same osmotic pressure as plasma then they are called isotonic. Where a fluid has a higher osmotic pressure than plasma, it is described as hypertonic. Where a fluid has a lower osmotic pressure than plasma, it is referred to as hypotonic. A hypotonic fluid will lose water to a hypertonic fluid until both fluids are isotonic, assuming that the permeability of the membrane does not change.

Electrolytes also exert an osmotic force on water molecules, preventing them from moving. Thus, if there is a high concentration of electrolytes then less water will be able to leave the solution.

Acid–base balance

The terms acidity and alkalinity refer to the concentration of hydrogen ions present within a solution and are expressed as a pH.

- Where the pH is <7, the solution is termed acidic.
- Where the pH is >7, the solution is termed alkaline.
- Where the pH is 7, the solution is termed neutral.

In order for the body to function properly, it needs to be kept within a narrow pH range. The normal pH of blood is 7.4 (range: 7.35–7.45) and the body strives to maintain this level.

Maintaining blood pH

When animals are ill (e.g. with diarrhoea or vomiting), the blood pH changes due to a loss of hydrogen or bicarbonate ions. Loss of hydrogen ions as a result of acute (short term) vomiting episodes leads to metabolic alkalosis. Loss of bicarbonate ions from the gut as a result of severe diarrhoea often leads to metabolic acidosis (see Chapter 20). Therefore, the body has mechanisms in place to maintain a pH of 7.4, which involves alterations to the activity of the respiratory and urinary systems and buffers, specifically:

- Respiration – carbon dioxide forms carbonic acid (a weak acid) when dissolved in water. If the pH of blood falls (becomes more acidic), an increased respiratory rate will increase the excretion of carbon dioxide, thereby reducing the concentration of carbonic acid in the blood. This is why animals in metabolic acidosis have increased respiration rates
- Sodium and hydrogen ion exchange – in the distal convoluted tubules of the kidneys, hydrogen rather than sodium ions can be excreted into the urine to increase the pH of blood
- Buffers – these are substances that can maintain the pH in the presence of increased or decreased levels of hydrogen ions; they include bicarbonate.

Cell structure

All organs of the body are made up of cells. The basic structure is the same for all cells, but they have specialized structures or forms depending upon their location and function. The basic cell comprises the following structures (Figure 3.6):

- Cell membrane – the outer covering of the cell composed of phospholipid. The cell membrane is semi-permeable and controls entry and exit of materials/molecules

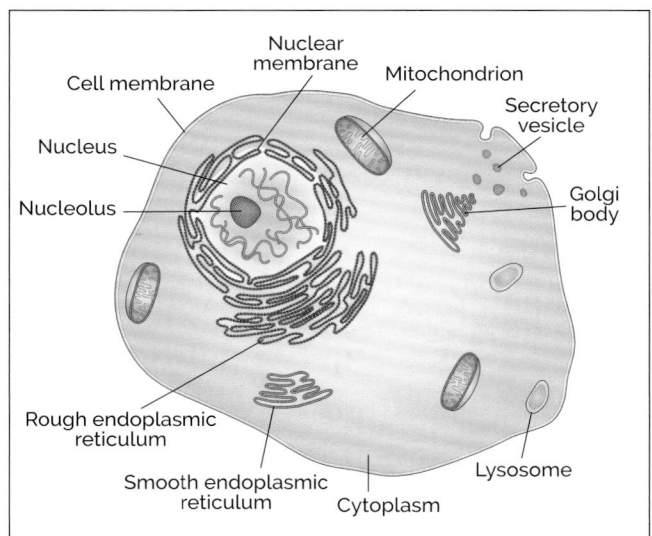

Cell membrane | Nucleus | Nucleolus | Nuclear membrane | Mitochondrion | Secretory vesicle | Golgi body | Rough endoplasmic reticulum | Smooth endoplasmic reticulum | Cytoplasm | Lysosome

3.6 The structure of the cell.

- Cytoplasm – the fluid within the cell, which contains the organelles
- Nucleus – the control centre of the cell. The nucleus contains DNA (deoxyribonucleic acid) in the form of chromosomes. The nucleolus forms part of the nucleus and contains RNA (ribonucleic acid). It is responsible for the manufacture of ribosomes.

Organelles

Organelles are smaller structures located within the cytoplasm of the cell and include:

- Centrosome – involved in cell replication and comprise two centrioles
- Mitochondria – produce energy for the cell by aerobic respiration
- Ribosomes – responsible for protein synthesis and are often attached to the rough endoplasmic reticulum
- Rough endoplasmic reticulum (RER) – synthesis and transport of proteins in conjunction with the attached ribosomes
- Smooth endoplasmic reticulum (SER) – synthesis and transport of lipids

- Golgi body/apparatus – consists of flattened membrane sacs. Involved in the production of lysosomes, secretory granules and plasma membrane. Responsible for the transport and modification of substances such as glycoproteins
- Lysosome – collection of digestive enzymes in membrane sacs. Forms part of the defence mechanism of the cell
- Vacuole – a membrane-bound organelle that can contain enzymes, foreign material or excretory compounds.

Cell division

Cells reproduce by a process of division. Two types of division can take place, mitosis and meiosis.

Mitosis (Figure 3.7) is the process by which most cells in the body divide: one parent cell divides into two identical daughter cells. The daughter cells have exactly the same number of chromosomes as the parent cell. There are five stages to mitosis:

- Interphase – cells are at rest and there is no division
- Prophase – chromosomes become apparent

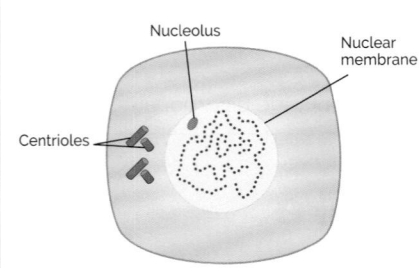

A Interphase
Cell has normal appearance of non-dividing cell condition: chromosomes too threadlike for clear visibility.

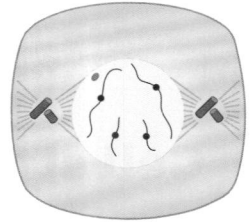

B Early prophase
Chromosomes become visible as they contract, and nucleolus shrinks. Centrioles at opposite sides of the nucleus. Spindle fibres start to form.

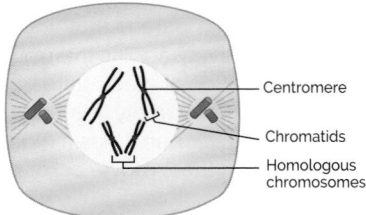

C Late prophase
Chromosomes become shorter and fatter – each seen to consist of a pair of chromatids joined at the centromere. Nucleolus disappears. Prophase ends with breakdown of nuclear membrane.

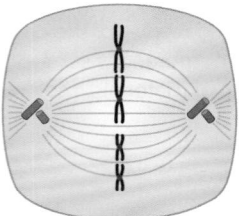

D Early metaphase
Chromosomes arrange themselves on equator of spindle. Note that homologous chromosomes do not associate.

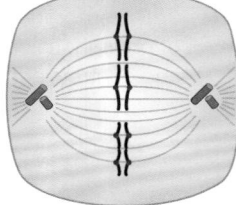

E Late metaphase
Chromatids draw apart at the centromere region. Note that the daughter centromeres are orientated toward opposite poles of the spindle.

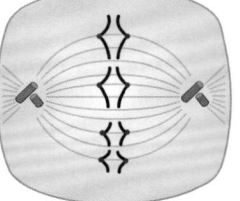

F Early anaphase
Spindle fibres contract and pull the chromatids apart, moving them to the opposite ends of the cell.

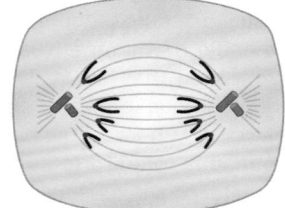

G Late anaphase
Chromosomes reach their destination.

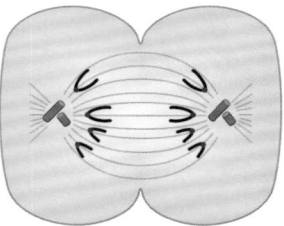

H Early telophase
The cell starts to constrict across the middle.

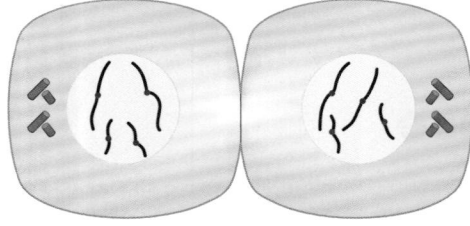

I Late telophase
Constriction continues. Nuclear membrane and nucleolus reformed in each daughter cell. Spindle apparatus degenerates. Chromosomes eventually regain their threadlike form and the cells return to resting condition (interphase).

Note that the daughter cells have precisely the same chromosome constitution as the original parent cell.

3.7 Cell reproduction: (mitosis). (Redrawn after M.B.V. Roberts (1986) *Biology: a functional approach, 4th edn*, Nelson)

- Metaphase – chromosomes line up along the middle of the cell
- Anaphase – chromatids separate
- Telophase – separation into two new cells.

Meiosis (see Chapter 4) is the process whereby one parent cell divides to produce four daughter cells. The daughter cells have half the number of chromosomes of the parent cell. This type of division takes place in the gonads (ovaries and testicles) to produce ova (eggs) or sperm.

Basic tissue types

Where similar cells are found in the one location, they are described as a tissue. The four types of tissue found in the body are:

- Epithelial – tissue that provides protection, absorption and secretion (e.g. squamous epithelium of the skin)
- Connective – tissue consisting of fibroblasts, fibres and a glycosaminoglycan matrix (e.g. bone and cartilage)
- Muscle – tissue that undergoes contraction and relaxation (e.g. skeletal, smooth and cardiac muscle)
- Nervous – tissue that receives and responds to stimuli from the environment and from within the body (e.g. brain, spinal cord, peripheral nerves).

Epithelial tissue

Epithelial tissue is found lining the outside of the animal (skin surface), the gastrointestinal tract, respiratory tract, reproductive tract and urinary tract, and lining the thoracic and abdominal cavities. The function of epithelial cells is to provide protection for underlying structures. Epithelial tissue can be classified depending on the appearance of the cells under a light microscope (Figure 3.8).

Connective tissue

Connective tissue can be fibrous or loose, depending on the specific cells and materials present. The basic structure of connective tissue comprises cells (fibroblasts, macrophages, mast cells, plasma cells, leucocytes), fibres (collagen, reticular fibres, elastic fibres) and a glycosaminoglycan matrix.

The main connective tissue types in the body are:

- Areolar (loose connective) tissue
- Dense connective tissue
- Reticular tissue
- Adipose (fat) tissue
- Cartilage
- Bone.

Muscle and nervous tissues

Muscle and nervous tissues form the basis of the muscular and nervous systems, respectively. These tissues and systems are discussed in greater detail later in this chapter.

Body cavities

Anatomically, the body in mammals can be divided into different compartments:

- Thorax
- Abdomen
- Pelvic cavity
- Mediastinum.

In birds and reptiles there is a single body cavity, called the coelom, as these species have no true diaphragm.

The body cavities are lined with connective tissue known as serosa. The lining of the cavity is known as parietal serosa; the lining of organs is known as visceral serosa.

Thoracic cavity

The thoracic cavity is the space bound by the ribcage and diaphragm; cranially it is bound by the thoracic inlet, caudally by the diaphragm, dorsally by the vertebrae, ventrally by the sternum and laterally by the ribs. The thoracic cavity is lined by a serous membrane known as the parietal pleura, and where it covers the surface of the lungs, it is known as pulmonary pleura (Figure 3.9). Between the lungs and the

Type of epithelium	Description/function
Simple squamous	Outer layer of cells. Composed of a single sheet of very thin, flat cells. The sheet of cells is thin and delicate, and is found in areas where diffusion occurs (e.g. alveoli of lungs, lining blood vessels, glomerular capsule)
Simple cuboidal	Cells have a square appearance. This type of epithelium is found lining many of the glands and their ducts, and also parts of the kidney tubules
Simple columnar	Cells are tall and rectangular. This type of epithelium is found lining the intestine, allowing the absorption of soluble food material
Ciliated	Cells are usually columnar in shape. Cilia or elongated structures, which can move, are present on the free surface of the cells. This type of epithelium lines tubes and cavities where materials must be moved (e.g. respiratory tract, oviducts)
Stratified	Layers of cells make it tough. It has a protective function. It is found in areas that are subjected to friction (e.g. oesophagus, mouth, vagina). In areas where it is subject to considerable abrasion, the cells are infiltrated with a tough protein called keratin, as seen in the epidermis of the skin
Transitional	Layers of cells which can stretch. A modified form of stratified epithelium. Found in structures that must be able to stretch (e.g. bladder, urethra)
Glandular	This type of epithelium has interspersed secretory cells, which secrete mucus/materials into the cavity or space they are lining. Folding of glandular epithelium results in the formation of a gland

3.8 Classification of epithelial tissue.

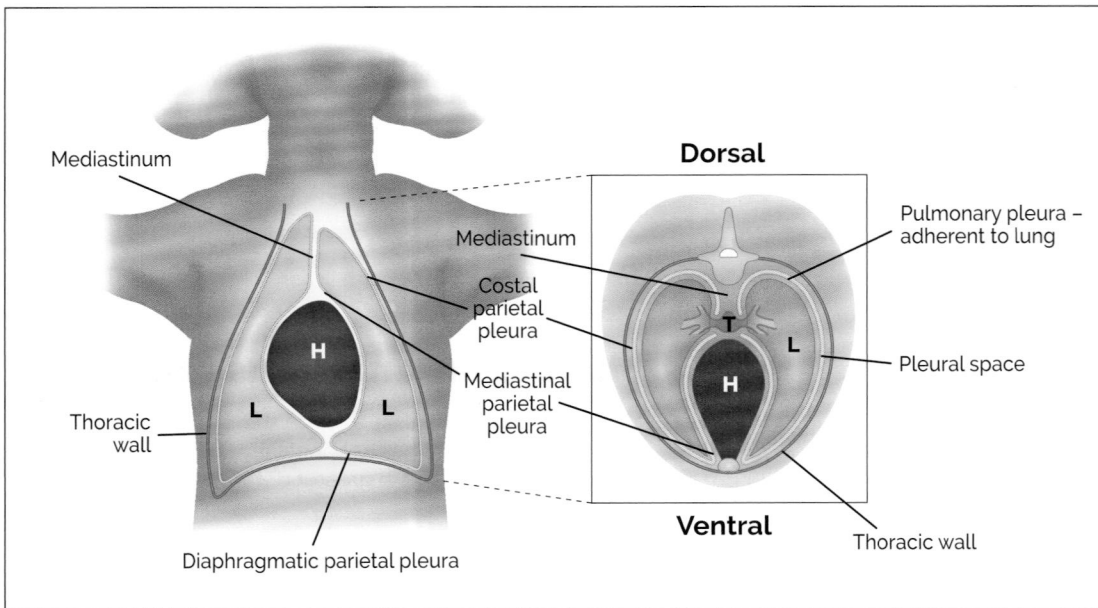

3.9 Thoracic cavity and serous membranes. **H** = heart; **L** = lungs; **T** = trachea. Inset: transverse cross section. (Reproduced from the *BSAVA Manual of Canine and Feline Thoracic Imaging*)

parietal pleura is the pleural space, which has a negative pressure in relation to atmospheric pressure. It is this negative pressure that keeps the lungs inflated. In addition, there is a very small amount of fluid in the pleural space, known as pleural fluid, which enables the lungs to move freely within the ribcage during inspiration and expiration.

Abdominal cavity

The abdominal cavity is defined cranially by the diaphragm, caudally by the pelvic opening, dorsally by the vertebrae and ventrally/laterally by the abdominal muscles. The organs within the abdomen are lined by a serous membrane known as the peritoneum. This membrane comprises a single layer of cells, which produce a very small amount of peritoneal fluid, to allow free movement of the organ surfaces against one another.

The part of the peritoneum that covers the abdominal organs is known as the visceral peritoneum; the parietal peritoneum covers the abdominal wall. The folds of peritoneum, which connect the parietal to the visceral part and suspend the small intestine, are known as the mesentery. Along the greater and lesser curvatures of the stomach, the serosa is continuous with a very thin connective tissue known as the omentum. The omentum has a lacy appearance due to the fat found therein.

Pelvic cavity

The pelvic cavity is not physically separated from the abdomen and therefore is purely an anatomical term rather than a truly separate cavity. Cranially the pelvic cavity is defined by the pelvic inlet, caudally by the pelvic outlet, dorsally by the pelvic bones and laterally by the muscles around the pelvic girdle.

Mediastinum

The mediastinum is the space in the anterior chest between the lungs, which contains the thymus, heart, aorta, trachea, oesophagus and various nerves and blood vessels.

Coelom

In mammals, the diaphragm separates the thorax from the abdomen. However, birds and reptiles do not possess a true diaphragm and therefore the terms thorax and abdomen cannot be accurately used when describing these species. The one cavity is instead known as the coelom or coelomic cavity.

Skeletal system

The skeleton has a number of different functions:

- To act as a framework for other structures to attach to
- To enable movement
- To protect softer tissues and organs within the body
- To play a part in haemopoiesis (production of blood cells)
- To store minerals such as calcium and phosphorus.

Bone

Structure

Bone is a living organ, which undergoes change throughout the life of the animal. It consists of cells, collagen and glycoproteins. The main mineral in bone is calcium hydroxyapatite, thus bone is a reservoir of calcium for the body. The principal cells found in bone are:

- Osteoblasts – immature cells that can synthesize osteoid (the bone matrix)
- Osteocytes – mature cells that maintain bone structure
- Osteoclasts – cells that can break down and remodel bone.

There are two main forms of bone: compact and cancellous.

Compact bone

This is found in areas that are prone to stress, such as the outer surfaces (cortices) of bones. It has a dense and regular structure almost entirely made of mineralized matrix. Compact bone comprises concentric circles of matrix called lamellae, which are arranged around a central canal (Haversian canal) that contains blood vessels, nerves and loose connective tissue (Figure 3.10). Gaps in the matrix are called lacunae and contain osteocytes. The whole system is known as the Haversian system or osteon.

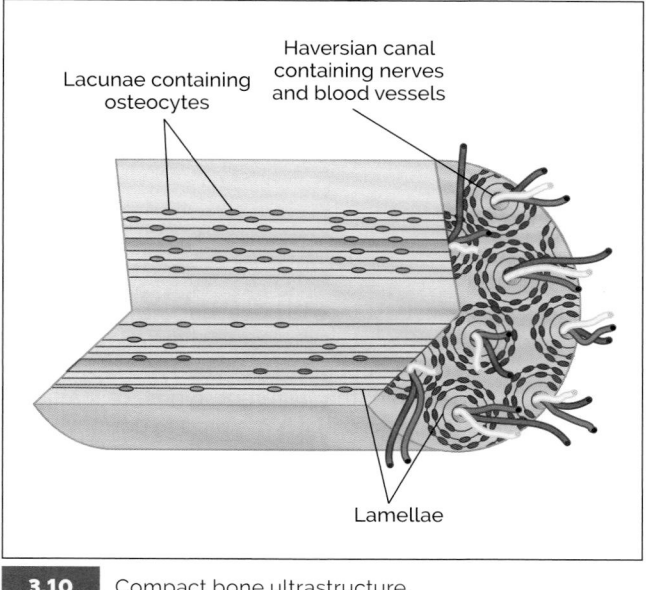

3.10 Compact bone ultrastructure.

Cancellous bone

This is more commonly found in vertebrae, flat bones and at the ends of long bones. Cancellous bone (also known as spongy bone) comprises trabeculae (interconnected 'bars' of bone) with spaces in between. This means that cancellous bone is not as strong as compact bone.

Types

- Long bones (such as the femur and humerus) consist of an outer cortex of bone and a central medullary cavity, which contains bone marrow. The outer part of the bone is covered in a connective tissue layer known as the periosteum. The blood supply to the bone enters at the periosteum and then branches to supply the bone tissue. Long bones have a central shaft known as the diaphysis and at each end an epiphysis (Figure 3.11). The area between the diaphysis and the epiphysis, which contains the epiphyseal growth plate, is known as the metaphysis and is an area of transition important in bone growth (see below).
- Short bones (such as the carpus) only have one section and develop from one centre of ossification. Sesamoid bones are a type of short bone.
- Flat bones (such as the bones of the skull) stretch out in two directions as they grow.
- Irregular bones do not fit easily into the other categories, as they are variable in shape. The bones of the pelvis and spine are in this category.
- Pneumatic bones are found in birds. The medullary cavity is largely replaced by air and is connected to the air sacs. The function is to make the skeleton lighter as an adaption to flight.

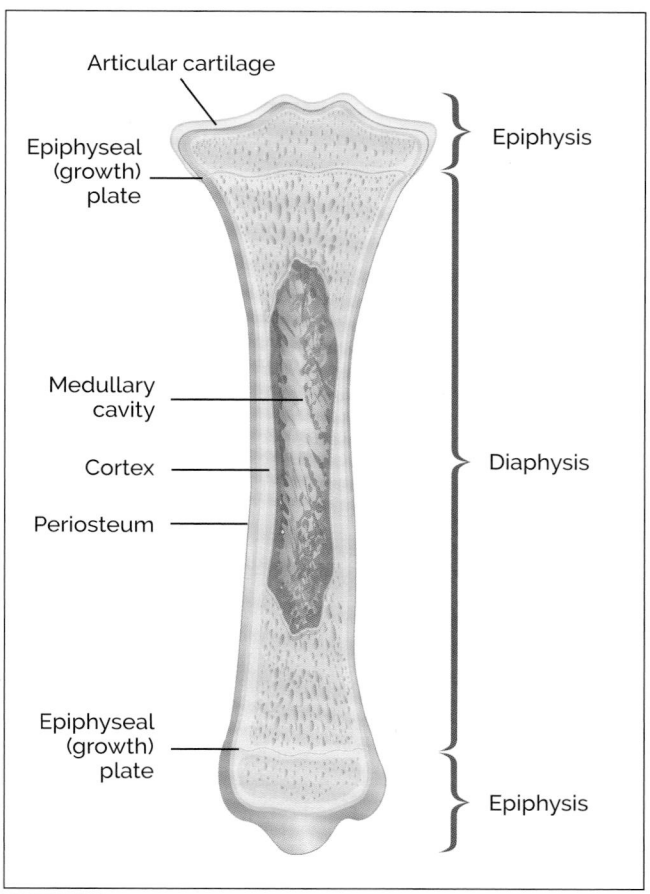

3.11 Structure of long bone.

Growth and development

In the very young animal the skeleton is predominantly cartilage. As the animal grows the amount of bone present increases as the cartilage is converted to bone. Bone development can take place by:

- Intramembranous ossification
- Endochondral ossification.

Intramembranous ossification

This is where bone is laid down to replace fibrous connective tissue. This occurs in the development of the bones of the skull, maxilla and mandible.

Endochondral ossification

This is where the initial hyaline cartilage is gradually replaced by osteocytes and calcium hydroxyapatite. This occurs in the long bones, vertebrae and pelvis in the following way:

1. The outline structure of the bone is formed first of cartilage.
2. Osteoblasts replace cartilage with bone:
   a. Primary ossification centres appear in the diaphysis of bones
   b. Secondary ossification centres appear at the ends (epiphyses) of bones (Figure 3.12).
3. The primary ossification centre in the diaphysis and the secondary centre in the epiphysis meet at a thick band of cartilage, known as the epiphyseal growth plate. The epiphyseal growth plate can be seen as a radiolucent 'gap' in the bone on radiographs of juvenile

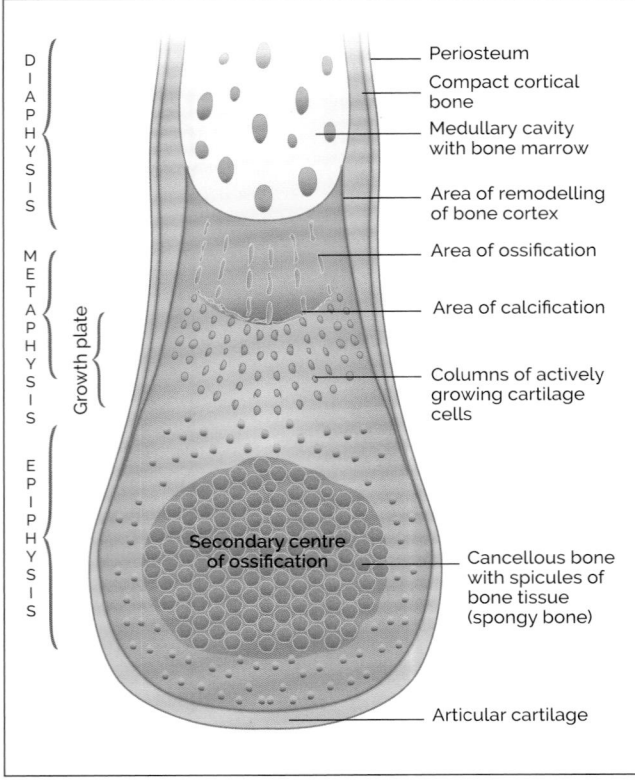

3.12 Endochondral ossification of a long bone.

animals. This is an area of weakness and can be easily damaged through trauma.

4. The epiphyseal growth plate produces new cartilage cells on the epiphysis side of the plate, thus elongating the bone at either end.
5. The cartilage cells on the side of the epiphyseal growth plate nearest the diaphysis are steadily converted to bone as they are ossified by osteoblasts.
6. Osteoclasts remodel the interior of the diaphysis and create the medullary cavity.
7. Once the bone has reached its final length, the cartilage cells stop dividing and all cartilage is ossified, thereby 'closing' the growth plate.

Physiology

Bones are living tissue and are constantly remodelling. They act as a source of calcium that can be added to, or utilized as the body needs (e.g. during lactation or egg laying in birds and reptiles). Parathyroid hormone and calcitonin control the amount of calcium present in bone (with help from calcitriol, the active form of the accessory hormone vitamin D3; see also 'Endocrine system', later).

Parathyroid hormone (PTH)

This is released by cells within the parathyroid gland and increases the activity of osteoclasts to break down bone and release calcium into the circulation. PTH inhibits the activity of osteoblasts, thus reducing calcium deposition in bone. PTH also increases the rate of excretion of inorganic phosphate by the kidneys, resulting in a drop in serum phosphate, leading to an increase in the release of both calcium and phosphate from bone. PTH works alongside and stimulates the production of calcitriol (1,25-dihydroxycholecalciferol) from the kidney.

Vitamin D3 and calcitriol

Vitamin D3 (hydroxycholecalciferol) is the inactive precursor of calcitriol (1,25-dehydroxycholecalciferol). Calcitriol promotes intestinal absorption of calcium, increases renal tubular resorption of calcium and stimulates osteoclast activity.

Calcitonin

This has the opposite effect to PTH and calcitriol. It decreases the activity of osteoclasts, thereby reducing the amount of calcium released from bone. It also increases the activity of osteoblasts, resulting in calcium deposition in bone. Calcitonin inhibits calcium absorption from the intestine.

Cartilage

Structure

Cartilage is a similar substance to bone, but without mineralization, and so is softer. It is predominantly composed of collagen produced by chrondrocytes. The type of collagen present varies between the different types of cartilage according to the functions that it is required to perform.

Types

The three different types of cartilage found in the body are:

- Hyaline cartilage
- Fibrocartilage
- Elastic cartilage.

Hyaline cartilage

This is the most common form of cartilage. It is bluish white in appearance and is found between the epiphysis and diaphysis of growing long bones, at the articular surfaces of moveable joints, the walls of the respiratory tract (from the nose to the bronchi) and at the ventral ends of the ribs.

Fibrocartilage

This has a structure somewhere between that of hyaline cartilage and dense connective tissue. It is found in intervertebral discs, the pubic symphysis and at the attachment points of ligaments and tendons. It is very strong in tension.

Elastic cartilage

This contains elastic fibres, which allow the cartilage to bend more than hyaline cartilage. It is found in the auricle of the ear, the external auditory canal, the Eustachian tube and epiglottis.

Skeleton

The skeleton in most vertebrate species is organized into three main portions:

- The axial skeleton consists of the skull, spine and pelvis
- The appendicular skeleton comprises the limbs, which attach to the axial skeleton
- The splanchnic skeleton is composed of those bones not attached to the appendicular or axial skeleton such as the os penis in the dog and cat.

The basic skeleton of the dog is shown in Figure 3.13, and of a bird in Figure 3.14.

Skull
Atlas
Axis
Cervical vertebrae (7)
Thoracic vertebrae (13)
Lumbar vertebrae (7)
Sacral vertebrae (3) or sacrum
11th anticlinal
Ilium
Ischium
Mandible
Hyoid
Scapula
Coccygeal vertebrae (variable in number)
Ribs (13)
Pubis
Humerus
Fabella
Femur
Costal arch
Sternum
Patella
Radius
Ulna
Tibia
Fibula
Carpus
Tarsus
Metacarpus
Metatarsus
Os penis
Proximal
Middle
Distal
Phalanx
Proximal
Middle
Distal
Phalanx

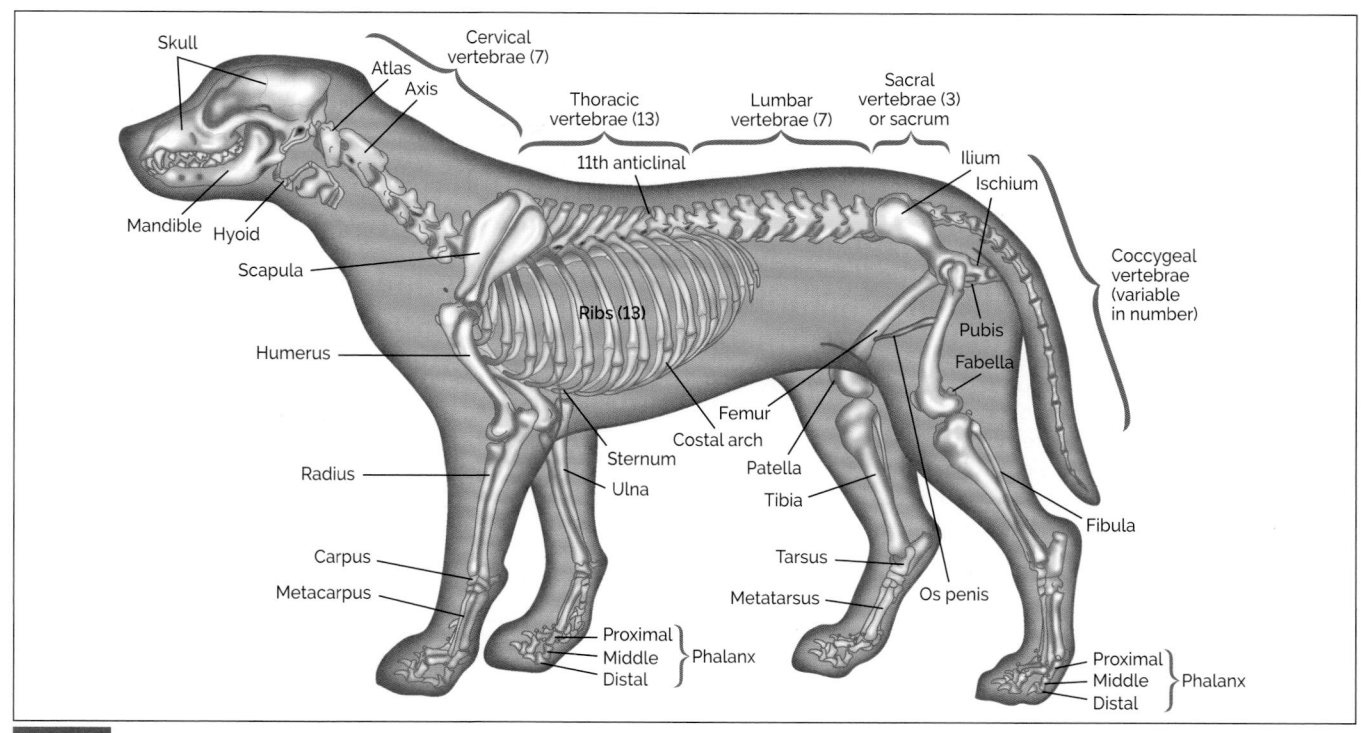

3.13 Skeleton of the dog.

Major digit
Minor digit
Carpometacarpus
Major metacarpal
Minor metacarpal
Alular digit
Radial carpal bone
Scleral ossicles
Craniofacial hinge
Ulnar carpal bone
Quadrate bone
Radius
Ulna
Pectoral crest
Elbow
Humerus
Mandibular ramus
Jugal bone
Palatine bone
Notarium
Cervical vertebrae
Glenoid cavity
Coracoid
Vertebral rib
Scapula
Uncinate process
Preacetabular ilium
Sternal rib
Femur
Carina
Trochanter
Patella
Antitrochanter
Femorotibial joint (knee)
Postacetabular ilium
Synsacrum
Sternum
Ilioischiadic foramen
Fibula
Ischium
Medial fenestra
Pygostyle
Tibiotarsus
Pubis
Intertarsal joint
Hypotarsus
P1
P2
Tarsometatarsus
P3
Digit IV
P4
Digit III

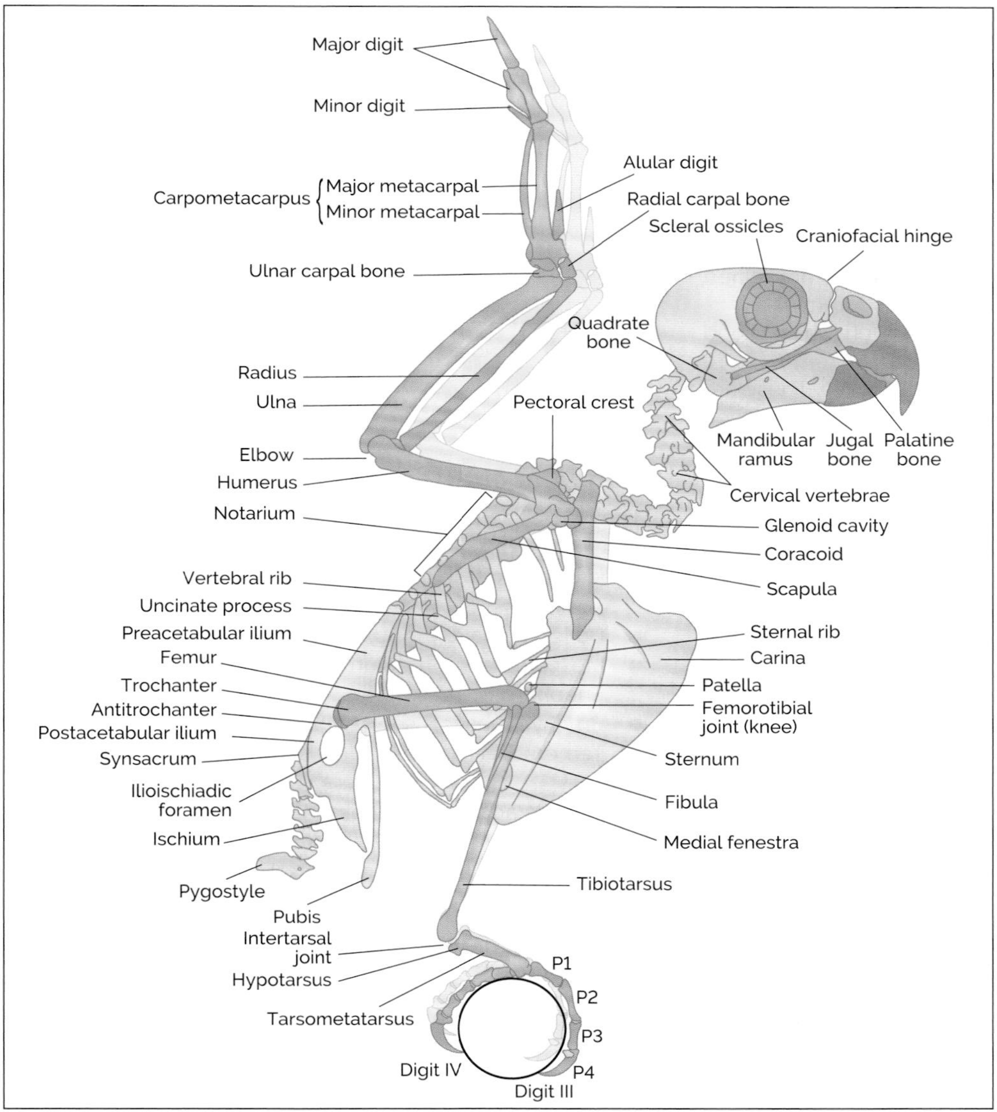

3.14 Skeleton of a psittacine bird. (Redrawn after Nigel Harcourt-Brown)

Terminology

Before examining the skeleton, it is useful to be aware of the terminology used to describe bones:

- Condyle – a rounded protuberance at the end of a bone
- Crest – a raised area of bone
- Foramen – a hole or opening within a bone
- Fossa – a depression within a bone where another structure is found
- Groove – a depression in a bone
- Medullary cavity – the centre of long bones, often where bone marrow is found
- Periosteum – the outer covering of bones
- Process – a thin, elongated projection
- Sinus – a narrow, hollow cavity
- Spine – the central part of a bone
- Trochanter – a prominent area of the femur that lies behind the head of the femur
- Tubercle – a small elevation on the surface of a bone
- Tuberosity – the area of the tubercle where tendons attach.

Axial skeleton

The axial skeleton is made up of the skull, vertebral column, ribs and sternum.

Skull

The skull consists of: an upper section called the cranium, which houses the brain; the maxilla (the upper jaw and nasal chambers); the mandible (the lower jaw); and the hyoid apparatus. These areas, particularly the cranium, are made up of many different bones (Figure 3.15), which are joined together by 'sutures'. Small holes known as foramina (singular: foramen) are present in the skull through which blood vessels and nerves pass.

Within the maxilla of the skull are the sinuses. These are hollow spaces that lighten the skull and provide resonance to the vocal chords. The sinuses are also attached to the upper respiratory tract and provide an area where air can be warmed and moistened.

Area of the skull	Composite parts
Cranium	Foramen magnum Frontal Occipital Orbit Parietal Sphenoid Temporal Tympanic bulla Zygomatic arch
Maxilla (upper jaw and nasal chambers)	Incisive Nasal Palatine
Mandible (lower jaw)	Alveoli (areas of tooth attachment) Condylar process Coronoid process Horizontal ramus Mandibular symphysis Vertical ramus

3.15 Parts of the skull.

The mandible consists of two halves, which are held together by connective tissue in the midline rostrally at the mandibular symphysis. Each mandible consists of a body (horizontal part) and a ramus (vertical part), which forms part of the hinge joint of the jaw.

The hyoid apparatus (Figure 3.16) comprises a series of small bones, which together suspend the tongue and larynx from the skull.

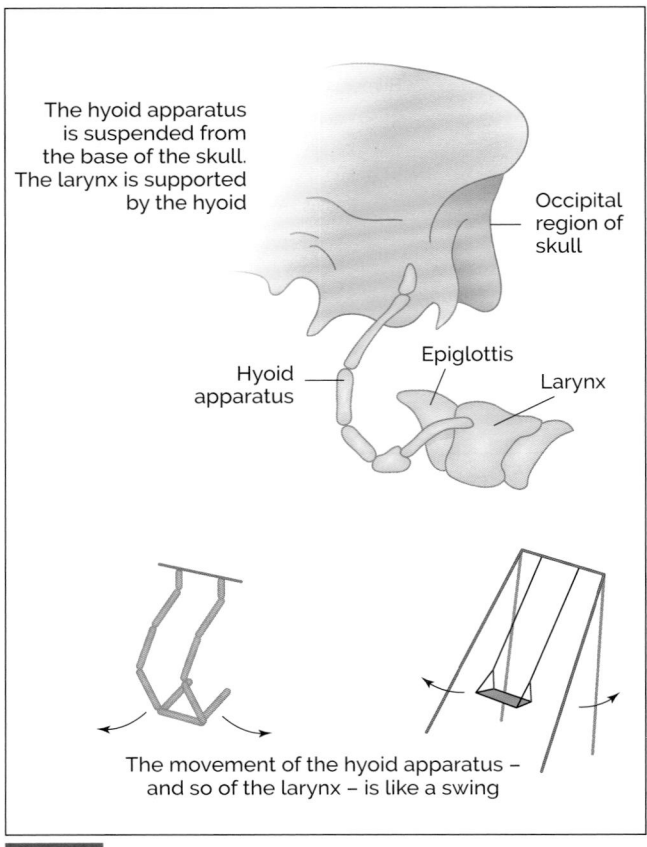

The hyoid apparatus is suspended from the base of the skull. The larynx is supported by the hyoid

Occipital region of skull

Hyoid apparatus

Epiglottis

Larynx

The movement of the hyoid apparatus – and so of the larynx – is like a swing

3.16 Hyoid apparatus.

Dogs and cats

The normal skull of the dog and cat is shown in Figures 3.17 and 3.18, respectively. In dogs, the wide range of breeds have three basic skull shapes:

- Dolicocephalic – long, narrow head (collies, Wolfhounds)
- Mesocephalic – medium-sized head ('normal'; German Shepherd Dogs, setters)
- Brachycephalic – short, wide head (Staffordshire Bull Terriers, Pekingese).

In dogs and cats (and other carnivores) the orbit is not a complete bony circle to allow attachment of the temporal muscle. The orbit is completed by a ligament, which connects the zygomatic process of the frontal bone to the zygomatic arch.

The main sinuses in dogs and cats are the frontal sinus and the maxillary sinus. The frontal sinus is found under the frontal bone and is divided into lateral, medial and rostral parts. The maxillary sinus is a large lateral diverticulum of the nasal cavity (located beneath the nasal and maxillary bones).

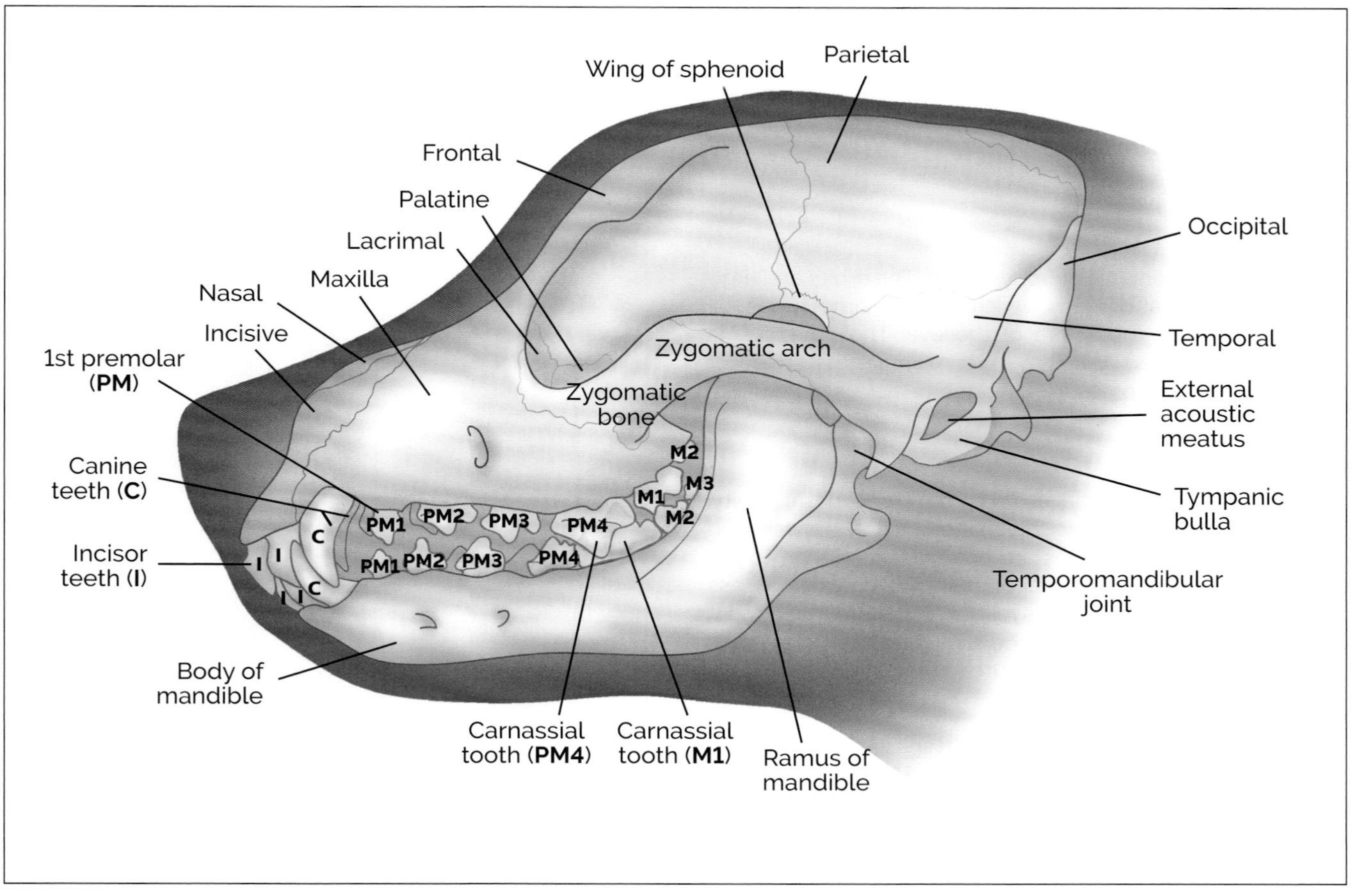

3.17 Lateral view of a dog skull showing tooth position.

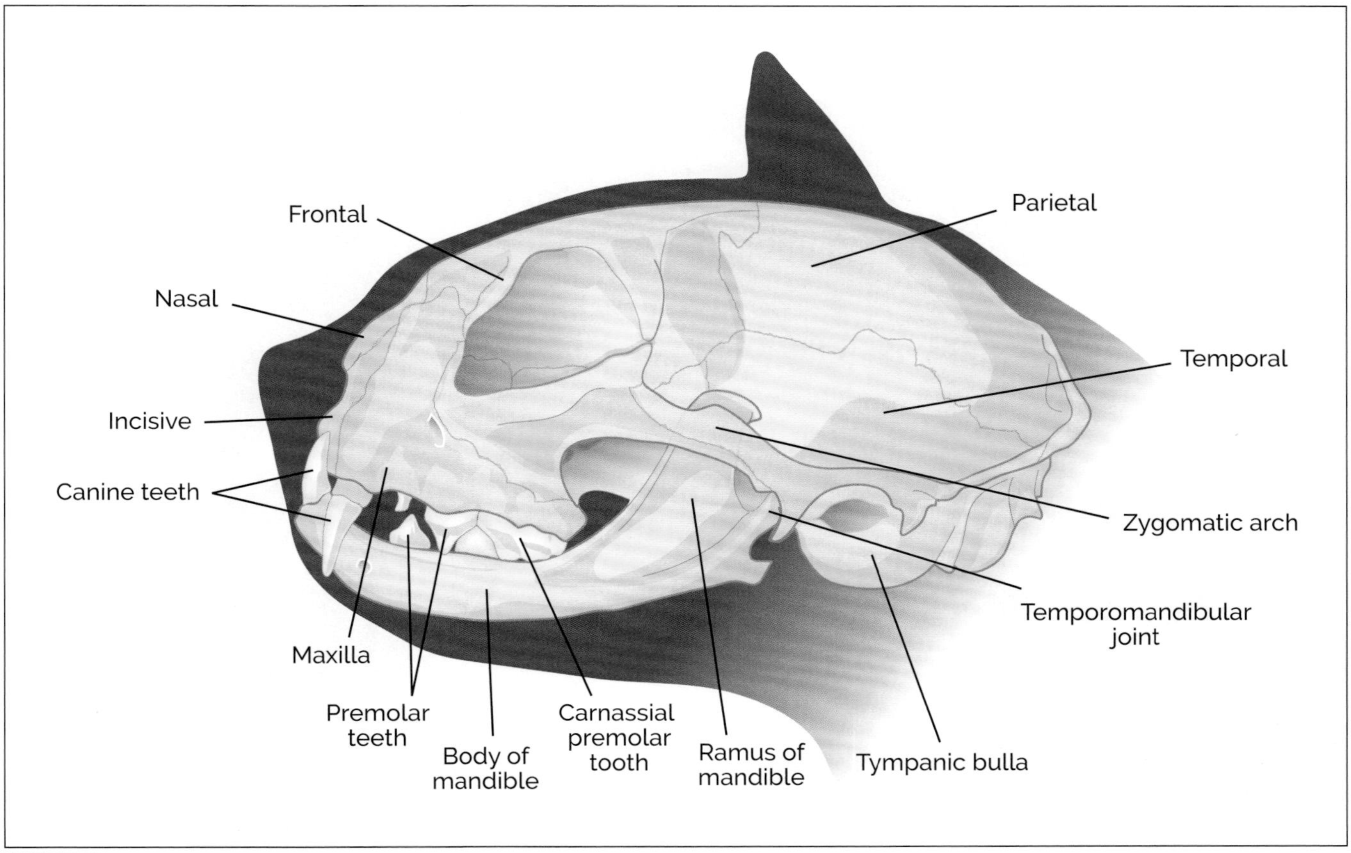

3.18 Lateral view of a cat skull showing tooth position.

Small mammals

In herbivores, the orbit is surrounded by a bony circle. In rabbits, the eyes are lateral giving an almost 360-degree view (Figure 3.19). The mandible is narrower than the maxilla, allowing lateral movement of the lower jaw to grind food. The chinchilla has well developed tympanic bullae, which may be observed on radiography.

Birds

The skull is light, only 1% of bodyweight. The orbits are large and contain scleral ossicles, which, as the name suggests, are embedded in the sclera of the eye. Their purpose is not fully understood, but they may maintain the shape of the eye, withstand pressure changes or act as a point for muscle attachment.

Reptiles

Snakes have a small cranial cavity but large nasal cavity. In order to eat large prey, the mandibular symphysis can separate and the mandibles are not fixed in relation to the skull. Instead of a temporomandibular joint, snakes possess a quadrate bone, which allows rostral and lateral movement of the mandible in relation to the skull. The skull of reptiles is more rigid and similar in structure to that of mammals.

Dentition

The teeth are embedded in the maxilla and mandible of mammals. The basic tooth structure is that of an upper crown above the level of the gum and a lower root, held in a socket or alveolus. The outer part of the crown is made of enamel, whilst the outer part of the root is made of cementum. The inner part of the tooth is made of dentine and in the centre of the tooth is the pulp cavity, which contains blood vessels, lymphatics and nerves (Figures 3.20 and 3.21). Teeth differ in shape, depending on their location within the mouth and their function (Figure 3.22; see Chapter 25).

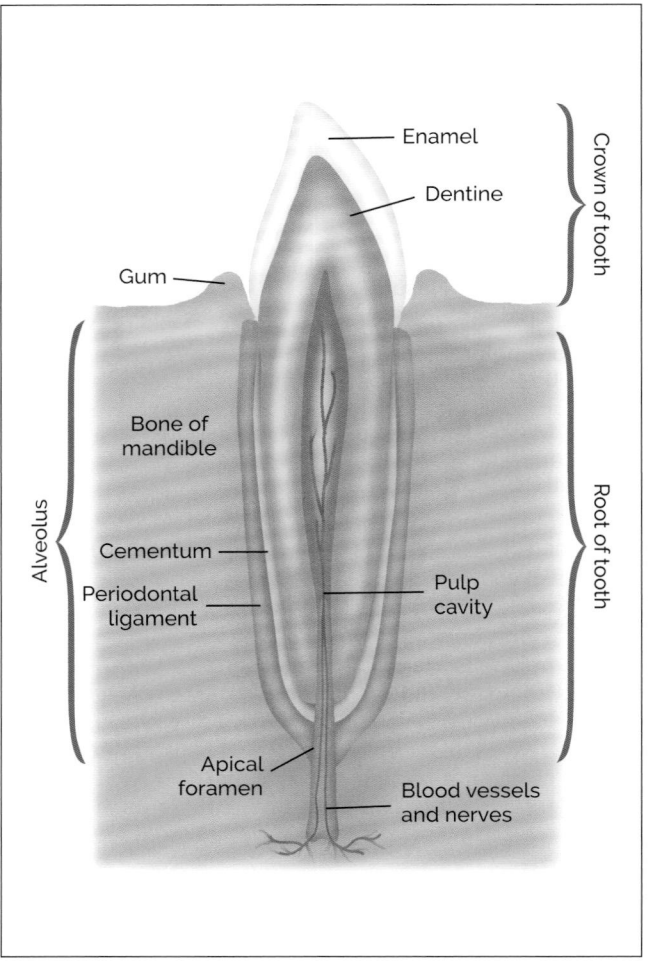

3.20 The structure of an incisor.

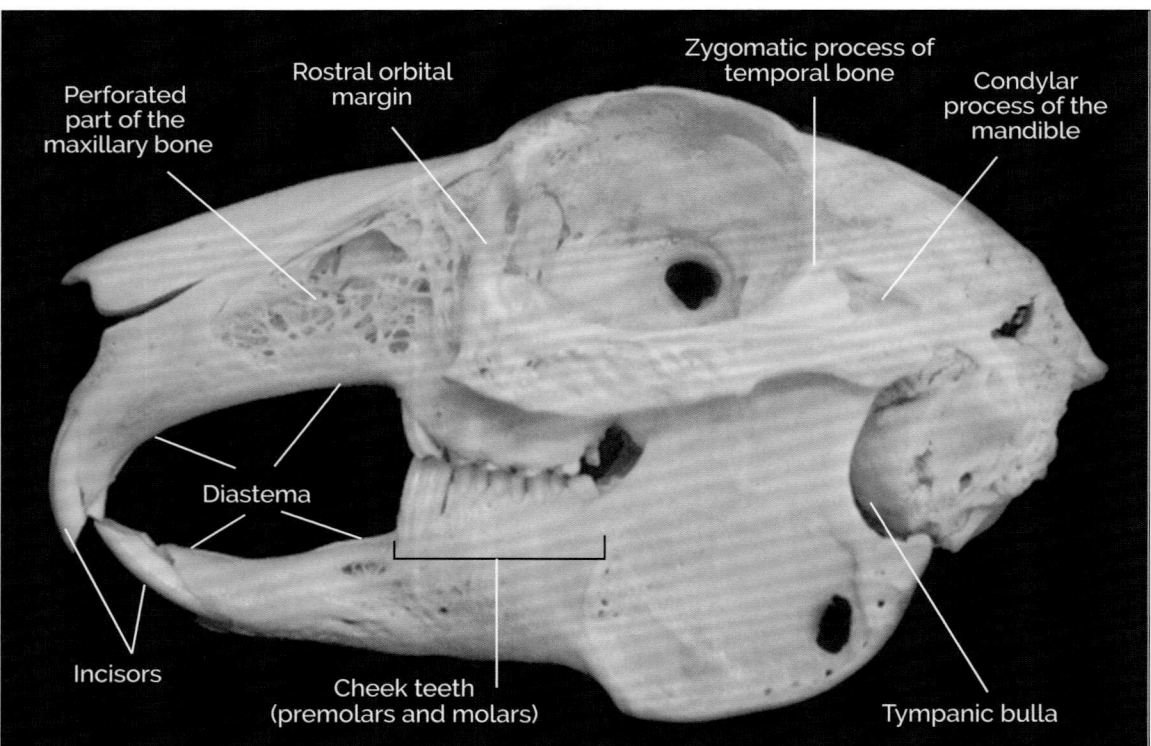

3.19 Rabbit skull. (Courtesy of Frances Harcourt-Brown and reproduced from the *BSAVA Manual of Rabbit Surgery, Dentistry and Imaging*)

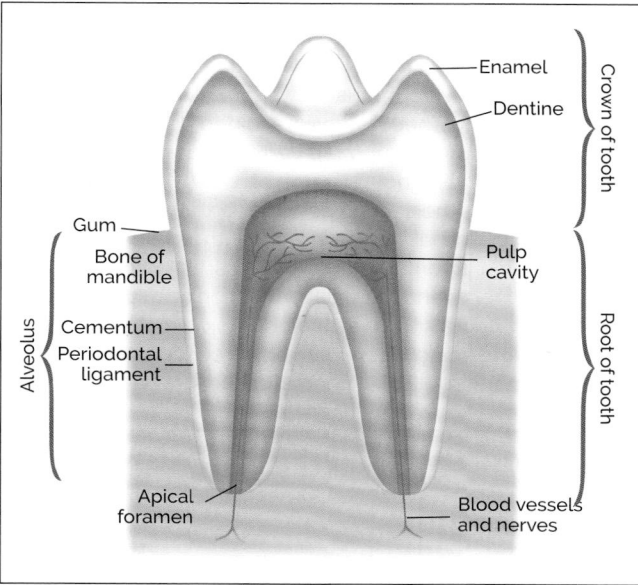

3.21	The structure of a molar.

Tooth	Function
Incisor	Nibbling of food, grooming
Canine	Piercing of food (e.g. for holding on to prey items)
Premolar	Shearing of food
Molar	Shearing and grinding of food (these teeth are flatter than premolars)

3.22	Functions of teeth.

Most mammals produce two sets of teeth. The first set of teeth, which are seen in the young animal and are known as deciduous or milk teeth, are shed before adulthood. Larger and more robust teeth, known as secondary teeth, replace the deciduous teeth.

Dogs

The dental formula for dogs is as follows:

Deciduous dentition

2x $\underline{\text{i3 c1 pm3}}$ = 28 teeth
     i3 c1 pm3

Secondary dentition (see Figure 3.17)

2x $\underline{\text{I3 C1 PM4 M2}}$ = 42 teeth
     I3 C1 PM4 M3

Where: C = canine; I = incisor; M = molar; PM = premolar. Lower case letters signify deciduous teeth (see Chapter 25 for further information).

Cats

The dental formula for cats is as follows:

Deciduous dentition

2x $\underline{\text{i3 c1 pm3}}$ = 26 teeth
     i3 c1 pm2

Secondary dentition (see Figure 3.18)

2x $\underline{\text{I3 C1 PM3 M1}}$ = 30 teeth
     I3 C1 PM2 M1

Small mammals

The dental formulae of various small mammals are as follows:

Ferrets – deciduous dentition

2x $\underline{\text{i1 c1 pm3}}$ = 18 teeth
        c1 pm3

Ferrets – secondary dentition

2x $\underline{\text{I3 C1 PM3 M1}}$ = 34 teeth
     I3 C1 PM3 M2

Rabbits – secondary dentition (see Figure 3.19)

2x $\underline{\text{I2 PM3 M3}}$ = 28 teeth
     I1 PM2 M3

Myomorph rodents (rats, hamsters, gerbils, mice) – secondary dentition

2x $\underline{\text{I1 M3}}$ = 16 teeth
     I1 M3

Hystricomorph rodents (chinchillas, guinea pigs, degus) – secondary dentition

2x $\underline{\text{I1 PM1 M3}}$ = 20 teeth
     I1 PM1 M3

In rabbits and rodents, deciduous teeth are often shed *in utero* and so these dental formulae are not listed. The roots of the cheek teeth (i.e. premolars and molars) in rabbits and rodents of the Hystricomorpha suborder (e.g. chinchillas and guinea pigs) grow continuously throughout life, with the teeth worn down by abrasive food material and the lateral movement of teeth grinding food. This is often referred to as open-rooted or elodent in nature. The way in which the teeth interlock and the uneven occlusal surfaces (lophs) enhances this abrasion. Myomorphs (rats, mice, gerbils and hamsters) also have incisors that grow continuously throughout life. Incisors are usually pigmented and have a chisel shape due to the lack of enamel on the lingual side. In rabbits and all rodents, the incisor teeth continuously erupt throughout life.

Rabbits and rodents do not have any canine teeth; instead, there is a space known as the diastema (see Figure 3.19).

Birds

The avian skull has a beak (rather than teeth held within a jaw). The beak varies between species, depending upon the type of food the bird eats. Adaptations include the powerful crushing beak of the parrot family (Psittaciformes) for cracking seeds and nuts. There is a kinetic hinge joint at the connection between the maxillary beak and the skull, which allows Psittaciformes to generate such power. Other avian adaptions include the hooked ripping beak of the raptors for tearing flesh, and the slender long beak of many wading birds used for probing soft mud for worms and crustaceans.

Reptiles

Chelonians (such as the spur-thighed tortoise and red-eared terrapin) possess a beak similar to that seen in birds, which forms a shearing surface for biting vegetation or flesh. Lizards possess fine simple peg-like teeth in four rows (two in the maxilla and two in the mandible). Depending upon the species, these teeth may be shed and replaced throughout life (e.g. iguanids with pleurodont dentition) or the lizard may have just one set of teeth for the whole of its life (e.g. agamids and chameleons with acrodont dentition). Some species have grooves in their teeth and venom glands (e.g. Gila monster).

Snakes possess fine simple curved teeth in six rows (average: four rows in the maxilla and two rows in the mandible). Some of the teeth in some species are adapted into fangs with venom glands. The teeth are often shed and regrow during the course of the snake's life. The teeth point caudally to encourage swallowing of prey.

Vertebral column

The vertebral column comprises a variety of different vertebrae: cervical, thoracic, lumbar, sacral and coccygeal. The basic structure of a vertebra consists of a body, transverse processes, a spinous process and a vertebral foramen (Figure 3.23). However, there are regional differences in the shape of the vertebrae (Figure 3.24).

- The first two cervical vertebrae are the atlas and axis:
  - The atlas is the first cervical vertebra and allows the head to nod. It articulates with the occipital condyles of the skull. It comprises two lateral wings with little or no body. These wings are joined dorsally and ventrally to surround the vertebral canal with a dorsal and ventral arch
  - The axis is the second cervical vertebra and allows a rotating or shaking movement of the head. It has a prominent dorsal spinous process. It also possesses a prominent ventral cranial projection from the body of the vertebra known as the odontoid process or 'dens'
  - The remaining 5 cervical vertebrae (dogs and cats) are more box-like in character.

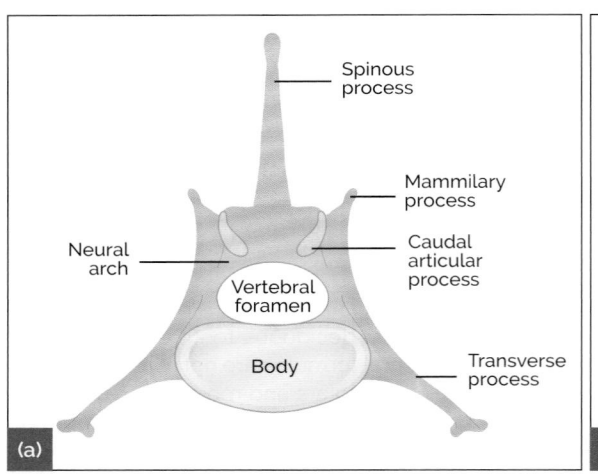
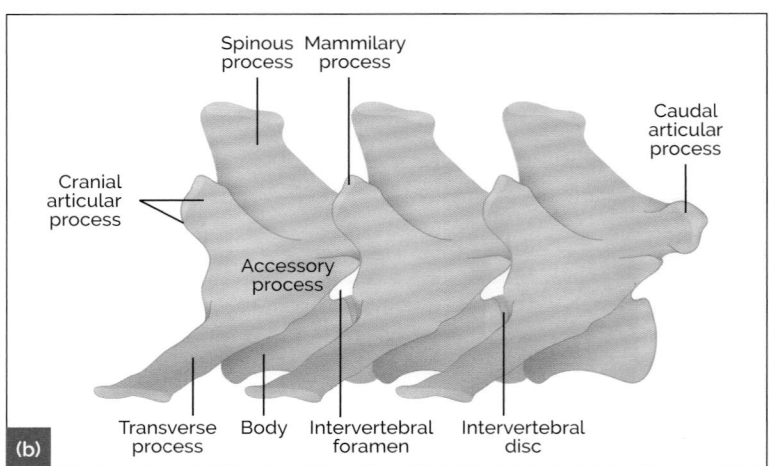

3.23 **(a)** Basic lumbar vertebra. **(b)** Part of the vertebral column showing three lumbar vertebrae (left lateral view).

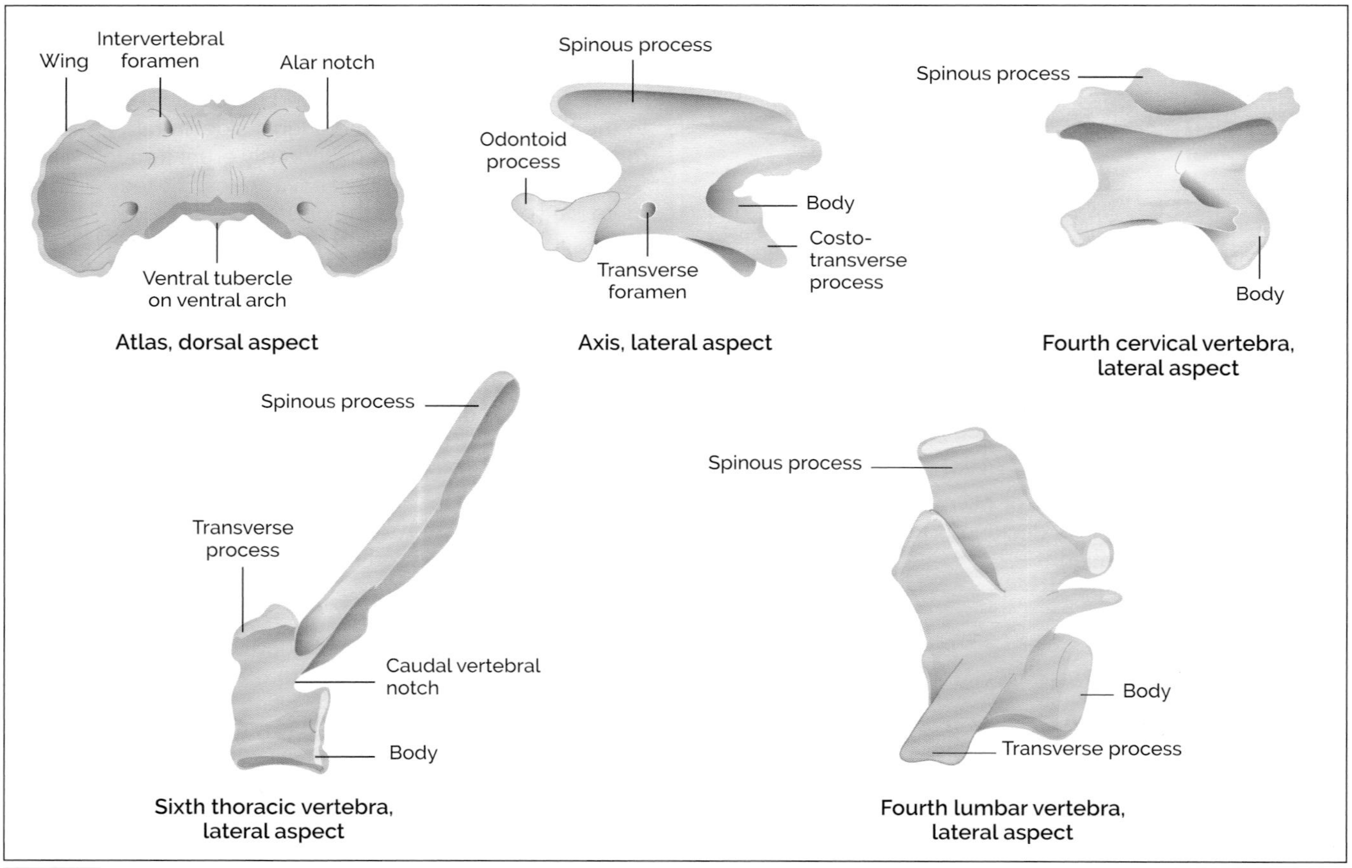

3.24 Regional differences in the vertebrae.

- The 13 thoracic vertebrae (dogs and cats) have a tall spinous process and very short transverse processes.
- The 7 lumbar vertebrae (dogs and cats) have a short spinous process but enlarged transverse processes. This allows the lumbar muscles to attach to the vertebrae.
- The 3 sacral vertebrae are fused in the dog and cat into the sacrum.
- The coccygeal vertebrae have very small transverse and spinous processes, making them almost cuboid in shape.

In addition, the number of different vertebrae (or the vertebral formula) varies between species (Figure 3.25).

Between the bodies of the vertebrae are intervertebral discs (see Figure 3.23b). These have two main parts: the nucleus pulposus and the annulus fibrosus. Intervertebral discs have a shock absorber effect, minimizing damage to the bones whilst allowing some flexibility and 'give' to the spinal column.

Reptiles

In some species of reptile (e.g. green iguanas; day geckos; smooth snakes), the caudal vertebral column ('tail') may be shed when grasped by a predator. Fracture planes in the muscle cartilage and between vertebrae allow easy and bloodless separation of the tail. In many cases, the tail may regrow – a process known as autotomy. When this occurs, the vertebral bodies are replaced with a cartilaginous cord and the scales of the skin covering the regrown tail are haphazard in arrangement.

Ribs and sternum

The basic rib structure (Figure 3.26) consists of a bony part, which articulates with the thoracic vertebrae dorsally at the head of the rib, also known as the body. Ventrally, the lower half of the rib comprises cartilage known as costal cartilage. The area where the bone meets the cartilage is the costochondral junction.

The ribs from the left and right sides meet ventrally at the sternebrae. The most cranial sternebra is known as the manubrium, and the most caudal sternebra is known as the xiphoid (or xiphisternum), the process of which can be felt

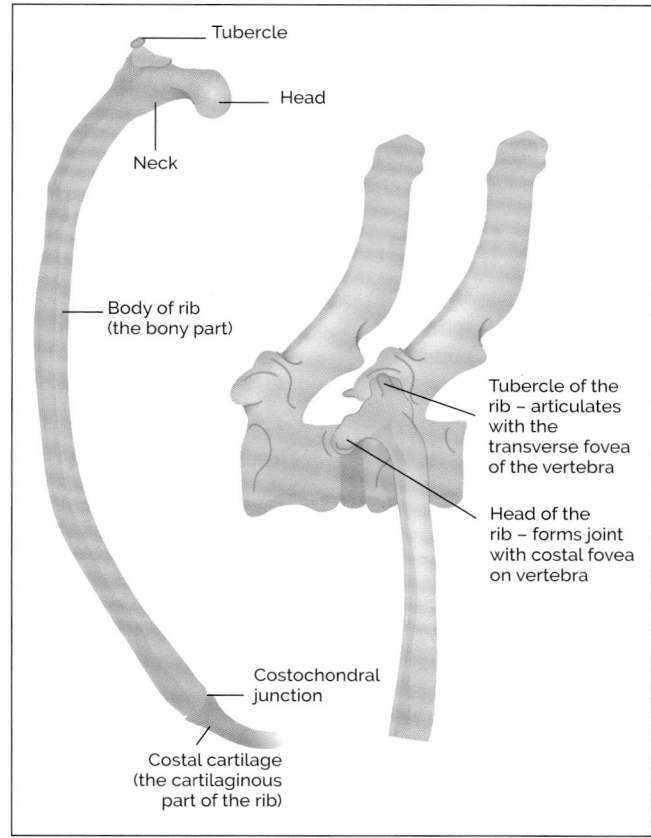

3.26 Structure of a rib and rib articulation.

protruding from the end of the sternum. Ribs 1–8 articulate with the sternum. Ventrally each rib curves cranially to touch the rib in front at its junction with the sternum.

Dogs and cats

In dogs and cats, ribs 9–12 curve cranially to touch the rib in front but do not touch the sternum, thus forming the costal arch. However, rib 13 does not curve cranially and the ventral point can be felt at the end of the ribcage; this is called the 'floating rib'.

Species	Type of vertebra				
	Cervical	*Thoracic*	*Lumbar*	*Sacral*	*Coccygeal*
Dog	7	13	7	3	20–23
Cat	7	13	7	3	20–23
Ferret	7	14–15	5–6	3–4	18
Rabbit	7	12–13	7	4	15–16
Guinea pig	7	13	6	3–4	4–6
Rat	7	13	6	4	27–31
Hamster	7	13	6	4	7–14
Birds	11–25 Large species variations	Often fused into one bone known as the notarium	Often one mobile lumbar vertebra. The rest are fused into the synsacrum	Fused together to form the roof of the pelvis known as the synsacrum	Large species variations. The last few vertebrae are fused together to form the pygostyle
Reptiles	Large species variations. Generally box-like	Chelonians: may be fused into the shell Lizards and snakes: mobile and box-like	Chelonians: may be fused into the shell Lizards and snakes: mobile and box-like	Chelonians: may be fused into the shell Lizards: may be fused to the roof of the pelvis or mobile	Large species variations Chelonians: may be few in number Lizards: significantly greater in number than chelonians

3.25 Vertebral formulae for different species.

Birds

These animals possess a keel bone over the sternum. This varies in prominence, being more important in species that are strong fliers as it provides the surface area for the attachment of the flight muscles. In species that float on water (e.g. ducks) the keel is flattened to create a boat-like hull shape.

Appendicular skeleton

The appendicular skeleton comprises the limbs, which attach to the vertebral column via the pectoral and pelvic girdles. For this reason, snakes do not have an appendicular skeleton, with the exception of the occasional vestige of the pelvis in some Boa species.

Forelimbs

The forelimb consists of the clavicle, scapula, humerus, radius, ulna, carpus, metacarpus and phalanges.

Clavicle

The clavicle is the collarbone, which is present to varying degrees in different animals (e.g. in dogs it is made of cartilage rather than bone and is not obvious on radiographs, whereas in cats it is fully formed and visible on radiographs).

Scapula

The scapula is a flat bone, which attaches to the body via muscles, not a joint. It consists of a cranial and caudal surface separated by a spine. The distal part of the spine is the acromion. In the dog, the acromion comprises one part, whereas in the cat it is split into two sections. The distal end of the scapula articulates with the humerus.

Humerus

The humerus is a simple bone comprising a head, which articulates with the scapula, and a greater tubercle, which makes up the shoulder. Distally there is a hole in the humerus known as the olecranon fossa, which is where the ulna articulates with the humerus to form the elbow joint. The humerus also expands distally into the medial and lateral condyles.

Radius and ulna

The lower part of the forelimb consists of the radius and ulna, which lie alongside each other. The radius is a short bone without any distinctive features. The ulna is longer than the radius and can be felt as the point of the elbow at the olecranon. The ulna articulates with the humerus where the anconeal process of the ulna fits into the olecranon fossa of the humerus. Distally the ulna tapers to a point known as the styloid process. Thus, the radius provides most of the proximal articular surface of the carpus.

Carpus

The carpus comprises a number of different bones (Figure 3.27). Proximally there are three carpal bones: the radial and ulnar, which articulate with the radius and ulna, respectively, and the accessory carpal bone, which can be felt to protrude laterally. Distal to this is another row of carpal bones, which articulate between the first row of carpal bones and the metacarpal bones. However, these distal carpal bones are only present next to the first four metacarpal bones. The fifth metacarpal bone articulates with the ulnar carpal bone.

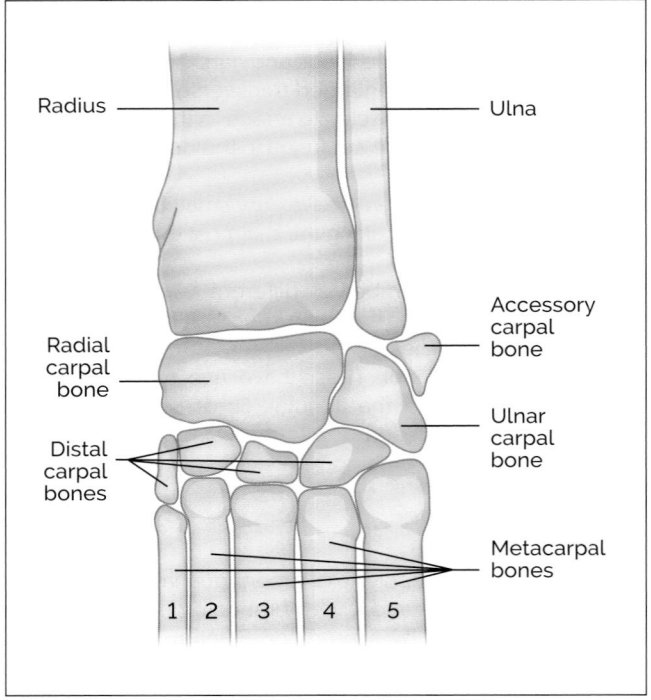

3.27 Structure of the left carpus.

Metacarpus and phalanges

Metacarpal bones are long and thin and join the carpus to the digits. The digits comprise smaller bones known as phalanges. The first digit has two phalanges (the dewclaw) and the other digits are made up of three phalanges. These are the proximal, middle and distal phalanges. The most distal phalange is modified to allow the nail to grow at the ungual process.

Small mammals

In ferrets, rabbits and most rodents the clavicle is present and obvious on radiographs. The scapula in small animals varies slightly between species; rabbits have a markedly hooked suprahamate process. In chinchillas, guinea pigs, hamsters and gerbils there are only four digits in the forelimbs.

Birds

The clavicles are well developed in birds and fused together to form the furcula or wishbone, which creates a spring-like effect to counteract the compressive forces generated on the downbeat of the wings. Birds also possess a coracoid bone, which projects ventrally from the shoulder joint to the keel bone and acts as a strut or support for the shoulder, allowing it to cope with the stress of rapid wing movements during flight.

The forelimbs are adapted to form wings, which results in a reduction in the overall number of bones. The scapulae are flattened and lie across the lateral surface of the ribcage. Each of the scapulae forms a shoulder joint with the humerus, the clavicle and the coracoid bones.

The radius is the smaller of the antebrachial bones in the bird. The secondary flight feathers attach directly to the periosteum of the stouter and more caudally placed ulna. The carpal bones are reduced to one major and one minor carpal bone. There are only three metacarpal bones: a vestigial first metacarpal bone known as the alula or 'bastard wing' (equivalent to the bird's thumb), and the major and minor metacarpal bones. The digits are similarly reduced to a single phalanx representing the first (minor) digit and two phalanges representing the major digit, which forms the tip of the wing. The primary feathers attach to the periosteum of the metacarpal bones and phalanges.

Reptiles

Lizards and chelonians possess well developed clavicles, although in the latter these are located within the ribcage. In addition, chelonians have a coracoid bone that projects dorsally from the shoulder joint to the inside of the dorsum of the carapace, which acts as a supporting strut for the shell and shoulder joint. The forelimbs in lizards and chelonians usually have five digits, although there is some species variation.

Hindlimbs

The hindlimb consists of the pelvis, femur, tibia, fibula, tarsus, metatarsus, phalanges, patella and fabellae.

Pelvis

The hindlimbs attach to the vertebral column via the pelvis. The pelvis comprises a number of different bones, which are fused together (Figure 3.28). Dorsally and cranially the ilium can be felt lying alongside the vertebral column. Ventrally the left and right sides of the pelvis meet at the pubis. Caudally the ischium can be felt on either side of the tail. Ventrally there is a large hole in either side of the floor of the pelvis known as the obturator foramen. The hindleg attaches to the pelvis via the acetabulum formed at the junction of the ilium, ischium and pubis.

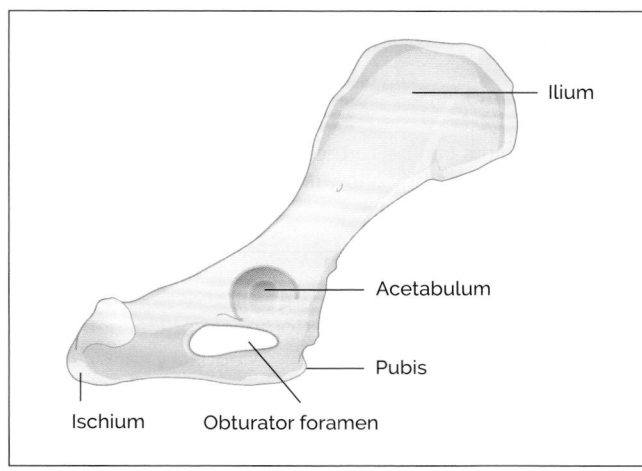

3.28 Structure of the pelvis.

Femur

The femur is the most proximal bone of the hindlimb. Structurally it is similar to the humerus. The round head articulates with the acetabulum of the pelvis (ball and socket joint). Laterally the greater trochanter can be felt on the proximal femur protruding alongside the hip joint. Distally the femur has a groove known as the trochlea, which forms part of the stifle (equivalent to the human knee joint).

Tibia and fibula

Distal to the stifle, making up the lower part of the leg, are the tibia and fibula. The tibia is the main weight-bearing bone, forming most of the distal articular surface of the stifle joint. Lateral to the tibia is the fibula, which is a long, thin bone. Distally the tibia and fibula articulate with the tarsus (or hock).

Tarsus

The tarsus is similar to the carpus in that it comprises rows of smaller bones (Figure 3.29). The tibia and fibula articulate with the talus in the proximal tarsus. Lateral to the talus is the calcaneus, which projects proximally to form the point of the hock. Distal to the talus is the central tarsal bone. Distal to the central tarsal bone are the smaller tarsal bones I, II and III. Lateral to this is tarsal bone IV (distal tarsal bone), which is larger than the other tarsal bones.

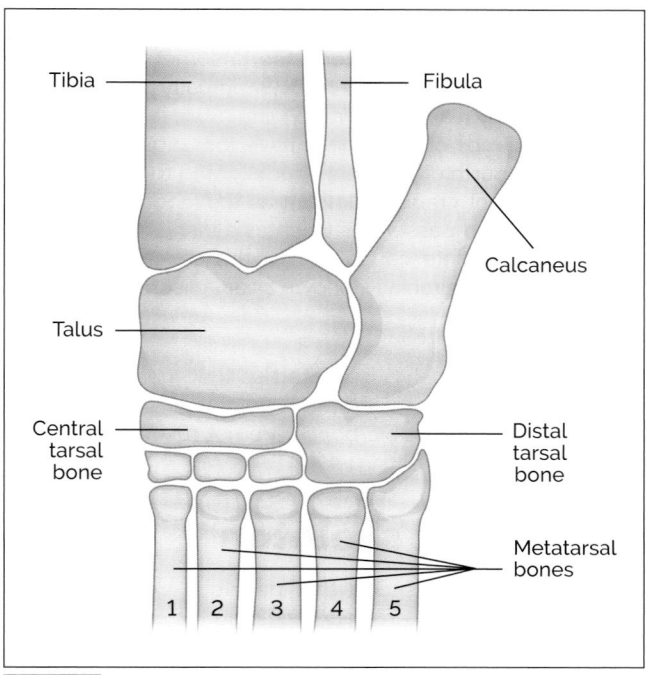

3.29 Structure of the left tarsus.

Metatarsus and phalanges

The metatarsal bones and phalanges of the hindlimb are similar to the metacarpal bones and phalanges of the forelimb.

Patella and fabellae

Sesamoid bones are found near to joints. Most are found in tendons, but some can be found in ligaments. The function of these bones is to protect the tendons. The patella (kneecap) is the largest sesamoid bone in the body. It is found on the cranial surface, and makes up the largest part, of the stifle. It sits in the trochlea of the femur and moves every time the knee is straightened or bent. Caudal to the stifle, smaller sesamoid bones known as fabellae can be found in the tendons of the gastrocnemius muscle.

Small mammals

The rabbit has a separate bone, known as the os acetabuli, which forms the structure of the hip joint. In addition, the femur is more flattened in the rabbit, making this bone less suitable for the intramedullary pin techniques used for fracture repair. In the guinea pig, a fibrocartilaginous suture line at the pubis and ischium allows separation of the pelvis prior to and during parturition. This suture line mineralizes as guinea pigs get older becoming less flexible, leading to problems at parturition in older guinea pigs. Because of this, guinea pigs who have not been bred before 1 year of age should not be used for breeding. In the majority of small mammals there are four digits in the hindlimb, with the exception of guinea pigs where there are three, and hamsters and gerbils where there are five.

Birds

The pelvis has separate pubis bones, which instead of meeting in the midline actually support the musculature of the ventral body wall. The pelvis fuses dorsally with the synsacrum.

The tibia in birds is fused with the proximal row of tarsal bones to form the tibiotarsus. The distal row of tarsal bones is fused with the metatarsal bones (which themselves are fused together into one bone) to form the tarsometatarsus. Thus, the avian equivalent of the hock is actually an intertarsal joint and is known as the suffrago joint.

The hindlimbs of most birds have four digits. In parrots, the first and fourth digits point caudally, and the second and third digits point cranially (known as a zygodactyl limb). In most raptors and passerines (such as canaries and finches), the first digit points caudally, and the second, third and fourth digits point cranially (known as an anisodactyl limb).

Reptiles

In chelonians, the pelvis is rotated so that the ilium is near vertical and the ischium and pubis point ventrally and cranially. In females, the pubic bones are not fused together, in order to allow egg laying.

Splanchnic skeleton

A splanchnic bone is one that develops within the soft tissues. In many male animals, including the dog, ferret, rat, mouse, hamster and gerbil, a bone is present within the penis. This is the os penis. It is absent or only partially present in male cats.

Joints

A joint occurs where two or more bones join or articulate. Different degrees of movement are present in different types of joint. Joints are classified as follows:

- Fibrous – little or no movement
- Cartilaginous – little or no movement
- Synovial – a wide range of movement.

Terminology

The range of movement of a joint is described using the following terms:

- Flexion – bending the limb by decreasing the angle of the joint
- Extension – straightening the limb by increasing the angle of the joint
- Adduction – moving the limb distal to the joint towards the midline/body
- Abduction – moving the limb distal to the joint away from the midline/body
- Gliding – flat surfaces moving over each other (e.g. in the carpus)
- Rotation – movement shown by a pivot joint
- Circumduction – moving one end of a bone (usually the end distal to the joint) in a circular motion →

Terminology *continued*

- Protraction – lengthening the limb by moving distal limb away from the body
- Retraction – shortening the limb by moving the distal limb towards the body
- Supination – turning the lower surface of the paw downwards
- Pronation – turning the lower surface of the paw upwards.

Fibrous joints

Fibrous joints are present as sutures in the skull, or syndesmoses between two areas of bone.

Cartilaginous joints

Cartilaginous joints can present as synchondroses, which are joints between the epiphyses and diaphyses in growing animals, or as symphyses, which are joints between the mandible bones of the lower jaw and the pubic bones of the pelvis.

Synovial joints

Synovial joints (diarthroses; Figure 3.30) are characterized by the presence of:

- Synovial membrane
- Fibrous joint capsule
- Articular surfaces
- Synovial fluid
- Ligaments
- Meniscus/menisci.

Synovial joints can be further described according to the range of movement they allow (Figure 3.31).

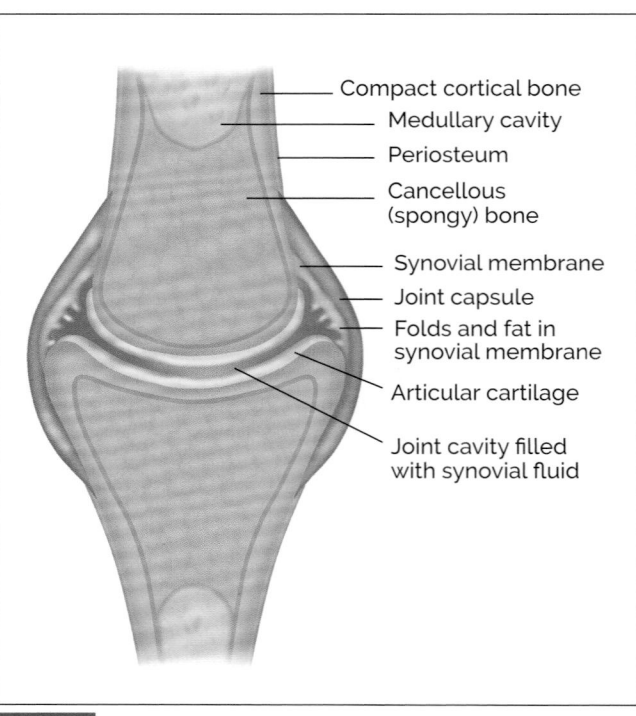

Compact cortical bone
Medullary cavity
Periosteum
Cancellous (spongy) bone
Synovial membrane
Joint capsule
Folds and fat in synovial membrane
Articular cartilage
Joint cavity filled with synovial fluid

3.30 A synovial joint.

Joint	Type of movement	Examples
Condylar	Convex surface which fits on to a concave surface to allow flexion and extension	Stifle (between femur and tibia; Figure 3.32)
Ellipsoidal	Sliding	Radiocarpal joint
Hinge	In one plane	Elbow (between humerus and radius/ulna)
Pivot	Rotational	Atlanto-axial joint; radius and ulna
Plane	Sliding	Between carpal and tarsal bones
Saddle	In one plane	Phalanges
Spheroidal (ball and socket)	Rotational	Hip (between femur and acetabulum)

3.31 Classification and range of movement of synovial joints.

Ligaments

Ligaments are thickened bands of fibrous tissue that connect bones and form the capsules of joints.

Stifle

The stifle comprises the femur, tibia, fibula and patella. These bones are held in place by four different ligaments (Figure 3.32):

- The medial collateral ligament joins the femur to the proximal tibia on the medial side of the stifle joint
- The lateral collateral ligament runs from the femur to the fibula on the lateral side of the stifle joint
- The cranial cruciate ligament runs from the lateral condyle of the femur to the caudal tibial plateau
- The caudal cruciate ligament runs at right angles to the cranial cruciate ligament, attaching the femur to the tibia.

In dogs, there are also two small sesamoid bones (fabellae) caudal to the stifle joint, situated in the origin of the gastrocnemius muscle. Located between the condyles of the femur and the tibia are menisci; wedge-shaped pieces of cartilage sitting both laterally and medially. These prevent some of the lateral movement of the femur in relation to the tibial plateau. The menisci also have nerve endings, which provide information to the nervous system about the pressure within and the position of the stifle joint.

Muscular system

There are three basic types of muscle: skeletal, smooth and cardiac (Figure 3.33).

Skeletal muscle

Skeletal (striated or voluntary) muscle is found in association with the skeleton. It consists of individual muscle cells known as muscle fibres, which are grouped together in bundles called fascicles by connective tissue called perimysium. Many perimysium-bound bundles are further grouped together, and the whole muscle is then surrounded by epimysium. Each muscle fibre contains many myofibrils. The basic unit of a myofibril is the sarcomere, which comprises actin and myosin filaments.

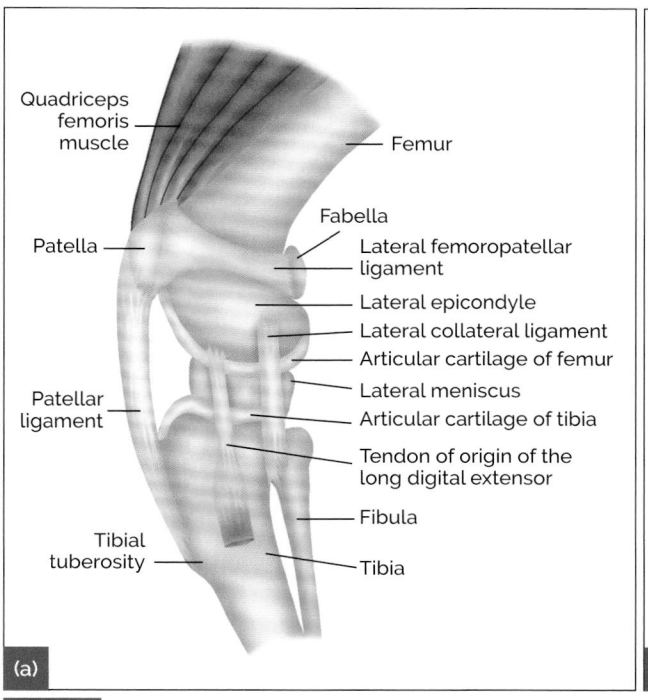

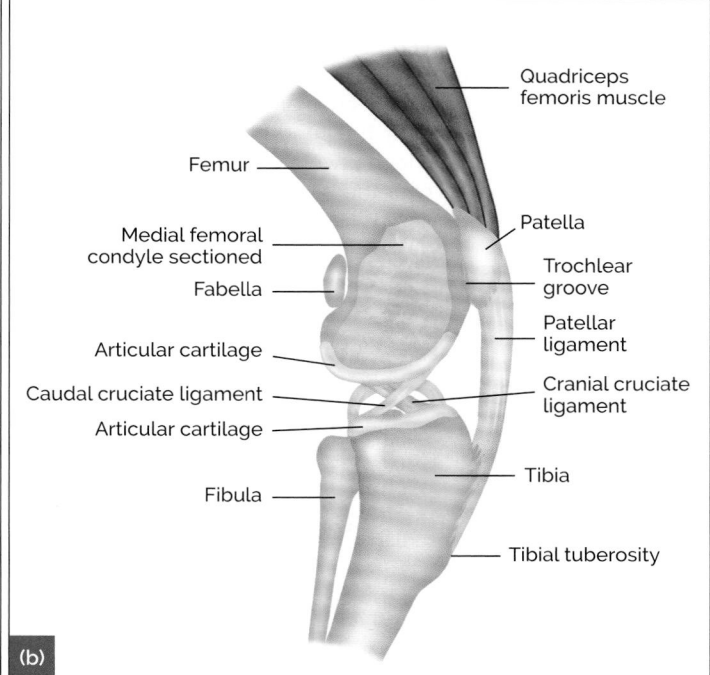

3.32 Structure of the canine left stifle joint. **(a)** Lateral view. **(b)** Medial view.

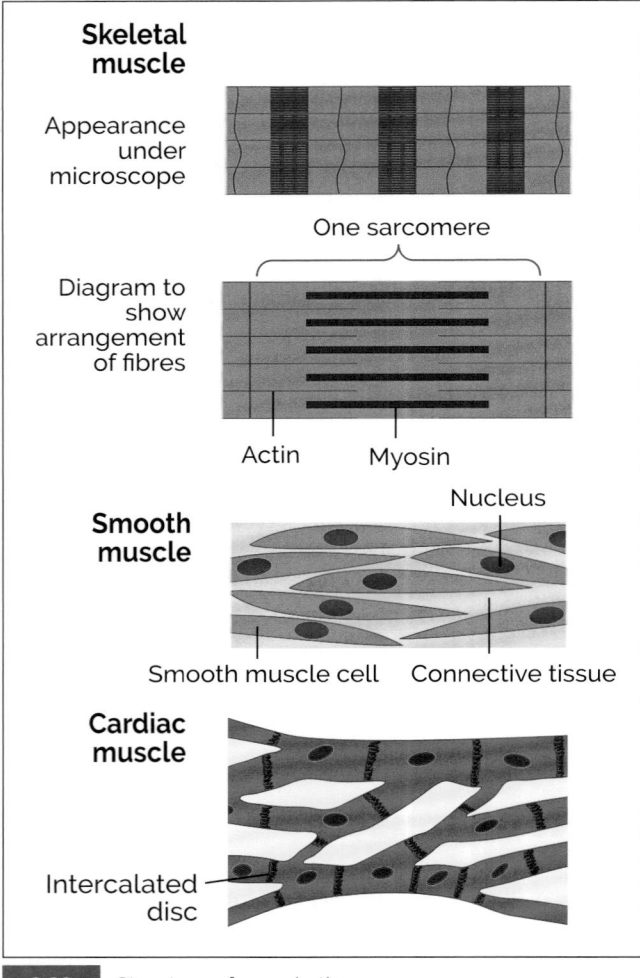

Skeletal muscle

Appearance under microscope

Diagram to show arrangement of fibres

One sarcomere

Actin   Myosin

Smooth muscle

Nucleus

Smooth muscle cell   Connective tissue

Cardiac muscle

Intercalated disc

3.33 Structure of muscle tissue.

The structure of skeletal muscle is shown in Figure 3.34. The muscle origin is the proximal attachment to the skeleton. The main part of the muscle is known as the muscle belly. The distal part of the muscle then attaches to the skeleton at the point of insertion. Muscles are attached to bones via tendons, which consist of connective tissue. Where a tendon is closely related to a bone, a bursa may be present to act as a protective cushion between the bone and the tendon. Surrounding the tendon is a connective tissue layer (the synovial sheath), which allows the smooth movement of the tendon over the bone and provides nutrients to the tendon. Some muscles have a broad area of

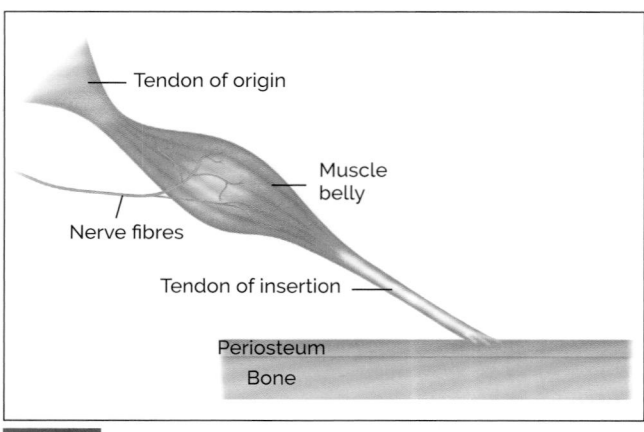

Tendon of origin

Muscle belly

Nerve fibres

Tendon of insertion

Periosteum
Bone

3.34 Muscle and tendon insertion.

attachment and utilize a sheet of connective tissue known as an aponeurosis.

Skeletal muscles are stimulated to contract by an impulse from a neuron. The first stage of contraction is initiated by an increase in the intracellular calcium concentration. This allows the actin and myosin filaments to move and overlap one another, resulting in contraction of the muscle.

Forelimb muscles

The muscles of the forelimb of the dog are shown in Figure 3.35 and described in Figure 3.36.

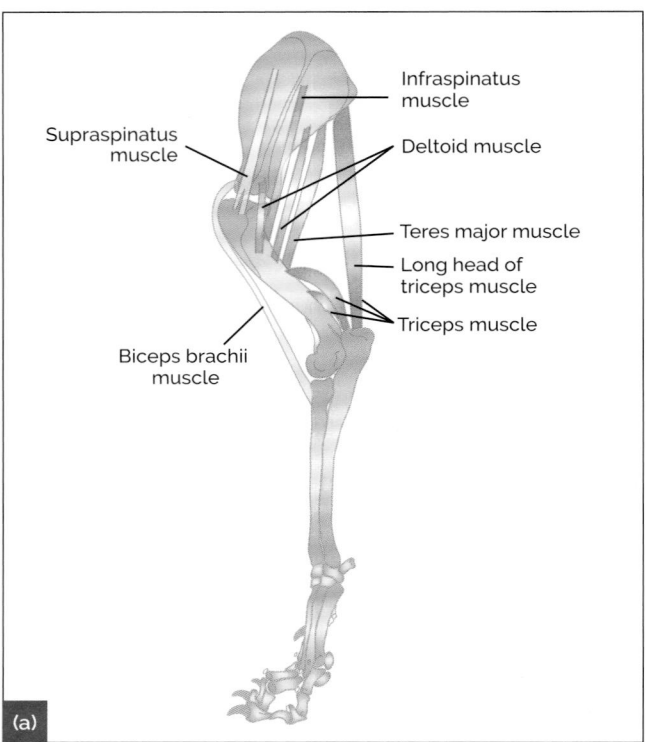

Supraspinatus muscle

Infraspinatus muscle

Deltoid muscle

Teres major muscle

Long head of triceps muscle

Triceps muscle

Biceps brachii muscle

(a)

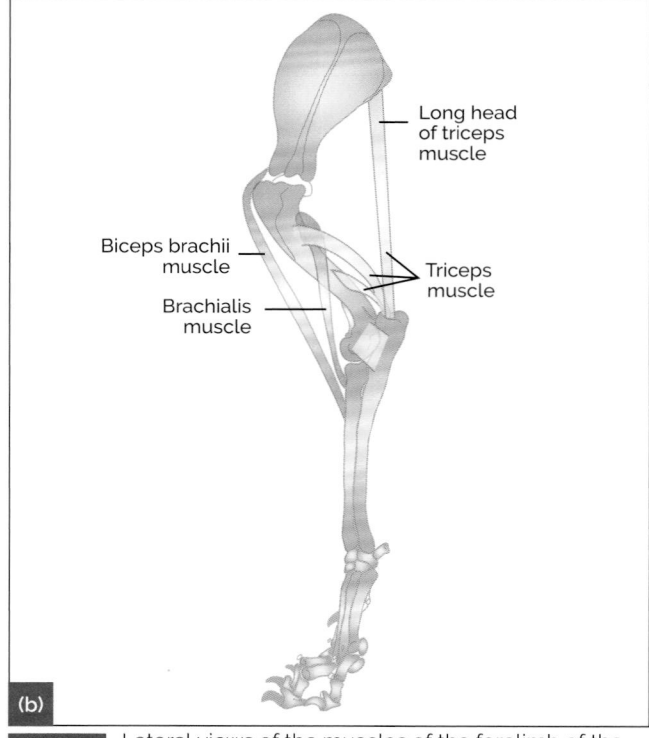

Long head of triceps muscle

Biceps brachii muscle

Brachialis muscle

Triceps muscle

(b)

3.35 Lateral views of the muscles of the forelimb of the dog. **(a)** Muscles that move the shoulder. **(b)** Muscles that move the elbow joint.

Muscle	Origin	Insertion	Function
Trapezius	Mid cervical and thoracic vertebrae	Spine of the scapula	Abductor of the forelimb

Brachiocephalicus:
  Cleidobrachialis
  Cleidocervicalis
  Cleidomastoideus
	Cervical region	Humerus	Advances the forelimb

Latissimus dorsi	Caudal thoracic and lumbar vertebrae	Medial humerus	Flexes the shoulder and retracts the forelimb
Supraspinatus	Supraspinous fossa	Proximal tuberosities	Stabilizes the shoulder
Infraspinatus	Infraspinous fossa	Lateral tubercle of the humerus	Stabilizes and abducts the shoulder
Triceps	Caudal border of the scapula and tricipital head of the humerus	Olecranon	Flexes the shoulder and extends the elbow
Biceps brachii	Supraglenoid tubercle	Radial tuberosity	Extends the shoulder and flexes the elbow
Brachialis	Proximal caudal aspect of the humerus	Radial tubercle	Flexes the elbow

Carpal flexors:
  Flexor carpi radialis
 	
  Flexor carpi ulnaris
 	
  Deep digital flexors
 	
  Superficial digital flexors
	
	Medial epicondyle of the humerus and medial radius
	Medial epicondyle of the humerus and caudal ulna
	Medial epicondyle of the humerus, caudal ulna and medial radius
	Medial epicondyle of the humerus
		
		Palmar side of metacarpal 2 and 3
		
		Accessory carpal bone
		
		Flexor surface of distal phalanges 1–5
		
		Palmar surface of phalanges 2–5
			Flex the carpus

Carpal extensors:
  Extensor carpi ulnaris
  Extensor carpi radialis
 	
  Common digital extensor
 	
  Lateral digital extensor
	
	Lateral ulna
	Lateral supracondylar crest of the radius
	Lateral epicondyle of the humerus
	Lateral epicondyle of the humerus
		
		5th metacarpal
		Tuberosities on 2nd and 3rd metacarpals
		Extensor processes of distal phalanges 2–5
		Proximal ends of all phalanges and distal ends of phalanges 3–5
			Extend the carpus

Digital flexors:
  Deep digital flexor
 	
  Superficial digital flexor
	
	Medial epicondyle of the humerus, distal radius (medial) and ulna (caudal)
	Medial epicondyle of the humerus
		
		Flexor surface of distal phalanges 1–5
		
		Palmar surface of phalanges 2–5
			Flex the digits

Digital extensors:
  Common digital extensor
 	
  Lateral digital extensor
	
	Lateral epicondyle of the humerus
	Lateral epicondyle of the humerus
		
		Extensor processes of distal phalanges 2–5
		Proximal ends of all phalanges and distal ends of phalanges 3–5
			Extend the digits

3.36 Muscles of the forelimb of the dog.

Hindlimb muscles

The muscles of the hindlimb are shown in Figure 3.37 and described in Figure 3.38. In addition, the Achilles tendon (common calcanean tendon) inserts on the point of the hock (the calcaneus; see Figure 3.29), allowing connection of the gastrocnemius muscle to the hock.

Epaxial muscles

The epaxial muscles lie dorsal to the transverse processes of the vertebrae. They are arranged in three parallel rows, which run from the neck to the lumbar area, and extend the vertebral column.

Hypoaxial muscles

The hypoaxial muscles lie ventral to the transverse processes of the vertebrae. The hypoaxial muscles cause flexion of the neck.

Intercostal muscles

The intercostal muscles are arranged in three layers: the external intercostal layer, internal intercostal layer and the subcostal layer. The external intercostal muscles run caudoventrally, from an origin on one rib to an insertion on another rib. Internal intercostal muscles run cranioventrally.

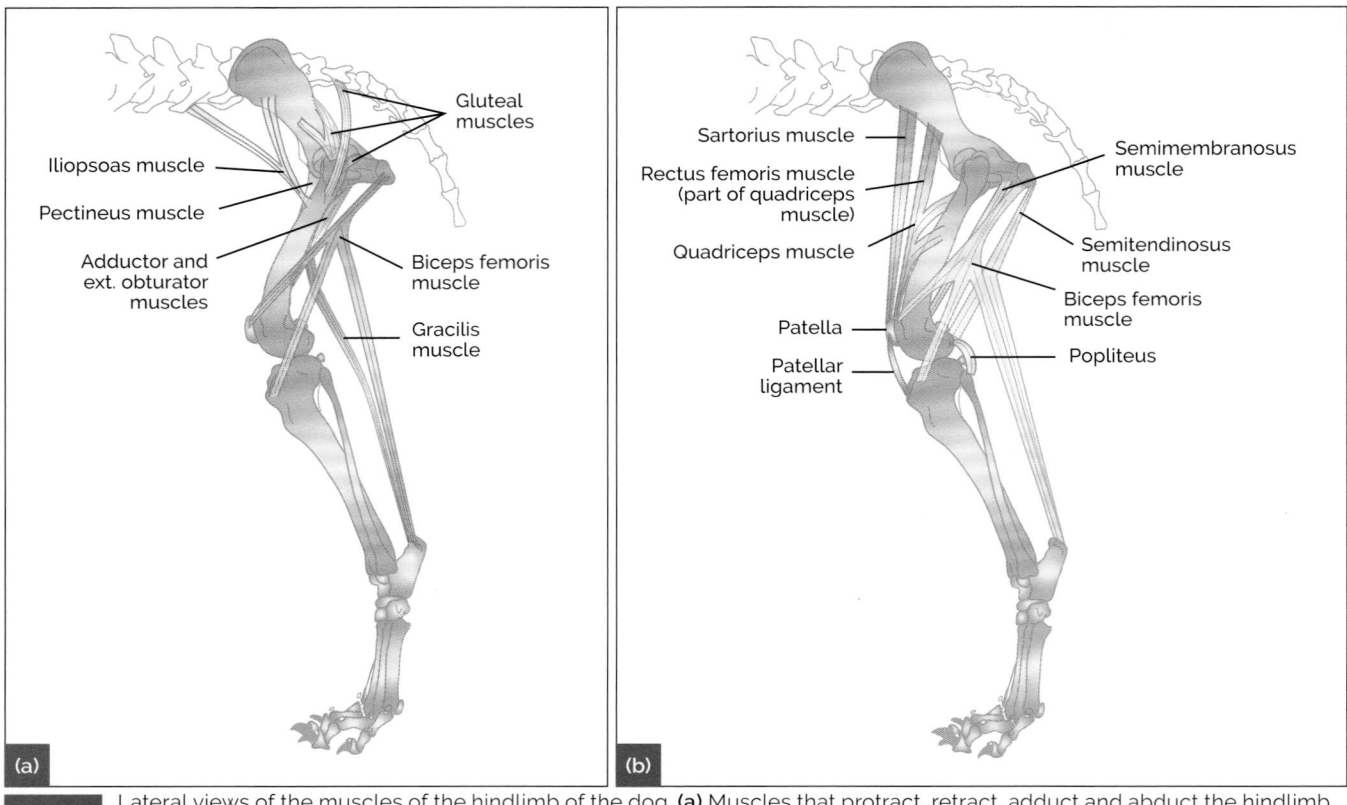

3.37 Lateral views of the muscles of the hindlimb of the dog. **(a)** Muscles that protract, retract, adduct and abduct the hindlimb. These muscles also flex and extend the hip. **(b)** Muscles that move the hip and stifle joint.

Muscle	Origin	Insertion	Function
Biceps femoris	Ischial tuberosity	Various insertions including the patella, tibial crest and calcaneus	Retracts the hip, flexes/extends the stifle and extends the hock
Semimembranosus	Ischial tuberosity	Medial distal femur and medial proximal tibia	Retracts the hip and flexes the stifle
Semitendonosus	Ischial tuberosity	Tibial crest and calcaneus	Retracts the hip and extends the stifle and hock
Quadriceps femoris: Vastus lateralis Vastus intermedius Vastus medialis Rectus femoris	 Proximal femur Proximal femur Proximal femur Ilium	Tibial tuberosity	Extends the stifle
Pectineus	Prepubic tendon and pelvis	Distal femur	Adducts the hip
Gastrocnemius	Caudolateral distal femur	Calcaneus	Flexes the stifle and extends the hock
Hock flexors: Long digital extensor Lateral digital extensor Cranial tibialis Fibularis brevis Fibularis longus	 Lateral epicondyle of the femur Proximal third of the fibula Proximal tibia laterally Lateral tibia and fibula distally Proximal tibia and fibula	 Dorsal surface of distal phalanges 2–5 Phalanges of 5th digit Metatarsal 1 and proximal end of metatarsal 2 Proximal end of metatarsal 5 Plantar surface of all metatarsals and 4th tarsal bone	Flex the hock
Hock extensors: Superficial digital flexor[a] Gastrocnemius Semitendinosis Biceps femoris	 Lateral supracondyle of the femur and sesamoid Medial and lateral supracondyles of the femur Lateral ischial tuberosity Sacrotuberous ligament and ischial tuberosity	 Tuber calcanei and distal metatarsophalangeal joints Via calcaneal (Achilles) tendon on tuber calcanei Medial tibia Tibial crest, tuberosity and merges into calcaneal (Achilles) tendon	Extend the hock

3.38 Muscles of the hindlimb of the dog. [a]Also flexes the digits.

continues ▶

Muscle	Origin	Insertion	Function
Deep digital flexor	Head of fibula	Bases of the distal phalanges	Flexes the digits
Digital extensors: 　Long digital extensor 　Lateral digital extensor 　Medial digital extensor	 Lateral epicondyle of the femur Proximal third of the fibula Medial aspect of the femur	 Distal phalanges 2–5 Digit 5 Digits 1 and 2	Extend the digits

3.38 *continued* Muscles of the hindlimb of the dog. [a]Also flexes the digits.

Diaphragm

The diaphragm separates the thoracic and abdominal cavities in mammals. It is dome-shaped, pointing toward the thorax, situated underneath the ribs. The central area is made of a tendon with muscle around the edge. Dorsally the diaphragm is divided into left and right crura (singular: crus). There are three openings in the diaphragm, that allow blood vessels and other organs to pass from the thorax to the abdomen. The aortic hiatus allows the aorta, azygous vein and thoracic duct to pass through the diaphragm. The oesophageal hiatus lies ventral to the aortic hiatus and allows the oesophagus and vagal trunks to pass through the diaphragm. The caval foramen is found in the central tendon and allows the caudal vena cava to pass through the diaphragm.

Birds

Significant adaptations to the skeletal muscles are present in birds in order to enable flight, including:

- No diaphragm
- Large superficial pectoral muscles for movement of the wings downwards
- Deep pectoral muscles (also known as the supracoracoideus muscles) beneath the superficial pectoral muscles, the tendon of which passes through the triosseal canal in the coracoids bone and attaches to the dorsal surface of the humerus, allowing upward movement of the wings.

Reptiles

Most of the body wall muscles in chelonians are reduced due to the presence of dermal bone, which forms the shell. In addition, although there is no true diaphragm in reptiles, chelonians may have partial muscular sheets which resemble this muscle.

Lizards have a similar muscular structure to mammals. Snakes have no limbs, but do have a strong segmented ventral body wall muscle used to create a wave of contraction from cranial to caudal, which raises the ventral scales propelling the snake forwards. This is enhanced by contraction of the intercostal body wall muscles, which makes the snake adopt a sinusoidal movement.

Smooth muscle

Smooth muscle is found in visceral structures such as the blood vessels, the gastrointestinal tract. the uterus and the bladder. The basic structure of the smooth muscle cell is different to that of skeletal muscle, with overlapping cells arranged in sheets or bundles. Smooth muscle lacks sarcomeres; this is obvious visually as they have no striations. However, the muscle cell still consists of actin and myosin filaments.

Contraction of smooth muscle is involuntary and controlled by the autonomic nervous system or hormones. As with skeletal muscles, contraction is initiated by an increase in the intracellular calcium concentration.

Cardiac muscle

Cardiac muscle is found in the heart and comprises branched muscle cells linked by intercalated discs, which support synchronized contraction of cardiac tissue. The basic structure is similar to that of skeletal muscle. Contraction of the heart muscle is controlled by a conduction system (see 'Heart' below).

Nervous system

Neurons

The main cell of the nervous system is the neuron (Figure 3.39). A nerve consists of many neurons. The neuron is a simple cell comprising:

- A cell body located at one end of the neuron containing the nucleus
- A series of thick dendrons or fine dendrites (short filaments of the cell body), which carry nerve impulses toward the cell body
- A single axon, which carries impulses away from the cell body toward other neurons. The axon may be a few millimetres or up to a metre in length
- Nerve endings at the end of the axon, which connect one neuron with another at a synapse or with a muscle cell at a neuromuscular junction.

The axon is often surrounded by an insulating cell, known as a Schwann cell. Such neurons are referred to as myelinated, as the Schwann cell produces a white lipoprotein sheath known as myelin around the axon, forming a neurolemmal membrane (neurilemma). Myelinated axons have a rapid rate of impulse transmission. The axon can still receive nutrients despite the myelin sheath as there are small gaps between adjacent Schwann cells, known as nodes of Ranvier.

Some axons do not have protective outer cells and are referred to as non-myelinated neurons. They are relatively uncommon and generally have slower rates of impulse transmission (e.g. neurons in the retina of the eye and in the grey matter of the brain and spinal cord).

Impulse conduction

At the synapse or neuromuscular junction there is a gap between the end of the axon and the next cell. In order for the electrical impulse to 'jump' across this gap, a chemical known as a neurotransmitter is released from the axon.

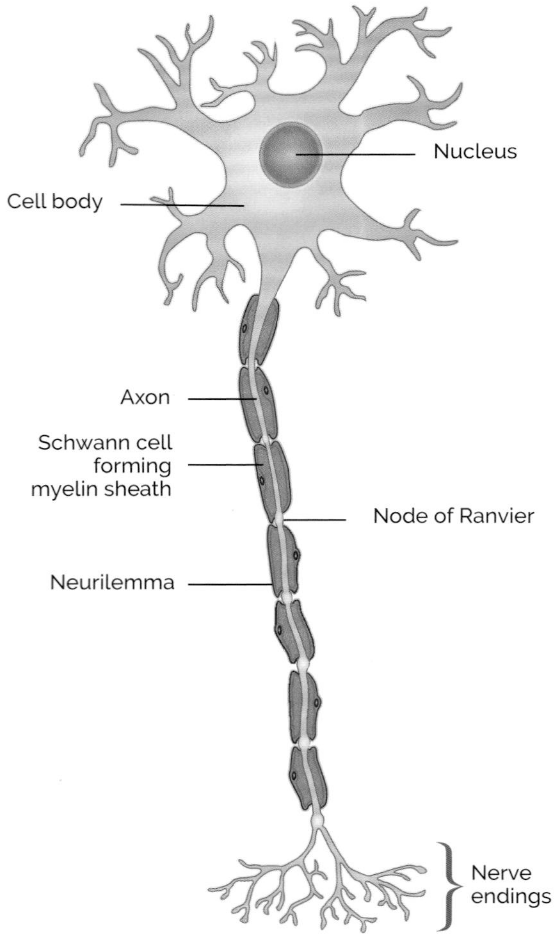
Nucleus
Cell body
Axon
Schwann cell forming myelin sheath
Node of Ranvier
Neurilemma
Nerve endings

3.39 Structure of a neuron.

The most common neurotransmitter is acetylcholine; however, both noradrenaline and adrenaline may be present in various neurons.

When the impulse reaches the nerve ending, voltage-sensitive calcium channels open, allowing calcium ions to enter the nerve ending from the extracellular and synaptic spaces. This influx of calcium ions causes the release of the chemical neurotransmitter into the synaptic gap or space, which then diffuses across the gap to the next neuron or muscle cell. The neurotransmitter binds to the adjacent cell, causing either more ion channels to open or further chemicals to be released, which results in continuation of the electrical impulse.

What happens in the postsynaptic neuron or muscle depends on whether the presynaptic neuron is inhibitory or excitatory. The presence of a synapse means that there is an 'all-or-nothing' phenomenon, in that either the impulse will cross the synapse or it will not; there is no gradation of response.

Structure

The nervous system is broadly divided into two parts:

- Central nervous system (CNS) – comprises the brain and spinal cord
- Peripheral nervous system (PNS) – comprises all nerves arising from the CNS.

Central nervous system

There are two components to the CNS: the brain and the spinal cord. Within the CNS, two types of tissue are found:

- Grey matter – peripherally located in the cortex of the cerebellum, but centrally located in the medulla of the spinal cord and cerebrum
- White matter – peripherally located in the cortex of the spinal cord and cerebrum, but laterally located in the medulla of the cerebellum.

The grey matter largely consists of non-myelinated neurons or those portions of the neuron that are not normally covered in myelin (e.g. the cell body). Accumulations of cell bodies are often referred to as nuclei. These nuclei act as relay centres for many subconscious neurological pathways from the brain to the spinal cord.

The white matter consists of myelinated neurons, or those portions of the neuron that are normally covered in myelin (e.g. the axon).

Brain

The brain (Figure 3.40) is divided into three areas:

- The forebrain – comprising the cerebrum (telencephalon) and the diencephalon
- The midbrain (mesencephalon) – comprising the tectum, tegmentum and the cerebral peduncle (crus cerebri)
- The hindbrain – comprising the medulla oblongata, pons and cerebellum.

Cerebrum

The cerebrum (telencephalon) consists of paired lateral cerebral hemispheres (often referred to as the neopallium), which are the most obvious external feature of the brain, as well as the paleopallium (the rostroventral part of the brain connected to the olfactory lobe) and the basal nuclei, which have connections to the olfactory and sensory motor centres.

The surface of the cerebral hemispheres is highly folded (the tops of the folds are known as gyri; the bottoms of the folds are known as sulci); this allows the brain to increase its surface area massively without increasing its overall size. The two hemispheres are separated by the longitudinal fissure into which the falx cerebri (a fold of the meninges) projects. The two hemispheres are connected by a band of white tissue known as the corpus callosum, which runs just beneath the dorsal surface of the cerebrum, forming the roof of the lateral ventricles (two fluid-filled areas, one in each hemisphere, located beneath the outer cerebral hemispheres).

The cerebrum can be further subdivided into cortical lobes, according to the overlying skull bone structure:

- Frontal lobe (rostral)
- Parietal lobe (dorsal)
- Occipital lobe (caudal)
- Temporal lobe (lateral)
- Olfactory lobe (ventrorostral; connected to the olfactory nerves via the olfactory bulb on the ventral surface).

Diencephalon

The diencephalon forms the most rostral part of the brainstem. Only the ventral part of this structure, known as the hypothalamus (see Figure 3.40), can be visualized. The diencephalon consists of three main parts:

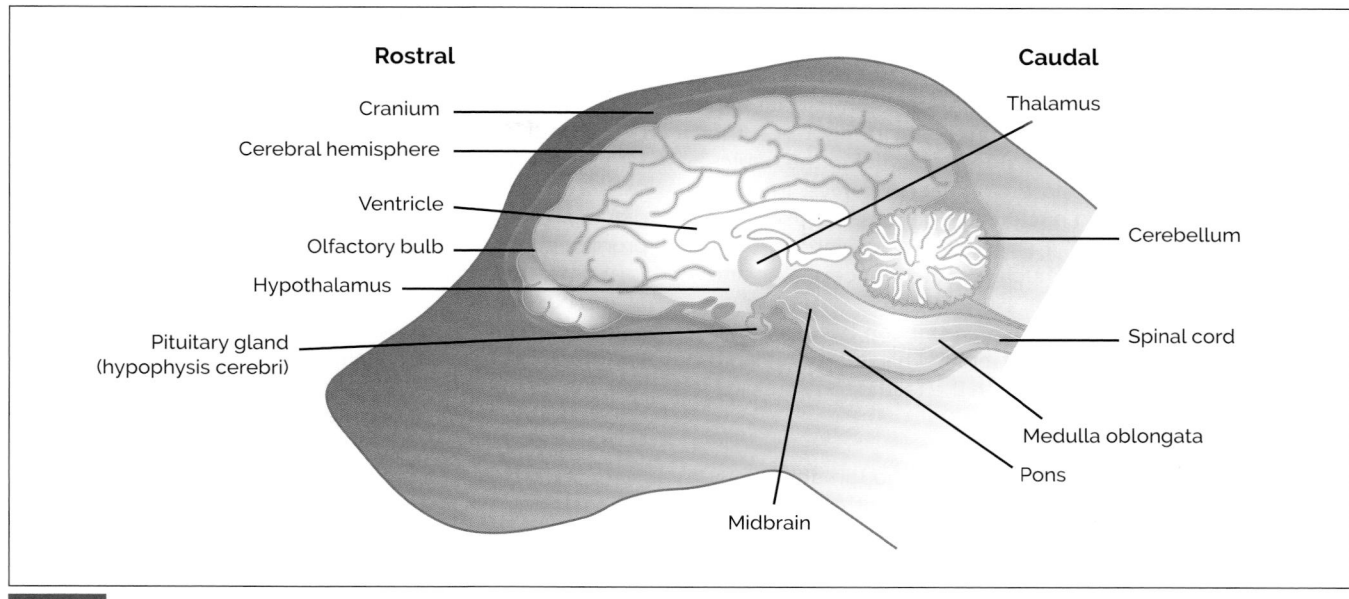

Rostral   **Caudal**

Cranium

Cerebral hemisphere

Ventricle

Olfactory bulb

Hypothalamus

Pituitary gland
(hypophysis cerebri)

Thalamus

Cerebellum

Spinal cord

Medulla oblongata

Pons

Midbrain

3.40   Structure of the brain of the dog.

- Hypothalamus
- Thalamus
- Epithalamus.

The hypothalamus forms the ventral and lateral walls of a cerebrospinal fluid-filled structure of the brain known as the third ventricle (Figure 3.41), which lies medially beneath the lateral ventricles. The hypothalamus contains a number of nuclei that are involved in hormonal regulation and connect the CNS with the autonomic nervous system (ANS). One of these connections is to the pituitary gland, which lies immediately ventral to the hypothalamus.

The pituitary gland (see Figure 3.40) consists of an anterior and a posterior lobe. The posterior lobe is an outgrowth of the hypothalamus and comprises neural tissue directly linked to the hypothalamus. It is responsible for the secretion of:

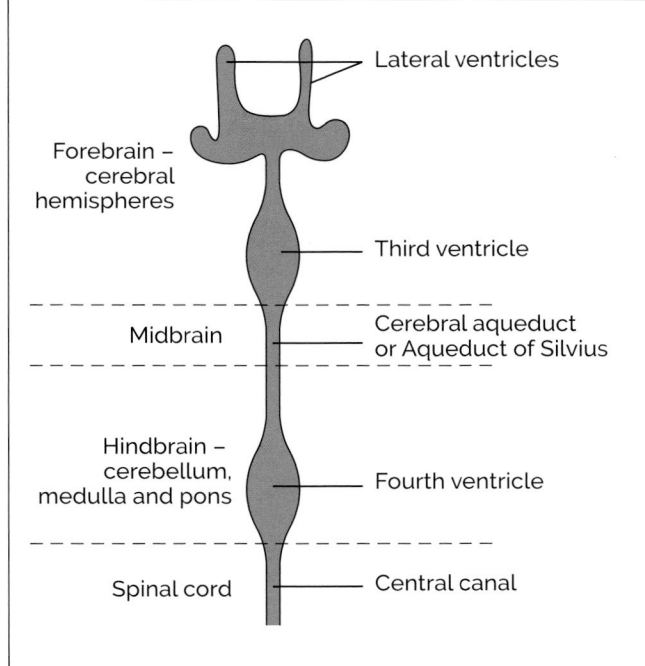

Lateral ventricles

Forebrain –
cerebral
hemispheres

Third ventricle

Midbrain

Cerebral aqueduct
or Aqueduct of Silvius

Hindbrain –
cerebellum,
medulla and pons

Fourth ventricle

Spinal cord

Central canal

3.41   General plan (dorsal view) of the ventricular system and its position within the brain.

- Oxytocin
- Antidiuretic hormone (ADH).

The anterior lobe is adjacent to the posterior lobe and is responsible for the secretion of:

- Follicle-stimulating hormone (FSH)
- Luteinizing hormone (LH)
- Growth hormone (GH)
- Thyroid-stimulating hormone (TSH)
- Prolactin (PRL)
- Adrenocorticotrophic hormone (ACTH).

These hormones are released by the anterior lobe in response to hormones secreted by the hypothalamus and posterior lobe. These hormones and their function are discussed more fully in the 'Endocrine system' (see below).

The thalamus is also surrounded by the third ventricle. The thalamus comprises a large number of nuclei. The role of the thalamus is to relay signals between the cerebrum and the brainstem. It receives incoming (afferent) signals from most sensory systems (with the exception of the nose, whose signals enter the forebrain through the olfactory bulbs and olfactory lobe) and acts as feedback control for most motor pathways.

The epithalamus is the most dorsal part of the diencephalon and contains the pineal gland, which is responsible for the regulation of reproductive activity as influenced by day length.

Mesencephalon

The ventral surface only of the mesencephalon (midbrain) can be seen in the intact brain. It has a lumen, known as the aqueduct of Silvius (see Figure 3.41), which joins the larger fluid-filled third and fourth ventricles. It has three parts (dorsal to ventral):

- Tectum
- Tegmentum
- Cerebral peduncle (crus cerebri).

The tectum lies dorsal to the aqueduct and consists largely of paired swellings, known as colliculi, which are connected to the thalamus and visual pathways (involved with the blink and pupillary reflexes) and are also spatial awareness integration centres.

The tegmentum is the main core of the midbrain and comprises the reticular formation, which contains the significant nuclei of the cranial nerves, including the oculomotor (III), trochlear (IV), and trigeminal (V) nerves. In addition, the nuclei of the red nucleus (so called because of its prominent vascular supply) are found here. These nuclei are connected to the basal nuclei of the telencephalon and also control motor movement.

The cerebral peduncle (crus cerebri) can be seen from the ventral surface of the intact brain. This is a nerve fibre tract connecting the brainstem with the telencephalon.

Medulla oblongata and pons

The medulla oblongata and the pons, although apparently grossly separate, are in fact continuations of one another, situated ventral to the cerebellum with the fluid-filled fourth ventricle (see Figure 3.41) lying between them and the cerebellum.

The pons is the most rostral part of the hindbrain and supports the middle cerebellar peduncles, bridging the two hemispheres of the cerebellum. It has many functions, including the control of respiration.

The medulla oblongata is caudal to the pons and continuous with the spinal cord. It has a series of decussating nerve fibres, forming significant tracts (e.g. the 'pyramids' tracts). In addition, many of the cranial nerves (see 'Cranial nerves' below) emerge from the CNS at this point, including the trigeminal (V), abducens (VI), facial (VII), vestibulocochlear (VIII), glossopharyngeal (IX), vagus (X), accessory (XI) and hypoglossal (XII) nerves. The olivary and pontine nuclei are also located in the medulla oblongata, along with the reticular formation; these are all important regulators of the feedback mechanisms controlling motor function. The reticular formation is also responsible for transmitting impulses that increase the animal's awareness of its surroundings when aroused. A decrease in the activity of the reticular formation tends to result in lethargy or sleep.

Cerebellum

The cerebellum is the spherical folded structure that sits immediately caudal to the cerebral hemispheres on the dorsal aspect of the pons and medulla oblongata. It has two main lateral hemispheres and a central body known as the vermis. The arrangement of white and grey matter is reversed in the cerebellum compared with the cerebrum and spinal cord, as the grey matter is located in the outermost cortical areas and the white matter in the central medulla. The cerebellum is attached to the brainstem by three paired peduncles: the cranial peduncle attaches it to the midbrain, the middle peduncle attaches it to the pons, and the caudal peduncle attaches it to the medulla oblongata. The cerebellum is responsible for CNS involvement with balance and coordination of postural and locomotive activities.

Birds

The avian brain is notable for its lack of folds (there are no gyri or sulci). Birds also have a reduced olfactory bulb and significantly enlarged optic nerve and optic lobes, which sit caudoventral to the cerebral hemispheres.

Reptiles

The reptilian brain is significantly smaller in relation to the whole body mass compared with small mammals and birds;

however, the basic structure of the brainstem is similar to the mammalian form. Reptiles have two cerebral hemispheres, but these are lyssencephalic (i.e. have no folds, gyri or sulci). A dorsal ventricular ridge (DVR) is present, arising from the lateral wall of the forebrain, which receives sensory input from the eyes, ears, nose and skin. The DVR relays the sensory information received to the cerebral hemispheres, diencephalon and efferent motor pathways. Snakes have prominent olfactory bulbs (as do some other species).

Some species have a parietal eye, which is a projection of the parietal part of the telencephalon connected to the pineal gland. This is well developed in species such as the green iguana and tuatara (which has a lens and a retina within the structure) and its function is to impart day length details to the brain to help regulate circadian rhythms and seasonal changes in metabolism and sexual behaviour.

Meninges

There are three membranes that protect the CNS and retain the cerebrospinal fluid:

- Dura mater
- Arachnoid mater
- Pia mater.

Dura mater

This is the outermost membrane and is largely attached to the periosteum of the inside of the cranium. In the spinal cord it is separated from the periosteum of the vertebral bodies by epidural fat deposits, creating an epidural space that can be used for anaesthesia (see Chapter 21).

Arachnoid mater

This is the next membrane and consists of large blood vessels supported by tough collagen fibres. The gap between the arachnoid mater and the dura mater (known as the subdural space) is filled with fat.

Pia mater

This is a thin fibrous membrane, which in the cranium is closely adherent to the surface of the brain. It contains small blood vessels that supply nutrients to the nervous tissue. The gap between the pia mater and the arachnoid mater (known as the subarachnoid space) is filled with cerebrospinal fluid.

Reptiles

There are only two membranes in reptiles: the pia arachnoid and the dura mater. The space between the membranes is referred to as the subdural space and is filled with cerebrospinal fluid.

Cerebrospinal fluid

The function of cerebrospinal fluid is to cushion and supply some nutrients to the nervous tissue. It is produced by a series of choroid (vascular) plexuses, which lie in the lumen of the ventricles. There are four main ventricles (see Figure 3.41):

- Two lateral ventricles in the forebrain (one in each hemisphere), just below the corpus callosum
- The third ventricle is situated around the thalamus in the centre of the brain
- The fourth ventricle is situated in the medulla oblongata.

The ventricles are connected: the lateral ventricles communicate across the midline with one another and caudally with the third ventricle. The third and fourth ventricles communicate via the cerebral aqueduct (aqueduct of Silvius), which runs through the midbrain. The fourth ventricle communicates with the central canal of the spinal cord.

Spinal cord

The spinal cord extends from the medulla oblongata, exiting the cranium via the foramen magnum of the skull, through the spinal column in the vertebral canal created by the meninges lining the linked lumens of the vertebral bodies. It terminates before the end of the spinal column in a series of fine nerves known as the cauda equina. A pair of nerves from the spinal cord exit at each intervertebral joint. These nerves carry both afferent (sensory) and efferent (motor) neurons to the musculoskeletal and visceral organs.

The spinal cord consists of an outer cortical layer of white matter and a central butterfly-shaped core of grey matter (Figure 3.42). The white matter is formed from myelinated neurons, which ascend to and descend from the brain. The grey matter consists of non-myelinated neurons and cell bodies, which connect afferent and efferent neurons. In the midline is the central canal, which connects the spinal cord with the ventricles of the brain and contains cerebrospinal fluid.

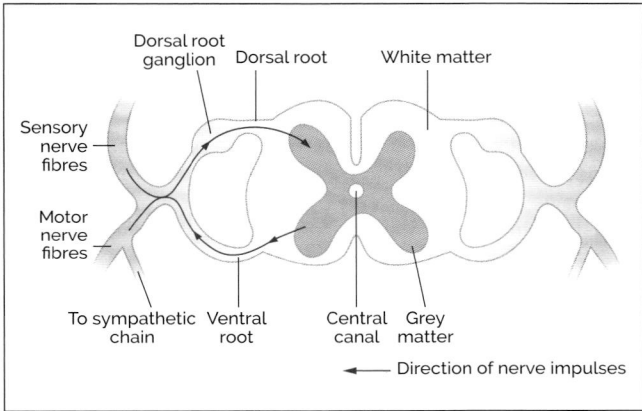

3.42 Cross-section through the spinal cord.

Peripheral nervous system

The PNS is how the CNS communicates with the organs and tissues of the body. Peripheral nerves comprise cranial and spinal nerves, which are made up of:

- Sensory or afferent nerve fibres, which collect information from the environment and transmit it to the CNS
- Motor or efferent fibres, which are responsible for carrying information from the CNS to the target tissues and organs, and control their activity.

Cranial nerves

Most cranial nerves (Figure 3.43) originate in the hindbrain and exit the cranium through various foramina. Many of these foramina, which can be seen on the skull, are situated around the base of the middle ear. Most have either a sensory or a motor function, but some such as the trigeminal, glossopharyngeal and vagus have a mixed motor and sensory function.

Spinal nerves

The spinal nerves are paired at each intervertebral junction (one left and one right) and exit through their respective

Nerve number	Nerve name	Function
I	Olfactory	Sensory nerve from the nasal mucosa (smell)
II	Optic	Sensory nerve connecting the eye to the sight centre of the brain
III	Oculomotor	Motor nerve supplying the muscles of the eye, eyelid and ciliary body
IV	Trochlear	Motor nerve supplying the dorsal oblique muscles of the eye
V	Trigeminal	Sensory nerve of the head/face. Very important nerve as it supplies a large number of structures within the head. Motor nerve supplying various muscles of the head/face
VI	Abducens	Motor nerve supplying the extrinsic muscles of the eye
VII	Facial	Motor nerve supplying various muscles (e.g. ears, eyelids, lips)
VIII	Vestibulo-cochlear	Sensory nerve for balance (from the semi-circular canals of the inner ear) and hearing (from the cochlea of the inner ear)
IX	Glosso-pharyngeal	Sensory nerve from the taste buds of the tongue and the pharynx. Motor nerve supplying the pharynx, root of the tongue, palate and some salivary glands
X	Vagus	Sensory nerve from the pharynx and larynx. Motor nerve supplying the larynx. It also carries parasympathetic motor fibres to the heart and other visceral organs (e.g. stomach and intestines)
XI	Accessory	Motor nerve supplying various muscles (e.g. trapezius and brachiocephalic)
XII	Hypoglossal	Motor nerve supplying the tongue

3.43 Cranial nerves.

intervertebral foramina. Each of the paired spinal nerves has a dorsal root and a ventral root (see Figure 3.42).

- The dorsal root is where the sensory nerves enter the spinal cord, relaying information from the sensory bodies to the cord. There is a small swelling where the cell bodies of the sensory neurons are located; where they form synapses is known as the dorsal root ganglion.
- The ventral root comprises motor nerves exiting the spinal cord on the way to the somatic muscles and visceral organs. The sympathetic nervous system is supplied by these motor nerve fibres. There is no corresponding ventral root ganglion.
- As the dorsal root has a sensory function and the ventral root has a motor function, a spinal nerve is a mixed nerve.

In the region of the forelimbs and hindlimbs, the spinal cord is thicker than normal. This is due to the large number of nerves passing into and out of the spinal cord. In addition, the spinal nerves anastomose (join together) to form the main nerves supplying the limbs. This anastomosis of spinal nerves is referred to as a plexus: the brachial plexus supplies the forelimb; the lumbosacral plexus supplies the hindlimb.

- The brachial plexus consists of the last three cervical and first two thoracic spinal nerves. It is located deep beneath the scapula and supplies the structures of the forelimb, with the exception of the trapezius, omotransversarius, brachiocephalicus and rhomboideus muscles, and the skin over the upper shoulder region.
- The lumbosacral plexus consists of the fourth lumbar through to the second sacral spinal nerves. It supplies the structures of the hindlimb, with the exception of a few proximal areas of skin.

  Significant nerves of the limbs include:

- The radial nerve, which derives from the caudal brachial plexus (C7–T1). It courses distally in the upper forelimb before moving between the long and medial heads of the triceps muscle, curving around the humerus to reach the craniolateral aspect of the forelimb. It innervates the triceps muscle, all carpal and digital extensor muscles and the skin; a branch innervates the craniolateral aspect of the antebrachium and carpus down to the dorsal aspect of the digits. Damage to this nerve can result in paralysis of the elbow extensor muscles, the carpal and digital extensor muscles and loss of skin tone and sensation
- The median nerve, which derives from the last cervical and first thoracic nerves (C8–T1). It courses along the medial surface of the upper forelimb and enters the antebrachium by the medial collateral ligament of the elbow joint. It innervates the flexor muscles of the carpus and digits and therefore overlaps (to some degree) with the innervation of the ulnar nerve. Due to this overlap, damage to the median nerve is often not easily identified in the movement of the animal
- The ulnar nerve, which is derived from the most caudal part of the brachial plexus (C8–T2). It follows the path of the median nerve until it moves towards the olecranon and crosses the elbow joint caudally. It innervates the skin over the lateral aspect of the forefoot and caudal aspect of the antebrachium, as well as the small muscles of the foot (e.g. the interosseous muscle) and the carpal and digital flexor muscles. Damage to this nerve is not often clinically obvious due to the overlap with median nerve function
- The sciatic or ischiadic nerve, which is derived from the most caudal aspect of the lumbosacral plexus (L6–S2). It courses through the middle and deep gluteal muscles, then it moves caudal to the greater trochanter, and runs distally between the biceps femoris and semitendinosus muscles. It divides into the peroneal and tibial nerves, which innervate the lateral and medial lower hindlimb. Damage to this nerve, therefore, is likely to affect the control of the entire lower hindlimb (caudal to the stifle), as well as sensory/skin control
- The femoral nerve, which derives from the cranial part of the lumbosacral plexus (L4–L6). It passes through the psoas muscles with the external iliac artery and vein, runs through the thigh between the sartorius and pectineus muscles, before becoming the saphenous nerve over the caudal femur, which then goes on to innervate the medial hindlimb. The femoral nerve innervates the quadriceps muscle principally, and so damage results in an inability to extend the stifle joint.

Spinal reflexes

Due to the dual sensory and motor function of the spinal nerves, they can form a reflex arc from sensory organ to spinal cord and then motor function, without going via the brain. Spinal reflexes (e.g. patellar reflex) can be used to ascertain whether there has been damage to the nerves at a local level. They do not indicate whether the spinal cord is intact above the reflex arc. However, if the animal vocalizes or turns to look at the site where the stimulus is being performed, this indicates that the sensation has been perceived at a higher, conscious level in the brain; therefore, the spinal cord above the reflex must be intact.

These reflex arcs are often referred to as:

- Monosynaptic – when there is only one synapse/connection and therefore only two nerves involved with the reflex
- Polysynaptic – when there is more than one synapse and therefore more than two nerves involved with the reflex.

Neurons in other segments of the spinal cord can also modify reflex arcs. If the modifying neurons are situated above the reflex arc, they are called upper motor neurons. If the modifying neurons are located below the reflex arc (rare), they are called lower motor neurons. When testing, if the reflex response is present but exaggerated, it may indicate that although the nerves responsible for the reflex arc are intact, the modifying nerves above or below that segment in the spinal cord may be damaged.

Reflex arcs can be overridden by the brain. For example, the local reflex may be to remove a limb from a noxious stimulus; however, the brain can override this reflex in order to keep the limb where it is. These are called conditioned reflexes and are learned.

Common reflex arcs

- **Pedal reflex:** This is also known as the flexor or withdrawal reflex in response to a painful stimulus. Pain receptors present in the skin are stimulated, resulting in flexion of the muscles to move the limb away from the stimulus
- **Panniculus reflex:** This is a twitch response of the skin over the back in response to a stimulus in that area
- **Patellar reflex:** Tapping the patellar ligament stretches the quadriceps muscle, which in turn results in contraction of the quadriceps muscle. This contraction causes the lower limb to be extended
- **Anal reflex:** This is a twitch response of the anal sphincter in response to a touch stimulus of the perianal skin

---

Autonomic nervous system (ANS)

This is the unconscious visceral nervous system, which supplies motor innervation to most of the vital organs (heart, gut, bladder) as well as to the endocrine and exocrine glands. There are two aspects to the ANS (Figure 3.44):

- Sympathetic nervous system
- Parasympathetic nervous system.

Sympathetic nervous system

This is the system of 'fright, flight and fight' and is responsible for a number of functions (Figure 3.45). The preganglionic

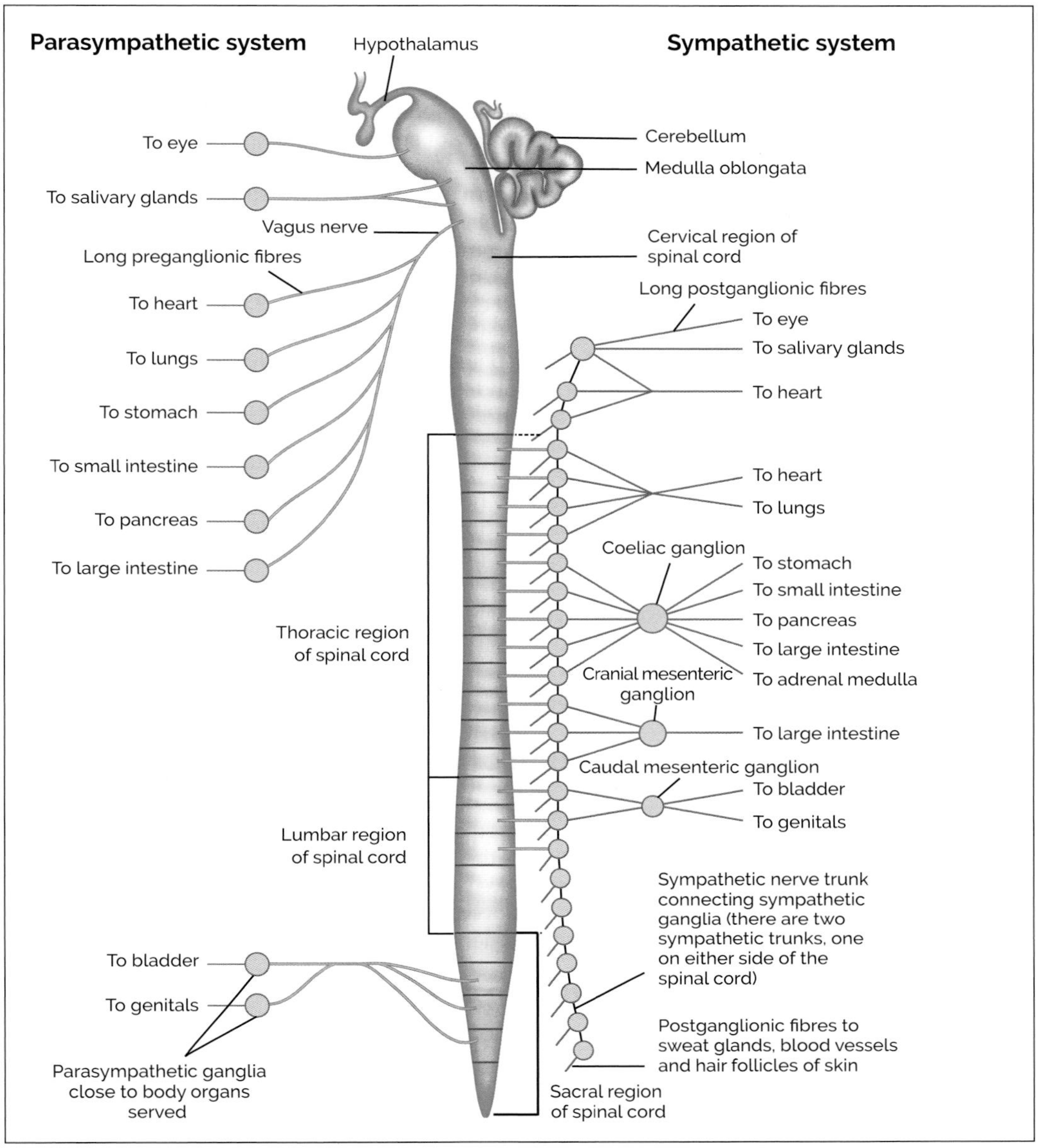

Parasympathetic system   **Sympathetic system**

Hypothalamus

To eye

To salivary glands

Vagus nerve

Long preganglionic fibres

To heart

To lungs

To stomach

To small intestine

To pancreas

To large intestine

Cerebellum

Medulla oblongata

Cervical region of spinal cord

Long postganglionic fibres

To eye

To salivary glands

To heart

To heart

To lungs

Coeliac ganglion

To stomach
To small intestine
To pancreas
To large intestine
To adrenal medulla

Cranial mesenteric ganglion

To large intestine

Caudal mesenteric ganglion

To bladder

To genitals

Thoracic region of spinal cord

Lumbar region of spinal cord

Sympathetic nerve trunk connecting sympathetic ganglia (there are two sympathetic trunks, one on either side of the spinal cord)

To bladder

To genitals

Postganglionic fibres to sweat glands, blood vessels and hair follicles of skin

Parasympathetic ganglia close to body organs served

Sacral region of spinal cord

3.44 The autonomic nervous system.

Structure innervated	Sympathetic effect	Parasympathetic effect
Bladder	Relaxes bladder muscle Increases bladder sphincter tone	Contracts bladder muscle Decreases bladder sphincter tone
Eyes	Dilates pupil Relaxes ciliary muscle (lens becomes flattened for far vision)	Constricts pupil Contracts ciliary muscle (lens becomes more convex for near vision)
Gastrointestinal tract	Reduces activity of the gut and stomach Inhibits secretions from the pancreas Dries salivary secretions	Increases activity of the gut and stomach Increases secretions from the pancreas Increases salivary secretions
Heart	Increases heart rate Increases contractility Increases conduction velocity of the atrioventricular node	Decreases heart rate Decreases contractility Decreases conduction velocity of the atrioventricular node
Lungs	Dilates bronchioles Increases respiratory rate Inhibits secretions	Constricts bronchioles Decreases respiratory rate Increases secretions
Skin	Causes piloerection Localized secretion from sweat glands (paws)	No effect on hairs Generalized secretion from sweat glands
Uterus	Gravid: contracts uterus Non-gravid: relaxes uterus	Variable response

3.45 Functions of the sympathetic and parasympathetic nervous systems.

nerves arise from the first thoracic through to the fourth lumbar vertebral space. They then pass into the ventral roots of the first thoracic to fourth lumbar spinal nerves, before exiting and joining the ganglia of the sympathetic trunk. The sympathetic trunk runs parallel to the spinal cord along the length of the neck and back, starting at the cranial cervical ganglion and ending in the diffuse splitting of nerves into the tail region (see Figure 3.44). For this reason, the preganglionic nerves of the sympathetic nervous system are short, whereas the postganglionic fibres are long.

Parasympathetic nervous system

The parasympathetic nervous system generally opposes the actions of the sympathetic nervous system (see Figure 3.45). The preganglionic neurons originate as discrete nuclei in the brainstem. They are often distributed within the cranial nerves (e.g. oculomotor, facial, glossopharyngeal and vagal). There is also a sacral outflow of the parasympathetic nervous system, which arises from S1–S2 and innervates the pelvic organs such as the bladder and genitals. The preganglionic nerves of the parasympathetic nervous system are long, whereas the postganglionic fibres are short.

Special senses

The special senses are smell, sight, hearing, taste and touch.

Smell

There are numerous sensory neurons (olfactory nerves) responsible for conducting the sensation of smell to the brain. The olfactory nerves traverse small holes in the cribriform plate of the ethmoid bone (the rostral part of the calvarium, the bone that immediately surrounds the brain) and pass directly into the olfactory lobe of the brain. The olfactory lobe is situated close to the nasal cavity. For a smell to be detected, molecules are trapped in the mucus lining the caudal nasal passages and dissolved. This creates a chemical reaction that stimulates the nerve endings. The vomeronasal organ (organ of Jacobson), which consists of two narrow parallel ducts in the rostral hard palate, also conducts the sensation of smell to the brain. The entrances to these two ducts sit immediately caudal to the incisors. The ducts are blind ending, covered in olfactory epithelium and communicate with the olfactory bulb of the brain. In mammals, they are thought to be associated with pheromone detection (lip curl or Flehmen reaction in domestic animals). In reptiles, they are particularly well developed and are also involved in prey detection in species such as snakes (see below).

Dogs

Dogs have some of the most tightly coiled nasal conchae of any animal, which increase the surface area of the nasal cavity and enhance the sense of smell.

Birds

Most birds have a reduced reliance on their sense of smell compared with mammals and reptiles. The nostrils are generally found at the base of the beak; however, in waterfowl they may be found more rostrally, and in birds such as the kiwi they may be found on the very distal tip of the beak.

Reptiles

Reptiles can detect smells via the sensory mucosa in the nasal passages in conjunction with the olfactory nerves. However, those reptiles (such as snakes) that particularly utilize their sense of smell for hunting also have an enlarged vomeronasal organ (organ of Jacobson) in the maxilla. The tongue darts out of the mouth and traps the scent molecules in the saliva coating its surface. The tongue is then withdrawn and the tip immediately pushed into this organ in the roof of the mouth. In addition to the identification and tracking of prey, the well developed vomeronasal organ is also used for sexual pheromone detection.

Some reptiles also appear to have additional 'nostrils' located around the maxilla. In the case of boid snakes, these pits are found around the upper lip; in the case of some vipers, there are two small pits that face cranially located between the eye and the true nares. These are heat-sensitive pores and not nostrils at all. In boids these pores are not very sensitive, but do allow the snake to locate prey in the dark. In pit vipers the pores are highly sensitive to heat differences and because they face forward have 'binocular' heat-sensing capabilities, allowing the snake to accurately judge how far the prey is in front of them.

Sight

Position of the eyes

In predators (e.g. cats and dogs) the eyes are to the front of the head, whereas in prey species (e.g. rabbits) the eyes are to the side of the head to give a greater field of vision. Cats, in particular, have excellent binocular vision (i.e. the field of view of each eye overlaps, allowing good depth perception). This is essential when hunting prey.

Structure of the eyes

The anatomy of the eye is shown in Figure 3.46.

Sclera and cornea

The sclera ('white' of the eye) is the opaque outer protective coating of the eye. The muscles responsible for movement of the eye (see below) originate at the sclera and attach to the periosteum.

The cornea is the transparent outer protective coating of the eye. The cornea does not normally contain any blood vessels; however, in some diseases blood vessels can enter the cornea, resulting in areas of opacity. Corneal cells receive their nutrition from the lacrimal fluid and aqueous humour. The cornea is very sensitive to stimuli due to the presence of numerous nerve endings (branches of the ophthalmic nerve). The closing of the eyelids in response to something touching the cornea is known as the corneal reflex.

The junction at which the sclera and cornea meet is known as the limbus.

Uvea

Beneath the outer connective tissue layer, is the vascular layer. This consists of:

- Choroid – found underneath the sclera, from the optic nerve to the limbus
- Ciliary body – found adjacent to the limbus
- Iris – found anterior to the ciliary body.

The choroid contains blood vessels. Situated in the dorsal part of the choroid is the tapetum lucidum, an area that

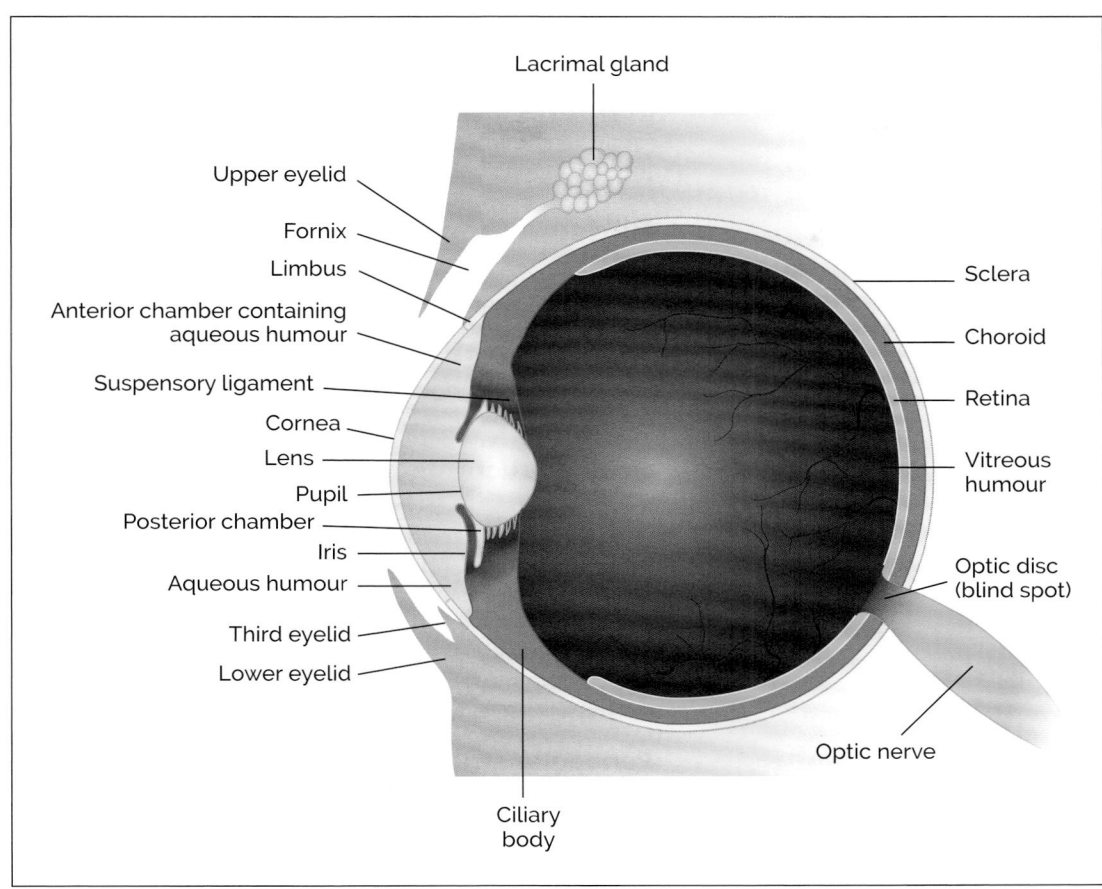

reflects light and aids vision in the dark. It is this structure that makes the eyes of dogs and cats shine in the headlights of a car. The colour of the tapetum lucidum varies according to age and breed in dogs. In puppies it has a blue/violet appearance, which changes to green/yellow as the animal gets older.

The ciliary body suspends the lens via zonular fibres, which collectively are known as the suspensory ligament. The ciliary muscle controls the shape of the lens.

The iris consists of pigment cells, which give colour to the eye, and smooth muscle, which controls the amount of light entering the eye by contracting and dilating the pupil.

The space between the lens and the cornea is filled with aqueous humour. This space is divided into an anterior chamber (between the iris and the cornea) and a posterior chamber (between the iris and the lens).

Retina

The retina contains light-sensitive cells and is connected to the brain via the optic nerve. The retina comprises different layers of cells:

- Pigmented cells (outer layer)
- Receptor cells (rods are responsible for black and white vision; cones are responsible for colour vision)
- Bipolar ganglion cells
- Multipolar ganglion cells.

Situated where the optic nerve exits the eye is the optic disc. There is no retina in the area of the optic disc, so this is a blind spot. A series of blood vessels run across the surface of the retina, arising from the retinal artery and radiating out from the optic disc. These blood vessels supply nutrients and oxygen to the cells of the retina.

The vitreous body is found caudal to the lens and consists of vitreous humour and connective fibres. The vitreous body maintains the shape of the eye.

Eyelids

The upper and lower eyelids join at the medial and lateral canthi (singular: canthus) and are secured by the palpebral ligaments. Each eyelid consists of a thin outer layer of skin, overlying a musculofibrous layer. At the edge of the eyelid (next to the eye) is a more fibrous area known as the tarsus, which gives structure to the eyelid. Along the margin of the eyelid are Meibomian glands (tarsal glands), which secrete an oily material. Located beside these glands are the eyelashes or cilia. The inner surface of the eyelid is lined by conjunctiva.

Located at the ventromedial aspect of the eye is the third eyelid. This is not a true eyelid but a T-shaped piece of cartilage, the nictitating membrane, covered by conjunctiva. The third eyelid provides protection for the eyeball and secretions from the Harderian gland.

Lacrimal gland

Situated dorsolaterally to the eye is the lacrimal gland. This is responsible for tear production. Lacrimal fluid is spread across the eye by blinking, and drains from the eye through the punctum lacrimale found at the medial aspect of the lower lid. The punctum lacrimale is connected to the nasolacrimal duct, which drains into the nasal cavity.

Movement of the eyes

Movement of the eyes is controlled by the muscles attached to the sclera, including:

- Retractor bulbi muscle
- Dorsal rectus muscle
- Ventral rectus muscle
- Medial rectus muscle
- Lateral rectus muscle
- Dorsal oblique muscle
- Ventral oblique muscle.

These muscles are supplied by a number of cranial nerves, including:

- Oculomotor nerve
- Trochlear nerve
- Abducens nerve
- Facial nerve
- Trigeminal nerve, which is responsible for transmitting sensory information from the eye.

Formation of an image

The formation of an image can be considered as a four step process:

1. Light rays from an object pass:
   a. Through the cornea and the pupil to hit the lens:
      - The cornea plays a part in focusing the light on to the retina
      - The iris alters in size and controls the amount of light entering the eye.
   b. Through the lens to be focused on to the retina:
      - The curvature of the lens is altered by the ciliary muscles and focuses the light rays on to the retina.
   c. Through the layers of the retina to the photoreceptor cells. Some light is reflected back to the retina by the tapetum lucidum to stimulate more receptor cells.
2. Resulting nerve impulses, generated by the photoreceptors, travel along the nerve fibres of the optic nerve to the brain.
3. On the ventral surface of the brain, a proportion of nerve fibres cross via the optic chiasma to opposite sides of the brain so that each cerebral hemisphere receives information from both eyes.
4. Information is carried to the visual cortex of the cerebral hemispheres, where it is interpreted as an image. The image formed on the retina is smaller than the original and inverted but the brain automatically modifies it.

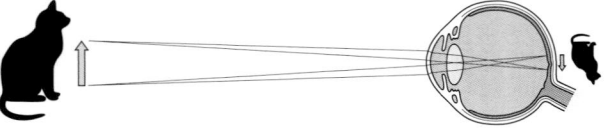

Small mammals

Most commonly kept small mammals are prey species and thus have laterally situated eyes. In the rabbit there is little binocular vision; each eye provides a separate image to the brain to be interpreted. This gives the rabbit a near 360-degree field of view. The third eyelid contains a large amount of lymphoid tissue, which can become reactive and swell when stimulated by antigens. The Harderian gland also enlarges in bucks during the breeding season. The single large punctum lacrimale in the lower lid is easy to cannulate for flushing the tear duct or for injecting radiopaque dye for the investigation of nasolacrimal duct disease.

Birds

Sight is the main sense in birds; therefore, they have relatively large eyes compared with body size. Birds have excellent colour vision. Predators (such as the raptors) tend to have more forward-facing eyes, which provide binocular vision; prey species tend to have more laterally placed eyes, enabling a wider field of vision.

Ocular structures

Birds have large pear-shaped eyeballs. Small bones (scleral ossicles) support the anterior globe at the junction of the sclera and cornea. The surface of the retina has no obvious blood vessels; instead there is a pecten oculi, a vascular plexus of capillaries near the optic disc, which provides nutrients to the inside of the eye. The iris comprises both skeletal and smooth muscle; therefore, constriction and dilatation of the pupil is partially under voluntary control.

Periocular structures

Birds have an infraorbital sinus, which has only soft tissue in the lateral wall. This means sinusitis results in puffing around the eye. The lower (main) eyelid is devoid of glands. There is a nictitating membrane that lies on the medial aspect of the eye. Ocular movement is limited as the globe is so large; however, it is possible for each eye to move independently. Occasionally, there is no bony septum between the eyes and the structures are so large that they touch one another.

Reptiles

The upper and lower eyelids in snakes are fused over the corneal surface, forming the transparent 'spectacle', which is shed with the rest of the skin each time the snake sloughs.

Some reptile species have a parietal or third eye, which plays a role in seasonal rhythms (e.g. sexual activity) (see 'Brain', earlier).

Hearing

The ear has two main functions: hearing and balance. The ear consists of three parts (Figure 3.47):

- Outer ear
- Middle ear
- Inner ear.

Outer ear

The outer ear consists of the auricle (pinna or ear flap) and the external acoustic meatus (ear canal). The auricle comprises cartilage (auricular cartilage) covered with skin. It is funnel-shaped, although this can vary between species and breeds, and can be moved toward the source of a sound. The ear canal is formed from cartilage and bone. It is lined with epithelium, which has a high concentration of ceruminous (wax secreting) and sebaceous glands. The ear canal is L-shaped, making treatment of external ear disease difficult in some cases.

3.47 Cross-section through the ear.

Diagram labels: Pinna (external ear); Petrous temporal bone; Stapes; Incus; Semicircular ducts (canals) surrounded by perilymph; Endolymphatic sac; Malleus; Vertical portion of ear canal; Vestibule; Saccule; External acoustic meatus; Horizontal portion of ear canal; Cochlear duct surrounded by perilymph; Tympanic membrane; Tympanic cavity; Auditory (Eustachian) tube (from pharynx)

Middle ear

The middle part of the ear is found within the temporal bone of the skull. Situated between the outer ear canal and the middle ear is the tympanic membrane (ear drum); this transmits sound vibrations to the middle ear. The middle ear contains the three auditory ossicles, known as the malleus (hammer; attached to the ear drum), incus (anvil) and stapes (stirrup).

The ventral part of the temporal bone expands into the tympanic bulla, which is very prominent in some species. It is thought that the tympanic bulla improves hearing ability. The auditory (Eustachian) tube connects the middle ear to the nasopharynx. It is responsible for ensuring equalization of air pressure between the middle ear and the atmosphere; it does this by opening slightly when the animal swallows (the sensation of ear 'popping' when you ascend in an aeroplane).

Inner ear

Located within the inner ear are the bony canals, which contain perilymph. Within these are the delicate membranous canals that contain endolymph. Together, these form semicircular ducts (canals), which allow the animal to maintain balance, and the cochlea, which is involved with hearing.

The endolymph in the semi-circular canals contains hairs and crystals. The crystals move in response to movement of the head, resulting in stimulation of the hairs. These minute hairs are connected to nerves, which coalesce to form the vestibulocochlear nerve, allowing transmission of movement to the brain. The three semi-circular canals are arranged at right angles to one another, thus providing a three-dimensional (3D) form, allowing the brain to determine the movement and position of the head more accurately.

The cochlea is shaped like the shell of a snail and is filled with fluid. This fluid allows the reverberation of sound to stimulate nerve endings. These impulses are transmitted via the vestibulocochlear nerve to the brain, which then interprets them as sound. Between the semi-circular canals and the cochlea are the utricle and saccule, which are principally responsible for interpretation of linear acceleration and thus help control posture and balance.

Small mammals

The rabbit has elongated pinnae, which have an excellent blood supply. The lateral/marginal ear vein is used for blood sampling and intravenous drug administration. Chinchillas have a very prominent tympanic bulla.

Birds

Birds have no pinnae, but often have a very short external ear canal before the tympanic membrane. The outer ear is frequently covered by short feathers. There is one auditory ossicle, the columella, attached medially to the vestibular window and laterally to the extracolumella cartilage, which in turn connects with the tympanic membrane. The cochlea is only slightly curved and has a blind-ending apex, known as the lagena, the function of which is not clearly understood.

Reptiles

Chelonians and lizards possess a tympanic membrane, but have only one auditory ossicle. Snakes do not have ears; the single auditory ossicle connects with the quadrate bone of the skull, allowing vibrations to be sensed and transmitted to the brain. Reptiles do not have a cochlea but do have a well developed semi-circular duct system. This suggests that the ears are mainly used for balance rather than hearing. However, it is clear that reptiles can 'hear' or detect both ground and air vibrations.

Taste

The taste buds are the primary organ for flavour detection. Dogs and cats have numerous taste buds scattered across the surface of the tongue, soft palate and epiglottis. As with the detection of smell, the chemical causing the 'taste' (gustation) dissolves in the mucus/saliva and stimulates the taste buds. Sensory signals are then sent via the facial, glossopharyngeal or vagus nerves, depending upon the location of the taste bud, to the brainstem.

Birds

Birds have a reduced number of taste buds, but can still readily discern different flavours.

Reptiles

Taste buds in a vestigial form have been found scattered across the oral mucosa and tongue in most reptiles.

Touch

Touch receptors are present in the skin (for details on the anatomy of the skin, see 'Integument', below) alongside receptors for pain, heat, pressure and cold.

- Pain receptors are present in the epidermis as free nerve endings.
- Bulbous corpuscle endings are present in the dermis and are stimulated by heat or cold. These nerve endings are encapsulated.
- Lamellar corpuscles comprise concentric layers of cells in the subcutis, which respond to pressure.
- Meniscoid corpuscles end in cup-shaped discs in the dermis and epidermis and act as touch receptors. Tactile hairs (vibrissae) on the muzzle and eyes are also responsible for the sensation of touch.

Small mammals

Many small mammals have tactile hairs around their muzzles and lower lips. For example, rabbits cannot see beneath the mouth and so rely on the tactile hairs to locate food.

Birds

Birds have tactile bristles around the beak and face.

Reptiles

Rudimentary corpuscles have been described in the skin of reptiles, particularly around the mouth and ventral aspect of the body (especially snakes). These corpuscles allow reptiles to interpret their surroundings. Reptiles do have heat receptors, but do not seem to respond to intense heat; therefore, they should be protected from heat lamps as severe thermal burns can result if the animal is too close to a heat source for a prolonged period of time.

Cardiovascular system

The cardiovascular system consists of the vessels and organs involved in the transport of blood around the body. The main components are the heart, arteries, veins and blood.

Heart

Anatomy

The heart (Figure 3.48) is responsible for pumping blood continuously around the body. It sits in the thorax within the mediastinum. Anterior to the heart in young animals is the thymus. The heart is surrounded by a sac known as the pericardium, which is attached to the base of the heart. This sac is also attached to structures surrounding the heart and keeps it in place in the thorax. The layer of pericardium in contact with the heart is known as the visceral pericardium; the outer layer is known as the parietal pericardium. The pericardium contains a small amount of pericardial fluid, which allows the heart to contract freely within the pericardium.

The heart has three layers of cardiac muscle: the epicardium (outer layer), the myocardium (thick middle layer) and the endocardium (thin and relatively smooth inner layer).

The heart consists of four chambers: right atrium, left atrium, right ventricle and left ventricle. The wall of the left ventricle is much thicker than that of the right ventricle; this can be appreciated on a visual examination of the heart. The right side of the heart is separated from the left side by a septum or wall of tissue that runs the length of the heart. Between the left and right atria this is known as the interatrial septum, and between the left and right ventricles it is known as the interventricular septum. On the outside of the heart, the atria and ventricles are separated by the coronary groove, which contains the major vessels of the coronary artery.

The atria and ventricles are also separated by atrioventricular (AV) valves. Valves are present in the heart to prevent blood from flowing backwards (i.e. from the ventricles into the atria). The AV valves are attached to papillary muscles (projections from the heart wall) via strands of tissue known as chordae tendinae. The chordae tendinae allow the AV valves to move, resulting in blood from the atria entering the ventricles. However, when the ventricles contract the chordae tendinae prevent the AV valves from swinging back into the atria, thus ensuring that the valves remain blood-tight. The combination of AV valves and chordae tendinae has the appearance of a parachute.

The AV valve between the right atrium and right ventricle is known as the tricuspid valve as it has three cusps or segments. The AV valve between the left atrium and left ventricle is known as the bicuspid or mitral valve and has two cusps. In addition to the tricuspid and bicuspid valves, there are also valves present where blood leaves the right ventricle and enters the pulmonary artery (pulmonary valve) and where blood leaves the left ventricle and enters the aorta (aortic valve). The pulmonary and aortic valves are also known as semilunar valves because of their half-moon shape.

Contraction

- Contraction of the heart is known as systole.
- Relaxation of the heart is known as diastole.

The heart contracts due to electrical activity in the cardiac muscle cells. A conduction system (Figure 3.49) allows the transmission of electrical impulses in a controlled

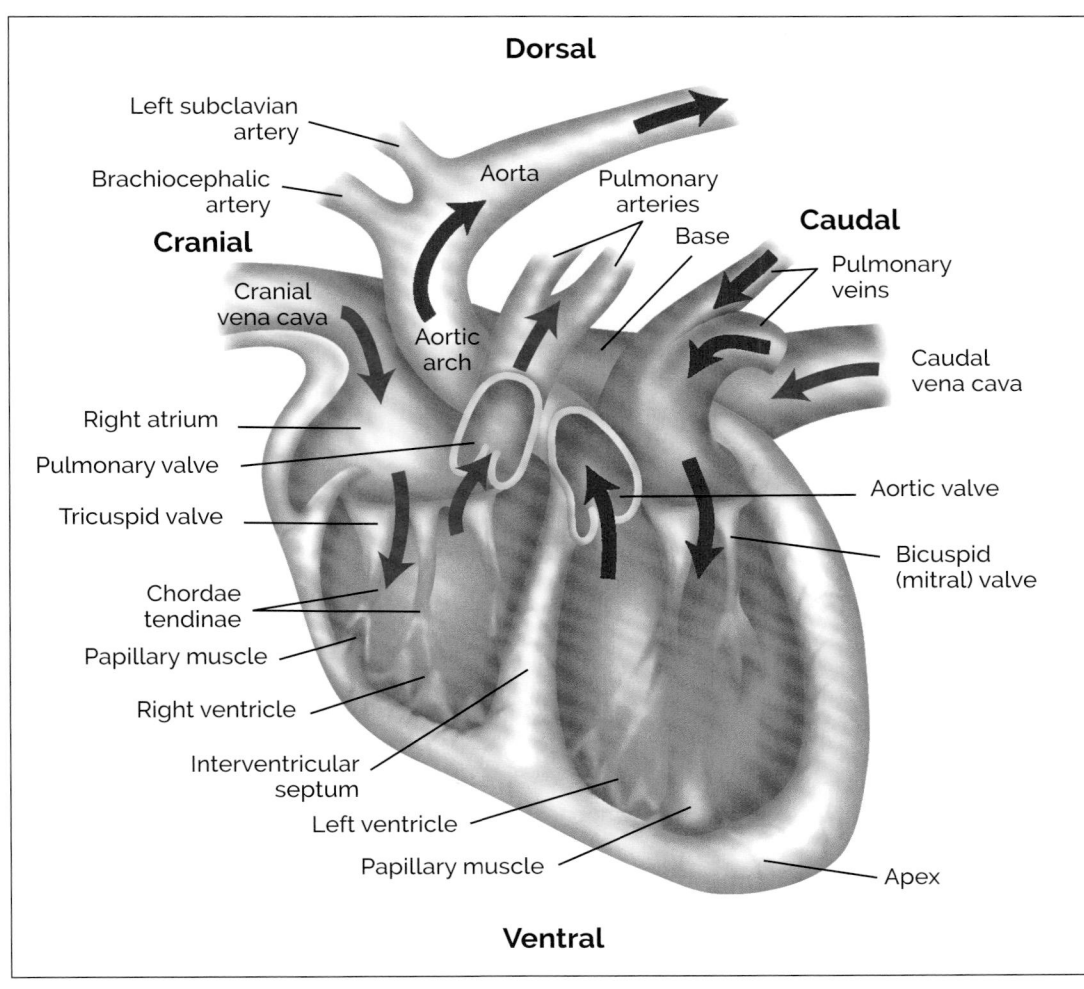

Dorsal

Left subclavian artery

Brachiocephalic artery

Cranial

Aorta

Pulmonary arteries

Base

Caudal

Pulmonary veins

Cranial vena cava

Aortic arch

Caudal vena cava

Right atrium

Pulmonary valve

Tricuspid valve

Aortic valve

Bicuspid (mitral) valve

Chordae tendinae

Papillary muscle

Right ventricle

Interventricular septum

Left ventricle

Papillary muscle

Apex

Ventral

3.48 The structure of the heart and direction of blood flow.

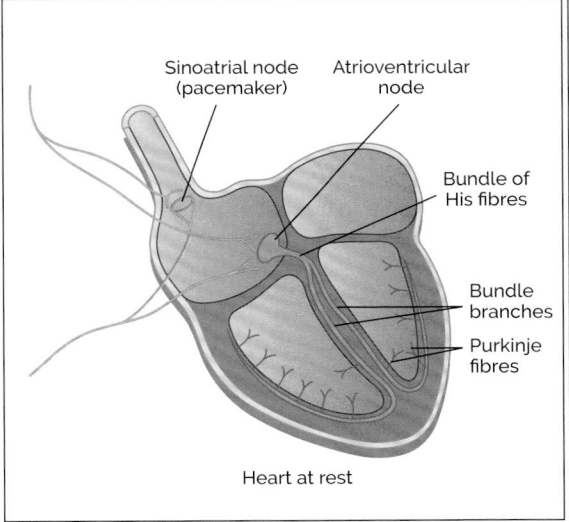

Sinoatrial node (pacemaker)

Atrioventricular node

Bundle of His fibres

Bundle branches

Purkinje fibres

Heart at rest

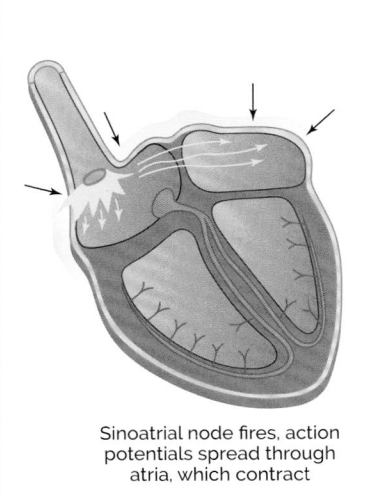

Sinoatrial node fires, action potentials spread through atria, which contract

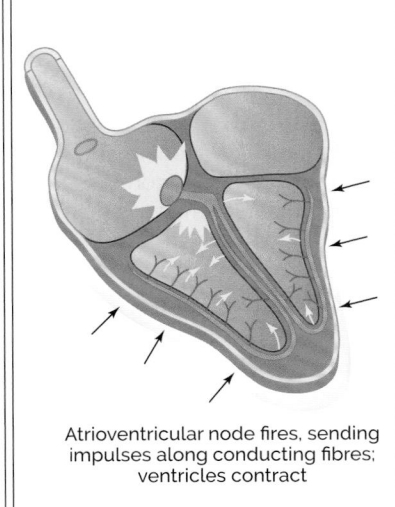

Atrioventricular node fires, sending impulses along conducting fibres; ventricles contract

3.49 The conduction mechanism of the heart.

manner, resulting in contraction of the heart. Abnormalities in the conduction system can lead to irregularities in the rhythm of contraction, known as arrhythmias.

Within the heart there are specialized areas of cells that control the rate at which the heart contracts. These areas are called pacemakers, and are predominantly located in the sinoatrial (SA) node (Figure 3.49a). The SA node is the beginning of the conduction system and initiates a wave of contraction in the atria (Figure 3.49b). The electrical impulse then passes to a second group of specialized cells located at the top of the interventricular septum. This area is called the atrioventricular (AV) node. From the AV node the impulse travels down the interventricular septum in the bundle of His (Figure 3.49c). The electrical impulse is then distributed to the ventricles in the part of the conduction system known as the Purkinje fibres/tissue. These structures are not apparent to the naked eye but can be seen under a microscope. The nerve fibres directly innervate the cardiac muscle cells.

There is a potential difference across the cell membrane of a cardiac muscle cell, with the inside of the cell being more negatively charged. When the cell is stimulated, the permeability of the cell membrane to potassium and sodium is altered; sodium moves into the cell and potassium moves out. This results in an electrical impulse and contraction of the cell.

Heart sounds

Closure of the AV valves due to contraction of the ventricles results in the first heart sound ('lub'), which can be heard on auscultation. In most animals, closure of the right and left AV valves cannot be heard separately; however, in conditions where this does arise it results in a 'split' first heart sound. Closure of the pulmonary and aortic valves (predominately the aortic valve) following contraction and emptying of blood from the ventricles results in the second heart sound ('dub'); this signals the end of systole.

Blood pressure

Due to contraction and relaxation of the heart, the pressure within the blood vessels is constantly changing. The pressure in the blood vessels when the heart contracts is known as the systolic pressure. The pressure when the heart relaxes is the diastolic pressure. Measurement of blood pressure using an inflatable cuff and Doppler probe on a distal limb determines only the systolic pressure.

Small mammals

In rabbits the heart is relatively small compared with overall body mass. In addition, the right AV valve has only two cusps.

Birds

In birds the heart is relatively large compared with body mass. It has a sinus venosus, which is formed at the confluence of the right cranial vena cava and caudal vena cava. The sinus venosus is separated from the right atrium by two muscular SA valves. The right AV valve has a single muscular flap and no chordae. The AV bundle gives off a fascicle, which encircles the AV opening and innervates the right AV valve. The pulmonary veins combine to form a single vessel before entering the left atrium. The entrance to the vein is guarded by a valve to prevent reflux.

Reptiles

In reptiles the heart has three chambers: two atria and a common ventricle. A fourth chamber is present in the form of the sinus venosus, which is separated from the right atrium by two valves. The pacemaker for the heart is believed to lie within the wall of the sinus venosus. The single ventricle functionally separates oxygenated and deoxygenated blood via a series of muscular ridges.

Arteries

Anatomy

The wall of an artery consists of three layers known as tunics (Figure 3.50).

- The internal tunic (tunica interna or tunica intima) is thin and consists of endothelium.
- The middle tunic (tunica media) is the thickest layer and comprises elastic tissue and smooth muscle.

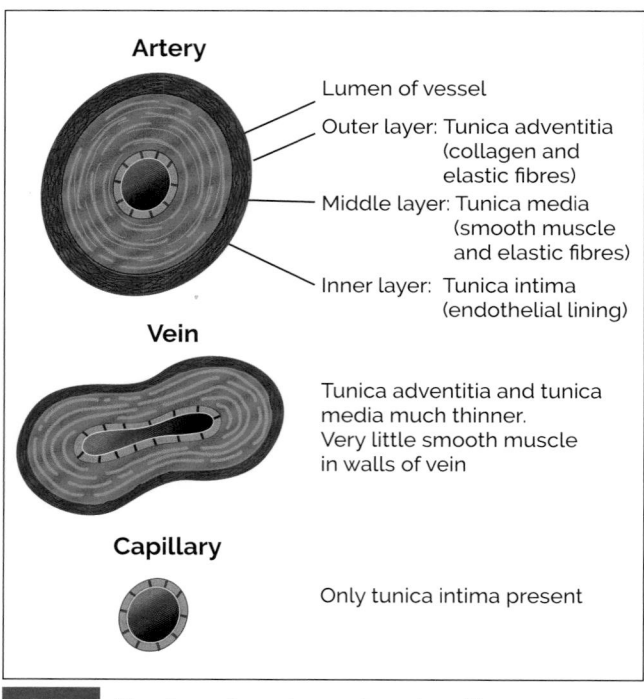

3.50 Structure of an artery, vein and capillary.

- The outer tunic (tunica adventitia) is made up of connective tissue. Within this layer in large arteries are small blood vessels, which supply nutrition to the artery itself. This is because it is not possible for large arteries to absorb nutrients directly from the bloodstream due to the thickness of the arterial wall.

The artery is designed to withstand the high pressure of blood from the heart. Elastic tissue is important in the arterial wall because it allows the artery to expand during systole, when blood is being forced around the body, and to recoil during diastole, when the heart relaxes. Recoil of the arteries also forces blood around the body. The smooth muscle controls the diameter of the artery and regulates the flow of blood to different organs. Due to the presence of elastic tissue and muscle, arteries do not need valves to control blood flow. As the arteries get smaller there is a larger proportion of smooth muscle to elastic tissue.

Arterial system

The main artery is the aorta, which arises from the left ventricle of the heart and travels in a caudal direction underneath the vertebrae dorsally. The aorta has many branches (Figure 3.51), which supply the major organs, including:

- The coronary artery, which supplies the heart muscle
- The brachiocephalic trunk, which divides into the common carotid and subclavian arteries
- There is a common carotid artery on the left and right side of the body. These vessels arise separately and travel up either side of the neck. The common carotid artery ends by dividing at the level of the larynx into the external and internal carotid arteries. These vessels supply the structures of the head
- The subclavian artery supplies the forelimb, neck and cervicothoracic area. There is a subclavian artery on the left and right sides of the body. The subclavian artery becomes the axillary artery and continues as the brachial artery as it passes down the forelimb

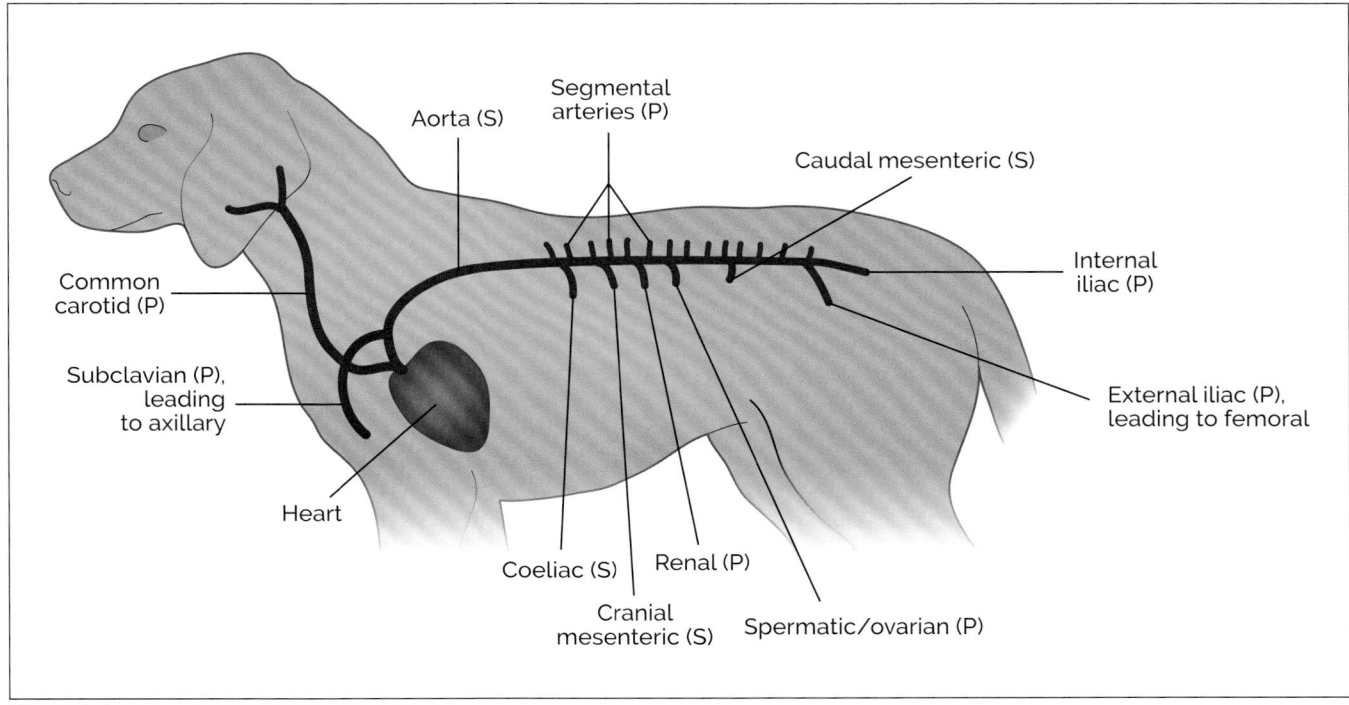

3.51 Diagrammatic representation of the major arteries of the dog. P = paired vessels. S = single vessel.

- The renal arteries, which supply the kidneys and adrenal glands
- The ovarian/testicular arteries, which supply the gonads
- The coeliac artery, which supplies the stomach, spleen and liver
- The cranial mesenteric artery, which supplies the small intestine
- The caudal mesenteric artery, which supplies the large intestine
- The external iliac artery, which branches into the femoral artery. The femoral artery supplies the hindlimbs
- The internal iliac artery, which supplies the pelvic organs.

Arteries continuously split into smaller and smaller vessels, like branches of a tree. As arteries become smaller they are known as arterioles.

Birds

In birds the aorta curves to the right rather than to the left as in mammals. The common carotid artery is very short and divides rapidly in the base of the neck to form the vertebral artery and the internal carotid artery. The subclavian artery provides a large pectoral trunk to the pectoral muscles. The kidneys are supplied by a cranial, middle and caudal artery. The pelvic limbs are supplied by an ischial artery, which continues in the thigh as the femoral artery. The ischiatic artery (larger than the femoral artery) also supplies the leg and divides distally into the popliteal and cranial tibial arteries.

Reptiles

In reptiles two aortas exit the heart (right and left), which merge to form a single abdominal aorta halfway down the body. The common carotid artery bifurcates in the neck region and connects to the carotid duct to form the right and left internal and external carotid arteries. There is a variable number of renal arteries in reptiles: 1–2 in snakes; up to 4–5 in agamids and chameleons.

Capillaries

When arterioles branch they divide into smaller vessels until the walls are only one cell thick: these vessels are known as capillaries (see Figure 3.50). The wall of a capillary comprises only the internal tunic (see above) and thus consists of endothelium. Capillaries form an interlacing network within the vital organs, allowing the exchange of fluid, gases and nutrients to and from the surrounding tissues. For this reason, capillaries are not watertight but are in fact full of small holes that allow molecules smaller than blood proteins to move by osmosis between the capillary lumen and the body cells.

Veins

Anatomy

Although similar in construction to arteries, the walls of veins are thinner (see Figure 3.50) and have valves along their length to prevent the backflow of blood. In addition, veins collapse in on themselves rather than holding their shape like arteries.

- The internal tunic is thin and does not have an elastic membrane. The main function of this layer is the formation of the valves. Each valve comprises two or three cusps. These valves are present in veins exposed to intermittent pressure and are greatest in number in veins leaving muscles and in the distal limbs. These valves aid the movement of blood back to the heart and are necessary due to the much lower blood pressure found in veins compared with arteries.
- The middle tunic is thinner in veins than in arteries and consists of more smooth muscle than elastic tissue.
- The outer tunic consists of connective tissue.

Venous system

Blood returns to the right atrium of the heart via the venous system (Figure 3.52), including:

- The coronary sinus, which returns blood from the heart wall
- The cranial vena cava, which is formed by the junction of the external jugular and subclavian veins. The cranial vena cava runs through the thorax in the mediastinum
- There are two pairs of jugular veins within the neck: the internal jugular vein, which is located beside the common carotid artery; and the external jugular vein, which runs from the angle of the jaw, down the neck and into the thorax. The external jugular vein drains the head
- The subclavian vein drains the forelimbs and receives blood from the cephalic, radial and ulnar veins
- The caudal vena cava, which is a large vein that traverses the abdomen dorsally just underneath the spinal vertebrae. The right and left internal iliac veins from the pelvic area join together to form the caudal vena cava. The external iliac veins (which drain the hindlimbs) then join the caudal vena cava. As it passes through the abdomen towards the thorax, the renal and hepatic veins also join the caudal vena cava. The vessel passes through the diaphragm and into the thorax via the caval foramen, which is located in the ventral part of the diaphragm. The caudal vena cava then travels forward and enters the right atrium of the heart
- The azygous vein is formed by the union of the first lumbar veins, and passes into the thorax through the aortic hiatus in the diaphragm, where it receives blood from the intercostal veins. The azygous vein then travels forward and enters the right atrium. However, the anatomy of the azygous vein can vary between different species.

Venous blood sampling

For venous blood sampling, the following vessels are used:

- Cephalic vein – important sampling site in dogs and cats. Can also be used in ferrets and rabbits. This vein is usually too small to obtain a diagnostic sample in other small mammals
- Jugular vein – important sampling site in dogs and cats. Can also be used in ferrets, rabbits, guinea pigs and chinchillas. However, it should be noted that in rabbits the jugular vein is the predominant drainage for the periorbital region, therefore if a thrombus forms significant periocular oedema may occur
- Saphenous vein – used in ferrets, rabbits and guinea pigs. This vein is usually too small to obtain a diagnostic sample in other small mammals
- Marginal lateral (auricular, lateral) ear vein – used in rabbits.

Birds

There are no brachiocephalic veins in birds, instead the left and right cranial venae cavae are formed by the union of the jugular and subclavian veins. The right jugular vein is dominant and often 2–3 times the size of the left. The brachial/basilic vein drains the wing and can be seen running along the ventral surface caudal to the humerus; it may be used for collecting a blood sample. The external iliac vein (rather than the sciatic vein) provides the main drainage for the leg. The external iliac vein is derived from the femoral vein, which in turn is derived from the popliteal and tibial veins.

In birds a renal portal system is present, whereby venous blood from the hindlimbs and caudal end of the body can travel back to the heart either by passing through the renal parenchyma or by being diverted through other vessels. This

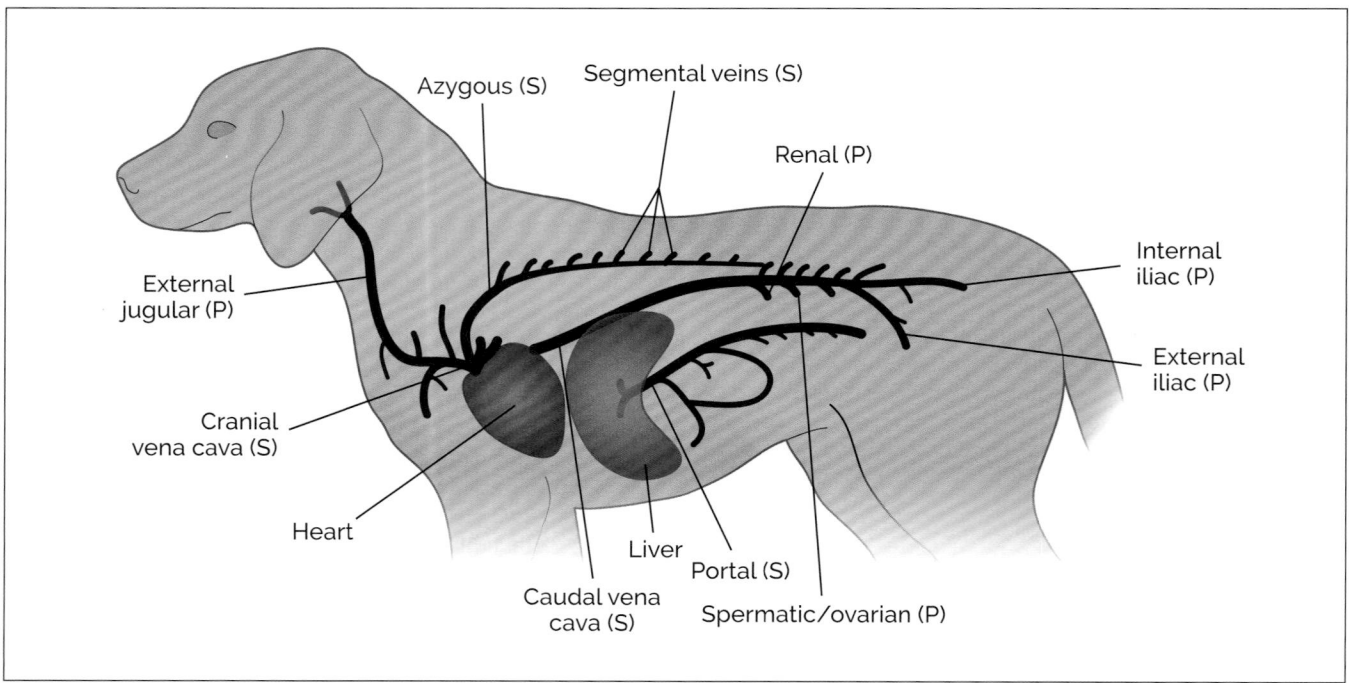

3.52 Diagrammatic representation of the major veins of the dog. P = paired vessels. S = single vessel.

means that any nephrotoxic drug injected into the legs or caudal half of the bird's body is likely to do more damage to the kidneys than if it were injected into the cranial half of the body.

Reptiles

In many reptiles, such as lizards, a midline ventral abdominal vein is present. The hepatic portal vein joins the ventral abdominal vein. A renal portal system is present and is a complex anastomosis of vessels, including the caudal and iliac veins. As with birds, the significance of the renal portal system is that blood from the caudal part of the body can pass through the kidneys prior to returning to the heart.

Blood

Blood comprises a cellular component and a fluid component. The cellular component consists of red blood cells, white blood cells and platelets. The blood cells have many different functions, including the carriage of oxygen, providing immunity and blood clotting. The fluid component consists of plasma, which contains many different proteins including albumin, globulins and nutrients.

Blood cells

Haemopoiesis

This is the process by which blood cells are produced from the bone marrow in the long bones, pelvis, sternum and skull in the young animal, and in the epiphyses of the long bones, pelvis, sternum and skull in the adult animal. The spleen and liver can also take part in production when there is an increased demand for blood cells.

Erythropoiesis

This is the process by which red blood cells (erythrocytes) are produced from the bone marrow (Figure 3.53). The process is stimulated by erythropoietin produced by the kidney. As red blood cells develop, the nucleus condenses and is present until the developing red cell becomes a reticulocyte. Reticulocytes are present predominantly in the bone marrow with only a few released into the circulation in the healthy cat and dog. However, in anaemia increased numbers of nucleated red blood cells and reticulocytes can be seen in the circulation.

Red blood cells

These are the most predominant type of blood cell. Mammalian red blood cells or erythrocytes are circular in shape with a depression in the centre, giving them a disc-like appearance. The depression in the centre on either side increases the surface area of the red blood cell and allows for a greater transfer of oxygen. Red blood cells contain haemoglobin, which is required to carry oxygen and gives the cells their red colour. Red blood cells are produced in the bone marrow (see above) and after entering the circulation survive for approximately 120 days. When the cells become damaged or die they are removed from the circulation by the spleen.

White blood cells

White blood cells or leucocytes (Figure 3.54) are involved in the cellular and humoral immune response (see Chapter 7) and comprise:

- Neutrophils
- Lymphocytes
- Eosinophils

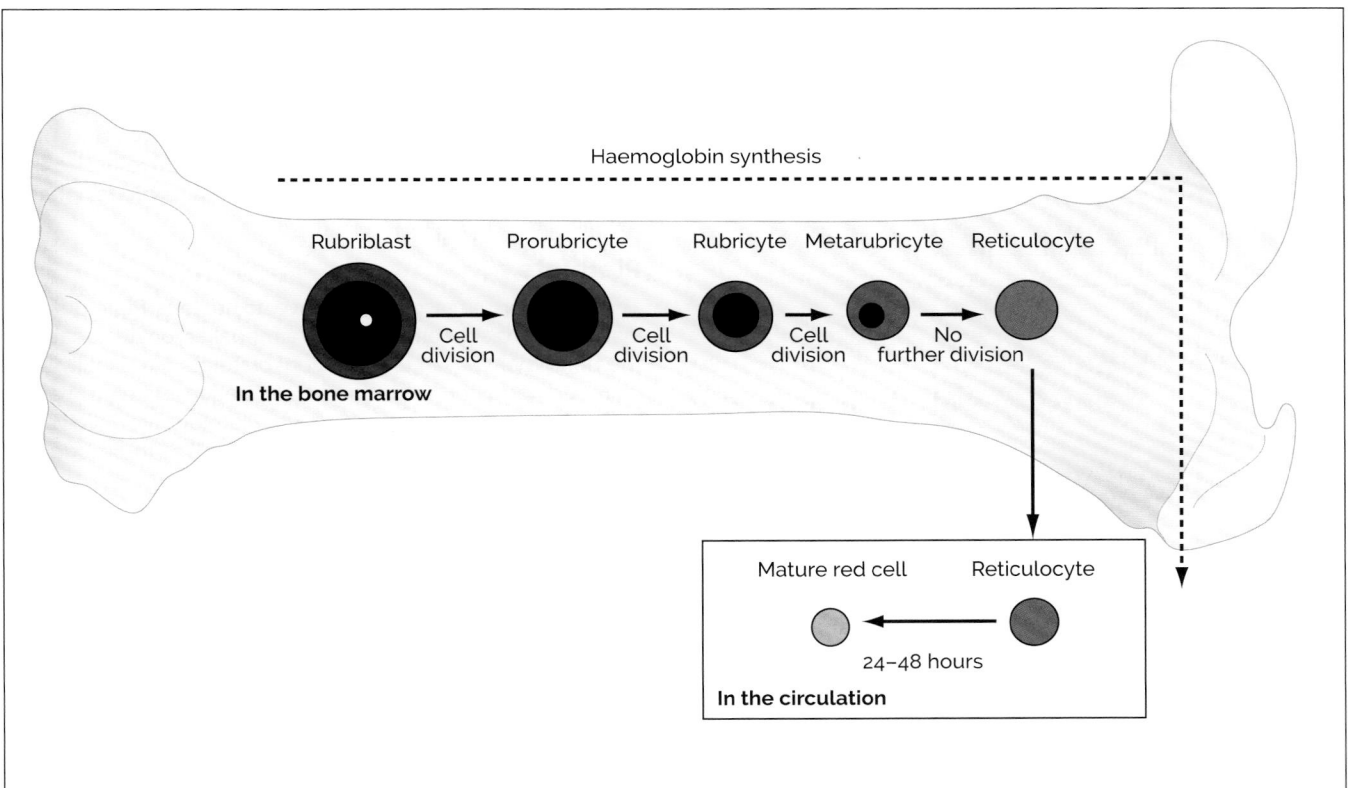

3.53 Erythropoiesis. The developing red blood cells become progressively smaller and accumulate haemoglobin. They are released in to the circulation as reticulocytes. (Reproduced from the *BSAVA Manual of Canine and Feline Clinical Pathology, 3rd edn*)

- Basophils
- Monocytes.

White blood cells are often seen as a white layer above the red blood cells when blood is centrifuged. This white layer is also known as the 'buffy coat'.

Neutrophils

In dogs and cats, neutrophils (polymorphonuclear leuco-cytes) make up the majority of white blood cells in the circulation. Roughly 70% of the white blood cells are neutro-phils and 30% are lymphocytes. The other white blood cells are present only in very small numbers.

Neutrophils are easily identified due to the large nucleus and numerous granules in the cytoplasm. The neutrophil nucleus consists of 2–5 lobes and appears segmented. Neutrophils are short-lived and usually only survive in the circulation for 1–4 days.

Blood cell	Appearance	Function
Neutrophil		Phagocytosis
Lymphocyte		Cellular immune response
Eosinophil		Immune response to allergens and parasites
Basophil		Immune response to allergies
Monocyte		Phagocytosis

3.54 Appearance and function of white blood cells. (May-Grunwald-Giemsa stain except basophil (Rapi-Diff); original magnification X1000). (Photographs reproduced from the *BSAVA Manual of Canine and Feline Clinical Pathology, 3rd edn*)

Neutrophils attack infectious agents; they phagocytose foreign material and release enzymes to digest any infecting organism (see Chapter 7). Neutrophils are also the predomi-nant cells present in pus. The presence of immature neutro-phils (also called band cells as the nuclei are less segmented than mature cells) and an increased number of neutrophils (neutrophilia) are suggestive of an infection.

Lymphocytes

There are two types of lymphocyte: T lymphocytes produced by the thymus and B lymphocytes produced by the bone marrow. These are very important cells in the immune response. Lymphocytes are larger than red blood cells and have a relatively large, dense, round nucleus; the cytoplasm of the cell can be stained pale blue for examination. The lifespan of lymphocytes can vary from a few days to years.

Eosinophils

These cells are much less common than neutrophils. The nucleus in eosinophils generally has two lobes and the cytoplasm contains numerous granules. Following standard staining (Romanowsky stains) these granules appear bright red on examination, making eosinophils very distinctive. The main function of eosinophils is to fight parasitic infections. Increased numbers of eosinophils can also be seen in allergic conditions.

Basophils

In cats and dogs, basophils make up only 1% of white blood cells and are difficult to locate in normal blood. The nucleus is separated into separate lobes and the cytoplasm con-tains numerous granules. Basophils appear similar to eosin-ophils, but the granules appear blue when stained with Romanowsky stains. Basophils are involved in inflammation and can contribute to allergic reactions.

Monocytes

These are the largest type of white blood cell and have an oval or horseshoe-shaped nucleus. Monocytes are pro-duced in the bone marrow and travel in the bloodstream to the connective tissue of the skin, spleen, brain and other organs. When monocytes enter the connective tissue they are known as macrophages and are responsible for phago-cytosis (see Chapter 7).

Platelets

These are very small cells and have no nucleus. Platelets orig-inate from a giant cell, known as a megakaryocyte, located in the bone marrow. On examination, platelets are usually seen clumped together. Once in the circulation platelets have a lifespan of approximately 10 days. Platelets are involved in the clotting mechanism and are also known as thrombocytes.

Small mammals

There are a couple of unusual white blood cells found in small mammals:

- Rabbits – pseudoeosinophil, which is really a neutrophil, but when stained for examination looks more like an eosinophil
- Guinea pigs – Kurloff cell, which is a circulating mononuclear cell with a large inclusion (Kurloff body), commonly seen in mature female guinea pigs during gestation.

In addition, there tend to be more lymphocytes than neutrophils.

Birds

The red blood cells are nucleated and oval in shape (Figure 3.55). Neutrophils are known as heterophils; they have a lobed nucleus and cigar-shaped granules in the cytoplasm, which appear red when stained for examination. Heterophils are the first line of defence during an infection. The avian platelet is also nucleated.

Reptiles

The red blood cells are nucleated and oval in shape (Figure 3.56). Neutrophils are known as heterophils; they have a lobed nucleus and cigar-shaped granules in the cytoplasm, which appear red when stained for examination. Heterophils are the first line of defence during an infection. Circulating plasma cells may be seen in cases of immunogenic stimulation. Snakes often have a circulating mononuclear cell, known as an azurophil, which may be found in small numbers in healthy individuals, but which can become elevated in chronic infections. The reptilian platelet is also nucleated.

Plasma

Plasma is the fluid part of blood and contains many different substances, including:

■ Proteins – albumin, fibrinogen and globulins are large molecules which contribute to the osmotic pressure of the plasma

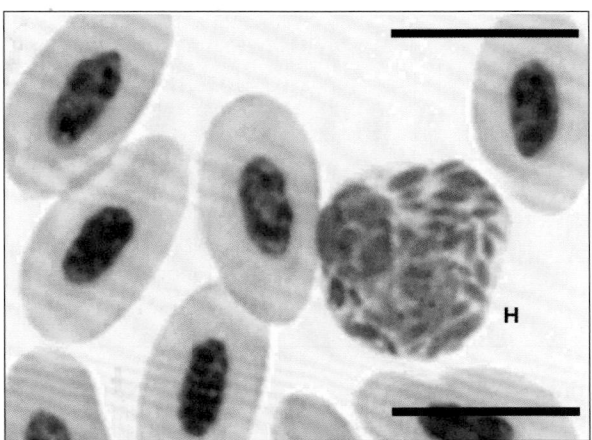

3.55 Appearance of red blood cells and heterophils from a bird. (Bar = 10 μm; Hemacolor stain) (Reproduced from the *BSAVA Manual of Psittacine Birds, 2nd edn*)

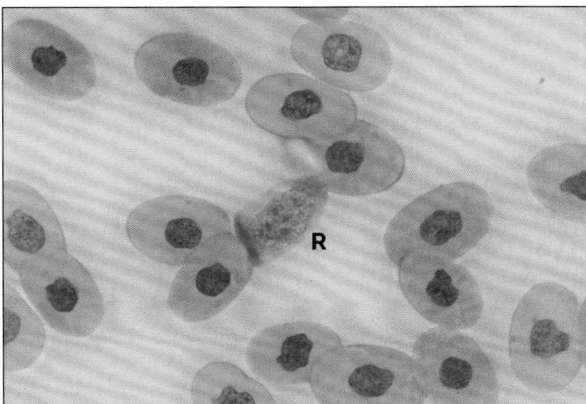

3.56 Appearance of red blood cells and a reticulocyte (**R**) from a reptile. (Wright-Giemsa stain; original magnification X1000). (Reproduced from the *BSAVA Manual of Reptiles, 2nd edn*)

■ Gases – oxygen and carbon dioxide
■ Electrolytes – sodium, potassium, calcium, magnesium, chloride and bicarbonate ions
■ Nutrients – amino acids, fatty acids and glucose are transported around the body in the plasma
■ Waste products – urea and creatinine are transported to the liver and kidneys for excretion
■ Hormones and enzymes – transported around the body in the plasma
■ Antibodies and antitoxins – form part of the immune system.

Circulation

Systemic

Blood returning from the body enters the heart via the cranial (left and right) and caudal venae cavae at the right atrium (Figure 3.57). This blood is venous and has a low concentration of oxygen and high concentration of carbon dioxide (deoxygenated). The blood then passes from the right atrium through the tricuspid valve and into the right ventricle.

From the right ventricle, blood is pumped to the lungs in the pulmonary arteries, where it becomes oxygenated and carbon dioxide is removed. The oxygenated blood then returns to the left atrium via the pulmonary veins. The blood passes from the left atrium through the bicuspid or mitral valve and into the left ventricle. Blood leaves the left ventricle in the aorta and is pumped around the body.

Pulmonary

Deoxygenated blood leaves the right ventricle in the pulmonary trunk, which then divides into the pulmonary arteries (these are the only arteries that transport deoxygenated blood). The pulmonary arteries then branch and enter the lungs. Within the lungs, the pulmonary arteries follow the bronchi and divide further into arterioles, where the blood becomes oxygenated in the alveoli. Oxygenated blood is transported to the left atrium of the heart in the pulmonary veins, which join before leaving the lungs. Valves are absent from these veins.

Hepatic portal system

Blood from the gastrointestinal system contains the products of digestion, which need transporting to the liver to be metabolized. The hepatic portal vein drains the spleen, abdominal digestive organs, caudal oesophagus and rectum. The three main vessels that form the portal vein are the cranial and caudal mesenteric veins (which drain the intestines) and the splenic vein. The hepatic portal system bypasses the heart.

Clotting

Blood clotting involves platelets and proteins known as clotting factors. Vitamin K is required by the liver to produce clotting factors, including II, VII, IX and X. A cascade or consecutive series of reactions occurs when blood clots.

1. Primary aggregation – when the endothelium (internal tunic) of blood vessels is damaged platelets are induced to clump together.
2. Secondary aggregation – the clumped platelets release chemicals, which induce further platelet aggregation.
3. Blood coagulation – factors present within the plasma, damaged blood vessels and platelets induce a cascade of reactions, resulting in the formation of fibrin from

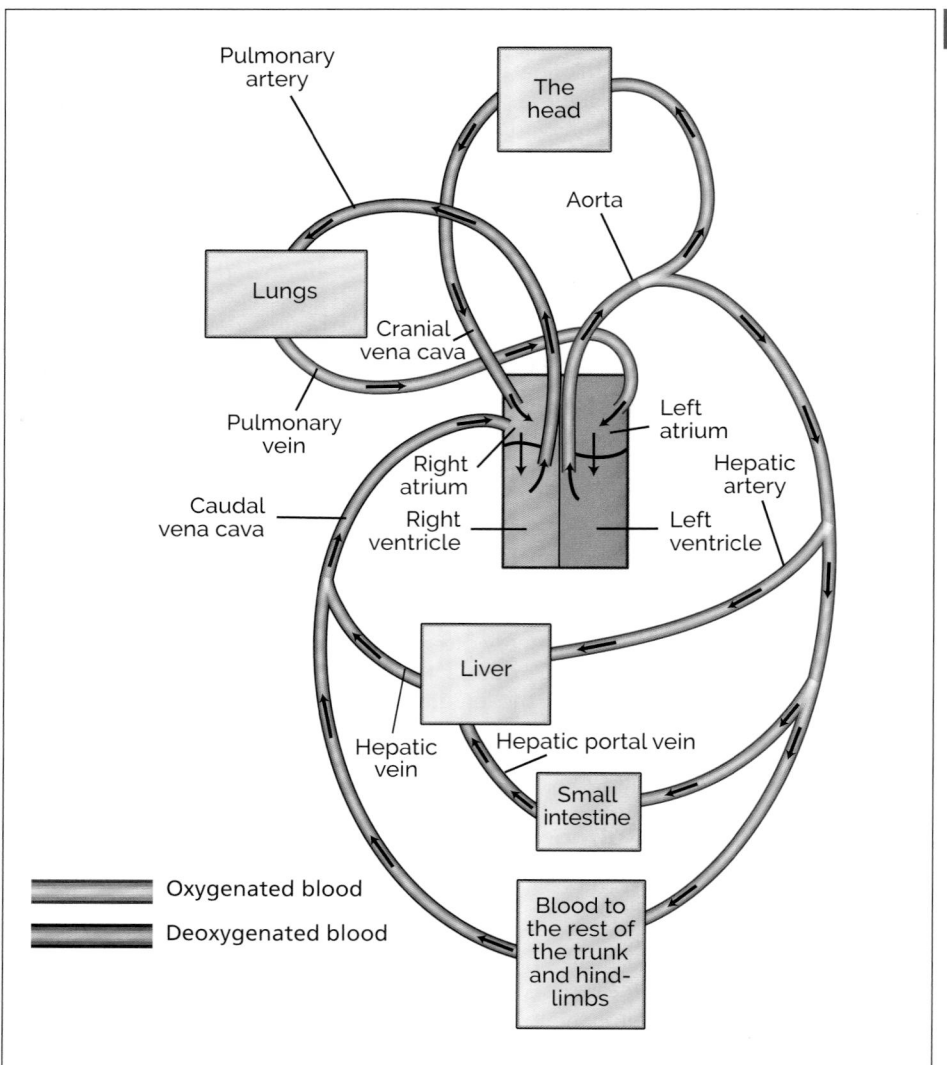

3.57 Circulation of blood around the body.

Oxygenated blood

Deoxygenated blood

fibrinogen (Figure 3.58), which is found circulating in the bloodstream.

a. Intrinsic pathway – the formation of fibrin is controlled by a protein present in the bloodstream known as Factor XII. The intrinsic pathway is initiated by damage to the endothelium and occurs whenever blood contacts any substance other than intact epithelium.

b. Extrinsic pathway – the formation of fibrin is initiated by thromboplastin, which is present on the cell membrane of most cells. The extrinsic pathway is activated when thromboplastin contacts blood, following damage to the vessel walls.

The activated factors produced by the intrinsic and extrinsic pathways join, resulting in the formation of thrombin, which in turn initiates the formation of fibrin. Fibrin forms a meshwork of fibres (skeleton of the clot), which traps more platelets and cells of the immune system. The clot is present to protect the tissue whilst healing takes place.

4. Clot dissolution – fibrinolytic mechanisms break up the clot.

5. Clot retraction – the clot contracts due to a chemical reaction, closing down the defect.

6. Clot removal – the clot is removed by an enzyme known as a plasmin.

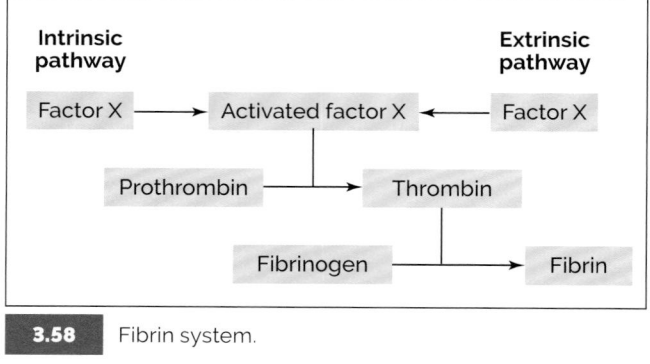

3.58 Fibrin system.

Lymphatic system

The lymphatic system is responsible for the transportation of fluid (lymph) from the cells to the right side of the heart. Fluid is transported to the body tissues in capillaries and forced out by the pressure from the left side of the heart to bathe the cells. However, as there is no pressure to force the fluid back into the capillaries, it has to enter the lymphatic system of vessels to return to the heart. In addition to the transportation of fluid, the lymphatic system is also involved with the immune system: the lymph nodes, spleen, thymus and sub-mucosal deposits of lymphoid tissue in the intestines, tonsils and pharynx play a role in this function. Lymphoid tissue acts as the first line of defence and helps control localized infections (see Chapter 7).

Lymphatic vessels

Lymphatic vessels have thin walls and pass through all the tissues in the body (Figure 3.59). They begin as blind-ending vessels, similar to capillaries, and consist of a thin endothelial lining, which is permeable to fluids and proteins. The lymphatic vessels join and drain into two main vessels:

- Thoracic duct – situated in the dorsal abdomen. The initial section of the thoracic duct is dilated and called the cysterna chyli
- Anterior vena cava – the thoracic duct passes cranially through the diaphragm at the aortic hiatus and opens into the anterior vena cava.

The lymphatic system also carries fat from the intestines to the bloodstream. In the intestines, there are blind-ending lymphatic ducts into which passes the fat that has been absorbed from the gut lumen. These lymphatic ducts are called lacteals.

Movement of fluid through the lymphatic system is aided by pulsating blood vessels situated alongside the lymphatic vessels, and by the contraction and relaxation of the surrounding muscles.

Lymph nodes

Lymph nodes are pale, bean-shaped structures situated intermittently along the length of the lymphatic vessels (see Figure 3.59). Each lymph node is enclosed in a capsule made from connective tissue. This connective tissue extends into the lymph node itself as trabeculae, along which the blood vessels travel. Lymphoid tissue fills the space between the outer capsule and in the connective tissue trabeculae. This tissue is divided into an outer cortex and an inner medulla. Within the cortex are follicles or germinal centres, which are areas of highly concentrated lymphocytes. These areas appear darker than the rest of the lymph node when examined under a microscope. Lymphatic vessels entering the lymph node are known as afferent vessels; those vessels leaving the lymph node are known as efferent vessels.

Lymph nodes found near the surface of the animal (superficial lymph nodes) can be palpated on clinical examination. The main lymph nodes that can be palpated in the dog and cat are:

- Submandibular – at the angle of the jaw
- Prescapular – anterior to the scapula
- Popliteal – just behind the stifle joint.

The parotid, axillary and inguinal lymph nodes may also be palpated in dogs, especially if they are enlarged.

Lymph nodes of small mammals are similar to those of cats and dogs, but may be difficult to detect due to the small size.

Ducks and geese possess a few internal lymph nodes, but these are not palpable. In other birds and reptiles, the lymphatic tissue is not condensed into obvious nodes, instead there are distinct areas of condensed lymphatic tissue within major organs.

Spleen

The spleen is a strap-shaped organ that sits on the left side of the body attached to the greater curvature of the stomach by the gastrosplenic ligament. The spleen looks similar to the liver in colour and texture. It has a tough outer connective tissue capsule, parts of which extend into the body of the

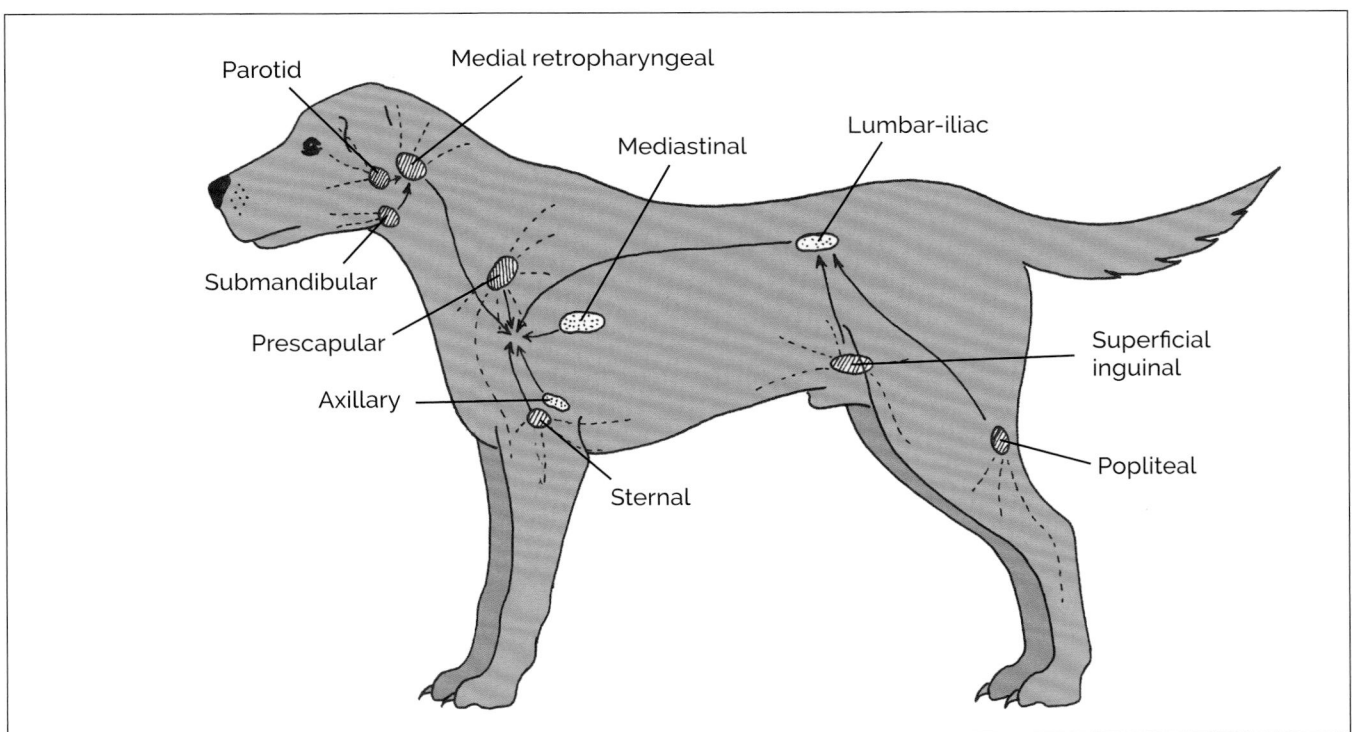

3.59 Lymph nodes and lymphatic vessels in a dog. (Reproduced from the *BSAVA Manual of Canine and Feline Oncology, 3rd edn*)

spleen. Follicles (concentrated areas of lymphoid cells) are found within the white pulp of the spleen, which appears pale when stained for examination. The more vascular areas of the spleen are referred to as the red pulp, and appear darker than the white pulp when stained for examination. The thick capsule that surrounds the spleen contains a large amount of smooth muscle. This allows the size of the spleen to vary greatly: as the muscle relaxes, the spleen becomes engorged with blood and so increases in size; as the muscle contracts, red blood cells are released into the circulation and the spleen becomes smaller. The functions of the spleen include immunity, removal of damaged cells from the blood-stream and the production and storage of red blood cells.

Thymus

The thymus is located in the thoracic cavity, cranial to the heart. It is at its largest in the young animal and decreases in size as the animal gets older, disappearing completely in dogs and cats by the time they reach reproductive maturity. The thymus has an outer cortex, which is densely populated with lymphocytes, and an inner medulla. The sole function of the thymus is to contribute to the immune system by producing T lymphocytes (see Chapter 7).

Submucosal deposits of lymphoid tissue

As well as being located in the thymus, spleen and lymph nodes, discrete collections of lymphoid tissue are found throughout the body. These collections are classified according to their location:

- Peyer's patches or gut-associated lymphoid tissue (GALT) – located throughout the intestines
- Skin-associated lymphoid tissue (SALT)
- Mucosa-associated lymphoid tissue (MALT).

Lymphoid tissue is also present in the tonsils and around the pharynx.

Small mammals

Small mammals have lymph nodes, a spleen and lymphatic tissue within the digestive tract (e.g. rabbits possess a so-called caecal 'tonsil'). The thymus is usually present in adult small mammals, as it does not markedly reduce in size with age.

Birds

Most birds do not have lymph nodes, with the exception of some waterfowl, which possess a single coelomic lymph node. Instead, the lymphatic tissue is often located within other organs such as the liver and kidneys. Birds do possess a spleen, but its size and shape varies with species: it is often spherical in psittacine birds and strap-like in passerine birds.

Thymic tissue is present (even in adults) as islands of cells throughout the cervical and cranial coelomic regions. In addition, birds have a unique type of lymphatic tissue located in the dorsal cloacal region, known as the bursa of Fabricius. This is the site of B lymphocyte production and reduces in size with age, disappearing in the adult bird.

Reptiles

Reptiles do not have discrete lymph nodes but instead have islands of lymphatic tissue within other organs such as the liver and kidneys. Some reptiles have a separate spleen, but in many (particularly snakes) the spleen fuses with the pancreas to form a splenopancreas. Thymic tissue is found in the cervical region and anterior coelomic cavity, and may persist in the adult.

Respiratory system

The respiratory system comprises the nose, pharynx, larynx, trachea, bronchi and smaller airways, lungs and diaphragm. Its function is to facilitate the passage of oxygen into the body and carbon dioxide out of the body.

Anatomy

The upper respiratory tract consists of the nose, nasal cavities, pharynx, larynx and trachea (Figure 3.60). The lower respiratory tract consists of the lungs, bronchi, bronchioles and alveoli.

Nose and nasal cavities

The external part of the nose is the nasal plate; the central fissure of the nasal plate is called the philtrum. The outer part of the nose is lined with epithelium, which continues into the entrance of the nares where it is gradually replaced with mucosa. The nasal cavities are lined with olfactory mucosa, which is well supplied with sensory nerves and serous olfactory glands. Secretions from the olfactory glands help to keep the mucosa moist. The two nasal cavities are separated by the nasal septum, which is made of cartilage. Located alongside the nasal septum is the vomeronasal organ (which is highly developed in some reptiles). This is responsible for the detection of phero-mones, and also plays a role in behaviour.

Situated within the nasal cavities are the dorsal, ventral and ethmoidal conchae.

- Dorsal and ventral conchae – these are folds of cartilage.
- Ethmoidal conchae – these are scrolls of cartilage located in the caudal part of the nasal cavities. The space between the cartilage scrolls is known as the ethmoidal meatus.

The dorsal, ventral and ethmoidal conchae provide a large surface area for the filtering (removal of dust and bacteria), moistening (with secretions from the olfactory glands) and warming (to near body temperature) of inspired air. Connected to the nasal cavities are the paranasal sinuses. In the dog, there are two main paranasal sinuses:

- The maxillary sinus – found in the maxillary bone of the skull
- The frontal sinus – found in the frontal bone of the skull.

The paranasal sinuses humidify and warm inspired air, and also help to lighten the skull. In addition, they have a role in voice resonance and so are generally larger in the male.

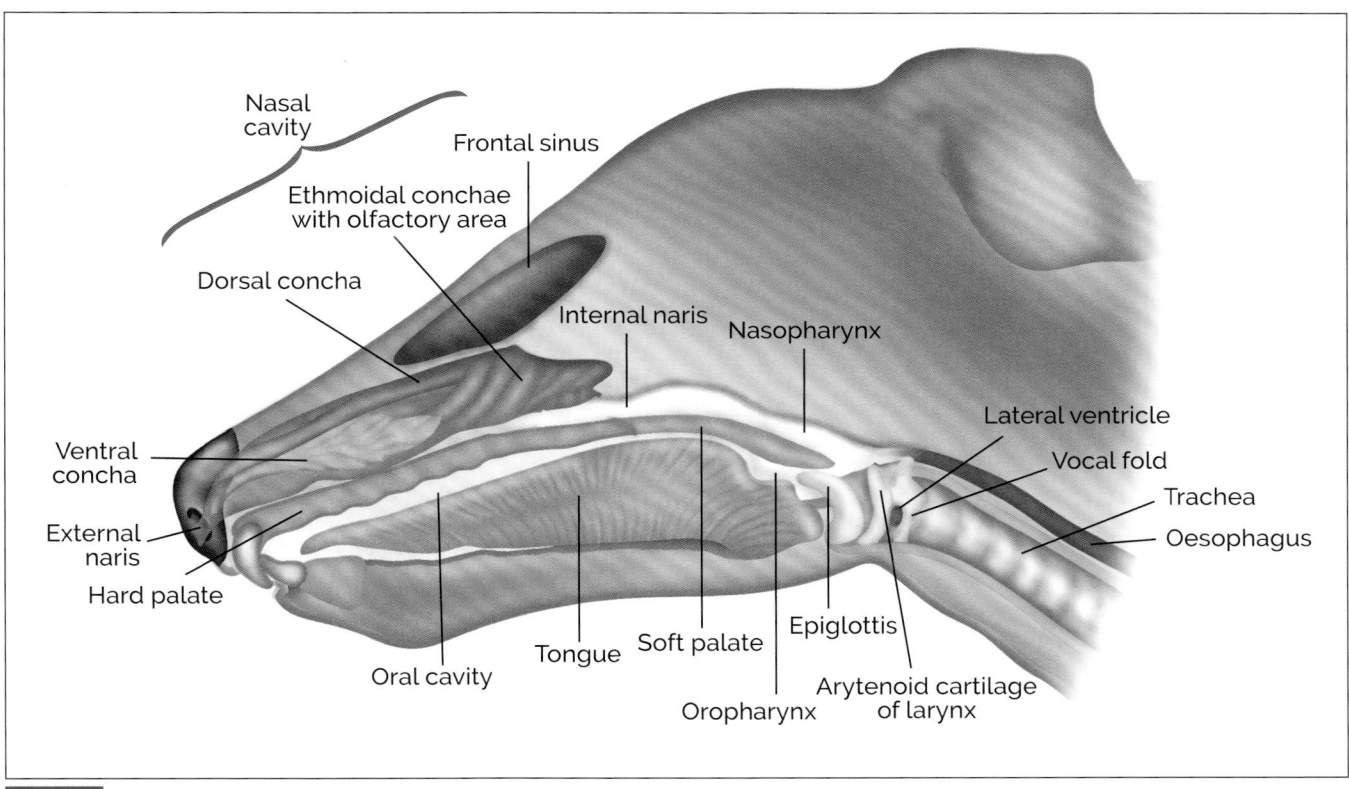

3.60 Midline section through a dog's head.

Pharynx

The pharynx is the part of the respiratory tract that connects the nasal cavities to the larynx. It also communicates with the mouth. The pharynx is divided by the palate into:

■ The nasopharynx – connected to the caudal nasal cavities
■ The oropharynx – connected to the caudal oral cavity.

Larynx

The larynx is a 'box' consisting of a group of cartilages (Figure 3.61):

■ Epiglottis – the most rostral of the cartilages. It is spade-shaped and attached to the tongue and thyroid cartilage

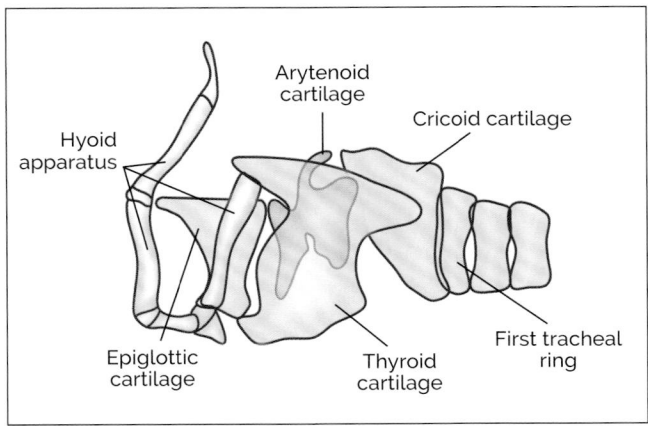

3.61 Structure of the larynx. (Reproduced from the *BSAVA Manual of Canine and Feline Head, Neck and Thoracic Surgery, 2nd edn*)

■ Thyroid – this is the largest of the cartilages and forms the floor of the larynx
■ Arytenoid – this forms the inside of the larynx and supports the vocal chords
■ Cricoid – a ring-like structure that articulates with the thyroid cartilage and trachea.

The functions of the larynx include:

■ Preventing the entry of foreign material into the respiratory tract during swallowing (deglutination)
■ Regulating the flow of gases into the respiratory tract
■ Contributing to vocalization.

Trachea

The trachea consists of C-shaped rings of cartilage connected by fibrous connective tissue and smooth muscle, and lined with ciliated epithelium. Dorsally the C-shaped rings are incomplete and the free ends are connected by soft tissue. The trachea passes into the thorax at the thoracic inlet and traverses the mediastinum. The mediastinum is the space between the lungs which is bound by the pleurae (see Figure 3.9) and where the heart, thymus and blood vessels are located. The trachea splits into two bronchi at the level of the heart base. The function of the trachea is to allow airflow from the larynx to the lungs.

Bronchi, bronchioles and alveoli

The bronchi are similar in structure to the trachea, but the cartilage rings are complete. The bronchi divide further into bronchioles. As the bronchioles become smaller the amount of cartilage present decreases, finally disappearing completely. The bronchioles continue to divide to the level of the terminal bronchioles and end in the alveolar ducts (Figure 3.62). Each alveolar duct terminates in a number of alveoli,

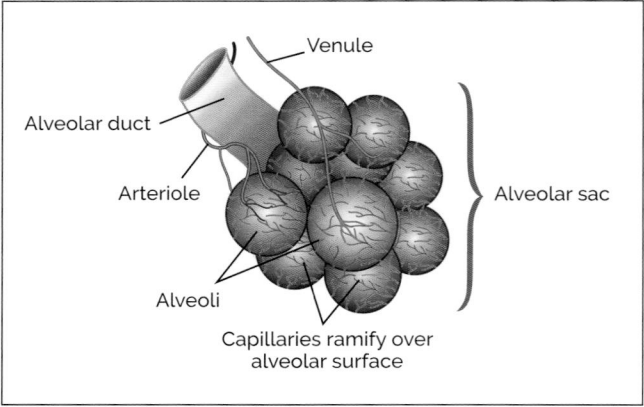

3.62 The terminal air passages.

the appearance of which can be likened to a bunch of grapes attached to their stalk. The alveoli are lined with a single cell thick pulmonary membrane covered in capillaries, across which gaseous exchange takes place.

Lungs

The lungs lie within the thoracic cavity, on either side of the mediastinum. Each lung is covered by a connective tissue layer known as the pulmonary pleura (visceral pleura). This is separated from the parietal pleura, which covers the inside of the thoracic cavity, by a small space known as the pleural space (see Figure 3.9).

The lungs consist of bronchi, bronchioles, alveoli, blood vessels and connective tissue (parenchyma). Each lung is divided into lobes (Figure 3.63): the left lung comprises the cranial, middle and caudal lobes; the right lung comprises the cranial, middle, caudal and accessory lobes.

Small mammals

Small herbivores are obligate nasal breathers. Many small rodents have a palatal ostium (an opening through the soft palate to access the trachea). The division of the lungs into lobes is generally less obvious. The diaphragm is more deeply domed and is the main impetus for inspiration.

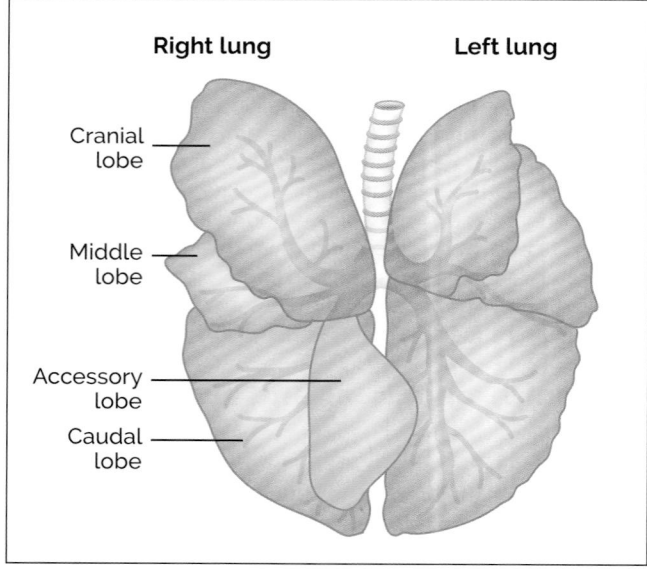

3.63 The lobes of the lungs in a dog.

Birds

Birds have one nasal concha per nasal passage. The main sinus is the infraorbital sinus (Figure 3.64), which sits below the eye and has no lateral bony wall. The nasal passages join and pass through the hard palate via the choanal slit, which sits at rest immediately above the glottis. The glottis lacks an epiglottis, thyroid cartilage and vocal folds. The glottis is held closed at rest. The trachea has complete signet ring-shaped cartilages supporting its structure. The trachea may be coiled inside the sternum in some waterfowl. Some birds (e.g. penguins) have a midline septum dividing the trachea in two as far cranially as the glottis. Male ducks have a diverticulum (bulla) of the trachea just inside the body cavity. The syrinx (avian voice box) may be found at the caudal end of the trachea.

The lungs are semi-rigid in birds and thus do not significantly inflate or deflate during inspiration and expiration. The lungs are attached to the underside of the dorsal body wall and protected by the notarium. There are nine air sacs in most species (Figure 3.64). There is no diaphragm in birds, and the common body cavity is referred to as the coelom.

Reptiles

There are salt glands present in the nares of some reptiles (e.g. green iguana) for excreting excess salt. Non-crocodilian reptiles do not possess a hard palate. The rings of cartilage in the trachea are O-shaped in chelonians, and C-shaped in lizards and snakes. The lungs are more alveolar and elastic than those in mammals. In many snakes (such as colubrids) the left lung becomes reduced, leaving only a major right lung (see Figure 3.74). There is no true diaphragm in reptiles.

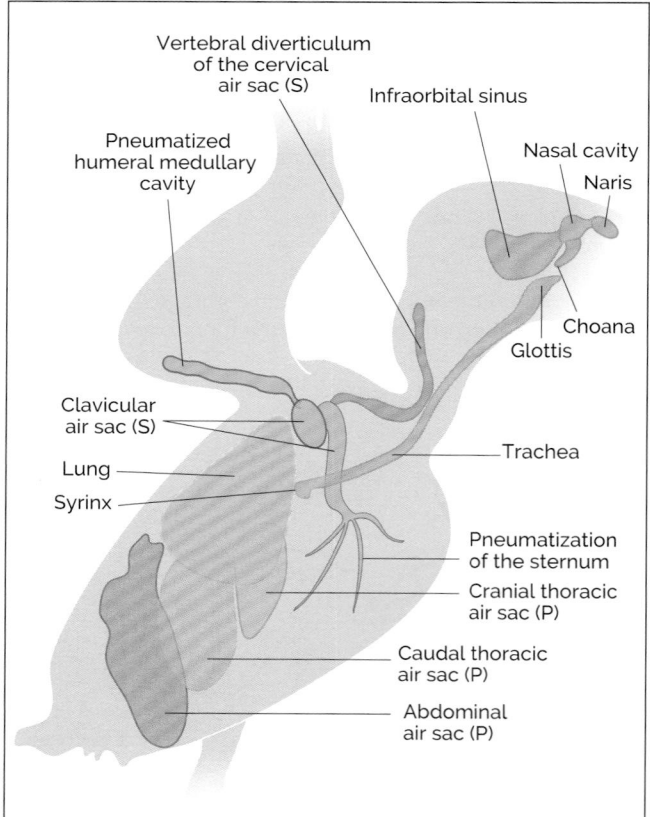

3.64 Respiratory system of the bird. P = paired air sacs. S = single air sac. (Redrawn after Nigel Harcourt-Brown)

Physiology of respiration

> ## Terminology
>
> - Total lung capacity – the total volume of air in the lungs
> - Tidal volume – the volume of air breathed in or out in one normal breath
> - Functional residual volume – the volume of air left in the lungs after one normal breath
> - Vital capacity – the maximum volume of air that can be forced out of the lungs
> - Residual volume – the volume of air left in the lungs after forced expiration
> - Anatomical dead space – the volume of air which does not reach the alveoli. This is equal to the volume of the trachea, bronchi and bronchioles
>
> The application of these terms with regards to general anaesthesia is discussed in Chapter 21.

Inspiration

During inspiration the diaphragm contracts, becoming flatter and moving in a caudal direction. At the same time the external intercostal muscles contract, lifting the ribcage outwards. These actions increase the volume within the thoracic cavity. Due to the negative pressure of the pleural space in relation to the atmosphere, when the volume within the thoracic cavity increases, the negative pressure increases, thus drawing air into the lungs and causing them to inflate.

Expiration

During expiration the diaphragm relaxes and the internal intercostal muscles contract, decreasing the volume of the thoracic cavity and forcing air out of the lungs.

Control of respiration

Inspiration and expiration are controlled by a number of different systems, including:

- Neural control
- Humoral control.

Neural control

When the lungs inflate, receptors in the bronchi and bronchioles send impulses to the respiratory centre in the medulla and pons of the hindbrain, which inhibit further inspiration and stimulate expiration. This is called the inflation reflex or Hering Breuer reflex. When the lungs deflate, the respiratory centre initiates the next inspiration. This is called the deflation reflex.

Humoral control

Respiration is also controlled by various chemicals in the blood, including carbon dioxide, which is monitored by the medulla of the hindbrain. When carbon dioxide levels in the blood increase, ventilation increases; when carbon dioxide levels in the blood decrease, ventilation decreases. The medulla only monitors carbon dioxide levels. Oxygen levels in the bloodstream are monitored by chemoreceptors in the carotid arteries and the aortic arch.

Birds

During inspiration the sternum moves downwards and the ribcage outwards, thereby increasing the volume of the coelom. This increased coelomic volume allows air to be drawn through the lungs and into the series of air sacs (see Figure 3.64), which act as passive bellows. The respiratory cycle is complex in birds and occurs over two inspirations and expirations.

- The first inspiration draws air into the lungs, much of it bypassing the areas of gaseous exchange and moving directly into the caudal air sacs (caudal thoracic and abdominal).
- During the first expiration, air in the caudal air sacs moves back through the neopulmonic part of the lungs and into the paleopulmonic sections (from caudal to cranial), where gaseous exchange occurs.
- The second inspiration allows air moving cranially from the first expiration to move into the cranial air sacs.
- The second expiration allows air in the cranial air sacs to be expelled through the secondary and primary bronchi.

Reptiles

The predominant stimulus for respiration in many reptiles is a lowered partial pressure of oxygen in the blood, rather than an elevated partial pressure of carbon dioxide, reflecting the fact that many reptiles have a low metabolic rate and can cope with high carbon dioxide environments. Reptiles such as chelonians are able to inspire by moving their head and limbs out of their shell, creating a negative pressure. Expiration is achieved by the reverse process. The structure of the reptilian lung is more open in nature, rather than alveolar, and so has a smaller surface area in comparison with an equivalent sized mammal.

Digestive system

Anatomy

The basic components of the digestive tract (Figure 3.65) are:

- Mouth
- Pharynx
- Oesophagus
- Stomach
- Small intestine
- Large intestine
- Liver and gallbladder
- Pancreas.

Although the general structure of the digestive system is similar, differences arise depending on whether the animal is a carnivore (meat eater), herbivore (plant eater) or omnivore (eats a mixture of meat and plants). Herbivores are of two broad types: ruminants (foregut fermenters, e.g. cattle) have highly developed stomachs; hindgut fermenters (e.g. rabbits, guinea pigs and chinchillas) have a highly developed large intestine and caecum.

Mouth

The mouth extends from the lips to the pharynx. It is divided into a cavity between the teeth and cheeks (buccal space or cavity) and the central cavity. The central cavity is bound by the hard palate, teeth (see 'Skull', above), gums and tongue.

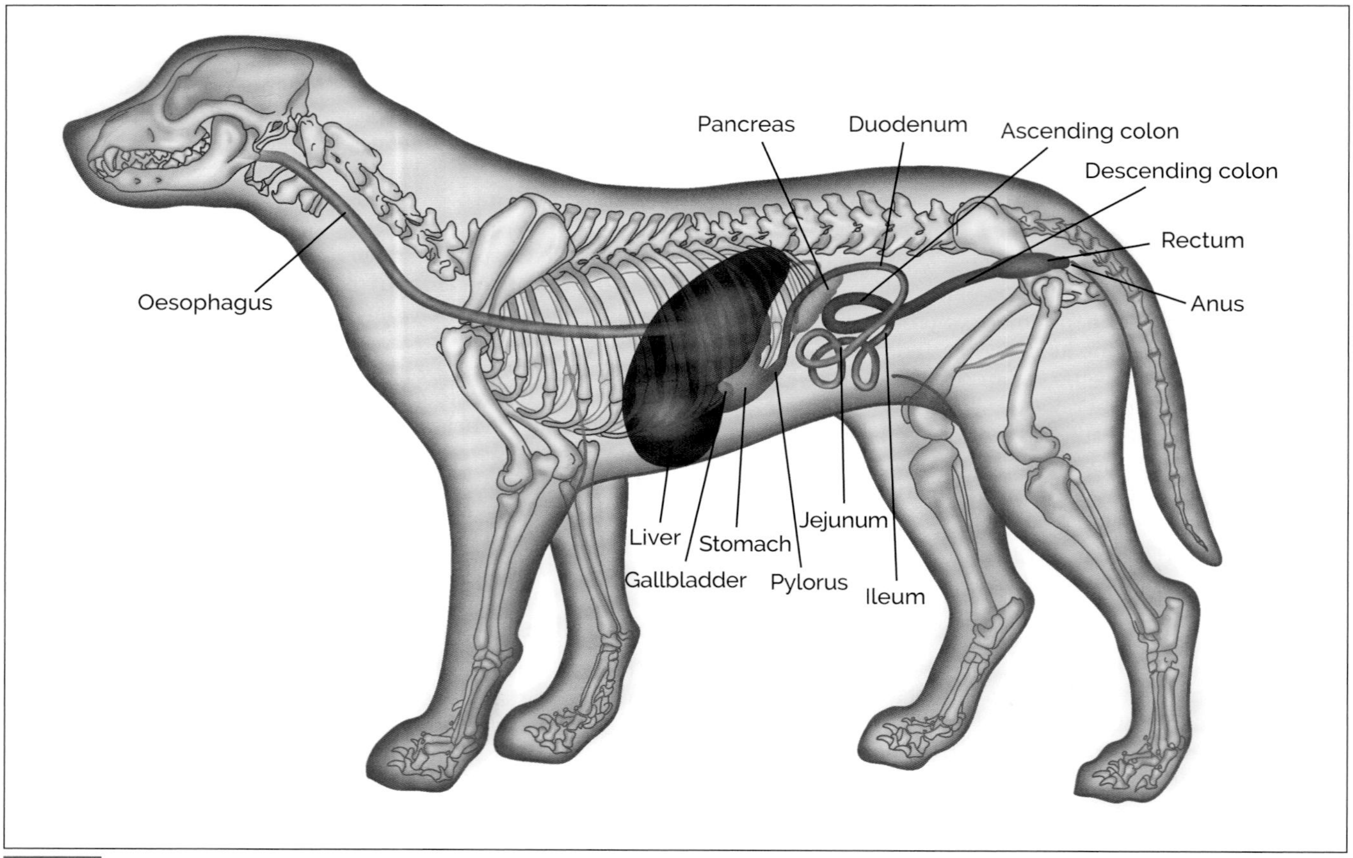

3.65 Digestive tract in the abdomen of a dog. The length of the intestines has been reduced in order to the simplify the diagram.

Lips

The lips comprise a covering of skin with underlying muscles and tendons and an inner layer of mucosa. The skin of the lips is well supplied with sebaceous glands, which provide waterproofing and scent. The facial nerve innervates the lips and controls movement. Some larger breeds of dogs have impressive lip folds, which may be prone to infection. The function of the lips is to bring food into the mouth (prehension). The degree to which the lips are involved in this process varies between species, being very important in herbivores such as rabbits, but less important in cats and dogs.

Cheeks

The cheeks are lined with stratified squamous epithelium (buccal mucosa). The cheeks or buccae are controlled by the buccinator muscle. The function of the cheeks is to move the food bolus from one side of the mouth to the other (along with the tongue) during chewing; this function is highly developed in herbivores.

Palate

The hard palate forms the roof of the mouth and consists of the incisive bone rostrally (which holds the incisors), maxillary bone laterally and palatine bone. The bones are covered in keratinized epithelium, which protects the underlying structures. Caudally the hard palate merges into the soft palate, which is lined with the same epithelium but comprises soft tissue rather than bone.

Tongue

The tongue consists of a number of different parts (Figure 3.66), including:

- Apex – tip of the tongue
- Body – main part of the tongue
- Root – where the tongue attaches to the mouth
- Median groove – central depression in the dorsal surface of the tongue
- Papillae – small projections on the surface of the tongue
- Frenulum – tissue that connects the tongue to the floor of the mouth
- Lyssa – an area of fibrous tissue present on the ventral surface of the tongue in dogs.

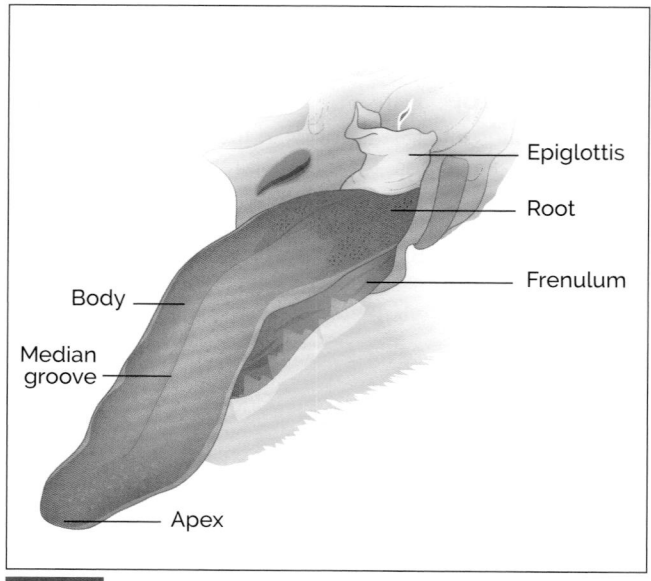

3.66 The structure of the tongue.

The tongue is attached to the hyoid bones and the mandible. It is covered in keratinized mucosa, which protects it from the trauma of mastication (chewing). Papillae are present to some degree on all tongues; they are well developed in cats, giving the tongue a rough appearance that can easily be seen with the naked eye. Some of the papillae contain taste buds. The tongue consists of skeletal muscle controlled by the hypoglossal nerve. The specific muscles present in the tongue are:

- Geniohyoideus
- Genioglossus
- Hyoglossus
- Styloglossus.

The tongue has many functions, including:

- Prehension
- Lapping
- Grooming
- Vocalization (in combination with the vocal folds)
- Heat loss through panting.

Salivary glands

Salivary glands are present in cats, dogs and other mammals. The four main salivary glands in the dog and cat are:

- Parotid – found at the base of the ear. The duct from the parotid gland exits rostrally and opens into the mouth opposite the upper fourth premolar tooth in the buccal space/cavity
- Mandibular – found at the angle of the jaw and is smaller that the parotid gland. The duct from the mandibular gland runs along the floor of the mouth and opens on the sublingual caruncle close to the frenulum of the tongue. The mandibular gland produces a mixture of serous and mucoid saliva
- Sublingual – found underneath the tongue. The sublingual gland drains via one single duct located alongside the mandibular duct, but has many smaller ducts which open alongside the frenulum. The sublingual gland also produces a mixture of serous and mucoid saliva
- Zygomatic – found near the eye in the dog.

Small salivary glands are also present on the lips, cheeks, tongue, soft palate and pharynx.

Saliva

This is required to moisten the mouth and provide lubrication. Saliva forms part of the non-specific immune system; it continuously washes the mouth and reduces the level of bacteria. Saliva is also required for the initial mechanical and chemical breakdown of food: the saliva of herbivores contains amylase, which breaks down starch. Whilst canine saliva is not generally thought to contain significant amounts of amylase, some research has found low levels of the enzyme (Contreras-Aguilar *et al.*, 2017). Feline saliva does not contain amylase. In addition, saliva is responsible for the excretion of minerals found in tartar.

Saliva is produced continuously, but the rate of production can be altered by the autonomic nervous system (ANS). Stimulation of the parasympathetic branch of the ANS can increase saliva production; stimulation of the sympathetic branch can decrease production. Eating food, or the anticipation of food (such as is seen in the classical Pavlovian reaction), can stimulate production of saliva. Fear and dehydration decreases the level of saliva and leads to a dry, tacky mouth.

Pharynx

The pharynx is defined by the base of skull, the mandible and the larynx. It comprises three parts:

- The nasopharynx – connected to the caudal nasal cavities
- The oropharynx – connected to the caudal oral cavity
- The laryngopharynx – connected to the oesophagus and lies alongside the larynx.

The act of eating involves three stages:

1. Prehension – taking food into the mouth.
2. Mastication – chewing food.
3. Deglutition – swallowing food.

The swallowing reflex is finely controlled to ensure that food does not enter the airway. A network of nerve impulses stimulates the nasopharynx and larynx to close, and the oropharynx to open, allowing the food bolus to pass into the oesophagus.

1. The soft palate is elevated to close off the nasopharynx.
2. The laryngeal muscles close the larynx; this means that the animal cannot breathe for a short time.
3. The tongue moves the bolus of food from the back of the mouth to the cranial oesophagus.
4. Peristaltic waves begin at the cranial end of the oesophagus to move the food bolus down into the stomach.

Oesophagus

The oesophagus consists of four layers:

- Outer layer – connective tissue
- Muscle layer – mainly striated muscle, changing to smooth muscle distally. In the dog the entire oesophagus comprises striated muscle. There are two layers of muscle: an inner circular layer and outer longitudinal layer
- Submucosa layer
- Inner layer – mucosa (stratified squamous epithelium).

The oesophagus passes down the left side of the neck. It enters the thorax and traverses the mediastinum, passing dorsal to the heart, through the diaphragm and into the abdomen, where it enters the stomach at the cardiac sphincter. A sphincter is a muscular valve, the cardiac sphincter controls the passage of food into the stomach. However, the cardiac sphincter is not a true sphincter as it opens with only the pressure of a food bolus: this allows passage of food into the stomach, and the return of food to the oesophagus when the animal regurgitates or vomits. The oesophagus is innervated by the vagus nerve, which controls peristalsis.

Stomach

The stomach has a curved appearance: the smaller cranial curve is known as the lesser curvature; the larger caudal curve is known as the greater curvature. The dorsal part of the stomach is the fundus (Figure 3.67a), which receives food from the oesophagus via the cardiac sphincter. The main part of the stomach is the body, where food is mixed with saliva and gastric secretions. From the body, ingesta moves to the antrum before entering the pylorus. From the pylorus food can either enter the duodenum via the pyloric sphincter, or return to the body of the stomach for further breakdown.

The stomach wall consists of six different layers:

- Serosa – outer layer
- Smooth muscle – three layers: longitudinal (top layer), circular (middle layer) and oblique (bottom layer)
- Submucosa
- Mucosa – inner layer consisting of glandular, columnar epithelium covered with mucus.

Different parts of the mucosa contain different types of gland (Figure 3.67b). The cardiac and pyloric mucosa contain mucus-secreting glands (goblet cells). The glands in the mucosa of the body (gastric glands) produce pepsinogen (chief cells) and hydrochloric acid (parietal cells). Pepsinogen is converted into its active form pepsin by hydrochloric acid in the lumen of the stomach. The hormone gastrin is also secreted by the stomach into the bloodstream. Gastrin stimulates the production of hydrochloric acid.

Gastric secretions (mucus, pepsinogen and hydrochloric acid) are stimulated by the sight or smell of food, the act of eating and the presence of food in the stomach. Inhibition of secretion occurs when the stomach contents reach a pH <2 or when the ingesta passes into the duodenum. The muscular layers of the stomach contract at different intervals to help break down food and move the ingesta towards the pyloric sphincter (e.g. the antrum contracts up to four times per minute, depending on the amount of food present). It should be noted that nutrients are not absorbed from the stomach.

Emptying of the stomach is carefully controlled by the nervous and endocrine systems. The speed at which the stomach empties also depends on the type of food consumed: high fat meals result in slower gastric emptying, so that fat breakdown can take place in the jejunum without it being overloaded. Blood is supplied to the stomach via the coeliac artery, which arises directly from the aorta. Branches of the coeliac artery initially supply the lesser and greater curvatures and then spread out to the rest of the stomach. Venous drainage is via the portal vein to the liver.

The functions of the stomach are:

- To act as a collecting chamber for food
- To initiate the mechanical breakdown of food
- To initiate the enzymatic breakdown of food.

Small intestine

The small intestine comprises the duodenum, jejunum and ileum. Ingesta from the stomach passes into the duodenum. This is a short section of intestine situated on the right side of the abdomen and fixed in position by tight connective tissue. The pancreatic duct and common bile duct are located here, allowing pancreatic enzymes and bile to enter the gastrointestinal tract.

From the duodenum, ingesta passes into the jejunum. This part of the intestine is very long and coiled within the abdomen. The final part of the small intestine is the ileum, which can be identified by the lack of villi on the mucosa. The ileum meets the large intestine at the ileocolic junction. The small intestinal wall consists of four layers (Figure 3.68a):

- Serosa – outer layer
- Smooth muscle
- Submucosa
- Mucosa – inner layer where the villi (finger-like projections; Figure 3.68b) are located. Along the villi are even smaller projections, known as microvilli, which are collectively termed the brush border (Figure 3.68c). The intestinal glands are also found in this layer.

Blood is supplied to part of the duodenum by the coeliac artery. The remainder of the duodenum along with the jejunum, ileum and the ileocolic junction is supplied by the mesenteric artery. Venous drainage is via the cranial and caudal mesenteric veins, which in turn drain into the portal vein. Lymphatic vessels from the small intestine drain into the cysterna chyli, which forms part of the thoracic duct and returns the lymphatic fluid to the venous bloodstream.

The functions of the small intestine are:

- Enzymatic digestion of food
- Absorption of nutrients following digestion of food.

Digestion of food within the stomach and small intestine takes place through the action of various secretions (Figure 3.69). The villi increase the surface area of the small intestine that the ingesta comes into contact with. Within each villus is a capillary that absorbs nutrients and lacteals that absorb chyle (a milky liquid containing digested fat).

Large intestine

The large intestine comprises the caecum, colon and rectum. The caecum is a blind-ending diverticulum found at the ileocolic junction. The size of the caecum varies between species. In the rabbit the caecum is a large organ, which is

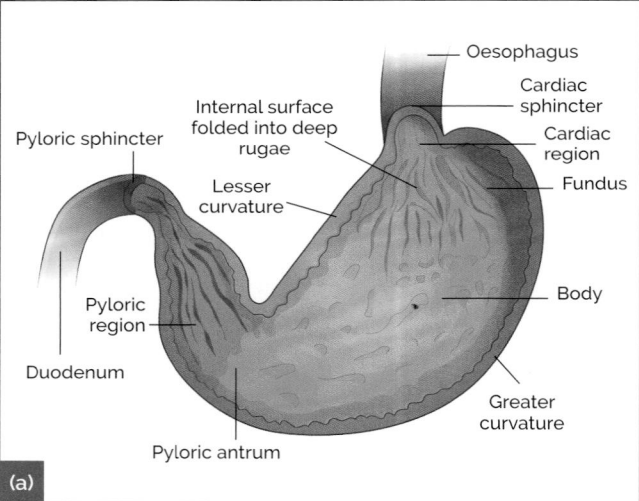

(a)

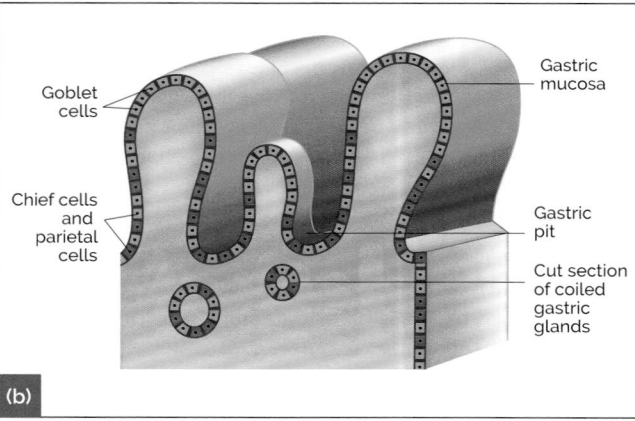

(b)

3.67 (a) Cross-section through the stomach wall. (b) Section showing the gastric pits.

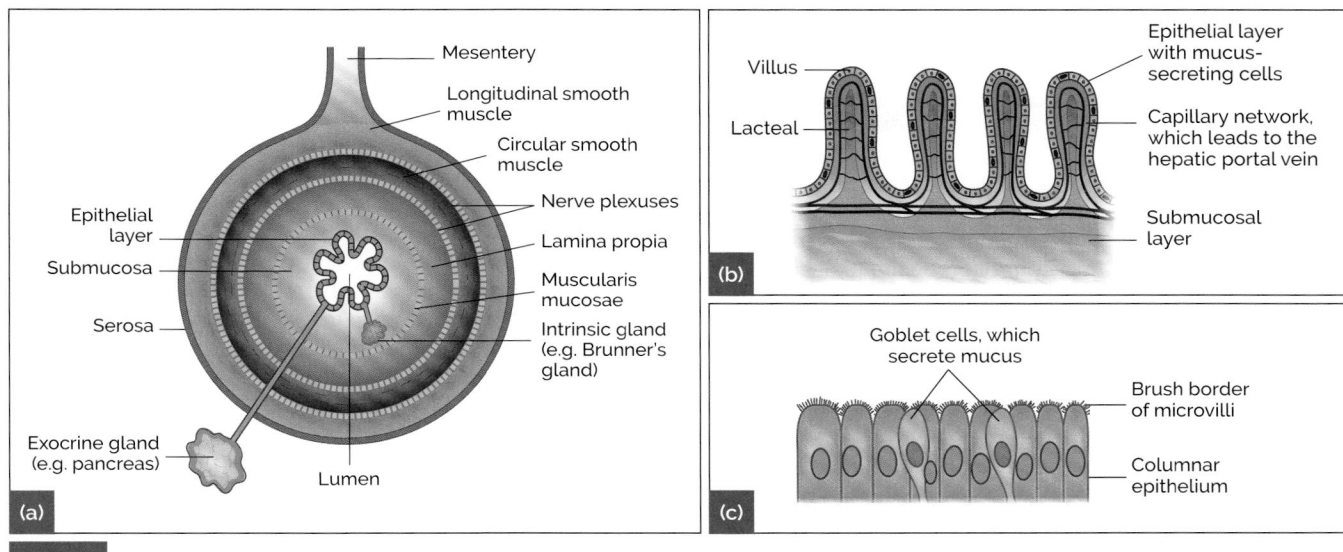

3.68 (a) Cross-section through the intestine wall. (b) Detail of the villus structure. (c) Detail of the epithelium.

Origin of secretion	Digestive juice	Contents	Action	Comments
Stomach				
Goblet cells	Gastric juices (the hormone gastrin is produced as food enters the stomach and stimulates the gastric pits to secrete gastric juices)	Mucus	No enzyme action. Lubricates food. Protects gastric mucosa from autodigestion	
Parietal cells		Hydrochloric acid (HCl)	Denatures protein. Creates a pH of 1.3–5. Converts pepsinogen to active pepsin	Protein digestion is made easier. Acid pH kills most pathogenic bacteria
Chief cells		Pepsinogen	When activated by HCl, pepsin converts protein to peptides	Peptides are small molecules
Small intestine				
Liver	Bile	Bile salts	Emulsifies fats to produce small globules. Activates lipases	As chyme enters the duodenum, the gallbladder contracts forcing bile along the bile duct
Exocrine pancreas	Pancreatic juice (produced in response to gastrin and the hormone cholecystokinin which is secreted by duodenal cells as chyme passes through the pyloric sphincter)	Bicarbonate	No enzyme action. Neutralizes the acid pH	Neutral pH stops action of pepsin and enables intestinal digestive enzymes to act
		Trypsinogen	Inactive	Converted to active trypsin by enterokinase present in succus entericus. Spontaneous conversion is prevented by a trypsin inhibitor
		Trypsin	Activates other enzyme precursors. Converts peptides and other proteins to amino acids	Amino acids are absorbed into the bloodstream
		Lipase	Converts fats to fatty acids and glycerol	Activated by bile salts
		Amylase	Converts starches to maltose	Starches are plant carbohydrates
Brunner's glands as succus entericus and crypts of Lieberkuhn	Intestinal juices (produced in response to the hormone secretin, which is secreted as chyme passes through the pyloric sphincter)	Maltase	Converts maltose to glucose	Glucose is absorbed by the blood capillaries
		Sucrase	Converts sucrose to glucose and fructose	Glucose and fructose are absorbed by the blood capillaries
		Lactase	Converts lactose to glucose and galactose	Glucose and galactose are absorbed by the blood capillaries
		Enterokinase	Converts trypsinogen to trypsin	Trypsin is activated
		Aminopeptidase	Converts peptides to amino acids	Amino acids are absorbed into the bloodstream
		Lipase	Converts fats to fatty acids and glycerol	Fatty acids and glycerol are absorbed into the lacteals

3.69 Processes involved in digestion.

required to break down fibre. In the dog and cat the caecum is vestigial, as vegetation only makes up a small part of the diet, or none at all.

Ingesta from the ileum passes into the colon. The colon consists of an ascending portion, a transverse portion (moving from right to left) and a descending portion (moving from the left flank to the pelvic cavity). From the colon, ingesta passes into the rectum. The rectum lies dorsally above the organs of the reproductive and urinary tracts. Movement of faeces out of the rectum is controlled by the anal sphincter. Located on either side of the anal sphincter are the perianal sacs, which are also known as the anal glands: this term is not strictly correct as they are not true glands. These sacs are lined with glandular epithelium, which secretes fluid used to scent mark territory. Each time the animal defecates, these sacs should empty.

Blood is supplied to the ascending and transverse colon by the cranial mesenteric artery. The descending colon and rectum are supplied by the caudal mesenteric artery. Venous drainage is via the cranial and caudal mesenteric veins.

The functions of the large intestine are:

- Microbial digestion
- Breakdown of fibre
- Production of essential amino acids
- Production of B vitamins and vitamin K
- Resorption of water and electrolytes.

As these functions take some time, gut transit is slower in the large intestine than in the small intestine.

Liver and gallbladder

The liver is a solid organ located between the stomach and the diaphragm. It is divided into lobes, the pattern of which varies between species. In the dog, six lobes are present:

- Left lateral
- Left medial
- Right lateral
- Right medial
- Quadrate
- Caudate.

The liver consists of cells, known as hepatocytes, arranged in hexagonal lobules. Located between the lobules are the bile canaliculi; this is where bile is secreted and then transported to the gallbladder. The liver receives blood from both the hepatic artery and the portal vein. The hepatic artery provides oxygenated blood from the aorta to the liver cells. The portal vein transports absorbed products of digestion from the gastrointestinal tract to the liver for metabolism. Venous drainage is via the hepatic vein.

The functions of the liver are:

- Metabolism of carbohydrate, protein and fat absorbed from the intestines
- Production of bile
- Neutralization and destruction of drugs and toxins
- Manufacture, breakdown and regulation of hormones
- Manufacture of enzymes and proteins (e.g. albumin)
- Removal of old red blood cells from the circulation
- Storage of iron and vitamins A, D, E and K.

The liver generates heat when carrying out these processes and is a major contributor to the maintenance of body temperature in endothermic animals.

The gallbladder is situated between the quadrate and right medial lobes of the liver. Its function is to store bile until it is required for digestion.

Pancreas

The pancreas is a glandular structure comprising an endocrine and an exocrine component. The endocrine section is responsible for the production of insulin and glucagon (see 'Endocrine system', below). The exocrine section produces bicarbonate and enzymes, which are required for digestion. Bicarbonate neutralizes acid from the stomach, ensuring that the ingesta entering the small intestines is less acidic. The digestive enzymes produced by the pancreas (see Figure 3.69) include:

- Trypsin – which breaks down protein
- Lipase – which breaks down lipids
- Amylase – which breaks down starch.

Small mammals

Many herbivores have a narrow oral cavity compared with dogs and cats. They have no canine teeth, but rather have a diastema (gap) between the incisors and premolars (see 'Dentition', above). The tongue is relatively immobile in rodents. Hamsters and chipmunks have well developed cheek pouches, which are used to store food.

The stomach in hamsters is divided into a glandular and a non-glandular part. Rabbits, guinea pigs and chinchillas have a capacious intestine and caecum designed to house bacterial and protozoal populations, which digest hemicellulose and cellulose (Figure 3.70). The caecum and colon are often folded into haustrae to improve fermentation by longitudinal bands of muscle known as taeniae. Ferrets have canine teeth, a simple stomach, no caecum and a short colon typical of other strict carnivores.

Birds

The tongue varies from muscular and mobile in psittacine birds to strap-like in passerine birds. Birds have a crop (Figure 3.71), a diverticulum of the oesophagus located at the base of the neck, which acts as a food storage chamber. Some species produce crop 'milk' from the crop lining, which is used to feed young animals (e.g. pigeons and doves).

Birds have two stomachs: an acid-secreting stomach (proventriculus), followed immediately by the ventriculus (gizzard). The ventriculus can be sac-like (e.g. raptors) or muscular (e.g. seed-eating birds) and helps to grind food. A significant duodenal loop is found in birds. Caeca (singular: caecum) are not present in all species (e.g. parrots do not have caeca), and where they do occur are often paired. Birds have a short large intestine, often referred to as a rectum.

Birds possess a cloaca, a communal chamber into which the gastrointestinal, urinary and reproductive tracts empty before exiting the body through the vent. The cloaca is split into three chambers:

- The coprodeum, which receives faeces from the gastrointestinal tract
- The urodeum into which the ureters and reproductive tract empty. It is separated from the coprodeum by a fold
- The proctodeum, which is the last chamber and in birds contains the bursa of Fabricius (the source of B lymphocyte production) in its dorsal wall.

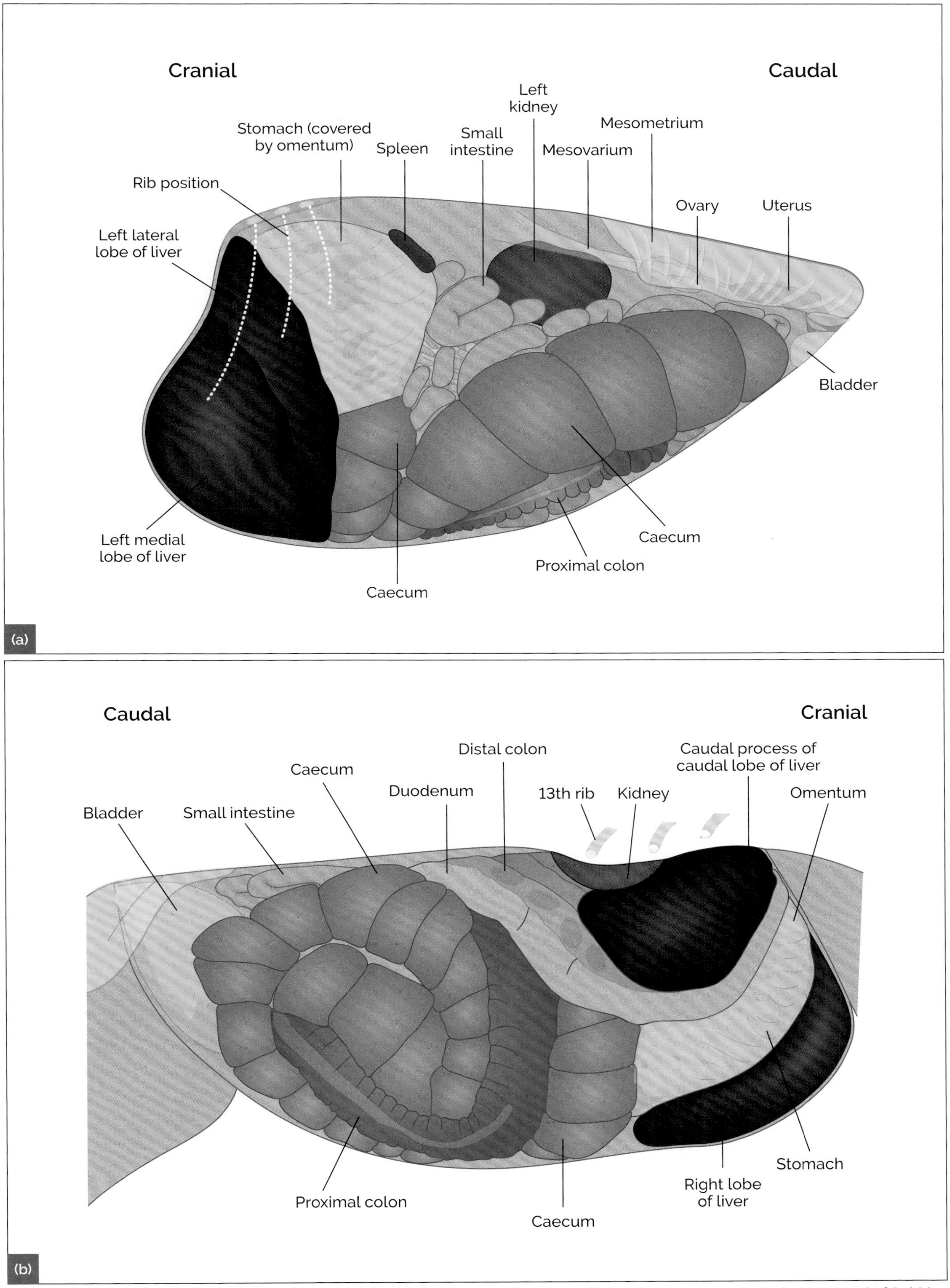

Cranial   Caudal

Left
kidney
Stomach (covered   Small   Mesometrium
by omentum)   Spleen   intestine   Mesovarium
Rib position   Ovary   Uterus
Left lateral
lobe of liver

Bladder

Left medial
lobe of liver
Caecum
Proximal colon
Caecum

(a)

Caudal   Cranial

Distal colon   Caudal process of
caudal lobe of liver
Caecum   Duodenum   13th rib   Kidney   Omentum
Bladder   Small intestine

Stomach
Proximal colon   Right lobe
of liver
Caecum

(b)

3.70 Rabbit viscera. **(a)** Left hand side of a rabbit. **(b)** Right hand side of a rabbit. (Reproduced from the *BSAVA Manual of Rabbit Surgery, Dentistry and Imaging*)

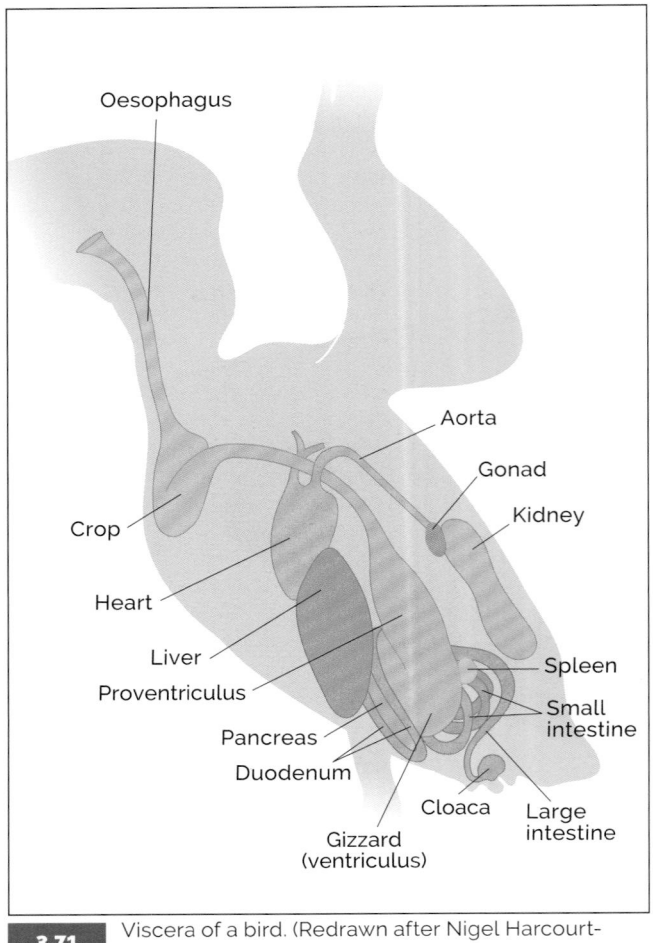

3.71 Viscera of a bird. (Redrawn after Nigel Harcourt-Brown)

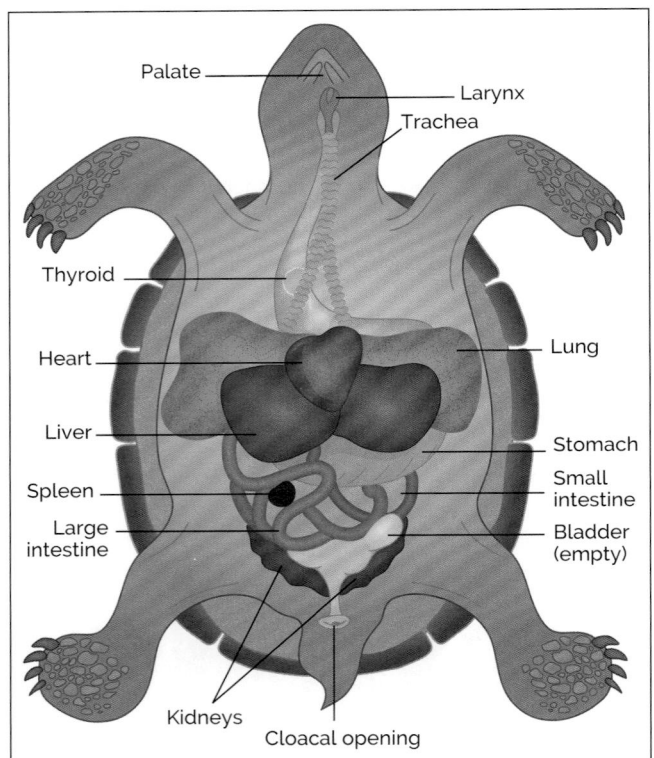

3.72 Main organs in the body cavity of a tortoise (plastron removed).

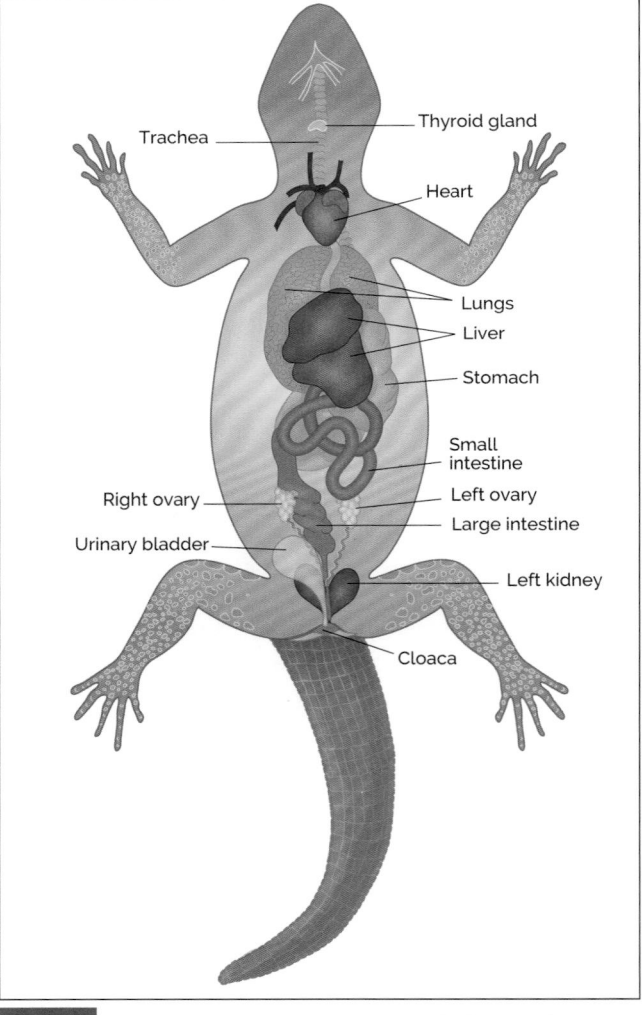

3.73 Main organs in the body cavity of a female lizard.

A bilobed liver is present. Some species have a gall-bladder; however, it is often absent in psittacine birds. Biliverdin is the main bile pigment in birds.

Reptiles

The tongue may be fleshy and immobile in chelonians; fleshy and mobile in many lizards; and strap-like and mobile in snakes. The lack of a diaphragm means that there is no division between 'abdominal' organs such as the liver and intestines, and 'thoracic' organs such as the heart and lungs. Instead there is a single coelomic cavity (Figures 3.72 to 3.74).

The large intestine may be multi-chambered in hindgut fermenters such as the green iguana. Reptiles possess a cloaca, which is similar in structure to that found in birds. The liver is generally bilobed and the main bile pigment is biliverdin. The pancreas may be fused with the spleen to form a splenopancreas, particularly in snakes.

Physiology of digestion

The functions of the gastrointestinal system are to receive and digest food so that the nutritional requirements of an animal can be met, and to excrete waste products. The process of digestion involves: the movement of ingesta along the gastrointestinal tract; mechanical breakdown of food; enzymatic breakdown of food; absorption of nutrients; and the excretion of waste.

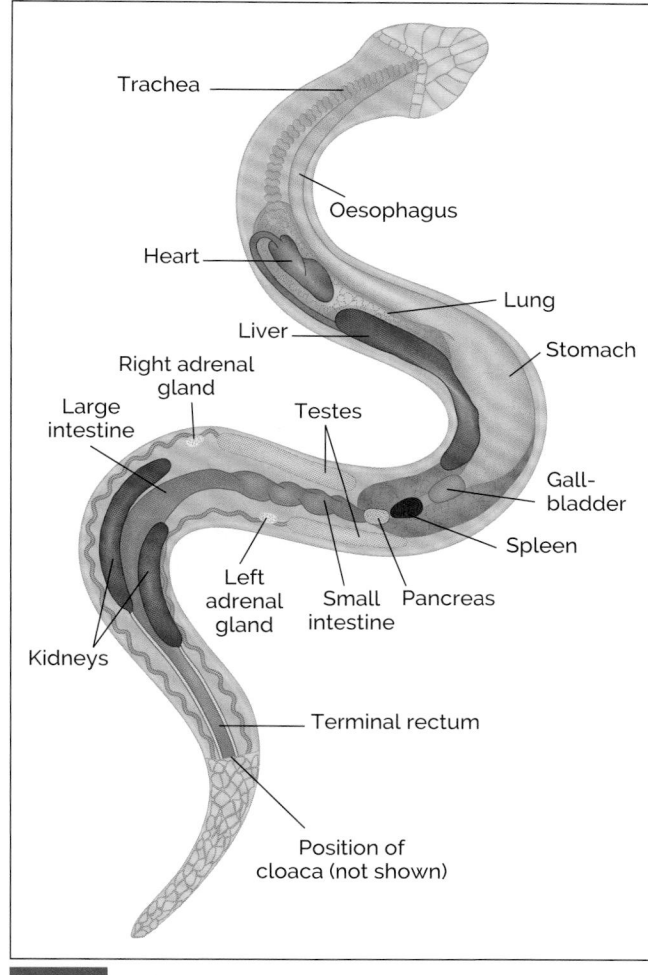

3.74 Main organs in the body cavity of a male snake.

Labels on figure:
Trachea
Oesophagus
Heart
Lung
Liver
Stomach
Right adrenal gland
Large intestine
Testes
Gall-bladder
Spleen
Left adrenal gland
Small intestine
Pancreas
Kidneys
Terminal rectum
Position of cloaca (not shown)

Nutritional requirements

The nutrients required by animals (see Chapter 13 for details) are:

- Water
- Proteins
- Fats
- Carbohydrates
- Minerals
- Vitamins.

Movement of ingesta

Waves of smooth muscle contractions (peristalsis) move ingesta along the gastrointestinal tract. Peristalsis is controlled by pacemakers situated throughout the gastrointestinal tract. Distension of the intestine can also stimulate muscular contractions. Even in a relatively empty gastrointestinal tract there are waves of peristaltic contractions, beginning at the stomach and moving caudally, pushing waste material and bacteria out of the rectum.

Mechanical breakdown

The mechanical breakdown of food is initially carried out by chewing, and continued by contractions of the stomach.

Enzymatic breakdown

Enzymatic digestion occurs from the stomach onwards (for further information, see Chapter 13).

- Pepsin begins the breakdown of proteins into peptides, which are further broken down to amino acids at the level of the brush border in the small intestine.
- Fats (triglycerides) are emulsified in the stomach and broken down in the small intestine by the action of pancreatic lipase. Bile acids act as a detergent and emulsify the fats for digestion.
- Carbohydrates are broken down to monosaccharides by pancreatic and intestinal disaccharides.

Absorption

Absorption of nutrients from the gastrointestinal tract into the bloodstream occurs from the duodenum onwards (see Figure 3.69). No absorption takes place in the oesophagus or stomach. The highest levels of absorption occur in the duodenum and jejunum. From the jejunum to the rectum, the level of absorption decreases with mainly water and electrolytes being absorbed from the large intestine.

Excretion of waste

Defecation is the process by which animals excrete solid waste products from the colon and rectum. The anal sphincter is the muscular end of the gastrointestinal tract. It is usually in a state of constriction, thus ensuring that the opening to the large intestine remains closed. Relaxation of the anal sphincter (usually under voluntary control) allows the passage of faeces. Contraction of the abdominal muscles whilst the glottis is closed increases the abdominal pressure and results in excretion. In dogs the entire rectum is emptied, which means that softer faeces will always be seen towards the end of defecation. This is normal and not suggestive of a gastrointestinal tract problem.

Neonatal gastrointestinal tract

The small intestine in neonates allows antibodies (large molecules) to pass directly into the bloodstream for a few hours after birth, rather than being broken down and absorbed. This results in a transfer of immunity from the dam to the offspring via the maternally derived antibodies (MDA) present in the colostrum. The extent to which this transfer occurs varies between species: it is minimal in humans where most of the MDA transfer occurs via the placenta; it is predominant in dogs, cats and ruminants, where colostral antibodies are an essential part of immunity (see Chapter 7).

Endocrine system

The endocrine system is a collection of ductless glands, which produce hormones and deliver them into the bloodstream, lymph or tissue fluid.

Terminology

- Hormones are chemicals that travel through the bloodstream until they reach their target organ and exert an effect
- Autocrine – of or relating to a hormone that has an effect on the original cell that produced it
- Endocrine – of or relating to a hormone that is transported in the bloodstream to the target organ
- Exocrine – of or relating to a hormone that is released through a duct or ducts
- Paracrine – of or relating to a hormone that has an effect on local cells

The secretion of many hormones is controlled by negative feedback. In simple terms, negative feedback is where increased levels of a hormone are detected by a gland and result in decreased levels of hormone production by that gland. Positive feedback has the opposite effect: increased levels of a hormone are detected by a gland and result in even more hormone being produced by that gland.

Hormones can be grouped according to their molecular structure:

- Proteins – growth hormone, insulin, adrenocorticotrophic hormone (ACTH)
- Peptides – thyroid-stimulating hormone (TSH), oxytocin
- Amines – dopamine, adrenaline
- Steroids – cortisol, progesterone.

Hypothalamus

The control centre of the endocrine system is the hypothalamus (see 'Central nervous system', above). The hypothalamus sits at the base of the brain and connects the endocrine system with the nervous system (see Figure 3.40). The hypothalamus produces releasing hormones, which in turn control the pituitary gland.

Pituitary gland

The pituitary gland (hypophysis) responds to the releasing hormones secreted by the hypothalamus by producing stimulating hormones, which are sent out to individual organs. The pituitary gland comprises an anterior and a posterior section, which produce different hormones.

Anterior pituitary gland

The anterior pituitary gland (adenohypophysis) produces the following hormones:

- Adrenocorticotrophic hormone (ACTH) – targets the adrenal gland cortex and stimulates the release of corticosteroids and mineralocorticoids
- Follicle-stimulating hormone (FSH) – targets the Sertoli cells in males causing spermatogenesis. In females it targets the ovaries stimulating growth of the follicles which contain the ova (eggs)
- Growth hormone (GH) – also known as somatotropin. It acts on all tissues of the body, stimulating growth by increasing the uptake of amino acids and protein production. Fat deposition is also increased by GH
- Luteinizing hormone (LH) – targets the Leydig cells in males and stimulates the release of testosterone. In females it targets the ovaries causing ovulation and the development of the corpus luteum. LH has various functions. It is released spontaneously in the bitch, but is only released in response to mating in the queen
- Prolactin (PRL) – targets the mammary glands to stimulate development during pregnancy and milk let down following parturition
- Thyroid-stimulating hormone (TSH) – targets the thyroid gland and stimulates the release of thyroxine. Thyroxine controls metabolic rate.

Posterior pituitary gland

The posterior pituitary gland (neurohypophysis) is connected to the hypothalamus and produces two hormones:

- Antidiuretic hormone (ADH) – also known as vasopressin. It is released in response to an increase in plasma osmotic pressure (as detected by baroreceptors). ADH targets the distal convoluted tubules in the kidney, increasing their permeability. This causes an increase in the resorption of water, thus increasing plasma volume and reducing the volume of urine produced
- Oxytocin – targets the uterus during parturition causing contraction of the smooth muscle. It also acts on the muscles lining the mammary glands, resulting in milk let down.

Pineal gland

The pineal gland is located within the brain and produces melatonin in response to daylight length. Melatonin is responsible for the functions of the body related to photoperiod such as reproduction, behaviour and coat changes.

Thyroid gland

The thyroid gland lies over the trachea, caudal to or at the level of the larynx. In dogs and cats the thyroid gland is divided into two lobes, which sit on either side of the larynx. The gland comprises follicles within a connective tissue capsule. Parafollicular cells (also known as C-cells) are located between the follicles. Parafollicular cells produce calcitonin, which is responsible for the control of blood calcium levels. Calcitonin decreases the blood calcium level by stimulating deposition of calcium in bone, decreasing calcium absorption from the gastrointestinal tract and increasing excretion of calcium in the urine.

Thyroid-stimulating hormone (TSH) targets the thyroid gland resulting in the secretion of thyroxine (T4) and triiodothyronine (T3). The secretion of these hormones is controlled by negative feedback: increased levels of thyroxine are detected by the anterior pituitary gland, resulting in a decrease in the secretion of TSH. Thyroid hormones act on virtually all cells in the body. They control metabolic rate and are essential for normal growth. Thyroid hormones have an effect on the skin, skeleton, cardiovascular system, neurological system and reproductive function.

Parathyroid glands

The parathyroid glands are found in close proximity to or sometimes embedded within the thyroid gland. There are two parathyroid glands associated with each lobe of the thyroid gland, resulting in a total of four parathyroid glands. They are much smaller and paler than the thyroid gland. The parathyroid glands produce parathyroid hormone (PTH), which is involved in the control of blood calcium levels. PTH has an antagonistic effect to that of calcitonin: it increases blood calcium levels by releasing calcium from bones, increasing calcium absorption from the gastrointestinal tract, accelerating vitamin D activation and decreasing excretion of calcium in urine by stimulating calcium resorption in the distal tubules of the kidneys. PTH also decreases blood phosphate concentrations by increasing phosphate deposition in bone.

Kidneys

The kidneys produce erythropoietin, which stimulates the bone marrow to produce red blood cells. The production and release of erythropoietin is regulated by the arterial oxygen concentration in a manner that is poorly understood.

Adrenal glands

The adrenal glands are small bean-like structures that lie in the dorsal abdomen craniomedial to the kidneys. They consist of an inner medulla and outer cortex, which is covered in a connective tissue capsule.

Cortex

The adrenal gland cortex is divided into three different zones:

- Zona glomerulosa (outermost)
- Zona fasciculata
- Zona reticularis.

Adrenocorticotrophic hormone (ACTH) from the anterior pituitary gland acts on the adrenal cortex, stimulating the production of mineralocorticoids and glucocorticoids. The adrenal gland cortex also produces sex hormones (androgens and oestrogens). However, the significance of these hormones is not clear as the majority of the sex hormones are produced by the gonads.

Mineralocorticoids

These are produced by the zona glomerulosa and include aldosterone, which controls the level of sodium and potassium in the body. Aldosterone is produced via the renin–angiotensin–aldosterone pathway (see 'Distal convoluted tubule' below).

Glucocorticoids

These are produced by the zona fasciculata and zona reticularis. Glucocorticoids, such as cortisol, are produced in a circadian rhythm (in dogs, levels of cortisol are higher in the morning and lower in the evening; in cats, levels of cortisol are lower in the morning and higher in the evening). Cortisol has diverse effects in the body. Its main functions are: metabolism of carbohydrates, proteins and fats; and the promotion of gluconeogenesis. Cortisol also reduces the inflammatory process and the immune response. Levels of cortisol increase if an animal is stressed.

Medulla

The adrenal gland medulla is connected to the nervous system and is responsible for the 'flight or fight' response via the release of adrenaline (epinephrine) and noradrenaline. The release of adrenaline is stimulated by hypoglycaemia, stress, decreased blood pressure and hypothermia. The adrenal glands have a good vascular supply, which allows adrenaline to be quickly released into the circulation. Adrenaline increases glucose production by the liver, increases blood glucose concentrations, increases blood supply to the skeletal muscles and increases heart rate. It also causes relaxation of the gastrointestinal smooth muscle, urinary retention, dilatation of pupils and sweat production.

Gastrointestinal hormones

Gastrin is released from G cells in the stomach, duodenum and pancreas. Secretion of gastrin occurs in response to the presence of peptides (from food) in the stomach. Gastrin stimulates hydrochloric acid release by the stomach lining. Cholecystokinin is released from I cells in the lining of the duodenum. It stimulates pancreatic and bile secretions to aid digestion. Secretin is released from S cells in the duodenum. It helps control the pH of gastrointestinal tract contents.

Pancreas

The pancreas is located in the mesentery of the duodenum. It has both exocrine and endocrine components. The exocrine section produces digestive enzymes which are secreted into the gastrointestinal tract (see 'Digestive system', above). The endocrine section comprises the islets of Langerhans. These islets consist of three different cells:

- Alpha cells – produce glucagon
- Beta cells – produce insulin
- Delta cells – produce somatostatin.

Glucagon production is stimulated by low blood glucose concentrations or stress. It acts on the liver to break down stored glycogen into glucose (glycogenolysis) and to increase the production of glucose (gluconeogenesis). Glucagon also increases lipolysis. Insulin production is stimulated by high blood glucose concentrations, as well as by the gastrointestinal hormones gastrin, cholecystokinin and secretin. Insulin stimulates the uptake of glucose into the cytoplasm of cells and the production of glycogen, triglycerides and proteins. Insulin has the opposite effect to glucagon. Somatostatin has a regulatory role inhibiting the release of both glucagon and insulin.

Reproductive glands

Follicle-stimulating hormone (FSH) and luteinizing hormone (LH) are gonadotrophins. They are released from the anterior pituitary gland (see above) and stimulate the reproductive organs. More detail on their actions is given in Chapter 24.

Testosterone

Testosterone is the predominant hormone in males. It is produced by the Leydig cells in response to LH.

Oestrogen

In males, oestrogen is produced by the Sertoli cells in the seminiferous tubules of the testes. In females, it is produced by the developing follicles during the oestrous cycle. It is responsible for the physical and behavioural signs of oestrus.

Progesterone

Progesterone is produced by the corpus luteum and is present in both pregnant and non-pregnant females. It is responsible for the maintenance of pregnancy and the signs associated with metoestrus.

Birds

Hormones such as prolactin and thyroxine help control the cycle of feather moulting and regrowth. The principal corticosteroid produced by the adrenal glands in birds is corticosterone rather than cortisol.

Reptiles

Reptiles produce vasotocin rather than oxytocin during egg production. The parietal eye (situated on the top of the head in reptiles such as the green iguana) and the pineal gland are responsible for the production of melatonin in reptiles. Melatonin controls seasonal variations in reproduction and activity. The thyroid gland plays an important role in the homeostatic mechanisms of hibernation.

Urinary system

Kidneys

The kidneys in dogs and cats are often described as bean-shaped. They are found in the retroperitoneum close to the dorsal body wall. The right kidney is positioned slightly more cranially than the left kidney. The cranial pole of the right kidney is located in a depression of the caudate process of the liver. The left kidney can be mobile, especially in cats.

The kidney is surrounded by a tightly adherent capsule and consists of three main areas (Figure 3.75):

- The outer cortex (often dark in colour as it is more vascular)
- The inner medulla (often light in colour as it is less vascular)
- The renal pelvis.

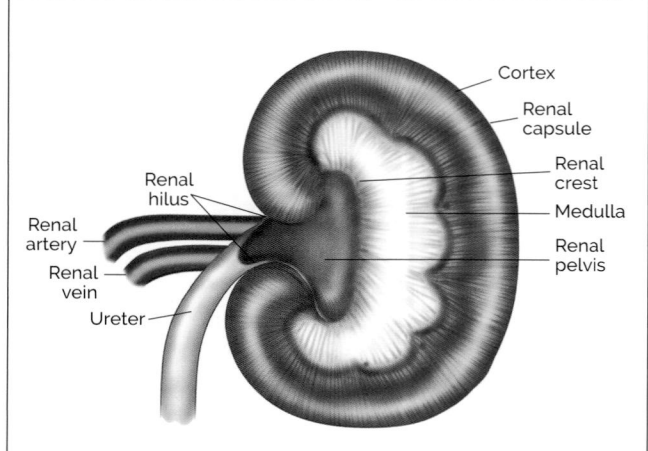

3.75 Longitudinal section through a kidney.

The nephron (Figure 3.76) is the functional unit of the kidney. It comprises a vascular plexus known as the glomerulus surrounded by the Bowman's capsule (glomerular capsule), located in the cortex. An afferent arteriole supplies the glomerulus and an efferent arteriole drains it. The Bowman's capsule leads to the proximal convoluted tubule, which in turn leads to the loop of Henle located within the medulla. The loop of Henle leads to the distal convoluted tubule situated within the cortex. The distal convoluted tubule then leads to the collecting duct, which is located in the medulla. The renal pelvis is where the collecting ducts merge into the neck of the ureter.

Physiology of urine formation

Glomerulus

The glomerular blood vessels tightly adhere to the basement membrane. Blood flows through the glomerulus and, due to the blood pressure, water, electrolytes and other substances, are forced through the holes in the wall of the glomerulus into the glomerular space. The holes are large enough to allow molecules such as urea, haemoglobin and simple sugars to leave the glomerulus, but will not allow larger molecules such as albumin to pass. This process is known as ultrafiltration and results in the production of urine.

Proximal convoluted tubule

The urine produced in the glomerulus moves into the proximal convoluted tubule. It is here that sodium and the

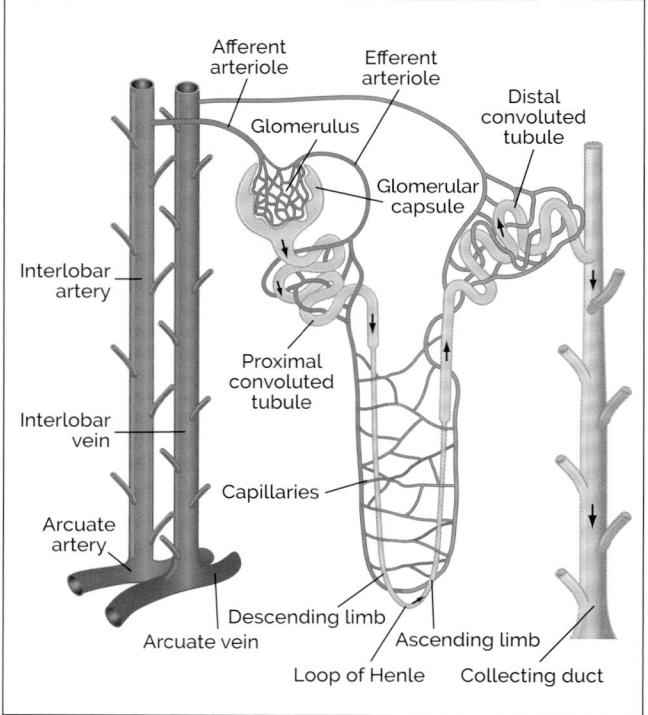

3.76 A kidney nephron. The arrows show the direction of urine flow.

majority of the water (around 75%) are reabsorbed. The resorption of sodium provides the osmotic potential for water resorption. In order to pump sodium out of the proximal convoluted tubule and into the peritubular blood vessels, it is exchanged for potassium. Thus, there is a net resorption of sodium and water and a net excretion of potassium. In addition, many drugs (e.g. penicillin) are actively excreted by the proximal convoluted tubule.

Loop of Henle

The urine passes from the proximal convoluted tubule into the descending limb of the loop of Henle. The descending limb has a thin wall and allows water to pass out of the lumen and into the interstitial tissue by osmosis. The urine then passes into the ascending limb of the loop of Henle. The ascending loop has a thick squamous epithelium, which prevents water from leaving the lumen. Sodium, potassium and chloride are pumped out of the ascending limb and into the interstitial tissue. This creates an osmotic gradient between the interstitial tissue (high osmotic concentration) and the descending limb (low osmotic concentration), allowing water to diffuse out of the lumen.

Distal convoluted tubule

From the loop of Henle the urine passes into the distal convoluted tubule. It is here that more sodium is reabsorbed, and potassium and hydrogen are excreted. Hydrogen excretion is important as it enables the body to maintain the acid–base balance. Aldosterone regulates sodium absorption and potassium excretion in the distal convoluted tubule. Aldosterone is produced via the renin–angiotensin–aldosterone pathway:

1. If an animal is dehydrated or suffers blood loss, the reduced blood flow to the glomerulus results in the release of the hormone renin from the granular cells in the juxtaglomerular apparatus of the kidney.

2. Renin acts on the plasma protein angiotensinogen to convert it to angiotensin I.
3. Angiotensin I is converted to angiotensin II by angiotensin-converting enzyme in the lungs.
4. Angiotensin II stimulates the production of aldosterone from the adrenal gland cortex. Angiotensin II also causes the afferent arteriole to constrict, reducing blood flow to the glomerulus and thus increasing blood pressure.
5. Aldosterone acts on the distal convoluted tubule to increase sodium resorption and potassium excretion. Water is consequently reabsorbed by osmosis, thereby increasing plasma volume.

Collecting duct

Urine passes from the distal convoluted tubule into the collecting duct. Each collecting duct collects urine from a number of nephrons. Antidiuretic hormone (ADH), released by the posterior pituitary gland in response to an increase in osmotic pressure or low blood pressure, acts on the collecting ducts to increase resorption of water. The urine then moves through the collecting ducts and into the renal pelvis, where it drains into the ureter.

Ureters

Each kidney has a single ureter, which drains the renal pelvis and transports the urine to the urinary bladder. The ureters are retroperitoneal and suspended within a fold of visceral peritoneum known as the mesoureter. The ureters are lined with transitional epithelium, which allows some expansion of the lumen. The transitional epithelium is supported by a sheath of smooth muscle, which helps propel urine from the kidney to the urinary bladder by peristaltic waves of contraction.

Urinary bladder

The bladder is situated within the retroperitoneum; although, when full it projects into the caudal abdomen. The bladder receives urine from the ureters, which enter through the trigone on the dorsal surface. The oblique angle at which the ureters enter the trigone prevents the reflux of urine from the bladder. The base of the trigone (triangle) lies between the two ureteral entrances with the apex at the urethral orifice. Urine is discharged from the bladder into the urethra at the level of the pelvic inlet.

A lateral ligament connects the lateral surface of the bladder to the lateral pelvic wall. A median ligament connects the ventral surface of the bladder to the symphysis of the pelvis and the midline of the body wall as far cranially as the umbilicus. In addition, there is a middle ligament which in the fetus contains the urachus. This is the stalk of the allantois, which disappears after birth leaving a peritoneal fold.

The urinary bladder is lined with transitional epithelium. The wall of the bladder comprises three layers of smooth muscle with a muscular sphincter at the bladder neck. These muscles are innervated by the pudendal nerve (somatic innervation), the hypogastric nerve (sympathetic innervation) and the pelvic nerve (parasympathetic innervation).

Urethra

The urethra is a simple structure lined with transitional epithelium, which is supported by a sheath of smooth muscle and connective tissue.

In male dogs the urethra runs from the neck of the bladder to the prostate gland, where it is joined by the deferent duct. The section of the urethra that runs through the prostate gland is called the prostatic urethra. As it exits the prostate gland, the urethra runs caudally through the pelvis to the pelvic brim. This part is called the membranous urethra. The urethra then moves ventrally, beneath the perineal surface, before travelling cranially to run through the penis on the ventral surface of the body. This part is termed the cavernous urethra and is surrounded by erectile tissue (Figure 3.77a). The external urethral orifice is found on the tip on the penis.

In tomcats, the course of the urethra diverges from that of male dogs once it has passed through the pelvis. In cats the urethra runs through the penis in the perineal region. Tomcats also have an additional urethral section: there is a short length of urethra cranial to the prostate gland, located between the opening to the bladder and the prostate gland. This is known as the pre-prostatic urethra. Tomcats also have a pair of bulbourethral glands, which open into the lumen of the urethra close to its caudal end (Figure 3.77b). The external urethral orifice is found on the tip of the penis.

The function of the urethra in males is to transport urine, sperm and spermatic fluid from the bladder and prostate gland to the penis for excretion.

In females the urethra runs from the bladder neck, through the pelvis, to the floor of the vagina. Its only function is to transfer urine from the bladder to the vagina for excretion. The external urethral orifice is located in the vestibule caudal to the vagina.

Small mammals

In small mammals that live in desert conditions, such as gerbils, the loop of Henle in the kidneys is comparatively longer than that of dogs. This means that gerbils can concentrate urine much more effectively.

Birds

Birds have long, thin trilobed kidneys (see Figure 3.71), which are attached to the ventral surface of the synsacrum. Approximately 50% of the nephrons in the kidney have no loop of Henle. The ureters empty directly into the urodeum section of the cloaca; thus, there is no urinary bladder in birds. The main waste product of protein metabolism is uric acid rather than urea. In addition, birds have a renal portal system (see 'Veins', above).

Reptiles

The kidneys in chelonians and lizards are compact (see Figures 3.72 and 3.73). The kidneys in snakes are long and thin (see Figure 3.74). The nephrons in the kidney have no loop of Henle. Some male reptiles have a sexual segment to the kidney, which is responsible for producing spermatic fluid. The ureters empty directly into the urodeum section of the cloaca. Many chelonians and lizards possess a urinary bladder, but snakes do not. As the ureters empty into the urodeum, urine is not sterile even when a urinary bladder is present. The main waste product of protein metabolism is uric acid rather than urea. Reptiles also have a renal portal system (see 'Veins', above).

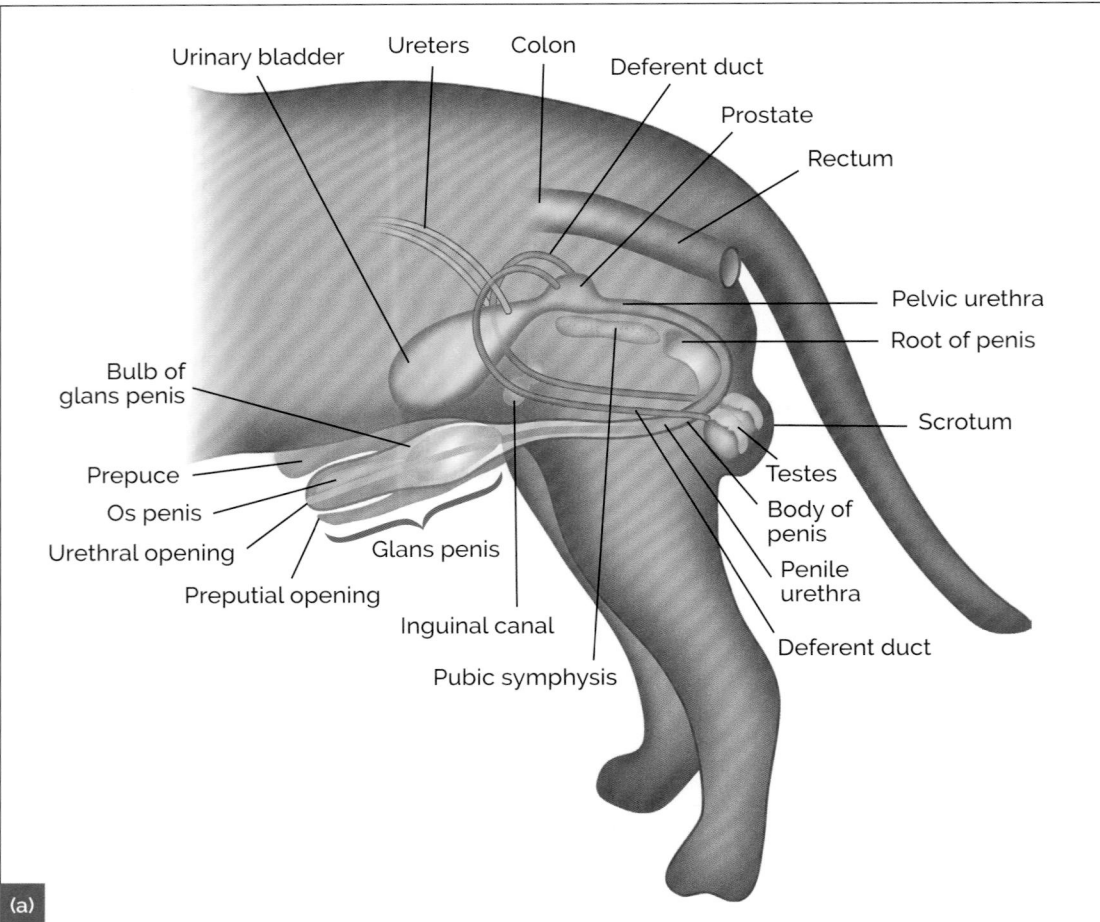

(a)

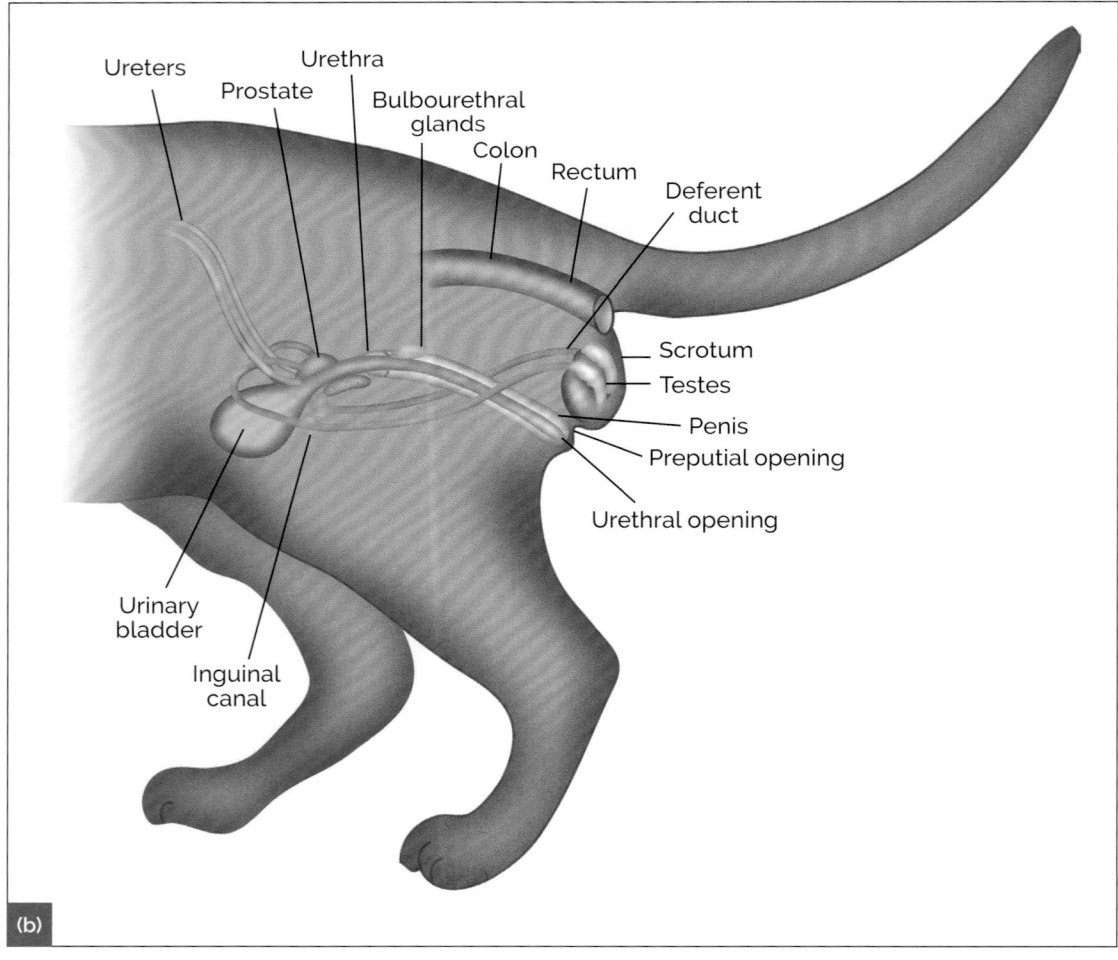

(b)

3.77

(a) Reproductive and lower urinary tract of a dog. (b) Reproductive and lower urinary tract of a tomcat.

3.77 (a) Reproductive and lower urinary tract of a dog. (b) Reproductive and lower urinary tract of a tomcat.

Reproductive system

For more information on the physiology of reproduction see Chapter 24.

Male reproductive system

Anatomy

The reproductive system of the male dog and tomcat are shown in Figure 3.77. The male reproductive tract comprises the testicles, epididymis, deferent duct, spermatic cord, urethra, penis, prostate gland and bulbourethral gland.

Testicles

The testicles are round to oval and found outside the abdomen in the scrotum. The temperature in the scrotum is slightly lower than core body temperature, and this is optimal for sperm production. The testicles consist of:

- Leydig cells (interstitial cells)
- Sertoli cells
- Spermatogenic cells.

Epididymis

The epididymis is part of the testicle, but appears grossly to be adhered to its outer surface. Sperm are produced in the main part of the testicle and then transported to the epididymis in ducts. The epididymis becomes narrower and tapers into the deferent duct.

Deferent duct

The deferent duct (also known as the vas deferens or ductus deferens) transports sperm from the epididymis to enter the urethra at the neck of the bladder.

Spermatic cord

The spermatic cord travels from the epididymis up into the abdomen. The spermatic cord and testicle are surrounded by a layer of connective tissue (an outpouching of the peritoneum) known as the vaginal tunic.

A number of structures can be found within the spermatic cord:

- Deferent duct
- Testicular artery and vein
- Lymphatic vessels
- Nerves
- Cremaster muscle – responsible for raising/lowering the testicle depending on the surrounding temperature.

Penis

The penis consists of erectile tissue, which has a profuse blood supply. In dogs the penis is present on the ventral abdomen, running from the ischial arch of the pelvis cranioventrally along the perineum. There is a small bone, known as the os penis, present dorsal to the urethra. In tomcats the penis is found under the tail, ventral to the anus. It points caudally (rather than cranially) and is covered in barbs, which are thought to be partly responsible for the induction of ovulation in the queen during mating.

Accessory glands

The accessory glands are responsible for the production of spermatic fluid. This fluid not only transports but also provides nutrition for the sperm and contains hormones that are important in fertilization. Various accessory glands are found along the male reproductive tract, including:

- Prostate gland – a single gland found around the urethra at the neck of the bladder. It is present in both dogs and tomcats
- Bulbourethral glands – paired glands located on the dorsal aspect of the urethra near the pelvic exit. These glands are absent in dogs and vestigial in tomcats.

Sperm

Sperm comprise four main parts:

- Acrosome – this is a cap-like structure found on the head of the sperm. It is derived from the Golgi apparatus
- Head – this is where the nucleus is located
- Mid-piece – contains mitochondria
- Tail – provides motion.

Small mammals
Ferrets

A male ferret is called a hob. The penis is located on the ventral abdomen. The os penis is J-shaped. Ferrets possess a prostate gland.

Rabbits

A male rabbit is called a buck. Mature males have obvious scrotal sacs, although it is possible for the testicles to move through the inguinal canal and into the abdomen. By applying pressure on either side of the urethral opening it may be possible to extrude the penis. The penis is conical and has no central slit. There is no os penis. Rabbits possess a prostate gland, vesicular glands, bulbourethral glands and coagulating glands. These accessory glands are found along the deferent duct and urethra, and produce seminal fluid.

Guinea pigs

A male guinea pig is called a boar. The inguinal ring is permanently open, through which a fat body from each testicle protrudes into the abdomen. A spicule-like os penis is present. Guinea pigs possess a prostate gland, vesicular glands and coagulating glands.

Rats and mice

Male rats have obvious testicles from approximately 5 weeks of age. However, the testicles may not always be present in the scrotum as the inguinal canal remains open throughout life. A spicule-like os penis is present. Rats possess ampullary, bulbourethral, preputial, prostate and vesicular accessory glands. Male mice have similar glands and a very pungent odour.

Hamsters and gerbils

Male hamsters and gerbils have obvious testicles and a spicule-like os penis. In addition, they have similar accessory glands to rats and mice.

Birds

A male bird is called a cock. Males possess two intra-abdominal testicles, located cranial to the kidneys, each with a separate vas deferens that empties into the urodeum portion of the cloaca. Most male birds do not have a penis, with the exception of some waterfowl and ratites (such as the ostrich). Instead semen is transferred from the male to the female via apposition of the cloacas. During the breeding season male birds may show up to a 10-fold increase in the size of the testicles.

Reptiles

Chelonians

Male tortoises possess intracoelomic paired testicles, located cranial to the kidneys, each with a separate vas deferens that empties into the urodeum portion of the cloaca. Male tortoises have one penis, which lies in the ventral cloaca. Male tortoises also have a longer tail and more distal vent than females. In addition, the plastron in males may have a concave appearance.

Lizards

Male lizards possess intracoelomic paired testicles, located cranial to the kidneys, each with a separate vas deferens that empties into the urodeum portion of the cloaca. Male lizards have two hemipenes located in the base of the tail, similar to those seen in snakes. For this reason, the base of the tail in males may appear wider than in females. Males may also have pores in the skin along the underside of the thighs (e.g. in agamids and iguanids) or in front of the vent (e.g. in geckos).

Snakes

Males possess intracoelomic paired testicles, located cranial to the kidneys (see Figure 3.74), each with a separate vas deferens that empties into the urodeum portion of the cloaca. Male snakes have a pair of hemipenes (singular, hemipenis), which are situated at the base of the tail. The hemipenes are inverted sacs at rest and only become obvious during mating. Snakes are sexed using a blunt-ended surgical probe, which is inserted through the vent and advanced cranially. In male snakes, the probe can be inserted a length equal to 8–16 subcaudal scales.

Physiology

The main hormones associated with the male reproductive tract are:

- Follicle-stimulating hormone (FSH) – targets the Sertoli cells causing spermatogenesis and the production of oestrogen
- Luteinizing hormone (LH) – targets the Leydig cells causing the production of testosterone
- Testosterone – influences spermatogenesis, development of the male reproductive tract and development of male secondary sexual characteristics.

Female reproductive system

Anatomy

The reproductive system of the bitch (Figure 3.78) and queen are similar in structure. The female reproductive tract comprises the ovaries, uterine tube, uterus, cervix, vagina and vulva.

Ovaries

The ovaries are paired and lie caudal to the kidneys. The ovary is suspended from the abdominal wall in the mesovarium, part of which is folded into the ovarian bursa. The ovarian bursa is a pouch-like structure that completely covers the ovary. The ovary is attached to the dorsal body wall by the ovarian ligament.

The ovaries are small and round or oval. However, the shape of the ovary changes during the oestrous cycle as follicles appear on its surface in response to follicle-stimulating hormone (FSH). Each follicle releases an ovum (egg) in response to a surge in luteinizing hormone (LH).

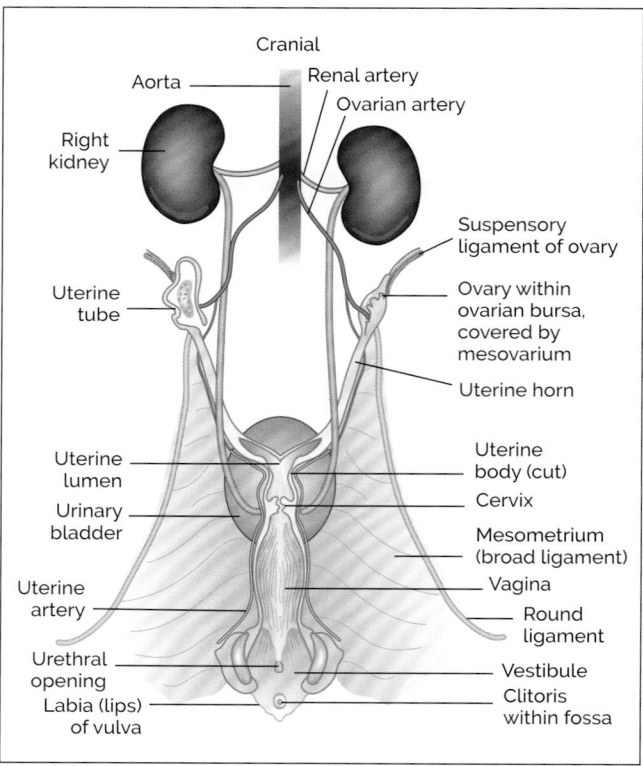

3.78 Ventrodorsal view of the urogenital system of a bitch.

Located close to each ovary is the infundibulum, which 'catches' the ovum when it is released and transports it through the uterine tube (also known as the Fallopian tube) to the uterus.

Uterus

The uterus comprises two horns, which join together at the uterine body. The length of the uterine horn varies depending on the species. Animals that have a large number of offspring per pregnancy (e.g. dogs and cats) have long uterine horns. Animals that have one or two offspring per pregnancy (e.g. cows) have shorter uterine horns.

The uterus consists of an outer layer of connective tissue, a central layer of muscle (myometrium) and a highly vascular inner layer (endometrium). Blood is supplied to the uterus via the uterine artery, which runs parallel to the uterine body from caudal to cranial on either side.

Cervix, vagina and vulva

The cervix is a short thick-walled sphincter, which separates the uterus from the vagina. It is closed most of the time but opens during oestrus and for parturition. The vagina extends from the cervix to the external urethral orifice, where the urinary tract joins the reproductive tract. The vulva is the external opening to the reproductive tract.

Mammary glands

These are modified skin glands that are found on either side of the midline in pairs. The number of mammary glands varies between breeds, but in general bitches have five pairs and queens have four pairs. Each gland consists of glandular epithelium lined with secretory epithelium. Milk from the sinuses drains into teat canals, which open on the surface at teat orifices (Figure 3.79). Milk is produced in response to progesterone and prolactin. Milk let down or excretion in response to suckling is due to muscular contractions induced by oxytocin.

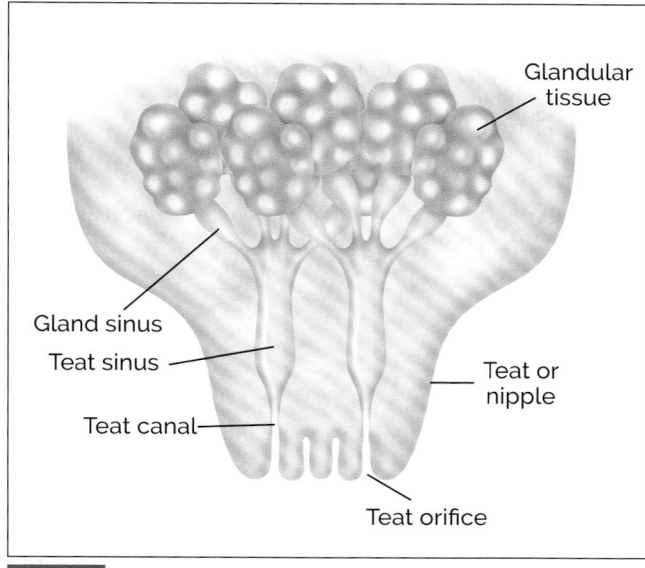

3.79 Structure of a mammary gland.

Labels: Glandular tissue, Gland sinus, Teat sinus, Teat canal, Teat orifice, Teat or nipple

Small mammals
Ferrets

A female ferret is called a jill. The urogenital opening is located ventral to the anus. Jills are seasonally polyoestrous and induced ovulators. This can lead to problems in unmated females as they do not ovulate, but instead remain in oestrus. This results in high levels of oestrogen, which can impair red blood cell production, leading to anaemia, which can be fatal in many cases. This is why it is important that a jill is either mated or injected with a progesterone or gonadotrophin-releasing hormone (GnRH) agonist to bring her out of oestrus. Normal gestation lasts 41–42 days. Pseudopregnancy lasts a similar length of time.

Rabbits

A female rabbit is called a doe. The ovaries lie caudal to the kidneys. The uterus has no uterine body: the two uterine horns each possess a cervix, which projects into the vagina. This arrangement is described as being duplex. Does have a high incidence of uterine tumours as they age, which is one of the main reasons for recommending routine neutering of female rabbits. The urethra also opens into the vagina. The vulva is rounded with a central slit. Does are induced ovulators and cycle every 12–16 days during the breeding season if they are not mated. The anogenital distance in females is shorter than in males.

Guinea pigs

A female guinea pig is called a sow. Guinea pigs have a bicornuate (heart-shaped) uterus, with two uterine horns, a single uterine body and a single cervix. Guinea pigs are non-seasonally polyoestrous and spontaneous ovulators. Each oestrous cycle lasts for approximately 16 days.

Following mating a copulatory plug forms, which falls out of the vagina after a few hours. It is thought that this plug may prevent further matings by other males. At the end of pregnancy, the release of relaxin and progesterone stimulates relaxation of the pelvic ligaments. This allows the pubis and ischium to separate to facilitate delivery of the young. However, this is usually only fully achieved in animals mated for the first time when they are young, before complete ossification of the pelvis. Guinea pig sows have two mammary glands.

Rats and mice

Rats and mice have a duplex uterus: the two parallel uterine horns each possess a cervix and join to the cranial vagina. However, from the external surface, the uterine horns appear to fuse cranially to the cervices, so some texts still refer to the uterus in rats as being bicornuate. The urethra and vagina have separate openings. Rats and mice are non-seasonally polyoestrous with an oestrous cycle of approximately 5 days. Gestation lasts 21–23 days in rats and 19–21 days in mice. Mammary tissue in rats and mice is extensive and covers the ventrum and lateral body walls.

Hamsters and gerbils

Female hamsters and gerbils are seasonally polyoestrous and spontaneous ovulators. They have a 4-day oestrous cycle and a gestation length of 15–18 days.

Birds

A female bird is called a hen. Egg production is the most obvious feature of avian reproduction. In most species only the left ovary is present, located cranial to the kidney. An oocyte is released from the ovary into the infundibulum during ovulation where, if mating has occurred, the oocyte is fertilized. The oocyte travels down the oviduct (a tube-like structure) towards the cloaca. The oviduct is divided into different sections: the infundibulum, magnum, isthmus and the uterus. In the infundibulum, the yolk supporting membrane is deposited (chalazion). In the magnum, the albumen or egg white is laid down. In the isthmus, the shell membranes are deposited. The uterus (shell gland) is where the egg shell is created. Once the egg is ready, the next section of the reproductive tract, the vaginal sphincter, relaxes so that the egg can be laid. It takes on average 20 hours for the oocyte to travel from the ovary to the cloaca.

Reptiles

Female reptiles have paired oviducts (see Figure 3.73). The oviducts comprise: the infundibulum, the magnum, the isthmus, the shell gland/uterus and the muscular vagina. The vagina opens into the urodeum portion of the cloaca.

Chelonians

Female tortoises have paired ovaries and can produce eggs twice a year. Some female tortoises have a hinge on the caudal part of the plastron to make egg-laying easier. They may also have longer hindlimb claws than males, which are used for digging holes in preparation for egg-laying. Eggs are produced in a similar manner to those in birds, but the shell is more leathery. The temperature at which the eggs are incubated determines the sex of the offspring (e.g. the spur-thighed tortoise produces males if the eggs are incubated at 29.5°C and females if the eggs are incubated at 31.5°C).

Lizards

Female lizards can be oviparous (egg-bearing), viviparous (bear live young) or ovoviviparous (eggs are produced internally, but when the young are 'born' they are not inside an egg). Sex determination in lizards is mainly chromosomal, with the exception of some geckos where the temperature at which the eggs are incubated determines the sex of the offspring: higher incubation temperatures result in males.

Snakes

Most species of snake have paired ovaries. Eggs travel from the ovary to the uterus via the oviduct. Female snakes can be oviparous (e.g. kingsnakes and pythons) or viviparous (e.g.

garter snakes and boa constrictors). Sex determination in snakes is chromosomal. Snakes are sexed using a blunt-ended surgical probe, which is inserted through the vent and advanced cranially. In female snakes, the probe can be inserted a length equal to 2–6 subcaudal scales.

Physiology

The normal activity of the ovaries is controlled by hormones (see also Chapter 24):

- Follicle-stimulating hormone (FSH) – produced by the anterior pituitary gland. It stimulates the ovary to develop follicles, which release oestrogen. Oestrogen has a negative feedback effect on the pituitary gland and decreases the amount of FSH released
- Luteinizing hormone (LH) – produced by the anterior pituitary gland. A surge of LH is released prior to ovulation and causes the release of the ovum from the follicle. Once the follicle has ruptured, scar tissue is formed. This scar tissue is known as the corpus luteum (yellow body). The corpus luteum is maintained by LH and produces progesterone
- Oestrogen – released from the follicles of the ovary. It is responsible for most of the physical and behavioural changes associated with the bitch or queen being 'in season' ('on heat')
- Progesterone – released from the corpus luteum. It is responsible for: preparing the uterus to receive fertilized ova (zygotes), maintaining pregnancy and causing mammary gland enlargement in pregnancy and pseudopregnancy. It is also present in pregnant and non-pregnant animals following oestrus.

Integument

The integument is the outer covering of the animal and comprises the skin, fur and claws.

Skin

Structure

The basic structure of the skin comprises the epidermis, the dermis (Figure 3.80) and the subcutaneous connective tissue. The thickness of each layer varies in different parts of the body and between species; for example, in areas prone to abrasion such as the footpads, the epidermis is thicker to protect the underlying structures. In dogs and cats, the skin is thicker dorsally and thinner ventrally. The thickness of the skin ranges from 0.5–5 mm in dogs and 0.4–2 mm in cats.

Epidermis

The epidermis consists of 4–5 layers of cells, which are constantly replaced from the basal layer:

- Stratum corneum
- Stratum lucidum
- Stratum granulosum
- Stratum spinosum
- Stratum basale.

Stratum corneum

This comprises many layers of cells known as corneocytes (47 layers have been described in skin from the flank of a dog). Corneocytes consist of keratin and provide a waterproof covering to the skin. These cells are dead. The outer corneocytes are continuously sloughed and replaced by cells from lower layers. On average, it takes 22 days for cells from the basal layer to reach to stratum corneum. However, this can vary depending on trauma and disease.

Stratum lucidum

This layer is only present on the nose and footpads of cats, dogs and small mammals. This is different to the skin of humans where the stratum lucidum is found throughout the epidermis. It consists of dead cells that contain lipid, which give the nose and footpads a glassy appearance.

Stratum granulosum

This is the granular layer. In this layer cells begin to die and are filled with keratin, which gives them a granular appearance under a light microscope. The nuclei of the cells are shrunken. This layer can be two cells thick in areas where hair is present, and up to eight cells thick in areas where hair is absent.

Stratum spinosum

The cells in this layer have a spiky appearance and are still alive and nucleated. This layer is one or two cells thick in areas where hair is present, and up to 20 cells thick in areas where hair is absent.

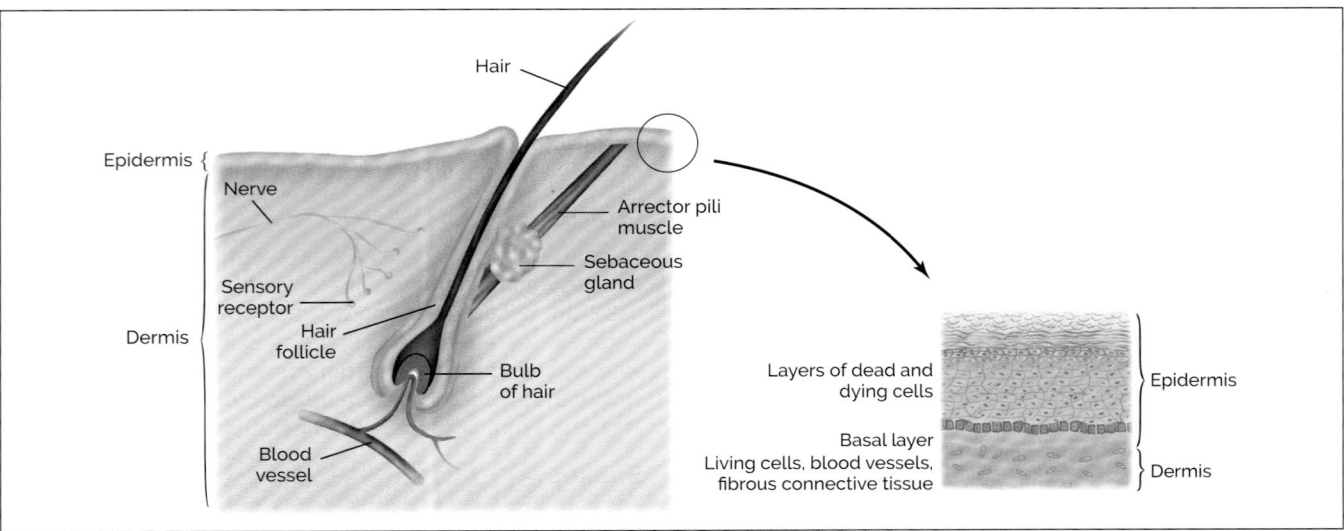

3.80 Cross-section through the skin to show its structure.

Stratum basale

This is the basal layer. It is the lowest layer of the epidermis and consists of a single layer of cells. The cells in this layer replicate by mitosis to replace those lost from other layers of the epidermis. Melanocytes, which give the skin its pigment, are present in this layer.

Dermis

This layer is where the blood vessels, lymphatic vessels, nerves, sweat glands, sebaceous glands and hair follicles are found, surrounded by a dense, elastic connective tissue. Arrector pili muscles (that cause hairs to stand on end) associated with hair follicles are also present in the dermis.

Hair

This is important for insulation, perception and to act as a barrier against injury. Hair comprises an inner medulla, an outer cortex and an overlying cuticle. Hairs that do not have a medulla (known as lanugo) are only found in fetal dogs and cats.

Hair follicles develop from epidermal cells. They can be single (simple follicles) or grouped (compound follicles). Hair follicles grow down into the underlying dermis to form a hair cone, which overlies a hair papilla. From the hair cone, keratinized cells grow to form a hair (Figure 3.81). The hair coat can be divided into primary hairs (outer coat) and secondary hairs (undercoat). Most hairs in dogs and cats are present as compound follicles, consisting of 2–5 primary hairs surrounded by secondary hairs. Each primary hair emerges through a separate pore and has an associated arrector pili muscle, sebaceous gland and sweat gland. Secondary hairs emerge through a common pore and only have an associated sebaceous gland.

Specialized hair cells can also be found in dogs and cats:

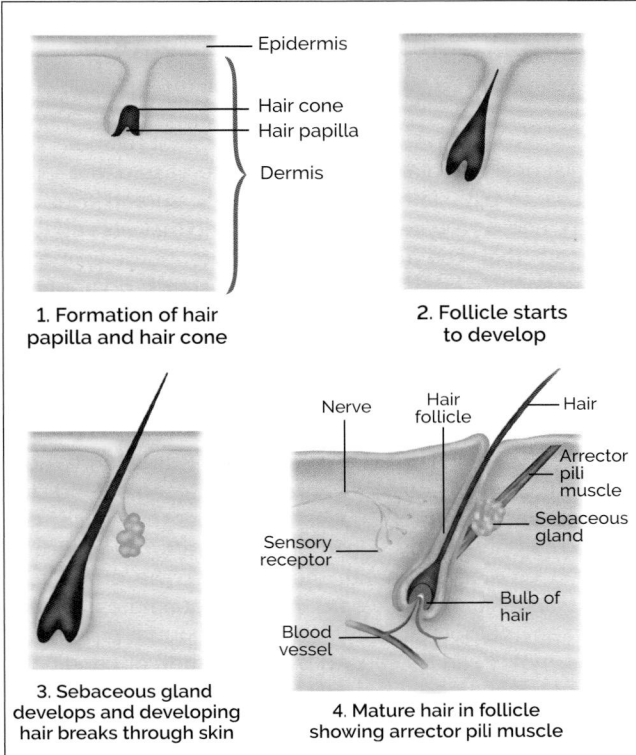

1. Formation of hair papilla and hair cone

2. Follicle starts to develop

3. Sebaceous gland develops and developing hair breaks through skin

4. Mature hair in follicle showing arrector pili muscle

Epidermis
Hair cone
Hair papilla
Dermis

Nerve
Hair follicle
Hair
Arrector pili muscle
Sebaceous gland
Sensory receptor
Bulb of hair
Blood vessel

3.81 The structure and formation of hairs.

- Sinus hairs – these are also known as whiskers or vibrissae and are found on the muzzle, eyelids, lips and face. In cats they are also located on the palmar aspect of the carpus. These hairs are very thick, stiff and have a profuse blood supply. Sinus hairs act as slowly adapting mechanoreceptors
- Tylotrich hairs – these are found scattered throughout the skin amongst the primary and secondary hairs. Tylotrich hairs are strong and thick and present as a single hair within a large follicle. Tylotrich hairs acts as fast-acting mechanoreceptors.

The direction in which the hairs grow gives rise to hair tracts. Hair in different parts of the body will grow in different directions. Hair growth can be divided into three phases:

- Anagen – rapid growth phase
- Catagen – transitional phase
- Telogen – resting phase when no growth takes place.

Hair growth is affected by seasonality, breed, sex, temperature, nutrition, genetics and hormones such as thyroxine and cortisol. Hair replacement in dogs and cats is usually in a mosaic pattern. Dogs and cats may shed more hair during the spring or autumn; however, this can be affected by central heating, thus they may shed hair all year round. The final length of the hair is determined by genetics. Once this predetermined length has been reached the hair enters a resting phase.

Sebaceous glands

Sebaceous glands are associated with hair follicles. There tends to be a larger number of sebaceous glands in areas where the hair follicle density is low (e.g. mucocutaneous junctions, interdigital spaces, chin and the dorsal neck, rump and tail). Sebaceous glands are not found on the footpads or nasal planum. Sebaceous glands produce sebum (a waxy/oily substance), which is secreted into the hair follicles. Sebum forms an emulsion over the surface of the skin that provides waterproofing, retains moisture and acts as an antimicrobial. The activity of the sebaceous glands is partly controlled by androgens, which cause glandular hypertrophy and hyperplasia, and oestrogens, which cause glandular involution.

Sweat glands

Sweat glands (also known as sudiferous glands) can be associated with hair follicles (apocrine or epitrichial) or can be found in areas where hair is absent, such as the footpads (eccrine or atrichial).

- Apocrine (epitrichial) sweat glands – the distribution of apocrine sweat glands is similar to that of sebaceous glands in that a greater number are found in areas of poor hair follicle density. Apocrine sweat glands are coiled and open into the hair follicle.
- Eccrine (atrichial) sweat glands – these are only found on the footpads and nasal planum. Eccrine sweat glands open on to the surface of the skin.

Specialized glands

Specialized glands are found throughout the skin, including:

- Anal sac glands – the anal sacs are found on either side of the anus. These sacs are lined with epithelium, which consists of specialized sebaceous glands that produce a strong smelling oily substance containing pheromones. When the animal defecates, the anal sacs empty, providing a means of scent marking

- Perianal (circumanal) glands – responsible for pheromone production
- Ceruminous glands – the external auditory canal of the ear is lined with ceruminous glands, which produce cerumin (ear wax)
- Tail (supracaudal or preen) gland – in dogs this oval gland is located at the level of the fifth to seventh coccygeal vertebrae. The hair coat in this area comprises stiff, coarse primary hairs. The surface of the skin can be yellow and waxy, and is more obvious in older, entire male dogs. In cats the tail gland runs the length of the tail on the dorsal surface.

Eyelid skin

Cilia or eyelashes are only present on the upper eyelids of dogs and cats. Meibomian (tarsal) glands are a type of sebaceous gland and open at the mucocutaneous junction. Zeis glands are sebaceous glands associated with the cilia. Moll's glands are apocrine sweat glands associated with the cilia. The Harderian gland is an accessory lacrimal gland, which produces tears. The lacrimal glands produce the watery part of the tear whilst the meibomian glands produce the oily portion which, along with the mucus from the conjunctiva, creates the protective tear.

Footpads

These consist of thickened epidermis, covering a fatty vascular structure called the digital cushion. Dogs and cats have seven footpads on the forepaws and five footpads on the hindpaws. There are three types of footpad (Figure 3.82):

- Digital – these footpads protect the distal interphalangeal joints
- Metacarpal/metatarsal – these footpads protect the metacarpal–phalangeal and metatarsal–phalangeal joints
- Carpal – these footpads are also known as stopper pads and lie distal to the carpus in the forepaw.

Small mammals

Many rabbits have a dewlap (ruff or fold of skin on the neck) and this, along with additional skin folds in breeds such as lops, can increase the susceptibility to dermatitis. Rabbits do not have footpads, but instead the palmar/plantar aspect of the foot is covered with dense fur. This can mean that with poor substrate husbandry and/or musculoskeletal disease, rabbits are at an increased risk of hock and lower hindlimb sores due to pressure ischaemia. The number of sweat glands in rabbits and rodents is much reduced, making them more prone to heat stress. Hamsters have lateral flank scent glands in the lower lumbar area, which may be raised and pigmented, particularly prominent in males. Gerbils have a ventral scent gland located near the umbilicus, which is more prominent in males, and this can be prone to infections and adenomas/adenocarcinomas. Gerbils also have fracture planes in the skin of the tail; this means that the skin is easily degloved if the tail is grasped firmly. The tail of rats is unfurred and may develop constrictions associated with low environmental humidity. This may result in ischaemic damage to the tail.

Birds

The epidermis and dermis are thinner in birds. Feather follicles, rather than hair follicles, are present and give rise to several types of feather:

- Primary or flight feathers – located on the manus of the wings. These are strong vaned feathers with a central rachis and interlocking barbs and barbules
- Secondary feathers – attach to the ulna of the wings. These feathers are similar in form to the primary feathers
- Down feathers – have a limited rachis and no interlocking barbs. These feathers are used for insulation
- Contour feathers – a smaller version of the primary feathers. They cover the down feathers and provide the overall shape and coloration of the bird
- Filoplume feathers – associated with the primary and contour feathers. They have a long thin unvaned rachis and a small tuft of barbs at the distal end. The root of these feathers is highly innervated, allowing the bird to subconsciously alter the position of the primary and contour feathers during flight
- Bristle feathers – usually found around the face. These feathers are innervated and allow sensory information to be relayed to the central nervous system.

Birds have a reduced number of sweat glands. The uropygial or preen gland is located at the base of the tail. It produces an oily substance which, when spread over the feathers, acts as a waterproofing agent and may also contain chemicals that can reduce ectoparasite burdens. Some species, such as emus, ostriches and bustards, do not have a uropygial gland.

Reptiles

The epidermis contains a large amount of keratin, which can be thrown into folds to create scales. Chelonians have intradermal bone, which forms the carapace. Lizards undergo a process known as ecdysis, where small patches of old skin are shed and replaced. Snakes also undergo ecdysis, but slough the entire body skin in one piece after the production of a new skin beneath the old one. The process of ecdysis takes around 2 weeks in most squamates. Dysecdysis is any pathological change to the normal process of ecdysis, which can be caused by a multitude of conditions including dehydration, ectoparasitism, wounds, septicaemia and organ failure.

Pigment cells may be prominent in some species (e.g. chameleons) and can be controlled by mood and neural stimulation. A parietal eye may be present in reptiles such as

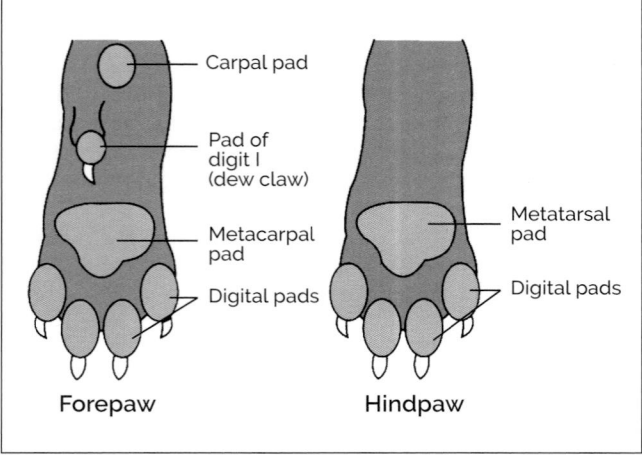

3.82 Ventral view of the forepaw and hindpaw showing the footpads in a dog.

the tuatara (see 'Nervous system' above). Some species of reptiles (e.g. green iguanas) have fracture planes in the tail, which allow the entire tail to be shed if it is grasped roughly by a predator. The tail often regrows in a process known as autotomy. Integumentary sensory organs are often found in the scales on the flanks of reptiles (e.g. crocodilians). These organs detect changes in water pressure associated with the movement of prey.

Function

The skin has many functions, including:

- Adnexa production – hairs and claws
- Antimicrobial – secretes antimicrobial agents
- Communication – alters appearance by raising the hairs if the animal is frightened
- Excretion of waste products in sweat (low levels)
- Indicator of general health (e.g. can be used to evaluate shock and jaundice)
- Motion and shape – flexible and elastic to allow movement
- Pheromone production
- Pigmentation – colour of the hair coat and skin helps prevent damage from solar radiation
- Prevents water and electrolyte loss
- Protection – provides a physical barrier, preventing chemicals and organisms from entering the body
- Sensation – heat, cold, touch, pressure, itch and pain
- Storage of fats, electrolytes, vitamins, carbohydrates and proteins
- Temperature regulation – hair coat, cutaneous blood supply (vasodilatation and constriction) and sweat glands
- Vitamin D production
- Waterproofing.

Claws

Claws are highly keratinized structures, which are continuous with the epidermis and dermis. The distal phalanx is located within the claw. The coronary band is found around the base of the claw, and it is from here that most nail growth occurs (Figure 3.83).

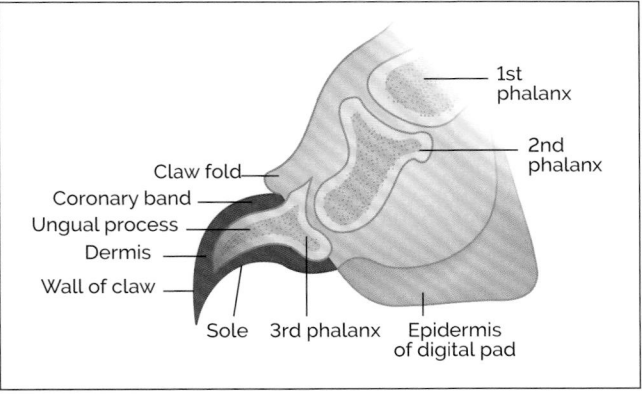

3.83 Longitudinal view of the toe in a dog, showing the claw.

References and further reading

Chitty J and Monks D (2018) BSAVA *Manual of Avian Practice*. BSAVA Publications, Gloucester

Colville TP and Bassert JM (2015) *Clinical Anatomy and Physiology for Veterinary Technicians, 3rd edn*. Mosby, St Louis

Contreras-Aguilar MD, Tecles F, Martinez-Subiela S *et al.* (2017) Detection and measurement of alpha-amylase in canine saliva and changes after an experimentally induced sympathetic activation. *BMC Veterinary Research* **13**, 266

Dobson JM and Lascelles DX (2011) *BSAVA Manual of Canine and Feline Oncology, 3rd edn*. BSAVA Publications, Gloucester

Gardiner A and Raynor M (2014) *The Dog Anatomy Workbook: A Guide to the Canine Body*. JA Allen, Wiltshire

Girling SJ and Raiti P (2004) *BSAVA Manual of Reptiles, 2nd edn*. BSAVA Publications, Gloucester

Girling SJ and Raiti P (2019) *BSAVA Manual of Reptiles, 3rd edn*. BSAVA Publications, Gloucester

Harcourt-Brown F and Chitty J (2013) *BSAVA Manual of Rabbit Surgery, Dentistry and Imaging*. BSAVA Publications, Gloucester

Harcourt-Brown N and Chitty J (2005) *BSAVA Manual of Psittacine Birds, 2nd edn*. BSAVA Publications, Gloucester

Holt D, ter Haar G and Brockman D (2018) *BSAVA Manual of Canine and Feline Head, Neck and Thoracic Surgery, 2nd edn*. BSAVA Publications, Gloucester

Keeble E and Meredith A (2009) *BSAVA Manual of Rodents and Ferrets*. BSAVA Publications, Gloucester

Klein BG (2012) *Cunningham's Textbook of Veterinary Physiology, 5th edn*. WB Saunders, Philadelphia

Meredith A and Lord B (2014) *BSAVA Manual of Rabbit Medicine*. BSAVA Publications, Gloucester

Schwarz T and Johnson V (2008) *BSAVA Manual of Canine and Feline Thoracic Imaging*. BSAVA Publications, Gloucester

Singh B (2018) *Dyce, Sack, and Wensing's Textbook of Veterinary Anatomy, 5th edn*. Elsevier, St Louis

Villiers E and Ristić J (2016) *BSAVA Manual of Canine and Feline Clinical Pathology, 3rd edn*. BSAVA Publications, Gloucester

Useful websites

Colorado State University – Virtual Canine Anatomy:
www.cvmbs.colostate.edu/vetneuro/

Hills Atlas of Veterinary Clinical Anatomy:
www.hillsvet.com/practice-management/atlas-of-veterinary-clinical-anatomy

Online Veterinary Anatomy Museum:
www.onlineveterinaryanatomy.net/

Self-assessment questions

1. Describe the positions of anatomical features on a diagram, or a live animal, using the following terms: cranial, caudal, medial, lateral, proximal, distal, ventral, dorsal, plantar and palmar.
2. Define the terms diffusion and osmosis.
3. Which organelles are found within a cell and what are their functions?
4. Name and describe the two types of cell division.
5. Name the body cavities in (a) a dog; and (b) a lizard.
6. In an immature animal how does a long bone grow?
7. What are the dental formulae for a mature dog, a kitten and a mature rabbit?
8. What is the difference between a tendon and a ligament?
9. List the cranial nerves (names and numbers).
10. Name the chambers and valves through which blood passes in the heart.
11. Explain the avian respiratory cycle.
12. The beta cells of the pancreas are responsible for the secretion of which hormone and what is its function?
13. What is the function of parathyroid hormone?
14. Leydig cells are responsible for the production of which hormone?
15. What is the name of the outermost layer of the skin?

Chapter 4

Genetics

James A.C. Oliver and Cathryn S. Mellersh

Learning objectives

After studying this chapter, readers will have the knowledge to:

- **Describe the structure of DNA**
- **Define the term gene and explain how a gene is composed**
- **Explain how genetic information results in protein formation**
- **Describe the main modes of sex determination in veterinary species**
- **Describe the cell cycle, cell division and meiosis**
- **Describe and understand the different modes of inheritance**
- **Describe how DNA profiling is used in parentage analysis**
- **Define inbreeding, line breeding, outcrossing and heterosis**
- **Describe the BVA/KC canine health schemes**
- **Describe the principles of DNA testing and give some examples of commonly performed DNA tests in the dog and cat**

Glossary

- **Alleles:** Alternative versions of the same gene
- **Amino acid:** An organic compound containing amine (–NH₂) and carboxyl (–COOH) functional groups, along with a side chain specific to each amino acid. Amino acids are the building blocks of proteins
- **Autosome:** The general name given to all chromosomes other than the two involved in determining the sex of an individual (the X and Y chromosomes in mammals)
- **Chromatid:** One copy of a newly copied chromosome that is still joined to the original chromosome
- **Codominant or incomplete inheritance:** The situation where two different alleles may be expressed in an individual heterozygote
- **Codon:** A sequence of three nucleotides that codes for a specific amino acid or indicates termination of translation (stop codon)
- **Diploid:** Somatic cells with two copies of every chromosome are known as diploid
- **Dominant inheritance:** Describes the relationship between alleles of one gene, in which the effect on phenotype of one allele masks the contribution of a second allele at the same locus. Dominant mutations can be expressed when there is only one copy of the mutation
- **Gene:** The basic unit of inheritance
- **Gene pool:** All of the genes that exist within an interbreeding population
- **Genome:** The name given to one complete set of chromosomes, and hence genes, within an organism
- **Genotype:** All of the genes found in the cells of an individual. The genetic make-up of an individual will influence the appearance or phenotype of that individual
- **Haploid:** Gametes have only one copy of every chromosome and are known as haploid
- **Heterosis:** The enhancement of traits in offspring as a result of mixing of the alleles derived from its parents
- **Heterozygous:** Individuals that have two different alleles of a gene for a particular characteristic. If one allele is recessive and one is dominant, the effect caused by the dominant allele will be apparent
- **Homozygous:** Individuals that have identical alleles for a particular characteristic. Recessive characteristics will only show if an individual is homozygous for that characteristic

→

Glossary *continued*

- **Inbreeding:** The mating of first degree relatives such as mother to son
- **Line breeding:** Breeding between closely related individuals
- **Locus:** The unique position of a gene on a DNA molecule
- **Meiosis:** Reproductive cellular division that gives rise to gametes (eggs and sperm), each of which contains half the amount of genetic material contained in the parent cell
- **Microsatellite:** A special region of DNA that possesses an unusual base sequence where two, three or four bases are repeated over and over again
- **Mitosis:** Vegetative cellular division during which each dividing cell gives rise to identical daughter cells both of which contain the same amount of genetic material as the parent cell
- **Mutation:** A permanent change in the base sequence of DNA
- **Phenotype:** The physical expression of an individual's genotype
- **Polymorphism:** The presence of more than one form of specific regions of DNA (alleles) within a given species or population
- **Protein:** A large molecule comprising one or more chains of amino acid residues
- **Recessive inheritance:** Describes the relationship between alleles of one gene, in which the effect on phenotype of one allele is masked by the contribution of a second allele at the same locus. Recessive mutations are only expressed when there are two copies of the mutation
- **Sex chromosomes:** Special chromosomes involved in determining the sex of an animal. In mammals, females possess two X chromosomes and males possess one X and one Y chromosome
- **Single nucleotide polymorphism (SNP):** A variation in a single nucleotide that occurs at a specific position in the genome where each variation is present to some appreciable degree within a population
- **Transcription:** The process by which a gene sequence in a single-stranded DNA template is copied into complementary single-stranded RNA
- **Translation:** The generation of a polypeptide derived from 'reading' of a strand of mRNA
- **X-linked inheritance:** Inheritance of characteristics that are determined by genes present on the X chromosome

Introduction

The physical appearance and overall health of an individual animal, be it a dog, a cat, a rabbit or a human being is a result of both that individual's genetic makeup and its environment. Whereas an animal's environment continuously changes throughout its life, in terms of the infectious pathogens it may encounter, the amount of exercise it has and its diet, its genetic makeup is determined at birth and remains more or less unchanged throughout its life. Examples of traits that are largely determined by genetics include physical characteristics (such as size, coat type and colour, ear shape), behavioural characteristics (such as the tendency of different breeds of dog to herd and retrieve) and the predisposition to develop certain diseases.

Technologies that are available to help scientists understand the genetic basis of physical, behavioural and disease traits are becoming ever more sophisticated. These technological advances are resulting in a quickly growing list of DNA tests that are available to probe the genetic makeup of dogs and cats. These tests help veterinary professionals understand the inherited disorders their patients might be at risk of, or are suffering from, and can reduce the unpredictability of breeding for dog and cat breeders.

Breeders can now use DNA tests to control certain cosmetic factors, such as the coat colour and coat length, of the animals they produce, but also, and more importantly from the animal's point of view, dramatically reduce the chances that they will develop particular diseases. DNA testing can also be used to confirm/elucidate parentage of a litter and, for dogs, shed light on the breed makeup.

It is probably nigh on impossible for a breeder (especially a dog breeder) to claim they are responsible and conscientious if they are not aware of any DNA testing available in their breed. Experienced breeders are typically well versed with the range of DNA tests available for their breed, but less experienced breeders may not be. These novice breeders may well turn to the veterinary profession for advice on which DNA tests they should consider prior to breeding and also how to interpret the results and make sensible breeding decisions. Genetic testing is rapidly moving into the mainstream and veterinary surgeons and veterinary nurses should have a robust grasp on at least the basic principles of genetics so they can best serve their patients and their owners.

Genetic material

DNA

The discovery of DNA (deoxyribonucleic acid) in 1953 by James Watson and Francis Crick marked a milestone in the history of science and gave rise to modern molecular biology, which is largely concerned with understanding how genes control the chemical processes within cells. DNA is the molecule that carries the genetic information in all cellular forms of life and is made up of long chains of nucleotides, called polynucleotides, with each nucleotide consisting of three components:

- A nitrogenous base: cytosine (C), guanine (G), adenine (A) or thymine (T)
- A five-carbon sugar molecule called deoxyribose
- A phosphate molecule.

DNA is formed of two strands of polynucleotides with each strand having a backbone of deoxyribose-phosphate groups. Each deoxyribose-phosphate group is linked to one of the four nitrogenous bases (Figure 4.1). The nitrogenous bases join each strand to each other by hydrogen bonds in a specific manner: C always pairs with G, and A always pairs

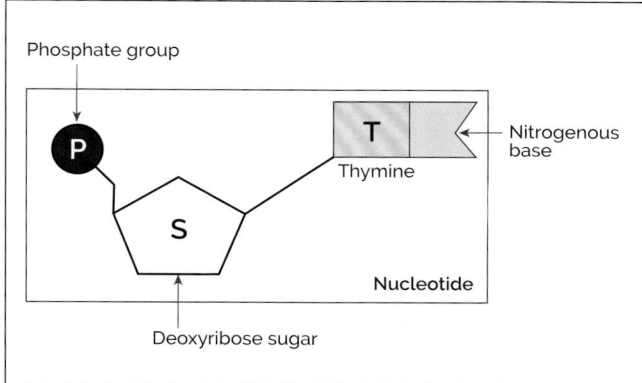

4.1 The structure of a DNA nucleotide. Each nucleotide is formed of a phosphate group, a deoxyribose sugar and a nitrogenous base.

with T. These are known as base pairs. There are two important factors that dictate this very specific pairing: first, a smaller base is always paired with a bigger one, which means the two strands are kept at a fixed distance from one another along the length of the strand; and, secondly, these particular pairs fit exactly to form very effective hydrogen bonds with each other. It is these hydrogen bonds that hold the two chains together. The two polynucleotide strands twist around each other to form a double-stranded helix (Figure 4.2).

Genes

The sum total of an organism's DNA located on all of its chromosomes is known as its genome and comprises genes (the basic structural and functional units of heredity) and intergenic regions. Each gene consists of three types of nucleotide sequence:

- Exons – the coding regions of a gene
- Introns – the non-coding regions between exons
- Regulatory sequences – involved in determining when, where and how much protein is made.

Each gene is positioned at a specific location on a specific chromosome known as its locus and the locus of an individual gene is the same for every member of the same species (apart from rare individuals with large structural mutations). Although genes are generally considered the most important constituents of DNA, they account for surprisingly little of it. In fact, genes only make up approximately 1% of the canine genome. The remaining 99% of DNA is non-coding. Although the precise function of much of the non-coding DNA has yet to be elucidated, it is known that non-coding DNA is involved with the overall control of gene expression, including important functions such as the regulation of transcription and translation (see below), and in DNA replication.

Protein synthesis

A protein is a large molecule consisting of one or more chains of amino acids. An amino acid is an organic compound containing amine ($-NH_2$) and carboxyl ($-COOH$) functional groups, along with a side chain specific to each amino acid. It is the precise order of nucleotide bases within the exons of a gene that determines the specific amino acid sequence of the protein that the gene encodes. The nitrogenous bases (A, T, G and C) form a four-letter alphabet that is used to 'write' different three-letter 'words' known as codons. Between

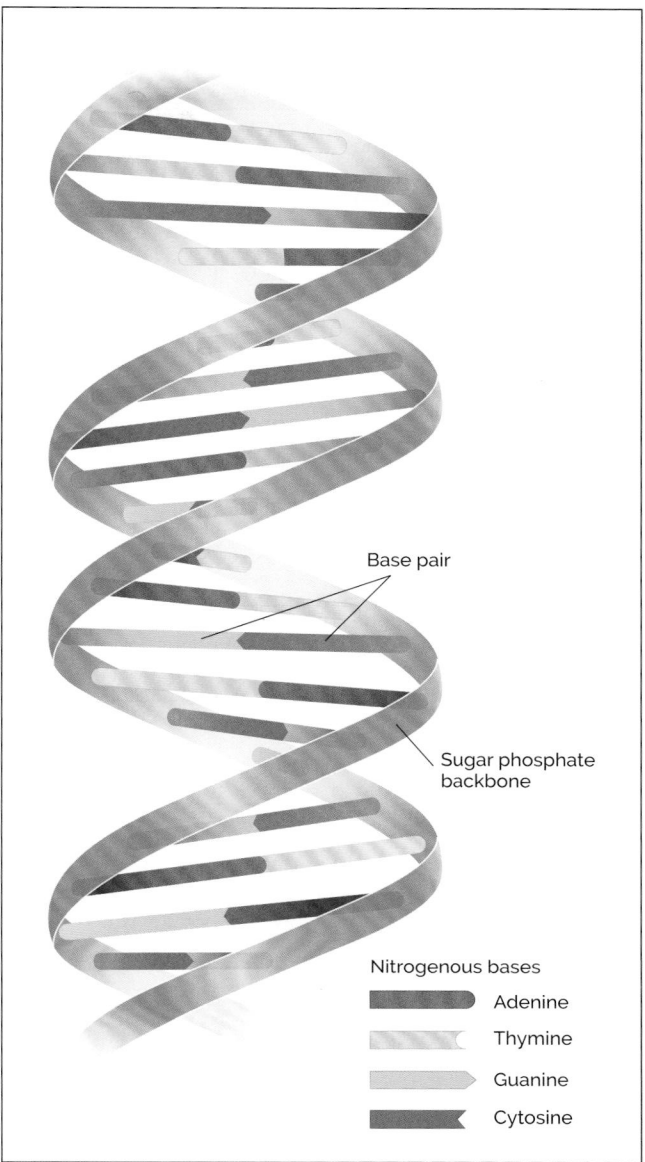

Base pair

Sugar phosphate backbone

Nitrogenous bases
- Adenine
- Thymine
- Guanine
- Cytosine

4.2 The double helical structure of DNA. The two polynucleotide strands are held together by hydrogen bonds between the nitrogenous bases and twist around each other to form a double-stranded helix.

them, the 64 possible codons encode the 20 different amino acids, with some amino acids being coded for by multiple codons (Figure 4.3). For the information encoded in a gene to be decrypted and turned into protein, two processes must occur: transcription and translation.

Transcription is the first step of gene expression and occurs in the nucleus of the cell. It is the process by which a gene sequence in a single-stranded DNA template is copied into complementary single-stranded RNA (ribonucleic acid) by the enzyme RNA polymerase (Figure 4.4). RNA is very similar to DNA but there are three key differences: RNA is single stranded; the five-carbon sugar is ribose (instead of deoxyribose); and the nitrogenous base uracil (U) replaces T. During transcription, each nucleotide in the DNA strand is transcribed into its complementary nucleotide. Thus, C is transcribed to G, G is transcribed to C, T is transcribed to A and A is transcribed to U. The newly synthesized RNA strand, known as messenger RNA (mRNA), then leaves the nucleus and passes to the cytoplasm, where it acts as a template for the next stage of gene expression, known as translation.

			Second letter				
		T	C	A	G		
First letter	T	TTT TTC }Phe TTA TTG }Leu	TCT TCC TCA TCG }Ser	TAT TAC }Tyr TAA **Stop** TAG **Stop**	TGT TGC }Cys TGA **Stop** TGG Trp	T C A G	Third letter
	C	CTT CTC CTA CTG }Leu	CCT CCC CCA CCG }Pro	CAT CAC }His CAA CAG }Gin	CGT CGC CGA CGG }Arg	T C A G	
	A	ATT ATC ATA }Ile ATG Met	ACT ACC ACA ACG }Thr	AAT AAC }Asn AAA AAG }Lys	AGT AGC }Ser AGA AGG }Arg	T C A G	
	G	GTT GTC GTA GTG }Val	GCT GCC GCA GCG }Ala	GAT GAC }Asp GAA GAG }Glu	GGT GGC GGA GGG }Gly	T C A G	

Key:

Ala	=	Alanine (A)
Arg	=	Arginine (R)
Asn	=	Asparagine (N)
Asp	=	Aspartate (D)
Cys	=	Cysteine (C)
Gin	=	Glutamine (Q)
Gly	=	Glycine (G)
His	=	Histidine (H)
Ile	=	Isoleucine (I)
Leu	=	Leucine (L)
Lys	=	Lysine (K)
Met	=	Methionine (M)
Phe	=	Phenylalanine (F)
Pro	=	Proline (P)
Ser	=	Serine (S)
Thr	=	Threonine (T)
Trp	=	Tryptophan (W)
Tyr	=	Tyrosine (Y)
Val	=	Valine (V)

4.3 The genetic code. The nitrogenous bases (A, T, G and C) form a four-letter alphabet which is used to 'write' different three-letter 'words' known as codons. Between them, the 64 possible codons encode the 20 different amino acids.

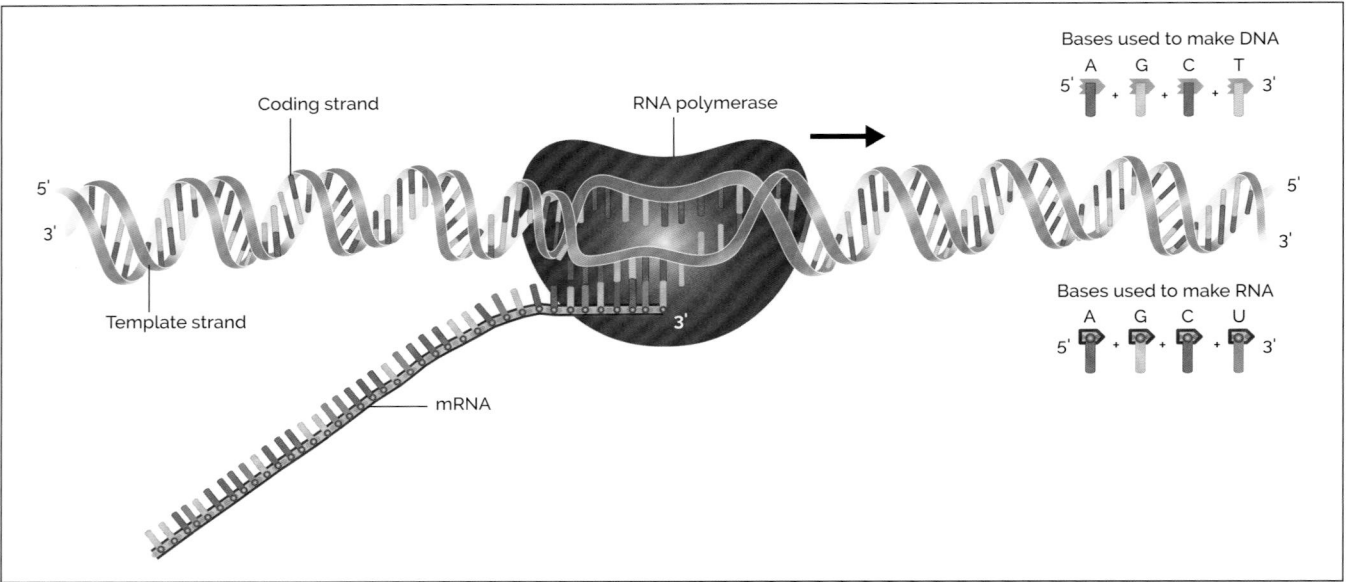

4.4 Transcription. The five carbon atoms in each deoxyribose/ribose molecule are numbered (1'–5', pronounced 1–5 prime). Each deoxyribose attaches to the next by connecting its 5' carbon to the 3' carbon of the other using a phosphate group. Each strand of DNA will end with a unbound free 5' carbon and the opposite end of the same strand will have an unbound free 3' carbon. The two complementary strands of a DNA molecule run in opposite 'directions', meaning one strand is 5' to 3' and the complementary strand is 3' to 5'. Conventionally, DNA is read 5' to 3'. The DNA template strand is copied into single-stranded messenger RNA (mRNA) by the action of RNA polymerase. The resultant mRNA strand is identical to the DNA coding stand, with the exception that U replaces T in the mRNA.

During **translation**, the nucleotide sequence of the mRNA molecule is 'read' by the cellular machinery to generate a sequence of amino acids (Figure 4.5). Translation proceeds in three stages: initiation, elongation and termination. During initiation, the ribosome assembles around the mRNA and a molecule called transfer RNA (tRNA) attaches to it at the start codon (AUG), transferring the amino acid mRNA to the ribosome/mRNA assembly. During elongation, the tRNA transfers an amino acid to the ribosome/mRNA assembly that corresponds to the next codon. The ribosome then moves along (translocates) the mRNA strand to continue the process and form a chain of amino acids, known as a polypeptide. Finally, termination occurs when the assembly arrives at a stop codon (UAA, UAG or UGA). At this point the ribosome releases the polypeptide, which may undergo further processing to result in the final protein.

Chromosomes

DNA is tightly packed into structures called chromosomes, which are located in the nucleus of the cell. Every cell of every animal (with the exception of gametes) has two copies of every chromosome: one pair of sex chromosomes and a variable number of pairs of autosomes (the non-sex chromosomes). One copy of each chromosome originates from the dam (mother) and one from the sire (father). Cells with two

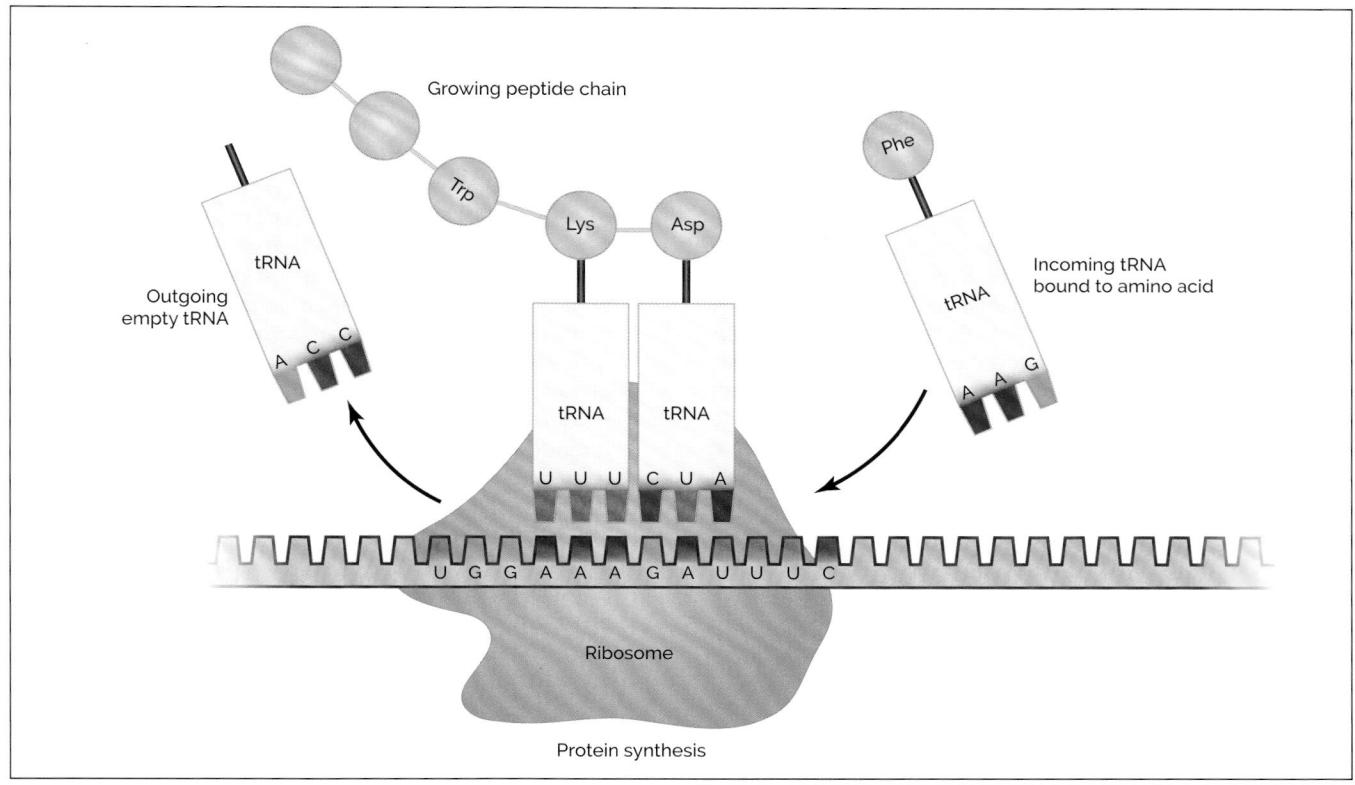

4.5 Translation. During translation, the nucleotide sequence of the mRNA molecule is 'read' by the cellular machinery to generate a sequence of amino acids. Transfer RNA (tRNA) first binds to the start codon (AUG), transferring the corresponding amino acid (methionine) to the ribosome/mRNA assembly. The ribosome then moves along (translocates) the mRNA strand to continue the process and form a chain of amino acids, known as a polypeptide until the assembly arrives at a stop codon.

copies of every chromosome are known as diploid, whereas gametes, which have only one copy of each chromosome, are said to be haploid.

The number of chromosomes varies between species, for example, the dog has a total of 39 chromosome pairs, the cat has 19 pairs and the rabbit has 22 pairs.

Chromosomes also determine an animal's sex. In mammals, the sex chromosomes are known as the X and Y chromosomes. Females are the homogametic sex having two X chromosomes (XX) and males are heterogametic having one X and one Y chromosome (XY). Birds (and some other species) follow an alternative mode of sex determination. In birds, the sex chromosomes are known as Z and W chromosomes. In the ZW mode of sex determination, and in contrast to mammals, males are the homogametic sex (ZZ) and females are heterogametic (ZW).

The cell cycle and cell division

The cells of an animal may undergo two different types of cell division: a vegetative division (mitosis) during which each dividing cell gives rise to identical daughter cells both of which contain the same amount of genetic material as the parent cell; and a reproductive division (meiosis) that gives rise to gametes (eggs and sperm), each of which contains half the amount of genetic material contained in the parent cell. Broadly speaking, mitosis occurs when more cells are required, such as during growth and repair, and meiosis occurs in the cells that give rise to gametes.

Interphase

Interphase is the stage of cell division that precedes both mitosis and meiosis and consists of three main stages: G1, S and G2 (Figure 4.6).

- G1 (first gap) phase. During this phase, cells that are intended for mitosis grow and carry out various metabolic activities.
- S (synthesis) phase. During this phase the cell duplicates its DNA. Each chromosome produces a copy of itself, called a sister chromatid. The two sister chromatids are joined together by a structure called a centromere, and resemble an X at this stage.
- G2 (second gap) phase. During this phase the cells continue to grow.

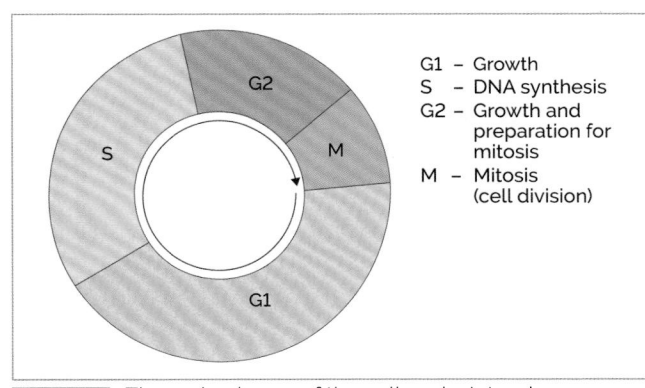

G1 – Growth
S – DNA synthesis
G2 – Growth and preparation for mitosis
M – Mitosis (cell division)

4.6 The main phases of the cell cycle. Interphase precedes both mitosis (M) and meiosis, and comprises three main stages: G1 (growth), S (DNA synthesis) and G2 (growth and preparation for mitosis).

Mitosis

From interphase, cells that are destined to divide vegetatively enter mitosis (known as the M phase), which occurs in four stages (Figure 4.7). The first stage of mitosis is known as **prophase**. The duplicated chromosomes are very compact at this stage and can be visualized using a microscope as sister chromatids. A network of protein filaments called the mitotic spindle emerges within the cell, from structures called centrioles. **Metaphase** follows prophase, during which the nuclear membrane dissolves and the mitotic spindle attaches to the sister chromatids at the centromere. By the end of metaphase, all the chromosomes are aligned along the mitotic spindle. The next stage of mitosis is **anaphase**, during which the sister chromatids are pulled apart and move towards opposite ends of the cell. **Telophase** is the final stage of mitosis, during which the chromosomes reach the opposite ends of the cell and the nuclear membrane forms again.

Meiosis

Cells that are destined to produce gametes progress from interphase to meiosis, which is divided into two distinct stages (Figure 4.8):

- **Meiosis I.** During this phase the two copies of each chromosome pair up, so both copies of chromosome 1 lie next to each other, as do both copies of chromosome 2 and so on. At this stage physical and reciprocal breakage and exchange can occur between homologous chromosomes, known as recombination, to generate recombinant chromosomes made up of genetic material that originated from the individual's two different parents. Homologous pairs of chromosomes align along the middle, or equator, of the cell and individual copies (each consisting of two chromatids) are pulled to opposite ends of the cell. The cell divides to form two new cells each with a haploid set of chromosomes, thus marking the end of meiosis I (see below). The chromosomes align at random and independently from one another, therefore it is random whether it is the maternal or paternal copy of each chromosome that enters a specific haploid daughter cell (see below).
- **Meiosis II.** Each of the two haploid daughter cells then enter the second stage of meiosis, during which the physical relationship between sister chromatids is broken, and the second stage of meiosis proceeds as for mitosis; the overall result being the formation of four cells each with the haploid number of chromosomes.

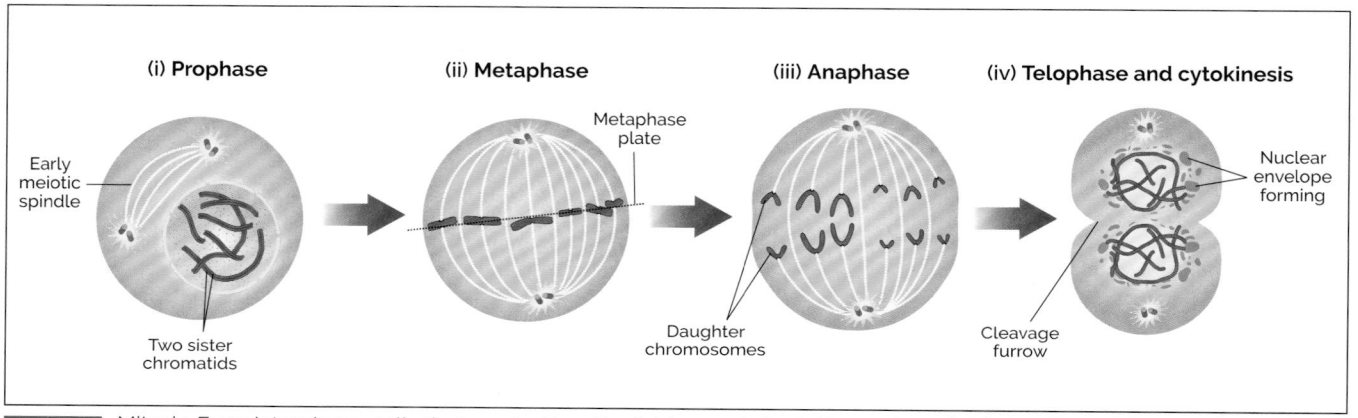

4.7 Mitosis. From interphase, cells that are destined to divide vegetatively then enter mitosis (known as the M phase), which occurs in four stages. **(i)** Prophase. **(ii)** Metaphase. **(iii)** Anaphase. **(iv)** Telophase and cytokinesis.

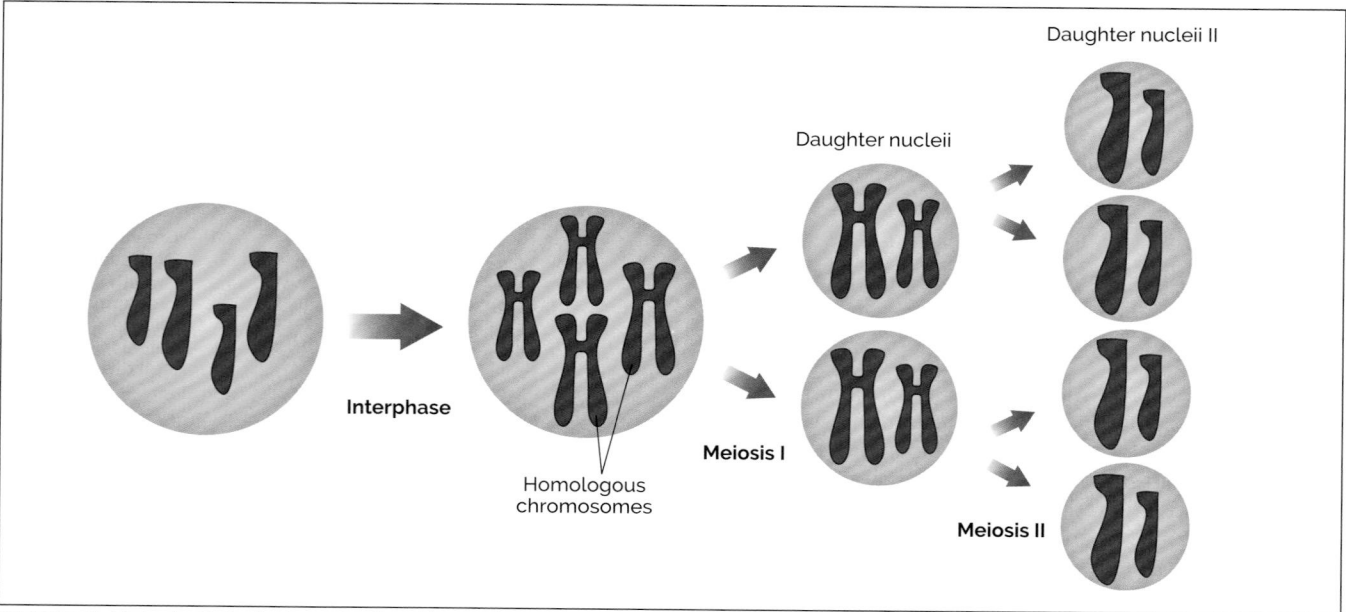

4.8 Meiosis. Cells that are destined to produce gametes progress from interphase to meiosis that is divided into two distinct stages (see main text).

Meiosis takes place in the reproductive tissues. In male animals, meiosis takes place in the testes and in females within the ovaries. The haploid cells that result from meiosis are known as **gametes**. Each gamete is genetically different, as a result of both **random alignment** of the homologous pairs of chromosomes (independent assortment of the chromosomes) and **recombination** between members of a homologous pair.

Mendel's laws of inheritance

Mendel's laws of inheritance are three statements regarding the way certain characteristics (phenotypes) are transmitted from one generation to another in an organism. These laws were deduced by the Austrian monk Gregor Mendel (1822–1884) based on experiments he conducted using pea plants. The characteristics that Mendel studied included flower colour, pod shape and colour, seed shape and colour and plant height. The Laws are as follows:

Law	Definition
Law of segregation ('First Law')	During gamete formation, the alleles for each gene segregate from each other so that each gamete carries only one allele for each gene.
Law of independent assortment ('Second Law')	Genes for different characteristics can segregate independently during the formation of gametes.
Law of dominance ('Third Law')	Some alleles of the same gene are dominant and others are recessive. An organism only needs one copy of the dominant allele to display the effect of that allele.

Inheritance

A mutation is a permanent alteration of the nucleotide sequence of DNA. Mutations are caused by errors in DNA replication or other types of DNA damage and give rise to different forms of the same gene, which are referred to as alleles. Although there may be more than two different alleles of each gene within a given species, each individual can only have two alleles (or 'copies') of each gene, one inherited from their mother (via the egg) and one inherited from their father (via the sperm). If an individual has two identical alleles of a specific gene it is said to be **homozygous**. If the two alleles of that gene differ from each other, it is said to be **heterozygous**. The term **genotype** refers to the genetic constitution of an individual at one or more loci. An individual's genotype determines the outward characteristic or trait, which is referred to by the term **phenotype**.

Once new alleles arise by mutation, meiosis and sexual reproduction combine different alleles in new ways to increase genetic variation. Genetic variation is, in general, good for a population because a population possessing a greater amount of genetic diversity has a greater probability of already possessing adaptive alleles that might be necessary to meet new environmental challenges. Occasionally, however, mutations can have a negative impact on gene function and cause disease.

Modes of inheritance

The terms dominant, recessive, codominant and incomplete inheritance describe the relationship between alleles at a given locus and how they determine the phenotype of the individual. In heterozygous individuals (those that carry two different alleles of a particular gene), one allele may be expressed at the expense of the other, suppressed allele. Such dominant alleles show their effect even if the individual is heterozygous for that allele (see above). In contrast, recessive alleles only show their effect if an individual is homozygous (carries two identical copies) for that allele. By convention, the dominant allele is referred to by upper case letters and the recessive allele by lower case letters. For example, albinism, a condition in which individuals lack pigment in the skin, hair and eyes (albinos), is caused by the recessive mutant allele, *a*, which is suppressed by the dominant normal allele, *A*. As each individual must have two alleles at a given chromosomal locus, the possible genotypes that exist for albinism are *AA* (homozygous for the dominant normal allele and phenotype of the individual is normal pigmentation), *aa* (homozygous for the recessive mutant allele and the phenotype of the individual is albino) or *Aa* (heterozygous with one copy of both the dominant normal and the recessive mutant alleles and the phenotype is normal pigmentation). If the genotypes of a given dam or sire are known, then it is possible to statistically predict, on average, what the genotypes of the offspring would be. A simple way of doing this is by the use of a matrix (Punnett square), as represented in Figure 4.9. For example, and as shown in Figure 4.9, if both the dam and the sire had the genotype Aa and they had four offspring, on average, two of the offspring would be Aa, one would be AA and one would be aa (albino).

Mode of inheritance can be further characterized depending on whether the mutant allele is autosomal or is carried on one of the sex chromosomes. The vast majority of mammalian sex chromosome mutations are located on the X chromosome. X-linked disorders affect males predominantly as, by having only one X chromosome, they lack the potential of having an alternative dominant allele to supress the expression of the mutant allele. An example of an X-linked disorder is haemophilia A (abnormal blood clotting) in the German Shepherd Dog. This disease is determined by a recessive gene on the X chromosome.

An example of autosomal dominant inheritance is seen in canine bobtail (short tail). In this condition (or phenotype) there are two alleles, the 'normal' allele that codes for tails of a normal length and the 'mutant' allele that codes for a short (bob) tail. The mutant bobtail allele, which we can call *B*, is dominant over the recessive, normal allele which we can call *b*. Only dogs with two copies of the normal allele (*bb*) will

		Heterozygous sire (*Aa*)	
		A	a
Heterozygous dam (*Aa*)	A	AA (homozygous dominant)	Aa (heterozygous)
	a	Aa (heterozygous)	aa (homozygous recessive)

4.9 A Punnett square showing the expected outcome of mating two heterozygous carriers of the allele for albinism, *a*. Each offspring has a 1 in 4 chance of inheriting the genotype *aa*, and expressing an albino phenotype.

have a normal length tail. For dogs to have a genetically short tail, only one copy of the dominant *B* allele is required (*Bb*). In fact, the genotype *BB* is lethal and puppies with two copies of the mutant allele die *in utero*. The matrix in Figure 4.10 illustrates the offspring that would statistically be expected to be derived from breeding dogs that are homozygous normal (clear), heterozygous (carrier) or homozygous mutant (affected) for an autosomal dominant allele.

Not all diseases are determined by dominant genes. An example of a recessive disease is progressive rod-cone degeneration (PRCD), an inherited form of retinal degeneration seen in multiple breeds of purebred dogs. For a dog to be affected it must have two copies of the defective *PRCD* gene. The matrix in Figure 4.11 illustrates the offspring that would statistically be expected to be derived from breeding dogs that are homozygous normal (clear), heterozygous (carrier) or homozygous mutant (affected) for an autosomal recessive allele.

Occasionally, alleles are codominant or incompletely dominant. In this situation, the heterozygote exhibits the effect of both alleles. An example is seen in the S series of alleles, which determine white markings in dogs. S is the allele for no white markings and sp is the allele for piebald – the situation in which white markings cover 50% or more of the body. Even though S is dominant to sp, an S/sp individual is not usually solid-coloured (i.e. no white markings) as the sp allele is still often partially expressed.

A final example of inheritance is polygenic inheritance. In this situation, multiple genes (and therefore alleles) contribute to the phenotype in question. This mode of inheritance is claimed to be responsible for the majority of characteristics, although there is often little evidence of which specific genes are actually involved. Examples of diseases and traits that have been associated with a presumed polygenic mode of inheritance in dogs include hip dysplasia, diabetes mellitus and behaviour.

Parentage analysis

In certain situations, it is necessary to prove the parentage of an individual animal. Usually, it is the identity of the sire that is in question as the dam's identity is normally known. Parentage can be either proved or disproved by comparing

	Homozygous unaffected male (aa)	Heterozygous affected male (Aa)		Homozygous affected male (AA)
Homozygous unaffected female (aa)	All puppies will be homozygous unaffected (aa)	50% chance of each puppy being homozygous unaffected (aa)		All puppies will be heterozygous affected (Aa)
		50% chance of each puppy being heterozygous affected (Aa)		
Heterozygous affected female (Aa)	50% chance of each puppy being homozygous unaffected (aa)	25% chance of each puppy being homozygous unaffected (aa)	25% chance of each puppy being homozygous affected (AA)	50% chance of each puppy being heterozygous affected (Aa)
	50% chance of each puppy being heterozygous affected (Aa)	50% chance of each puppy being heterozygous affected (Aa)		50% chance of each puppy being homozygous affected (AA)
Homozygous affected female (AA)	All puppies will be heterozygous affected (Aa)	50% chance of each puppy being heterozygous affected (Aa)		All puppies will be homozygous affected (AA)
		50% chance of each puppy being homozygous affected (AA)		

4.10 Autosomal dominant inheritance. The matrix illustrates the offspring which would statistically be expected to be derived from breeding dogs that are homozygous unaffected (clear), heterozygous affected or homozygous affected for an autosomal dominant allele (A).

	Homozygous unaffected male (AA)	Heterozygous unaffected male (Aa)		Homozygous affected male (aa)
Homozygous unaffected female (AA)	All puppies will be homozygous unaffected (AA)	50% chance of each puppy being homozygous unaffected (AA)		All puppies will be heterozygous unaffected (Aa)
		50% chance of each puppy being heterozygous unaffected (Aa)		
Heterozygous unaffected female (Aa)	50% chance of each puppy being homozygous unaffected (AA)	25% chance of each puppy being homozygous unaffected (AA)	25% chance of each puppy being homozygous affected (aa)	50% chance of each puppy being heterozygous unaffected (Aa)
	50% chance of each puppy being heterozygous unaffected (Aa)	50% chance of each puppy being heterozygous unaffected (Aa)		50% chance of each puppy being homozygous affected (aa)
Homozygous affected female (aa)	All puppies will be heterozygous unaffected (Aa)	50% chance of each puppy being heterozygous unaffected (Aa)		All puppies will be homozygous affected (aa)
		50% chance of each puppy being homozygous affected (aa)		

4.11 Autosomal recessive inheritance. The matrix illustrates the offspring which would statistically be expected to be derived from breeding dogs that are homozygous unaffected (clear), heterozygous unaffected (carrier) or homozygous affected for an autosomal recessive allele (a).

DNA of the offspring with that of the proposed parent by a technique called DNA profiling.

DNA profiling relies on two well-founded principles of genetics – genetic variation and inheritance.

- **Genetic variation** exists as a result of the presence of more than one form of specific regions of DNA to exist within a given species. This polymorphism not only exists in the protein-coding genes but also occurs in other regions of the genome. Polymorphic regions can serve as useful 'markers' in DNA profiling.
- **Inheritance.** As discussed above, each individual has two copies of every piece of DNA – one copy inherited from the dam and one from the sire. If DNA is available from the known dam as well as the offspring, then the maternally-derived makers can be accounted for and the alternative markers must be derived from the sire. If the same pattern of markers, or 'DNA profile', is not present in the suspected sire, then paternity can be excluded. Alternatively, if all the non-maternally derived markers of the offspring match alleles carried by the presumed sire then it is highly likely this male is the biological father, although that is impossible to state with absolute certainty (due to the theoretical possibility that another male has the same genotype as the suspected sire).

In parentage analysis, the polymorphic markers usually employed are called **microsatellites**. Microsatellites are tandem repeats of base pairs (e.g. CACACACACA) found at the same site along the genome in different animals of the same species. Polymorphism in microsatellites occurs as a result of differences in the number of repeats between individuals. Those microsatellites with a greater variety in the number of possible tandem repeats in the population are the most useful. Furthermore, increasing the number of microsatellite markers in a DNA profile 'panel' used in parentage analysis will increase the reliability of results, with most laboratories using standard panels of around 18–23 universally recognized markers for canine parentage analysis. A similar standardized panel has been developed for cats and it has been shown that 11 markers are sufficient for parentage, gender determination and identification testing of random bred, purebred and some wild bred feline species (Lyons, 2012).

Breeding strategies

Breeding strategies are used both to retain and increase the frequency of desirable traits within a given breed and to reduce or eliminate undesirable traits from a given breed. Examples of traits that breeders may wish to modify by selective breeding include head and body conformation, coat colour, behaviour and disease. The frequency of an inherited trait within a population can be increased by increasing its homozygosity (and thus removing its variability) within a population. Once a trait is homozygous in every individual of a particular breed or population, that trait is said to be 'fixed' in that breed. The most efficient way of achieving this is by inbreeding.

Inbreeding

Inbreeding is the mating of related individuals. The closest form of inbreeding involves mating between full siblings and between first-degree relatives (parents and their offspring). Inbreeding is an extremely efficient way of increasing the homozygosity of alleles within a population and the chance of outwardly identifiable traits being passed on from parents to offspring.

The inbreeding coefficient of an individual may be defined as the probability that the two alleles of a given gene in that individual have been inherited by an ancestor common to both the sire and dam. The inbreeding coefficient is calculated using pedigree data and is a reflection of homozygosity – the lower the inbreeding coefficient, the lower the degree of inbreeding. The United Kingdom's Kennel Club offers a free inbreeding coefficient calculation service accompanied by an annual breed average to enable breeders to put the inbreeding coefficient of their dog(s) into perspective (www.the kennelclub.org.uk/health/for-breeders/inbreeding/).

A major disadvantage of inbreeding is that by increasing the overall level of homozygosity (to fix desirable traits), the frequency of recessive disease mutations is also increased, resulting in more recessive diseases in highly inbred breeds or populations.

Line breeding

Line breeding is a form of inbreeding that aims to maximize the genetic influence of a common ancestor on a given population. In this situation, a particular ancestor considered to have desirable characteristics, as the case may be, for example, with a show champion, occurs more than once in a pedigree of an individual. Each occurrence of the ancestor in the pedigree provides an independent opportunity for that individual to have inherited the ancestor's genes. Mated individuals, although still closely related, are not as closely related as first-degree relatives and, as a result, it is hoped that offspring will be homozygous for the desirable alleles and heterozygous for possible undesirable alleles.

Outcrossing

Outcrossing, or outbreeding, is the method of introducing unrelated genetic material into a breeding line. By outcrossing, recessive alleles tend to be masked in the offspring because it is unlikely that unrelated individuals from the outcross population will share the same recessive alleles. In certain situations, offspring may also demonstrate hybrid vigour – also known as heterosis. Heterosis occurs when the traits of the offspring are enhanced as a result of mixing of the alleles derived from its parents. In purebred dogs, the most efficient means of outcrossing and increasing heterozygosity of the offspring would be to mate individuals from two unrelated breeds. This would obviously be an unpopular strategy for many breeders who wish to maintain 'purity' of their breed. Instead, outcrossing within breeds is likely to be preferred, with the mating of two individuals less closely related than the population as a whole. This is best achieved using inbreeding coefficients as previously discussed.

Breed variation

The domestic dog (Canis familiaris) is the most diverse mammalian species known in terms of shape, structure, size and colour. All domestic dog breeds can trace their ancestry back to the grey wolf (Canis lupis). Wolf domestication is thought to have commenced 15,000–30,000 years ago as dogs became used for hunting, shepherding, guarding and companionship. The majority of today's approximately 400 dog breeds were developed much more recently – over the last 200–300 years. Breed creation was largely driven by the selection of various phenotypic characteristics such as skull and body conformation, size, coat colour and behaviour. Selection involved inbreeding and backcrossing to allow fixation of the desirable traits, which led to a much increased level of homozygosity in these canine breeds compared with their lupine (wolf) ancestors.

Dog breed development has come with the cost of significant health and welfare problems. First, the selected trait itself may be associated with health problems (for example, brachycephalic breeds have a high incidence of obstructive airway disease). Secondly, the intermittent homozygosity within the genome that exists within a breed may expose the deleterious effect of a single pathogenic mutation.

Genomic analyses using microsatellite and single nucleotide polymorphism (SNP) markers have enabled researchers to determine the genetic distinctions that separate most popular dog breeds, leading to the commercial availability of various different DNA tests that owners can use as a tool to understand the breed ancestry of their dog (Parker, 2012).

The domestic cat (*Felis catus*) demonstrates much less variation, reflecting their more recent ancestry and less well-defined barriers between breeds (Menotti-Raymond *et al.*, 2008). Nevertheless, at the time of writing, The International Cat Association (TICA) recognizes 58 cat breeds and there is significant interbreed variation in terms of body size and conformation, skull shape, coat and temperament.

Hereditary diseases, testing for hereditary conditions and health schemes

Hereditary diseases are caused by mutations in genes that are transmitted between generations by reproduction. Mutations responsible for inherited disorders occur spontaneously and at random in animals and are only passed on to offspring and subsequent generations if that animal reproduces. A disease is usually first suspected of being inherited when it appears particularly prevalent in dogs of the same breed or extended pedigree. Pedigree analysis offers a relatively straightforward means of demonstrating heredity and determination of the mode of inheritance of simple (single gene) disorders. The downside to pedigree analysis is that it requires detailed clinical examination and/or laboratory tests of a large number of related individuals, which is often impractical. Furthermore, some hereditary diseases are late in onset, and so there is a possibility that genetically affected animals will go undetected if examination is performed before a certain age.

Health schemes are designed with the aim of identifying animals affected by hereditary diseases, allowing them to be removed from the breeding population and thus reducing disease prevalence over time. In theory, control of dominant mutations is straightforward as all animals that possess the mutant allele will be clinically affected and easily identifiable, as long as the disease manifests before breeding. If the mutation is recessive, clinically affected animals are only produced when inbreeding has occurred and carriers cannot be identified by examination. Traditionally, carriers were identified by test matings in which they were backcrossed to clinically affected, and therefore, recessive individuals. Fortunately, the advance of molecular diagnostic techniques has allowed for a much superior and ethical means of carrier identification.

For polygenic diseases, control is particularly challenging. Examples of suspected polygenic diseases include hip and elbow dysplasia and syringomyelia/Chiari-like malformation. For these diseases, the relevant health scheme makes use of diagnostic imaging techniques to score the severity of the disease in question. The breeders may then use the score to make an informed choice on suitability for breeding.

Testing for hereditary conditions

The increased sophistication, accessibility and affordability of molecular tools for genetics research has led to an explosion in disease-associated mutation discovery and the commercial availability of DNA tests in the dog and cat. Breeders have become increasingly aware of which inherited diseases affect their breed and turn more and more to DNA tests to ensure the health of their breed, using the resultant information to make informed decisions about breeding. DNA tests also represent an important tool for the veterinary surgeon in achieving a definitive aetiological diagnosis for numerous clinical conditions. DNA tests can usually be performed on buccal mucosal swabs, allowing owners to take and submit samples themselves; although some tests require EDTA blood samples, which must be taken by a registered veterinary surgeon or nurse. Details of some of the most common commercially available DNA tests for canine and feline inherited disorders are presented in Figures 4.12 and 4.13, respectively. The reader is directed to online resources for more detailed and current information on DNA testing, such as those of the University of Pennsylvania (www.vet.upenn.edu/research/academic-departments/clinical-sciences-advanced-medicine/research-labs-centers/penngen) and the Kennel Club (www.thekennelclub.org.uk/health/for-breeders/dna-testing-simple-inherited-disorders/worldwide-dna-tests).

Providing breeding advice based on DNA test results is usually relatively straightforward for scientists and veterinary surgeons. For autosomal recessive disorders, essentially all dogs can be safely bred from as long as they have been genotyped (DNA tested). To prevent the production of affected offspring, carriers (heterozygotes) and genetically affected dogs (homozygous mutants) must only mated to dogs genetically clear of the mutation (homozygous normal). Although many breeders may be reluctant to breed from carriers, their initial inclusion in any breeding programme can be extremely important in maintaining genetic diversity within a breed, particularly when the disease in question is particularly prevalent in that breed. Exclusion of all carriers for a common mutation would lead to a significant reduction of the gene pool for that breed and would come at the risk of exposing other, previously silent, recessive mutations.

Furthermore, in order for a breeder to reach a decision on the merit of an individual DNA test, it is important that they understand the clinical importance of the disorder being tested for, along with having access to up-to-date information on the prevalence of the disorder in their breed (Mellersh, 2016).

Disorder	Mode of inheritance	Gene(s) involved	Most commonly affected breed
Autosomal dominant progressive retinal atrophy	AD	*RHO*	Bullmastiff, English Bullmastiff
Bobtail	AD	*T-box*	Australian Shepherd, Boxer, Brittany Spaniel, Pembroke Welsh Corgi, Polish Lowland Sheepdog, Schipperke, Spanish Water Dog, Swedish Vallhund
Collie eye anomaly (choroidal hypoplasia)	AR	*NHEJ1*	Border Collie, Rough Collie, Shetland Sheepdog, Smooth Collie
Degenerative myelopathy	AR	*SOD1*	Boxer, Chesapeake Bay Retriever, German Shepherd Dog, Rhodesian Ridgeback
Hereditary cataract	AD	*HSF4* (2 different mutations)	Australian Shepherd
	AR		Boston Terrier, French Bulldog, Staffordshire Bull Terrier
Multidrug resistance	AR	*MDR1*	Australian Shepherd, Border Collie, Old English Sheepdog
Primary lens luxation	AR	*ADAMTS17* (single mutation)	Chinese Crested Terrier, Lancashire Heeler, Miniature Bull Terrier, Parson Russell Terrier, Sealyham Terrier, Tibetan Terrier
Primary open angle glaucoma	AR	*ADAMTS10* (2 breed-specific mutations) *ADAMTS17* (4 breed-specific mutations)	Beagle, Norwegian Elkhound / Basset Fauve de Bretagne, Basset Hound, Petit Basset Griffon Vendeen, Shar Pei
Progressive rod-cone degeneration	AR	*PRCD* (single mutation)	American Cocker Spaniel, Cocker Spaniel, Labrador Retriever, Miniature Poodle, Toy Poodle, Yorkshire Terrier
von Willebrand's Disease (types I, II and III)	AR	*VWF* (3 different mutations)	Bernese Mountain Dog, Boxer, Coton De Tulear, Dobermann, German Pinscher, German Shorthaired Pointer, German Wirehaired Pointer, Kerry Blue Terrier, Papillon, Pembroke Welsh, Scottish Terrier, Shetland Sheep Dog, Welsh Corgi (Cardigan and Pembroke)
X-linked progressive retinal atrophy	XR	*RPGR* (2 different mutations)	Samoyed, Siberian Husky

4.12 Common commercially available DNA tests for inherited canine disorders. AD = autosomal dominant; AR = autosomal recessive; XR = X-linked recessive.

Disorder	Mode of inheritance	Gene(s) involved	Most commonly affected breed(s)
Gangliosidosis 1	AR	GBL1	Korat, Siamese
Gangliosidosis 2	AR	HEXB	Burmese, Korat
Glycogen storage disease	AR	GBE1	Norwegian Forest
Hypertrophic cardiomyopathy	AD	MYBPC	Maine Coon, Ragdoll
Hypokalaemia	AR	WNK4	Burmese
Progressive retinal atrophy (early onset)	AD	CRX	Abyssinian
Progressive retinal atrophy (late onset)	AR	CEP290	Abyssinian
Polycystic kidney disease	AD	PKD1	Persian
Pyruvate kinase deficiency	AR	PKLR	Abyssinian, Somali, Domestic Shorthaired
Spinal muscular atrophy	AR	LIX1-LNPEP	Maine Coon

4.13 Common commercially available DNA tests for inherited feline disorders. AD = autosomal dominant; AR = autosomal recessive.

Health schemes

The British Veterinary Association (BVA) and the Kennel Club (KC) operate in partnership to offer a number of health screening programmes for dogs, collectively known as the canine health schemes. The canine health schemes enable breeders to screen their dogs for inherited diseases so that they can make informed decisions regarding suitability for breeding. Data collected by the health schemes also allow disease prevalence within each breed to be estimated on an annual basis. The ultimate aim of the health schemes is to reduce disease prevalence over time by selective breeding.

Hip Dysplasia Scheme

Hip dysplasia is a common inherited orthopaedic problem of dogs caused by abnormal development of the structures that make up the hip joint. The resultant joint deformity leads to secondary changes such as osteoarthritis, osteoarthrosis and degenerative joint disease, which manifest as varying degrees of lameness and/or pain. Hip dysplasia is more common in larger dog breeds, examples include the Labrador Retriever, Golden Retriever, German Shepherd Dog, Rottweiler, Bernese Mountain Dog and Newfoundland.

The BVA/KC Hip Dysplasia Scheme has operated since 1975 and currently surveys 175 different dog breeds, although the scheme is open to all breeds and cross-breeds. The basis of the scheme is radiographic examination of young adult dogs (at least 12 months of age) prior to breeding. Ventrodorsal radiographs of the pelvis are taken under sedation or general anaesthesia by a local veterinary surgeon and then submitted to the BVA where they are interpreted by a panel of scrutineers and scored (see Chapter 16). The hip score is the sum of the points accrued for each of nine radiographic features in each hip joint (Dennis, 2012). The lower the score the less the degree of hip dysplasia present. The minimum (best) score for each hip is zero and the maximum (worst) is 53, giving a range for the total score of both hips from 0 to 106. Breeders are generally advised to only breed from dogs with scores lower than the breed median score, which is calculated and published on an annual basis. It is also strongly recommended that hip scores of parents, grandparents, siblings and any previous progeny are considered to give the most accurate assessment of an individual dog's hip status. By following these recommendations, the aim is to gradually reduce the breed median score over successive generations.

Elbow Dysplasia Scheme

Elbow dysplasia, or abnormal development of the elbow joint, may be caused by one or more primary lesions, including an ununited anconeal process, a fragmented or ununited medial coronoid process and osteochondritis dissecans. These conditions then induce a secondary osteoarthritic process, which causes pain and lameness. Some common breeds at risk are the Basset Hound, Bernese Mountain Dog, Dogue de Bordeaux, German Shepherd Dog, Great Dane, Irish Water Spaniel, Irish Wolfhound, Large Munsterlander, Mastiff, Newfoundland, Otterhound, Golden Retriever, Labrador Retriever, Rottweiler and St Bernard.

As with the Hip Dysplasia Scheme, the basis of the Elbow Dysplasia Scheme is the interpretation of radiographs taken by a local veterinary surgeon. Two radiographic views of each elbow joint are required and a simple scoring system is employed (see Chapter 16):

- 0 = Normal
- 1 = Mild elbow dysplasia
- 2 = Moderate elbow dysplasia or presence of a primary lesion
- 3 = Severe elbow dysplasia.

Each elbow is given a score and the highest score is used to grade that dog. Ideally only dogs with normal (grade 0) elbows should be bred from, but for breeds in which elbow dysplasia is particularly prevalent, dogs with mild elbow dysplasia may need to be used initially to maintain genetic diversity within the breed. For these breeds such advice will only be effective in reducing prevalence of elbow dysplasia if it is continued over a number of generations.

Eye Scheme

The BVA and KC have operated a hereditary eye disease scheme in conjunction with the International Sheep Dog Society (ISDS) since the 1960s. The main purpose of the BVA/KC/ISDS Eye Scheme is to ensure the dog has no evidence of an inherited eye problem prior to breeding and thus, with time, disease prevalence can be reduced. Adult dogs are usually examined from 1 year of age and before they are used for breeding. Thereafter, annual examination is recommended. For breeds in which congenital/early onset hereditary ocular problems are known to be a problem, litter screening is performed between the age of 5 and 12 weeks. Following examination, a Certificate of Eye Examination is issued, on which conditions relevant to the breed in question are marked as either 'clinically affected' or 'clinically unaffected' (a grading system exists for pectinate ligament abnormality). Currently, the Scheme allows for Certification of 12 different inherited eye diseases across 62 different dog breeds. Under the Eye Scheme examination, however, all ocular abnormalities are recorded, which allows for monitoring of new and emerging inherited eye diseases, and the Scheme is open to all breeds and cross-breeds. Ophthalmic examination is performed by trained veterinary ophthalmologists using a combination of diagnostic techniques and equipment to examine the eye and adnexa. To examine the lens, vitreous and fundus of the eye, pupil dilation must first be performed with a topical ophthalmic mydriatic agent such as 1% tropicamide, which is effective within 20–30 minutes and lasts 6–8 hours. In breeds in which primary closed angle glaucoma is recognized, this routine clinical examination is preceded by examination of the drainage angle of the eye, using a technique called gonioscopy. Gonioscopy is used to assess the drainage angle for an inherited abnormality called pectinate ligament abnormality (also known as goniodysgenesis), which is considered to be a risk factor for glaucoma, and is usually advised every 3 years in predisposed breeds.

Chiari-like malformation/syringomyelia Scheme

Syringomyelia (SM) is a neurological condition most commonly seen in the Cavalier King Charles Spaniel in which it has high heritability (Lewis et al., 2010). It is characterized by fluid-filled cavities, called syrinxes, within the spinal cord and usually occurs in association with a deformity of the brain known as Chiari-like malformation (CM). Both conditions may be diagnosed by magnetic resonance imaging (MRI), which is the basis of the BVA/KC CM/SM Scheme. MR scanning of the brain and upper spinal cord is performed after 1 year of age under general anaesthesia. MR images are then assessed by qualified scrutineers to allow scoring of the degree of CM/SM.

Panel DNA testing

Following technological advances, new methods have become available that enable the assay of multiple DNA variants simultaneously. This means that from a simple buccal cheek swab sample, hundreds of variants can be assessed across a dog's genome in a single experiment. Several canine DNA testing providers have used these new platforms to develop custom assay sets (panel tests) that can, in parallel, test the dog's DNA for:

- Disease-associated mutations
- DNA variants associated with particular traits (e.g. coat colour)
- An assessment of the genetic diversity/coefficient of inbreeding for that dog
- A panel of DNA variants that enable estimation of the dog's breed makeup.

The latter two tests are dependent on the provider possessing comprehensive and relevant reference datasets for comparison.

Most of the disease-associated mutations tested by 'one size fits all' panel tests are not relevant to the breed being tested, which may lead to misinterpretation of results. Most autosomal recessive diseases in the dog are unique to an individual breed or closely related breeds. This means that, unless there has been some outcrossing, other breeds are extremely unlikely to carry that particular mutation. Just to complicate matters further, there are also many disorders in the dog that appear clinically very similar but are caused by different mutations in the same or different genes. For example, with progressive retinal atrophy (PRA) over 25 PRA-associated mutations have now been identified, each of which causes PRA in a specific breed or breeds (Downs et al., 2014). Thus, just because a dog from one breed is tested free of all 25 mutations, the results are only relevant if one (or more) of those PRA-causing mutations is known to be present and cause PRA within that particular breed; otherwise the result is meaningless. In fact, the dog may well be affected by (a new form of) PRA, it is just that the causative mutation has not yet been identified in that breed.

Testing all dogs (regardless of their breed) for all mutations can, occasionally, lead to important findings – a breed closely related to the breed in which the mutation was first discovered ('discovery breed') may share the same mutation, and so once that breed has been investigated clinically to ensure correlation of genotype with disease, the same DNA test can be formally extended to that breed. The PRA example can again be used to illustrate this point. The most common form of canine PRA is progressive rod-cone degeneration (PRCD), which is caused by a single mutation in the *PRCD* gene (Zangerl et al., 2006). This form of PRA is known to affect multiple canine breeds because the mutation is ancestral to their formation. Thus, if this mutation were to be discovered in a new breed and specialist veterinary verification of clinical disease was achieved, then the *PRCD* DNA test may also become applicable to this new breed.

In summary, panel DNA testing offers an extremely efficient and affordable means of screening dogs for a large number of variants in a single test. The vast majority of the tests, however, will not be relevant to the dog being tested and so careful interpretation of the results is required.

Kennel Club

The Kennel Club, in partnership with Weatherbys, has introduced Combibreed® Health Test Packages, which can be purchased for certain breeds of dog. The package is an 'all in one' test for multiple genetic disorders. From a single buccal swab, the test identifies whether the dog has any genetic material linked to a range of significant inherited conditions specific to that breed. The resulting information can be used by the dog owner to make decisions regarding the types of mates that would be genetically compatible. More information is available on the Kennel Club website (www.thekennelclub.org.uk/health/forbreeders/dna-testing-simple-inherited-disorders/combibreed-health-test-packages/)

Estimated breeding values

Estimated breeding values (EBVs) are another tool to help breeders reduce disease prevalence. EBVs allow breeders to determine the relative genetic risk of an individual for a certain trait that will be passed on to their offspring by mating. EBVs are calculated using the results of health screening that exist for the individual dog and all its relatives. The calculated EBV of an individual can then be compared with the breed average, which is always set as 0. Negative EBVs represent a lower genetic risk and positive EBVs a higher genetic risk than the breed average.

The KC currently offers an EBV calculator service for hip and elbow dysplasia, which computes hip and/or elbow scores from the above detailed schemes, for breeds where sufficient data have been collected. Using EBVs to make mating decisions will be more accurate than using the observed hip or elbow score and will lead to faster progress in reducing the prevalence of disease. The results from the BVA/KC CM/SM Scheme are also used to generate EBVs. It must be emphasized, however, that EBVs are complementary to the relevant health scheme(s) and are not a replacement for them and rely on the collection of accurate population-wide data.

References and further reading

Dennis R (2012) Interpretation and use of BVA/KC hip scores in dogs. *In Practice* **34**, 178–194

Downs LM, Hitti R, Pregnolato S et al. (2014) Genetic screening for PRA-associated mutations in multiple dog breeds shows that PRA is heterogeneous within and between breeds. *Veterinary Ophthalmology* **17**, 126–130

Lewis T, Rusbridge C, Knowler P et al. (2010) Heritability of syringomyelia in Cavalier King Charles Spaniels. *The Veterinary Journal* **183**, 345–347

Lyons LA (2012) DNA testing in domestic cats. *Molecular and Cellular Probes* **26**, 224–230

Mellersh CS (2016) DNA testing man's best friend: roles and responsibilities. *The Veterinary Journal* **207**, 10–12

Mellersh CS (2012) DNA testing and domestic dogs. *Mammalian Genome* **23**, 109–123

Menotti-Raymond M, David VA, Pflueger SM et al. (2008) Patterns of molecular genetic variation among cat breeds. *Genomics* **91**, 1–11

Parker HG (2012) Genomic analyses of modern dog breeds. *Mammalian Genome* **23**, 19–27

Zangerl B, Goldstein O, Philp AR et al. (2006) Identical mutation in a novel retinal gene causes progressive rod–cone degeneration in dogs and retinitis pigmentosa in humans. *Genomics* **88**, 551–563

Useful websites

University of Pennsylvania – Canine and Feline Hereditary Disease (DNA) Testing Laboratories:
www.vet.upenn.edu/research/academic-departments/clinical-sciences-advanced-medicine/research-labs-centers/penngen

Kennel Club – Worldwide DNA tests:
www.thekennelclub.org.uk/health/for-dna-testing-simple-inherited-disorders/worldwide-dna-tests.

Kennel Club – Inbreeding – using COIs (coefficients of inbreeding):
www.thekennelclub.org.uk/health/for-breeders/inbreeding/.

British Veterinary Association (BVA)/Kennel Club Canine Health Schemes:
- Chiari Malformation/Syringomyelia (CM/SM)
  www.bva.co.uk/Canine-Health-Schemes/CM-SM-Scheme/
- Elbow Dysplasia
  www.bva.co.uk/Canine-Health-Schemes/Elbow-Scheme
- Hereditary eye disease
  www.bva.co.uk/Canine-Health-Schemes/Eye-Scheme/
- Hip Dysplasia
  www.bva.co.uk/canine-health-schemes/hip-scheme/

Self-assessment questions

1. Describe the components of a DNA nucleotide.
2. What are the three main phases of the cell cycle?
3. Name the two processes required for the nucleotide sequence of a gene to be converted into protein.
4. What is the name of the type of genetic marker used in parentage analysis?
5. Define the term inbreeding coefficient.
6. What is meant by the term line breeding?
7. What is the main purpose of the canine health schemes?
8. DNA testing is usually performed on what type of tissue sample(s)?
9. Give an example of an autosomal dominant and an autosomal recessive disorder in the cat for which DNA tests exist.

Principles of microbiology

Maggie Fisher

Introduction

The microorganisms described in this chapter represent a very small proportion of all microorganisms and are those that interrelate with animal hosts in some way. They vary in size (Figure 5.1) from the relatively large ringworm fungi to viruses that can only be seen with an electron microscope. The major similarities and differences between the different types of microorganism are shown in Figure 5.2.

There are several ways in which microorganisms can relate to hosts (Figure 5.3). Some microorganisms may be beneficial or neutral in effect; however, the focus of this chapter will be upon those that have the potential to harm their hosts by causing infection or disease of dogs, cats and exotic pets. A few important organisms that are carried by cats and dogs without clinical signs but are capable of causing disease in humans (i.e. are zoonotic) are included.

Microorganisms obtain their nutrition from a variety of sources and some have more specific nutritional requirements than others (see Figure 5.2).

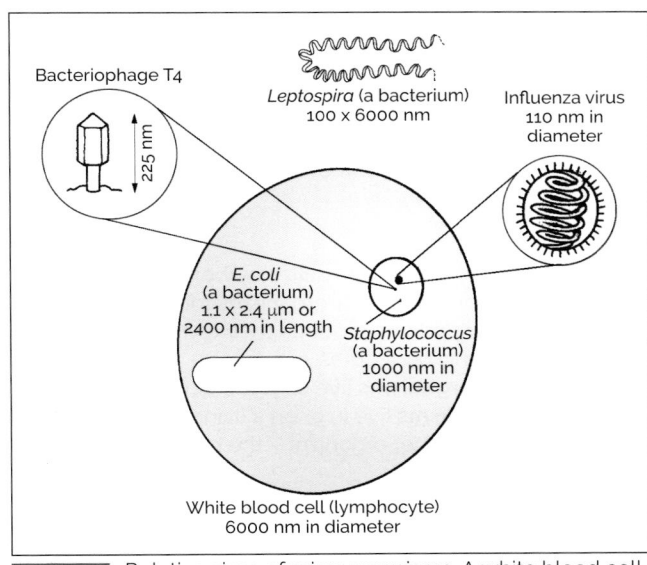

5.1 Relative sizes of microorganisms. A white blood cell (lymphocyte) is shown for comparison.

Characteristic	Bacteria	Viruses	Fungi	Protozoa	Algae
Size	0.5–5 µm	20–300 nm	3–8 µm (yeasts)	10–200 µm	Approximately 20 µm
Cell arrangement	Unicellular	Non-cellular	Unicellular or multicellular	Unicellular	Unicellular or multicellular
Cell wall	Present; mainly peptidoglycan	Absent	Present; mainly chitin	Absent	Present; mainly cellulose
Nucleus	No true membrane-bound nucleus	Absent	Membrane-bound nucleus	Membrane-bound nucleus	Membrane-bound nucleus

5.2 Major similarities and differences between different types of microorganism.

continues ▶

Characteristic	Bacteria	Viruses	Fungi	Protozoa	Algae
Nucleic acids	DNA and RNA	DNA or RNA	DNA and RNA	DNA and RNA	DNA and RNA
Reproduction	Asexual by binary fission	Replicate only within another living cell	Asexual and sexual by spores, budding in yeast	Asexual and sexual	Asexual and sexual
Nutrition	Mainly heterotrophic – can be saprophytic or parasitic; a few are autotrophic	Obligate parasites	Heterotrophic – can be saprophytic or parasitic	Heterotrophic – can be saprophytic or parasitic	Autotrophic
Motility	Some are motile	Non-motile	Non-motile except for certain spore forms	Motile	Some are motile
Toxin production	Some form toxins	None	Some form toxins	Some form toxins	Some form toxins

5.2 *continued* Major similarities and differences between different types of microorganism.

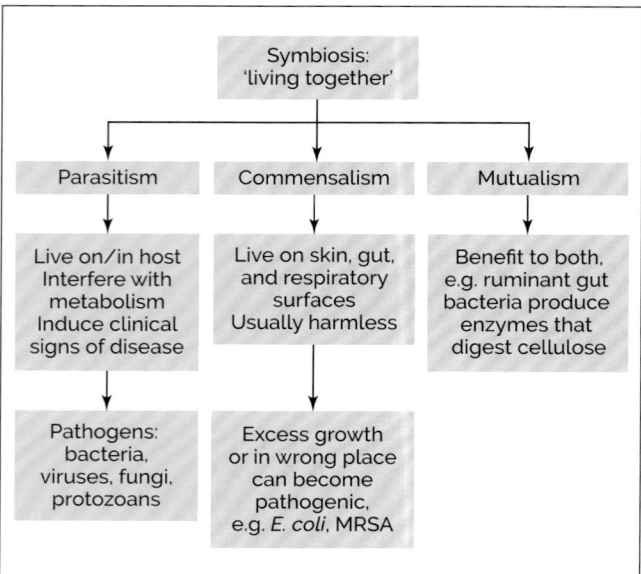

5.3 Relationships between microorganisms and animal hosts.

- **Heterotrophic organisms** utilize carbon in the form of organic carbon from other organisms for growth.
- **Autotropic organisms** produce their own food from simple inorganic molecules.
- **Saprophytic organisms** live off dead or decaying matter.
- **Parasitic organisms** live in or on a living organism at the expense of the other organism – the host.

Viruses

Structure and naming

Viruses are extremely small and are sometimes not classified as living organisms as they are incapable of reproduction without a host cell. A virus particle, or virion, is little more than a package containing instructions for the recreation of further virus particles. Each virus particle is composed of two parts (Figure 5.4):

- *Nucleic acid* – RNA or DNA (never both) forming a **central core**
- *A protein coat* – **the capsid**.

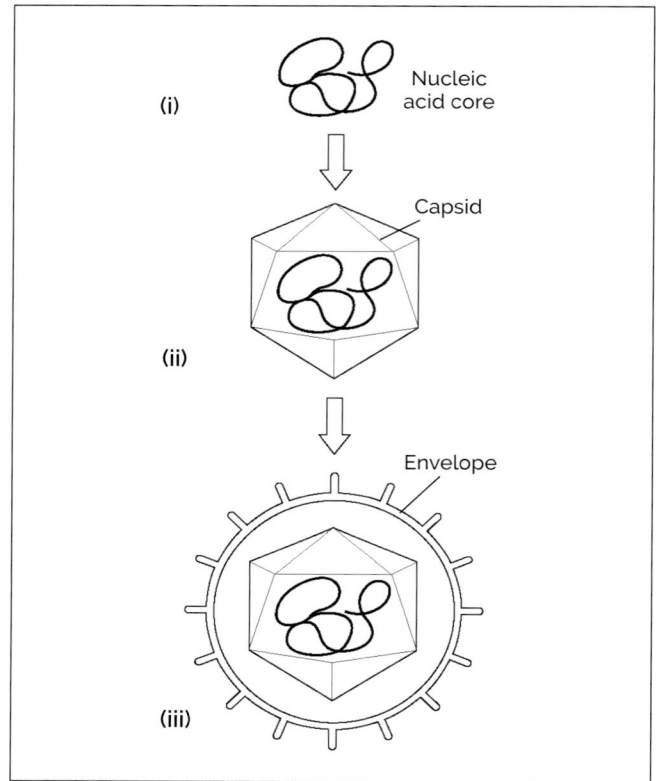

5.4 General virus components: **(i)** central core of nucleic acid; **(ii)** capsid surrounding the nucleic acid to form a nucleocapsid (with icosahedral symmetry); **(iii)** in addition, some viruses possess an outer envelope.

Together, these two parts form the **nucleocapsid**. For some viruses, this is all that an individual virus particle will comprise. Various shapes of virus nucleocapsid have been identified:

- Helical
- Icosahedral
- Complex (poxvirus)
- Composite (some bacteriophages).

Some viruses have an additional envelope around the outside, often formed of the host cell membrane (see Figure 5.4iii). Each of the helical or icosahedral shapes of the nucleo-capsid can be enveloped or non-enveloped (Figure 5.5), giving four possible basic shapes for viruses. In fact, there are no animal viruses (only plant viruses) that are helical and

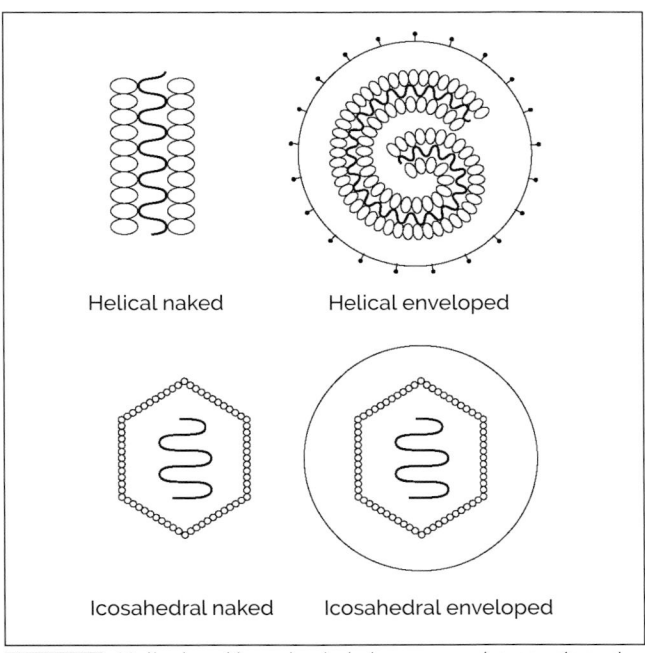

Helical naked   Helical enveloped

Icosahedral naked   Icosahedral enveloped

5.5 Helical and icosahedral viruses may be enveloped or non-enveloped (naked).

non-enveloped, so viruses of dogs and cats can be grouped by and large into the other three types. Viruses have been classified together on the basis of structural similarities. For example, the group of viruses causing true 'flu are the influenza viruses.

Viral replication

A virus is only able to attach to cells that carry a compatible receptor. For example, influenza viruses can only attach to ciliated epithelial cells in the respiratory tract. This specificity

of viruses for specific tissues is known as tissue tropism. Viruses normally have only one or two host species that they are able to infect (e.g. parvovirus in dogs does not infect cats, and measles virus will only infect humans and apes). Once attached, virus particles are taken into the host cell (Figure 5.6) by fusing the virus envelope with the host cell membrane or, in the case of non-enveloped viruses, by causing the host cell to engulf the virus particle into the cell. Once inside the cell, the virus is able to switch the cell's normal metabolism to obey the instructions of the virus. The virus may cause this to happen immediately, so that the cell begins to produce the constituents of new virus particles within hours of infection. Alternatively, as in the case of feline leukaemia virus (FeLV), the virus may join to the host cell's own nucleic acid for an extended period before making any changes to cell metabolism. New virus particles are then assembled and released from the cell. Depending on the virus, this may leave the host cell intact or may cause its rupture and destruction.

Transmission

Viruses are transmitted from host to host either directly (e.g. by a cat licking feline calicivirus in nasal secretions from the face of another cat) or indirectly (e.g. a dog licking the floor of a kennel that had been occupied by a dog with parvovirus infection and had not been adequately cleaned). Different viruses have adapted their means of transmission according to their structure (which affects their ability to survive in the environment) and their location in the host. For example, a respiratory tract virus is often transmitted by virus particles being sneezed from one host into the air breathed in by another host. This is ideal for influenza virus, as these enveloped viruses are not very robust and do not survive for extended periods in the environment. An ability to survive in the environment for longer periods is beneficial for canine parvovirus. The virus must be licked up and ingested by another dog for infection of the gastrointestinal tract to occur.

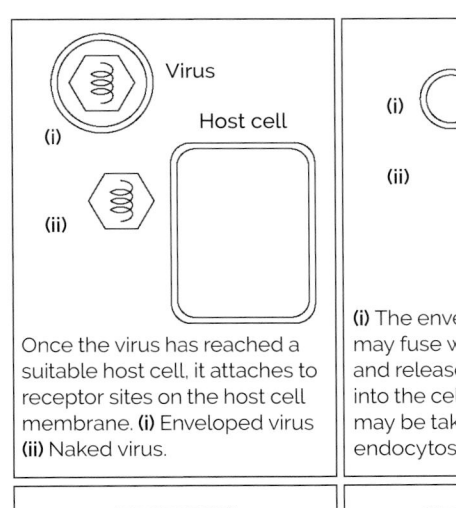
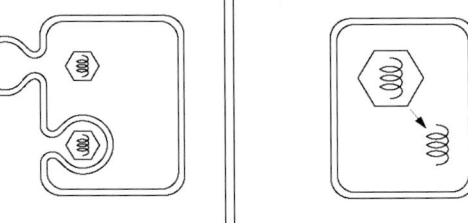
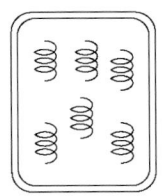

Once the virus has reached a suitable host cell, it attaches to receptor sites on the host cell membrane. **(i)** Enveloped virus **(ii)** Naked virus.

(i) The envelope of the virus may fuse with the cell wall and release the nucleocapsid into the cell or **(ii)** the virus may be taken into the cell by endocytosis.

The virus enters the host cell and the protein coat (capsid) breaks down to release the viral nucleic acid.

The viral nucleic acid replicates (either in the host cell cytoplasm or nucleus) and directs the host cell metabolism to make new virus material.

5.6 Replication of animal viruses.

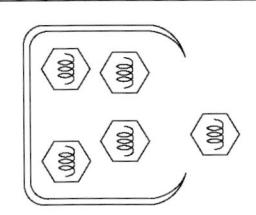
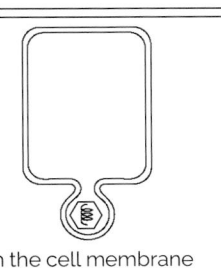

The new viruses are assembled.

They leave the host cell either by rupture of the cell membrane (naked viruses); or

through the cell membrane (enveloped viruses).

Incubation

Once a host animal has been infected with a small number of virus particles, there is a time lag before the clinical signs that are associated with the infection are seen; this is the **incubation period**. During this time, the virus reaches the cells that it can invade and initially infects a small number of cells in order to increase the number of virus particles. Clinical signs are seen once large numbers of virus particles infect a large number of cells.

Viral diseases

Some infections in dogs and cats that are caused by viruses are shown in Figures 5.7 and 5.8, respectively. Some examples of viral infections of exotic pets are shown in Figure 5.9. It should also be noted that some viruses of companion animals are zoonotic (Reperant *et al.*, 2016). More medical details of viral diseases in small animals can be found in Chapter 18.

Name of virus	Disease caused	Clinical signs	Nucleic acid type	Shape of nucleocapsid	Enveloped
Parvovirus	Parvovirus	Vomiting, haemorrhagic diarrhoea, anorexia, dehydration, may be fatal	DNA	Icosahedral	No
Canine adenovirus 1 (CAV-1)	Infectious canine hepatitis	May be rapidly fatal, vomiting, abdominal pain and diarrhoea	DNA	Icosahedral	No
Canine adenovirus 2 (CAV-2)	Infectious canine tracheobronchitis – part of kennel cough syndrome	Bouts of severe coughing	DNA	Icosahedral	No
Canine distemper virus	Distemper	May be mild or severe. Conjunctivitis, cough, depression, anorexia, vomiting, diarrhoea	RNA	Helical	Yes
Canine parainfluenza virus	Canine influenza – part of kennel cough syndrome	Bouts of severe coughing	RNA	Helical	Yes
Rabies virus	Rabies	Classically subtle behavioural changes followed by restlessness and aggression. May be followed by a short paralytic stage before death	RNA	Helical	Yes
Canine herpesvirus	'Fading puppy syndrome'	Disease and death in very young puppies	DNA	Icosahedral	Yes
Canine coronavirus	Canine coronavirus infection	Vomiting and diarrhoea	RNA	Helical	Yes

5.7 Some viral diseases of dogs.

Name of virus	Disease caused	Clinical signs	Nucleic acid type	Shape of nucleocapsid	Enveloped
Feline parvovirus (panleucopenia)	Feline infectious enteritis	Fever, anorexia and depression	DNA	Icosahedral	No
Feline herpesvirus	Feline rhinotracheitis; cat 'flu	Depression, sneezing, anorexia, pyrexia followed by ocular and nasal discharges	DNA	Icosahedral	Yes
Feline calicivirus	Cat 'flu	Clinical signs vary in severity. Pyrexia, oral ulceration, respiratory and conjunctivitis in the mild and most common form	RNA	Icosahedral	No
Feline coronavirus	Feline infectious peritonitis (FIP)	Clinical signs variable: can include pyrexia, weight loss, decreased appetite, depression and abdominal enlargement,	RNA	Helical	Yes
Feline leukaemia virus (FeLV)	Feline leukaemia	Variable clinical signs including anaemia, immunosuppression and premature death	RNA	Icosahedral	Yes
Feline immunodeficiency virus (FIV)	FIV infection	Clinical signs variable and non-specific including fever, enteritis and respiratory disease	RNA	Icosahedral	Yes
Rabies virus	Rabies, although cats are less susceptible to infection than dogs	Behavioural changes with erratic activity and anxious appearance in the eyes. Followed by a paralytic stage	RNA	Helical	Yes

5.8 Some viral diseases of cats.

Name of virus	Host species	Disease caused	Clinical signs	Nucleic acid type	Shape of nucleocapsid	Enveloped
Canine distemper virus	Ferret	Canine distemper	Severe illness with fever, lethargy, ocular and nasal discharges, death	RNA	Helical	Yes
Hamster polyomavirus	Hamster	HaPV infection	Loss of weight and condition, maybe internal lump-like swellings and wart-like lumps on the skin	DNA	Icosahedral	No
Herpesvirus	Tortoise	Herpesvirus infection	Anorexia, runny nose and drooling, maybe gurgling whilst breathing	DNA	Icosahedral	Yes
Myxoma (a poxvirus)	Rabbit	Myxomatosis	Nasal and ocular discharge, pyrexia, depression and anorexia	DNA	Brick-shaped, slightly pleomorphic	Yes
RHDV viruses	Rabbit	Rabbit haemorrhagic disease	Depression, loss of appetite, incoordination, difficulty breathing, bloody discharge from the nose or mouth	RNA	Icosahedral	No

5.9   Examples of viral infections of exotic pets.

Diagnosis of viral infections

Viral infections may be diagnosed on the basis of clinical signs and the animal's clinical history. Often there are several infections that may cause similar signs and it may be important to be able to confirm the particular virus present. This may be carried out in a number of ways, including the following:

- Virus particles are too small to be seen with a light microscope but they may be seen with an electron microscope
- Large numbers of virus particles may clump together in cells; the clump may then be seen with a light microscope. Large groups of rabies virus particles are seen in cells of animals infected with rabies; these are known as Negri bodies. An animal can only be examined for these and a number of other virus-related changes at post-mortem
- Serology may be carried out to detect the specific antibody produced by the host in response to infection (e.g. FIV). In some cases, the virus protein (antigen) can be detected directly in serum (e.g. FeLV)
- Polymerase chain reaction (PCR) can be used to amplify and detect the nucleic acid of the virus (e.g. canine distemper).

Treatment of viral infections

Viral infections can be combatted in a number of ways. Treatment of viral infections in animals normally involves supportive nursing, for example:

- Fluids (oral and intravenous) (see Chapter 20) to prevent dehydration in the case of canine parvovirus infection
- Tempting foods for cats with cat 'flu
- Antibacterials to limit secondary bacterial infection.

Animals may also be vaccinated in order to stimulate an immune response (see Chapters 7 and 8).

There are now treatments for some viral infections, these were originally introduced for human use against, for example, HIV (human immunodeficiency virus), the shingles form of chickenpox and for herpes simplex virus (the cause of cold sores).

Increasingly, antiviral treatments are used in companion animals, though the products such as aciclovir, famciclovir, ganciclovir, lamivudine and zidovudine are licensed for human use and are used by veterinary surgeons under the Cascade (see Chapter 8).

Prevention of viral infection

As viral infections are difficult to treat once the animal is infected, control has been aimed at preventing infection, particularly of severe viral diseases. This can be done at a number of levels:

- A country can have a border policy to prevent entry of diseases that are not present in that country (e.g. countries seek to prevent entry of rabies by quarantine or vaccination policies) (see Chapter 7)
- Accommodation can be designed to avoid or limit the spread of infection (e.g. catteries may be designed so that airborne viruses are not readily transmitted from cat to cat) (see Chapter 14)
- Suitable disinfectants can be used to kill viruses that may be present in animal cages between occupants (e.g. to prevent the transmission of parvovirus between dogs) (see Chapter 14)
- Individual animals may be protected by vaccination (e.g. canine distemper, canine parvovirus, feline leukaemia). More details about vaccination may be found in Chapters 7 and 8.

Prions

Prions are very small proteinaceous particles that cause infections within the central nervous system, leading eventually to the death of the animal. The incubation period is usually long; it takes from 2 months to 20 years before signs of disease become apparent. Until relatively recently, the study of prion diseases was highly specialized work carried out by only a few people. Researchers have investigated scrapie, which is a transmissible spongiform encephalopathy of sheep, caused by a prion, and has been recorded in Europe for the last 200 years. Interest and research in prion infections increased greatly following the outbreak of bovine spongiform encephalopathy (BSE), which was first identified in the UK in the mid-1980s. BSE transmission to humans was shown to be due to eating infected cattle products. Over 150 deaths have been attributed to such infection resulting in variant Creutzfeldt–Jacob disease (vCJD), a form of the human encephalopathy, Creutzfeldt–Jacob disease (CJD). Transmission to humans was controlled by measures such as the introduction of a slaughter scheme and removal of specified bovine offal from the food chain. Transmission to cattle was controlled through a ban on the feeding of processed animal protein. Around 20 cases of a similar disease, feline spongiform encephalopathy (FSE), in cats and other felids have been recorded since 1990. Affected cats exhibit nervous signs and incoordination. Much research effort is now aimed at being able to confirm disease in the live animal. Diagnosis using lymph node samples in the live animal is now possible, offering an alternative to diagnosis based on the appearance of brain tissue at post-mortem examination.

Bacteria

Size and shape

Bacteria (singular: bacterium) are single-celled organisms and most range in size from 0.5 μm (micrometres or microns; 10^{-6} m) to 5 μm in length, though there are some exceptions. The shape and physiology of bacteria present in infections are used to identify their species and thus assess prognosis and suitable treatments.

Three basic shapes are generally recognized and these are sometimes used as a means of classification and naming of bacteria:

- Cylindrical or rod-shaped cells (Figure 5.10a) are called **bacilli** (singular: bacillus). Some bacilli are curved (Figure 5.10b) and these are known as **vibrios**
- Spherical cells are called **cocci** (singular: coccus). Some cocci exist singly while others remain together in pairs

after cell division and are called **diplococci**. Those that remain attached to form chains are called **streptococci** (Figure 5.10c) and if they divide randomly and form irregular grape-like clusters they are called **staphylococci** (Figure 5.10d)
- Spiral or helical cells are called **spirochaetes**.

Structure

Some of the structures shown in the generalized bacterial cell depicted in Figure 5.11 are common to all cells; others are only present in certain species or under certain environmental conditions.

Bacteria are commonly stained with the Gram stain, which differentially stains many bacteria either purple (Gram-positive) or pink (Gram-negative) depending on the structure of their cell wall.

Naming bacteria

All bacteria, in common with plants and animals, are named according to the binomial system. The first word starts with a capital letter and indicates the genus (plural: genera) to which they belong (e.g. *Escherichia*). This is followed by the species name all written in lower case (e.g. *coli*). Thus, *Escherichia coli* is one of the species of the genus *Escherichia*, just as *Homo sapiens* (modern humans) is one of the species of the genus *Homo*. The generic name is frequently shortened to an initial letter, e.g. *Escherichia coli* becomes *E. coli*; *Staphylococcus aureus* may be seen written as *Staph. aureus*. Both generic and specific names are written in *italics*. The genus name can also be used with the abbreviation sp. (for one species) or spp. (denoting multiple species of the same genus), e.g. *Staphylococcus* spp.

Endospores

Some species of bacteria produce dormant forms called endospores (or simply **spores**), which can survive in unfavourable conditions. They are formed when the vegetative (growing) cells are deprived of some factor (e.g. when the

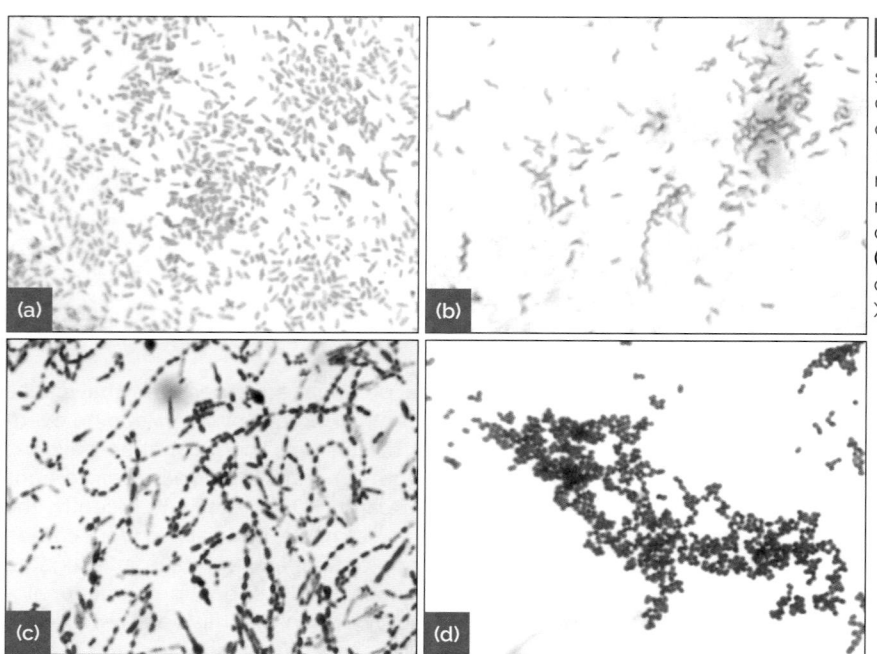

5.10 Classification of bacteria by shape. These preparations have all been stained with Gram stain: Gram-negative organisms appear pink; Gram-positive organisms appear purple. **(a)** Rods. **(b)** *Campylobacter* sp. rods appear bent; single rods appear banana-shaped and pairs resemble flying seagulls. **(c)** *Streptococcus* sp. cocci showing chain formation. **(d)** *Staphylococcus* sp. cocci showing characteristic clumping. (Original magnification X500) (© Andrew Rycroft)

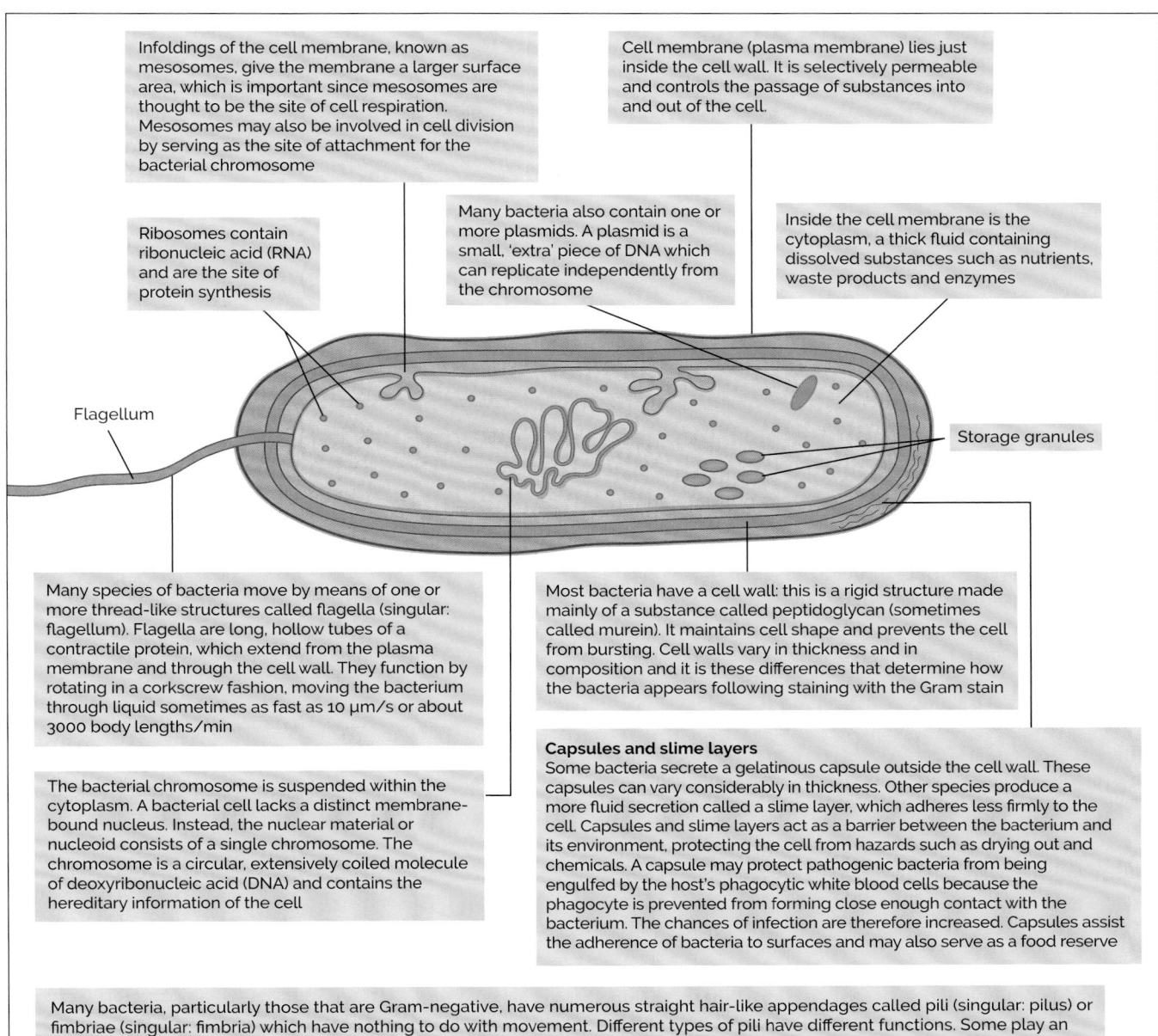

Infoldings of the cell membrane, known as mesosomes, give the membrane a larger surface area, which is important since mesosomes are thought to be the site of cell respiration. Mesosomes may also be involved in cell division by serving as the site of attachment for the bacterial chromosome

Cell membrane (plasma membrane) lies just inside the cell wall. It is selectively permeable and controls the passage of substances into and out of the cell.

Many bacteria also contain one or more plasmids. A plasmid is a small, 'extra' piece of DNA which can replicate independently from the chromosome

Inside the cell membrane is the cytoplasm, a thick fluid containing dissolved substances such as nutrients, waste products and enzymes

Ribosomes contain ribonucleic acid (RNA) and are the site of protein synthesis

Flagellum

Storage granules

Many species of bacteria move by means of one or more thread-like structures called flagella (singular: flagellum). Flagella are long, hollow tubes of a contractile protein, which extend from the plasma membrane and through the cell wall. They function by rotating in a corkscrew fashion, moving the bacterium through liquid sometimes as fast as 10 μm/s or about 3000 body lengths/min

Most bacteria have a cell wall: this is a rigid structure made mainly of a substance called peptidoglycan (sometimes called murein). It maintains cell shape and prevents the cell from bursting. Cell walls vary in thickness and in composition and it is these differences that determine how the bacteria appears following staining with the Gram stain

The bacterial chromosome is suspended within the cytoplasm. A bacterial cell lacks a distinct membrane-bound nucleus. Instead, the nuclear material or nucleoid consists of a single chromosome. The chromosome is a circular, extensively coiled molecule of deoxyribonucleic acid (DNA) and contains the hereditary information of the cell

Capsules and slime layers
Some bacteria secrete a gelatinous capsule outside the cell wall. These capsules can vary considerably in thickness. Other species produce a more fluid secretion called a slime layer, which adheres less firmly to the cell. Capsules and slime layers act as a barrier between the bacterium and its environment, protecting the cell from hazards such as drying out and chemicals. A capsule may protect pathogenic bacteria from being engulfed by the host's phagocytic white blood cells because the phagocyte is prevented from forming close enough contact with the bacterium. The chances of infection are therefore increased. Capsules assist the adherence of bacteria to surfaces and may also serve as a food reserve

Many bacteria, particularly those that are Gram-negative, have numerous straight hair-like appendages called pili (singular: pilus) or fimbriae (singular: fimbria) which have nothing to do with movement. Different types of pili have different functions. Some play an important part in enabling bacteria to stick to host cells. For example, in infection, pili help pathogenic bacteria to attach to the cells lining the respiratory, intestinal or urinary tracts, thus preventing them from being washed away by body fluids. Other pili, sometimes called sex pili, are involved in the transfer of genetic material from one bacterial cell to another during bacterial conjugation (see Figure 5.13). Some microbiologists now use the term fimbriae to refer to the appendages involved in attachment and restrict the term pili to those involved in the transfer of DNA during conjugation

5.11   Components of a generalized bacterial cell and their functions.

supply of nutrients is inadequate). It is important to note that endospore formation (or **sporulation**) is not a method of reproduction: one vegetative cell produces a single spore which, after germination, is again just one vegetative cell. Spore formation is most common in the genera *Bacillus* and *Clostridium*. These genera contain the causative agents of tetanus, anthrax and botulism. These diseases are zoonoses, affecting domestic pets, farm animals and humans. Species susceptibility to each disease varies; for example, dogs only infrequently suffer from tetanus, whilst humans are very susceptible and require routine vaccination.

Many endospore-forming bacteria are inhabitants of the soil, but spores can exist almost everywhere, including in dust. They are extremely resistant structures that can remain viable for many years. They can survive extremes of heat, pH, desiccation, ultraviolet radiation and exposure to toxic chemicals, such as some disinfectants. The reason why endospores are so resistant is not completely understood, but heat resistance is thought to be due to the fact that a dehydration process occurs during spore formation, which expels most of the water from the spore. The spore develops within the bacterial cell, and under the microscope it appears as a bright, round or oval structure.

The fact that spores are so hard to destroy is the principal reason for the various sterilization procedures that are carried out in veterinary practice. Common techniques employed to kill spores include:

- Autoclaving (moist heat, 121°C under pressure 6.9 kPa for more than 15 minutes)
- Tyndallization (repeated steaming)
- Dry heat (160°C for at least 2 hours).

Conditions necessary for bacterial growth

Bacteria can grow and reproduce only when environmental conditions are suitable. The essential requirements for growth include:

- A supply of suitable nutrients
- The correct temperature (the temperature at which a species of bacterium grows most rapidly is the optimum growth temperature; most mammalian pathogens grow best at normal body temperature)
- The correct pH (the majority of mammalian pathogens grow best at pH 7–7.4)
- Water
- The correct gaseous environment (many species of bacterium can grow only when oxygen is present).

Bacteria that must have oxygen for growth are called strict or **obligate aerobes**. Some, known as **obligate anaerobes**, can only grow in the absence of oxygen, while others, the **facultative anaerobes**, grow aerobically when oxygen is present but can also function in the absence of oxygen. A few species, the **microaerophiles**, grow best when the concentration of oxygen is lower than in atmospheric air (e.g. *Campylobacter* spp.).

Reproduction of bacteria

If the environment is suitable, bacteria can grow and reproduce rapidly. The time interval between successive divisions is called the **generation time**. In some bacteria the generation time is very short; for others it is quite long. For example, under optimum conditions the generation time of *E. coli* is 20 minutes, whereas for the tuberculosis bacterium *Mycobacterium tuberculosis* it is approximately 18 hours. Given appropriate conditions, growth is exponential, i.e. one bacterium produces two, then two produce four, and so on.

Bacteria reproduce asexually by simply dividing into two identical daughter cells, a process called **binary fission** (Figure 5.12). Prior to cell division, the cell grows; once it has reached a certain size, the circular chromosome or nucleoid replicates to form two identical chromosomes. As the parent cell enlarges, the chromosomes are separated and the cell membrane grows inwards at the centre of the cell. At the same time, new cell wall material grows inwards to form the septum and this divides the cell into two daughter cells. These may separate completely, but in some species (e.g. streptococci, staphylococci) they remain attached to form the characteristic chains or clusters. Replication of pathogenic bacteria usually takes place outside the host's cells – unlike pathogenic viruses, where reproduction is intracellular.

Conjugation

The process of conjugation (Figure 5.13) involves the passage of DNA from one bacterial cell (the donor) to another (the recipient) while the two cells are in physical contact. The cells are pulled together by an appendage called the **sex pilus**, which is formed by the donor cell. Once contact has been made, the pilus retracts so that the surfaces of the donor and recipient are very close to each other. The cell membranes fuse, forming a channel between the two cells, and DNA then passes from the donor to the recipient.

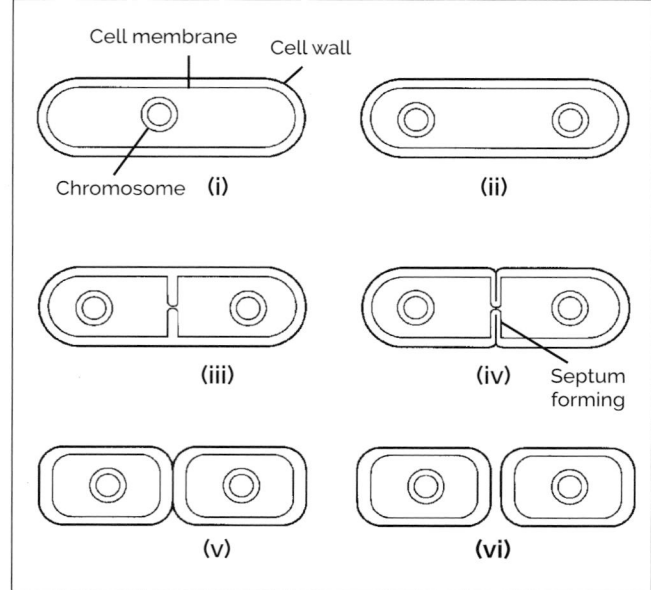

5.12 Replication of bacteria by binary fission. **(i) (ii)** The cell grows and the chromosome replicates to form two identical chromosomes. **(iii)** As the cell enlarges, the chromosomes are separated and the cell membrane grows inwards at the centre of the cell. **(iv)** At the same time, new cell wall material grows inwards to form the septum. **(v) (vi)** The cell divides into two daughter cells.

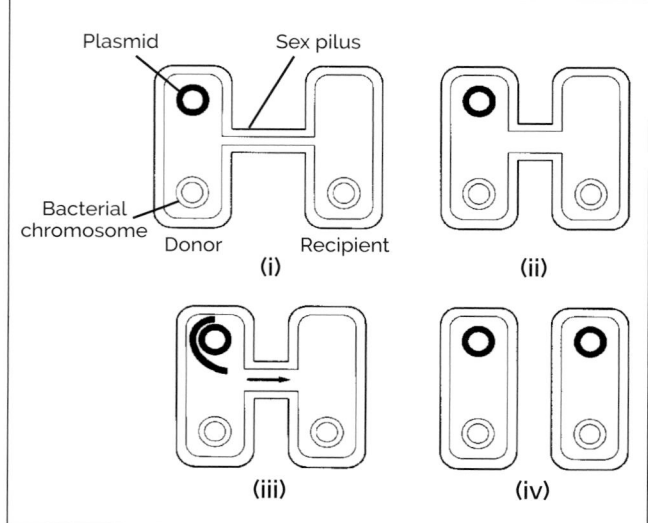

5.13 Sequence of events in conjugation. **(i)** Donor and recipient cells are pulled together by the sex pilus, which is formed by the donor cell. **(ii)** The pilus retracts, bringing the two cells very close to each other, and the cell membranes fuse to form a channel between the two cells. **(iii)** The plasmid replicates and one strand passes through the channel to the recipient. **(iv)** The two cells separate. The recipient becomes a potential donor, because it now has the plasmid.

Frequently, a plasmid (see Figure 5.11) is transferred from the donor to the recipient but sometimes part of the donor cell chromosome, or even the whole chromosome, is transferred. Conjugation is important because the recipient acquires new characteristics. For example, one plasmid, the R plasmid, carries genes for resistance to antibiotics.

Conjugation is rare among Gram-positive bacteria but common among those that are Gram-negative. It is sometimes regarded as a primitive type of sexual reproduction but this is misleading because, unlike sexual reproduction in other organisms, it does not involve the fusion of two gametes to form a single cell.

Identification of bacteria

It can be important to identify the bacteria causing an infection, for example so that appropriate antibacterials can be selected for treatment. The simplest and quickest way to identify bacteria is to make a smear and stain it with Gram stain, which involves a sequence of steps. As well as indicating whether the bacterium is Gram-positive or Gram-negative, this also allows the structure of the bacterial cell to be observed.

There are often several bacteria that look alike at this stage and so it may be necessary to culture the bacterium so that the identity can be determined more precisely. Figure 5.14 shows how this process might occur for the investigation of an infection causing otitis externa in a dog's ear.

Practically, samples are often cultured initially in order to obtain quantities of a pure growth of the bacterium responsible for the infection. The characteristics of the colony can then be observed and there is enough bacterial material to carry out any further tests that are necessary. Culture also allows an experienced microbiologist to differentiate important colonies from those of bacteria that are normally present or otherwise insignificant in the infection.

Bacterial cultivation in the laboratory

The cultivation of bacteria in the laboratory requires an appropriate nutrient material or culture medium (see Chapter 17). The culture medium must contain a balanced mixture of the essential growth requirements – carbon, nitrogen and water. Culture can also be used as a method of bacterial identification, as many bacteria have specific individual requirements for optimal growth.

Respiratory requirements

The different oxygen requirements of bacteria, described above, can be used in helping to identify bacterial pathogens, as can the detailed biochemical pathways that they use to provide energy. Bacteria that will grow in the amount of oxygen in the air may be cultured in an incubator. For anaerobes and microaerophiles (including most *Campylobacter* species), Petri dishes containing appropriate culture medium can be placed in an anaerobic jar to minimize atmospheric oxygen and encourage the growth of the bacteria. If the appropriate conditions for a particular organism are not provided, its presence may not be recognized as it will not grow in the laboratory. Respiratory mechanisms of any particular bacterium can be identified by testing for the presence of enzymes that are involved in oxidative processes, such as catalase and cytochrome oxidase.

Diseases caused by bacteria

A variety of bacteria are capable of infecting dogs, cats and exotic pets; in these species some can cause signs of infection. Examples of some important disease-causing bacteria are given in Figures 5.15 and 5.16. Sometimes the same bacterium is responsible for causing disease in a number of species; other infections are more species-specific. Some bacteria are primary pathogens and so can cause disease on their own. Other bacteria are secondary and will usually only cause disease when animals are already debilitated due to other disease.

The clinical signs of infection may be:

- Directly associated with the presence of the bacterium
- Related to damage caused to local tissue by the presence of the infection
- Related to the inflammatory reaction stimulated by the infection
- Due to toxins produced by bacteria.

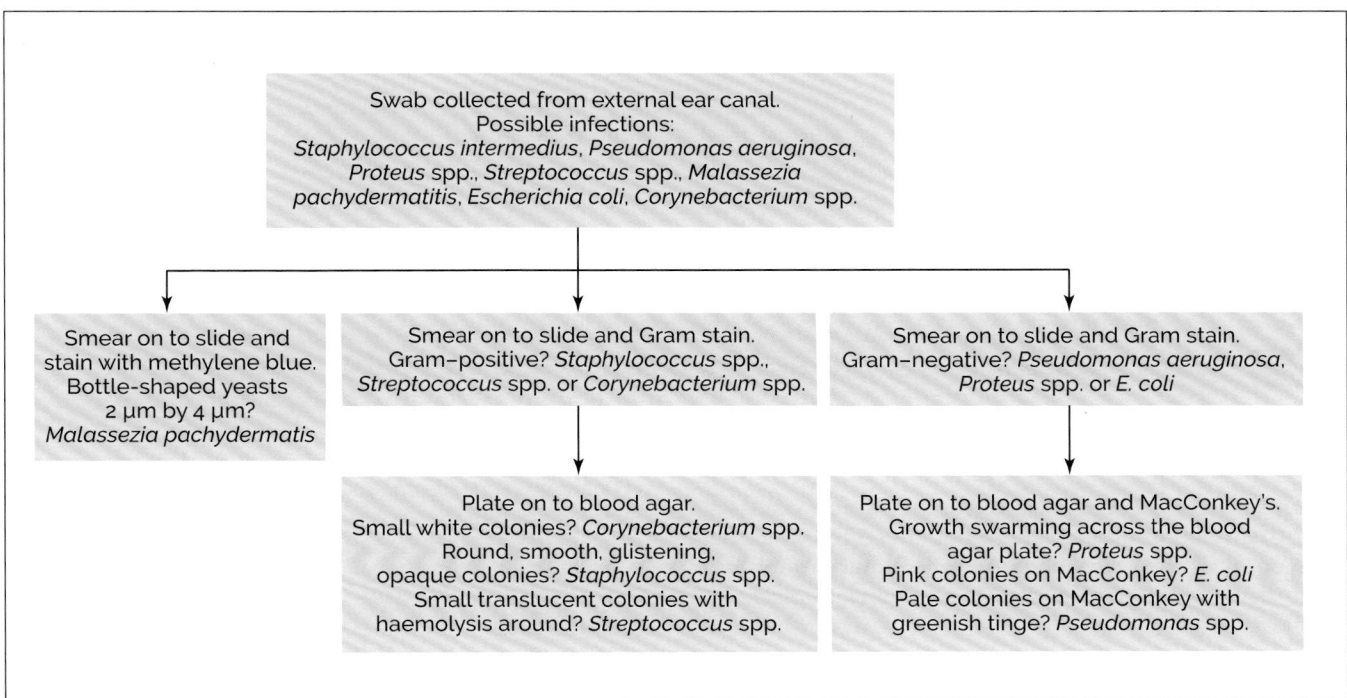

5.14 Flowchart for the identification of bacteria or the fungus *Malassezia pachydermatis* from a dog with chronic otitis externa. Further identification and sensitivity testing should be carried out.

Name of bacterium	Susceptible species	Disease caused	Clinical signs	Shape	Gram staining	Aerobic
Salmonella spp.	Dog	Salmonellosis	Diarrhoea	Rods	Negative	Yes
Campylobacter spp.	Dog	Campylobacteriosis	Diarrhoea	Curved rods (see Figure 5.10b)	Negative	Yes (but prefer less oxygen than in air)
Bordetella bronchiseptica	Dog	Kennel cough	Bouts of severe coughing	Short rods	Negative	Yes
Leptospira spp.	Dog	Leptospirosis	Variable but include fever, sudden death, diarrhoea and vomiting	Helically coiled (spirochaete)	Negative	Yes
Borrelia burgdorferi	Dog	Lyme disease	Variable but include fever and polyarthritis	Helically coiled (spirochaete)	Negative	Yes
Streptococcus spp.	Dog	Streptococcal infection	Infection, particularly in puppies, occasionally otitis externa, metritis	Cocci (arranged in chains) (see Figure 5.10c)	Positive	Yes
Staphylococcus spp.	Dog	Staphylococcal infection	Pyoderma or wound infection	Cocci (arranged as bunches of grapes) (see Figure 5.10d)	Positive	Yes
Clostridium tetani	Dog	Tetanus (rare)	Begins with stiffness close to the site of a wound, becoming more extensive over time	Long rods	Positive	No
Mycoplasma felis	Cat	Mycoplasmal conjunctivitis	Conjunctivitis	Pleomorphic as there is no rigid cell wall	Negative	Yes
Pasteurella spp.	Cat	Cat-bite abscess (other organisms may also be involved)	Typically subcutaneous swelling	Rods or coccobacilli	Negative	Yes

5.15 Some bacterial diseases of dogs and cats.

Name of bacterium	Susceptible species	Disease caused	Clinical signs	Gram staining	Shape
Chlamydia psittaci	Birds, zoonotic	Psittacosis	Signs include: weight loss, anorexia, difficulty breathing, depression and sudden death	Negative (require specialized stains)	Cocci
Mycobacterium avium	Birds	Avian tuberculosis	Signs include weight loss, depression, weakness and reduced egg production.	Positive (but stain very poorly so alternative 'acid-fast' stains used)	Rods
Pasteurella multocida	Rabbits and other species	Pasteurellosis (including respiratory disease)	'snuffles' in rabbits	Negative	Rods or coccobacilli
Salmonella spp.	Range of reptiles, zoonotic	Salmonellosis	Many reptiles asymptomatic but risk of infection to humans	Negative	Rods
Staphylococcus aureus	Ferrets, hamsters, mice, rats	Staphylococcal infection	Pyoderma and ulcerative dermatitis	Positive	Cocci

5.16 Examples of bacterial infections of exotic pets.

Rickettsias and chlamydias

Both rickettsias and chlamydias possess a cell wall like other Gram-negative bacteria but both need to live inside other cells, i.e. they are **obligate intracellular organisms**. These bacteria are responsible for a number of diseases in animals.

Rickettsias

■ These are transmitted by vectors such as ticks, lice, fleas and mites.

■ A particularly pathogenic species is the tick-transmitted infection *Ehrlichia canis*, which is endemic in France and the Mediterranean basin.

■ Rickettsias are often seen on cytological examination of blood smears during clinical pathology examinations.

Chlamydias

■ Various strains of *Chlamydia psittaci* are the cause of psittacosis in psittacine birds (parrots, parakeets and wild birds such as pigeons) and mammals. Psittacosis is a zoonotic infection that humans can acquire by inhaling the organism in the airborne dust or from cage contents of infected birds.

■ Feline pneumonitis is caused by *Chlamydia felis*, which may also cause conjunctivitis in the cat. The bacteria are transmitted by inhalation of infectious dust and droplets and by ingestion. There is also evidence to suggest that vector-borne infection may occur.

Identification

Generally, the identification of rickettsias and chlamydias is more difficult and thus more specialized than that of most bacteria. Diagnosis of infection may be based on demonstration of the organisms themselves or on the demonstration of increased antibody titres in paired serum samples. Rickettsias are smaller than most bacteria and are barely visible using a light microscope. They can only be cultivated in tissue culture or in the yolk sac of embryonated eggs. Typically, they are rod-shaped and measure about 0.8–2.0 µm.

Mycoplasmas

Mycoplasmas are tiny bacteria-like organisms but they do not possess a cell wall. Examples include: *Mycoplasma felis*, a cause of chronic conjunctivitis in cats; *Mycoplasma hyopneumoniae*, the cause of enzootic pneumonia in pigs; and *M. cynos* in dogs. Damage caused by *Mycoplasma* spp. infection of the respiratory tract may predispose the animal to secondary bacterial infection.

Mycoplasmas will grow on agar-based media (Figure 5.17) but, as they are so fragile, isolation and identification are specialized skills.

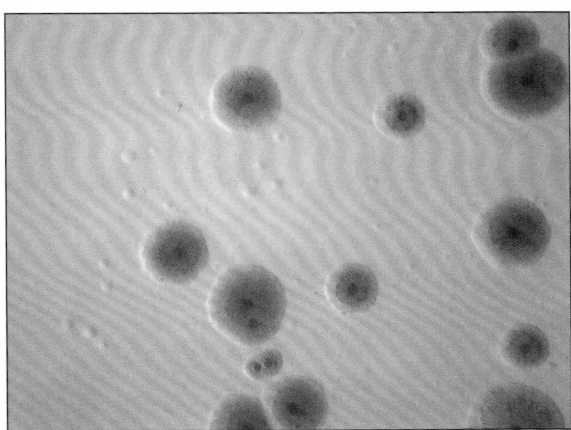

5.17 *Mycoplasma* spp. growing on specialized culture medium. (© Andrew Rycroft)

Toxins

Toxins are poisonous substances that have a damaging effect on the cells of the host. The effects of the toxin are felt not only in the affected cells and tissues but also elsewhere in the body as the toxin is transported through the tissues. Two types of toxin are recognized: exotoxins and endotoxins.

Exotoxins

Exotoxins are proteins produced mainly by Gram-positive bacteria during their metabolism. They are released into the surrounding environment as they are produced. This can be into the circulatory system and tissues of the host (e.g. *Clostridium tetani* introduced into a wound produces tetanus toxin, a neurotoxin) or, as in food poisoning, into food that is then ingested (e.g. botulism is caused by ingestion of a neurotoxin produced by *Clostridium botulinum*). Microbial toxins include many of the most potent poisons known and may prove lethal even in small quantities. The body responds to the presence of exotoxins by producing antibodies called **antitoxins**, which neutralize the toxins, rendering them harmless.

As proteins, exotoxins are destroyed by heat and by some chemicals. Chemicals such as formaldehyde are used to treat toxins so that they lose their toxicity but not their ability to elicit an immune response. These treated toxins are called **toxoids** and will stimulate the production of antitoxins if injected into the body. For example, tetanus toxoid is used widely as the vaccine to induce immunity to tetanus.

Endotoxins

Endotoxins are a part of the cell envelope of Gram-negative bacteria (lipopolysaccharide) and are released mainly when cells die and disintegrate. Compared with exotoxins, they are less toxic, cannot be used to form toxoids and are able to withstand heat. Blood-borne endotoxins are responsible for a range of non-specific reactions in the body, such as fever, loss of appetite and apathy. A bacterial infection such as mastitis or pneumonia may be present. At higher levels they can sometimes result in a serious drop in blood pressure (a condition commonly called **endotoxic shock**).

Aflatoxin

Toxins are not made exclusively by bacteria. The saprophytic fungus *Aspergillus flavus* produces a toxin called aflatoxin. The fungus grows in warm, humid conditions and contaminates a variety of agricultural products such as peanuts, cereals, rice and beans. Aflatoxin has been implicated in the deaths of many farm animals that have been fed on mouldy hay, corn or on peanut meal.

Effects of toxins

The effects of toxins are usually very specific. For example, when spores of the anaerobic tetanus bacillus *Clostridium tetani* get into a wound that provides favourable conditions, they may germinate and grow in the tissues. The bacteria do not spread through the tissues but secrete an exotoxin that travels along peripheral nerves to the central nervous system, where it interferes with the regulation of neurotransmitters that control the relaxation of muscle. This leads to uncontrollable muscle spasms and paralysis. Tetanus toxin is called a neurotoxin because of its activity in the nervous system.

Unlike tetanus, which is caused by exotoxins produced while the organism is growing within the host, botulism, caused by the saprophytic bacterium *Clostridium botulinum*, is the result of ingestion of food containing the toxins. In botulism, the exotoxin affects the nervous system, leading to paralysis; it too is therefore a neurotoxin.

Other exotoxins formed outside the body include those produced by *Staphylococcus aureus*, the bacterium that causes staphylococcal food poisoning. This is an **enterotoxin** because it functions in the gastrointestinal tract, causing vomiting and diarrhoea.

Commensal bacteria carried by cats and dogs

There are a number of bacteria (known as commensals) that are normally carried by cats and dogs without causing any clinical signs. However, in certain circumstances, disease can result from infection. Both of these examples are potential zoonoses:

- *Bartonella henselae* is a small Gram-negative bacterium present in a proportion of the cat population and is not normally pathogenic to cats. It may be transmitted to a human in the course of a cat scratch and may result in a local or more general infection in the person, so-called cat-scratch disease
- Some *Staphylococcus aureus* strains developed resistance to the antibacterial meticillin (meticillin-resistant *Staphylococcus aureus*, or MRSA) in the 1960s. Since then some strains have developed resistance to many antibacterials. These resistant bacteria can live on the skin or in the nasal passages of dogs, cats or humans without clinical signs. However, if infection establishes in a wound or other organ, severe damage can be caused. As the organism is resistant not only to meticillin but also to other antibacterials, the infection can be very difficult to treat. The presence of infection in a veterinary hospital ward may necessitate the closure of the ward and thorough cleaning until the infection is eliminated (see Chapter 7).

Treatment of bacterial infections

Bacterial infections can occur in many different locations within an animal and so the treatment will depend on the location and the type of bacteria present (see Chapter 7).

Bacterial sensitivity testing

It is important to identify the antibacterials to which the bacteria causing an infection will respond in order that the infection may be cured efficiently with the least amount of antibacterial possible. A bacterial sensitivity test can be conducted where, for example, the bacteria are spread on an agar plate and discs containing different antibacterials are placed on top. After incubation, the patterns of growth around the discs are examined:

- If the growth occurs right up to a disc, that antibacterial will not be effective
- If there is a wide zone of inhibition of bacterial growth around a disc, the antibacterial contained in that disc is likely to be effective (see Chapter 17).

Fungi

There are many different fungi but only a few are able to infect animals. Fungi grow aerobically (using oxygen) and gain their energy from the organic substances on which they grow. They can be divided into two categories and the fungal pathogens seen in small animal veterinary practice include both types.

- Moulds (Figure 5.18) are multicellular (examples include the 'ringworm' dermatophytes)
- Yeasts (Figure 5.18) are unicellular (examples include *Malassezia pachydermatis* and *Candida albicans*).

Choice of treatment

- With increasing antimicrobial resistance, there is a drive to use antibacterials judiciously. Some antibacterials, for example colistin, may be withdrawn from animal use in an effort to preserve them for human disease (Rhoume *et al.*, 2016; Al-Tawfiq *et al.*, 2017)
- Bacterial infections should be treated locally wherever possible for example: a surface infection or a cat-bite abscess might be treated with local cleaning with an antibacterial wash (e.g. chlorhexidine)
- Systemic antibacterials should be used only where indicated and specific antibacterials classified as critically important antibiotics should not be used empirically in veterinary medicine so may be used where indicated by sensitivity results
- Where possible narrow range antibacterials, effective against a narrow range of organisms, should be selected; therefore, it is necessary to have an idea of the infectious organism present, and preferably the organisms sensitivity in order to choose an appropriate antibacterial agent (see 'Bacterial sensitivity testing', above)
- Where systemic antibacterial treatment is indicated, treatment may be administered by mouth or by injection. Some antibacterials can be administered intravenously when speed of activity is essential
- Antibacterials effective against a range of Gram-positive and Gram-negative organisms are termed broad-spectrum: these should be used only where indicated by the infection present
- Choice of an antibacterial also requires an understanding of where the drug will reach in the body. For example, if treatment of bacterial cystitis is required, an antibacterial that is not broken down before it reaches the urinary tract should be selected
- Some antibacterials can destroy the microflora necessary for normal functioning. This is a particularly important consideration when choosing a treatment for small mammals such as rabbits, gerbils and hamsters
- Some infections, particularly in reptiles, are secondary to poor husbandry conditions or management and so conditions should be improved, and such improvements may be adequate to avoid the necessity for treatment
- Numerous organizations, including the Food and Agriculture Organization (FAO, 2016), have produced guidance on the use of antimicrobials. Best practice is summarized in the British Veterinary Association poster *Responsible use of antimicrobials in veterinary practice. The 7-point plan* (BVA, 2017)

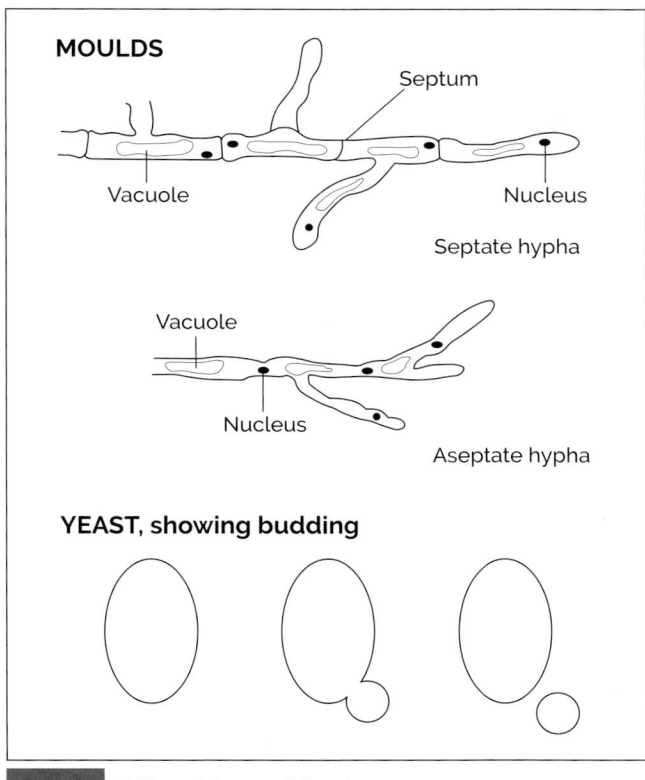

5.18 Different forms of fungi.

Dermatophytes

Fungal infections of keratin (the horny tissue that forms nail, hair and skin) can affect cats, dogs, rabbits and guinea pigs. The condition broadly known as ringworm is caused by dermatophytes such as the species *Trichophyton mentagrophytes* (in the dog, cat, rabbit and guinea pig) and *Microsporum canis* (in the dog and cat) amongst others.

In its most obvious form, ringworm appears as circular areas of hair loss with active fungal infection around the edge of the lesion (Figure 5.19). The lesions may be small and discrete or large and coalescing, with an irregular outline. Some are not very inflamed and cause little irritation, whilst others may show severe inflammation. A more marked reaction is common in dogs.

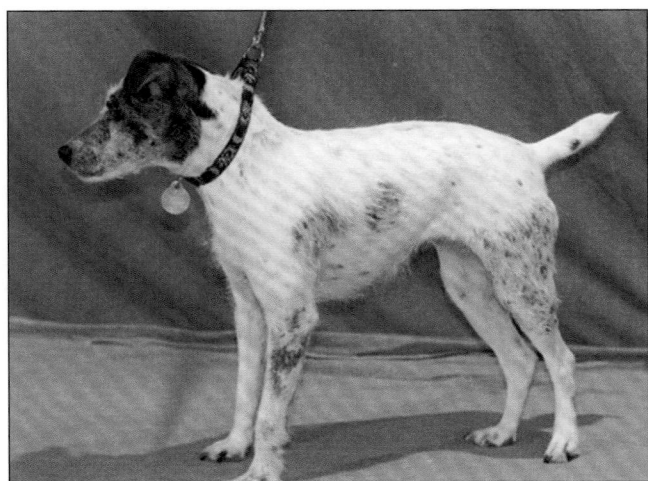

5.19 Ringworm lesions on a Jack Russell Terrier. (Courtesy of David Duclos)

Transmission may be directly from affected animal to animal, or to humans (many dermatophytes are zoonotic). Long-haired cats, in particular, may appear normal but may be carriers of infection. There may also be indirect transmission via bedding, cages, rugs, grooming tools, etc. Ringworm spores can remain viable in the environment for prolonged periods.

Diagnosis

This can be performed by staining hair pluck or skin scrape samples, by examining for fluorescence with a Wood's lamp (for species that fluoresce) and/or by culture on specialist media (see Chapter 17).

Treatment

Topical

Treatments include a fungicidal wash (such as enilconazole). Topical treatment is usually repeated after an interval to effect a full cure. It may be possible to treat the area of a discrete lesion only, or it may be necessary to wash the whole animal. In severe or non-responsive cases (e.g. some long-haired cats), it will be necessary to clip the affected part or even the entire animal to facilitate treatment.

Systemic

Itraconazole can be administered orally for the treatment of dermatophytes.

Candida albicans

The yeast *Candida albicans* is often present in the intestinal tract of animals without causing disease but it can become pathogenic in certain circumstances. *Candida* infections are usually opportunistic, i.e. they take advantage of a young, debilitated or immunocompromised animal and cause disease. Infection may also be seen after prolonged antibacterial treatment or following skin damage such as that incurred in a burn. The infection is known as 'thrush' and is commonly seen on mucous membranes (e.g. in the mouths of puppies or kittens). Rarely, it can occur at mucocutaneous junctions or systemically. Humans can acquire the infection but transfer of infection would be highly unlikely unless the person were immunocompromised in some way (e.g. a person with HIV).

- Infection of the skin of a dog may appear as an ulcer that does not respond to antibacterial therapy.
- Infection of the mouth may appear as a white growth and ulceration of the affected area in a puppy or kitten and may be associated with unwillingness to suck.
- In birds, *C. albicans* can infect the crop, particularly after prolonged antibacterial treatment.

Treatments for candidiasis include clotrimazole or miconazole (topically), or fluconazole (systemically).

Malassezia pachydermatis

Malassezia pachydermatis is a yeast that may be found on normal skin. In some situations, particularly seborrhoeic conditions, overgrowth may cause pruritic dermatitis (localized or generalized) or otitis externa, usually in dogs, but cats are sometimes infected. Infection occurs most commonly in warm summer months. Lesions may appear greasy and may have a distinct odour.

Suspected lesions can be sampled by pressing adhesive tape to the area (see Chapter 17). The strip is stained with methylene blue, attached to a microscope slide and examined microscopically. *Malassezia* appear as small, blue, bottle-shaped yeasts (see Chapter 17). As they are present on normal skin in low numbers, significant infection is indicated by an increase in numbers, perhaps when multiple organisms are seen in each high-power field of view under the microscope. Infection can be treated with a shampoo containing chlorhexidine and miconazole.

Other fungal infections

Occasionally, dogs, cats and other companion animals develop internal fungal infections. A number of different fungi can be responsible. For example, *Aspergillus fumigatus* can infect the nasal passages of the dog and the respiratory system of birds. Fungi such as *Saprolegnia* spp. can infect fish and may cause severe disease and death.

Zoonoses

A number of viral and bacterial infections are potentially zoonotic. Zoonotic viruses include tick-borne encephalitis (which is transmitted by tick bites) and rabies (transmitted by saliva). Zoonotic bacteria include *Salmonella* spp. from animal-derived food products and *Borrelia burgdorferi*, the cause of Lyme disease (which is tick transmitted) and *Bartonella henselae*, the cause of cat scratch disease. Vector-borne infections are receiving increasing attention, accompanied by concerns of their spread particularly with pet travel and climate change (Vayssier-Taussat *et al.*, 2015; Dantes-Torres and Otranto, 2016). A One Health Concept has been introduced to better understand the links between, for example, disease in humans and animals and impacts on the environment (Sikkema and Koopmans, 2016).

Acknowledgement

Andrew Rycroft is acknowledged and thanked for his constructive comments on this chapter.

References and further reading

Al-Tawfiq JA, Laxminarayan R and Mendelson M (2017) How should we respond to the emergence of plasmid-mediated colistin resistance in humans and animals? *International Journal of Infectious Diseases* **54**, 77–84

BVA (2017) *Responsible use of antimicrobials in veterinary practice: The 7-point plan*. Available at: www.bva.co.uk

Dantes-Torres F and Otranto D (2016) Best practices for preventing vector-borne diseases in dogs and humans. *Trends in Parasitology* **32**, 43–55

FAO (2016) *The FAO action plan on antimicrobial resistance 2016 – 2020*. Available at: www.fao.org

Gillespie S and Bamford K (2012) *Medical Microbiology and Infection at a Glance*. Wiley-Blackwell, Chichester

Heritage J, Evans EGV and Killington RA (2008) *Introductory Microbiology*. Cambridge University Press, Cambridge

Meredith A and Johnson-Delaney C (2010) *BSAVA Manual of Exotic Pets, 5th edn*. BSAVA Publications, Gloucester

Meredith A and Lord B (2014) *BSAVA Manual of Rabbit Medicine*. BSAVA Publications, Gloucester

Paterson S (2006) *Skin diseases of Exotic Pets*. Blackwell Publishing, Oxford

Quinn PJ, Markey BK, Leonard FC *et al.* (2011) *Veterinary Microbiology and Microbial Disease*. Wiley-Blackwell, Chichester

Reperant LA, Brown IH, Haenen OL *et al.* (2016) Companion animals as a source of viruses for human beings and food production animals. *Journal of Comparative Pathology* **155**, S41–S53

Rhoume M, Beaudry F, Thériault W and Letellier A (2016) Colistin in pig production: chemistry, mechanism of antibacterial action, microbial resistance emergence, and One Health perspectives. *Frontiers in Microbiology* **7**, 1789

Sikkema R and Koopmans M (2016) One Health training and research activities in Western Europe. *Infection Ecology and Epidemiology* **6**, DOI: 10.3402/iee.v6.33703

Vayssier-Taussat M, Kazimirova M, Hubalek Z *et al.* (2015) Emerging horizons for tick-borne pathogens: from the one-pathogen – one disease vision to the pathobiome paradigm. *Future Microbiology* **10**, 2033–2043

Self-assessment questions

1. Define the terms 'parasitic', 'commensal' and 'symbiotic'.
2. What distinguishes a virus from other organisms?
3. Give ten examples of viral infections in dogs, cats and exotic pets.
4. Describe the structure of a bacterial cell.
5. How do bacteria replicate?
6. Give ten examples of bacterial infections in dogs, cats and exotic pets.
7. What does MRSA stand for and why is it an important infection?
8. What are the considerations in choosing a suitable antimicrobial drug?
9. What are bacterial toxins?
10. How can ringworm be identified?

Chapter 6

Principles of parasitology

Maggie Fisher and John McGarry

Learning objectives

After studying this chapter, readers will have the knowledge to:

- **Describe the biology and life cycles of internal and external parasites of dogs, cats and common exotic pets**
- **Identify common parasites on the basis of their morphology and location on or in the host**
- **Explain how these parasites affect their animal host, and identify those which can also infect people**
- **Describe the routes of transmission for parasites**
- **Identify when prevention of infection (prophylaxis) is necessary and situations for optional control**
- **Advise clients on programmes of preventative treatment appropriate to species**

Glossary

- **Parasite:** A eukaryotic organism advantageously living off its host
- **Ectoparasites:** Parasites which usually live on or burrow into the surface of the host's epidermis
- **Endoparasites:** Parasites that live in the internal organs of the host
- **Eukaryote:** Organism in which the chromosomes are enclosed in a nucleus (this includes animals, plants and fungi)
- **Direct life cycle:** Transmission of infective stages occurs from one animal host to the next without the need for an intermediate host
- **Indirect life cycle:** The parasite requires one or more intermediate hosts to complete its life cycle
- **Definitive host:** The primary host in which the parasite develops to the adult stages
- **Intermediate host:** A host in which the parasite can undergo some stage(s) of its development, but without sexual reproduction
- **Paratenic host:** An organism that the parasite can use during part of its life cycle, but which is not essential for completion of the life cycle
- **Vector:** An organism such as a tick or blood-feeding fly that transmits a parasite
- **Sporulation:** The process by which immature (non-infective) coccidian oocysts develop into the mature, infective form
- **Sporozoite:** A motile spore-like stage in the life cycle of some parasitic sporozoans, that is typically the infective agent introduced into a host

Ectoparasites

Ectoparasites belong to the Phylum Arthropoda in the animal kingdom. They have a chitinous outer shell or exoskeleton, a segmented body and paired jointed limbs. They include:

- Insects, where the adult has three pairs of legs and the body is divided into three parts: head, thorax and abdomen (e.g. lice, fleas)
- Arachnids, where the adult has four pairs of legs and the body is divided into two parts only: cephalothorax (a fused head and thorax) and the abdomen (e.g. mites, ticks).

Ectoparasite morphology is illustrated for specific ectoparasites in the following sections.

Insects

The identification, diagnosis of infestation and control of insect ectoparasites are described in Figure 6.1. Further information on medical treatments is given in Chapter 8.

Parasite	Diagnosis	Control
Lice	Demonstration of the eggs attached to hairs. Visualization of the adult louse. The adult lice may be seen with the naked eye on close examination of an animal's haircoat or may be seen in a skin scrape/brush	Thorough cleaning of environment, bedding and grooming equipment, etc. Topical treatment of all pets in the household with a product licensed for louse treatment containing, e.g. imidacloprid, fipronil or selamectin. Formulations include sprays and spot-ons
Fleas	Demonstration of an adult flea or their faeces in the coat of a dog or cat by combing the coat thoroughly, preferably with a very fine-toothed comb (e.g. a human louse comb). The animal may be brushed over a sheet of damp white paper. Flea faeces will be seen on the paper as small black dots. Since they contain a large amount of undigested blood, a ring of red is seen around the black spot when moistened. There is also a skin test for allergy to fleas	Control of the environmental stages: ■ Daily vacuuming, particularly around where the pet sleeps ■ Applying an environmental insecticide and/or an insect growth regulator such as methoprene or pyriproxyfen, for example, to kill the immature stages. Depending on the formulation, these products may be applied to the animal or directly to the environment. the chitin synthesis inhibitor (lufenuron) is given orally to the dog or cat or by injection to the cat. It prevents eggs hatching and/or larval development
		Control of adult fleas on the animal: ■ Thorough grooming, e.g. using a human louse comb ■ Applying an insecticide in the form of, for example, a spray, impregnated collar, powder, shampoo or spot-on. Several new compounds have been recently introduced to the range of insecticides used as flea adulticides, including spinosad, oxadiazines (indoxcarb) and isoxazolines (afoxalaner, furalaner and sarolaner). These add to the existing range that includes chemicals in the class phenylpyrazole (fipronil), neonicotinoids (such as nitenpyram and imidacloprid), avermectins (selamectin) and the synthetic pyrethroids which include permethrin
Fly larvae	An affected animal will often stop eating and appear restless and later depressed. The animal should be thoroughly examined to find the larvae and thus diagnose the problem	In order to treat the infestation, the first step is to remove the larvae: ■ Wash the affected area with a mild antiseptic solution, ensuring that the larvae are removed in the process ■ Lightly towel-dry the area. Apply antiseptic ointment Any underlying problem (e.g. diarrhoea) that may have predisposed the animal to becoming 'fly-blown' should be investigated and treated, and an antiparasitic agent such as cyromazine applied

6.1 Diagnosis and control of insect ectoparasites.

Lice

Heavy infestations of lice cause a disease known as pediculosis, which may affect a range of animals including dogs, cats, rabbits, rodents and birds. Lice are subdivided into chewing (biting) lice (Figures 6.2 and 6.3) and blood-sucking lice (Figure 6.4), reflecting their manner of feeding. Chewing lice infest both mammals and birds, whereas sucking lice infest only mammals. Chewing lice feed off surface debris and tissue fluid, whilst sucking lice have modified mouthparts to permit them to pierce through the skin into blood vessels to suck blood.

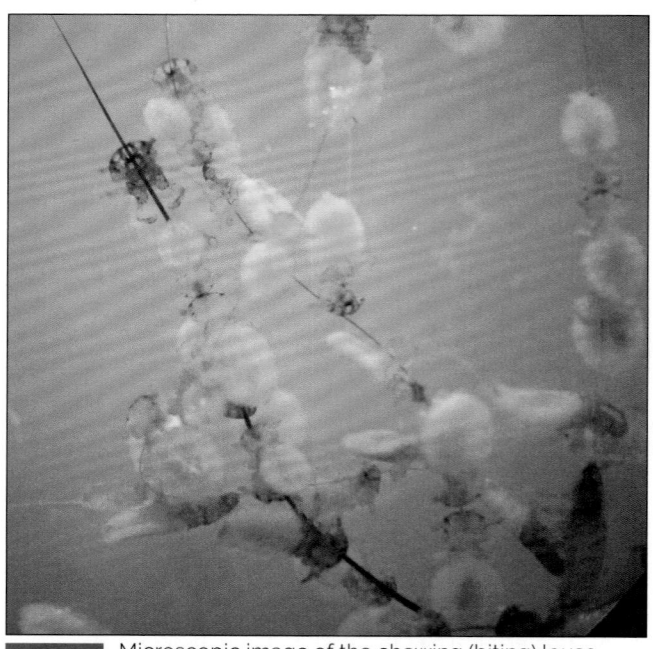

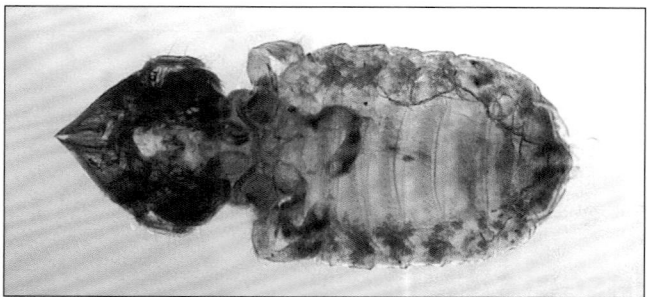

6.2 Microscopic image (dorsal view) of the chewing (biting) louse *Felicola subrostratus*. Found on cats, it is approximately 2 mm long. If viewed from the side, the louse would appear dorsoventrally flattened.

6.3 Microscopic image of the chewing (biting) louse *Trichodectes canis*. Found on dogs, it is a small louse approximately 2 mm in length. Chewing lice tend to have shorter, broader heads than sucking lice. (© J McGarry)

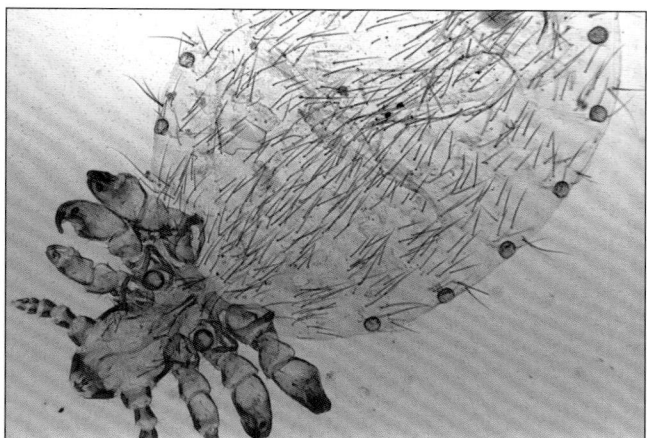

6.4 Microscopic image (ventral view) of the sucking louse *Linognathus setosus*. Found on dogs, it is approximately 2 mm long. Sucking lice tend to have elongated, narrow heads.

Lice are transmitted by close contact, as the louse spends its entire life cycle on the host, but fomites (e.g. grooming equipment) may carry louse eggs or lice themselves on hair removed from an infested individual. Lice, however, do not survive for long periods off their host. Individual louse species are highly host-specific, thus dog lice do not affect cats, and people do not acquire lice from their pets.

Large numbers of lice cause intense irritation and concomitant self-inflicted injury. In addition, sucking lice may cause anaemia if they are present in large enough numbers. Young or debilitated animals are often the worst affected. The chewing louse is also the intermediate host for the tapeworm *Dipylidium caninum* (see below), and dogs and cats become infected when they swallow tapeworm-infected lice during grooming.

Life cycle

Adult female lice lay their eggs individually and cement them to hairs. The eggs ('nits') are just visible to the naked eye, being about 1 mm in size (Figure 6.5). When these hatch, immature lice that are identical in appearance to the adult emerge and, after several moults, become adults. The whole life cycle takes about 2–3 weeks.

Fleas

Adult fleas bite their host in order to take a blood meal. The areas that have been bitten often show an inflammatory reaction and can cause intense irritation. Like chewing lice, fleas can transmit *Dipylidium caninum* (a tapeworm; see below) and may also transmit the infectious agents that cause feline leukaemia (FeLV) and feline infectious anaemia. Fleas are also involved in the spread from cat to cat of *Bartonella henselae*, the bacterium responsible for cat scratch disease in humans (see Chapter 5). It is believed that the cat's claws may be contaminated with the bacteria, probably derived from the cat grooming infected flea faeces out of its coat.

Some animals become sensitized to flea allergens; reacting to salivary proteins that induce harmful and exaggerated immunological reactions in susceptible cats and dogs due to repeat flea bites. Severe dermatitis can develop after just a few bites, causing a condition known as flea allergic dermatitis (FAD).

Most fleas on cats and dogs are the 'cat flea' *Ctenocephalides felis* (Figure 6.6), but dogs in permanent kennels (e.g. Greyhound kennels) may be infected with the 'dog flea' *Ctenocephalides canis*. Infrequently, other flea species, e.g. hedgehog fleas (*Archaeopsylla erinacei*), are found on cats or dogs.

Rabbits can be infested with *C. felis*, particularly if they are living in a household with dogs or cats. Wild rabbits, however, are often infested with *Spillopsyllus cuniculi*, a species of flea that tends to stay attached in one place (often the face). Rats, mice and ferrets can also be infested with fleas. Birds have their own species of flea, the immature stages of which live in the birds' nests.

The species of flea present may be identified by the appearance of its head (see Figure 6.6), in particular the presence or absence of spines in the form of a comb on the cheek (genal comb) or collar (pronotal comb) and the number and shape of spines in each comb.

Life cycle of the cat flea

The life cycle of the cat flea (*C. felis*) is shown in Figure 6.7. The adult is laterally compressed, which allows it to move readily between the host's hairs. The female flea feeds on blood, then mates on the host and lays eggs. These are smooth, pearly white and fall off into the environment, particularly in the area around where the animal usually lies. Depending on the environmental temperature, after 2–14 days the eggs hatch out into larvae that look like small maggots. These larvae feed on skin debris, the faeces of

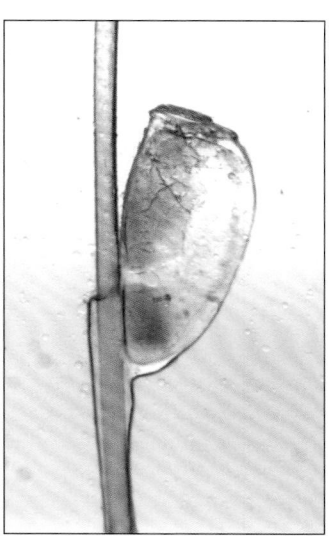

6.5 Microscopic image of a louse egg ('nit') attached with 'cement' to the shaft of hair.

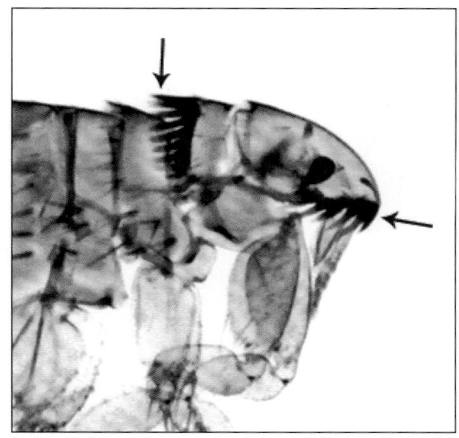

6.6 Microscopic image (lateral view) of the head of the cat flea, *Ctenocephalides felis*, showing the characteristic combs (arrowed). (© J McGarry)

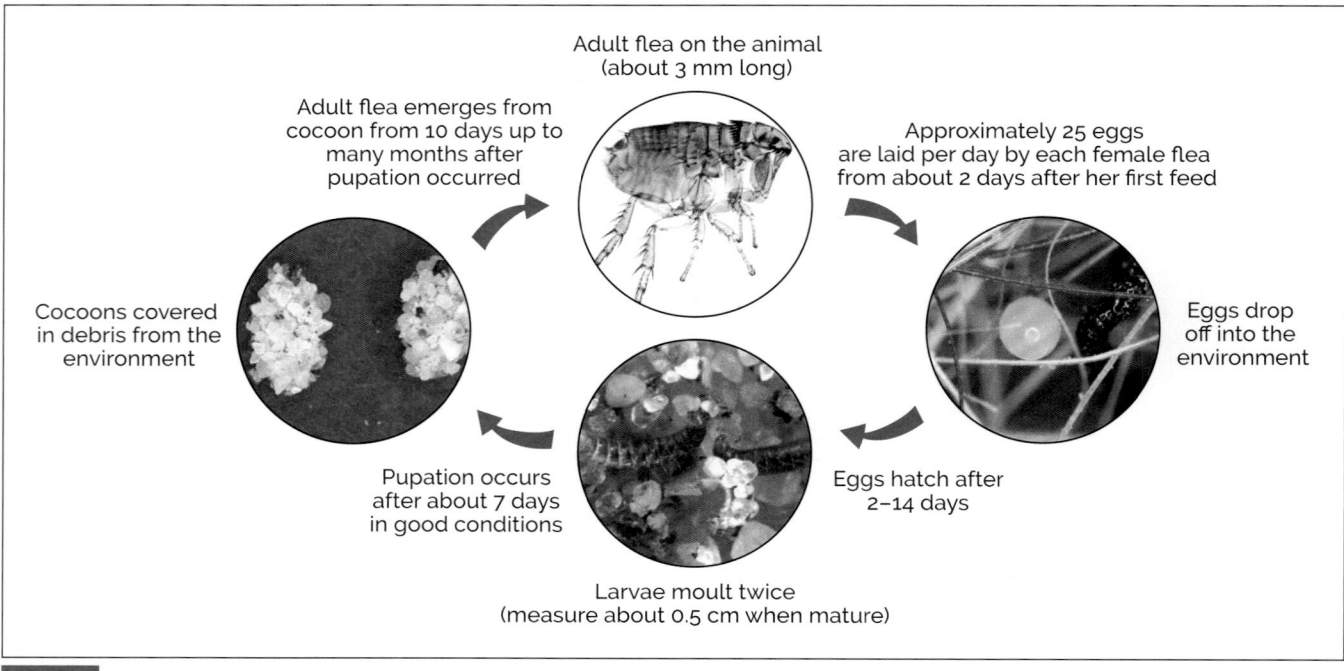

6.7   Life cycle of the cat flea. (Photographs © J McGarry)

adult fleas and other organic matter in the environment. After about a week, each mature larva spins a cocoon and pupates. The outside of the cocoon is sticky and so bits of debris from the environment adhere to it, affording protection. After a further 10 days (although this can be considerably longer in cold or dry conditions), the adult flea is fully developed inside the pupa. Before it emerges, it waits for signs of a host being available, e.g. pressure on carpets, noise and other vibrations (this is one explanation for the experiences of new occupants going into an empty house and being bitten by fleas within hours). Once emerged from the pupal case, the flea will locate a host and jump on to it. Treatment of fleas should ideally be aimed at all stages of the life cycle (i.e. adult fleas on the pet and stages in the environment; see Figure 6.1). However, it should be borne in mind that the pupal stage can be difficult to treat because of the location of the cocoon within bedding, carpets, etc., and the fact that the pupa is enclosed and thus protected from chemical treatments. Hoovering the animal's bedding/carpets and washing at high temperatures is an effective mechanical approach to eradication in conjunction with chemical methods.

Myiasis flies

Myiasis ('fly strike') is the invasion of living tissue by the larvae of dipteran flies (blowflies), usually green bottles (genus *Lucilia*), in late spring or summer. In severe cases, blue bottles (*Calliphora* spp.) may be involved as secondary myiasis species, attracted to the smelly skin caused by *Lucilia*. The life cycle is shown in Figure 6.8. In cases of skin myiasis, flies are attracted to hosts in order to lay their eggs, mainly on a rear end contaminated with faeces (i.e. around the perineal

6.8   Life cycle of the blowfly.

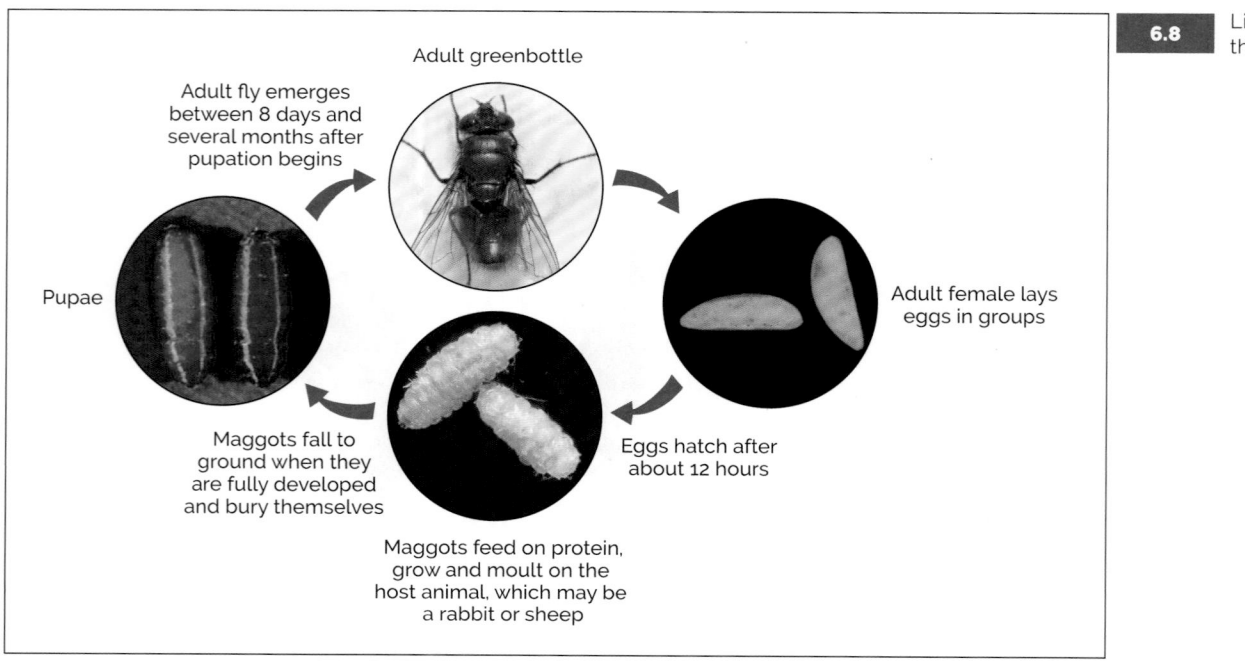

area of a rabbit), but in fact any skin in poor condition is attractive to flies. Flies are particularly attracted to a smelly animal, e.g. one soiled by diarrhoea, and 'strike', the colloquial name for this type of myiasis, can be minimized by ensuring that animals are kept clean and healthy. The larvae (maggots) hatch from deposited eggs after as little as 12 hours and begin to traumatize the skin surface and feed off the damaged tissue. After two moults, the mature larvae drop to the ground. Adult fly emergence is temperature-dependent and several waves of blowflies may occur during the summer. The larvae and pupae can survive over winter in the environment, and it is important to note that these flies can develop in carrion (decaying flesh of dead animals) as well as in living tissue. Any animal in poor condition, including neglected cats and dogs, can be affected by these flies. Larval development can be prevented by treating the animal with a larval growth inhibitor such as cyromazine.

Biting and nuisance flies

Flies may act as vectors in the transmission of infections (see Chapter 7). For example, sandflies can transmit the protozoal parasite responsible for the disease leishmaniosis (leishmaniasis) in southern Europe, and certain mosquitoes may carry the heartworm *Dirofilaria immitis* and the cutaneous worm *Dirofilaria repens*, which, although not presently endemic in the UK, are an important consideration when pets travel to and from warmer countries, such as southern France, Italy and Spain; there is the real chance that these diseases may become established in the future in the UK. Sandflies and mosquitoes suck blood. Animals may also be affected by nuisance flies that seek secretions, and of note is a particular type of fruit fly (*Phortica*) that can transmit an eye worm (*Thelazia*); cases in the UK so far have involved dogs imported from Europe.

Ticks and mites

Ticks and mites are arachnids; they are morphologically distinct from insects. Ticks are of huge veterinary importance. The larvae that emerge from the eggs of these ectoparasites look like smaller versions of the adult, except that they have only three pairs of legs; the nymph and adult stages each have four pairs of legs.

Mites

Mites cause a range of skin problems, and severe dermatitis is known as 'mange'. Most parasitic mites are permanent ectoparasites (i.e. they spend their entire life cycle on the host); the main exceptions are *Dermanyssus gallinae* (the red mite of poultry that lives in bird accommodation), which takes several blood meals, and *Trombicula autumnalis* (the 'harvest mite'), with only the larval stage being parasitic during the autumn.

Mites may be subdivided into skin burrowing mites and surface-feeding mites. The dermatitis caused by both these groups of mites often causes pruritus (itchiness). Diagnosis is usually by inspection of coat brushings under a low power stereomicroscope or by examination (at higher power) of skin scrapes or hair plucks (see also Chapter 17). Specific guidance on the diagnosis and treatment of each mite is given in Figure 6.9; further information can also be found in Chapters 8 and 17.

Burrowing mites

Burrowing mites create small tunnels within the surface layers of the skin, laying their eggs within small 'pockets'. There are four main species of burrowing mites seen in domestic pets: *Sarcoptes scabiei* var. *canis* (mainly dogs); *Notoedres* (cats, rodents, hedgehogs); *Cnemidocoptes* spp. (cage birds); and *Trixacarus caviae* (guinea pigs). *Demodex* (dogs and hamsters) is also classed as a burrowing mite; it lives in hair follicles and sebaceous glands, and is usually quite harmless.

Sarcoptes scabiei var. *canis*

This round mite, bearing scales and projections on the dorsal surface (Figure 6.10) affects dogs (foxes and other canids) and, very rarely, cats. The disease this mite causes is known as sarcoptic mange or scabies. Other host-adapted strains of this ectoparasite cause mange in rodents, and a form of scabies exists in humans (although this is clinically very different to animal scabies, which may also affect people). Animals become infected by close contact with infected animals, or by acquiring mites or eggs that are present in bedding or the environment (Figure 6.11). *S. scabiei* is a permanent ectoparasite; however, mites may be shed by heavily infected individuals and in optimal conditions can survive in the environment for several days. Often the tips of the ears (Figure 6.12a), elbows and hocks (Figure 6.12b) and then the face (Figure 6.12c) are the first areas affected, but large areas of the body (Figure 6.12d) may be infected in severe cases. Affected areas become hairless, thickened and inflamed. This is partly due to the effect of the mites themselves and partly due to the trauma that the animal causes by rubbing and scratching the affected area – the condition is very pruritic. The disease in foxes can be extensive and debilitating. Sarcoptic mites from dogs will irritate human skin, but normally the lesions are small and self-limiting (this feature helps distinguishes the zoonotic condition from the human form mentioned above, which is known as Norwegian scabies).

Parasitic	Diagnostic samples	Treatment
Sarcoptes scabiei	Skin scrapes or blood test	Mite infections may be treated with a suitable acaricide such as amitraz, selamectin, sarolaner or moxidectin. Where no authorized product is available, treat with e.g. fipronil consistent with the Cascade and published recommendations. Also treat the environment in *Cheyletiella* spp. infection
Notoedres spp.	Skin scrapes	
Cnemidocoptes spp.	Skin scrapes	
Demodex spp.	Skin scrapes or hair plucks	
Cheyletiella spp.	Coat brushings or sellotape strips (adult mite and/or eggs)	
Otodectes cynotis	Ear wax	Clean the ear canal; instil ointment containing suitable acaricide, often in combination with antibiotic. Also treat in-contact animals to clear potential reservoirs of infection. Alternatively, selamectin or moxidectin spot-on may be used: these are typically applied to the back of the neck or behind the shoulder blades

6.9 Diagnosis and treatment of mites.

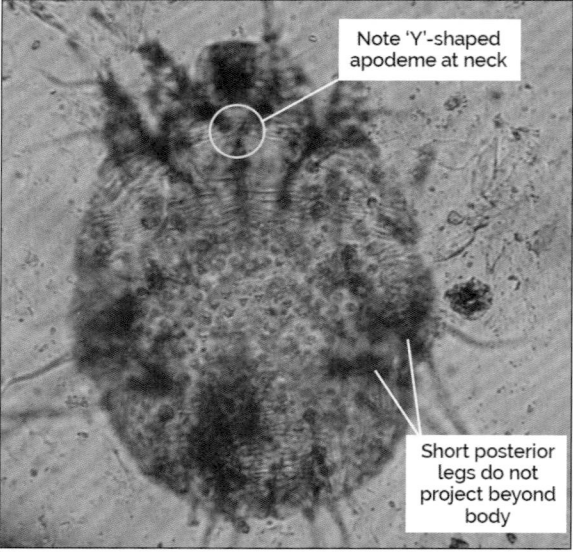

Note 'Y'-shaped apodeme at neck

Short posterior legs do not project beyond body

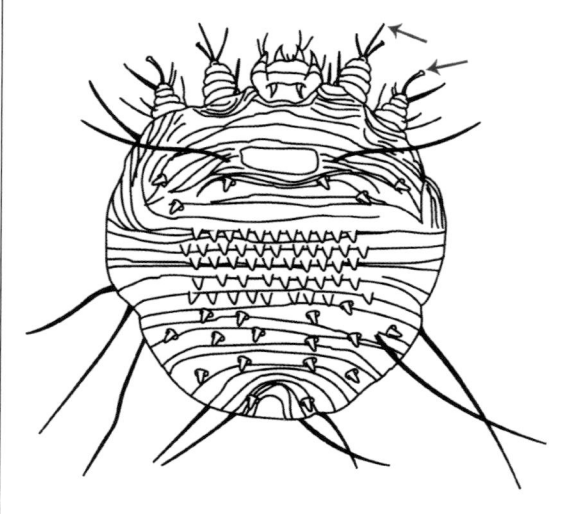

6.10 Microscopic image (dorsal view) of an adult *Sarcoptes* mite (0.4 mm long). The illustration shows the short, stubby legs that barely project beyond the body, spines and pegs, terminal anus, and pedicles with suckers (arrowed) at the ends of the legs. (Photograph © J McGarry)

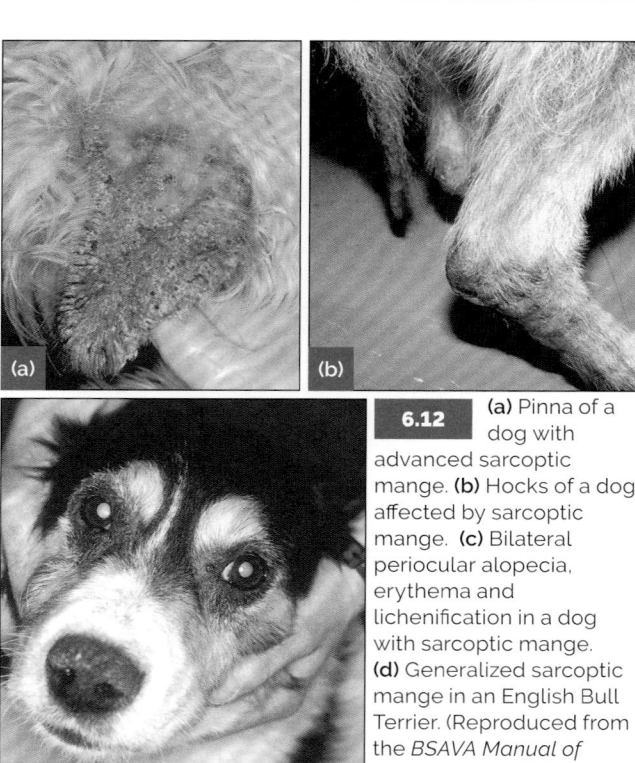

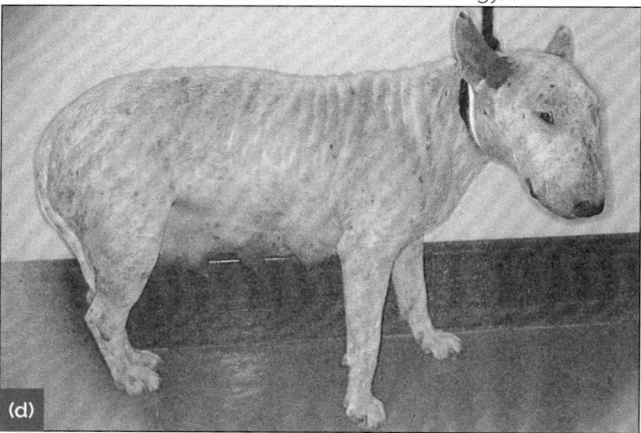

6.12 (a) Pinna of a dog with advanced sarcoptic mange. (b) Hocks of a dog affected by sarcoptic mange. (c) Bilateral periocular alopecia, erythema and lichenification in a dog with sarcoptic mange. (d) Generalized sarcoptic mange in an English Bull Terrier. (Reproduced from the *BSAVA Manual of Canine and Feline Dermatology, 3rd edn*)

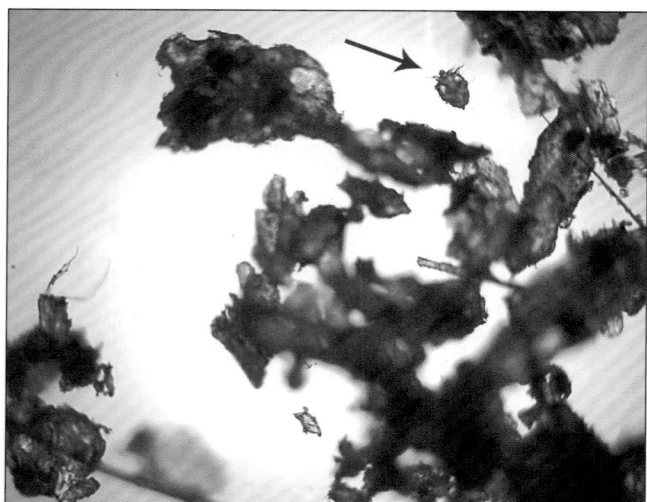

6.11 Microscopic image of a *Sarcoptes* mite (arrowed) in sweepings taken from a pen that housed an infected fox. (Courtesy of E Mullineaux)

Notoedres spp.

The burrowing mite of the cat (Figure 6.13) is very rarely seen in the UK but it causes similar signs to *Sarcoptes scabiei* in the dog. *Notoedres* infestation also occurs in rats.

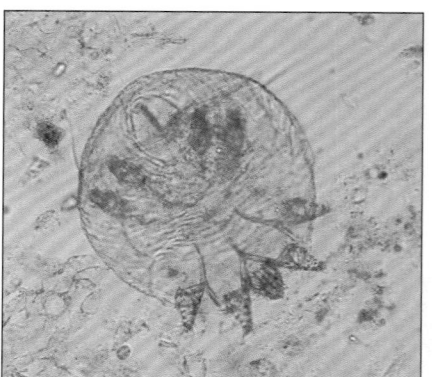

6.13 Microscopic image (dorsal view) of an adult female *Notoedres* mite (0.36 mm long) showing concentric circles on body and the dorsal anus. (© J McGarry)

Cnemidocoptes spp.

These mites are the cause of 'scaly leg' and 'scaly face' in birds, particularly budgerigars and chickens.

Demodex spp.

This small cigar-shaped mite (Figure 6.14) is not a typical skin burrowing mite, rather, it has evolved to inhabit and reproduce in hair follicles and sebaceous glands without necessarily causing any problems to the host. *Demodex* are found on a range of mammalian hosts; each has its own highly host-specific species. In companion animals, clinical signs associated with infection are most commonly seen in dogs and hamsters. In young dogs with an apparent genetic predisposition and in older dogs with immunosuppression, the population of *Demodex* can increase dramatically and cause a dermatitis that is characteristically an area of non-pruritic alopecia. In localized demodicosis (Figure 6.15a), where lesions are small, the face is often affected, particularly around the eyes or mouth. Affected animals may appear to be wearing spectacles. Generalized demodicosis (Figure 6.15b) can affect any area, with involvement of the feet being especially painful and problematic. *Demodex* can be trickier to find (and control) than other burrowing mites, as it is smaller and dwells deep within the hair follicle; hair plucks are often useful.

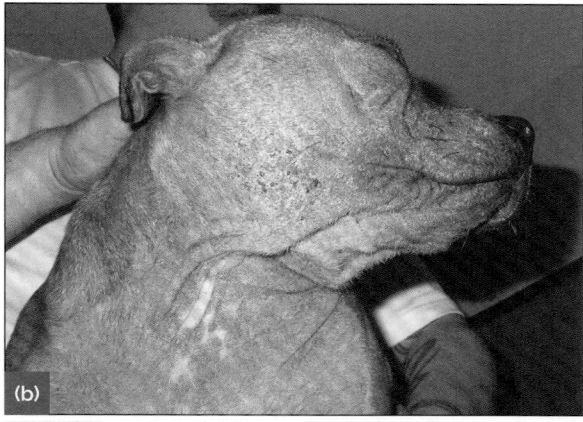

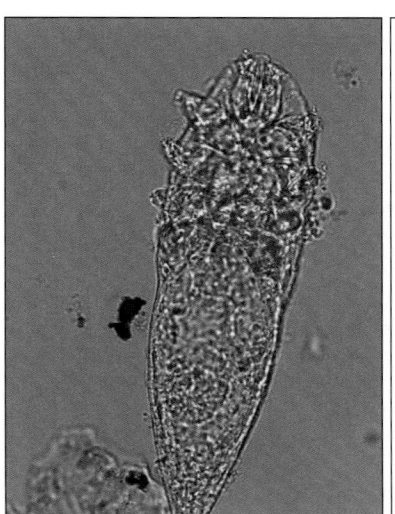 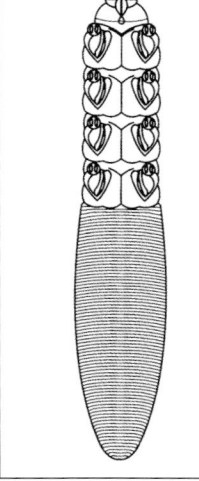

6.15 *continued* **(b)** Generalized demodicosis caused by *Demodex canis*. (Reproduced from the *BSAVA Manual of Canine and Feline Dermatology, 3rd edn*)

Surface-feeding mites
Otodectes cynotis

These oval-shaped mites cause a type of mange inside the ears of dogs, cats and, occasionally, ferrets (Figure 6.16). They live quite deep within the ear canal, often stimulating a dark brown waxy discharge, particularly in cats. The mites may be

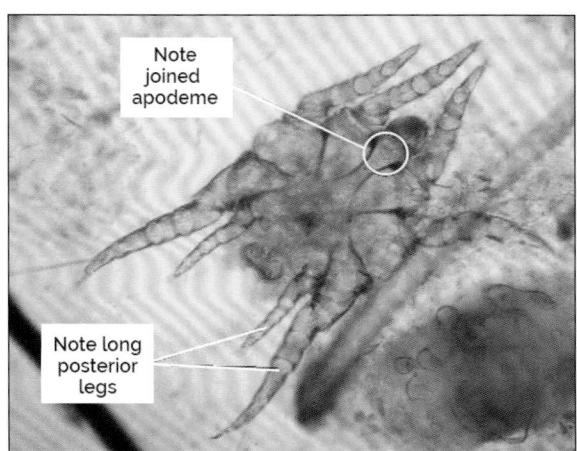

6.14 Microscopic image (dorsal view) of a *Demodex* mite, showing its typical cigar-shaped body (0.2 mm long). The illustration shows the four pairs of legs, closely grouped at the anterior end of the mite. (Photograph © J McGarry)

Note joined apodeme

Note long posterior legs

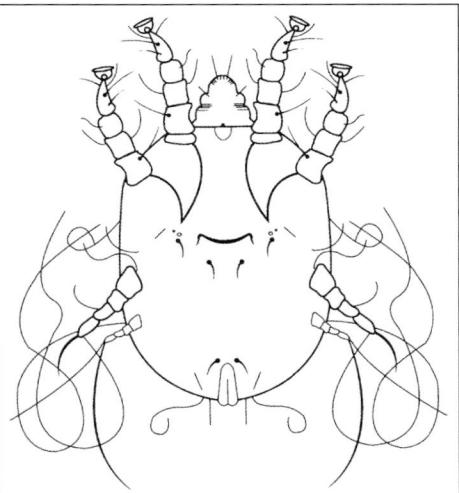

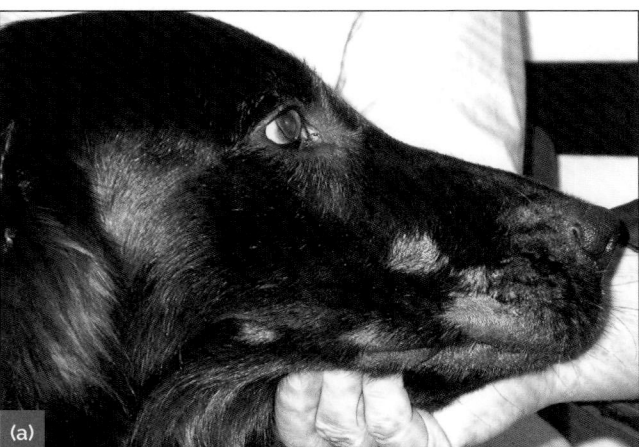

6.15 **(a)** Localized demodicosis caused by *Demodex canis*. (Reproduced from the *BSAVA Manual of Canine and Feline Dermatology, 3rd edn*) *continues* ▶

6.16 Microscopic image (dorsal view) of a male *Otodectes* mite (0.4 mm long). The illustration shows the long legs protruding from the body and the unjoined pedicles (stalks) with suckers on the end. Note the apodemes (thickenings of the exoskeleton) of legs 1 and 2 are joined. (Photograph courtesy of Donald Mactaggart)

seen on the surface as small white moving dots, and secondary bacterial infection can result in a pus-like discharge. However, some dogs, and many cats, show no clinical signs. Animals, particularly dogs, will often shake their heads and rub their ears when infection is present, resulting in trauma to the ears and haematoma formation in the ear flap.

Psoroptes spp.

Ear 'canker' in rabbits is caused by an oval-shaped, surface-feeding mite, *Psoroptes cuniculi*. The mites cause crusting on the inside of the pinnae of affected rabbits (Figure 6.17).

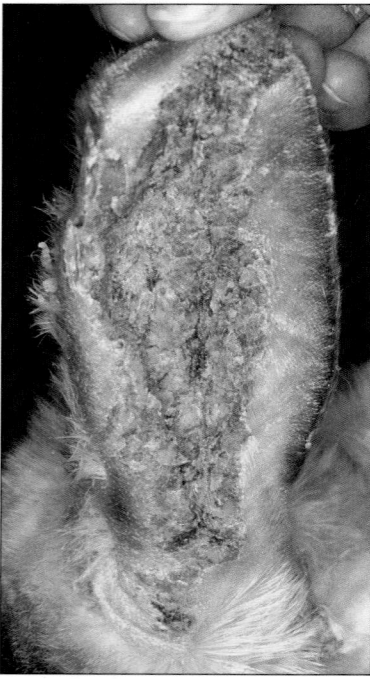

6.17 *Psoroptes cuniculi* infection in the ear of a rabbit. (Courtesy of D Scarff and reproduced from the *BSAVA Manual of Rabbit Medicine*)

Cheyletiella spp.

Dogs, cats or rabbits infested with this fur mite may be described as having 'walking dandruff', since infection often leads to the production of excess scale (Figure 6.18) noticed on the dorsal surface. The mites (Figure 6.19) are large enough to be just visible to the naked eye when hair and skin debris from the animal is brushed off and viewed against a dark background. Infection does not usually cause any marked loss of hair. The mites often move on to humans handling the infested animals, and their activity causes a transient dermatitis which presents as small raised red spots and pruritus. These signs resolve once the animal is effectively treated.

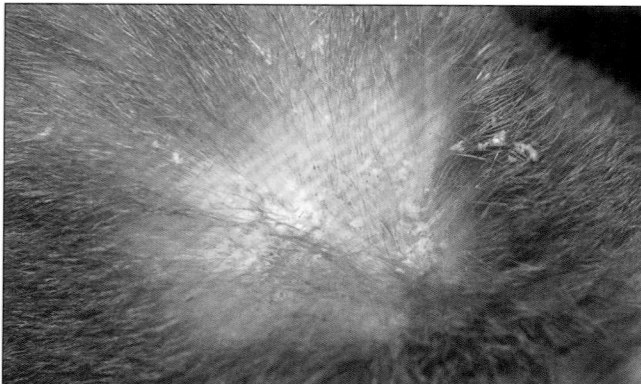

6.18 *Cheyletiella parasitovorax* in a rabbit. This mite typically causes scaling of the skin with minimal pruritus. (Reproduced from the *BSAVA Manual of Rabbit Medicine*)

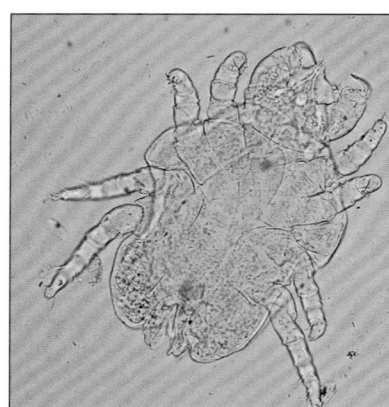

6.19 Microscopic image (dorsal view) of a *Cheyletiella* mite (0.4 mm long). The illustration shows the 'comb' on the end of each leg and the large palps on either side of the head, each with a large claw. (Photograph © J McGarry)

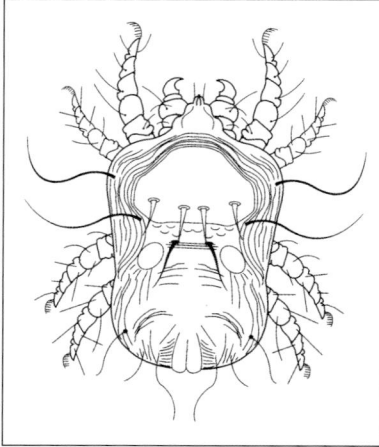

Trombicula autumnalis

This mite, as its name suggests, normally becomes a problem in late summer and autumn, and was formerly associated with specific geographical areas such as the Cotswolds. Now, however, it is considered common in many woodlands throughout the UK. The orange larval mites (Figure 6.20) attach themselves to the legs and feet of any passing animal (dogs, cats) in order to cluster and feed, which takes 2–3 days, and results in a very intense irritation.

Dermanyssus gallinae

This is the 'poultry red mite', which notoriously sucks the blood of chickens and very occasionally other animals. All stages live off the host (e.g. in the eaves of poultry houses), but the mites visit chickens at night to feed and hide away during the day. Chronic infection causes irritation and debility,

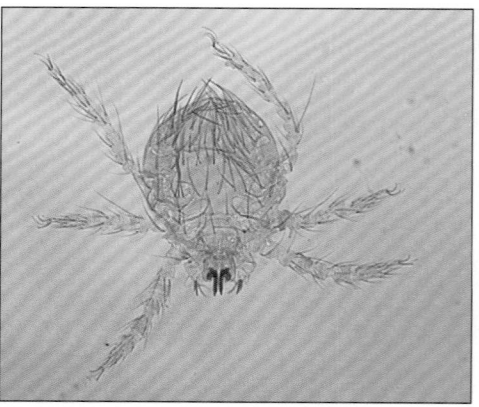

6.20 Microscopic image (dorsal view) of a *Trombicula autumnalis* (harvest mite) larva (1 mm long, orange–brown in colour). Note that there are only three pairs of legs.

with anaemia in heavy infections. Control is by cleaning the henhouse and treatment with an acaricide (a treatment effective against acari).

Ticks

A variety of tick species may attach to domestic animals. Each stage (adult, nymph and larva) is an obligate blood-feeding parasite, which remains on the host for several days and engorges with blood as it feeds. This is the mechanism by which they act as vectors for disease pathogens (viral, protozoal or bacterial organisms capable of causing disease in a host). The identification of tick species is a specialized skill and is important in recognizing vectors for a specific disease.

Species

Ixodes ricinus (Figures 6.21 and 6.22), the sheep tick found in rural areas of woodland, upland and rough grass and scrub, is by far the most common tick species attaching to companion animals in the UK. In small animal practice it is usual to encounter just one or two ticks on a cat or dog, and an owner who is concerned about how to get rid of them. Although not appealing, they usually present little problem to the host. The main health risk relating to ticks is in their potential to transmit infections, such as the Lyme disease agent *Borrelia burgdorferi*.

Other species of tick affect dogs in the UK and one of these, *I. canisuga*, is host-specific to the dog and may infest kennels. The hedgehog tick, *I. hexagonus*, is also encountered in small companion animals in an urban setting, particularly in hunting cats.

Identification and removal

Initially, all that is visible when a tick attaches to an animal is a small greyish firmly attached swelling. Inspection reveals pairs of legs close to the attachment with the host; the mouthparts (Figure 6.23) are buried into the animal's flesh. As the tick ingests the host's blood it increases in size and once fully fed (in days) will drop off its host.

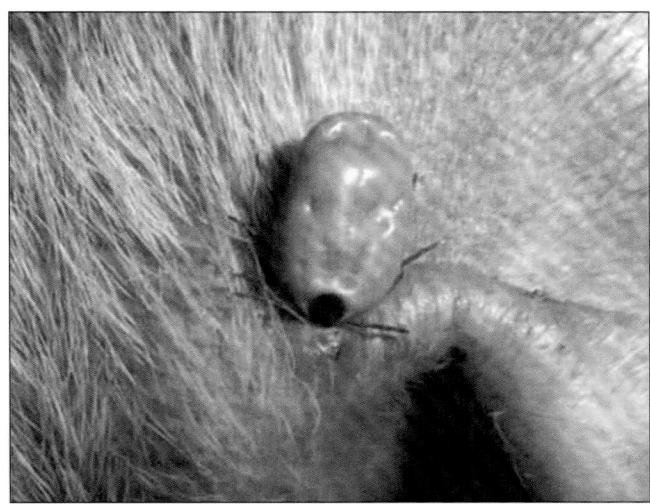

6.22 Engorged adult female sheep tick, *Ixodes ricinus*, measuring approximately 7 mm. Note the small dark brown scutum or plate near to the head. (© J McGarry)

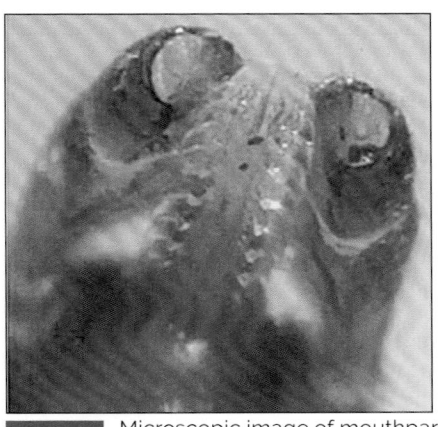

6.23 Microscopic image of mouthparts of a tick. (© J McGarry)

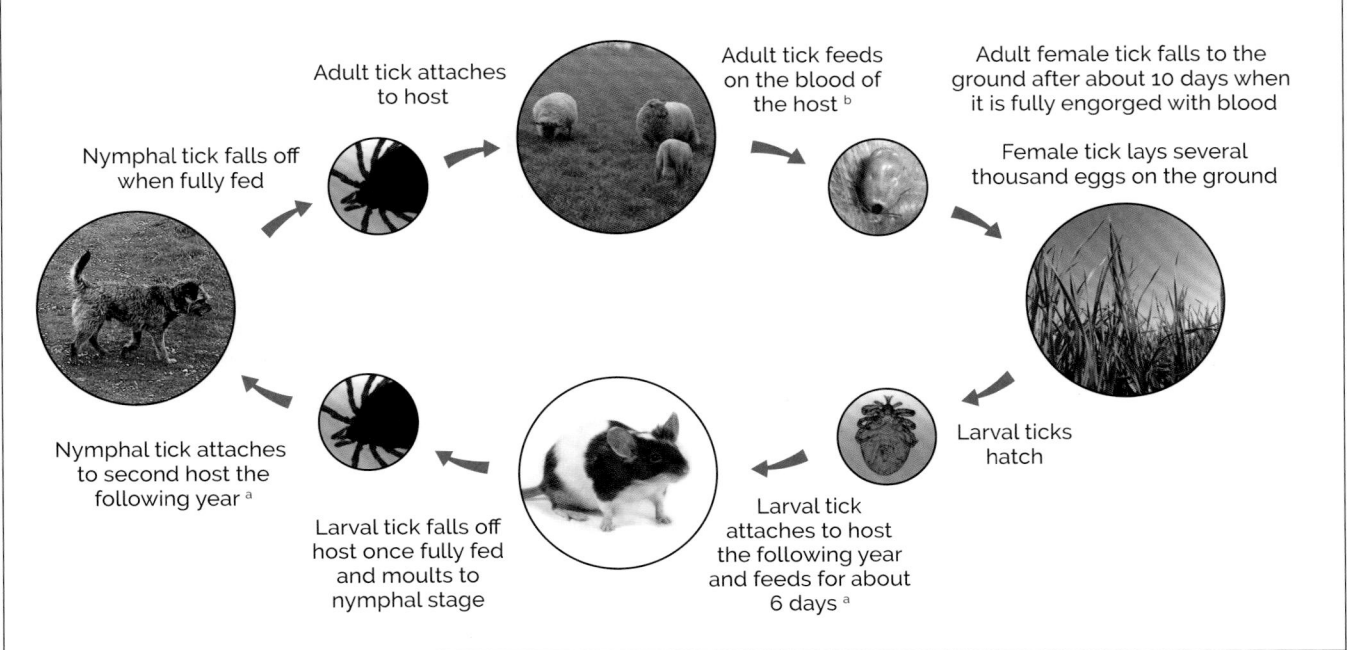

Adult tick attaches to host

Adult tick feeds on the blood of the host [b]

Adult female tick falls to the ground after about 10 days when it is fully engorged with blood

Female tick lays several thousand eggs on the ground

Nymphal tick falls off when fully fed

Larval ticks hatch

Nymphal tick attaches to second host the following year [a]

Larval tick attaches to host the following year and feeds for about 6 days [a]

Larval tick falls off host once fully fed and moults to nymphal stage

6.21 Life cycle of the sheep tick (*Ixodes ricinus*). The life cycle involves three hosts: each stage feeds on a different animal, which may be the same or a different host species. [a] Larvae and nymphs tend to feed on small mammals (e.g. mice and dogs); [b] adults tend to feed on larger animals (e.g. sheep or deer). (Adult female tick photograph © J McGarry)

Individual ticks should be removed as soon as possible using a special tick removal device; they can then be killed by dabbing them with a cotton wool bud that has been treated with an acaricide. At times of tick challenge, it is worthwhile carrying out prophylactic treatment to ensure that any ticks are repelled from the dog or cat and that any that do attach are killed soon afterwards. There are a number of products available containing a variety of acaricides (pyrethroids: permethrin, flumethrin and deltamethrin; fipronil; pyriprole; isoxazolines: fluralaner, afoxalaner, sarolaner) in a range of formulations (including spot-ons, collars, sprays and tablets for oral administration) to achieve this aim, some of which will protect against flea infestation at the same time.

> **WARNING**
>
> - Never try to pull off a live tick without using an effective 'tick remover' as the mouthparts may be left embedded in the animal and the lesion may become a focus for infection
> - Avoid local application of a spot-on acaricide to remove a tick close to an animal's mouth

Emerging diseases

Since the advent of the Pet Travel Scheme there has been an increased opportunity for some of the tick-transmitted pathogens endemic in mainland Europe to be introduced into the UK. In order to prevent infected ticks from entering the UK, it was, until 2012, mandatory for dogs and cats to be treated with an approved acaricide before their return to the UK. As this provision has now been removed, veterinary surgeons in UK practices need to be aware of diseases such as canine babesiosis in travelled dogs and advise clients of the clinical signs to be aware of and appropriate preventative treatments. Canine babesiosis can be fatal and is transmitted by ticks such as the brown dog tick, *Rhipicephalus sanguineus*, which is common in most of southern Europe. Details of the latest requirements can be found on the UK government website (www.gov.uk). In addition, canine babesiosis appears to have taken hold in local tick populations, following a report of cases of canine babesiosis in Essex in dogs that had never travelled outside the UK (de Marco *et al.*, 2017). More information can be found on the ESCCAP (European Scientific Counsel Companion Animal Parasites) and ESCCAP UK websites (www.esccap.org; www.esccapuk.org.uk).

Endoparasites

Endoparasites can be divided into helminths and protozoa.

- Helminths are the 'worms' and are subdivided into three types:
  - Flukes (trematodes) (common in ruminants but do not normally affect dogs or cats in the UK)
  - Tapeworms (cestodes)
  - Roundworms (nematodes).
- Protozoal parasites are small unicellular organisms.

Figure 6.24 lists the species in each category of significance in dogs and cats in veterinary practices in the UK.

Parasite group	Species	Host
Helminths		
Cestodes (tapeworms)	*Echinococcus granulosus granulosus* (sheep strain)	Dogs
	Echinococcus equinus	Dogs
	Echinococcus multilocularis [a]	Dogs and cats
	Dipylidium caninum	Dogs and cats
	Taenia spp.	Dogs and cats
Nematodes (roundworms)		
Ascarids	*Toxocara canis*	Dogs
	Toxascaris leonina	Dogs and cats
	Toxocara cati	Cats
Hookworms	*Uncinaria stenocephala*	Dogs
	Ancylostoma tubaeforme [b]	Cats
	Ancylostoma caninum	Dogs
Whipworm	*Trichuris vulpis*	Dogs
Heartworm	*Dirofilaria immitis* [c]	Dogs and cats
Capillaria	*Capillaria plica*	Dogs
	Capillaria hepatica	Dogs
Lungworms	*Aelurostrongylus abstrusus*	Cats
	Angiostrongylus vasorum	Dogs
	Oslerus osleri (formerly *Filaroides osleri*)	Dogs
Protozoa		
Coccidia	*Isospora* sp.	Dogs and cats
	Cryptosporidium parvum	Dogs and cats
	Sarcocystis spp.	Dogs and cats
	Toxoplasma gondii	Cats
	Neospora caninum	Dogs
	Hammondia sp.	Cats
Flagellates	*Giardia* sp.	Dogs and cats
Piroplasm	*Babesia* sp. [d]	Dogs

6.24 Species of endoparasite commonly seen in dogs and cats in veterinary practices in the UK. [a] Mainland Europe only. [b] Hookworm infection occurs rarely in cats in the UK. [c] Not in the UK – endemic in the Mediterranean area. [d] Not in the UK, although infected dogs may be imported from the southern part of mainland Europe.

Helminths

Cestodes (tapeworms)

Cestodes are tape-like and lack an alimentary tract. They are composed of three parts: the head or scolex; an area behind this where segments form; and finally the mature segments (proglottids) (Figure 6.25). Tapeworms are hermaphrodites, i.e. they have a set of male and female reproductive organs in each segment. As the segment matures, reproduction takes place and eggs then develop within the segment, so a fully mature proglottid is simply an egg-containing structure. Eggs find their way into the environment when the mature segments break off and are excreted in faeces. Tapeworms have an immature 'larval' stage (the metacestode) that develops in an intermediate host; the given name and exact nature of the larval structure varies according to the species of tapeworm.

Tapeworms found in cats and dogs in the UK (see Figure 6.24) include:

- *Dipylidium caninum* – common in both dogs and cats; the intermediate host is an arthropod

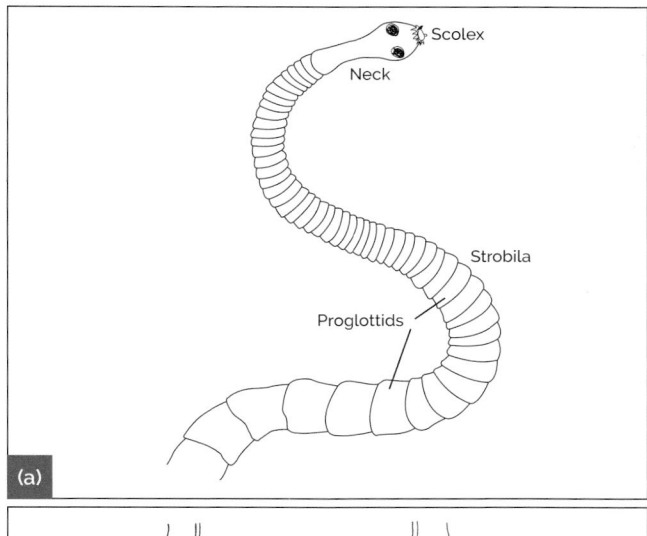

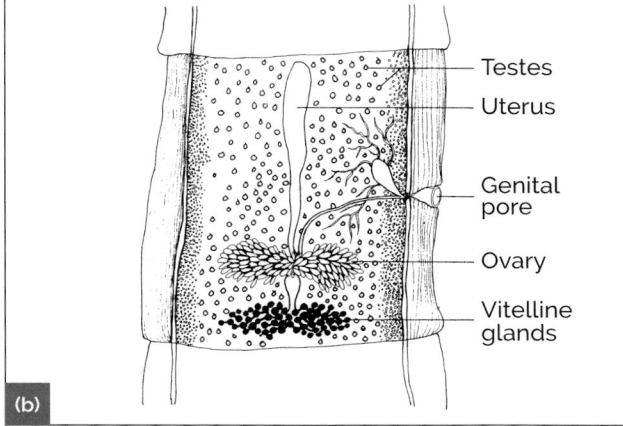

6.25 (a) A typical adult cestode. (b) A mature proglottid. (Reproduced from Urquhart *et al.*, 1996, with permission of Blackwell Publishing)

- *Taenia* species – one species in cats and several species in dogs
- *Echinococcus granulosus* – rare and usually seen in rural dogs; humans can be infected through ingestion of the eggs, resulting in dangerous liver cysts.

Adult tapeworms are found in the small intestine and are not normally a clinical problem to the small animal definitive (final) host; however, the sight of tapeworm segments in faeces is repugnant to pet owners. Larval infection of the intermediate host (see Figure 6.29), either because the larval tapeworms manifest as cysts causing clinical disease (e.g. hydatid disease in humans due to *E. garnulosus*) or because affected meat is condemned as unfit for human consumption, is of greater significance.

Tapeworm definitions
Adult tapeworms:
- Scolex: Head of a tapeworm – used for attachment to the host's small intestinal mucosa using suckers and the rostellum (where present) for attachment
- Rostellum: The anterior part of the scolex, present in most tapeworms; it is a protrusible cone and is armed with hooks in some species
- Strobila: The chain of individual segments (proglottids)
- Proglottid: Name for each individual segment that makes up the strobila. →

Tapeworm definitions *continued*
Immature larval tapeworms (metacestodes):
These are found in intermediate hosts and have one of four names:
- Cysticercoid: Single evaginated scolex. This is the larval form for *Dipylidium* and is found in fleas and lice
- Cysticercus: Fluid-filled cyst containing a single invaginated scolex attached to the cyst wall. This is the larval name for certain *Taenia* spp. (e.g. the human tapeworm, *Taenia saginata*, where the cyst stage is found in cattle)
- Coenurus: A cyst with many invaginated scolices attached to the cyst wall. This is the larval name for certain Taenia spp. (e.g. *Taenia multiceps*)
- Hydatid cyst: Large cyst containing many scolices, some loose in the fluid inside and some contained within 'brood capsules'. This is the larval name used for *Echinococcus* spp.

Dipylidium caninum

This is probably the most common tapeworm of cats and dogs in the UK. The intermediate host is a flea, as well as the chewing louse *Trichodectes canis* in the case of the dog. These insects contain the cysticercoid and infection occurs when the pet ingests an infected flea or louse during grooming. Infection is normally diagnosed by the presence of motile segments (shaped like rice grains) containing 'egg packets' (Figure 6.26) in the faeces or around the anus. The full life cycle is shown in Figure 6.27. Control depends on treating the existing infection and eliminating any flea or louse problem to break the transmission cycle.

Taenia spp.

Dogs and cats may be infected when they eat raw meat, either in the form of uncooked meat or offal containing larval cysts (usually dogs), or through catching and eating prey containing the intermediate larval tapeworm stages (usually cats). The life cycle of *Taenia hydatigena* is shown in Figure 6.28. The definitive (final) and intermediate hosts of a range of *Taenia* species are given in Figure 6.29. Diagnosis is based on seeing segments passed by the animal. More rarely, eggs liberated from the segments are seen during microscopic examination of a faecal sample. *Taenia* eggs (Figure 6.30) are half the size of eggs of *Toxocara*, a common roundworm

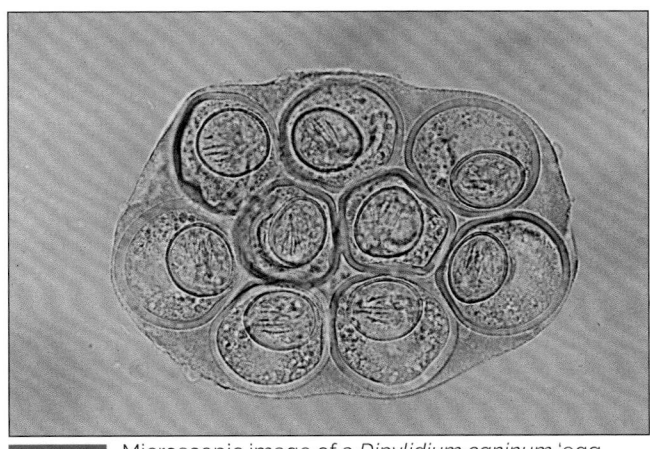

6.26 Microscopic image of a *Dipylidium caninum* 'egg packet' (approximately 160 µm in length).

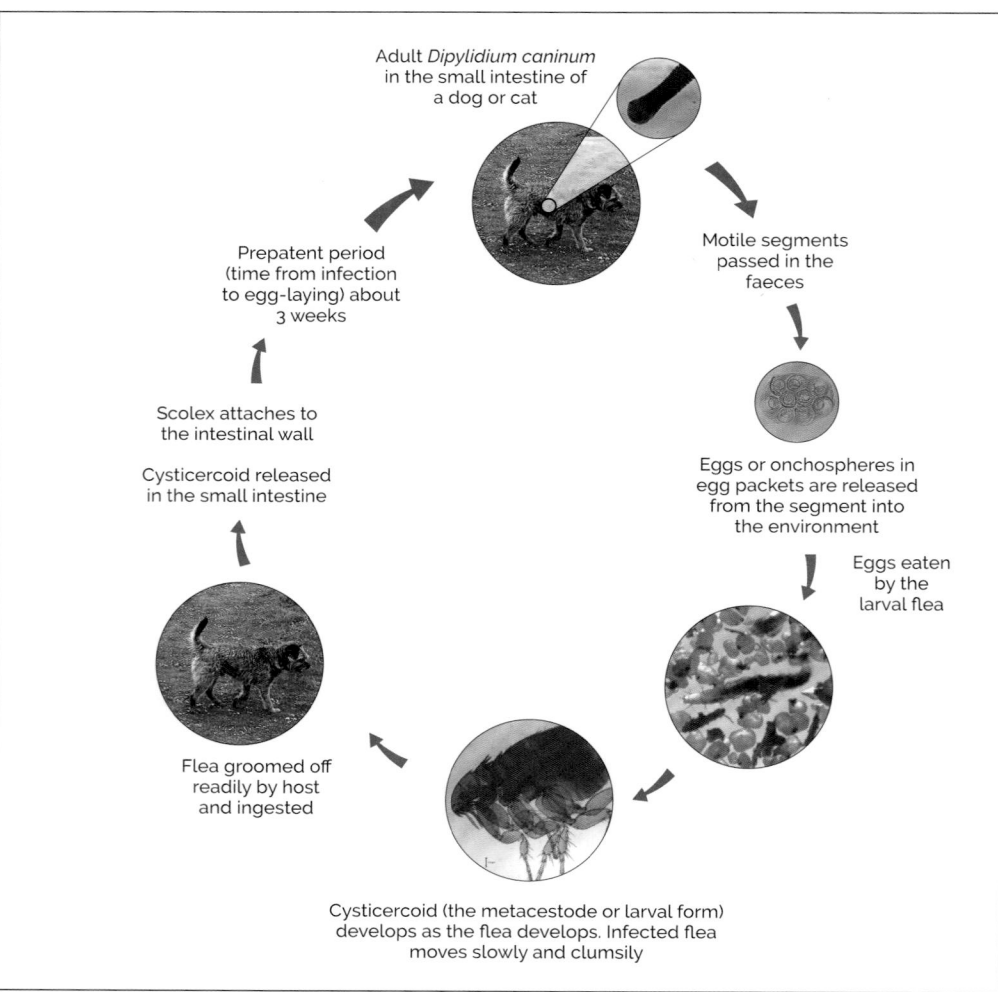

Adult *Dipylidium caninum* in the small intestine of a dog or cat

Motile segments passed in the faeces

Eggs or onchospheres in egg packets are released from the segment into the environment

Eggs eaten by the larval flea

Cysticercoid (the metacestode or larval form) develops as the flea develops. Infected flea moves slowly and clumsily

Flea groomed off readily by host and ingested

Cysticercoid released in the small intestine

Scolex attaches to the intestinal wall

Prepatent period (time from infection to egg-laying) about 3 weeks

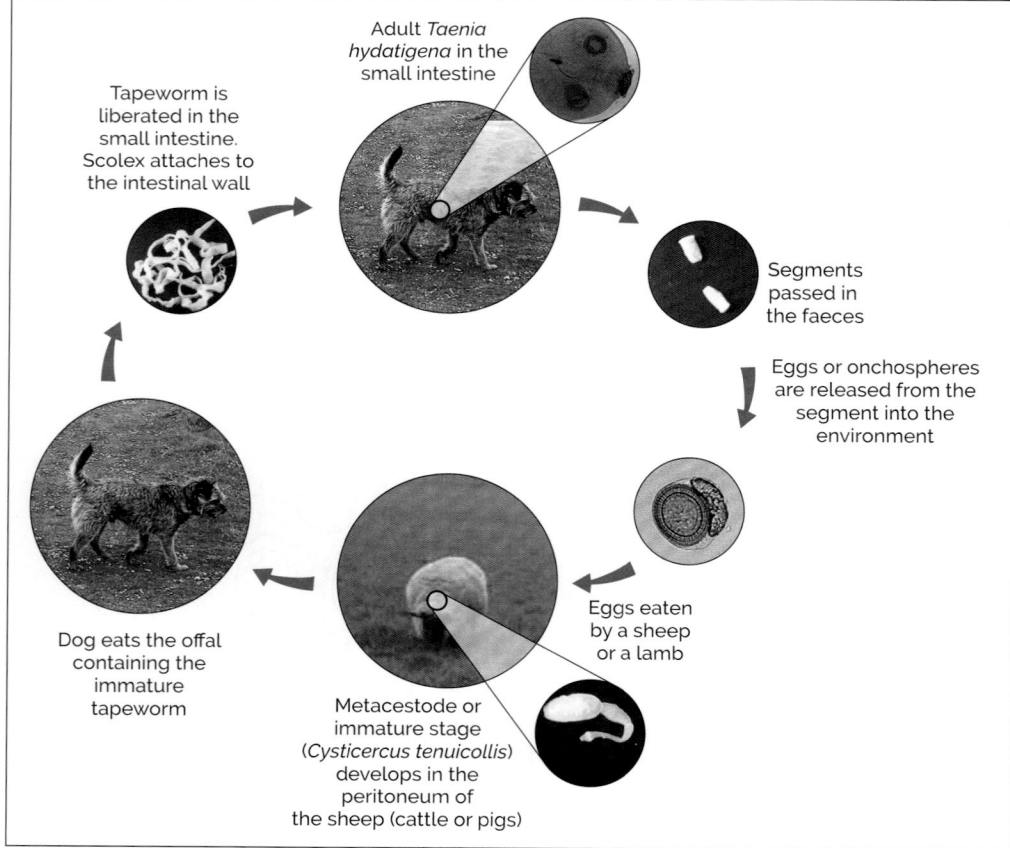

Adult *Taenia hydatigena* in the small intestine

Tapeworm is liberated in the small intestine. Scolex attaches to the intestinal wall

Segments passed in the faeces

Eggs or onchospheres are released from the segment into the environment

Eggs eaten by a sheep or a lamb

Metacestode or immature stage (*Cysticercus tenuicollis*) develops in the peritoneum of the sheep (cattle or pigs)

Dog eats the offal containing the immature tapeworm

Taenia species	Definitive (final) host	Intermediate host
T. taeniaeformis	Cat	Rat or mouse (*Cysticercus fasciolaris* in the liver)
T. serialis	Dog	Rabbit (*Coenurus serialis* in connective tissue)
T. pisiformis	Dog	Rabbit (*Cysticercus pisiformis* in the peritoneum)
T. ovis	Dog	Sheep (*Cysticercus ovis* in muscle)
T. hydatigena	Dog	Sheep/cattle/pig (*Cysticercus tenuicollis* in the peritoneum)
T. muliticeps	Dog	Sheep/cattle (*Coenurus cerebralis* in the central nervous system)

6.29 Hosts of *Taenia* tapeworms.

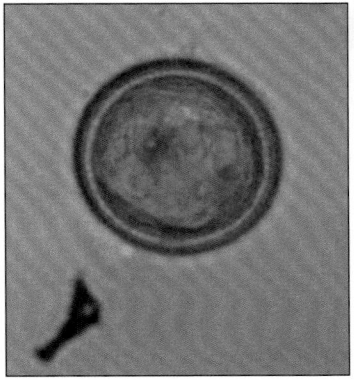

6.30 Microscopic image of a *Taenia* spp. egg, approximately 40 μm in diameter. (© J McGarry)

of dogs and cats (see Figure 6.34), measuring about 40 μm in diameter. Control is based on treating the current infection and then preventing the animal having access to uncooked flesh, something that is easy to do where the animal is fed by the owner but more difficult if the infection is due to hunting prey.

Rabbits are the intermediate hosts of *Taenia serialis*. Infection may occur as a result of grass eaten by rabbits being contaminated with eggs passed by dogs or foxes. Larval cysts (*Coenurus serialis*) are normally located in connective tissue and can appear similar to a subcutaneous abscess. Affected animals may show other clinical signs, including decreased appetite. Treatment involves the surgical removal of cysts.

Echinococcus granulosus granulosus

This organism has a dog-to-sheep life cycle (Figure 6.31). It is an important zoonotic pathogen that occurs in the UK but is fortunately fairly rare. It is endemic in two areas of the UK (Wales and the Hebrides), where dogs have the opportunity to feed on sheep carcasses on the hills.

The adult parasite is very small, only about 6 mm long, and several thousand may be present in the small intestine. This parasite has been the focus of several control programmes in the past (e.g. Powys, Wales), whereby at-risk dogs have been regularly treated with an effective anthelmintic and denied access to sheep carcasses in order to break the transmission cycle. If a human accidentally ingests a proglottid or individual eggs, then a hydatid cyst may develop in the liver or lungs in the same way as it develops in the sheep. This forms a space-occupying lesion that may grow to some considerable size. Treatment of affected people is based on anthelmintics followed by draining the cyst and then surgically removing the wall of the cyst. This is a hazardous procedure for the patient.

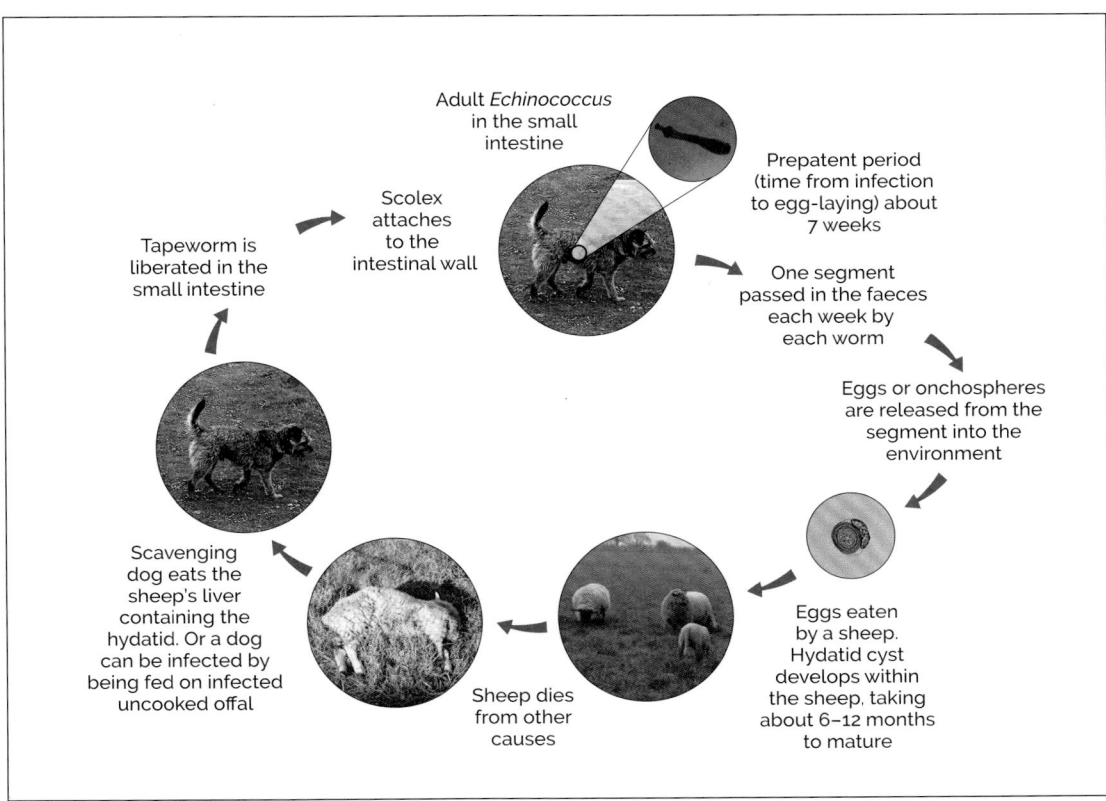

6.31 Life cycle of *Echinococcus granulosus granulosus*.

Adult *Echinococcus* in the small intestine

Prepatent period (time from infection to egg-laying) about 7 weeks

Scolex attaches to the intestinal wall

One segment passed in the faeces each week by each worm

Tapeworm is liberated in the small intestine

Eggs or onchospheres are released from the segment into the environment

Scavenging dog eats the sheep's liver containing the hydatid. Or a dog can be infected by being fed on infected uncooked offal

Sheep dies from other causes

Eggs eaten by a sheep. Hydatid cyst develops within the sheep, taking about 6–12 months to mature

Echinococcus granulosus equinus

This species of tapeworm has a dog-to-horse life cycle. It occurs particularly where hounds are fed on horse offal. Horses are infected when they graze pasture contaminated with tapeworm eggs. It is not believed to pose a zoonotic risk.

Echinococcus multilocularis

This tapeworm is found in continental Europe and was of particular concern and attention in Switzerland; it has now spread into a wide area of central Europe, including Germany and much of France. This parasite is of major concern because the larval stage (a multilocular invasive cyst, normally found in rodents) can cause infection in humans that ingest the eggs shed by dogs, foxes and, less likely, cats, which are the definitive (final) hosts. With regard to the Pet Travel Scheme, the threat this parasite poses to human health is the reason why there is a mandatory tapeworm treatment (praziquantel) for animals returning to the UK. Up-to-date information about this and other requirements of the Pet Travel Scheme may be found on the UK government website (www.gov.uk/take-pet-abroad).

Cestode infections in exotic pets

Birds and other animals, such as rabbits, mice, rats and hamsters, may all be infected with adult tapeworms specific to the host species. In most cases, infection has no clinical effect on the host. Occasionally, a heavy tapeworm burden in hamsters may be associated with weight loss and, rarely, intestinal blockage. In each case the intermediate host is an invertebrate such as a beetle or mite.

Treatment of cestode infections

Adult tapeworms can be killed by a number of anthelmintics. These may be products that have activity only against tapeworms, in which case they are known as cestocides. Alternatively, the preparation (usually a drug combination) may have activity against both nematodes and tapeworms; these are known as broad-spectrum anthelmintics (see Chapter 8). It is much more difficult to kill immature tapeworm infections in intermediate hosts and this is not usually carried out; hence surgical removal is the treatment of choice in affected sheep and rabbits, but is not routine practice. Unfortunately, there are no specific prophylactic treatments available for dogs; however, where *Echinococcus* spp. are endemic, regular treatment at 4- or 6-weekly intervals (depending on species) will remove adult worms before they begin egg laying, and hence will reduce environmental contamination with eggs and the associated zoonotic risk.

Nematodes (roundworms)

Nematode worms are cylindrical, elongated and have a digestive tract. Most have a direct life cycle but some (e.g. lungworms) have a slug or snail as an intermediate host. Others may be carried by a paratenic host.

Ascarids

An important nematode group seen in small animal veterinary practice are the ascarids (especially *Toxocara canis*, *Toxascaris leonina* and *Toxocara cati* in dogs and cats). These relatively large, white, fleshy worms (Figure 6.32) are most numerous and frequently seen in young animals.

Ascarids also occur commonly in exotic pets, including reptiles (e.g. tortoises) and birds (especially parakeets). In each case, the ascarid species is host-specific and heavy burdens may be associated with poor growth or intestinal impaction.

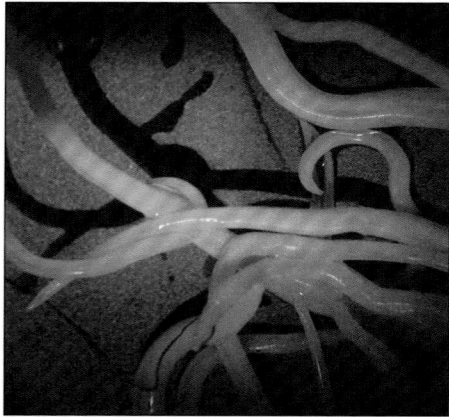

6.32

Typical appearance of adult ascarids (up to 10 cm long). (© J McGarry)

Toxocara canis

This is a very important worm, as it is a zoonotic pathogen (infects people) and can also cause disease in young puppies. Its life cycle is shown in Figure 6.33.

Puppies are first infected before birth by larvae that pass from the bitch's muscles to her uterus after about the 42nd day of pregnancy. These larvae migrate through the liver and lungs of the young puppies and are then coughed up and swallowed. They remain in the small intestine, where they develop to adult worms by the time the puppies are 3 weeks old. Puppies can receive further infection from infective eggs in the environment and by infective larvae that pass in the mother's milk, but the majority of the infection will usually have occurred across the placenta. Puppies that have a heavy *Toxocara* burden will typically be stunted, with distended bellies; they may vomit and/or have diarrhoea, and severe infections may lead to a total blockage of the intestine. As immunity develops following exposure, and possibly related to an increase in age, puppies begin to expel their *Toxocara* infection spontaneously from about 7 weeks of age. Most have expelled all of their adult worms by 6–7 months of age. Normally, further larvae that are ingested pass from the intestine to muscle, where they enter a resting state.

Adult worms pass large numbers of eggs; as many as several thousand eggs per gram of faeces in a 3-week-old puppy. Each egg is surrounded by a thick wall (Figure 6.34), which is very resistant to physical and chemical damage. The eggs are not immediately infective but require time for a larva to develop inside. In ideal conditions this takes about 14 days, but it takes much longer in low temperatures. Since the larva remains in the shell until eaten by an animal, the eggs may remain infective in the environment for up to 2 years. If the animal that ingests the eggs happens to be a bitch, the larvae remain in this resting state until she becomes pregnant; some of the larvae will migrate to infect her puppies; others will remain to infect her subsequent litters.

Control of *Toxocara canis*

The aims are:

■ Control of infection in the dog, to prevent disease in puppies and to prevent eggs being put into the environment
■ Prevention of infection in children.

Control in dogs is based on the following:

■ Prenatal infection in puppies may be controlled by treating the bitch, prior to whelping, with a

Control of *Toxocara canis* continued

product that will kill the migrating larvae, e.g. fenbendazole, from the 40th day of pregnancy to 2 days' post whelping
- Alternatively, puppies may be treated at regular intervals with a suitable anthelmintic, starting from 2 weeks of age. The bitch should be treated at the same time
- Reducing the number of eggs in the environment is very difficult once the eggs are present. Environmental control is best achieved by education of the dog-owning public to pick up and correctly dispose of dog faeces.

The most important methods of preventing children from becoming infected are to ensure that:
- Dogs defecate in specified areas in parks
- 'Pooper scoopers' or other means of appropriate faecal disposal are used
- Children wash their hands before eating and after handling puppies
- Children are discouraged from handling young puppies unless the animals have been thoroughly wormed.

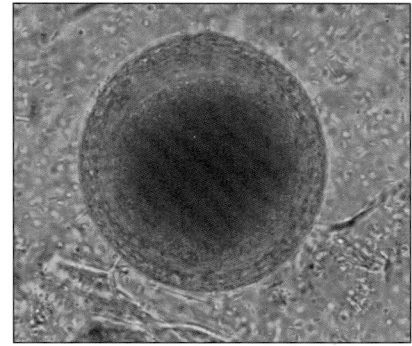

6.34 Microscopic image of a *Toxocara canis* egg (approximately 80 μm diameter). Note the dark contents and dark shell with pitted edge. (© J McGarry)

Larvae that are accidentally eaten by other animals (including humans) migrate from the intestine and enter a resting state in other tissues. If a human ingests a large number of infective eggs and these all migrate together through the body, a condition known as visceral larva migrans may develop, associated with signs of damage to the organs through which the larvae are migrating. If only a few larvae are ingested, they will usually migrate through the human body without any signs of illness. However, in the rare case where they come to rest in the eye, sight dysfunction or even blindness may result. Infection is usually seen in children, as they are the most likely to have unhygienic habits. To perpetuate their life cycle, dormant larvae in the tissues of birds or animals other than dogs depend upon their paratenic host being eaten by a dog.

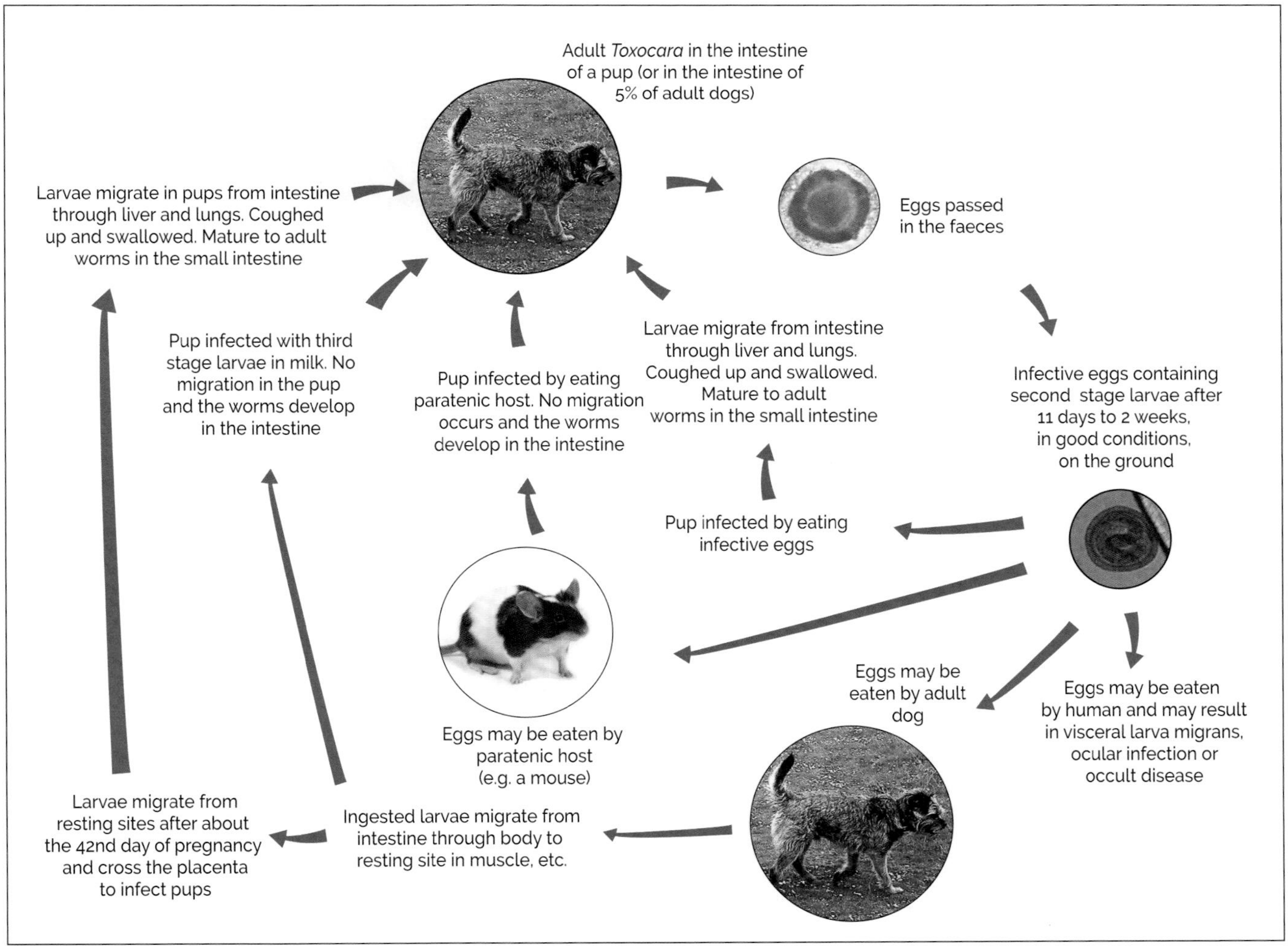

Adult *Toxocara* in the intestine of a pup (or in the intestine of 5% of adult dogs)

Larvae migrate in pups from intestine through liver and lungs. Coughed up and swallowed. Mature to adult worms in the small intestine

Eggs passed in the faeces

Pup infected with third stage larvae in milk. No migration in the pup and the worms develop in the intestine

Pup infected by eating paratenic host. No migration occurs and the worms develop in the intestine

Larvae migrate from intestine through liver and lungs. Coughed up and swallowed. Mature to adult worms in the small intestine

Infective eggs containing second stage larvae after 11 days to 2 weeks, in good conditions, on the ground

Pup infected by eating infective eggs

Eggs may be eaten by paratenic host (e.g. a mouse)

Eggs may be eaten by adult dog

Eggs may be eaten by human and may result in visceral larva migrans, ocular infection or occult disease

Larvae migrate from resting sites after about the 42nd day of pregnancy and cross the placenta to infect pups

Ingested larvae migrate from intestine through body to resting site in muscle, etc.

6.33 Life cycle of *Toxocara canis*.

In some adult dogs, especially where there is a low level of challenge, adult worms will develop in the small intestine. Lactating bitches are particularly likely to have a patent (egg-producing) infection, probably due to the change in their hormonal status. Their infection may come from a number of sources, including young worms passed by the puppies that the bitch ingests as she cleans up around the whelping area. Usually the bitch expels her remaining infection shortly after the puppies are weaned.

In the UK, approximately 2% of dogs are infected; in developing countries prevalence may be much higher. Infected dogs are not necessarily consistently the same individuals.

Toxocara cati

This organism is responsible for ascarid infection in cats, particularly kittens. It is transmitted to kittens via their mothers' milk; infection also occurs through infective eggs in the environment and ingestion of paratenic hosts (Figure 6.35). Unlike *T. canis*, it is **not** transmitted via the placenta. A heavy infection may cause stunting of growth in kittens and a pot-bellied appearance.

The adult worm can be distinguished by the appearance of the alae or 'wings' either side of the head end (Figure 6.36), but the egg is grossly indistinguishable from that of *T. canis*.

Control is by regular treatment of kittens from about 3 weeks of age until they are several months old. Kittens are infected via the milk and so they will be about 6 weeks of age before the first infection becomes patent. This is a zoonotic parasite whose relative importance for human health has yet to be determined.

Toxascaris leonina

Toxascaris leonina is found in both cats and dogs. Its life cycle is shown in Figure 6.37. There is no prenatal infection; infection is therefore usually first seen in adolescent animals. The worm is not normally associated with clinical signs, since large burdens are reasonably well tolerated. The shape of the alae can be used to differentiate adult worms from *T. cati* (see Figure 6.36). The egg (Figure 6.38) can be distinguished by the smooth outer wall to its shell. *T. leonina* has rarely been implicated as a zoonosis.

Hookworms

Hookworms are short stout worms with hooked heads (Figure 6.39). *Uncinaria stenocephala* and *Ancylostoma caninum* occur in the small intestine of the dog. Of the two species, *U. stenocephala* is far more common in the UK and is known as the northern hookworm; it is particularly seen in Greyhounds or in hunt kennels and is common in urban foxes, which may be a source of infection for domestic dogs. *Ancylostoma braziliensis* infects the skin and intestinal tract of dogs and cats in tropical and subtropical regions; its larvae may also be zoonotic. The species may be distinguished by the appearance of the head: *A. caninum* has three pairs of large teeth; *A. braziliensis* (Figure 6.40) has two pairs of similar teeth; and *U. stenocephala* has plates in the mouth cavity.

The life cycle of *U. stenocephala* is shown in Figure 6.41. The worms attach to the small intestinal mucosa via their mouthparts (the buccal cavity), using their teeth to damage the surface and then feed off the tissue fluids; blood in the case of *A. caninum*. A heavy burden of *Uncinaria* may cause emaciation and in the case of *Ancylostoma*, anaemia.

Eggs produced by the female worms are passed in the faeces. The infective larvae of both worms may penetrate the skin. Larvae of *Uncinaria* spp. simply cause dermatitis, as

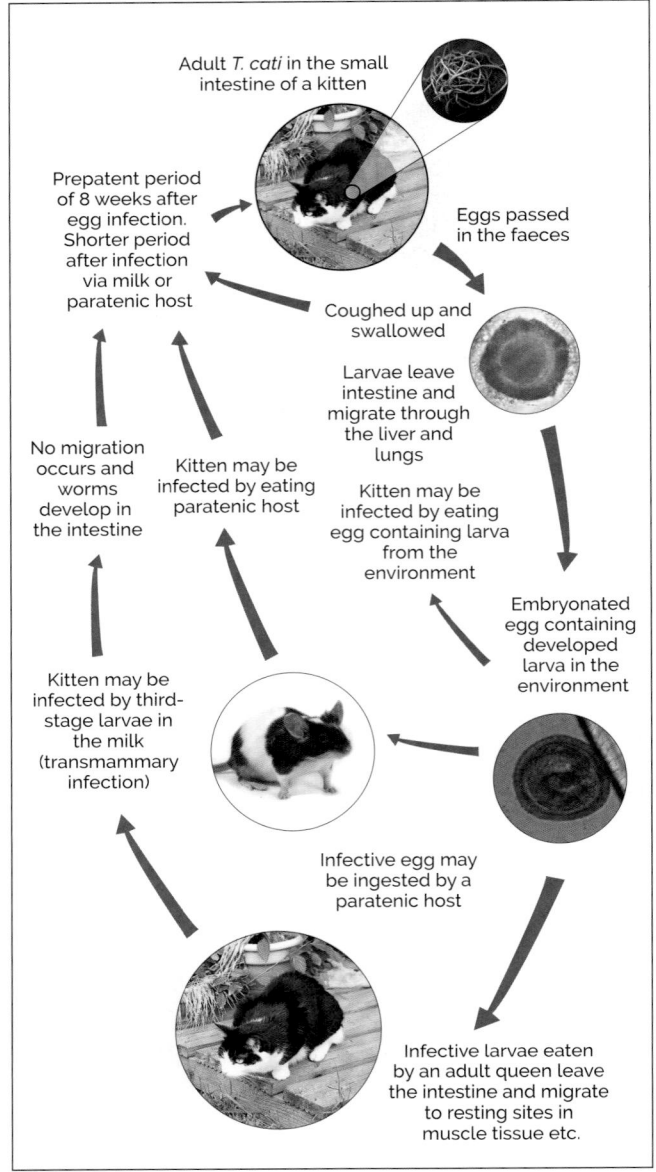

6.35 Life cycle of *Toxocara cati*.

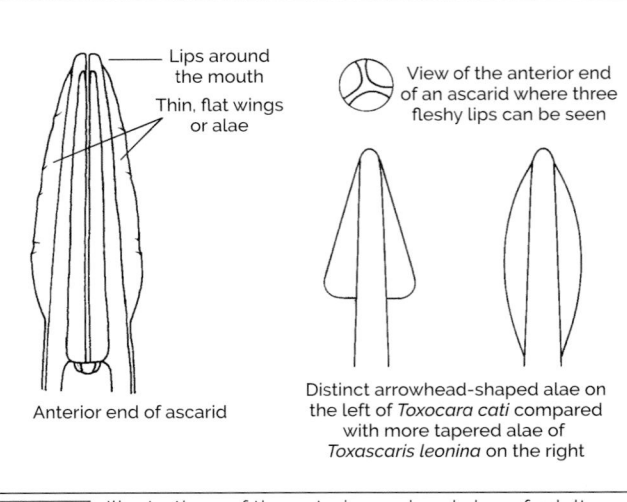

6.36 Illustrations of the anterior end and alae of adult ascarids.

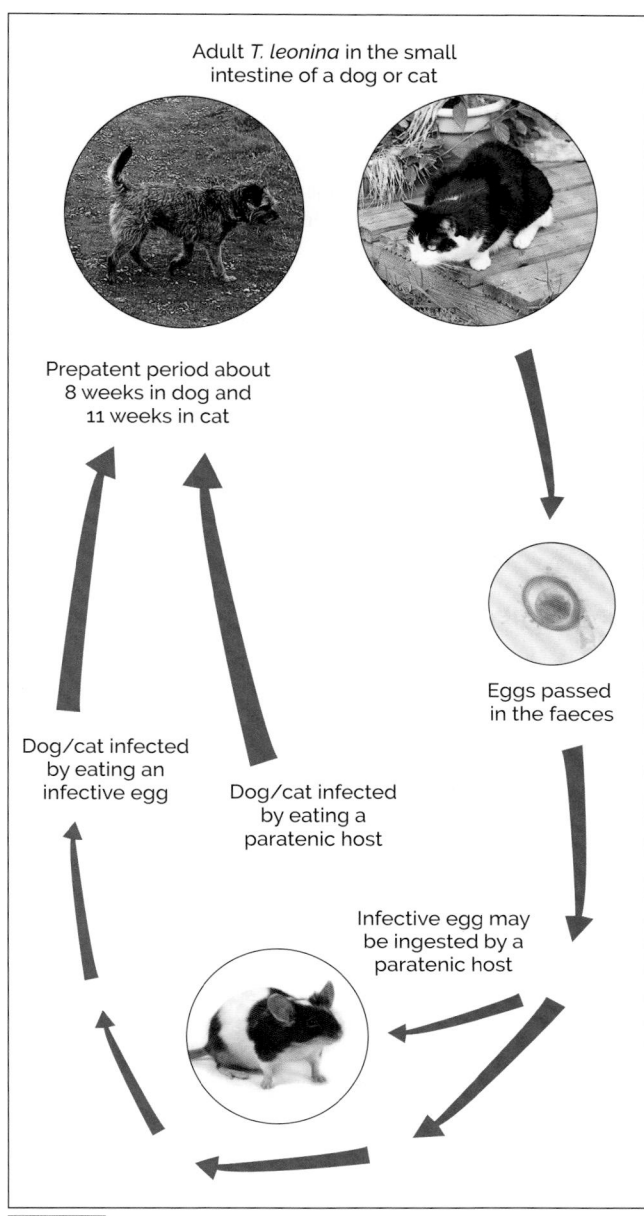

Adult *T. leonina* in the small
intestine of a dog or cat

Prepatent period about
8 weeks in dog and
11 weeks in cat

Eggs passed
in the faeces

Dog/cat infected
by eating an
infective egg

Dog/cat infected
by eating a
paratenic host

Infective egg may
be ingested by a
paratenic host

6.37   Life cycle of *Toxascaris leonina*.

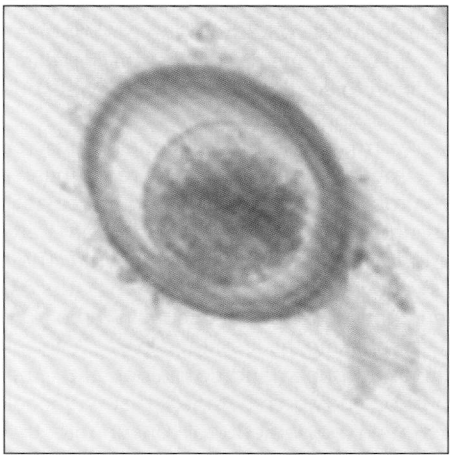

6.38   Microscopic image of a *Toxascaris leonina* egg
(approximately 85 μm long). Note the smooth outer
wall. Contents are paler than those of *Toxocara* species.

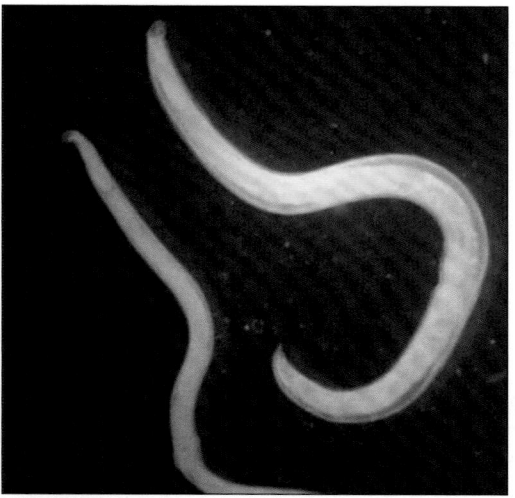

6.39   Adult hookworms measuring just over 1 cm in
length. (© J McGarry)

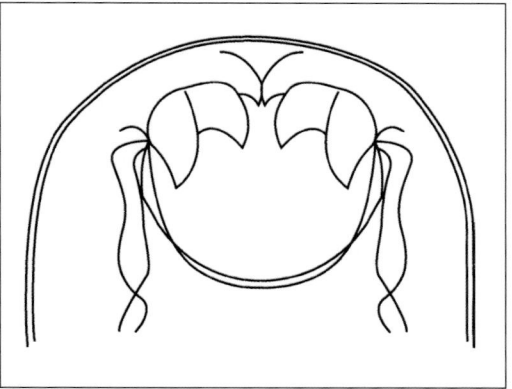

6.40   Illustration of the head of *Ancylostoma brazilienis*
showing two pairs of teeth at the entrance to the
buccal capsule. *Uncinaria stenocephala* has a similarly sized
buccal capsule but with cutting plates instead of teeth.
A. caninum has three pairs of teeth.

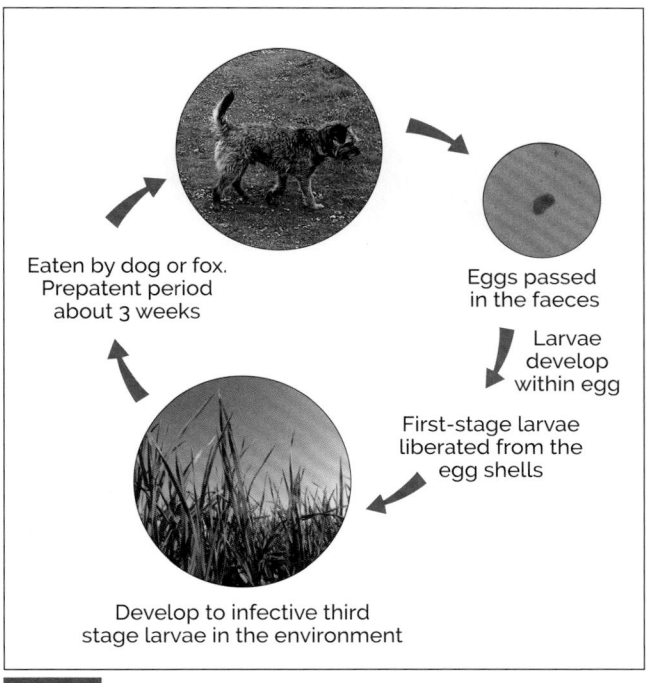

Eaten by dog or fox.
Prepatent period
about 3 weeks

Eggs passed
in the faeces

Larvae
develop
within egg

First-stage larvae
liberated from the
egg shells

Develop to infective third
stage larvae in the environment

6.41   Life cycle of *Uncinaria stenocephala*.

they are incapable of tissue migration, whereas those of *Ancylostoma* spp. may travel to the intestine and develop into adults. Bitches may also infect their puppies with *Ancylostoma* spp. larvae via their milk. Cats can be infected with hookworms, but this appears to be rare in the UK.

Whipworm

Trichuris vulpis has a whip-like appearance (Figure 6.42). The worms burrow into the mucosa of the large intestine, leaving the thicker caudal end in the intestinal lumen. A low burden is well tolerated but a heavy infection may be associated with bloody mucus-filled diarrhoea. The eggs have characteristic polar plugs (Figure 6.43) and are covered in a thick shell, which makes them resistant to environmental extremes. Eggs containing infective first stage larvae may survive for several years in the ground and thus *T. vulpis* tends to cause recurrent problems when dogs have access to permanent grass runs. Clinical disease due to this parasite is rarely seen in the UK.

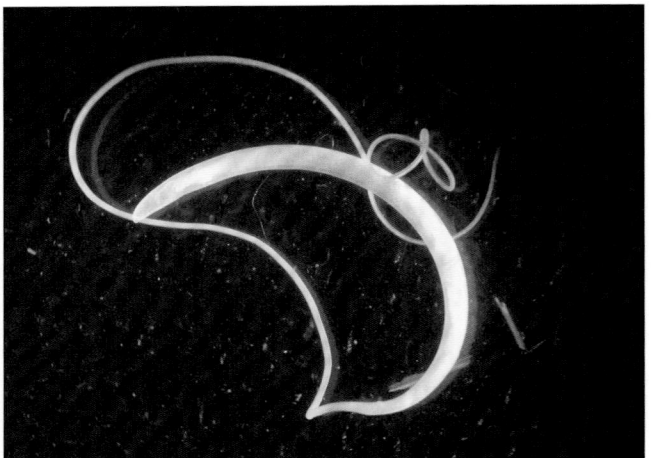

6.42 Typical appearance of *Trichuris vulpis*. Note the wide posterior end and the narrow anterior end normally buried in the mucosa of the large intestine (1–3 cm long). (© J McGarry)

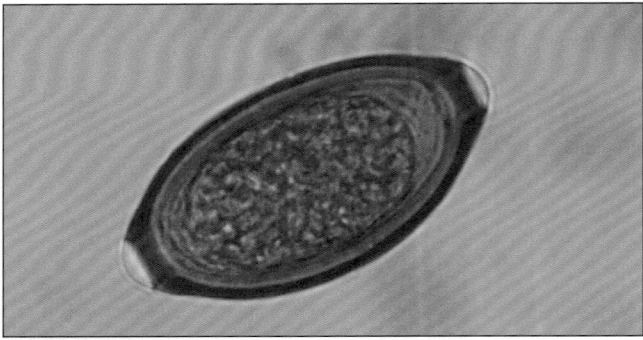

6.43 Microscopic image of a *Trichuris vulpis* egg (approximately 70 μm long). Note plugs at both ends. (© J McGarry)

Heartworm

Dirofilaria immitis does not occur in dogs in the UK, but may be seen in dogs imported from warmer countries. The adult worms live in the heart and produce first stage larvae known as microfilariae. These are dispersed in the host's blood and transmission occurs when a mosquito feeds and takes up the microfilariae, which then develop to the infective third stage

before being transferred to another dog when the mosquito feeds again. A light infection may be well tolerated but a larger burden can lead to right-sided heart failure. Infection in cats is somewhat less common, but the clinical effects of just a single worm can be severe.

This is another parasite to consider when owners are planning to take their pet to mainland Europe, as heartworm is endemic from the Mediterranean area of France southwards. Prophylactic treatment should be carried out by owners, using one of the licensed treatments recommended by their veterinary surgeon, following datasheet instructions. Adults of a related worm, *Dirofilaria repens*, are found under the skin. Transmission occurs in the same way as *D. immitis* and again this is an infection found in mainland Europe.

Eyeworm

Thelazia callipaeda are found on the surface of the eye and can cause lacrimation and other local signs. Infection is present in several countries across Europe, and this parasite was reported in dogs imported into the UK for the first time in 2016.

Oesophageal worm

Spirocerca lupi is found in the wall of the oesophagus of dogs and can cause cancerous changes to local tissue.

Bladder, respiratory tract and liver worms

Capillaria plica lives in the bladder and hence the eggs are passed in the urine of affected dogs. The eggs appear very like those of *Trichuris* (see Figure 6.43), but are smaller and have less distinct plugs, which are asymmetrically opposed. Infection is rarely seen in the UK.

Capillaria aerophila worms infect many wildlife hosts (mainly foxes and hedgehogs) and are found in the lower respiratory tract of cats and dogs; *Eucoleus boehmi* worms (a related species) infect the upper respiratory tract of dogs.

Capillaria hepatica is principally a parasite of brown rats. The adult worm lives in the liver of the host, where it lays its eggs. These are only released when the rat dies or is eaten by another animal. Cats, dogs and humans may be infected, but this occurs very rarely.

Other *Capillaria* species that are specific to birds may cause diarrhoea in pigeons.

Lungworms

Dogs (and foxes) tend to acquire the highly pathogenic nematode, *Angiostrongylus vasorum*, through eating slugs and other molluscs containing the infective third larvae (L3), but other routes not involving molluscs are also thought possible (e.g. ingestion of the free infective L3 from the environment (slime, water bowls, grass)). Transmission of this infection before 1990 was confined to south Wales and Cornwall, but it is now being seen in most of the country.

The slender adult worms live in the pulmonary artery of the dog, hence it is sometimes referred to as French heartworm. Adult females produce eggs that travel to the alveoli, where they develop and hatch; the larvae then penetrate the alveolar walls and travel through the parenchyma. They are coughed up, swallowed and passed in the faeces. Development to the infective stage (L3) occurs in a mollusc that has fed on faeces containing the first stage larvae. Clinical signs include coughing, dyspnoea and coagulopathies. The diagnosis is confirmed by finding first stage larvae in faecal samples (using Baermann equipment to concentrate the larvae from samples overnight), by radiography, by examining a bronchoalveolar lavage (BAL) sample or by performing a blood test which detects *A. vasorum* antigens.

Crenosoma vulpis, the fox lungworm, has a similar life cycle and pathogenesis to *A. vasorum*, although is far less common in both foxes and dogs. Another (rarer) lungworm, *Oslerus osleri*, may be found in small nodules at the bifurcation of the trachea (in dogs, particularly Greyhounds). The nodules can be seen on endoscopy; they may cause coughing in some dogs, but others tolerate their presence without showing clinical signs. The adult female worms produce larvae that are coughed up and swallowed. For this parasite, the life cycle is direct and the bitch may infect her puppies as she grooms them.

Cats become infected with *Aelurostrongylus abstrusus* (cat lungworm) by eating a slug or snail containing the infective larvae. The adult worm lives within the lung tissue of the cat. Infection with many worms may cause coughing, but a few worms often go unnoticed. Adult female worms produce larvae (rather than eggs) that are coughed up and swallowed. Diagnosis is confirmed by finding larvae in the faeces, using the Baermann technique (see Chapter 17).

Diagnosis of nematode infections

To confirm the diagnosis of nematode infection, worm eggs and larvae need to be identified in the faeces of companion animals (this is called coproanalysis). For coproanalaysis, it is very important that faecal samples are fresh and are quickly picked up from the ground, otherwise the sample can become contaminated with soil, as well as invaded by free-living nematodes and their eggs from the environment. The main diagnostic methods are modified McMaster techniques to detect and quantify nematode eggs in faeces and the Baermann technique (see Chapter 17) to detect larvae. Wet smears (in saline) can also be useful as an initial screening tool.

Treatment of nematode infections in dogs and cats

Treatment of nematode infections is carried out in three main situations.

Regular or routine treatment

A broad-spectrum anthelmintic with additional cestocidal activity is often used to remove any infections that may have accumulated since the animal was last wormed. Adult dogs and cats will usually be treated at intervals ranging from 1 month (in high-risk situations) to 3 months (in low-risk situations), depending on the likelihood of infection. There is now an option to control nematodes and fleas at the same time by using selamectin or imidacloprid plus moxidectin in cats and dogs, or lufenuron plus milbemycin in dogs; all of which are administered at monthly intervals (see Chapter 8). Like cestodes, there is no prophylactic treatment available, although some treatments are effective against immature nematodes and thus will prevent maturation of infections.

Toxocara infections in puppies and kittens

Since these infections occur in the vast majority of litters, it is normal to control them by treating all puppies and kittens regularly (from 2 weeks of age in puppies and 3 weeks in kittens until weaning), following the datasheet instructions for the product being used (see also 'Control of *Toxocara canis*', above).

Diagnosed nematode infection

Where the presence of a nematode infection has been diagnosed as the cause of a clinical problem, the product with the best activity against that infection will usually be chosen for treatment of the animal. Where regular treatment is not conducted, regular faecal examinations followed by treatment as required, is an alternative option.

Protozoal parasites
Coccidia

Coccidia may cause marked diarrhoea in young animals, particularly lambs, birds and rabbits.

Isospora

Two pathogenic species infect cats and another two pathogenic species infect dogs. The animals are infected when they ingest either sporulated oocysts (oocysts take a few days in the environment to reach this infective stage after they have been passed in the faeces) or infected intermediate hosts. Reproduction occurs in the cells lining the small intestine. Infection is usually associated with few clinical signs, but there may be transient diarrhoea. Heavy infection may cause severe diarrhoea in puppies and kittens. Toltrazuril has been reported to be an effective treatment and may be used under the Cascade (see Chapter 8).

Eimeria

Rabbits may be infected with three significantly pathogenic *Eimeria* species:

- *Eimeria intestinalis* and *E. flavescens* infect the caecum, causing diarrhoea and emaciation
- *E. stiedae* infects the bile ducts in the liver, causing wasting, diarrhoea and excess urine production.

Diagnosis is based on finding oocysts in the faeces (Figure 6.44). Treatment such as sulphonamide may be given in rabbits' drinking water, or to pet rabbits on an individual basis. Control is based on making sure that the rabbits have clean bedding and that droppings or diarrhoea are not allowed to build up in the feeding area.

Chickens, in common with other species of bird, are susceptible to several species of coccidia (*Eimeria* spp.), which in commercial flocks may be the cause of poor weight gain and/or mortality (depending on the *Eimeria* species involved) in young birds. The most common species affecting chickens are:

- *Eimeria tenella*: Pathogenic coccidian located in the caecum. Young chicks are most commonly affected, with high morbidity and mortality. Faeces from affected birds may contain visible blood

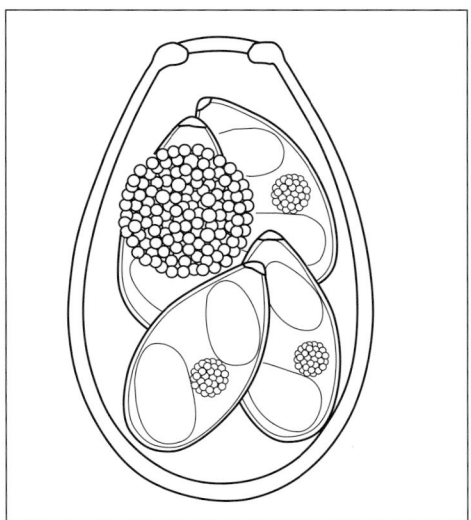

6.44 Illustration of a sporulated oocyst of *Eimeria* spp. (Reproduced from Urquhart *et al.*, 1996, with the permission of Blackwell Publishing)

- *E. necatrix:* Develops in the small intestine and caecum and may be associated with morbidity and mortality
- *E. acervulina* and *E. maxima:* Both develop in the upper part of the small intestine. Infection is typically associated with weight loss.

Prevention of disease can be achieved by careful attention to hygiene, although this can be difficult (e.g. with frequently used runs, wooden chicken houses), and anticoccidial treatments (medication, anticoccidial chemicals and ionophores) may be required. Dietary modification and the use of nutraceuticals have been investigated to reduce the effects of coccidial infection in chickens.

Cryptosporidium parvum

This small protozoan parasitizes epithelial cells in the small intestine. Both asexual and sexual reproduction occur in the intestine; and small oocysts, the result of sexual reproduction, are passed in the faeces. Infection occurs by ingesting sporulated oocysts; this has been associated with diarrhoea in young puppies and kittens and the young of other domestic animals including foals. Humans may be infected, usually only causing a transient diarrhoea, although severe diarrhoea may be associated with infection in immunocompromised individuals. Diagnosis is based on finding the oocysts (4.5–5 μm diameter) in the faeces. Identification may be assisted by staining with Ziehl–Neelsen, as the oocysts are acid-fast, or by using pet-side faecal antigen detection tests. There is currently no authorized treatment for the infection in small animals.

Toxoplasma gondii

The definitive (final) host for *T. gondii* is the cat (Figure 6.45). Sexual reproduction occurs in the epithelial cells of the small intestine. Large numbers of ocysts are produced that are passed in the faeces. The cat usually shows no sign of infection and normally, after excreting oocysts for about 10 days, becomes immune and stops production.

Asexual reproduction can occur in the extra-intestinal (outside the intestine) tissue of almost any animal. Following ingestion of oocysts or asexual stages, the sporozoites leave the intestine and travel to tissue, particularly muscle or brain. Here they divide to form tachyzoites. Once an immune response is initiated by the host, these undergo slower division; they are then known as bradyzoites, which remain in the tissue ready for consumption by the cat (the definitive (final) host). The tissue cysts are minute and cause few problems except in certain circumstances:

- Where a ewe is infected for the first time during pregnancy, as a result of eating feed contaminated with cat faeces, the normal immune responses are compromised in the placenta and the cysts are able to replicate. This may result in abortion, stillbirth or weak lambs
- Where a woman is infected for the first time during pregnancy, perhaps by eating meat containing bradyzoites or accidentally swallowing sporulated oocysts shed from a cat, infection of the fetus may result. Depending on the stage of pregnancy, this may result in abortion or severe abnormalities or in no clinical signs at all. Fortunately, infections during human pregnancy are not common. Further information and leaflets can be obtained from Tommy's website (www.tommys.org)
- Infection in humans may be associated with malaise and 'flu-like symptoms that vary in severity from individual to individual
- Cysts in immunosuppressed individuals may begin to undergo rapid division and cause severe tissue lesions.

6.45 Life cycle of *Toxoplasma gondii.*

Cat infected by eating intermediate host

Oocysts passed in large numbers in the faeces

Sexual reproduction in the cat's intestine

Bradyzoites

Cat infected by eating sporulated oocyst

Oocysts become infective i.e. sporulated, after about 3 days

Other host (sheep, human, mouse, dog, etc.) infected by eating sporulated oocyst

Tachyzoites

Other animals may be infected by eating meat containing bradyzoites

Asexual reproduction occurs in the tissues of non-cat host

In order to try to prevent these infections occurring:

- Farmers are advised to prevent cats, particularly young cats, from getting into food stores intended for sheep
- Sheep can be vaccinated against *Toxoplasma gondii*
- Pregnant women are advised to take precautionary measures. For example, they should not clean out cat litter trays, they should wear gloves when gardening, they should not assist with lambing ewes, and they should ensure that all meat is thoroughly cooked before eating it.

There is no effective treatment to prevent cats shedding the oocysts. Children who have been infected prenatally (before birth) are treated with antiprotozoals to prevent any long-term effects.

Sarcocystis

This organism has a complex life cycle. The intermediate hosts are ruminants, pigs or horses. Large unsightly cysts are formed in muscle and so infected meat is condemned. In addition, infection may result in marked illness in the infected animal, including reduced weight gain, anaemia, myositis, abortion and neurological signs. The definitive (final) host for each species is the dog or the cat; the definitive host is unlikely to show any overt signs of infection. For example, *Sarcocystis tenella* (also known as *S. ovicanis*) is a parasite of sheep and dogs. Reproduction occurs in the small intestine of the definitive host without clinical signs. The oocysts, measuring approximately 10–15 µm, are already sporulated when passed.

Neospora caninum

This parasite causes incoordination in young dogs and abortion in cattle. In the past, infection was normally ascribed to *Toxoplasma gondii*. The dog is the definitive (final) host for this parasite. Treatment of affected puppies may be necessary. Breeding bitches can be screened serologically for signs of infection.

Hammondia

This is a lesser known protozoan parasite where the cat is the definitive (final) host. Infection is not normally associated with clinical signs. Sexual reproduction occurs in the intestine of the cat and the oocysts produced appear similar to those of *Toxoplasma*. Rodents are the intermediate hosts for *Hammondia* and so the presence of oocysts does not present a zoonotic risk.

Giardia spp.

This flagellate protozoan may parasitize the small intestine of humans and domestic animals. The species found in most mammals is *Giardia intestinalis*, also known as *G. duodenalis* and *G. lamblia*. It is still unknown how important *Giardia* infection in pet animals is as a source of human infection, although some strains of *G. intestinalis* have been identified as potential zoonoses, whilst others are not. The species in mice and other small rodents is *G. muris*. Infection with *G. psittaci* may cause death in cage birds such as cockatiels and budgerigars.

Infection may be asymptomatic or may be associated with transient or chronic diarrhoea. Puppies are at greatest risk. Diagnosis is based on demonstration of the cysts (Figure 6.46), which are small (approximately 10 µm) and may be passed intermittently in the faeces. Even when a sample is

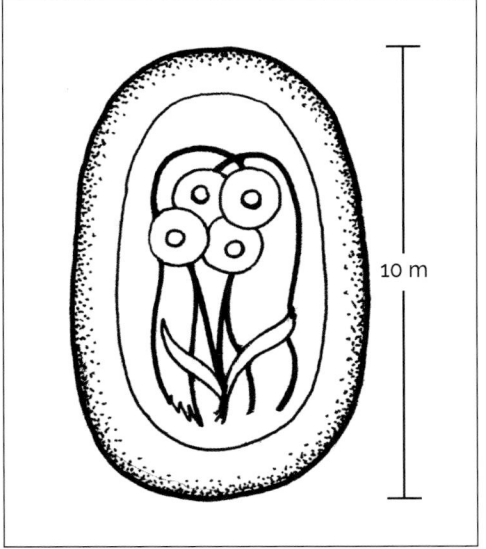

10 m

6.46 Illustration of a cyst of *Giardia* spp.

positive, cysts may be present in low numbers, so a sensitive microscopic detection technique is required. It has been suggested that collecting faecal samples for 3 days and pooling the sample may increase the chance of detecting the cysts. Other diagnostic methods based on the identification of antigens can also be used to confirm infection. Treatment can be carried out with repeat doses of benzimidazoles, such as fenbendazole, or with metronidazole. Cleaning and hygiene, to eliminate cysts and hence prevent re-infection, are important parts of controlling an outbreak.

Encephalitozoon cuniculi

E. cuniculi is a microsporidian parasite of rabbits that can also affect humans and a variety of other animals. Microsporidia were classified as Protozoa, but their classification is currently under review. Rabbits are infected by ingestion of spores from the environment or from infected rabbit urine. Between 7.5% and 68.1% of rabbits have seroconverted, i.e. have antibodies in the blood, which is indicative of exposure to infection. However, disease only develops in a proportion of these animals. Signs of disease are varied and include head tilt, ill-thrift (failure to grow, gain weight or maintain weight in the presence of apparently adequate food supplies), weight loss and renal failure, as infection localizes in a number of organs, particularly the nervous system and kidneys. Treatment consists of symptomatic treatment and administration of fenbendazole to eliminate the infection. There is also evidence that treatment with fenbendazole may be useful to eliminate the parasite in infected but asymptomatic animals.

Tritrichomonas foetus

Tritrichomonas foetus is a unicellular flagellate protozoan that can cause chronic diarrhoea in cats. Since it was first recognized as a pathogen in cats (it is the same organism that causes sexually transmitted disease in bulls) in 2003, it has been the subject of substantial research aimed at understanding its pathology, epidemiology and treatment. It can occur as a co-infection with other pathogens. Diagnosis is by direct visualization of the parasite in a smear or by using diagnostic kits (Yao and Köster, 2015).

Babesia spp.

Babesia spp. are parasites that infect the red blood cells of dogs, thereby causing anaemia. This is a tick-transmitted infection endemic in central and southern Europe. An outbreak of apparently locally transmitted babesiosis has been reported in dogs from Harlow in Essex (de Marco *et al.*, 2017). Infection can result in acute disease with fever, jaundice and even death if the infection is particularly severe or is not treated rapidly.

Leishmania spp.

Leishmaniosis is caused by a flagellate protozoan (*Leishmania* spp.) and is transmitted by sandflies in many warmer parts of the world, including the Mediterranean area. The incubation period (time between exposure to the causative pathogen and the first appearance of clinical signs) can be particularly long and it is often extremely difficult to clear the infection completely with drug treatment. Dogs, particularly rescued animals, infected with *Leishmania* are not infrequently imported into the UK and may be increasingly seen in veterinary practices. Signs of infection are various and can include dermatological signs, such as localized alopecia, and systemic signs including weight loss.

Additional information on exotic pets

Examples of parasites in exotic pets have been included throughout the main text and are further summarized in Figure 6.47. The range of parasites in these species is large, however, and the relevant species-specific BSAVA Manuals and other books should be consulted for more complete details. There are few authorized treatments for exotic pets, but a wider variety are available under the Exemptions for Small Pet Animals (ESPA) scheme. More information can be found on the Veterinary Medicines Directorate website, and in the *BSAVA Small Animal Formulary, Part B: Exotic Pets.*

References and further reading

De Marco MDMF, Hernández-Triana LM, Phipps LP, Hansford K, Mitchell ES *et al.* (2017) Emergence of Babesia canis in southern England. *Parasites and Vectors* **10**, 241

Eatwell K and Hedley J (2019) Parasitology. In: *BSAVA Manual of Reptiles, 3rd edn*, ed. S Girling and P Raiti, pp. 411–422. BSAVA Publications, Gloucester

Host	Parasite group							
	Ectoparasites					**Endoparasites**		
	Lice	**Fleas**	**Flies**	**Mites**	**Ticks**	**Cestodes**	**Nematodes**	**Protozoa**
Rabbits	*Haemodipsus ventricosus*	*Spilopsyllus cuniculi* *Ctenocephalides felis*	*Lucilia* spp.	*Psoroptes cuniculi* *Cheyletiella parasitivorax* *Listrophorus gibbus*	Various	*Cysticercus pisiformis* *Coenurus serialis*		*Eimeria intestinalis* *E. flavescens* *E. stiedae*
Mice	*Polyplax serrata*	*Ctenocephalides felis*		*Myobia musculi* *Myocoptes musculinus*				
Rats	*Polyplax spinulosa*			*Radfordia ensifera* *Notoedres muris*				
Hamsters		*Ctenocephalides felis*		*Demodex* spp.				
Guinea pigs	*Gliricola porcelli*			*Trixacarus caviae*				*Eimeria caviae*
Ferrets		*Ctenocephalides felis*		*Otodectes cynotis* *Sarcoptes scabiei*	*Ixodes* spp.			
Parrots				*Dermanyssus gallinae*			*Ascaridia* spp.	*Giardia* spp. *Eimeria* spp.
Budgerigars				*Cnemidocoptes* spp. *Dermanyssus gallinae*			*Ascaridia* spp.	*Giardia* spp. *Eimeria* spp. *Trichomonas* spp.
Tortoises			Various		Various spp.		*Ascaridia* spp.	*Hexamita* spp.
Bearded dragons				*Ophionyssus natricis*	Various spp.		*Ascaridia* spp.	*Isospora* spp.

6.47 Key parasites found in exotic pets. The dark grey shading indicates those parasites that are of important clinical significance. The lighter grey shading indicates where there are also parasites in a group that are of less clinical significance in that exotic pet species. Data compiled from Eatwell and Hedley (2019); Harcourt-Brown (2007); Harcourt-Brown and Chitty (2005); Keeble and Meredith (2009); Meredith and Johnson-Delaney (2009) and Paterson (2006).

Harcourt-Brown F (2007) *Textbook of Rabbit Medicine.* Butterworth Heinemann, London

Harcourt-Brown N and Chitty J (2005) *BSAVA Manual of Psittacine Birds, 2nd edn.* BSAVA Publications, Gloucester

Jackson HA and Marsella R (2012) *BSAVA Manual of Canine and Feline Dermatology, 3rd edn.* BSAVA Publications, Gloucester

Jacobs D, Fox M, Gibbons L and Hermosilla C (2015) *Principles of Veterinary Parasitology.* Wiley Blackwell, Oxford

Keeble E and Meredith A (2009) *BSAVA Manual of Rodents and Ferrets.* BSAVA Publications, Gloucester

Meredith A (2015) *BSAVA Small Animal Formulary – Part B: Exotic Pets, 9th edn.* BSAVA Publications, Gloucester

Meredith A and Johnson-Delaney C (2009) *BSAVA Manual of Exotic Pets, 5th edn.* BSAVA Publications, Gloucester

Meredith A and Lord B (2014) BSAVA *Manual of Rabbit Medicine.* BSAVA Publications, Gloucester

Paterson S (2006) *Skin Diseases of Exotic Pets.* Blackwell Publishing, Oxford

Taylor MA, Coop RL and Wall RL (2015) *Veterinary Parasitology, 4th edn.* Wiley Blackwell, Oxford

Varga M (2013) *Textbook of Rabbit Medicine, 2nd edn.* Elsevier, Oxford

Yao C and Köster LS (2015) *Tritrichomonas foetus* infection, a cause of chronic diarrhea in the domestic cat. *Veterinary Research* **46**, 35

Zajac AM and Conboy GA (2012) *Veterinary Clinical Parasitology, 8th edn.* Wiley Blackwell, Oxford

Useful websites

BSAVA Position Statement and supporting information – Parasite control:
www.bsava.com

European Scientific Counsel Companion Animal Parasites (ESCCAP) – provides guidelines for parasite control in dogs and cats:
www.esccapuk.org.uk
www.esccap.org

National Office of Animal Health (NOAH) compendium – datasheets for ectoparasiticides and endoparasiticides:
www.noahcompendium.co.uk

Tommy's – information about toxoplasmosis in pregnancy:
www.tommys.org

UK Government – Bringing your pet dog, cat or ferret to the UK: Pet passport and other documents:
www.gov.uk/take-pet-abroad

Veterinary Medicines Directorate (VMD) – information about authorized medicines and the Exemption for Small Pet Animals (ESPA) scheme:
www.gov.uk/government/organisations/veterinary-medicines-directorate

Self-assessment questions

1. Define the terms 'ectoparasite' and 'endoparasite'.
2. Describe how you could differentiate between an insect and an arachnid.
3. Describe how you could differentiate between a burrowing and a surface mite.
4. List the zoonotic ectoparasites and zoonotic endoparasites of dogs and cats.
5. Define the terms 'permanent' ectoparasite and 'direct life cycle'.
6. State the four ways in which dogs can become infected with *Toxocara canis*.
7. Compare and contrast the transmission routes of *T.canis* with those of *Toxocara cati*.
8. Based on the transmission routes of the two species, identify prevention and treatment options for both *T. canis* and *T. cati*.
9. State the most common cestode of the dog and cat and describe how this tapeworm is transmitted.
10. Name the cestode that has to be treated for under the Pet Passport Scheme and the treatment given. Why is this parasite particularly important?
11. Give two examples of pathogens that can be transmitted by ticks.
12. Give one example of a pathogen transmitted by sandflies.

Chapter 7

Principles of infection and immunity

Susan Dawson and Barbara Cooper

Learning objectives

After studying this chapter, readers will have the knowledge to:

- **Define common terms associated with disease transmission**
- **Describe relationships between microorganisms and host in health and disease**
- **List factors that may influence the occurrence, onset and severity of disease**
- **List routes of entry of infectious agents into the host, providing examples**
- **Describe how pathogens establish, spread and multiply within the host, triggering disease**
- **Identify which infectious agents may be shed and transmitted**
- **Apply the principles involved in the control of infectious disease**
- **Describe the functional components of the immune system**
- **Explain the underlying principles of vaccines and vaccination**
- **Discuss the principles of hypersensitivity and other immune disorders**

Principles of infection and infectious disease

Definitions

- **Infection** is the **colonization** of an individual (host) by a foreign microorganism. Infectious agents that cause harm are termed **pathogens**; these can live within or on the host and disrupt physiological function
- **Disease** occurs when normal bodily functions are sufficiently impaired to reduce performance, leading to specific recognizable clinical signs. Though infection is a common cause of disease, there are many other potential causes
- Infectious diseases may be **contagious**, i.e. spread through **contagion** directly or indirectly from one individual host to another. They may be caused by organisms such as bacteria, viruses, fungi or parasites. Important examples of contagious diseases are given in Chapter 18. The ability of a pathogen to spread varies and is dependent on:
  - **Transmissibility:** the capacity to pass from one host to another, typically determined by the ability of the pathogen to survive outside the body
  - **Infectivity:** the ability to penetrate host defences
- **Pathogenicity** is the ability of a pathogen to cause disease, and it is dependent on both its capacity to spread and its ability to harm the host, or virulence (Figure 7.1)
- **Epidemiology** is the study of the occurrence, spread and distribution of disease in populations and is of vital importance in the design and monitoring of effective control policies
- **Endemic** refers to a disease present at a normal level in a country or region. For example, myxomatosis is now **endemic** in wild rabbits in the UK and feline calicivirus (FCV) is **endemic** in the domestic cat population
- **Epidemic** refers to a disease where a pronounced increase in incidence has been observed within a country or geographical region. The foot-and-mouth **epidemic** in the UK in 2001 led to controls on movement and widespread slaughter of infected and at-risk livestock

➔

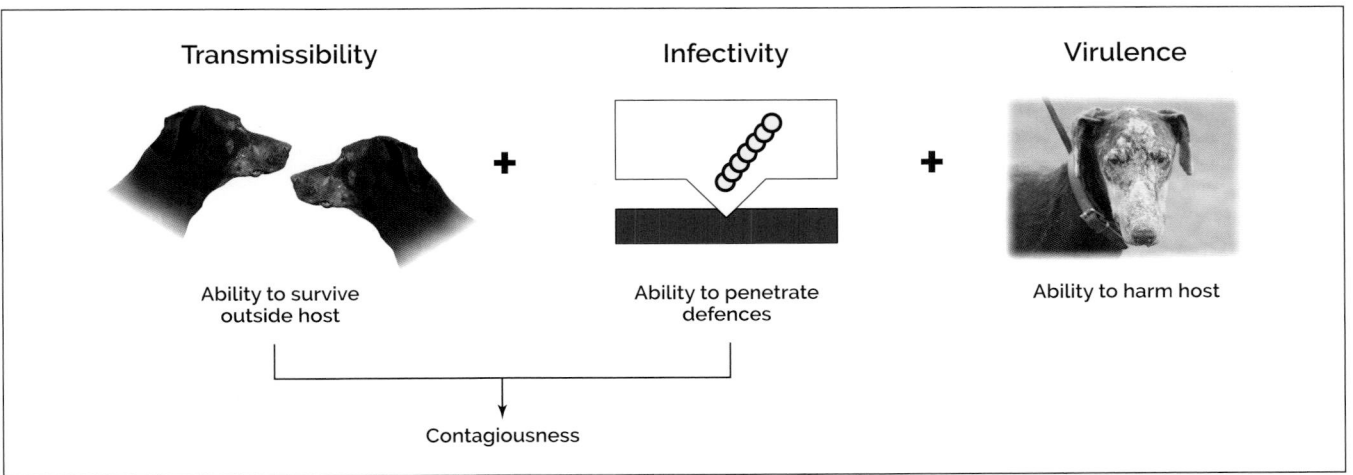

7.1 Factors influencing pathogenicity.

The resident microflora

Most microorganisms, or microbes (see Chapter 5), are useful to people and animals and may even be vital for life; relatively few are associated with ill health. The skin, oral cavity, conjunctiva, gastrointestinal tract and distal urogenital tracts all house a varied resident microflora, consisting of billions of microbes – principally bacteria. These organisms are described as commensal, because they share the body and usually do no harm; furthermore, their presence may help to prevent colonization by more harmful organisms.

Non-contagious disease

Microbes that normally live benignly on or within the host or environment can cause disease. Such infections, most commonly bacterial, are less likely to lead to disease in other in-contact individuals, but gain advantage in the affected host because normal innate immunity (see 'Innate immunity', below) is weakened or bypassed, or abnormal local conditions favour infection. Common examples include:

- Cat-bite abscesses
- Wound infections
- Bacterial skin infection (pyoderma) (Figure 7.2)
- Bladder infection (bacterial cystitis).

Factors influencing occurrence and severity of disease

In order to trigger disease, pathogens need to:

- Penetrate host defences and establish themselves
- Multiply on or within host tissues

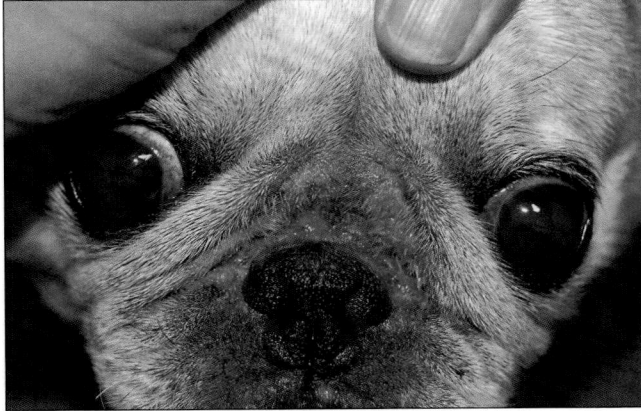

7.2 Erythema and mild exudation in intertrigo (skin fold pyoderma). (Reproduced from the *BSAVA Manual of Canine and Feline Dermatology, 3rd edn*)

- Overcome the initial natural defence mechanisms within the host
- Harm the host in some way.

The expression of disease in an individual depends on a balance between the nature of the infectious challenge and the resistance of the host. The capacity of an infection to cause disease is determined by:

- The infective dose, i.e. the number of agents, such as bacteria or viral particles
- The virulence of the agent; this may vary between different strains.

Host susceptibility may be increased by:

- YOPI (young, old, pregnant, immunosuppressed)
- Stress (e.g. transport, novel environment)

- Concurrent disease (e.g. chronic disease in older individuals)
- Genetic factors (e.g. inbreeding, breed predispositions)
- Lack of or reduction in immunity (e.g. immunosuppressive illness such as feline immunodeficiency virus)
- Medication (e.g. immunosuppressive drugs such as corticosteroids)
- Malnutrition.

Based on the balance between the infectivity of an agent and host susceptibility, a number of outcomes are possible:

- The pathogen may be eliminated by the immune system without consequence to the host
- Subclinical infection may occur, i.e. an animal is infected but does not show any clinical signs of disease. There is a possible risk of transmission to other animals
- Disease may occur, associated with infection and risk of transmission to others.

The **incubation period** for an infectious disease is the time interval elapsing between exposure to the causative pathogen and the first clinical signs appearing. For many diseases this period is a few days, but it may be weeks, months or even years. Dose and virulence of the infecting pathogen, as well as host susceptibility, can affect both incubation period and the severity of disease, so that within a group of infected individuals both the severity and onset of clinical signs can vary markedly.

Routes of entry

Pathogens infect new hosts via a variety of routes

- Ingestion (taken in via the mouth): in contaminated food or water; during hunting or mutual grooming; through coprophagia (ingestion of faeces); through contact with infected items (fomites; see 'Mechanical vectors', below)
- Inhalation (breathing in) of infected particles (droplet infection) (e.g. kennel cough in dogs, *Bordatella bronchiseptica* infection in guinea pigs)
- Direct contact with saliva/nasal secretions (e.g. FCV, rabbit haemorrhagic viral disease (RHVD) viruses)
- Through the skin: through bite or surgical wounds; via vectors such as fleas, ticks or mosquitoes (e.g. Lyme disease (borreliosis), *Dirofilaria immitis* (heartworm), myxomatosis)
- Via skin contact (e.g. ectoparasites, ringworm)
- Across mucous membranes: gastrointestinal and respiratory epithelia are frequent entry routes; *Leptospira* bacteria may penetrate intact mucosae as well as damaged skin
- Across the placenta or during birth (e.g. *Toxocara canis*, feline panleucopenia, feline leukaemia virus)

Spread within the host

Pathogens commonly establish and multiply at the point of entry. For many viral pathogens, this is in the epithelial cells of the gastrointestinal or respiratory tracts. From these initial entry points spread to local lymph nodes may then occur. Infection may remain localized in response to a rapid immune response and/or because of a preference (predilection, tropism) for certain cell types. Alternatively, the agent may spread into the blood circulation. The occurrence of virus within the blood is called **viraemia**. Bacterial infection may also remain localized, but serious infections can spread systemically via the bloodstream (**bacteraemia**). **Septicaemia** occurs if bacteria actively multiply in the bloodstream leading to sepsis.

How pathogens trigger disease

Harm may be caused in a variety of ways.

- The cells within tissues may be destroyed by the pathogen itself. For example, in order to reproduce and propagate, viruses 'hijack' the normal metabolic processes of the host cell, finally rupturing and destroying the cell as new virus particles leave to infect other host cells (see Chapter 5).
- Biological poisons (toxins) may disrupt normal physiological function. The presence of toxins in the circulation is called toxaemia. In severe sepsis, circulatory collapse caused by endotoxic shock is a potentially life-threatening consequence. (See Chapter 5 for more discussion on microbial toxins.)
- The response of the immune system to infection may cause damage. For example, in patients with feline infectious peritonitis (FIP), which is caused by a coronavirus, the actual damage occurs as a result of the body's immune response attempting to eliminate the virus. This may damage organs, commonly including the kidneys, eyes and central nervous system ('dry' form of FIP), or may lead to exudation of large quantities of fluid into the chest or abdominal cavity ('wet' form of FIP). See also 'Allergy and hypersensitivity reactions', below.

Transmission

For pathogens to succeed and propagate they need to both infect a host and have the capacity to spread to other susceptible individuals.

Direct transmission

This involves the spread of pathogens by direct contact. Direct transmission is particularly important for fragile pathogens such as feline leukaemia virus (FeLV) and feline immunodeficiency virus (FIV), because they are unable to survive for long outside the host. Examples of direct transmission include bites, scratches and droplet spread.

Indirect transmission

This occurs if infection is acquired from a contaminated environment or via a vector.

Mechanical vectors

Also known as fomites, these may be inanimate objects such as bedding, grooming kits, feed buckets/bowls and litter trays. People may also act as vectors by transporting infection on skin, clothing or shoes. For example, canine parvovirus persists for many months or years in the environment and is susceptible to few disinfectants. Virus is excreted by infected puppies for only a few days. Due to the survival ability of the virus, indirect spread via ingestion from an environment contaminated by the faeces of infected dogs is the most significant route. Direct ingestion of the faeces of an infected dog (coprophagia) would also be a possible route of transmission.

Biological vectors

These are organisms that may not cause disease in their own right but may convey infectious agents from one host to another. A number of significant canine diseases, for which dogs travelling to Europe and beyond may be at risk, are transmitted by biological vectors. Important examples of such vectors include: sandflies, which transmit leishmaniosis; ticks, which may transmit a number of serious infections including Lyme disease (borreliosis), babesiosis and ehrlichiosis; and mosquitoes, which may carry the *Dirofilaria immitis* heartworm.

Horizontal transmission

This term is sometimes applied to direct or indirect spread of infections between individuals of the same generation.

Vertical transmission

In some infections, transmission occurs from dam to offspring, either before or during birth. Possible effects of fetal infection include:

- Fetal death, resorption, mummification, abortion or stillbirth
- Birth of individuals showing clinical signs of disease
- Poor viability (e.g. fading kittens or puppies)
- Birth of infected carriers showing no disease signs (i.e. animals that are subclinically infected and asymptomatic).

Different infective agents may be excreted or 'shed' by a variety of routes. Careful consideration of likely routes of transmission enables appropriate disease control measures to be implemented.

Routes of transmission

- In saliva, via bites (e.g. rabies, FIV)
- In nasal or ocular discharges (e.g. feline upper respiratory tract disease: feline calicivirus, feline herpesvirus; *Chlamydia felis* conjunctivitis in cats; RHVD in rabbits)
- In urine (e.g. leptospirosis; infectious canine hepatitis)
- In faeces or vomitus (e.g. canine parvovirus; bacterial enteritis; panleucopenia; salmonellosis)
- In blood, via a biological vector (e.g. feline infectious anaemia caused by *Mycoplasma haemofelis* is transmitted by fleas)
- In milk (e.g. FeLV; FIV; *Toxocara*)
- Across the placenta (transplacentally) to the fetus *in utero* (e.g. *Toxocara canis*; panleucopenia)
- By aerosol, i.e. airborne (e.g. 'kennel cough'; canine distemper; *Bordatella bronchiseptica*)
- By skin contact (e.g. ectoparasites; ringworm)
- During coitus or parturition (e.g. panleucopenia; FIV; myxomatosis)
- In water contaminated with animal faeces or urine
- Via fomites such as bedding, towels, water and feed bowls and toys

---

Carriers

In some diseases, infected animals, known as carriers, may continue to shed infective agents despite showing minimal or no signs of disease.

- Cats infected with feline herpesvirus (FHV) carry infection throughout their lives and may 'shed' virus intermittently, throughout life, with or without signs of disease, usually following episodes of stress. Between periods of shedding, the infection remains latent (dormant) and the virus cannot be isolated on swabs.
- In contrast, cats infected with FCV shed virus continuously, following apparent recovery from disease. Unlike FHV infection, most FCV-infected individuals eliminate the infection completely within weeks or months; however, a small proportion of cats can remain subclinically infected for years.

Controlling infection and disease

A range of measures must be taken in order to contain the potential spread of infection between animals and from animals to humans (see 'Zoonoses', below) and to reduce the risk of disease occurring. Hygiene measures in hospital wards are discussed further in Chapter 14 and include:

- Efficient cleaning and appropriate use of disinfection of accommodation, paying attention to potential fomites
- Careful cleaning and disposal of faeces, urine, body fluids and discharges; appropriate disposal of contaminated waste
- Good hygiene in all stages of storage, handling and preparation of pet food. High-quality tinned and dry diets are available and avoid the potential hazards of offering raw meat, which can potentially present a source of food-poisoning bacteria and parasites.

Animal management risks should be considered:

- Quarantine animals with suspected contagion and newly introduced animals of unknown health status (see 'Isolation and quarantine', below)
- 'Barrier nurse' cases of suspected infectious disease.

To manage disease risk factors, the following actions should be considered.

- Wear suitable protective clothing whenever handling animals; change clothing if it becomes soiled.
- Observe regular hand hygiene – wash/disinfect hands between patients (Figure 7.3) and before touching any potential fomites (consider pens, clinical notes, cigarettes, door handles, food, cups, etc.).
- Ensure good draught-free ventilation and low stocking rates in multi-animal facilities, such as kennels and catteries. Avoid mixing animals in large groups and in the same airspace.
- Rest accommodation following occupation for as long as practicable, depending on the likely persistence of the infectious agent(s) of concern, to reduce the risk of residual environmental contamination.

How to Handwash?

WASH HANDS WHEN VISIBLY SOILED! OTHERWISE, USE HANDRUB

🕐 **Duration of the entire procedure:** 40-60 seconds

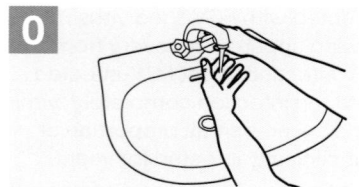

0 Wet hands with water;

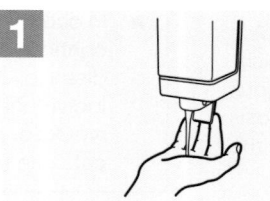

1 Apply enough soap to cover all hand surfaces;

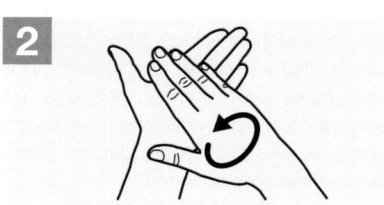

2 Rub hands palm to palm;

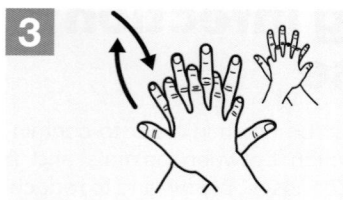

3 Right palm over left dorsum with interlaced fingers and vice versa;

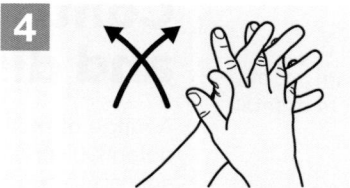

4 Palm to palm with fingers interlaced;

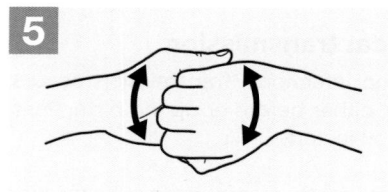

5 Backs of fingers to opposing palms with fingers interlocked;

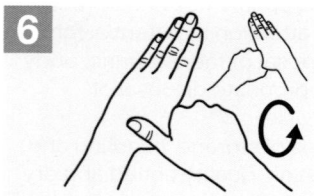

6 Rotational rubbing of left thumb clasped in right palm and vice versa;

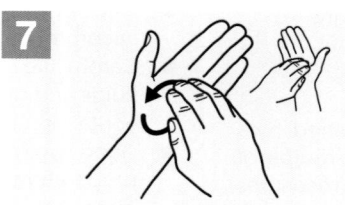

7 Rotational rubbing, backwards and forwards with clasped fingers of right hand in left palm and vice versa;

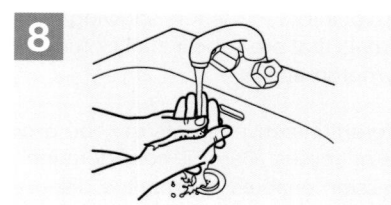

8 Rinse hands with water;

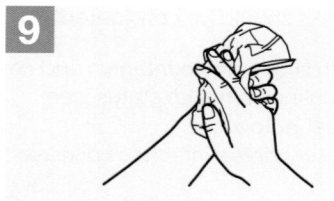

9 Dry hands thoroughly with a single use towel;

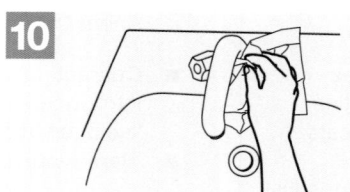

10 Use towel to turn off faucet;

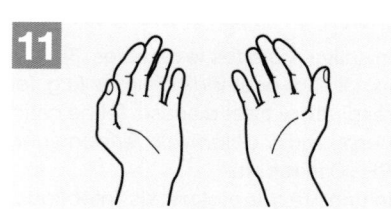

11 Your hands are now safe.

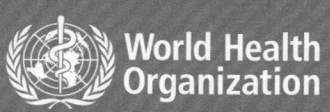

World Health Organization | **Patient Safety** A World Alliance for Safer Health Care | **SAVE LIVES** Clean **Your** Hands

7.3 World Health Organization (WHO) poster providing instructions on how to hand wash. (© World Health Organization 2009)

- Minimize stress through good husbandry. Ensure optimum nutrition and prompt attention to any ancillary health problems.
- Control disease vectors, such as external parasites. Where appropriate, reduce populations of stray animals, via rescue centres and neutering programmes.
- Immunize against infectious agents where possible and appropriate. Use appropriate vaccines in animals (and people), both routinely and targeted where specific disease risks are identified.
- Consider animals more at risk of infection due to the presence of underlying disease.
- Prepare food safely: meat and fruit/vegetables should be prepared separately.
- Avoid sharing of food/water bowls, bedding and toys.
- Avoid unnecessary travel/movement of animals.

Owners should also be educated regarding disease risks, hygiene and good husbandry, including endo- and ectoparasite control and vaccination.

Apparently healthy animals may harbour infection and it may be unclear that an animal carries a zoonosis, so care should always be exercised. In addition to the general risk reduction measures listed above, some special precautions should be taken.

Hand hygiene

- Effective hand hygiene and disinfection should be practised between all patients
- A handwashing procedure, such as that recommended by the World Health Organization (WHO; see Figure 7.3) should be followed
- Hands should be washed:
  - Before and after touching a patient
  - Before and after touching a patient's surroundings or any potential fomites
  - Before gloving
  - Before any clean or aseptic task
  - After any risk of exposure to contaminated fluids or tissue (even if gloves have been worn)
  - Between patients

Precautions against the spread of zoonotic infections

- Do not allow animals to lick people (particularly on the face and mouth). Children are particularly at risk as they have higher susceptibility and lower awareness of basic hygiene
- Facilities and utensils for animal food preparation and washing up should be separate from those for human use
- Avoid unnecessary exposure to infections: reduce unnecessary animal handling and ensure that handling technique minimizes risk (e.g. from bites/scratches)
- Pregnant women and immunocompromised individuals should be especially vigilant about personal hygiene after animal contact, since infection risks are greater
- Always seek medical advice if human infection is suspected
- Tetanus immunization is advisable for all veterinary nurses. If working with wild animals, zoo animals or captive primates, vaccinations against rabies, tuberculosis and hepatitis should also be considered
- Avoid unnecessary animal travel
- Regularly clean and disinfect the animal environment
- Cook meat and eggs thoroughly, and wash raw fruits and vegetables
- Appropriate disposal of faeces, urine and other body excretions
- Prevent bites from ticks, fleas and mosquitoes

Zoonoses

Zoonoses (singular: zoonosis) are diseases that are transmissible from animals to humans. Some are potentially life-threatening (e.g. rabies, leptospirosis), while others may pass unnoticed unless an individual is particularly susceptible; toxoplasmosis, for example, is mainly a risk in pregnant or immune-suppressed individuals. Figure 7.4 lists some important examples of zoonotic infections.

Nosocomial infections

Infections acquired by patients in hospital are termed nosocomial infections and are of particular concern because the patient's immunity may be compromised by underlying disease, drugs, surgery, invasive supportive care (e.g. intravenous or urinary catheters), malnutrition or stress. Poor hygiene and transfer of pathogens between patients, combined with the potential for build-up of antimicrobial

Disease/infection	Risk source
Major enteric infections	
Campylobacter spp.	Contaminated food (esp. poultry meat); faeces of livestock, poultry, dogs, cats, wild birds
Salmonella spp.	Contaminated food; faeces of carrier mammals including livestock and pets, and of birds, reptiles and fish
Eschericia coli (Strain VTEC O157)	Contaminated food; faeces of healthy carrier livestock and birds
Cryptosporidiosis	Contaminated water; livestock (esp. calves, lambs)
Notifiable animal diseases in the UK	
Anthrax	Cutaneous form from contact with imported infected hide (very unlikely)
Avian influenza (fowl plague)	Airborne from infected poultry

7.4 Some important examples of zoonoses. [a] Disease currently absent from the UK. [b] *Echinococcus granulosus* tapeworm in UK; *E. multilocularis* is currently absent from the UK but present in mainland Europe. *continues* ▶

Disease/infection	Risk source
Notifiable animal diseases in the UK continued	
Bovine spongiform encephalopathy (causes variant Creutzfeld-Jakob disease in humans)	Ingestion of contaminated beef
Bovine tuberculosis (TB)	Unpasteurized milk (now unlikely in the UK). Most cases due to human TB
Brucellosis	Contact with infected aborting cattle
Rabies[a]/European bat lyssavirus (EBL-2)	Mammalian hosts (esp. dogs) via bites. Risk in UK of EBL from bites from infected bats
West Nile Virus (WNV)[a]	Mosquito transmission – wild birds, horses
Other important zoonoses	
Hydatid disease[b]	Dog faeces
Leptospirosis	Water-borne; urine of infected rats, dogs, cattle
Orf	Viral skin infection of sheep
Pasteurellosis	Animal bites – cats and dogs
Psittacosis	Infected birds (esp. psittacines)
Ringworm	Contact with infected dogs, cats, livestock and wildlife (e.g. hedgehogs)
Toxocariasis	Dogs, cats (roundworms)
Toxoplasmosis	Cat faeces; uncooked meat

7.4 continued Some important examples of zoonoses. [a] Disease currently absent from the UK. [b] *Echinococcus granulosus* tapeworm in UK; *E. multilocularis* is currently absent from the UK but present in mainland Europe.

resistance, lead to increased risk of exposure and of more severe consequences if infection occurs. These infections can be endogenous, arising from an agent present within the body of the animal, or exogenous, being transmitted from another source within the practice.

Examples of nosocomial infections include:

- Urinary tract infection following repeated catheterization
- Wound infection following surgery (e.g. meticillin-resistant *Staphylococcus aureus* (MRSA), see below)
- Diarrhoea due to overgrowth of antibiotic-tolerant microbes (e.g. clostridia)
- Multiple drug resistant *Escherichia coli*.

Effective biosecurity

Nosocomial infections may be minimized by effective bio-security (a set of preventative measures designed to reduce the risk of disease transmission).

- Cleaning and disinfection of kennels/housing between patients.
- Good barrier nursing technique.
- Reducing infection risk:
  - Good wound management (e.g. changing soiled bandages)
  - Correct management and hygiene of indwelling catheters and drains
  - Good antibacterial stewardship.

Antibacterial agents, although helpful in treating susceptible infections, may select for resistant microorganisms. An increase in antimicrobial resistance (see Chapter 8) has reduced the ability to treat some formerly treatable infections in humans and animals. To reduce the build-up of resistance, antibiotics should be used only when strictly necessary and never as a substitute for good patient care and practical infection control measures.

Screening of animals, staff and the environment should take place periodically to check microbiological standards.

Meticillin-resistant bacteria

MRSP: meticillin-resistant *Staphylococcus pseudintermedius*

MRSP is considered a major pathogen in dogs, typically involved in skin, mouth, nose and ear infections, urinary tract and gastrointestinal infections, and postoperative infections. *Staphylococcus pseudintermedius* is also part of the normal flora of healthy dogs. It is an opportunistic pathogen causing infection and illness in animals and people that are immunocompromised. MRSP is diagnosed based on culture and sensitivity testing. It is highly resistant to many antibiotics, which can make MRSP a challenging infection to treat. High standards of clinical practice and hygiene are essential to prevent the spread of MRSP. Responsible antimicrobial use will help slow the development of resistance and help preserve the efficacy of antimicrobial drugs for the future.

MRSA: meticillin-resistant *Staphylococcus aureus*

Staphylococcus aureus is a commensal bacterium of the skin and nasal passages of humans. In certain situations, especially where patients are hospitalized, the bacterium can cause disease including gastrointestinal disease, septicaemia, skin infections and post-surgical wound infections. Some *Staphylococcus* species are commensal on the skin and in the oral cavity and nasal passages of animals, although *S. aureus* is less common in animals than in people. However, it has been shown that cats that have contact with people are more likely to have *S. aureus* present on their skin, and the isolation of identical isolates from an in-contact cat and human suggest that interspecies transmission may occur.

MRSP and MRSA resistance

Of major concern to veterinary practices is the development of resistance to a wide range of antibacterial agents, including meticillin. MRSP is a concern for veterinary practices and hospitals, and MRSA continues to be a concern in human hospitals and healthcare units, causing high morbidity and mortality during outbreaks. Although MRSA isolates are, by definition, resistant to all the groups of penicillin drugs, via the *MecA* gene, they can still be sensitive to other antibacterial drugs. However, there is an increasing tendency for resistance to build up against other antibacterial drugs, and treatment in some cases is becoming very problematic. Healthy nasal carriers occur in the human population, making elimination of the organism difficult. There are also community-acquired infections, with MRSA isolates increasingly recognized in people.

A useful reference source is the BSAVA practice guidelines on reducing the risk from MRSA and MRSP, which can be found on the website (www.bsava.com).

Prevention of spread

Routine measures to prevent the spread of MRSA and MRSP include:

- Scrupulous hand hygiene
- Clean environment
- The appropriate use of antimicrobials (including antibiotics) to minimize overuse and reduce microbial resistance
- Compliance with all of the above biosecurity measures.

Sterilization and disinfection

- **Sterilization is the complete elimination of microorganisms from equipment and surfaces.** To achieve this, surgical equipment is typically subjected to high temperatures and pressure within an autoclave (see Chapter 22).
- **Disinfection is the physical or chemical destruction of microorganisms** (see Chapter 14). A range of chemical disinfectants is available in order to achieve this aim.

Because pathogens vary in their structure and properties, their susceptibility to different disinfectants also varies; true sterilization may be difficult to achieve by chemical means. For optimum effect, an appropriate disinfectant needs to be selected, instructions for the correct dilution should be carefully followed and the product should be used in a physically clean environment.

Good wound management

All wounds, whether clean or contaminated (see Chapter 23), need proper care to reduce the risk of complications:

- Sterile gloves should be worn at all times
- All swabs, cotton buds or instruments entering the wound should be sterile
- Irrigation fluids used for flushing should be sterile
- Bandaging materials should be sterile
- Dressings should always be changed regularly and whenever they become soiled or wet
- Self-trauma should be prevented if necessary by using an Elizabethan collar and providing adequate pain relief
- Careful disposal of soiled dressings, bandages, swabs, etc., is required (see Chapter 2)
- Barrier nursing precautions should be followed as indicated (see Chapter 14).

Isolation and quarantine

Isolation

This is the physical segregation of an animal or group of animals suspected of having, or proven to have, a contagious disease, so as to eliminate the potential for transmission to other susceptible individuals. Isolation is also required for the exclusion of infections from 'high health status' animals, such as specific pathogen-free (SPF) animals used in research.

A self-contained isolation ward should be established and clearly labelled when in use to prevent the admittance of other animals and to restrict staff access. No visitors should be permitted into the isolation ward at any time. The isolation ward should have its own facilities for washing and waste disposal, as well as a range of equipment and stock solely for use within the unit. This should include:

- Personal protective equipment (PPE):
  • Gloves and overshoes
  • Gowns and masks
- Food and water bowls
- Disposable bedding
- Litter trays and different types of cat litter
- Cleaning equipment – such as a mop and bucket, as well as detergents and disinfectants
- Medications, syringes and needles
- Appropriate diagnostic and monitoring equipment.

Ideally, the entrance to the ward and its ventilation should be separate from those of the main practice. A footbath at the entrance, for disinfecting footwear, and the allocation of different personnel to the isolation unit are useful precautions.

Potential routes of transmission (see 'Transmission', above) should be carefully considered when designing procedures to avoid the spread of infection. The risk of spread of airborne pathogens can be minimized by reducing the number of animals in the same airspace and ensuring a good rate of air exchange. Within buildings, positive pressure ventilation may be used to encourage airflow from cleaner to potentially contaminated zones.

For further information on isolation facilities within a hospital ward, the reader is referred to Chapter 14.

Barrier nursing

Barrier nursing is the term used to describe the precautions followed when nursing an animal kept in isolation due to a suspected or confirmed infectious disease. The principles of using appropriate nursing adaptations to prevent cross-contamination should be adopted. For further information on barrier nursing and isolation protocols, the reader is referred to Chapter 14.

Quarantine

This is the segregation of individuals of unknown disease status for a period prior to entry to a new premises or country, to limit the risk of disease introduction.

In the UK, quarantine is most commonly associated with preventing the entry of rabies. The UK has been free from terrestrial rabies since 1922, although endemic European bat lyssaviruses (EBLV-1 in a Serotine bat and EBLV-2 in Daubenton's bats) have been identified and can be responsible for causing 'bat rabies' in humans. Prior to the PETS travel scheme, 6 months of compulsory quarantine for all pet dogs and cats entering the UK successfully prevented reintroduction of terrestrial rabies.

Pet Travel Scheme (PETS)

The Pet Travel Scheme for dogs, cats and ferrets replaced the 6-month quarantine requirement for dogs and cats entering the UK from designated countries, including European Union (EU) member states, the USA, Japan, Australia, New Zealand and many rabies-free islands. The scheme operates via certain carriers and designated entry points within the UK, including Eurotunnel, major ports and airports. For animals that fail to comply with PETS rules, the 6-month quarantine rule still applies.

'Pet Passports', recognized throughout the EU, hold all the relevant certification in booklet form and double as entry documents for many EU countries, simplifying export procedures (see also Chapter 10).

To qualify for entry or return to the UK, a number of criteria have to be met. For an animal new to the Scheme, these are (in chronological order):

1. Microchip implantation.
2. Rabies vaccination.
3. For pets travelling to the UK from non-approved countries, a blood sample (taken at least 30 days after vaccination) with serological testing to show adequate rabies immunity.
4. A correctly completed Pet Passport, with the relevant identification, vaccination and blood testing details.
5. A waiting period after vaccination. For travel to the UK from EU member states and 'listed' Third countries this is 21 days. For entry to the UK from non-approved countries, the waiting period is currently 3 months from the date of blood testing before animals can be considered for entry.
6. A visit to a veterinary surgeon 24–120 hours (5 days) prior to the return to the UK for tapeworm treatment and certification to that effect.

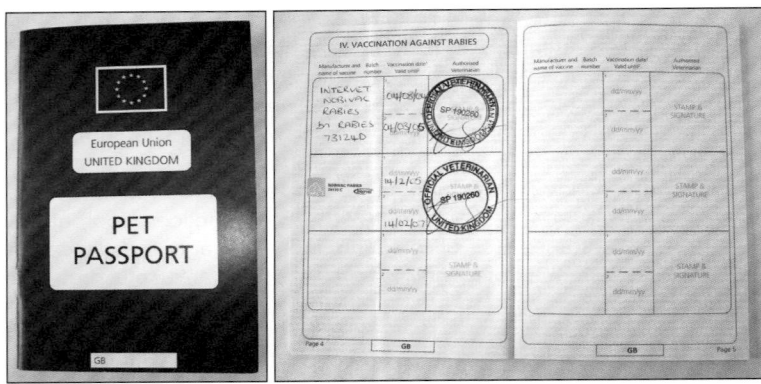

In order to keep 'passports' valid, rabies boosters must be repeated within the duration of immunity of the particular vaccine used.

At the time of writing it is unclear whether the UK will remain part of the PETS scheme when it leaves the EU or become regarded as a 'Third country' outside of the EU. Clients should be advised to start the process of applying for certification well in advance of travelling (at least 4 months). **The up-to-date requirements of the Department for Environment, Food and Rural Affairs (Defra) should be checked before travel: www.defra.gov.uk.**

The immune system

This is the defence system by which the body protects against disease by detecting and resisting microbial or parasitic invasion. The immune system must distinguish invasion of these pathogens from the host's own healthy cells and tissues in order to function properly.

The immune system functions on three basic levels: physical barriers, innate immunity and acquired immunity. Throughout life, individuals are continuously exposed to a range of foreign antigens. These are delivered to the immune system, such that over time the individual can become resistant to a wide range of pathogens.

Physical barriers

Physical barriers to invasion (the skin and the surfaces of the gastrointestinal, respiratory and urogenital tracts) provide an initial obstacle. The movement of mucous secretions up the respiratory tract, coughing, sneezing, urine flow, vomiting and diarrhoea all aid in clearing pathogens.

Innate immunity

Innate immunity constitutes the next layer of defence. Components of innate immunity are either pre-existing or rapidly activated:

- **Pre-existing:** e.g. enzymes such as lysozyme in tears and saliva, and various proteins that can bind to bacteria and hasten their destruction
- **Rapidly activated:** cells such as macrophages and neutrophils can recognize molecules on the outside of invading microbes before engulfing (by phagocytosis) and destroying them (Figure 7.5). Inflammation allows blood flow to increase to areas of damaged tissue, bringing such cells to the site of injury.

Innate immunity is a vital and effective layer of defence, but many pathogens successfully overcome it, and more sophisticated and specific approaches are therefore required.

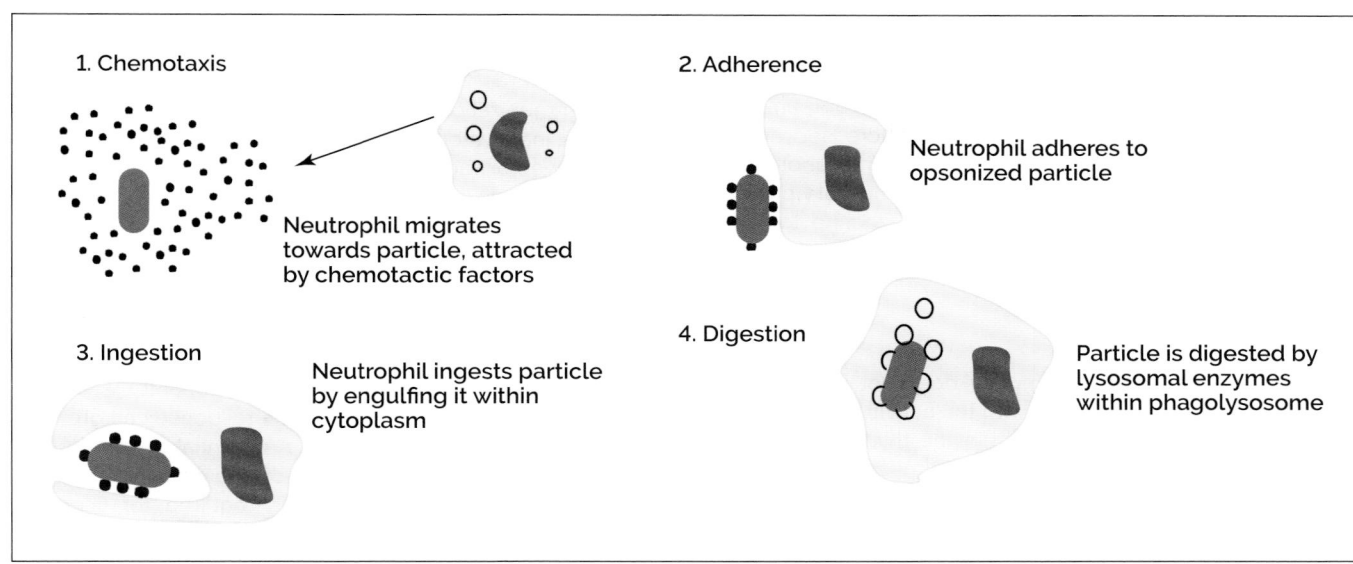

7.5 The process of phagocytosis. **(1) Chemotaxis:** neutrophils are attracted to areas of infection by chemical factors from bacteria or damaged cells. **(2) Adherence** of the neutrophil is facilitated by presence of opsonins such as antibodies or protein components known as complement. **(3) Ingestion:** the neutrophil engulfs the particle within its cytoplasm. **(4) Digestion:** the particle is digested within a phagolysosome by lysosomal enzymes.

Acquired immunity

Acquired immunity recognizes and responds to specific foreign pathogens. Following infection, the immune system learns to produce specific cells and antibodies directed against the particular pathogen involved. In contrast to the rapid response of innate immunity, this active immunity takes several days to begin to act against infections not previously encountered by the host. However, because specific memory cells are formed following initial exposure, a much more rapid response may be expected if challenged by the same pathogen again.

Active immunity is initiated when components of foreign substances and microbes that trigger immune recognition (antigens) are collected by antigen-presenting cells (e.g. dendritic cells and macrophages) and delivered to lymph nodes, where they are presented to lymphocytes. Some lymphocytes specifically recognize the antigen and become activated.

There are two major divisions of acquired immunity: humoral and cellular.

Humoral immunity

Humoral immunity (Figure 7.6) is associated with B lymphocytes (B cells), which mature within bone marrow. Activated B lymphocytes develop into plasma cells, which manufacture proteins called **antibodies** (composed of immunoglobulins). Antibodies lock on to specific foreign antigens and neutralize them, or facilitate the binding of other components of the immune system. Humoral immunity can be measured by assessing the level of specific antibodies in the blood. Such tests are commonly used as diagnostic tests for specific infections, e.g. FeLV (see Chapter 17).

Humoral immunity can be acquired via passive transfer of antibodies. In nature, this is by passage of **maternally derived antibodies** (MDA) across the placenta and in the first milk (colostrum) from a dam to her offspring. Whereas in humans the vast majority of MDA pass across the placenta before birth, in dogs and cats few MDA are received in this way and the vast majority are present in the colostrum. The intestine of neonatal animals is initially permeable to

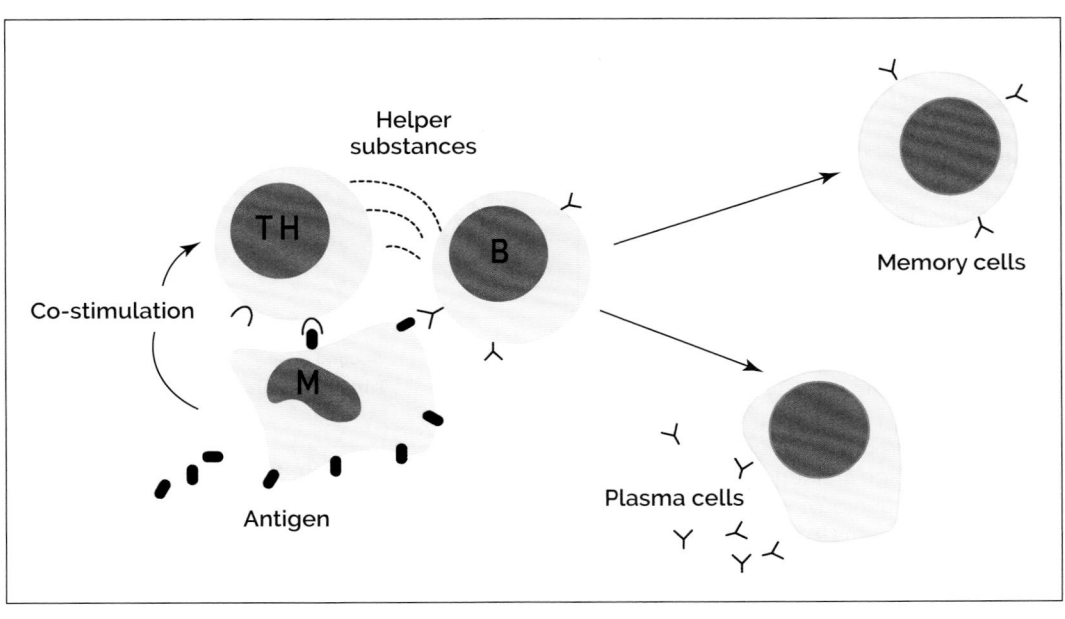

7.6 B cells differentiate into antibody-producing plasma cells and memory cells. Interaction with, and stimulation by, antigen-presenting cells such as macrophages (M) and helper T cells (TH) is needed for this to occur.

the passage of these antibodies, allowing an efficient transfer into the circulation. However, the efficiency of this transfer declines rapidly within hours of birth and this means that significant delays to colostral intake by young animals may lead to poor passive immunity and increased risk of infection. Whereas active immunity invokes immunological memory, passive immunity confers only temporary protection. Within a few weeks of birth, MDA decline to non-protective levels, whereupon young animals become more susceptible to disease.

Cellular immunity

Cellular or cell-mediated immunity does not involve antibodies, instead it is associated with the activity of T lymphocytes (T cells), which mature within the thymus. Activated T lymphocytes manufacture chemical messengers called cytokines, which help to direct immune cell functions and responses. There are a number of different types of T lymphocyte:

- **Helper T cells** recognize processed antigen and coordinate macrophages and B cells in the immune response, promoting immune function (see Figure 7.6)
- **Cytotoxic T cells** destroy cells infected with intracellular pathogens such as viruses
- **Suppressor T cells** keep the immune system in check by suppressing immune reactions within tolerable limits. Decreased activity of these cells is one mechanism by which the immune system may begin to damage the body's own tissues and organs (see 'Autoimmune disease', below).

Principles of vaccination

The purpose of a vaccine is to stimulate an active immune response in the recipient against one or more specific pathogens, to improve the immunological response in infection. Resulting immunity varies, depending on the pathogen and vaccine, from full protection of the host against clinical disease, infection and shedding (sterilizing immunity) to simply a reduction of clinical signs following infection. The contribution made by vaccination towards preventing and reducing the incidence of major infectious diseases in humans and animals is, without doubt, enormous. Many serious contagious diseases are seldom seen today, but continued widespread vaccination is essential if this is to remain so.

Immunization may be passive or active.

- **Passive immunization:** This involves administration of antisera or antitoxins containing concentrated antibodies against either a pathogen or a toxin, respectively. Used in the treatment of disease or at the time of possible exposure, passive immunization cannot give long-term protection because the levels of antibody decline over several weeks. An important example is the therapy of animals with clinical tetanus.
- **Active immunization:** Most vaccines stimulate immunity by exposing the immune system to foreign antigens associated with specific infections. Immunological memory stimulated by such exposure means that, if challenged by the same infections, acquired immunity quickly neutralizes or minimizes the threat.

Types of vaccine

There are three broad categories of vaccine designed for active immunization (see also Chapter 8): attenuated (live) vaccines; inactivated (killed) vaccines; and subunit, recombinant and vector vaccines.

Attenuated (live; 'infectious') vaccines

Live vaccines usually contain weakened (attenuated) strains of the infectious pathogen, i.e. strains that cannot cause disease in the host. The immune response following vaccination with such products mimics what occurs following natural infection. Good cellular and humoral immunity is usually stimulated, and a protective immune response can often be expected rapidly after one dose. A potential concern when using live vaccines is reversion of the vaccine strain to virulence, although stringent trials required for licensing make this an unlikely scenario.

Inactivated (killed; 'non-infectious') vaccines

Inactivated vaccines remove the potential for reversion to virulence by containing pathogens that have been inactivated or killed to make then non-infectious. Many inactivated vaccines contain an **adjuvant**. An adjuvant is an agent that stimulates (irritates) the immune system to find and react to the vaccine agent. Killed vaccines often require two or more doses to stimulate an effective response (Figure 7.7) and are usually better at stimulating humoral than cell-mediated responses. In some cases, the immunity acquired from a killed vaccine may not be as durable or complete as that from a live equivalent.

Inactivated toxins used as vaccines are known as toxoids. Most commonly used in horses, tetanus toxoid stimulates active immunity to give longer-term protection in contrast to antitoxins, which are for short-term treatment and prophylaxis only.

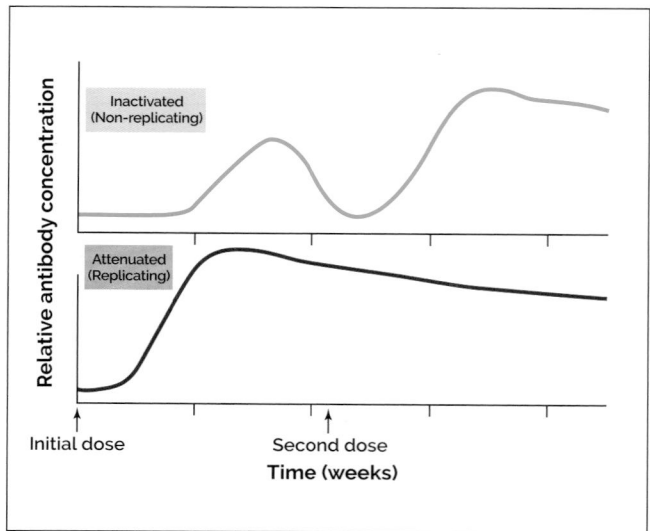

7.7 Comparison of antibody responses following inoculation with an inactivated vaccine (top) and a live attenuated vaccine (bottom). In this example, two doses of inactivated vaccine are required to stimulate a protective 'anamnestic' response, whereas only one dose of live vaccine is required to stimulate active immunity.

Subunit, recombinant and vector vaccines

Subunit vaccines contain a small fragment or fragments of pathogen containing the necessary antigens. Some are termed **recombinant vaccines** because they are manufactured using genetic engineering techniques. One advantage of recombinant vaccine technology is that there is virtually no chance of the vaccine becoming infectious and the host becoming ill from the agent, since the vaccine contains just a single protein, not the organism itself. Traditional vaccine risks come from the organism not being totally weakened (attenuated), or reversion to a virulent form, both of which may be potentially infectious and cause disease. Adjuvants may be one vaccine component responsible for some expected adverse effects such as local swelling at the injection site, malaise and fever.

Vector vaccines try to combine the potential advantages of live vaccines with some of the advantages of using an inactivated subunit vaccine. In vector vaccines, the useful subunits are incorporated into a different non-pathogenic live virus. In this case, the vector is 'infectious' but does not cause disease in the species being vaccinated. One feline leukaemia vaccine currently available in the UK uses a canarypox virus, genetically modified to contain important FeLV antigens, to stimulate immunity. An advantage of vector vaccine technology is that an adjuvant may not be needed to stimulate the immune response adequately.

Administering vaccines

Vaccine antigens available for use in dogs and cats at the time of writing are listed in Figure 7.8.

Some vaccines contain single components (e.g. parvovirus alone) but, for convenience, a number of different components are often packaged together as a **multivalent** vaccine, conferring immunity against more than one pathogen. Recommendations for use of different vaccines vary and are detailed within product datasheets. Live vaccines are often freeze dried, requiring reconstitution with a diluent prior to use (Figure 7.9).

Not all vaccines are administered by injection. Figure 7.10 shows a *Bordetella* vaccine being administered intranasally to a cat. Intranasal administration stimulates the rapid formation of specific antibodies on the lining of the respiratory tract, which neutralize infection at the point of entry. Intranasal vaccines typically work within a few days and can be effective in the face of MDA, allowing some products to be used to protect even very young animals.

Approach to vaccination

Over the last few years there have been some changes to the way vaccines are used in domestic animals. Best practice, as outlined in the World Small Animal Veterinary Association (WSAVA) guidelines (Day *et al.*, 2016, Day, 2017), focuses on vaccinating the animal according to the infection needs of the individual and the population within which it lives. Vaccines may be categorized as 'core' (essential for every dog or cat) or 'non-core' (may be used in those dogs and cats whose geographical location or individual lifestyle places them at risk of exposure to infection) (see Figure 7.8).

Core vaccines should be administered to all dogs and cats when first vaccinated (see 'Primary vaccination', below), usually as puppies and kittens. The decision to use a specific non-core vaccine is based upon disease risk in the local area and on the lifestyle of the individual pet (e.g. indoor *versus* outdoor, urban versus rural environment, working *versus* companion activity, travel and boarding). Serology (measurement of antibody levels) should then be used to determine when the next vaccine (see 'Booster vaccinations', below) is needed.

For dogs
Core vaccinations (essential for every dog)
■ Canine adenovirus-2 (CAV-2) (MLV; parenteral)   ■ Canine distemper virus (CDV) (MLV; parenteral)   ■ Recombinant canine distemper virus (rCDV) (parenteral)   ■ Canine parvovirus-2 (CPV-2) (MLV; parenteral)   ■ *Leptospira interrogans* (killed bacterin; parenteral). Should be restricted to use in geographical areas where a risk of exposure has been established or for dogs whose lifestyle places them at risk. In the UK, this is considered a core vaccination   ■ Rabies (killed; parenteral). Core where required by statute, in areas where the disease is endemic or for travel
Non-core (optional) vaccinations (may be used in those dogs whose geographical location or lifestyle (e.g. indoor versus outdoor living, rural versus urban environment, working versus companion activity, boarding or travelling) places them at increased risk of exposure to infection)
■ *Bordetella bronchiseptica* (live avirulent bacteria; intranasal, oral). Available as a single product or in combination with CPiV or with both CPiV and CAV-2. Must not be delivered by parenteral injection as this may lead to severe adverse reactions, including death   ■ *Bordetella bronchiseptica* (killed bacterin, cell wall antigen extract; parenteral). Intranasal or oral products are preferred to the killed parenteral product   ■ *Borrelia burgdorferi* (killed whole bacterin, recombinant-outer surface protein A; parenteral). Generally recommended only for use in dogs with a known high risk of exposure, living in or visiting regions where the risk of vector tick exposure is considered to be high or where disease is known to be endemic   ■ Canine influenza (CIV) (killed adjuvanted; parenteral). Licensed only in USA. Consider for at-risk groups of co-housed dogs such as those in kennels   ■ Parainfluenza virus (CPiV) (MLV; parenteral, intranasal). Use of CPiV (MLV intranasal) is preferred to the parenteral product as the primary site of infection is the upper respiratory tract
Not recommended
■ Canine adenovirus-1 (CAV-1) (MLV, killed; parenteral). Not recommended where CAV-2 (MLV) is available   ■ Canine coronavirus (CCoV)   ■ Canine parvovirus-2 (CPV-2) (killed; parenteral). Not recommended where MLV is available

7.8 Disease antigens currently available as vaccines for dogs and cats. MLV = modified live virus. (Data from Day *et al.*, 2016)

continues ▶

For cats

Core vaccinations (essential for every cat)

- Feline calicivirus (FCV) (MLV non-adjuvanted, killed adjuvanted, killed non-adjuvanted; parenteral, intranasal). Usually found in combination with FHV-1 vaccine
- Feline herpesvirus-1 (FHV-1) (MLV non-adjuvanted, killed adjuvanted; parenteral, intranasal). Usually found in combination with FCV vaccine
- Feline parvovirus (FPV) (MLV, MLV non-adjuvanted, killed adjuvanted, killed non-adjuvanted; parenteral, intranasal)
- Rabies (canarypox virus-vectored recombinant non-adjuvanted, killed adjuvanted; parenteral). Core in areas where the disease is endemic or for travel

Non-core (optional) vaccinations (may be used in those cats whose geographical location or lifestyle (e.g. indoor versus outdoor living, rural versus urban environment, boarding or travelling) places them at increased risk of exposure to infection)

- *Bordetella bronchiseptica* (avirulent live non-adjuvanted; intranasal). Vaccination may be considered in cases where cats are likely to be at specific risk of infection
- *Chlamydia felis* (avirulent live non-adjuvanted, killed adjuvanted; parenteral). Vaccination is most appropriately used as part of a control regime for animals in multi-cat environments where infections associated with clinical disease have been confirmed
- Feline immunodeficiency virus (FIV) (killed adjuvant; parenteral)[a]
- Feline leukaemia virus (FeLV) (canarypox virus-vectored recombinant non-adjuvant, killed adjuvant, recombinant protein subunit adjuvant; injectable, parenteral). Only FeLV-negative cats should be vaccinated

Not recommended

- Feline infectious peritonitis (FIP) (MLV non-adjuvanted; intranasal)[a]

Serology may be used to inform decision-making regarding the frequency of use of some (but not all) core vaccines

7.8 *continued* Disease antigens currently available as vaccines for dogs and cats. [a]Not available in the UK. MLV = modified live virus. (Data from Day *et al.*, 2016)

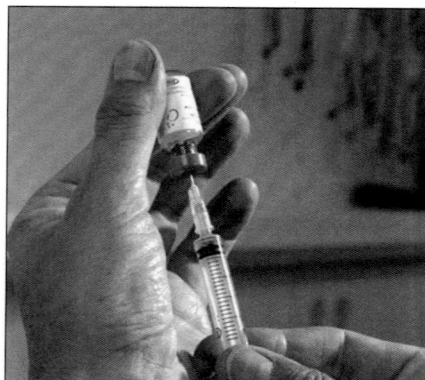

7.9 Preparing a vaccine for use.

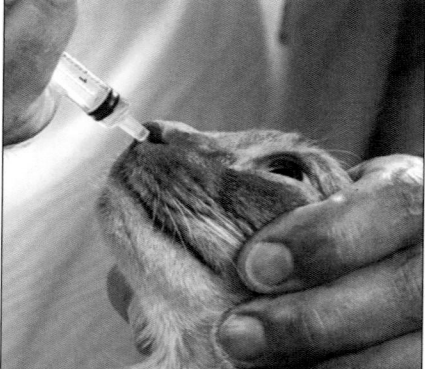

7.10 Intranasal vaccination in a cat.

Unfortunately, the way vaccines are produced and sold often means that the WSAVA guidance is practically difficult to follow and many veterinary practices vaccinate the majority of pets in a standard, rather than an individual, way following the vaccine manufacturers' guidelines.

Primary vaccination

Primary vaccination describes the initial administration or course of administrations that establishes immunity. Significant levels of passive antibodies (e.g. MDA) can interfere with the immune response to the vaccine. The recommendations for timing of primary vaccine course doses are based on an understanding of when MDA will decline to levels that will not interfere with the immune response (Figure 7.11).

- Vaccines currently in use in the UK typically have recommendations for the final dose of the primary course to be given at 10 weeks of age in dogs and 12 weeks in cats. However, some vaccine guidelines now recommend a later longer course, especially in puppies in areas where canine parvovirus is common.

A **turnout period** (often around 7–14 days) should be carefully observed following final vaccination before protective immunity is established and individuals can be exposed to risk; during this time, animals should not be allowed outside or in contact with others that may pose a disease risk.

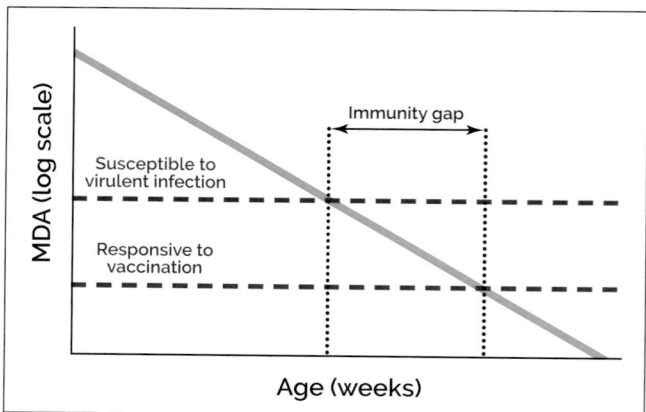

7.11 The fall in maternally derived antibodies (MDA) is depicted by the solid line. As MDA interfere with response to vaccination, the final vaccination is timed to coincide with the expected decline in MDA to a point where a response is possible. The period between the decline in MDA to non-productive levels and vaccinal immunity developing is known as the **immunity gap**. Animals exposed to infection during this period will not be protected.

Booster vaccinations

Booster vaccinations are required in those individuals where immunity may decline to non-protective levels. Ideally this immunity is assessed by serological testing, but in many instances boosters are given routinely following the vaccine manufacturers' recommendations. For most UK canine vaccines against distemper, hepatitis and parvovirus, the recommended licensed intervals are every 3 or 4 years (although recommendations vary with manufacturer). Available evidence shows that annual boosters against other diseases, such as leptospirosis, are often essential to maintain optimal immunity. A similar approach is taken with cats and it is therefore important to check manufacturer's guidelines.

Immune-mediated disorders

Allergy and hypersensitivity reactions

Allergy is a state of exaggerated immune sensitivity induced by exposure to a particular, usually otherwise harmless, antigen (or allergen), resulting in harmful immunological reactions on subsequent exposures (Figure 7.12). Allergies may be localized problems in one organ (e.g. skin, intestinal tract, respiratory tract) or can result in systemic and potentially life-threatening reactions.

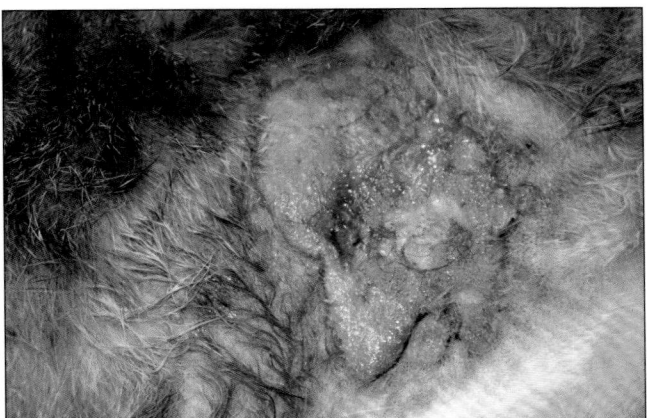

7.12 Close-up view of an eosinophilic plaque on the ventrum of a cat, secondary to chronic pruritus caused by flea allergy dermatitis. (Reproduced from the *BSAVA Manual of Canine and Feline Dermatology, 3rd edn*)

Hypersensitivity reactions are the inappropriate immune responses that result from exposure to a foreign antigen. They are the underlying mechanisms for allergies as well as a number of other important autoimmune diseases (see below) and rare drug and vaccine reactions. Different forms occur. A type I (immediate-type) hypersensitivity reaction is perhaps the most common and is the classical underlying mechanism for allergic reactions such as hay fever in humans, urticaria (wheals) and atopic dermatitis. Clinical signs vary from mild and localized (hay fever) through to systemic and life-threatening (anaphylactic shock).

Other hypersensitivity reactions are underlying mechanisms for a number of diseases, including autoimmune disease. Figure 7.13 summarizes the different types of hypersensitivity reactions seen in animals and gives examples of diseases where such reactions are noted.

Autoimmune disease

Autoimmunity occurs if the immune system reacts to one or more of the body's own tissues as foreign. Although rare, such conditions can prove life-threatening and difficult to manage. Examples include: pemphigus complex, where the immune system specifically attacks the skin and/or mucocutaneous junctions; rheumatoid arthritis; and immune-mediated haemolytic anaemia (IMHA), which is characterized by the breakdown of red blood cells, resulting in anaemia. Some types of endocrine disease, such as diabetes and hypothyroidism in dogs, may also arise as a result of an immune-mediated destruction of glandular tissues.

Graft rejection

Transplanting organs and tissues is a regular occurrence in human surgery and there is now some interest in the veterinary field. A potential problem is rejection of the graft or implant because the recipient's immune system may recognize transplanted tissue as foreign and attack it (see Chapter 23). Careful tissue matching reduces such risks; nevertheless, lifelong use of immunosuppressive drugs by the recipient is usually necessary.

Acknowledgement

The authors would like to acknowledge the contribution of John Helps and Karen Coyne to the chapter in the previous edition of the *BSAVA Textbook of Veterinary Nursing*.

Hypersensitivity reaction	Type	Components	Disease examples
I	Immediate-type	Antigen binds to IgE antibodies on mast cells, which release histamine and other inflammatory mediators	Atopy; hay fever; urticarial; anaphylactic shock
II	Antibody-dependent or cytotoxic	Antibodies attach to antigens on the body's own cells (e.g. red blood cells), triggering their destruction	Immune-mediated haemolytic anaemia; transfusion reactions; pemphigus complex; babesiosis
III	Immune complex	Immune complexes of antibody and antigen form in tissues (e.g. joints, kidneys, blood vessels), precipitating damage	Immune-mediated polyarthritis; glomerulonephritis; vasculitis
IV	Delayed-type	A cell-mediated reaction involving cytotoxic T cells, helper T cells and macrophages	Tuberculosis; allergic contact dermatitis; feline infectious peritonitis (FIP)

7.13 Hypersensitivity reaction types.

References and further reading

Day MJ (2012) *Clinical Immunology of the Dog and Cat, 2nd edn.* Manson Publishing, London

Day MJ (2017) Small animal vaccination: a practical guide for vets in the UK. *In Practice* **39**, 110–118

Day MJ, Horzinek MC, Schultz RD and Squires RA (2016) WSAVA guidelines for the vaccination of dogs and cats. *Journal of Small Animal Practice* **61**, E1–E45

Jackson H and Marsella R (2012) *BSAVA Manual of Canine and Feline Dermatology, 3rd edn.* BSAVA Publications, Gloucester

Sykes J and Greene C (2011) *Infectious Diseases of the Dog and Cat, 4th edn.* Elsevier, Philadelphia

Thrusfield MV and Christley R (2018) *Veterinary Epidemiology, 4th edn.* Wiley Blackwell, Oxford

Tizard IR (2017) *Veterinary Immunology – An Introduction, 10th edn.* Elsevier, Philadelphia

Useful websites

Bella Moss Foundation:
www.thebellamossfoundation.com

BSAVA practice guidelines – reducing the risk from MRSA and MRSP
www.bsava.com/Portals/0/resources/documents/BSAVA_MRSA_Guidelines_0711.pdf?ver=2016-09-27-103833-567

NOAH Compendium of Datasheets for Veterinary Products:
www.noahcompendium.co.uk

Pet Travel Scheme:
www.defra.gov.uk/wildlife-pets/pets/travel/index.htm

World Health Organisaiton – hand washing guidelines:
www.who.int/gpsc/clean_hands_protection/en/

WSAVA – vaccine guidelines:
www.wsava.org/Guidelines/Vaccination-Guidelines

Self-assessment questions

1. Using specific examples, describe the main routes of entry for pathogens into hosts.
2. Using specific examples, describe how pathogens can be transmitted between hosts.
3. What three levels does the immune system function on?
4. How do physical barriers provide obstacles to pathogen invasion?
5. What is the difference between innate immunity and acquired immunity?
6. Define a zoonotic infection and list five pathogens of cats that are zoonotic.
7. Describe three different types of vaccines available.
8. Which types of patients are at the highest risk of nosocomial infections?
9. Describe the precautions required whilst nursing a patient with MRSA infection.
10. Why is the timing of puppy and kitten vaccinations important?

Chapter 8

Medicines: pharmacology, therapeutics and dispensing

Elizabeth Wright

Learning objectives

After studying this chapter, readers will have the knowledge to:

- **Describe the principles of pharmacokinetics, pharmacodynamics and pharmacological terminology**
- **List the main classes of drugs used in veterinary medicine**
- **Dispense medicines correctly and responsibly in accordance with veterinary surgeon direction, legislation and the latest guidance**
- **Ensure safe and legal handling and management of drugs, including medicine storage, ordering and receipt of goods, record keeping requirements, and disposal of all classes of medicines, including Controlled Drugs and cytotoxic drugs**
- **Administer oral, topical, parenteral, ophthalmic and aural medicines safely and effectively**
- **Recognize suspected adverse reactions, be aware of the Suspected Adverse Reaction Surveillance Scheme (SARSS), and alert the veterinary surgeon when appropriate**
- **Recognize health and safety regulations with respect to medicines. Manage risk to self and others associated with particular substances**
- **Advise clients on safe and correct routes of administration, potential side effects, and on the storage and disposal of medication**
- **Demonstrate to clients safe techniques for administering medication**
- **Calculate drug doses appropriately**
- **Access the appropriate sources of data on licensed medicines**

Medicines and nomenclature

Veterinary medicinal products

A veterinary medicinal product (VMP) may be defined as:

- Any substance or combination of substances presented as having properties for treating or preventing disease in animals
- Any substance or combination of substances that may be used in, or administered to, animals with a view either to restoring, correcting or modifying physiological functions by exerting a pharmacological, immunological or metabolic action, or to making a medical diagnosis (Veterinary Medicines Regulations (VMR) 2013 (www.legislation.gov.uk/uksi/2013/2033/contents/made)).

Summary of product characteristics (SPCs) for all authorized veterinary medicines in the UK may be found on the Veterinary Medicines Directorate's (VMD's) product information database (www.vmd.defra.gov.uk/ProductInformation Database/). The NOAH Compendium (www.noahcompendium.co.uk/) also lists many, but not all, UK authorized veterinary medicine SPCs. Datasheets for medicines licensed for use in humans may be found at www.medicines.org.uk/emc.

Medicine names

Veterinary medicines are generally referred to using two names:

- The **generic** (or non-proprietary) name is the description of the active ingredient (e.g. cefalexin)
- The **trade** (or proprietary) name is unique to each manufacturer (e.g. Therios®, Cephacare®, Cefaseptin®, Rilexine™, and Ceporex™ are all brands of cefalexin).

Generic drugs used to be referred to using the British Approved Name (BAN); however, European law now dictates that we use the Recommended International Non-proprietary Name (rINN). This description is recognized internationally and is used throughout this chapter.

Pharmacology

Pharmacology is the science of medicines and how they affect living organisms. Any medicine has the possibility of causing harm rather than healing, particularly if used at the wrong dose. To enable veterinary surgeons to determine what dose is appropriate, there must be knowledge and understanding of the pharmacokinetic and pharmaco-dynamic properties of the drug.

- **Pharmacokinetics** is the study of how the body acts on a drug when it is administered; how drugs are absorbed, distributed, metabolized and eliminated.
- **Pharmacodynamics** is the study of how a drug acts on the body after administration.

The ADME process

ADME is an acronym for the pharmacokinetic processes of absorption, distribution, metabolism and elimination.

Absorption

After a dose is administered, it takes time for the drug to be absorbed into the systemic circulation (bloodstream). If a drug is administered intravenously, there is no absorption phase because the drug has been administered directly into the circulation. The chemical properties of some drugs will affect the required absorption site. For example, acidic drugs such as meloxicam are best absorbed in the stomach, while others such as omeprazole, are best absorbed in the intestines. Small molecules diffuse more rapidly than larger molecules, so are absorbed more rapidly.

Distribution

This is the process by which drugs are moved through the body and transferred from tissue to tissue. Drug distribution is affected by factors such as blood flow, natural barriers such as the blood–brain barrier, and the properties of the drug itself. Drugs that are lipid-soluble are widely distributed throughout the body.

Metabolism

This is the breaking down of a drug compound to allow it to be removed from the body. Most drug metabolism occurs in the liver and inactivates the drug. However, some drugs such as codeine and enalapril require metabolism to become effective. These are called prodrugs. Another factor affecting the metabolism of drugs by the liver are the cytochrome P450 (CY450) enzymes. These enzymes are involved in drug metabolism and can be affected by certain medicines. Enzyme-inducing medicines, which increase the amount of CYP450 and therefore increase the rate of drug metabolism, include phenobarbital and rifampicin. Enzyme inhibitors, which reduce the amount of CYP450 and therefore reduce the rate of drug metabolism, include cimetidine and diltiazem. Understanding which drugs are enzyme inducers and inhibitors is very important because using these drugs alongside others will either increase or decrease expected drug levels in the body. Drug metabolism is also affected by liver disease, which can prevent animals from metabolizing drugs effectively.

Excretion

This is the removal of drugs from the body. Excretion usually occurs via the kidneys, although it can also occur through bile into the digestive tract, and occasionally via tears, sweat, breath and saliva. Drugs can be excreted unchanged or as metabolites. Patients with renal disease may have a reduced ability to excrete drugs. Depending on the severity of disease, doses may need to be reduced, or a drug avoided altogether. Drug information sheets or SPCs are the best places to look for information about the appropriate use of a particular drug in patients with liver or renal disease.

Intravascular and extravascular administration

There are two categories of drug administration site: intravascular and extravascular.

Intravascular administration

There are two methods of intravascular drug administration: intravenous and intra-arterial injection. With intravascular drug administration, the drug has an almost immediate onset of action because it does not need to be absorbed into the systemic (general) circulation – it is already there. The entire dose is available to produce a pharmacological effect, so doses are often lower than with other forms of administration. This type of administration is often used in life-threatening situations because of its fast onset of action, but one disadvantage is that adverse reactions are difficult to reverse or control. This makes accuracy in calculating and administering the correct dose critical. Intra-arterial injection is rarely used. Intra-arterial access is more commonly used to monitor blood gases and blood pressure during surgery and for patients under intensive care.

Extravascular administration

Any route of administration other than intravenous and intra-articular injection is considered extravascular (e.g. oral, topical, rectal, inhalation, ophthalmic, intranasal, or subcutaneous and intramuscular injection). With extravascular administration, the drug has to be absorbed from the site of administration into the systemic circulation before a pharmacological effect can occur. This means there is a delay between the dose being administered and it taking effect. For example, when administered orally, a dose of potentiated amoxicillin takes between 1.5 and 2 hours to be absorbed to maximum concentration into the systemic circulation of dogs. In addition, any drug that is absorbed via the gastrointestinal (GI) tract will be subject to **first pass metabolism**, which can decrease the amount of drug available to the systemic circulation.

First pass metabolism

Drugs absorbed via the GI tract enter the portal circulation before reaching the systemic circulation. The portal circulation is a system consisting of the heart, liver, hepatic portal vein, small intestine, stomach and large intestine. Before it reaches the systemic circulation and the heart, any drug absorbed from the GI tract is taken to the liver for processing (metabolism) via the hepatic portal vein. This processing can decrease the amount of active drug available for absorption into the general circulation, so the initial required dose for oral medications is often higher than for other routes of administration.

Birds and reptiles also have a renal portal system, whereby venous blood from the caudal half of the body drains through a network of veins to the kidneys. It has long been argued that drug injections should be administered into the cranial half of the reptile patient to avoid first pass metabolism by the kidney prior to reaching the systemic circulation and to minimize potential drug nephrotoxicity. Research into the significance of the renal portal system in reptiles is conflicting and it is not clear if all species are affected, but by tradition most clinicians will inject reptiles in the anterior muscle groups. Pharmacokinetic studies and observation suggest the renal portal system does not clinically affect drug administration in avian species.

Drug receptors

Drugs usually exert their effect on the body by binding to a receptor. Receptors are proteins located in or on a cell wall that bind to the drug molecules. This binding reaction sends a signal to the cell and the cell acts accordingly (Figure 8.1).

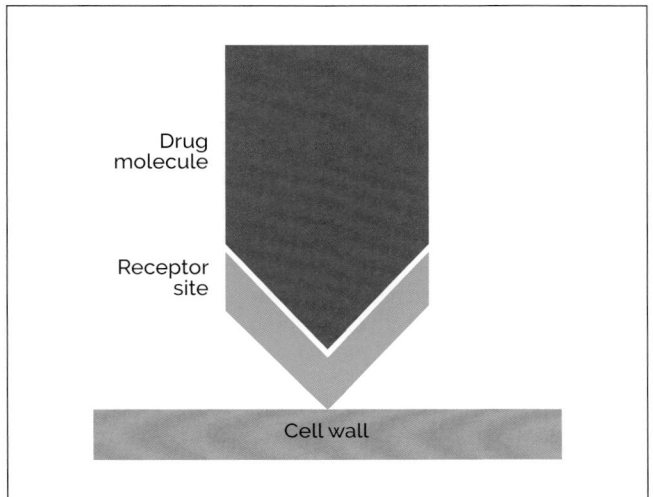

8.1 Drug molecule binding to a receptor site on the cell wall.

An **agonist** is a drug that binds to a receptor and elicits a response. An **antagonist** is one that binds to a receptor but elicits no response and blocks access to the receptor by an agonist. Ideally, a drug would only bind to the receptor required for the desired effect. Unfortunately, no drug is able to do this, which leads to side effects. Some drugs are more selective than others in their binding sites; generally, the more selective the better.

Medicine formulations

Tablets and caplets

Medicines are most commonly formulated as tablets or caplets (Figure 8.2). A caplet is an oblong-shaped tablet and is often easier to administer due to its shape. The active drug is mixed with various excipients (inert substances used to enhance the formulation in some way) before being pressed into a tablet shape. These excipients can include diluents, colourings, flavourings, binding agents (products to make the tablet stick together more easily), glidants and lubricants (products to help the powdered drug flow easily through tablet-making machines) and preservatives. Some tablets are scored to make them easier to break into halves or quarters for more accurate dosing. Others may be sugar-coated to help disguise an unpleasant tasting drug, making the tablet more palatable.

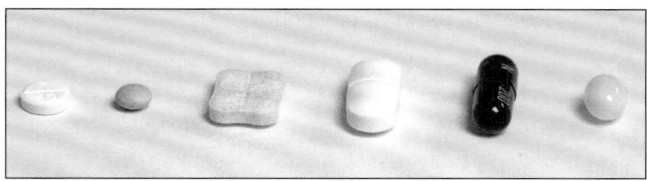

8.2 Selection of tablets, caplets and capsules.

- **Enteric coating (EC):** Some drugs may have an enteric coating. These tablets are designed to pass through the stomach without causing irritation or drug degradation, for absorption in the intestines.
- **Modified-release (MR):** These drugs can also be called controlled-release (CR) or sustained-release (SR). Some drugs are formulated in such a way that the absorption is slowed, or avoided completely, until the tablet reaches a specific site in the body (often the small intestine). This allows a higher strength to be administered and for the tablets to be given less often. It is useful for drugs that would otherwise need to be administered very frequently (e.g. diltiazem) and for those that would be denatured in the acidic contents of the stomach (e.g. omeprazole).

> **WARNING**
>
> Modified-release preparations should not be split or crushed. To do so would destroy their modified-release properties and could result in either a large dose being administered immediately or could denature the drug. Enteric coated tablets should not normally be crushed or split without consulting the SPC or the manufacturer directly

Capsules

The outer case of a capsule is generally made from gelatine and can be hard or soft. Soft gelatine capsules are used to encapsulate liquids, suspensions and semi-solids. They can be round, oval or oblong in shape, and are always sealed during the manufacturing process. Hard gelatine capsules can be used to encapsulate powders, granules, beads or tablets. In addition to the active drug, they contain excipients similar to those found in tablets. Hard gelatine capsules vary in size and are tasteless, odourless and can be coloured to improve their appearance. They are useful for administering drugs with an unpleasant taste or odour. Gelatine capsules are not suitable for use with hygroscopic drugs (those that absorb water), because they will absorb the water present in the capsule shell and disintegrate.

Oral liquids

These are very useful for:

- Animals that do not easily accept tablets and capsules
- Medicines that require very accurate dosing
- Species such as small mammals, birds and reptiles that require a very small dose.

The main components of these medications are the solvent (the liquid base) and the solute (the drug). Oral liquids also contain excipients such as colourings, flavourings, preservatives, viscosity enhancers (used to thicken the liquid) and surfactants (used to increase solubility of some drugs).

There are four types of oral liquid.

- **Solution:** The solute is completely dissolved in the solvent.
- **Suspension:** The solute is not dissolved in the solvent, or is only partially dissolved. When shaken, the solute will mix with the solvent, but soon after it will settle into two parts (Figure 8.3); the liquid solvent at the top and the solid solute at the bottom. Large particles do not stay in suspension for long, they settle to the bottom of the bottle very quickly after mixing. Smaller particles stay in suspension longer, but even these may need the addition of a suspending agent or viscosity enhancer to help the drug mix thoroughly in the solvent long enough for an accurate dose to be withdrawn.

> **WARNING**
>
> Suspensions must be shaken gently before use. Failure to do so may result in the dose being drawn up from the top layer of liquid which contains only the solvent

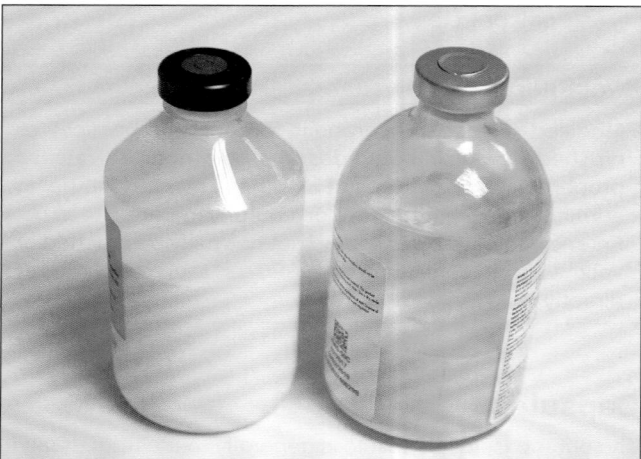

8.3 Separated suspension of an antibacterial product.

- **Syrup/linctus/elixir:** These are viscous (thick), sugary liquids in which the solute is dissolved.
- **Emulsions:** A mixture of two or more immiscible liquids (i.e. liquids that do not mix, such as oil and water). Either or both of the liquids may contain a dissolved drug. Emulsions need to be gently shaken to mix the two liquids and will settle upon standing. Emulsifying agents can be added to help stabilize the emulsion.

Granules, powders and pastes

These formulations are generally used for anthelmintics, laxatives and food supplements. Granules and powders can be added to food for easy administration, while pastes are very palatable and are a useful way of administering medicines to animals that are difficult to pill with a tablet or capsule.

Topical formulations

Topical formulations are designed to be applied directly to the skin, eyes, ears and mucous membranes. They generally have a local effect, but some are absorbed through the skin or mucous membranes into the systemic circulation.

> ## Types of topical medications
>
> - **Creams:** The base is a mixture of oil and water, with the active drug dissolved or evenly dispersed throughout. They are used for drug delivery on to or into the skin
> - **Ointments:** An oily or greasy semi-solid that may contain a surfactant to allow it to be washed off more easily. They are used as emollients (moisturisers), or for drug delivery either to the skin surface or for deeper penetration
> - **Lotions:** Aqueous (water-based) suspensions or solutions that cool inflamed skin and deposit a protective layer of solid particles over the skin
> - **Shampoos:** May be medicated or non-medicated. Shampoos often contain chlorhexidine, antimicrobials and/or antifungals
> - **Ear drops:** Solutions or suspensions of medicines in solvents such as water, glycerol, diluted alcohol or propylene glycol. For ear drops to be effective, sufficient contact time should be provided
> - **Eye drops:** Active ingredient in a vehicle (usually aqueous), along with an antimicrobial preservative to maintain sterility
> - **Spot-on medications:** Liquid preparations mainly used as anthelmintics and pesticides. Spot-on medications are applied between the shoulder blades, where the patient is not able to lick the product. They generally have a prolonged action and can be delivered throughout the body, either through the lipid layer of the skin or absorbed into the systemic circulation
> - **Aerosols (inhalers):** These are a mixture of active drug as a solution or suspension mixed with an inert propellant. The mixture is contained under pressure in a small metal canister with a valve designed to deliver the appropriate dose
> - **Transdermal gels and patches:** Some drugs can be effectively administered through the skin for systemic effect. The drug may be formulated as a gel (e.g. an unlicensed product used under the Cascade containing methimazole gel is administered on to the thin skin of a cat's inner ear to treat hyperthyroidism) or as a patch (e.g. fentanyl patches, which may be applied to a clean, non-hairy patch of skin for pain relief). Patches generally release the drug slowly over a number of days

Implants

These are solid dosage forms that are inserted under the skin. They are not commonly used in veterinary practice, but one example is deslorelin, an implant used to temporarily chemically castrate entire male dogs and ferrets. Release of the drug from implants is generally slow so long-term therapy can be achieved.

Injections

These are sterile formulations that can be administered into the body by injection or infusion (see later for more details). They can be of large or small volume, and can be packaged into:

- **Single-dose ampoules:** Either glass or plastic with a snap or twist-off cap. Snap-top glass ampoules may have a dot to indicate a weak point where the top should be snapped. If any liquid is sitting in the neck of the ampoule, it can be gently tapped to move it down before opening

- **Multi-dose and single-dose vials:** Glass bottles with a rubber membrane over the neck, held in place with an aluminium seal. Many formulations in this type of packaging will be multi-dose, but some may be for single use only
- **Pre-filled syringes:** These are syringes of injectable drug ready prepared for administration. Not common in veterinary practice due to the great variation of doses required
- **Collapsible bag:** Contains a large volume of the drug, generally for infusion. Made from plastic that collapses as the bag is emptied to prevent air being infused into the patient.

Figures 8.4 and 8.5 show a range of multi-dose vials, ampoules and collapsible bags. Single-dose ampoules are designed for **single use**, and any drug remaining in the ampoule after the required dose has been withdrawn should be disposed of. Multi-dose vials are designed for multiple use (i.e. the rubber membrane may be pierced more than once to withdraw the required dose).

> **WARNING**
>
> Some manufacturer information sheets instruct that even multi-dose vials should be broached no more than 20 times, with the remainder of the drug discarded

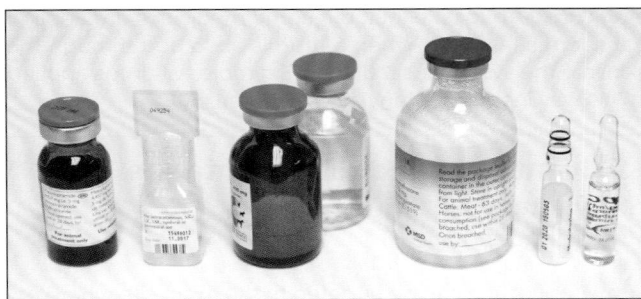

8.4 Selection of ampoules and vials.

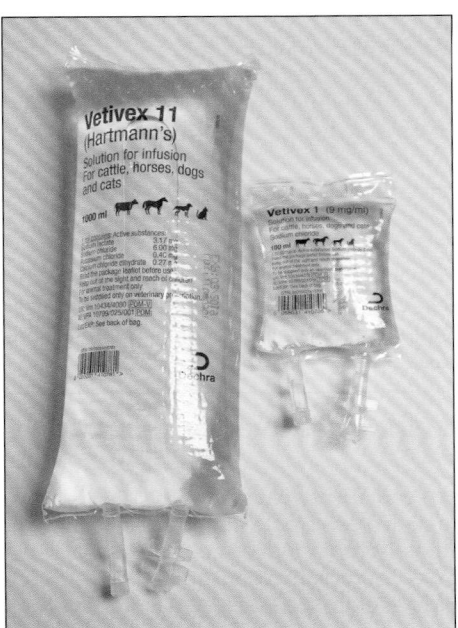

8.5 Collapsible bags.

Suppositories

Solid dosage forms designed for insertion into the rectum are called suppositories. Drugs delivered by this method can be for local or systemic action.

Inhalers

Drugs used in the treatment of lung diseases may be effectively administered by inhalation. This delivers the drug directly to the site of action.

Routes of medicine administration

The route of administration is the way through which a medicine is administered into the body for the treatment or prevention of disease. Drug administration routes can be classified into two main categories: enteral and parenteral.

- **Enteral administration** involves the GI tract and includes oral, buccal and rectal.
- **Parenteral administration** does not involve the GI tract and is often taken to mean injections, such as intravenous and subcutaneous, but also includes topical and inhaled administration.

The route of administration chosen depends on a number of factors:

- The properties of the active drug
- The disease state to be treated
- The temperament and condition of the patient
- The confidence and ability of the owner to administer the medication.

Enteral drug administration

Oral

> ### Advantages and disadvantages
> #### Advantages:
> - Cheap – no need to sterilize; machine produced in large quantities
> - Generally easy for owners to administer at home
> - Variety of dosage forms available.
>
> #### Disadvantages:
> - Onset of action is relatively slow
> - Absorption from the GI tract may be irregular
> - Some drugs are destroyed by enzymes in the GI tract
> - Not suitable for vomiting, seizuring or unconscious patients
> - Food can affect the absorption of some drugs (e.g. pimobendan should always be administered 1 hour before food).

The oral route is the most commonly used method of medicine administration. The medicine, formulated as either a solid or liquid, is absorbed via the GI tract (Figure 8.6).

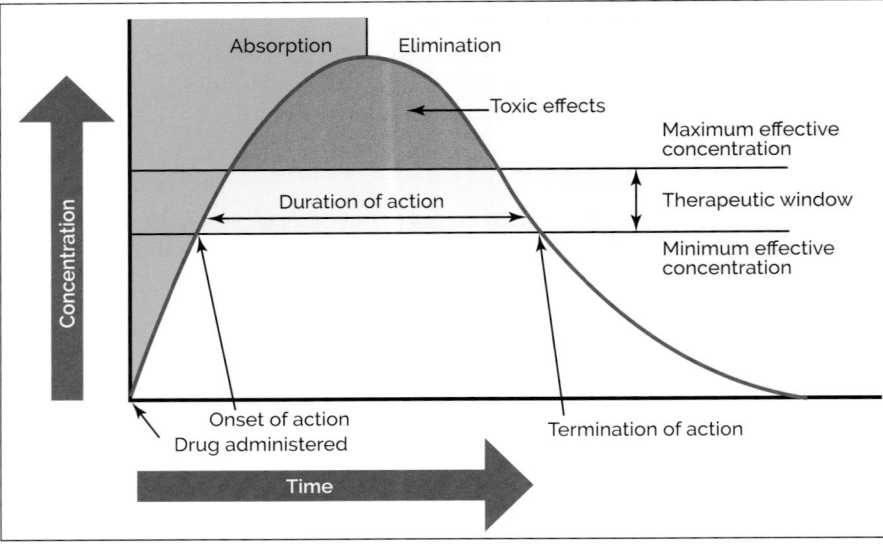

Typical absorption and elimination of a drug following oral administration.

Minimum effective concentration: The minimum concentration of drug in the body for an effect to be felt.

Maximum effective concentration: If drug levels in the body go above this level, toxicity will result.

Therapeutic window: Drug levels should ideally be maintained within the therapeutic window for a therapeutic effect to be achieved with no toxic effects.

Buccal and sublingual

Medicines delivered by the buccal and/or sublingual route have a fast onset of action. This is because of the highly vascular nature of the tongue and buccal cavity, and the presence of saliva, which facilitates the dissolution of the drug. For buccal absorption, the tablet is placed between the cheek and the gum where it dissolves and is absorbed. For sublingual absorption, the tablet is placed under the tongue.

Advantages and disadvantages
Advantages:
- Quick onset of action
- Can be administered to unconscious patients
- Can be useful if patient is vomiting because the medication is not swallowed
- Drugs are absorbed directly into the systemic circulation, thereby avoiding first pass metabolism.

Disadvantages:
- Variability in absorption between species. For example, buprenorphine is well absorbed in cats following sublingual administration, but not in dog
- Few drugs are available in formulations suitable for buccal and sublingual absorption
- Some drugs taste unpleasant.

Rectal

Less commonly used in practice, but many drugs that are given orally can also be used rectally, either as a liquid or a suppository.

Advantages and disadvantages
Advantages:
- Can be used when the oral route is inappropriate (e.g. diazepam for a seizuring patient)
- Useful when the drug causes GI tract irritation.

Disadvantages:
- Absorption can be irregular and unpredictable, leading to variable effect
- Less convenient than the oral route and low owner acceptability for home use.

Parenteral drug administration
Topical

For the topical route, the skin, eyes, nasal passages and ears are used as sites of administration. The skin is the largest organ of the body, although in most species hair is a barrier to topical administration. Medicines applied topically are generally used for local effect, but some medicines are applied transdermally. This is when a drug is absorbed through the skin into the systemic circulation. Examples of drugs applied in this way include fentanyl and methimazole.

Advantages and disadvantages
Advantages:
- Easy to apply
- Non-invasive
- Application can be targeted to the exact site where it is required.

Disadvantages:
- Slow absorption
- Ophthalmic preparations must be applied frequently due to the continuous production of tears
- Most drugs have a high molecular weight and are poorly lipid-soluble, so are not absorbed via the skin or mucous membranes.

Inhalational

Medicines can be inhaled either through the mouth or the nose using inhalers with a spacer device, or a nebulizer (Figure 8.7). Medicines administered by this method are generally for local use.

Advantages and disadvantages
Advantages:
- Fast absorption and onset of action
- Medicines are delivered directly to the site of action
- No first pass metabolism, so doses can be lower than with the oral route, with a consequent reduction in side effects. →

Advantages and disadvantages
continued

Disadvantages:

- Administration can be difficult in animals that do not tolerate a spacer device well
- Nebulizers are expensive.

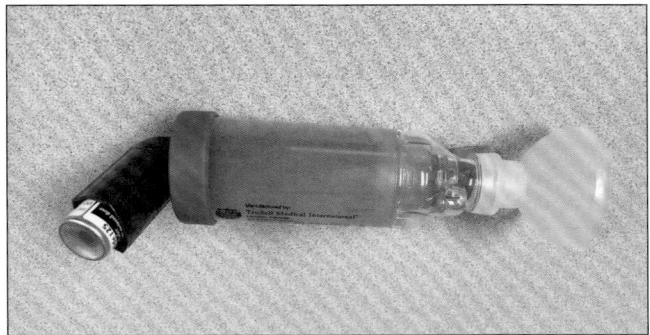

8.7 AeroKat® spacer device and inhaler for the provision of inhalational medications.

Injectable

There are a number of available of routes for injecting medications, including:

- Intravenous (i.v.)
- Subcutaneous (s.c.)
- Intradermal
- Intramuscular (i.m.)
- Intra-arterial
- Intra-articular
- Intraosseous (i.o.)
- Epidural
- Intrathecal
- Intraperitoneal
- Intracardiac
- Intratracheal
- Subconjunctival.

Intravenous

This involves the administration of a medicine directly into the venous blood. Common sites for administration include the cephalic vein and the lateral saphenous vein. Administration can be direct by needle and syringe or after placement of an intravenous catheter, which is useful if administering intravenous medicines frequently or over a number of days. Intravenous catheters should not normally be kept in place for longer than 3 days. Good aseptic technique must be employed and the catheter should be maintained carefully; daily monitoring is required to check for signs of infection and catheter patency (see Chapter 20).

Advantages and disadvantages

Advantages:

- Drugs act quickly because they are delivered directly into the systemic circulation
- 100% bioavailability is achieved because no drug is lost to first pass metabolism
- Drugs irritant to tissues can be given by this method (e.g. cytotoxic drugs). ➔

Advantages and disadvantages
continued

Disadvantages:

- May require catheter placement
- More expensive and time-consuming than other methods of administration
- Drug must be in solution as small particles in a suspension may occlude blood vessels
- Intravenous injection of drugs may cause local irritation
- Intravenous catheters are prone to infection and require regular maintenance (see Chapter 20).

Subcutaneous

This involves the injection of a drug under loose skin, usually the scruff of the neck in small animals as this is where nerve supplies are low and there are no large blood vessels. Only non-irritant fluids can be injected by this method.

Advantages and disadvantages

Advantages:

- Generally pain-free, although it does depend on the drug being administered (e.g. maropitant is known to sting; keeping the bottle in the fridge can reduce this effect)
- Can be used for large volumes (if volume to be injected is very large multiple sites should be used).

Disadvantages:

- Local reactions can occur, leading to swelling and inflammation
- Slower onset of action than intravenous injection, typically 30 minutes. This is due to the lack of large blood vessels.

Intradermal

This is the injection of very small volumes into the dermis. Used in intradermal skin testing for allergies.

Intramuscular

This method commonly uses either the quadriceps muscle of the hindlimb or the paralumbar area (see Figure 8.18). Alternating sides can prevent repeated injections causing one muscle group to become very sore. Care must be taken not to injure the nerves and blood vessels in the area, such as the sciatic nerve.

Advantages and disadvantages

Advantages:

- Drugs are absorbed more quickly and more consistently than with the subcutaneous route
- Drugs in suspension can be given by intramuscular injection.

Disadvantages:

- Painful injection
- Only small volumes can be injected in each site (up to 2 ml in cats and 5 ml in dogs).

Intra-arterial

The arterial route is not used to administer medicines; however, it can be used to monitor blood gasses and arterial blood pressure.

Intra-articular

Used to administer drugs, such as antibiotics and corticosteroids, directly into a joint cavity.

Intraosseous

The injection of a medicine directly into the bone marrow of a long bone. This route may be used when intravenous access is compromised or in small mammals, birds or chelonians. Strict aseptic technique must be used.

Epidural

The administration of a drug into the vertebral canal outside the dura mater. This route is used to administer analgesics and local anaesthesia preoperatively in spinal surgery, and can provide analgesia for up to 8 hours.

Intrathecal

Injections are made into the subarachnoid space. Excellent aseptic technique is required and patients must be monitored carefully for respiratory depression. This route is most commonly used for contrast media administration for myelography.

Intraperitoneal

If intravenous access is compromised, this route can be used to administer fluids and is occasionally used to administer pentobarbital for euthanasia. Absorption can be variable and there is a risk of puncturing an internal organ. A strict aseptic technique is required.

Intracardiac

This route is used in cardiac resuscitation and is where a drug (e.g. adrenaline) is administered directly into the heart.

Intratracheal

This method is also used during cardiac resuscitation and is where drugs are administered directly into the trachea.

Subconjunctival

Not commonly used in small animal practice; this is when a drug is injected into the conjunctival membrane of the eye.

Equipment and techniques used to administer medicines

Administration of enteral medicines

Tablets and capsules

1. Hold the patient's head from the top with your non-dominant hand. If the patient has a long nose, hold the top jaw between your thumb and index finger. Gently fold the top lip over the teeth so if the patient bites down it will bite its lip and not your fingers.

2. Hold the tablet or capsule between the thumb and index finger of your dominant hand.
3. Tilt the head back and use the middle finger of your dominant hand to gently pull down the lower jaw. Keep your finger on the small middle incisor teeth, avoiding the canines. A cat's mouth will automatically open when its head is tilted back.
4. Place the tablet or capsule as far back on the patient's tongue as you are able (Figure 8.8). If you do not manage to get the tablet far enough back, the patient may spit it out.
5. Hold the mouth closed and stroke the patient's throat to encourage swallowing.

> **WARNING**
>
> Some tablets and capsules can cause oesophageal ulceration if they stick in the throat (e.g. doxycycline). A syringe of water or a small amount of food should be given immediately after administration to aid the passage into the stomach

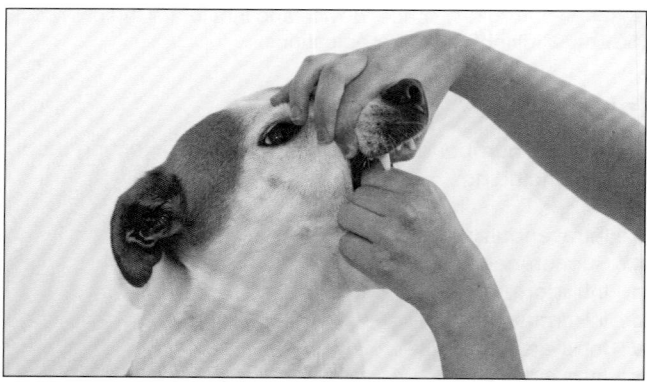

8.8 Oral tablet administration.

Oral liquids

1. Oral liquids are administered into a pouch between the cheek and teeth. With the patient's mouth closed, use the thumb of your non-dominant hand to gently pull back the side of the mouth.
2. Using your dominant hand, squirt the medication into the pouch that is formed between the cheek and teeth (Figure 8.9).
3. Hold the patient's mouth closed and massage the neck to encourage swallowing.

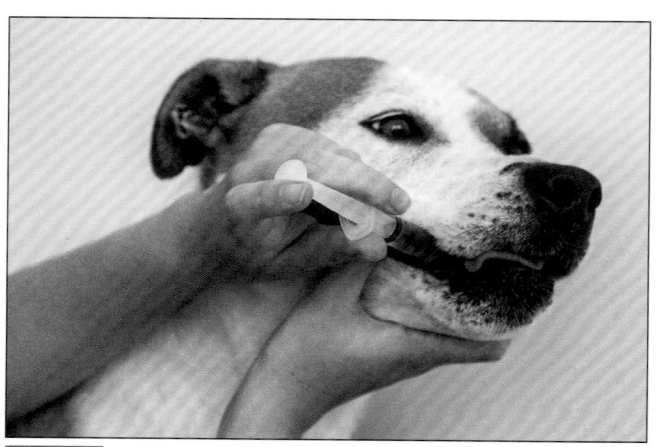

8.9 Oral liquid administration.

WARNING

Liquids are more likely to accidentally enter the windpipe compared with tablets or capsules. To avoid the patient inhaling liquid into the windpipe, do not tilt the head backward

---

Aids to administering oral medications

To help with administration to difficult animals, it may be useful to disguise the medication in some way. Some liquid or powder medications can (and should) be administered on food, but it may also be possible to wrap tablets and capsules in a small amount of something tasty, such as a wet food, ham or a hotdog. Commercial products are also available (e.g. Easypill® Cat Putty, Easypill® Dog Putty and Webbox® Lick-e-Lix), which can be used to disguise medication. If a patient is still unwilling to take the medication, a pet pilling device can be used to directly administer the tablet or capsule (Figure 8.10). These devices are used in the same way as described above, but instead of holding the tablet, it is placed in the tip of the pilling device to enable the tablet to be placed at the very back of the tongue without putting a hand inside the patient's mouth and potentially being bitten.

It may be possible to crush or split tablets using a pill crusher or splitter for easier administration. The SPC should always be checked beforehand to ensure this is appropriate.

In some cases, a patient may require a particular dose that is not readily available in commercial form. In these cases, a medication may need to be compounded into a strength that is appropriate for the patient. Very basic compounding can be performed at the practice using empty gelatine capsules; however, the VMD and Royal College of Veterinary Surgeons (RCVS) recommend that all compounding is performed by a specialist compounding pharmacy. This ensures accuracy of dosing and that an appropriate shelf-life is set for the compounded medicine.

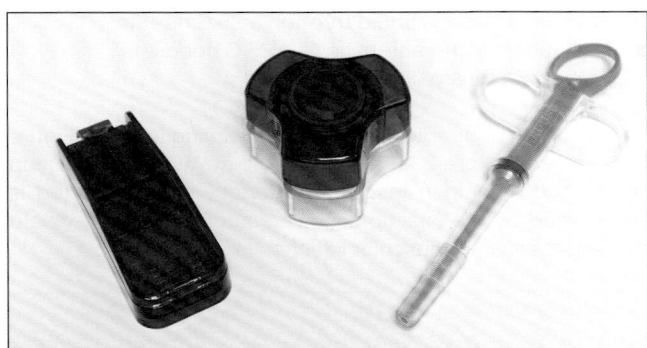

8.10 Equipment that may be useful for administering oral medications: (left to right) tablet splitter, tablet crusher and pilling device.

Administration of parenteral medicines

Topical medications

When applying topical medications, it is important to know when it is essential to wear gloves. Some topical products contain immunosuppressants or steroids, which can cause thinning of the skin with repeated contact. Prolonged or repeated contact with such products can cause some of the drug to be absorbed into the systemic circulation.

Administering a spot-on product

1. Wear gloves or wash hands immediately after use.
2. Check you have the correct pipette size for the patient's weight.
3. Hold the pipette upright. Tap the narrow part of the pipette to ensure that the contents are within the main body of the pipette. Break the snap-off top of the spot-on pipette along the scored line, or remove cap.
4. Part the patient's coat between the shoulder blades until its skin is visible. Place the tip of the pipette directly against the bare skin and squeeze gently several times to empty its contents. Repeat this procedure at one or two different points along the patient's back if a large volume is to be administered.
   It is important to make sure that the product is applied to an area where the animal cannot lick it off, and to make sure that animals do not lick each other following treatment.
5. Care should be taken to avoid excessive wetting of the hair with the product as this will cause a sticky appearance of the hairs at the treatment spot. However, should this occur, it will disappear within 24 hours following application.

Administering eye drops and ointment

1. Wash hands and get medication ready. TAKE CARE: you may need to wear gloves with some products.
2. Clean eye of any discharge using a sterile eye cleaning solution.
3. With your non-dominant hand, cradle the animal's head and use your thumb to pull down the lower eyelid to form a pouch (the conjunctival sac).
4. Hold the drops or ointment in your dominant hand, resting it on the animal's forehead so that if it should jerk, your hand will move with it and you will not injure the patient with the tip of the bottle (Figure 8.11).
5. Holding the bottle or tube close to the eye, apply the required number of drops or a line of ointment into the conjunctival sac. This is a good place to apply treatment as it helps disperse the product and prevents it from running out straight away. Take care not to let the tip of the bottle or tube touch the eye.
6. Continue to hold the patient for a few seconds to give the product time to disperse before they shake their head. If the product is an ointment, gentle massage of the eyelid can aid dispersal.

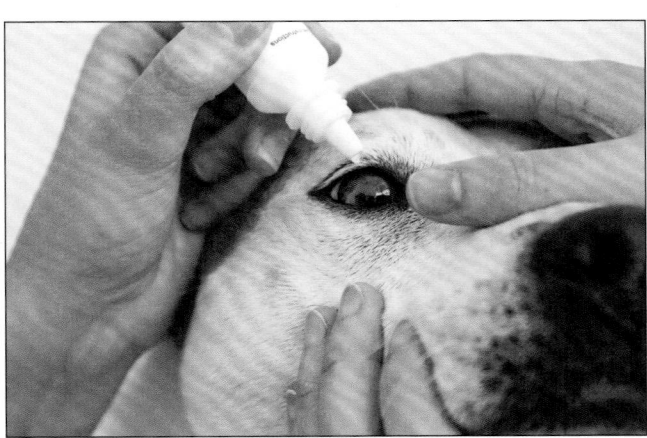

8.11 Eye drop administration.

Administering aural medications

To allow aural medication to be effective, ears must be free of wax and debris. Cleaning of the ears is therefore recommended before commencing treatment for any infection. It is important not to clean the ears directly before applying ear treatment, however, as any ear cleaner present in the canal would dilute the ear treatment. There should be at least 20 minutes between ear cleaning and treatment, to allow the patient to shake its head and for all discharge to be wiped away. Alternatively, ear cleaning and treatments may be administered morning and night, respectively.

Cleaning

1. Position the patient either between your legs or hold it against your chest on a table if the patient is small in size.
2. The ear cleaner should be at room temperature.
3. Hold the ear flap up and backwards using your non-dominant hand and pour the cleaner into the ear canal opening. You should administer enough cleaner to fill the canal (Figure 8.12).
4. Continue to hold the ear flap up and backwards so the cleaner does not leak out of the canal. Massage the base of the ear near the neck with your dominant hand for 15–30 seconds to encourage the cleaner to reach the bottom corners of the ear canal and dislodge any deep wax or debris.
5. Use a cotton ball or swab to remove any debris that has floated up to the surface of the cleaner. Never insert a cotton bud or Q-tip® into the ear canal.
6. Inspect the ear and repeat cleaning if significant dirt and debris are still visible.

Treatment

1. Hold the medication in your dominant hand.
2. Gently pull the animal's infected ear flap up and backwards, exposing the ear canal. With smaller animals, you can do this with the last two fingers of the same hand that is holding the ear medication, placing the non-dominant hand under the dog's jaw to support its head.
3. Administer the prescribed number of ear drops, placing the dropper a short way into the ear canal.
4. Rub the base of the ear against the head in a circular motion. Be cautious and gentle as the patient may object to this procedure. You should hear a 'squishing' sound as you massage the medication deep into the ear canal.
5. Release the ear and allow the patient to shake its head.
6. Use a cotton ball or swab to gently wipe away any accumulated debris or drops from the ear flap.

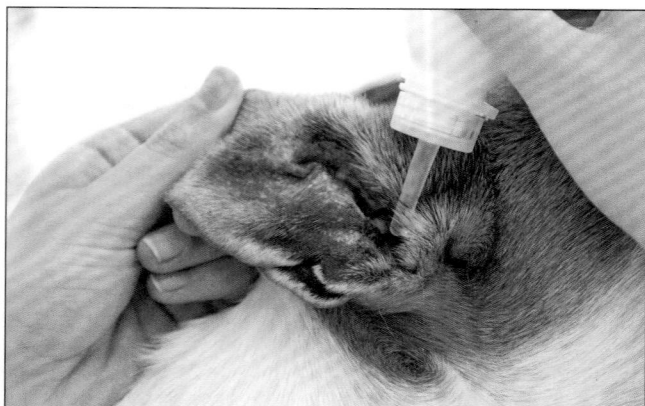

8.12 Ear cleaner administration.

Inhalers and spacer devices

Spacers consist of a chamber with a mask at one end and a hole in the other for inserting the mouthpiece of the inhaler (see Figure 8.7). The patient's nostrils should be covered by the mask and the mouth should be held closed. Depress the canister to deliver the required number of puffs, and hold the mask in place for 5–6 breaths to allow the drug to be inhaled into the lungs. If the patient is nervous of the sound of the inhaler, hold the chamber away from them while you depress the canister, then immediately place the mask over their nose. Spacers should be washed periodically in warm soapy water, taking care not to damage the membrane, and allowed to drip dry. **Do not** use a towel to dry the chamber because this can cause a build-up of static energy, which makes the drug particles stick to the wall of the spacer instead of being breathed into the lungs.

Injections and infusions

The administration of drugs by injection or infusion (generally defined as an injection lasting longer than 15 minutes) requires the use of a hypodermic needle and syringe, and possibly an intravenous cannula, infusion pump or syringe pump.

Hypodermic needles

These consist of a hollow stainless steel tube called a **shaft**, which is cut at an angle at one end to make a sharp point or bevel for easy penetration of the skin. Attached to the other end of the shaft is the needle **hub**, which allows attachment to a syringe. Needle hubs come in various shades, each universally signifying the width, or **gauge** (G), of the needle. Hypodermic needles are available in sizes ranging from 6 G to 31 G, with the smaller number signifying a wider diameter needle. In small animal medicine, the needle sizes most commonly used are 21 G, 23 G and 25 G (Figure 8.13). The appropriate gauge to use is determined by:

- The properties of the drug to be injected – it is difficult to draw up a viscous liquid through a 25 G needle
- The patient's characteristics – a 25 G needle is preferable for small exotic species.

Hypodermic needles also come in varying lengths (Figure 8.13). For example, a 23 G needle may be available in a ⅜ inch length and a 1¼ inch length. The length to be selected is determined by the injection site (e.g. a longer needle would be used for an intramuscular injection in a large dog).

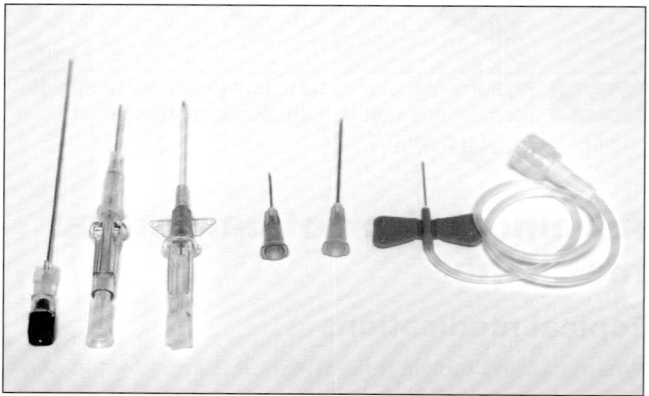

8.13 Selection of needles. Left to right: 22 G, 3.5 inch spinal needle; 24 G, 3/4 inch intravenous catheter; 20 G, 1.25 inch winged intravenous catheter; 23 G, 5/8 inch hypodermic needle; 21 G, 1.5 inch hypodermic needle; 27 G butterfly needle.

Hypodermic syringes

These are made up of a transparent plastic **barrel** that is graduated to indicate the volume. A plunger moves up and down the barrel to measure the volume. With 3-part syringes, a rubber stopper at the top of the plunger ensures that no liquid leaks out, whilst in 2-part syringes, the plunger is designed for a precise fit that stops any leakage. The 3-part syringes generally have a smoother feel when in use. The tip of the syringe is open, with a **Luer fitting** for attachment to a needle or Luer connector. Syringes are available in sizes ranging from 1 ml to 60 ml, with different tips depending on their use (Figure 8.14).

- A Luer slip tip is the standard tip, which slips into a needle hub.
- A Luer lock tip has a screw on attachment for needles and connectors for a secure fit. These are used for chemotherapy administration.
- A catheter tip is longer than a Luer tip, and can be attached directly on to catheters and feeding tubes.

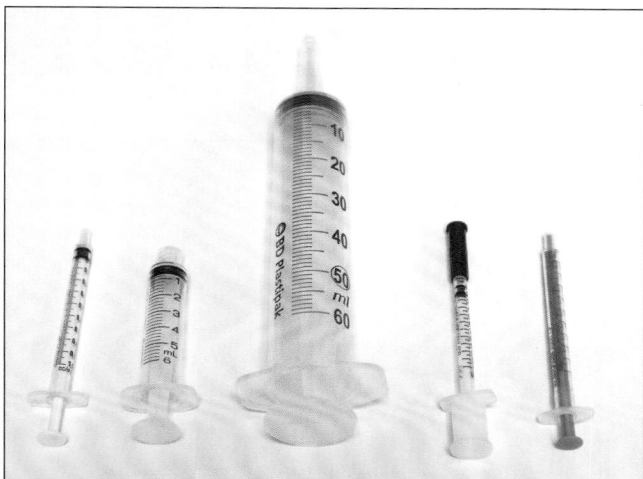

8.14 Selection of syringes. Left to right: 1 ml Luer slip syringe; 5 ml Luer lock syringe; 50 ml catheter tip syringe; 40 IU/ml 0.3 ml insulin syringe; 1 ml low dead space syringe.

The size of syringe selected depends on the volume to be administered. It should be the smallest available that will allow the dose to be accurately measured (i.e. do not use a 10 ml syringe to measure a dose of 3.5 ml, for greater accuracy a 5 ml syringe should be used instead).

> **WARNING**
>
> Some drugs, such as diazepam, are absorbed into the plastic of a syringe and should not be drawn up in advance. Refer to manufacturer's SPC for advice if the product is not for immediate use

Low dead space syringes are also available. These come with a plunger designed to extend into the hub of the needle/syringe to avoid wastage of the drug. They are particularly useful for avoiding wastage of Schedule 2 Controlled Drugs.

Insulin syringes are used for precise measurement of insulin doses. They are graduated in international units (IU) rather than in millilitres and are available as 40 IU/ml or 100 IU/ml in sizes from 0.3 ml to 1 ml. Insulin syringes come with a needle already attached and have no needle hub to avoid wastage of insulin (see Figure 8.14).

> **WARNING**
>
> It is vitally important to ensure that the correct type of insulin syringe is selected for the type of insulin being administered. Even small errors in an insulin dose can have severe consequences

Intravenous cannulae

These are for peripheral use (see Figure 8.13) and consist of a flexible nylon catheter surrounding a stainless steel trochar (needle), and a hub that may or may not have wings for secure attachment to the patient. The cannula has a Luer fitting for attachment of a syringe, port, infusion set or adaptor (see Chapter 20 for more details).

Infusion drivers and syringe pumps

The reader is referred to Chapter 20 for discussion of infusion drivers and syringe pumps.

Withdrawing a dose from a multi-dose vial

1. Gather the required equipment: medicine vial, needle and syringe, alcohol pad and sharps container.
2. Wash your hands.
3. Check the medicine and dosage are correct.
4. Wipe the rubber top clean with an alcohol pad and leave to dry for 30 seconds.
5. Hold the syringe in your hand like a pencil, with the needle pointed upwards.
6. With the cap still on, pull back the plunger to the line on the syringe for your dose. This fills the syringe with air.
7. Insert the needle into the rubber top. Do not touch or bend the needle.
8. Slowly push the air into the vial. This prevents a vacuum from forming. If too little air is put in, it is hard to draw out the medicine. If too much air is put in, the medicine may be forced out of the vial.
9. Turn the vial upside down and hold it up in the air. Keep the needle tip in the medicine.
10. Pull back the plunger to the line on the syringe for your dose.
11. Tap the syringe with your finger to move air bubbles to the top. Then push gently on the plunger to push the air bubbles back into the vial.
12. If there are a lot of bubbles, push the plunger to push all the medicine back into the vial. Draw the medicine out again slowly and tap the air bubbles out. Double check that you still have the right amount of medicine drawn up.
13. Remove the syringe from the vial and recap the needle using the one-handed technique (Figure 8.15).
14. Draw back slightly on the syringe plunger before removing the needle and replacing with a new one and carefully expelling the air bubble.
15. Check you still have the appropriate dose.
16. If the medicine is not to be administered immediately, label the syringe with the drug name and strength, date, and time.

When reconstituting a powder in a multi-dose vial, care should be taken to select the correct diluent and appropriate diluent volume. Some products come with a separate vial of diluent, but sterile water or sterile sodium chloride may have to be used for injection. Inject the diluent into the vial, keeping the needle above the level of the vial contents. To relieve pressure in the vial, release the syringe plunger occasionally to allow air to escape into the syringe.

Recapping needles: The 'one-handed' technique

Many accidental needlestick injuries occur when staff are recapping needles. Recapping is a dangerous practice: if at all possible, needles should be disposed of immediately without recapping them.

If it does become necessary to recap a needle (for example, to avoid carrying an unprotected sharp when immediate disposal is not possible), do not bend or break the needle and do not remove the hypodermic needle from the syringe by hand.

To safely recap needles, use the one-handed technique:

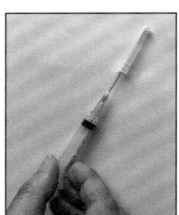

Step 1
Place the cap on a flat surface, then remove your hand from the cap.

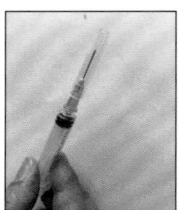

Step 2
With one hand, hold the syringe and use the needle to 'scoop up' the cap.

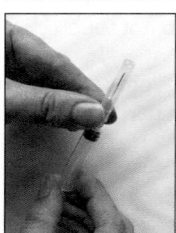

Step 3
When the cap covers the needle completely, use the other hand to secure the cap on the needle hub. Be careful to handle the cap at the bottom only (near the hub).

8.15 Recapping needles safely using the one-handed technique.

Withdrawing a dose from a snap-top ampoule

1. Gather the required equipment: medicine ampoule, needle and syringe, gauze pad and sharps container.
2. Wash your hands.
3. Check that the medicine and dosage are correct.
4. Tap the ampoule with your finger to move the liquid down from the ampoule neck.
5. Wrap the top of the ampoule with a gauze pad and snap. The ampoule may be marked with a dot or small line to indicate the weakest part of the neck. This is where the ampoule should be broken.
6. Place the ampoule top into a sharps container.
7. Check the ampoule contents for glass fragments. If any are visible, discard the ampoule.
8. Tilt the ampoule. Surface tension will prevent the liquid from running out, even if fully inverted.
9. Using a needle and syringe withdraw the appropriate dose, ensuring the needle does not touch the neck of the ampoule.
10. Tap the syringe with your finger to move air bubbles to the top. Then push gently on the plunger to expel the air bubbles.
11. Check you have the required dose; invert the ampoule and draw up further medication if required.

12. If you plan to put the syringe down, put the cover back on the needle using the one-handed technique (see Figure 8.15).
13. If the medicine is not to be administered immediately, label the syringe with the drug name and strength, date and time.
14. Place the ampoule into a sharps container.

Intravenous injection

In the dog and cat, the most common site for intravenous drug administration is the cephalic vein (Figure 8.16). Other injection sites include the saphenous vein and the jugular vein. Administration of drugs through the jugular vein requires placement of a central line and is used when patients require intensive care (see Chapter 20). Ideally, an intravenous catheter would be placed for repeated intravenous injections, but single injections may be given using a needle and syringe.

Where multiple drugs are being administered through the same intravenous cannula using a Y-site connector or multiway adaptor, it must be confirmed that they are compatible with other medicines and fluids. If two or more injections are to be given through a fluid line, the line must be flushed well in between. Incompatibilities between drugs can cause crystals to form, which would be harmful if administered to the patient.

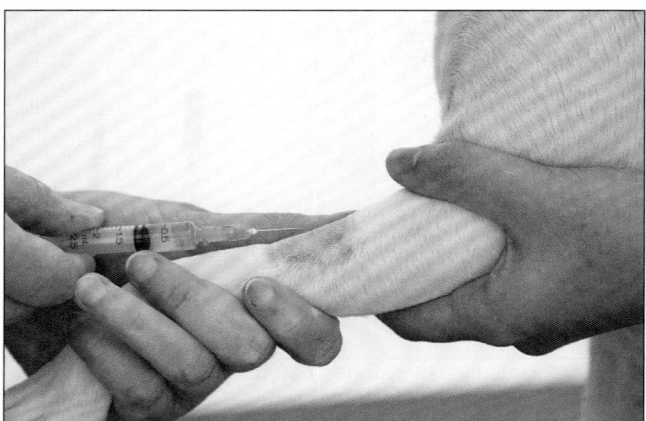

8.16 Intravenous injection into the cephalic vein.

Giving an intravenous injection into the cephalic vein

1. Gather the required equipment: needle and syringe loaded with the appropriate drug and dose, swab soaked in alcohol, clean dry swab and microporous tape.
2. Wash your hands.
3. The patient should be sitting or in sternal recumbency. An assistant should restrain the animal's head with one hand and use the other to extend the leg (see Chapter 11).
4. The operator should clip the area of intended venepuncture and clean the area with the alcohol-soaked swab. The skin should be left to dry for 30 seconds.
5. The assistant should raise the vein by applying pressure around the elbow joint.
6. Remove the needle cap and insert the needle into the vein with the bevel facing upwards. If the needle is in the vein, blood should flow into the syringe if the plunger is withdrawn gently.
7. When the needle is in the correct position, the assistant should remove pressure from the vein and the injection may be administered by slowly depressing the syringe plunger.

8. If large volumes are to be given, regular checks should be made to ensure the syringe is still in the vein.
9. Once the injection has been administered, withdraw the needle and immediately apply pressure to the injection site for 30 seconds using a dry swab to prevent haemorrhage.
10. Use tape to secure the swab in place.

Subcutaneous injection

The loose skin from the back of the neck to the rump is the most common site for subcutaneous injection in small animals (Figure 8.17). This area is suitable because there are relatively few nerves and large blood vessels.

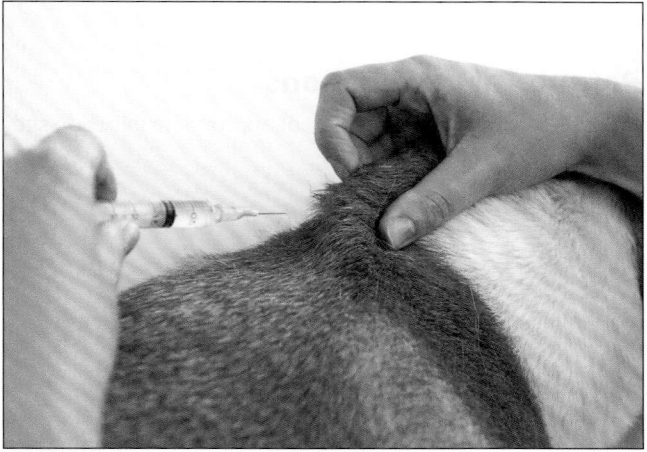

| 8.17 | Subcutaneous injection. |

Giving a subcutaneous injection

1. Gather the required equipment: needle and syringe containing the appropriate drug and dose.
2. Wash your hands.
3. With the non-dominant hand, gently raise a fold of skin at the back of the patient's neck (the scruff).
4. Insert the needle under the skin, taking care to ensure the needle does not go all the way through the fold.
5. Once the needle has been inserted, pull back on the plunger only. If blood is seen, remove the needle and try a different location. If there is no blood, push the plunger forward to empty the syringe.

Intramuscular injection

An assistant will be needed to restrain the animal because intramuscular injections are generally painful.

Giving an intramuscular injection

1. Gather the required equipment: needle and syringe containing the appropriate drug and dose.
2. Wash your hands.
3. Locate the area for injection (e.g. the lumbar or quadriceps muscles in a dog).
4. Holding the syringe at a right angle to the injection site, insert the needle through the skin and into the muscle (Figure 8.18).
5. Once the needle has been inserted, pull back on the plunger. If blood is seen, remove the needle and try a different location using a new needle. If not, push the plunger forward to empty the syringe and then remove the needle.

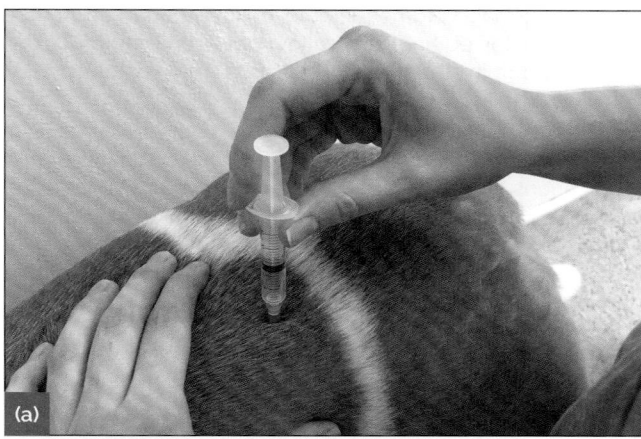

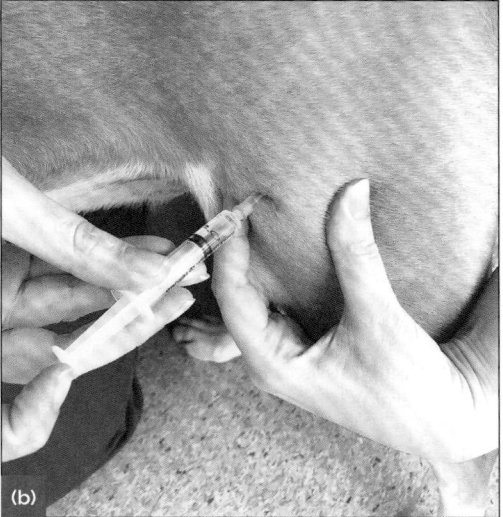

| 8.18 | Intramuscular injection. **(a)** Injection into the epaxial muscle. **(b)** Injection into the quadriceps muscle. |

Administration of medicines to exotic species

The majority of medicines for exotic species are administered either as oral liquids or by injection. Oral liquids should be administered carefully, with as small a volume used as possible. Larger volumes should be administered via crop/feeding tube to avoid the patient aspirating the drug. Some medicines may need to be diluted due to the very small volumes to be administered. Sterile water can be used to dilute most solutions; suspensions should not be diluted. Patients may willingly take oral medications if mixed with something sweet, such as banana or yoghurt (check that any food used is suitable for the species in question). Oral medications may also be mixed into drinking water; however, this has the disadvantage of it being difficult to monitor whether the entire dose has been administered, and is not suitable for use at home where more than one animal shares the water supply.

Oral medications

Small mammals

Small mammals may be given oral medications by gently syringing the liquid into the side of the mouth. For fractious rabbits, wrapping them in a towel 'burrito' can be helpful. Medication should be syringed as far back in the mouth as possible to ensure that the patient does not spit it out, but not directly down the throat which may cause aspiration of the medicine. Small volumes should be used and the patient should be allowed time to swallow between mouthfuls; this can make administering oral medicines time-consuming.

Birds

For avian patients, a crop tube can be used to administer oral medications, fluids and food. Metal crop tubes are preferred to plastic or silicone, but care should be taken not to perforate the oesophagus with a rigid tube. To reduce the risk of inadvertently placing the tube in the trachea, a tube with a diameter greater than the tracheal diameter should be used.

Crop tube (gavage) feeding

1. Restrain the bird's body and head, holding the bird in a vertical position with the neck extended.
2. Ensure the crop tube is lubricated.
3. Insert the tube from the left side of the mouth, moving it backwards and across the mouth, past and to the right of the glottis, sliding it into and down the oesophagus on the right side of the neck and into the crop.
4. Confirm the tube is in the oesophagus/crop by visual inspection and/or gentle palpation of the neck.
5. Slowly deliver the medication, fluid or feed formula, monitoring for fluid appearing in pharynx. If this occurs, stop and continue at a slower rate.

Reptiles

Oral medication for reptiles may also be administered by gavage. This is particularly appropriate where large volumes (>1 ml/kg) are to be administered. Depending on the species and size of the patient, a range of tubes may be used, from intravenous catheters to intravenous giving set tubing. Suggested maximum volumes are 5–15 ml/kg for chelonians, 15–30 ml/kg for snakes and 10–20 ml/kg for lizards.

Topical medications

Topical products are of limited value in birds and reptiles, although they are used in small mammals. Reptile skin has a thick, impermeable keratinized layer, and the feathers of avian species make topical application difficult. Exceptions to this are for the treatment of surface lesions and ectoparasitic infections.

When administering aural medicines to rabbits, the ear should be held whilst applying the drops, in order to prevent immediate shaking of the medication out of the ear canal post-application. Massaging the base of the ear when administering ointments improves the rabbit's tolerance of being medicated. Care must be taken to ensure the patient cannot groom the site of application of dermal products. The ideal application site for spot-on products is between the shoulder blades.

Inhaled medications

A nebulized solution of F10, diluted 1:250 with water may be used in rabbits with chronic respiratory disease and is very well tolerated. Other products, such as antibacterials and antifungals, can be nebulized in birds.

Parenteral medications

Figure 8.19 provides a summary of appropriate injection sites for a variety of exotic species.

Safe handling and disposal of equipment

Gloves should be worn when directly handling any loose medicinal product. Particular care should be taken by those at risk, such as pregnant women, the immunosuppressed or those with allergies to medicines such as penicillin. It may be appropriate for such individuals to avoid certain tasks within the pharmacy and a risk assessment should be performed before medicines are handled.

Some medicines, such as cytotoxic drugs, should be prepared and administered in a separate location to the main pharmacy, using equipment with needle-free systems (Figure 8.20) or fume cupboards (Figure 8.21).

Special care should be taken when handling sharps. Snap-top ampoules should be placed immediately in the sharps bin after the required dose has been withdrawn. Needles should only be recapped using the appropriate

Patient type	Intravenous	Subcutaneous	Intramuscular	Intraperitoneal	Intraosseous
Small mammals	Marginal ear vein; cephalic vein; lateral tail vein	Dorsal body; 'scruff'	Lumbar	Off midline, caudal to umbilicus	Proximal femur; proximal tibia; proximal humerus
Birds	Brachial vein; medial metatarsal vein	Inguinal; axillary; interscapular	Pectoral (in very large birds, the quadriceps is used)	Not applicable	Distal ulna; proximal tibiotarsus
Snakes	Ventral coccygeal vein	Dorsal lateral third, over ribs	Intercostal	Cranial to vent on lateral wall (intracoelomic)	Not applicable
Lizards	Ventral tail vein	Loose lateral skin, over ribs	Triceps	Ventral, off midline, caudal to ribs	Proximal/distal femur; proximal tibia
Amphibians	Femoral vein; midline abdominal vein	Dorsal area over shoulders	Triceps	Ventrolateral quadrant (intracoelomic)	Not applicable
Chelonians	Dorsal tail	Distal limb	Triceps; pectoral	Ventral, cranial to hindlimb in fossa	Bridge between plastron and carapace; femur
Fish	Caudal vein	Not applicable	Dorsal lateral epaxial musculature	Rostral to ventral on lateral surface (intracoelomic)	Not applicable

8.19 Appropriate injection sites for the administration of medications in exotic pets.

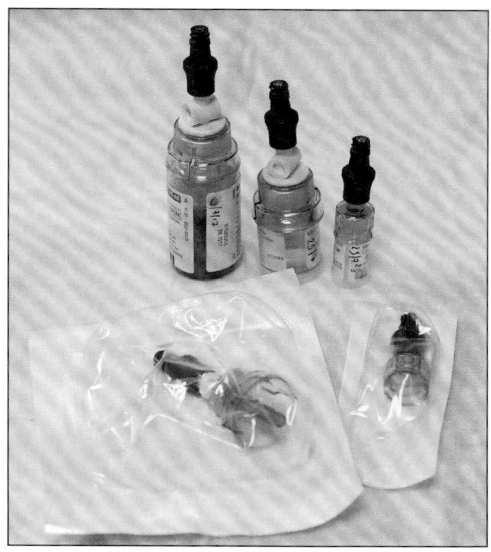

Needle-free system.

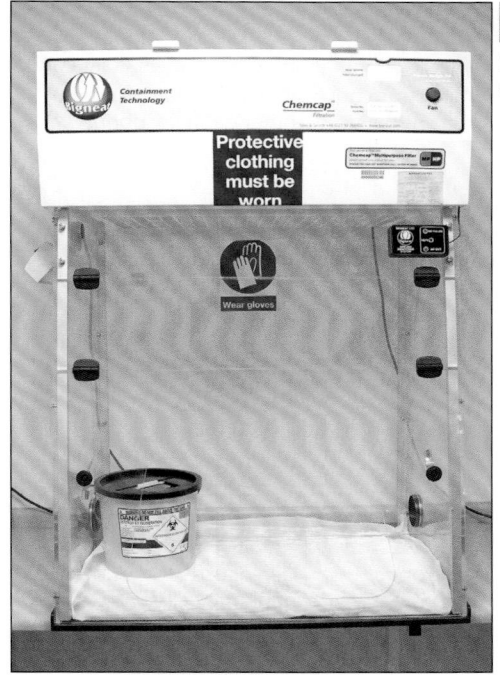

Fume cupboard.

one-handed technique (see Figure 8.15) and if not capped, they should be placed directly into a sharps bin after use. Uncapped needles should not be transported around the practice.

Disposal of equipment used in the dispensing process (see Chapter 2) should be as follows:

- Gloves into clinical waste bin
- Snap-top ampoules and needles into yellow lidded sharps bin. It is not recommended that the needle be separated from the syringe
- Contaminated syringes into a blue pharmaceutical waste bin
- Empty medicine containers into a blue pharmaceutical waste bin.

Contaminated counting apparatus such as triangles and measures should be washed in warm soapy water, dried and reused.

Classes of drugs used in veterinary medicine

Information on medicines used in veterinary practice can be found in a variety of sources, from textbooks and formularies, to websites and datasheets. Most drugs administered are licensed for use in animals, but some are not. It is important to recognize the difference between licensed and unlicensed indications and doses in the reference sources you consult (see 'Legal aspects of veterinary medicines' for more information on the requirement to use medicines licensed for use in animals where available (the Cascade)). The source of information should also be considered. Some websites may contain information based on a lay person's knowledge, not on evidenced-based medicine and clinical trials. The following information is a guide to the most common classes of drugs used in veterinary medicine. It contains information on medicines that are licensed and unlicensed for use in animals.

Antimicrobial drugs

- An **antimicrobial** is any substance of natural, semi-synthetic or synthetic origin that kills or inhibits the growth of microorganisms but causes little or no damage to the host.
- An **antibacterial** is a substance that has an inhibitory or lethal effect on bacterial organisms (see Chapter 5). It may be of natural, semi-synthetic or synthetic origin.
- An **antibiotic** is a low molecular weight substance produced by a microorganism that at a low concentration inhibits or kills other microorganisms. Strictly speaking, antibiotics do not include antimicrobial substances that are synthetic (sulphonamides and quinolones) or semi-synthetic (meticillin and amoxicillin).

Antibacterial drugs

Antibacterials are classified in several ways, including:

- Spectrum of activity
  - Broad-spectrum antibacterials are active against both Gram-positive and Gram-negative organisms.
  - Narrow-spectrum antibacterials have limited activity and are primarily only useful against particular species of microorganisms.
- Effect on bacteria
  - Bactericidal drugs are those that kill target organisms.
  - Bacteriostatic drugs inhibit or delay bacterial growth and replication.
  - Some antibiotics can be both bacteriostatic and bactericidal, depending on the dose, duration of exposure and the state of the invading bacteria.
- Mode of action
  - Inhibitors of cell wall synthesis.
  - Inhibitors of cell membrane function.
  - Inhibitors of protein synthesis.
  - Inhibitors of nucleic acid synthesis.
  - Inhibitors of other metabolic processes.

Figure 8.22 provides a summary of the main classes of antibacterial drugs used in veterinary medicine.

There are a number of factors to consider when choosing the most appropriate antibacterial for any given infection.

Class of drug	Mechanism of action	Examples	Spectrum of activity	Additional information
Beta-lactam: Penicillins	Cell wall inhibitor Bactericidal	Penicillin	Narrow-spectrum penicillins: Gram-positive	Hypersensitivity reactions in humans can occur
		Amoxicillin Ampicillin	Extended activity penicillins: improved activity against Gram-negative bacteria	Amoxicillin is often potentiated with clavulanic acid to inhibit the enzyme beta-lactamase
		Cloxacillin	Anti-staphylococcal penicillins: highly effective against *Staphylococcus aureus*	Rarely used in veterinary medicine
		Ticarcillin	Anti-pseudomonal penicillins: especially effective against *Pseudomonas aeruginosa*	Rarely used in veterinary medicine except for ears infected with *Pseudomonas*
Beta-lactam: Cephalosporins	Cell wall inhibitor Bactericidal	Cefalexin	1st generation: Gram-positive	Often used for *Staphylococcus* infections
		Cefuroxime	2nd generation: weaker activity against Gram-positive bacteria but have a wider Gram-negative bacteria spectrum	Used for surgical prophylaxis
		Ceftazidime	3rd generation: limited Gram-positive spectrum but have a wide Gram-negative spectrum	Better penetration into cerebrospinal fluid than other cephalosporins
		Cefixime	4th generation: highly effective against both Gram-positive and Gram-negative bacteria	Must be administered intravenously. Not commonly used in veterinary medicine
Beta-lactam: Carbapenems	Cell wall inhibitor Bactericidal	Imipenem	Highly effective against Gram-negative bacteria and Gram-positive bacteria. Use restricted to prevent resistance	Not used in veterinary medicine
Beta-lactam: Monobactams	Cell wall inhibitor Bactericidal	Aztreonam	No activity against Gram-positive or anaerobic bacteria but highly effective against certain Gram-negative bacteria	Not used in veterinary medicine
Aminoglycosides	Interfere with protein synthesis Bactericidal	Amikacin Gentamycin	Gram-negative aerobes	Can cause ototoxicity, nephrotoxicity and neuromuscular blockade
Fluoroquinolones	Inhibit nucleic acid synthesis Bactericidal	Enrofloxacin Marbofloxacin Pradafloxacin	Broad-spectrum, especially Gram-positive and Gram-negative bacteria	Resistance occurs rapidly with older fluoroquinolones. Can be neurotoxic
Tetracyclines	Interfere with protein synthesis Bacteriostatic	Oxytetracycline Doxycycline	Broad-spectrum. Gram-positive and Gram-negative bacteria	Do not give to pregnant or young animals due to effects on bones and teeth. Give with food or water bolus to avoid irritating the oesophagus
Macrolides	Interfere with protein synthesis Bactericidal or bacteriostatic	Erythromycin Azithromycin Tylosin	Gram-positive and anaerobes	Pain and swelling can occur after injection; more commonly used orally
Potentiated sulphonamides	Inhibit the bacterial enzyme which converts TH4 into folic acid, which is required for DNA synthesis Bactericidal	Trimethoprim/ Sulfadiazine	Broad-spectrum. Gram-positive, Gram-negative and some protozoal organisms	Do not give alongside antacids. Adverse effects generally due to hypersensitivity reactions

8.22 Summary of the main classes of antibacterial drugs.

continues ▶

Class of drug	Mechanism of action	Examples	Spectrum of activity	Additional information
Lincosamides	Interfere with protein synthesis Bactericidal or bacteriostatic	Clindamycin	Particularly effective against anaerobes	Can cause gastrointestinal disturbances
Nitroimidazoles	Inhibits nucleic acid synthesis Bactericidal	Metronidazole	Anaerobes	Do not use in pregnant animals. May cause red/brown discoloration of urine. Useful for protozoal infections
Chloramphenicols	Interfere with protein synthesis Bacteriostatic	Chloramphenicol Florfenicol	Broad-spectrum. Gram-positive, Gram-negative, anaerobes	Use of chloramphenicol is restricted to emergency use in humans except for ophthalmic use

8.22 *continued* Summary of the main classes of antibacterial drugs.

- The properties of the infecting bacteria (e.g. anaerobe, aerobe, Gram-positive, Gram-negative) (see Chapter 5).
- The spectrum of activity of the drug must be understood, to allow for selection of an antibacterial likely to be effective against the known, or suspected, organism. Ideally, culture and sensitivity tests should be performed to identify which antibacterials will be effective.
- The site of infection must be considered. For example, not all antibacterials can cross into the cerebrospinal fluid (CSF) so are ineffective against infections of the central nervous system (CNS).
- Host factors such as liver or kidney disease, age, allergies or pregnancy mean some antibacterials may have to be excluded or doses altered.
- Any potential side effects of the drug.
- Drug interactions with any concurrent treatments.

Antimicrobial resistance

Antimicrobial resistance occurs when microorganisms (e.g. bacteria, fungi, viruses and parasites) change when they are exposed to antimicrobial drugs (e.g. antibiotics, antifungals, antivirals, antimalarials and anthelmintics). As a result, the medicines become ineffective and infections persist in the body, increasing the risk of spread to others. Examples of resistant bacteria include *Escherichia coli* and meticillin-resistant *Staphylococcus pseudintermedius* (MRSP). To help prevent increasing antimicrobial resistance, the BSAVA and the Small Animal Medicine Society (SAMSoc) have produced a set of guidelines (Figure 8.23).

PROTECT ME

P rescribe only when necessary
- Consider non-bacterial disease (e.g. viral infections, nutritional imbalance, metabolic disorders)
- Remember that some bacterial diseases will self-resolve without antibacterials
- Offer a non-prescription form

R educe prophylaxis
- Perioperative antibacterials are **NOT** a substitute for surgical asepsis
- Prophylactic antibacterials are only appropriate in some immunocompromised patients ➜

8.23 BSAVA and SAMSoc PROTECT ME.

O ffer other options
- Consider therapeutic alternatives (lavage and debridement of infected material, cough suppressants, fluid therapy, nutritional modification)
- Using topical preparations reduces selection pressure on resident intestinal flora (the microbiome)
- Use effective hygiene techniques and antiseptics to prevent infections

T reat effectively
- Consider which bacteria are likely to be involved
- Consider drug penetration of the target site
- Use the shortest effective course and avoid underdosing
- Ensure compliance with appropriate formulation and provide clear instructions

E mploy narrow spectrum
- Unnecessarily broad-spectrum antibacterials could promote antibacterial resistance
- The use of narrow-spectrum antibacterials limits effects on commensal bacteria
- Use culture results to support de-escalation (switching to a narrower spectrum antibacterial)

C ulture appropriately
- A sample for culture should be collected before starting antibacterial therapy wherever possible
- Culture is essential when prolonged (>1 week) treatment courses are anticipated, when resistance is likely (e.g. hospital acquired infections) and in life-threatening infections
- If first-line treatment fails, do not use another antibacterial without supportive culture and sensitivity results (avoid cycling antibacterials)

T ailor your practice policy
- A customized practice policy can guide antibacterial selection to address the bacterial infections and resistance patterns that you encounter, minimizing inappropriate use
- Complete the tick boxes in this poster to highlight your practice's first-line approach to each condition

M onitor
- Track and record culture profiles and update your practice policy accordingly
- Monitor for preventable infections (e.g. postoperative) and alter practices if needed
- Audit your own antibacterial use, particularly of critically important antibacterials (floroquinolones/cefovecin), e.g. using mySavsnet AMR

E ducate others
- Share this important message to reduce the threat from multi-resistant strains of bacteria and improve the health of pets and people

Antifungal drugs

Superficial fungal infections of the skin are common, with topical treatment being the most usual therapy. Systemic infection may be severe and life-threatening, and may require oral or occasionally parenteral therapy. Fungal infections are often difficult to clear completely and treatment can be prolonged. Owners should be informed to continue treatment for some time after the clinical signs have cleared up to ensure that all fungi present have been treated, or relapse may occur. Hair may need to be clipped to allow sufficient contact by topical agents with the skin. Figure 8.24 lists the antifungals used in veterinary medicine.

Antiviral drugs

Ideally, infection by viruses should be prevented by vaccination; however, this is not always possible. Unfortunately, the way viruses replicate makes them difficult to treat. With antiviral drugs being of limited use, treatment of viral infections is generally supportive. There are a small number of antivirals available:

- Interferon omega is licensed for the treatment of canine parvovirus, feline immunodeficiency virus (FIV) and feline leukaemia virus (FeLV)
- Aciclovir is not licensed for use in animals but can be useful in the treatment of feline herpesvirus
- Zidovudine may be of some use in FIV, although it is also not licensed for use in animals.

Vaccines

A vaccine is a biological preparation that improves immunity to a particular disease. Traditional vaccines contain either parts of microbes or whole microbes that have been killed or weakened so that they do not cause disease. These are termed **killed** or **inactivated** vaccines. **Live attenuated** vaccines produce a better and longer acting immune response than inactivated vaccines. These are made from live viruses

or bacteria which replicate in the patient, but because they have been weakened, they cause no, or only subclinical, disease. **Toxoid vaccines** are made from a toxin (poison) that has been made harmless and work by eliciting an immune response against the toxin. They are based on the toxins produced by certain bacteria (e.g. tetanus or diphtheria). The toxin invades the bloodstream and is largely responsible for the clinical signs of the disease. The protein-based toxin is rendered harmless (now called a toxoid) and used as the antigen in the vaccine to elicit immunity. (See also Chapter 7.)

Vaccines comprise two main parts: the **antigen** and the **adjuvant**.

- Antigens are the components derived from the structure of disease-causing organisms, which are recognized as 'foreign' by the immune system and trigger a protective immune response to the vaccine.
- Adjuvants are added to stimulate the production of antibodies against the vaccine to make it more effective.

Figure 8.25 lists the main vaccines available for companion animals in the UK.

Antiparasitic drugs

Parasites are organisms that live on or in another organism, deriving their nourishment from their hosts. Drugs used for the treatment of parasitic infections can be separated into three main classes: antiprotozoals, anthelmintics and ectoparaciticides.

Antiprotozoal drugs

Protozoans are single-celled organisms, many of which infect the GI system. Examples include *Giardia duodenalis*, *Babesia canis*, *Leishmania infantum* and *Toxoplasmosa gondii*. Protozoan infections can be treated with antibiotics such as metronidazole and potentiated sulphonamides. Other drugs are available for specific infections (e.g. fenbendazole for *Giardia*).

Class of drug	Mechanism of action	Examples	Spectrum of activity	Additional information
Polyene macrolide antibiotics	Interfere with cell membrane Fungicidal	Nystatin (Canaural® ear drops); Amphotericin B (no licensed veterinary products available)	Broad-spectrum	Amphotericin B is toxic if given by injection. It should only be used in severe, life-threatening infections due to toxic effects. Nystatin is not absorbed into the systemic circulation after oral administration. It is used topically, or orally for infections of the mouth, and must come into direct contact with the organism to be effective
Imidazoles	Alter cell membrane permeability Fungistatic	Clotrimazole (Aurizon®, Marbodex® and Otomax® ear drops); Econazole; Miconazole (Malaseb® shampoo, Easotic® and Surolan® ear drops); Ketoconazole (Fungiconazole® tablets); Itraconazole (Itrafungol® oral solution); Fluconazole; Climbazole	Broad-spectrum	Itraconazole, ketoconazole and fluconazole are used systemically; the other imidazoles are primarily used topically
Terbinafine	Interferes with cell membranes Fungicidal	Terbinafine (Osurnia® ear gel)	Dermatophytes and yeasts	Do not use topically or systemically in dogs with generalized demodicosis or in pregnant or breeding animals

8.24 Summary of the main classes of antifungal drugs.

Infectious Agent	Species	Vaccine type	Additional information
Canine distemper virus (CDV)	Dogs	Live attenuated	Initial course: two doses, 2–4 weeks apart Revaccination: every 1–3 years depending on the manufacturer's recommendation
Canine parvovirus (CPV)	Dogs	Live attenuated	Initial course: two doses, 2–4 weeks apart Revaccination: every 1–3 years depending on the manufacturer's recommendation
Canine adenovirus (CAV-1)	Dogs	Live attenuated (CAV-2)	Initial course: two doses, 2–4 weeks apart Revaccination: every 1–3 years depending on the manufacturer's recommendation
Leptospira spp.	Dogs	Inactive, bacterial	Initial course: two doses, 2–4 weeks apart Revaccination: every 12 months
Canine parainfluenza virus	Dogs	Live attenuated	Initial course: two doses, 2–4 weeks apart Revaccination: every 12 months
Bordetella bronchiseptica	Dogs	Live, bacterial	Vaccination reduces the severity of the infection and the shedding of infectious particles, but does not necessarily prevent infection. Intranasal use. Single dose, given annually
Canine herpesvirus (CHV)	Dogs	Subunit vaccine	Used in breeding bitches to prevent disease in puppies. Mineral oil vaccine. Accidental self-injection is extremely harmful First injection: either during heat or 7–10 days after the presumed date of mating Second injection: 1–2 weeks before the expected date of whelping Revaccination: during each pregnancy, according to the same schedule
Rabies virus	Dogs, cats and ferrets	Inactivated or recombinant [a] vaccine	Single dose every 1–3 years depending on manufacturer's recommendation
Chlamydia felis	Cats	Live attenuated or inactivated depending on manufacturer	Initial course: two doses, 3–4 weeks apart Revaccination: every 12 months
Feline calicivirus (FCV)	Cats	Live attenuated or inactivated depending on the manufacturer	Initial course: two doses, 3–4 weeks apart Revaccination: every 12 months
Feline rhinotracheitis herpesvirus (FHV)	Cats	Live attenuated or inactivated depending on the manufacturer	Initial course: two doses, 3–4 weeks apart Revaccination: every 12 months
Feline leukaemia virus (FeLV)	Cats	Inactivated or recombinant [a] vaccine	Initial course: two doses, 3–4 weeks apart Revaccination: every 12 months
Feline panleucopenia virus	Cats	Live attenuated or inactivated depending on the manufacturer	Initial course: two doses, 3–4 weeks apart Revaccination: every 12 months
Myxomatosis	Rabbits	Live attenuated	Single dose every 12 months
Viral haemorrhagic disease (VHD) (two strains: RVHD1 and RVHD2)	Rabbits	Inactivated	Single dose every 9 or 12 months depending on vaccine manufacturer

8.25 Vaccines available for companion animals in the UK. Note that the dosing schedule and vaccine type varies between manufacturers. [a] Recombinant vaccine is produced using genetic engineering using specific genetic material from a pathogen to produce proteins which stimulate an immune response when the animal is vaccinated.

Anthelmintics

Anthelmintics are drugs used to treat internal (endo)parasites such as roundworm, tapeworm and lungworm. The 'ideal' anthelmintic would have a wide safety margin, a broad spectrum of activity, be active against both mature and immature parasites, be easy to administer and prevent reinfection for prolonged periods of time. Many modern anthelmintics come close to this ideal.

Parasite resistance is increasingly becoming a problem with anthelmintics, although this is less of an issue with companion animals than with food-producing species. It is important to ensure an appropriate dose is given because subtherapeutic doses can lead to increased resistance.

Figure 8.26 details anthelmintic classes, examples and spectrum of activity.

Ectoparasiticides

Ectoparasiticides are drugs used to treat and prevent infection by external parasites, such as fleas, ticks and mites. There are a great number of products available on the market, many of which contain a combination of ingredients to treat different ectoparasites and endoparasites. As ectoparasites can live in the animal's local environment, some products contain environmental control agents, which prevent reinfection of the animal from parasites emerging from an infected home. Figure 8.27 shows the available ectoparasiticides, their duration of action and spectrum of activity.

Class of drug	Mechanism of Action	Examples	Spectrum of activity	Additional information
Benzimidazoles	Inhibit tubulin polymerization	Febantel	Roundworms, whipworms, hookworms	Often used in combination with praziquantel and pyrantel. **Do not give with piperazine, levamisole or cholinesterase inhibitors**
		Fenbendazole	Roundworms, whipworms, hookworms, tapeworms (*Taenia* spp. only), some lungworms	Also used for *Giardia* (extended course of treatment). Various formulations available
Cyclic octadepsipeptides	Bind to latrophillin receptor to interfere with nerve transmission	Emodepside	Roundworms, tapeworms, some lungworms	Only licensed for cats in the UK Women of child-bearing age should avoid contact with the drug
Macrocyclic lactones	Interfere with nerve transmission	Selamectin	Adult roundworms, whipworms, heartworms	Also has activity against ectoparasites. Take care with collies and related breeds as toxicity can occur with excessive doses
		Milbemycin	Roundworms, whipworms, lungworms	Always in combination with other agents. Take care with collies and related breeds as toxicity can occur with excessive doses
		Moxidectin	Roundworms, whipworms, hookworms	Always in combination with imidacloprid. Licensed for flea and heartworm treatment in ferrets. Also has activity against ectoparasites
Tetrahydropyrimidines	Interfere with nerve transmission	Pyrantel	Roundworms	Often used in combination with febantel and praziquantel
Miscellaneous	Interfere with energy production	Nitroscanate	Roundworms, tapeworms	Tablets should not be broken or divided
	Cause flaccid paralysis	Piperazine	Adult roundworms	Very safe, available as AVM-GSL
	Increases cell permeability to calcium, which induces contraction of the parasites, resulting in paralysis	Praziquantel	Tapeworms	Generally given in combination with another anthelmintic

8.26 Anthelmintics used in small animal practice.

Class of drug	Mechanism of Action	Examples	Oral or Topical?	Duration of action	Spectrum of activity
Formamidines	Bind to octopamine receptors	Amitraz	Topical	Treat every 5–7 days until no live mites or viable eggs are present	Demodectic and sarcoptic mange
Insect growth regulators	Inhibit the development of immature stages of insects	Methoprene	Topical	Used in combination with fipronil to give up to 8 weeks protection against fleas	Fleas,
		Lufenuron	Oral	Monthly	Fleas
Isoxazolines	Block ligand-gated chloride channels	Afoxolaner	Oral	5 weeks for fleas, 4 weeks for ticks	Fleas, ticks
		Fluralaner	Oral and topical	12 weeks	Fleas, ticks
		Lotilaner	Oral	1 month	Fleas, ticks
		Sarolaner	Oral	At least 5 weeks	Fleas, ticks
Macrocyclic lactones	Cause paralysis by binding to glutamate-gated chloride channels in the parasites' nervous system	Moxidectin	Oral	4 weeks	Fleas, lice, mites
		Selamectin	Topical	1 month	Fleas, lice, sarcoptic mites

8.27 Ectoparasiticides licensed for use in small animal practice.

continues ▶

Class of drug	Mechanism of Action	Examples	Oral or Topical?	Duration of action	Spectrum of activity
Neoni-cotinoids	Cause paralysis and death by inhibiting cholinergic transmission	Imidacloprid	Topical or (collar in combination with flumethrin)	4 weeks	Fleas, biting lice
Oxadiazines	Block the voltage-gated sodium ion channels in insects	Indoxacarb	Topical	4 weeks	Fleas
Phenyl-pyrazoles	Bind to gamma-aminobutyric acid and glutamate-gated receptor sites of insect nervous systems	Fipronil	Topical	Up to 4 weeks for ticks, up to 8 weeks for fleas	Fleas, ticks
		Pyriprole	Topical	Minimum of 4 weeks for fleas, 4 weeks for ticks	Fleas, ticks
Pyrethrins	Cause paralysis by disrupting sodium and potassium ion transport in nerve membranes	Deltamethrin	Topical (collar)	5–6 months for ticks and sandflies, 6 months for mosquitos	Ticks, sandflies, mosquitos
		Flumethrin	Topical (collar)	7–8 months (when combined with imidacloprid)	Fleas
		Permethrin	Topical Often used in products in combination with other insecticidal agents	4 weeks	Fleas, ticks Do not use permethrin in cats
Spinosyns	Target binding sites on nicotinic acetylcholine receptors leading to involuntary muscle contractions, prostration with tremors and paralysis	Spinosad	Oral	4 weeks	Fleas

8.27 *continued* Ectoparasiticides licensed for use in small animal practice.

Drugs acting on the respiratory system

Control of bronchial smooth muscle tone is complex and involves a number of sensory receptors. Stimulation of these receptors by chemical, physical or mechanical means, results in bronchoconstriction, tachypnoea and cough. Airways can also be occluded by mucus and oedema, or by chemical mediators released during infection. Drugs used to treat these clinical signs may be given systemically, but direct administration of such drugs by inhalation allows high doses to be administered to the site of action. This local delivery, either by using a nebulizer or inhaler and spacer device, can reduce systemic side effects. Commonly used drugs for respiratory diseases are shown in Figure 8.28.

Drugs acting on the cardiovascular system

Cardiovascular drugs act on the heart, blood vessels, kidneys or the blood clotting system. They are used to treat a variety of conditions from hypertension to chronic heart failure. Many drugs in this group have more than one indication; for example, furosemide may be used for hypertension and feline dilated cardiomyopathy. For details on cardiovascular drugs see Figure 8.29.

Class of drug	Examples	Effects and uses
Antitussives	Codeine Butorphanol Dextromethorphan	Suppresses the cough centre in the brain
Bronchodilators	Beta-adrenergic agonists: salbutamol, salmeterol, terbutaline	Relaxes bronchial smooth muscle to dilate the airways. May contribute towards mucous clearance by the respiratory tract cilli
	Methylxanthines: theophylline, propentophylline	Relaxes bronchial smooth muscle to dilate the airways
	Anticholinergics: atropine, glycopyrronium	Block cholinergic stimulation to prevent bronchoconstriction
Corticosteroids	Prednisolone Fluticasone	Reduces inflammation of the airways
Mucolytics and expectorants	N-acetylcysteine Bromhexine Guaifenesin	Reduces viscosity of mucous to make it easier to cough up
Respiratory stimulants	Doxapram	Acts on the respiratory centre of the brain to stimulate respiration

8.28 Drugs that affect the respiratory system.

Class of drug	Examples	Effects	Clinical use
Cardiac glycosides	Digoxin	Increases myocardial contractility, slows ventricular heart rate	Congestive heart failure, atrial fibrillation and supraventricular tachycardia
Phosphodiesterase inhibitors	Pimobendan	Increases myocardial contractility, dilates blood vessels	Congestive heart failure
Angiotensin-converting enzyme (ACE) inhibitors	Enalapril Benazepril Ramipril Imidapril	Vasodilation and reduces sodium and water retention	Congestive heart failure, reduction of proteinuria associated with chronic kidney disease in cats
Calcium channel blockers	Amlodipine Diltiazem	Reduces contractility of the heart, slows heart rate, dilates blood vessels	Amlodipine is used for hypertension in cats. Diltiazem is used for atrial fibrillation, ventricular tachycardia, hypertrophic cardiomyopathy and hypertension
Antiarrhythmics	Lidocaine	Controls abnormal cardiac rhythm	Emergency treatment of ventricular arrhythmias
Nitroglycerides	Glyceryl trinitrate	Dilates blood vessels	Emergency treatment of congestive heart failure
Diuretics	Loop diuretics: furosemide, torasemide Thiazide diuretics: hydrochlorothiazide Potassium-sparing diuretics: spironolactone	Increases urine production by the kidney. Different classes of diuretic act of different parts of the kidney	Congestive heart failure

8.29 Drugs that affect the cardiovascular system.

Drugs acting on the gastrointestinal tract

Drugs affecting the GI system may be used to increase appetite, control nausea, inhibit or induce vomiting, control diarrhoea, treat colitis (inflammation of the gut), as a laxative, to protect the GI tract or to affect digestive function. The main drugs used are summarized in Figure 8.30.

Drugs acting on the endocrine system

The endocrine system is made up of the pituitary gland, thyroid gland, parathyroid glands, adrenal glands, pancreas, ovaries (in females) and testicles (in males) (see Chapter 3 for further information). Disorders of the endocrine system generally occur as a result of over- or underproduction of

Class of drug	Examples	Effects and uses
Appetite stimulants	Cyproheptadine Diazepam Mirtazapine	Acts on satiety centre of the brain to stimulate appetite
Emetics	Apomorphine Xylazine	Used to stimulate vomiting after consumption of a toxin
Antiemetics	Maropitant Metoclopramide Ondansetron	Used to prevent vomiting in patients receiving chemotherapy and for motion sickness
H2 antagonists and proton pump inhibitors	Cimetidine Ranitidine Famotidine Omeprazole	Reduces gastric acid secretion
Gastroprotectants	Sucralfate Misoprostol	Protects the GI mucosa and encourages healing of ulcers and erosions
Prokinetics	Metoclopramide Cisapride Ranitidine	Increases the movement of ingested material through the GI tract
Anti-diarrhoeals	Loperamide	Reduces gut peristalsis and increases intestinal transit time
Laxatives	Osmotic laxative: lactulose Bulk-forming laxatives: sterculia and macrogol Stimulant laxatives: bisacodyl	Draws water into the colon Increases bulk of faeces Increases the motility of the intestine

8.30 Drugs that affect the gastrointestinal tract.

continues ▶

Class of drug	Examples	Effects and uses
Bowel cleansing solutions	Klean-Prep® Fleet® enema	Used rectally to 'clean' the bowel prior to colonoscopy
Drugs used in colitis	Tylosin Sulfasalazine Metronidazole	Reduces inflammation
Adsorbants	Activated charcoal Kaolin	Activated charcoal is used to adsorb toxic substances and diarrhoea causing enterotoxins. Kaolin is often used to treat diarrhoea but there is little evidence to prove its effectiveness
Drugs affecting digestive function	Pancreatic lipase	Contains the enzymes amylase, lipase and protease. Used to treat dogs with pancreatic insufficiency
Drugs used in hepatic disease	Ursodeoxycholic acid (ursodiol)	Reduces cholesterol synthesis and secretion by the liver and decreases intestinal absorption of cholesterol. Used to treat gallstones

8.30 *continued* Drugs that affect the gastrointestinal tract.

endogenous hormones from these glands. Drug therapy aims to enhance or replace missing hormones, or to reduce the production of excess hormones. Figure 8.31 provides more information on endocrine diseases and their treatment.

Drugs acting on the central nervous system

Drugs acting on the CNS include:

■ Local anaesthetics
■ General anaesthetics

Gland	Over or underproduction of endogenous hormone	Endogenous hormone involved	Condition	Drug treatment		
Adrenal	Over	Adrenocorticotrophic hormone (ACTH)	Hyperadrenocorticism (Cushing' disease)	Trilostane		
	Under	Cortisol (primary Addison's disease), or ACTH (secondary Addison's disease)	Hypoadrenocorticism (Addison's disease)	Desoxycortone pivalate (mineralocorticoid), fludrocortisone (mineralocorticoid) and prednisolone (glucocorticoid)		
Endocrine pancreas	Over	Insulin	Hyperinsulinaemia	Dextrose, glucocorticoids		
	Under	Insulin	Diabetes mellitus	Insulin (see below)		
				Type of insulin	*Example*	*Duration of action in the dog (shorter in the cat)*
				Short-acting	Neutral insulin	Onset: 0–30 min Peak: 0.5–5 h Duration: 1–8 h
				Intermediate-acting	Lente, isophane	Onset: 30–60 min Peak: 1–10 h Duration: 4–24 h
				Long-acting	Protamine zinc, glargine	Onset: 1–4 h Peak: 4–14 h Duration: 6–28 h
Pituitary	Under	Antidiuretic hormone (ADH) also called vasopressin	Diabetes insipidus	Desmopressin		
Thyroid	Over	Triiodothyronine (T3) and thyroxine (T4)	Hyperthyroidism	Carbimazole, methimazole, thiamizole		
	Under	Triiodothyronine (T3) and Thyroxine (T4)	Hypothyroidism	Levothyroxine		

8.31 Endocrine diseases and drug treatments.

- Analgesics
- Sedatives
- Muscle relaxants
- Antiepileptics
- Behaviour-modifying agents.

Local and general anaesthetics, analgesics, sedatives and muscle relaxants are discussed in Chapter 21.

Antiepileptic drugs

Epilepsy is the most common neurological condition in dogs, it is more common in dogs than in cats. It is not a curable disease; managing epilepsy, therefore, requires a lifetime commitment by the pet owner. The aim of therapy is to reduce the frequency of seizures, whilst minimizing side effects from the medication. Antiepileptic drugs should not be stopped abruptly because this may lead to seizures.

To allow rapid availability in the CNS, drugs used in status epilepticus are generally given by intravenous injection or infusion, although diazepam can also be given rectally. It should be noted that oral medications are unsuitable for seizuring patients. Drugs used include benzodiazepines, such as diazepam and midazolam, and phenobarbital. If the seizure is refractory to these drugs, anaesthesia may be induced with an agent such as propofol. This should only be performed in an intensive care setting because of the need for continuous blood pressure monitoring and, ideally, central venous pressure monitoring. General anaesthesia prevents tonic–clonic movements and allows manual control of respiration.

Phenobarbital

This is the oldest and most commonly used antiepileptic medication in veterinary practice. It acts on the gamma-aminobutyric acid A (GABA$_A$) receptors, which are responsible for reducing electrical activity between nerve cells. This partial activation of the GABA receptors is believed to reduce electrical activity and help prevent seizures. Phenobarbital may also inhibit calcium channels, resulting in a decrease in excitatory transmitter release.

Side effects of phenobarbital include sedation, ataxia and anxiety. Occasionally, polyphagia, polyuria and polydipsia have been reported, but these effects are usually transitory and disappear with continued medication. Damage to the liver has also been reported at high plasma concentrations.

It is recommended that:

- Hepatic function is evaluated prior to initiation of therapy (e.g. measurement of serum bile acids)
- Therapeutic phenobarbital serum concentrations are monitored to enable the lowest effective dose to be used. Typically, concentrations of 15–45 µg/ml are effective in controlling epilepsy
- Hepatic function is re-evaluated on a regular (6 to 12 month) basis
- Seizure activity is re-evaluated on a regular basis.

Phenobarbital is an enzyme inducer, so can increase the metabolism of other drugs. Care must be taken with doses of other medicines.

Potassium bromide

This may be used alone or in conjunction with phenobarbital. It has a similar mode of action to phenobarbital, but should not be used in patients with severe renal failure. In animals with mild renal failure, the dose should be reduced.

Imepitoin

This antiepileptic drug works in a similar way to phenobarbital and potassium bromide. It has an effectiveness similar to phenobarbital, but is associated with fewer side effects. Of particular importance is that imepitoin does not cause hepatotoxicity, so regular liver function tests are not required.

Other drugs

Although unlicensed in animals, using the Cascade veterinary surgeons may prescribe other, newer antiepileptic drugs for refractory patients. Examples include levetiracetam, topiramate and zonisamide.

Behaviour-modifying drugs

Anxiolytics, antipsychotics, antidepressants and mood stabilizers are commonly used to treat human behavioural disorders, and are increasingly being used in veterinary medicine for clinical signs such as aggression, noise phobia, separation anxiety, inappropriate elimination (defecation and urination) and destructive behaviour.

There are three licensed veterinary behaviour-modifying drugs:

- Clomipramine
- Selegiline
- Fluoxetine.

Clomipramine

This has a broad-spectrum of action in blocking the neuronal reuptake of both serotonin (5-HT) and noradrenaline, neurotransmitters known to have an effect on mood. It is licensed for use in dogs as an aid in the treatment of separation-related disorders manifested by destruction and inappropriate elimination and only in combination with behavioural modification techniques. It is also used in the management of a wider range of anxiety related disorders in dogs and cats.

Selegiline hydrochloride

This is an inhibitor of monoamine oxidase, an enzyme involved in removing the neurotransmitters noradrenaline (norepinephrine), serotonin and dopamine from the brain. It is licensed for use in depression and anxiety, and in association with behaviour therapy, the treatment of signs of emotional origin observed in behavioural conditions such as over activity, separation problems, generalized phobia and unsociable behaviour.

Fluoxetine

This is newly licensed for use in dogs in the UK (although at the time of writing has not yet been released on to the market). Its licensed indication is similar to that of clomipramine, and it works by blocking the reuptake of serotonin.

Other drugs

Behaviour-modifying drugs used in veterinary medicine, which are not currently licensed for use in animals include the tricyclic antidepressant amitriptyline, the antipsychotic trazodone, and anxiolytics such as diazepam and alprazolam.

Anti-inflammatory drugs

There are three main classes of anti-inflammatory drug: corticosteroids, non-steroidal anti-inflammatory drugs (NSAIDs) and antihistamines. These drugs can be used for a number of inflammatory processes and have analgesic, antipyretic and anti-inflammatory effects.

Corticosteroids

Corticosteroids are primarily used for their anti-inflammatory effects, and at high doses will decrease the immune response. They all have both mineralocorticoid and glucocorticoid activity, but to varying degrees. Mineralocorticoid activity controls sodium/potassium and water balance, while glucocorticoid activity affects the metabolism, inflammatory and immune response.

Long-term corticosteroid therapy should not be stopped abruptly, or withdrawal signs relating to an Addisonian-like crisis such as weakness, nausea and vomiting, diarrhoea, hypotension and hypoglycaemia can occur. Severe cases of withdrawal can result in circulatory shock, which is life-threatening. Doses should be gradually tapered off over a period of between 2 and 5 weeks, depending on how long the patient has been receiving steroid treatment. Short courses of up to a week can be discontinued abruptly because the adrenal glands have not had time to reduce the amount of corticosteroids they produce.

Side effects of corticosteroid therapy occur particularly with long-term treatment and with high doses. They include:

- Increased susceptibility to infections
- Hyperglycaemia and diabetes mellitus
- Loss of muscle mass
- Osteoporosis
- Atrophy of the skin and hair loss
- Decreased ability to heal
- Gastric ulceration
- Polyuria and polydipsia
- Behavioural changes
- Iatrogenic Cushing's syndrome
- Water and sodium retention and potassium loss
- Corneal ulceration.

Side effects can be reduced by decreasing the dose or by switching to alternate day dosing. Figure 8.32 details the available corticosteroids, their relative glucocorticoid and mineralocorticoid activities and duration of action. In comparing the relative potencies of corticosteroids in terms of their anti-inflammatory (glucocorticoid) effects, it should be borne in mind that high glucocorticoid activity in itself is of no advantage unless it is accompanied by relatively low mineralocorticoid activity. For example, the mineralocorticoid activity of fludrocortisone acetate is so high that its anti-inflammatory activity is of no clinical relevance.

Non-steroidal anti-inflammatory drugs

NSAIDs inhibit fewer inflammatory pathways than corticosteroids, which means they have the potential to reduce pain and inflammation without some of the side effects common to steroid therapy. NSAIDs primarily inhibit prostaglandin synthesis by inhibiting cyclooxygenase (COX). There are two forms of COX: COX-1 and COX-2. COX-2 is involved in inflammatory pathways and inhibition of this mediator results in the antipyretic and anti-inflammatory actions of NSAIDs. Inhibition of COX-1, which occurs in virtually every tissue in the body, results in side effects such as:

- Vomiting
- Diarrhoea
- GI ulceration, leading to iron deficiency anaemia if bleeding is severe
- Renal toxicity
- Hepatic toxicity.

NSAIDs vary in their degree of COX-1 and COX-2 inhibition, with those that target COX-2 being termed COX-2 selective or COX-2 specific. These drugs provide anti-inflammatory and antipyretic effects without causing the common NSAID side effects.

> **WARNING**
>
> Corticosteroids should not be administered alongside NSAIDs due to the increased rick of gastric ulceration, which is a common side effect of both drugs

Figure 8.33 gives further information on the available NSAIDs.

Drug	Relative mineralocorticoid activity	Relative glucocorticoid activity	Duration of action
Hydrocortisone	1	1	Short-acting
Fludrocortisone	120	15	Short-acting
Prednisolone	0.8	5	Intermediate-acting
Methylprednisolone	0.5	5	Intermediate-acting
Dexamethasone	0	25	Long-acting

8.32 Corticosteroids: relative mineralocorticoid and glucocorticoid activity and duration of action.

Drug	Selectively inhibits COX-2	Treatment duration	Additional information
Cimicoxib	Yes	Perioperative pain: 3–7 days Osteoarthritis: 6 months	Licensed only for dogs. Oral tablets only
Fircoxib	Yes	Postoperative: 3 days Osteoarthritis: long-term but monitor if over 90 days	Licensed only for dogs. Oral tablets only
Ketoprofen	No	Injection: 3 days Oral tablets: 30 days	Injection and oral

8.33 Non-steroidal anti-inflammatory drugs (NSAIDs). *continues* ▶

Drug	Selectively inhibits COX-2	Treatment duration	Additional information
Mavacoxib	Yes	Two doses 14 days apart, then dosing interval increases to monthly. Treatment cycle should not exceed seven consecutive doses	Rate of clearance from the body is very slow so treatment is monthly. Licensed only for dogs. Oral tablets only
Meloxicam	Yes	Cats: up to 14 days Dogs: long-term with appropriate monitoring	Available as injection, oral tablets and oral suspension. Double dose given on day 1. Commonly used in rabbits and guinea pigs, which require a much higher dosage than cats and dogs
Robenacoxib	Yes	Orthopaedic surgery: one dose at least 30 minutes prior to surgery, then continued for a further 2 days postoperatively Acute musculoskeletal disorders: up to 6 days	Available as injection and oral tablets. If given perioperatively, administer alongside butorphanol
Tolfenamic Acid	No	Acute use: single injection repeated once after 24 hours; treatment continued by the oral route, once daily for 3 days repeated every 7 days (i.e. 3 days of medication followed by 4 days without medication)	Injectable and oral tablets. Licensed for dogs and cats

8.33 *continued* Non-steroidal anti-inflammatory drugs (NSAIDs).

Antihistamines

Histamine is produced as part of a local immune response and causes inflammation. It also performs several important functions in the bowel and acts as a neurotransmitter or chemical messenger that carries signals from one nerve to another. Drugs have been developed to inhibit two specific types of histamine: H1 and H2. An H1 antagonist (anti-histamine) blocks the action of histamine responsible for increased capillary permeability, redness and swelling. H2 antagonists (e.g. cimetidine) block histamine associated with gastric acid secretions and are discussed in the section on gastrointestinal drugs.

There are currently no veterinary licensed H1 antagonists available in the UK. Under the Cascade, veterinary surgeons may prescribe antihistamines such as chlorphenamine and cetirizine for inflammation associated with allergic reactions. Chlorphenamine is available in injectable form and is used in anaphylactic reactions.

Drugs acting on the reproductive system

Most drugs used to treat disorders of the reproductive system are hormones. Figure 8.34 gives details of the main drugs and their uses (see Chapter 24 for more information).

Drugs acting on the urinary tract

The process of urination is controlled by the sympathetic and parasympathetic nervous systems.

- Sympathetic nerves cause the upper section of the bladder to relax and the bladder neck to contract, allowing storage of urine. They also cause the internal urethral sphincter to tighten, helping to hold stored urine in the bladder. Drugs that act on the sympathetic nerves are called **sympathomimetics**.
- Parasympathetic nerves cause the upper part of the bladder to contract and the bladder neck to relax, assisting in the process of micturition (urination). They also cause the urethral sphincter to relax to allow urine to pass out of the bladder. Drugs that act on the parasympathetic nerves are called **parasympathomimetics**.

Drugs used in the treatment of urinary dysfunction are described in Figure 8.35.

Drug	Effects and indications for use
Proglisterone	Suppression and postponement of oestrus and treatment of false pregnancy
Cabergoline	Treatment of false pregnancy and suppression of lactation in bitches
Megestrol	Suppression and postponement of oestrus in bitch and queen, control of undesirable behaviour in male dogs (e.g. aggression, mounting, territorial marking)
Chorionic gonadotrophin	Induction of ovulation, prolonged pro-oestrus and anoestrus in bitches
Delmadinone	Treatment of hypersexuality in male dogs and cats, and prostatic hypertrophy in male dogs
Osaterone	Benign prostatic hypertrophy
Deslorelin	Induction of temporary infertility (chemical castration) in entire, sexually active male dogs and ferrets
Aglepristone	Induction of abortion up to 45 days after mating

8.34 Drugs that affect the reproductive system.

Condition		Drug class	Examples	Additional information
Urinary incontinence		Oestrogen	Estriol	Used in neutered bitches
		Sympathomimetic	Phenylpropanolamine	Used in neutered bitches
Urinary retention		Alpha-blocker	Prazosin	Decreases urethral sphincter tone
		Cholinergic	Bethanechol	Increases detrusor urinary muscle tone and contraction
Urinary obstruction		Alpha-blocker	Prazosin	Promotes urine flow and treats functional urethral obstruction
Cystitis and pyelonephritis		Broad-spectrum antibiotics	Amoxicillin Potentiated sulphonamides	Higher doses required for pyelonephritis
Chronic kidney disease		Angiotensin receptor blockers	Telmisartan	Telmisartan is only licensed for use in cats. It reduces arterial blood pressure and reduces proteinuria in cats with chronic kidney disease
		Angiotensin-converting enzyme (ACE) inhibitors	Enalapril Benazepril	Dilate blood vessels and help support blood flow through the kidneys
		Phosphate binders	Aluminium hydroxide, supplements such as Ipaketine and Pronefra	Controlling blood phosphate levels appears to have a good protective effect on the kidneys
Urolithiasis	Struvite	Urinary acidifier	Methionine	More commonly managed with specialized diets
	Calcium Oxalate	N/A	N/A	Medical dissolution has not been established and surgery is recommended
	Urate	Xanthine oxidase inhibitor	Allopurinol	More commonly managed with specialized diets
		Urinary alkalinizer	Sodium bicarbonate or potassium citrate	

8.35 Drugs that affect the urinary tract.

Drugs used to treat malignant disease

Drugs for malignant disease are of particular importance for neoplasms that are not amenable to surgery, such as lymphoma and leukaemia. They may also be used before or after surgical removal of a tumour or radiotherapy. Depending on the type of cancer and the kind of drug used, chemotherapeutic agents may be administered by different methods. They can be administered orally, or given by intravenous, intramuscular or subcutaneous injection.

The two UK veterinary drugs licensed to treat malignant disease are **toceranib phosphate** and **masitinib**. Both are tyrosine kinase inhibitors (TKIs). TKIs have both antitumour and antiangiogenic properties, which means they can work against both the tumour itself and the blood vessels that supply it. They are licensed for the treatment of mast cell tumours in dogs.

Although not licensed in the UK, there is a vaccine available to treat canine melanoma that can be imported from America under license by the VMD. Conventional vaccines (for other common diseases) stimulate an immune response directed against foreign proteins. Tyrosinase, a protein present on canine melanoma cells, is not usually targeted by the dog's immune system because it is also present on normal canine cells. The melanoma vaccine is used following surgery to remove the primary tumour, and trains the dog's immune system to recognize this cancer-associated protein as a threat to its health.

Other drugs used in pets are licensed only for human use and include:

- **Alkylating agents:** These act directly on the DNA (deoxyribonucleic acid), causing cross-linking of DNA strands, abnormal base pairing or DNA strand breaks, thus preventing the cell from dividing. Examples include cyclophosphamide, chlorambucil and lomustine
- **Antimetabolites:** These replace natural substances as building blocks in DNA molecules, thereby altering the function of enzymes required for cell metabolism and protein synthesis. In other words, they mimic the nutrients that the cell needs to grow, tricking the cell into consuming them, so it eventually starves to death. Examples include methotrexate and cytarabine
- **Antitumour antibiotics:** These act by binding with DNA and preventing RNA (ribonucleic acid) synthesis, a key step in the creation of proteins, which are necessary for cell survival. They are not the same as antibiotics used to treat bacterial infections. Rather, these drugs cause the strands of genetic material that make up DNA to uncoil, thereby preventing the cell from reproducing. Doxorubicin, mitoxantrone and actinomycin D are some examples of antitumour antibiotics
- **Vinka alkaloids:** These are derived from the Madagascar periwinkle plant. They disrupt the formation of a structure called a spindle, which provides the framework for dividing the copied genetic material between the intended new cells (see Chapter 3). Examples include vincristine and vinblastine
- **Platinum compounds:** These work by binding together the strands of the DNA to stop cell replication. Examples include carboplatin and cisplatin.

Drugs acting on the eyes

Few drugs used in the treatment of ophthalmic disorders are licensed for use in animals. There are many drugs that may be used on the eye (see below). Topical drugs are usually in the form of an ointment or drop. Systemic drugs may also reach therapeutic concentration in the eye if they are lipid-soluble.

Aids to ophthalmic examination

The local anaesthetic proxymetacaine is used to facilitate ophthalmic examination of the painful eye. Mydriatics are drugs used to dilate the pupil, often for ophthalmic examination. There are two types of mydriatics: antimuscarinics such as **atropine** and **tropicamide**, and sympathomimetics, such as **phenylephrine**.

Eye infections

Antimicrobials such as **fusidic acid**, **gentamicin** and **cloxacillin** are used in the treatment of conjunctivitis and other eye infections. **Chloramphenicol** and **ofloxacin** are also used but are not licensed for use in animals.

Glaucoma

Glaucoma is a condition that causes damage to the optic nerve and gets worse over time. It is often linked to a build up of pressure inside the eye. Drugs used to treat glaucoma include the miotic **pilocarpine**, the beta-blocker **timolol**, the carbonic anhydrase inhibitor **dorsolomide**, and the prostaglandin analogue **travoprost**. All of these drugs work by reducing the amount of fluid in the eye, thereby reducing the pressure.

All these drugs work by reducing the amount of fluid in the eye, thereby reducing the pressure on the optic nerve. Pilocarpine, timolol and dorsolomide work by reducing the production of intraocular fluid, whilst travoprost works by increasing the outflow of fluid form the eye. Combination products are also available (e.g. dorzolamide and timolol (Cosopt®)).

Dry eye

Treatment for dry eye syndrome helps to control the clinical signs, but there is no cure. Mild to moderate cases of dry eye syndrome can usually be treated using lubricants that consist of a range of drops, gels and ointments. Ointments are generally used only at night because they can blur vision and tend to be effective for a longer period of time. The immunomodulator **ciclosporin** is often used for the treatment of severe dry eye syndrome that does not respond to lubricants. It is licensed for use in animals for the treatment of:

- Chronic, recurrent conjunctivitis resulting from autoimmune disease of the eye
- Keratoconjunctivitis sicca (KCS, 'dry eye')
- Chronic superficial keratitis ('pannus') in the dog.

Inflammatory eye conditions

Steroids such as prednisolone and dexamethasone are used to treat inflammatory eye conditions. They should not be used if there is a corneal ulcer. Steroids are also available in combination with antibiotics (e.g. dexamethasone, neomycin and polymyxin B).

NSAIDs such as ketololac and diclofenac may also be used to treat ocular inflammation and are useful when topical corticosteroids are contraindicated (e.g. in ulcerative keratitis). Topical NSAIDs have the potential to increase intraocular pressure and should be used with caution in patients predisposed to glaucoma.

Drugs acting on the ear

Ear cleaners

Healthy ears should not need cleaning. Patients who regularly experience ear infections should have their ears cleansed once or twice weekly. There are four main types of aural discharge:

- Waxy and adherent – dark brown in colour and associated with ceruminous otitis
- Waxy to seborrheic – pale brown to grey and is associated with *Malassezia*
- Seborrheic to purulent – pale brown to yellow and associated with staphylococci
- Purulent – yellow to green and associated with *Pseudomonas*.

It is important to choose an ear cleaner targeted to the particular type of discharge present.

Ear treatments

Drugs administered to the ear are generally designed to treat infection and reduce inflammation. Most ear preparations are combination products containing more than one ingredient.

- Antimicrobials (e.g. gentamicin and marbofloxacin). Some antimicrobials such as the aminoglycosides are ototoxic and can cause vestibular signs or irreversible deafness.
- Antifungals (e.g. miconazole and clotrimazole).
- Steroids (e.g. dexamethasone, hydrocortisone and prednisolone).

Following culture and sensitivity testing, and if appropriate, recurrent ear infections in the dog can be treated with a gel formulation of terbinafine, florfenicol and betamethasone acetate. This product requires only two treatments, 7 days apart, and is effective for up to 45 days. Treatments for ear mites may be administered into the ear or as a spot-on on the skin as previously described.

Drugs acting on the skin

Skin conditions can be treated with either systemic or topical drugs. Topical treatments are formulated as a cream, ointment, spray, mousse, shampoo, gel or lotion. The formulation selected depends on:

- The site to be treated (e.g. areas with a lot of hair are best treated with a foam or lotion)
- How large an area is to be treated (e.g. foams and shampoos may be better for large areas)
- The depth to which penetration of the drug is required (e.g. if a condition affects the deeper layers of the skin, a systemic treatment may be more appropriate)
- The moisture level in the skin (e.g. ointments are greasier and more occlusive than creams).

Although symptomatic treatment is relatively straightforward, understanding and treating the underlying cause can be complex. Even if a trigger is identified, it may not be possible to eliminate it completely. For example, if a patient suffers from an allergy to grass pollen, it is probably not possible to avoid grass altogether, although washing the skin after contact with grass may lessen the severity of signs.

Figure 8.36 summarizes the most common skin diseases of cats and dogs and gives examples for their treatment.

Condition	Class of drug	Systemic or topical	Example
Pyoderma	Antimicrobial	Systemic	Clindamycin
		Topical	Mupiricin
Dermatophytosis	Antifungal	Systemic	Terbinafine
		Topical	Clotrimazole
Malassezia dermatitis	Antifungal	Topical	Miconazole, chlorhexidine
Demodicosis (*Demodex* mite infestation)	Insecticide (octopamine receptor agonist)	Topical	Amitraz
	Neonicotinoid/macrocyclic lactone combo	Topical	Imidacloprid/moxidectin
	Macrocyclic lactone	Systemic	Ivermectin
	Isoxazoline	Systemic	Sarolaner
Cheyletiella	Isoxazoline	Systemic	Sarolaner Fluralaner
	Macrocyclic lactone	Topical	Selamectin
	Neonicotinoid/macrocyclic lactone combo	Topical	Imidacloprid/moxidectin
	Phenylpyrazole	Topical	Fipronil
Sarcoptic mange	Macrocyclic lactone	Topical	Selamectin
	Neonicotinoid/macrocyclic lactone combo	Topical	Imidacloprid/moxidectin
	Isoxazoline	Systemic	Sarolaner
Seborrhoea	Keratolytics	Topical	Selenium sulphide
Inflammatory and immune-mediated disorders	Corticosteroids	Topical	Hydrocortisone
		Systemic	Prednisolone
	Immunosuppressants	Systemic	Ciclosporin
	Immunotherapy	Systemic	Allergen-containing vaccine
	Janus kinase inhibitors (JAK) inhibitors	Systemic	Oclacitinib

8.36 Drugs used for skin disease.

Legal aspects of veterinary medicines

Veterinary Medicines Directorate

The use of veterinary medicines in the UK is governed by the VMD on behalf of the Department for Environment, Food and Rural Affairs (Defra). The VMD is the executive agency of Defra (i.e. they write the legislation and ensure that it is followed). They operate the licensing system for animal medicines with the aim to safeguard public health, animal health and the environment. The VMD ensures the **safety**, **quality** and **efficacy** of medicines within the UK, and runs surveillance and information schemes such as MAVIS (the Marketing Authorisations Veterinary Information Scheme) and SARSS (the Suspected Adverse Reaction Surveillance Scheme; see later for more information on SARSS). One piece of legislation written by the VMD, the Veterinary Medicines Regulations 2013 (VMR), covers the manufacture, sale and supply, importation, storage, marketing, advertising and disposal of medicines.

Veterinary Products Committee

The Veterinary Products Committee (VPC) offers advice to the VMD on behalf of the Secretary of State, in respect of new and renewal Marketing Authorisations (MAs), Provisional MAs, variations to MAs and Animal Test Certificates (ATCs). They also set up working groups to advise on many topics such as SARSS, antibiotic resistance and the use of hormone growth promoters.

Royal College of Veterinary Surgeons

The RCVS is the statutory regulator for the veterinary profession and is responsible under the Veterinary Surgeons Act 1966 for keeping the register of veterinary surgeons eligible to practice in the UK, setting standards for veterinary education and regulating the professional conduct of veterinary surgeons and nurses. They also hold the register for registered veterinary nurses and veterinary practice premises. Registered veterinary nurses and surgeons are required to comply with the Code of Professional Conduct, as written by the RCVS. The RCVS also produce additional guidelines and recommendations for veterinary practice.

British Veterinary Association

The British Veterinary Association (BVA) is the national representative body for veterinary professionals in the UK. They champion veterinary surgeons and speak for the profession at government meetings. The BVA also produce guidelines and recommendations to help veterinary surgeons and nurses comply with the VMR.

British Small Animal Veterinary Association

The British Small Animal Veterinary Association (BSAVA) was founded in 1957 as a professional body to serve veterinary surgeons who treat companion animals. Members of the association may be veterinary surgeons or veterinary nurses. The BSAVA works on behalf of its members to encourage vets and nurses to improve their professional skills. They run regular continuing education (CE) courses and seminars throughout the UK, and publish books, manuals and videos on a range of small animal topics.

The BSAVA also provides a forum for the discussion of issues of importance to veterinary surgeons and nurses in small animal practice and submits evidence on their behalf to the BVA and the RCVS, as well as to government departments. As part of this remit, the BSAVA hosts the *BSAVA Guide to the Use of Veterinary Medicines* (www.bsavalibrary.com/), which provides information to help navigate the minefield of issues, changes and regulations associated with veterinary medicines, and to promote best practice.

Legal categories of medicines

In the UK, licensed veterinary medicines are separated into several legal categories, which determine who can prescribe and supply them. There are four classes of veterinary medicines: POM-V, POM-VPS, NFA-VPS and NFA-GSL (Figure 8.37 provides further details).

POM-VPS and NFA-VPS products can be prescribed by a Registered Qualified Person (RQP), who may be a:

- Veterinary surgeon
- Registered pharmacist
- Suitably Qualified Person (SQP) – in some cases this may be a veterinary nurse, but anyone who has been trained by the Animal Medicines Training Regulatory Authority (AMTRA) and is registered with the VMD may prescribe POM-VPS and/or NFA-VPS products, as long as they prescribe within their sphere of competence. Veterinary surgeons and pharmacists

are allowed to prescribe for any species, but SQPs might only be registered to prescribe for certain species. Figure 8.38 details the different types of SQP and the species they are allowed to prescribe for.

It should be noted that according to the Veterinary Surgeons Act 1966, only a veterinary surgeon may diagnose an animal with a particular condition. Pharmacists and SQPs may prescribe medication for a particular condition upon request (including the prevention of disease), but they must not diagnose.

SQP category	Comments
QA-SQPS	SQPs qualified to supply VPS medicines for the treatment of avian species only
QC-SQPS	SQPs qualified to supply VPS medicines for the treatment of companion animals only
QCA-SQPS	SQPs qualified to supply VPS medicines for the treatment of avian species and companion animals only
QE-SQPS	SQPs qualified to supply VPS medicines for the treatment of equines and companion animals only
QEA-SQPS	SQPs qualified to supply VPS medicines for the treatment of avian species, equines and companion animals only
QG-SQPS	SQPs qualified to supply VPS medicines for the treatment of equines and farm animals only
QJ-SQPS	SQPs qualified to supply VPS medicines for the treatment of equines only
QK-SQPS	SQPs qualified to supply VPS medicines for the treatment of farm animals and companion animals only
QL-SQPS	SQPs qualified to supply VPS medicines for the treatment of farm animals only
QR-SQPS	SQPs qualified to supply VPS medicines

8.38 Types of SQP and the species they are allowed to prescribe medicines for.

Class of medicine	Notes
Prescription Only Medicine – Veterinarian (POM-V)	These can be prescribed by a veterinary surgeon only after clinical assessment of the animal or herd. If the supplier is also the prescriber, the prescription may be oral, otherwise a written prescription is required. A veterinary medicinal product (VMP) is generally classified in this way because it contains a new active ingredient, has safety issues, a narrow safety margin, due to government policy or because specialized veterinary knowledge required for its use. Controlled Drugs are a subcategory of POM-V (see text for details)
Prescription Only Medicine – Veterinarian, Pharmacist, Suitably Qualified Person (POM-VPS)	Generally for food-producing species. Can be prescribed by veterinary surgeon, pharmacist or suitably qualified person. No clinical assessment is required, the prescriber must be sure the owner is competent to administer the product. A VMP is generally included in this category when it is used to reduce or prevent endemic disease in herds, flocks or individual animals. There is some risk for the user, consumer, animal or environment but users can be made aware of the risks by verbal or written advice, and adequate training can be given for regular use
Non-Food Animal – Veterinarian, Pharmacist, Suitably Qualified Person (NFA-VPS)	Similar to POM-VPS but must be for non-food animals
Authorised Veterinary Medicine – General Sales List (AVM-GSL)	No restrictions on its supply. These drugs have a wide safety margin and specialist advice is not required

8.37 Legal categories of veterinary medicines.

For a vet to prescribe a POM-V medicine, they must have performed a clinical assessment and have the animal under their care. No legal definition exists for these terms, but the RCVS has taken them to mean:

- **Clinical assessment** – an assessment of relevant clinical information, which may include an examination of the animal
- **For animals under my care**
  - The veterinary surgeon must have been given the responsibility for the health of the animal or herd by the owner or the owner's agent
  - That responsibility must be real and not nominal
  - The animal or herd must have been seen immediately before prescription or,
  - Recently enough or often enough for the veterinary surgeon to have personal knowledge of the condition of the animal or current health status of the herd or flock to make a diagnosis and prescribe
  - The veterinary surgeon must maintain clinical records of that herd/flock/individual.

What constitutes 'recently or often enough' must be a matter for the professional judgement of the veterinary surgeon in the individual case.

Prescribing Cascade

Veterinary surgeons, pharmacists and SQPs are required by law to prescribe a medicine licensed for the treatment of that particular condition, in the particular species of animal affected. If no such medicine exists, to avoid unacceptable suffering, a veterinary surgeon may prescribe an unlicensed medicine in the following order (Cascade):

1. A product licensed in the UK for another condition in the same species or a product licensed for another animal species with the same condition.
2. i. A human product licensed in the UK or
   ii. In accordance with a Special Import Certificate, a medicine authorized for veterinary use in another European Union (EU) member state.
3. A product prepared extemporaneously by a veterinary surgeon, a pharmacist or a person holding a manufacturer's authorization, as prescribed by the veterinary surgeon.
4. In exceptional circumstances, a veterinary medicine can be imported from outside the EU or a human medicine can be imported from any other country with a Special Import Certificate.

It should be noted that only a veterinary surgeon may use the Cascade to prescribe an unlicensed medicine. Pharmacists and SQPs may only prescribe medicines licensed for the species and condition to be treated.

Records must be kept for 5 years and should include: date of examination; name and address of owner; number and identification of animal(s) treated; diagnosis; product details, including batch number; doses; duration of treatment; and withdrawal period recommended.

When using the Cascade to prescribe medications, veterinary surgeons are required to obtain **written** consent from the animal's owner or keeper. This consent form must name the unlicensed drug and the reason for using it. The consent must be informed (see Chapter 9). General consent for the use of unlicensed medicines is only appropriate when a patient is hospitalized, in emergency situations and for exotic patients where there are very few drugs licensed for the species to be treated.

Prescriptions and labels

A prescription is a means of defining the product, its dose and other relevant instructions. It must be provided in writing, unless the medication is being supplied by the person issuing the prescription or by someone at the same premises. A client may request a written prescription for a POM-V or POM-VPS medicine if they do not wish to purchase the medicine from the prescriber. For POM-V medications, only a veterinary surgeon may write the prescription, but it may be supplied by another veterinary surgeon or a pharmacist. For a POM-VPS or NFA-VPS medicine, an RQP may prescribe it and it may be supplied by any other RQP. Written prescriptions are valid for 6 months and must contain the following:

- Name, address and phone number of prescriber
- Qualifications of the prescriber (RCVS or SQP number)
- Name and address of the owner or keeper of the animal
- A description of animal(s) (i.e. name and breed)
- Premises the animals are kept if not at owner's address
- Name and amount of product prescribed
- Dose and administration instructions
- Withdrawal period, if relevant
- 'For use under the Cascade', if relevant
- Date
- Written in indelible format
- Signature of prescriber
- The statement 'For animals under my care'
- Repeat instructions, if relevant.

When writing a prescription, decimals should be avoided (so 500 mg should be used instead of 0.5 g). If decimals cannot be avoided, ensure a zero is included before the decimal place (so 0.5 mg, not .5 mg). Micrograms, nanograms or units should not be abbreviated.

Many prescribers use Latin abbreviations for speed. Latin abbreviations commonly used include:

- o.d. – omni die (once daily)
- s.i.d – semel in die (once daily)
- b.i.d – bis in die (twice daily)
- t.i.d – ter in die (three times daily)
- q.i.d – quarter in die (four times daily)
- p.c. – post cibum (after food)
- a.c. – ante cibum (before food)
- p.r.n – pro re nata (when required)
- o.m. – omni mane (in the morning)
- o.n. – omni nocte (at night)
- stat – immediately.

All medicines supplied by the practice must be labelled in accordance with the VMR. When not prescribed under the Cascade (i.e. the product is licensed for that species with that particular condition), the original manufacturer's packaging and package insert will contain information on appropriate doses, warnings and side effects. In these cases, no additional labelling is required; however, both the VMD and the RCVS consider it is good practice to attach a dispensing label to the packaging. When supplying a medicine in its original packaging, additional labels must not obscure any of the pre-existing information, particularly the batch number and expiry date. Whilst there are no specific labelling require-ments, the RCVS PSS requirements for labelling POM-Vs is helpful:

- Name and address of the animal owner
- Name and address of the veterinary practice supplying the medicine
- Date of supply
- Name, strength and quantity of the product
- Dosage and directions for use
- 'For animal treatment only'
- For topical preparations 'For external use only'.

If the medicine is prescribed under the Cascade or the product has been decanted from its original container, it must legally be labelled with the following information:

- Name and address of the animal owner
- Name and address of the veterinary practice or pharmacy supplying the medicine
- Name (or initials) of the prescribing veterinary surgeon
- Identification of the animal(s), including species
- Date of supply and product expiry date, if applicable
- Name, quantity and strength (if applicable) of product
- Dosage and administration instructions
- Any special storage precautions
- Any necessary warnings for the user, target species, administration or disposal of the product
- Withdrawal period, if relevant
- 'For animal treatment only'
- 'Keep out of the reach of children'
- 'For external use only', if relevant
- If the product if for a food-producing species, the batch number.

Ideally, labels should be computer generated and medi-cines should be dispensed in their original container. If this is not possible or practical, written information on the safe and effective use of the product, such as package leaflet or SPC should be supplied. The BSAVA produces a range of Client Information Leaflets for use by its members that can be used when dispensing unlicensed medicines prescribed under the Cascade. This is particularly useful because in these instances the SPC is designed for when the medicine is being dispensed to a human patient, so it would not be appropriate to supply the SPC that comes in the medicine packet. Examples of BSAVA Client Information Leaflets include omeprazole, allopurinol and gabapentin, although there are many more available for members to download from the BSAVA library (www.bsavalibrary.com/).

Instalments and repeat prescriptions

An example of a repeat prescription is when the prescriber has written a prescription for 60 tablets which can be repeated three times. This means that the supplier should initially dispense 60 tablets, and the owner can request another batch of 60 tablets a further three times (i.e. 240 tablets in total).

An example of instalment of a prescription is when the prescriber has written a prescription for 240 tablets, with the directions stating the owner should administer one tablet twice daily. The prescriber can state that the supplier should dispense 60 tablets every 30 days. This is useful for pain medication because it prevents the owner from requesting too much medication at once

---

Record keeping

For POM-V and POM-VPS medicines, incoming and out-going transactions should be recorded and kept for 5 years. Information that needs to be recorded includes:

- Date and nature of transaction
- Identity of the product
- Quantity received or supplied
- Name and address of supplier or recipient
- Copy of the prescription and the name and address of the person who wrote the prescription
- Batch number of the product.

If retailing or supplying veterinary medicines, an audit must be carried out annually. This audit must detail all the incoming and outgoing transactions and this must tally with current stock levels. Records must enable an individual to track the product name and batch number in terms of dates, quantities, name and address of clients supplied and current stock levels.

Special Import Scheme and Special Import Certificates

Where there is no suitable veterinary medicinal product (VMP) authorized in the UK, a veterinary surgeon may seek to import a medicine under the Special Import Scheme.

- Importing a veterinary medicine licensed in another EU member state for use with any animal species requires a Special Import Certificate and is considered use under the Cascade.
- Importing a veterinary medicine licensed in a country outside the EU or a human medicine from any country other than the UK also requires a Special Import Certificate but is considered outwith the Cascade and will only be granted in exceptional circumstances.

Applications may be made online via the VMD website and must include details of the animal to be treated, the medicine required, the supplier and the justification for importing the medicine.

Exemption scheme for small pet animals

Some veterinary products can be marketed for small pet animals without a marketing authorization and, therefore, are not required to prove safety, quality or efficacy (but must be manufactured to certain standards). The active ingredient, species it is to be used for and how the product is to be used must be approved, and products must be labelled clearly to show that they are being marketed under this scheme. Species covered include aquarium fish, cage birds, homing pigeons, terrarium animals, small rodents, ferrets and rabbits. Products containing antibiotics, narcotics or psycho-tropic agents are not included in the scheme. Products intended for parenteral, ophthalmic or aural administration may not be included in the scheme.

Controlled Drugs

Controlled Drugs for veterinary use are regulated in the same way as Controlled Drugs for humans, not under the VMR. The

Misuse of Drugs Act (1971) prohibits the possession, sale or supply of Controlled Drugs except in accordance with The Misuse of Drugs Regulations (2001). Controlled Drugs are divided into three classes for criminal purposes (Class A, B and C) and are divided into five Schedules for medicinal purposes.

Schedule 1

- Veterinary surgeons have no authority to possess or prescribe these drugs, except with a special licence from the Home Office.
- These drugs have no therapeutic value.
- Examples include cannabis and lysergic acid diethylamide (LSD).

Schedule 2

- There are special requirements for the requisition, prescribing, record keeping, storage and disposal of these drugs (see below).
- These drugs have therapeutic value but are highly addictive.
- A requisition form must be supplied in writing to the supplier and signed by the veterinary surgeon.
- These drugs must be stored in a Home Office approved, locked receptacle – a Controlled Drugs cabinet (with the exception of secobarbital).
- These drugs must be destroyed in the presence of a person authorized by the Secretary of State.
- Examples include morphine, methadone, pethidine, ketamine, fentanyl and secobarbital.

Schedule 3

- Subject to the same prescription and requisition requirements as Schedule 2 Controlled Drugs.
- Do not need to keep a record in a register, unlike for Schedule 2 Controlled Drugs.
- Most Schedule 3 Controlled Drugs should be kept in a locked receptacle; an exception is tramadol which is exempt.
- Examples include pentobarbital, phenobarbital, buprenorphine, tramadol and midazolam.

Schedule 4

- Exempt from most of the restrictions of Controlled Drugs.
- Examples include benzodiazepines and anabolic substances.

Schedule 5

- Exempt from most of the requirements, except that invoices need to be kept for 2 years.
- Examples include certain preparations containing codeine, cocaine and morphine in low concentrations.

Requisitioning Controlled Drugs

To requisition (order) a Schedule 2 or 3 Controlled Drug from a supplier, the practice must complete a Home Office approved Controlled Drug requisition form. The requisition form is split into three sections:

- Section A: Complete the supplier details, including company name and address
- Section B: Complete the drugs required, including the drug name, strength, form, quantity required and purpose for which drugs are to be used. In a veterinary practice, box 6 (Other) should be circled and annotated with 'For animals under my care'
- Section C: Complete details of the veterinary surgeon requesting the medication, including their name, MRCVS number, full practice address including phone number and postcode, wholesaler account number, professional occupation (veterinary surgeon), signature in indelible ink and the date.

The original copy of the requisition form must be sent to the supplier before the drugs can be despatched. Veterinary wholesalers must retain Controlled Drug requisition forms for inspection.

Prescribing Controlled Drugs

Written prescriptions for Controlled Drugs are only valid for 28 days. In addition to the requirements for any veterinary written prescription they must:

- Have the total quantity prescribed in words and figures (e.g. sixty (60) tablets)
- State the strength and form of the product
- Have specific directions (i.e. 'give as directed' is not adequate, the prescriber should say 'give one tablet twice daily')
- Have the statement 'For animals under my care'
- Not have any repeats for Schedule 2 and 3, although instalment dispensing is allowed
- Recommendation – the veterinary surgeon should only prescribe 30 days' supply at a time, except for patients on long-term medication, such as phenobarbital for epilepsy, when longer courses can be supplied.

Record keeping for Controlled Drugs

For Schedule 2 Controlled Drugs:

- Record on obtaining:
  - Date
  - Name and address of supplier
  - Amount obtained.
- Record on supplying:
  - Date
  - Name and address of person supplied
  - Veterinary surgeon's name
  - Amount supplied (and wasted, if relevant).
- If the drug is to be supplied to an owner for taking home, the following must also be recorded:
  - Name of person collecting the drug
  - Was proof of identification of the person collecting the drug requested? (Yes/No)
  - Was proof of identification of the person collecting the drug supplied? (Yes/No).

Although not required by law, other useful information to include in a Controlled Drugs Register could be:

- The name of the person withdrawing the dose from the Controlled Drugs cabinet
- The batch number of each drug
- The wholesaler invoice or delivery note number for all Controlled Drugs received. This is useful for tying up any discrepancies.

The Controlled Drugs Register must be either a computerized system or a bound book with separate sections for each drug, form and strength. Entries must be made in indelible ink, in chronological order and must be made within 24 hours of drug administration. They should be signed by the prescribing veterinary surgeon and registers should be kept for 2 years from the date of last entry. Amendments should be made in the margin and signed by a veterinary surgeon; it is not acceptable to score out any entry made in a Controlled Drug Register. Current legislation recommends that a running tally of stock is maintained. However, the RCVS requires running balances to be completed and will inspect these as part of their Practice Standard Scheme inspection process. Figure 8.39 is an example of the entries required for maintaining a Controlled Drugs Register.

Wastage from multi-dose vials and ampoules

Due to the nature of the packaging of Controlled Drugs, not all medication taken from the cabinet will be administered to the animal. If the drug is packaged in a single-use ampoule, the required dose should be recorded in the register and the remainder of the ampoule recorded as wastage (e.g. for a 1 ml ampoule: '0.4 ml given, 0.6 ml wastage'). If the drug is packaged in a multi-dose vial, wastage can come from two sources: the hub of the needle and syringe, and the small volume left in the vial when all possible doses have been withdrawn. Practice staff must do everything possible to minimize wastage. It is not possible to quantify exactly how much wastage will arise from the use of multi-dose vials, but

fewer doses of a large volume will result in less wastage than a greater number of small volume doses. Manufacturers of needles and syringes can provide information on the exact volume of 'dead space' in their products. Generally, the smaller the syringe and needle gauge, the less dead space. Special syringes with no dead space are available and could be used to minimize wastage. Good technique when withdrawing the required dose can also minimize wastage (e.g. the process of expelling air from a syringe can lead to loss of product).

Storage of Controlled Drugs

Controlled Drugs must be held in a Home Office approved locked cabinet, which is secured to the fabric of the building (Figure 8.40). The veterinary surgeon in charge must ensure that there is no unauthorized access to Controlled Drugs. The room housing the Controlled Drug cabinet should be lockable, tidy and not normally accessible to clients. The Controlled Drug cabinet keys must either be kept on the responsible veterinary surgeon's person at all times, or locked in an appropriate key safe. This key safe should be fitted with a combination lock and bolted to the wall. Controlled Drug cabinets are also available with combination locks and these could be considered in larger practices where multiple people require access to Controlled Drugs. The following procedures should be maintained for both a key box and combination Controlled Drug cabinet:

Drug name: Methadone Hydrochloride | Schedule: 2 | Strength: 10 mg/ml | Form: Book 1, Injection vials

Date	Name and address of supplier	Quantity obtained	Client's name and number	Quantity given	Quantity wasted/not given	Administered by: (veterinary surgeons signature)	Comments	Balance
02/12/2011							Balance b/f	0 ml
02/12/2011	VMD Wholesale Ltd. KT15 3LS	1 x 10ml	–	–	–	–	–	10 ml
02/12/2011			Bobby Jones (J145)	1.8 ml	–	Vet 1	Vial A	8.2 ml
10/12/2011			Rex Davis (D418)	3.1 ml	–	Vet 3	Vial A	5.1 ml
12/12/2011	VMD Wholesale Ltd. KT15 3LS	2 x 10ml	–	–	–	–	–	25.1 ml
13/12/2011			Cats Trust, Chobham	4 x 0.2 ml	–	Vet 5	Vial A	24.3 ml
15/12/2011			Archie Smith (S489)	2.8 ml	1.5 ml	Vet 3	Vial A – no usable vol remaining	20 ml
15/12/2011			Kelly Evans (E365)	3.8 ml	–	Vet 5	Vial B	16.2 ml
31/12/2011			Jake Price (P982)	2.5 ml	–	Vet 4	Vial B	13.7 ml
31/12/2011			–	–	Vet 1		Stock audit	13.7 ml
06/01/2012			Queenie Clarke (C145)	1.2 ml	–	Vet 2	Vial B	12.5 ml
07/01/2012			Buster Stenson (S482)	3.2 ml	0.8 ml	Vet 1	Vial B emptied, vial C opened	8.5 ml
09/01/2012	VMD Wholesale Ltd. KT15 3LS	1 x 10ml		–	–	–	–	18.5 ml
17/01/2012			Pixie James (J354)	1.8 ml	–	Vet 2	Vial C	16.7 ml
22/01/2012			Cats Trust, Chobham	3 x 0.2 ml	–	Vet 1	Vial C	16.1 ml
27/01/2012			Skip Marsden (M741)	2.9 ml	–	Vet 4	Vial C	13.2 ml
05/01/2012			–	–	3.2 ml	Vet 3	Vial C expired. Denatured and destroyed	10 ml

8.39 Example of entries required for maintaining a Controlled Drugs Register, both on receipt and when supplying/prescribing/administering. (Contains public sector information licensed under the Open Government Licence v3.0.)

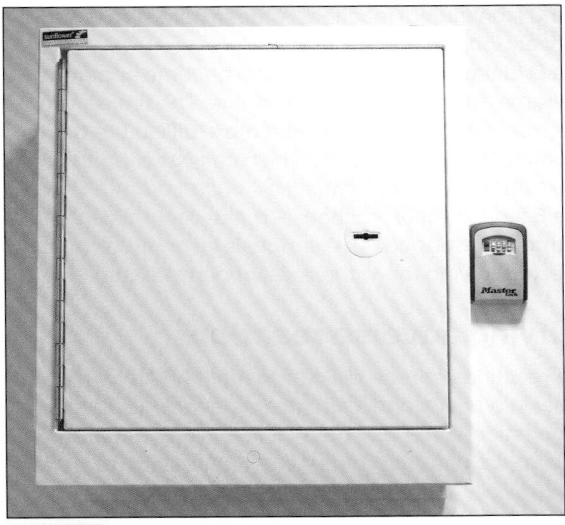

8.40 Controlled Drugs cabinet and key box.

- Combinations should not be written down
- Combinations that are issued to individual members of staff should not be shared with anyone else, including colleagues
- All combinations should be changed regularly, or at least every 6 months as a minimum, to prevent the locks from being compromised
- Combinations should be changed whenever there are grounds to suspect that they may have become known to an unauthorized person
- Regardless of whether a combination is shared by a group of people or issued to an individual, it should be changed whenever a member of that group or the individual to whom it was issued leaves the business or otherwise no longer requires access to the lock.

Disposal of Controlled Drugs

Any out-of-date Controlled Drugs, or those returned by clients, should be held in a segregated section of the Controlled Drugs cabinet ready for disposal. Out-of-date Controlled Drugs are classed as stock until they are denatured and disposed of. The process of denaturing Controlled Drugs must be witnessed by:

- An inspector authorized by the VMD (this can be an RCVS Practice Standards Scheme inspector)
- A veterinary surgeon who has no connection to the practice and receives no financial payment
- A police Controlled Drugs Liaison Officer.

If a client returns a Schedule 2 Controlled Drug, it should be recorded in a 'patient returns logbook', which records the date, the patient to whom the drug was prescribed, the name of the drug, strength and form, and the amount returned. Patient returns may be disposed of without being witnessed.

Procedure for denaturing Controlled Drugs

1. Identify any Schedule 2 and 3 Controlled Drugs that are obsolete, expired, unwanted or that have been returned by an owner.
2. Make sure that an authorized person is present to witness the destruction of the Controlled Drugs (this can be the responsible veterinary surgeon for patient returns; for stock Controlled Drugs, it must be a person authorized by the Home Office, a police officer or a veterinary surgeon who has no connection to the practice).
3. Update the records of any patient-returned Schedule 2 Controlled Drugs that have been destroyed in the back of the patient returns register. Record:
   - The drug name, form and strength
   - The quantity destroyed
   - The date of destruction
   - Signature of the authorized person
   - Signature of the witness.
4. Record the destruction of any stock Schedule 2 Controlled Drugs (i.e. non-patient returns) in the relevant section of the Controlled Drugs Register. Record:
   - The drug name, form and strength
   - The quantity destroyed
   - The date of destruction
   - Signature of the authorized person
   - Signature of the witness.
5. All stock of the Schedule 2 Controlled Drug in question must be manually counted to ensure that the amount of stock held corresponds to the balance in the stock record.
6. Gloves, an apron and goggles should be used if required.
7. Denature the Controlled Drugs by:
   - Crushing in a tablet crusher or mortar and pestle and placing in the denaturing kit (Figure 8.41)
   - Opening the capsule and sprinkling the contents into the denaturing kit
   - Opening ampoules and shaking the contents into the denaturing kit
   - Drawing up liquid from multi-dose bottles and placing it in the denaturing kit
   - Folding patches in on themselves and placing in the denaturing kit
   - Filling the denaturing kit to the line with water.
8. Place the filled denaturing kit in the Controlled Drugs cabinet and then wash your hands.
9. After 24 hours, remove the filled denaturing kit and place in a pharmaceutical waste bin.
10. Do not store waste in quantities in excess of 5 cubic metres or for longer than 6 months.
11. After waste collection, file the collection dockets issued by the waste contractor and retain for 5 years.

Any medicine left in an ampoule or vial, which is deemed unusable, is considered to be a waste product. There is no legal requirement to have the disposal of the waste product witnessed. As disposal of the waste product happens so frequently, using denaturing kits would prove very costly. In these cases, the waste product should be placed in a container of wood-based cat litter mixed with washing up liquid to denature the drugs. Once full, the container should be placed in the pharmaceutical waste bin for disposal.

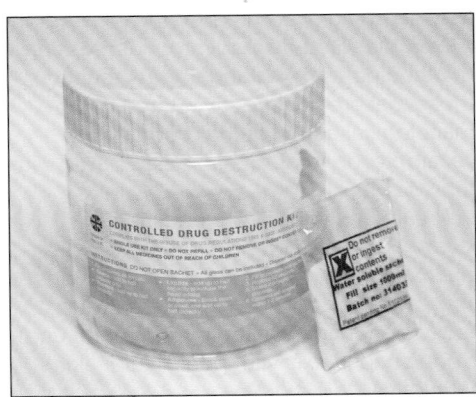

8.41

Controlled Drug denaturing kit.

Suspected Adverse Reaction Surveillance Scheme (SARSS)

This is a national surveillance scheme run by the pharmacovigilance unit of the VMD, which aims to record and monitor reports of suspected adverse reactions (or lack of effect) to licensed and unlicensed veterinary medicines in both animals (any species) and humans. It also collates information on adverse reactions to human licensed medicines used in animals and adverse reactions to microchipping. Adverse reactions in humans administering human licensed medicines to animals should be reported to the Medicines and Healthcare Products Regulatory Agency (MHRA) under the 'yellow card scheme'.

Reports should be made to the VMD online via their website. The person reporting will require basic information such as:

- The name of the product which caused the suspected adverse reaction or lack of efficacy
- The animal(s) or person(s) in which the adverse reaction or lack of efficacy occurred
- The signs observed of the adverse reaction or lack of efficacy that is suspected
- The contact details of the reporter of the adverse reaction or lack of efficacy.

Anyone can report an adverse reaction, although veterinary nurses may wish to alert the prescribing veterinary surgeon before making a report. All adverse reactions should be reported, even if they are only suspected reactions or it is not clear which drug caused the reaction. The VMD will collate the reports and send them to the VPC, who will make an assessment and decide whether any action is required. Actions required by manufacturers can vary from a minor amendment of the SPC to include a new side effect or interaction, to the complete withdrawal of the product from the market.

Classifying adverse drug reactions

Adverse reactions can be classified according to the system below:

- **Type A** (augmented) reactions – these result from an exaggeration of a drug's normal pharmacological actions when given at the usual dose range and are normally dose-dependent (i.e. the higher the dose the greater the clinical signs). Examples include respiratory depression with opioids or bleeding with warfarin. Type A reactions also include those that are not directly related to the desired pharmacological action of the drug but are expected; for example, dry mouth that is associated with tricyclic antidepressants
- **Type B** (bizarre) reactions – these are unusual responses that are not expected from the known pharmacological actions of the drug. These reactions are less common and may only be discovered after a drug has already been made available for general use. Examples include anaphylaxis with penicillin or skin rashes with antibiotics

- **Type C** (continuing) reactions – these persist for a relatively long period of time
- **Type D** (delayed) reactions – these become apparent sometime after the use of a medicine. The timing of these reactions may make them more difficult to detect. An example is leucopoenia, which can occur up to 6 weeks after a dose of lomustine
- **Type E** (end-of-use) reactions – these occur when a treatment is stopped. An example is insomnia and anxiety following the withdrawal of benzodiazepines.

Identifying adverse reactions

Adverse reactions can be difficult to identify. An owner may not perceive a new sign as an adverse effect, so it is important to question when any new clinical signs began to see if they tie in with starting treatment. Other signs to be alert for include:

- Abnormal physical parameters (e.g. temperature, pulse, blood pressure, respiratory rate and blood glucose levels)
- Abnormal biochemistry or haematology results
- Medication being started that is being used to treat an adverse effect (e.g. cimetidine to treat gastrointestinal upset due to NSAID therapy).

Pharmacy management

Storage of medicines

To enable the VMD to fulfil its obligations under European law to maintain and improve traceability of, and accountability for, veterinary medicines, all premises from which medicines are prescribed and supplied must be registered as Veterinary Practice Premises (VPP) with the RCVS. All registered premises are inspected by the VMD, except those practices that are members of the RCVS Practice Standards Scheme (PSS), which are inspected by the RCVS as part of this scheme. Veterinary practice premises must be a permanent building or part of a permanent building, be clean, well maintained and vermin proof. Premises where medicines are held should be capable of being secured to deter intruders. Controlled Drugs and injection equipment are attractive not only to drug misusers but also to professional criminals. Professional advice should be obtained on the suitability of the premises, as well as locks, shutters and security alarms.

Areas of the practice used for the storage or supply of medicines must not be residential, and public access should be denied or controlled to areas where POM-V, POM-VPS and NFA-VPS medicines are held (i.e. they should be 'staff only areas'). There should be no smoking, food consumption or storage of food in areas where medicines are stored or supplied, with notices in place informing staff and clients accordingly. Particular attention should be taken with fridges; the storage of medicines alongside food or laboratory samples must be avoided. To avoid contamination, medicines should not be stored in toilet or washing areas or laboratories. Medicines to be supplied to clients should not be stored in areas where animals are kept, such as kennels, except those medicines already dispensed.

Flammable products must be stored in an appropriate flammables cabinet specifically designed for this purpose, preferably on the floor to prevent breakages. Shelving should be of sturdy construction and well designed to reduce the possibility of breakage and spillage. It should be designed in such a way to ensure medicines are easy to locate with areas suitable for small and bulk storage.

A record must be kept at the practice main premises of all other locations where medicines may be stored (e.g. practice cars or homes where medicines are kept for on-call purposes).

Consulting rooms

Medicines stored in consulting rooms should be kept to a minimum and should be placed out of sight in drawers or cupboards. There is no requirement for these cupboards to be locked but it could be considered good practice to do so if clients are left in consulting rooms unsupervised. Medicines subject to abuse should not be held in consulting rooms.

Practice cars

Medicines held in vehicles should be kept to a minimum. Only those used frequently and only sufficient for immediate use should be carried routinely because the temperature within the car may fluctuate greatly, causing reduced efficacy of the products. Any medicines that are kept in vehicles should be clean and well organized. Cars should be fitted with refrigerated units and the temperature of these should be monitored to ensure they are maintained between 2°C and 8°C. Precautions against theft, such as not storing medicines in the car for long periods of time or overnight, not leaving medicines on display and parking vehicles in secure areas, should be considered. Controlled Drugs should be stored in either a locked glove box or a locked container fixed within the boot of the car which must meet the requirements of the Safe Custody Regulations, or in a constantly attended separate locked bag, box or case that is removed from the vehicle if it is left unattended.

Storage requirements

In addition to security, there are also a number of other factors that can affect the stability of medicines, which must be taken into account when designing the area that medications are stored:

- Temperature
- Humidity
- Light
- Oxygen
- Time.

Temperature

The temperature of the pharmacy and any area where drugs are stored must be monitored and kept within:

- Fridge: 2–8°C
- Room: ambient temperature, approximately 18–25°C.

The temperature should be checked daily and recorded at least weekly. If the thermometer does not keep a log of temperature recordings, it is good practice to record daily. Data loggers can be used, which record the temperature of the room or fridge at set intervals. This information is then periodically downloaded on to a computer. These should only be used if they have an audible alarm to warn staff members when the temperature goes outside the required range.

There should be written procedures in place describing the action to be taken in the event of loss of control over the storage conditions of temperature-sensitive products; for example, the accidental disconnection or breakdown of a refrigerator. These procedures should identify any action that needs to be taken and should include:

- What temperature deviation requires an action
- Where to move products to temporarily
- Which products may be reused and which must be disposed of (this will depend on whether the temperature dropped too low, too high, to what temperature, and for how long)
- Where to find information on which products may be safely used (the manufacturer, SPC or medicines information pharmacists at your local NHS hospital)
- Who to contact for repairs or to inform of any products to be disposed of.

Regular cleaning, servicing and stock control of refrigerators should be performed as for other storage areas.

Humidity

Medicines should not be stored anywhere near autoclaves, washing machines or in any area where steam may be generated. Medicines should always be stored in their original packaging; if they have a desiccant the drug will be as well protected as possible. Some blister packs are specially formulated to keep moisture out.

Light

The pharmacy should be sited in the middle of the building with no windows, so it is not in direct sunlight. Most light-sensitive drugs come in brown bottles, but not all (e.g. metronidazole and furosemide), so should always be kept in their boxes.

Oxygen

Poorly fitting or damaged lids can cause excessive exposure to oxygen, leading to oxidation and degradation of fat or wax-based products.

Time

When new deliveries arrive, always stock in date order with the longest expiry dates on the bottom of the pile/back of the shelf. It is an offence to administer any drug after its expiry date, including the in-use expiry date, or to obscure the expiry date on the packaging of any medicine. The in-use expiry date tells the user how long the bottle may be kept open after first broaching. It is usually, but not always:

- 28 days for multi-dose vials
- 6 months for oral liquids
- 1 year for tablets and capsules
- 3 months for creams (6 months for ointments)
- Immediately for snap-top ampoules.

Extra care should be taken with powders for reconstitution; some have to be discarded straight away, whilst others such as marbofloxacin for injection can be kept for 28 days after reconstitution. Some creams, oral liquids and tablets may have a much shorter in-use shelf-life. The standards stated above should be used only if no specified in-use shelf-life is specified in the SPC or product packaging. All open products should be marked with the date of first use and the specified in-use expiry date. Bright stickers can be useful to draw attention, but all multi-dose vials with an in-use shelf life now have a space to write this information. Any drug left in the vial after the specified time must be discarded.

Each item in the pharmacy must be date checked at least once every 3 months and short-dated stock marked. A named person should be responsible for ensuring that date checking occurs. Some computer systems can batch control all pharmaceutical stock and record exactly what is in stock at any time. These systems can identify items that will shortly go out-of-date, so there is no need to manually check every bottle, with the exception of open bottles to check the in-use shelf-life.

Dispensing and packaging medicines

Many medicines come packaged conveniently in blister packs, which aids the dispensing process and avoids direct contact with the product by the dispenser. However, some products are packaged in bottles of loose tablets or capsules, which need to be counted out according to the prescriber's requirements. When counting such medicines, there are a number of aids available such as a counting triangle, capsule counter or electronic scales. Liquid medicines may be measured using a syringe or conical measure (Figure 8.42).

All dispensed medicines need to be supplied to the client in appropriate packaging. The ideal container should be:

- Robust enough to protect the contents from crushing during handling and transport
- Easy to open and close (but child proof for safety)
- Constructed of inert materials that do not interact with the medicine
- Be sufficiently transparent to allow the contents to be seen.

Medicines should be dispensed in their original packaging, where possible, because such packaging has been specifically designed to maintain the medicine in the ideal storage conditions (e.g. it may contain a desiccant for medicines sensitive to moisture). If the quantity required differs from the original packaging, medicines should be dispensed into:

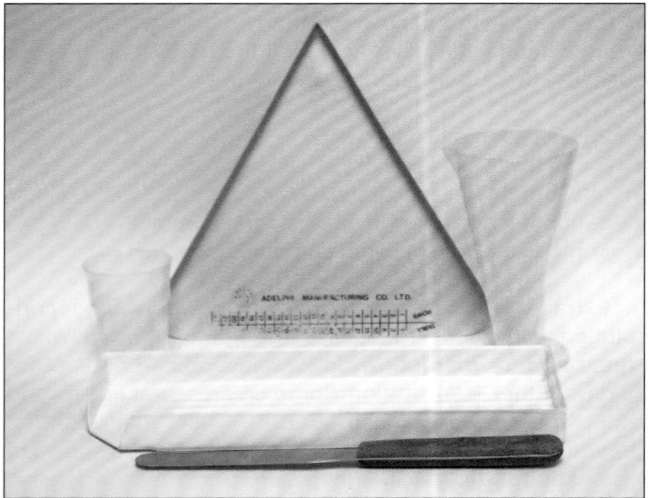

8.42 Aids for dispensing medications.

- Click lock amber bottles for loose tablets and capsules (must be crush and moisture proof) (Figure 8.43)
- Paper cartons or envelopes for blister packs (these are not appropriate for loose tablets)
- Leak proof amber bottles for oral liquids
- Ribbed amber bottles for topical liquids (these are becoming increasingly difficult to obtain).

Child-resistant caps must be used unless specifically requested otherwise (e.g. if the owner has dexterity problems and cannot open childproof bottles).

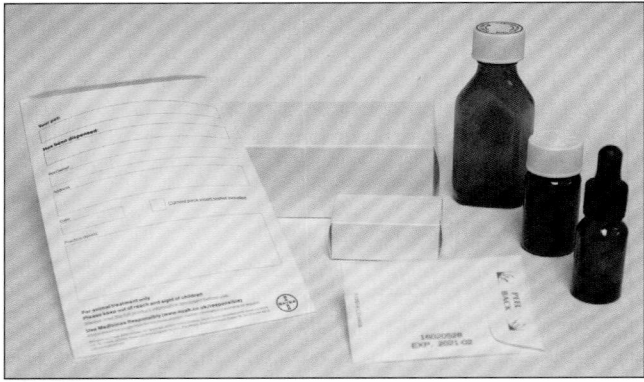

8.43 Packaging for medications.

Stock control

Key points

- Stock control processes must be in place to ensure medicines are used or disposed of within their shelf-life (including their in-use shelf-life)
- Good stock control will reduce waste and save money
- Medicines returned by owners should be disposed of
- It is an offence to supply or administer an out-of-date medicine

Efficient stock control allows the right product to be at the right place at the right time. It ensures that capital is not tied up unnecessarily and protects against problems arising in the supply chain. It is good practice to:

- Set stock levels to allow accurate stock holding
- Have a named person responsible for stock control
- Store products in original packaging, in a logical order
- Supply a product leaflet or SPC with all products dispensed
- Dispense products with the shortest expiry date first
- Store products with different batch numbers together.

Dates of deliveries and items delivered from manufacturers or wholesalers should be recorded, unless this information is on the invoice or delivery note which is retained. Packs with damaged or defaced packaging and out-of-date stock should be stored separately while awaiting disposal.

Stocking levels

In order to perform stock control effectively, maximum and minimum levels must be set for every product. This can be done using a small card placed on the products at the correct place, a sticker on the shelf, or a fully automated system. Any system will require information such as product description, order up to level (OUTL), re-order point (ROP), supplier and item code.

The amount of stock to be kept can be calculated using the basic equation:

OUTL = D x L   (D = daily demand, L = lead time)

In practice, however, average daily demand is very difficult to calculate accurately and does not take into account weekends, public holidays or periods of exceptional use. Thus, it may be better to work on a principle of 2 or even 4 weeks cover, so the average daily demand becomes the average demand for 2 or 4 weeks. This will allow sufficient stock to cover for any emergencies. It may be wise to keep 4 weeks cover of any drugs used in emergency situations, but only 2 weeks of routine products where the consequences of not having a bottle in stock are not so great. If the item is seasonal, extra consideration will be needed to set an OUTL, which may be different for specific times of the year.

'Rep' orders (orders place directly with a company representative, which are usually a special offer, e.g. buy 10 get 2 free) can be a cost-effective way of ordering stock for frequently used products. It must be recognized, however, that the product will have been bought and paid for within a month and that until enough stock has been sold to cover what has been paid, the practice will be out of pocket. If just 2–4 weeks supply is ordered, the stock should always have been sold on by the time the wholesaler is paid for it; this helps with cash flow.

Products subject to intermittent use will not fit into the OUTL calculation. For example, some emergency drugs are used infrequently but when required, large volumes may be used. This needs to be factored in when OUTLs are set.

Stock control is an ongoing process. Stock levels should be altered as new products are brought to the market or preferences change.

Stock rotation

Products with the shortest expiry should be dispensed first to reduce the number of products going out-of-date. This can generally be achieved by ensuring that all new stock from deliveries is placed at the bottom or back of current stock, but it is useful to double check that the expiry dates of the newly delivered stock are longer than the current stock, particularly if orders are placed with different companies.

Stock loss and annual stocktake

There are a number of reasons for stock loss within a veterinary practice. These include:

- Products going out-of-date
- Broken or damaged stock
- Items mistakenly not charged for
- Items charged for by wholesalers but not received
- Wholesaler credit for goods returned or missing not received
- Consumable wastage
- Theft.

Products going out-of-date means money lost to the practice. Setting appropriate ROPs and OUTLs will reduce stockholding and lead to fewer products going out-of-date. Monthly date checking should be performed to ensure products are used before they expire (where clinically appropriate).

The VMD requires all practices to perform an annual stocktake, where incoming and outgoing medicinal products are reconciled. Any missing items must be accounted for. Out-of-date products are still considered 'stock' until they are removed from the stock file. In the annual stocktake, all products that have gone out-of-date must be accounted for or they will be assumed to be missing. Broken or damaged stock should also be recorded for stocktaking purposes. A system should be put in place to ensure all items used are charged for appropriately. This will ensure not only that the practice maximizes their income, but that purchases and sales of each product can be reconciled for the annual stocktake.

To prevent the theft of medicines, food and pet products such as leads, clients should not have access to medicine cupboards when left alone in the consulting room and any waiting room displays should be within sight of the reception staff. Regular stocktakes of vulnerable items should be performed to check for discrepancies.

Medicines received from wholesalers should always be checked against delivery notes and any missing or damaged goods claimed for at the time of receipt. Once a claim has been made, ensure the credit is received by reconciling credit notes against returns books.

It is advised that practices set up a dummy client called 'Disposal' on their practice management system and record all medicines that are unusable. This can help the practice identify where medicines are being wasted and also help with reconciling stock during audits.

Medicine returns

As the correct storage conditions (and therefore safety and effectiveness) of medicines returned by owners cannot be guaranteed, such products should be disposed of and not accepted back into stock. Products dispensed for animals on the premises that have not left the practice can be accepted back into stock providing the storage conditions are known to be acceptable and they are not contaminated in any way (e.g. by using the same syringe to withdraw multiple oral doses from a bottle of liquid medicine). Unwanted or mistakenly ordered medicines should be returned to the wholesalers as soon as possible. There may be restrictions on such returns as returned medicinal products may be destroyed.

Batch recording

All practices are required to keep a log of the batches of medicine used. For non-food producing species, the date of first use of an item must be recorded. For example, if a bottle of prednisolone tablets is opened on the 1st January and dispensed on the 3rd, 4th and 5th of January before opening a new bottle on the 7th January, as long as the date each batch number started to be used is recorded, if there is a product recall it is possible to work out who received the affected batch. This allows for a basic batch tracking capability in case of a product recall.

Dispensary management

Key points

- A single person should be responsible for dispensary management
- A dispensary manual should be written detailing standard operating procedures (SOPs) and risk assessments
- All staff involved in medicines handling should be suitably trained

One person should be responsible for ensuring the legal requirements, safety assessments and best practice procedures are carried out. This person should be responsible for ensuring:

- The layout of the dispensary is efficient and appropriate shelving is used
- The dispensary is always clean and tidy
- Date checking is performed and recorded regularly
- Staff are suitably trained
- SOPs are written and implemented
- Stock control is efficient to reduce stock loss
- Storage conditions (particularly temperature) are monitored in the dispensary and practice cars.

Dispensary manual

A dispensary manual should be prepared containing SOPs, risk and Control of Substances Hazardous to Health (COSHH) assessments, blank forms and other useful information (e.g. on special suppliers and unusual products). This should be available to and read by all those involved in dispensing medicines.

Staff training

All those involved in the supply of medicines should be suitably trained. To prevent both contamination of the medicinal products and to protect the staff member, training should include the requirement for a high standard of personal cleanliness, with regular hand washing seen as essential and open wounds covered at all times. Staff should also be trained on how to avoid direct contact with medicines, such as wearing gloves or using a tablet counting triangle and spatula.

Although there is no legal requirement for staff members working in the dispensary to have formal training, all staff members should have read the dispensary manual and be aware of practice SOPs and risk assessments. It is required under the RCVS PSS that practices with hospital status have at least one member of staff who has completed a dispensing course in the last 4 years. This can be an external course (such as the BSAVA Dispensing Course), a webinar or an online course. The National Proficiency Test Council (NPTC) provides competency testing in the safe use of veterinary medicines. It should be considered best practice for the person responsible for dispensary management to have completed one of these courses in the last 5 years.

Standard operating procedures

An SOP is a written document describing routine procedures carried out in veterinary practice. Well written SOPs provide direction, improve communication, reduce training time and improve work consistency. SOPs should be:

- Provided for all staff members
- Regularly reviewed
- Designed according to practice policy.

The use of SOPs may be taken, along with relevant training and continuing professional development (CPD), as sufficient evidence that staff are regarded as 'competent' under the requirements of the VMR. The benefits of implementing SOPs include:

- Assurance of the quality of the service
- Ensures the achievement of good practice

- Enables veterinary surgeons to delegate and so free time up for other duties
- Avoids confusion about who does what
- Provides advice and guidance to locums and part-time staff
- Provides a useful tool for training new staff members
- Contributes to the audit process
- Provides financial benefits
- Most importantly, SOPs protect staff and clients.

SOPs can be written in four different formats: simple steps, hierarchical steps, graphic procedures or a flowchart. The most appropriate format to use will depend on the number of steps involved in the process and how many decisions the user has to make during the procedure. For more information on writing SOPs, see the *BSAVA Guide to the Use of Veterinary Medicines*.

Advice to owners

For a medicine to be effective, it must be correctly administered. It is the prescriber's legal responsibility to ensure that the person who will administer the product understands how to do so safely and effectively. Good advice is key to ensuring this happens.

There are a number of barriers to client understanding (see Chapter 9 for more information on client communication), which relate to the safe and effective use of medicines:

- Use of technical terms
- Hearing impairment
- Sight impairment
- Problems with reading (words/numbers/fractions/decimals)
- Dyslexia.

It is vitally important that the client's understanding of how any medicine prescribed should be used is checked before they leave the practice.

The supplying practice **must** provide written information about the medicine. Information written on a dispensing label may be enough, but manufacturer information leaflets, package inserts and SPCs will provide a greater depth of information. Information leaflets, in particular, are written specifically for clients using lay terms and pictures, which make them easy to understand.

It is particularly important that the client is made aware of any warnings associated with the product. These may be warnings for the person administering the product; for example, wear gloves, wash hands after use or do not handle during pregnancy. Warnings can also relate to how the medicine should be stored; for example, shake well before use or store in the fridge. There may be warnings relating to the animal being treated; for example, side effects to watch out for, whether to give with food or not, and what to do if the medicine is not working. It is important to check with clients whether they have any allergies to medicines, such as a penicillin allergy, which would mean they cannot administer such drugs.

It may be necessary to demonstrate how to administer the medicine and ask the client to demonstrate back, in order that their understanding can be checked. It is helpful for clients of a newly diagnosed diabetic cat, for example, who are not confident giving injections to come to the practice a few times to inject insulin under supervision.

Owners should be counselled on the importance of giving the medicine exactly as it was prescribed, and what to do when the supplied medication is finished (i.e. is the course completed, or should they come in to request further supplies). They should specifically be informed of the importance of completing a course of antibiotic treatment to reduce the risks of antimicrobial resistance. Owners should also be informed what to do with any unused medicines (i.e. return them to the practice for safe disposal).

When dispensing repeat prescriptions of medicines, or when animals are presented for a recheck, the client should be questioned to ensure that they are able to administer the medicine easily. If a client's cat runs away every time it sees her because it is scared when medicines are administered, the client will soon become unhappy and possibly stop giving the medication altogether. Clients will be grateful for any suggestions on how to help administer the medication, whether it requires a change in formulation from tablet to liquid, something tasty to disguise a tablet, or a complete change in drug choice (to be decided by the prescribing veterinary surgeon).

Disposal of medicines: unused, expired and damaged stock

To ensure the safety of humans, animals and the environment, it is important that waste medicines are disposed of safely. They should never be disposed of into the sewerage system where they will contaminate the water, or into general household waste. When dispensing medicines for owners to administer at home, it is important to make them aware that any leftover medicines should be returned to the veterinary practice for safe disposal. Chapter 2 contains detailed information about waste management.

England and Wales, Scotland and Northern Ireland have their own sets of laws and regulations for the disposal of waste medicines, which differ slightly from each other but are broadly similar (see Chapter 2). Medicinal waste can be classified as hazardous (called 'special' in Scotland) or non-hazardous, and may be made up of whole or residual pharmaceuticals. Medicinal waste must be segregated according to the European Waste Catalogue (EWC), with hazardous waste being further classified by its hazardous properties:

- HP6 – toxic teratogenic
- HP7 – carcinogenic
- HP9 – infectious
- HP10 – toxic for reproduction
- HP11 – mutagenic.

Prior to collection by a waste contractor, medicinal waste should be placed in rigid containers with the appropriate colour of lid (Figure 8.44). In the case of medicines in foil blister packs, the outer paper carton may be removed and recycled, but the tablets or capsules should be kept in the blisters. Loose tablets, capsules and liquids should be kept in the outer packaging to prevent any of the medicines coming into direct contact with each other. Such contact may cause a chemical reaction, which could lead to a fire.

Colour code	Type of waste
Blue	Non-hazardous medicinal waste
Purple	Hazardous medicinal waste
Purple	Sharps contaminated with hazardous waste
Yellow	Non-hazardous medicinally contaminated sharps
Orange	Non-medicinally contaminated sharps (e.g. needles used to take blood samples)

8.44 Medicinal waste should be separated into containers with the appropriate coloured lid prior to collection.

Hazardous pharmaceutical waste

- Must be placed into a purple lidded container.
- May be made up of:
  - Out-of-date medicines
  - Medicines returned from clients
  - Damaged medicines
  - Empty pots, bottles and vials (note: snap-top ampoules are classed as sharps and should be placed in a sharps bin).
- Consists of medicines which are:
  - Cytotoxic
  - Cytostatic
  - Immunosuppressant
  - Antiviral
  - Hormonal (only some hormones are classified as hazardous; for example, prostaglandins such as delmadinone and aglepristone).
- European Waste Catalogue code 18 02 07.

Non-hazardous pharmaceutical waste

- Includes any whole or residual pharmaceutical waste, other than those in the previous hazardous waste section.
- Should be placed into a rigid blue (or blue lidded) container.
- May be made up of:
  - Out-of-date medicines
  - Medicines returned from clients
  - Damaged medicines
  - Used syringes
  - Denatured Controlled Drugs (see 'Disposal of Controlled Drugs' for procedure)
  - Empty pots, bottles and vials (note: snap-top ampoules are classed as sharps and should be placed in a sharps bin).
- European Waste Catalogue code 18 02 08.

Medicine contaminated sharps

- Should be placed in a yellow lidded rigid sharps bin.
- May be made up of:
  - Open snap-top glass ampoules
  - Contaminated needles.
- It is not recommended that syringe bodies be separated from needles, although waste is usually charged by

227

volume so this can lead to vastly increased costs for disposal. If a risk assessment and an SOP are in place, it may be appropriate to the separate needle and syringe, with the syringe body being disposed of as pharmaceutical waste.
- Sharps contaminated with hazardous medicines should be separated and placed in a purple lidded sharps bin.
- European Waste Catalogue code 18 02 02.

Management of health and safety at work

Health and safety in the dispensary requires identification of **hazards** and **risks**.

- A **hazard** is anything that may cause harm, such as chemicals, electricity, working at height or an open drawer.
- The **risk** is the chance (high or low) that somebody could be harmed by these and other hazards, together with an indication of how serious the harm could be.

Control of Substances Hazardous to Health

The 2002 COSHH Regulations require employers to control substances that are hazardous to health. The exposure of workers to hazardous substances may be prevented or reduced by:

- Finding out what the health hazards are
- Deciding how to prevent harm to health (risk assessment)
- Providing control measures to reduce harm to health and making sure they are used
- Keeping all control measures in good working order
- Providing information, instruction and training for employees and others
- Providing monitoring and health surveillance in appropriate cases
- Planning for emergencies.

Every employer or self-employed person is legally required to make an assessment of the health and safety risks arising from their work. The purpose of the assessment is to identify what needs to be done to control the health and safety risks. If a practice employs five or more people, the assessment(s) must be recorded in writing. Failure to adequately control hazards can lead to prosecution under the COSHH Regulations and civil action from injured or ill employees.

Hazardous substances include:

- Substances used directly in work activities and classified as dangerous to health under the **R**egistration, **E**valuation, **A**uthorisation and restriction of **CH**emicals (REACH) legislation 2007 (recognizable by their warning symbols) (e.g. cleaning agents)
- Substances generated during work activities (e.g. waste fumes from anaesthesia equipment)
- Naturally occurring substances (e.g. dust from litter trays if concentrations in the air exceed levels specified in the COSHH Regulations)
- Biological agents, such as bacteria and other microorganisms

- Other substances that may pose a risk to health, but not covered by the Classification Labelling and Packaging (CLP) Regulations for technical reasons (e.g. medicines).

To comply with COSHH Regulations the following eight steps must be followed:

1. Assess the risks.
2. Decide what precautions are needed.
3. Prevent or adequately control exposure.
4. Ensure that control measures are used and maintained.
5. Monitor the exposure.
6. Carry out appropriate health surveillance.
7. Prepare plans and procedures to deal with accidents, incidents and emergencies.
8. Ensure employees are properly informed, trained and supervised.

Risk Assessments

Risk assessment involves five steps:

1. Identify the hazards.
2. Decide who might be harmed and how.
3. Evaluate the risks and decide on precautions.
4. Record significant findings.
5. Review assessment and update if necessary.

Areas of work in the dispensary requiring risk assessment include:

- General medicines handling
- Handling cytotoxic drugs
- Spillage of medicines
- Manual handling (accessing high shelves, moving drug order, etc.)
- Trip hazards
- Waste disposal.

Risk assessments should be carried out for all of these tasks and reviewed annually. SOPs should be written detailing the required control methods, and all staff should be required to sign to acknowledge the SOPs have been read and understood.

When working with veterinary medicines there is a wide variation in risk. Many medicines can be classified as low- or medium-risk but others pose a very serious risk to health.

Low- and medium-risk substances

Risks associated with handling low- and medium-risk medicines can be adequately controlled by performing assessments by therapeutic group/type/route of administration. For example, the practice may produce standard methods for the control of exposure to:

- Injectable anaesthetics
- Inhalation anaesthetics
- Pour-on anthelmintics
- Steroidal compounds
- Vaccines
- Antibiotics
- Disinfectants.

Within these groups, practices must identify specific risks, such as penicillin allergy.

High-risk substances

Specific and detailed assessments, along with the resulting control methods, should be made for high-risk substances including:

- Cytotoxic drugs
- Tilmicosin (for use in cattle and sheep)
- Hormones
- Oil-based vaccines (e.g. Eravac inactivated vaccine against rabbit haemorrhagic disease type 2 virus (RHDV2) in injectable emulsion)
- Gluteraldehyde disinfectants
- Etorphine (large animal Immobilon).

Summary

In general, when handling medicines members of staff must:

- Treat all medicinal products as potentially harmful
- Be aware of the hazards associated with medicines and know the results of the COSHH and risk assessments
- Wear disposable gloves when handling any open or loose products
- Be familiar with the practice SOP for handling medicines and use additional protective clothing and equipment as and when specified
- Inform the Health and Safety Officer if they are or expect to become pregnant. In the case of pregnancy, be aware of and avoid handling teratogenic drugs (see *BSAVA Small Animal Formulary* for a listing) likely to harm the unborn child or drugs likely to cause miscarriage
- Inform the Health and Safety Officer if they experience any allergies or adverse effects thought to be caused or made worse by the handling of, or exposure to, VMPs
- Wash their hands after handling medicines, even if disposable gloves have been worn.

Summary of product characteristics

To perform risk assessments, employers require information on the safe use of medicines, chemicals and disinfectants. Manufacturers are no longer required to provide safety data-sheets for medicines. Instead, information on the safe use of each medicine can be found in the SPC. The VMD Product Information Database (www.vmd.defra.gov.uk/ProductInformationDatabase) has a full list of veterinary SPCs for:

- Currently authorized products
- Expired products
- Suspended products
- Registered homeopathic products
- Specified feed additives.

For non-veterinary authorized drugs (e.g. human prescription-only medicines) used under the Cascade, SPCs can be found on the electronic Medicines Compendium (eMC) website (www.medicines.org.uk/emc/).

Chemicals and disinfectants are required under the REACH Regulations 2007 to have a safety datasheet and appropriate warning symbols on the product packaging.

Calculation of drug doses
Weights, volumes and concentrations

The amount of active ingredient in a drug is expressed in terms of weight. Standard units for weight are kilogram (kg), gram (g), milligram (mg) and microgram (mcg or µg; although, it is good practice not to abbreviate the word micrograms).

- 1 kilogram = 1000 grams.
- 1 gram = 1000 milligrams.
- 1 milligram = 1000 micrograms.

Standard units for volume are litre (l) and millilitre (ml); where 1 litre = 1000 millilitres. The amount of active drug in liquid medicines can be expressed in milligrams per millilitre (mg/ml) or as a percentage (%) solution. Percentage solutions give the weight of a drug (w) per volume of liquid (v). If 1 g of drug is dissolved in 100 ml of liquid, this gives a 1% solution. This fact allows the easy conversion of any % w/v solution into mg/ml. For example, a 15% w/v solution contains 15 g in 100 ml, or 15,000 mg in 100 ml, or 150 mg in 1 ml (i.e. 150 mg/ml). It is important to use the correct units and to always convert weights into mg for calculating drug doses.

Exceptions to the rule

Some drugs, such as insulin, oxytocin and heparin, have strengths expressed in International Units (IU). The volume or mass that makes up one International Unit is dependent on the concentration or potency of the substance and, therefore, varies from substance to substance depending on what is being measured. Drugs that use International Units come in standard strengths (e.g. insulin comes in 40 IU/ml and 100 IU/ml).

Dosages

Doses are usually expressed in milligrams of drug per kilogram of bodyweight (mg/kg), although some drugs such as chemotherapy agents are dosed per square metre of body surface area. The following examples illustrate the basic principles of dosage calculations.

Example 1

An 18 kg dog requires potentiated amoxicillin at a dose rate of 12.5 mg combined actives per kg bodyweight twice daily. The patient should be dispensed enough tablets for a 7 day course. Potentiated amoxicillin is available in 500 mg tablets (containing 400 mg amoxicillin and 100 mg clavulanic acid), 250 mg tablets (containing 200 mg amoxicillin and 50 mg clavulanic acid) and 50 mg tablets (containing 40 mg amoxicillin and 10 mg clavulanic acid). The tablets may be halved for accurate dosing. What strength and quantity of tablets should be dispensed?

- Number of mg per dose is 18 (weight of patient) x 12.5 (dose rate) = 225 mg.
- Closest tablet size available is 250 mg.
- 7 days x 2 times daily dosing = 14 x 250 mg tablets.

→

Example 2

A 400 g bearded dragon requires a combined 25 mg/kg dose of trimethoprim/sulfamethoxazole once daily by mouth for 7 days. Using a paediatric suspension containing 200 mg sulfamethoxazole and 40 mg trimethoprim in 5 ml = 48 mg/ml. What volume should be dispensed?

- Weight of the bearded dragon is 400 g = 0.4 kg.
- Dose required per day is 25 x 0.4 = 10 mg/ml.
- The concentration of the suspension is 48 mg/ml (240/5).
- Volume in ml required per dose per day is calculated by dividing the dose in mg by the concentration of the suspension in mg/ml = 10/48 = 0.21 ml.
- Total volume required for 7 days is 0.21 x 7 = 1.47 ml.

Due to the amount of wastage caused by dispensing the medication into even the smallest bottle, the product should be dispensed to the owner in pre-drawn up syringes.

Example 3

A 16 kg dog requires buprenorphine for pain relief. The dose to be administered is 0.02 mg/kg and the preparation is available in a strength of 0.3 mg/ml. What volume should be administered?

- Total dose required in mg is 16 (bodyweight in kg) x 0.02 = 0.32 mg.
- The concentration of the preparation is 0.3 mg/ml.
- The volume required is the total dose required divided by the concentration = 0.32 divided by 0.3 = 1.07 ml.

Example 4

A 5 kg cat requires bupivacaine for a nerve block. The required dose is 0.1 mg/kg and the concentration available is 0.25% w/v. What volume needs to be drawn up?

- Total dose required in mg is 5 (bodyweight in kg) x 0.1 = 0.5 mg.
- A 0.25% w/v solution = 0.25 g in 100 ml = 250 mg in 100 ml = 2.5 mg/ml.
- The volume required is the total dose required divided by the concentration = 0.5 divided by 2.5 = 0.2 ml.

Example 5

A 20 kg dog is to be given furosemide by intravenous infusion at a dose rate of 5 mg/kg/h. The fluid rate required is 50 ml/h. How much of the 5% furosemide solution should be added to a 500 ml bag of fluids to give the correct dose?

- Dose required per hour is 20 (bodyweight in kg) x 5 = 100 mg/h.
- A 5% w/v solution of furosemide = 5 g in 100 ml = 5000 mg/100 ml = 50 mg/ml.
- The fluid rate required is 50 ml/h, so a 500 ml bag will last 10 hours.
- The patient requires 100 mg/h for 10 hours = 1000 mg total dose.
- The concentration of the furosemide solution is 50 mg/ml, so the volume required to be added to the bag is the total dose divided by the concentration = 1000 divided by 50 = 20 ml.

An alternative way of working this out is:

- Dose required per hour is 20 (bodyweight in kg) x 5 = 100 mg/h.
- A 5% w/v solution of furosemide = 5 g in 100 ml = 5000 mg/100 ml = 50 mg/ml.
- So, 50 ml of fluid needs to contain 100 mg of furosemide, which means a 2 mg/ml solution is required (i.e. 100 divided by 50).
- The amount of furosemide needed in the whole fluid bag = 2 mg x 500 (the volume of the fluid bag) = 1000 mg. The volume of furosemide to be added to the bag = dose required divided by the concentration = 1000 divided by 50 = 20 ml.

References and further reading

Girling SJ (2013) Veterinary Nursing of Exotic Pets, 2nd edn. Wiley-Blackwell, Chichester

Jambhekar S and Breer PJ (2012) Basic Pharmacokinetics, 2nd edn. Pharmaceutical Press, London

Kahn CM (2016) Merck Veterinary Manual, 11th edn. Merck and Company Inc., New Jersey

Marriott J, Wilson K, Langley CA and Belcher D (2010) Pharmaceutical Compounding and Dispensing, 2nd edn. Pharmaceutical Press, London

Meredith A (2015) BSAVA Small Animal Formulary, 9th edn: Part B – Exotic Pets. BSAVA Publication, Gloucester

Merton Boothe D (2001) Small Animal Clinical Pharmacology and Therapeutics. WB Saunders, Philadelphia

Nind F and Mosedale P (2019) BSAVA Guide to the Use of Veterinary Medicines. BSAVA Publications, Gloucester

Ramsey I (2017) BSAVA Small Animal Formulary, 9th edn: Part A – Canine and Feline. BSAVA Publications, Gloucester

Varga M, Lumbis R and Gott L (2012) BSAVA Manual of Exotic Pet and Wildlife Nursing. BSAVA Publications, Gloucester

Winfield A, Rees J and Smith I (2009) Pharmaceutical Practice, 4th edn. Churchill Livingstone, London

Useful websites

BSAVA Guide to the Use of Veterinary Medicines:
www.bsavalibrary.com/content/book/10.22233/9781905319862

Health and Safety Executive:
www.hse.gov.uk/

- **Control of Substances Hazardous to Health Regulations 2002:**
www.hse.gov.uk/coshh/index.htm

- **Registration, Evaluation, Authorisation and restriction of Chemicals (REACH):**
www.hse.gov.uk/reach/index.htm

- **Risk assessments:**
  www.hse.gov.uk/risk/index.htm
- **Suspected Adverse Reaction Surveillance Scheme (SARSS):**
  www.hse.gov.uk/foi/internalops/ocs/300-399/oc394_1.htm

National Office of Animal Health (NOAH) Compendium:
  www.noahcompendium.co.uk

Royal College of Veterinary Surgeons – Requirements for handling of controlled drugs and medicines:
  www.rcvs.org.uk/news-and-views/features/a-reminder-from-the-rcvs-and-vmd-of-the-requirements-for

Veterinary Medicines Directorate:
  www.gov.uk/government/organisations/veterinary-medicines-directorate
- **Guidance Notes:**
  www.gov.uk/government/collections/veterinary-medicines-guidance-notes-vmgns
- **Product Information Database:**
  www.vmd.defra.gov.uk/ProductInformationDatabase

Veterinary Medicines Regulations 2013:
  www.legislation.gov.uk/uksi/2013/2033/contents/made

Self-assessment questions

1. What do the letters ADME stand for in relation to pharmacokinetics?
2. What are the advantages of intravenous drug administration?
3. What is antimicrobial resistance?
4. What are the side effects of corticosteroid therapy?
5. Who should suspected adverse reactions be reported to?
6. What are the four legal categories of veterinary medicines?
7. Describe the steps of 'The Cascade'
8. Who can witness the destruction of Schedule 2 Controlled Drugs?
9. What factors affect the stability of medicines?
10. What are the five steps to risk assessment and how do they relate to medicines?

Chapter 9

Client communication and practice organization

Jill Macdonald

Learning objectives

After studying this chapter, readers will have the knowledge to:

- State the skills required for effective communication in veterinary practice when communicating with clients, colleagues and other professionals
- List the skills of verbal and non-verbal communication
- Specify the components of a formal interaction with a client, and how to apply a commonly used framework to interactions such as consultations
- Describe the skills needed for different interactions with clients, including managing difficult situations such as anger, grief, uncertainty and financial discussions
- Describe the key components and skills used during admission and discharge appointments, including obtaining informed consent
- Identify what makes an effective team and review processes to ensure that there is good team communication
- Describe what good customer service is
- Specify the skills required to market the practice and use social media
- Carry out the role of reception, including welcoming clients, telephone skills, making appointments and taking payments
- State the key legislation that applies to veterinary practice management

Principles of communication

Communication is of vital importance for the everyday effective functioning of veterinary practice, from receiving and conveying messages, to building and maintaining relationships with clients and colleagues in the veterinary team. Communication takes many forms, but the basic premise is that it is a two-way process whereby a message is sent, received and responded to. Communication is, of course, not all about verbal (spoken) communication. Much of the message received during communication involves non-verbal cues, and it is well known that whilst words are important, the non-verbal aspects of communication can affect the message considerably.

Verbal communication skills

Many consider verbal communication to include written communication, since this also uses words (or *verbatim*), but

for the purposes of this chapter, verbal communication is taken to refer to spoken or oral communication only, and written communication is addressed separately.

First, consider the verbal skills we use when communicating. Our choice of words is crucial, whether we are giving important information or helping a distressed client. Whilst day-to-day life in practice is ever-changing and no two days are the same, many of the interactions that we have with clients follow the same pattern and cover the same topics. Communication with clients takes practice and experience, and listening in on colleagues' consultations (with their consent) will help you to gather skills in this area and create a 'bank' of words and phrases that are appropriate at specific times, whilst also developing your own style.

Non-verbal communication

There are several aspects of non-verbal communication, including:

- Posture and body position ('body language')
- Eye contact

- Facial expressions
- Paralanguage
- Proxemics and haptics
- Appearance.

Posture and body position ('body language')

Effective communication is best achieved by demonstrating an open body posture and facing your client with appropriate eye contact. Try to avoid habits such as folded arms, crossed legs and turning sideways to the person you are talking to. There are three main barriers to an open posture in the practice environment – the consulting room table, the reception desk and the computer station. Standing behind an object closes down an open posture, and there are obvious disadvantages if you turn away from the client and focus on a computer. Aim to stand to one side of these physical barriers; it really does make a difference. When using the computer, tell your client what you are doing, so they know that you are still focused on them; for example, 'I'm just going to write up some notes on Bobby's record and then I'll take a look at him – is that OK?'

Eye contact

Eye contact is a component of body language; it is important to maintain 'appropriate' eye contact, ensuring that the other person knows you are engaging with them, but without it becoming uncomfortable. It is also important that you maintain contact even when the person who is talking looks away, as when they look back to you, they will be seeking eye contact, and if it is not there, it may seem as if you were not listening. Staring and blinking are important non-verbal behaviours. If a person encounters another person or things they like, the rate of blinking increases and pupils dilate. The way a person looks at another person can indicate a range of emotions including interest, attraction and hostility. Eye contact can be a challenge for some people, and it is important to practise this skill.

Facial expression

Facial expressions can change the message we convey considerably and, whilst sometimes difficult to control (especially if surprised, shocked or upset), it is important to be aware of our expressions. It is important to be open and friendly to our clients, and a relaxed, smiling welcome will stand you in good stead when greeting a client. Expressions must be appropriate to the situation, for example, conveying concern when the client is telling you about something that is worrying them. A simple smile can indicate our approval of a message, while a scowl might signal disagreement. Understanding facial expressions and their meaning is an important part of communication with clients.

Paralanguage

Paralanguage relates to the aspects of speech outside the words themselves. How we say things has an impact on the message conveyed, so it is important to be aware of tone and volume of voice, speed of speech, clarity, intonation and emphasis on certain words. Whilst it may feel uncomfortable, it can be really helpful to record interactions with others (with their consent) and listen back to this at a later time. Very often the way we think we sound or come across is not necessarily what the other person hears. Managing tone

and pace can be especially challenging when under pressure, and practising these skills is vital to enable you to become a confident communicator even under difficult circumstances. Paralanguage also includes 'non-lexical' aspects that we add to speech, including marks of encouragement such as 'ah', 'hmmm' and 'uh-huh', which can be useful when encouraging someone to keep speaking. This is also an important component of 'listening skills' (see below).

Proxemics and haptics

Proxemics and haptics relate to the proximity to a person and touch, respectively. They should be tailored depending on your own style and what you are comfortable with, as well as the client's preference, and may also be related to factors such as culture. Most people have 'personal space' parameters and it is important to 'read' the client's response to you; for example, if the client is trying to move away from you then you are too close, so move back a little. A typical amount of space to have between you and another person during a casual conversation is about 0.5 to 1 m, compared with the distance when speaking to a crowd of people that you do not know, which is about 3 m.

Touch can be used to communicate affection, familiarity, sympathy and other emotions. Touch is a contentious subject and many say that we should never touch clients in a clinical environment; however, if touch is part of your communication style, it may just come naturally and feel 'right', especially with a client who is worried or upset. It is important to be aware that touch may not always be appropriate and that some clients will not respond well to being touched. There may also be important cultural issues around touch that need to be understood.

Appearance

The choice of colour, what someone wears, their hairstyle and other factors can affect appearance and are considered a means of non-verbal communication. The wearing of a uniform or a white coat can affect physiological reactions, judgements and interpretations. Colours are also recognized as evoking different moods.

> ### Exercise
>
> Ask a colleague to come into a few consultations with you and take notes on your non-verbal skills (e.g. facial expressions, body language, and vocal tone and pace). Ask them to provide feedback after the consultation about your non-verbal communication. This exercise can also be performed in reverse so that you can offer mutual feedback

Communicating with clients

Our communication skills directly affect the client experience in the practice, from the moment they enter reception (or even from when they call to make an appointment) to the moment they leave the practice. When considering communication with clients, empathy is especially pertinent. Many of us are animal owners ourselves, and appreciate the emotion that is synonymous with pet ownership. Whilst the human–animal bond felt by different clients will vary, most clients usually have an emotional attachment to their pet and will be worried about their healthcare, alongside other pressures such as financial worries and potential difficulties in understanding their pet's condition.

Using a consultation framework

In more formal interactions with clients, it is extremely useful to have a standard 'framework' to refer to, and for many years it has been the Calgary-Cambridge model (Munson and Willcox, 2013) (adapted for veterinary use) that has been used to teach, evaluate and practise veterinary communication skills (Figure 9.1), although other frameworks are available. This framework can be used for any interaction with a client (including telephone calls) but here it is discussed in terms of a consultation or clinic. The most common underlying cause for a client complaint is poor communication.

Preparation

Good preparation is essential in order to provide a professional and safe service, and may include:

- **The environment:** ensuring the clinical area is clean, tidy, safe and private
- **Patient history:** checking the patient details, name, sex and previous history, including notes of any adverse reactions (to drugs or veterinary staff!)
- **Equipment:** ensuring you have the necessary equipment, paperwork and drugs ready will show good organization skills and also help with time management
- **Self:**
  - Appearance: veterinary nurses should be smartly and professionally presented (it is important to have spare practice uniforms available)
  - Emotions: sometimes it can be difficult to smile when faced with the challenges of everyday practice, but it is important to put previous consultations or upsetting experiences behind you and re-focus afresh for each client.

Opening the consultation

Having a clear and professional opening to a consultation will set the scene for the rest of that interaction. Several components should be used, including a warm and friendly facial expression, a clear greeting (to the client and the animal) and an introduction if you have not met the client previously. It is important to establish a rapport. Introducing yourself may feel awkward at first, but it is important that the client knows who you are and what your role is. A good

Preparation
- Establish context
- Create a professional, safe and effective environment

Initiating the consultation
- Preparation
- Establish initial rapport with client and animal
- Identify the reason(s) for the consultation

Gathering information
- Explore the client's presenting complaint(s) to discover:
  – the clinical perspective (disease – short-term history)
  – the client's perspective (include animal's purpose)
  – essential background information (long-term history)

Physical examination

Explanation and planning
- Provide the appropriate amount and type of information
- Aid accurate understanding and recall
- Achieve a shared understanding: incorporate the client's perspective
- Plan: appropriate shared decision-making

Closing the consultation
- Summarize
- Forward planning

OBSERVATION

Providing structure to the consultation
- Make organization overt
- Attend to flow

Building the relationship with the client
- Non-verbal behaviour
- Develop rapport
- Involve the client
- Involve the animal(s)

9.1 A guide to the veterinary consultation based on the Calgary-Cambridge model (Munson and Wilcox, 2013).

example would be 'I don't think we've met before – my name is Jill and I'm one of the veterinary nurses and I'll be giving Bobby his second vaccination today – is that OK?' Some brief 'chatter' can help build a rapport with the client and put them at ease, even if it is something as simple as a comment on the weather (the classic British conversation opener!) or complimenting them on how well their pet looks. The consultation should start off with an open question such as 'How are things with Bobby?' This gives the client a chance to provide general information and, depending on the client, can yield some very useful details. It is important to allow the client to speak and not interrupt them.

Gathering information (taking a history)

Effective history-taking will enable us to get the most detailed and accurate picture of a pet's problem and background possible, and is vital in identifying problems and working out how to progress (see Chapter 10). Asking open questions, effective listening and using questions effectively to gather more precise information are the main skills used during history-taking. An open question, such as 'So, tell me, how has Bobby been doing since I last saw you?' will give the client an opportunity to offer plenty of information. Effective listening and using techniques such as reflecting back information the client has given in order to clarify or offering a summary to check back with the client that you have the information right, will help you obtain accurate information whilst helping to build a relationship with the client. By adapting the two frameworks (i.e. the disease framework (biomedical perspective) and the illness framework (client's perspective)), effective history-taking with shared understanding and decision-making will take place.

Types of questions

Open questions

Questions without a definite or simple answer (e.g. 'How are things with Treacle?'). They encourage the client to open up and offer more information.

Closed questions

Questions that have a specific answer (e.g. 'How many times has she vomited?'). They help us to focus in on specific information.

The open—closed funnel

This technique is used when moving from open questions (to gather overall information) to closed questions (to gather more specific information). Open questioning can be returned to at any time.

Listening skills

Attentive listening requires four main components – time to respond, facilitative responses (mirroring, nodding, eye contact), non-verbal skills, and picking up on verbal and non-verbal cues.

- Maintaining appropriate eye contact.
- Appropriate facial expression (e.g. smiling if the client is telling you good news).
- Body language (open and receptive, nodding).
- Paralanguage ('hmmm', 'ah', 'uh-huh'). →

Listening skills *continued*

- Resisting interruptions and allowing silence when needed. If there is a pause, do not jump in – let your client fill the space.
- Reflective statements (e.g. 'So you were saying that you think Bobby has lost weight and seems a little less bright than normal, so let's just find out more about that.').
- Summarizing – giving a quick summary of recent information. This shows that you have been listening, helps you to bring together the information, helps the client to consider if there is anything they want to add and helps you think of anything extra you need to know.

Physical examination

Examination of the animal may begin whilst you are still gathering the history or can wait until the history has been taken: there are advantages and disadvantages to both approaches. If time permits, then it usually works better to finish taking a history before beginning to examine the patient, so that you can give each element your full attention. It is important to 'signpost' this stage, for example, 'OK, so I'm just going to give Bobby a little check over now – do you think he'd feel more relaxed on the table or on the floor?' The client can also be included and engaged in the examination by, for example, letting them feel a lump you have found or showing them how clean their pet's ears are.

Giving information, explaining and planning

We should always aim to achieve client concordance (see 'Compliance *versus* concordance', below) in order for treatment plans to be successful, and this will largely be affected by how we present information, how well it is understood and whether we have involved the client in the treatment decision and plan. This is the premise behind the positive effect that good communication has on clinical outcome. Without concordance, and therefore adherence to the plan, the treatment is meaningless. When giving information to clients it is important to ensure that:

- Information is clear and succinct, and offered in an appropriate order
- We do not give too much information at once and that we break this down into sections and try to ensure that each piece of information is understood
- Information is pitched at the correct level for the client (including using or avoiding terminology or scientific terms depending on the knowledge and/or experience of the client)
- We use appropriate tools to aid understanding (such as diagrams, models or demonstrations)
- We incorporate 'shared decision-making' into our approach (see below), if appropriate for the situation and client
- We motivate the client as much as we can to want to comply with the treatment or programme
- We respect and take into account the client's cultural and socio-economic status.

Closing the consultation

A professional closure to the consultation is as important as the opening, and a final summary of the discussion and plan should be offered. We should always check that there are no further concerns, and if we have been thorough then we should ameliorate any last minute comments such as 'Oh, there was something else – he has itchy ears!' The client should always be asked whether they have any final questions.

Safety netting

This involves providing the client with an idea of what to expect and clear guidance on what to do if anything unexpected occurs. For example, if we have provided a weight loss diet, then during the consultation we should have explained in what quantity this should be fed, aligned with the client's wishes (such as providing food in a feeding toy) and discussed any side effects (such as increased faecal output). Safety netting may look something like 'So let's see how he does on the new food, and if you have any worries at all, or if you're not happy with the food, then just give me a call straight away.'

Follow-up

There should always be some follow-on from any consultation; for example, an appointment in 3 weeks, a phone call to check progress or the annual booster in 3 months. We should try to ensure that any recommendations are followed through. It can sometimes help to 'walk' the client to the reception desk, so that you can relay the message to the receptionist; this interaction should have a supportive and friendly feel to it (rather than being pressured). You could consider designing some 'recommendation cards' that

outline the 'next step', so that the client has this information to take away, and the next appointment details could be added to this card.

Building a relationship with the client

Creating trust between you and your client is a vital skill that will help you to consult more effectively, achieve client concordance and adherence to treatment plans (and therefore improved clinical outcomes and patient welfare) and feel a heightened sense of satisfaction from your client interactions. Clients often come to highly value the relationship that they have with veterinary nurses at the practice, and there are many skills and activities that can contribute to building this relationship. Clients (and their pets) will sense and appreciate you being genuinely interested in your patients (Figure 9.2). Showing we care, for example, by greeting the pet on arrival, by asking open questions such as 'How is Bobby doing?' and showing empathy for any concerns, will go a long way. As mentioned previously, body language (including eye contact) can markedly affect communication and rapport.

Client perspective

It is important that we always consider the client's perspective, and this includes understanding the relationship between the client and their pet (e.g. whether it is a working dog that lives outside, a show animal, or their only remaining link with a deceased relative), as this relationship (the human–animal bond) may have an impact on treatment decisions. For example, assistance dogs (such as guide dogs or animals that help children or adults with mental or physical disabilities) can be of enormous value to their owners and this should be considered when discussing management options and recovery times. It is also important to ask what the client thinks may be wrong with their pet; this can offer really insightful information. The client knows their pet better than you, and they may have noticed something that is significant. Owners may have taken the trouble to research the problem themselves, and this should be commended rather than seen as a 'threat'. Culture and religion may also have an impact on both how we interact with the client and on treatment, and it is important to be aware and respectful of any cultural or religious beliefs and ethics.

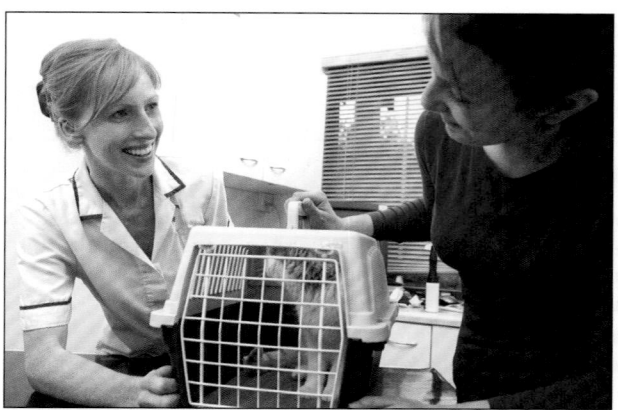

9.2 Clients appreciate veterinary staff showing a genuine interest in their pets. (Monkey Business Images/Shutterstock.com)

Shared decision-making

Shared decision-making (SDM) is a phrase used to describe the process whereby medical professionals seek the opinions, goals and wishes of their patients/clients and work with them to try and achieve these goals. It is important with SDM to ensure that treatment options are fully explored, along with risks and benefits, the choices available and that decision-making is reached together with the client and the veterinary professional. Compared with the rather 'old fashioned' paternalistic (or directive) approach, where it is assumed that clients simply want to be 'told' what to do (since we are the experts), you can see how SDM may help to build relationships more effectively. However, some clients still prefer a more directive style, so it is important to gauge this, or even ask the client what they would prefer.

An example of SDM in action might be something along the lines of: 'So, I wanted to talk to you about flea control. Let's just look at what Bobby does on a day-to-day basis, where you go with him, that sort of thing, how easy you find it to use different treatments, and then we can both take a look at what we have available and decide on the best option for you – how does that sound?' A directive approach may look more like: 'I know you said you take Bobby to Wales sometimes, so I'm going to ask the vet to prescribe some treatment that is effective against ticks, as this is important.'

Mirroring

It has been shown that 'mirroring' another person's body language and choice of words can help to demonstrate assent. This often occurs naturally, for example, if you are talking to someone you respect, you will probably inadvertently copy their body language. We can use this technique with language with clients; for example, if they use a phrase, then we can use the same phrase to show that we are 'on the same level'.

Empathy

Empathy is a key aspect of effective communication. It can be defined as being able to 'put yourself in another's position', or imagine what a situation is like for another person and appreciate the difficulties that this may bring them. You are then able to adapt your communication to what will be the most effective for the interaction. It is important to understand that empathy is not in any way saying you 'know how they feel', as you will probably not. Empathy does not only have to be reserved for clients who are emotionally distraught, but can be used at a 'low level' for many situations. It serves to show that you are approachable, caring and considerate of the client's and animal's needs and fears. Empathic statements are a useful way of demonstrating this, but it is important that they are natural, so as with many aspects of communication this is a skill that should be practised. For example, say Fluffy has come in for a nail clip, we may consider this a routine appointment, but the client may be worried due to a previous experience or one that has been relayed to them. They may say that 'she hates having her nails clipped' and this is a 'cue' from the client that there is a level of anxiety. We could respond by saying 'Oh, poor Fluffy; well let's see if we can do this as easily as possible so we don't stress her. What do you think will work best?' This is a good example of an empathic statement, alongside gaining the client's perspective and opening up shared decision-making. Tune into the emotional cues. Listen well, and also pay attention to non-verbal communication, picking up subtle cues almost subconsciously. Show sensitivity,

and understand others' perspectives. Veterinary nurses with this skill respect and relate well to everyone, regardless of their background.

Empathy

The ability to 'put yourself in another person's situation' and imagine how they may feel (Figure 9.3). Demonstrating empathy may include:

- Body language – open, welcoming, leaning in to the client, eye contact, (touch?)
- Facial expression and gestures (e.g. cocking head to one side, putting hand out to client)
- Soft tone and slower pace of speech
- Empathic statements (e.g. 'I can see you're really upset')
- Listening without interruption and leaving pauses
- The location or time when you communicate.

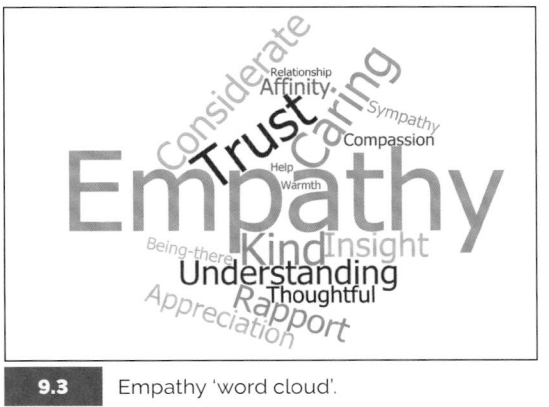

9.3 Empathy 'word cloud'.

Non-verbal 'cues'

It is important to pick up on the client's (and patient's) cues and respond to them. A client may be feeling distressed and demonstrate this in their facial expressions, body language and what they are saying. Listening to your client and responding to them can help build your client's confidence and trust in you. Empathic communication is not just adapting your language; it is considering all of the variables for what happens when you send a message.

Low stress handling

Patient handling is covered in Chapter 11; however, it is important to note that using techniques that are as stress-free as possible will promote patient welfare. This will also communicate to the client that we want their pet to have as good an experience in the clinic as possible, helping considerably with our client relationships. For example, clients will often say 'I want to see (a particular staff member) next time, as s/he was really gentle with Fluffy', but are less likely to ask to see the veterinary surgeon or nurse who used forceful restraint whilst struggling to administer an injection.

Motivational interviewing

This is a technique that involves finding a client's motivation for wanting to make a change in their pet's healthcare, and is especially useful for situations such as a weight management clinic. Rather than *telling* ➜

the client that their pet is overweight, we can try to explore the motivations that may exist within the client (e.g. getting the pet back to their original health and activity levels, being able to go on long walks or jump on to the bed without effort again). We can use open questions such as 'Have you seen any changes in Max?' and look for cues from the client for the changes they wish to make. Once these motivators have been established, we can then use shared decision-making to work out a plan together

Breaking bad news

Sometimes we will be called upon to break bad news to a client, and this is never easy. Empathy is key in this situation. It is important to offer a 'warning shot' to help prepare clients and this can be something as simple as 'I'm sorry, I'm afraid I have some bad news for you.' Try to be as concise as you can, without being blunt. The use of pauses and silences are very important as they give the client time to think and collect themselves, and they demonstrate that you are giving them time to do this. Try and ensure that you have a chair for the client to sit on and a box of tissues to hand.

Supporting clients through euthanasia

Euthanasia of a pet can be a very difficult time in a person's life, and people experience the same grieving process for animals as they do for fellow humans (Figure 9.4). The responsibility is enormous. These are the last moments that this person will spend with their pet, and ensuring that it is handled as thoughtfully as possible is paramount. The emotion is also somewhat heightened because the decision has been made by the client to end their pet's life, adding a stronger component of guilt, uncertainty and distress. There are many reasons why euthanasia may be elected, from not being able to afford treatment to alleviating suffering of a terminally ill pet, and emotions will vary depending

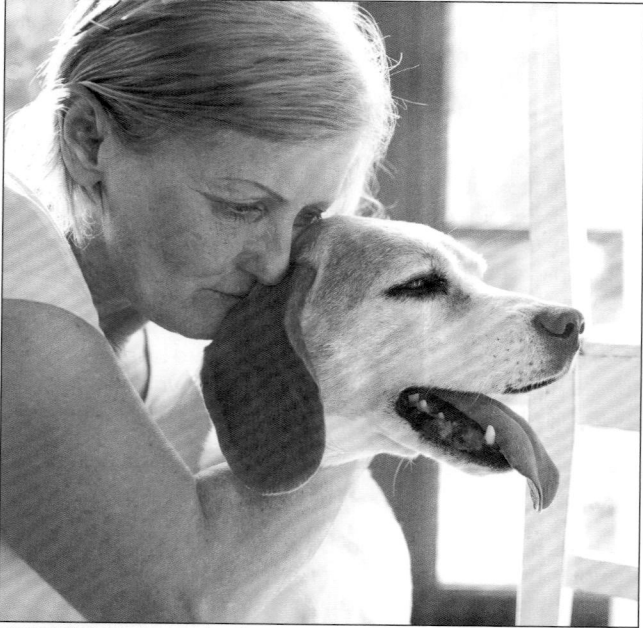

Euthanasia of a pet can be a very difficult time in a person's life. (Halfpoint/Shutterstock.com)

on the client, their relationship with the pet, and the illness that has resulted in this decision. They may be feeling angry and resentful, especially when finance is the major factor. They may feel guilt; they may even feel relieved if the pet has been suffering, and this in turn can lead to guilt. Bereavement is a very complex psychological process, and beyond the remit of those in the profession to understand fully without specific training; however, it can help to appreciate the different emotions that clients may experience. The client may not display their emotions outwardly, or may mask them (e.g. by appearing indifferent when in fact they are falling apart inside), and empathy is absolutely the key in every euthanasia appointment, whatever the client's 'cues' are telling you.

It is important to afford the client privacy, respect and as much time as needed, and these appointments should be scheduled at the end of surgery and clients allowed to wait in a private room with their pet. It can help to just talk to the client if they seem to want to – let them tell you about their pet, the worries that they have had, and the happy times too. Make sure that there are tissues available and a chair for the client to sit on.

It is vital that the procedure has been explained clearly to the client, so they know what to expect. This includes:

- Who will perform the procedure
- How the drug is administered
- How long it takes for the pet to pass away
- What to expect following the procedure
- That the animal will not be aware or suffer any pain
- That they can stay with their pet before, during and after the procedure
- That they do not need to be present for the procedure, but can see their pet afterwards, if preferred
- What happens afterwards and the options available.

Many practices now offer a 'pre-euthanasia appointment' to explain the process and discuss options, so that when the animal is brought in for the procedure, the client is able to dedicate their attention fully towards their pet.

Safety should be observed at all times and this may include appropriate handling of a fearful animal (with sedation if necessary), ensuring that the euthanasia drug does not pose a risk to handlers or the owner (placement of an intravenous catheter is useful both for safety and in reducing stress in the animal), and correct disposal of the animal's body (see Chapter 2). Some owners may prefer to bury their pet at home and appropriate advice should be given if this is the case, but most owners use the cremation services offered through the practice. The two main options are a 'communal cremation' (where several animals are cremated together) and a 'private cremation' (where animals are individually cremated and the ashes can be returned to the owner); most crematoriums now also offer other options such as a choice of scatter tubes or caskets.

Payment for euthanasia

The payment aspects of euthanasia must be handled sensitively. If the client is not known to the practice, and depending on practice policy, it is usual to take the payment beforehand when the client first arrives. It challenges us with a harsh emotional contrast between not wanting to upset the client and understanding that services must be paid for. If the client is distraught and alone, it is helpful to offer to call a relative or friend, and dissuade them from driving or walking out of the practice alone.

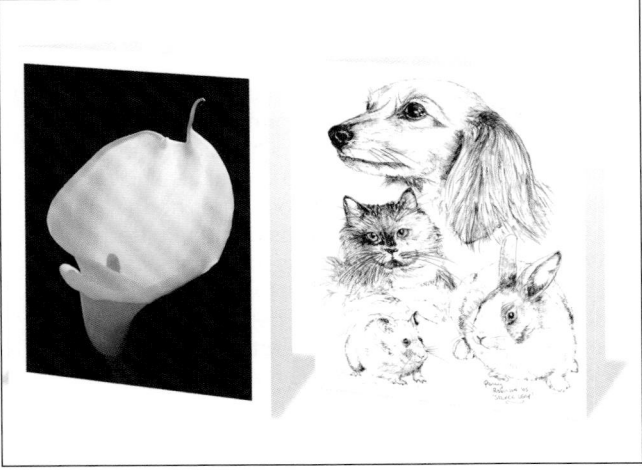

9.5 PetSavers sympathy cards.

Sending a practice sympathy card (Figure 9.5) is a thoughtful touch and many clients are very grateful for this gesture. It can help if the card is personalized (e.g. with a memory of the pet held by the practice). Practices often have books or 'walls' of remembrance where clients can write something or display a photograph of their pet. Other keepsakes include pendants containing a pet's ashes or a mould of the pet's paw print.

Support services

Whilst it is vital that practice staff support clients through euthanasia, it is as important that they are able to recognize when the needs of the client are beyond the scope of staff expertise; for example, if the client is very distressed or is unable to come to terms with the loss of their pet after some time. There are support services available such as the Samaritans and Blue Cross (the latter of whom provide a pet bereavement support service), and it may be appropriate to offer all clients this information so that they can seek help if they need it. It is also really important that practice staff are supported, as the strain of supporting owners can present a heavy emotional burden; staff wellbeing is considered briefly later in the chapter and in Chapter 1.

Key points for euthanasia appointments

- Offer privacy, respect and time
- Empathy, and the ability to demonstrate empathy, is vital in helping clients to feel supported
- Explain the procedure so that they know what to expect
- Discuss any options clearly and slowly
- Provide support before, during and after the procedure
- Offer follow-on support, such as a sympathy card and telephone call
- Know when to signpost to additional help
- Consider offering pre-euthanasia ('end of life') appointments
- Discuss with the owner the impact that may be felt by other animal companions in the family. They may have been closely bonded with the animal who has died. It may be considered helpful to provide the opportunity to see and smell the deceased companion's body

---

Admission and discharge procedures

The responsibility for admitting and discharging animals for procedures is often delegated to the veterinary nurse. Both situations demand accuracy, competence and the skills for helping clients who may be emotional, worried or have a lot of questions. It is important to understand your limitations and be prepared to obtain assistance from a colleague if required.

Admission procedure

For admission procedures, it may be useful to follow a consultation structure. This may include the following key points:

- General points
  - Signpost the order in which the admission process will be carried out – this will help the client feel informed and less anxious
  - Remember clients will probably be worried – empathy is a key aspect in admitting a patient
- Preparation
  - Check patient history
  - Prepare admission form
  - Prepare inpatient sheet if used in the practice
- Gathering information
  - Confirm client's identity (or if they are an agent)
  - Confirm animal's identity (use identity tag if practice policy)
  - Confirm client contact details, including contact number for throughout the duration of the pet's stay
  - Check that the feeding/watering guidelines have been followed
  - If patient is on medication, confirm when last dose was given
  - Check patient's current clinical condition with the client: if the animal is being admitted for an elective procedure, check that the patient is well; if non-elective, check whether the patient has improved or become worse
  - Confirm procedure to be performed and double check this with patient history
  - Confirm vaccination status
- Physical examination
  - Perform a clinical examination (if this is practice protocol) or explain when this will be carried out
- Giving information
  - Explain procedure and obtain informed consent. A consent form needs to be signed by a person over 18 years of age
  - Confirm costs of procedure and payment method
  - Note/label any patient possessions
  - Obtain client's signature on the consent form
  - Provide contact details
- Planning and closure
  - Advise the client on the next steps in terms of the patient, when to contact for progress and when the patient can be collected.

Informed consent

Informed consent involves gaining permission from the client to perform procedures on or administer treatments to their pet, whilst ensuring that the client understands the procedure that their pet will be undergoing, any risks involved (including any possible postoperative complications) and the aftercare that will be required.

- Informed consent for the procedure and the financial 'contract' are two distinct aspects and should be discussed separately.
- Someone over 16 years old can give consent for their pet's treatment; however, they must be over 18 to enter into a financial contract. Where the person seeking veterinary services is 16 or 17 years of age the veterinary surgeon should, depending on the extent of the treatment, the likely costs involved and the welfare implications for the animal, consider whether consent should be sought from parents or guardians before the work is undertaken.
- The procedure should be explained in detail and the terminology should be geared towards the client. For example, if you are speaking to a GP, then using 'glucose curve' may be appropriate; if not, then saying 'taking blood samples to check the glucose (or sugar levels) throughout the day' may be more appropriate.
- It is important to be overt about words such as 'castrate' or 'spay', making it clear what that surgery entails, and that it means the pet cannot be used for breeding after this point.
- The admission form should also reflect this language and not contain any acronyms such as 'GA' or 'IVFT', or practice code such as 'Dental 3'.
- If there are optional aspects, such as pre-anaesthetic blood tests, then these options, and their benefits and risks, should be discussed. It is usually the remit of the veterinary surgeon to discuss more complex options such as whether to choose medical or surgical intervention, but more experienced veterinary nurses will also need to be competent in handling these discussions.
- Any risks associated with the anaesthesia and surgery, as well as possible postoperative complications, should be clearly stated, and the worst case scenario should be offered, but without over-worrying the client. The worst case scenario under anaesthesia (or sedation) is death, and the client has the right to know that whilst very unlikely, there is still a very small risk. Even procedures such as blood sampling carry some risk. Postoperative complications, even for routine procedures such as an ovariohysterectomy, can be quite significant, so it is important that these are highlighted.
- Avoid coercion – if the client seems unsure or unhappy about the procedure, then pause the admission procedure, find out what is troubling them, and seek help from a colleague if necessary.
- Make sure any special requests, if plausible, are noted on the record and communicated to other staff. For example, the client may want a particular veterinary surgeon or nurse to deal with their pet.
- Clients must have the 'capacity' to give informed consent – if they are under the influence of alcohol or drugs, in emotional distress, have mental health challenges or have a disability that may affect their ability to give consent, then an 'agent' on their behalf may need to be called upon such as a family member or translator and/or you may need to seek advice from a colleague.

- Any conversations or important points must always be noted on the patient or client record, and also on the admission documents, if appropriate.
- Whilst it is important to obtain the client's signature, the overriding factor is that informed consent has been obtained rather than the signature itself.
- Consent can also be obtained verbally (e.g. over the telephone) when extra procedures need to be performed after the animal has been admitted.
- Where it appears a client lacks the mental capacity to consent, the RCVS Code of Professional Conduct advises that one should try to determine whether someone is legally entitled to act on that person's behalf, such as someone who may act under an enduring power of attorney. If not, staff should act in the best interests of the animal and seek to obtain consent from someone close to the client, such as a family member who is willing to provide consent on behalf of the person (RCVS, 2018).

For further information on consent, the reader is referred to Chapter 1 and the *BSAVA Guide to the Use of Veterinary Medicines* (www.bsavalibrary.com/content/book/10.22233/9781905319862).

Discharge appointments

As with admission procedures, it can help to follow a consultation structure when discharging pets. Whilst the elements of 'gathering information' will not really apply, except to confirm the identity of the client, all other aspects may be relevant, including:

- Preparation
  - Ensure you are clear about the procedure that the pet has undergone, any complications that have occurred and any prior communication with the client from colleagues
- Gathering information
  - Check that the client pairs with the patient you are about to discharge
- Physical examination
  - Depending on practice policy, the patient will need to be checked to ensure that they are ready for discharge. Sometimes it can help to show the client wounds or other areas of treatment, so they can ask questions whilst still in the practice; although, it is always best to not return the patient to the owner until after you have given them important information, so that they are not (understandably) distracted by their pet's presence
- Giving information
  - This is the key component of the discharge appointment and many of the tips covered in the giving information, explaining and planning section of the consultation framework (see above) can be used. Breaking down information and gauging understanding are paramount. It is imperative to also give the client some written information (such as a homecare plan) to take away with them and refer to, as they may not remember all that you have said
  - Safety netting is paramount with the discharge appointment, so that if there are any problems, the client contacts the practice straight away. Out-of-hours contact details should also be provided.

Written communication

There are many situations which involve the use of written communication, including:

- Writing up clinical notes (see section on 'Clinical records', below)
- Letters to clients (e.g. inviting them to an event or clinic, or advising of an outstanding debt)
- Emails to clients and colleagues
- Official documentation such as laboratory submission forms, insurance claim forms, admission/discharge forms and vaccine records
- In-house forms such as hospitalization sheets, patient handover sheets and anaesthetic monitoring charts
- Flyers, handouts and other promotional or supporting material
- Notes and memos (e.g. on a notice board or sticky notes).

Some key points should be observed:

- Any form of written communication from the practice should be on headed paper, preferably printed rather than handwritten, and signed/clearly annotated with the individual's name and role in the practice
- Emails should be written with the same care and thought as letters, with correct use of grammar and punctuation
- Vaccine cards, laboratory submission/insurance claim/admission/discharge forms, hospitalization sheets, anaesthetic monitoring charts and any other form of documentation should be fully, accurately and legibly completed (see Chapters 14, 15, 17 and 21)
- Written communication with colleagues should be professional, considered and thoughtful, and disputes should never be carried out by email, text, memos or social media
- Flyers and other promotional materials produced by the practice should be well considered, involve input from different members of the team and be proofread before printing.

Discussing finances

In veterinary medicine we are often faced with the challenge of balancing best veterinary care with the financial scope and preferences of the client. Several aspects can help us to manage this situation effectively and tactfully.

- Discuss options and their associated costs openly. Be overt about any costs that may not be obvious (e.g. long-term diets).
- Break down costs and provide a written estimate for each option (see below).
- Never 'X-ray clients' pockets' and judge their ability or inability to pay for a certain level of care. All options should always be given and the relative costs clearly communicated.
- When there is a problem with a client's ability to pay (either prior to treatment or at time of discharge), there are two overriding factors to consider:
  1. This is a difficult emotional situation for the client, and empathy and understanding are vital.
  2. The practice can only survive as a business if debt is managed well.

- These two factors clearly have a high level of conflict, and it is important that veterinary staff are clear on practice finance policy and know which colleague to go to for help and advice should an issue arise.

Financial estimates

It can help clients considerably if the costs associated with the different options are written down, so that they can digest the information in their own time and discuss the options with other family members, rather than having to make an on-the-spot decision. This can be done using estimate forms generated by practice software. It is important to go through the estimate with the client, explaining what each of the options and costs are, and to record the estimate on the clinical notes. It is important to make a distinction between a 'quote' (an exact figure) and an 'estimate' (a guideline figure). We should only ever aim to offer estimates since the actual requirements will change depending on the (sometimes unforeseen) circumstances.

Pet insurance

Many clients now have health insurance for their pets and this information must be noted on the clinical records, including the policy information (and any exclusions) and if a 'direct claim' is permitted. Whilst insurance means that treatment options may be more affordable, it is important that when having conversations with clients of insured and uninsured pets that the same treatment options are offered and discussed and that the pricing structure is identical (see Chapter 1).

Insurance policies can be complicated and confusing to clients, and whilst the client's policy is a contract between them and their insurance company, it is useful to have a general understanding of how policies function, what exclusions and excesses apply and what may not be covered by pet insurance. Veterinary staff should also be aware of a system called the 'Referral Vet Network' where certain insurance policies' underwriters have created a list of referral practices where, in a non-emergency, clients are encouraged to take their pets. Should clients choose a referral practice that is not on this list, an extra fee may be incurred.

Seeking charity assistance for clients

There are certain situations where the client simply does not have the ability to pay due to their economic status, and seeking charity assistance is required. There are usually two routes for this:

1. Referring the patient to the charity and the charity taking over the case and administering treatment.
2. Referring the costs to the charity and the original practice providing treatment and then invoicing the charity.

There are certain criteria that have to be met in order for charities to agree to treatment, such as benefit status of the client, and it is important that this is handled sensitively. It can help to have a print out of the charity's requirements so that you and the client can work through this together and ascertain whether the client qualifies for support. Many of the charities will only provide veterinary services to pets where the owner is on certain means tested benefits (e.g. housing benefit, income support, pension credit, council tax benefit, working tax credit, job seekers allowance, child tax credit or universal credit).

Referral to a specialist or paraprofessional services

When animals are referred to specialist services, it is often the duty of the veterinary nurse to communicate the necessary information to enable continuity of care and so that the other parties have accurate and up-to-date clinical records. It is important to establish exactlywhat information is needed (this may include clinical notes, results of diagnostic tests and imaging, and client information) and in what format this information is required. It is now more common to send information via email, so it is vital that the email address you have is correct in order to protect data. Sometimes X-rays (if not digital) need to be sent by post or with the client, and these must be clearly identifiable. It is good practice to call the other party to ensure that the information has been received. Remember that whenever you are dealing with a referral centre or other service, you are responsible for the impression you give of your practice to the 'outside world'.

Clients can often be very worried or stressed when their pet is referred, since it usually means that the pet's condition is serious or more complicated. They will also be going to a strange practice or premises, often having to travel some distance, dealing with professionals that they do not know, and liable to pay much higher costs than in first-opinion practice, so it is important to be understanding and to explain as much of the process to the client as you can. It can really make a difference to offer support with things such as making sure they have the centre's address and telephone number, that they know who the consultant is that they will be seeing, and helping them to make the appointment.

Communicating with colleagues

Effective and professional communication within the team and with other professionals is an important component to the effective, safe and enjoyable running of a practice or veterinary environment.

Examples

Examples of colleague communication include:

- Verbal (spoken) – during every day work to communicate patient's needs and status, client information and practice information. Includes use of in-house telephone system
- During meetings or discussions
- During emergency situations, where quick relay of information is required
- On a one-to-one basis
- When referring patients (e.g. to an out-of-hours clinic or specialist referral centre)
- Written – in the form of clinical notes on patient care sheets (see Chapter 14) and on clinical records
- Patient handover – to ensure that the next person caring for the patient has all the necessary information (verbal and written)
- In emails, memos and via social media.

Patient safety and client service are paramount, and these can only be achieved by veterinary colleagues communicating at the correct level and with the right information. Teamwork is the cornerstone of successful practices and involves the desire and ability of a team to exhibit cohesive and respectful communication with each other at all times.

Staff wellbeing

We should always be mindful of the emotional, mental and sometimes physical strain that can be experienced by veterinary professionals (Figure 9.6). Supporting clients through euthanasia, difficult decision-making in situations where the stakes are high, uncertainty, long working hours, increasing client demands, and the tendency historically for professionals to function in a rather isolated manner are all components that affect staff wellbeing. Fortunately, over recent years, mental health and stress have become much more openly discussed and addressed, and awareness and understanding has improved. It is important to be aware of your own vulnerabilities and to seek help if you feel overwhelmed. It is also important to be aware of any changes in your colleagues that may indicate they are having difficulties. It can be difficult to know what to do in this situation. Having a mentor in practice can be helpful for many reasons, and practices often follow this system of colleague support. Further advice can be obtained from the services listed in Figure 9.7.

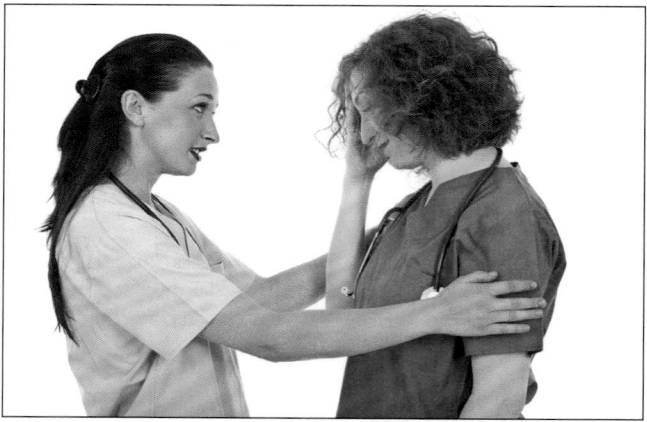

9.6 It is important to support each other in the challenging environment of veterinary practice. (Blaj Gabriel/Shutterstock.com)

- **Vetlife**
  Vetlife offers support to all members of the veterinary profession, including students and support staff
  Telephone: 0303 040 2551
  Email: info@vetlife.org.uk (anonymous email service also available)
- **Samaritans**
  Samaritans is a charity that offers telephone, email, text, written or face-to-face support
  Telephone: 116 123
  Email: jo@samaritans.org
- **Mind Matters**
  An initiative funded and run by the RCVS that aims to improve the mental health and wellbeing of all those in the veterinary team
  Website: www.vetmindmatters.org/

9.7 Organizations or initiatives that provide support for veterinary professionals.

Emotional boundaries

Supporting clients and exhibiting empathy and care have been mentioned throughout this chapter – and rightly so, as this is the cornerstone of our role as veterinary nurses – but we do have to apply 'emotional boundaries' in order to protect ourselves. If we do not protect ourselves, then we cannot continue to help others; rather like the principle in an aircraft emergency where parents are instructed to put their own oxygen mask on before attending to children. In the context of client care, we need to ensure we have boundaries in our mind that we will not cross, and this is an aspect of being a healthy professional. Personal communication with clients should be avoided, and it is sensible not be become 'friends' with clients on social media or offer any advice or support outside of the remit of your practice role. Being able to 'switch off' after work and having interests beyond work that are different from your everyday role are also factors in a healthy life balance.

Patient handover

It is likely that during the care of a patient, a colleague will take over the care provision from you at some point (e.g. at a shift change), and a clear process for patient handover can help to ensure that this goes smoothly and that all information has been relayed. It is good practice to have some time set aside for this process, so that it is not hurried, and communication should be both verbal and written (in the form of a handover sheet). It can help to go through the patient's hospitalization sheet together, and if there are any particular observations (e.g. wounds, mobility, neurological or behavioural signs) then these should be examined and discussed.

Meetings

Meetings are a vital aspect of practice and team development. They provide an opportunity to disseminate important information, discuss practice developments and ideas, resolve problems, and allow the whole team to have an input into the ongoing goals and aspirations of the practice. As a member of the practice team, it is important to have an input when this is required, even though it may seem daunting at the time. A well run meeting will encourage and nurture input from attendees, but sometimes meetings can be dominated by the more senior members of the team, so it is useful to be prepared for this. If you have an opinion that you wish to share, it works well to ask if you can offer it; for example, 'I have an idea for this, is it OK if I share it?' As your confidence as a veterinary nurse grows you will find it easier to have an input into practice matters, and as a senior nurse will yourself manage meetings. There are several different types of meeting, ranging from formal (with a chair leading the meeting, presenting ideas and controlling input) to very informal (where people openly air their views or where input is gathered from attendees writing on a whiteboard).

Reflective practice

Reflective practice is an integral part of being a professional and involves considering experiences and using this reflection to progress and develop (see Chapter 12). It is a process that all professionals subconsciously perform every day (e.g. thinking about an encounter with a client and considering how you could have handled it differently, or when you forget something important, thinking of a solution to help you be more organized). Sometimes we should perform this process in a more conscious and structured way, as this is when we get best results. Figure 9.8 shows a 'reflective cycle' that can be used to reflect on an experience in practice and help you learn from it. Concerns regarding fellow colleagues may be the most challenging to deal with, and more guidance on this and 'whistleblowing' can be found in Chapter 1.

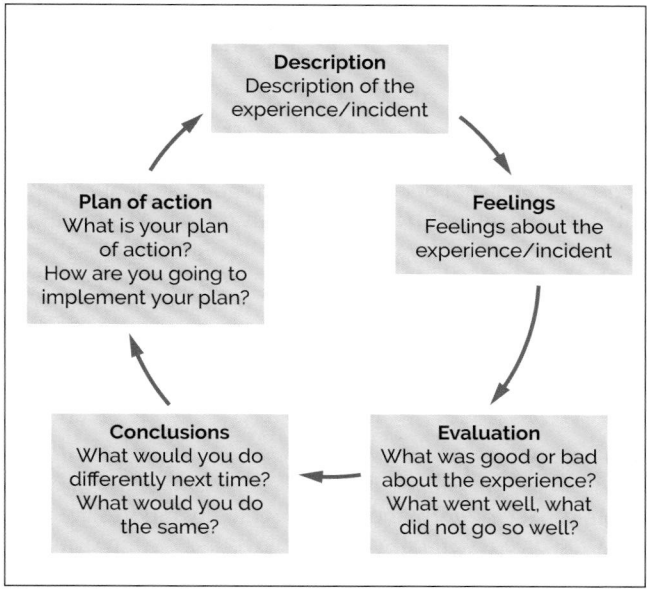

| 9.8 | Reflective cycle to promote learning from experiences (Gibbs, 1988). |

Clinical audit

One of the ways that practices can reflect on performance is by performing a 'clinical audit', which helps to check where things are being done well and where improvements may need to be made. It involves deciding on the area that requires audit or where review of practice may be useful, collecting data, comparing this with current research ('best practice') and making decisions based on the outcomes (i.e. ascertaining whether everything is being done to the correct standard, or whether changes need to be made).

Communicating problems to colleagues

Sometimes things go wrong, and we need to inform a colleague or senior member of staff to ensure that any issues are dealt with. Making mistakes is part of everyday practice and whilst they need to be avoided wherever possible, it is how they are dealt with and learnt from that is important. It is best to be upfront as soon as possible if you have made or noticed a mistake, so that it can be addressed before it is allowed to escalate. The veterinary profession is moving away from a 'blame-culture' and more towards a collaborative approach, where mistakes can be discussed openly so that everyone can learn from them and use them to develop.

Morbidity and mortality meetings

When an unexpected patient death occurs it can be extremely difficult, especially for the team members involved. Morbidity and mortality meetings (MMMs) offer a structured, non-blame approach to reflecting on what happened, why it happened, and how it may possibly be avoided if the same circumstances arise. They can also serve to provide team members with the reassurance that whilst mistakes should be averted as much as possible, they do happen, and learning from them is a vital part of the process. It is good practice to hold a similar team meeting whenever any adverse event occurs.

Evidence-based veterinary medicine

Evidence-based veterinary medicine (EBVM), in basic terms, is the use of current evidence (or research) to inform clinical decisions, whilst aligning these with the individual patient/client circumstances. As more work is done in this relatively new area of veterinary medicine, a repository of information will be built that veterinary surgeons and nurses can use as a reference point when making clinical decisions. Many clients are aware of EBVM and quite rightly want to know that the treatment or approach for their pet's condition is based on the best available evidence (see Chapter 1).

Appraisals

Appraisals or 'performance reviews' are an opportunity for a two-way discussion between employers and employees to clarify roles and responsibilities, discuss performance, strengths and weaknesses, and identify practice and employee goals and how these can be worked towards. Prior to the appraisal, a 'pre-appraisal form' is usually offered, and you should take your time to fill this in as comprehensively as you can so that you can get the best out of your appraisal. It is important to remember that the process is for the benefit of both parties and, at the end of the meeting, work with your appraiser to agree a mutual plan that aligns the aspects and goals discussed during the interview. Appraisals may be scheduled by the practice yearly, or the practice may have a more flexible approach, allowing employees and employers to review progress whenever it is felt necessary. Whilst career planning options have not historically been a strength in veterinary practice, as management skills become more prevalent, it is likely that veterinary nurses will be able to consider and plan a career more effectively with the aid of their practice; this is one of the benefits of appraisals. Appraisals are also a tool that may feed into management decisions regarding pay review, promotion, training needs and taking on new responsibilities.

Customer service and the value of clients

A high level of customer service is integral to any successful veterinary establishment. The equation is simple. Veterinary practices can only provide care to patients (and create income from this) if clients continue to return to the practice, and clients will only do this if they are satisfied with the service that they receive. Clients will also leave the practice when they move away or when they no longer have pets, so it is important that new clients are gained and become 'bonded' to the practice, and this can only be achieved if relationships are built and a high level of service maintained.

More and more practices are opening in the UK, and many of them run as large groups or corporations, so competition for business is high. Clients quite rightly expect to be treated with respect and integrity, and much of this can be achieved with effective communication. Timeliness and adhering to assurances, such as having a prescription or insurance form ready when you said it would be, or calling a client back when this has been promised, are also essential. Asking clients for feedback on practice performance not only yields important information to aid practice development, but also demonstrates to clients that you value their opinion. So, it is extremely useful to have a system for requesting client feedback forms in reception.

Complaints and conflicts

As customers of the business, there will be times when clients are dissatisfied with the service they have received and will wish to make either a formal or informal complaint. How this complaint is dealt with can have an impact on the client's impression of (and whether they decide to leave) the practice and staff wellbeing (a badly handled complaint can have negative effects on the staff who are involved).

There are some key points that should be considered when dealing with 'on-the-spot' complaints or conflicting views. These principles also apply to conflicts with staff.

- Any complaint or conflict should be acknowledged immediately and addressed as soon as possible.
- Conversations should be carried out in private when at all possible.
- Stay calm and professional, be confident and assertive, but open to listening and resolution.
- Allow the other person to have their say, employ impeccable listening skills and ensure that it is clear you are taking their concerns seriously.
- Try and pinpoint exactly what the problem is (e.g. a complaint about a bill may not be about the bill in its entirety, but about a specific component of the bill).
- Obtain any extra information if the details you have are incomplete.
- Use shared decision-making to attempt to find a solution that is acceptable to both parties.
- Do not be afraid to ask for help from another staff member.
- If the situation is or becomes threatening, then seek help immediately.
- Assure the other party that the issues raised will be shared with the team in order to work out a new practice approach and ensure that the situation does not happen again.
- Ensure that all details of the complaint are recorded in full in the appropriate manner.

Formal complaints, such as a written complaint or a complaint that has been received via the Royal College of Veterinary Surgeons (RCVS), should be dealt with according to practice procedures and following guidance from the RCVS. The practice indemnity insurer, for example The Veterinary Defence Society (VDS), may be consulted for advice if required.

Reception duties

Whilst many practices have dedicated reception staff, veterinary nurses are often required to cover reception. In addition, there are instances when it is beneficial for a member of nursing staff to deal with a particular query or problem. Reception staff are the first (and last) point of contact for clients, so ensure you make a good first impression (Figure 9.9). A clear, timely and friendly greeting of the client and animal, professionalism, and dealing with their query promptly and efficiently are essential.

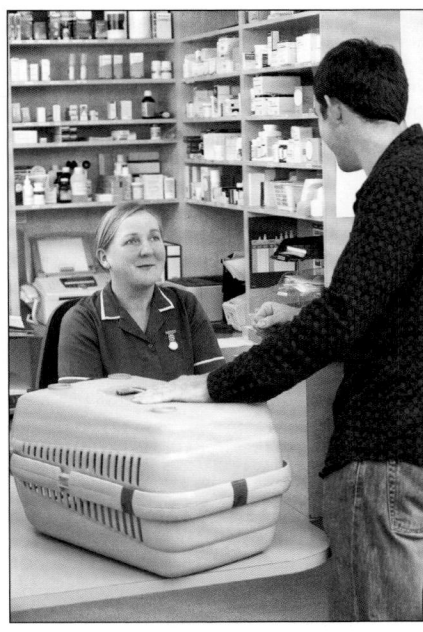

9.9

Reception staff are the first (and last) point of contact for clients. (Monkey Business Images/ Shutterstock.com)

Key components of reception duty

- Being the 'front of house' for the practice – exhibiting a professional, helpful and welcoming manner
- Greeting clients in the waiting area and dealing with their needs
- Answering the telephone
- Dealing with queries, requests, and making and amending appointments
- Dealing with complaints or problems, and knowing when it is necessary to refer to another member of staff
- Processing payments and organizing payment plans if appropriate
- Handing out medications (that have been prescribed and prepared by clinical staff)
- Supporting clients at difficult times (e.g. when clients have received bad news or during euthanasia appointments)
- Being aware of practice and staff schedules
- Knowledge of what constitutes an emergency, and how to prioritize appointments

---

Telephone communication

Communication via telephone brings its own challenges, as we are not able to rely on certain elements of non-verbal communication, and the person we are talking to can only receive information from what we say and how we say it. There are many circumstances in practice where we need to use telephone communication, such as taking query calls and making appointments, offering updates on patients and following-up on patient progress.

When using the telephone it is important to:

- Always offer your name and who you are, so that the client knows who they are speaking to and has a point of contact for the future. Try to have a bright, happy voice when answering the phone, as this will help get the conversation off to a good start
- Speak slowly and clearly. This takes practice, as often what we think is a suitable pace of speech is actually too fast and the client will not take in or hear what you have said
- Use language that is appropriate for the recipient. Avoid technical jargon or abbreviated words that may not be understood
- Have access to the patient notes if possible, so that you can refer to these if necessary
- Allow the client to speak without interruption
- Repeat important points during a call
- Take notes so that you have something to refer back to
- Always ask another team member if you are not sure about something
- Ensure that any messages are passed on to the appropriate team member, no matter how insignificant they may seem.

Appointment organization

Each practice will have its own system for organizing consulting and surgical duties. Depending on the number of staff, there may be several consulting and operating lists running simultaneously, which can make management of appointments quite challenging! When taking calls to book appointments, you will need to know when consultations are available and the veterinary surgeon or nurse who is on duty so that the client can book in with the appropriate team member. Quite often the practice is not able to offer the client the appointment slot that they would prefer, so it is important to manage this tactfully and try to find a compromise. Knowing what constitutes an emergency and how to deal with this is a vital skill when answering the telephone, as is knowing when to ask a colleague for advice. The practice should have a protocol for managing the booking of procedures, including those involving anaesthesia. Ensure that you understand this in order to handle booking these types of appointments efficiently.

Processing payments

For most services and goods offered through a veterinary practice, there will be a charge. Any fees should have been explained clearly to the client prior to them arriving at the reception desk to make payment; however, it is always wise to check this with the client (e.g. 'has the vet explained the fees for today to you?'). Invoices generated by the practice management system during the consultation or procedure should offer detail as to what the charges are for, and these should be outlined to the client at the point of payment.

Payments are usually taken by cash or payment card, and it is important to ensure that the payment is paired with the correct client account. At the end of the working day or other defined period, 'reconciliation' will be carried out. This involves matching payments taken with those recorded on client's records, so any discrepancies will be highlighted at this stage, but it is much easier if they do not occur in the first place! Value added tax (VAT) is payable on veterinary services and most medications and products.

Second opinions

Clients at your practice may seek an opinion (known as a second opinion) from either another veterinary surgeon at the practice or, more commonly, from another practice. Conversely, clients may attend your practice requesting a second opinion. There are a few rules that help to ensure proper and safe treatment, as well as 'etiquette' towards other practices and veterinary surgeons, and these are covered in the RCVS Code of Professional Conduct (Supporting Guidance 1 – Referrals and Second Opinions). Key points include:

- Clients should never be dissuaded from obtaining a second opinion or referral to another practice, and practices should be helpful to clients in assisting with the process
- When a new client presents at the practice, it should always be ascertained whether the animal is under treatment at another practice and, if so, that that practice is informed and any relevant clinical history is obtained
- If a client refuses to disclose their previous practice, the case should be declined
- It is normal practice for both referral and second-opinion clients to return to their original practice after the presenting problem has been addressed. Taking over second-opinion or referral clients as your own clients is classed as 'supersession' and is not acceptable practice
- If the client expresses that they wish to change to your practice, then this is their decision and their previous practice should be informed
- In the case of an emergency, it is acceptable to administer essential treatment before contacting the client's usual veterinary practice.

Advertising and promotion

Whilst veterinary practices are permitted to promote their goods and services, it is important that any advertising or promotion complies with professional conduct guidelines, UK advertising codes and data protection law. Further guidance on this topic can be found in the RCVS Code of Professional Conduct and from the Advertising Standards Authority and the Information Commissioner's Office. Particular caution should be exercised when making comparisons with other practices or competitors.

Practice websites are the online 'shop-front' for the practice, so it is very important that they reflect the ethos of the practice and are kept up-to-date with contact information, services offered and current team members. Your practice website can be a very useful tool for promoting the work that you do.

Social media

Most veterinary practices use social media as a method of communicating with their clients and for promotion of their work. Most practices have a Facebook page and this can be an excellent tool for engaging your clients, distributing important information, celebrating practice successes and gaining positive reviews; however, if your Facebook page is poorly managed, at best it will not have a positive impact and at worst it could damage your reputation or public presence. It is advisable to have at least one dedicated practice team member who manages the page, gaining regular input from the veterinary team, if possible.

Using Facebook

- Ensure that the page is set up as a business 'page' and not a 'profile'
- Ensure that the page is secure, with only those requiring administrator access having the password
- Have a clear message displayed that states anyone requiring veterinary assistance must contact the practice directly
- Obtain explicit permission for any posts/pictures of pets from their owner. For example, this should not just be a 'tick-box' on an admission form but a distinct request
- Try to engage followers by asking questions, offering quizzes and inviting input
- Try to educate clients on topics that you, as a practice, feel are important
- Advise clients accurately on any new information on pet healthcare
- Ensure that any comments or messages are promptly and appropriately responded to

Your personal online presence

Our professional responsibilities lie beyond the confines of the practice and as part of a profession we are always representing the profession in everything we do and say. It is important to remember these responsibilities (as outlined in the RCVS Code of Professional Conduct) and that we must not 'engage in any activity or behaviour that would be likely to bring the profession into disrepute or undermine public confidence in the profession'. Social media is a good example of where the lines between professional responsibilities and personal opinions and freedoms can become blurred, and it is always sensible to consider whether what you are saying, even if to personal friends and family, offers a positive impression. Veterinary nurses should be familiar with the *Fitness to Practise* – a guide for UK providers of veterinary nursing education and student veterinary nurses (RCVS, 2016).

Practice organization
Structure of the veterinary team

Practice team structures can vary considerably, depending on practice size, type and setup. Many practices are part of a larger 'group' or company, with support offices and directors making decisions outside of the practice itself. All members of the team have value, and all team members need other members of the team in order to work effectively, from the manager or practice owner to the kennel assistant.

An overview of a typical or traditional basic veterinary practice staff structure is given in Figure 9.10. It is important that all team members understand their role and feel confident to perform the duties assigned to them in order for the team to be effective. This can be clarified and adapted by using robust appraisal systems (see 'Appraisals' above).

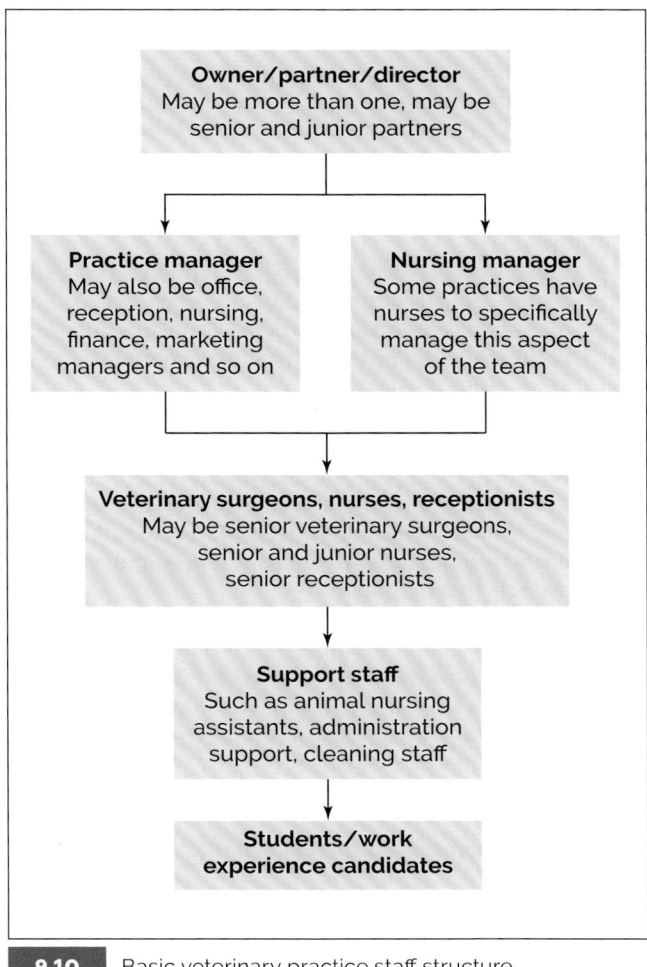

9.10 Basic veterinary practice staff structure.

Legislation and regulation

All activity undertaken within or related to veterinary practice is governed by the law and it is a criminal offence to practise outside of this legislation. The RCVS regulates the profession in accordance with the Veterinary Surgeons Act (VSA) 1966 (at time of writing) and this law outlines the legalities regarding all aspects of practising veterinary medicine and the registration of veterinary surgeons and veterinary nurses.

Following a supplemental Royal Charter, which came into effect on 17th February 2015, confirming the RCVS as regulator of veterinary nurses, only veterinary nurses who are entered on to the RCVS register have the right to practise veterinary nursing in the UK (see Chapter 1). The Schedule 3 Amendment Order to the VSA outlines the medical treatment and minor surgical procedures that are permitted to be performed by veterinary nurses and veterinary nurse students (who are registered with the RCVS) under the direction and/or supervision of the veterinary surgeon in charge of the animal's care.

Employment law

Employment law governs the relationship between employers and their employees, what employers can expect and the protection offered to employees. These laws relate to recruitment, contracts, discrimination and equality, working time regulations, disciplinary processes and termination,

and whilst an employee does not need to know the law, it is wise to be aware of the employee rights that exist so that these can be referred to and exercised if necessary.

Data protection

The General Data Protection Regulation (GDPR) was implemented in the UK on 25 May 2018 and replaced the previous data protection legislation, the Data Protection Act 1998 (DPA). Further information is available from the Information Commissioner's Office (ICO) (https://ico.org.uk/for-organisations/guide-to-data-protection/guide-to-the-general-data-protection-regulation-gdpr/).

There are many forms of data that will be created and stored by a veterinary practice, relating to both patients and clients, as well as practice staff. The GDPR does not apply to data from which you can identify an animal. Examples of data that may be handled and/or kept by the practice that do come under GDPR include:

- Client records
  - Name, address, contact details including email address, financial and payment records, and correspondence including disputes
- Patient records
  - Clinical history, hospitalization charts and nursing care plans, anaesthetic records, imaging records and laboratory data
- Personnel/staff data
  - Contact details, attendance and sickness data, health information, appraisal records, salary information, training records, emails and disciplinary information
- Financial data
  - Practice finances and credit card/bank statements, invoices and payments, payroll and supplier accounts
- Health and Safety
  - Risk assessments and accident records
- Monitoring data
  - Closed circuit television (CCTV), recorded telephone calls (e.g. for 'mystery shopping' data), customer feedback data, emails and social media activity. It is important to ensure that all data held complies with the GDPR.

The RCVS has also published frequently asked questions on GDPR (www.rcvs.org.uk/setting-standards/advice-and-guidance/gdpr--rcvs-information-and-qandas/).

Veterinary practices must ensure that they comply with the GDPR. The principles stipulate that personal data must be:

1. Processed fairly and lawfully and in a transparent manner.
2. Collected for a specific, explicit and legitimate purpose.
3. Adequate, relevant and limited to what is necessary (data minimization).
4. Accurate and, where necessary, kept up to date.
5. Reasonable steps should be taken to rectify data that are inaccurate.
6. Kept for no longer than is necessary (storage limitation).
7. Kept so that appropriate technical and organizational measures are taken to prevent unauthorized/unlawful processing, loss or damage.
8. Processed in accordance with the rights of the person whose data are held.
9. Not transferred to a country or territory outside the European Economic Area (unless that country or territory ensures an adequate level of protection for the data).

Subject access

Data subjects have the right to be informed and provided with information in clear and plain language as to how their data are processed. Individuals have the right to access this data. Practices should meet such requests within 1 month and without charging a fee. Data controllers may withhold disclosure where a request is excessive. The ICO website has guidance that will assist practices regarding considerations on receipt of a subject access request and includes a helpful checklist (https://ico.org.uk/). The practice should ensure that its privacy notices are clear, concise and easily accessible, and that clients know how their personal data are processed.

Right of rectification

Data subjects are entitled to have their personal data rectified if it is inaccurate or incomplete (right of rectification) and in some cases to have it deleted (right of erasure or 'right to be forgotten'). If the data have been disclosed to a third party, the veterinary practice must inform the third party of the rectification (or erasure), where possible. The individual must also be informed about the third party to whom their data have been disclosed.

Data breach

The GDPR requires mandatory notification of a data security breach to the ICO, no later than 72 hours after becoming aware of it, unless it is unlikely to result in a risk to the relevant individuals' rights and freedoms. Late notification requires justification. If there is a breach that is likely to result in a high risk to a person's rights and freedoms, e.g. physical harm, discrimination, identity theft or fraud, reputational damage, financial loss, loss of confidentiality and any other significant economic or social disadvantage, you must also inform the individual(s) concerned without undue delay. A record of all breaches must be kept and the actions noted. Further information can be found on the ICO website (https://ico.org.uk/for-organisations/guide-to-data-protection).

Sharing patient information with another veterinary practice

Information relating to animals is not affected by the GDPR. The practice will, however, need a lawful basis for transferring a client's data, such as consent. Clients must be made aware of the data on file that the practice has consent to transfer to a new practice. A client may not want you to transfer personal data relating to their bills and/or invoices and payment history.

Clinical records

Patient clinical records are an essential aspect of patient care, since they provide information on the patient's medical history that will need to be referred to at every visit. It is vital that clinical notes are accurate and coherent, so that they can be understood by anyone who may need to access them in the future (e.g. another staff member at your practice, another practice or a referral centre). Whilst they should be comprehensive, they should be easy to refer to and not contain any unnecessary information. Personal comments about clients should never be contained within the clinical notes; first, this is unprofessional and, secondly, the client has the right to access the notes, which could also be potentially

used as evidence in any court case or RCVS hearing. Some practices may use abbreviations to signify certain clinical traits, and this is also very unwise practice. Clients have the right to access their pet's clinical records under the RCVS guidelines, as long as the records pertain to the animal whilst under the client's ownership.

Clinical records should be:

- Timely
  - Clinical notes/records should be written up as soon as possible after the consultation or procedure (preferably immediately or, if this is not possible, from notes taken during the consultation shortly afterwards) (Figure 9.11)
- Accurate
  - It is vital that records are accurate. This may be with reference to: the animal; the disease, injury, procedure or treatment; diagnostic tests/imaging and results; advice given or issues discussed; the client's requests, preferences or abilities; or any other aspects that may arise
- Comprehensive
  - The more comprehensive the clinical notes, the more information is available to refer back to. However, it is important to maintain a balance between enough information and so much information that it becomes unmanageable
  - Notes should include details on the presenting complaint or issue being dealt with, as well as routine information such as current diet
- Professional
  - As mentioned previously, defamatory remarks should never feature in the clinical notes, whether they relate to the client, the animal or the condition
  - Ideally, clinical information should be recorded separately from personal information (such as financial information), so that should another party (such as another practice) require the patient's clinical information, this can be provided without disclosing private matters
  - It is good practice to initial clinical notes so that anyone looking back can see who has created them. As most practices now have computerized records, this is usually done by the system, but this is not fail-safe as sometimes (although this should be avoided) notes may be made under another staff member's log in

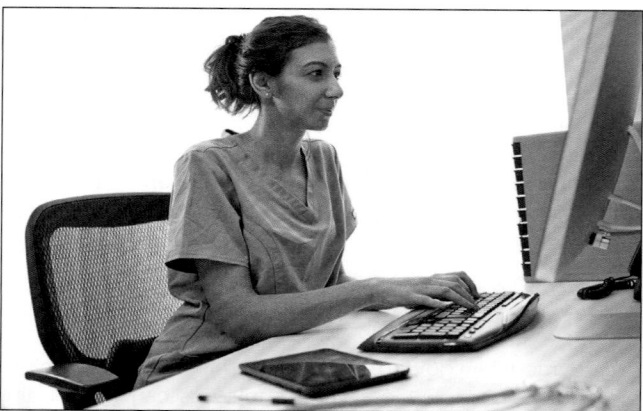

9.11 It is important that clinical notes/records are written up as soon as possible after the consultation or procedure. (Monkey Business Images/Shutterstock.com)

- Useful
  - Some additions to the notes can offer really useful information, such as the nature of the animal and their handling tolerance, client preferences and goals
  - It is important to note any follow-up on the record; for example, 'check-up in 3 months'
  - Any communication with client (e.g. advice given or discussed) should be included for future reference.

Filing paperwork and other documents

While most data are now held digitally, there may be some that are still stored as 'hard copies'. This may include insurance claim forms, traditional X-rays and vaccination cards. Whatever filing system your practice uses, it is imperative to understand the system and stick to this rigidly, as misfiled documents can be difficult, if not impossible, to locate.

Disposal of records

The guidelines regarding the retention of records are complex but, in general, they should be kept no longer than required and when destroyed, this must be done securely (e.g. by cross-shredding). Indemnity insurers have historically advised retention for 7 years (6 years is the maximum limitation period for a civil claim plus 1 year). Practices must also meet the record keeping requirements set out within the Veterinary Medicines Regulations. Records for the retail supply (including administration) of POM-V and POM-VPS medicines must be kept for 5 years. Current employment legislation requires certain records to be kept for 3 years (such as accident reports); salary details should be kept for 6 years. The GDPR do not specify retention periods for personal data.

Data management

Most digital practice management software has the ability to monitor data from the practice, so that certain information can be collected and used for practice management purposes. This can include data such as appointment attendance, number of procedures carried out and sales of products. These data can be especially useful when evaluating the success of a certain clinic (see Chapter 10), deciding whether or not to set up a new service, or if carrying out a clinical audit (see above).

Client confidentiality

Veterinary professionals have a legal and ethical duty to ensure client confidentiality is maintained at all times. With reference to the RCVS Code of Professional Conduct guidance on client confidentiality, in basic terms this means:

- Under normal circumstances, a veterinary surgeon or nurse should not disclose to any third party any information about a client or their animal
- Information may be disclosed under certain circumstances (e.g. if the client has consented or when there is a welfare issue)
- The client's permission may be express (i.e. directly given) or implied (e.g. when a new practice or an insurance company requests a patient's history), but express permission should always be sought if possible

- Registration of a dog with the Kennel Club permits a veterinary surgeon who carries out a Caesarean section on a bitch, or surgery to alter the natural conformation of a dog, to report this to the Kennel Club
- Specific guidance is offered by the RCVS regarding client confidentiality in the context of social media.

Finance management

Effective control of the practice finances is an essential aspect of practice management and ensures the ongoing success of any business. There are several key components that feed into this equation, including:

- Effective stock control (see below)
- Cost-effective stock sourcing, so that the best price is found for stock and equipment
- Budgeting and planning to ensure that any (non-essential) equipment purchased is justified by the revenue that it will bring back to the practice, and that other costs such as salaries and bonuses are managed appropriately and fairly
- Suitable pricing/fee structure for both goods (items) and services (consultations, surgical procedures)
- Efficient pricing so that items/charges do not get overlooked
- Effective debt management.

Whilst practice financial matters are usually the responsibility of the practice owners/partners and senior or financial staff, it is important to be aware of this aspect of practice, to be mindful that practices must run as a business and to have an input if required (e.g. team decisions on a fee change or on introducing a new service).

Debt management

Most practices operate on a non-credit basis, meaning that the client pays for any goods or services at the time the cost is incurred. This is the most effective way to avoid non-payment of fees; however, practice policies will vary and it is important to be aware of any special circumstances that may exist.

As mentioned above, there will be circumstances where the client is unable to pay, and one option is to provide a payment agreement. It is important that this is set up and administered in a formal and organized manner so that there is no ambiguity about when payments should be made and the amount required, and that any non-payments are followed up promptly. Most practices will outsource unpaid debts to a debt recovery service, but due to the cost of this service, this is normally reserved for larger debts.

Without doubt, the best way to avoid unpaid debt is to prevent client debts in the first instance. This is best achieved by clear communication of fees and how these must be paid in the initial and ongoing discussions with clients.

Stock control

Practices need to hold a wide range of stock items in order to function effectively. These include:

- Drugs and medications
  - Includes those used in practice and those dispensed to clients for their animals
  - Examples: vaccines, antibiotics and parasiticides

- Consumables
  - Items used in everyday practice to provide treatment, care and cleaning/disinfection of the practice
  - Examples: syringes, needles, bandages, suture materials, disinfectants and veterinary diets
- Over-the-counter (general sale) items
  - Items available for clients to purchase without being under the care of the veterinary practice
  - Examples: toys, life-stage diets, leads and grooming tools
- Office and staff consumables
  - Examples: paper, pens, practice stationery and beverages.

If you consider the number and variety of items that fall within each of these categories, it is easy to see how important it is to have an effective stock control system, as items being out of stock can have serious ramifications for the provision of care and customer service (Figure 9.12).

Whilst most, if not all, practices now have a computerized stock control system, many still use a manual ordering system, which involves having a record of stock in hand and placing an order when stock becomes low. Computerized stock control is preferable in many ways, since it will hold a record of all stock held at the practice and as items are sold through the system, they will be taken out of stock and automatically ordered when stock falls below a pre-defined level.

With regard to stock control it is important that:

- There is a clear and consistent stock control system and that everyone in the practice is aware of and adheres to the system
- Stock is not excessive or depleted (the former causes issues with cash flow and items becoming out-of-date; the latter causes issues for the provision of care and customer service)
- The stock data on the system or on the stock list are accurate and kept up-to-date
- Items that are consumed within the practice (i.e. not charged to a record) are 'de-stocked' using a consistent method
- Items that are used in procedures or for treatment are all charged for or 'sold' at a zero fee (or are 'de-stocked' as above) to ensure that they are accounted for
- Items used out-of-hours and on visits are accounted for.

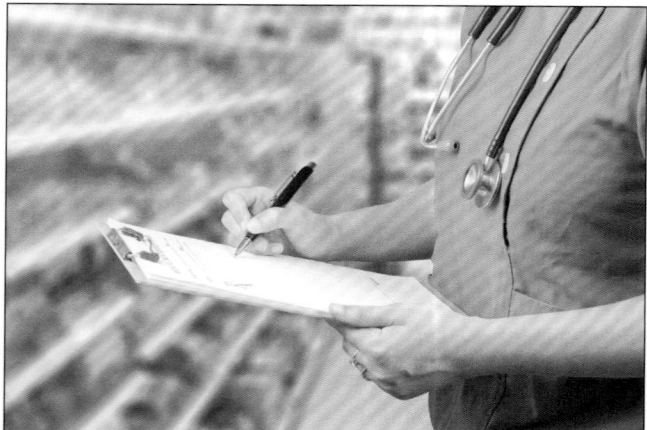

9.12 Effective stock control is a vital component of practice organization. (Have a nice day Photo/Shutterstock.com)

Ordering and receiving stock

Most practices will have a preferred or main supplier, but usually there are items that are ordered from elsewhere due to lack of availability or price differences with the main supplier. Orders can usually be placed via an online system, by telephone or by email. It is sensible practice to have one or two people in charge of the stock system and ordering; however, the remit for this task often falls to whoever is on duty at the time.

The ordering of Controlled Drugs requires that a generic prescription written and signed by a veterinary surgeon is provided to the supplier at the time of ordering, so it is important to plan ahead when ordering these items (see Chapter 8). When stock is received, it must be carefully checked to ensure that the stock provided matches the order note and any discrepancies must be reported immediately to a senior colleague and/or the supplier.

Equipment

Practices will own or lease a variety of equipment and this will vary enormously depending on the type and size of the practice. Small practices may only possess the most basic of equipment, whereas referral hospitals may possess a large range of equipment of staggering value.

Knowledge about the equipment you are required to use is imperative and may include use, cleaning, maintenance (including sourcing relevant consumables and spares) and troubleshooting. Information on this should be provided by the person in charge of your training, but it is, as with many aspects of the nursing role, important to appreciate your limitations and to ask for help if you are unsure, as failing to do so may render the equipment unusable or dangerous, which could be disastrous for a patient or another staff member.

Problems with equipment or practice facilities should be reported as soon as possible, since malfunctioning equipment could put animals, staff and clients in danger. If necessary, a notice can be placed on a piece of equipment to alert that there is an issue until the appropriate person has been notified.

Rota management

The staff rota outlines which staff are on duty at certain times, the duties they are assigned and incorporates staff absence due to sickness and leave. The size of the practice and the services offered will affect the relative complexity of the rota system. The responsibility for organizing the rota (not usually an envied task as it can be notoriously difficult!) usually lies with the practice manager or other senior member of staff, but it is important to have an awareness of other staff duties, as well as your own, as this will help with basic practice running such as making appointments and booking in procedures. Rotas usually run to a pre-set 'formula' so that they can be repeated easily, are fair and incorporate all staffing requirements encountered.

References and further reading

Ackerman N (2012) The role of the nurse in the veterinary practice: the consultation. In: *The Consulting Veterinary Nurse*. Wiley-Blackwell, Oxford

Ashall V, Millar K and Hobson-West P (2018) Informed consent in veterinary medicine: ethical implications for the profession and the animal patient. *Food Ethics* **1(3)**, 247–258

Belshaw Z, Robinson NJ, Dean RS and Brennan M (2018) Owner and veterinary surgeon perspectives on the roles of veterinary nurses and receptionists in relation to small animal preventive healthcare consultations in the United Kingdom. *Veterinary Record* **183(9)**, 296

Clarke C and Chapman M (2012) *BSAVA Manual of Small Animal Practice Management and Development.* BSAVA Publications, Gloucester

Dickinson D, Wilkie P and Harris M (1999) *Taking medicines: concordance is not compliance.* [Available at: www.ncbi.nlm.nih.gov/pmc/articles/PMC1116621/]

Esterhuizen P (2019) *Reflective Practice in Nursing, 4th edn.* Sage Publications, Exeter

Gibbs G (1988) *Learning by Doing: A guide to teaching and learning methods.* Further Education Unit, Oxford Polytechnic, Oxford

Gray C and Moffett J (2016) *Handbook of Veterinary Communication Skills.* Wiley-Blackwell, Oxford

Hewson C (2015) Grief for pets – Part 2: Avoiding compassion fatigue. *Veterinary Nursing Journal* **29**, 388–391

Macdonald J and Gray C (2014) 'Informed Consent' – how do we get it right? *Veterinary Nursing Journal* **29**, 101–103

Munson E and Willcox A (2013) Applying the Calgary-Cambridge model. *Practice Nursing* **18(9)** DOI: doi.org/10.12968/pnur.2007.18.9.27158

Pullen S and Gray C (2006) *Ethics, Law and the Veterinary Nurse.* Elsevier Science, Oxford

Radford AD, Stockley P, Silverman J et al. (2006) Development, teaching and evaluation of a consultation structure model for use in veterinary education. *Journal of Veterinary Medical Education* **33**, 38–44

RCVS (2016) *Fitness to practise – a guide for UK providers of veterinary nursing education and student veterinary nurses.* [Available at: https://www.rcvs.org.uk/news-and-views/publications/]

RCVS (2018) *GDPR – RCVS information and Q&As.* [Available at: www.rcvs.org.uk/setting-standards/advice-and-guidance/gdpr--rcvs-information-and-qandas/]

Rollnick S, Miller W and Butler C (2008) *Motivational Interviewing in Healthcare: Helping Patients Change Behavior.* Guildford Press, New York

Shilcock M and Stutchfield G (2008) *Veterinary Practice Management: A Practical Guide, 2nd edn.* Saunders-Elsevier, Philadelphia

Wager C (2013) Informed consent: what do veterinary nurses need to know? *The Veterinary Nurse* **2(7)** DOI: doi.org/10.129681 vetn.2011.2.7.344

Useful websites

ACAS – provide help and advice for employers and employees: www.acas.org.uk

Animal Samaritans Pet Bereavement Service: www.animalsamaritans.org.uk

Association of Private Pet Cemeteries and Crematoria: www.appcc.org.uk

Blue Cross Pet Bereavement Support Service: www.bluecross.org.uk

Cats Protection Bereavement Support: www.cats.org.uk/grief

EASE Pet Loss Support Services: www.ease-animals.org.uk

Information Commissioner's Office (ICO) – provides several online articles and checklists to help veterinary practices with the GDPR overview: ico.org.uk/for-organisations/guide-to-data-protection/guide-to-the-general-data-protection-regulation-gdpr/

Mind Matters: www.vetmindmatters.org/

Royal College of Veterinary Surgeons (RCVS) Code of Professional Conduct for Veterinary Nurses: www.rcvs.org.uk/advice-and-guidance/code-of-professional-conduct-for-veterinary-nurses/

Samaritans: www.samaritans.org/

Society for Companion Animal Studies (SCAS): www.scas.org.uk

SupportLine: info@supportline.org.uk

The Veterinary Surgeons Act 1966: www.legislation.gov.uk/ukpga/1966/36/contents

Vetlife: www.vetlife.org.uk/

Self-assessment questions

1. Why is 'client compliance' important, and how can we help to achieve it?
2. What aspects of non-verbal communication are important in demonstrating empathy to clients?
3. Explain how you might support a client who has brought their pet to the practice for euthanasia.
4. List the key principles when obtaining informed consent.
5. What is reflective practice, and how can we use reflective practice to aid professional development?
6. Describe how you might handle a complaint from a client in reception about the care of their pet.
7. What are the key duties performed in the role of receptionist?
8. Explain the importance of maintaining professionalism and confidentiality, and the guidelines that should be followed with respect to practice and personal use of social media.
9. What are the key principles of client confidentiality?
10. List the key considerations required in order to achieve effective stock control.
11. How does the GDPR impact veterinary practices?
12. What is paralanguage and how might you apply this when dealing with a client that is upset about their pet's health?

Chapter 10

Nurse-led clinics

Nicola Ackerman

Learning objectives

After studying this chapter, readers will have the knowledge to:

- **Set up and effectively run nurse-led clinics**
- **Use consultation models in the performance of nurse-led clinics**
- **Undertake the roles delegated by the veterinary surgeon in nurse-led clinics**
- **Educate owners in preventative healthcare and aid in compliance**
- **Support clients and their animals with chronic conditions**

Setting up and running veterinary nurse clinics

There has been an increase in the number of veterinary nurse-led clinics in recent years, improving the care of patients and providing opportunities for role development for nurses within the veterinary practice. Whilst the veterinary nurse-led clinics may vary in the way they are set up, there are some common characteristics.

- When considering whether or not to introduce a veterinary nurse-led clinic, the nurse must be able to demonstrate that there is a clear business need, explaining why the service is required and what will be offered to clients (e.g. puppy clinics, weight management clinics, diabetic clinics, behavioural management clinics and geriatric clinics).
- The format of the clinics will need to be considered (e.g. a walk-in or drop-in service for guidance on nutrition versus fixed appointments for weight management).
- The aims and objectives of the veterinary nurse-led clinic need to be clear and effectively communicated to both clients and the other members of the veterinary team.
- Marketing and promotion. The clinic will not succeed if owners are not aware of its existence. Some practices produce leaflets to promote the services offered through nurse-led clinics. Publicity should begin during the planning stage as it may prompt discussion that leads to

adjustment of the proposed clinic service. Posters, leaflets, practice website information, social media channels, group discussions and visits to the local communities can all highlight what the service is about and how it can be accessed.

Other factors that should be considered when planning a nurse-led clinic include:

- Is there computer access and a room to carry out the work effectively?
- Is there likely to be any opposition or difficulties with using the facilities required?
- Is administrative support required or can the clinic be managed by the nurse alone (e.g. drafting letters, instructions and booking appointments)?

Although the term 'veterinary nurse-led' implies a strong degree of independence, the service provided by the clinic is, of course, part of the patient's broader veterinary care and should be considered in conjunction with the care being provided by the whole veterinary team.

Prior to instigating any nurse-led clinic, the veterinary nurse should talk to the rest of the practice team, as they will be instrumental in referring clients to the service, as well as suggesting additional opportunities for education, advice and support. The sharing of knowledge and experience is an important part of professional development for veterinary nurses.

The business case is invaluable in making clear arguments regarding the need and viability of veterinary nurse-led clinics. One of the most important elements of veterinary nurse-led clinics is professional development, as it underpins a competent service. It is important, therefore, to put structures in place to evaluate and identify any professional development requirements.

Basic history taking

Client communication is equally important to consulting as to other areas of veterinary practice (see Chapter 9 for information on principles of communication). Several frameworks for consulting have been developed for medical education; however, none have been developed specifically for veterinary use. The Cambridge–Calgary consulting model (see Chapter 9) was adapted by the National Unit for the Advancement of Veterinary Communication Skills and therefore is the most relevant for veterinary professionals undertaking consultations.

Part of the model considers history-taking in order to gather information relevant to the consultation. The reason for the nurse consultation will somewhat dictate the nature of the questions being asked, alongside the previous clinical history. Good questioning and listening skills are vital to draw out the information required. Utilizing different questioning styles (Figure 10.1) can aid in obtaining the required information.

History-taking during a nurse consultation is different to when triaging an emergency patient. History-taking can be taught using many methods, including videos, online courses and hands-on approaches (e.g. small group workshops, feedback with role play or simulated clients), as well actual practice and experience. Checklists can also complement the history-taking process by minimizing human error through enhanced communication and facilitation of better teamwork (Olin and Tolbert, 2016) (Figure 10.2). All these details should be recorded in the clinical history of the animal.

Questioning Style	Examples	Comments
Open questions	What, Where, When, Who, Why, How	Ensures that the client gives answers that open up discussion
Closed questions	Did, Can, Was, Were, Is	Used to confirm facts and close down discussion
Probe questions	"Why did that happen?" "How did that affect you?"	Give understanding behind the first answer
Reflective questions	"You mentioned, he couldn't exercise as much; are there specific activities he finds harder?"	Reflects back to the client's answer and leads to further questions. Demonstrates active listening
Leading questions	Do you prefer X or Y?	Can be useful, but should be avoided
Multiple questions	Asking a question that asks for two-part answers	Should be avoided as can cause confusion

10.1 Examples of different questioning styles.

Outline goals of visit

Use open-ended questions to identify:
- Chief complaint
- Owners' biggest concerns
- Additional problems and concerns

Expand presenting complaint

- Describe current problem
- Duration of problem?
- When did it first start?
- Has the problem changed or progressed since it started?
- Have any treatments been used to treat the problem?
- What was the response to treatment?
- When was the animal last normal?

Basics

- Vomiting?
- Diarrhoea?
- Coughing?
- Sneezing?
- Behavioural changes?
- Pain?

Input/output

- Changes in appetite?
- Perceived or noted weight loss?
- Diet type, amount, frequency of feeding:
  - Normal diet
  - Recent diet, if different from normal
  - Treats
- Changes in water intake?
- Changes in urination?
- Defecation?

Other medical conditions

This should be included in the clinical history. If the patient is new to the practice, ensure previous history has been requested

Lifestyle

- Indoor/outdoor?
- Check husbandry – will depend on species
- Travel outside of UK?
  - If yes, where? When?

10.2 Questions used in history taking. (Adapted from Olin and Tolbert, 2016)

Basic clinical examination

When performing a physical examination, a systematic approach should be adopted; having a set routine and using an examination checklist (Figure 10.3) will help ensure that a comprehensive examination is completed. For detailed information on how to perform a clinical examination, the reader is referred to Chapter 14. The main points for consideration are summarized below:

- Prior to the examination:
  - Be aware of the clinical history of the animal (e.g. if the animal is known to have arthritic joints, care must be taken not to exacerbate any discomfort during the examination)
  - Scan the animal if it is new to the owner or the practice and make a note of any microchip details (see 'Scanning technique' below)

Examination	Body system	Parameters assessed
Observe from a distance		
Primary survey	Cardiovascular	■ Heart rate ■ Pulse quality any pulse deficits) ■ Mucous membrane colour ■ Capillary refill time ■ Cardiac auscultation ■ Evidence of severe (arterial) haemorrhage
	Respiratory	■ Rate ■ Effort ■ Mucous membrane colour ■ Thoracic wall injuries
	Neurological	■ Consciousness ■ Mentation ■ Gait/movement ■ Cranial nerve responses
Secondary survey	Head and neck	■ Head position ■ Eye position and general ocular examination ■ Ears ■ Jaw (crepitus, malalignment, asymmetry) ■ Teeth (wear, fractures, missing) ■ Beak (apposition, length, wear) ■ Superficial lymph nodes
	Abdominal	■ Body wall trauma (bites, punctures) ■ Distension ■ Herniation
	Genitourinary	■ Cloaca ■ Vulva ■ Anus ■ Mammary glands ■ Prepuce ■ Scrotum
	Musculoskeletal	■ Palpate length of limbs or wings ■ Palpate tail ■ Manipulate all joints
	Skin and integument	■ Epidermis ■ Feathers ■ Coat ■ Evidence of bruising, bleeding, wounds, etc.
	Lymphatic system	■ Palpate superficial lymph nodes
Additional observations	Hydration status Temperature Pain	

10.3 Example of a clinical examination checklist.

- Consider how the patient should be handled and restrained for the examination (see Chapter 11) and whether any adaptations are required (e.g. larger dogs may be more comfortable being examined on the floor; cats may be more amenable if cat-friendly techniques, such as examining the head, ears and mouth last, are adopted)
■ Observe the animal from a distance – how is the animal moving? Is it interacting? Does it appear lame or ataxic? Are the head, jaws and rest of the body, including the muscle groups, symmetrical? Is there any nasal discharge?
■ Primary survey – assess the cardiovascular, respiratory and neurological systems
■ Secondary survey – evaluate the head and neck, abdomen, skin and integument, along with the genitourinary, musculoskeletal and lymphatic systems.

Five vital assessments need to be performed at the end of the clinical examination – heart rate, respiratory rate, temperature, pain and nutrition. Pain can be measured using a pain scoring system or grimace scales (see Chapter 21). A nutritional assessment, comprising bodyweight, body condition score (BCS) and muscle condition score (MSC) should be completed. These measurement form a baseline against which subsequent assessments can be measured.

Pet selection advice

Ideally, all potential new pet owners should seek advice from veterinary professionals before they go out and select a new pet. Owners need to take several aspects into consideration. These include: their own lifestyle (time, working hours), the household environment (including outdoor space), the financial impact of owning a pet and their own preconceptions (rescue animals are all badly behaved; reptiles are cheap and easy to keep). There are many websites that work through all of these aspects and give appropriate suggestions to the type of pet to get.

The Kennel Club has resources that help with breed selection and finding the right breeder when purchasing a pedigree dog. Helping owners with breed selection does need to include discussion of the potential health risks of certain breeds, and the recognition that with crossbreeds the health issues can be associated with the breed of either parent. There are many genetic tests that are now available for dogs and cats, some of which are required by The Kennel Club to be undertaken prior to breeding, others are recommendations from the individual breed societies. Details on the requirements for each breed should be sought prior to breeding (see also Chapter 4).

Selection of exotic species needs to be undertaken with great care. Client education surrounding the husbandry of the chosen species is paramount. Different animals, even of the same species, will have different requirements concerning space, company (or not) of other animals, heat, humidity, ultraviolet (UV) light and diet.

Pet identification

As of the 6th April 2016, all dogs older than 8 weeks of age are required by law to be microchipped in England, Scotland and Wales (local rules should always be checked as differences may occur). If not, owners face a fine of up to £500. Thus, all puppies require microchip implantation by 8 weeks of age. The breeder is considered the first keeper of their litter of puppies and it is their legal responsibility to get their puppies microchipped and recorded on a database compliant with the new regulations. The breeder may not record the new owner as the first keeper of a puppy instead of themselves; it is an offence if they are not listed as the first keeper of their puppies on a microchipping database compliant with the regulations. A puppy may only be passed to its new keeper once it has been microchipped. With recent technology, smaller chips are now available and these are ideal for implantation in small animals, especially small exotic species and puppies.

It is vital that all parties that implant and check microchips, scan all animals to establish that they have not been stolen or lost – this includes puppies, kittens, rabbits, birds and tortoises. When microchips are detected, many readers just display the microchip number; however, some readers also display whether the pet has been reported lost or stolen. The Royal College of Veterinary Surgeons (RCVS) has produced excellent flowcharts that should be used when a client presents an animal registered in another person's name, which detail where to seek further guidance (www.rcvs.org.uk/document-library/client-confidentiality-and-micro-chipped-animals-flow-chart/). Dogs are also required to be registered on a government-approved microchip database. A list of these databases can be found at www.gov.uk/get-your-dog-microchipped.

Who can implant a microchip?

Section 9 of the Microchipping of Dogs (England) Regulations 2015 stipulates that no person may implant a microchip in a dog unless:

- They are a veterinary surgeon or veterinary nurse acting under the direction of a veterinary surgeon
- They are a student of veterinary surgery or a student veterinary nurse, and in either case acting under the direction of a veterinary surgeon
- They have been satisfactorily assessed on a training course approved by the Secretary of State for that purpose
- Before the day on which these Regulations came in to force, they received training on implantation which included practical experience of implanting a microchip.

The Department for Environment, Food and Rural Affairs (Defra) can advise on training courses that have been approved for the teaching of microchip implantation and holds a list of qualified non-veterinary microchip implanters. Registered Veterinary Nurses (RVNs) and enrolled student nurses working under the direction of a veterinary surgeon do not have to undertake an additional course as adequate training should occur in-house as part of the student nurse's training.

Scanning technique

When scanning a pet, it is important to use a methodical standardized pattern in order to ensure that the full area is scanned (Figure 10.4).

- Hold the scanner over the surface of the animal so that the scanning 'hot spot' is in contact with the fur.
- **Scan slowly.** The scanner needs time to transmit the signal and the microchip needs time to respond. The scanner should be **gently rocked** from side to side during the examination; this action helps to maximize the potential for success by allowing for slight deviation in chip positioning.
- If the microchip is not present in the usual area (Figure 10.4a), then the rest of the animal should be thoroughly scanned. **Scan in a slow S-shaped** pattern down the back of the animal starting from the left shoulder (Figure 10.4b).

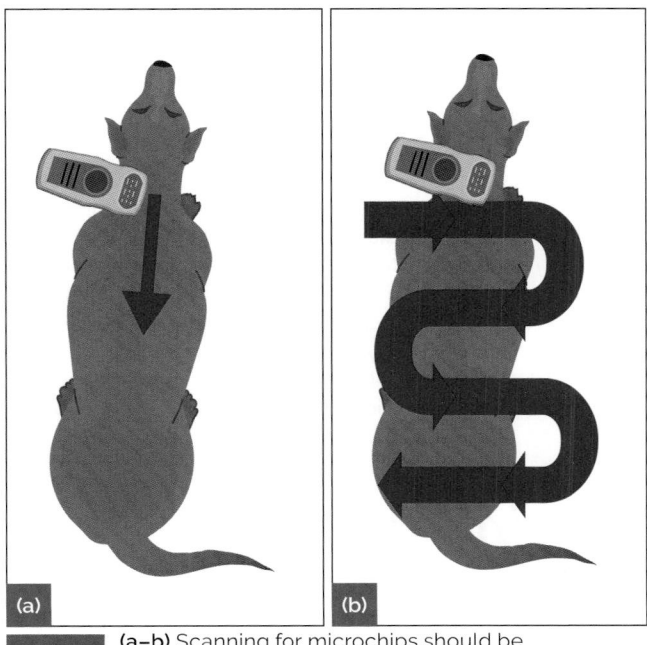

(a)   (b)

10.4 **(a–b)** Scanning for microchips should be systematic in pattern. *continues* ▶

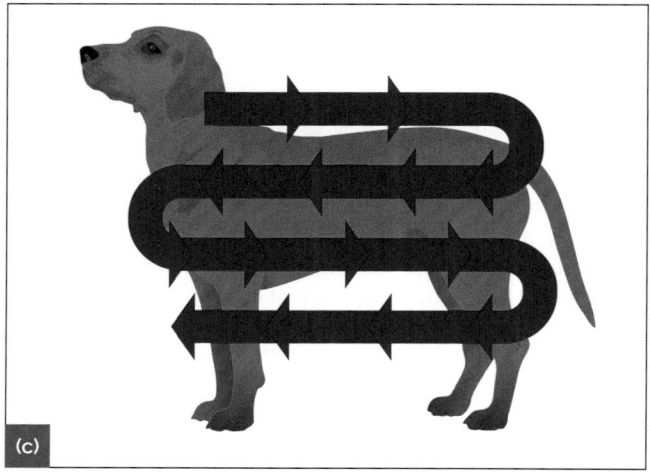

(c)

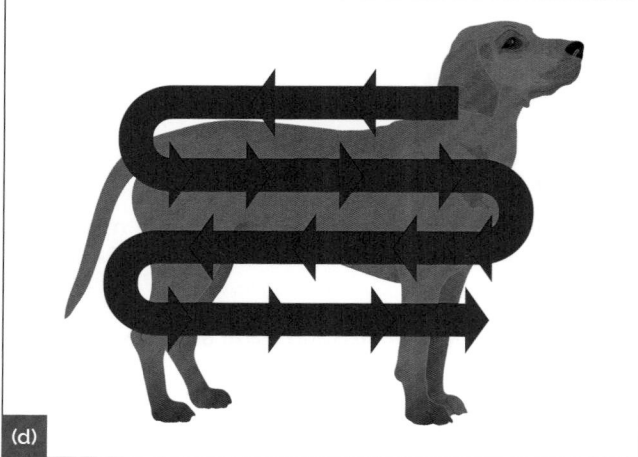

(d)

10.4 *continued* **(c–d)** Scanning for microchips should be systematic in pattern.

- Repeat the **slow S pattern** on both sides of the animal from head to tail (Figure 10.4cd).
- If a microchip is still not found, slowly scan the chest and abdomen using a slow S pattern from head to tail.

Where microchips have migrated, it is the responsibility of the veterinary nurse to inform the owner.

Microchip Adverse Event Reporting Scheme

Veterinary surgeons and veterinary nurses should report an adverse reaction to a microchip or the failure of a microchip to the Veterinary Medicines Directorate (VMD). Further information about the Microchip Adverse Event Reporting Scheme is available from the Pharmacovigilance Unit at the VMD and reports can be submitted online (www.vmd.defra.gov.uk). The VMD closely monitors all reports to identify emerging issues and will feed back any concerns to the chip manufacturer and Microchip Trade Association (MTA).

Vaccination

Vaccinations are the mainstay of preventative healthcare in companion animals. Under Schedule 3 of the Veterinary Surgeon's Act 1966, the administration of vaccinations to companion animals can be delegated to RVNs and student veterinary nurses, providing that certification is not required. To give a first vaccination with a prescription-only medicine (veterinary) (POM-V), the animal must be under the care of the prescribing veterinary surgeon and a full clinical assessment must be carried out. The veterinary surgeon may then administer or, under his or her direction, an RVN or supervised student veterinary nurse may administer, the vaccination.

The subsequent vaccination approximately 2–4 weeks later (i.e. close in time to the first vaccination) should be authorized by the veterinary surgeon at the time of the first vaccination; this allows the administration of the second vaccination to be undertaken by an RVN or a supervised student veterinary nurse at the practice, provided that the veterinary surgeon is not intending to certify the vaccination. Nevertheless, it is advisable for a veterinary surgeon to be on the premises at the time the vaccine is administered to the animal, to be able to assist in the event of the animal suffering an adverse reaction.

RVNs need an understanding of the different types of vaccine and their modes of action. Client education can prove very important in compliance with lifelong vaccination of the animal (see Chapter 7).

Pet Passport Scheme

The current European Union (EU) Pet Passport Scheme will remain in place until further notice. At present, in order to travel within the EU and those non-EU countries that are listed on the government website, the following are required:

- A microchip
- A rabies vaccination (make sure the pet is microchipped first or the vaccination will be invalid)
- A Pet Passport or official third country veterinary certificate
- Tapeworm treatment (for dogs only) for re-entry into the United Kingdom (UK). The treatment must have been given no less than 24 hours and no more than 120 hours (5 days) before re-entering the UK. Treatment for tapeworms is not required if the dog is coming in directly to the UK from Finland, Ireland, Malta or Norway. The treatment must be approved for use in the country in which it is being given and have praziquantel or an equivalent as its active ingredient.

Some elements of the passport require Official Veterinarian (OV) signature. An OV is a private practice veterinarian who performs work on behalf of an EU member state. The work performed by the OV is normally of a statutory nature (i.e. is required by law) and is often undertaken at public expense. Full details are available on the Defra website, but in short the passport must be filled out as follows:

- Sections I–III: can be completed by practice support staff or a veterinarian. The owner may affix the photograph in Section II
- Section IV: the first two boxes can be completed by a practice veterinarian. The final box (authorized veterinarian) must be completed by a Panel 2 Official Veterinarian (Local Veterinary Inspector)
- Section V: must be completed by a Panel 2 Official Veterinarian
- Sections VI–IX: can be completed by a practice veterinarian.

Where appropriate, the passport should be stamped and signed by a Panel 2 Local Veterinary Inspector appointed by Defra, the Scottish Executive Environment and Rural Affairs Department or National Assembly for Wales as an OV for export purposes. The passport must be signed and stamped with the OV stamp in any ink colour other than black.

Flea and worm control

Discussion of preventative health regimes is an important aspect of nurse consultations. Underpinning knowledge of parasite life cycles is required in order to explain parasite control and how different active ingredients effect each aspect of the life cycle (see Chapter 6). Accurate weighing of all animals needs to be undertaken regularly in order for the correct dosage of parasite control to be dispensed. Weight should be recorded in the clinical history each time the pet is weighed.

In the UK, there are four main categories of authorized veterinary medicinal products (VMPs) (see Chapter 8):

- Prescription-only medicine – veterinarian (POM-V)
- Prescription-only medicine – veterinarian, pharmacist, suitably qualified person (POM-VPS)
- Non-food animal – veterinarian, pharmacist, suitably qualified person (NFA-VPS)
- Authorized veterinary medicine – general sales list (AVM-GSL).

Practice protocols will dictate which parasite control is preferred. Those that are POM-Vs will require a prescription from the veterinary surgeon. A prescription can be written annually by the veterinary surgeon and then dispensed throughout the length of the prescription by a competent individual. Many RVNs have additional qualifications as a Suitably Qualified Person (SQP) in order to dispense prescription-only medicines. Prescription-only medicines – veterinarian, pharmacist, SQP (POM-VPS) can be prescribed by a veterinary surgeon, pharmacist or SQP. Non-food animal medicines – veterinarian, pharmacist, SQP (NFA-VPS) do not require a require a prescription but must be supplied by a veterinary surgeon, pharmacist or SQP.

Parasite control in all species (including exotic pets) is an important aspect of husbandry. Pre-hibernation checks of tortoises should include faecal flotation analysis and worming, if required (see Chapter 6 for more details). Examination of the animal for external parasites can be performed by combing through the hair with an appropriate comb or via tape impressions for those with scales.

Socialization of puppies and kittens

Owners should be encouraged to attend monthly puppy or kitten clinics from the time their pet is vaccinated through to at least 6 months of age. There are many advantages of these clinics, including the opportunity to bond the client to the practice, and for preventative healthcare and socialization, as well as parasite control and prevention. Adolescent health checks at (on average) 6 months of age can also be performed by the veterinary nurse.

The role of the veterinary nurse in educating clients in the importance of puppy and kitten socialization is paramount. Veterinary practices should openly promote puppy and kitten clinics, puppy parties and puppy socialization groups. Nurses need to understand how puppies and kittens assimilate these learning processes in order to fully convey to owners why their pets display certain behaviours.

The socialization period begins at 3 weeks of age and is a period of rapid brain development that coincides with the maturation and myelination of the spinal cord. At this age the puppy/kitten becomes fully aware of, and able to respond to, its environment. There are many features of socialization that occur in the main socialization period (between 4 and 14 weeks in puppies; shorter in kittens), but the features of most long-term behavioural significance are:

- Development of anticipatory responses as a result of an increased ability to attend to the environment
- Emergence of social behaviour, including determination of relative rank
- Ability to form primary social relationships with conspecifics and with other animals (including people).

In puppies there is a rapid increase in the tendency to approach unfamiliar people up to the age of 5 weeks old. After 5 weeks of age, puppies can become increasingly cautious of unfamiliar individuals or situations, but social motivation to approach and interact outweigh fear up to the age of 8 weeks old. From the age of 12–14 weeks, puppies can become easily frightened, and it has been concluded that after 12–14 weeks the growing tendency to react fearfully to novelty puts an end to effective socialization. During the juvenile period (14 weeks to sexual maturity), gradual improvement in motor skills occurs, and refinement of behaviour patterns in both relevance and context are seen. During this period there is an increased tendency to explore the environment. At about 4 months of age, the speed of formation of conditioned reflexes begins to slow down, as associations made previously probably interfere with new learning. There is evidence for a second period of heightened sensitivity to fear-provoking stimuli just before puberty at around 4–6 months (Riemer et al., 2014).

The role of the veterinary nurse in aiding clients with the socialization of puppies must start from a very early age. Greater results can be achieved if socialization is started whilst the puppy is still with the bitch. This can only be achieved if breeders are welcome to ideas and take on the responsibility of socialization of the puppies. Feeding behaviour when with litter mates can greatly influence feeding behaviour in adulthood. Puppies when with litter mates should have their own food bowl; puppies that have to share bowls are more likely to bolt food down (this can result in vomiting if food is eaten too quickly) and guard their food, resulting in aggression towards food.

When puppies are presented to the veterinary practice they are usually 8 weeks old, an age where socialization is exceptionally important. Nurse clinics are an ideal opportunity to educate owners on why socialization is required and how to achieve it. Monthly clinics are a useful opportunity to ensure that worming regimes are being adhered to and that appropriate socialization is taking place. Veterinary surgeons are vital in their role during the primary vaccination course to highlight to clients the importance of socialization and of attending puppy socialization parties. It is also important to remember that this visit to the practice is usually the puppy's first visit and therefore needs to be as atraumatic as possible and positively pleasant for the puppy.

Puppy parties (Figure 10.5) are mainly run by veterinary nurses and are vital in educating owners how to socialize their puppy. Many organizations, including the Kennel Club, Dogs Trust and PDSA, have information and have socialization charts that can be followed by owners and these provide a good indication of the things that they should be looking at achieving with their puppy. It is important to instil in owners that puppies should be socialized in a vast variety of different ways: circumstances can change and therefore puppies should be socialized in everything that they may possibly encounter during their lives. People that live in rural areas should take their puppies into the city, and vice versa, for socialization. Owners that do not have children still need to socialize their puppy with children. A new baby may come into the house later on in the dog's life; it is impossible to predict the future and this should be highly emphasized to owners.

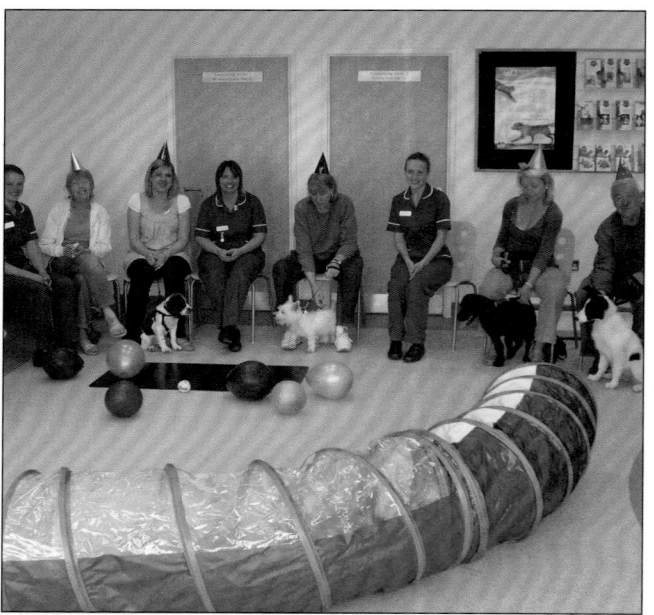

| 10.5 | Veterinary nurses can provide important client education in the form of puppy parties. (Reproduced from the *BSAVA Manual of Canine and Feline Advanced Veterinary Nursing, 2nd edn*) |

Recognition and prevention of behavioural problems

Understanding what is normal behaviour in cats, dogs and commonly encountered exotic species is required. When behaviours are displayed outside the norm, referral to the veterinary surgeon should be instigated. Prevention of behavioural problems is part of the veterinary nurse's role in owner education. Commonly encountered problems include house-training puppies, aversion to fireworks, abnormal feeding behaviours and stress in cats. A basic understanding of these problems is required. It is also important that veterinary nurses can take a behavioural history from the client so that they can guide the owner to useful sources of information, including leaflets and websites.

PetSavers client information leaflets

PetSavers has developed a range of client information leaflets on topics such as caring for elderly pets, advice on caring for pets with diabetes and behavioural problems.

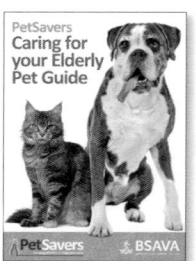 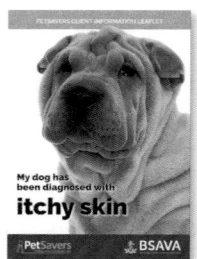 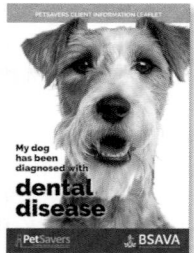
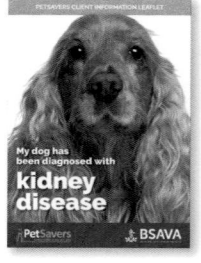 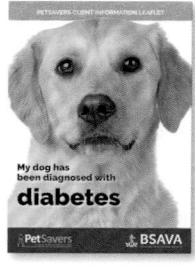 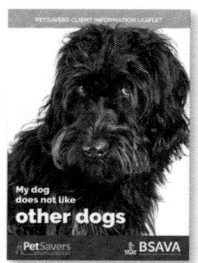

Nutritional consultations

Nutritional consultations should be offered for all animals, both healthy and unwell. For healthy animals, consultations should include discussion about lifestage diets, feeding behaviours and how to calculate feeding quantities. An accurate bodyweight and body condition score (BCS) should be obtained as part of the consultation. Client education at certain times, for example, when metabolic changes occur (i.e. following neutering or at the end of the growth stage), can help to prevent obesity. Those animals that are unwell need a nutritional assessment, which alongside the clinical history and any diagnostic findings, can help guide a nutritional recommendation (see Chapter 13 for more details).

Weight management

The weight management of pets is an element of preventative healthcare that needs to be advocated by veterinary nurses. Obesity is on the rise within the pet population and is believed to be the biggest health and welfare concern. It obesity can be prevented in the first place, the welfare of the pet will be greatly improved.

The conditions associated with obesity are both life-limiting and life-threatening, so it is important that there is a clear understanding of the risks. There are a number of endocrine diseases associated with obesity, including diabetes mellitus, hypoadrenocorticism and hypothyroidism. Orthopaedic disease is also associated with obesity, with overweight dogs more likely to be treated for lameness and ruptured cruciate ligaments. Obesity and cardiovascular disease are heavily linked in human medicine and have been more recently reported in dogs (Tropf *et al.*, 2017). Obesity can also have a profound effect on respiratory function, increasing the risk of tracheal collapse in small dogs (German, 2006). It has been shown that expiratory airway resistance is greater in obese dogs compared with animals of a normal weight during periods of hyperpnoea (e.g. during exercise) (Bach *et al.*, 2007).

Veterinary nurses can play a key role in educating clients about having a healthier pet as a result of weight loss. It is important that there is a clear strategy for targeting and supporting owners of overweight pets by providing a well thought out and delivered weight management service.

- Establish the animal's bodyweight at the beginning of the clinic. As there is significant breed variation in frame size and conformation, ideal breed weights can be inaccurate. A BCS (see Chapter 13) should be used alongside the animal's weight in order to ensure that an accurate picture of the animal's overall condition is recorded before a weight loss programme is initiated.
- Establish the animal's calorific needs at its ideal bodyweight. This is important at this stage and should be calculated using the resting energy requirement (RER) equation ($70 \times$ ideal bodyweight $(kg)^{0.75}$). Calculating the RER for the animal at its ideal bodyweight is often the best way to start any weight loss programme.
- A 20% reduction from the current intake can be a good starting point. This may be a dramatic reduction in food and should not occur all in one go. Regular and effective communication with the owner is necessary during the programme to ensure that the weight loss does not occur too quickly or that the owner becomes disillusioned with the process.
- It may be possible to reduce bodyweight by feeding less of the animal's original food; however, there has been research that suggests that this may result in a reduction in vital nutrients (German *et al.*, 2007). It has also been suggested that a weight loss programme that uses the animal's own food is less likely to be successful than one using a commercial weight loss diet. There are many different diets aimed at the correction of obesity, with different nutrient specifications. Finding the best one for the animal will very much be on an individual basis. Increasing the fibre content of diets for dogs can potentially increase the feeling of satiety, and this may lead to a reduction in begging and scavenging behaviour. However, it is thought that this is a behavioural problem and not one related to nutrition (German *et al.*, 2012). Behaviour is a really important aspect in obesity control and prevention and feeding patterns, and how we present the food (e.g. puzzle feeders) is potentially more important than what is fed.

Breeding and neutering

Ideally, all clients should seek veterinary advice prior to breeding from their pet. When discussing neutering with owners, veterinary nurses need to refer to evidence-based medicine. The British Small Animal Veterinary Association (BSAVA) and British Veterinary Association (BVA) recommend that pet cats are neutered from 16 weeks of age. In the case of feral and rescue kittens, it may be necessary to neuter earlier than 16 weeks, due to the age at which they were trapped. In these circumstances, neutering at 8–12 weeks of age is considered safe and appropriate compared with the harm of not neutering. The BVA believes that there is no current scientific evidence to support the view that spaying of bitches should take place after the first 'season' and that there is insufficient data available to form a position of the early neutering of dogs and bitches (www.bva.co.uk/take-action/our-policies/neutering-of-cats-and-dogs/). Changes to advice and practice protocols should be regularly discussed within the practice with other veterinary professionals. For further information, the reader is referred to Chapter 24.

Dental home care

It is important that all veterinary professionals provide the same advice regarding dental healthcare; a practice protocol on this aspect can be very useful. Puppy and kitten consultations should involve habitualization of handling the animal's mouth and gradual introduction of dental hygiene treatment, leading up to brushing. Tooth brushing is the gold standard of dental hygiene care and should be advocated in all patients. Mechanical removal of plaque from the tooth surface and the gingival sulcus is most effectively achieved with a toothbrush, as the bristles can sweep subgingivally and remove the plaque (Bloor, 2015). The introduction of tooth brushing can take weeks and the offer of support throughout the process can help to provide motivation and ensure compliance.

The aim of dental homecare is to reduce plaque formation and hence prevent the development of periodontitis, or after periodontitis has occurred to slow the destruction of the periodontal ligament and thus save the tooth. There are two main ways in which plaque control can be achieved:

- Physically (tooth brushing, chews and diets)
- Chemically (chlorhexidine, xylitol additives; note that caution should be exercised with the use of xylitol additives as they can be toxic to dogs).

The best homecare plans usually involve more than one form of treatment. No single product or technique is 100% effective and, like people, pets still need regular examinations with a veterinary professional.

Veterinary nurses should be involved in the post-procedure consultations for all animals that have undergone a dental procedure (cats, dogs and rabbits) to discuss dental homecare and diet (see also Chapter 25). Nutrition plays an integral role in dental homecare; discussion of appropriate food that will not damage the teeth is important. Owners need to be educated about unsuitable toys, stone chewing and sticks in order to prevent any damage to the teeth and mouth.

Mobility clinics

An owner's perception of mobility in older pets can be difficult to ascertain, as many think that their pet is sleeping more or not playing as much due to age rather than a reduction in mobility. Careful questioning of the owner, alongside use of a chronic pain score (e.g. the Helsinki Chronic Pain Index or the Liverpool Osteoarthritis in Dogs (LOAD) questionnaire), can be useful in identifying whether there is an issue and helping owners acknowledge the problem. A clinical diagnosis will need to be made by the veterinary surgeon and medication may also need to be prescribed. Nurse clinics are the ideal situation in which to discuss nutritional support, nutraceutical supplements, reaching and maintaining an ideal BCS and MCS, exercise and the pet's environment with the owner. Adaptations to the existing environment may include the provision of ramps, rather than steps, low-sided litter boxes, non-slip flooring and padded bedding.

Diabetes clinics

A diagnosis of diabetes mellitus (see Chapter 18) can be very overwhelming for an owner and support from the veterinary nurse, in what can be a difficult time, is important. Owners will need guidance on the administration, storage and use of insulin, monitoring of the pet, exercise and feeding regimes and what to do if the pet becomes unwell. Having a written practice protocol for these clinics can be useful to ensure that standardized advice is given. Some practices have moved away from long-term monitoring of patients using glucose curves, and nurse clinics are ideally placed to take blood samples for fructosamine levels, blood pressure monitoring, urine testing and clinical examination. Guidelines on care for diabetic patients needs to follow the requirements of the veterinary surgeon in charge of the case. Good communication between the veterinary nurse and veterinary surgeon is needed to ensure good care of the patient and client.

Renal clinics

Early identification of patients with chronic kidney disease is helpful in the long-term management of these cases. Screening programmes for adult and senior pets can aid early identification. The mainstay of treatment for patients with renal disease is nutritional management; phosphate should be restricted and excess protein should be controlled. Owners will need guidance on nutritional management with a renal diet, advice of transitioning to a renal diet, and how to monitor their pet at home. In many renal clinics, the veterinary nurse is also responsible for the measurement of blood pressure at required intervals, blood testing and urine testing. Management of renal disease can be difficult and may include discussion of quality of life (QoL) at some point. Use of QoL measurement scales (such as the HHHHHMM scale; see Chapter 1) can help owners in the quantification of QoL.

Nail clipping

Many animals are presented to the practice for nail clipping, including exotic species (see Chapter 14). Nail clipping for cats, dogs and small mammals can be performed during a nurse consultation. Nail clipping in cats does require extra time as discussion with the client about normal feline behaviour is required. If the cat's nails are overgrown, then discussion is required regarding why the cat is not scratching; the potential for arthritis should be considered. It should also be

remembered that senior cats can sometimes lose the ability to fully retract their claws, so they can appear longer than they actually are. In these cases, it is important not to clip the claws too closely. Referral to the veterinary surgeon may be required.

Nail clipping in fearful dogs needs to be performed empathetically. Forceful restraint of a fearful dog will not improve the situation. Slow habitualization of the dog with the veterinary practice, handling and nail trimming will be required. Discussion of the case should occur with a veterinary surgeon. Handling and grooming are important aspects of husbandry that should be discussed with clients during puppy and kitten clinics, and when exotic species are presented to practice.

Postoperative checks

Postoperative checks can be completed by veterinary nurses and good clinical details should be recorded in the patient history at each stage. Clients should be advised that their pet may be a little quieter than normal immediately following surgery, but should never be sent home if drowsy. They should be encouraged to provide their pet with a comfortable bed or basket, away from draughts and noise. Young children and other animals should be discouraged from disturbing the pet.

Animals should be fed in the postoperative period once they have sufficiently recovered. A highly digestible low-fat food is recommended, as it will reduce the potential for vomiting. Exercise may need to be restricted, depending on the procedure performed. Each practice should have a written protocol providing details for instructions for staff to give out the same correct advise to clients. Clients should be advised about the signs of discomfort to look out for and what analgesics should be given. Wounds should be checked daily and bandages kept client and dry (see below). All information should be given both verbally and in a written format such as handouts or in an electronic form.

Bandage checks and changes

Bandages should be frequently checked and changed. The frequency of these changes should be determined by the clinical condition, although every 3–4 days is normally acceptable if the correct placement technique has been used (see Chapter 15). Records relating to bandaging changes and wound management should include details about the appearance of the wound (including measurements and photographs), so that progress can be monitored.

Prior to patient discharge, veterinary nurses should educate clients regarding the signs of bandage-related problems and their implications, and provide written details on bandaging care. Follow-up appointments to check and change or remove bandages should also be made.

There are numerous reasons why a patient may develop further injuries following bandage application. The two main causes can be classified as primary and secondary ischaemic injury.

■ Primary ischaemic injury occurs whilst the bandage is still in place. This may be due to interruption of the blood flow to the tissues, which causes direct pressure necrosis.
■ Secondary ischaemic and reperfusion injury occurs 24–48 hours after the removal of the bandage. This is due to the return of blood to tissue that has suffered a

period of ischaemia or lack of oxygen. An inflammatory reaction results, which causes deterioration of wound even after the bandage has been removed.

Inappropriate bandage application includes those that are placed too tightly or become constrictive after the affective area swells or the dressing becomes wet. Soft tissue abrasions can occur if the bandage slips from its original location as a result of being applied too loosely. Insufficient padding may also result in inadequate protection or skin damage. Further information can be found in Chapter 15.

Suture removal

When the wound has healed so that it no longer needs the support of non-absorbable suture material, skin sutures must be removed. The length of time the sutures remain in place depends upon the rate of healing and the nature of the wound, but is typically 10–14 days. Sutures should be removed using a clean or aseptic technique.

- The area should be cleansed with an antiseptic. Hydrogen peroxide can be used to remove dried serum encrusted around the sutures.
- One end of the suture should be picked up with either the thumb and index finger or thumb forceps and cut as close as possible to where it enters the skin.
- The suture strand should be gently pulled out through the side opposite the knot using forceps.
- To prevent infection, the suture material should be removed without pulling any portion that has been outside the skin, back through the skin.

Advice on the care of senior pets

It is recommended that all pets are seen annually by a veterinary surgeon for their health check and vaccination; 6 months later these animals should see a veterinary nurse for an interim health check. These interim clinics should be tailored to the meet the needs of the individual patient. For dogs and cats over 7–8 years of age, attending a geriatric clinic should be recommended.

Setting up and running geriatric clinics that are valued by the client, pet and the veterinary practice is an essential part of building a client relationship. These clinics may be promoted via the practice newsletter, social media, practice website or on reminder letters (e.g. booster vaccinations). The underlying message should be of health monitoring, not of finding a problem. Engaging pet owners in screening and monitoring programmes helps promote preventative healthcare, and clients that are educated about the signs of illness are more likely to notice and report problems earlier, making treatment more effective in many cases.

All consultations should comprise a full clinical history, clinical examination, urine testing and blood pressure monitoring, especially in cats. A detailed clinical history needs to be obtained from each owner and should include information relating to behaviour and feeding patterns. Nurses are in an ideal position to question owners about their pets, and some owners may speak more freely with a veterinary nurse than a veterinary surgeon. Appropriate questioning and scoring against pain management criteria can assist in the early identification of changes required to the existing analgesia or medication provision. Blood testing can be a useful screening tool for age-related changes, but can be cost prohibitive in some cases.

Nutrition in senior pets is very much dependent on the individual. The prevalence of obesity increases with age in dogs, whereas in cats after the age of 8 years old bodyweight may decrease. Weight management should be considered in any age of pet, as quality of life is greatly affected by obesity (Yam *et al.*, 2016). Some senior cats have an energy and protein requirement similar to that of the growth phase in kittens. Senior rabbits still require *ad libitum* amounts of fresh hay, water and greens on a daily basis. Many food companies now offer extruded nuggets, specifically manufactured for the dietary needs of senior rabbits. Senior rabbits should be weighed weekly so that the volume of food provided can be adjusted based on their weight and energy levels. This highlights the importance of undertaking a nutritional assessment at each consultation.

Discussion in these consultations should cover commonly encountered problems in older age, but again this will be dependent on the species and the individual. Conditions that are more likely to be seen in older aged animals include:

- Degenerative joint disease
- Dental disease
- Hyperthyroidism (cats)
- Chronic kidney disease
- Liver disease
- Heart disease.

Diagnostic testing for these conditions can be undertaken during nurse consultations (Figure 10.6). A practice protocol for how each condition should be managed will provide guidance as to what tests need to be performed in each nurse consultation for each individual animal. Consensus statements are regularly produced by specialist societies and can be used to help shape practice protocols (for example, the International Society for Feline Medicine (ISFM) Consensus Statement on the diagnosis and treatment of chronic kidney disease; Sparkes *et al.*, 2016).

The topics of quality-of-life and euthanasia are a lot easier to approach if the veterinary nurse has an established relationship with the client (see also Chapters 1 and 9).

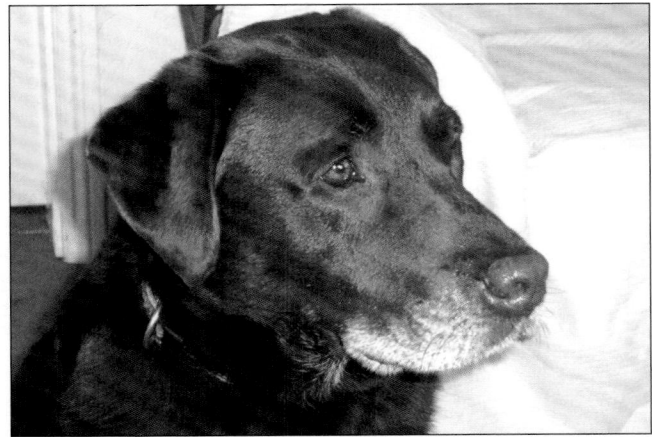

10.6 A healthy senior pet makes an ideal candidate to attend a screening clinic to ensure it is not at risk of suffering from an undiagnosed condition. (Reproduced from the *BSAVA Manual of Canine and Feline Advanced Veterinary Nursing, 2nd edn.*)

References and further reading

Ackerman N (2012) *The Consulting Veterinary Nurse.* Wiley Blackwell, Oxford

Bach JF, Rozanski EA, Bedenice D, Chan DL, Freeman LM *et al.* (2007) Association of expiratory airway dysfunction with marked obesity in healthy adult dogs. *American Journal of Veterinary Research* **68(6)**, 670–675

Bard AM, Main DCJ, Haase AM, Whay HR, Roe EJ *et al.* (2017) The future of veterinary communication: partnership or persuasion? A qualitative investigation of veterinary communication in the pursuit of client behaviour change. *PLoS One* **12(3)**, e0171380

Bloor C (2015) Oral homecare regimens and products. *Veterinary Nurse* **6(9)**, 522–530

British Veterinary Association (BVA) (2016) Pet obesity epidemic is top welfare concern for vets. Available from: www.bva.co.uk/news-and-blog/news-article/pet-obesity-epidemic-is-top-welfare-concern-for-vets/

German AJ (2006) The growing problem of obesity in dogs and cats. *Journal of Nutrition* **136(7)**, 1940S–1946S

German AJ, Holden SL, Bissot T, Hackett RM and Biourge V (2007) Dietary energy restriction and successful weight loss in obese client-owned dogs. *Journal of Veterinary Internal Medicine* **21**, 1174–1180

German AJ, Holden SL, Morris PJ and Biourge V (2012) Long-term follow-up after weight management in obese dogs: the role of diet in preventing regain. *The Veterinary Journal* **192(1)**, 65–70

Hielm-Bjorkman AK and Tulamo RM (2009) Psychometric testing of the Helsinki chronic pain index by completion of a questionnaire in Finnish by owners of dogs with chronic signs of pain caused by osteoarthritis. *American Journal of Veterinary Research* **70(6)**, 727–734

Hotston Moore A and Rudd S (2008) *BSAVA Manual of Canine and Feline Advanced Veterinary Nursing, 2nd edn.* BSAVA Publications, Gloucester

Mader DM (2015) Physical examination: the cornerstone of veterinary medicine. *Clinician's Brief* 13–17

Olin SJ and Tolbert MK (2016) Starting off right: checklists are essential for a good history. *Veterinary Team Brief* 13–16

Pet Food Manufacturer's Association (PFMA) (2019) Pet obesity: 10 years on (2009–2019). Available from: www.pfma.org.uk

Riemer S, Muller C, Viranyi Z, Huber L and Range F (20014) The predictive value of early behavioural assessments in pet dogs – a longitudinal study from neonates to adults. *PLoS ONE* **9(7)**, 1–13

Sparkes AH, Caney S, Chalhoub S, Elliott J, Finch N *et al.* (2016) ISFM Consensus Guidelines on the Diagnosis and Management of Feline Chronic Kidney Disease. *Journal of Feline Medicine and Surgery* **18(3)**, 219–239

Tropf M, Nelson OL, Lee PM and Weng HY (2017) Cardiac and metabolic variables in obese dogs. *Journal of Veterinary Internal Medicine* **31(4)**, 1000–1007

Walton MB, Cowderoy E, Lascelles D and Innes JF (2013) Evaluation of construct and criterion validity for the 'Liverpool Osteoarthritis in Dogs' (LOAD) clinical meterology instrument and comparison to two other instruments. *PLoS One* **8(3)**, e58125

Weber M, Bissot T, Servet E, Sergheraert R, Biourge V and German AJ (2007) A high-protein, high fiber diet designed for weight loss improve satiety in dogs. *Journal of Veterinary Internal Medicine* **21(6)**, 1203–1208

Wortinger A and Burns K (2015) *Nutrition and Disease Management for Veterinary Technicians and Nurses, 2nd edn.* Wiley Blackwell, Oxford

Yam PS, Butowski CF, Chitty JL, Naughton G, Wiseman-Orr ML *et al.* (2016) Impact of canine overweight and obesity on health-related quality of life. *Preventive Veterinary Medicine* **127**, 64–69

Useful websites

Animal and Plant Health Agency (APHA) – Official Veterinarian:
http://apha.defra.gov.uk/official-vets/index.htm

British Veterinary Association (BVA):
- Advice for pet owners:
www.bva.co.uk/pet-owners-and-breeders/advice-for-pet-owners/
- Neutering of cats and dogs:
www.bva.co.uk/take-action/our-policies/neutering-of-cats-and-dogs

Defra – Get your dog microchipped:
www.gov.uk/get-your-dog-microchipped

Kennel Club – I'm looking for a puppy or dog:
www.thekennelclub.org.uk/getting-a-dog-or-puppy/

PDSA – Get PetWise:
www.pdsa.org.uk/taking-care-of-your-pet/choosing-a-pet

Royal College of Veterinary Surgeons Code of Professional Conduct for Veterinary Nurses:
www.rcvs.org.uk/advice-and-guidance/code-of-professional-conduct-for-veterinary-nurses/

Veterinary Medicine Directorate – Pharmacological Unit:
www.gov.uk/guidance/veterinary-pharmacovigilance-your-responsibilities

Self-assessment questions

1. When performing a nutritional assessment what three factors should you include?
2. What are the legal requirements for veterinary nurses performing second vaccinations in nurse consultations?
3. What are the steps within the Cambridge-Calgary consultation model?
4. What advice would you give the client of an obese dog requiring weekly weight loss?
5. What are the differences between open and closed questioning techniques?
6. What are the legal requirements of prescribing and dispensing preventative flea control?
7. At what age should puppies be microchipped in the UK? Who is legally responsible for this?
8. What six factors should be considered for the elderly patient?
9. What three factors should you include in a dental care protocol for an owner with a young dog?
10. What five factors should be included in the written protocol for owners of a diabetic cat?

Chapter 11

Animal handling, restraint and transport

Clare Wilson with exotic pets by Simon Girling

Learning objectives

After studying this chapter, readers will have the knowledge to:

- Describe how to handle and restrain dogs, cats and exotic pets correctly for examination, transportation and treatment
- Adopt canine and feline communication strategies and behaviour as a foundation for an approach to animal capture, handling and restraint that is both ethologically appropriate and causes minimal stress
- Identify why animals might show anxiety or fear behaviour at the veterinary practice and use methods of approach, catching, handling and restraint that recognize and minimize anxiety and fear
- Discuss basic learning theory in animals and how this applies to the veterinary context
- Describe approaches used to interact with, handle and restrain dogs, cats and exotic pets to ensure human safety whilst providing excellent patient welfare
- Adopt techniques to manage the handling of aggressive or potentially aggressive patients, including the use of relevant equipment
- Apply the principles of handling and restraint to use in everyday veterinary practice

Introduction

Veterinary nurses are commonly required to handle and restrain animals for various reasons and must learn how to do so for the safety of the animals, staff and clients. Appropriate handling of animals allows tasks to be completed efficiently and with minimal distress to the patient. Stress has detrimental consequences such as triggering defensive aggressive behaviour or escape attempts, as well as adverse effects on healing, immunity and health. Client perceptions must also be considered; if respect and care is shown towards their animal, the client-practice relationship will improve, providing long-term benefits.

Aims of handling and restraint:

- To ensure high standards of patient welfare and minimize distress
- To allow efficient examination, treatment or procedures
- To ensure safety of all involved (patients, staff and clients), particularly in relation to using sharps or instruments, as well as in relation to the responses of the animal, both of which risk causing injury
- To ensure that existing injuries, pain or distress are not exacerbated.

This chapter discusses not only handling techniques but also how to identify emotional states of patients through observation of behaviour and ways in which animals learn. This information is crucial for ensuring appropriate handling, in addition to creating long-term successful relationships between patients and the veterinary staff. When handling non-tame animals of any species, alternative techniques may be required due to the necessity to medically treat these patients. However, it must be noted in all cases that learning will affect future behavioural responses and, in cases where animals are excessively fearful, the use of chemical restraint (sedation or general anaesthesia) is preferable. It is also the case that all species, domesticated and non-domesticated, can be trained to allow minimally invasive handling techniques.

Canine and feline communication

Ethology is the study of animals' behaviour, in particular in their normal environment. Interacting with patients in an ethologically appropriate manner aims to ensure their wellbeing, whilst keeping the veterinary surgeon and veterinary nurse safe. Understanding normal behaviour and the strategies that animals use for communication is a crucial foundation for appropriate interaction. This enables staff to adapt techniques depending on the response of the patient and thus minimize fear and distress. Fear and pain are the most common underlying causes of aggressive behaviour in the veterinary context. Therefore, minimizing fear and being aware of potential pain reduces the risk of animals exhibiting aggressive behaviour.

Avoidance of conflict

Physical conflict is potentially dangerous in dogs and cats due to the risk of serious injury, so strategies for both species aim to minimize this risk. The strategies used in each species are different due to significant differences in their evolutionary and domestication history and are addressed separately (see below). In both species, one of the primary aims of communication is to avoid confrontation and physical conflict, so a thorough understanding of this is crucial for effective handling.

Canine communication

Dogs are highly adapted to social living and have well developed, complex means of communicating to ensure avoidance of conflict. They use visual, vocal, olfactory and tactile strategies, but those of primary relevance in a handling context are the visual signals of body language, including posture and facial expressions. It is essential to recognize subtle signs of anxiety and fear, and to identify the triggers for those responses in order to avoid the expression of aggressive behaviour.

Figure 11.1 illustrates the escalating responses of dogs that are seen when they feel under threat. Lower level signals (e.g. turning the head away, licking the nose and lifting a paw) are seen in response to low intensity threat. If the threat intensity increases, dogs will escalate their signalling in an effort to avoid physical confrontation. Only when dogs are feeling very threatened will they resort to biting. If a threat is suddenly very intense, dogs may bite without having the opportunity to show lower level signalling. Each individual will show unique responses as their perception of what is deemed a threat depends on several factors, such as genetics, early experience and physical illness/pain. Responses also vary depending on prior experience. If dogs have experience that lower level signalling is ignored, they may escalate more rapidly to growling, snapping and biting. It is therefore crucial that these communication signals are recognized and respected when interacting with patients.

Feline communication

The ancestor of the domestic cat was a highly territorial and solitary wild cat. Although the domestic cat has adapted to social living and is capable of making strong social bonds,

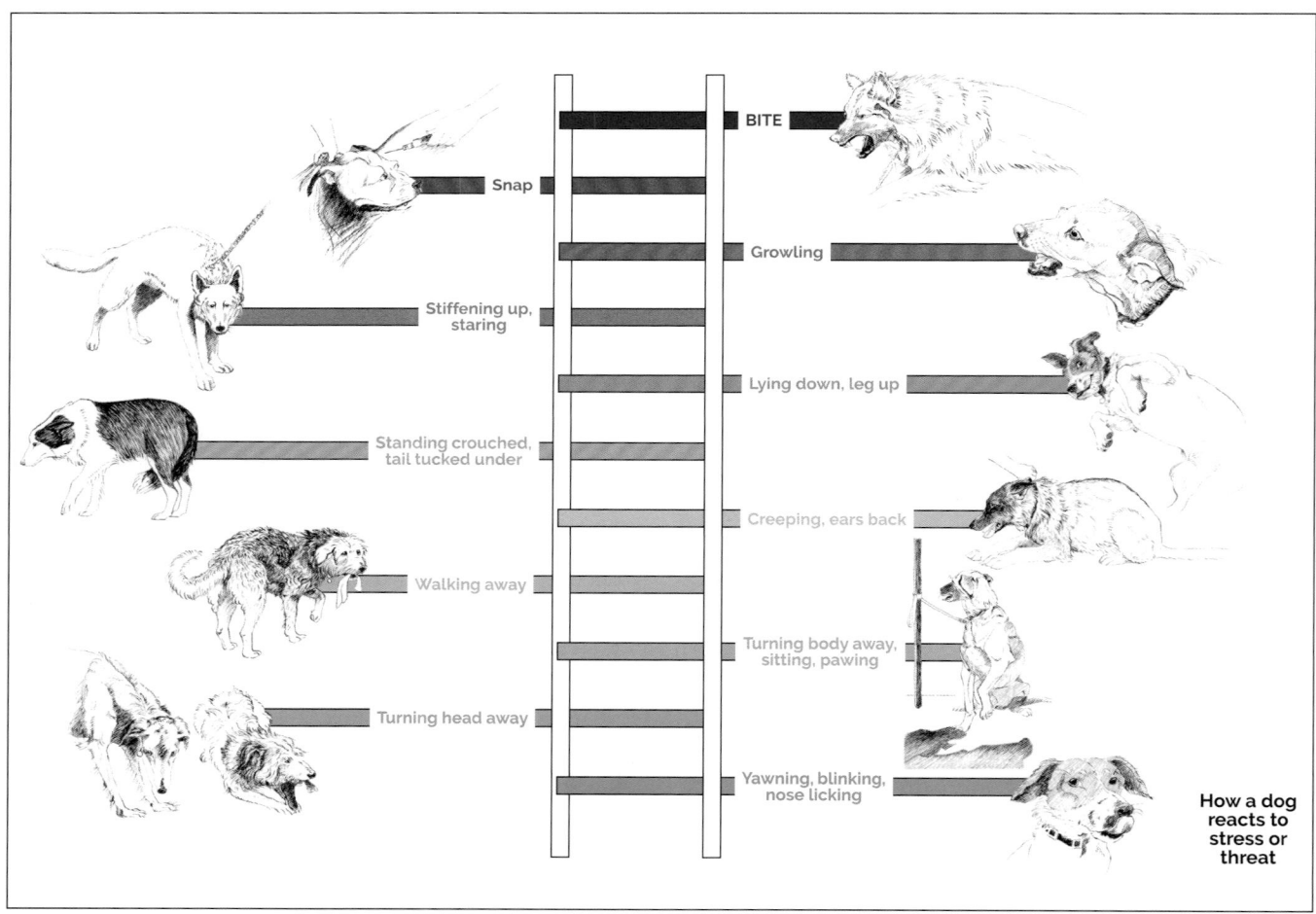

11.1 The Ladder of Aggression. (© Maggy Howard and Kendal Shepherd)

much of their communication is still based on their evolutionary history of solitary living and territorial behaviour. Cats have not developed an intricate system of escalating signals to appease threatening behaviour like dogs. Their system of communication is primarily based on using distance-maintaining strategies to avoid coming into close proximity with unfamiliar cats, in combination with using affiliative behaviours towards those within their social group. If these distance-maintaining strategies fail, cats have very limited communication skills for resolving conflict and, in this context, fights and injuries are common. Therefore, the veterinary professional needs to ensure that cats feel safe when handled in order to avoid defensive aggression and the risk of serious injury. Observing facial expressions and body posture provides a great deal of information about how a cat is feeling. Figure 11.2 illustrates changes in body posture and facial expressions that occur during different emotional states in cats.

Learning theory and its practical application to the veterinary context

Understanding how animals learn is crucial for working effectively with them in both short-term situations, such as in a 10-minute consultation, and for the long-term consideration of future surgery visits. The general processes discussed below occur not only during active training but also in everyday life in relation to all the environmental and social stimuli experienced.

Habituation

This is the process whereby the animal 'gets used to' a stimulus such that it no longer shows an active response to it. The purpose of such learning is to avoid overwhelming the sensory systems with information that is not useful. This is the process we should use when socializing young animals to stimuli we wish them to ignore in the future (e.g. traffic, fireworks, people and other dogs walking by).

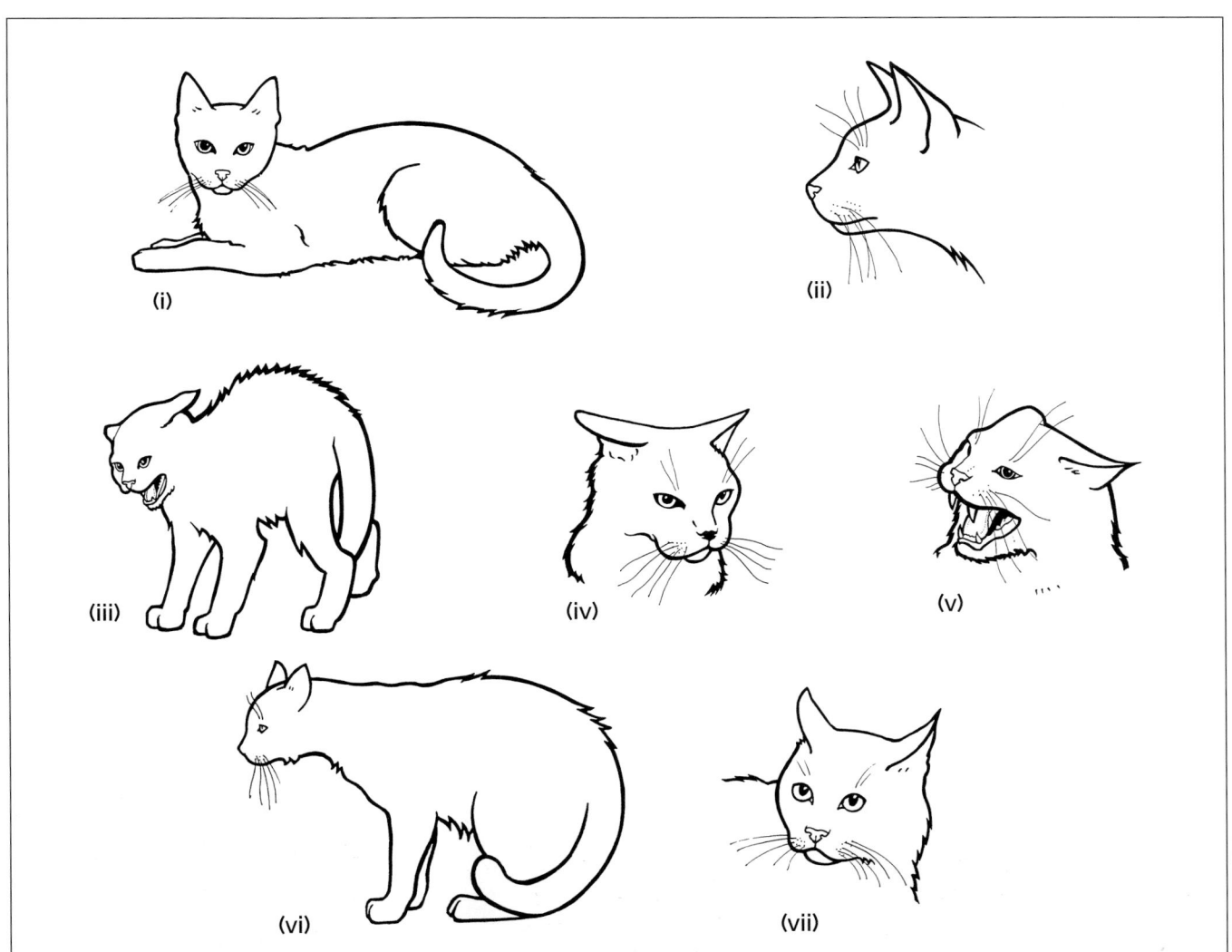

11.2 Feline visual communication signals help to differentiate between **(i–ii)** an alert non-threatened cat, **(iii–v)** a fearful and defensive cat and **(vi–vii)** a confident aggressive cat. (Reproduced from *An Ethogram for Behavioural Studies of the Domestic Cat (Felis silvestris catus L.)* by the UK Cat Behaviour Working Group (1995); plates 3, 4, 5, 6, 7, 16 and 17, by permission of Universities Federation for Animal Welfare (UFAW), Wheathampstead)

Sensitization

Sensitization is the opposite of habituation and results in the animal becoming more responsive to a stimulus over time. This is the basis of the development of sound phobias but is equally relevant to aversive experiences at the veterinary surgery, which can lead to increasingly fearful and anxious behaviour over time. This process needs to be avoided.

Associative learning

When two previously unrelated stimuli become relevant to each other, associative learning has occurred.

Classical conditioning

In this type of conditioning, an association is formed between two stimuli that were previously unrelated, based on instinctive responses. No 'thinking' is involved in this process. The purpose is to create predictive cues to make the world easier to understand and live in. It is happening all the time; for example, dogs make an association between their lead being picked up and going for a walk. This learning makes the world more predictable and therefore less stressful. This process must be used to prevent fear responses from developing by ensuring that handling, examination and treatment are paired with good consequences. For example, clipping nails or applying eardrops can be associated with food treats by doing the procedure then giving a treat. The timing of this is crucial, as the action must predict the food.

Operant conditioning

Operant conditioning is related to consequences of behaviour rather than just a simple association. There is an increase in the behaviour if it has positive (good) consequences and a decrease in the behaviour if the consequences are negative (bad) or neutral. As veterinary professionals, if we are aware of this learning process, situations can be created whereby the dog is set up to behave appropriately and is rewarded for that behaviour. For example, rewarding a dog for sitting as we pass a kennel door in the hospital will increase the frequency of sitting occurring in the future, as the dog learns that sitting predicts a beneficial outcome. If this form of learning is ignored in the clinic, dogs may inadvertently learn inappropriate responses, such as kennel guarding, as the frightened dog learns that aggressive responses keep people away from the kennel.

Desensitization

During this process, the animal's perception of a stimulus that results in sensitization is altered such that it shows a neutral response to it. This process can be used to reverse sensitization by very carefully exposing the animal to a stimulus they are sensitized to at a low intensity and allowing them to habituate to it. Over time, the intensity is increased at a rate the animal can cope with, so that when this process is complete the animal will ignore the stimulus when it is presented at a normal intensity.

Counter-conditioning

This process can be used to create a positive (good) association with a stimulus that previously caused a negative (bad) association. This is a crucial process to understand when working with animals who have developed fear responses to handling, restraint, examination and treatment. As with desensitization, the aim must be to present the stimulus (e.g. otoscope, syringe, nail clippers) at a low intensity so that the animal is relaxed in its presence and then to associate that experience with something positive (e.g. food, play, verbal praise, physical interaction).

Context specificity of learning – importance of generalization

Many dog owners will have done at least some basic training with their pets, either in the context of classes, at home or when out walking. However, their pets are unlikely to have practised responding to cues in the context of the veterinary surgery, or learned cues associated with a clinical examination or treatment. Learning occurs in a context-specific manner and, therefore, owners should be encouraged to practice responses to various cues in various different situations. The use of learned cues during veterinary examination and treatment can vastly aid handling (Figure 11.3).

Effects of stress on learning and response to learned cues

There are many emotional states that can lead to a stress response, including frustration, fear, anxiety and pain. Mild stress benefits the learning process but higher levels of

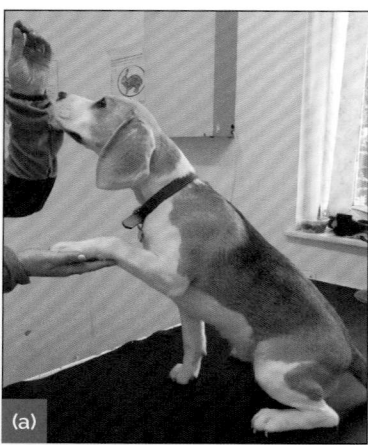
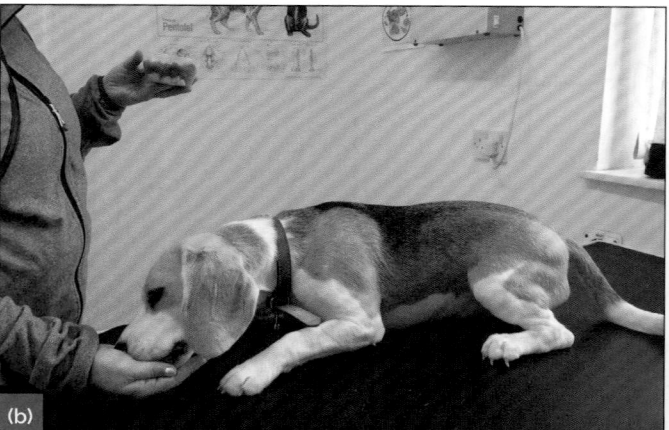
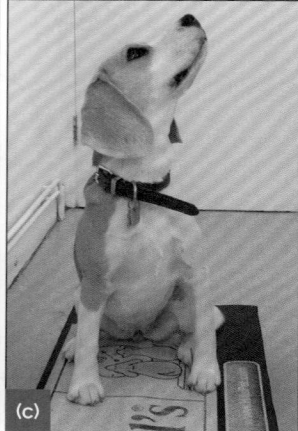

11.3 (a) Food lures, (b) rewards and (c) cued behaviours can aid examination of veterinary patients. (© C. Wilson)

stress, such as stress that may occur in some patients at the surgery, may adversely affect learning. Stress can reduce an animal's ability to learn new responses or respond to previously well-trained cue words such as 'sit'. However, stress also heightens the animal's ability to learn about negative (bad) experiences and, therefore, stressed animals are even more at risk of learning to show avoidance or defensive aggression if they are not interacted with appropriately. Just one aversive experience can have a powerful effect, particularly in young animals in their early visits to the surgery. Thus, it is always better to err on the side of caution and consider whether an individual patient is resilient enough to cope with the planned procedure or whether an alternative strategy might be more appropriate.

Initial approach and handling of dogs and cats

The manner in which animals are approached and handled will have a long-term effect on the client–practice relationship, affect the behaviour and welfare of the animal, and influence risks of aggressive and/or escape responses. Animals must therefore be treated with respect and handled gently and calmly. When the owner is present, not only is their opinion of how you treat their animal to be considered, but also their safety. Owners can be involved in assisting with handling, but the risks must always be assessed and other practice staff utilized if an owner is at risk of being injured. Owner behaviour should also be considered, as an overly anxious owner or an owner using forceful techniques on their animal may adversely influence the animal's behaviour. For some animals, particularly puppies, it is best to ensure that the owner is present as they provide important emotional security.

Fear and anxiety

Fear is the most common underlying reason for pets showing aggressive behaviour in the veterinary context (as discussed above). Animals become anxious or fearful for many reasons, for example ill health, pain, an unfamiliar environment, pre-existing fear of unfamiliar people, previous experience, owner anxiety about their pet's health or behaviour, aversive scents and stress during transport to the surgery. The concept of 'trigger stacking' must be considered (see Figure 11.4); this is where several small stressors have a cumulative effect and result in an animal going over their threshold for coping. Educating owners in how to reduce potential stressors (e.g. cat box training) can help pets to arrive at the surgery in a more relaxed state. Management of the waiting room, for example separate rooms for cats and dogs, partitions between dogs and avoiding long waiting times, can all reduce the build-up of stress.

Trigger stacking

There are many potential triggers that can cause stress at the surgery, one or two of which in isolation may not adversely affect the patient. However, if several triggers co-exist in a relatively short space of time, their ➡

Trigger stacking *continued*

cumulative effects can have severe consequences on the patient's ability to cope (Figure 11.4). The entire process of a surgery visit must be considered: the client getting the animal ready for transport, the journey itself, entry to and time spent in the waiting room, and every other aspect of the surgery visit. Addressing as many of these triggers as possible that affect an individual patient will be of significant benefit to subsequent handling and restraint

---

History-taking

Taking the history before examining the animal allows time for them to adjust to the situation in which they find themselves. It also provides for distant observation of the animal, for both behavioural and clinical purposes. Dogs and cats without a history of aggression can be allowed to explore the consulting room, dogs with their lead trailing and cat carriers opened to allow them the opportunity to exit should they choose to. Allowing cats to explore their three-dimensional (3D) environment is very beneficial and owners should be encouraged to allow them to do this rather than trying to contain them on the consulting table. During this time, some patients may choose to approach and initiate interaction, which can be welcomed with calm and gentle responses. In addition to asking the general clinical and pre-anaesthetic questions, owners should also be asked for behavioural information about their pet. This is of primary importance for patients that are to be hospitalized but is also relevant for consultation appointments (see also Chapters 10 and 14).

Distant observation

In addition to noticing specific communication signals in cats and dogs, observing general muscle tension and posture are also relevant to identifying emotional state. These can be observed from a distance when an animal first enters the surgery or consulting room, or is resting in a hospital cage, to provide an initial assessment. Identifying signs of anxiety or fear allows the type of approach to be tailored to the individual animal. Observing the distribution of bodyweight in the animal reveals whether they want to move away or towards us. Activation of the sympathetic nervous system in anxious or fearful animals results in various physical changes that can be observed at a distance. The respiratory rate may be elevated in anxious animals, resulting in panting in dogs, although dogs may pant for a variety of other reasons including increased environmental temperature and respiratory compromise. Cats only pant if severely stressed or if they have a compromised respiratory system. Widely dilated pupils, which are often non-responsive to pupillary light reflex testing, in combination with either staring or hypervigilance may indicate fear.

Environment observation

Animals have four basic responses when they are feeling frightened: freezing, flight (running away), fight (defensive aggression) or 'faffing about' (showing displacement behaviours such as sniffing, scratching, grooming). As discussed above, animals generally prefer to avoid conflict but, if

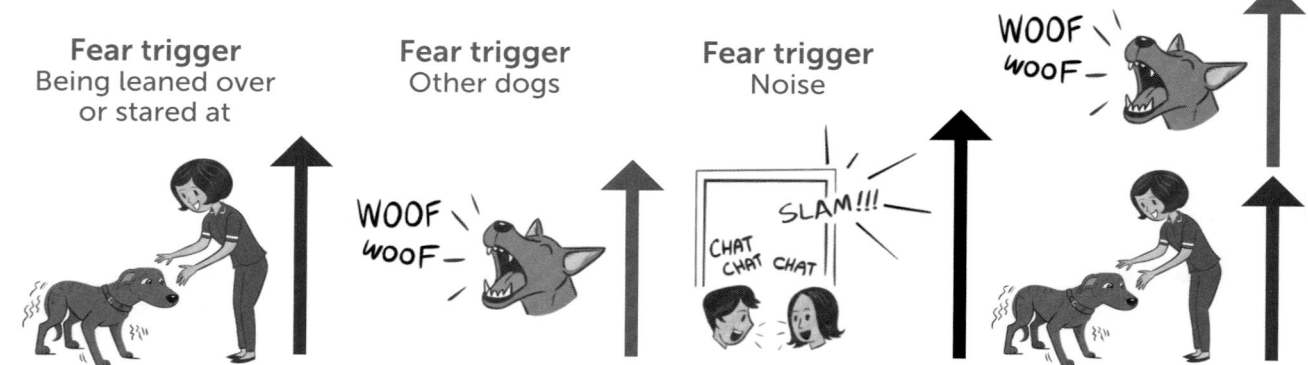

11.4 Trigger stacking. (© APBC, images by Lili Chin)

options are restricted, they are more likely to show aggressive behaviour. The environment must be taken into account when initially approaching animals in the veterinary surgery as confinement, whether in the consulting room, a hospital cage, being physically restrained or on a lead, can cause animals to show defensive aggression when, if given the choice, they would have used avoidance.

In addition to the physical environment, the social environment should also be considered. The owner–pet relationship should be considered; for example, observing whether the owner is providing important support for their pet or whether they are inadvertently exacerbating anxious responses. The presence of other animals in the consulting room may affect the behaviour of the patient; for example, some anxious dogs may benefit from having their canine housemate with them if the other dog is relaxed at the surgery. However, if both dogs are anxious this might aggravate the situation and they may be better seen separately. Dogs and cats who have a good relationship at home may not provide the same support to each other in an unfamiliar environment; this is particularly true for cats who, having been brought out of their familiar home territory, may find the presence of the dog an additional stressor.

Interacting with the dog

When approaching dogs, the veterinary professional must bear in mind what a dog may perceive as confrontation. Dogs do not approach each other head-on during friendly greetings, but from the side and circle around each other. A head-on approach is seen as confrontational and may inadvertently cause even a friendly dog to feel under threat, so a side-on approach is preferred (Figure 11.5a). Direct eye contact can also be misinterpreted as a threat, so avoiding eye contact will help put an anxious dog at ease. Where the dog is touched during an examination should also be considered; starting with the front of the chest is a non-threatening approach. Reaching over the head or leaning over the dog should be avoided (Figure 11.5b). If possible, allowing the dog to approach voluntarily is preferable to the staff approaching the dog. The use of previously learned cued behaviours should be used to the veterinary professional's advantage (see Figure 11.3). Nervous dogs often relax if they are given cue words or hand signals that they recognize and expect rewards for. Appetite is often inhibited by stress, so the willingness of a dog to eat treats in the consulting room can be a good measure of anxiety levels, which provides important information for deciding how best to interact with that patient.

Interacting with the cat

The use of a towel pre-sprayed with feline facial pheromones on the consulting table may help some cats feel more relaxed. Cats may willingly exit their carrier when the door is opened, but others may prefer to remain inside, as hiding is one of the cat's main coping strategies when worried. The information below explains how best to approach cats that are unwilling to exit their carriers. Forceful

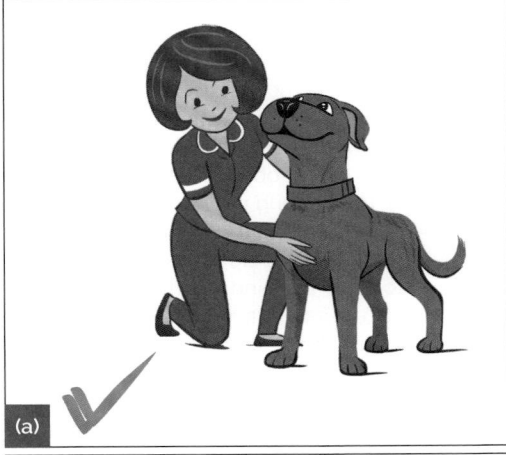

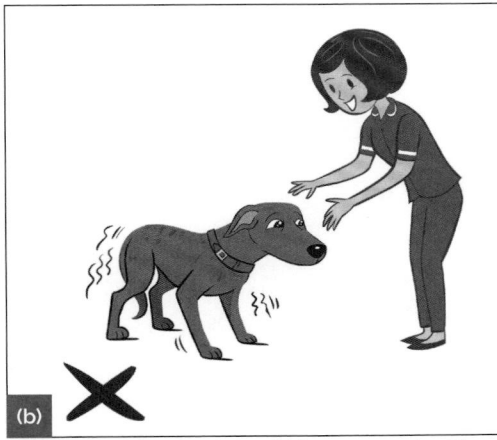

11.5 **(a)** Animal should be approached from the side. **(b)** Leaning over or reaching over the head of an animal should be avoided.

extraction must be avoided at all costs, as this is likely to frighten the cat and make handling difficult. Allowing cats to choose where they feel safe reduces the chances of them attempting to escape or showing defensive aggression during examination. Therefore, owners should be discouraged from attempting to control their cat's movement if the animal prefers to move around the consulting room. Cats use elevation and hiding for safety and may, for example, feel more secure being examined on a window sill or hiding in the lower half of their cat box. Nervous cats should be approached slowly and quietly. As with dogs, direct eye contact should be avoided. Cats, generally, are more likely to accept touch around their cheeks and under their chin, and are less likely to tolerate touch along their lower back and around their tail. Therefore, the clinical examination and handling should reflect this. Fussing a cat around the cheeks and under the chin helps to release facial pheromones, which can help the cat to relax, and this can be used effectively during examination and restraint.

Extracting a cat from a carrier

- After ascertaining from the clinical notes and owner reports that the cat is usually tolerant of being handled at the surgery, the cat box door can be opened
- The cat should be given the opportunity to exit the carrier in their own time whilst a history is taken →

Extracting a cat from a carrier
continued

- If the design of the carrier does not allow examination without removing the cat and the cat does not exit of their own accord:
  - If the carrier can be dismantled, quietly remove the top half and allow the cat to remain in the bottom half for examination
  - If the carrier cannot be dismantled and has a top opening, the cat can be gently lifted out ensuring they are well supported and any potentially painful areas are avoided
  - If the carrier cannot be dismantled and has a front opening, gently tilting the carrier can encourage the cat to exit
- Once the cat is out of the carrier, put the carrier out of the way to avoid repeated attempts by the cat to return to the safety of the carrier in order to prevent the risk of frustration or increased fear

Moving, transporting and lifting dogs and cats

Escape either within the surgery or into the external environment must be prevented through careful management of patients. Dogs must always be on secure leads attached to fixed size, sturdy, well-fitted collars or harnesses. For patients who are remaining at the surgery, it may be beneficial to use collars and leads owned by the practice to ensure they are in good condition and to prevent accidents such as snapped clips. Although slip leads can be useful as a back-up, used in addition to a normal collar and lead, these are best avoided due to the risk of overtightening, which not only compromises the respiratory and circulatory systems but also aggravates fear and anxiety. If slip leads are used, the tab should be moved to the inner side of the metal ring to prevent overtightening (Figure 11.6). Cats and other small animals should be contained in carriers when being moved and this may also be appropriate for small dogs.

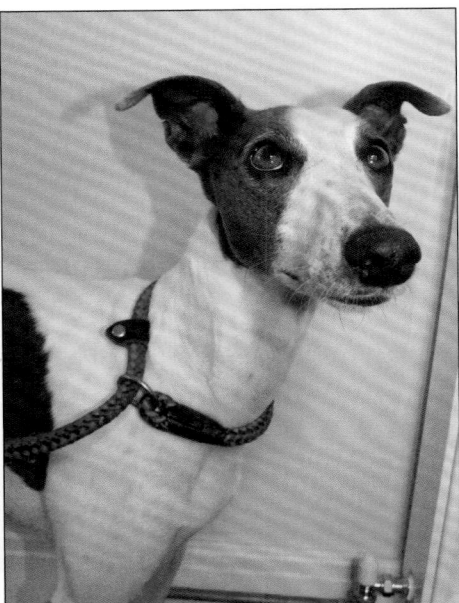

11.6 Avoiding over tightening of slip leads by moving the tab to the inner side of the metal ring. (© C. Wilson)

Moving dogs

Dogs should never be forced to move if they are unwilling, as this will aggravate fear responses, risking defensive aggressive behaviour. Dogs attending for a consultation who are unwilling to enter the surgery or consulting room can be examined in the car park or the waiting room. Such patients would most likely benefit from a behavioural referral to assist with future visits. For inpatients, if dogs are reluctant to leave their owners, asking the owner to accompany their pet to the hospital area can be considered. This approach, allowing the owner to see where their pet will be housed, will also help owners to feel more comfortable about leaving their pet at the surgery. Alternatively, if the owner leaves first whilst the dog remains in the consulting room with the member of staff, the dog will then often keenly exit the consulting room, hoping to follow the owner.

Lifting and carrying

The aim of lifting and carrying an animal must be to ensure that it feels safe and secure so that it does not make attempts to struggle free or show defensive aggression. Excessive restraint should be avoided as this may trigger defensive behaviour if the animal feels under threat. It is important before lifting an animal to assess for areas of discomfort or injury, which may be aggravated during handling. Painful areas are best held on the side away from the handler's body to avoid accidental pressure. The animal should be made aware of the presence of the handler before any attempt to lift it is made, so that it is not taken by surprise. Health and safety guidelines must also be adhered to (see Chapter 2).

- Small to medium-sized dogs may be lifted by one person, although assistance may be required if intravenous fluids are being administered or cage doors need to be opened. The hind legs can be supported and held against the handler's body using their elbow and upper arm, whilst their hand and forearm support under the animal's chest. Their second arm can support the front of the chest and, potentially, hold the head gently against their body should the dog struggle (Figure 11.7a).
- Cats may be lifted and carried in a similar way, but with the handler's hand also used to hold the front legs against their body. Cats often respond well to the second hand rubbing the cheeks or under the chin to help them relax (Figure 11.7b).

- Larger dogs (>20 kg) should be lifted by two people, preferably of a similar height to ensure the dog is kept level and feels secure. Safe lifting techniques (see Chapter 2) must be observed at all times. One person should support the front of the dog with one hand around the chest, holding below the neck area to ensure that the airways and circulation are not obstructed, and the other arm below the chest. The second person should have one arm under the abdomen and the other supporting the hind legs (Figure 11.7c). Some dogs may feel sufficiently relaxed to allow the hind legs to hang loosely, but other animals will feel safer having them supported.
- Some animals may be best transported on stretchers (Figure 11.8a) or blankets (Figure 11.8b); for example, if they have serious injuries or surgical wounds.
- Trolleys should be used to transport sedated or anaesthetized animals and their position should be checked and monitored to ensure maintenance of the airways.

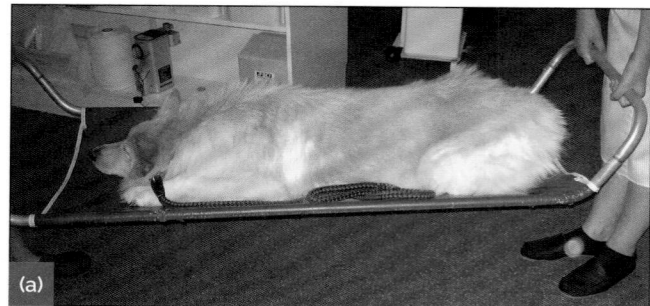
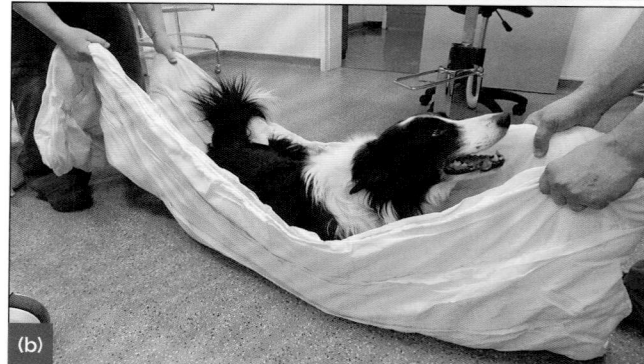

11.8 (a) Carrying a dog on a stretcher. (b) Lifting a dog with a duvet. There should be enough staff available to ensure that the dog is safely restrained as it is lifted. Relevant health and safety protocols regarding manual handling (i.e. lifting with bent arms and legs) should be observed at all times. (a, Courtesy of E. Mullineaux; b, © Kate Chitty)

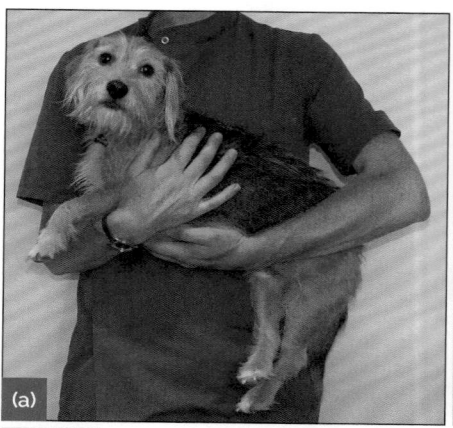
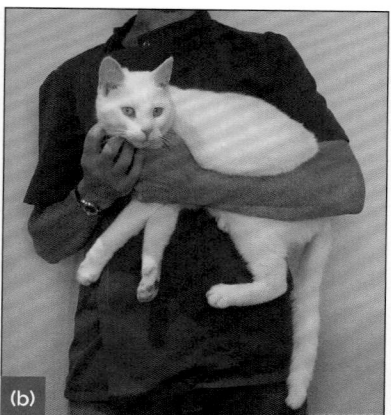
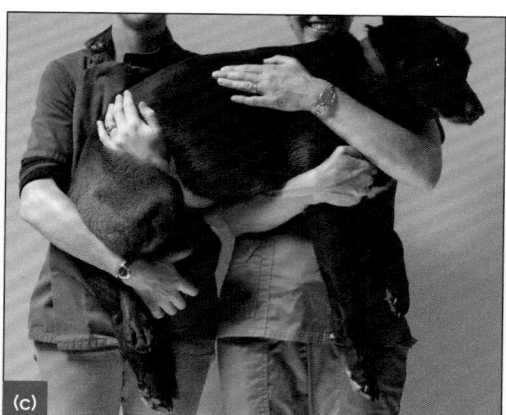

11.7 Techniques for carrying (a) a small dog, (b) a cat and (c) a large dog. (© C. Wilson)

Restraint of dogs and cats for examination or treatment

Dogs and cats tend to respond best to low intensity handling techniques, where they experience minimal restraint and feel safe to use avoidance strategies if they become frightened. Excessive restraint risks the development of aggressive behaviour due to the animal's avoidance responses being constrained. This gentle restraint should be carried out in a manner that is flexible, i.e. allows increased restraint if safety requires it (e.g. during venepuncture), or quick, considered, reduction of restraint if an animal is becoming distressed (e.g. panicking to escape). The type of restraint that is appropriate will vary and each individual situation must be considered in isolation.

Factors to consider include:

- The emotional state of the animal (recognized via body language and behaviour)
- The procedure to be carried out (e.g. are sharps involved?)
- The duration of the procedure (e.g. does it all need to be done in one go?)
- The environment (social and physical)
- The previous experience of the animal
- The health status of the animal
- The experience and the emotional state of the staff (and client if they are present).

Animals in respiratory distress should be provided with first aid treatment with minimal examination and restraint until they are in a more stable condition (see Chapter 19). This is particularly important in cats, as they are usually seriously compromised by the time they reach a state of respiratory distress. Animals that are in pain may require analgesia and/or sedation or anaesthesia prior to full examination, and restraint must take into account the areas of the body that may be painful. The use of appropriate doses of premedication drugs and analgesia (see Chapter 21) can significantly benefit the subsequent need for restraint during venepuncture for general anaesthesia. The appropriate use of benzodiazepines at home prior to practice visits is beneficial for patients that are generally anxious about attending the surgery.

Minimal handling involves not only using minimal physical contact and pressure but also the minimum number of staff. Crowding an animal with several members of staff (Figure 11.9) can significantly add to the stress of that individual, and animals that require significant levels of restraint should be sedated or anaesthetized rather than subjected to such inappropriate handling.

Restraint of dogs

Wherever possible, dogs should be given cues and/or hand signals to request pre-trained behaviours to aid a cooperative, low stress approach. When holding dogs for restraint, if they usually enjoy physical interaction then gentle stroking or ruffling of the fur can help keep them calm. Talking in a calm manner may also be of benefit; in particular using the dog's name and any relevant cue words the dog has been previously taught, such as 'wait' or 'stay'. Figure 11.10 illustrates restraint of a dog for presenting the forelimb to clip the fur

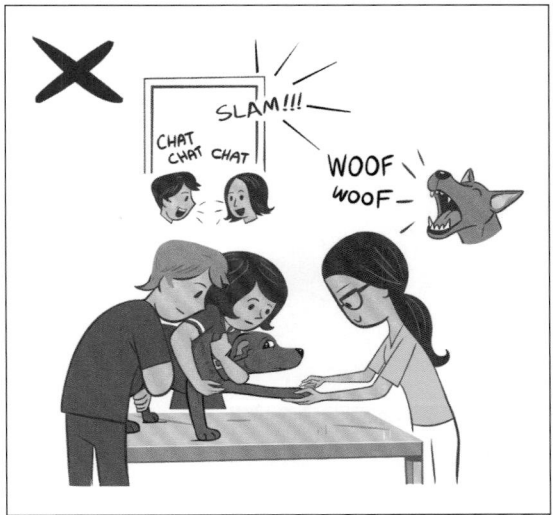

11.9 Overcrowding animals during restraint for examination should be avoided.

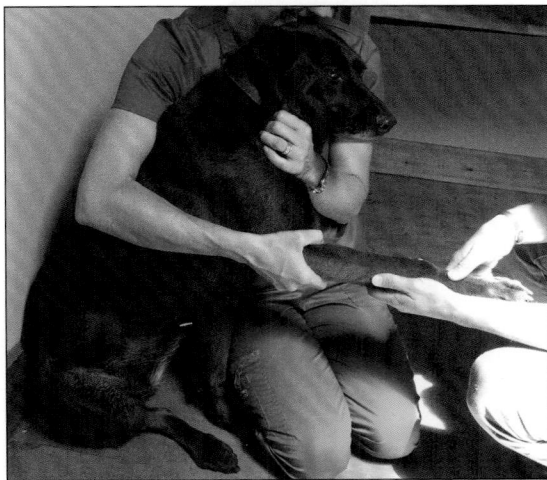

11.10 Restraint of a dog to obtain a blood sample from the cephalic vein. Note that the wall is being used to help prevent the dog from moving backwards and this is preferable to using additional staff, which may inadvertently overwhelm a nervous dog. (© C. Wilson)

and obtain a blood sample via the cephalic vein, or for other purposes such as bandaging of the forelimb. In Figure 11.10, the wall is used to help prevent the dog from moving backwards and this is preferable to using extra staff which may inadvertently overwhelm a nervous dog. Figure 11.11 shows two methods of steadying a dog's head. The rolled-up towel method is particularly useful with small brachycephalic breeds and can be used to prevent a dog from turning round to bite, in some instances avoiding the need for a muzzle.

If a dog needs to be examined or treated lying down, then providing a comfortable surface to encourage the dog to lie down on cue is beneficial for any patient, particularly elderly dogs suffering from joint pain (Figure 11.12). The dog may then be willing to roll over or be gently manoeuvred on to its side. Once lying on its side, the limbs closest to the floor or table can be gently held to keep the dog in place (Figure 11.13) and, again, giving verbal cues to 'wait' or 'stay', along with the dog's name, can be of great benefit. This is a good position for obtaining a blood sample from the saphenous vein. Dogs may also be gently restrained for sampling from the jugular vein by asking the dog to sit, the nurse standing to the side of the dog and then gently elevating the chin (Figure 11.14).

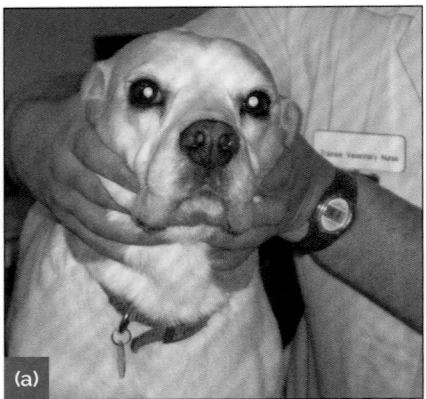

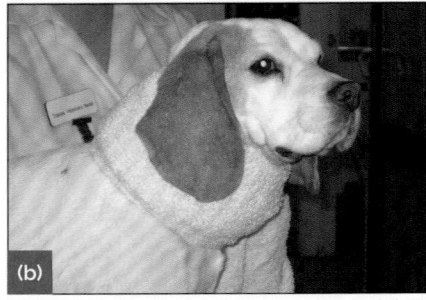

11.11 Restraining a dog's head. **(a)** The hands are placed either side of the neck and the head is gently pushed forwards with the fingers. **(b)** A rolled-up towel is held firmly but gently around the dog's neck. (Courtesy of E. Mullineaux)

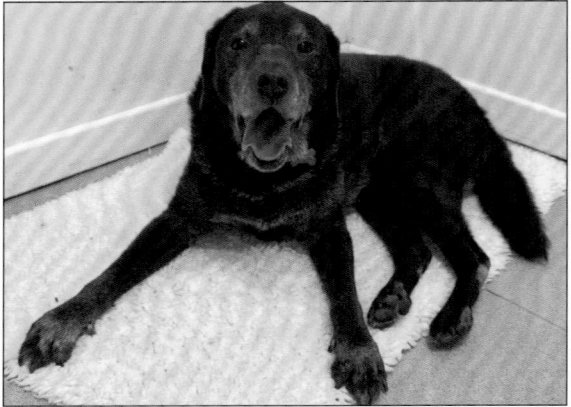

11.12 Provision of comfort to aid examination. (© C. Wilson)

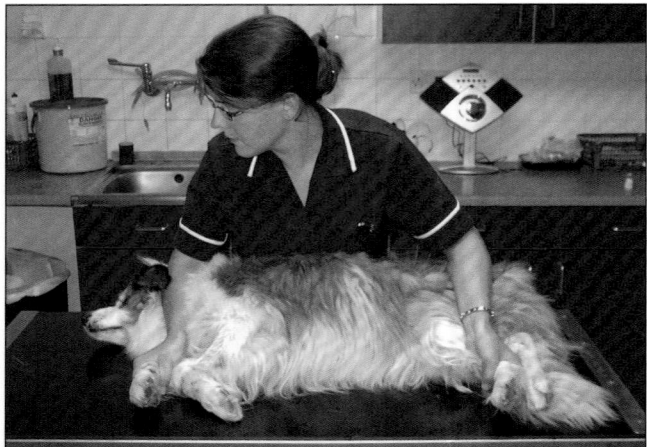

11.13 Restraining a dog on its side. (Courtesy of J. Niehoegen)

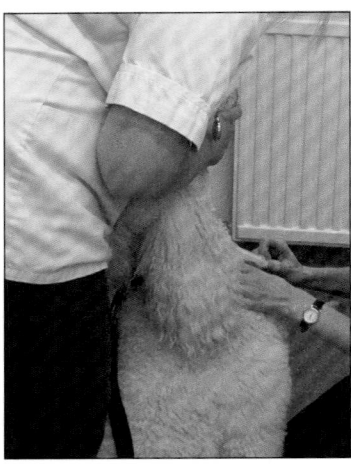

11.14 Restraint of a dog for jugular blood sampling. (Courtesy of E. Mullineaux)

Restraint of cats

Cats respond best to minimal restraint. When obtaining a blood sample from the cephalic vein, a similar method to that for restraining dogs (see Figure 11.10) can be used but with the cat on a table and the body of the handler being used to prevent the cat from moving backwards. Fussing the cat around the cheeks and under the chin can aid relaxation and reduce the risk of struggling (Figure 11.15). Jugular vein venepuncture is often best tolerated in cats. Having the cat in a sitting position with one hand gently resting in front of the forelegs, as a barrier to them being lifted up, whilst the other is used to raise the chin is the best method. Similar restraint can be used for examination or treatment of the head area (Figure 11.16). It is often recommended to hold both forelegs in one hand (Figure 11.17), but this extra restraint often causes cats to struggle so is better used as a last resort.

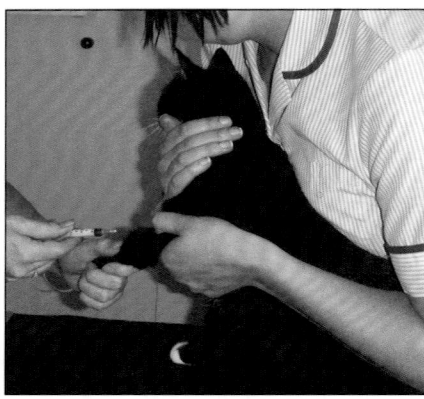

11.15 Raising a cat's cephalic vein or restraint for examination of foreleg.

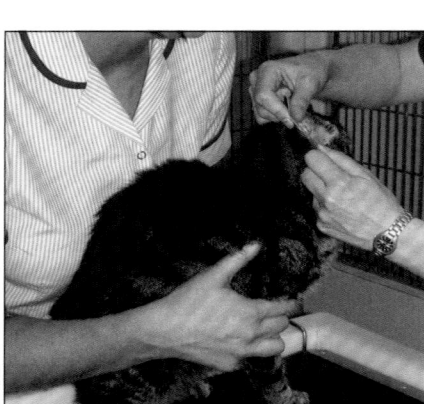

11.16 Restraint of a cat to allow treatment or examination of the head, including the ear.

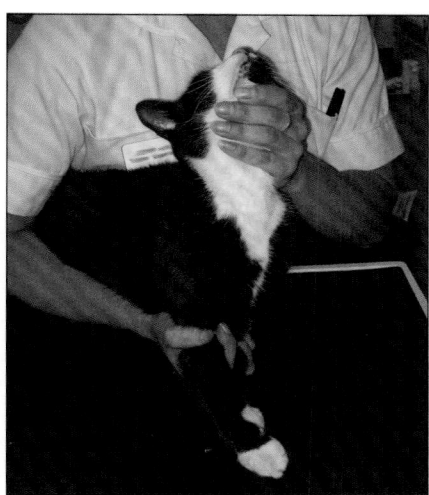

11.17 Restraint of a cat for jugular blood sampling. (Courtesy of E. Mullineaux)

Handling difficult or aggressive dogs and cats

The overall aim when interacting with patients should be to ensure that they do not feel the need to show aggressive or avoidance behaviour. In reality, however careful we are, some animals will react adversely to veterinary interventions whether due to anxiety, fear, pain or frustration. In the first instance, taking a good history, observing the animal and checking the clinical notes will give forewarning of expected problems. Whilst taking the history, the animal should be allowed some time to settle in the room but potentially aggressive dogs should not be permitted to wander without lead restraint and cats should be contained in their boxes until the time of examination. In cases where examination or treatment is non-urgent, the opportunity for behavioural referral must be considered. Some dogs and cats may have learned that aggressive behaviour is effective at keeping people away and may appear very confident. However, it is important to realize their original motivation for showing this behaviour was most likely fear and they just have confidence in aggression keeping them safe. Dogs who have learned contextual cues which exacerbate their anxiety may be better examined in the car park or another environment where they feel safer. At all times the safety of staff, clients and the animals must be paramount (see Chapter 2).

Options for aggressive animals

It is important to consider why an animal has felt the need to show an aggressive response so that the approach can be altered.

- Is the animal in pain?
  - Use of opiates may aid examination if needed immediately.
  - Use of non-steroidal anti-inflammatory drugs for a few days may aid future examination.
- Is the procedure essential?
  - If yes, then sedation or general anaesthesia should be considered.
- Does the procedure need to be carried out now or can it be postponed to a later date?
  - If it needs to be carried out now, then sedation or general anaesthesia should be considered. ➜

Options for aggressive animals
continued

  - If the procedure can be postponed for a day or more, the use of anxiolytic benzodiazepines 30–60 minutes before the next appointment should be considered.
  - If the procedure can be postponed for longer, referral to a clinical animal behaviourist is advisable.
- Can the approach be altered to help the animal feel safer?
  - The methods of restraint, the type of approach, the manner of interaction, the presence or absence of the owner, and the environment should be considered.
  - Frightened animals respond much better to a minimal restraint approach as they feel able to use avoidance rather than aggression.

Difficult cats

Removing difficult cats from a carrier

Cats that either have a history of problematic handling or are already aroused must be treated with caution. Inappropriate reactions from staff or the owner may exacerbate the cat's arousal state and render handling impossible. Figure 11.18 shows a technique for safely removing a fractious cat from a carrier by placing a towel between the top and bottom halves, covering the cat and wrapping it as a means of safe restraint.

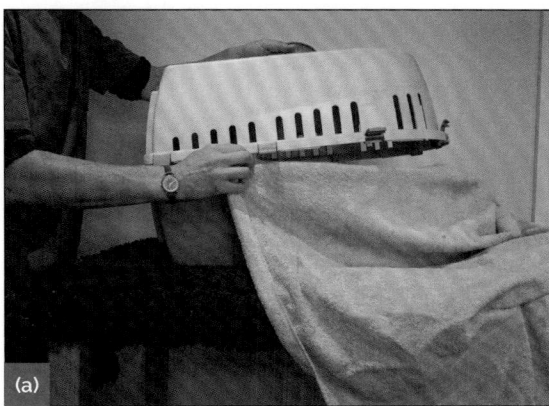

(a)

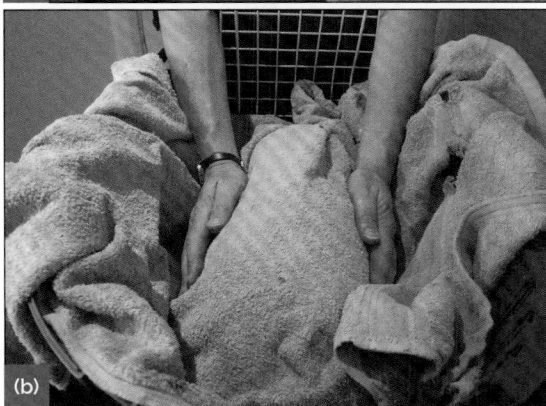

(b)

11.18 Technique for removing a fractious cat from a carrier. **(a)** Place a towel between the two halves of the carrier and **(b)** position over and around the cat before removing the animal from the box. (© C. Wilson)

Restraining cats in large towels or blankets

Cats generally respond far better to minimal restraint as they feel safer and therefore less in need of showing defensive aggression or escape responses. Forceful restraint is highly likely to further aggravate an aroused cat and should be avoided at all costs. Scruffing cats is rarely warranted as a restraint method due to the physical restrictions on the airway and blood supply, which is clinically inappropriate but also serves to increase fear and arousal. Figure 11.19 demonstrates the appropriate use of towels as restraint for accessing different body areas of cats that are difficult to handle. Cats in which it would be unsafe to access the jugular vein (Figure 11.19a) for blood sampling can be fully enclosed in a towel and a rear leg exposed for sampling from the saphenous vein (Figure 11.19b). Cat bags may be used, but a towel is preferable as this allows the cat to hide and feel safer.

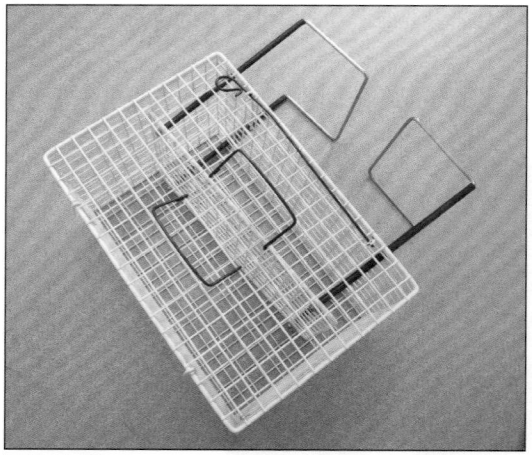

11.20 A crush cage used for cats. (© C. Wilson)

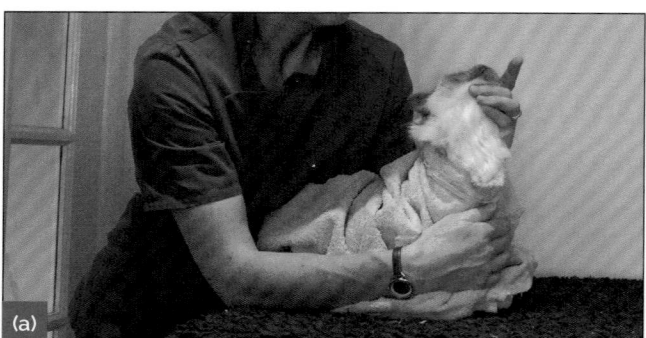

(a)

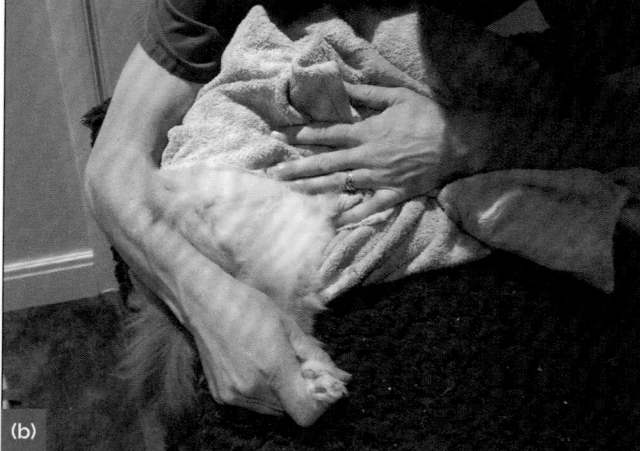

(b)

11.19 Restraining a cat in a towel for **(a)** jugular vein and **(b)** saphenous vein access. (© C. Wilson)

Crush cages for cats

A crush cage has a sliding partition that allows the cat to be physically restrained for injection of sedatives or anaesthetic drugs (Figure 11.20). These are very useful for cats that are dangerous to handle but are generally only used for feral cats as most pet cats respond well to the other methods described.

Cat muzzles

Cat muzzles are not widely used in the UK and, although they are available, it is more appropriate to use blankets and sedation/anaesthesia. Cat muzzles usually cover the eyes and mouth (Figure 11.21), which may be useful for brief procedures such as jugular blood sampling. Cats that require regular muzzling (e.g. frequent blood tests) should be trained to accept the muzzle in much the same way as dogs (below).

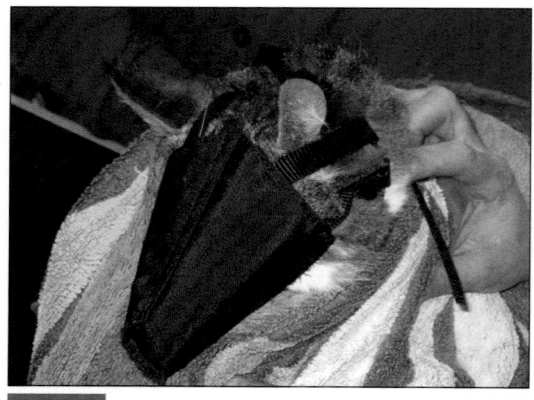

11.21 Cat muzzle.

Muzzling dogs

Muzzling of dogs must be used appropriately and be proportionate to the risks involved. It is vital when dogs are muzzled that the emotional state of the animal is still observed and considered. Fearful dogs often respond better to muzzling than to being excessively restrained and, therefore, for an urgent procedure, muzzling is preferable to heavy-handed restraint. Dogs that require muzzling for regular surgery visits should be trained at home (see 'Useful websites') by the owners in order to feel relaxed wearing a muzzle. Veterinary staff should avoid inadvertently making aversive associations with muzzles, as this can be counterproductive for future muzzle training.

A variety of fabric, plastic and leather muzzles are available (Figure 11.22). Basket style muzzles (Figure 11.22a) are the best as they allow the dog to pant, crucial for thermoregulation, to show warning signs such as a curled lip or bared teeth, and to be fed food treats. Once the dog is trained, basket muzzles can be placed on the dog before entering the surgery.

Although an open-ended fabric muzzle (Figure 11.22d) may be useful, dogs may still nip with their incisors and this design restricts the dog's ability to show important communication signals and compromises panting. Panting is a common sign of stress and, therefore, fabric muzzles that do not allow panting are not appropriate for anything other than a very brief procedure. Using a tape muzzle (Figure 11.23) can be useful in an emergency but must only be used for very brief procedures due to compromised respiration and signalling. An inability to pant is likely to increase the stress response and consequentially increase the difficulty of handling.

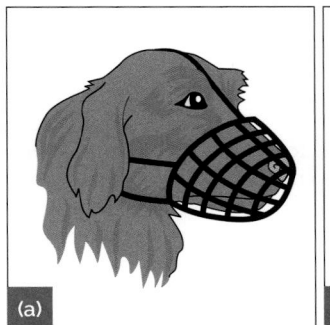
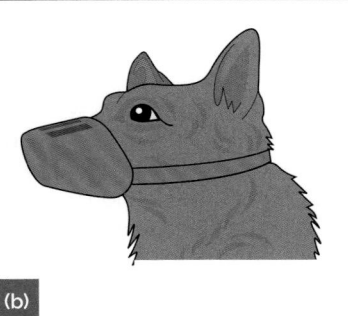
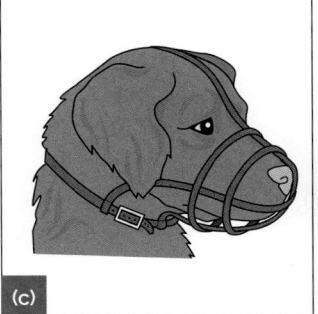
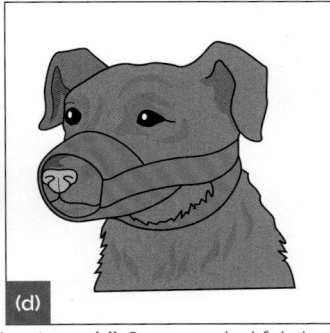

11.22 Examples of muzzles. **(a)** Closed basket type. **(b)** Closed plastic type. **(c)** Semi-closed leather type. **(d)** Open-ended fabric type.

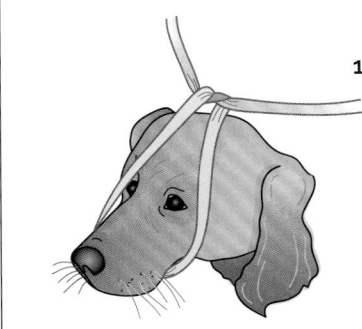

1. Form a loop by tying a loose square knot without tightening. With the dog suitably restrained, drop the loop over the dog's nose, with the knot uppermost.

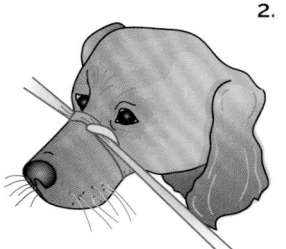

2. Pull the ends quickly to tighten the knot and so 'muzzle' the dog.

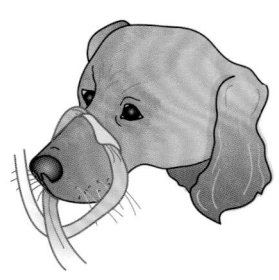

3. Cross the ends under the dog's jaw.

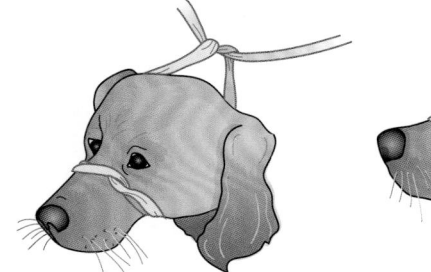

4. Tie at the back of the dog's head, using a 'quick-release' bow.

11.23 Applying a tape muzzle. Use a length of tape or non-stretch bandage at least 100 cm long for a medium-sized dog.

Feeding treats from a muzzle builds a good association (Figure 11.24) and encourages the dog to choose to place their nose into it. Often dogs better tolerate their owner placing a muzzle on them, but the safety of the owner must be considered; if there is a risk of injury, muzzling should be carried out by the staff. When approaching a dog to place a muzzle, it is best to approach from the side or from behind (Figure 11.25) as a head-on approach is confrontational and will increase the fear response. Occasionally, a dog may be too scared of a muzzle to allow it to be safely placed, in which case a loop of bandage can be used (Figure 11.23). However, this should only be used as a last resort as it is not comfortable for the dog and does not allow panting. It can be helpful to allow time to inject a dog with an intramuscular sedative; the tape can then be immediately released.

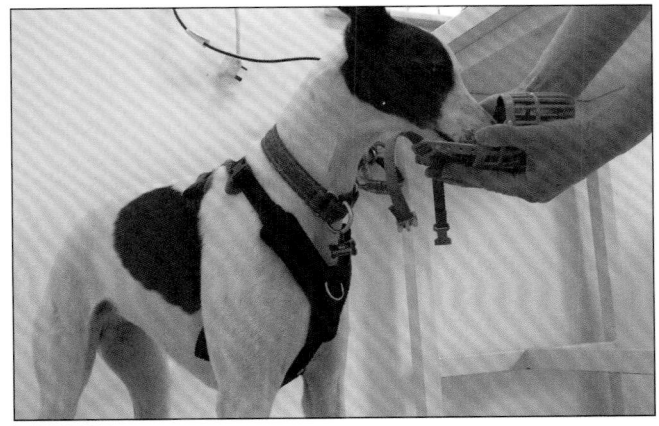

11.24 Feeding from a muzzle. (© C. Wilson)

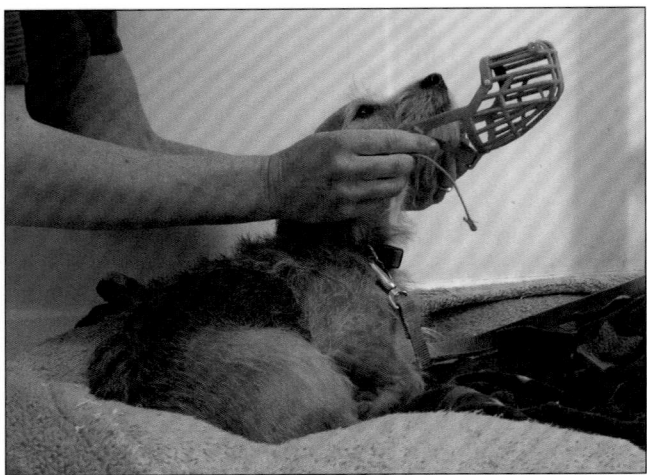

11.25 Dogs should be approached from behind when placing a muzzle. (© C. Wilson)

Appropriate responses to aggressive behaviour

If an animal starts to show signs of aggression or trying to escape, the style of interaction and handling must be adapted to ease its distress and reduce its need to show such responses. Confrontation or an increase in restraint is very likely to escalate the animal's behaviour. The Ladder of Aggression (see Figure 11.1) shows the risk of escalation of aggressive responses if lower level stress signals are ignored. However, in conjunction with reducing distress, the handler must also consider the safety of the animal and the safety of the people in the vicinity. For example, if a restrained dog is becoming highly aroused, the restraint must be reduced to allow the dog to relax, but consideration as to how that dog may behave once the restraint is reduced is also critical, both in terms of exacerbating the patient's existing injuries and risk of injury to people. Each situation is unique, so a risk assessment must be made based on the individual circumstances; options for diffusing a situation include calmly returning a dog to his kennel to allow him to settle, asking the owners to take the dog out of the surgery via a back door to avoid distressing waiting patients, reducing the number of people in the room, removing a muzzle if muzzling has caused the distress or placing a muzzle if required to allow loosening of other restraint. A highly aroused cat may have to be returned to a carrier or kennel before reducing restraint to ensure it does not become loose in the room.

Postponing a procedure

In some cases, the most appropriate decision is to postpone a procedure if the animal is struggling to cope with handling. The veterinary surgeon will need to make a clinical judgement as to whether this is appropriate and must inform and explain to the owner the basis of this judgement to ensure the animal receives the necessary care. Depending on the reason for handling, the animal may have time for referral to a clinical animal behaviourist prior to the next appointment, or other shorter-term strategies may be required in the interim, such as the use of anxiolytic medication at home prior to the visit and changes in the interaction style of the staff to ensure the animal does not feel so threatened.

Removing a reactive dog from a hospital cage

Kennel guarding may occur even in previously friendly dogs and the underlying fear associated with this behaviour must be respected. Dogs are unable to use avoidance strategies in this context and, if fearful, are more likely to show aggressive responses. Enquiring about previous crate training or kennelling and about responses to unfamiliar people during the history-taking can provide important information (see Chapter 14).

If a dog is at risk of kennel guarding, a longline lead should be attached and trailed out of the kennel door (Figure 11.26). If dogs show aggressive or avoidance behaviour from within a kennel, a direct approach must be avoided, as must eye contact. Instead, the longline should be approached and held, the kennel door opened, and the handler should then turn to the side and allow the dog space to come out of its own accord. In most cases, once the dog is out of the confined area and able to use avoidance strategies, the need to show defensive aggression subsides. If a dog unexpectedly kennel guards and, therefore, does not have a lead attached, a slip lead may be used to noose the dog as it comes out through a small gap as the door of the cage is opened. If a dog is kennel guarding when being discharged from the hospital, it may be prudent to involve the owner, as the dog may feel much safer and not demonstrate the same behaviour towards them.

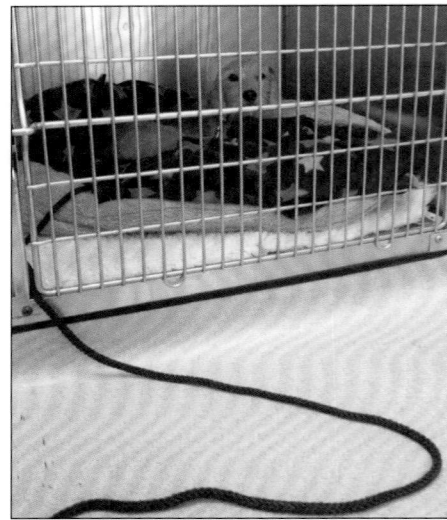

11.26

A longline attached to a collar should be used for dogs at risk of kennel guarding. (© C. Wilson)

Removing a reactive cat from a hospital cage

All cats should be given hiding and perching opportunities in their hospital cages to ensure they feel safe. If space allows, and the design of the carrier is appropriate, then placing the cat's own carrier inside the cage, with familiar bedding and scents, is ideal. Frightened cats will invariably choose to hide when given the opportunity and, therefore, offering them their carrier to voluntarily enter removes the need for handling. If the cage is too small to allow this, or the cat is unwilling to enter the carrier, a towel or blanket can be placed over the animal and wrapped underneath, and the cat picked up inside the towel/blanket as shown in Figure 11.18b.

Dog catchers and cat grabbers

These tools (Figure 11.27) should only be used in an emergency as a last resort as they are highly traumatic for the animal.

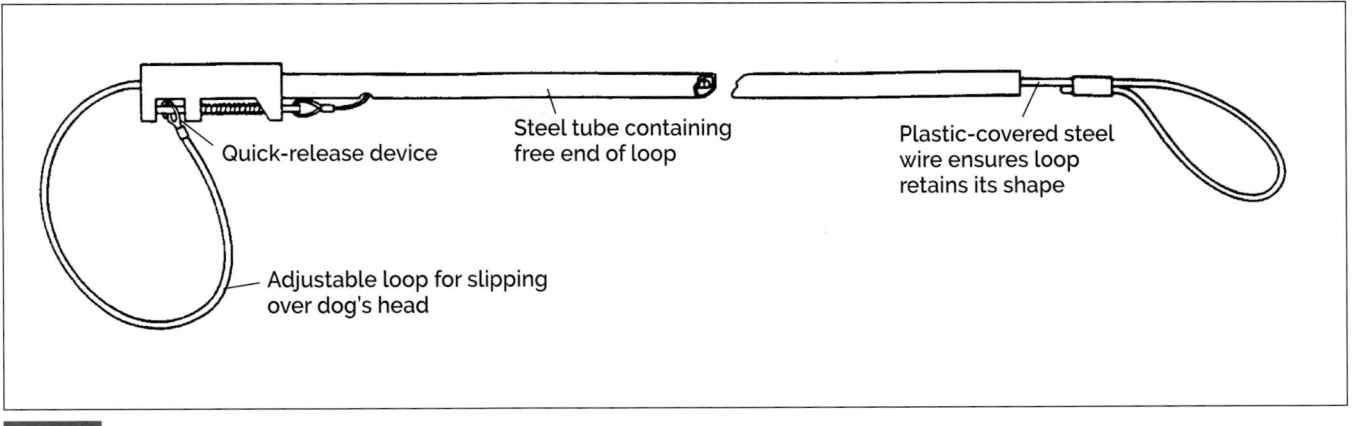

11.27 A dog-catcher.

Referral to a clinical animal behaviourist

Animals that show excessive fear responses at the surgery, or that are difficult to handle, should be referred to an appropriately qualified behaviourist, an RCVS Specialist in Behavioural Medicine, a Diplomate of the European College of Behavioural Medicine, an Association for the Study of Animal Behaviour (ASAB) Certificated Clinical Animal Behaviourist or an Animal Behaviour Training Council (ABTC) registered Clinical Animal Behaviourist.

Handling and restraint of exotic pets

Travelling boxes

Exotic pets should be fully assessed before any attempt is made to remove them from their cages or boxes. Often significant clinical information can be obtained through 'hands off' observation of both the patient and its cage.

Removing exotic pets from their travelling boxes for examination can be a challenge in itself and depends to a certain extent on the type of carrying box the animal has arrived in and the species. Examples of dealing with different types of pets in differing boxes are given below; however, these should be considered in conjunction with the species-specific advice that follows. In all cases, it is easier to remove the patient when the handler is at roughly the same level; therefore, picking the box up and placing it on to a table with a non-slip mat is preferred. In some cases with larger rabbits, it may be preferable to kneel down and remove the patient from its box on the floor, particularly where nervous or aggressive individuals are concerned.

Top-loading boxes

In most cases, it is best to consider sliding a towel in underneath the lid before the lid is fully opened to ensure that the patient does not suddenly leap out, in the case of a rabbit or ferret, or fly out, in the case of a parrot. The towel may then be allowed to cover the animal whilst the lid is carefully opened and the animal scooped out of the carrying box. In the case of ferrets and rabbits that are fractious or nervous, it may be advisable to grasp the scruff of the neck with one hand through the towel, whilst reaching underneath and restraining the hindlegs around the hocks. The rabbit or ferret may then be carefully lifted out and placed on to a non-slip surface.

Side-front-loading boxes

For rabbits and other small mammals in this type of box it is preferable to remove the door where possible, as this increases the opening available for removal of the patient. A towel may then be introduced and the scruff of the neck grasped, to enable the patient to be moved forward enough to allow the hindlegs to be grasped and the animal removed as described above.

In the case of a parrot or other larger cagebird, a towel should be carefully introduced to prevent escape of the bird past the towel. This should then be draped over the head and body, and the head grasped from behind, transferring the thumb and fingers underneath the lower mandible to control the beak. The rest of the towel is then used to drape over the wings and body, and the other hand is used to wrap the bird in the towel to prevent it flapping and hurting itself. The bird may then be removed from the box.

Bird cages

Many smaller cage birds are transported to the practice in their everyday cage. This can be useful to assess the local environment and the type of droppings the bird has been passing recently, assuming it has not been cleaned out prior to the visit. However, such cages may present a problem in removing the bird safely from the cage as many small cagebirds have plentiful perches, toys (e.g. mirrors, bells) and food items that provide cover to hide behind and that could potentially cause damage. The first aim is therefore to remove the majority of these obstructions carefully from the cage.

In the case of highly nervous and flighty individuals, it may be sensible to transfer the cage into a darkened room, preferably with a red light as diurnal (day-active) birds do not see well in red light; this makes catching the patient easier. Once the cage has been depopulated of toys etc., a small hand towel or paper towel may be introduced through the largest opening to aid the catching of the bird. This presents a larger surface area than the hand alone, and so tends to make the bird less likely to dodge around the towel and escape. It also provides something for the patient to bite on whilst trying to control the head and beak, and allows some passive restraint of the wings as well (Figure 11.28).

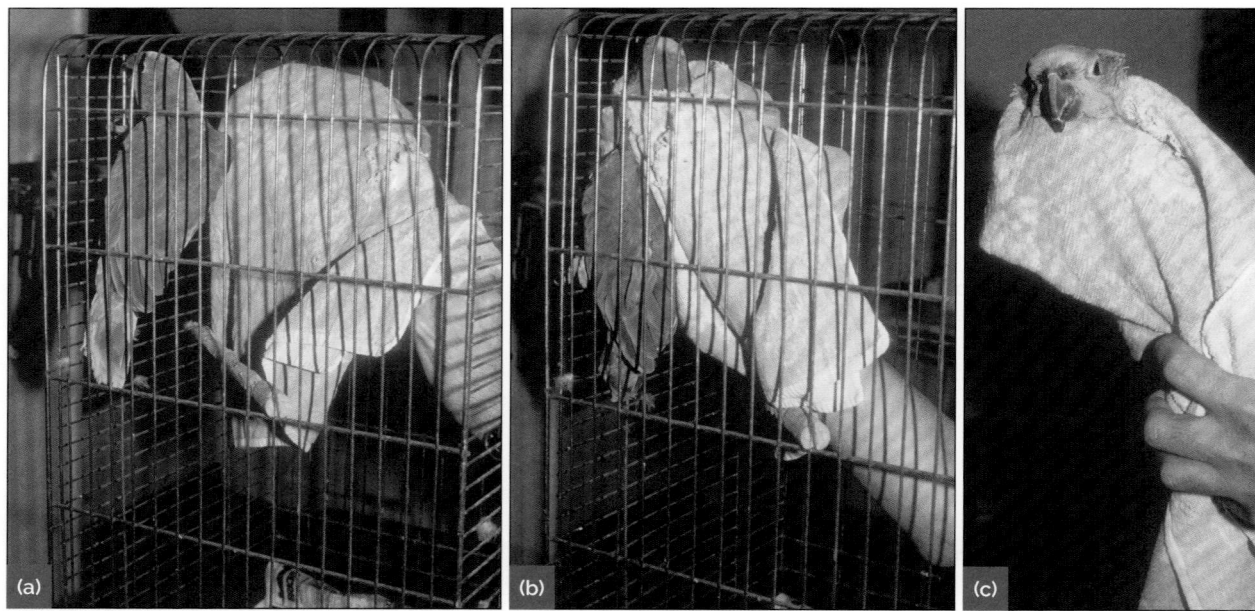

11.28 Removing a parrot from its cage. **(a)** The towel and hand are introduced into the cage. **(b)** The bird is firmly but gently grasped from the back. The head must be located first, to allow the thumb and forefingers to be positioned underneath the lower beak, in order that it can be pushed upwards, thus preventing the bird from biting. The rest of the towel is then used to wrap around the bird to gently restrain its wing movement. This will avoid excessive struggling and wing trauma. **(c)** The patient may then be cocooned in the towel, with the head still held extended from behind through the towel, and the rest wrapped loosely around the bird's body.

Rodent cages

As with bird cages, there may be a lot of cage furniture inside these enclosures and the majority should be removed to allow free access. Hamsters in modular housing should be encouraged to move into their sleeping quarters, which may then be detached from the maze of tunnels.

Once the cage is cleared of excess furniture, a light hand towel or paper towel may be introduced and draped over the rodent to initially restrain it. The scruff of the neck may then be firmly grasped, as described below for more active and aggressive animals such as hamsters. Alternatively, the thumb and forefingers may be slid under the forelimbs and the other hand introduced to support the rear end of more docile rodents such as chinchillas and rats.

Handling and restraint of small mammals

Pet mammals come in many different shapes and sizes, and from many different backgrounds – from those more adapted to human co-habitation, such as mice and rats, through to the animals more recently adopted as pets, such as chipmunks, which are still semi-wild in nature.

The behavioural characteristics of each animal should be considered before handling. Most of these species are 'prey' animals and will be stressed if not familiar with human handling. In order to avoid making the animal's clinical condition worse, and to avoid human injury, careful assessment is required (see 'Assessment before handling'). Further information on behavioural traits in exotic pets is given in the relevant BSAVA manuals (see 'References and further reading').

Rabbits

Understanding rabbit behaviour is key to their handling (Figure 11.29); further information is given in the BSAVA rabbit manuals (see 'References and further reading').

Assessment before handling

1. Is the patient severely debilitated and/or in respiratory distress?
   Examples include the pneumonic rabbit, with obvious oculonasal discharge and dyspnoea, or older rats with chronic lung disease. Excessive or rough handling of these patients is contraindicated and the journey into the veterinary practice may already have caused stress.
2. Is the species tame?
   Examples of the more unusual small mammals that may be kept include chipmunks, marmosets and other small primates, opossums and raccoons. All of these are potentially hazardous to handlers and themselves, as they will often bolt for freedom when frightened, or turn and fight. Even the more routinely kept small mammals (such as hamsters) may be aggressive.
3. Is the small mammal suffering from a metabolic bone disease?
   This is often seen in small primates, young rabbits and guinea pigs. The diet may have been inadequate with regard to calcium and vitamin D3, and exposure to natural sunlight may be absent. Hence, long-bone mineralization during growth will be poor, leading to spontaneous or easily fractured bones.
4. Does the small mammal patient require medication/ physical examination?
   If so, handling is often essential.

The majority of domestic rabbits are docile, but the odd aggressive doe or buck, usually those not used to being handled, does exist. The potential dangers to the veterinary nurse arise from the claws, which can inflict deep scratches rivalling those inflicted by cats, and the incisors, which can produce deep bites. Aggression is frequently worse at the

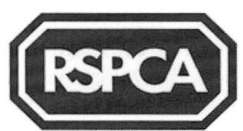

Understanding rabbit behaviour
YOUR RABBIT'S BODY LANGUAGE CAN HELP YOU TO UNDERSTAND HOW THEY ARE FEELING

A happy rabbit
These rabbits are relaxed and happy.

Rabbits 1-3 show ears close together, facing slightly backwards and pointing outwards. Eyes may be partially closed.

 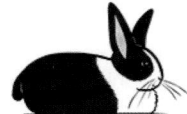 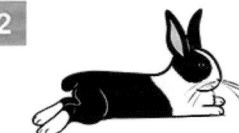 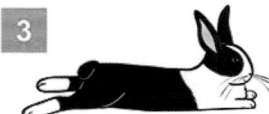 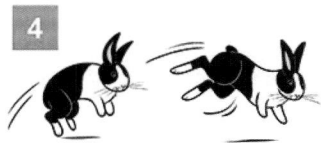

Rabbit is lying down, with a relaxed body posture and legs tucked under the body.

Rabbit is lying down, with front paws pointing forward and rear legs stuck out sideways. Body is relaxed and extended.

Rabbit is lying down with a fully extended, relaxed body. Back legs are stretched out behind the body and the front paws are pointing forward.

Rabbit jumps into the air with all four paws off the ground and twists in mid-air before landing.

A worried rabbit
These rabbits are telling you that they are uncomfortable and don't want you near them.

Rabbit is in a crouched position, muscles are tense, head held flat to the ground, ears wide apart and flattened against the back, pupils dilated.

 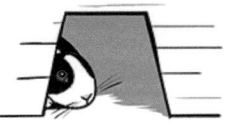

Rabbits who are worried or anxious may hide.

An angry or very unhappy rabbit
These rabbits are not happy and want you to stay away or go away.

 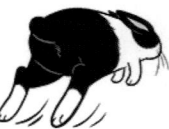   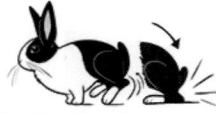 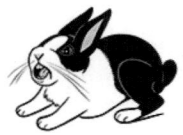

Rabbit turns and moves away flicking the back feet. Ears may be held against the back.

Rabbit is sitting up on back legs with front paws raised displaying boxing behaviour. Ears pointed upwards and facing outwards, rabbit may be growling.

Rabbit is standing tense, with back legs thumping on the ground. Tail raised, ears pointing upwards and slightly turned outwards, facial muscles are tense and pupils dilated.

Rabbit is standing tense with body down and weight towards the back, head tilted upwards, mouth open and teeth visible. Ears held back and lowered, tail raised, pupils dilated.

Royal Society for the Prevention of Cruelty to Animals
Wilberforce Way, Southwater, Horsham, West Sussex RH13 9RS
www.rspca.org.uk facebook.com/RSPCA twitter.com/RSPCA_official
The RSPCA helps animals in England and Wales. Registered charity no: 219099 The RSPCA only exists with the support of public donations.
Illustrations: Lili Chin, © 2015. All rights reserved. With thanks to Julie Bedford, certified clinical animal behaviourist.

11.29 Understanding rabbit behaviour. (Reproduced with permission from the RSPCA; illustrations © Lili Chin)

start of the breeding season in March/April. In addition to the damage they may cause the handler, a struggling rabbit may lash out with its powerful hindlimbs and fracture or dislocate its spine. Severe stress can even induce cardiac arrest in some individuals. Rapid and safe restraint is therefore essential.

To this end, if aggressive, the rabbit may be grasped by the scruff with one hand whilst the other hand supports underneath the rear legs. If the rabbit is not aggressive, then one hand may be placed under the thorax, with the thumb and first two fingers encircling the front limbs, whilst the other is placed under the rear legs to support the back.

When transferring the rabbit from one room to another, it must be held close to the handler's chest. Non-fractious individuals may also be supported with their heads pushed into the crook of one arm, with that forearm supporting the length of the rabbit's body; the other hand is then used to place pressure/grasp the scruff region (Figure 11.30).

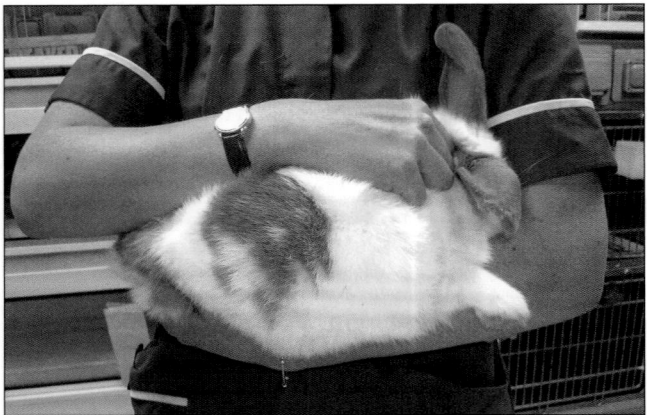

11.30 Carrying a docile rabbit, with its head in the crook of the elbow. Most rabbits find this method of restraint settling. (Reproduced from the *BSAVA Manual of Rabbit Medicine and Surgery, 2nd edn*)

Once caught, the rabbit may be calmed further by wrapping it in a towel, similar to the method used for cats, so that just the head protrudes in a 'bunny burrito' (Figure 11.31). There are also specific rabbit 'papooses' available that zip up along the rabbit's dorsum, leaving the head/ears free for blood sampling, but confining the limbs to prevent escape or self-harm. It is important not to allow rabbits to overheat in this position, as they, like a lot of small mammals, do not have significant sweat glands and do not actively pant. They can therefore quickly overheat if their environmental temperature exceeds 23–25°C, with fatal results.

Covering a rabbit's eyes will often help to calm it, but care should be taken not to damage the prominent ocular globes (Figure 11.32).

Trancing and turning

The method of restraint commonly known as 'trancing' (more accurately, creating a state of tonic immobility), whereby a rabbit is induced to become immobile after lowering it into a dorsal recumbency, should not be used. Contrary to popular belief, rabbits in a state of tonic immobility are not relaxed, hypnotized or insensitive to pain. Scientists believe that this is a defence mechanism employed once a rabbit has already been 'caught' by a potential predator. By remaining very still the rabbit may appear already dead, thereby causing the attacker to release its grip momentarily and allow the rabbit to escape. Research has shown that in this state rabbits show increased heart and respiratory rates plus elevated plasma corticosterone levels, indicative of fear-induced stress. The stress caused by this procedure may prove fatal, especially for rabbits suffering from respiratory or cardiovascular disease, and the sudden transition from the passive state to one of very active escape can be instantaneous and unpredictable and may result in significant injury to the patient.

Enlisting the help of an assistant to raise the rabbit's forelimbs off the ground, whilst keeping the rabbit's hindlimbs in contact with a solid surface, allows for ventral examination of rabbits.

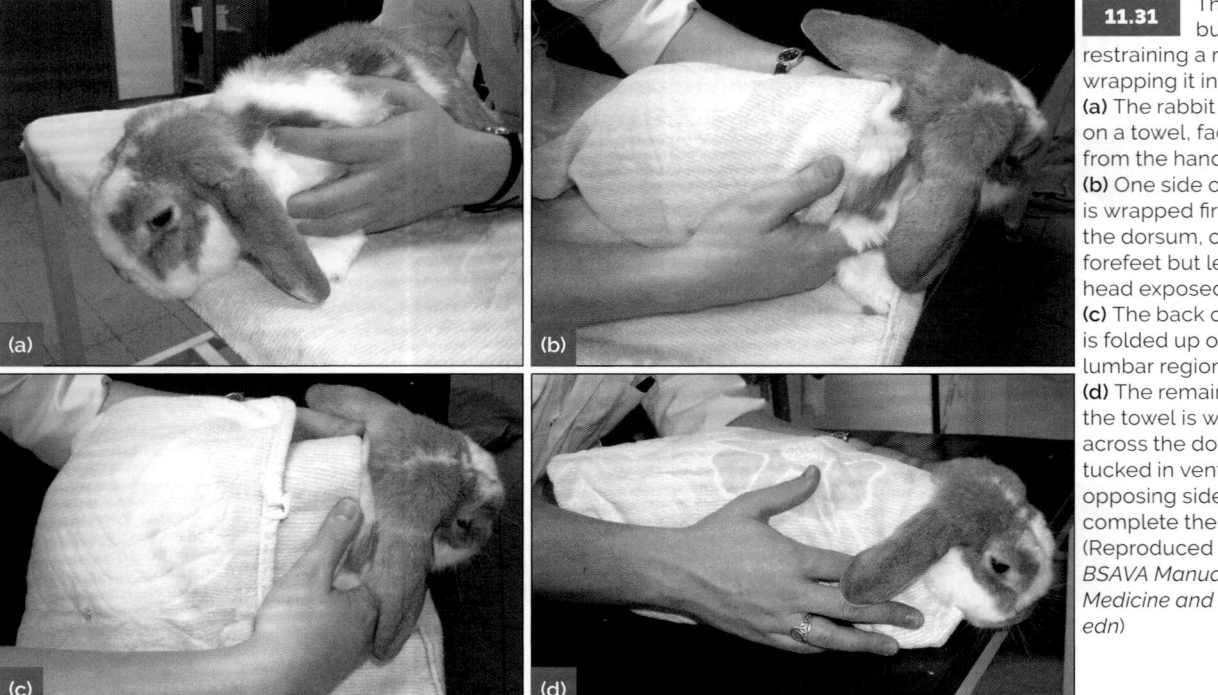

11.31 The 'bunny burrito': restraining a rabbit by wrapping it in a towel. **(a)** The rabbit is placed on a towel, facing away from the handler. **(b)** One side of the towel is wrapped firmly across the dorsum, covering the forefeet but leaving the head exposed. **(c)** The back of the towel is folded up over the lumbar region. **(d)** The remaining side of the towel is wrapped across the dorsum and tucked in ventrally on the opposing side to complete the wrap. (Reproduced from the *BSAVA Manual of Rabbit Medicine and Surgery, 2nd edn*)

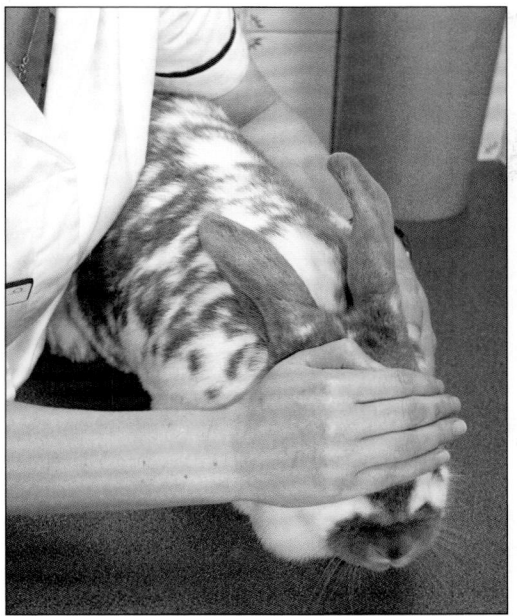

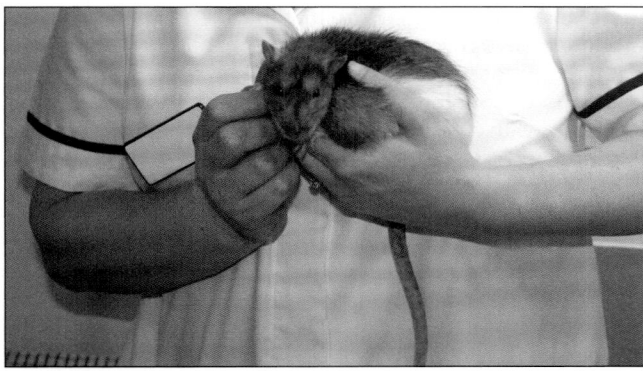

11.34 Holding a tame rat. (Courtesy of C. Clarke)

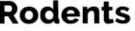

11.32 A hand over the rabbit's eyes helps to keep the animal calm. (Courtesy of C. Clarke)

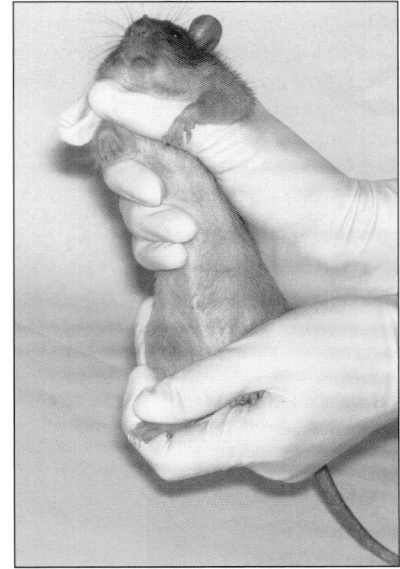

11.35 Restraining a rat. (Reproduced from the *BSAVA Manual of Exotic Pets, 4th edn*)

Rodents

Mice and rats

Mice will frequently bite an unfamiliar handler, especially in strange surroundings. It is first useful to grasp the tail near to the base and then place the mouse on a non-slip surface (Figure 11.33a). Whilst still holding the tail, the scruff may now be grasped firmly between the thumb and forefinger of the other hand (Figure 11.33b), allowing the mouse to be turned and examined as necessary (Figure 11.33c).

Rats will rarely bite unless roughly handled (Figure 11.34). They are best picked up by encircling the pectoral girdle, immediately behind the front limbs, with the thumb and fingers of one hand whilst bringing the other hand underneath the rear limbs to support the rat's weight (Figure 11.35). The more fractious rat may be temporarily restrained by grasping the base of the tail before scruffing it with thumb and forefinger.

Hamsters and gerbils

Hamsters can be relatively difficult to handle as, being nocturnal, they are never pleased at being awoken and picked up during daylight hours. If the hamster is relatively tame and used to being handled, simply cupping the hands underneath the animal is sufficient to transfer it from one cage to another.

Some breeds of hamster are more aggressive than others, with Russian, Djungarian or hairy-footed hamsters being notorious for their short temper. In these cases, the hamster should be placed on to a firm, flat surface and gentle but firm pressure placed on to the scruff region with the finger and thumb of one hand. As much of the scruff as possible should then be grasped, with the direction of pull

> **WARNING**
>
> Under no circumstances should mice or rats be restrained by the tips of their tails, as de-gloving injuries to the skin in this area will easily occur

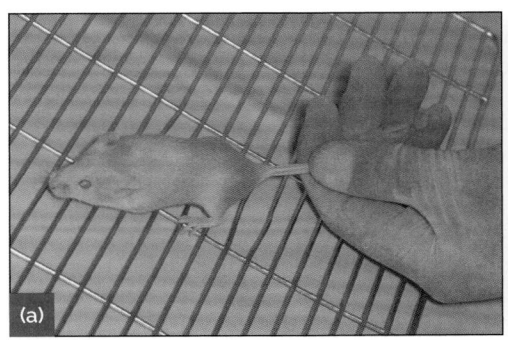
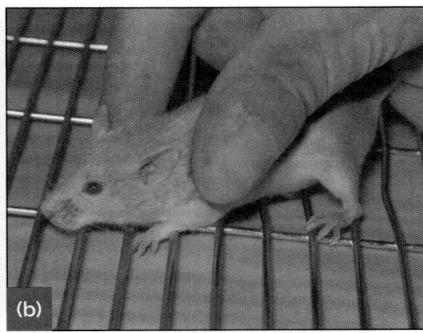
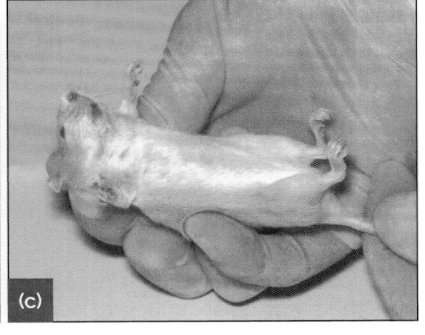

11.33 (a–c) Handling techniques for mice. (Reproduced from the *BSAVA Manual of Exotic Pets, 4th edn*)

in a cranial manner to ensure that the skin is not drawn tight around the eyes (Figure 11.36); hamsters have a tendency for ocular proptosis if roughly scruffed. If a very aggressive animal is encountered, the use of a small glass/perspex container with a lid for examination and transport purposes is useful.

Gerbils are relatively docile but can jump extremely well when frightened and may bite if roughly handled. For simple transport, they may be moved from one place to another by cupping the hands underneath the gerbil. Small mammals should always be approached from the side and at low levels, as when they are descended upon from a great height, the handler's hands mimic the swooping action of a bird of prey, startling the rodent.

For more rigorous restraint, the gerbil may be grasped by the scruff between the thumb and forefinger of one hand after placing it on to a flat level surface. It is vitally important not to grasp a gerbil by the tail as this will lead to stripping of the tail's skin, leaving denuded coccygeal vertebrae. This will never regrow and the denuded vertebrae will themselves undergo avascular necrosis and drop off later. Jirds and jerboas are related species, and handling techniques are the same.

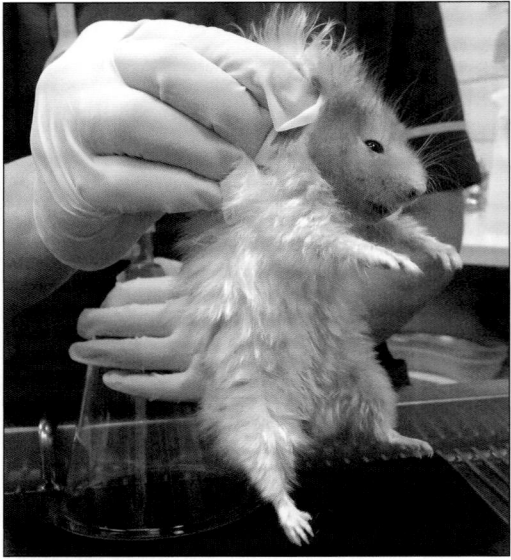

11.36   Handling a hamster. (Courtesy of A. Raftery)

Guinea pigs, chinchillas and degus

Guinea pigs are rarely aggressive, but they become highly stressed when separated from their companions and normal surroundings. This makes them difficult to catch, as they will move at high speed in their cage. To aid restraint, dimmed lighting can be used and environmental noise restricted to reduce stress levels. Restraint is also easier if the guinea pig is already in a small box or cage, as there is less room for it to escape. To restrain a guinea pig, it should be grasped behind the front limbs from the dorsal aspect with one hand, whilst the other is placed beneath the rear limbs to support the weight (Figure 11.37). This is particularly important as the guinea pig has a large abdomen, but slender bones and spine that may be easily damaged.

Chinchillas are equally timorous and rarely, if ever, bite. They too can be easily stressed; dimming room lighting and reducing noise can be useful during capture. Some chinchillas, when particularly stressed, will rear up on their hindlegs and urinate at the handler, with surprising accuracy.

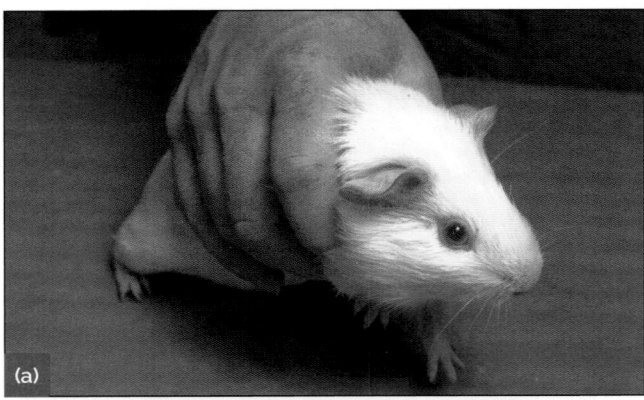

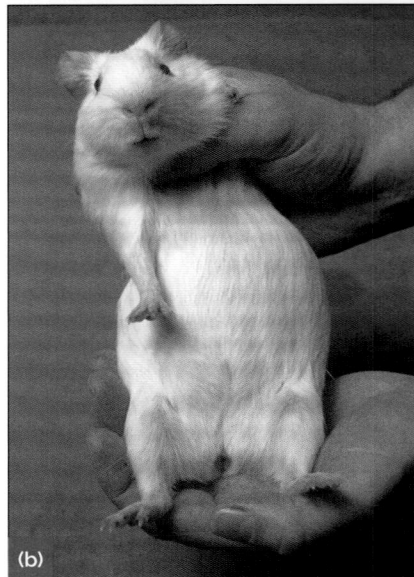

11.37   Restraining a guinea pig. **(a)** The animal is first grasped around its shoulders. **(b)** It can then be lifted, with the hindquarters supported.

It is therefore essential to pick up the chinchilla calmly and quickly, with minimal restraint, placing one hand around the pectoral girdle from the dorsal aspect just behind the front legs, with the other hand cupping the hindlegs and supporting the chinchilla's weight.

Degus may be handled in a similar way to chinchillas.

> **WARNING**
>
> Chinchillas must not be scruffed under any circumstances, as this will result in the loss of fur at the site held. Chinchillas may actually lose some fur due to the stress of the restraint, even if no physical gripping of the skin occurs. This 'fur slip', as it is known, will leave a bare patch which will take many weeks to regrow

Chipmunks

There are more than 24 species of chipmunk, with the most common species seen in the UK currently being the Siberian, although smaller North American species are also kept. Chipmunks are extremely highly strung and the avoidance of stress is essential to avoid fatalities. Generally, they are very difficult to handle without being bitten, unless hand-reared when they may be scruffed quickly or cupped in both hands. The easiest method to catch them in their aviary-style enclosures is to use a fine-meshed aviary/butterfly net, preferably made of a dark material. The chipmunk may then be safely netted and quickly transferred to a towel for manual restraint, examination or injection/induction of chemical restraint.

Ferrets

Ferrets can make excellent house pets and many are friendly and hand-tame. Some ferrets kept as working animals, to hunt rabbits, may be less frequently handled and more aggressive.

For excitable or aggressive animals, a firm grasp of the scruff, high up at the back of the neck, should be made. The ferret may be suspended from this whilst stabilizing the lower body with the other hand around the pelvis (Figure 11.38). In the case of more hand-tame animals, they may be suspended with one hand behind the front legs, cupped between thumb and fingers from the dorsal aspect, with the other hand supporting the rear limbs (Figure 11.39a). This may be varied somewhat in the livelier individuals by placing the thumb of one hand underneath the chin, pushing the jaw upwards, and the rest of the fingers grasping the other side of the neck (Figure 11.39b). The other hand is then brought under the rear limbs as support.

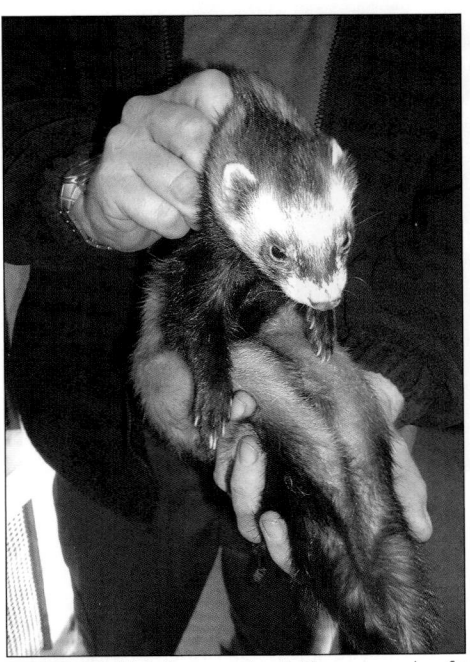

11.38 Holding a potentially aggressive ferret, using the scruff. (Courtesy of S. Redrobe)

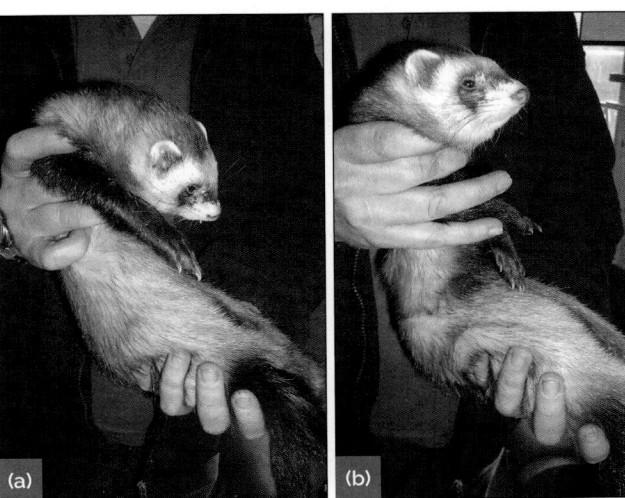

11.39 **(a, b)** Holding a less aggressive ferret. (Courtesy of S. Redrobe)

Handling and restraint of birds

As with small mammals, the veterinary nurse needs to make a decision on whether the bird in question is safe to restrain. This is not only because of the danger to the nurse's welfare (in the case of an aggressive or potentially dangerous bird of prey), but also because of the medical aspects of the patient's health.

Assessment before handling

1. Is the bird in respiratory distress, and is the stress of handling therefore going to exacerbate this?
2. Is the bird easily accessible, allowing quick stress-free and safe capture?
3. Does the bird require medication via the oral or injectable route, or can it be medicated via nebulization, food or drinking water?
4. Does the bird require an in-depth physical examination at close quarters, or is cage observation enough?

It is not always necessary to restrain the bird. It is important to remember that many avian patients are highly stressed individuals, so any restraint that is performed should involve minimal periods of handling and capture.

Initial approach

The majority of avian patients seen in practice (with the obvious exception of the owl family) are diurnal (active during the daylight hours), so reduced or dimmed lighting in general has an extremely calming effect. This can be used to the veterinary nurse's advantage when catching a flighty or stressed bird. In the case of Passeriformes (perching birds such as canaries and finches) and Psittaciformes (members of the parrot family, which includes budgerigars, cockatiels and the larger parrots), turning down the room lights or drawing the curtains or blinds is enough.

For birds of prey, there may well be access to the practice's, or the bird's own, 'hoods'; these are leather caps that slot over the head, leaving the beak free but completely covering the eyes. These are mainly used for falcons and eagles, but the bird has to be trained to accept the hood in the first instance (Figure 11.40). They are used to calm the bird when on the hand or during handling or transporting.

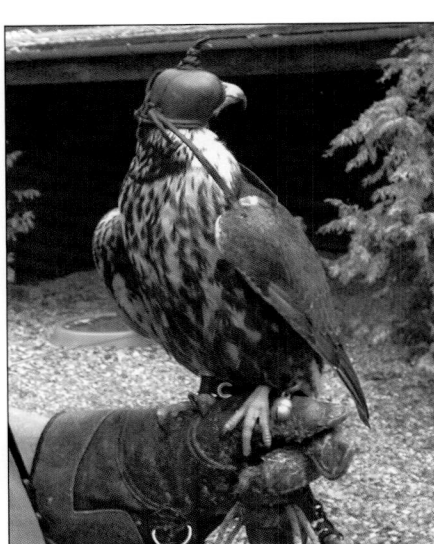

11.40 A hood keeps a raptor calm. (© John Chitty)

It is also advisable to keep the noise levels to a minimum when handling avian patients, as the acuity of their hearing is second only to the acuity of their vision. With these two initial approaches, stress and time for capture can be greatly reduced.

Prior to capture, all obstructing items should be removed from the cage or box (e.g. toys, water bowls, food bowls). This helps to avoid self-induced trauma by the bird and reduces the time needed to capture the patient. Once these initial arrangements have been made, the avian patient can be approached.

Birds of prey

There are two main categories of birds of prey commonly seen in practice: Falconiformes (includes falcons, hawks and eagles) and Strigiformes (the owl family). Falconiformes are mainly diurnal (daylight active) and they make up the most commonly seen group of birds of prey in practice. Strigiformes are generally nocturnal (active during the hours of darkness) and so use of hoods and darkening the room will not quieten these birds. However, they generally tend to be relatively docile.

Several pieces of specific handling equipment are often used for birds of prey. Hoods (see Figure 11.40) are used to calm many falcons and hawks, and many of these birds will also have jesses on their legs. These are the leather straps attached to their 'ankles' (lower tarsometatarsal area) and they allow the falcon to be restrained whilst on the owner's fist. Jesses may also be connected to a leash (via a metal swivel), which can be used to tether the bird to a perch when it is not being handled.

Leather gauntlets (see Figure 11.40) should be worn by all handlers for all birds of prey, as their talons and the power of the grasp of each foot can be extremely strong. The feet of birds of prey represent the major danger to the handler and not the beak (with the exception of some of the larger species of eagle). It is important to note that when the bird of prey is positioned on the gauntleted hand, the wrist of this hand (traditionally the left hand in European falconers) is kept above the height of the elbow. If not, the bird has a tendency to walk up the arm of the handler, with serious and painful results. The type of gauntlet should be either a specific falconer's gauntlet or one of the heavier duty leather pruning gauntlets available from garden centres.

1. Place the gauntleted hand into the cage or box or beside the bird's perch.
2. Grasp the jesses with the thumb and forefinger of the gauntleted hand and encourage the bird to step up on to the glove.
3. Once on the hand, retain hold of the jesses and slip the hood over the bird's head (assuming that the bird has been trained to accept the hood).

The bird of prey may then be safely examined 'on the hand' and is frequently docile enough to allow manipulation of wings and beak and for small injections to be administered or for oral dosing to occur.

If the bird of prey does not have jesses on but is trained to perch on the hand it may well step up on to the gauntlet of its own accord, otherwise the room lighting needs to be reduced for Falconiformes. A blue or red light source could also be used, allowing the handler to see the bird but preventing the bird of prey from seeing normally. There are then two possible approaches:

- The bird may be grasped from behind in a thick towel; the handler should ensure that they are aware of where the bird's head is (this is known as casting the bird (Figure 11.41)). The bird is restrained across the shoulder area with the thumbs pushing forward underneath the beak to extend the head away from the hands. The hood can then be placed over the bird's head and the bird placed on to a gauntleted hand (if the bird is trained to accept the hood). The majority of birds are happier and struggle less when their feet are actually grasping something, rather than being held in a towel with their feet freely hanging
- Alternatively, the hooded bird may be held from behind with the middle and fourth finger of each hand grasping the leg on the same side and directing the feet away from the handler. This method of holding the legs prevents the raptor from grasping one foot with the other, which causes severe puncturing of the skin, leading to secondary infections known as 'bumblefoot'.

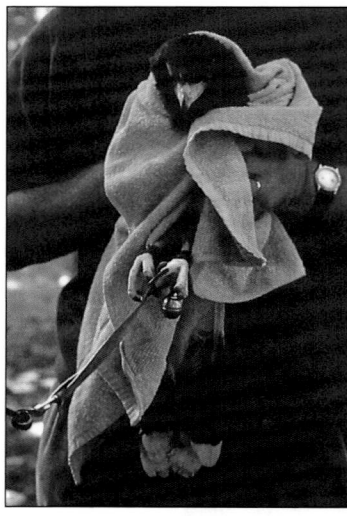

11.41 Casting a Harris' hawk. (© John Chitty and reproduced from the *BSAVA Manual of Exotic Pets, 5th edn*)

If the bird is not trained to accept the hood, then the procedure should be carried out as described above but minus the hood. In these cases, the examination/restraint should be kept as brief as possible to avoid distressing the bird.

For the majority of raptors, if they are loose in their aviary, it is best to catch them at dusk/night. Nocturnal species of owl should be caught during the day. The use of nets and towels is often required.

Finally, it is important to remember that the majority of birds of prey are regularly flown, so it is vital to preserve the integrity of their flight and tail feathers. Unfortunately, few falconers will thank you for saving their bird's life if they then cannot fly that bird until after the feathers have been replaced at the next moult; moulting usually occurs in the autumn. This means that during hospitalization, the tail feathers should be protected from fraying by taping pieces of light-weight card around their ends or using a commercial tail protector. Care should also be taken when handling birds to avoid damaging both the tail feathers and the primary and secondary wing flight feathers.

Parrots and other cagebirds

Parrots are often trained to step up on to the hand. If the owner does not have the bird already trained to do this, he/she should be encouraged to do so. A tasty treat can be held in front of the bird, with the other hand just in front and above the internal perch. The treat should be at such a distance that the bird must step on to the hand to get the treat. It is important to be aware that nervous birds may reach down to the hand, as it is normal for many parrot species to use the beak as a third limb to help balance. The novice handler may mistake this for an attempt to bite and pull away, making matters worse as the bird is now even less sure about stepping on to the hand and may grab at the hand in a desperate attempt to pull itself on to the hand, biting in the process. All of these birds will also benefit from subdued, blue or red light to calm the bird and to allow restraint with minimal fuss.

- In psittacine birds (e.g. African grey parrots, macaws, Amazon parrots and cockatoos), the main weapon is the beak and a powerful bite is possible.
- In passerine birds (e.g. mynah birds, starlings and orioles), the main weapon may again be the beak. Although this is less damaging as a biting weapon, it may still be a sharp stabbing weapon.

Wearing heavy gauntlets is not recommended for restraint of either family group as it will not allow easy judgement of the strength of the handler's grip on the patient. Instead, it is better to use dish or bath towels for the larger species and paper towels for the smaller ones as these provide some protection from being bitten without masking the true strength of the grip. The towel technique is also more beneficial than gloves alone because it presents a larger surface area for the bird to try and evade. The bird is then less likely to try and bolt for freedom, whereas a single hand can be a much smaller target and encourages escape attempts. After removal of the bird from its cage (see Figure 11.28), the limbs may then be removed from the towelling one at a time for examination or medication.

> **WARNING**
>
> Birds do not have a diaphragm and so rely solely on the outward movement of their ribcage and keel bone for inspiration. Restriction of this movement with too tight a grip can be fatal

For smaller cagebirds:

1. A piece of paper towel may be used and then the bird transferred to the hand. Nitrile gloves may be worn.
2. The neck of the bird should be held between the index and middle fingers (Figure 11.42).
3. The thumb and forefinger can then be used to manipulate legs or wings.
4. The rest of the hand should gently cup the bird's body to resist struggling.
5. Care should be taken not to over-constrain as this could cause physical harm.

In the case of particularly aggressive parrots that are very difficult to handle, leather gauntlets may be employed. It should be noted that too strong a grasp around the bird's body can prove fatal.

Young and hand-tame parrots

In the case of hand-reared and very tame young parrots, these may be removed from their containers by scooping them up between the palms of both hands before being placed into a towel-lined cardboard box or shallow dish. They should never be left unattended as they could still

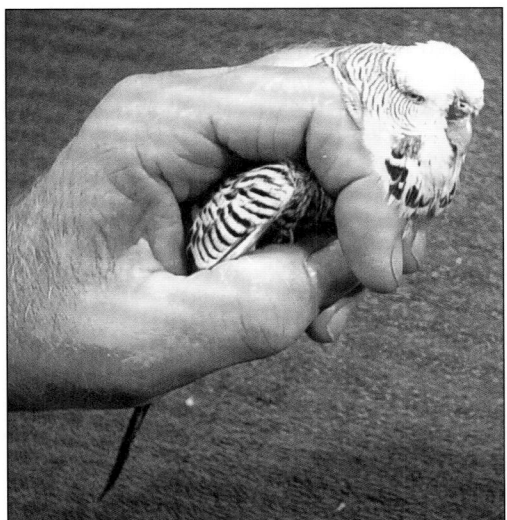

11.42 Holding a budgerigar for examination. (Reproduced from the *BSAVA Manual of Psittacine Birds, 2nd edn*)

jump out of the container and injure themselves; however, this technique may allow sufficient restraint to allow a clinical examination.

For fully feathered immature parrots it may still be necessary to towel restrain the bird to examine the vent, feet and other sensitive areas without the bird biting or flapping its wings and escaping.

Waterfowl

Ducks, geese and swans are often kept in farm situations, but are also kept by smallholders and so may well be brought in for treatment. Restraint of these species is relatively straightforward but may become hazardous with the larger species of swan and goose.

1. The first priority is to concentrate on capturing the head. This can be done manually, by grasping the waterfowl around the upper neck from behind.
2. Make sure that your fingers curl around the neck and under the bill whilst the thumb supports the back of the neck and the potentially weak area of the atlanto-occipital joint. Failing this, a swan or shepherd's crook or other such adapted smooth metal or wooden pole attached hook can be used to catch the neck – again high up under the bill.
3. Next, it is essential that the, often powerful, wings are controlled before the bird has a chance to damage itself or you. This can be most easily achieved by using a towel, thrown or draped over the avian patient's back and loosely wrapped under the sternum. Some practices may have access to more specialized goose or swan cradle bags, which wrap around the body, containing the wings but allowing the feet and head and neck to remain free.
4. The bird may now be safely carried or restrained by tucking its body (contained within the towel or restraint bag) under one arm and holding this close to the torso. With your other hand, the neck can be loosely held from behind just below the bill.

Toucans and hornbills

Another group of birds increasingly kept in private collections are the toucans and hornbills. These have an extremely impressive beak, with a serrated edge to the upper bill.

Provided the head is initially controlled using the towel technique described above for parrots, an elastic band or tape may be applied around the bill, preventing biting. The handler still needs to be careful of stabbing manoeuvres and it may be a good idea to work with a second handler. Otherwise, restraint is the same as for Passeriformes.

Escaped birds

Where a bird is loose in a room or in an aviary flight cage, a number of methods can be applied. Again, darkening the room for diurnal species and reducing its area, if possible, are both very helpful to calm and confine the bird.

- In the case of larger parrots, throwing a heavy bath towel over the bird can confine them for long enough to allow the handler to restrain the head from behind and then wrap the patient in the towel.
- For very small birds, the investment in a fine aviary or butterfly net (preferably made of dark, very fine mesh) is extremely useful to catch the bird safely, either in mid-flight or against the side of the cage or room. Larger nets are available from specialist retailers for catching the larger species of birds.

Handling and restraint of reptiles

Reptiles tend to be less easily stressed than birds and so restraint of the debilitated animal may be performed according to the degree of risk. It is still worthwhile considering one or two aspects that may make restraint dangerous to animal and veterinary nurse alike.

Assessment before handling

1. Is the patient in respiratory distress?
   Examples include pneumonic cases, where mouth breathing and excessive oral mucus may be present, and where excessive manual manipulation can exacerbate the condition.
2. Is the species of reptile a fragile one?
   The small day geckos (*Phelsuma* spp.), for example, are extremely delicate and very prone to shedding their tails when handled. Similarly, some species such as green iguanas (*Iguana iguana*) are prone to conditions, such as metabolic bone disease, whereby their skeleton becomes fragile and spontaneous fractures are common.
3. Is the species an aggressive one?
   Some are naturally so, for example, alligator snapping turtles (*Macroclemys temminckii*), Tokay geckos (*Gekko gecko*), and rock pythons (*Python sebae*).
4. Does the reptile patient require medication/physical examination?
   In these cases, restraint is essential.

Reptiles are ectothermic and so rely on their environmental temperature to maintain their body temperature. Handling periods should therefore be minimized as much as possible to prevent undue cooling of the reptile. Most reptiles commonly seen in veterinary practices require an optimum temperature range of 22–32°C.

WARNING

It should be borne in mind that many species of reptile have a bacterial flora in their digestive systems that frequently includes *Salmonella* spp. Personal hygiene is therefore very important when handling these patients, to prevent zoonotic disease transmission. Disposable gloves may be worn. Hands must always be washed thoroughly with hot water and liquid soap after handling

---

Chelonians

This group includes all land tortoises, terrapins and aquatic turtles. Size differences in this order are not as great as those for lizards and snakes, but it is still possible to see chelonians varying from the small Egyptian tortoises (*Testudo kleinmanni*), weighing a few hundred grams, all the way up to adult leopard tortoises (*Stigmochelys pardalis*), at 40 kg, and the Galapagos tortoises, which can weigh several hundred kilograms. The majority of chelonians are harmless, although surprisingly strong. The exceptions include the snapping turtle (*Chelydra serpentina*) and the alligator snapping turtle (*Macrochelys temminckii*), both of which can give a serious bite. Most of the soft-shelled terrapins have mobile necks and can also bite; even red-eared terrapins (*Trachemys scripta elegans*) may give a nasty nip.

For the mild-tempered chelonians, such as the Mediterranean *Testudo* species, the tortoise may be held with both hands, one on either side of the main part of the shell behind the front legs (Figure 11.43a). For examination, to keep the tortoise still, it may be placed on top of a cylinder or stack of tins. This ensures that the legs are raised clear of the table and the tortoise is balancing on the centre of the underside of the shell (plastron).

For aggressive species, it is essential that the shell is held on both sides behind and above the rear legs to avoid being bitten (Figure 11.43b). In order to examine the head region in these species, it is necessary to chemically restrain them.

For the soft-shelled and aquatic species, soft cloths and nitrile gloves should be used in order not to mark the shell.

Lizards

Lizards come in many different shapes and sizes, from the 1.2 m long adult green iguana to the 10–12 cm long green anole (*Anolis carolinensis*). They all have roughly the same structural format, with four limbs (although these may become vestigial, for example in the case of the slowworm) and a tail. The potential danger to the veterinary nurse includes their claws and teeth, and in some species such as iguanas, their tails, which can lash out in a whip-like fashion.

Geckos, other than Tokay geckos, are generally docile, as are lizards such as bearded dragons (*Pogona* spp.). Iguanas may be extremely aggressive, particularly sexually mature males. They may also be more aggressive towards female owners and handlers as they are sensitive to human, as well as reptile, pheromones.

Restraint is best performed by grasping the pectoral girdle with one hand from the dorsal aspect, so controlling one forelimb with the forefinger and thumb, and controlling the other forelimb between the middle and fourth fingers. The other hand is used to grasp the pelvic girdle from the dorsal aspect (Figure 11.44), controlling one limb with the thumb and forefinger, and the other limb between the middle and fourth fingers. The lizard may then be held in a vertical manner with the head uppermost and the tail out of harm's way

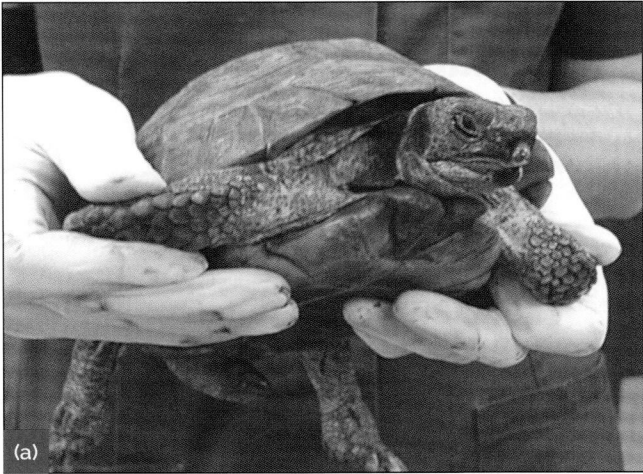

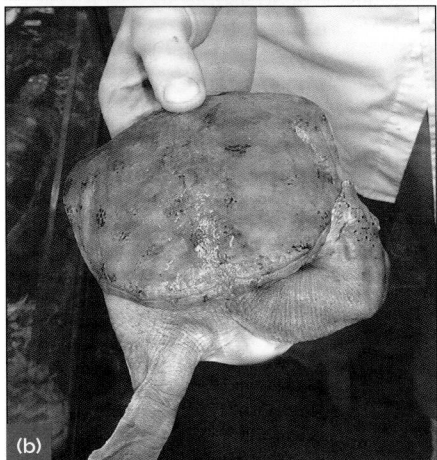

11.43 Handling chelonians. **(a)** Lifting a docile species. **(b)** Handling an aggressive species by grasping the caudal part of the carapace. (Reproduced from the *BSAVA Manual of Reptiles, 3rd edn*)

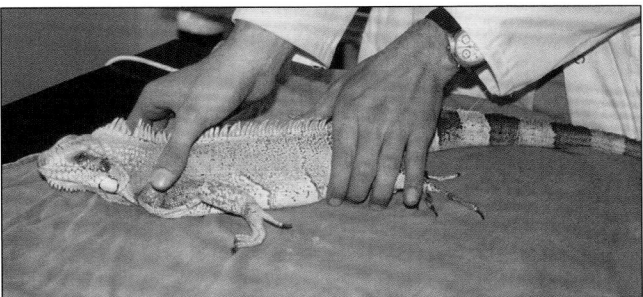

11.44 Holding the forelimbs and hindlimbs against the thorax and tailbase, respectively, restrains medium to large lizards such as this iguana. (Courtesy of S. Redrobe)

underneath the handler's arm. When holding a lizard in this manner, the handler should allow some flexibility as the lizard may wriggle, and if the restraint is overly rigid the spine can be damaged. It is then possible to present the head and feet of the lizard away from the handler to avoid injury.

Some of the more aggressive iguanas may need to be pinned down prior to this method of handling. Here, as with avian patients, the use of a thick towel to control the tail and claws is often very useful. In some instances, gauntlets are necessary for particularly aggressive large lizards and for those which may have a venomous bite, such as the Gila monster (*Heloderma suspectum*) and the beaded lizard (*H. horribilis*). It is important not to use too much force when

restraining the lizard, as those with skeletal problems, such as metabolic bone disease, may be seriously injured. Lizards, like other reptiles, do not have a diaphragm, and so over-zealous restraint will lead to the digestive system pushing on to the lungs and compromising respiration.

Geckos can be extremely fragile and the day geckos, for example, are best examined in a clear plastic container rather than physically restraining them. Other gecko species have skin that is easily damaged; nitrile gloves and soft cloths should be used and the gecko cupped in the hand rather than restraining it physically.

Small lizards may have their heads controlled between the index finger and thumb to prevent biting.

> **WARNING**
>
> It is important that lizards are never restrained by their tails. Many will shed their tails at this time, but not all of them will regrow (show autotomy). Green iguanas, for example, will only regrow their tails as juveniles (under 2.5–3 years of age); once they are older than this, they will be left tail-less

Vago-vagal reflex

There is a procedure that may be used to place members of the lizard family into a trance-like state. It involves closing the eyelids and placing firm but gentle digital pressure on both eyeballs. This stimulates the parasympathetic autonomic nervous system, which results in a reduction in heart rate, blood pressure and respiration rate (the vago-vagal reflex). To maintain pressure on the eyeballs, a cotton-wool ball may be placed over each closed eye and a bandage wrapped around the head, holding these in place. Provided there are no loud noises or environmental stimuli, after 1–2 minutes the lizard may be placed on its side, front, back, etc., allowing radiography to be performed without using physical or chemical restraint. Loud noises or physical stimulation, however, will immediately bring the lizard back to its normal wakeful state. A similar procedure may be performed with larger snakes by placing cotton wool balls over the eyes and lightly taping them in place.

The 'trancing' of rabbits (see above) has been reviewed on welfare grounds, based upon recent scientific research. Such scientific evidence is not currently available for lizards and snakes. It is not yet known whether the physiological response of the lizard or snake differs from that of a tranced rabbit or if the same welfare concerns arise. The procedure in lizards and snakes should therefore currently be viewed with an open mind.

Snakes

There is a wide range of sizes, from the enormous anacondas (*Eunectes murinus*) and Burmese pythons (*Python molurus bivittatus*) (Figure 11.45), which may achieve lengths of up to 10 m or more, down to the thread snake family (Leptotyphlopidae), which may be a few tens of centimetres long. They are all characterized by their elongated form with an absence of limbs. The potential danger to the veterinary nurse is from the teeth (and in the case of the more venomous species, such as the viper family, the fang teeth) or, in the case of the constrictor and python family, the ability to asphyxiate the prey by winding themselves around the victim's chest or neck. With this in mind, the following restraint techniques may be employed.

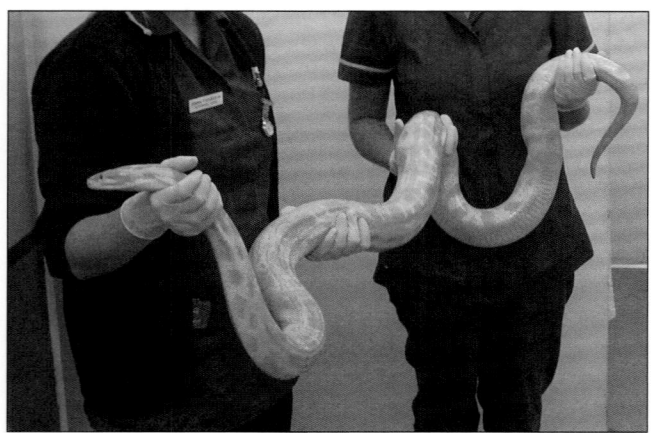

11.45 Carrying a large snake requires support from more than one handler. (Reproduced from the *BSAVA Manual of Reptiles, 3rd edn*)

Non-venomous snakes

Non-venomous snakes can be restrained initially by controlling the head. This is done by placing the thumb over the occiput and curling the fingers under the chin. Reptiles, like birds, have only one occipital condyle and so the importance of stabilizing the atlanto-occipital joint cannot be overstated. It is also important to support the rest of the snake's body, so that not all of the weight of the snake is suspended from the head. With smaller species, this is best achieved by allowing the snake to coil around the handler's arm, so that it is supporting itself.

In the larger species (those longer than 3 m), it is necessary to support the body length at regular intervals (see Figure 11.45). Indeed, it is vital to adopt a safe operating practice with the larger constricting species of snake. For this reason a 'buddy system' should be operated, whereby any snake longer than 2.5–3 m in length should only be handled by two or more people. This is to ensure that if the snake were to enwrap the handler, the 'buddy' could disentangle them by unwinding from the tail end first. Above all, it is important not to grip the snake too hard as this will cause bruising and the release of myoglobin from muscle cells that will lodge in the kidneys, causing damage to the filtration membranes.

Venomous and aggressive snakes

Venomous reptiles should only be handled by those who have the training and experience to do so safely. Venomous snakes (such as vipers and rattlesnakes) and very aggressive species (such as the green anaconda (*Eunectes murinus*), reticulated python (*Python reticulatus*) and rock python (*P. sebae*)) may be restrained initially using snake hooks. These are 0.5–0.75 m steel rods with a blunt shepherd's hook at one end. They are used to loop under the body of a snake, to move it at arm's length into a container. The hook may also be used to trap the head flat to the floor before grasping it with the hand. Once the head is controlled safely the snake is rendered harmless – unless it is a member of the spitting cobra family. Fortunately, it is rare to come across spitting cobras in general practice, but staff who do handle them must wear plastic goggles or a plastic face visor as they may spit venom into the handler's eyes and mucous membranes, causing blindness and paralysis. Using a specialist veterinary centre with both the experience and appropriate equipment is preferable to these species being seen in general practice.

Handling and restraint of amphibians

Examination of the amphibian patient should be performed at the species' optimum body temperature. A rough guide is between 21 and 24°C, which is lower than the more usual 22–32°C reptile housing conditions.

The examination table should be covered with paper towels (unbleached) soaked in dechlorinated, preferably purified, water. Additional purified water should be on standby to be applied to the amphibian patient to prevent dehydration during the examination.

It is useful not to restrain the patient until the extent of any problem is assessed, as many have severe skin lesions that are extremely fragile.

Once an initial assessment has been made, the patient may be restrained manually. It is advisable to use a pair of nitrile gloves. This minimizes irritation to the amphibian's skin caused by the normally acidic human skin. The wearing of gloves is also essential for handling members of the toad family or the arrow tree frogs, which can secrete irritant or even potentially deadly toxins from their skin. These toxins can be absorbed through unprotected human skin. It may be necessary to wear goggles when handling some species of toad. The giant toad (*Bufo marinus*) can squirt a toxin from its parotid glands over a distance of several feet.

When handling the amphibian patient, the method of restraint will obviously depend on the animal's body shape.

- The elongated form of salamanders and newts will require similar restraint to that of a lizard: one hand grasps the pectoral girdle from the dorsal aspect, with the index finger and thumb encircling one forelimb and the second and third fingers the other, while the opposite hand grasps the pelvic girdle, again from the dorsal aspect in a similar manner. Some salamanders will shed their tails if roughly handled and so care should be taken with these species.
- Large anurans (members of the frog and toad family) can be restrained by cupping one hand around the pectoral girdle immediately behind the front limbs, with the other hand positioned beneath the hindlimbs (Figure 11.46). Care should be taken with some species that have poison glands in their skin, as mentioned above. Care should also be taken with species such as the Argentinian horned frog (*Ceratophrys ornata*) as these can bite.
- Aquatic urodeles (newts and salamanders) should be examined only in water, as removal from the water results in skin damage. Some of the larger urodeles, such as the hellbender species (*Cryptobranchus* spp.), can also inflict unpleasant bite wounds on handlers.

Smaller species and aquatic species may be best examined in small plastic or glass jars.

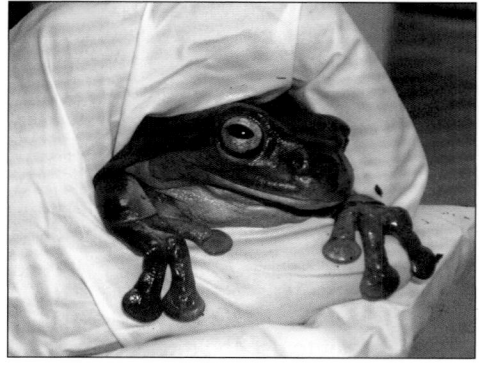

11.46

Handling a frog. (Courtesy of G. Goodman)

Handling and restraint of invertebrates

The species involved will naturally determine the methods by which the patient can be safely, for handler and invertebrate alike, restrained.

Many invertebrates present no direct threat to the handler. Examples include giant land snails, stick insects and cockroaches. These may be gently picked up and cupped in the hand, or allowed to walk on to a towel or similar non-slip surface.

Other species, such as those in the mygalomorph spider family, may present multiple hazards. These may flick setae (the small hairs that cover their abdomens) at the handler if stressed or if they feel threatened. These setae are highly irritant on the skin and are particularly dangerous if they come into contact with the conjunctiva/cornea. In addition, many of these spiders have a nasty bite. The bites are rarely fatal but still cause pain and potential harm, similar to the pain associated with a bee or wasp sting. These species should be transferred into a Perspex, glass or plastic container (Figure 11.47), and only ever handled with nitrile gloves. If it is necessary to pick up such a spider, it may be either cupped in paired hands or grasped with atraumatic forceps or fingers, immediately behind the cephalothorax, around its 'waist'. Protective goggles should be worn if the spider is to be removed from its container.

Scorpions present a similar problem, with the tail sting being the most obvious danger. The majority of scorpions kept in captivity, such as the imperial scorpion, are not seriously dangerous, although the sting may be likened to a wasp or bee sting. To restrain these species safely, they may be transferred into a Perspex, plastic or glass container, or alternatively a sheet of clear plastic may be gently but firmly laid over the top of the scorpion to confine it for examination or to allow a better grasp. They may also be lifted gently by the tip of the tail using atraumatic forceps, with a sheet of card or plastic supporting the body from underneath.

Aquatic invertebrates should be examined and moved in water, using either their own tank or a clean plastic, Perspex or glass container.

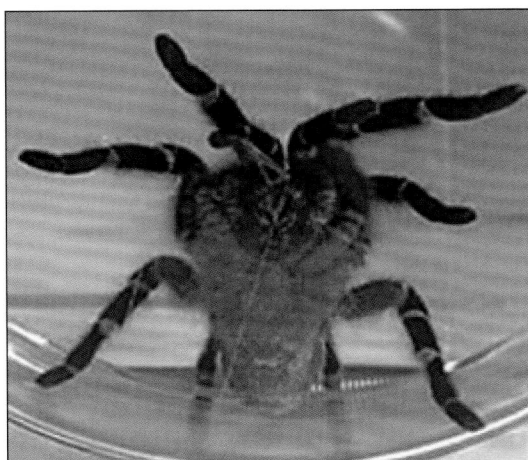

11.47 Placing a spider in a transparent container allows it to be examined easily. (Courtesy of E. Morgan)

References and further reading

Buseth ME and Saunders RA (2015) *Rabbit Behaviour, Health and Care.* CABI, Oxfordshire

Chitty J and Monks D (2018) *BSAVA Manual of Avian Practice.* BSAVA Publications, Gloucester

Ellis S and Sparkes A (2016) *Feline Stress and Health: Managing Negative Emotions to Improve Feline Health and Wellbeing.* International Society of Feline Medicine, Tisbury

Fowler ME (2008) *Restraint and Handling of Wild and Domestic Animals, 3rd edn.* Wiley-Blackwell, Iowa

Fraser M and Girling S (2009) *Rabbit Medicine and Surgery for Veterinary Nurses.* Wiley-Blackwell, Oxford

Girling SJ (2013) *Veterinary Nursing of Exotic Pets, 2nd edn.* Wiley-Blackwell Publishing, Oxford

Girling SJ and Raiti P (2018) *BSAVA Manual of Reptiles, 3rd edn.* BSAVA Publications, Gloucester

Harcourt-Brown F and Chitty J (2013) *BSAVA Manual of Rabbit Surgery, Dentistry and Imaging.* BSAVA Publications, Gloucester

Hedges S (2014) *Practical Canine Behaviour for Veterinary Nurses and Technicians.* CABI, Oxfordshire

Horwitz DF and Mills DS (2009) *BSAVA Manual of Canine and Feline Behavioural Medicine, 2nd edn.* BSAVA Publications, Gloucester

Keeble E and Meredith A (2009) *BSAVA Manual of Rodents and Ferrets.* BSAVA Publications, Gloucester

McBride EA (2017) Small prey species' behaviour and welfare: implications for veterinary professionals. *Journal of Small Animal Practice* **58**, 423–436

McBride EA, Day S, McAdie T *et al.* (2007) Hypnosis: a state of fear or pleasure? *Proceedings of CABTSG Study Day 2007: Emotional Homoeostasis, Stress, the Environment and Behaviour,* pp. 38–40

Meredith A and Flecknell P (2006) *BSAVA Manual of Rabbit Medicine and Surgery, 2nd edn.* BSAVA Publications, Gloucester

Meredith A and Johnson-Delaney C (2010) *BSAVA Manual of Exotic Pets, 5th edn.* BSAVA Publications, Gloucester

Meredith A and Lord B (2014) *BSAVA Manual of Rabbit Medicine.* BSAVA Publications, Gloucester

Mills D, Dube MB and Zulch H (2013) *Stress and Pheromonatherapy in Small Animal Clinical Behaviour.* Wiley-Blackwell, Chichester

Varga M, Lumbis R and Gott L (2012) *BSAVA Manual of Exotic Pet and Wildlife Nursing.* BSAVA Publications, Gloucester

Yin S (2009) *Low Stress Handling, Restraint and Behaviour Modification of Dogs and Cats: Techniques for Developing Patients who Love Their Visits.* Cattledog Publishing, California

Useful websites

Animal Behaviour and Training Council: www.abtcouncil.org.uk

Association for the Study of Animal Behaviour – Register of Certified Practitioners: www.asab.org/ccab-register

Association of Pet Behaviour Counsellors:
- Appropriate way to approach a dog www.youtube.com/watch?v=lpecvb9Q7QY
- Cat carrier training www.youtube.com/watch?v=tSp8nl9xK3g

Barbara's Force Free Animal Training – Force free training of all species for veterinary interventions: https://barbarasffat.com

Blue Cross – Muzzle training: www.bluecross.org.uk/pet-advice/dogs-and-muzzle-training

British Small Animal Veterinary Association (BSAVA) – Position Statement on Aversive Training Methods: www.bsava.com/Resources/Veterinary-resources/Position-statements/Aversive-training-methods

RSPCA – Understanding rabbit behaviour: www.rspca.org.uk/adviceandwelfare/pets/rabbits/behaviour/understanding

Self-assessment questions

1. What are the four main aims of the veterinary nurse when restraining an animal?
2. What are the signs that could indicate that a dog or cat may be fearful and/or potentially aggressive?
3. What actions should and should not be taken when initially approaching and handling a dog or cat?
4. What are the important behaviours to adopt when handling a dog that is demonstrating aggressive behaviour?
5. How is a tape muzzle applied and when should one be used?
6. How should an aggressive rabbit be restrained?
7. How should rodents be handled? Which species of rodent should not be routinely grasped by the scruff of the neck to restrain them?
8. What are the common methods of handling birds? What type of bird will not be quietened by moving it into a darkened room?
9. How should small cage birds be restrained? When restraining a bird, what should the handler be careful not to do too firmly?
10. How should reptiles be handled? What important zoonotic bacteria may be carried by reptiles?
11. What are the principles of handling invertebrates? What defence mechanism might mygalomorph spiders employ to avoid being handled?

Chapter 12

The nursing process, nursing models and care plans

Andrea Jeffery
with clinical application of models by Stuart Ford-Fennah

Learning objectives

After studying this chapter, readers will have the knowledge to:

- Describe what the nursing process is and how its use ensures a systematic approach to nursing care
- List the differences between the Medical (Biomedical) Model and the Nursing-focused Models of nursing care
- Explain the key principles of a range of nursing models, including the Roper, Logan and Tierney and Orem human-centred models and the Orpet and Jeffery Ability Model developed for veterinary patients
- Use an appropriate model of care to deliver the nursing process and create care plans for a range of disorders and diseases
- Interpret nursing care plans and carry out appropriate nursing interventions

Introduction

In defining a professional role for veterinary nurses, one of the first steps has been to introduce the nursing process and models of nursing care into the Royal College of Veterinary Surgeons (RCVS) Day One Competencies and Skills for Veterinary Nurses, emphasizing the importance of developing up-to-date evidence-based nursing practice through the implementation of care plans, in which the nursing care of veterinary patients is systematically planned and delivered by veterinary nurses. The effectiveness of the care given is then evaluated by the whole team, including the veterinary surgeon.

The history of nursing

Florence Nightingale, as long ago as 1859, was of the opinion that medicine and nursing should be clearly differentiated from each other, and yet in the 1990s veterinary surgeons were still being asked to lecture to veterinary nurses about nursing. Today, in the 21st century, the number of lectures delivered by veterinary surgeons to veterinary nurses about nursing has reduced significantly. This is an important change within the profession, as Peplau in 1987 argued that those who teach control the content of the occupation. It is therefore important that veterinary nurses deliver education to other veterinary nurses regarding patient care, as this is their area of expertise.

The Medical (Biomedical) Model

According to Aggleton and Chalmers (2000), within the Medical Model (also referred to as the Biomedical Model) (Figure 12.1) the patient is seen as a complex set of anatomical parts and physiological systems. This model emphasizes anatomical, physiological and biochemical malfunctions

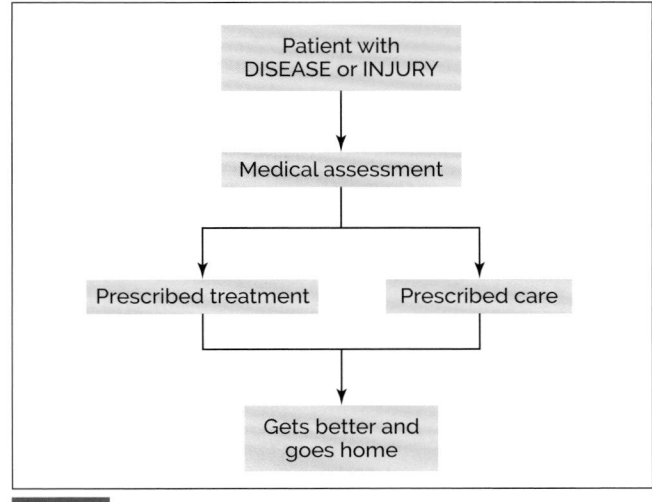

12.1 The Medical Model (Aggleton and Chalmers, 2000).

as the causes of ill health and, by doing so, it encourages a disease-oriented approach to the patient. The primary role of the veterinary surgeon is to diagnose and treat disease, and they may therefore have a disease-oriented approach to a patient. The veterinary team, and veterinary nurses in particular, however, should see their patients as unique individuals and take a holistic (nursing each animal as a 'whole' individual rather than the disease it has been admitted with) patient-oriented approach to the nursing care they deliver. Veterinary nurses should still be fully aware of, and have a good understanding of, the clinical problem that the patient has, as this will inform the care delivered.

The nursing process

The nursing process is the key to professional nursing, as it enables nurses to provide organized, structured and holistic care to patients. By nursing in this way it is hoped that the care provided addresses the individual patient's needs, rather than focusing on the disease or clinical problem the patient has been admitted with (Lock, 2011; Nelson and Welsh, 2015).

The nursing process is a cyclical process, which provides a structure to the way in which nursing care for the patient is planned. The 'process of nursing', as currently used to plan and deliver patient care, is encapsulated in Figure 12.2.

In contrast, Figure 12.3 illustrates the 'nursing process'. There is very little difference between the diagrams, but one difference is the insertion of the additional stage that occurs between Assessment and Planning: the 'nursing diagnosis'. This was introduced later in the development of the nursing process and refers to the nursing decision that is made, with

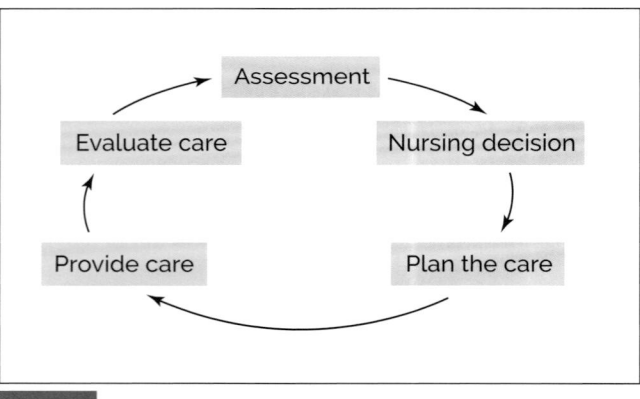

12.2 The process of nursing.

12.3 The nursing process (Lock, 2011).

regard to what care is given to patients. The nursing diagnosis is an important element of the nursing process; after all, the care of a patient cannot be planned if no decision has been made on what that care should be. In this way the nurse is making a diagnosis of the patient's individual needs based on its care requirements, which are ascertained by using a systematic approach involving a detailed patient assessment.

Following the nursing process will ensure that nurses have a systematic approach to the delivery of care.

Assessment

Assessment will clearly establish the individual needs of the patient. It is only once a patient assessment has been carried out that effective care can be given.

1. Collect the necessary information systematically from your own observations, from the client and from other team members.
2. Review the collected information.
3. Identify actual and potential nursing problems.
4. Identify priorities among the problems.

It is important to remember at this point that the nursing process and models of care can be used to provide holistic nursing care to all species seen within general practice. However, for the purpose of this chapter the majority of examples given are either canine or feline patients.

Patient example: Ben – a dog with polyuria/polydipsia

Ben Jones is an 11-year-old male neutered Golden Retriever. He has been admitted for hospitalization by the veterinary surgeon for investigation of lethargy, polydipsia and polyuria, which he has had for several days. The veterinary surgeon has requested that he is kennelled for observation and that preliminary urine and blood tests are carried out to investigate the cause of the problem.

The admitting veterinary surgeon may have asked questions taking a disease-focused approach. Using a more detailed assessment approach may allow for more comprehensive information to be gathered. Gathering information about a patient is very important as it sets the scene for any action to be taken:

- Wrong information ⟶ wrong action
- Lack of information ⟶ inadequate action.

There may not always be the opportunity to do this during the admission of the patient (or it may not feel like the right time). If a face-to-face conversation with the owner does not take place, it may be possible to telephone the owner at a later time on the day of admission, as a follow-up. Better still, would be to ask the client to complete an assessment questionnaire and bring it with them or email it to the practice before the patient is admitted, in order for informed decisions to be made regarding any patient from the point of admission.

At whatever point the nurse decides to carry out the interview, it is important that the owner understands that the nurse is asking these additional questions to help them to assess the pet's individual needs and plan the pet's care accordingly.

The information from the owner, along with the information from the admitting veterinary surgeon, is essential as it is important to know what is 'normal' for each patient. Knowing what the patient's 'normal' routines, behaviour and preferences are will ensure that the nurse's approach to the care of patients is as individualized as possible. Gathering this information could make a significant difference to the care delivered. The information from the patient assessment is also key to the home care plan drawn up by the practice for the owner to follow, and helps improve compliance after discharge as it determines the client's limitations (Orpet, 2011).

Patient example: Ben – assessment

It is already known from the admitting veterinary surgeon that Ben has exercise intolerance, polydipsia and polyuria. However, if a veterinary nurse had spoken to the dog's owners, they would have ascertained that Ben is deaf in his left ear, eats one meal per day, in the evening, and will only urinate and defecate on concrete and not on grass. All of this information is important for Ben's hospitalization.

Nursing diagnosis

As discussed earlier, a nursing diagnosis differs from a medical diagnosis in that it is not concerned with making a judgement about disease, but rather with the nursing intervention needed to provide the patient with the most appropriate nursing care.

There may occasionally be some overlap but it is extremely important to understand the difference between a clinical veterinary diagnosis, which is not within the remit of nursing, and a nursing diagnosis, which obviously is.

Planning

After the assessment phase of the nursing process (when all the information is gathered) comes the planning stage. This involves making plans to overcome the nursing problems that have been identified.

Planning may begin by considering the aims of nursing:

- To solve identified actual problems
- To prevent identified potential problems becoming actual
- To alleviate any problems that cannot be solved
- To help the patient and client cope positively with problems that cannot be solved or alleviated
- To prevent recurrence of a treated problem
- To help make the patient as comfortable as possible, even when death is inevitable.

Patient example: Ben – planning

The veterinary surgeon has made a diagnosis of diabetes mellitus. Planning Ben's nursing can now be carried out, using all the information that has been collected.

The **actual problems** identified for Ben are:
- Exercise intolerance
- Polydipsia/polyuria due to unstable diabetes mellitus
- Unilateral deafness due to age-related degeneration

The **potential problems** identified if the actual problems are not solved include:
- Weight loss
- Dehydration
- Hypoglycaemia

Setting goals

A goal must be set for each actual and potential problem identified during the initial assessment, and a distinction should be made between short-term and long-term goals. It is important that any goals set should be stated in terms of outcomes that can be observed, measured or tested, so that effective evaluation can then be carried out.

Patient example: Ben – short-term goals while his diabetes is stabilized

Problem	Short-term goal/outcome	Timing	Nursing intervention
Polydipsia	Prevent dehydration	At all times	Provide measured volumes of fresh drinking water and record
Polyuria	Ensure Ben has the opportunity to urinate regularly	Every hour	Take Ben into an outside concrete run to allow him opportunity to urinate and record

The nursing plan

A plan should be made including all the proposed nursing interventions needed to achieve the goals. This plan should be written in enough detail that any nurse reading it will know what care is required. For example, in order to achieve the short-term goal of ensuring that Ben does not urinate in his kennel, the nursing intervention would be to take him outside, on concrete, every 60 minutes.

Implementation

Implementing the nursing plan is the doing stage of the nursing process, otherwise known as the nursing intervention. It is important that nurses make it clear what decision-making has taken place, in order to justify the nursing intervention. All of this information should be recorded clearly and indelibly on the patient care plan.

Evaluation

This is a vital part of the nursing process. It is difficult to justify planning and implementing nursing interventions if the outcomes cannot be shown to have benefited either the patient or the client in some way. Evaluation involves reflecting upon the nursing process and the outcomes achieved by it. Evaluation is a difficult process. As a nurse, one hopes that the evaluation will show that all the nursing goals have been achieved. If this is not the case, the following questions need to be asked (adapted from Luker, 1989):

- Has the goal set for the patient been partially achieved?
- Is more information from the veterinary surgeon or the client required to decide the next step in the nursing care?
- Is a specific problem unchanged and should the nursing intervention be changed or stopped?
- Is there a worsening of the problem and should the goal and nursing intervention be reviewed?
- Was the goal inappropriate when first set?
- Does the goal require interventions from other members of the veterinary team (e.g. veterinary surgeon or physiotherapist)?

By asking these questions, a re-evaluation of the patient is taking place, leading to a revision of the original nursing plan, where needed, in order to address the issues that have become apparent. Any changes required are recorded on the care plan and the whole process begins again.

Models of nursing

The nursing process offers a systematic approach to care but is limited in its function unless it is integrated into a model of nursing.

According to Aggleton and Chalmers (2000) the nursing process:

- Encourages nurses to assess but does not tell them what to look for
- Advocates planning but does not say what form the care plan should take
- Talks of intervention but does not specify what might be appropriate interventions
- Calls for evaluation without specifying the standards against which comparisons should be made.

This is where nursing models come in. Nursing models provide the nurse with key pointers regarding patient assessment, care planning, the type of interventions that are appropriate and, finally, evaluation. Together with the nursing process, they provide detailed guidance for the steps that need to be taken when delivering nursing care.

Models are systematically constructed. This means that they have been developed logically and can be adapted to meet specific patient requirements. They also act as guides for nursing practice by providing a framework in which to deliver nursing care.

There are a number of published nursing models developed by human-centred nursing theorists, two of which are discussed below; these are the Roper, Logan and Tierney Model, which focuses on the 12 activities of living, and the Orem Self-care Model, which focuses on the patient's self-care requisites (how much the patient can still do for itself).

The Ability Model is currently the only model of care for veterinary patients and is an adaptation of both of these human-centred models, with the assessment phase focusing on the 'abilities' of the individual animal, no matter which species it belongs to.

The Roper, Logan and Tierney Model

The Roper, Logan and Tierney Model of nursing is based primarily on activities of living (Roper *et al.*, 1993). It is often used to assess how the life of a patient has changed due to illness, injury or admission to hospital, rather than as a way of planning for increasing independence and quality of life.

The Roper, Logan and Tierney Model of nursing is made up of five parts:

1. Activities of living.
2. The patient's lifespan.
3. Dependence–independence continuum.
4. Factors influencing the activities of living.
5. Individuality in living.

Relationship between the component parts of the model

Figure 12.4 shows how the component parts relate to one another and the significance of each in the construction of the Roper, Logan and Tierney Model of nursing.

Part one: Activities of living

According to Roper, Logan and Tierney these are the central components of the model (Roper *et al.*, 1993). There are twelve activities of living.

The twelve activities of living

- Maintaining a safe environment
- Communicating
- Breathing
- Eating and drinking
- Eliminating
- Personal cleansing and dressing (grooming)
- Controlling body temperature
- Mobilizing
- Working and playing
- Expressing sexuality
- Sleeping
- Dying

If a client were asked to describe what each day involved for their pet, most people would include some or all of the functions listed above. This is why they are called 'activities of living' (ALs).

Roper reports that when this model was first introduced in 1980, the inclusion of 'expression of sexuality' as an AL was greeted by surprise, but is less likely to cause a problem within the veterinary field. The fact that 'dying' was considered an AL was also unusual at this time, but in veterinary science euthanasia is something that a client can opt for when and if it is needed, which makes this an important activity when this model is applied to veterinary patients.

Part two: Lifespan

Each animal has a lifespan from birth to death and is likely to have stages along the way of neonate, kitten/puppy, adolescent, adult, senior (geriatric). Some may die before they reach old age.

Within the care plan, the 'lifespan' is represented as a diagram showing a unidirectional arrow from birth to death:

Neonate ⟶ Geriatric

It is added at the beginning of the care plan in order that a particular patient's position can be plotted on it, and their age can be seen at a glance. It is important that nurses have a visual reminder of the patient's age when they consider each of the ALs for any particular patient.

Part three: Dependence–independence continuum

This part of the model is closely related to lifespan and to the ALs:

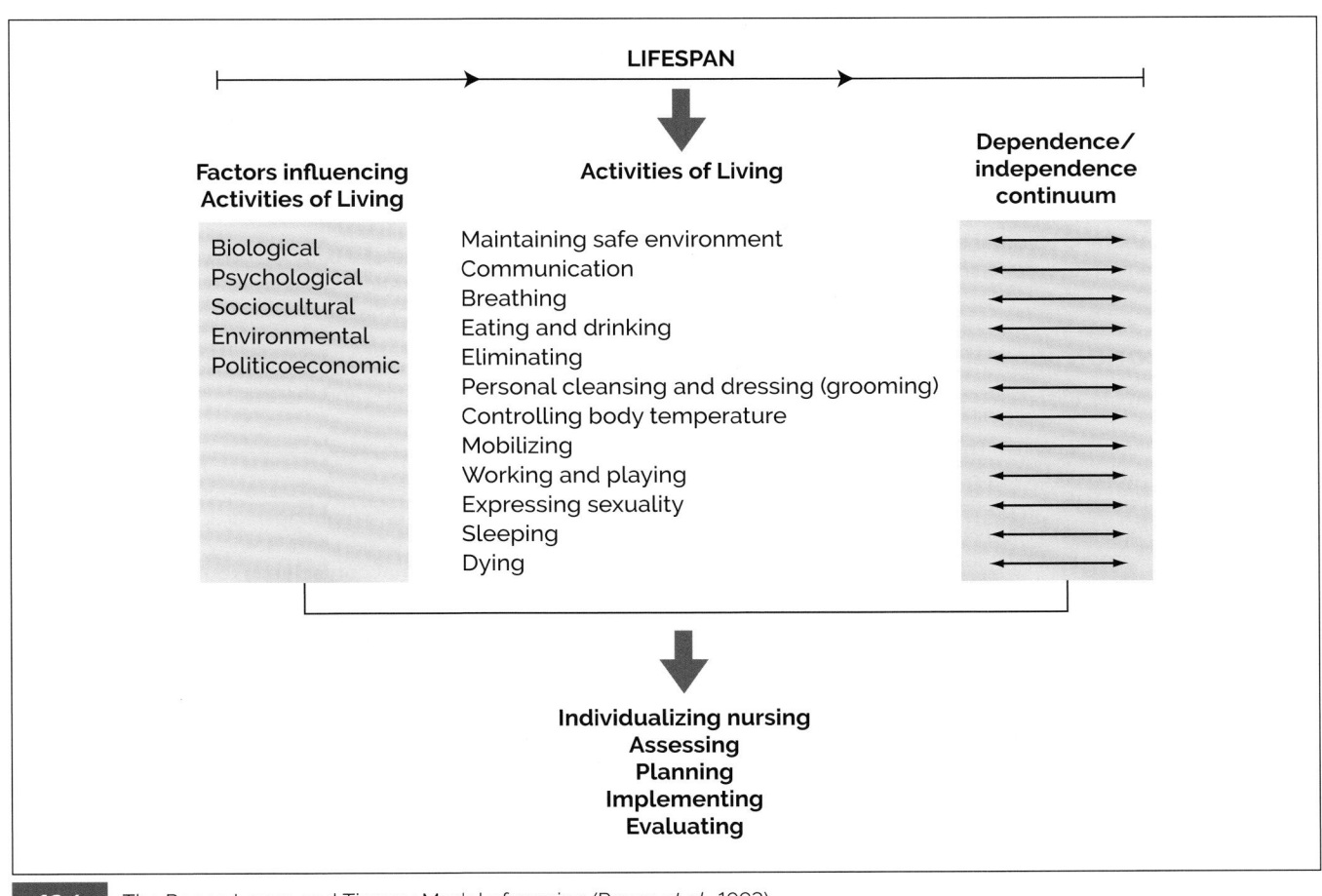

12.4 The Roper, Logan and Tierney Model of nursing (Roper *et al.*, 1993).

Total dependence (D) ⟶ Total independence (I)

It acknowledges that there are times in life when a patient cannot perform certain ALs independently. Each patient will have a dependence–independence continuum for each AL and the patient's position can be plotted on each of these to provide an impression of that patient's degree of dependence or independence. Throughout the patient's stay, its position on each continuum will be plotted more than once; the patient should become less dependent during their stay at hospital, as the problem for which it has been admitted resolves.

An example of how the Roper, Logan and Tierney Model can be applied to a rabbit patient, Bruce, is given at the end of this chapter.

Part four: Factors influencing the activities of living

Five main factors influence the ALs and should be considered when preparing a care plan for each individual patient:

- Biological
- Psychological
- Sociocultural
- Environmental
- Politico-economic.

Biological

It is important to be aware of the biological state of the patient's body and how this might influence any of the ALs.

The veterinary nurse must be familiar with the anatomy and physiology of both the healthy and sick animal in order to understand the impact of a disease on an animal within their care.

Psychological

The impact of psychological stresses on the ALs can be significant. For example, a veterinary patient that is separated from its owner may become withdrawn, refuse to eat and drink and be unable to sleep, all of which will have a detrimental effect on its health and an impact on the ALs.

Sociocultural

It is important that nurses have knowledge of sociocultural factors and how they may influence ALs. It may appear on first reading that this is not appropriate when nursing veterinary patients, but the relevance becomes apparent when considered in the context of the owner:

- The client – cultural idiosyncrasies of the client need to be considered in relation to the ALs
- The patient – some animals are herd animals.

Environmental

The environment in which the patient is housed (see Chapter 14) may influence its ALs.

- The atmosphere – light and sound waves. For example, bright light can be very tiring for an ill patient, as can the noise of a busy ward with the radio on. Both of these may even prevent the patient from resting or sleeping.

- The atmosphere – organic and inorganic. For example, dust may irritate an atopic patient and pathogenic microorganisms are a risk to all patients, in particular those who are elderly, immunosuppressed or recovering from major surgery.
- The built environment. For example, the veterinary practice kennels and all other areas must be safe in order that the first AL ('maintain a safe environment') can be achieved.

Politico-economic

There are two parts to this:

- Health and economic status. This relates to the client more than the patient in a veterinary context; it is likely that the economic status of the client may influence the ALs
- Health and world economy. Recession will have an impact on the amount that clients will spend and that veterinary surgeons will invest in staff and equipment; this may impact on the care of the veterinary patient.

Part five: Individuality in living

The ALs are the main concept of this model. Although every patient is likely to carry out these activities, each patient may do them differently, thus expressing themselves as an individual. For example, a cat may eat in a very different way to a dog.

Orem's Model

Dorothea Orem's views on nursing science are the basis for understanding how empirical nursing evidence is gathered and interpreted. Her quest for greater understanding of the nature of nursing focused on three questions:

1. What do nurses do, and what should nurses do, as practitioners of nursing?
2. Why do nurses do what they do?
3. What are the results of nursing interventions?

Orem's Model of nursing focuses on the key idea that an individual is self-caring if they can manage the following effectively:

- Support of life processes and normal functioning
- Maintenance of normal growth and development
- Prevention and control of disease and injury
- Prevention of, or compensation for, disability
- Promotion of wellbeing.

According to Cavanagh (1991), central to Orem's concept of self-care is the concept that care is being initiated voluntarily and deliberately by an individual. Self-care is the practice of activities that will maintain life and health and will promote wellbeing.

Universal self-care requisites

Essential to Orem's Model are the eight 'universal self-care requisites', which are activities that must be performed in order to achieve self-care.

Orem's universal self-care requisites

- The maintenance of a sufficient intake of air
- The maintenance of a sufficient intake of water
- The maintenance of a sufficient intake of food
- Satisfactory elimination functions
- The maintenance of a balance between activity and rest
- The maintenance of a balance between solitude and social integration
- The prevention of hazards to life, wellbeing and functioning
- The promotion of functioning and development within social groups and the desire to be normal (normality)

These self-care requisites are essential tasks that an individual must be able to manage in order to care for themselves. As with Roper, Logan and Tierney's ALs, these are all requisites that an animal can achieve, but some of the self-care requisites may be easier for wild animals than for domesticated ones. For example, intake of food may be difficult if the domesticated animal is reliant on an owner to feed it and it has no freedom to scavenge or hunt.

The idea of balancing demands and abilities (Figure 12.5) is central to Orem's Model.

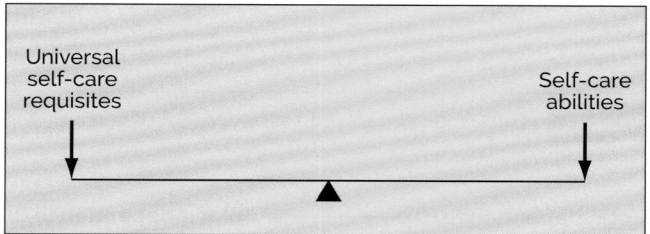

| 12.5 | The Orem Model of nursing. A healthy individual: the self-care abilities meet self-care requisites (Cavanagh, 1991).

Developmental self-care requisites

Orem identified a second kind of requisite found in special circumstances associated with development.

Orem's specific developmental self-care requisites

- Intrauterine life and birth
- Neonatal life
- Infancy
- The developmental stages of childhood (for which substitute puppy, kitten, etc.), adolescence and early adulthood
- The developmental stages of adulthood
- Pregnancy

It is at this point that Orem differs from Roper, Logan and Tierney, as the lifespan within the Roper, Logan and Tierney Model begins with the neonate and does not consider intrauterine life, as the Orem Model does. Orem argues that at each of these stages universal self-care requisites must also be considered (Figure 12.6). An example of a specific

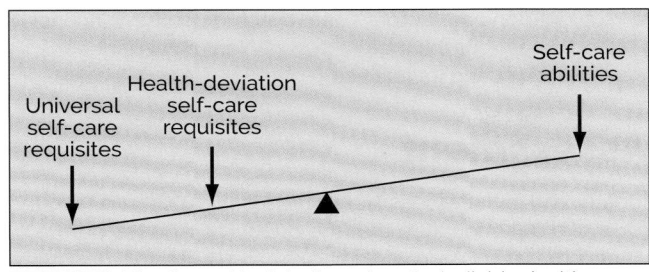

12.6 The Orem Model of nursing. An individual with additional developmental self-care requisites is in need of intervention (Cavanagh, 1991).

developmental self-care requisite would be temperature regulation in a neonate. An adult may be able to control its own body temperature but a neonate may not.

Health-deviation self-care requisites

There are times when an individual is ill, becomes injured, has disabilities or is under medical care. In these circumstances, the following additional healthcare demands are placed upon them:

- Seeking and securing appropriate medical assistance
- Being aware of and attending to the effects and results of pathological conditions and states
- Effectively carrying out medically prescribed treatment
- Being aware of, and attending to, the discomforting and deleterious effects of medically prescribed treatment
- Modifying self-image in accepting oneself as being in a particular state of health
- Learning to live with the effects of pathological conditions and states.

The owner may act for the animal in order that some of the additional healthcare demands are achieved, and an individual animal may experience a change in the status of their health but still be able to meet the universal and health-deviation self-care requisites (Figure 12.7).

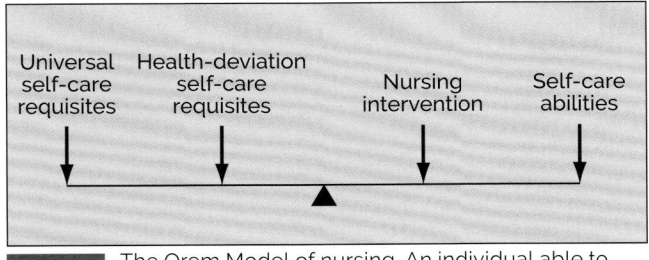

12.7 The Orem Model of nursing. An individual able to meet all requisites with nursing assistance (Cavanagh, 1991).

However, a situation could exist where the total demand placed on an animal exceeds its ability to meet it. In this situation an individual will need nursing intervention in order to enable it to meet its self-care needs. The nurse needs to assess which interventions are needed immediately and which might be needed in the future. An example would be a cat with a fractured jaw and lacerated tongue, this patient would be unable to eat and drink by itself due to the nature of its injuries, and as such the cat would need a nursing intervention in order for it to meet its need for sufficient water and food.

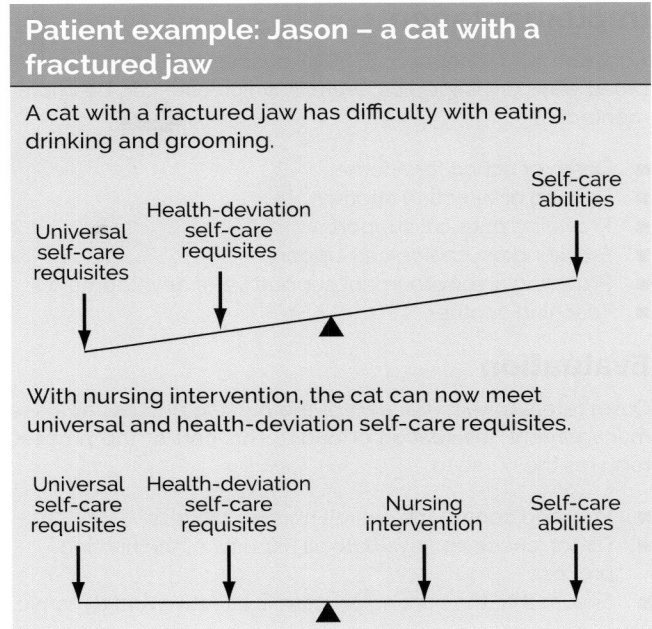

Putting the theory into practice

Cavanagh (1991) suggested that there is no single 'correct' way of setting out a care plan based upon Orem's Model. Instead, the nurse must take the ideas that Orem presents and develop a plan to meet the needs of each patient. This relies on the confidence of the nurse; however, this is a model that can be adapted to meet the needs of veterinary practice while still individualizing care of the patient. If this is the model that is used in practice, it is vital that each stage is recorded to ensure all who read the plan are able to understand and follow it. The nursing process is a vital part of the model and is the basis of the care plan for any individual patient. An example of a completed care plan, demonstrating the application of the model to the patient example, Jason, is given at the end of this chapter.

Interpretation of language used within Orem's Model

Assessment

Orem does not often refer to 'assessment' but chooses to use 'nursing history' instead.

Planning

Once the nursing history has been taken, the 'planning' stage of the nursing process begins. At this stage, the nurse will be in discussion with the owner and other professionals within the team regarding the extent to which the nurse will support the patient with their self-care requisites. The following degrees of nursing intervention might be considered:

- Wholly compensatory – the patient and client are completely dependent on the veterinary nurse (e.g. a unconscious dog)
- Partially compensatory – the nurse, patient and client work together to meet the self-care requisites (e.g. a dog with a long bone fracture)
- Supportive/educative – the nurse is there for support/reassurance (e.g. teaching an owner how to inject their pet with insulin).

Implementation

Aggleton and Chalmers (2000) believe that there are six broad ways envisaged by Orem in which care can be implemented:

- Doing or acting for another
- Guiding or directing another
- Providing physical support
- Providing psychological support
- Providing an environment supportive of development
- Teaching another.

Evaluation

Orem refers to this vital part of the nursing process as 'case management' (evaluation or audit). This part of the process requires the nurse to:

- Plan and control the overall nursing process
- Direct, check and evaluate all aspects of the nursing process
- Ensure that the nursing process is effective and dynamic.

The Ability Model

The human models of nursing, whilst useful as a basis for veterinary nursing, are not ideal for animals and their owners. For this reason, a specific model for veterinary patients, the Ability Model was developed and forms the basis for developing nursing care plans. Figure 12.8 provides a visual representation of the Ability Model, showing the three key components:

- The 10 abilities – Orpet and Jeffery (2007) believe that if the animal is able to achieve these it can be deemed 'healthy'
- Lifespan – this will be an influencing factor; it is important to know where, within the lifespan, the patient sits when carrying out an assessment

- Key influencing factors – these include cultural, financial and owner compliance factors, which may impact on the patient and its abilities.

Assessment

Ideally, the initial assessment of the patient should take the form of a questionnaire that the owner completes before or during the admission of their animal. Giving the questionnaire to the client prior to admission provides them with the opportunity to think clearly about their answers and often makes them feel that the practice values their pets and the care given to them. If done at the point of admission, ensure the client has time to complete the information in detail.

The information needed for the assessment is based on the 10 abilities of the animal (Figure 12.9).

It is important to remember that the way in which questions are asked and the environment in which questioning takes place is very important. Open questions are likely to gain more information about the patient than closed questions (see also Chapter 9). For example, with Ben the Golden Retriever, 'Does Ben eat adequately?' would probably result in a yes/no answer. However, 'What does Ben normally eat? How much does he eat and at what times?' should provide a more detailed response, which will help to inform the nursing team of the patient's normal routine during the time that they are hospitalized. It is important to consider where the assessment is done, e.g. on the phone before admission or in a room away from the busy reception area, so that attention can be focused on the owner and what they are saying, without any distractions. If the information is completed via an online form or emailed to the practice, this will give the nurse time to read through it and formulate any other questions they may need to ask the client regarding the patient at the point of admission.

A further example of a completed patient assessment form (Jess) can be found at the end of this chapter.

The next stage of the nursing assessment concerns what the animal is able or not able to do once it has been admitted. This uses the same 'checklist' of 10 abilities from the model.

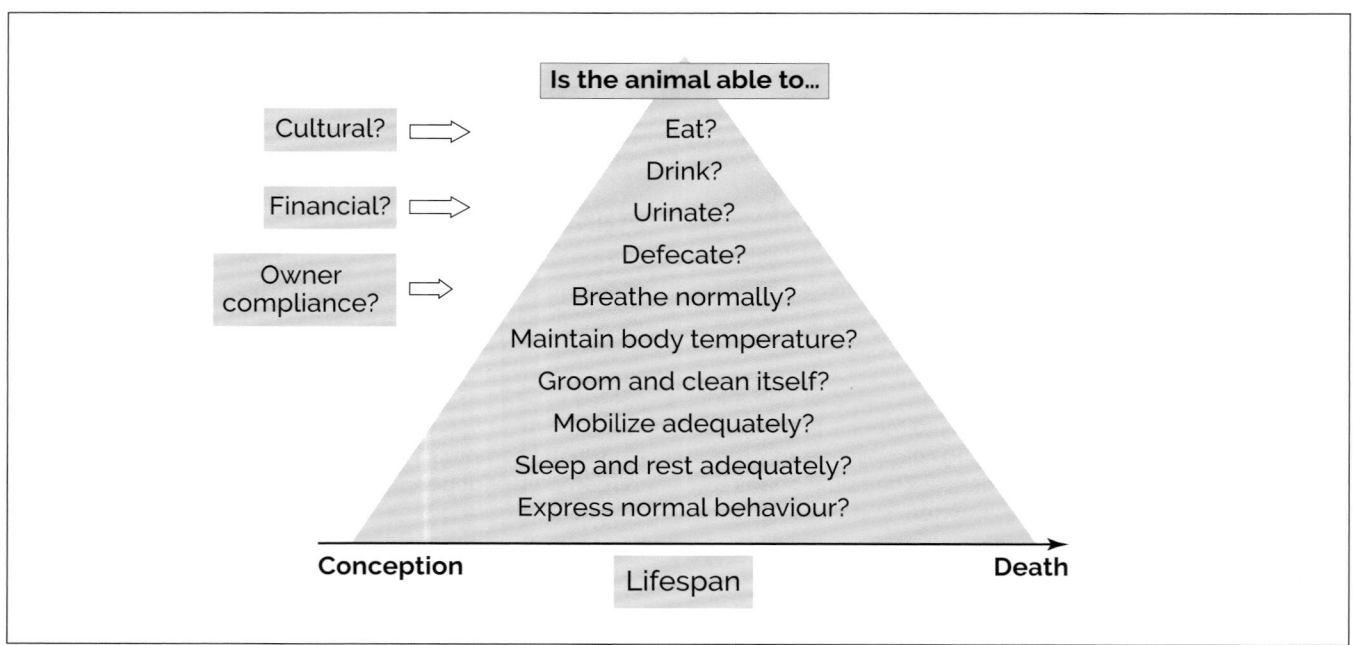

12.8 The Orpet and Jeffery Ability Model. (Reproduced from Orpet and Welsh (2011) with permission)

Is the animal able to....	Questions to ask the owner	Rationale for question
Eat adequate amounts?	What does the patient normally eat?	To get the patient back to eating their normal food
	How much, how often and when?	Calculation of resting or maintenance energy requirement may be necessary to maintain bodyweight (see Chapter 13)
	Does the patient prefer any particular type of bowl?	Brachycephalic cats (e.g. Persians) often prefer flat bowls. Cats generally prefer china or ceramic rather than plastic bowls
Drink adequate amounts?	How much does the patient normally drink?	This will vary from animal to animal. It may depend on whether the animal's normal diet is wet or dry
	Does the patient often drink water from containers outside, e.g. collected rain water?	The type of water can be important. Cats may drink from a dripping tap. Rabbits and other small mammals may drink from a bottle or bowl
Urinate normally?	Where does the patient normally urinate?	Patients may show different preferences. Inside or outside? Does a cat use a litter tray? What type of litter? Does a dog urinate on walks? Always on grass or on concrete?
	Does the owner use any commands for urination?	Used in well trained animals
	Does the patient have any problems urinating?	Does the patient have arthritis? Joint stiffness can affect how the animal urinates
Defecate normally?	How often does the patient defecate per day and when?	How often the animal defecates can depend on its diet
	Where is this usually done and on what?	Some dogs have preferences on where they urinate/defecate. Likewise, cats may have a preference for the type of substrate used in their litter tray
Breathe normally?	Does the patient have any problems breathing?	This may be linked to exercise. There may be underlying disease, including allergy
	Does the patient often snore while sleeping?	Facial conformity of the animal may result in breathing difficulties, e.g. Persians or Pugs
Maintain body temperature?	Do you think the patient feels the cold? Do they wear a coat in colder weather?	Very young and old animals may not be able to regulate their temperature effectively
	Where does the animal normally sleep?	Animals may show preferences, for example for warmer or cooler places (e.g. kitchen floor)
Mobilize adequately?	Does the patient have any problems walking?	Difficulties in mobility may affect care routines. These may be identified by simply watching the animal walk. With cats sitting in baskets, however, it may not be possible to assess
	Can they get into the car easily or get upstairs?	Older animals may suffer from stiff joints and arthritis, which limits their normal routine
Groom and clean itself?	Does the patient normally groom itself?	Cats often spend a long time grooming and washing themselves
	Do you normally groom or bath the patient? If so, how often?	Long-haired animals are often groomed regularly by their owners. It is important to know how often and with what
Sleep and rest adequately?	How much sleep does the patient have during a 24-hour period?	Dogs spend a lot of time sleeping despite what owners think. Cats are often nocturnal, hunting at night and sleeping all day. Sleeping, however, is not something the owner will usually monitor
Express normal behaviour?	Is the patient neutered? If female, when was her last season?	Un-neutered animals can display certain behaviours associated with sex hormones
	How does the patient behave toward strangers or other animals?	It is important to try and ascertain whether the animal displays any aggressive behaviour. Be aware that you may not always get accurate information on this from owners
	Does the patient have any favourite toys, chews, etc.?	Toys can help settle the animal into the hospital environment
	Does the patient respond to any particular commands for certain activities?	Police dogs and guide dogs may have certain commands – it may be necessary to know these in advance. Many dogs have a command for urinating or defecating – this may also be useful for dogs in strange environments away from the owners
	Does the animal suffer from any sight or hearing impairment?	Often associated with old age – important to know as the animal will be unsettled even more in a strange environment

12.9 Assessment framework for the Ability Model. These are questions to ask the owner when admitting the animal. It is important to remember that these questions can be asked of the owner of any species kept as a pet, including exotic pets, although they may need to be adapted slightly depending on the species.

Patient example: Ben – patient assessment form

Date of Admission: 15 February 2020	**Date of nursing assessment:** 15 February 2020
Case No.: 1900210	**Patient Name:** Ben **Breed:** Golden Retriever **Sex:** Male, neutered

Owner: Andrew Non
Address: 195 Cromwell Street, Gloucester
Contact No.: 01234 567890

Clinical summary (reason for admission): Investigation into polyuria and polydipsia, lethargy, inappetence	**Owner's perception of problem:** Excessive drinking and urination, no energy and not eating

Previous history (surgery, disease, vaccination status, allergies):
Castrated 2010, vaccinations up-to-date

Temperature: 38°C	**Current medication:** None yet – to be prescribed by veterinary surgeon once blood tests and urinalysis carried out
Pulse: 80 beats/min	
Respiration: 20 breaths/min	
Mucous membrane colour: pale pink	
Capillary refill time (CRT): <2 s	
Weight: 37 kg	

Life stage:
Age: 11 years

neonate — adult — geriatric (marker positioned between adult and geriatric)

Assessment of abilities

Ability	Usual routine	Actual problems	Potential problems
Eat adequate amount	Eats 1 tin of Chappie with mixer in evenings; favourite treat is warm cooked chicken	Not eating	Weight loss
Drink adequate amounts	Approx. 500 ml/day	Drinking 1–2 litres/day	Dehydration if water not replenished
Urinate normally	Outside 3 times a day on concrete. Trained not to urinate on grass	Increased to 7–8 times a day	Urination in kennel if not taken out hourly
Defecate normally	Outside once daily, early morning. Trained not to defecate on grass	Has not yet defecated, though not eating	May become constipated
Breathe normally	Normal	None	None expected
Maintain body temperature	No problems – sleeps on memory foam dog bed on tiled kitchen floor	None at present	Patient may be too warm in hospital kennels
Groom itself	Owner grooms weekly with a rake brush	None	Matted coat if not groomed
Mobilize adequately	Goes for walks at 7am and 4pm, about 40 minutes each	Has not wanted to walk, very slow and not interested in anything	Reduced mobility
Sleep/rest	No problems – indoors mostly	Very lethargic, has not wanted to get up for walks	May become less mobile if balance of sleep and exercise is not maintained
Express normal behaviour	Normally active. Use a whistle to call him as he is deaf in left ear	Deafness. Not willing to exercise	Not able to hear staff approaching. Boredom

The care plan

The information gained from the assessment can be used to identify actual problems. It is also important to consider potential problems that may occur, to mitigate against them. Once the problems have been identified and prioritized, the goals and nursing interventions can be decided.

Implementing the care plan

Detail in the care plan is important; everyone needs to know exactly what the nursing intervention is, how often care should be implemented and the nature of the care required.

This should be clearly documented, legible and in a language that everyone understands and cannot be misinterpreted. The use of abbreviations is acceptable if everyone reading the care plan knows what these mean.

Evaluation

In order to evaluate effectively, the assessment phase should be carried out again. For each of the 10 abilities, the animal should be assessed on what it can now do or still not do by itself. Hopefully the nursing interventions have worked and the animal is now more 'able' than when admitted. If not, the care given should be reviewed and the plan adjusted as necessary.

Care plan for Ben

Patient Name: Ben | **Date:** 15 February 2020

Date	Problem	Short-term goal	Nursing intervention	Reassess/ evaluation	Review time/date
15 February	Not eating	To eat 1 tin of Chappie per day	Tempt to eat by hand-feeding, warming food. If disinterested in Chappie, tempt with small amounts of chicken	Has eaten half a tin of Chappie	16 February
15 February	Drinking excessively	Ensure hydration status is maintained	Assess hydration status and check hourly that water bowl is full. Measure and record volume drunk	Hydration status maintained	16 February
15 February	Excessive urination	Ensure patient has opportunity to urinate regularly	Take dog out hourly into concrete run and record whether urinated and volume	Urinated 8 times, no soiling of kennel	16 February
15 February	Normal behaviour affected by condition	Encourage as far as possible normal behaviour	Regular contact with nursing staff, not just when feeding or medicating. Assess pain relief requirements	Pain score completed and no change in level of pain	Ongoing during stay

Ben was diagnosed with diabetes mellitus and his condition was stabilized using insulin. The problems he had on admission associated with the disease were solved once the treatment began.

Influencing factors

The life stage

The assessment and consequent nursing care that is carried out may be affected by other factors. The life stage of the animal is an important factor to consider. Even healthy neonates are unable to feed, drink, maintain their body temperature or mobilize by themselves. Geriatric animals may have weaker senses purely because they are old, and mobility may be decreased due to arthritis.

Cultural differences

These may affect the care given to the animal. It is important to consider the role that the pet plays in the owner's life, e.g. whether it is a working animal, a family pet or used for breeding. It may be that the owner does not believe in euthanasia or their religious beliefs may stop them consenting to a blood transfusion. It is important to understand and respect these beliefs, remembering that the welfare of the animal should remain the number one concern.

Financial implications

Financial implications may prevent the required care from taking place. In this situation, alternatives should be explored. For example, where full physiotherapy and hydrotherapy is recommended but is too expensive for the client, the veterinary nurse may be able to teach the owner some basic care techniques or rehabilitation methods.

Owner compliance

Nursing involves not only caring for the patient, but also liaising with the owner regarding the nursing care given. The veterinary nurse's role is vital in maintaining the communication between the client and the practice (see Chapter 9). Veterinary nurses often speak to clients to reassure them of how their pet is progressing in the hospital. Once the animal goes home, the veterinary nurse must ensure the owner is competent at administering any further care required.

Alternative solutions to a problem may need to be explored. For example, it may be unrealistic for a Dobermann with a hindlimb amputation to negotiate four flights of stairs in a block of flats with a 70-year-old owner. The influencing factors should always be considered when creating the care plan for the animal, and adjustments made appropriately for when the animal is to return home (see Figures 12.8 and 12.9).

Development of the nurse–patient interpersonal relationship

In 1952, Hildegard Peplau (1909–1999) published a book entitled *Interpersonal Relations in Nursing* in which she introduced the idea of a theoretical framework that nurses could use to look systematically at the care they provide. This related particularly to the area of mental health nursing. Peplau saw illness as a potential learning experience, and that through a meaningful nurse–patient relationship both the patient and the nurse would grow and develop. Peplau believed that patients would have a greater opportunity to learn from the nurse about their illness, and so gain greater insight into themselves and their condition. Once this had been achieved, the patient could begin to manage their feelings and actions in relation to their mental health problems. Peplau believed that the nurse should work with, as well as for, the patient to achieve changes in their mental health.

Peplau saw that health can fail for a number of reasons:

- Lack of knowledge
- The patient is incapable of thinking healthily because they have been ill for so long
- The provision of healthcare is restricted by limited resources
- The inability of health professionals to organize themselves properly
- A poor working relationship between the nurse and the patient.

By addressing these problems, Peplau believed that health could be achieved, particularly if the nurse had the necessary skills to help the patient communicate their feelings and thoughts, and could identify gaps in the information the patient had about their illness and their ability to manage it. More information on general communication in veterinary practice is given in Chapter 9.

Peplau defined nursing as a significant, therapeutic, interpersonal (interaction between two or more individuals with a common goal) process and saw the nursing role as both educative and therapeutic. Her belief was that nurses needed to be aware of the roles they undertake, and the short- and long-term consequences of these roles for their patients.

Sequential phases in interpersonal relationships

Peplau identified four sequential phases in interpersonal relationships, which can be related to the four stages of the nursing process (Figure 12.10):

1. Orientation.
2. Identification.
3. Exploitation.
4. Resolution.

Phase	Focus	Nursing process
Orientation	Problem defining phase	Assessment
Identification	Selection of appropriate professional assistance	Planning
Exploitation	Use of professional assistance for problem-solving alternatives moving towards goals	Implementation
Resolution	Termination of professional relationship	Evaluation

12.10 Phases of the Peplau Model and how they relate to the nursing process (Peplau, 1952).

According to Peplau, each phase overlaps, interrelates and varies in duration as the process evolves towards a solution.

Different nursing roles are assumed during the various phases:

- Stranger
- Teacher: gives knowledge
- Resource: provides specific information to aid understanding
- Counsellor: defined as someone who, through use of certain skills, aids another in recognizing, facing, accepting and resolving problems that are interfering with the other's ability to live happily and effectively
- Leader: helps patient to maintain goals
- Technical expert: someone who provides physical care by delivering clinical skills and operating equipment
- Surrogate: one who takes the place of another (e.g. nurse in role as surrogate)

In the sections below, Peplau's references to 'the patient' have been translated into 'patient and client' in order for the model to be contextualized from a veterinary nursing perspective.

Orientation

- Initially – two strangers.

The veterinary nurse should work together with the patient and client to recognize, clarify and define the existing problem. This is similar to the assessment phase in the nursing process described above. The orientation phase is directly affected by the patient's and nurse's attitude about giving or receiving aid from a reciprocal person (Figure 12.11).

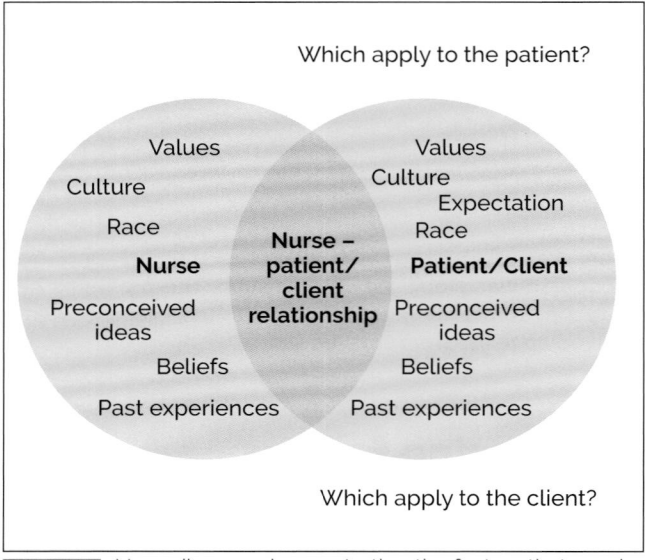

12.11 Venn diagram demonstrating the factors that need to be considered when developing a nurse–patient/client relationship.

In this beginning phase, the nurse needs to be aware of his or her personal reactions to the patient; for example, a veterinary nurse may react differently to a 3-year-old Golden Retriever that has been admitted for castration which is boisterous and friendly, as opposed to a dog that is aggressive. It should also be borne in mind that the client may have stereotyped the nurse as being able to perform only technical skills and may not see the nurse as someone who can define problems.

- Beginning of orientation ⟶ Strangers
- End of orientation ⟶ Striving to identify problems and becoming comfortable with one another

Identification

Identification is similar to the planning phase in the nursing process described above. The patient/client responds selectively to the people who can meet their needs.

- The dog/cat associates the veterinary nurse with feeding.
- The dog/cat may associate the veterinary surgeon with pain/fear.

The patient/client response to the nurse is three-fold:

1. Participate with and be interdependent with the nurse.
2. Be autonomous and independent from the nurse.
3. Be passive and dependent on the nurse.

Patient example: Ben – nurse–patient/client relationship

Ben was diagnosed with diabetes mellitus and prescribed insulin injections to manage his condition.

- Ben cannot be independent as he requires the nurse or client to provide him with food and insulin injections. However, the client could be independent from the nurse.
- Ben could be considered to participate with and be interdependent with the nurse (i.e. submissive when injected; however, this could also be interpreted as passive and dependent). The client could also be dependent on the nurse.

During the identification phase, the perceptions and expectations of the patient/client and nurse are more complex than during the orientation phase. For example, a patient needs to lose weight. The owner agrees, but during its weekly weigh in, the dog's weight is not reducing. The nurse explores the reason for this and the owner admits to not being able to read and therefore was unsure about the volume of food to be given. The nurse demonstrates using a scoop and the problem is resolved. Working through the identification phase, the patient/client should begin to feel a sense of belonging and a capacity to deal with problems; there should be a decrease in feelings of helplessness and an increase in optimistic attitude.

Exploitation

- The patient moves into the exploitation phase in which they (and the client) take advantage of all the services available.

- The degree to which these services are used is based upon the needs and interests of the individual patient (ranging from vaccinations to amputation).
- The individual (patient/client) begins to feel as though he or she is an integral part of the environment and begins to take control of the situation by extracting help from the services offered.
- During this phase, some patients may make more demands than they did when they were seriously ill. They may make many minor requests or may use other attention-seeking techniques (e.g. a dog that has previously been very ill now barks when left in the kennel by itself).
- Clients may also make demands, as well as become involved in the care of the patient, therefore, relying less on the nursing staff.

Resolution

Resolution is equivalent to the evaluation phase of the nursing process. The patient's needs have been met. The patient (and client) and nurse now need to terminate their therapeutic relationship and dissolve the links between them. Sometimes the nurse and patient (and client) have difficulty dissolving these links. The client (rather than the patient) may feel that it is not yet time to end the relationship, particularly if there has been a long-term problem with their animal. During successful resolutions the patient drifts away from identifying with the nurse.

It was Peplau's suggestion that as the nurse works with the patient to resolve problems in everyday life, the nurse's practice becomes increasingly more effective, and therefore the kind of person the nurse is and becomes has a direct influence on their skill in developing a therapeutic, inter-personal relationship with patients.

Patient example: Dexter – a stray cat

Presentation

Stray animal, which is being rehomed. It is infested with fleas, its fur is badly matted and there was an injury noted to the flank. The animal was very nervous/aggressive.

Orientation

What are the existing problems?
How can the nurse get to know the patient and gain its trust?

Beginning of the phase = strangers ⟶ End of the phase = becoming comfortable with each other

Use this stressful situation as a learning experience, so that a new pattern of behaviour and changes can be instigated

Identification

The patient responds to people who meet its needs
The patient responds to the nurse in three different ways:

- Participates with and is interdependent with the nurse
- Autonomous and independent from the nurse
- Passive and dependent on the nurse

The patient may move through these different responses as the nurse learns about the patient and the patient learns more about the nurse

Exploitation

Patient takes advantage of all the services available

- Eating
- Warmth
- Bedding
- Treatment making the animal comfortable
- TLC

Resolution

Patient and nurse terminate their relationship and dissolve the links when the animal is rehomed

Using models of nursing in a clinical veterinary environment

The use of a nursing model in which the nursing process is embedded is vital when delivering nursing care to patients. It ensures that all nurses within the practice are following the same set criteria for any one patient and that there are recorded goals and coordinated interventions. As the goals set are able to be measured or observed, it means that reflection and subjective evaluation can be made of the nursing care given, providing a clear evidence base for nursing practice.

When initially introducing care plans into the veterinary nursing clinical environment, it may be seen to be producing yet more paperwork for nurses to complete on a day-to-day basis. It is therefore important to emphasize the rationale for nurse care planning and the nursing process.

Some nurses will argue that they perform care planning and evaluation automatically; for example, if a patient does not eat one type of diet attempts are made at tempting them with another. However, in a clinical setting in which numerous nurses may be caring for a single patient, there may be a lack of continuity of this care.

Following on from the diet example, a nurse may find that a patient refuses to eat diet 1, but will eat diet 2. However, if this information is not recorded anywhere and the nurses then change shifts, a second nurse may give diet 1, and unsurprisingly find that the patient does not eat this. This lack of communication is likely to compromise patient care. A lack of communication may impede the progress of the patient's nursing care and also have a demoralizing effect on the nursing team.

If a care plan had been implemented in this situation, with documentation of the nursing process, the second nurse would be aware that the patient does not eat diet 1 and instead prefers diet 2. The use of a care plan will ensure there is continuity of care throughout conventional 'hand-overs', with individual nurses and the nursing team as a whole providing a high level of care tailored to a patient's individual needs. Where care plans are implemented, clinical outcomes may be improved and recovery time from illness shortened.

Patient admission is usually the time when the nurse asks the client questions about their pet and is the most effective time for an initial assessment to be carried out.

More patient examples

Patient Details: Bruce – a 1-year-old male Dutch rabbit due to have an elective castration

Patient's position on lifespan: Neonate ———————▶ Geriatric

Activity of living	Nursing assessment of patient ability to carry out activity of living	D = dependent I = independent	Patient problem potential/actual	Nursing goals	Nursing interventions	Evaluation
Maintaining a safe environment	The rabbit is unable to do this himself and must be provided with a quiet kennel containing a bed, hay, food and a water bottle or bowl	D ▼——┼—— I	Potential	To ensure that the rabbit has a safe and comfortable cage in a quieter area away from other noisy animals, to minimize stress and allow recovery from anaesthesia	Place the rabbit away from dogs, cats and excess noise, to minimize stress	A safe and comfortable environment was maintained and no problems occurred
Communicating	The rabbit is able to use physical ways of communicating, which are interpreted by the nurse based on information provided by the owner	D ▼——┼—— I	Potential	To be able to understand the signs shown by the rabbit	Observe and record patient behaviour to ensure there are no changes	On recovery, the rabbit showed signs of being distressed and an increased respiration rate. A towel was placed over the front of the cage to darken it and to make the rabbit feel safer. The patient was observed every 15 minutes until distress subsided
Breathing	The rabbit is young and healthy with a normal respiratory pattern	D ▼——┼—— I	Potential	To ensure that respiratory function is maintained within normal parameters	To monitor respiration rate in the perioperative period and to ensure that it remains within normal parameters	The respiratory rate stayed within normal parameters with no complications whilst in surgery. During initial stages of recovery it did increase but returned to normal within 30 minutes
Eating and drinking	The rabbit was able to eat and drink normally on admission	D ▼——┼—— I	Potential	To ensure on recovery that the rabbit eats and also passes faeces normally	In line with current guidelines, food was not withheld prior to surgery. Encourage eating. Offer dandelions to stimulate feeding, or syringe feed if required	After surgery, the rabbit recovered and ate with encouragement. No faeces passed
Eliminating	The rabbit was fit, healthy and had no difficulties in toileting or any previous history of problems	D ▼——┼—— I	Potential	To ensure that toileting remains normal during stay	Observe and record faecal output to show that the gut is functioning correctly. Inform veterinary surgeon if not and administer faecal stimulant as directed	The rabbit had not passed faeces, so a gut stimulant was administered
Personal cleansing (grooming)	The rabbit was in good condition and was able to groom itself	D ▼——┼—— I	Potential	To ensure that the rabbit stays clean and dry throughout his stay and coat remains in good condition	Clean any eliminations accordingly to reduce contamination of the surgical wound	No contamination of the coat occurred during the hospital stay and the wound remained clean

continues ▲

Nursing care plan for a rabbit, Bruce, using the Roper, Logan and Tierney Model.

Patient Details: Bruce – a 1-year-old male Dutch rabbit due to have an elective castration

Patient's position on lifespan: Neonate ———+———▶ Geriatric

Activity of living	Nursing assessment of patient ability to carry out activity of living	D = dependent I = independent	Patient problem potential/actual	Nursing goals	Nursing interventions	Evaluation
Controlling body temperature	Prior to surgery the rabbit's temperature was within normal limits	D ◀—+——▶ I	Potential	To ensure that normal parameters are maintained throughout the surgery and postoperatively	Monitor temperature, pulse and respiration rate every 15–30 minutes during the perioperative period (as directed by veterinary surgeon) to ensure that they are maintained within normal ranges and that the rabbit does not become hypothermic. Supply external heat sources if required	The rabbit maintained normal body temperature throughout the surgery and postoperatively. However, external heat sources were supplied until he had fully recovered from anaesthesia
Mobilizing	The rabbit has no mobility problems	D ◀—+——▶ I	Potential	To ensure that the rabbit recovers well and gains full mobility following surgery	Provide a padded environment for the rabbit to recover in and to avoid any bumps or knocks. Ensure patient is able to mobilize fully	The rabbit recovered well without any injuries
Working and playing	A young active rabbit with no problems in playing, etc.	D ◀—+——▶ I	Potential	To ensure that the rabbit recovers well, but limit activity following surgery	Provide a less active environment to discourage play	The rabbit was lethargic following the surgery and did not show any interest in wanting to play. He was less active
Expressing sexuality	The rabbit was showing evidence of sexual activity prior to surgery	D ◀—+——▶ I	N/A	N/A	N/A	The rabbit had an elective procedure to eliminate this
Sleeping	The rabbit needs to be provided with a quiet environment to enable him to sleep	D ◀—+——▶ I	Potential	To ensure that a comfortable environment is provided in a quiet area away from noise and distraction, to enable rabbit to rest and sleep	A quiet, dark bed and a heat pad were provided so that the rabbit could rest and recover from surgery in a warm comfortable environment	The rabbit was stressed following surgery, but a quiet cage was provided, allowing him to sleep
Dying	On admission the rabbit was young, fit and healthy	D ◀—+——▶ I	(Potential) Although the rabbit is young, there is a risk with any general anaesthesia, and handling can cause stress levels to rise	To ensure that the rabbit is monitored closely whilst under anaesthesia to avoid any potential problems arising, and to ensure the rabbit makes a full recovery	The patient was monitored every 5 minutes using anaesthetic monitoring equipment (e.g. oesophageal stethoscope, pulse oximetry, electrocardiography), to ensure that its vital signs remained within normal ranges during the surgical procedure	The patient was stable during anaesthesia and recovered well

continued Nursing care plan for a rabbit, Bruce, using the Roper, Logan and Tierney Model.

Patient details: Jason – a 12-month-old neutered male, Domestic Shorthaired cat

Reason for admission: Fractured jaw

Universal self-care requisites	Self-care abilities	Self-care limitations	Patient actions	Nursing actions
Maintain intake of air	Breathes without difficulty	Unable to groom/clean, therefore, food sticks to nose	Breathes well when nostrils clear	Ensure nostrils remain clear during and after feeding Assess respiratory ventilation and temperature, pulse and respiration (TPR) measurements q6h initially
Maintain intake of water	Can put mouth down to water bowl and lap water	Difficulty in drinking from a high-sided bowl	Drinking Swallowing	Provide water in a shallow bowl Keep a fluid balance chart Observe for signs of dehydration
Maintain intake of food	Can put mouth down to food bowl	Unable to prehend food	Can swallow when food in mouth	Ensure food is in manageable form Assist with feeding Maintain a record of food eaten
Manage elimination	All	Normally urinates outside in soil	Use litter tray to urinate and defecate	Provide litter tray containing soil Keep a record of urinary/faecal output frequency
Balance activity and rest	Is able to rest and sleep	Unable to have free access	Walk around kennel Rest and sleep on appropriate bedding (e.g. Vetbed®)	Provide a large kennel Provide an environment for rest/sleep when required
Balance solitude and social intergration	Is able to communicate through body language	Unable to purr or meow due to fracture Unable to communicate with brother		Provide regular nursing attention Organize for family, including children, to visit
Prevention of hazards to life, wellbeing and functioning	Possesses pain sensation Can hear and see	Cannot maintain safety of environment		Monitor vital signs and assess patient for changes in physical and psychological condition
Normalcy	Is able to communicate through body language	Unable to vocalize	Interact with staff, family and other animals	Provide an environment in which he feels at ease Provide grooming opportunities

Nursing care plan for a cat, Jason, using Orem's Model.

Date of Admission: 4/2/20	Date of nursing assessment: 5/2/20
Case No.: 12345	Patient Name: Jess Breed: Basset Hound Sex: Female, entire

Owner: Sue Donym

Address: 230 Montrose Avenue, Bristol

Contact No.: 0987 6543210

Clinical summary (reason for admission): Road traffic accident. Subsequent fractured pelvis and growth plate fracture	Owner's perception of problem: Owners are aware how serious the injuries are and are expecting Jess to have a long recovery

Previous history (surgery, disease, vaccination status, allergies):
Up-to-date vaccines and preventive parasite treatment. No other known problems

Temperature: 38.7°C	Current medication:
Pulse: 88 beats/min	Methadone
Respiration: 28 breaths/min	Meloxicam
Mucous membrane colour: pink	Amoxicillin/clavulanic acid
Capillary refill time (CRT): >2 s	IVFT – Hartmann's 2 ml/kg/h (maintenance)
Weight: 15.3 kg	

Life stage:
Age: 7 months

neonate — adult — geriatric

Assessment of abilities

Ability	Usual routine	Actual problems	Potential problems	Long-term goals
Eat adequate amount	Fed twice daily	Anorexic	Unable to maintain body condition	Provide nutrition to prevent loss of body condition
Drink adequate amount	Water available at all times	Unable to move to water bowl	Inadequate fluid intake	Provide access to oral fluids at all times
Urinate normally	Goes out four times a day. Has command 'Go toilets'	Fractures prevent Jess walking, therefore, difficult to take out	Urine retention, discomfort	Enable Jess to carry out normal routine
Defecate normally	As above. Usually passes am and pm	Fractures prevent Jess walking, therefore, difficult to take outside	Methadone may cause reduced gut motility and constipation	Freedom from constipation and provide normal routine
Breathe normally	Normal for breed	None at present	Methadone may alter respiratory rate and depth	Maintain normal
Maintain body temperature	Usually sleeps in kitchen at home	Temperature high end of normal	Warmer in hospital than at home, may increase body temperature	Monitor and maintain normal range
Groom itself	Owner grooms weekly, occasional baths	Damage to coat from incident	Wounds and sores where no fur covering	Keep coat clean and enable wounds to heal
Mobilize adequately	Normally walked twice daily	Fractures impede movement of hindquarters	Decubitus ulcers (pressure sores), constipation, hypostatic pneumonia	Prevent, reduce potential problems occurring
Sleep/rest	Normally sleeps afternoons and night-time	Hospital active throughout day, so Jess unable to have quiet time	Jess cannot sleep in active noisy environment	Allow rest time between medications and checks
Express normal behaviour	Usually playful puppy	Unable to play due to injuries	May become depressed	Ensure adequate pain relief is provided at all times. Provide stimulation between rest periods

Patient assessment form for the Ability Model. Completed as for patient example, Jess.

References and further reading

Aggleton P and Chalmers H (2000) *Nursing Models and Nursing Practice, 2nd edn*. Palgrave, Basingstoke

Benner P (1984) *From Novice to Expert: Excellence and Power in Clinical Nursing Practice*. Addison-Wesley, Menlo Park, CA

Cavanagh SJ (1991) *Orem's Model in Action, 3rd edn*. Macmillan, Palgrave, Basingstoke

Chin PL and Kramer MK (1995) *Theory and Nursing: A Systematic Approach, 4th edn*. Mosby, St Louis

Holland K (2003) *Applying the Roper-Logan-Tierney Model in Practice: Elements of Nursing*. Churchill Livingstone, Edinburgh

Jeffery A (2006) Moving away from the medical model. *Veterinary Nursing Journal* **21**, 9

Jeffery A and Orpet H (2007) Holistic Nursing. *BSAVA Congress Scientific Proceedings: Nursing Programme*, pp. 4–5

Joiner T (2000) An holistic approach to nursing. *Veterinary Nursing* **15**, 4

Lock K (2011) Reflections on designing and implementing a nursing care plan. *The Veterinary Nurse* **2(5)**, 272–277

Luker KM (1989) Evaluating nursing care. In: *The Nursing Process*, ed. CR Kratz, pp. 124–146. Baillière Tindall, London

McGee P (1998) *Models of Nursing in Practice: A Pattern for Practical Care*. Stanley Thornes Ltd, Cheltenham

Murray ME and Atkinson LD (1994) *Understanding the Nursing Process, 5th edn*. McGraw–Hill, New York

Nelson D and Welsh P (2015) Using the ability model to design and implement a patient care plan. *The Veterinary Nurse* **6(3)**, 141–149

Orpet H (2011) How well do you know your patient? The need for nursing assessment. *Veterinary Nursing Journal*, **26(7)**, 242–245

Orpet H and Jeffery A (2006) Moving towards a more holistic approach. *Veterinary Nursing Journal* **26**, 5

Orpet H and Jeffery A (2007) Implementing the ability model. Teaching notes from: *Week Three Applied Clinical Nursing, Graduate Diploma in Professional and Clinical Veterinary Nursing*. Royal Veterinary College, London

Orpet H and Welsh P (2011) *Handbook of Veterinary Nursing, 2nd edn*. Wiley-Blackwell, Oxford

Pearson A, Vaughan B and Fitzgerald M (2004) *Nursing Models for Practice*. Butterworth-Heinemann, Oxford

Peate I (2006) *The Compendium of Clinical Skills for Student Nurses*. Wiley, Oxford

Peplau H (1952) *Interpersonal Relations in Nursing*. GP Putnam and Sons, New York

Roper N, Logan W and Tierney A (1993) *The Elements of Nursing: A Model for Nursing Based on a Model for Living*. Churchill Livingstone, Edinburgh

Roper N, Logan W and Tierney A (2002) *The Elements of Nursing, 4th edn*. Churchill Livingstone, Edinburgh

Walsh M (1997) *Models and Critical Pathways in Clinical Nursing: Conceptual Frameworks for Care Planning*. Baillière Tindall, London

Wilkinson J (1996) *Nursing Process: A Critical Thinking Approach*. Addison-Wesley, California

Self-assessment questions

1. What are the key components of the Medical (Biomedical) Model?
2. Name the five stages of the nursing process.
3. At which stage of the nursing process does the nurse plan the patient care?
4. Why is it important to set goals for patients that can be measured in some way?
5. What are the key questions that the nurse needs to ask themselves during the evaluation stage of the nursing process?
6. List the five components of the Roper, Logan and Tierney Model.
7. With regard to the Roper, Logan and Tierney Model, what is the purpose of the dependence–independence continuum?
8. Orem refers to the patient's 'self-care requisites'; how many of these are there?
9. List the three key components of the Orpet and Jeffery Ability Model.
10. With regard to the Orpet and Jeffery Ability Model, why is the initial patient assessment important in patient care delivery?

Chapter 13

Nutrition and feeding

Isuru Gajanayake with exotic pets by Simon Girling

Learning objectives

After studying this chapter, readers will have the knowledge to:

- Describe the process and control of digestion and absorption of nutrients
- Recognize the constituents of a balanced diet
- Identify and calculate the nutritional needs for a range of species
- Describe the differences in energy and macronutrient requirements during the different life stages
- Describe the key nutrients in various disease processes
- Describe the pros and cons of various feeding tubes
- Understand the broad principles of nutritional requirements for common exotic pets

---

Introduction

Nutrition is fundamental to good health, performance and longevity. In addition to maintaining a healthy state, nutrition can also play a key role in the management and prevention of disease. For these reasons, it is essential that veterinary nurses have a sound knowledge of this continually evolving field of veterinary medicine. This is particularly important because nurses are often responsible for feeding hospitalized animals and giving nutrition advice to clients .

The formulation of a balanced diet for dogs and cats requires consideration of a number of interlinking factors, including nutrient content, energy content, digestibility and palatability. A balanced diet must maintain a state of metabolic equilibrium, without net gain or loss of nutrients from the body. This is achieved through the supply of key nutrients needed to meet daily requirements, together with the quantity of energy required to sustain the animal's physiological state.

Energy

Energy is essential to sustain life. An animal's energy requirement is met through the metabolism of food, so dietary intake should be sufficient to meet the needs for maintenance, growth, reproduction, etc. and should lead to minimal changes in the energy stored by the body. This energy balance is only possible by matching energy input and output over an extended period of time. When caloric intake exceeds energy expenditure (positive energy balance), excess energy will be stored primarily as fat in the adipose tissue, leading to bodyweight (BW) gain and obesity. Conversely, if caloric intake is less than the animal's requirements, a negative energy balance results and weight loss ensues. In order to feed an animal the correct amount of energy (food), knowledge of its energy requirements and energy expenditure is required.

Common measurements of energy

Energy can be measured in kilocalories (kcal) or kilojoules (kJ), with 1 kcal equating to 4.2 kJ. Energy in food is provided by the three macronutrients: carbohydrate, fat and protein. The energy content derived from these macronutrients can be estimated using modified Atwater factors; i.e. fat provides 8.5 kcal/g, protein provides 3.5 kcal/g and carbohydrate provides 3.5 kcal/g. These values can be used to calculate the relative number of calories provided by the three macronutrients in any given diet (Figure 13.1).

Gross energy (GE) is the total energy released by complete oxidation of food and is usually measured by burning food in pure oxygen in a calorimeter (an instrument that accurately measures the heat released on combustion). No animal is able to utilize the gross energy content of its food (i.e. some energy is lost in the faeces); the extent to which food can be digested and absorbed is known as the **digestible energy (DE)**.

BSAVA Textbook of Veterinary Nursing, sixth edition. Edited by Barbara Cooper, Elizabeth Mullineaux and Lynn Turner. ©BSAVA 2020

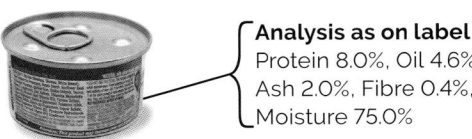

Analysis as on label
Protein 8.0%, Oil 4.6%,
Ash 2.0%, Fibre 0.4%,
Moisture 75.0%

1. The label is read and the percentage of the energy-producing nutrients noted.
   The percentage of carbohydrate is not usually stated in the typical analysis, unlike protein and fat (oil or lipid) content. It is therefore calculated by adding the percentages of the ingredients given and subtracting this from 100.

   8.0 + 4.6 + 2.0 + 0.4 + 75 = 90

   Therefore, % carbohydrate is 100 – 90 = 10%

2. The percentage content of the nutrients is converted to calorie content.

   Energy produced from fat is 8.5 kcal/g
   Energy produced from protein is 3.5 kcal/g
   Energy produced from carbohydrate is 3.5 kcal/g

   Thus:

   kcal from the fat (oil) per 100 g of the pet food
   = 4.6 × 8.5 = 39 kcal

   kcal from the protein per 100g of the pet food
   = 8.0 × 3.5 = 28 kcal

   kcal from the carbohydrate per 100g of the pet food
   = 10 × 3.5 = 35 kcal

3. The total energy density is calculated by totalling the kcal from the fat, protein and carbohydrate.
   39 + 28 + 35 = 102 kcal per 100 g

4. The energy provided by each nutrient as a percentage of the total energy content is calculated.

   t% calories from fat = 39/102 × 100 = 38%
   % calories from protein = 28/102 × 100 = 27%
   % calories from carbohydrate = 35/102 × 100 = 34%

13.1 Calculation of the energy density of a pet food and the energy of each nutrient as a percentage of the total energy content.

The **digestibility** of any nutrient is a measure of the difference between the amount eaten and the amount lost in the faeces. Only some of the digestible energy is made available to the tissues. The remainder is lost in urine and gas (e.g. methane). The remaining portion of energy that is utilized by the tissues is the **metabolizable energy (ME)**. Heat is produced following the intake of a meal as a result of digestion and absorption. This process is known as **meal-induced thermogenesis** or heat increment. **Net energy (NE)** is the metabolizable energy minus the heat increment and is used primarily for maintenance and production (i.e. growth, lactation, reproduction). If there is insufficient energy left after maintenance needs are satisfied, production will not take place.

The digestible and metabolizable energy contents of food vary according to species and individual metabolic efficiency. Animals eat food to meet their energy requirements, not the requirements for other nutrients (e.g. protein). Thus, the energy requirement of the animal, together with the energy density of the food, determines the quantity of food eaten each day and in turn the amount of nutrients ingested. Nutrient requirements are usually expressed in

terms of ME concentration (e.g. mg per 100 kcal), so that the values are applicable to any type of food or diet regardless of water content, nutrient content or overall energy value.

Energy in relation to other nutrients

Energy density

Animals consume sufficient food to meet their energy requirements (provided the food is palatable). To ensure that other essential nutrients are eaten in adequate amounts, they should be considered in relation to the energy content or energy density of the diet. Ideally, when an animal finishes eating the food provided, sufficient energy should have been consumed and the animal should have *met all* other nutritional needs.

Bulk-limited *versus* energy-limited diets

If a diet has a low energy density, the animal will continue to eat until its stomach is so full that no further food can be consumed. The animal will stop eating then, even if its energy needs have not been met. It is likely that the diet will also be deficient in other nutrients. Such a diet is said to be bulk-limited. Weight loss diets are formulated in this way; however, non-energy nutrient concentrations are higher so that their requirements are met with a reduced energy intake.

If an animal has an adequate diet and can eat to meet its energy requirements, the diet is said to be energy-limited. If the diet is then supplemented with additional energy (e.g. feeding of treats), the animal will eat less of the balanced diet and so may become deficient in certain nutrients. In general, treats should comprise no more than 10% of the daily calorie provision.

Energy requirements of animals

The energy requirements of animals can be either measured using laboratory equipment or estimated using mathematical calculations. Energy requirements can be measured using calorimetry (direct and indirect) and other techniques (e.g. double labelled water method). With direct calorimetry, animals are housed in closed chambers and their heat production is used to calculate energy requirements. With indirect calorimetry, oxygen consumption and carbon dioxide production are measured and used to estimate energy requirements.

Calculating the energy requirements of animals has been achieved using a variety of methods, including charts, allometric formulae (linking size and energy requirement), linear equations and body surface area (BSA). Ultimately, all of these provide an estimation of energy needs and will require adjustment based on the animal's weight, breed, health status, life stage, environmental conditions and activity levels.

Resting energy requirement (RER)

An animal's resting energy requirement (RER) is the amount of energy required for maintaining homeostasis while the animal rests quietly in a stress-free, non-fasted, thermoneutral environment. The RER is best calculated using the exponential formula (see below), which is conserved in animals ranging from mice to elephants. The linear formula (also below) is only accurate in animals weighing between 2 kg and 30 kg.

Calculating RER

- RER is calculated using the following formula:
  RER = 70 x (BW in kg)$^{0.75}$
- For animals weighing between 2 and 30 kg, the following linear formula gives a good approximation of energy needs:
  RER = (30 x BW in kg) + 70

The RER is the basic unit of energy requirement. This calculated amount can be multiplied by various factors, depending on the specific requirements of the animal (e.g. growth, exercise). Traditionally, the RER was multiplied by illness factors to account for increases in metabolism associated with different disease conditions and injuries. Recently, there has been a move away from these illness factors and the current recommendation is to use more conservative energy estimates to avoid overfeeding of sick animals, which can result in metabolic and gastro-intestinal complications, hepatic dysfunction and increased carbon dioxide production, amongst other complications. Of the metabolic complications, the development of hyperglycaemia is most common, and possibly the most detrimental.

Maintenance energy requirement (MER)

Maintenance energy requirement (MER) is the energy requirement of a moderately active adult animal in a thermoneutral environment. It includes the energy needed for obtaining, digesting and absorbing food in amounts to maintain BW, as well as energy for spontaneous exercise. It does not include the energy required for additional activity (work), gestation, lactation, growth and repair. The MER can be calculated as a factor of the RER (e.g. the MER for an adult neutered dog is 1.6 x RER) or using other formula (e.g. MER = 140 x (BW)$^{0.75}$). See also Figures 13.14 and 13.15, and 'Nutrion for different life stages in dogs and cats', below.

Nutrients

The health and viability of an animal is dependent upon an adequate supply of nutrients that the body utilizes for energy or as parts of its metabolic machinery. Knowledge of these nutrients, their function, requirements and availability, and the consequences of deficiencies and excesses, is essential in order to feed animals correctly and to give advice about nutrition and feeding. An essential nutrient is one that is required in the diet and not synthesized in the body.

Energy-producing nutrients (also called **macronutrients**):

- Carbohydrate
- Fat
- Protein.

Non-energy-producing nutrients:

- Water
- Minerals
- Vitamins.

Macronutrients

Carbohydrate

Carbohydrates are composed of carbon, hydrogen and oxygen and have the basic formula CH_2O. The primary function of carbohydrates is to provide energy, but they may also be converted to body fat and stored. The quality of carbohydrate sources can vary, and cooking can significantly improve the digestibility of certain carbohydrates. Meat is a poor source of carbohydrate.

Functions of dietary carbohydrate

- Provision of energy (3.5 kcal/g)
- Synthesis of other essential body compounds such as RNA and DNA
- Source of fibre

Carbohydrates can be classified as:

- Monosaccharides
- Disaccharides
- Polysaccharides.

Monosaccharides, commonly referred to as simple sugars, are the basic form and include glucose, fructose (fruit sugar) and galactose (milk sugar). Glucose circulates in the bloodstream and is the primary form of carbohydrate used for energy.

Disaccharides are composed of two molecules of monosaccharide linked together. Examples include lactose, maltose and sucrose. Digestion of disaccharides is controlled by the activity of specific enzymes (disaccharidases), e.g. sucrase for sucrose, lactase for lactose. The activity of lactase decreases with age in the dog and cat; therefore, older animals that consume an excessive amount of milk and other lactose-containing products may develop diarrhoea.

Polysaccharides are more commonly referred to as complex carbohydrates and consist of vast numbers of linked monosaccharide molecules. Polysaccharides are found widely. Examples include starch, glycogen and fibre. Starch is used for energy storage. Dietary fibre or roughage (see below) includes the polysaccharides cellulose, pectin and lignin.

When food is digested, it is mixed with saliva; this contains the enzyme amylase, which hydrolyses starch. This is of particular importance in humans but less important in dogs. Feline saliva lacks amylase and feline pancreatic amylase activity is only 5% of that of dogs. Pancreatic amylase in the dog breaks down polysaccharides to oligosaccharides and disaccharides. The enterocytes of the small intestine contain four enzymes (disaccharidases). These enzymes break down carbohydrates into smaller particles (Figure 13.2), which are then absorbed by enterocytes and rapidly released into the capillaries and transported to the liver. No enzymes capable of hydrolysing complex plant carbohydrate (cellulose) are found in dogs and cats. Consequently, cellulose does not provide energy to dogs and cats.

Dietary fibre

Fibre differs from starch in that it resists enzymatic digestion in the small intestine of dogs and cats. It is, however, subject to bacterial fermentation in the colon. Depending on the type, fibre can be partly or completely fermented, producing

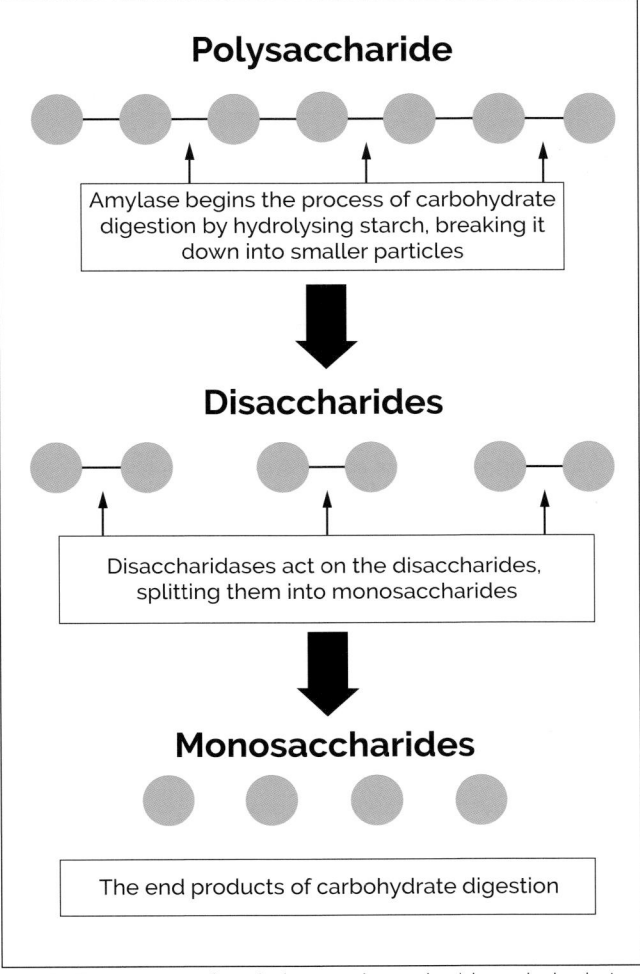

Polysaccharide

Amylase begins the process of carbohydrate digestion by hydrolysing starch, breaking it down into smaller particles

Disaccharides

Disaccharidases act on the disaccharides, splitting them into monosaccharides

Monosaccharides

The end products of carbohydrate digestion

13.2 Enzymes break down polysaccharide carbohydrates into progressively smaller units.

gases (e.g. carbon dioxide, methane and hydrogen) and short-chain fatty acids (SCFAs). SCFAs are a significant energy source for enterocytes and colonocytes.

Functions of dietary fibre

- Increase bulk and water of intestinal contents
- Reduce energy density of food to promote weight loss
- Regulation of gut transit time
- Production of short-chain fatty acids that help to maintain the health of the colon
- Maintenance of the structural integrity of the gut mucosa
- Therapeutic uses in the treatment of fibre-responsive diseases
- Alteration of nutrient absorption and metabolism

Fibre can be classified as soluble (e.g. pectins) or insoluble (e.g. cellulose and lignin). Whilst fibre is not considered an essential dietary component, both soluble and insoluble dietary fibre are important and influence the health and function of the gastro-intestinal tract. Sources of insoluble fibre can act as bulking (laxative) agents and help prevent constipation. Sources of soluble fibre can help regulate blood glucose and, thus, may be of importance in diabetic animals. Whilst it is important for animals to consume adequate

amounts of fibre, excessive amounts can have negative effects, including flatulence and borborygmi, increased bowel movements, increased faecal output, and constipation due to the bulking effect.

Fat

Dietary fat is part of a group of compounds known as lipids. Lipids are termed 'fats' if they are solid at room temperature, and 'oils' if they are liquid at room temperature. The most common form of dietary fats are triglycerides, which are composed of one molecule of glycerol and three molecules of fatty acids. The specific types of fatty acid determine the physical and nutritional characteristics of the fat. Fatty acids may vary depending on their length (i.e. short-, medium- and long-chain), presence and number of double bonds (i.e. saturated, monounsaturated, polyunsaturated), and the location of the first double bond (e.g. omega-3 and omega-6 fatty acids).

Functions of dietary fat

- Provision and storage of energy (8.5 kcal/g)
- Essential fatty acids (EFAs)
- Aid absorption of fat-soluble vitamins A, D, E and K
- Metabolic and structural functions
- Insulation
- Enhance food palatability
- Synthesis of hormones (especially steroids)

Dietary fats do not dissolve in the watery content of the gastrointestinal tract. As a result, they are not easily broken down by lipase, a water-soluble digestive enzyme produced by the pancreas. Thus, fats take longer to digest than carbohydrates or proteins. Digestion begins with the emulsification of fat, which is accomplished under the influence of bile secreted by the liver. The fat globules are split into smaller particles, allowing lipase to act on the globule surfaces and break the fats down into glycerol and fatty acids (Figure 13.3). In the absence of bile secretion, enzymes are less efficient at this process.

Bile salts are also essential for fat digestion and help to separate the fat droplets from the surrounding water. Fats are insoluble in water, unlike glycerol and fatty acids, which can be easily absorbed into the body. The fat molecules that are too large to be absorbed into the intestinal cells are split by the pancreatic enzyme lipase. They then enter the lacteals and pass via the lymphatic duct into the venous blood supply. Some fat is utilized immediately to release energy and some is stored in adipose tissue for future use. When required, the stored fat is transported to the liver where it is converted and used for energy production.

Essential fatty acids

Dietary fat provides a source of essential fatty acids (EFAs), including linoleic acid (LA) and arachidonic acid (ARA). The functions of EFAs include acting as constituents of cell membranes, in prostaglandin synthesis during inflammation, and in control of water loss through the skin. In most animals, alpha-linolenic acid (ALA) and ARA can be synthesized from LA. The exception to this is the cat which, regardless of the amount of LA present in the diet, requires a dietary source of ARA. Fatty acid deficiency can impair wound healing and cause a dry coat and scaly skin. This often occurs as a result of consumption of low-fat food or dry food that has undergone prolonged storage, leading to rancidity.

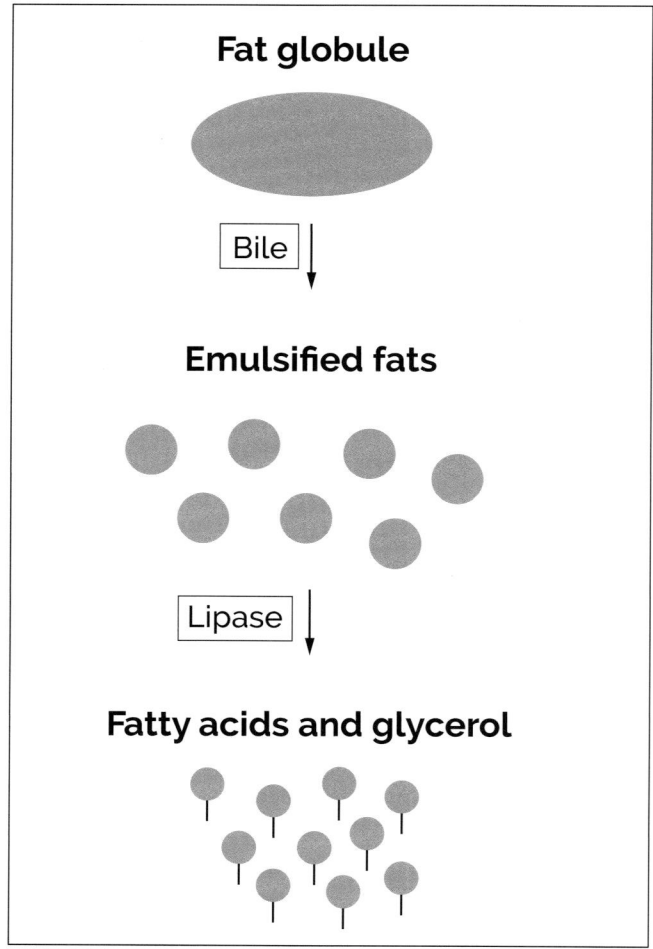

Fat globule

Bile

Emulsified fats

Lipase

Fatty acids and glycerol

13.3 Digestive breakdown of fats.

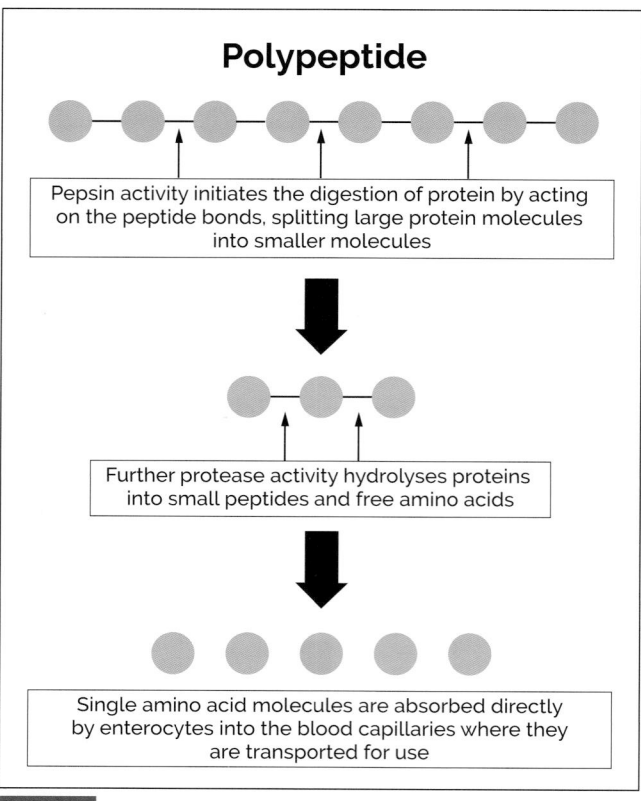

Polypeptide

Pepsin activity initiates the digestion of protein by acting on the peptide bonds, splitting large protein molecules into smaller molecules

Further protease activity hydrolyses proteins into small peptides and free amino acids

Single amino acid molecules are absorbed directly by enterocytes into the blood capillaries where they are transported for use

13.4 Digestive breakdown of proteins.

Protein

Dietary proteins are large, complex molecules composed of long chains of amino acids bound together by peptide linkages. Amino acids joined together are called peptides; two peptides joined together are a dipeptide, three linked together are a tripeptide, and more than three bonded together are a polypeptide. Essential amino acids cannot be synthesized by the body in sufficient quantities and therefore must be supplied in dietary form. The essential amino acids include arginine, histidine, isoleucine, leucine, lysine, methionine, phenylalanine, threonine, tryptophan, valine and, in cats, taurine. Non-essential amino acids can be synthesized by the body from other precursors.

Functions of dietary protein

- Tissue growth and repair
- Manufacture of hormones and enzymes
- Source of energy (3.5 kcal/g)
- Protection against infections
- Transport of oxygen
- Regulation of metabolism
- Structural role in cell walls

Most protein digestion occurs in the upper small intestine, i.e. in the duodenum and jejunum. Pepsin, the peptic enzyme of the stomach, begins the digestion of protein molecules by converting them into smaller polypeptides and peptides (Figure 13.4). This splitting of proteins occurs as a result of hydrolysis of the peptide linkages between amino acids. Hydrochloric acid in the stomach combined with stomach contents and secretions from glandular cells, creates an acidic environment that is highly favourable for pepsin activity. Constant protein digestion results in continuous amino acid production. Any surplus amino acids cannot be stored and are therefore excreted via the liver and kidneys in the form of urea.

Protein quality

The quality of a protein is determined by its biological value (BV), which is defined as the percentage of absorbed protein that is retained by the body. This figure will vary according to the amount and number of essential amino acids that it contains, and is dependent on how acceptable, digestible and utilizable the protein is. Of the common pet food ingredients, egg is known to be one of the highest quality protein sources. Other high-quality sources include casein (found in cheese), beef, lamb, pork, chicken and liver. Lower-quality sources include soybean, barley, wheat, corn and collagen.

The digestibility and quality of the protein is critical to the body for effective utilization of the food. Highly digestible proteins that contain a sufficient quantity of essential amino acids to satisfy an animal's needs, are considered to be of high quality. Those that are either low in digestibility or lacking any of the essential amino acids are considered to be of low quality.

Water

Water is vital to life and is considered the most important nutrient in terms of the ability to survive. The mammalian body consists of 60–70% water. Deficits of more than a few percent of total body water are incompatible with good health, and large water deficits (15–20% of BW) can prove fatal. Water deprivation can lead to death within days, whereas healthy animals can survive without food for a period of weeks. Excessive consumption of water is rare in normal healthy animals but may occur in animals offered water ad libitum following prolonged dehydration.

Functions of water in the body

- Electrolyte balance
- Temperature regulation
- Removal of waste
- Transport medium for nutrients
- Major component of blood and lymph
- Required for chemical reactions involving hydrolysis
- Regulates oncotic pressure, helping to maintain body shape

Animals consume water to meet a variety of needs, including physical and social, and individual differences influence the absolute requirement. Factors affecting requirements for water include:

- Polyuria/polydipsia
- Environmental temperature
- Body temperature
- Type and amount of food ingested
- Stress
- Illness or disease and general state of health
- Diarrhoea/vomiting
- Exercise
- Lactation
- Water losses through excretion or evaporation.

Water losses can be replaced either through water derived from metabolism of nutrients or by consumption of water as a liquid or as a component of food. Dry foods contain on average 6–10% moisture, and canned or moist foods contain on average 80% moisture. Provided that fresh clean water is freely available to drink and the correct quantity of a complete and balanced diet is fed, most dogs and cats will be able to meet their water requirements and self-regulate their water balance through voluntary oral intake.

Micronutrients

Minerals

Based on the quantities needed, minerals can be subdivided into macrominerals (needed in amounts more than 100 mg per megacalorie) or trace minerals (needed in amounts less than 100 mg per megacalorie). The macrominerals include calcium, phosphorus, sodium, chloride, potassium and magnesium.

The absorption and utilization of minerals from the diet is dependent on many factors, including the:

- Amount and form of the mineral in the diet
- Age, sex and species of the animal
- Physiological demand for the mineral
- Environmental factors.

Minerals serve three major functions in the body:

- Structural components, e.g. calcium in bone and teeth
- Body fluid constituents, e.g. sodium in blood
- Catalysts and cofactors for enzymes and hormones, e.g. iodine in thyroid function.

Calcium

Animal products containing bone are good sources of calcium. Dietary calcium is absorbed via an active process in the duodenum and proximal jejunum, and via a passive process in the distal intestine. The absorption, metabolism and excretion of calcium are tightly regulated in the body by parathyroid hormone, vitamin D and calcitonin. Vitamin D in particular acts to promote calcium absorption in the proximal duodenum (see Chapter 3). It is not involved in the passive absorptive process in the distal intestine. Parathyroid hormone is secreted when blood calcium levels are low and leads to the resorption of calcium from the bone, reduced excretion of calcium in the urine and the activation of vitamin D (which then increases calcium uptake in the gut). Calcitonin has an opposing role to reduce the absorption of calcium from bone when the blood concentration of calcium is high. Calcium serves both structural roles (in bones and teeth) and functional roles (cellular messaging, blood clotting, muscle and nerve function). Calcium deficiency can lead to growth retardation, reduced bone mineralization and loose teeth. Excessive calcium intake can lead to kidney damage, orthopaedic disease (especially in young large breed dogs) and uroliths containing calcium.

Phosphorus

All meats are high in phosphorus. This nutrient is absorbed from the intestine by a saturable, carrier-mediated process and a non-saturable concentration-dependent process. As with calcium, the absorption and excretion of phosphorus is under the control of parathyroid hormone and vitamin D. In particular, vitamin D enhances the absorption of phosphorus from the gut (see Chapter 3). However, in contrast to calcium, parathyroid hormone promotes the excretion of phosphorus in the urine rather than reducing its excretion. Phosphorus, like calcium, serves important structural roles in bones and teeth. It is a vital component of nucleic acids (e.g. DNA), cell membranes and ATP (adenosine triphosphate, the basic energy-producing compound). Phosphorus is also necessary for acid–base regulation and oxygen delivery. Phosphorus deficiency can lead to decreased growth, reduced fertility, a dull coat and poor bone mineralization. Excessive phosphorus can cause urolithiasis, soft tissue calcification and secondary hyperparathyroidism.

Magnesium

Foods rich in magnesium include bones, oilseed (e.g. flaxseed) and grains/fibres (e.g. bran). Up to 70% of dietary magnesium is absorbed in the intestine by a carrier-mediated process (when the dietary concentration is low) or by simple diffusion (when the dietary concentration is high). Certain dietary factors (e.g. diets high in fat, protein and calcium) can reduce magnesium absorption. Once absorbed, the kidneys play a central role in magnesium metabolism. For this reason, certain medications (e.g. diuretics) and diseases (e.g. diabetes mellitus) can cause magnesium to be lost through the kidneys as a result of excess urine production. Magnesium has many structural and functional roles in the body. It is the third most common mineral in bone and also serves vital roles in processes such as carbohydrate and lipid metabolism, catalysing enzyme reactions, promoting cellular energy production and in neuromuscular function. Signs of magnesium deficiency include muscle weakness, growth retardation, reduced bone mineralization, neuromuscular hyperactivity (e.g. tetany and seizures) and anorexia. Excess dietary magnesium has been linked to struvite urolithiasis.

Potassium

Foods rich in potassium include grains and fibres (e.g. wheat bran), yeast and soybean. The majority of potassium is absorbed in the upper small intestine by simple diffusion but it is also absorbed to a lesser degree in the lower small intestine and in the large intestine. Potassium is not stored in the body to an appreciable degree and is readily excreted in the urine. The body can therefore become depleted in potassium (hypokalaemia) when excessive potassium is lost by the kidneys (e.g. in polyuric renal failure); conversely, potassium excess (hyperkalaemia) can occur when the kidneys fail to excrete it (e.g. in advanced renal failure).

Potassium is the most important intracellular cation (K^+). It also has many roles in maintaining osmotic and acid–base balance, in nerve function, in muscle (including heart) contraction and in various enzyme systems. Potassium deficiency usually occurs due to excessive (gastrointestinal or renal) loss or reduced intake. The most common signs of potassium deficiency include anorexia, lethargy, weakness, heart rhythm disturbances and neck ventroflexion (in cats). Dietary potassium toxicity is unlikely if kidney function is normal (see Chapter 3).

Sodium and chloride

Sodium and chloride are absorbed and metabolized in tandem. Good sources of sodium and chloride include fish, eggs, poultry and whey. The absorption of sodium and chloride occurs primarily in the upper small intestine and is very efficient. Excessive amounts of sodium and chloride are excreted in urine. The absorption of calcium and some water-soluble vitamins is linked to sodium absorption. Sodium and chloride are normally tightly regulated in the body via mechanisms that monitor the blood pressure and the tonicity (concentration) of blood (see Chapter 3). In general, the kidneys are capable of regulating sodium excretion in accordance with the dietary intake. The primary role of sodium and chloride in the body is maintaining the osmotic balance in blood. Additional vital roles include regulation of acid–base and water balance, transmission of nerve impulses and muscle contraction. Deficiency is rare but signs include anorexia and lethargy. Signs of excessive sodium and chloride include thirst, pruritus, constipation and seizures.

Trace minerals

Of the numerous trace minerals, six are considered essential: iron, copper, zinc, manganese, selenium and iodine (Figure 13.5).

Vitamins

All vitamins have five basic characteristics:

- Organic compounds but distinct from the macronutrients
- Components of the diet
- Essential for normal physiological function
- Absence causes a deficiency syndrome
- Not synthesized in the body to a degree that supports normal function.

Vitamins can be subdivided into those that are fat-soluble (vitamins A, D, E and K) and those that are water-soluble (vitamins B and C). Fat-soluble vitamins require bile for their absorption, whereas water-soluble vitamins are absorbed via active transport. Fat-soluble vitamins are stored in body fat, making them less prone to deficiencies but more prone to toxicity. In contrast, water-soluble vitamins are not stored and as a result the body can become depleted in situations such as polyuric renal failure.

Fat-soluble vitamins

Vitamin A

Good sources of vitamin A include fish oils, liver, eggs and dairy products. Plant sources of the vitamin are usually in the form of carotenes (a provitamin that requires activation in the body). Cats are unable to convert beta-carotene to vitamin A and thus require the vitamin in their diet. The absorbed vitamin is transported to and stored in the liver and then transported in the bloodstream in the form of an ester. Vitamin A is necessary for vision, reproduction, immunity and bone and muscle growth. The classical signs of vitamin A deficiency (hypovitaminosis A) are night blindness and xerophthalmia (dryness of the conjunctiva). In contrast, an excess of vitamin A (hypervitaminosis A) classically manifests in skeletal malformations, including fusion of vertebrae in cats.

Vitamin D

Marine fish and fish oils are particularly good sources of vitamin D. Plants also contain vitamin D but in the form of ergocalciferol, rather than the cholecalciferol form found in animals. Cholecalciferol can be produced in the skin of mammals by ultraviolet (sun) light activation of the provitamin. However, this process is inefficient in cats and dogs and a dietary source is necessary. Vitamin D is absorbed from the small intestine by a passive, non-saturable process that is dependent on bile. The absorbed vitamin D is transported in the bloodstream in combination with vitamin D-binding

Trace mineral	Dietary sources	Functions	Signs of deficiency	Toxicity
Iron	Organ meats	Oxygen transport (haemoglobin), electron transport, enzymes	Anaemia, poor coat, ill-thrift	Anorexia, weight loss
Zinc	Meat, fibres	Metabolism of nucleic acids and carbohydrate, protein synthesis, immune system	Anorexia, ill-thrift, parakeratosis, alopecia	Not dietary
Copper	Organ meats	Haemopoiesis, neurotransmitters, connective tissue	Anaemia, reproductive failure, depigmentation	Liver damage
Manganese	Fibre, fish-meal	Enzyme activator, reproduction	Skeletal deformities, reproductive problems	Not reported
Iodine	Fish, eggs	Thyroid hormone	Hypothyroidism	Reduced appetite, rough coat
Selenium	Fish, eggs, liver	Antioxidant, immune system	Not reported	Not reported

13.5 Details of six of the essential trace minerals.

protein that then facilitates distribution of the vitamin to the peripheral tissues. Vitamin D is essential for calcium and phosphorus metabolism and in particular it enhances absorption from the intestine and protects against loss of these elements from bone. Clinical signs of vitamin D deficiency include poor bone mineralization (i.e. rickets in young animals, osteomalacia in adults). Decreased serum calcium and phosphorus levels are also noted. Vitamin D excess leads to hypercalcaemia, soft-tissue mineralization and renal failure.

Vitamin E

Vitamin E is only produced in plants and can be found in high concentrations in vegetable oils, seeds and grains. This vitamin is absorbed by a passive and non-saturable process in the intestine. Its absorption is enhanced by simultaneous absorption of fat. The vitamin circulates in the bloodstream bound to lipoproteins and is deposited equally in all tissues of the body. Vitamin E functions primarily as an antioxidant. There are several forms of vitamin E, of which alpha-tocopherol is the most biologically active form. Vitamin E together with selenium is postulated to be the first line of defence against oxidative damage in cells (with the glutathione system forming the second line of defence). Signs of vitamin E deficiency in dogs include degenerative skeletal muscle disease, impaired male reproductive function and failure of gestation. In cats, signs include steatitis and myositis. Vitamin E toxicity is rare but high doses can impair the absorption of other fat-soluble vitamins.

Vitamin K

Vitamin K is present in green leafy vegetables in two forms, both of which require activation in the body. Bacteria in the large intestine can also synthesize vitamin K. The vegetable forms of the vitamin (phylloquinone and menaquinone) are absorbed in the small intestine and then transported to the liver, where they are concentrated. The vitamin produced by the bacteria in the colon is absorbed by passive diffusion across the colonic wall. The main function of vitamin K is in the activation of several blood clotting factors and its deficiency leads to signs of coagulopathy. Excessive dietary vitamin K is unlikely to cause signs of toxicity.

Water-soluble vitamins

Vitamin C (ascorbic acid)

Dogs and cats, unlike humans, are able to synthesize vitamin C in their liver; this means that it is not strictly considered to be a vitamin in these species. The absorption of vitamin C in dogs and cats is via a process of passive diffusion. Vitamin C has many functions in the body: it acts as an antioxidant and a free-radical scavenger and also plays roles in collagen synthesis, immunity and in drug and steroid metabolism. Deficiency does not occur in dogs and cats and the risk of toxicity is low.

The B vitamins

These include thiamine (B1), riboflavin (B2), niacin (B3), pyridoxine (B6), pantothenic acid, folate, biotin and cobalamin (B12) (Figure 13.6). Additional information on the B vitamins with recognized clinical deficiency syndromes in dogs and cats is given below.

Thiamine is very labile and is susceptible to destruction by food processing. It can also be inactivated by antagonists such as thiaminases, which can be found in high concentrations in raw fish and shellfish. Thiaminases are destroyed by cooking. Commercial diets are supplemented with the synthetic form of the vitamin. Thiamine is absorbed in the jejunum and transported in red blood cells and dissolved in the plasma. Thiamine is involved in energy production and is necessary for normal nervous system function. Clinical signs of thiamine deficiency include anorexia, ill-thrift, muscle weakness, ataxia and paresis, ventroflexion of the neck (in cats) and cardiac hypertrophy (in dogs). Deficiency states can be confirmed by blood tests (erythrocyte transketolase activity or measurement of blood metabolites).

Vitamin	Dietary sources	Absorption	Functions	Deficiency	Signs of deficiency	Toxicity
Thiamine (B1)	Whole grains, liver, yeast	Jejunum (carrier-mediated)	Enzymatic reactions	Food processing; thiaminases	Anorexia, ill-thrift, muscle weakness, neurological deficits	Very rare
Riboflavin (B2)	Dairy products, meat, eggs, green vegetables, yeast	Upper gastrointestinal tract	Energy metabolism; enzymatic reactions	Uncommon	Cats: dermatitis, erythema, weight loss, cataracts, anorexia, impaired reproduction	Not reported
Niacin (B3)	Yeast, meat, fish, cereals, legumes	Stomach and small intestine	Oxidoreductive reactions; tryptophan metabolism	High corn/grain diet	Pellagra, diarrhoea, dementia, death	Not reported
Pyridoxine (B6)	Meat, whole grain, vegetables, nuts. Widely available	Small intestine	Amino acid, glycogen and lipid metabolism; neurotransmitter biosynthesis; taurine, carnitine and porphyrin biosynthesis	Uncommon	Ill-thrift, muscle weakness, neurological signs (e.g. ataxia), anorexia	Neural damage in experimental studies
Pantothenic acid	Meat, rice, wheat bran, yeast. Widely available	Intestine (energy-dependent)	Energy production and biosynthesis of fatty acids, steroid hormones and cholesterol	Uncommon	Inappetence, poor growth, fatty liver, coma, poor immunity	Non-toxic

13.6 Summary of B vitamins.

continues ▶

Vitamin	Dietary sources	Absorption	Functions	Deficiency	Signs of deficiency	Toxicity
Folate	Liver, egg yolks, green vegetables	Proximal intestine	Nucleotide, phospholipid and methionine biosynthesis; amino acid metabolism; neurotransmitter production; creatinine formation	Gastrointestinal disease	Weight loss, anaemia, anorexia	Not reported
Biotin	Egg yolks, liver, yeast	Intestine	Metabolism of lipids, glucose and amino acids	Very rare: antibiotic therapy; feeding raw egg whites	Dermatitis, poor growth, lethargy, neurological abnormalities	Not reported
Cobalamin (B12)	Meat, milk	Ileum, mediated by pancreatic intrinsic factor	Carbon metabolism; methionine biosynthesis	Gastrointestinal disease	Poor growth, anaemia, neuropathies	Dietary toxicity not reported

13.6 *continued* Summary of B vitamins.

Folate (folic acid) and cobalamin (vitamin B12) are linked in their metabolism. Folic acid refers to the oxidized form of the vitamin (found in supplements) whereas folate refers to the reduced form (found naturally in foods). Cobalamin is the largest and most complex B vitamin and contains acentral cobalt ion. Folate is necessary in the daily diet whereas intestinal bacteria can produce cobalamin. Common signs of folate deficiency include weight loss, anaemia and anorexia, whilst cobalamin deficiency is reported to cause poor growth and neuropathies. Deficiencies of these vitamins commonly occur in cats and dogs with enteropathies (e.g. inflammatory bowel disease) or with reduced pancreatic function (e.g. exocrine pancreatic insufficiency). Both of these vitamins can be readily measured in blood to demonstrate deficiency states. In addition to this, serum or urine methylmalonic acid concentration can also be used indirectly to identify cobalamin deficiency. Toxicity has not been reported.

Vitamin-like substances

These include substances that can be considered conditionally essential, i.e. their requirement is dependent on the metabolic state of the animal. Choline and L-carnitine fall into this category, as do carotenoids and bioflavonoids.

Choline

This is synthesized in the liver, and is needed in comparatively larger amounts (compared to vitamins). Egg yolks and glandular organs are rich sources. Absorption of choline takes place in the jejunum and ileum by a carrier-mediated process. Choline functions as a structural component in biological membranes, promotes lipid transport and acts as a neurotransmitter (i.e. acetylcholine). Signs of choline deficiency include growth retardation, hepatic lipidosis and renal degeneration. Adverse effects may be possible with over-supplementation.

L-Carnitine

This is necessary in cells to facilitate fatty acid oxidation. This is especially important in cardiac and skeletal muscle. Several compounds including the vitamins pyridoxine and niacin are involved in L-carnitine metabolism. Clinical signs of deficiency include muscle weakness, hypoglycaemia and cardiomyopathy.

Feeding dogs and cats

When feeding dogs and cats, their energy, macronutrient and micronutrient requirements must be considered. These components can vary when feeding both healthy animals (depending on their physiological state, such as growth, reproduction) and during illness (depending on the underlying cause of illness).

Carbohydrate requirements of healthy dogs and cats

Whilst dogs and cats do not have a minimum dietary requirement for carbohydrate (i.e. it is not an essential nutrient), animals do require adequate glucose or glucose precursors (e.g. amino acids and glycerol) in order to provide essential fuel for cells. When energy requirements are high, readily digestible carbohydrates and starches should be fed to maximize the efficiency of glucose production. It is worth noting that sugars in pet food may also serve to increase palatability for dogs, but less so for cats. Consequences of excessive and inadequate carbohydrate intake are shown in Figure 13.7.

The metabolic differences between cats and dogs support the classification of cats as obligate carnivores and dogs as omnivores. Cats have low levels of the hepatic enzymes glucokinase and hexokinase, both of which act to trap glucose in the liver following delivery from the intestine. In contrast, they have a strong capability for gluconeogenesis, i.e. the production of glucose from amino acids and

Excessive dietary carbohydrate intake
■ Obesity
■ Irregular bowel movements (diarrhoea)

Inadequate dietary carbohydrate intake
■ Protein will be used to meet energy needs, thus decreasing the amount available for tissue repair and growth
■ Lack of energy
■ Irregular bowel movements (constipation)

13.7 Consequences of excessive and inadequate carbohydrate intake in dogs and cats.

other compounds. Cats are also deficient in certain digestive enzymes required for carbohydrate absorption (e.g. the lower levels of lactase results in impaired digestion of sugars such as lactose, which is found in milk). For these reasons, the ability of cats to utilize a large amount of dietary carbohydrate is somewhat limited, yet they can maintain normal blood glucose levels when fed low-carbohydrate, high-protein foods.

Fat requirements of healthy dogs and cats

Fat can be considered an essential nutrient because it provides essential fatty acids. Of the three macronutrients, fat is the most energy dense (it provides 2¼ times more calories compared with protein and carbohydrate). This may be of particular importance when food consumption is reduced (e.g. due to illness) or when trying to reduce excessive BW. Dogs and cats require dietary fat to enhance absorption of the fat-soluble vitamins A, D, E and K. High fat concentration in a diet requires increased antioxidant protection, such as added vitamin E. If there are inadequate antioxidants, dietary fats will soon become rancid, resulting in oxidation, reduced palatability and reduced vitamin activity. Consequences of excessive and inadequate fat intake are shown in Figure 13.8.

Excessive dietary fat intake
■ Obesity
■ Pansteatitis (yellow fat disease)
■ Metabolic and gastrointestinal complications
■ Hepatic dysfunction
■ Increased carbon dioxide production

Inadequate dietary fat intake
■ Fatty acid deficiency
■ Lack of energy
■ Poor growth
■ Poor skin condition
■ Impaired fertility
■ Anaemia

13.8 Consequences of excessive and inadequate fat intake in dogs and cats.

Protein requirements of healthy dogs and cats

The protein component of the diet is vital to provide essential amino acids. A deficiency in any amino acid leads to clinical signs. Cats and dogs are particularly sensitive to a deficiency of the amino acid arginine. Following consumption of an arginine-deficient meal, the highly active catabolic enzymes in the liver produce ammonia. Without arginine, ammonia cannot be converted to urea and subsequent ammonia toxicity occurs within hours, leading to death.

Cats have a high requirement for taurine. Most mammals have the ability to synthesize this amino acid from methionine and cysteine, but cats have a limited capacity to do so and therefore it is required in the diet. Thus, commercial pet foods for cats are typically supplemented with taurine. Taurine can only be sourced in significant quantities from materials of animal origin, thus homemade vegetarian diets and cereal-based dog food can cause taurine deficiency in cats. Taurine is important for normal retinal, cardiac, reproductive, platelet and immune function. Inadequate intake can lead to irreversible blindness, heart problems and impaired reproduction and fetal development.

Cats require a higher level of protein for maintenance than dogs because their ability to regulate amino acid catabolism is limited. Additional protein may be required by both species during growth, pregnancy, lactation and tissue repair. If more protein is consumed than required, the excess cannot be stored. Deamination occurs in the liver; the resulting 'amino' part is converted to urea and excreted by the kidneys, whilst the 'acid' part is converted to glycogen or fat and stored in adipose tissue. The consequences of excessive and inadequate protein intake are shown in Figure 13.9.

Excessive dietary protein intake
■ May be detrimental to the health of older animals
■ May speed growth
■ May be a causal factor in the development of orthopaedic problems in young and large canine breeds

Inadequate dietary protein intake
■ Poor growth or weight loss
■ Dull hair coat
■ Muscle atrophy
■ Increased susceptibility to disease
■ Anaemia
■ Infertility
■ Oedema
■ Emaciation

13.9 Consequences of excessive and inadequate protein intake in dogs and cats.

Water requirements of dogs and cats

Water requirements are related to maintaining water balance. In a healthy animal, water losses occur due to:

- Urine (20 ml/kg/day)
- Faeces (10–20 ml/kg/day)
- Respiration (20 ml/kg/day).

The minimum daily requirement for dogs and cats is considered to be between 40 and 60 ml/kg and can be calculated using the formula: 50 ml x BW (kg).

Pet food types

Veterinary surgeons and veterinary nurses have a key role to play in ensuring that owners are given accurate and impartial advice about feeding their pet dogs and cats. On many occasions, lay people with no nutrition or veterinary training (e.g. breeders) are consulted by owners for dietary advice, especially if the veterinary team fails to provide this information. With the wide variety of pet diets and types of food available (Figure 13.10), it is imperative that owners receive comprehensive dietary advice. In order to provide effective information on this topic, veterinary nurses must have knowledge of the specific nutrient requirements of each species (cat *versus* dog) and life stage (i.e. maintenance, growth, reproduction and senility), together with a familiarity of different food types and their ability to meet these nutritional demands.

Homemade diets

It is becoming increasingly common for clients to enquire about feeding their pets a homemade diet rather than commercial pet food. Making a balanced homemade diet is time-consuming, demanding and requires a level of

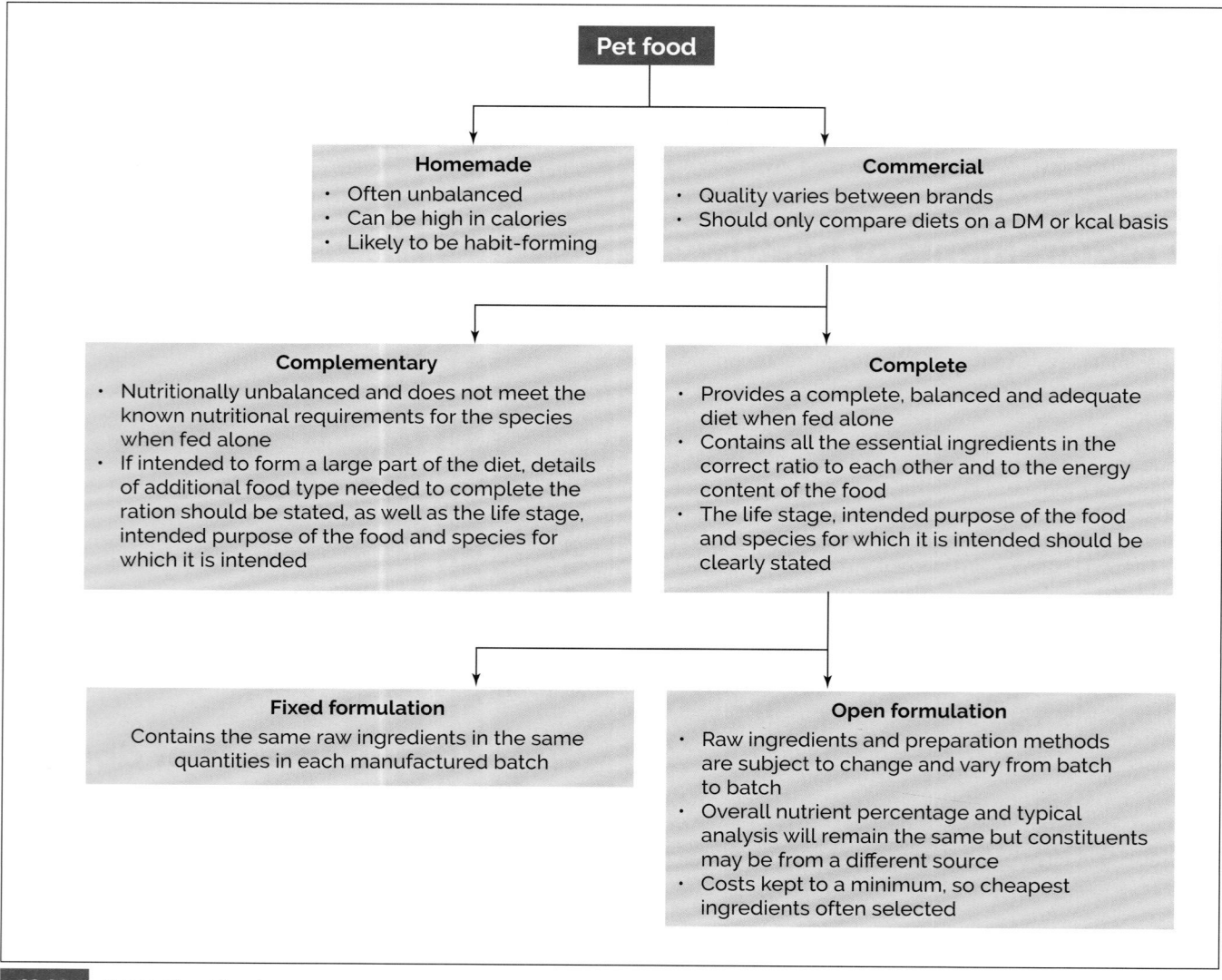

13.10 Types of pet food.

nutritional knowledge. Cooking has been shown to alter much of the nutrient content, making some dietary components more readily available (e.g. starches) and others less so (certain vitamins, minerals and proteins). Thus, micronutrient supplementation is required before homemade diets can be offered as the sole diet. Finding the appropriate balance is not simple and can easily result in the consumption of an unbalanced diet. Recipes derived from books and websites are rarely balanced (with both deficiencies and excesses of nutrients noted), and these unbalanced diets are likely to be particularly harmful during nutritionally demanding physiological states (e.g. growth, reproduction) and illness.

Despite the difficulties in producing a balanced homemade diet, there are circumstances when one may be recommended (e.g. for a dog or cat that refuses to eat commercial food). In some sick animals, concurrent medical conditions necessitate a home-cooked diet because there may be no commercial diets to meet certain criteria (e.g. both fat- and protein-restricted diets). If such a diet is recommended for long-term use, a veterinary nutritionist should be consulted to ensure it is a balanced diet.

Alternative diets

In recent years there has been great interest in using unconventional diets, such as vegetarian, grain-free and raw diets,

for companion animals. Raw diets have a particularly strong following, which include some veterinary advocates and special interest groups. For these reasons, veterinary nurses must be aware of the concerns and controversies surrounding these diets.

Raw diets

The pros and cons of raw diets are discussed in detail by Freeman *et al.* (2013). Raw feeding advocates claim that these diets mimic the food consumed by ancestral wild dogs and cats and as such are superior to commercial pet food. The claims made in favour of raw diets include that these diets:

- Are free of chemicals found in commercial food
- Contain reduced amounts of carbohydrate
- Lead to reduced incidence of dental disease
- Improve digestion and faecal quality
- Have other effects (e.g. improved coat quality).

Despite several anecdotal success stories about the use of raw diets, scientific studies showing a benefit over commercial food are currently lacking. In addition, the use of raw diets has raised some concerns among veterinary nutritionists. Chiefly, that many home recipes for raw diets are not balanced for micronutrient requirements. Feeding such unbalanced diets, particularly to the nutritionally vulnerable (e.g. puppies, kittens), can have devastating consequences (such as nutritional secondary hyperparathyroidism). However, there are now commercially produced raw diets that should be balanced for the appropriate life stages.

Proponents of raw diets advise against feeding commercial food due to the risk of contamination (e.g. melamine and cyanuric acid contamination in 2007 in the USA) of these diets. However, raw diets also carry a significant risk of contamination, in the form of microbes and parasites. Salmonella is commonly found in raw diets; studies show that dogs fed these diets are up to seven times more likely to shed *Salmonella* in their faeces (Lefebvre *et al.*, 2008). Some of the *Salmonella* strains exhibit resistance to multiple antibiotics, which has important pet and human health implications. There have been reported cases of systemic salmonellosis caused by a strain traced back to the raw diet of the animal (Fauth *et al.*, 2015). Many other pathogens have also been isolated from raw diets, including *Mycobacterium bovis* which caused an outbreak of tuberculosis in cats following the ingestion of a particular raw diet (O'Halloran *et al.*, 2019). For these reasons, feeding of raw diets to inpatients in veterinary hospitals should be discouraged. Increasingly, government authorities in some countries advise against raw feeding of pets belonging to vulnerable people (e.g. those with immune-compromising diseases).

Grain-free diets

Grain-free diets have also become very popular within the last few years. The main reasons given by those who advise against the feeding of grains are that they cause allergies, provide unnecessary carbohydrate and do not have any other nutritional value. Although not an essential nutrient, carbohydrate is important to provide readily available calories for animals and also to avoid excessive feeding of protein and fat. Contrary to what is clamed, grains (in particular whole grains) provide protein, fatty acids and micronutrients, in addition to digestible carbohydrate. Although allergies to grains are possible, these are comparatively uncommon compared with other food items such as meat (discussed later).

Vegetarian and vegan diets

The practice of feeding vegetarian and vegan diets to pets usually originates from owners who follow such diets themselves. Although there are commercially available vegetarian diets, there is a real risk of nutrient deficiencies (particularly with amino acids) with this feeding practice (Kanakubo *et al.*, 2015). For this reason, the feeding of vegan and vegetarian diets, especially to cats, should be strongly discouraged.

Human foods that are toxic to dogs and cats

Some food items that may be given to dogs and cats as treats (e.g. grapes, chocolate) or as part of home-cooked diets (e.g. onions, garlic) can have harmful effects. Dogs and (especially) cats can develop Heinz body anaemia and methaemoglobinaemia secondary to sulfoxides found in onions and garlic (see Chapter 19). Acute kidney injury is now well recognized in dogs following ingestion of grapes and raisins, but the causative agent is unknown. Methylxanthines found in chocolate can cause gastrointestinal signs (e.g. vomiting) and cardiac signs (e.g. tachycardia). The artificial sweetener xylitol (as found in human diabetic cakes) can cause severe hypoglycaemia and liver necrosis in dogs. Further information is available in Chapter 19 and in the *BSAVA/VPIS Guide to Common Canine and Feline Poisons* (BSAVA/VPIS, 2012).

Commercial diets

The market positioning of pet foods is segmented into generic, private label, grocery and speciality/premium brands. Manufacturers may label their products with terms such as premium, ultra-premium, natural and holistic. Such terms currently have no official definitions. However, pet foods made using high-quality ingredients and manufactured in accordance with a formula that remains unchanged from one production to the next ('fixed formulation' diets) are considered superior pet foods and are often recommended. In conjunction with strict quality standards for raw materials, this approach ensures quality and consistency by minimizing nutrient variability. These diets often provide balanced nutrition for each life stage.

Veterinary therapeutic diets

Veterinary therapeutic (or prescription) diets are usually supplied through veterinary surgeons and are designed for the dietary treatment or management of medical problems and pathological conditions, or to achieve a specific dietary requirement (discussed later). Therapeutic diets generally undergo many tests to ensure that specifications are met. However, because certain medical conditions require nutritional adjustments that may not be appropriate for healthy animals (e.g. protein restriction), it is important to use therapeutic diets only as directed by a veterinary surgeon. It is also important to appreciate that some of these diets may lack palatability, particularly when the animal is in the advanced stages of illness.

Comparison of different food types

Animals consume enough food to meet their energy requirements (assuming the food is palatable). To ensure that essential nutrients are eaten in adequate amounts, they should be considered in relation to the energy content or energy density of the diet (see above). The nutrient content of different foods is usually expressed in one of the following ways:

- As-fed basis
- Dry matter basis
- Energy (i.e. kilocalorie) basis.

These methods provide different values for the same diet as they depend on the moisture content of the diet. In order to guarantee correct nutritional management, it is vital to identify which method has been used to calculate the nutrient content.

Dry matter comparison

If two different foods are to be compared, the nutrient percentages must first be converted to dry matter (DM) figures:

$$\frac{\% \text{ Nutrient}}{\% \text{ Dry matter}} \times 100 = \% \text{ nutrient on a DM basis}$$

The moisture content of diets varies from 3% in some dry diets, up to over 87% in some moist diets (Figure 13.11). For example, if a diet contains 25% moisture, it will contain 75% dry matter (DM).

Classification	Moisture (%)	Dry matter (%)	Packaging and presentation
Moist	60–87+	13–40	Stainless steel cans, aluminium and plastic trays, sachets, plastic and compressed tubes
Semi-moist	25–35	65–75	Cellophane wraps, sachets
Dry	3–11	89–97	Bags and boxes

13.11 Moist *versus* dry pet foods.

Energy basis comparison

Comparison of nutrient content on an energy basis will provide greater accuracy than comparison on a dry matter basis (Figure 13.12).

Diet A = 250 kcal ME per 100 g of food, containing 3% protein as fed

Diet B = 500 kcal ME per 100 g of food, containing 3% protein as fed

These diets both appear to contain the same amount of protein; however, closer evaluation reveals a disparity in energy content. Consequently the animal will ingest different amounts of protein.

This can be calculated as follows:

Diet A

Grams of food per 100 kcal $= \dfrac{100}{250} \times 100 = 40$

Each 40 g of food contains 3% protein as fed

Grams of protein per 100 kcal ME $= \dfrac{40}{100} \times 3 = 1.2$

Diet A contains 1.2 g protein per 100 kcal ME

Diet B

Grams of food per 100 kcal $= \dfrac{100}{500} \times 100 = 20$

Each 20 g of food contains 3% protein as fed

Grams of protein per 100 kcal ME $= \dfrac{20}{100} \times 3 = 0.6$

Diet B contains 0.6 g protein per 100 kcal ME

13.12 Comparison of the nutrient content of two diets on a kilocalorie/energy basis. As diet B has a higher energy density, the pet eats less food and so consumes less protein.

Proximate analysis

Proximate analysis is the most accurate method of determining the nutrient content of a food product because it utilizes laboratory analysis. By subjecting the diet to a series of tests, the percentage of moisture, fat, protein, soluble carbohydrate, fibre and ash can be determined (Figure 13.13). European regulations dictate that the concentrations of protein, oil, fibre and ash must be declared as percentages in the product. The Feeding Stuffs Regulations 1991 also requires details of the percentage moisture content in the product, if over 14%.

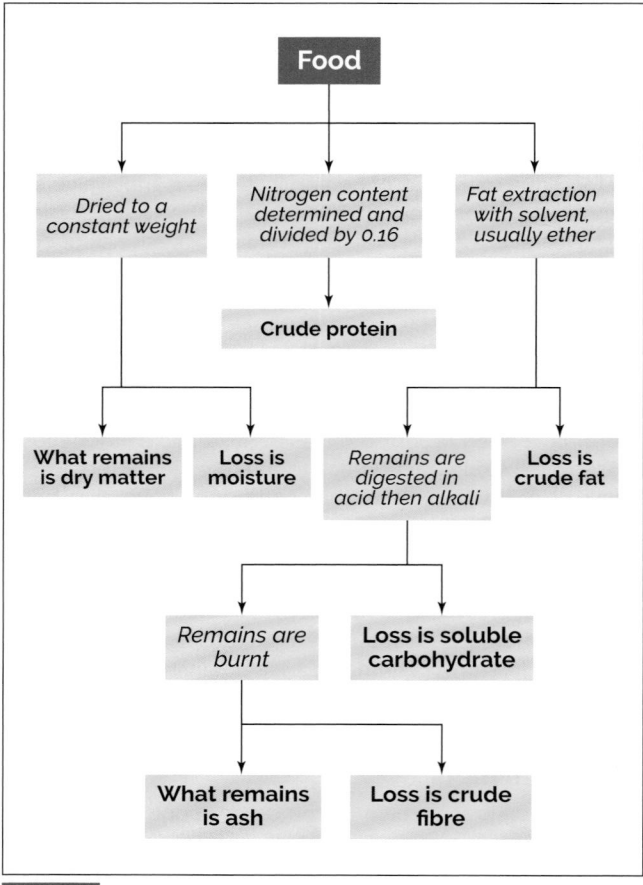

13.13 Proximate analysis process.

Understanding pet food labels

The pet food label is the primary means by which product information is communicated between a manufacturer or distributor and the purchaser. Consumer interest in human food label information has led to an increased awareness of the information available on pet food labels. Owners are now referring to these to assist them in making an informed decision about whether a food will be suitable for their pet. Similar to food intended for human consumption, animal foods must be correctly labelled. Pet food labels in Europe are divided into two main sections, although the distinction between the two is not as stringent as in the USA. Initial assessment of a particular diet is best determined by looking initially at the principal display panel (section 1). This attracts the buyer's attention and immediately communicates the product's identity:

- Product name
- Manufacturer's name
- Brand name
- Statement of intent
- Nutritional/marketing claim(s)
- Graphics and pictures.

The second section is the information panel (statutory statement) and usually includes the following:

- Directions and description of the product, including the species of animal for which the food is intended and an indication of whether the product is a complete or complementary one

- List of ingredients
- Details of additives – preservatives, antioxidants, colours
- Typical analysis (the average percentage of the nutrient level calculated from several samples) of crude protein, crude fat, crude fibre and ash (moisture must also be stated if it exceeds 14%)
- Address of company responsible for the product
- Best-before date
- Batch number
- Net weight.

Reading and interpreting a pet food label is one way of obtaining information about a pet food; however, labels do not provide information about factors such as digestibility and biological value. Contacting the manufacturer or nutrition experts for additional information is the best way to compare the quality of pet foods. Manufacturers often produce manuals and leaflets providing information about their diets. This is usually one of the most accessible sources of information freely available to all members of the veterinary practice team.

Ingredients

Ingredients must be listed on the label in descending order of their predominance by weight according to the product's formulation. Typical analysis assures that minimum or maximum amounts of the nutrients named can be found in the food but theactual amounts can vary widely. It is often difficult to assess the quality of the ingredients from the label but, as a general rule, cheaper pet foods will often use corn, wheat, soy, byproducts, and meat and bone meal. These ingredients are inexpensive. The material of animal origin used by the pet food industry comprises those parts of animals that are either deemed surplus to human needs or are not normally consumed by people in the UK. Byproducts are basically defined as 'parts other than meat'. These may include internal organs not commonly eaten by people, such as lungs and spleen.

Calculating cost per day

A seemingly cheaper food can be more expensive to feed on a daily basis than one that appears more expensive. It is easy for owners to compare the unit price (cost per weight); however, feeding costs are directly related to the energy provided by a given volume of food and the cost of that food volume. True costs of feeding are best reflected by the cost of the food per day or per year or the cost per calorie.

Nutrition for different life stages in dogs and cats

When feeding healthy animals, it is useful to consider the different stages of life separately:

- Pre-weaning
- Juvenile (growth)
- Adult
- Reproduction (including pregnancy and lactation)
- Senior.

The system of life stage nutrition tailors feeding to optimize longevity and performance and to prevent disease. This encompasses consideration of energy, macronutrient and micronutrient requirements for each physiological state.

As discussed previously, the basic calculation of energy requirement is the resting energy requirement (RER). The daily energy requirement of a healthy animal in different life stages can then be expressed as a factor of the RER (Figures 13.14 and 13.15). It must be stressed that these simplistic formulae should serve only as rough guidelines and the energy provision should be monitored and adjusted for each individual animal. Factors other than the physiological state, e.g. exercise level and ambient temperature, can have a significant impact on the energy requirements of animals.

Requirements for orphaned puppies and kittens

Newborn animals have high energy demands; kittens and puppies require approximately 13–18 kcal per 100 g of BW. The ideal method for rearing orphaned animals is to foster them to another lactating bitch or queen (when the age difference between the neonates does not exceed 14 days) (see Chapter 24). Failing this, hand-rearing is possible with the aid of species specific milk replacers; cow or goat milk does not meet the nutritional requirements of puppies and kittens as they contain inadequate protein, fat and calories. Orphans should ideally be fed every 2–4 hours when very young but can be fed less often (i.e. every 6 hours) when older. Nursing kittens should gain 18–20 g of BW per day, whilst puppies should gain 2–4 g of weight per kg of adult weight per day.

When caring for orphaned puppies and kittens, the provision of heat, humidity, immunity, elimination, sanitation, security and social stimulation also needs to be considered. The physical environment of the puppy and kitten should be warm, draught-free and reasonably humid (50%). Social stimulation should be provided with regular handling. In animals <3 weeks of age, elimination needs to be encouraged by swabbing the perineal region with a warm, moistened cotton ball. As most orphaned kittens and puppies are deprived of colostrum, it is also essential to maintain stringent hygiene practices to prevent infections (see Chapters 7 and 14).

Requirements for growth

The key requirements for growing kittens and puppies include energy, protein, calcium, phosphorus and fatty acids. These requirements can be safely and effectively met using a commercial diet balanced for the specific requirements of each species. Such diets can be introduced at 3–4 weeks of age.

The energy requirements for growing puppies are usually determined by age: 3 x RER from weaning to 4 months of age, then 2 x RER thereafter until adult weight is reached. In contrast, the energy provision for growing kittens is more constant: 2.5 x RER from weaning to adult weight. Although the provision of a high quality and palatable diet is essential for growing animals, excessive calorie intake can be detrimental. This can manifest as obesity and developmental orthopaedic disease (e.g. hip and elbow dysplasia) in large-breed dogs. Meal feeding, as opposed to *ad libitum* feeding, can help slow the rate of growth in large dogs.

Life stage	Energy requirement	Comments
Adulthood		
Entire	1.8 x RER	Dogs housed outside in cold temperatures may require up to 90% additional energy
Neutered	1.6 x RER	Reduced activity levels and possibly increased appetite
Sedentary	1.0 x RER	
Light exercise	2.0 x RER	
Moderate exercise	3.0 x RER	
Heavy exercise	4–8 x RER	Highly athletic dogs such as sled dogs may need up to 15 x RER
Obese-prone	1.4 x RER	
Senior (small breed >11–12 years, large breed >9 years)	1.4 x RER	Reduced lean body mass, metabolic rate and body temperature. Increased body fat content
Breeding		
Pregnancy – first two-thirds	1.8 x RER	
Pregnancy – final third	3.0 x RER	Most fetal growth takes place in the final third of pregnancy, at which time energy demands are high
Lactation	(1.9 x RER) + 25% per puppy	Depends on lactation period and number of puppies
Growth		
<4 months of age	3.0 x RER	Most of a puppy's growth takes place in the first 6 months and then plateaus as the puppy reaches adulthood
50–80% of adult weight	2.5 x RER	
>80% adult weight	1.8–2.0 x RER	

13.14 Energy requirements of healthy dogs during different life stages as a factor of the resting energy requirement (RER).

Life stage	Energy requirement	Comments
Adulthood		
Entire	1.4–1.6 x RER	
Neutered	1.2–1.4 x RER	
Obese-prone/sedentary	0.8–1.0 x RER	
Senior (>7–8 years)	1.1–1.4 x RER	Energy needs decrease in mature cats compared to younger cats
Geriatric (>10–12 years)[a]	1.6 x RER	Energy needs increase again in older age
Breeding		
Early pregnancy	1.6 x RER	
At parturition	2.0 x RER	Weight gain (and thus energy requirement) is linear throughout the pregnancy
Lactation	2.0–6.0 x RER	Peak energy needs occur 6–7 weeks post partum
Growth		
Growth	2.5 x RER	

13.15 Energy requirements of healthy cats during different life stages as a factor of the resting energy requirement (RER). [a] Tend to have a lower capacity to digest fat.

Protein, fatty acids, calcium and phosphorus are key nutrients in growing animals. Puppies and kittens have higher protein requirements compared with adult animals, and this difference is more notable in dogs. Specifically, the National Research Council's (NRC) recommended allowance of crude protein for kittens is 5.6 g per 100 kcal, compared with 5 g of crude protein per 100 kcal for adult cats. In contrast, the recommended crude protein allowance for puppies is 5.6 g per 100 kcal compared with 2.5 g per100 kcal for adult dogs. In addition, the fat requirements for kittens and adult cats are similar; however, puppies require more dietary fat compared with adult dogs (the NRC recommended allowance is 2.1 g per 100 kcal for puppies and 1.4 g per 100 kcal for adult dogs).

In addition to the essential fatty acids LA and ARA (see above), both kittens and puppies also require a source of the omega-3 fatty acid docosahexaenoic acid (DHA) for normal brain and retinal development. A correct calcium/phosphorus balance is vital in growing animals in general, and in large-breed puppies in particular. Both inadequate and excessive amounts of either or both of these nutrients can cause skeletal disease (a deficiency in calcium can lead to nutritional secondary hyperparathyroidism, whereas over-supplementation can lead to developmental orthopaedic disease). For these reasons, not only must the absolute amounts of calcium and phosphorus be considered but also the ratio between these two nutrients, particularly in large breed dogs.

Requirements for adult animals

The main consideration when feeding adult animals is their energy provision. Evidence shows that lean dogs are likely to live longer compared with their heavier counterparts (Kealy *et al.*, 2002). Both neutering and sedentary lifestyles have been linked to obesity, so these factors should be considered when calculating an appropriate energy provision for an adult dog or cat. Typically, an energy provision of 1.8 x RER is recommended for entire dogs and 1.4 x RER for entire cats; whereas neutered dogs should be fed approximately 1.6 x RER and neutered cats 1.2 x RER. Sedentary dogs and cats are likely to need less energy than this (e.g. 1.4 x RER for dogs and 1.0 x RER for cats). In contrast, working dogs (e.g. sled dogs) may need huge amounts of energy to sustain their workload.

Requirements for pregnancy and lactation

Pregnancy and lactation are particularly demanding physio-logical states, necessitating high energy and nutrient require-ments. The energy requirement during the first two-thirds of the pregnancy in the bitch is identical to that of the adult maintenance level; however, in the last third of the pregnancy a higher energy provision (3 x RER) is recommended. In cats, during gestation up to a 50% increase in energy may be nec-essary, but there is a gradual rise in the energy requirement compared with dogs. In cats, protein deficiency during preg-nancy can have a negative impact on kitten health, including lower BW and increased mortality, as well as poor immune function, learning behaviour and locomotor development.

The energy requirement during lactation is dependent on the period of lactation and the number of offspring in the litter. The process of lactation demands an increased energy intake and energy is also lost by the mother in the milk. Peak milk production occurs at about 3–5 weeks of lactation, during which an energy provision of up to 8 x RER may be nec-essary. This energy demand on the bitch and queen can be minimized by introducing food to the young at 3 weeks of age.

The most significant increase in protein requirement is during lactation. This is especially true for bitches, as their milk is high in protein (more than twice that of cow milk). For this reason, a protein provision of 5 g/100 kcal is recom-mended during lactation in bitches. Lactation also produces a heavy demand for dietary protein in cats, as a queen in peak lactation produces up to 19 g of milk protein per day. A protein provision of 5.3 g/100 kcal is recommended during gestation and lactation in queens.

The highest water requirement is during lactation, where up to 5–6 litres/day may be necessary. This excessive require-ment is especially pertinent to bitches, as they produce com-paratively more milk than their human counterparts.

Although there are no specific levels of carbohydrate required in dogs, during pregnancy and lactation a carbo-hydrate allocation of at least 23% of DM is recommended by some. Similarly, pregnant and lactating cats require a mini-mum of 10% DM carbohydrate, as this is thought to have a protective effect against weight loss during lactation. In addi-tion, the lactose content of milk is higher when some carbo-hydrate is fed to the bitch or queen.

The demand for calcium and phosphorus increases with gestation, due to fetal skeletal development. However, excessive calcium supplementation during pregnancy can predispose to the development of eclampsia and fetal abnormalities. Therefore, during pregnancy calcium supple-ments are not recommended and instead a diet balanced for gestation and lactation should be fed.

Requirements for elderly dogs and cats

The nutritional recommendations for senior dogs and cats have evolved somewhat with improved understanding of the physiological effects of ageing. The energy requirements of elderly dogs are thought to decrease with increasing age, which may be related to lowered metabolic rates and activity levels. If this reduced energy requirement is not addressed by a reduced calorie provision, obesity may develop. In contrast, cats >10–12 years of age have increased energy requirements compared with mature adult animals. Thus, inadvertent calorie restriction may lead to weight loss in geriatric cats. Both senior dogs and cats must undergo regular body condition scoring to maintain an ideal weight (see Figures 13.16 and 13.17).

The protein requirement of elderly dogs and cats is also very important. Like people, elderly dogs and cats are suspected to undergo the process of age-related muscle wasting called sarcopenia (as opposed to cachexia, which is the form of muscle wasting associated with disease). Aged cats and dogs are thought to have higher protein require-ments compared with their younger counterparts, and a higher dietary protein provision may slow the loss of muscle with ageing. Historically, the protein provision to elderly animals has been less than adult maintenance levels, on the assumption that these patients may have protein intolerance due to reduced renal function. However, protein restriction should only be implemented when there is confirmed renal disease because inappropriate restriction is likely to be detrimental. Elderly dogs may have an increased water requirement for medical reasons. Cats meet the majority of their water requirements from their food, but tend to be less sensitive to thirst stimuli.

Clinical nutrition in dogs and cats

Balanced nutrition is vital in disease states because these patients are likely to be more vulnerable to nutrient deficien-cies and excesses. In addition, modulation of specific nutri-ents can be used to treat and prevent disease. Comparative studies in people have shown that nutrition plays a vital role in reducing morbidity, complications and duration of hospitalization. Evidence suggests that nutrition can play a significant role in patient outcome in hospitalized dogs and cats (Brunetto *et al.*, 2010).

Nutritional assessment

The first step in planning a nutritional intervention is to assess the patient's current nutritional status. This is to iden-tify not only the patients who are already malnourished but also those at risk of malnutrition. The assessment should take into consideration historical information (e.g. duration of clinical signs, previous diet, etc.), physical exam-ination findings (e.g. lean body mass) and laboratory para-meters (e.g. serum albumin concentration). Patients may not be malnourished at the time of assessment but may still be at high risk of malnourishment. In these cases, a nutritional intervention should be implemented (e.g. feeding tube placement).

Indicators of malnutrition include:

- Unintentional weight loss (>10% of BW)
- Poor coat
- Muscle wasting
- Poor wound healing
- Hypoalbuminaemia.

Risk factors for malnutrition include:

- Anorexia for >3 days
- Severe underlying disease (e.g. trauma, sepsis, pancreatitis)
- Large protein losses (e.g. due to gastrointestinal disease, peritonitis).

Body condition scoring

Body condition score (BCS) systems utilize both visual and tactile (i.e. palpation) assessment of the body fat content (Figures 13.16 and 13.17). Such systems avoid the pitfalls of using BW as the sole assessment of weight gain or loss. Generally, 5-point and 9-point scoring systems are in use; with a score of 3/5 and 5/9, respectively, considered ideal (a score of 4/9 is ideal for large sized dogs). In the 9-point system, each score corresponds to an approximate 10% increase or decrease from the ideal condition (e.g. a BCS of 6/9 would be considered 10% overweight, whereas a score of 3/9 would be considered 20% underweight). Although the 9-point scoring system is preferred, as it is validated against the gold standard of body fat assessment (dual X-ray energy absorptiometry or DEXA scanning), it is important to use the same system consistently.

More recently, the concurrent use of muscle condition scoring has been recommended (www.wsava.org/nutrition-toolkit). This system specifically assesses the lean body tissue (i.e. muscle mass) of a cat or dog at four different sites. Muscle loss due to illness is termed cachexia and this most commonly occurs with heart failure, kidney disease and cancer.

Nutrition and specific conditions

Nutritional modulation is the cornerstone of the management of many diseases. However, some of these modulations can be detrimental to health in some scenarios (e.g. severe protein restriction in puppies and kittens). For this reason, any dietary modulations should be carefully planned, instituted and monitored.

Adverse reactions to food

Adverse reactions to food usually manifest as dermatological and/or gastrointestinal signs. These signs can be categorized as those with an immunological basis (food allergies) and those with a non-immunological basis (food intolerances). Dermatological reactions to food are most commonly due to food allergies. These usually result in pruritic skin disease, which is sometimes accompanied by concurrent gastrointestinal disease. The five most common food allergens in dogs are beef, dairy, wheat, egg and chicken; whereas in cats they are beef, dairy, fish, lamb and poultry (Verlinden et al., 2006). Gluten sensitivity (termed coeliac disease in people) is very rare in dogs and has only been reported in Irish Setters (causing gastrointestinal signs) and Border Terriers (causing canine epileptoid cramping syndrome).

Unfortunately, blood testing (i.e. serum immunoglobulins) is unreliable and should not be used to confirm or rule out food sensitivities (Foster et al., 2003). Suspected food sensitivities should be investigated by performing a food elimination trial. The diet fed during this period should consist of a single novel protein source or a hydrolysed protein diet. Many single-source protein diets and hydrolysed diets are commercially available for this purpose. The duration of a food trial for skin disease is usually 12 weeks; however, with food-responsive gastrointestinal signs, a reaction is usually seen sooner than this (i.e. 3–4 weeks).

Nutrition and orthopaedic disease

Nutrition in early life plays a key role in certain developmental orthopaedic diseases. For example, canine hip dysplasia and osteochondrosis are both diseases with a nutritional component to their pathogenesis. The pathological role of nutrition in these diseases is prior to growth plate closure, especially in large and giant breeds. Two nutritional constituents have been proposed as factors in these disorders, i.e. excessive energy provision during growth and excess calcium in the diet. The provision of a large amount of energy causes rapid skeletal growth, and this can lead to orthopaedic disease via increased biomechanical stresses. Based on these observations, feeding ad libitum and feeding excessively energy-dense food in large- and giant-breed dogs is not recommended. A calcium level of 0.7–1.2% DM and a calcium to phosphorus ratio of 1.2:1 should also be maintained during growth. Excess calcium intake is known to disrupt endochondral ossification (the process by which bone grows).

Nutrition is also directly involved in some rare but well characterized skeletal diseases. Nutritional secondary hyperparathyroidism refers to osteopenic skeletal disease and occurs due to diets deficient in calcium, excessive in phosphorus or with an inappropriate calcium to phosphorus ratio. For example, feeding puppies and kittens meat-only diets may lead to secondary hyperparathyroidism, as meat is low in calcium and high in phosphorus. This combination stimulates excessive parathyroid hormone secretion, which in turn causes the resorption of bone. Rickets in young animals (and osteomalacia in adults) are similar skeletal mineralization disorders. These occur due to inadequate dietary calcium, phosphorus or vitamin D.

Nutrition and cardiovascular disease

Taurine and L-carnitine are two nutrients implicated in the development of cardiomyopathy in cats and dogs. Feline taurine deficiency-induced dilated cardiomyopathy was first described in 1987. Since then, commercial diets have been supplemented with taurine and the incidence of this condition has drastically reduced; although it is still occasionally noted in cats fed taurine-deficient (e.g. vegetarian) diets. Taurine-deficient dilated cardiomyopathy has also been reported in dogs fed diets with very low protein levels. It is well recognized that L-carnitine is necessary for the heart to metabolize fatty acids (its primary energy source). Cardiomyopathy due to L-carnitine deficiency is suspected to occur in certain breeds (e.g. Boxers).

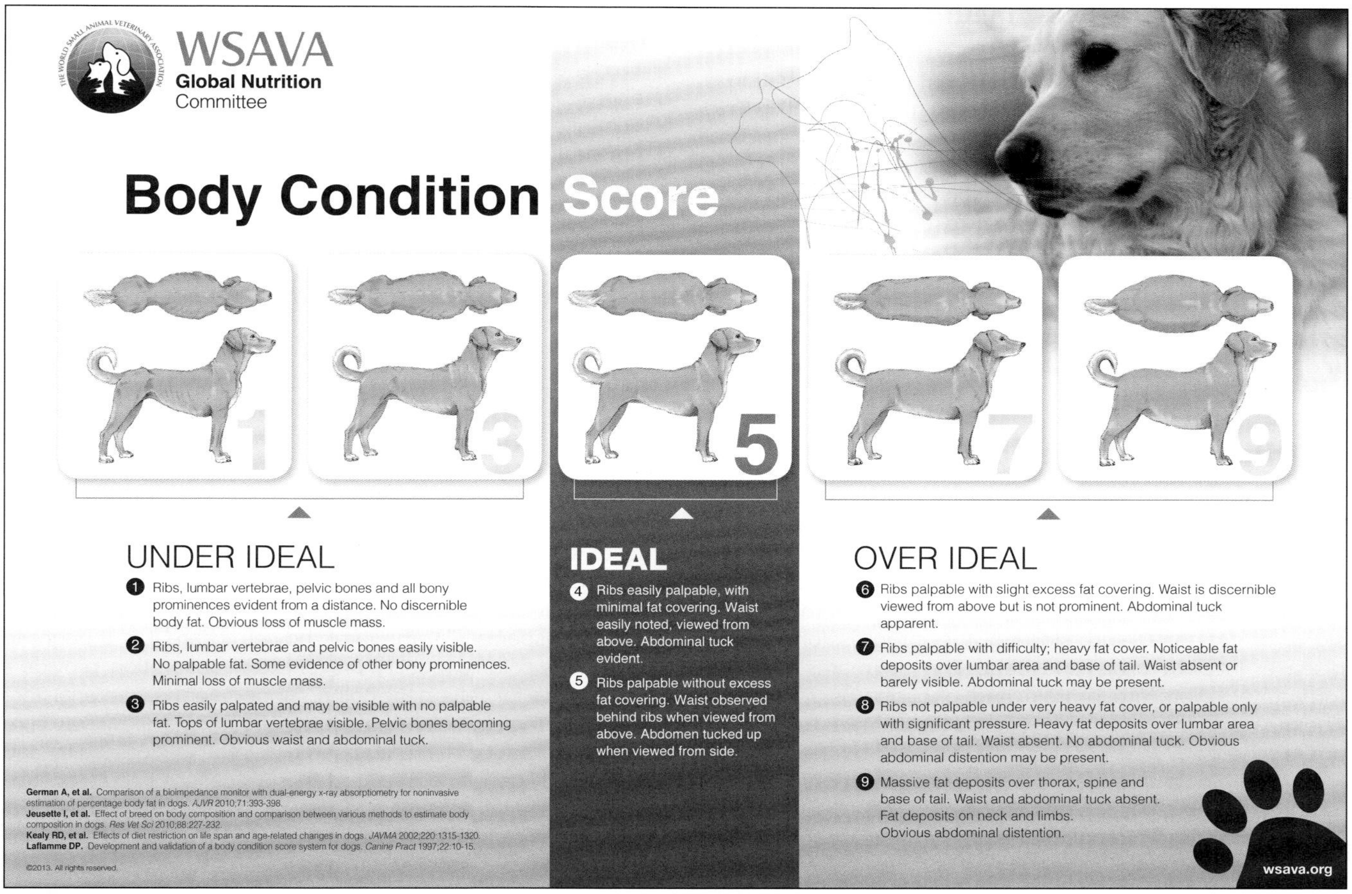

WSAVA
Global Nutrition
Committee
THE WORLD SMALL ANIMAL VETERINARY ASSOCIATION
Body Condition Score
1
3
5
7
9
UNDER IDEAL
1 Ribs, lumbar vertebrae, pelvic bones and all bony prominences evident from a distance. No discernible body fat. Obvious loss of muscle mass.
2 Ribs, lumbar vertebrae and pelvic bones easily visible. No palpable fat. Some evidence of other bony prominences. Minimal loss of muscle mass.
3 Ribs easily palpated and may be visible with no palpable fat. Tops of lumbar vertebrae visible. Pelvic bones becoming prominent. Obvious waist and abdominal tuck.
IDEAL
4 Ribs easily palpable, with minimal fat covering. Waist easily noted, viewed from above. Abdominal tuck evident.
5 Ribs palpable without excess fat covering. Waist observed behind ribs when viewed from above. Abdomen tucked up when viewed from side.
OVER IDEAL
6 Ribs palpable with slight excess fat covering. Waist is discernible viewed from above but is not prominent. Abdominal tuck apparent.
7 Ribs palpable with difficulty; heavy fat cover. Noticeable fat deposits over lumbar area and base of tail. Waist absent or barely visible. Abdominal tuck may be present.
8 Ribs not palpable under very heavy fat cover, or palpable only with significant pressure. Heavy fat deposits over lumbar area and base of tail. Waist absent. No abdominal tuck. Obvious abdominal distention may be present.
9 Massive fat deposits over thorax, spine and base of tail. Waist and abdominal tuck absent. Fat deposits on neck and limbs. Obvious abdominal distention.
German A, et al. Comparison of a bioimpedance monitor with dual-energy x-ray absorptiometry for noninvasive estimation of percentage body fat in dogs. AJVR 2010;71:393-398.
Jeusette I, et al. Effect of breed on body composition and comparison between various methods to estimate body composition in dogs. Res Vet Sci 2010;88:227-232.
Kealy RD, et al. Effects of diet restriction on life span and age-related changes in dogs. JAVMA 2002;220:1315-1320.
Laflamme DP. Development and validation of a body condition score system for dogs. Canine Pract 1997;22:10-15.
©2013. All rights reserved.
wsava.org

13.16 Body condition scoring chart for dogs. (Courtesy of the WSAVA)

WSAVA
Global Nutrition
Committee
THE WORLD SMALL ANIMAL VETERINARY ASSOCIATION
Body Condition Score
1
3
5
7
9
UNDER IDEAL
1 Ribs visible on shorthaired cats. No palpable fat. Severe abdominal tuck. Lumbar vertebrae and wings of ilia easily palpated.
2 Ribs easily visible on shorthaired cats. Lumbar vertebrae obvious. Pronounced abdominal tuck. No palpable fat.
3 Ribs easily palpable with minimal fat covering. Lumbar vertebrae obvious. Obvious waist behind ribs. Minimal abdominal fat.
4 Ribs palpable with minimal fat covering. Noticeable waist behind ribs. Slight abdominal tuck. Abdominal fat pad absent.
IDEAL
5 Well-proportioned. Observe waist behind ribs. Ribs palpable with slight fat covering. Abdominal fat pad minimal.
OVER IDEAL
6 Ribs palpable with slight excess fat covering. Waist and abdominal fat pad distinguishable but not obvious. Abdominal tuck absent.
7 Ribs not easily palpated with moderate fat covering. Waist poorly discernible. Obvious rounding of abdomen. Moderate abdominal fat pad.
8 Ribs not palpable with excess fat covering. Waist absent. Obvious rounding of abdomen with prominent abdominal fat pad. Fat deposits present over lumbar area.
9 Ribs not palpable under heavy fat cover. Heavy fat deposits over lumbar area, face and limbs. Distention of abdomen with no waist. Extensive abdominal fat deposits.
Bjornvad CR, et al. Evaluation of a nine-point body condition scoring system in physically inactive pet cats. AJVR 2011;72:433-437.
Laflamme DP. Development and validation of a body condition score system for cats: A clinical tool. Feline Pract 1997;25:13-18.
©2013. All rights reserved.
wsava.org

13.17 Body condition scoring chart for cats. (Courtesy of the WSAVA)

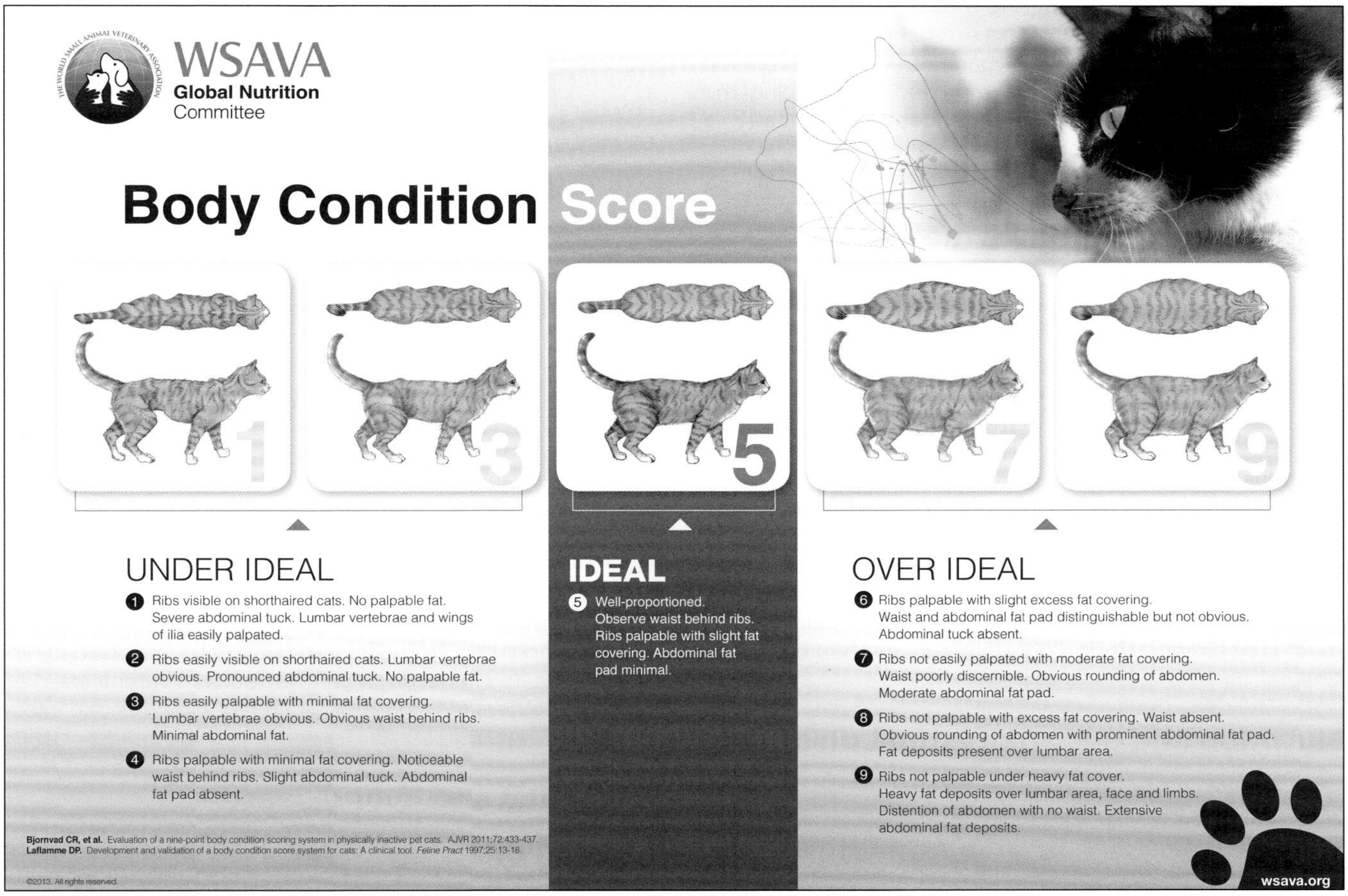

Diet in congestive heart failure

In congestive heart failure (CHF), dietary sodium is an important nutrient of modulation. The current recommendation is for moderate sodium restriction (50–80 mg/100 kcal) in mild to moderate CHF and more pronounced sodium restriction (<50 mg/100 kcal) in severe heart failure. In asymptomatic heart disease, mild sodium restriction (<100 mg/100 kcal) is advisable, as excessive sodium restriction when unnecessary can lead to activation of the renin–angiotensin–aldosterone system, which can lead to deleterious effects. Low-salt foods are also less palatable. Pet treats (commonly used to administer medication) are usually high in sodium and their salt content must be taken into consideration in heart failure cases (see Chapter 18).

Nutrition and kidney disease

Chronic kidney disease (CKD) is a disease where nutritional modulation can have a significant impact on the clinical signs as well as the prognosis (see Chapter 18). Veterinary studies comparing maintenance diets to those designed for renal failure have shown a positive effect on the clinical signs of uraemia, and slowing the progression of this disease, in both dogs and cats. The hallmarks of renal formulated diets are protein and phosphorus restriction. The main aim of protein restriction is to minimize the load of urea in the body that needs to be excreted by the kidneys. Increased blood urea (due to poor renal excretion) can lead to some of the clinical signs associated with CKD, such as inappetence and vomiting. Phosphorus restriction goes hand in hand with protein restriction because the majority of phosphorus in the diet is in the protein (meat) source. Phosphorus restriction has been shown to reduce progressive renal disease by minimizing the deleterious effects of parathyroid hormone activation (i.e. renal secondary hyperparathyroidism). The main drawback of renal diets is their poor palatability. This can be improved by warming the food or adding (low salt) flavouring agents. Alternatively, a balanced homemade diet can be formulated by consulting a nutritionist.

Nutrition and diabetes mellitus

Arguably the most important recommendation when feeding diabetic dogs is that a consistent amount and type of food is fed, divided into two equal meals given at each insulin administration. The feeding plan is less important in cats and 'grazing' can be instituted instead of meal feeding, as this more closely mimics their normal feeding behaviour. Diets designed for diabetic cats differ from those for dogs in that these have a reduced carbohydrate content and increased protein. Feline diabetic diets have been shown to reduce the insulin requirement and also to increase the possibility of achieving diabetic remission. This is in contrast to the situation in dogs, where diabetic remission is rarely achieved, irrespective of the diet, and a reduction in the insulin requirement is not seen with the equivalent (high-fibre) diets (see Chapter 18).

Nutrition and gastrointestinal disorders

Gastrointestinal disorders are the most common situations where dietary therapy is considered. In dogs and cats with acute-onset vomiting or diarrhoea, water and electrolytes (such as sodium, chloride and potassium) are the key nutrients of concern. Deficits are best addressed by providing intravenous fluid therapy.

In animals with gastrointestinal disorders, consumption of even a small amount of food (e.g. one quarter of the RER) may be beneficial because the enterocytes derive most of their energy from the lumen. Although an increased fat content enhances the energy density of diets, a high fat content may not be tolerated by animals with gastrointestinal disorders and thus a moderate fat provision is recommended. A novel protein source diet is ideal; however, these are usually reserved for more chronic gastroenteropathies. In general, dogs and cats with acute gastrointestinal disturbances are fed a diet of highly digestible protein and carbohydrate (also known as low-residue or intestinal diets). Alternatively, bland home-cooked diets (e.g. boiled rice with boiled chicken or cottage cheese) can be offered for short-term feeding.

Fibre can also be important in managing certain gastrointestinal diseases. Fibre can be classified into soluble and insoluble forms. Soluble fibre (e.g. psyllium, oats, barley) forms a gel in solution, delays gastric emptying, slows intestinal transit and is fermented in the colon. Insoluble fibre (e.g. cellulose, wheat, rye) does not form a gel and does not affect gastric emptying, but hastens intestinal transit and increases faecal bulk. Dietary fibre may have beneficial gastrointestinal effects, especially in the large bowel, where it is thought to normalize colonic motility, prevent toxin absorption, provide a fuel source for cells in the colon, support normal bacterial flora and alter the viscosity of the luminal contents. However, fibre may also reduce nutrient absorption, protein digestibility and the energy density of the food. In most cases of acute gastroenteritis, a small amount of fermentable fibre is recommended. With chronic colitis, fibre may be used to slow transit, whereas in constipation a stool softening effect may be desired.

Nutrition and pancreatic disorders

Although historically low-fat diets have been recommended in canine acute pancreatitis (because high-fat diets may worsen pancreatitis), there is no evidence to suggest that a moderate fat content is harmful. In addition, low-fat diets are generally less palatable, especially when there is a reduced appetite due to the underlying disease. For these reasons, careful selection of a palatable diet with moderate to low fat content is advisable. Pancreatitis is a common indication for a nutritional intervention, such as a feeding tube or parenteral nutrition (see later). Following a single bout of pancreatitis, most dogs can be transitioned back to their regular balanced diet. Long-term fat-restricted diets are only indicated in dogs with hypertriglyceridemia (e.g. Miniature Schnauzers) because this metabolic derangement is a risk factor for recurrent pancreatitis. Obesity is also a risk factor for pancreatitis, thus obese dogs once recovered from pancreatitis should be transitioned on to low calorie (low fat) weight loss diets. Anecdotally, some dogs with chronic pancreatitis may benefit from dietary fat restriction, however, there is no scientific evidence to support this recommendation. Pancreatitis in cats usually occurs secondary to intestinal disease and fat restriction is not necessary. There is no specific dietary recommendation for exocrine pancreatic insufficiency in dogs or cats (some dogs can be fed a maintenance diet, whereas others may improve when fed a low-residue intestinal diet) (see Chapter 18).

Nutrition and liver disease

Historically, protein restriction has been the cornerstone of the management of liver disease. However, unnecessary protein restriction can lead to protein malnutrition, which is particularly harmful in young growing animals. For this reason, protein restriction should be carefully planned and instituted, and the maximum tolerated amount of protein should be fed to animals with liver disease. There is also some evidence to suggest that vegetable protein sources (e.g. soya) may be less likely than meat protein sources to cause encephalopathic signs (see Chapter 18).

Nutrition and urolithiasis

Certain types of uroliths (struvite, urate and cystine) are amenable to dissolution via dietary and medical management. In addition, the recurrence of some types of uroliths can be prevented by feeding a specific diet. Diets designed for struvite dissolution are acidifying and have reduced contents of magnesium, phosphorus and protein. Diets to prevent oxalate urolithiasis are non-acidifying, have adequate magnesium and phosphorus, and are reduced in protein. Urate dissolution diets are reduced in protein and are alkalizing, whilst cystine stone dissolution diets are reduced in protein and sodium and are also alkalizing. A factor common to all urolith dissolution and preventive diets is to increase urine production by increasing water consumption. This can be achieved by feeding wet diets (as opposed to dry food) and/or by increasing the dietary sodium content (which will cause thirst and encourage drinking). Some diets designed for urolith dissolution are severely protein-restricted (e.g. urate dissolution diets) and these are not appropriate for growing animals or for long-term use in adults.

Obesity

The incidence of obesity in pet cats and dogs is increasing. Obesity should be considered a form of malnutrition, because increased BW can have serious repercussions on the health of animals. Human studies have shown that obesity can cause or worsen respiratory, metabolic, cardiac, gastrointestinal, orthopaedic and neoplastic disease. In dogs and cats, obesity can have a significant impact on diseases such as diabetes mellitus, chronic bronchitis, osteoarthritis, tracheal collapse and pancreatitis. Studies have shown that obese dogs live on average 2 years less than their ideal-weight counterparts (Kealy et al., 2002).

Strategies to manage obesity

A successful weight loss programme should involve careful consideration of the diet, exercise regimen and client education. Feeding a smaller amount of a maintenance diet is unlikely to achieve satisfactory weight loss and may lead to nutrient deficiencies. For this reason, diets designed for weight loss are recommended, because they provide restricted calories but are also supplemented with increased levels of micronutrients to prevent such deficiencies. Diets designed for weight loss tend to be high in fibre and/or protein, both of which are thought to have a satiating effect.

Client education begins with them accepting that their dog or cat is overweight and that this has detrimental effects on their pet's health. It is also vital to motivate the pet owner with the weight loss goals for their animal. Finally, realistic goals should be set to achieve the target body condition. An ideal rate of weight loss is approximately 1–2% of BW per week; so a dog or cat that is 20% overweight (e.g. with a condition score of 7/9) would take approximately 5 months to achieve its target weight. Monitoring during weight loss programmes is key to their success. Regular (e.g. fortnightly) body condition scoring and weighing enables close monitoring of the weight loss so that any alterations required to the programme can be made quickly and effectively.

Key elements of a weight management programme

- Prior to starting a weight loss programme, it is important to assess how overweight the patient is by using a body condition scoring system
- A complete dietary history to establish the number, quantities and types of meals and treats offered should be obtained
- Based on this information, an appropriate energy allocation can be made. In general, a safe starting energy allocation is the resting energy requirement (RER) at the actual BW. The daily amount of food can then be divided into the usual number of meals the dog or cat is given. A small part of the daily allowance can be allocated for treats during the day
- It is important to reassess the progress of weight loss with fortnightly weight checks
- A target weight loss of 1–2 % of the BW per week is ideal. If weight loss is less than this, further calorie restriction is recommended
- It is also important to instigate an exercise plan to promote weight loss. This may require 'playtime' with cats and non-traditional approaches such as hydrotherapy in dogs
- A key aspect in a successful weight loss programme is client education. The health benefits of weight loss must be clearly outlined and owners should be forewarned that the target weight loss may not be achieved for 6–12 months. Diaries and graphs outlining the progress of weight loss may be helpful in maintaining client motivation

Nutrition and critical illness

Providing adequate nutrition during hospitalization is known to have a significant positive effect on outcome in human patients. Likewise, in dogs and cats consideration should be given to addressing the nutritional needs of the animal, once its hydration, electrolyte and acid–base imbalances have been addressed. Providing adequate calories is essential to prevent catabolism of the lean body mass, maximize healing and immunity and prevent muscle weakness. It is a misconception that overweight or obese animals are better able to tolerate malnutrition due to their abundant body fat stores because during illness the body preferentially catabolizes lean body mass, rather than body fat stores.

Unless the underlying disease dictates otherwise, hospitalized dogs should be provided with 4–6 g of dietary protein per 100 kcal of energy (i.e. 15–25% of total energy requirement) and hospitalized cats should be provided with at least 6 g protein/100 kcal (25–35% of total energy requirements). Other nutritional requirements depend upon the patient's underlying disease, clinical signs and laboratory parameters. The energy goal for hospitalized patients is to provide the resting energy requirement (RER). This target amount should be gradually met over 2–3 days, depending on the duration of anorexia and tolerance to this provision. A continual decline in BW or body condition with this level of provision should prompt the clinician to reassess and modify the feeding plan (e.g. increasing the calories provided by 25%). Previous recommendations to provide increased energy in certain disease states (termed illness factors) are no longer recommended due to the risk of associated metabolic complications such a hypergly-caemia, hepatic dysfunction and hypertriglyceridaemia.

Re-feeding syndrome is a rare yet potentially devastating complication caused by providing rapid and excessive nutrition in patients following prolonged periods of anorexia. In this condition, the sudden provision of food leads to metabolic imbalances such as hypokalaemia and hypophosphataemia, which can then lead to severe cardio-vascular (arrhythmias), neurological (seizures) and haemato-logical (anaemia) consequences. Re-feeding syndrome can be prevented by slow introduction of nutrition where prolonged anorexia has been present and by closely monitoring and correcting any electrolyte disturbances.

Dietary supplements

In recent years, various nutritional supplements have come in and out of favour in both the human and veterinary markets. Supplementation of the omega-3 fatty acids doco-sahexaenoic acid (DHA) and eicosapentaenoic acid (EPA) has gained particular attention. These fatty acids are also termed fish oils, because fish such as sardines, mackerel and salmon are rich in these omega-3 fatty acids. It is important to highlight that plant-based omega-3 fatty acids (e.g. found in linseed oil) contain alpha-linolenic acid (ALA), which is very poorly converted to EPA and DHA. There is some evidence in the veterinary literature that omega-3 fatty acids are beneficial in certain kidney, heart and joint diseases. Human omega-3 fatty acid supplements and veterinary preparations can be used.

Glucosamine and chondroitin have been reported to be useful in orthopaedic diseases such as osteoarthritis. Glucosamine may serve both a structural role (as a component of the cartilage glycosaminoglycan layer) and a functional role (in mediating joint inflammation) in osteoarthritis. Chondroitin is thought to have a synergistic role with gluco-samine in reducing osteo-arthritic change and ameliorating cartilage damage. A large study investigating the potential role of these nutrients in osteoarthritis found only a benefit for fish oil supplements in dogs (Vanderweerd et al., 2012).

Oxidative damage is important in various diseases, but may also occur due to ageing, trauma and with other stresses. Vitamin E, selenium, vitamin C, beta-carotene and thiols such as S-adenosylmethionine are all reported to have antioxidant properties. Coenzyme Q10 has received particular attention from cardiologists, as its deficiency may lead to cardio-myopathy and because this compound is thought to have an antioxidant role in the heart. Although some of these anti-oxidants have shown beneficial effects in the laboratory, a beneficial effect in patients (e.g. improved outcome) has yet to be proven.

Probiotics are live organisms (e.g. *Lactobacillus acido-philus*) that provide a beneficial role in health. Prebiotics are carbohydrates (e.g. lactulose, fructo-oligosaccharides) that act as substrates for beneficial bacteria and thus promote their growth over harmful bacteria. Probiotics and prebiotics are believed to antagonize harmful gut bacteria and also modulate the immune system of the gut.

Nutritional interventions

Once a nutritional intervention is deemed appropriate for a patient, a decision has to be made as to the most appropriate type and route of delivery. Even when parent-eral (i.e. intravenous) nutrition is available, enteral (i.e.

gastrointestinal) nutrition is preferred due to its beneficial effects on the gastrointestinal tract, fewer complications and reduced cost. Feeding tubes are used widely in general veterinary practice; however, parenteral nutrition is generally confined to referral institutions.

Appetite stimulants

Force-feeding of dogs and cats is usually poorly tolerated and can lead to food aversion or more serious complications, such as aspiration pneumonia. For these reasons, feeding tubes are preferred (see below). Appetite stimulants have traditionally been used to combat anorexia, especially in cats. Older generation appetite stimulants, such as diazepam and cyproheptadine, may stimulate the appetite briefly, but the effects are short-lived and can be associated with serious adverse reactions. Newer generation appetite stimulants, such as mirtazapine, have been shown to be effective, ulti-mately leading to weight gain in animals with medical conditions such as chronic kidney disease (Quimby and Lunn, 2013). Side effects to these newer appetite stimulants are possible; however, they appear to be dose-dependent and so can be prevented by accurate dosing.

Feeding tubes

The provision of enteral nutrition via feeding tubes is widely utilized in veterinary practice. The four main types of feeding tube are:

- Naso-oesophageal
- Oesophagostomy
- Gastrostomy
- Jejunostomy.

Each has distinct features with regard to their placement, use and complications.

Choice of feeding tube

- Patient factors:
  - Duration of intended intervention
  - Underlying disease, including the treatment and prognosis
  - Necessity and safety of anaesthesia
  - Tolerance of tube.
- Technical factors:
  - Clinician's experience
  - Risk of complications
  - Invasiveness
  - Type of diet to be used.
- Owner factors:
  - Cost
  - Willingness to use at home.

Complications

While feeding tubes are generally highly beneficial to anorexic patients, no technique is entirely without risk of complications. These aspects need to be considered when deciding how to proceed and patients should be monitored closely so that significant complications are not overlooked.

Naso-oesophageal feeding tubes

Naso-oesophageal (N-O) feeding tubes are placed via the nasal cavity into the oesophagus or stomach. These are the least technically challenging to place and can be placed with the aid of topical (nasal) anaesthesia and/or light sedation (Figure 13.18). N-O tubes are usually well tolerated in the short term (i.e. 3–5 days) but their use is limited by the small diameter of the tube (and thus the type of diet that can be used). They are useful in patients that can tolerate gastro-intestinal feeding but are not sufficiently stable to undergo general anaesthesia. In such patients, N-O feeding can provide nutrition for 3–5 days, after which another feeding tube can be placed, if necessary. N-O tubes are generally contraindicated in animals that are vomiting or have reduced mentation. The tubes used are usually 5–6 Fr in cats and 8–10 Fr in dogs. Due to the small bore of these tubes, liquid diets must be used. Until recently, there have been limited available options for liquid diets.

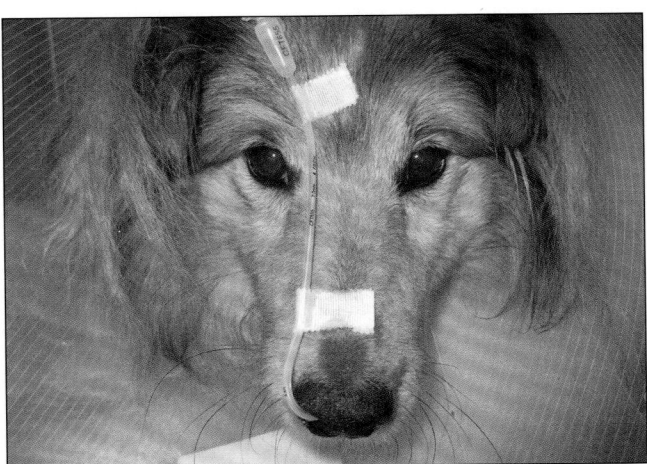

13.18 Dog with a naso-oesophageal feeding tube in place that has been secured with tape and glue (sutures can also be used).

Oesophagostomy feeding tubes

Oesophagostomy (O) tubes have revolutionized enteral feeding in dogs and cats due to their versatility, patient tolerance and relative ease of placement. General anaesthesia is necessary to place an O tube; however, the placement technique is not challenging and no specialized equipment is needed (Figure 13.19). O tubes are usually well tolerated by patients (especially cats) and do not hamper voluntary consumption of food (Figure 13.20). They are generally used for

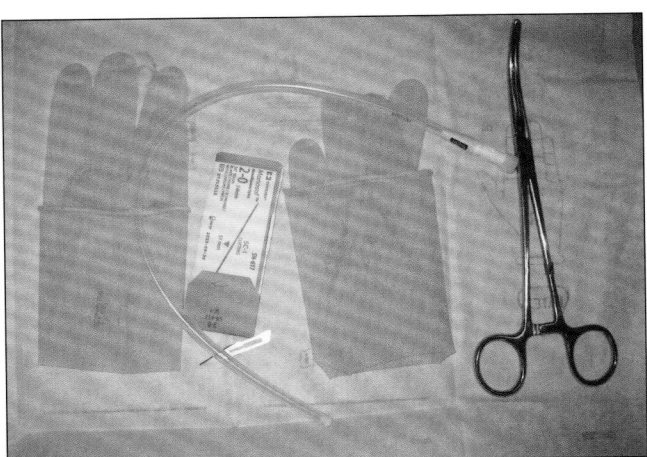

13.19 The equipment needed for placement of an oesophagostomy feeding tube includes: curved forceps (e.g. Carmalt), scalpel blade, tube (14–19 Fr), sterile gloves and suture material.

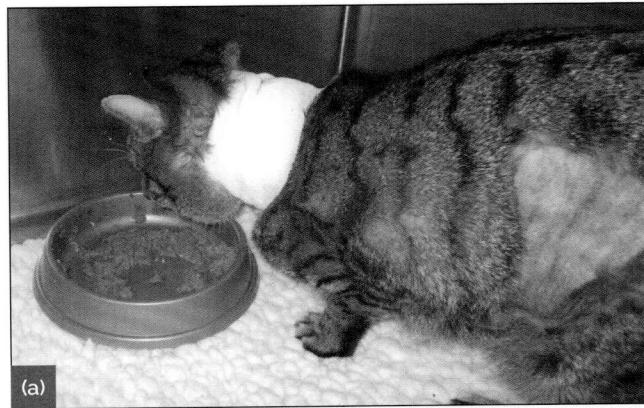

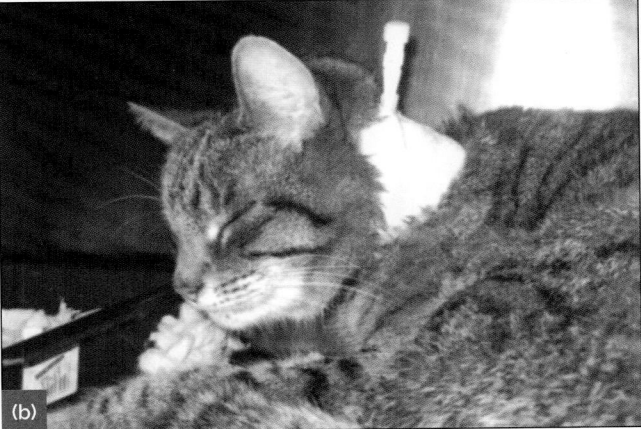

13.20 (a,b) A cat with an oesophagostomy feeding tube in place. These tubes are usually very well tolerated and cats will eat and rest without hindrance from the tube.

short- to mid-term nutritional intervention (i.e. 3–4 weeks) but can be used for prolonged periods (including for at home feeding). O tubes are contraindicated in animals with oesophageal diseases such as megaoesophagus and oesophagitis.

Although O tubes made from different materials are commercially available, silicone tubes are recommended for their flexibility and biocompatibility. One of the main advantages of O tubes is the relatively large diameter (typically 14 Fr for cats and 19 Fr for dogs), which enables the use of many different types of diets. Liquid diets, instant powdered diets or even liquidized canned diets can be used with these tubes. To prevent blockages, it is recommended that an extra exit hole is made in the side of the tube prior to placement. O tubes can be used immediately after placement (although the patient should fully recover from anaesthesia before feeding), and they can be removed at any time. Most owners can be taught how to feed their pet at home using these tubes (Figure 13.21).

As mentioned above, due to the relatively large diameter of these tubes, liquidized canned diets can be used. This is particularly helpful in situations where the specific dietary requirements of a patient (e.g. chronic kidney disease) cannot be met by liquid or instant diets. The canned diet must be liquidized in a blender with a defined amount of water to produce slurry that will easily pass through the tube. It is important to strain the slurry prior to feeding to prevent tube blockages.

Complications associated with O tubes are most commonly due to stoma site infection and abscessation. This can be prevented and/or managed by meticulous checking and cleaning of the stoma on a regular basis. Routine antibiotics are not indicated to prevent stoma infection. Severe

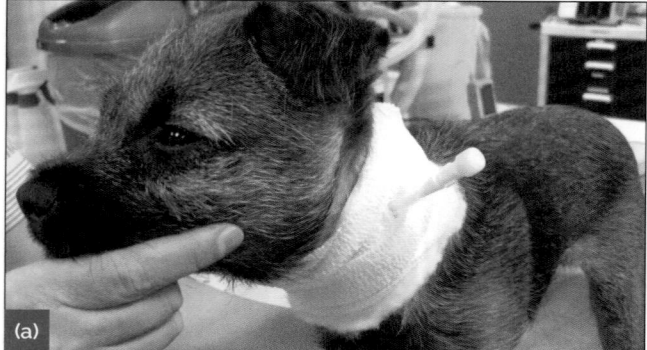

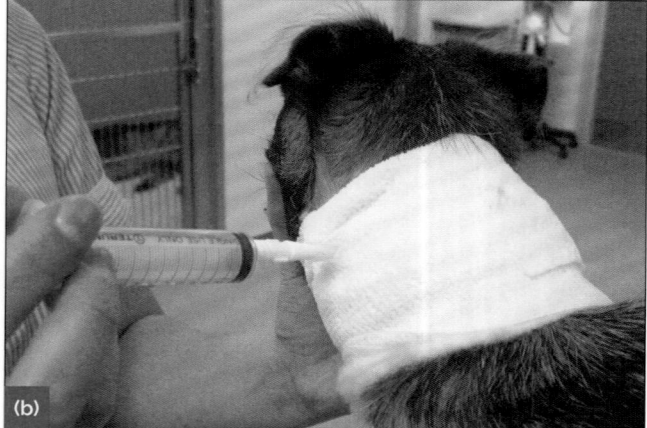

13.21 (a,b) A Border Terrier puppy with an oesophagostomy feeding tube in place. To feed using these tubes: 1) the cap is removed; 2) the tube is flushed with a small volume (5–10 ml) of water; 3) the liquid food is fed slowly over 20–30 minutes; 4) the tube is flushed again with a small volume of water; and 5) the cap is replaced.

complications can occur during tube placement (e.g. damage to blood vessels and nerves, inadvertent feeding tube placement into the trachea); however, these can be easily avoided by following safety protocols (e.g. by placing the feeding tube on the lateral aspect of the neck to avoid the nerves and blood vessels that are located ventrally or by placing an endotracheal tube during anaesthesia to prevent inadvertent feeding tube placement into the trachea). Kinking and vomiting up of tubes is also possible. Once placed, the position of the O tube should be checked via thoracic radiography (Figure 13.22).

Gastrostomy feeding tubes

Gastrostomy feeding tubes can be placed surgically or via endoscopy (the latter are called percutaneous endoscopic gastrostomy or PEG tubes). PEG tubes require flexible video-endoscopy and some skill to place (Figure 13.23). Typically, gastrostomy tube sizes are 15 Fr for cats and small dogs and 19 Fr for medium to large dogs. PEG tubes can be bought as a complete kit or can be modified from a surgical gastrostomy tube. Although oesophagostomy feeding tubes are safer and easier to place, there are clinical situations (e.g. megaoesophagus or oesophagitis) where gastrostomy feeding is preferred.

Once placed, PEG tubes must not be removed for at least 10–14 days (or longer in hypoproteinaemic or immuno-compromised patients) so that a seal can form between the gastric and abdominal walls. Removal of the tube prior to this (intentionally or due to self-trauma) can result in septic peritonitis. Due to the large bore of the tubes, both instant convalescence diets and liquidized canned diets can be used. As with oesophagostomy tubes, PEG tubes can also be used by the owner at home. In cases of prolonged use, the gastrostomy tube can be modified to a low-profile device. In small to medium sized dogs, PEG tube removal may require endoscopy to retrieve the 'stopper' from the stomach, whereas in larger dogs this can be left to pass with the faeces.

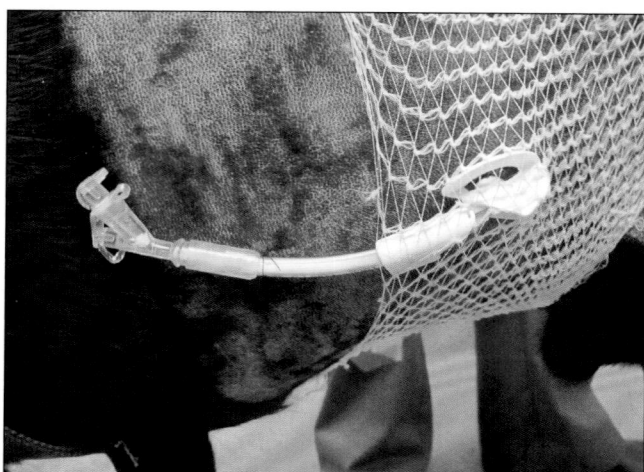

13.23 A percutaneous endoscopic gastrostomy (PEG) tube secured in a dog using a body stockinet.

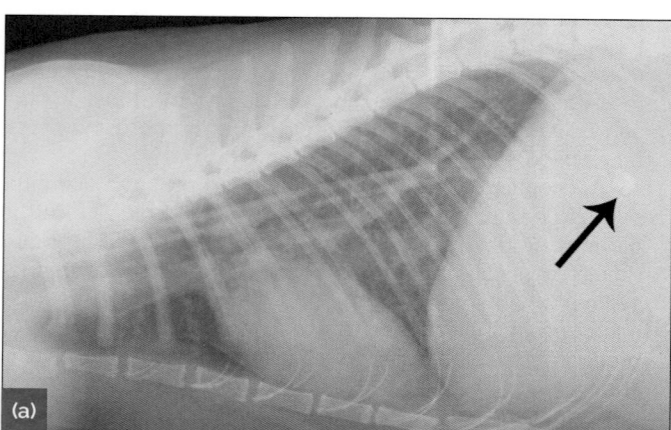

13.22 A thoracic radiograph should always be taken after placement of an oesophagostomy feeding tube to confirm that it is in the correct position. (a) The tube is too far caudal (i.e. in the stomach; arrowed). (b) The tube is in the ideal position (i.e. in the caudal oesophagus; arrowed).

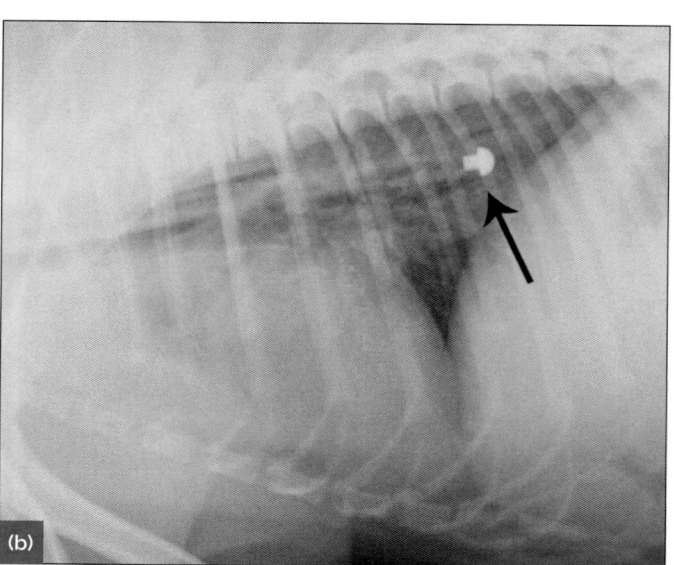

Jejunostomy feeding tubes

Jejunostomy (J) tubes bypass the oesophagus and stomach and are placed directly into the small intestine. These are usually placed during open abdominal surgery, although endoscopic placement techniques have been described. J tubes are technically challenging to place and can be associated with serious complications. The indications for use of these tubes are limited to situations such as following major pancreatic, proximal gastrointestinal or biliary tract surgery. Feeding via J tubes should be performed as a continuous rate infusion (rather than as a bolus) with a partially digested (i.e. elemental) liquid diet to mimic the normal physiology of the intestine.

Administering food

In general, the full provision of food (100% of the RER) is gradually reached over 3 days, i.e. a third of the RER is fed on the first day, two-thirds on day 2, and then 100% of the RER is fed from day 3 onwards. If bolus feeding is used, the total daily food volume is divided into 4–6 meals per day. Tube feeding should be performed slowly over 20–30 minutes. The tube should be flushed with a small volume of water (5 ml) prior to and after use to ensure patency and positioning. A larger flush volume (e.g. 10 ml) should be used for thicker diets (e.g. liquidized canned food). Each individual meal size (including the flush volumes) should not exceed 10–12 ml/kg. When starting feeding (especially after a long period of starvation), the first few meals should be <5 ml/kg per meal.

Administering medications

Drugs can also be administered via feeding tubes, but some steps should be taken to avoid drug interactions or tube complications:

- Ideally give medications separately to food
- Give one medication at a time and flush the tube in between
- Use a liquid form of the medication whenever available
- Tablets must be crushed to a fine powder and mixed with water
- Some medications (e.g. sucralfate, aluminium hydroxide) should never be delivered via feeding tubes.

Tube blockages and obstructions

Prevention of tube blockages is key to good management. Diets should be carefully prepared (e.g. canned diets adequately liquidized and strained) and the tube flushed with the recommended amount of water before and after feeding in order to prevent blockages and obstructions. Minor blockages can be managed by repeated flushing and suction with warm water or by instilling a carbonated soft drink in the tube for about 1 hour followed by flushing. In cases where tube blockages cannot be rectified, replacement of the tube is likely to be necessary.

Stoma site care

A non-adhesive dressing with antibiotic ointment can be used to cover the stoma site of oesophagostomy, gastrostomy and jejunostomy tubes. The tube exit site is covered with a light bandage. For gastrostomy tubes, stockinet can be used instead of a bandage, provided the animal cannot reach the tube. Elizabethan collars may be necessary to prevent damage to the tube. For the first few days after tube placement, daily bandage changes are recommended; after this time, bandage changes every 2–3 days are sufficient in most cases.

Feeding at home

Most owners can be taught to feed their pets at home using feeding tubes. In these situations, it is necessary to provide detailed written instructions on food preparation and administration, as well as a clear demonstration of the feeding protocol prior to discharge. Owners should be advised to monitor their pet for signs of vomiting, regurgitation, coughing, discomfort, dyspnoea, abdominal distension or discharge from the stoma and to contact the veterinary practice if any of these occur.

Parenteral nutrition

Parenteral nutrition (PN) is the provision of an animal's nutritional requirements intravenously. This technique is being used more frequently, especially in referral centres. PN solutions usually contain sources of carbohydrate (glucose), protein (amino acid) and fat (lipid), which can be formulated to meet some or all of the patient's energy requirements. PN solutions are usually administered using a central line (i.e. via a jugular catheter), but can be administered peripherally if the osmolality is not excessive (see Chapter 20). PN solutions are usually tailor-made to a patient's nutritional requirements and require proficiency in formulation and administration. Readymade PN solutions (usually containing protein and carbohydrate sources only) are also available in some countries.

The administration of PN requires proficiency in catheter placement (i.e. jugular catheter or long-stay peripheral catheter) and the capability for monitoring these patients. Catheters for PN should be placed and managed aseptically. Although complications are possible with PN, this form of nutrition has been unfairly criticized for being associated with a high complication rate. The complications can be classified as metabolic (e.g. hyperglycaemia, electrolyte disturbances), mechanical (e.g. thrombophlebitis) and septic. Many of these complications can be prevented or addressed by good technique and close monitoring of patients.

Feeding exotic pets
Small mammals

Basic energy and macronutrient requirements for rabbits and rodents are given in Figures 13.24 and 13.25.

Rabbits

Rabbits are herbivores with a high dietary requirement for fibre. Many commercial rabbit pelleted diets are available (Figure 13.26) but it is still vitally important that rabbits are encouraged to consume significant quantities of freshly grazed grass or dried grass products and hay. This is to ensure that the correct fibre levels (crude fibre levels of >18% with indigestible fibre levels of >12.5% have been quoted) are achieved to encourage normal gastrointestinal motility and dental wear. The silicates present in grasses are particularly abrasive and help to ensure sufficient dental wear. Supervised browsing on other plants may also be encouraged but grass cuttings should not be fed as these may ferment.

Rabbits have an unusual metabolism of calcium, whereby they cannot downregulate the absorption of calcium from their gut. Instead excess calcium is excreted via

	Rabbits	Guinea pigs	Hamsters	Gerbils	Rats and mice
Bodyweight (BW)	0.5–7.0 kg	0.75–1.0 kg	85–140 g	50–60 g	20–800 g
Maintenance	110.00	110.00	110.00	110.00	110.00
Growth	190–210	145.00	145.00	145.00	145.00
Gestation	135–200	145.00	145.00	145.00	145.00
Lactation	300.00	165.00	310.00	440.00	440.00

13.24 Basic energy requirements for rabbits and rodents (ME kcal/day) = 110–440 BW$^{0.75}$ where BW is in kg.

	Rabbits	Guinea pigs	Hamsters	Gerbils	Rats and mice
ME (kcal/g)	2–2.4	1.7–2.9	2.5–3.9	2.5–3.7	2.2–3
Protein (%)	12–18	18–20	18–22	17–18	13–20
Fat (%)	2–4	2–4	4–5	6–9	1–5
Fibre (%)	13–24	10–18	4–8	4	4

13.25 Basic macronutrient requirements for rabbits and rodents.

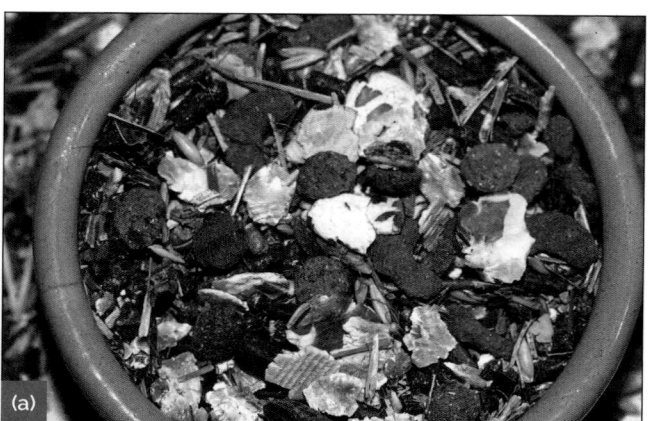

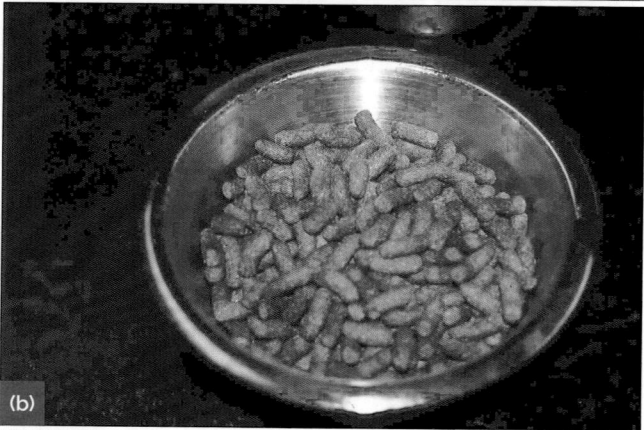

13.26 Commercially available rabbit diets. **(a)** Coarse mix. **(b)** Pelleted diet – this prevents selective feeding. (Reproduced from *BSAVA Manual of Rabbit Medicine and Surgery, 2nd edn*)

of these can produce a diet that is seriously deficient in calcium, vitamin D and other nutrients. Owners should encourage rabbits to eat all ingredients in the ration by offering smaller quantities and refilling the container only when all food has been consumed. Many now believe that pelleted foods, whilst important to provide some of the nutrients that may be absent from forages, should be both homogeneous so the rabbit cannot pick and choose what it wants to eat, and rationed. The rationing of pelleted food is important for several reasons. It ensures that the rabbit turns to forages such as dried grass or hay, which is better for gut and dental health, and it avoids the rabbit being exposed to excess calorie and mineral levels that may lead to obesity (see Figure 13.27), atherosclerosis and urolithiasis. Small volumes of leafy greens and root vegetables such as carrot may be fed but not so much that the rabbit significantly reduces the amount of hay/grass it consumes. Fruit should be avoided as the soluble carbohydrates can lead to osmotic and bacterial diarrhoea.

Rabbits tend to adjust their food intake according to their energy requirements and the energy content of the diet, but adults are likely to eat approximately 30–60 g of dry food per kg of BW per day. Free access to clean water in bowls should be provided and adults may drink 50–100 ml/kg BW per day. Suspended water bottles may be provided as an alternative but care should be taken to ensure that individuals drink enough, if water is only provided in this way, as evidence suggests they may drink significantly less than from open water bowls.

Guinea pigs

Guinea pigs are herbivorous hindgut fermenters and require a dietary source of vitamin C. A deficiency can result in clinical signs of scurvy that include loss of fur, dental disease, swollen painful joints, lethargy and death. The main types of feed available are pelleted foods or coarse mixes, but these should be formulated specifically for guinea pigs, i.e. have additional vitamin C in them. Rabbit feeds are unsuitable, since they are lower in protein and are not supplemented with vitamin C; also some products contain coccidiostats, which can cause liver or kidney damage in guinea pigs. Some pelleted feeds for guinea pigs contain vitamin C at levels that only just meet the minimum requirements, and prolonged storage (over 3 months) can deplete vitamin C levels in the

the kidneys. Excessive dietary calcium can give rise to urolithiasis and renoliths (usually calcium carbonate), whereas dietary deficiency (often exacerbated by a vitamin D deficiency) is a common cause of osteodystrophy, with associated skeletal and tooth defects. Problems can arise in some rabbits fed 'rabbit mixes' because they are selective feeders and may reject the higher-fibre items (often the pellets and hay) in the ration. Most vitamin and mineral supplements are incorporated in the pelleted portion of the diet and rejection

Rabbit Size-O-Meter

Size-O-Meter Score:

Characteristics:

1 Very Thin
More than 20% below ideal body weight

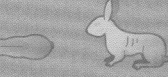

- Hip bones, ribs and spine are very sharp to the touch
- Loss of muscle and no fat cover
- The rump area curves in

2 Thin
Between 10-20% below ideal body weight

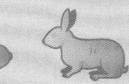

- Hip bones, ribs and spine are easily felt
- Loss of muscle and very little fat cover
- Rump area is flat

3 Ideal

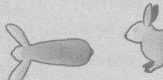

- Hip bones, ribs and spine easily felt but are rounded, not sharp – Ribs feel like a pocket full of pens!
- No abdominal bulge
- Rump area is flat

4 Overweight
10-15% above ideal body weight

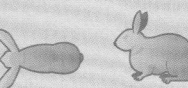

- Pressure is needed to feel the ribs, spine and hip bones
- Some fat layers
- The rump is rounded

5 Obese
More than 15% above ideal body weight

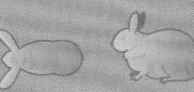

- Very hard to feel the spine and hip bones – Ribs can't be felt!
- Tummy sags with obvious fat padding
- Rump bulges out

☐ Your pet is a healthy weight

☐ Seek advice about your pet's weight

☐ Seek advice as your pet could be at risk

Please note

Getting hands on is the key to this simple system. Whilst the pictures in the Rabbit Size-O-Meter will help, judging whether your pet is the right weight purely by sight alone has its difficulties. A long coat can disguise ribs, hip bones and the spine, while a short coat can make a rabbit's appearance more irregular and highlight these areas. You will need to gentle feel your pet which can be a pleasurable bonding experience for both of you!

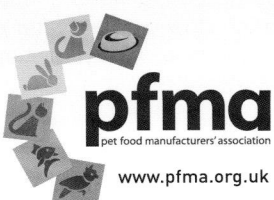

www.pfma.org.uk

Rabbit Size-O-Meter

Results:

Check out our top 5 tips for feeding your rabbit.

1. Always provide access to fresh water from a bowl or metal tipped feeding bottle, check the bottle regularly to make sure it's working properly.
2. Ensure your rabbit has an unlimited supply of good quality hay or grass which are an essential form of fibre for rabbits. They are great for their teeth, digestive system and keep them occupied. Lawnmower clippings should be avoided as they ferment rapidly and can cause digestive disturbances.
3. Buy specialist rabbit food – ask your vet or pet shop for advice.
4. Feed leafy vegetables which are good for their teeth and provide variety. Root vegetables including carrots aren't good for rabbits, so only use them as occasional treats.
5. Rabbits can get fat quickly if they're not eating the right food or not taking enough exercise. Use our Rabbit Size-O-Meter every four weeks or so to check your rabbits body condition.

Remember to make the most of advice on weight management offered by many vet practices and pet care professionals.

Your Rabbit is score **Very Thin** **1**
Your pet is very likely to be underweight. Your pet may have a naturally lean physique but we recommend you speak to your local vet to rule out any underlying medical reasons such as dental or kidney disease. If your pet is healthy but otherwise underweight, your vet is likely to advise some dietary and lifestyle changes.

Your Rabbit is score **Thin** **2**
Your pet is thin and potentially underweight. Your pet may have a naturally lean physique but we recommend you speak to your local vet for a health check up. If your pet is healthy but otherwise underweight, your vet may advise some dietary and lifestyle changes.

Your Rabbit is score **Ideal** **3**
Congratulations your pet is in ideal body condition! This is great news, as being at its ideal weight increases the chances of your pet living a long and healthy life. To keep your rabbit in tip top shape, monitor its weight and body condition on a regular basis (eg. once a month) and be careful what you and everyone else in the family feeds it. Remember any changes in lifestyle (eg. reduced exercise, recent surgery, extra treats, or even factors such as stress) can result in weight change.

Your Rabbit is score **Overweight** **4**
Your pet is potentially overweight. Being overweight is unhealthy for pets as it can lead to a shortened life-span, high blood pressure, heart disease, arthritis, cystitis and other health complications. Speak to your local vet for advice and a thorough health check-up. The vet will look for any underlying medical reasons as to why your pet may be too heavy. If there are no underlying health issues, a change of diet and lifestyle is likely to be suggested. Many vet practices run free weight management consultations, ask about these services when you ring to book an appointment.

Your Rabbit is score **Obese** **5**
Your pet is likely to be obese and this can have serious medical implications. Being overweight is unhealthy for pets as it can lead to a shortened life-span, high blood pressure, heart disease, arthritis, cystitis and other health complications. Speak to your local vet for advice and a thorough health check-up. The vet will look for any underlying medical reasons as to why your pet may be too heavy. If there are no underlying health issues, a weight loss programme will probably be individually developed for your pet and should include diet and lifestyle changes.

For more information on the Rabbit Size-O-Meter and tips on how to prevent weight gain visit **www.pfma.org.uk**. In addition to providing useful tips on how to keep your pet healthy and happy, a team of veterinary nutrition experts are on hand to answer your pet nutrition questions in the 'Ask the Expert' section.

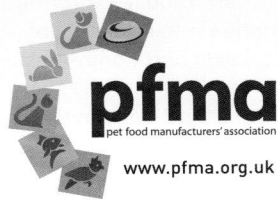

www.pfma.org.uk

13.27 Body condition scoring chart for rabbits, designed for use by pet owners. (© Pet Food Manufacturers' Association)

food. Supplementary vitamin C may be administered in the drinking water (1 g/l), or fresh fruit and leafy vegetables, which contain high levels of the vitamin, may be added to the diet. Any dietary changes should take place gradually to avoid gastrointestinal upset. The minimum dietary requirement for vitamin C in the guinea pig is 10 mg/kg/day. This will dramatically increase in situations such as pregnancy, growth and disease.

Relatively high levels of fibre are required and a shortage can lead to dental disease and fur chewing, which may result in the formation of hairballs. Gastrointestinal hypomotility may also occur on diets insufficient in crude fibre and lead to bloat. An adequate supply of good quality hay or dried grass products can usually prevent these conditions. Malocclusion can prevent feeding, drinking and swallowing of saliva (slobbers) and can prove fatal, as guinea pigs often develop metabolic ketoacidosis when they cease feeding, as well as developing hypovitaminosis C (scurvy).

Guinea pigs may eat 5–8 g/100 g BW per day. Food may be provided in open bowls on the cage floor but may become contaminated with excreta. Average daily water intake is 10 ml/100 g BW but this may increase if no succulent foods are fed. Free access to water should be provided. Open water bowls may allow greater water consumption than sip feeders, but are more easily contaminated with substrate and faecal matter.

Chinchillas

In the wild, chinchillas eat a wide range of vegetables, but their diet is composed mainly of grasses and seeds. Commercial diets are available but good-quality rabbit or guinea pig diets are also suitable. Good-quality hay should be available *ad libitum* as dental disease due to lack of dental wear is common in chinchillas. The diet may be supplemented with small quantities of dried fruit, nuts, carrot, washed green vegetables and fresh grass. Supplements should be provided in moderation to prevent obesity, bloat, diarrhoea or other gastrointestinal upsets.

Adults may eat approximately 20–40 g/day. Free access to water should be provided from hanging water bottles and it may be advisable to offer an additional water dish until the animal is used to drinking from a bottle.

Gerbils

Gerbils are herbivorous and their natural diet is based on grains and seeds, supplemented with fresh vegetables and roots when these are available. Commercial pelleted foods or seed and grain diets are available for gerbils, or adult gerbils can be fed good-quality rat or mice diets. Some mixes may contain large amounts of sunflower seeds, which have a high fat and low calcium content; these may be eaten at the expense of other dietary ingredients, resulting in obesity, hypercholesterolaemia (with resultant arterial disease) and calcium deficiency, with associated skeletal problems. The diet should be supplemented with chopped green vegetables, roots and fruit, and if pelleted food is given an appropriate seed mix should also be provided. Average food consumption in the adult is 10–15 g daily.

Like other rodents, gerbils need some hard foods or pieces of wood in their environment to gnaw and so prevent problems with tooth malocclusion. Food dishes should be ceramic, since plastic dishes may be eaten.

Gerbils conserve water efficiently through their ability to concentrate their urine. Most of their water requirement is met from succulent foods and from metabolism of the diet, but free access to clean water should always be provided. Water containers with drinking tubes are best placed outside the cage and should be checked regularly to ensure that they are working. Care should be taken to avoid using water feeders that leak as this leads to increased humidity in the environment, which can encourage skin disease such as red nose in gerbils.

Hamsters

Hamsters are omnivorous. Specific diets are available but most good-quality rat or mouse diets will meet the requirements of the hamster. Commercial pelleted diets or coarse mixes can be supplemented with treat foods such as washed vegetables, seeds, fruits and nuts. Diets rich in simple sugars (glucose, lactose, sucrose, fructose) are best avoided.

Most adults will eat 5–15 g of pelleted feed and drink 15–20 ml of water per day, but free access to water should be offered. Food and water should be provided in heavy dishes that are not easily overturned or contaminated; alternatively, hoppers may be used. Stale food should be removed from the cage to prevent hoarding by the hamster.

Rats and mice

Rats and mice are omnivorous. Their nutritional requirements are well documented and commercial pelleted foods or coarse mixes are widely available. The basic ration may be supplemented with small quantities of a variety of foods, particularly vegetable-based materials, and offering these may encourage handling by the owner. Most rats and mice will adjust their energy intake to match their requirements, but overfeeding of highly palatable soluble carbohydrate foods can lead to obesity. As a guide, adult rats require 10–20 g/day of dry food, whereas adult mice require 5–10 g/day.

Free access to water should be available from small bowls or suspended water bottles. Adult rats may drink 25–45 ml/day and adult mice may drink 5–7 ml/day.

Ferrets

Ferrets are strict carnivores with high protein and fat requirements. High-fibre diets should be avoided. Ferrets require 35% protein and 20% fat on a dry matter basis, which is higher than for adult cats. Pelleted diets for ferrets are commercially available. Whole carcasses (mice, rabbits, day-old chicks) or chicken heads may occasionally be offered to provide variety or to supplement the diet. If vegetable proteins are fed, urolithiasis and hyperammonaemia with resultant fitting may ensue.

Deficiencies are uncommon if a commercial ferret diet is fed, but some home-mixed diets may result in problems. Examples include a diet based purely on meat, which can lead to calcium deficiencies with resultant skeletal and kidney problems. Ferrets, like cats, require preformed arachidonic acid, vitamin A and taurine in their diets, all of which are found in whole meat-based foods and commercial cat and ferret diets.

Food preferences are established early in life and some individuals may resent dietary change. Ferrets should be fed *ad libitum*, as they have high metabolic rates and are prone to conditions such as insulinomas in later life. For this reason, and also because dental disease is common in ferrets, feeding a predominantly dry diet is advisable. Water intake is approximately 75–100 ml/kg per day.

Birds

Cage birds

Passerine bird species, such as the canary and zebra finch, eat a wide variety of fruit and small seeds to obtain a balanced diet in the wild. Captive birds should be fed a mixture of seeds and fruit that mimic the bird's natural feeding ecology. Similarly, psittacine birds (such as parrots, budgerigars, cockatoos, cockatiels, macaws and parakeets) seek out a natural diet containing a wide range of fruit, shoots and seeds, but in captivity they are commonly fed only seed mixes that are composed predominantly of sunflower seeds, which are high in fat but low in calcium and vitamin A. This type of diet may predispose the bird to obesity or nutritional disorders and the problem is compounded in some individuals that become addicted to sunflower seeds. A particular condition is seen in African Grey parrots (*Psittacus erithacus*) where such a calcium and Vitamin D3-deficient diet can lead to hypocalcaemic episodes with collapse and fitting.

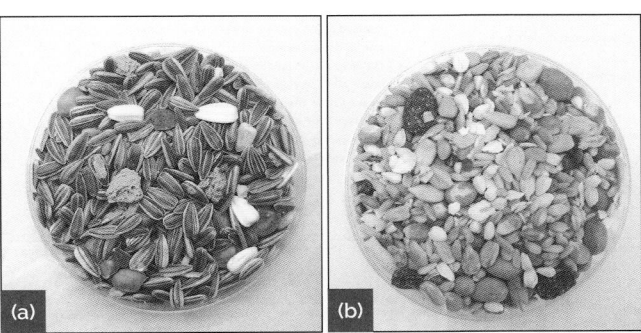

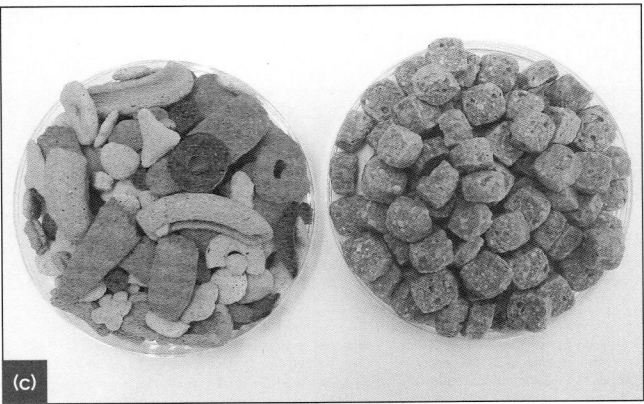

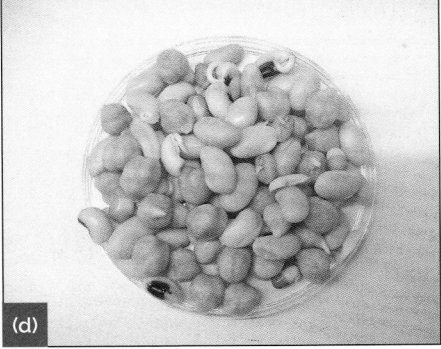

13.28 Commercial cage bird diets. **(a)** Traditional seed diet, with a high proportion of sunflower seed. **(b)** Dehusked seed diet – nutritionally poor. **(c)** Two modern pellet feeds for parrots. **(d)** Pulse diet, best used as a supplement. (Reproduced from *BSAVA Manual of Psittacine Birds, 2nd edn*)

Commercial diets formulated to meet the needs of different types of bird are available (Figure 13.28) but should still be supplemented with fresh fruit and vegetables. All-seed diets are unlikely to be nutritionally complete for birds and careful vitamin/mineral supplementation will be required. Suitable vegetables include romaine lettuce, chickweed, parsley, watercress, sprouted seeds and root vegetables. Suitable fruits include apples, plums, oranges, grapes (in small amounts), tomatoes, melon, mango, papaya and pears. Many parrots also relish sprouted seeds such as mung beans or barley/rye grass seeds (owners should ensure that these have not been treated with arsenic, as many commercial lawn seeds are treated with this as an antifungal agent). Millet sprays are often fed to adult budgerigars but should be limited, as they are extremely high in fat and encourage obesity (see Figure 13.29).

Small birds have high metabolic rates and energy requirements, so it is important that a continuous supply of food is available. Empty husks should be blown from the top of the food on a frequent basis to avoid mistakes in judging how much the bird has actually eaten. Food may be provided in seed hoppers but young birds may be fed from the floor of the cage until they are familiar with alternative feeding systems.

Two types of mineral grit, insoluble and soluble, are frequently offered to companion birds as a dietary supplement. Insoluble grit, such as quartz or other forms of silica, remains in the gizzard where it may assist in the mechanical digestion of food and thus improve digestibility of the diet. Some evidence suggests that captive birds such as parrots that dehusk seeds prior to eating them do not actually require insoluble grit in their diets. Indeed, if the diet is deficient in calcium (as so many all-seed diets are) the parrot may over-consume the insoluble grit in an attempt to correct the deficiency and so develop an impaction of the gizzard. Soluble grit, such as oyster shell or cuttlefish, is usually completely digested by birds and provides a valuable supplementary source of minerals, including calcium and phosphorus. Fresh water should be available at all times in open bowls.

Birds of prey

Birds of prey are carnivores and in captivity they are usually fed whole chicks or occasionally rodents. This diet provides a complete source of nutrition (as it includes the bones and gut contents), although problems may still arise as day-old chicks are often high in fat and low in calcium. For this reason, the removal of the yolk sac prior to feeding is advised.

Birds of prey are usually 'worked' by their owners in the summer months and should be weighed at least once a week to ensure that they maintain a steady BW. In general, the larger the bird of prey, the less prey should be fed as a percentage of the bird's BW.

Some falconers feed wild-caught prey to their raptors. Care should be taken, as two main problems can occur:

- Lead poisoning, from any lead shot remaining in the carcass
- Trichomoniasis or capillariasis from feeding wild-bird prey, such as pigeons, which can be infected with the parasites *Trichomonas* and/or *Capillaria*.

The freezing and thawing before feeding of any wild-caught pigeons helps to reduce the risk of transmission of these parasites, but there is still some risk and of course freezing does not remove the dangers of lead poisoning.

Bird Size-O-Meter

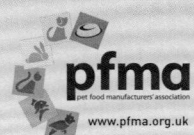
www.pfma.org.uk

Size-O-Meter Score: Characteristics:

viewed from above   skyline view of breast bone and muscle

1 Very Thin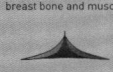
- Breast bone is very sharp to the touch
- Loss of breast muscle and no fat cover

2 Thin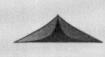
- Breast bone is easily felt and sharp
- Loss of breast muscle and little or no fat cover

3 Ideal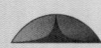
- Breast bone easily felt but not sharp
- Breast muscle rounded

4 Overweight
- Pressure is needed to feel the breast bone
- Well rounded breast muscle and some fat cover
- May see some fat below where breast bone ends

5 Obese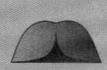
- Very hard or not possible to feel the breast bone
- Very rounded muscle and possible to feel or see fat moving under the skin.
- Fat also obvious below where the breast bone ends

Produced with assistance and advice from Anna Meredith MRCVS

☐ Your pet is a healthy weight
☐ Seek advice about your pet's weight
☐ Seek advice as your pet could be at risk

How to check your birds shape

- Getting hands on is key. Not all birds are used to being handled but it is difficult to judge if your bird is the right weight by sight. You will need to gently feel your bird, using restraint if necessary.
- Use bare hands and not gloves to handle birds as then you can judge the tightness of grip. If you need to protect yourself – use a cloth or towel.
- Small birds can be held in one hand with the neck between the first and second finger and the bird's back against the palm so that the wings and body are gently restrained in the closed hand.
- Larger parrots may take two people, one to hold the bird and the other to assess its body condition. A towel or cloth is used over the open hand to grasp the bird firmly behind its head and neck. The towel is then wrapped around the wings and body to prevent flapping. Gently stroking the top of the head and talking to the bird gently will help to calm it.
- Gently run your fingertips down the centre of the front of the bird in the midline over the breast area. You should be able to feel a bony ridge (known as the keel or breast bone). This should be easy to feel but not too prominent.
- Next, run your fingers at right angles to the keel across the breast muscles. If these feel shrunken so that the keel sticks out prominently your bird is too thin. If the breast muscles are just rounded but you can still feel the keel your bird is in good condition. If you cannot feel the keel and the muscles are very rounded or you can feel or see fat moving underneath the skin your bird is overweight.
- The breast muscle can also vary in size depending on how much exercise your bird gets – so if it flies a lot it will have larger firmer breast muscles than a bird who does not fly. However, the same criteria still apply in assessing body condition – prominence of the bony keel and presence of fat underneath the skin.

Bird Size-O-Meter

Results:

Feeding tips:

- Pet birds can get obese (fat) quickly if they are fed an improper diet, and especially in combination with lack of exercise.
- The most common cause of obesity in parrots is feeding a diet that is too high in seeds (e.g. sunflower seeds) – these are high in fat and cholesterol and low in many essential vitamins and minerals, and lead to many health problems.
- Although some smaller birds such as finches, canaries and budgerigars, will do well on a largely seed-based diet, larger parrots do not. Complete pelleted diets that are nutritionally balanced are widely available for most species of pet parrots and can be supplemented with a variety of fruits, vegetables and nuts. Different species will have differing nutritional requirements.
- Consult your vet for dietary advice for your bird.

Increasing Exercise:

- It is ideal to let your bird out of the cage at least twice a day to fly freely. Pet parrots can easily be trained and should never need to have their wings clipped. Flying is a key part of a bird's normal behaviour. Always make sure the area is secure. i.e. close all windows and doors, away from other pets that may harm them (e.g. cats and dogs).
- Where appropriate free flight in a large aviary outdoors is ideal. Exposure to natural sunlight is also very important for birds, as long as they do not get too cold. Indoors special UV lights for birds can be used.
- Parrots enjoy playing with toys and these should be used to provide mental stimulation as well as physical exercise.

Your Bird is score **1** Very Thin
A score of one suggests that your bird is very likely to be underweight. Your bird may have a naturally lean physique but we would recommend you speak to your local vet to rule out any underlying medical reasons such as kidney disease. If your pet is healthy, but otherwise underweight, your vet is likely to advise some dietary and lifestyle changes.

Your Bird is score **2** Thin
A score of two means your bird is thin and potentially underweight. Your bird may have a naturally lean physique but we recommend you speak to your local vet for a health check up. If your bird is healthy but otherwise underweight, your vet may advise some dietary and lifestyle changes.

Your Bird is score **3** Ideal
Congratulations your bird is in ideal body condition! This is great news, as being at ideal weight increases the chances of your bird living a long and healthy life. To keep your bird in tip top shape, monitor its weight and body condition on a regular basis (e.g. once a month) and be careful what you and everyone else in the family feeds it. Remember any changes in lifestyle (e.g. reduced exercise, extra treats or other factors such as stress) can result in weight-change. To help you keep on track – check out our feeding and exercise tips.

Your Bird is score **4** Overweight
A score of four means your pet is potentially overweight. Being overweight is unhealthy for birds as it can lead to a shortened life-span, atherosclerosis, heart and liver disease and other health complications. Please speak to your local vet for advice and a thorough health check-up. The vet will look for any underlying medical reasons as to why your bird may be too heavy. If there are no underlying health issues, a change of diet and lifestyle is likely to be suggested. Many vet practices run free weight management consultations led by the veterinary nurse, ask about these services when you ring to book an appointment.

Your Bird is score **5** Obese
A score of five means your bird is likely to be obese and this can have serious medical implications. Being overweight is unhealthy for pets as it can lead to a shortened life-span, shortened life-span, atherosclerosis, heart and liver disease and other health complications. Please speak to your local vet for advice and a thorough health check up. The vet will look for any underlying medical reasons as to why your pet may be too heavy. If there are no underlying health issues, a weight loss programme will probably be individually developed for your bird and should include diet and lifestyle changes.

For more information and details of how to perform the assessment and check your bird's shape please visit **www.pfma.org.uk**. In addition to providing useful tips on how to keep your pet healthy and happy, a team of veterinary nutrition experts are on hand to answer your pet nutrition questions in the 'Ask the Expert' section.

13.29 Body condition scoring chart for birds, designed for use by pet owners. (© Pet Food Manufacturers' Association)

Reptiles

Chelonians

Most land tortoises are herbivores, whereas terrapins and many of the soft-shelled turtles are carnivores and scavengers. Newly hatched tortoises start to feed properly once the yolk sac has been absorbed and may be offered a variety of finely chopped fruits, vegetables and pre-soaked specific tortoise pellets. This diet can be supplemented with vitamins and minerals, and food should be offered *ad libitum*. Juvenile and adult tortoises may be fed the same range of foods, but the items do not need to be chopped up and the animals can be housed outdoors in summer, with access to grass and other plants. Food intake is reduced or will stop for up to several weeks prior to hibernation, which occurs when ambient temperature and daylight hours begin to decrease.

Although most water requirements are met from their food, tortoises should be provided with regular access to water. The bowl should be deep enough for them to submerge their nose as well as mouth, as they have no hard palate and so must do this to create suction.

Young terrapins feed in water and it is therefore advisable to have a separate feeding tank from their main housing tank, due to the levels of detritus that can build up. Their diet includes small insects, small crustaceans and amphibian eggs and larvae. There are several companies that produce commercial aquatic chelonian pelleted diets. Adult terrapins eat amphibians and fish in the wild and so in captivity whole fish or chopped portions of whole fish should be fed to prevent nutritional imbalance. Herring, sprat, whitebait, sardines, minnows, sand eels, tadpoles or froglets, fresh prawns, shrimps and snails are all suitable foods. It is also possible to feed tinned cat or dog foods, hard-boiled eggs, cheese, earthworms or fresh liver or kidney rubbed in a vitamin/mineral supplement occasionally.

The main deficiencies seen in land-based chelonians are in calcium and vitamin D3. These deficiencies are often exacerbated by diets high in protein and by low environmental humidity, which have been implicated in the development of shell deformities such as pyramiding. Tortoises should be provided with a vitamin D3 and calcium supplement, and access to a source of ultraviolet (B) light. In carnivorous chelonians the main deficiencies are associated with vitamin A and calcium, chiefly in individuals fed an all-meat diet with no supplementation. This can result in shell deformities, kidney damage, and xerophthalmia.

Lizards

Lizards eat a wide variety of foods: different species may be insectivorous, carnivorous, herbivorous, frugivorous or omnivorous, and some species may change their feeding requirements as they mature, e.g. bearded dragons (*Pogona vitticeps*) start out in life as insectivores and become progressively more herbivorous as they mature in the wild. Insectivores (geckos, chameleons, skinks, anoles, lacertids) feed mainly on mealworms, silk-moth larvae, crickets, locusts and wingless fruit flies. These insects are deficient in calcium and must first be fed an appropriate nutritional supplement to ensure an adequate intake of supplement by the lizard. Monitors and tegus eat raw eggs, meat, dog food or rodents such as mice or rats. Biotin deficiency can occur due to the avidin content of raw, unfertilized eggs, which can act as an anti-vitamin to biotin; therefore, care must be taken when feeding hens' eggs.

Vitamin and mineral supplementation is usually required in diets for captive lizards, particularly calcium and vitamin D3 supplementation in lizards such as iguanas, basilisks, chameleons, agamids and water dragons. Access to ultraviolet lighting is also essential, UV-B being necessary to facilitate vitamin D3 synthesis in the lizard's skin (Figure 13.30; see Chapter 14). All lizards should have access to fresh water. Some, such as chameleons and a lot of green iguanas, will only drink from water droplets on plants and it is important to mist the tank several times a day. Most lizards should be regularly sprayed with water to prevent skin problems associated with low humidity.

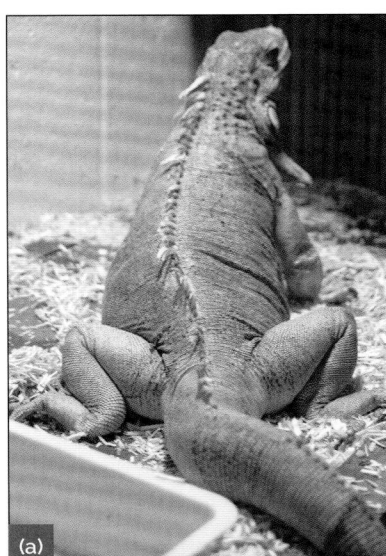

(a)

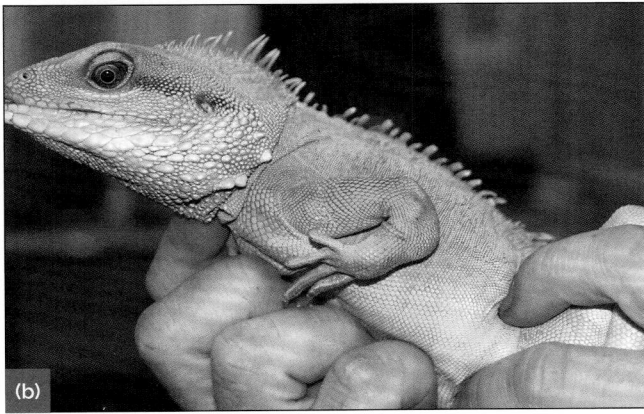

(b)

13.30 A deficiency of vitamin D3 can lead to osteodystrophy in lizards. Note the malformed **(a)** tail and **(b)** forelimb. (Courtesy of Oaklands College, Hertfordshire)

Snakes

Snakes are carnivorous and in captivity will eat rabbits, rats, mice, gerbils, chicks, earthworms, fish, amphibians, lizards or other snakes. The whole carcass is fed, to provide a balanced diet. For humane reasons and to prevent injury to the snake, food is generally offered as dead prey, which may be freshly killed or thawed from frozen.

Certain types of fish, including whitebait, have high thiaminase activity and therefore prolonged feeding without thiamine supplementation can result in thiamine deficiencies. This is particularly common in the fish-eating garter snakes (*Thamnophis* spp.). Supplementation may be given at 35 mg thiamine per kg of food. Cooking the fish to 80°C for 5 minutes will destroy the thiaminases. A garter snake can be converted on to rodent prey by smearing the rodent with the previous fish prey to fool the snake until it regularly accepts the new food.

The quantity of food and frequency of feeding depend on the BW of the snake and surface area of the prey. For example, small garter snakes may require feeding on a daily basis, whereas a large python may require a rabbit feed once every 2–3 weeks. As a guideline, adult snakes should be fed as often as is required to maintain normal BW. Snakes may not eat for long periods of time and although this is normal at certain times of the year or before a slough, it can result in inanition. Regular weighing is advisable and excessive weight loss may indicate that nutritional support is required. Fluids and easily assimilated foods can be administered by stomach tube. Water requirements of snakes are low but water bowls should always be provided.

Amphibians

All adult amphibians are carnivores and, since feeding is initiated by the movement of prey, live prey is usually required. Some species may adapt to feeding on dead prey, meat, tinned dog food or even commercial pelleted diets. Raw meat must be supplemented with calcium (10 mg per gram of meat). Captive amphibians should be fed two to three times a week.

Adult frogs and toads feed on insects such as fruit flies, crickets and mealworms; large toads will also eat mice. Aquatic species may eat fish and prepared fish diets. It should also be noted that any amphibian being fed on insects should also receive calcium and vitamin D3 supplementation, preferably by prefeeding mineral/vitamin powders to the insect to prevent metabolic bone disease.

Salamanders eat earthworms, bloodworms, slugs, insects and prepared fish diets. Larval stages are herbivorous and feed on algae initially, or food sprinkled on the water. As they mature, aquatic prey (small crustaceans such as the water flea, *Daphnia* spp.) and then larger insects or animals are eaten.

Ornamental fish

One of the difficulties in feeding ornamental fish is that, with a few exceptions such as the goldfish, they are rarely kept in a single-species environment. Anatomical differences and variations in feeding strategies complicate the formulation of a single diet that will meet all the requirements of a mixed community, which may include representatives of herbivorous, omnivorous and carnivorous fish species.

An adequate delivery of nutrients is essential for the optimum health of the fish, but in a closed aquatic environment overfeeding and poor diet formulation can have a detrimental effect on conditions in the aquarium. Waste, in the form of uneaten food, undigested food and the excreted metabolic breakdown products of protein, will directly pollute the living environment and can pose a serious threat to the health of aquarium fish. To minimize the risk of pollution-induced stress, the diet must be palatable, easily digested, nutritionally balanced and of high biological value. A number of commercial diets are available for ornamental fish. Nutritionally complete diets are marketed as pellets, flakes and granules; other (complementary) foods include certain pond foods and frozen insect larvae, bloodworms and cockles.

Live aquatic food, such as *Daphnia* or *Tubifex* spp., is sometimes offered but may represent a disease risk and pre-frozen packs are considered safer. Fish kept in an established pond may feed on the pond's natural flora and fauna, and so complete diets are seldom required. Species that are kept in relatively bare display ponds, such as koi carp, will require a complete diet.

Of the complete diets available, flake formats offer versatility in that they can be floated on the water for surface feeders or submerged to sink slowly for middle and bottom feeders. Since the flakes are easily broken up into smaller pieces, they provide an excellent single food for a range of species and sizes of fish. Granules offer lower leaching of nutrients, because their surface area to volume ratio is larger, and different granule sizes and densities may be used to target different groups of fish in the aquarium.

As a general guideline, fish kept in a community tank should be fed to satiation two or three times per day. This allows close inspection of the fish and the tank on a regular basis. Feeding to satiation involves the continuous addition of small amounts of food to the aquarium until the fish stop feeding eagerly, and is normally achieved in a few minutes or less, depending on the tank size and stocking density.

It should be emphasized that pollution from nitrogenous waste is a considerable threat to the health of fish held in a closed volume of water. Correct diet formulation and feeding regimen can improve protein utilization and help to minimize pollution, but water quality should be maintained through regular water changes or, in the larger aquaria, through the use of filter systems, which must be properly maintained.

References and further reading

BSAVA/VPIS (2012) *Guide to Common Canine and Feline Poisons.* BSAVA Publications, Gloucester

Brunetto MA, Gomes MOS, Andre MR *et al.* (2010) Effects of nutritional support on hospital outcome in dogs and cats. *Journal of Veterinary Emergency and Critical Care* **20**, 224–231

Chan DL (2015) *Nutritional Management of Hospitalised Small Animals.* Wiley Blackwell, Chichester

Fascetti AJ and Delaney SJ (2012) *Applied Veterinary Clinical Nutrition.* Wiley Blackwell, Chichester

Fauth E, Freeman LM, Cornjeo L *et al.* (2015) Salmonella bacteriuria in a cat fed a Salmonella-contaminated diet. *Journal of the American Veterinary Medical Association* **247**, 525–530

Foster AP, Knowles TG, Moore AH *et al.* (2003) Serum IgE and IgG responses to food antigens in normal and atopic dogs, and dogs with gastrointestinal disease. *Veterinary Immunology and Immunopathology* **92**, 113–124

Freeman LM, Chandler ML, Hamper BA *et al.* (2013) Current knowledge about the risks and benefits of raw-meat based diets for dogs and cats. *Journal of the American Veterinary Medical Association* **243**, 1549–1558

Girling S (2013) *Veterinary Nursing of Exotic Pets, 2nd edn.* Wiley Blackwell, Oxford

Harcourt-Brown F and Chitty J (2005) *BSAVA Manual of Psittacine Birds, 2nd edn.* BSAVA Publications, Gloucester

Kanakubo K, Fascetti AJ and Larsen JA (2015) Assessment of protein and amino acid concentrations and labelling adequacy of commercial vegetarian diets formulated for dogs and cats. *Journal of the American Veterinary Medical Association* **247**, 385–392

Kealy RD, Lawler DF, Ballam JM et al. (2002) Effects of diet restriction on life span and age-related changes in dogs. *Journal of the American Veterinary Medical Association* **220**, 1315–1320

Lefebvre SL, Reid-Smith R and Boerlin P (2008) Evaluation of risks of shedding Salmonellae and other potential pathogens by therapy dogs fed raw diets in Ontario and Alberta. *Zoonoses and Public Heath* **55**, 470–480

Meredith A and Flecknell P (2006) BSAVA *Manual of Rabbit Medicine and Surgery, 2nd edn.* BSAVA Publications, Gloucester

O'Halloran C, Ioannidi O, Reed N *et al.* (2019) Tuberculosis due to *Mycobacterium bovis* in pet cats associated with feeding a commercial raw food diet. *Journal of Feline Medicine and Surgery* **21(8)**, 667–681

Quimby JM and Lunn KF (2013) Mirtazapine as an appetite stimulant and anti-emetic in cats with chronic kidney disease: a masked placebo-controlled crossover clinical trial. *Veterinary Journal* **197**, 651–655

Vandeweerd JM, Coisnon C, Clegg P et al. (2012) Systematic review of efficacy of nutraceuticals to alleviate clinical signs of osteoarthritis. *Journal of Veterinary Internal Medicine* **26**, 448–456

Verlinden A, Hesta M, Millet S *et al.* (2006) Food allergy in dogs and cats: a review. *Critical Reviews in Food Science and Nutrition* **46**, 259–273

Useful websites

WSAVA Global Nutrition Toolkit:
www.wsava.org/nutrition-toolkit

European Pet Food Industry Federation – Nutritional Guidelines for Complete and Complementary Pet Food for Cats and Dogs:
www.fediaf.org/images/FEDIAF_Nutritional_Guidelines_Update_December_2018.pdf

Self-assessment questions

1. Explain the meaning of the resting energy requirement of an animal.
2. How do the protein and energy requirements during growth compare with that of adulthood?
3. When would a hydrolysed protein diet be used in cats and dogs?
4. Name two key nutrients that should be restricted in chronic kidney disease.
5. Briefly describe the process of fat digestion and absorption.
6. What are the contraindications for oesophagostomy feeding tube placement?
7. What are the indications for parental nutrition and what are the possible complications?
8. Which species requires vitamin C in its diet and what is the minimum daily requirement in mg/kg?
9. Which species are prone to hypercholesterolaemia and other cardiovascular problems when fed high levels of seeds such as sunflower?

Chapter 14

Managing the hospital ward and basic patient care

Victoria Bowes

Introduction

The Animal Welfare Act 2006, Animal Health and Welfare (Scotland) Act 2006 and Welfare of Animals Act (Northern Ireland) 2011 state that anyone responsible for a captive animal, including owners and temporary and permanent keepers, must ensure that the welfare 'needs' of that animal are met. These needs follow on from the 'Five Freedoms' (see Chapter 1) and are expressed in the Acts as follows:

- The need for a suitable diet – by ready access to food and fresh water in order to maintain full health and vigour

- The need for a suitable environment – by providing an appropriate environment, including shelter and a comfortable resting area
- The need to be protected from pain, suffering, injury and disease – by prevention and/or rapid diagnosis and treatment
- The need to be able to exhibit normal behaviour patterns – by providing sufficient space, proper facilities and appropriate enrichment
- The need to be housed with, or apart from, other animals – by providing, where necessary and appropriate, company of the animal's own kind.

Each individual patient that is admitted to the hospital ward must have its basic needs fulfilled at all times.

Inpatient accommodation

Dogs and cats

Ward accommodation is specifically designed for short-stay patients that require nursing and veterinary care. The kennels are restricted in size to ensure strict rest and allow staff clear observation of the patient. Under the Royal College of Veterinary Surgeons (RCVS) Practice Standards Scheme (PSS), the requirements for kennels depend on the stated tier of the veterinary practice (RCVS, 2018).

- Core tier – The practice must have at least one kennel suitable for a large breed of dog or have a plan in place for this facility if the need arises.
- General practice tier – There must be a range of accommodation of suitable size for the number and species routinely treated.
- Veterinary hospital tier – There must be a minimum of six kennels or cages for the hospitalization of patients.

The RCVS PSS also states that the inpatient facilities must be secure and of a suitable size, and that they must be durable and escape proof. Ideally, they should be made of non-permeable materials so they can be easily cleaned and disinfected (Figure 14.1).

There must be adequate heating, lighting and ventilation of the hospitalization area (see below). A range of bedding materials must be provided (see below) and there should also be the provision of appropriate food and fresh water.

There should be a full range of accommodation to meet the needs of the various breeds and size of dogs and cats that are routinely admitted (Figures 14.2 and 14.3). Consideration should be given to the predator–prey scenario when choosing appropriate accommodation for the range of species commonly seen in the veterinary practice, therefore, separate dog and cat wards are preferred. In addition, there must be the provision of a walk-in kennel to provide accommodation for large-breed dogs (Figure 14.4).

Separate accommodation for boarding animals and animals for grooming is recommended and obligatory under the RCVS PSS. There should also be a written isolation protocol to include the appropriate accommodation suitable for contagious patients (see Chapter 7).

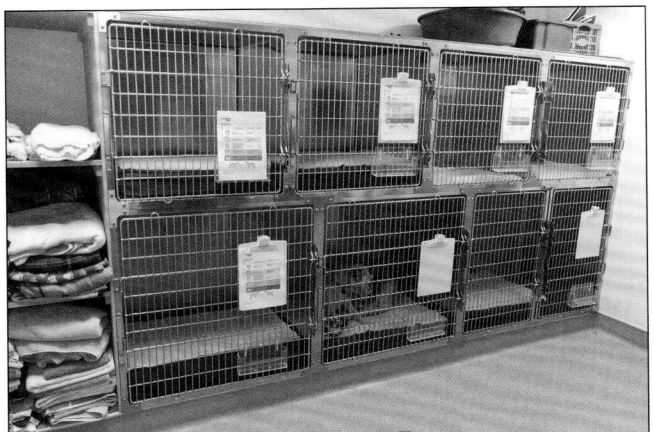

14.1 Ward for small dogs with stainless steel kennels. These are durable, escape proof and easily cleaned and disinfected.

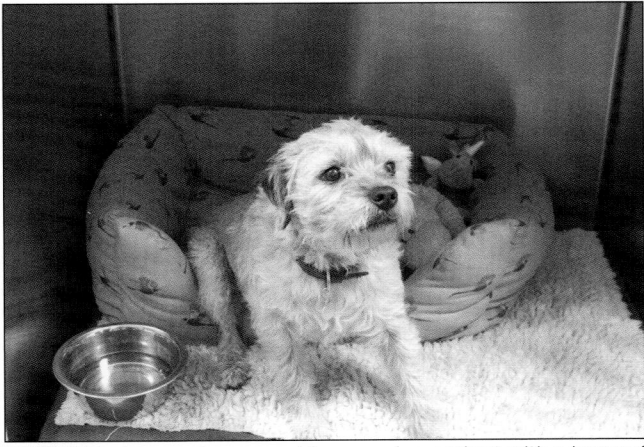

14.2 A kennel prepared for a canine patient with a layer of newspaper, incontinence pad and Vetbed®. The dog has also been provided with synthetic padded bedding for comfort.

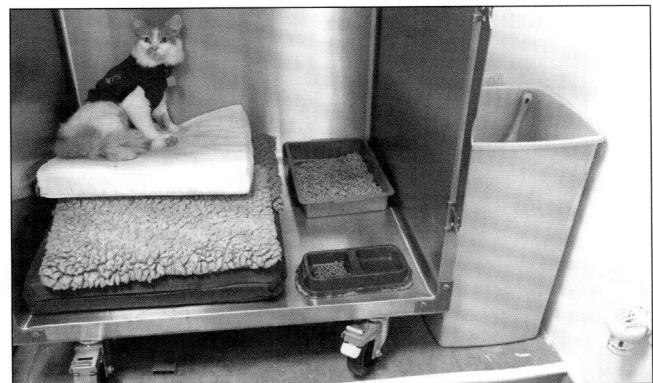

14.3 A kennel provided for a feline inpatient. The kennel has been prepared with a layer of newspaper, an incontinence pad and Vetbed®. The cat has also been provided with synthetic padded bedding for comfort.

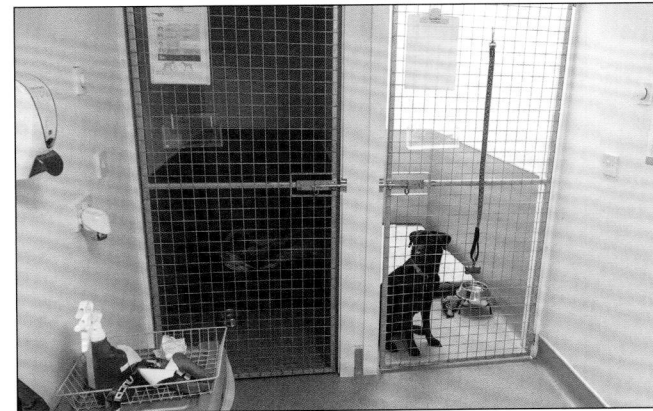

14.4 A walk-in kennel for large-breed dogs. These kennels are durable, escape-proof and easily cleaned and disinfected. The patient is also clearly visible from outside the kennel area.

Bedding

Appropriate bedding should be provided for all dogs and cats (see Figures 14.2, 14.3 and 14.5). It should be noted that under the RCVS PSS, newspaper on its own is not considered a suitable bedding material for overnight patients.

Type of bedding	Disposable or reusable	Advantages	Disadvantages
Fleece bedding (e.g. Vetbed®)	Reusable	Absorbable, warm, soft, durable, washable	Expensive, chewable
Blanket, towels	Reusable	Warm, washable	Expensive to buy
Covered foam wedges	Reusable	Washable cover, support and warmth for recumbent patients	Chewable
Newspaper	Disposable	Cheap and readily available, provides minimal warmth	Hard to lie on, ink leaks
Incontinence pads	Disposable	Provides some warmth, absorbable	Hard, expensive
Bean bags	Reusable	Insulating, warm, comfortable	Cover only washable

14.5 Suitable bedding materials for dogs and cats that can be used in the veterinary practice.

Environmental requirements

All animal accommodation must be well constructed to ensure the safety and security of the patient, but also provide suitable temperature, humidity and ventilation. All animals should be kept clean, dry and comfortable at all times.

Temperature

The ambient temperature for hospital ward accommodation for most animals should be kept at 18–22°C; the preferred ambient temperature for each species needs to be maintained. Animals must be protected from extreme changes in temperature and ideally all animal accommodation should have temperature control facilities to both

warm and cool the environment (Figure 14.6). Animals that are very sensitive to temperature changes, such as geriatric and young animals, may require additional supportive heating or cooling. A supported environmental temperature is especially important for animals recovering from general anaesthesia or sedation, as their ability to thermoregulate can be compromised. Additional heat sources, such as warm air blankets or insulation in the form of extra blankets or bubble wrap, can be provided to prevent or treat hypothermia (see also Chapters 19 and 22).

Animals suffering from hyperthermia usually require active cooling methods. One of the most effective methods for cooling the environmental temperature is air-conditioning; alternatives such as fans can be used for direct cooling of the

Type	Advantages	Disadvantages
Central heating	■ Easily controlled ■ Use of thermostats ensure minimum temperature kept constant ■ Economical	■ Expensive to install ■ Requires regular maintenance ■ Additional heat in individual kennels may be necessary ■ Requires suitable wall space for fitting ■ Difficult to clean and disinfect
Electric fan-assisted heating/fan heaters	■ Convenient ■ Rapid heating effect	■ Heater should not be placed too close to the animal as overheating may occur ■ Noisy ■ Expensive to run ■ Spread of airborne diseases risk increased ■ Moves dust around
Air conditioning/ heating	■ Temperature easily controlled ■ Humidity can also be controlled ■ Animals have no potential contact with heating source ■ Wall space not a problem	■ Expensive to install ■ Expensive to run
Underfloor heating	■ Floors dry quickly ■ Very comfortable for animals to lie on	■ If insulation is poor floors can become very hot ■ Faecal material difficult to remove ■ Expensive to install and repair
Portable radiators	■ Mobile ■ Cheap to purchase	■ Take a long time to heat an area ■ Supervision required ■ May be knocked over in a busy area ■ Surface temperature may injure staff or animals if they come into contact ■ Cables must be protected from animals ■ Switches and sockets should be waterproof ■ Sockets in kennels must be covered when not in use
Portable electric fan heaters	■ Good for boosting the temperature rapidly ■ Useful as emergency back-up if heating system fails ■ Can be controlled individually ■ Heat can be directed towards animals	■ Heater should not be placed too close to an animal's kennel (overheating) ■ Noisy ■ Expensive to run ■ Spread of airborne diseases risk increased ■ Move dust around ■ Fire risk

14.6 Examples of types of heating that may be used in the veterinary practice.

patient. Brachycephalic breeds, in particular, may struggle with extreme temperatures; these animals must be monitored carefully and appropriate cooling provided.

Neonatal puppies and kittens (commonly until 10–14 days old) are unable to maintain their own body temperature and should be kept in an incubator set at 25°C and carefully monitored (see also Chapter 24).

Lighting

Lighting should mimic the natural conditions of the species as realistically as possible. Daylight is preferred, if possible, for birds and mammals, but a shaded area should also be provided. Artificial lighting is needed to ensure thorough cleaning and provision of nursing care. Daylight-simulating bulbs are available; these provide a more natural lighting effect with the emittance of a yellow glow. It is also recommended to have a night glow bulb in the hospital ward to allow observation of animals without the need for a full bright light, which can disturb sleep, which in turn can have an effect on the animal's recovery.

Ventilation

Ventilation should be adequate not only to prevent damp, stale odours and draughts, but also to reduce the risk of nosocomial infections (hospital-acquired infections, e.g. kennel cough). Fans can be situated around the animal accommodation ward, but should not be placed directly in front of the patient in order to prevent drying of the eyes, or in front of a window as this will hinder the circulation of air. Minimum recommendations for air changes are 4–8 changes per hour; however, this can increase with temperature, number of inpatients and disease states (e.g. isolation facilities, see below). Adequate ventilation systems will be effective in reducing the effects and infection risks of respiratory disease.

Exotic pets

Many exotic pets commonly admitted to the veterinary hospital accommodation are naturally prey species and, ideally, should be housed in quiet areas away from dogs and cats to reduce the exposure to noise and olfactory stressors. Some veterinary practices have dedicated exotic wards, which allow the heating, lighting and ventilation to be manipulated to suit the species.

Ferrets

Ferrets can be housed in the same type of hospital accommodation used for cats or small dogs. A small locker type kennel can be provided. Ferrets are best housed away from the exotic ward as they are a natural predator of rabbits and other small mammals, and their presence in the ward could cause stress. Ideally they should be placed away from dogs and cats as well, but this is not always possible. Towels and blankets, which the ferret can use to sleep in or under, should be provided. The environmental temperature should be between 21 and 23°C for most patients.

Rabbits

Rabbits can be hospitalized for a short period of time in a small locker type kennel with newspaper on the floor, straw for bedding and hay for nutrition (Figure 14.7). Acrylic veterinary bedding can be provided; however, this can be chewed. A box should be provided for the rabbit to hide in; this allows natural prey species to hide and can reduce stress levels.

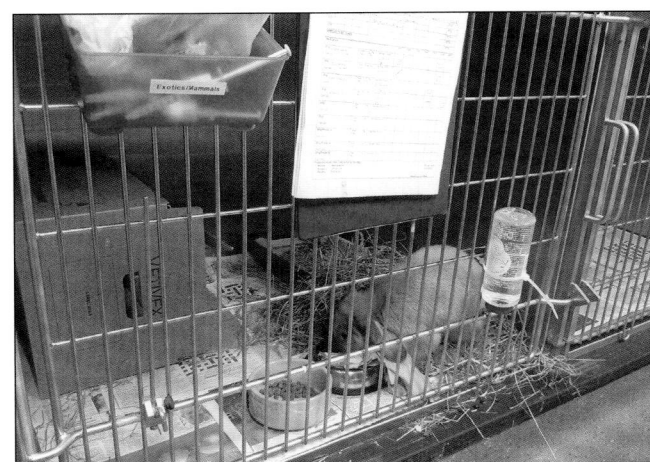

14.7 A typical rabbit hospital cage containing an appropriate sized hide box, a bundle of hay 1–2 times the size of the rabbit, a litter tray, and food and water provision. (Reproduced from the *BSAVA Manual of Rabbit Medicine*)

It should be noted that the box should be stable and safe within the environment (e.g. no sharp edges or staples). Rabbits should not be kept too warm as they are unable to sweat, 21–23°C is the maximum temperature recommended.

Guinea pigs

Guinea pigs are very sensitive to changes in housing and the resulting stress can cause problems and delay recovery. Guinea pigs require a slightly warmer environment than rabbits. They should be provided with a box to hide in when feeling threatened; this box should have hay inside it (Figure 14.8). It is best to provide additional hay in a receptacle located higher up the side of the cage to encourage stretching, if appropriate.

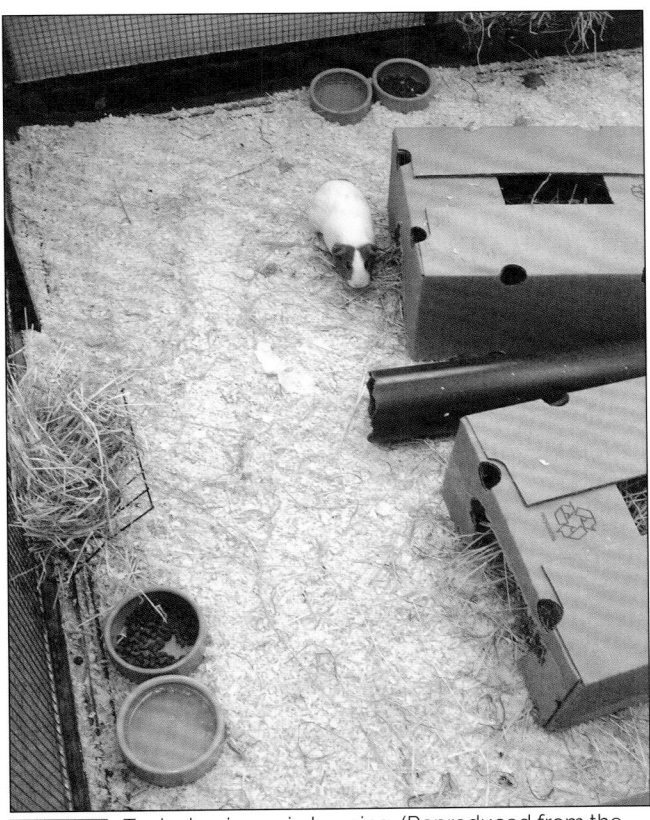

14.8 Typical guinea pig housing. (Reproduced from the *BSAVA Manual of Rodents and Ferrets*)

Chinchillas

Chinchillas should be housed in accommodation that provides different heights to encourage exercise. If appropriate, they should also be provided with non-toxic branches (e.g. fruit tree branches) and wooden toys for chewing. A dust/sand bath should be provided for hygiene and enrichment. As chinchillas are unable to sweat, they should not be kept in temperatures higher than 21–23°C.

Rats, mice, hamsters and gerbils

These animals are best housed in their own cages, which provide them with familiar smells and their own bedding. The cages should be purpose built to avoid patient escape. Only gerbils should be housed in plastic or glass tanks, as the poor ventilation can cause respiratory problems in other species. Hamsters can climb wire cages and may fall, so deep plastic cages are the best option for these species. Depending on the reason for admittance to the practice, it may be appropriate to provide shredded paper rather than shavings to reduce wound contamination and prevent exacerbation of respiratory disorders. Cardboard boxes may be provided as hiding places to reduce stress. The temperature should be approximately 21–23°C. Small species, such as hamsters, are particularly susceptible to hypothermia due to their high surface area to bodyweight ratio, and measures must be in place to prevent heat loss. These smaller mammalian species are also very susceptible to damp and drafts.

Chipmunks

Chipmunks are best housed in their own cages, which will provide them with familiar smells and their own bedding. The cages should be purpose built to avoid escape. Chipmunks need to be housed in a very quiet environment, as they can be disturbed by extraneous sounds (e.g. the radio). Hiding places should be provided to reduce stress.

Birds

Birds may be housed within veterinary incubators; these can be moved to the most appropriate area in the practice to reduce stress. For larger birds, or those that do not need confinement, the cage should be large enough for the bird to spread its wings. Stainless steel cages are suitable for most species; however, smaller species such as finches will need to be housed in purpose built cages. Most species should be provided with a perch, which should be sited away from food and water. Stainless steel bowls can be used to provide food. If the bird is suspected to be suffering from psittacosis it will require isolation. Larger birds (e.g. poultry) may be best accommodated in a dog or cat kennel.

Reptiles

All reptile species should be housed in vivaria, which should have a heat lamp and an ultraviolet (UV) lamp or a combined lamp (Figure 14.9). Tortoises may be housed in open top enclosures, as long as UV and heat lamps are provided. Furniture placed in the accommodation should reflect the habitat of the species. It is also important to know the humidity and temperature requirements for each individual species. Day length should be reflected by having the lights on a timer. If the reptile is suspected of harbouring an infectious disease, it will require isolation.

Semi-aquatic reptiles and amphibians

Semi-aquatic reptile species and amphibians should be provided with a water source, such as a litter or plastic tray (Figure 14.10). The water should be treated appropriately or be left to stand to allow the chlorine to be removed. Furniture should be provided to support the species getting in and out of the water tank. Amphibian species need a damp environment; this can be provided using peat or moss which is sprayed regularly to ensure it is kept moist (Figure 14.11). These species should not be fed in their housed environment they should be fed in a feeding tank.

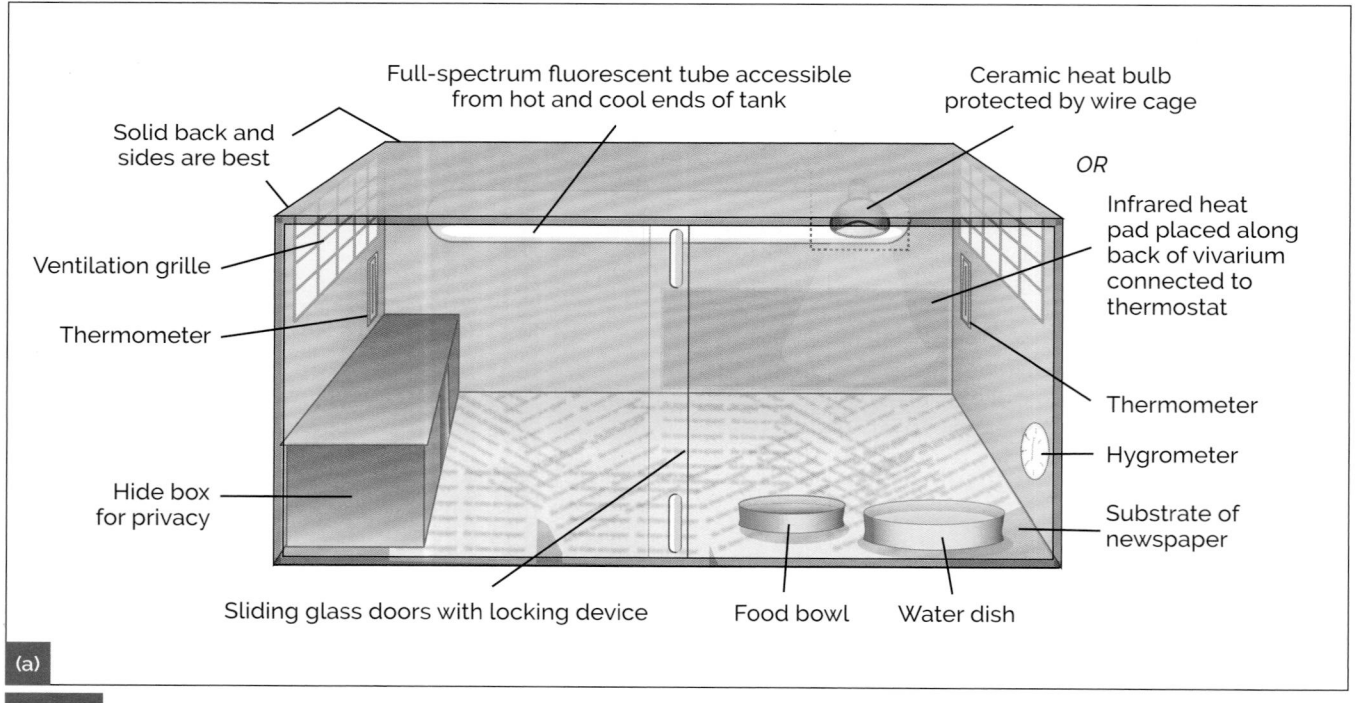

Full-spectrum fluorescent tube accessible from hot and cool ends of tank

Ceramic heat bulb protected by wire cage

Solid back and sides are best

OR

Infrared heat pad placed along back of vivarium connected to thermostat

Ventilation grille

Thermometer

Thermometer

Hygrometer

Hide box for privacy

Substrate of newspaper

Sliding glass doors with locking device

Food bowl   Water dish

(a)

14.9 Reptile environments: **(a)** clinical.

continues ▶

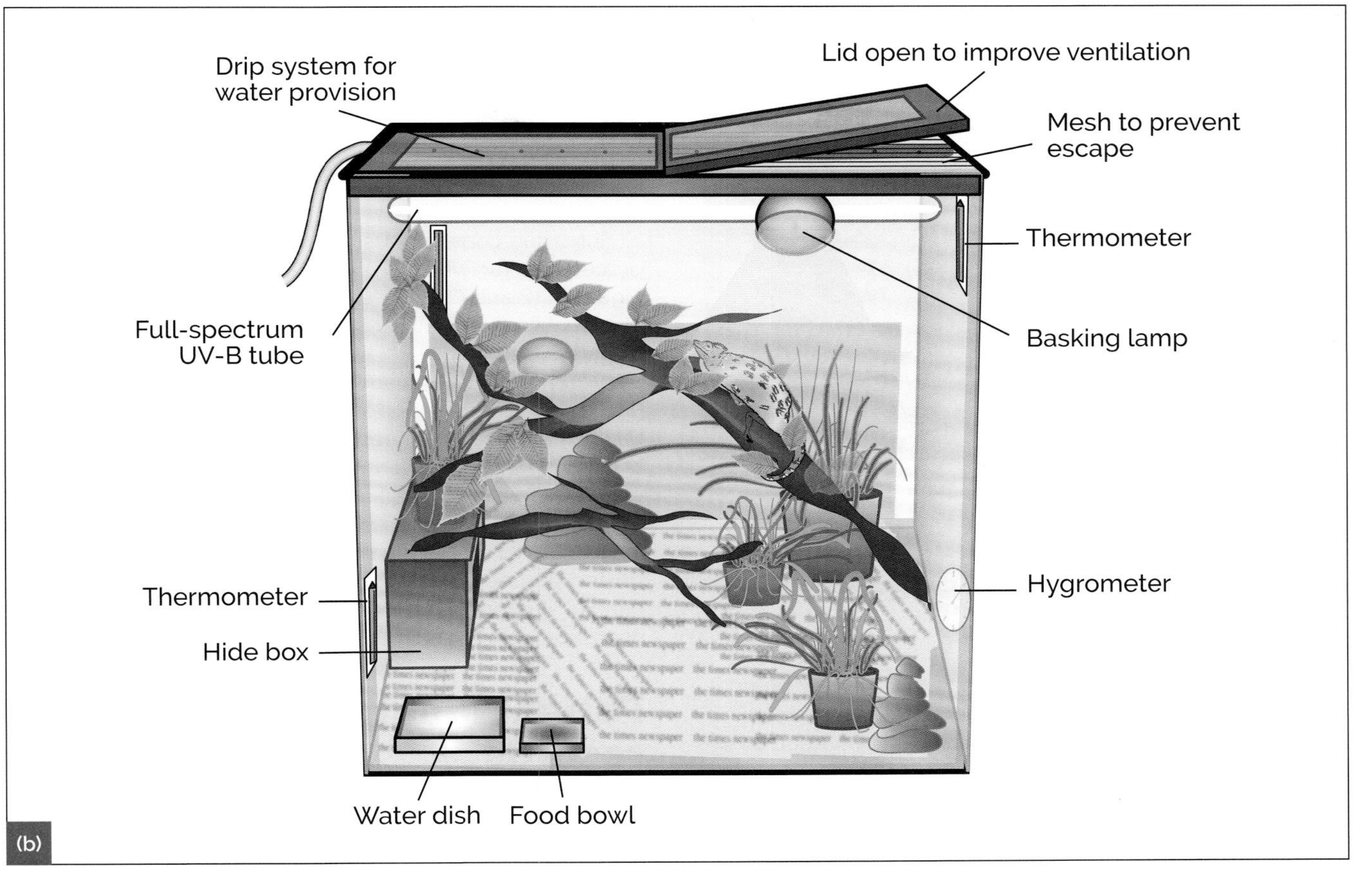

14.9 *continued* Reptile environments: **(b)** arboreal.

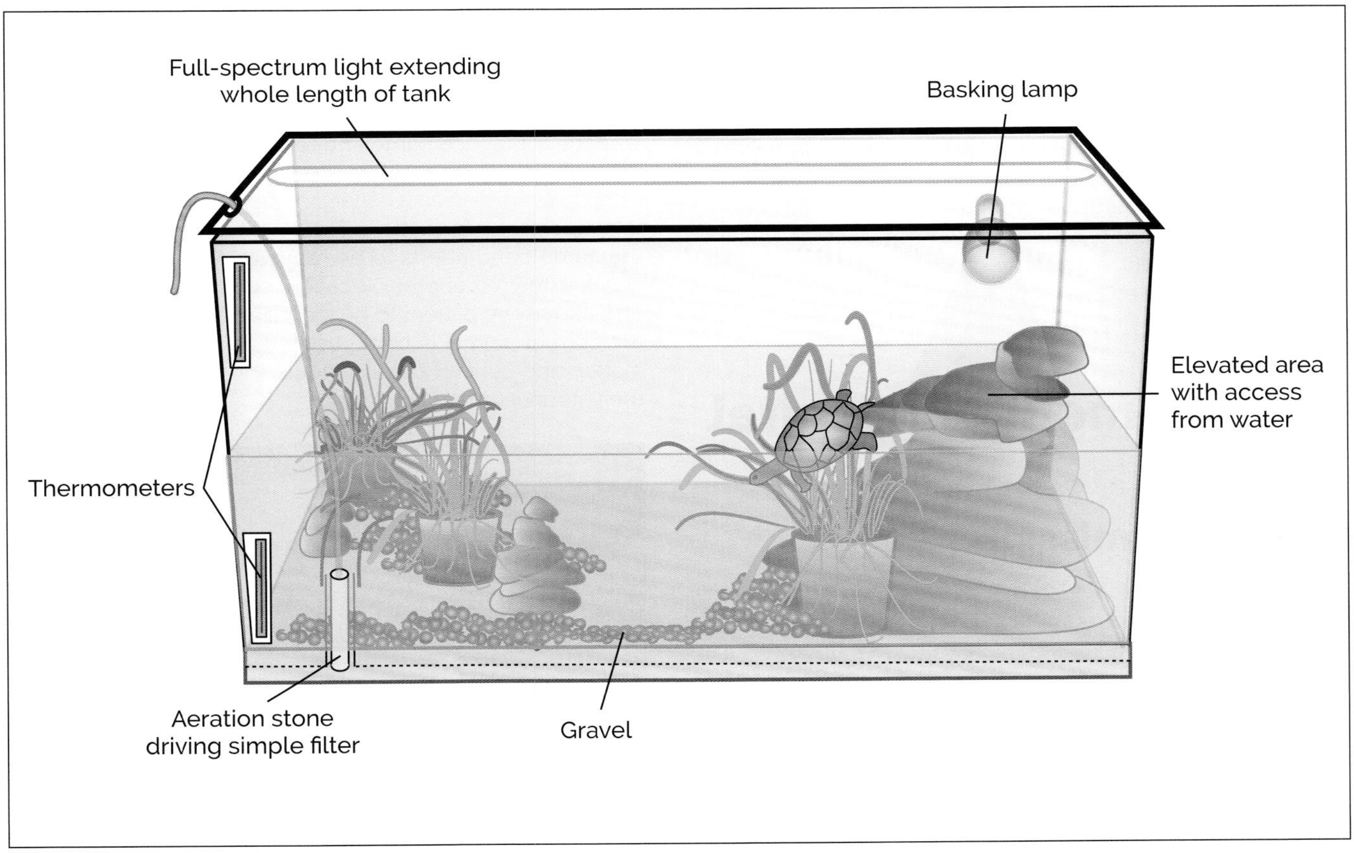

Labels: Drip system for water provision; Lid open to improve ventilation; Mesh to prevent escape; Thermometer; Basking lamp; Full-spectrum UV-B tube; Hygrometer; Thermometer; Hide box; Water dish; Food bowl; (b)

14.10 Semi-aquatic reptile environment.

Labels: Full-spectrum light extending whole length of tank; Basking lamp; Elevated area with access from water; Thermometers; Aeration stone driving simple filter; Gravel

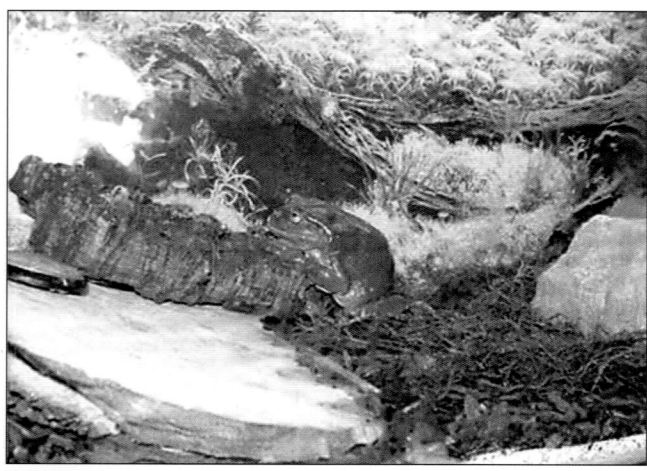

14.11 Frogs require an aqua-terrarium.

Patients requiring special medical care

Some patients admitted to the hospital ward may be critically ill or have conditions that require them to be hospitalized in a separate area. Isolation protocols will need to be followed if the patient has an infectious disease and barrier nursing protocols should be put in place to prevent the spread of disease (see 'Veterinary isolation and barrier nursing', later).

Patients admitted with seizures, either status epilepticus or intermittent, should be hospitalized in an area that is quiet and preferably dimly lit. Frequent or continuous monitoring of the patient will be required and the area should not be too remote from other personnel and assistance.

Patients requiring, or potentially requiring, oxygen support need to have accommodation that is located near to an oxygen source, this could be piped or cylinder method (see Chapter 19).

Seriously ill patients and those with potentially life-threatening conditions (e.g. pneumothorax or gastric dilatation–volvulus (GDV)) should be admitted into an area where immediate treatment can be given. These patients require one-to-one constant nursing as changes in status can be rapid and intense (see Chapter 19).

Management of hospital wards

Patient admission

It is always best practice to complete a thorough patient assessment prior to admittance and to provide each patient with a nursing care plan (see Chapter 12) to ensure delivery of personalized care. Careful questioning of the owner during patient assessment will provide useful information about the individual animal; owners notice the slight changes in their pet's normal behaviour and will be able to provide key details on their daily routine. This information can be collected as part of an admission and consent form (Figure 14.12) or via specific Client questionnaires (see examples at the end of the chapter).

Other forms of documentation may need to be reviewed when a patient is admitted to the hospital ward (e.g. vaccination certificates and pet passports). Vaccination status is required in some instances, as it provides key information that may assist in differential diagnosis. This will also aid in determining the location in which the patient is housed in cases where an infectious disease is suspected or there is a need for reverse isolation.

Informed consent must be sought from the owner for all procedures for which the animal has been admitted (see Figure 14.12 and Chapter 9). The patient should have a positive identification method at all times whilst on the veterinary premises (see below).

When admitting all species, and exotic species in particular, there needs to be careful consideration of the fine balance between the need for hospitalization and the stress of moving the animal into an inpatient accommodation environment. It is often preferable to discharge surgical exotic pet patients the same day, rather than keeping them in hospital accommodation for extended periods. There may be the requirement for owners to have information about hand or syringe feeding (see Chapter 13) and this can also be of assistance if the animal requires medication at home.

Patient identification and records

For the safety and security of animals on practice premises, all animals should be clearly identified. It is also vital that hospitalized patients are easy to distinguish from other animals; this is to avoid any confusion.

Name bands and tags

Paper and plastic name bands can be used effectively in both dogs and cats. If using this method, the name band should be placed on the patient (normally around the neck) as soon as it is admitted to the inpatient ward. This should contain information such as the patient's full name and the veterinary practice name and telephone number, written in indelible ink (Figure 14.13). The patient's own identification methods (e.g. disc on a collar) can be difficult to read or contain incorrect information. If, during surgery or treatments, the name band needs to be removed, it must be replaced immediately on another location, such as above the hock. This allows the patient to be identified at all times to ensure the correct animal is being treated and provides key information and contact details should the patient escape from the veterinary practice.

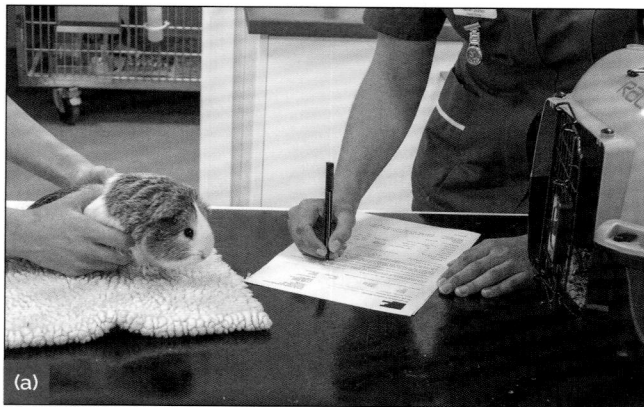

14.12 (a) A guinea pig being admitted to the veterinary practice. *continues* ▶

Admission form

Owner name: Client A

Owner address: 256 Borrow Drive, Coventry CV5 9XD

Home/landline telephone number: 01234567890

Mobile telephone number: 07123456789

Animal number:	51683011	Date:	2nd August 2019
Name:	Reggie	Colour:	Cream
Species:	Guinea Pig	Sex:	Male
Breed:	Guinea Pig	Date of birth:	30/07/2018 Age: 1

Details of operation and related procedures where appropriate: General anaesthetic to examine the mouth and perform any necessary dental procedures

The cost of the procedures described above will be: £ _____ OR within the range: £ 110 to £ 150

I hereby give permission for the administration of an anaesthetic or sedative to the above animal and to the surgical or other procedures detailed on this form together with any other procedures which may prove necessary.

The nature of these procedures and of other procedures as might prove necessary has been explained to me.

I understand that there are some risks involved in all anaesthetic techniques and surgical procedures.

I accept that the likely cost will be as detailed in the estimate above and that in the event of further treatment being required or of complications occurring which give rise to additional costs, I shall be contacted as soon as practicable so that my consent to such additional treatment and costs maybe obtained.

In the event that the veterinary surgeon is unable to contact me on the numbers provided, I understand that the veterinary surgeon will act in the best interests of my animal.

Blood test required   Yes/(No)

Signature of owner/guardian Client A

All fees are due at time of collection

Admission

Weight 0.59 kg

Vaccinated —

Blanket: —

Check sex M

Microchip: Yes/(no)/microchip today

Admit TPR: T – 38.0 C   P – 100 bpm   R – 25 bpm

Medication: none at

Cage/basket/box: grey RAC box

Last heat:

Admitted by: Harriet

Last eaten: This am

Collar/lead/choke: none

Other prep: —

Date: 2/8/19

Notes: (including own diet, toilet behaviour, exercise behaviour) Eats from bowl, drinks from bottle, exercises outside, urinates on paper.

Booked by: V. Bowes

(b)

14.12 *continued* **(b)** Completed admissions form.

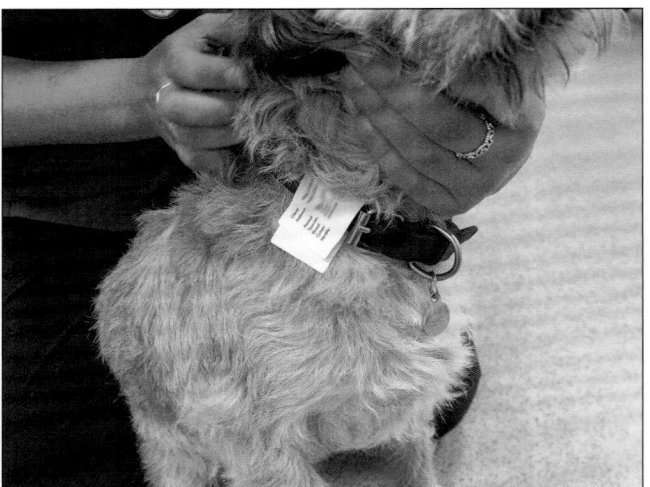

14.13 Identification tag used in a veterinary hospital. This is completed with the patient's name, identification number, species and owner details.

Microchips

Microchips have a unique identification number that cannot be lost or altered once implanted under the skin of an animal. In dogs and cats, the microchip is typically placed in the subcutaneous skin layer between the scapulae in the area of the dorsal midline (Figure 14.14). Microchipping is required by law for dogs in the UK, as of April 2016. It is also required for the PETS travel scheme prior to rabies vaccination (see Chapter 10). Microchipping may also be required for some canine health schemes; since 2010, the British Veterinary Association (BVA) canine health schemes for hips, elbows and eyes require that the animal is permanently identified (see Chapter 4). Microchip placement in most mammals is midline between the scapulae.

In exotic species, microchipping is commonplace and forms part of the legal restrictions for the importation of these animals. Microchips are required for exotic species falling under CITES (the Convention on International Trade in Endangered Species of Wild Fauna and Flora) legislation. Microchip placement in birds is normally in the pectoral muscle (commonly the left) and in chelonia the left hindleg is usually used. The acceptable sites vary between species and should be checked with the regulatory authorities or microchip suppliers prior to placement.

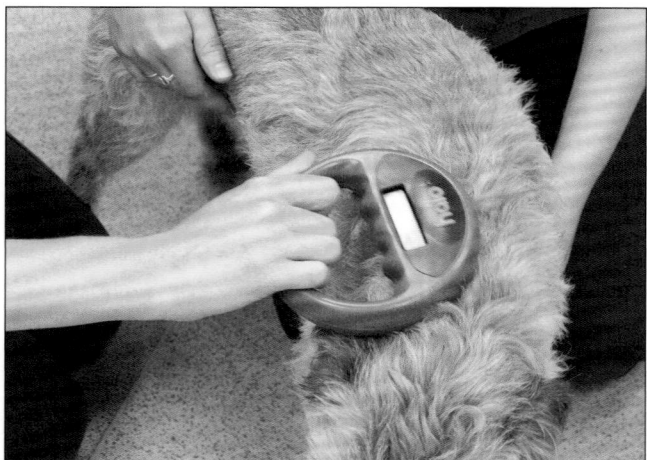

14.14 Scanning for the presence of a microchip in a dog. The microchip is commonly placed in between the scapulae. When scanning for the microchip, the scanner should be moved over this area and down both the front legs.

There are several brands of microchips available; it is important to know that only those of recognized international standard (ISO) are suitable and acceptable for pet importation and exportation schemes (such as the PETS travel scheme, see Chapter 10).

Many owners consider the main purpose of a microchip is to aid in the recovery of a pet if it is lost or stolen. The individual microchip number, together with patient and owner information, is held in a databank, which allows animals to be traced back to their owners. With the new microchip legislation, owners could face a fine for non-compliance with the new requirements.

Verification of microchips may be required prior to a procedure being performed to ensure full identification of the animal, if other forms of identification, such as a collar, are not clearly visible or available.

Tattoos

Tattoos are not a routine method of identification in domesticated species in the UK. However, they may be used with laboratory animals and racing Greyhounds. Animals imported from outside the UK may have tattoos on their right ear, containing information on where they were bred and their identification. Verification of tattoos may be required prior to a procedure being performed to ensure full identification of the animal.

Other physical methods of identification

Other forms of identification may be used in exotic pets. These include: leg rings in birds and rabbits, leg bands in birds, and wing tattoos in pigeons.

Individual breeds and markings

Different breeds of dogs, cats and small pets should be recognized by the veterinary nurse (see Appendix 1). The staff should have no confusion about the different breeds. Additional information on specific colour and any identifying marks should be recorded on consent forms and within the patient's notes. This may be important if two sibling cats that are almost identical are admitted for procedures on the same day; nurses must be able to distinguish between the cats to ensure accurate records are kept for each patient.

Record keeping

There are many different records that the veterinary practice may keep; it is essential that these records are efficiently kept to maintain good communication within the veterinary practice (see Chapter 9). It must always be remembered that what is not recorded is deemed not to have happened. Record keeping is a paramount role in the clinical care of a patient. Accurate and detailed records aid in patient care, protect the practice from legal challenges and are vital for efficient stock and financial control. Records can be paper-based (e.g. hospital forms) or electronic, and may include other types of media such as X-rays.

Records should be accurate and clear, as this can increase client confidence in the veterinary practice. Clarity, legibility and accuracy are vital; incorrect name spelling, inability to read writing or untidy writing may not present a good impression to the client. Records must also be kept and stored in a way that fulfils the General Data Protection Regulations (GDPR) (see Chapter 9).

Suitable records should be kept for all patients to record at least basic inpatient care information (Figure 14.15).

Types of records a veterinary practice may keep

- Client records with contact details
- Medical records, including hospitalization charts, ward notes, anaesthetic charts, laboratory results, images of slides, radiographs, digital images and recordings
- Personnel records, including salary records, recruitment information and staff reviews/appraisals
- Financial records, including bank statements and invoices
- Payment records and electronic payment information sheets
- Training records, such as student college reports, professional behaviour logs, nursing progress logs and tutorial records. These can either be electronic or printed out in hard copy
- Monitoring (e.g. CCTV)
- Clinical audits and meeting minutes
- Health and safety records, including accident records, risk assessments, Control of Substances Hazardous to Health (COSHH) datasheets and local rules

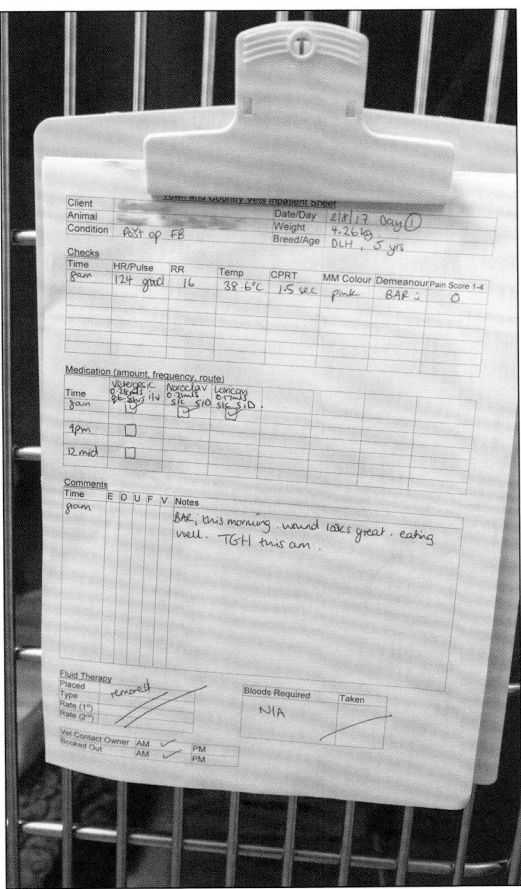

14.15 Inpatient record card, attached to a kennel door, containing information regarding the patient's temperature, pulse and respiration. There is ample space to record any key changes in the patient's behaviour or health and to make key medical notes. It provides the details of both the patient and the owner.

Some patients may require more detailed hospital sheets that include further clinical information (see Figure 14.49). Any additional checks or care should be documented on these sheets.

Basic equipment in the veterinary practice ward

Every veterinary practice ward requires a range of clinical and non-clinical equipment, which must be maintained and checked on a regular basis.

Common practice equipment held within the ward area includes:

- Personal protective equipment (PPE; see Chapter 2) – e.g. gloves, aprons, masks and safety googles
- Diagnostic equipment – e.g. stethoscopes, thermometers, auriscopes, ophthalmoscopes and patient-side monitoring equipment such as glucometers
- Animal restraint equipment – e.g. muzzles, leads including slip leads, cat catchers and dog catchers (see Chapter 11)
- Electrical equipment – e.g. clippers, heat pads, syringe drivers, electrocardiography (multi-parameter) machine and drip pumps
- Cleaning equipment, including brushes, mops and buckets. These should be specifically colour-coded (see Figure 14.16) or labelled so they are not used in other areas of the practice.

Common stock kept within the ward area includes:

- Consumables used in the course of any treatment, such as cotton wool, syringes and needles, as well as disposable gloves, aprons and masks
- Bandaging material
- Drugs dispensed in a course of treatment such as tablets and oral pastes
- Standard drugs used within the hospital ward
- Food and disposable bedding for hospitalized patients
- Non-disposable bedding, such as Vetbed® and blankets
- Food/water bowls and litter trays
- Cat litter (different types should be available)
- Bedding material such as wood shavings, hay and straw for exotic pet species.

Cleaning and disinfection

The routine cleaning of the hospital ward should be undertaken daily. Kennels should be cleaned even if they are not soiled as this promotes a clean sanitary environment. Soiled bedding should be disposed of as non-hazardous 'offensive waste', unless considered infectious when it should be disposed of as 'hazardous waste' (see Chapter 2) or washed at a temperature appropriate to kill the infectious agents (see Chapter 7). Items which could be potential fomites (e.g. food bowls, toys, leads and harnesses) should be washed and disinfected. Routine sterilization of equipment should be completed at least monthly. Communal areas should be kept tidy, waste should be segregated (see Chapter 2) and bins should be emptied regularly; if they contain any odorous waste, they should be emptied even when not full.

When cleaning different accommodation the principles of infection control will be very similar. Cleaning and disinfection are just two key infection control methods; others are listed below.

Methods for preventing the spread of infection

- Cleaning and disinfection
- Barrier nursing
- Isolation
- Quarantine
- Protective clothing
- Treatment
- Sterilization
- Vaccination
- Hygiene
- Ventilation
- Owner compliance

Key definitions

- **Disinfection** is the removal of microorganisms, but not necessarily all pathogens and their spores. There is a reduction in the number of microbes
- **Sterilization** is the removal of all microorganisms, including bacterial spores (e.g. by using an autoclave)
- A **disinfectant** is a chemical agent that kills or prevents the breeding of microorganisms on inanimate objects such as worktops
- An **antiseptic** is a disinfectant that is commonly used on living tissue (often termed a skin disinfectant because it is safe to use on the skin)
- **Antisepsis** is the prevention of sepsis or infection, which is achieved by disinfection. It is a common term used to describe the prevention of infection in living tissues by the use of an antiseptic
- **Asepsis** is the complete removal of all microorganisms and spores, resulting in a complete sterile state. This is usually achieved by sterilization
- **-cide** is the suffix defining that something is killed (e.g. a virucide kills viruses)
- **-stat** is the suffix defining the prevention of growth or multiplication of something (e.g. a bacteriostat prevents the growth or multiplication of bacteria)

Disinfection is the process by which pathogenic microorganisms are destroyed or removed from inanimate objects (e.g. cleaning the work surface after handling an animal). This is a very important method of controlling the spread of disease and can be achieved using both physical and chemical methods. The physical actions of scrubbing and cleaning are just as important as the correct use of a disinfectant and its chemical actions.

Organic matter, such as blood and faeces, encourages the growth of microorganisms and can dramatically affect the efficacy of the disinfectant. Disinfectants must have direct contact with microorganisms in order to work effectively and destroy them, so organic matter must be removed prior to disinfection. Once the organic matter has been removed, the disinfectant will be more effective.

The most efficient method of disinfection is to use a chemical disinfectant following mechanical cleaning. The efficacy of chemical disinfectants that require dilution can usually be increased by mixing them with warm, rather than cold, water. Heating is another method of disinfection and a way of achieving asepsis, as microorganisms are destroyed by high temperatures (e.g. by steam cleaning and machine washing of bedding). (See also Chapter 7.)

Cleaning a clinical environment

Each area of the practice should be assessed for the risk of potential cross-infection. Standard operating procedures should then be created for the cleaning and disinfection of each area according to its individual risk (see Chapter 2). All staff should be aware of the standard operating procedures and potential risks. The veterinary practice should have separate cleaning equipment for the key areas of the practice. Colour coding the cleaning equipment can be the best method to reduce the risk of cross-contamination (Figure 14.16).

Classification of infection risks by area

- Low-risk areas include offices and corridors
- High-risk areas include any area that may have become contaminated with body fluids (e.g. theatres, preparation rooms and kennels)

There are areas in the veterinary practice that may be considered low-risk but where the potential for cross-infection is high. A key example is the reception area or waiting room, as every animal that enters the practice will use these communal areas. Control measures should be put in place for these areas; any animal that is considered to have a contagious disease should be immediately isolated in a separate area of the practice whilst waiting to be seen. New puppies should not be placed on the floor of the veterinary practice or allowed to mix with other animals.

If puppy parties are hosted at the practice, conscientious cleaning protocols should be completed before and after each party to ensure prevention of disease. This should include a deep clean of the rooms in which the puppy parties are hosted. Time of the day and exposure to other patients should also be considered; it may be best to hold these parties when

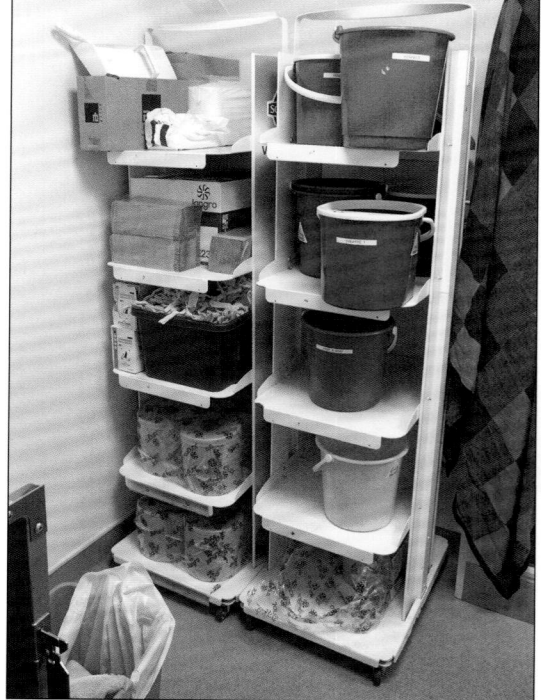

14.16 Key areas of the practice should have separate cleaning equipment. Colour coding the equipment, in this case using different coloured buckets, helps to prevent cross-contamination.

the practice is closed to routine appointments. A discussion should be had with all owners before attendance to ensure that their puppy is in good health and has typically received a first primary vaccination (see Chapter 7).

Low-risk areas require a disinfectant that is easy to use and a standard operating procedure that combines cleaning with disinfection. High-risk areas should be thoroughly cleaned and disinfected daily (Figure 14.17). This should be completed using a fast action broad-spectrum disinfectant.

- Surfaces and floors should first be cleaned using a detergent to ensure the removal of organic material and then cleaned using an appropriate fast action broad-spectrum disinfectant.
- Walls should be cleaned regularly to a height of 1.5 m with both detergents and disinfectants.
- Mop heads should be machine washed daily at 60°C, allowed to dry and replaced regularly.
- Any surfaces that may have come into contact with patients should be disinfected after use; any other potential sources of infection (e.g. equipment) should be cleaned and disinfected appropriately between patients.
- Clippers and clipper blades should be cleaned and disinfected appropriately between patients.
- Any soiled areas or surfaces should be spot cleaned throughout the day.

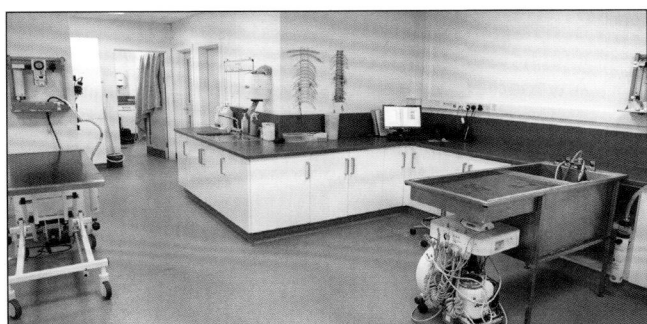

14.17 Areas of the veterinary practice at high risk for cross-infection, such as the 'prep' room should be cleaned and disinfected on a daily basis.

Cleaning kennel areas

- Remove the patient from the kennel into a clean kennel or enlist another member of staff to walk the patient whilst the kennel is cleaned
- Remove all soiled items from the kennel and place into the laundry as appropriate
- Any food bowls, litter trays and water bowls should be placed for cleaning in the separate food preparation area. These should be cleaned using the products detailed in the practice policy
- Orthopaedic mattresses should be removed from the kennel and any dirt or debris should be removed from the kennel with a paper towel or a brush
- The kennel should then be cleaned using the correct method, dilution of detergent/disinfectant and colour-coded equipment, as per the practice protocol. This includes the walls, ceiling, floor and door bars. The kennel should be allowed to air dry
- The mattress should be wiped using a cleaning cloth and allowed to air dry
- Once dry, the mattress, fresh bedding and the patient can be returned to the kennel

Veterinary isolation and barrier nursing

When nursing potentially infectious or infectious patients, cleaning and disinfection are of the upmost importance. In addition, strict isolation procedures should be followed for the nursing and care of these animals, including the cleaning and disinfection of the isolation facility, to ensure the safety of all animals and staff within the practice.

If at any point, there is concern that a patient may be infectious, then it should be assumed that it is infectious and treated as such. This is key to reduce the risk of exposure of the infectious animal to other areas within the practice and potentially contaminate areas, staff and increase the risk of infection to other animals.

It is extremely important that all staff are adequately trained to recognize the clinical signs of different transmissible diseases. It may be practice policy that any animal admitted with vomiting and diarrhoea should be isolated until the veterinary surgeon is able to see them, as these are key signs for many infectious diseases. Practices may carry out daily isolation risk assessments to determine individual requirements for barrier nursing.

Key definitions

- **Isolation** is the physical separation of an animal, reducing the risk of contamination from proven or suspected infectious disease
- **Quarantine** is the compulsory isolation with very strict protocols of animals with, or with suspected exposure to, infectious diseases. Quarantine kennels are used to isolate animals entering the UK that do not comply with the PETS travel scheme (see Chapter 7). Ordinary kennels and veterinary practices use the term quarantine to describe the isolation of animals with a suspected contagious disease or an animal with an unknown health status (see Chapter 7)
- **Barrier nursing** creates a 'physical' barrier between the infectious animal and the veterinary staff and other animals in the practice (e.g. wearing protective clothing (see Figure 14.18) or using separate equipment). This is usually completed as part of an isolation protocol. It can also be a technique where the patient is treated by specific and minimal staff to aid in bonding and continual support of the patient, as well as to minimize staff exposure
- **Protective isolation** or **reverse isolation** is the isolation of very susceptible animals (e.g. young, old or immune-suppressed) in an attempt to protect them from sources of infection

Isolation facilities

When an animal is admitted to the veterinary practice ward with a suspected infectious disease, it should be isolated immediately. The isolation facilities should be labelled effectively as 'in use' to prevent admittance of other animals and ensure access to staff is restricted. Visitors should never be allowed into the isolation unit and the isolated patient should have no contact with other animals. Colour-coding protocols should be in place to ensure that all staff are aware that a contagious case has been admitted, and they should also be aware of the standard operating procedure(s) to be used for that disease.

The facility is best self-contained; this limits the number of times staff have to enter/leave the isolation area. The area should be clearly labelled with appropriate isolation notices. Ventilation is extremely important within the isolation facility. The isolation unit should be under mild negative pressure (meaning that air will move into the unit when the door is opened, rather than air rushing out through the door and into other areas of the practice). This can be achieved by the use of extractor fans, with the fan in the isolation area set to extract and others in the practice to draw air in. If active ventilation is installed, the number of air changes per hour should be set to a minimum of 12.

Isolation facilities should have separate equipment, PPE, cleaning equipment and waste segregation (Figure 14.18). Equipment should be collected together, so that it is only used in the isolation area. It can be useful to have most, if not all, equipment colour-coded, so that it is easily identifiable as belonging to the isolation unit.

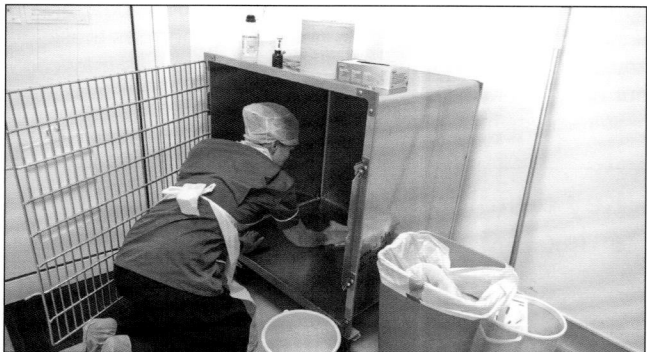

14.18 Isolation facilities should have their own colour-coded equipment. Staff should wear the protective clothing provided before entering the isolation facility.

Equipment that may be required in the isolation facility

- PPE – coveralls, aprons, hoods, clogs/wellington boots, shoe covers, hats, facemasks (for cleaning purposes and for nursing animals with airborne zoonoses such as psittacosis) and gloves
- Colour-coded food and water bowls, as well as feeding equipment such as cutlery and scales
- Litter trays and different types of cat litter
- Thermometer
- Cleaning equipment, including a mop and bucket, detergents and disinfectants
- Incontinence pads
- Newspaper
- Disposable bedding (i.e. bedding that should never be reused)
- Bags for hazardous waste
- Monitoring equipment (e.g. stethoscope)
- Drip pumps
- Clinical equipment (e.g. needles and syringes)

Isolation protocols

Barrier nursing is one of the best protocols to use in isolation facilities. One or two members of staff should be allocated to nurse patients in the unit. If possible, they should only provide care for an individual animal to minimize the risk of indirectly passing infections from one animal to another. If individual nursing is not possible, then it must be ensured

that the infectious animal is nursed and treated last. Under no circumstances should isolated animals and high-risk patients (i.e. the very young, very old and immuno-suppressed) be nursed together.

- A footbath containing an appropriate and suitable disinfectant for the disease should be placed at the entrance to the isolation facility. Shoes should be dipped on entering and leaving the isolation ward. Separate shoes for the isolation unit are the preferred alternative, as submersing shoes in water baths is not as effective as a complete change of shoe; the main reason being that the contact time of the disinfectant is not met.
- PPE should be put on when entering the ward and discarded immediately after use.
- Hands should be thoroughly washed using the World Health Organization (WHO) technique (see Chapter 7) with an appropriate antibacterial hand wash on entering and leaving the ward, and disposable hand towels should be used to dry hands.

After the infectious case has been discharged, a strict cleaning and disinfection regime should be followed.

Cleaning isolation units

- Once the patient has left isolation, remove all soiled bedding and other material and dispose of as infectious hazardous waste (see Chapter 2)
- Any food bowls, litter trays and water bowls should be washed at 60°C and then soaked in an appropriate disinfectant for the likely or confirmed infectious agents, or disposed of as infectious hazardous waste
- The unit should be swept and wiped to remove all dirt and debris
- The unit should then be mopped and wiped thoroughly using an appropriate disinfectant and the correct concentration for the likely or confirmed infectious agents. All surfaces, walls, floor, ceiling and doors, must be disinfected
- Cleaning equipment should be soaked in an appropriate disinfectant for the likely or confirmed infectious agents and washed as appropriate at 60°C, or thrown away as infectious hazardous waste

---

Observation and assessment of the patient

Patient observation

Veterinary nurses are extremely important members of the veterinary team that provide care for the patient within the veterinary practice. Nursing observations on the patient's health status at admission, during its adaptation to the hospital environment and throughout the course of treatment all provide valuable information to the veterinary surgeon on the animal's clinical condition, wellbeing and progress. It is a key component of the role of the veterinary nurse to recognize normal and abnormal appearance, demeanour and behaviour of any species of animal in their care. Observation should commence as soon as the animal attends the veterinary practice.

Initial observations

- Dogs that enter the reception area can be observed for interaction with all the changes that they experience in the practice (e.g. smells, people, unfamiliar areas and other animals)
- Information gained from this observation can identify valuable characteristic traits such as excitement, aggression and anxiety
- Observations from afar may reveal key information about the presenting condition, such as lameness. It also allows time for triage of patients; for example, if a patient has difficulty breathing or is bleeding they may require prompt veterinary attention
- Cats or small animals that are transported in secure carriers are more difficult to visualize. If possible, it is best to try and observe them in the carrier to ensure they are not exhibiting signs of excessive stress due to travelling or the presenting illness
- Mouth breathing in cats and small animals may indicate stress or severe respiratory distress and these animals need to be given immediate attention

---

Adaptation to the hospital environment

Different species and animals respond in different ways to the stress of the veterinary environment. Every patient needs to be considered as an individual and must have their own care plan (see Chapter 12). Rabbits, small mammals and birds will require special consideration, as many are 'prey' species and may be stressed outside their normal environment. This experience of vulnerability and stress due to the change of environment can cause the animal to behave differently; well behaved animals can become difficult to handle or display unnatural behavioural characteristics, such as aggression or submission. Some patients may exhibit traits such as kennel guarding.

Stress reduction

Veterinary practices can be very stressful environments for patients; changes in routine and situation can cause additional stress. It should be part of the nursing consideration to reduce the stress for a patient. It has been shown that stress and anxiety may have detrimental effects on patient health during hospitalization and can result in inappetence, altered biochemical parameters and can prolong recovery times, as well as make the patient restless or unsettled (Asres and Amha, 2014).

An unsettled patient should undergo an assessment to determine the reason for the changes in behaviour. Some dogs may become vocal if they want to urinate or defecate; others will vocalize if they are in pain. If the patient becomes unsettled and causes disruption, this could affect all patients within the ward. A noisy ward of barking dogs can be stressful for both patients and staff alike. There are many ways the veterinary nurse can help to minimize stress in the veterinary environment; a key way would be to segregate the animals appropriately and promote normal behaviour. Each animal needs to be considered as an individual and careful questioning of the owner (see below and Chapter 12) may

provide key guidance for stress reduction (e.g. hiding boxes for rabbits, relaxing music within the dog and cat wards and comfort provided by nursing staff).

Prey species, such as rabbits, rodents and birds, will benefit from being housed away from predator species, such as dogs and cats. It should be remembered that prey species rely heavily on their fight or flight response when in potentially dangerous situations. They may become anxious if in close proximity to the noise and smells of other patients and may be stressed due to the fact that they have no means of escape or hiding. Housing small mammals or birds in their own cages may be beneficial if they allow observation of the patient and reduce stress levels.

Geriatric and very young patients may require additional support as they may not be able to adapt to changes in routine and environment as easily as other patients. Having separate 'quiet' wards for these individuals can be useful.

Promotion of normal patient behaviour
Client questionnaires

At the time of admission, it is extremely important to obtain any specific commands the animal responds to from the owner. Most dogs, for example, will be trained to commands for eating, exercising, urination and defecation. This information should be gained and then input into the patient's individual nursing care plan. The use of familiar commands and equipment will help provide an element of normality for the patient within a strange environment and can also be useful for nurses when handling and restraining patients.

Questionnaires can be designed to determine the needs of each individual species of patient that may be admitted (see 'Examples of client questionnaires', at the end of the chapter). There are some additional key questions that need to be asked for small mammals and other exotic pets:

- Types of water bottles or bowls normally used
- Usual bedding material
- Normal and favourite foods
- How easy the pet is to handle.

The information gathered from these assessments can be used by the nursing team to prepare the animal's individual environment and make them as comfortable as possible in the hospital environment. For example, a patient assessment of a cat may reveal that it does not eat all of its dry food in one go, but rather grazes on the food throughout the day. It may also show that the cat likes to eat whilst being hidden; this requirement could be met by providing a box within the accommodation. Further information on nursing care plans is given in Chapter 12.

Inpatient behaviour

Animals will sense the mood and attitude of staff working with them, so it is extremely important to maintain a calm and quiet environment at all times.

Cats

The following should be considered when trying to achieve calm and happy cat wards:

- No dogs
- Avoid cats facing each other
- Reduce noise (e.g. banging doors and lots of people)
- Avoid kennels at floor level
- Place cats in baskets on higher levels and place a towel on top

- Use boxes or covered beds to provide areas of shelter
- Encourage gentle handling
- Calm atmosphere, quiet radio and calm nurses
- Use of feline pheromones.

The use of pheromones to modify the behaviour of animals within the hospital environment (pheromona-therapy) can be useful to reduce stress in the cat. Synthetic versions of two naturally occurring facial pheromones (F3 and F4) are commercially available as a spray or plug-in diffuser (Figure 14.19). Sprays may be applied directly on to objects (e.g. bedding or cat baskets) prior to admission. The diffuser can provide full environmental cover. The environmental use of pheromones may improve the demeanour, appetite and ability to adapt to the stresses that a strange situation can cause to the feline patient.

Dogs

Dog-appeasing pheromone (Adaptil®) diffusers are available for use in canine wards. The synthetic pheromone can help to reduce stress and anxiety within the kennel environment, making the dogs feel more calm and safe. DAP sprays and collars are also available.

Exotic pets

Exotic species are best kept in separate wards, away from dogs and cats. Predator and prey species should be separated (considering sight, sounds and smell). For information on appropriate exotic pet accommodation to promote normal behaviour, see earlier in the chapter.

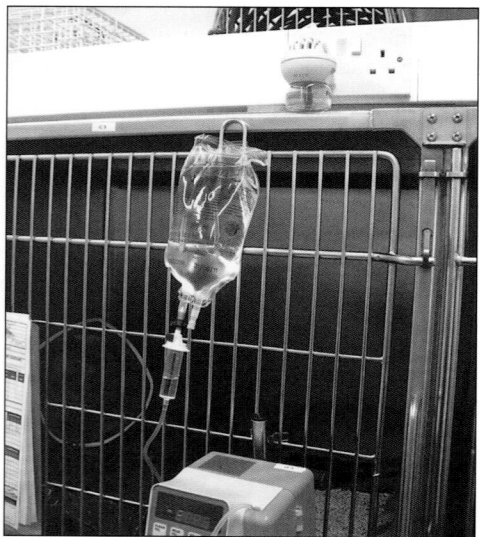

14.19 Plug-in pheromone diffuser above a kennel in a cat ward.

Assessment of the patient

On admission to the veterinary practice, the patient will normally have had a full history gathered from the owner. A member of the practice team will complete a thorough physical examination (see below); this allows useful information to be gathered on the animal's physical status and provides baseline parameters such as temperature, respiration rate, heart rate and pulse quality. During the patient's hospitalization period, these will be reviewed at regular times. All observations should be recorded and will form part of the patient's hospital record card. Patients with an apparently obvious disease should still undergo a full examination and assessment of every body system, as concurrent problems may be identified. Treatment and nursing plans based on these assessments should address all aspects of patient care, not just the specific illness or injury identified (see Chapter 12).

Initial observation

The patient should initially be observed from afar – mental alertness, response to surroundings, body posture, gait, body condition and coat quality can all be assessed this way. During this time, the patient's respiratory rate and effort can be assessed; this is best completed prior to restraint, as the restraint process can cause stress and excitement, which in turn can produce inaccurate results. This is due to the autonomic response of the body to stressful situations. Measuring the respiration rate of cats, rabbits and small mammals may be best completed with the animal still in its carry basket.

Patient mentation

The patient's mental state should be considered as much as the physiological parameters. Although this assessment is subjective, improvement or deterioration of the patient's condition may be detected. Bright alert responsive (BAR) and quiet alert responsive (QAR) are key terms that can be used when recording the patient's mentation on hospital records. It must be remembered that some patients may become withdrawn or quiet in the kennel environment; there are many reasons for this, including fear, pain and stress.

Variations in species, age and breed also need to be considered when evaluating mentation:

- Dogs may have different behaviour and mentation depending on their breed (e.g. working breeds such as Border collies are commonly very mentally alert)
- Normally active and alert cats may be very quiet and subdued in a hospital environment
- Younger and geriatric animals will commonly sleep for longer periods in the hospital environment and often require special care (see 'Essential patient care', below).

Additionally, in exotic pets:

- Observation of mentation in exotic pets, such as reptiles, is hard to assess because interactions with humans are usually limited
- Small mammals, such as hamsters, rabbit and guinea pigs, as well as birds, are usually more used to social interactions and changes in demeanour and behaviour may be more easily recognized.

The patient's response to stimuli should also be assessed.

Response to stimulation

- Does the animal respond to the observer's presence?
- Does the animal respond to verbal communication (if appropriate to species)?
- Is the animal more responsive outside the kennel?
- Does the animal become more responsive when food is offered?
- Does the animal respond to contact such as grooming?

With clear analysis of the patient's response to these situations, more information about the animal's mental state can be gained. This information should be reassessed at least daily and any changes noted. Patients with neurological conditions such as head trauma or brain tumours must be assessed for changes in mentation more frequently, as subtle changes could indicate fatal deterioration (see Chapter 19).

Environmental observations

Prior to cleaning out patient accommodation, the cage or kennel should be observed for any key signs of abnormalities; this can be especially beneficial in exotic pets. These include obvious signs such as vomit or diarrhoea in gastrointestinal cases, to less obvious signs such as disturbed bedding, tipped bowls or litter trays in neurological cases. When observing the environment, the presence of faeces, urine, uneaten food and the volume of remaining water should all be recorded. Any abnormalities (e.g. blood, mucus) in urine, faeces or vomit should also be noted.

Physical examination

When undertaking a physical examination, a systematic approach should be followed to ensure that a thorough examination is performed and a full patient record is completed. First, there should be an overview of the patient, then the hands-on assessment should start at the head area and finish in the tail region. A physical examination checklist (Figure 14.20) can be used as a visual reminder to ensure all areas of the patient are assessed and the information is recorded accurately.

Handling and restraint

Handling techniques for dogs, cats and exotic pets are described in Chapter 11. These should be implemented for the safety of the handler and animal. Small mammals, birds and reptiles require special consideration regarding physical handling techniques, as they may not be used to regular contact. These patients will also be susceptible to stress from travelling to the practice, changes in the environment, and being handled by unfamiliar handlers using different techniques.

Head and oral cavity

Head

The patient's head posture should be upright with no evidence of a head tilt. The musculature of the head should be symmetrical and normal for the species and breed being examined. The surface of the skull, preorbital area, zygomatic arches, maxilla and mandible (see Chapter 3) should all be palpated to monitor for any abnormalities, such as masses or swelling. Patients who have suspected head trauma should undergo limited palpation, if any, as inadvertent decompression of a skull fracture may result in brain compression. Cheek pouches of hamsters should be examined to ensure they are not impacted.

Nares and upper respiratory tract

The nares should be slightly moist with no discharge. Air flow should be observed for patency of each nostril; this is undertaken by placing a few cotton fibres in front of each nostril and monitoring for movement. Cats and rabbits are obligate nasal breathers, thus if mouth breathing is ever observed in these species, it is indicative of severe respiratory compromise.

Upper respiratory noise, **stertor** (noise on inspiration) and **stridor** (noise on expiration), can often indicate partial obstruction of the airway. Some breeds of dogs, in particular brachycephalic breeds such as the Pug or Bulldog, often have stenotic nares and an elongated soft palate and will commonly make upper respiratory noises at all times.

Oral cavity

The jaws should be able to be opened without difficulty and examined for any misalignment. The tongue, teeth and oral cavity should then be inspected.

The tongue should be assessed for any marks, cuts or ulcers; ulcerated areas on the tongues of rabbits can be indicative of malocclusion. Gentle examination of a rabbit's

Area examined	Normal findings	Examples of abnormal findings
Mentation	Bright, alert, responsive	Depressed, non-responsive, distressed
Body condition score and weight	Animal within normal weight range for species and breed Normal body condition	Animal not within normal weight range and/or has too low or high body condition score (i.e. over- or underweight)
Behaviour and body posture	Normal behaviour for species displayed Not scared/stressed Eating/drinking normally	Scared, stressed, shivering Aggressive/submissive behaviour displayed Not eating and/or drinking
Head position	Upright and central	Head tilt
Nares	Clear and clean	Discharge (e.g. blood), dry, crusty, sneezing
Mouth and teeth	Clean, no smell, no broken teeth, pink mucous membranes Capillary refill time <3 seconds	Broken teeth, tartar, inflamed (red) gums, bad breath (halitosis), bleeding tongue/gums Mucous membrane colour: brick red, pale or blue Capillary refill time >3 seconds
Eyes	Bright, clear, clean	Discharge, cloudy, redness/inflammation Bloodshot eyes Glaucoma, cataracts
Lymph nodes	Submandibular, periscapular and popliteal nodes palpable but small	Peripheral lymph nodes large; axillary and inguinal nodes palpable

14.20 A clinical examination checklist can help provide a logical sequence for a physical examination. *continues* ▶

Area examined	Normal findings	Examples of abnormal findings
Ears	Clean, clear, no smell	Smell, discharge, wounds on ear flap Signs of ear mites
Skin and coat	Glossy, clean, no parasites, no dandruff, no wounds	Dull, dirty, parasites, dandruff, wounds, animal scratching, hair loss (alopecia)
Limbs	No wounds, animal not lame (no difficulty walking), no swelling, no pain	Wounds, cuts, bleeding, swelling, limping/lame (showing difficulty walking), pain Lameness classification
Feet and nails	Clean, nails at a good length and not broken, no smell, no wounds	Smelly, swollen, wounds, broken nails, overgrown nails, bleeding, frayed nails (common road traffic indicator in some species)
Thorax	Normal respiratory rate and effort Normal on auscultation	Increased respiratory rate and effort Abnormal on auscultation
Abdomen	No distension Non-painful	Distended Painful
Tail	Held normally Non-painful No wounds	Tail held abnormally Evidence of tail damage (e.g. wounds) or autotomy (self-shedding of tail) Tail painful
Anus and perineum	Clean, no soiling	Soiling, discharge Anal furunculosis
Reproductive organs	No discharge Both testes present in males No mammary gland enlargement	Vaginal discharge, preputial discharge Undescended testes Mammary enlargement, discharge or pain

14.20 *continued* A clinical examination checklist can help provide a logical sequence for a physical examination.

mouth can be performed using an auriscope to identify any lacerations, ulcerations or dental disease (Figure 14.21).

The teeth should be examined for any evidence of dental disease, such as tartar, bleeding or receding gums, odour and fractured or missing teeth. The hard and soft palate should be inspected for any congenital abnormalities such as cleft palate in neonates, wounds and foreign bodies.

The skin and hair around the mandible should be examined for signs of excess salivation; this is a key sign of dental problems in small mammals. Dental disease and its treatment in small mammals is discussed in Chapter 25.

Skin fold pyoderma may be seen in larger breeds or breeds with excessive skin folds, such as St Bernards and Bullmastiffs, especially around the head and mouth area.

Mucous membranes

The mucous membranes are a very good tool for monitoring many different body systems in the patient. Usually the gums (oral mucous membranes) are used, but the mucous membranes of the eyelids, prepuce and vulva can also be used. The gums and the inside of the lips should be moist; dry tacky gums may be indicative of dehydration (Figure 14.22).

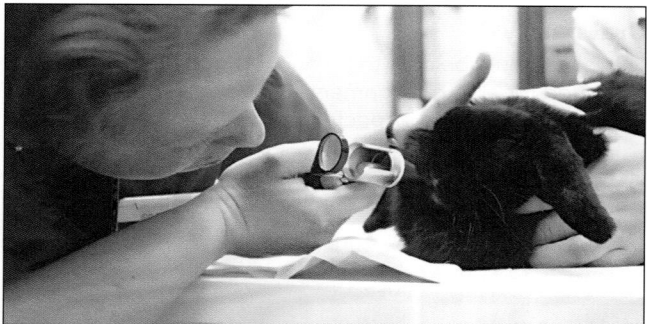

14.21 Using an auriscope to examine the mouth in a conscious rabbit. (Photograph by J Bosley; © Quantock Veterinary Hospital)

Estimation of dehydration (% bodyweight)	Moisture status mucous membranes	Skin turgor	Capillary refill time	Eye position	Heart rate
<5%	Moist	Normal	1–2 seconds	Normal	Normal rate
5–8%	Tacky	Slight tenting	Slightly prolonged ~ 2	Slightly sunken	Normal to slight tachycardia
8–10%	Dry	Moderate tenting	Prolonged >2 seconds	Sunken within orbit	Tachycardia
10–12%	Dry	Tenting remains in place	Prolonged 2–3 seconds	Sunken within orbit	Marked tachycardia and signs of shock (see Chapter 19)
12–15%	Dry	Tenting remains in place	Prolonged >3 seconds	Sunken within orbit	Marked tachycardiaq (may eventually lead to shock (see Chapter 19), cardiac arrest and death)

14.22 Typical physical examination parameter findings used to estimate hydration status. Note that combinations of signs may differ between individual patients.

Mucous membrane colour

- Normal oral mucous membranes should be pink in colour (Figure 14.23)
- Pale membranes are indicative of poor perfusion; this may be seen in patients with circulatory collapse, anaemia, haemorrhage or severe vasoconstriction
- Red (congested) membranes (Figure 14.24) may indicate sepsis, fever, congestion, causes of extensive tissue damage or excitement
- Blue or purple membranes (cyanosis) indicate severe hypoxaemia (lack of oxygen in the blood). This could be caused by respiratory difficulty and immediate action must be taken to increase the patient's oxygen saturation
- Yellow membranes (icterus/jaundice) may be due to liver disease, bile flow obstruction or an increase in red blood cell destruction and circulating bilirubin
- Chocolate brown membranes in dogs and cats are indicative of paracetamol poisoning. Cats are unable to metabolize paracetamol and thus toxicity can occur after the consumption of even low doses
- Cherry red membranes are seen in patients suffering from carbon monoxide poisoning (e.g. following exposure to car exhaust or smoke fumes)

Petechiae may be observed on the mucous membranes of patients with clotting disorders such as von Willebrand's disease or rodenticide poisoning. These appear as pinpoint, round purplish spots that are caused by submucosal haemorrhage (Figure 14.25).

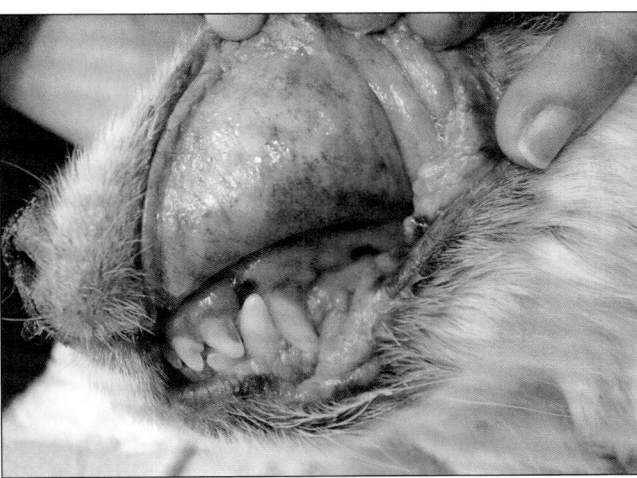

14.25 Petechial haemorrhages on the mucous membranes of a dog. (Courtesy of I Battersby)

Capillary refill time

Capillary refill time (CRT) is a very useful guide to a patient's circulation status. To assess the capillary refill time, a clean finger is used to apply pressure to the mucous membranes of the mouth, usually the gum area above the canine tooth (Figure 14.26). This pressure causes blanching of the tissues; the time taken for the pink colour to return to the area is the CRT. A normal CRT should be 1–2 seconds. If it takes longer than this, it can be indicative of poor perfusion, which has many causes including: hypovolaemia; dehydration (see Figure 14.22); heart failure; and shock. Patients with severe sepsis and fever may demonstrate a faster than normal CRT.

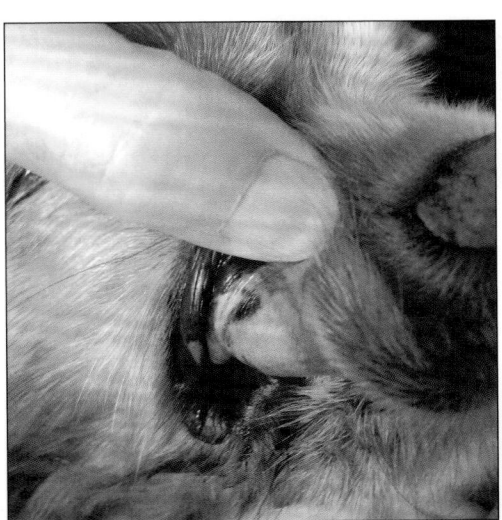

14.23 Physical examination of a canine patient's oral mucous membranes; in this case, they are a normal salmon pink colour.

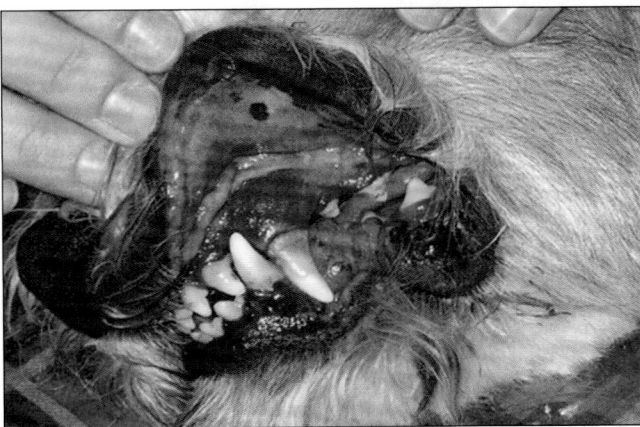

14.24 Congested mucous membranes due to polycythaemia. (Courtesy of N Whitley)

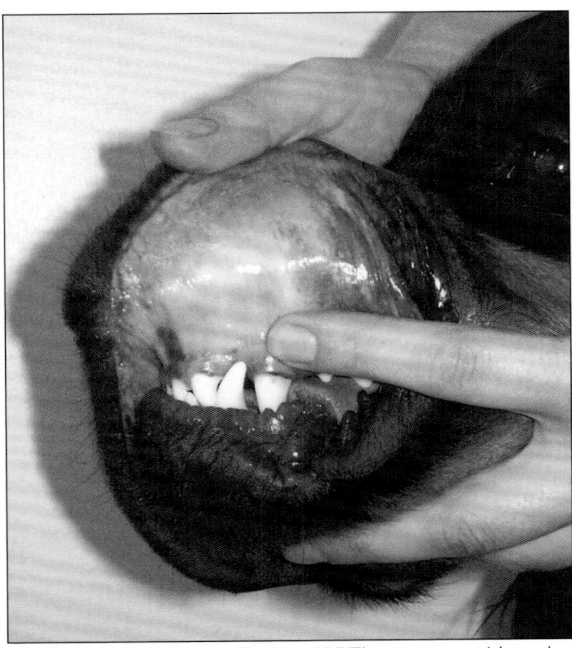

14.26 Capillary refill time (CRT) assessment in a dog. Pressure is applied the gum and then released. The time taken (in seconds) for the normal pink colour to return to the area is the CRT.

Eyes

The ocular surface is very delicate and the smallest scratch can develop into a painful ulcer. When examining the eyes, this must be undertaken carefully and gently and the cornea must not be touched.

The patient's eyes should be open, with no squinting of the eyelids (blepharospasm). Both eyes should be of the same size and neither eye should protrude more than the other; an enlarged globe may be indicative of glaucoma. This is a condition where the intraocular pressure is raised. Eyes that are sunken within the orbits may be seen in patients suffering from dehydration (see Figure 14.22) or in patients with excessive muscle wastage (as seen in cachexic patients).

Exophthalmos is a condition that results in abnormal protrusion of the globe; it may be seen in patients with an orbital mass or small mammals with dental disease. Proptosis (prolapse of the globe) is a commonly occurring problem in brachycephalic breeds, such as Pugs. This is a condition that requires immediate attention in order to preserve the globe (see Chapter 19).

Any discharge from the eye, the colour of any discharge and the content/consistency of the discharge need to be recorded. It is also important to note which eye is affected. In all species, conjunctivitis may be caused by a range of pathogens (viral, bacterial, parasitic and fungal). The presence of foreign bodies such as grass seeds can also cause ocular discharge and inflammation. Cleaning of the eye and discharge (see Figure 14.54) may be postponed until the veterinary surgeon has seen the patient. This is extremely important if the patient has undergone recent intraocular surgery, as a clear discharge may indicate leakage of fluid from the anterior chamber of the globe. Ocular discharge in small mammals may be the result of dental problems. Abnormal growth of the cheek teeth and incisor roots can affect the tear ducts, resulting in an abnormally increased or decreased tear flow and possibly causing purulent discharge from the tear ducts.

Irritation to the ocular surface can be caused by the abnormal anatomy of the eyelids. Entropion is the inward rotation of the eyelid margins, usually at the medial canthus. Ectropion, the outward rotation of the eyelids, is commonly seen in dogs with 'droopy' facial features, such as Bassett Hounds. Both of these eye conditions may cause inflammation of the cornea, which is known as keratitis. Corneal ulceration can be caused by the presence of distichiasis (an additional row of eyelashes that rub against the globe).

The 'third eyelid' or nictitating membrane should always be assessed; this fold of conjunctiva is attached to the medial canthus and moves across the eye when the eyelids are closed. In normal healthy patients, it is not normally visible, but may become obvious if the globe is depressed within the orbit (as can be seen with dehydration). Unwell cats often have a visible nictitating membrane and this is a non-specific sign of ill health. Damage to the nerve pathways of the eye can also be a reason for the nictitating membrane to be visible (see Figure 14.27).

The size and location of the pupil should be assessed; pupils should be the same size. Aniscoria (Figure 14.27) is the term used to describe unequal pupils. This is a neurological sign and can indicate intracranial trauma. Pupils should be examined for a pupillary light reflex; normal pupils will constrict when a bright light is shone into them and then return to normal when the light is withdrawn.

The ocular conjunctiva (Figure 14.28) can be used to observe mucous membrane colour and this is especially useful in animals which have pigmented oral membranes, such as the Chow Chow. The ocular sclera should also be examined for colour changes such as those associated with pallor or icterus (Figure 14.29).

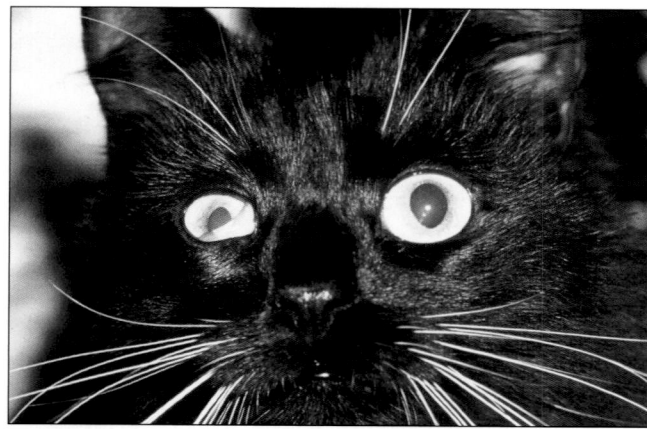

14.27 Aniscoria in a cat with Horner's syndrome. The right eye has a more constricted pupil than the left and the nictitating membrane is visible. (Courtesy of D Gould)

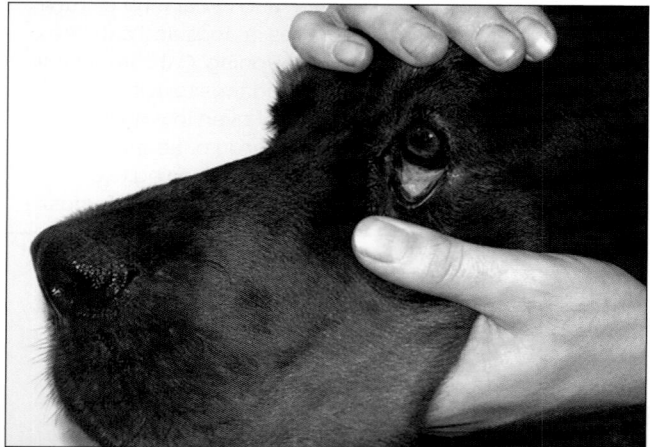

14.28 Normal pink conjunctival mucous membranes in a dog.

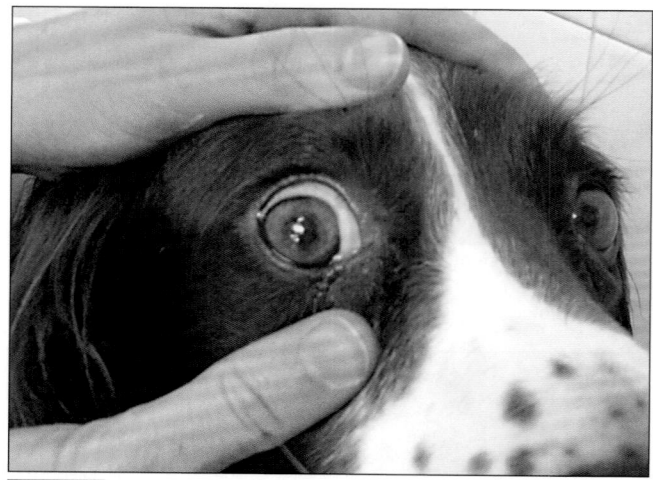

14.29 Icteric sclera in a dog. (Courtesy of I Battersby)

Lymph nodes

Peripheral lymph nodes (see Chapter 3 for location of lymph nodes) should be palpated for enlargement. Submandibular, periscapular and popliteal nodes can normally be located in the dog and cat; axillary and inguinal nodes may only be palpated when enlarged. Lymphadenopathy (disease of the lymph nodes) results in enlargement and may indicate infection or neoplasia, which may be localized or systemic.

Rabbits have smaller lymph nodes than dogs and cats; typically, only the periscapular, submandibular and popliteal lymph nodes are palpable. Most bird species and reptiles do not have palpable or recognizable lymph nodes; rather they possess lymphatic tissue within organs.

Ears, skin, hair and feathers

Ears

The ear pinnae should be examined for scratches, wounds and swellings, such as haematomas. The vertical ear canal can be checked for signs of inflammation (Figure 14.30), discharges, foreign bodies and ectoparasites such as ear mites (see Chapter 6). Fungal infections within the ear may be noted and can be associated with a significant odour (examples include *Malassezia* and *Pseudomonas*). Rabbits are prone to ear mites (*Psoroptes cuniculi*), which may result in a large accumulation of exudative crusts within the ear canal.

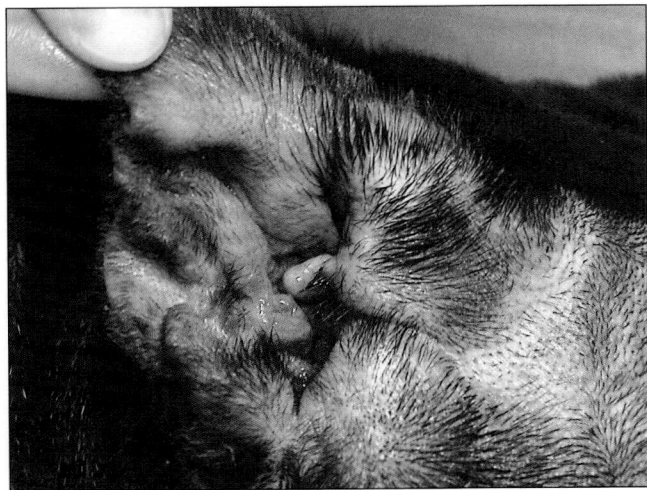

14.30 Otitis externa in a dog. (Courtesy of J Bray)

Skin

In most animals, the overall hair, coat or feather condition can be assessed from afar. In mammals, alopecia, the thinning or loss of hair (usually in patches), may be identified and can be indicative of endocrine diseases. Syrian hamsters can have dark pigmented areas on their flanks due to glandular secretions; older animals may also have alopecia in this area, which is normal. The skin should be examined for dryness, scaliness, greasiness and evidence of macroscopic ectoparasite infestation by fleas (flea dirt may also be evident), lice and ticks (see Chapter 6).

Microscopic ectoparasites, such as demodectic, chorioptic and sarcoptic mites, may cause skin lesions that require further diagnostic procedures (see Chapter 6).

Hydration status can be assessed by skin elasticity (see Figure 14.22). The skin of a normally hydrated animal will fall back into place when pinched and released. Skin tenting indicates a degree of hydration; as dehydration increases, the ability of the skin to return to its normal position is reduced.

Feathers

In birds, the plumage should be examined for evidence of feather damage, areas of missing feathers and irregular moulting. The skin should be examined for wounds, inflammation and signs of infection, such as pustules and redness. Chickens are particularly susceptible to infestations of mites.

Forelimbs

The degree of movement and gait may indicate areas that need further investigation. In small animals, the range of movement, flexion, extension and rotation of the forelimbs should be noted. Assessment of both limbs for symmetry will allow for observation of any differences, including any sign of muscle wastage (atrophy). The limbs and joints should be gently palpated for heat, signs of discomfort, swelling and abnormal sounds (crepitus); this may indicate dislocation or fracture. The feet, pads and claws should be examined for wounds, abrasions and foreign bodies. Frayed and torn nails may indicate involvement in road traffic accidents. Proprioception tests may be performed to evaluate the animal's neurological functions.

Thorax

Respiration rate and effort can be recorded if not assessed prior to the physical examination. Examination of the thorax should include palpation of the thoracic vertebrae, sternum and ribs. Palpation of the thorax and the ease of reaching the ribs will enable a body condition score to be determined (see Chapter 13). The heartbeat can be located between ribs three and six on the left side of the ventral chest. Auscultation of the heart and lungs can be performed using a stethoscope (see also 'Monitoring: temperature, pulse and respiration', below). Palpation of the heart rate can be completed on smaller mammals, cats and small dogs with narrow chests. Auscultation of the lung fields should be performed to detect abnormal lung sounds (such as crackles and rales), which may indicate thoracic pathology such as pneumonia, pulmonary oedema and bronchitis.

Abdomen

First, the abdomen should be assessed visually for any signs of distension. Ascitic fluid or haemorrhage within the abdominal cavity, gas within the stomach, a gravid (pregnant) uterus, a very full bladder, constipation and obesity (excessive fat) may cause distension of the abdomen.

In small mammals, gentle palpation can be performed to evaluate the cause of the distension. Light pressure is applied using flattened fingers, with one hand on either side of the abdomen; internal structures may be located. Abnormal structures, masses and painful or tender areas may also be detected this way. Deeper internal organs, such as the kidneys, liver and intestines, can also be palpated, although care should be taken with the amount of pressure applied. Patients that are tense or overweight may be difficult to assess. Mammary tissue should also be palpated.

Care needs to be taken when handling the abdomen of birds, as the respiratory muscles are located in the abdomen (as birds lack a diaphragm, see Chapter 3). Thus, tight compression of the abdomen during examination should be avoided, where possible, as this may affect the bird's ability to breathe.

Pelvis and hindlimbs

The patient's gait and range of movement of its hindlimbs should be observed. Musculature, flexion, extension and rotation of the limb should be noted. The hindlimbs should be assessed in the same manner as the forelimbs, with specific reference to excessive heat and symmetry. The popliteal lymph nodes can be palpated on the caudal aspect of the limb within the gastrocnemius muscle caudal to the stifle. The femoral pulse can be palpated on the medial aspect of the hindlimb, as the femoral artery passes over the proximal femur. The skin of the medial hindlimbs and ventral abdomen should be examined for signs of irritation that could be associated with ectoparasites or soiling.

The limbs of birds should be examined for evidence of raised keratinous scales or swollen toes, which may indicate diseases such as 'scaly leg' or 'bumblefoot', that require treatment.

Tail

The tail should be examined to ensure that there is voluntary movement; it should also be checked to identify any wounds or damage to the tail tip. Autotomy is the shedding of the tail and is seen in lizards that are handled by the tail. The tail tips of rats, mice and gerbils can also be damaged by inappropriate handling (see Chapter 11). Some small mammals and birds have a glandular area just above the tail that can appear greasy; this is normal for some species.

Anus and perineum

The anus should be examined for signs of soiling, discharge or disease, such as masses or furunculosis. Anal glands are situated on both sides of the anus in carnivores and are involved in scent marking. These glands can become impacted or infected. The area of the perineum needs to be examined for inflammation and swelling; this may indicate perineal rupture. Hamsters with 'wet tail' will have evidence of wetness and diarrhoea around the perineal area. This can be the result of stress or an inappropriate diet. The patient's rectal temperature can also be assessed at this time (see 'Monitoring: temperature, pulse and respiration', below).

Reproductive organs

The external genitalia should be examined; small mammals should be supported correctly during the examination to prevent any spinal injuries. Entire male animals should have two descended testes within the scrotum and the penis should be examined for any injuries or discharge. Phimosis is the inability to protrude the penis out of the sheath. Paraphimosis is the inability to retract the penis into the pre-putial sheath.

Female animals should be examined for discharge or swelling of the vulva. In the bitch, vaginal discharge is associated with the reproductive cycle and swelling of the vulva can be seen in various stages of the oestrus cycle. Abnormal discharges should be noted. Purulent discharge in mature middle-aged bitches may be associated with infection of the uterus (pyometra). Imminent parturition can be indicated by the presence of a clear or blood-stained discharge in the bitch and a brown discharge in the queen; a green or black odorous discharge could indicate death of the unborn fetus or postpartum infection (see Chapter 24).

Swelling of the anal and genital openings is commonly seen in rabbits with myxomatosis. In birds that are egg-bound, palpation of the egg may be possible if it is located within the lower region of the reproductive tract. Prolapse of the cloaca may indicate egg-binding in snakes.

Physiological assessment

Normal functions should be observed and assessed for variations and abnormalities.

Changes in urination

The patient's urine should be examined for colour, smell, turbidity and volume, and the results noted on their record card.

Urine samples should be obtained for laboratory analysis when any form of dysfunction is evident (see Chapter 17). Urinalysis can also be performed on samples of avian urine, but care must be taken to avoid contamination with the faecal component of the dropping.

Urine production

Urine should be passed freely with no straining or discomfort.

- Adult dogs and cats with normal renal function should produce 1–2 ml/kg/h, although this does reduce slightly overnight.
- Reduced urine production (oliguria) may be due to conditions such as dehydration, hypovolaemia and acute renal failure. A volume of <0.5 ml/kg/h should be investigated and intravenous fluid therapy should be initiated if necessary.

To enable accurate measurement of urine production, an indwelling urinary catheter with a closed collection system may need to be placed. The lack of urine production (anuria) can be very serious; causes include damage to the urinary tract, a ruptured bladder, a urinary obstruction (e.g. urinary stones and/or calculi) and acute renal failure. These conditions can lead to metabolic difficulties and abnormalities that can be life-threatening. Patients may be observed to have difficulty urinating (dysuria).

Urine appearance

The colour and consistency of the urine produced should be noted (for further information, see Chapter 17).

- Blood in the urine (haematuria) may be visible; cystitis, trauma to the urinary tract, neoplasia and infection may all be possible causes.
- Rabbit urine contains plant pigments (porphyrins) that cause the colour of normal urine to be a very dark yellow to red; this is commonly mistaken for haematuria.
- Guinea pig urine is yellow and cloudy, as is the urine of female chinchillas.

Changes in water intake

Increased urine production (polyuria, PU) is usually accompanied by increased thirst (polydipsia, PD). Many conditions present with clinical signs of both PU and PD (e.g. diabetes mellitus, diabetes insipidus, Cushing's disease and pyometra). Pyrexia and panting can also increase water intake. Some medications may also cause an increased intake of fluid and increased urination.

Voluntary water intake varies with species and the diet being fed. The maintenance water intake required by dogs and cats is approximately 50 ml/kg/24h, and for rabbits is approximately 100 ml/kg/24h. This calculation should be used to estimate how much water should be consumed per day. Dogs and cats drinking in excess of 100 ml/kg/24h are considered to be polydipsic.

Worked maintenance water intake calculation

The maintenance water intake for an 11-year-old Cavalier King Charles Spaniel that weighs 10 kg can be calculated as follows:

10 kg x 50 ml/kg/24h = 500 ml per 24 hours

All patients should have their water intake measured by subtracting the volume of water remaining (i.e. not consumed) from the volume provided over a set period of time. This volume should then be recorded on the patient's hospital record. Periods of exercise, and the quality and type of food eaten should be taken into consideration when noting water intake. In addition, the environmental conditions (e.g. the potential for evaporation) also need to be considered. Information on the provision of food and water is given in the sections below.

Changes in defecation

The amount, consistency and colour of the faeces passed by the patient should be observed and recorded.

Faecal appearance

Normal faeces vary between species, especially in exotic pets (Figure 14.31). Macroscopic examination of the faeces can be undertaken to determine the colour, smell, shape and consistency (for further information see Chapter 17).

- Black faeces (melaena) can indicate bleeding into the upper gastrointestinal tract.
- Fresh blood in the faeces (haematochezia) is indicative of bleeding from the lower bowel.

Further microscopic investigation may be required to assess the presence of microorganisms and parasites (see Chapters 6 and 17).

Diarrhoea

This is an increase in the liquidity of faeces, which are normally passed more frequently. Some patients show no other systemic signs of disease. There are many causes of diarrhoea, including irritation of the mucosa, dietary imbalances, inflammation, bacterial infections (e.g. *Escherichia coli*, *Campylobacter*), endoparasites and viral diseases (e.g. parvovirus). Patients suspected of having an infectious or zoonotic disease should be isolated from other animals.

Patients with diarrhoea should be given plenty of opportunities to go outside, as many animals will be trained not to soil their bedding; soiling of the bed may cause stress for these animals. Patients need to kept clean from any soiling. Barrier creams can be applied to prevent faecal burning.

Longhaired cats and dogs may benefit from having their fur trimmed or tails wrapped in bandage. Good hygiene measures should be in place.

Dehydration can occur due to the increased fluid loss associated with diarrhoea; fluid therapy may be required in small mammals such as rabbits and neonates, as well as analgesia and spasmolytic agents for patients with abdominal pain.

Constipation

This is difficulty in passing faeces. There are many causes of constipation, including ingestion of foreign bodies and dehydration; the resulting affect is unproductive straining (tenesmus). Hard and dry faecal matter may build up within the colon or rectum, causing impaction.

Environmental factors, such as changes in routine for dogs and outdoor cats, may also stop the animal defecating. Cats can be very specific about the type of litter they pass faeces in, especially if it has been used. It is important to gain the appropriate information from the owner on admission.

Additional causes of constipation are discussed in detail in Chapter 18.

Changes in appetite

A change in the patient's appetite (see also 'Monitoring food intake', below) is indicative of ill health; however, it should be remembered that stress can also have an effect on the animal's appetite. There may be many reasons for inappetence:

- Dental disease is one of the most common causes of inappetence and can affect all species
- Difficult in eating (dysphagia) may be due to trauma (e.g. mandibular symphysis separation)
- Nausea and loss of smell can have a significant impact on appetite, especially in the cat.

Key definitions
- **Anorexia** is the term for not eating. This can be a result of many different conditions
- **Pica** is the term given to the craving of unnatural foodstuffs (e.g. carpet lining) →

Patient type	Appearance of normal faeces	Appearance of abnormal faeces	Possible causes of abnormality
Rabbits	Round dry pellets or soft, mucus covered caecotrophs	Presence of dark and sticky caecotrophs around the anus; diarrhoea or loose faeces	Enteritis; changes in diet; obesity; other disorders that may cause the accumulation of caecotrophs.
Guinea pigs	Oval pellets (medium to dark brown) or caecotrophs (aromatic green brown pellets)	Clumped pellets; smaller pellets; pitted pellets; diarrhoea	Reduced food intake; intestinal bacteria overgrowth; parasitic or bacterial infection
Hamsters	Small, oval, brown pellets, moist to dry	Soft consistency; diarrhoea around anus and/or abdomen	Insufficient foods high in moisture, such as greens or fruit; wet tail (this can also be a result of stress)
Birds	Three components: urine (clear, watery portion); solid urates (white); faeces (colour dependant on diet but ranges from light brown to black, liquid or tubular form)	Colour change of urate portion to yellow/green or diarrhoea	May indicate malnutrition or liver disease; change in diet; endoparasites
Reptiles	Formed faeces with chalky, solid urates (urinary waste)	Soft consistency; diarrhoea	*Salmonella*; endoparasites

14.31 Characteristics of normal and abnormal faeces in some exotic pet species.

Vomiting and regurgitation

It is important to determine whether a patient is vomiting or regurgitating, and to continually monitor those patients as the risk of aspiration pneumonia is high.

- Vomiting is the forceful ejection of the stomach contents through the mouth; this may be accompanied by active retching. Prior to vomiting, the patient may exhibit signs of nausea, such as hyperventilation, lip smacking and, in the case of cats, a different toned meow. Common causes of vomiting include gastric foreign bodies, gastric dilatation, poisons and systemic diseases such as renal failure or pancreatitis.
- Regurgitation is the passive movement of food or liquid into the mouth with no warning. Regurgitation may occur due to megaoesophagus, oesophagitis, oesophageal strictures or vascular ring anomaly (see Chapter 18).

Many small animal and exotic patients are unable to vomit.

- Rabbits, guinea pigs and rats are unable to vomit.
- The movement of food from a hamster's pouch may be mistaken for regurgitation.
- Birds can both vomit partially digested or digested food from the proventriculus and regurgitate food from the crop. Vomiting is abnormal for birds, whereas regurgitation is normal behaviour.
- Lizards are able to regurgitate and/or vomit food; this may occur due to illness, because the food particles are too large or spoiled, or due to stress (e.g. when moving after eating).

The vomiting patient needs frequent monitoring and the volume and content of the vomitus should be recorded; the presence of blood or material should be noted. Vomitus that contains blood is called haematemesis. Forceful projectile vomiting without retching is indicative of pyloric obstruction. The vomiting of faecal matter is termed stercoraceous vomiting and can be caused by intestinal obstruction.

Excessive vomiting can be extremely stressful and tiring for the patient; it is paramount that the nursing staff are present to reassure the patient and clean and continually wipe or wash their face. Vomiting can cause severe electrolyte disturbances and patients will often require intravenous fluid and electrolyte therapy. Patients that are regurgitating require careful monitoring to detect whether there is a pattern associated with the episodes of regurgitation. The management of the vomiting patient is described further in Chapter 15 and the causes of vomiting are discussed in Chapter 18.

Occurrence of coughing

Patients that are presented with coughing must first be investigated to ensure that they are not harbouring an infectious disease; if at any point there is suspicion that the patient may have an infectious disease, they must be isolated (see above). The cough reflex is initiated by sensitivity of the respiratory mucosa and is used for clearing the respiratory passages. Inflammation and irritation can also induce the cough reflex.

There are many conditions that are associated with coughing, such as heart failure, canine distemper, kennel cough and a collapsing trachea (see Chapter 18). It is important to assess whether the cough is moist and productive, harsh or dry. Patients that develop a cough during hospitalization must be recorded and reported immediately to the clinical team, especially if they are receiving intravenous fluid therapy or suffering from regurgitation. Pulmonary oedema and inspiration pneumonia may be possible causes of unexpected coughing. Coughing may also be associated with other changes in respiration.

Pain assessment

The stress that may be experienced by an animal in a hospital setting has been discussed above. Uncontrolled pain is one of the key reasons that patients may appear to be unsettled. Patients exhibit pain in many different ways; for example, prey species may appear 'stoic' and unmoving, seeming almost to freeze. The age of the animal may also affect the way it demonstrates pain. The site of the pain can also affect the clinical signs that are seen; for example, an animal with chest pain may have altered respiratory function, an animal with a flank drain may struggle with movement which in turn can affect its breathing, and abdominal pain may result in the animal being tense and demonstrating the 'praying' position.

It should be remembered, that each patient has an individual response to pain and it is the role of the veterinary nurse to recognize and interpret the presenting signs; this can be not only challenging but also subjective. The detrimental effects of pain will prolong a patient's recovery and the return to normal behaviour and function

Providing pain relief (analgesia) is an ethical and responsible action under the RCVS Code of Professional Conduct. Identifying pain in animals and monitoring the response to analgesic drugs can be challenging, but some general indicators can be used. For further information, the reader is referred to Chapter 21.

In all species, good standards of nursing care may help to alleviate pain and stress (see also 'Essential patient care', below:

- Bedding should be dry and comfortable and be shaped to areas of the body as required
- Padding should be used to reduce pressure on painful areas; this will also reduce the probability of decubitus ulcer formation
- Mental stimulation is essential for the patient's wellbeing and for reducing stress levels. A recumbent patient may benefit from being moved to an active area of the practice
- Discharges from the eyes and nose should be cleaned, and animals that cannot groom themselves should be washed and groomed regularly. Grooming can also prove effective at stimulating the patient to eat

Physiotherapy can be provided to ensure good circulation and lymphatic draining (see Chapter 15). It also promotes movement of the joints and allows for the provision of TLC ('tender loving care').

Monitoring: temperature, pulse and respiration

The vital clinical signs of temperature, pulse and respiration should be monitored regularly and recorded when the patient is hospitalized; these should be compared with the references ranges for that species (Figures 14.32 to 14.34). When obtaining the measurements, consideration must be given to the stress of the patient, as this can elevate the readings.

Temperature

Temperature measurement in conscious patients is usually taken rectally. There has been research into the use of aural temperatures (Lamb and McBrearty, 2013) and although non-rectal temperature readings are not as reliable as rectal temperatures, some practices are adopting this technique. This approach can be especially useful if completing night observations with limited staff. Specific aural thermometers are available and provide a fast reading (Figure 14.35).

Digital rectal thermometers are safe and robust; disposable covers are available to maintain infection control (Figure 14.36). The use of glass mercury thermometers has

Species	Body temperature (°C)	Heart rate (beats/min)	Respiratory rate (breaths/min)
African Grey Parrot	40–42	100–300	15–45
Cockatiel	40–42	150–350	40–50
Lovebird	40–42	250–400	60–100
Budgerigar	40–42	260–400	60–100

14.33 Reference ranges of vital signs seen in some common bird species. (Values taken from Girling (2013), the *BSAVA Manual of Exotic Pets, 5th edn* and the *BSAVA Manual of Canine and Feline Advanced Veterinary Nursing, 2nd edn*)

Species	Preferred optimal temperature range (°C)	Heart rate (beats/min)	Respiratory rate (breaths/min)
Cornsnake	25–30	40–50	6–10
Royal python	25–30	30–50	6–10
Green iguana	26–36	30–60	10–30
Leopard gecko	23–30	40–80	20–50

14.34 Reference ranges of vital signs seen in some common reptile species. (Values taken from Girling (2013), the *BSAVA Manual of Exotic Pets, 5th edn* and the *BSAVA Manual of Canine and Feline Advanced Veterinary Nursing, 2nd edn*)

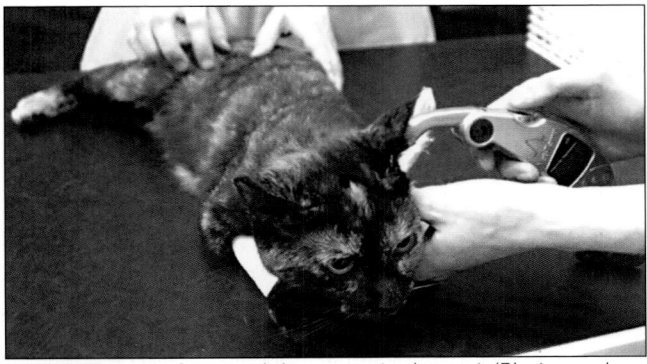

14.35 Use of an aural thermometer in a cat. (Photograph by J Bosley; © Quantock Veterinary Hospital)

Species	Body temperature (°C)	Heart rate (beats/min)	Respiratory rate (breaths/min)
Dog	38.3–39.2	70–140	10–30
Cat	38.2–38.6	100–200	20–30
Ferret	37.8–40	200–250	33–36
Domestic rabbit	38.5–40	130–325	30–60
Chinchilla	37–38	200–350	40–80
Guinea pig	37.2–39.5	230–380	90–150
Chipmunk	38 (during torpor, a few degrees above ambient)	264–296 (during torpor, may drop to 3–6)	75 (during torpor, may drop to <1 and is barely detectable)
Gerbil	37.4–39	260–600	85–160
Hamster (Russian)	36–38	300–460	60–80
Hamster (Syrian)	36.2–37.5	300–470	40–110
Rat	38	310–500	70–150
Mouse	37.5	420–700	100–250

14.32 Reference ranges of vital signs in the dog, cat and some common small mammal pets.

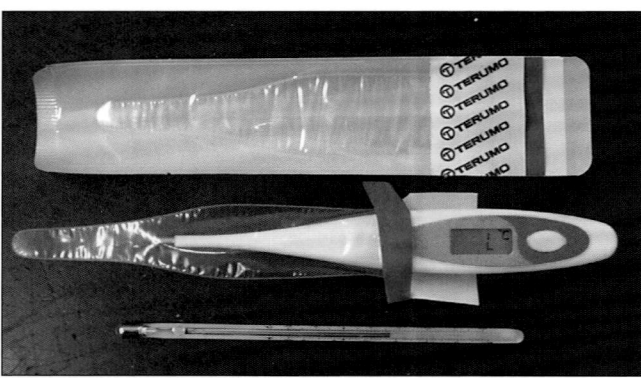

14.36 Different types of thermometers. From the top: thermometer cover; digital thermometer with cover; mercury thermometer.

Temperature conversion

To convert Celsius to Fahrenheit – multiply by 9, divide by 5 and add 32. For example 38.5°C = 101.3°F:

- 38.5°C x 9 = 346.5
- $\dfrac{346.5}{5}$ = 69.3
- 69.3 + 32 = 101.3°F

To convert Fahrenheit to Celsius – subtract 32, multiply by 5 and divide by 9. For example 102.5°F = 39.2°C:

- 102.5°F – 32 = 70.5
- 70.5 x 5 = 352.5
- $\dfrac{352.5}{9}$ = 39.2°C

been phased out in most veterinary practices due to health and safety concerns and the difficulty in preparing the thermometer for use. Thermometers should be cleaned thoroughly before and after use; storing the thermometer in a jar of disinfectant with cotton wool is not acceptable as it will evaporate and need replacement daily.

- Care should be taken when obtaining rectal temperatures in small mammals; adequate restraint must be used to avoid struggle and injury from the thermometer.
- Birds have very delicate cloacal openings and trauma to the gastrointestinal/urogenital tract must be avoided.
- Reptiles are exothermic and therefore rely on environmental temperature to determine their body temperature.

Procedure to record rectal temperature using a digital thermometer

1. Clean the thermometer prior to use; antibacterial wipes or dilute chlorhexidine-soaked cotton wool swabs can be used.
2. Apply a disposable thermometer cover (if available).
3. A small amount of sterile lubricant should be applied directly to the bulb of the thermometer.
4. Ask an assistant to restrain the patient; this will prevent inaccurate readings and thermometer trauma.
5. Insert the thermometer into the rectum, using a gentle twisting motion, and position the tip against the dorsal rectal wall to avoid insertion into faecal matter.
6. Hold the thermometer in place for 30–60 seconds, depending on the manufacturer, or until the bleeping indicates removal. Never release the thermometer during the procedure.
7. Gently remove the thermometer from the rectum.
8. Read and record the temperature; any anomalies or temperature changes must be immediately reported to the clinical team.
9. Remove and dispose of the cover and clean the thermometer ready for next use.

Interpretation of temperature measurements

Temperature should be measured in Celsius (°C) or Fahrenheit (°F). Both values may be used; however, Celsius is now the standard unit of measurement in the UK.

An elevated temperature may be due to fever (pyrexia), pain or hyperthermia.

- Fever (pyrexia) – this can be caused by infectious diseases, drug reactions, medical illness and neoplasia; these conditions result in the release of pyrogens that raise the thermoregulatory set point in the hypothalamus.
- Hyperthermia – this occurs when the hypothalamic thermoregulatory set point is not changed, but mechanisms of heat loss are unable to respond to the temperature rise. Hyperthermia may be seen in many situations, such as heat stroke, increased environmental temperature, increased muscle activity from seizures and exercise, and increased metabolic rate as a result of pain and stress.

A lowered temperature (hypothermia) can be seen in patients with:

- Chronic disease or illness
- Heat loss during anaesthesia and recovery (see Chapter 21).
- Environmental exposure and drowning.

Hypothermia is also seen in neonatal and paediatric patients that cannot regulate their own body temperature; this is termed poikilothermic. It can also occur in depressed, moribund and unconscious patients.

Pulse

Assessment of pulse rate and quality will help provide an overall evaluation of the efficiency and condition of the animal's cardiovascular system. Pulse waves can be palpated at areas where an artery runs close to the peripheral tissue. The rhythmical wave corresponds to blood being ejected from the left ventricle of the heart and travelling through the arterial circulation. In the dog and cat, it can be assessed at various sites (Figure 14.37). The number of pulses in a minute is termed the pulse rate and should be recorded as part of the patient's clinical record. Palpation and recording of pulse rates can be difficult in some patients, especially those that are trembling. Small mammals and some cats have higher pulse rates than dogs; in these patients, auscultation with a stethoscope may be useful.

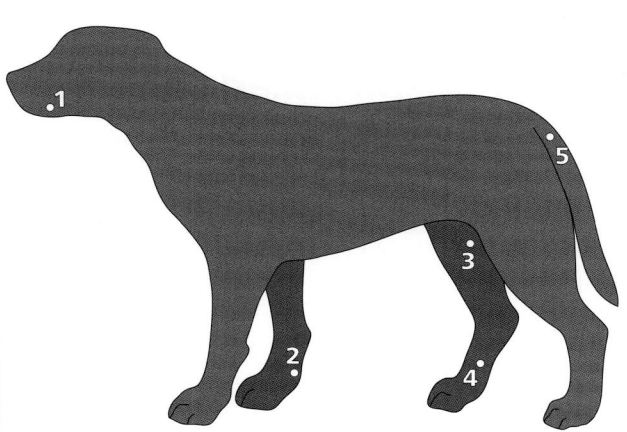

1. Lingual artery – ventral surface of the tongue (not advised in the rabbit as excessive palpation of the tongue may cause swelling).
2. Carpal artery – palmar aspect of the carpus.
3. Femoral artery – medial aspect of proximal femur.
4. Dorsal metatarsal artery – medial aspect of the tarsus (Figure 14.38).
5. Coccygeal artery – ventral aspect of the tail base.

14.37 Common pulse point locations in the dog.

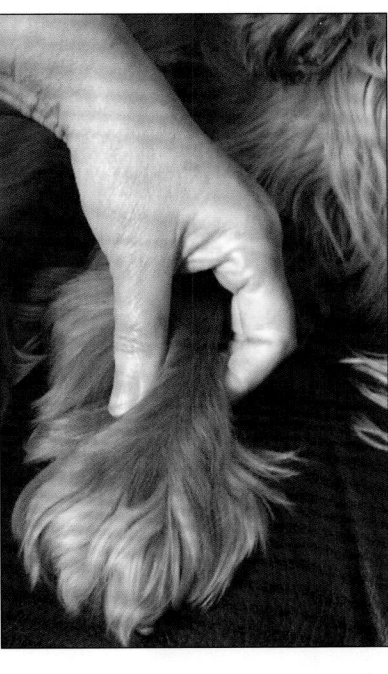

14.38 Palpation of the pulse in a dog using the carpal artery which is on the palmar aspect of the carpus.

It is useful to assess the pulse quality, including strength, speed and duration, as well as the pulse rate to detect any abnormalities.

- Sinus arrhythmia – normal variation in pulse rate; the pulse speeds up on inspiration and decreases on expiration.
- Tachycardia – increased heart and pulse rates. This may be seen with exercise, stress, disease, hypovolaemia and drug administration.
- Bradycardia – reduced heart and pulse rates. This can be either drug-induced or seen in animals that are asleep, very fit or suffering from cardiac arrhythmias. Exotic animals that hibernate have a low pulse rate during the winter months.

- Weak pulses – may indicate reduced circulating blood volume or cardiac disease.
- Strong and jerky pulses – can indicate temporary compensatory mechanisms for reduced circulating volume or congenital cardiac anomalies such as patent ductus arteriosus.

A pulse rate that does not correspond to the heart rate indicates a pulse deficit is present. Electrocardiography (ECG) should be performed to gain more information regarding he abnormal rhythm.

Respiration

The natural movement of the chest is to expand on inspiration and to contract on expiration. This is controlled by complex systems within the body and by the movement of the diaphragm. The number of breaths the animal takes per minute is termed the respiratory rate. This can be counted on either inspiration or expiration. The respiratory rate should be recorded on the patient's record card. This measurement is sometimes best undertaken by observing the animal from afar. A patient in respiratory distress may exert more effort on inspiration and the movement of the chest will be exaggerated; abdominal movement may be noted in animals in severe respiratory distress. If observed, the clinical team must be informed immediately.

Abnormal respiration

- Tachypnoea – an increase in respiration rate, which may be observed in patients that are excited or following exercise. Thoracic pathology, such as pneumothorax, stress and pain may also cause tachypnoea.
- Bradypnoea – a reduction in respiration rate, which may be seen in relaxed and/or sleeping patients. Brain and neck trauma can also affect the ability of the animal to ventilate, as can some medications and poisons.
- Dyspnoea – difficulty breathing. This may be caused by a number of different conditions, including obstruction, respiratory tract disease, lung pathology, increased pressure from the abdominal organs on the diaphragm and trauma to the thorax.
- Paradoxical breathing – this is when the breathing pattern is different to what is expected and movement may result in severe traumatic injury to the chest (e.g. where ribs are broken and moving freely from the rest of the rib cage).

Auscultation using a stethoscope

Auscultation is the process of listening for sounds produced in the body; it is an important skill that a veterinary nurse must have in order to complete a full physical examination. Auscultation may be performed on the heart, lung fields and abdomen. A stethoscope is routinely used to amplify the subtle sounds and allow detailed information to be gathered. Abdominal auscultation can be used to assess intestinal peristalsis. In rabbits in particular, the absence of gut sounds can be indicative of gut stasis.

Stethoscopes

The earpieces of stethoscopes should sit within the ears of the operator in a forward-facing direction. Binaural or ear tubes connect the earpieces to the tubing that transmits sounds from the head of the stethoscope to the earpieces. Stethoscopes come in various types: combined diaphragm, single diaphragm or double-sided diaphragm (Figure 14.39).

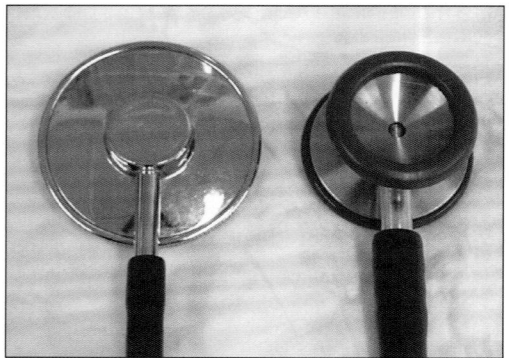

14.39 Single-sided (left) and double-sided (right) stethoscope heads.

Digital stethoscopes are also available that record the heart rate on the front digital interface. When using a single or combined diaphragm stethoscope, the pressure applied indicates the types of sounds that will be heard. Light pressure detects low pitch sounds; whilst firmer pressure detects higher pitched sounds. Stethoscopes can be very expensive and the diaphragm is fragile and can be easily damaged. Stethoscopes should be cleaned with anti-bacterial wipes after use; they should never by submersed in water.

Procedure for auscultation

1. Locate the heartbeat between the third and sixth ribs on the left side of the ventral chest.
2. Hold the diaphragm of the stethoscope gently against the patient's chest and move it cranially, caudally and ventrally to cover the base and apex of the heart. The heart rate should be monitored over at least 1 minute to establish a beats per minute reading. Note the rate, rhythm, intensity and clarity of the heartbeat.

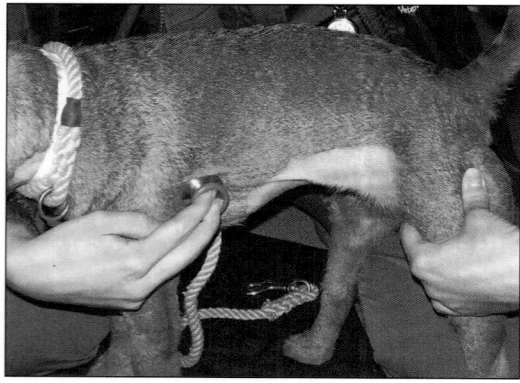

3. If physically possible, palpate the patient's pulse simultaneously to ensure that there is no pulse deficit (heart sounds with no accompanying pulse produced), as this could indicate that the patient has a cardiac arrhythmia.
4. Auscultation should also be performed from the right side of the chest – although auscultation may not be as clear, different heart sounds or murmurs may be heard.
5. Then auscultate the cranial and caudal lung fields, dorsally, medially and ventrally at inspiration and expiration, to detect abnormal lung sounds.

Essential patient care

Care of hospitalized patients

Patients that have been admitted to the veterinary practice for investigation or treatment may be hospitalized for a few hours up to a few weeks. No matter how long the stay is for the patient, all their essential needs must be addressed. A nursing care plan should be formulated and followed for each patient (see Chapter 12).

Comfort

On admittance, each patient should be assigned appropriate accommodation (see 'Inpatient accommodation' above). When selecting the accommodation, the species, breed and the reason for admission should be taken into consideration. There must be sufficient space to allow the animal to move around within the enclosure and for food and water bowls, as well as litter trays (if applicable), to be placed away from the bedding. Suitable bedding should be provided in the first instance (see above), but a range of materials should also be available to meet the potentially changing needs of patients.

- Metal kennels should be lined with insulating materials to avoid the patient coming into contact with the cold surface of the kennel.
- Arthritic patients should be provided with thick comfortable bedding.
- Recumbent patients may benefit from additional padding, such as a waterproof foam mattress (Figure 14.40; see also Figures 14.2 and 14.3); this helps to prevent pressure sores and decubitus ulcer formation. Duvets and pillows should be used as positioning aids and to provide support for the patient's head.
- Veterinary fleece bedding (e.g. Vetbed®) is soft and comfortable and allows fluid to pass through and be absorbed in the base layer; this will help to keep the patient dry.

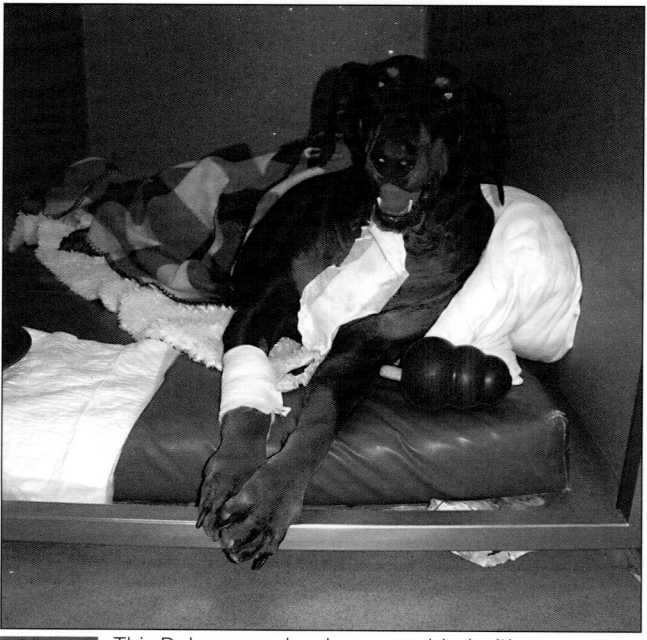

14.40 This Dobermann has been provided with a supportive mattress, warm bedding and a chew toy.

Patients with fractured limbs, wounds or that have sustained trauma should be provided with sufficient and appropriate bedding. Affected limbs should be positioned uppermost and supported with additional padding to stop rotation. Paraplegic patients may feel anxious and distressed if their lack of mobility has an acute onset. If appropriate, the patient may benefit from their head being raised to allow them to look at their surroundings.

Warmth

Wards should be kept at a constant temperature of 18–22°C. However, some patients, such as the very young, very old or immunocompromised, may require an elevated environmental temperature on admission. An initial temperature of 25–30°C is recommended for these patients, which can subsequently be reduced to 22°C, as long as it is kept constant and measures are in place to reduce any draughts. Healthy patients that are admitted for routine procedures may also require supplementary warmth (e.g. during premedication or recovery from general anaesthesia). Methods for providing additional warmth to hospitalized patients are described in Figure 14.41 and illustrated in Figures 14.42 to 14.45.

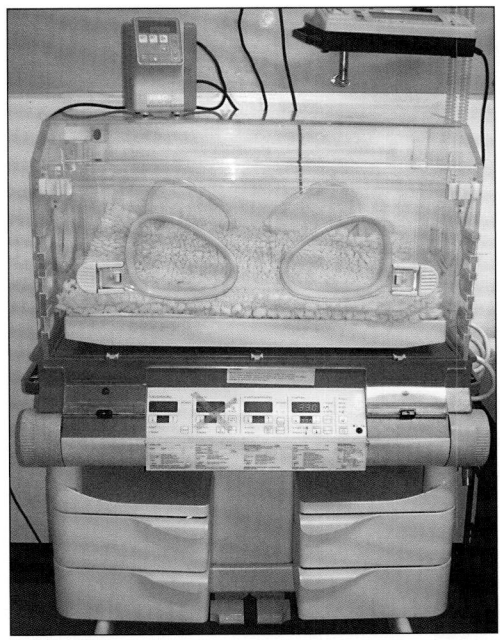

14.42 An incubator suitable for warming veterinary patients.

Heat source	Comments
Blankets, towels and bedding	Can be used to provide an insulated area for the patient to lie on. Patients can be covered with additional bedding to prevent heat loss, but this is not an effective way to replace heat in a patient that is already cold. Care should be taken to ensure that the patient is not lying on bedding that has become wet due to urination
Incubators (Figure 14.42)	Are thermostatically controlled to provide the desired level of warmth; they are ideal for smaller patients and provide a warm, confined area that allows easy observation of the patient. This can be very useful for patients recovering from anaesthesia and those that are critically ill and need constant supervision.
Heat pads (Figure 14.43)	Are water resistant electrically heated flat pads that warm up to a pre-set temperature (often quite hot); care should be taken that they are always well covered with bedding so that the patient cannot come into direct contact with the pad. They should be used with caution with recumbent patients as they can cause thermal burns; any patient should be turned frequently whilst heat pads are being used. The electrical wire is a potential electrocution hazard and should not be used with animals that have a tendency to chew items.
Hot water bottles	Can be used for small mammals and for puppies and kittens. They are cheap and easy to use, although care should be taken not to use boiling water and to ensure that the seal is fully watertight before use. Cooling of the contents will occur and so regular refilling will be required. The bottle should always be covered with a towel and bedding to prevent thermal burns and there is a risk of leakage and scalding if the bottle should burst or if it is chewed.
Microwaveable pads and bags	Can be of use as they will stay warmer for a longer period of time than hot water bottles. Care should be taken not to overheat them as they can become very hot and risk burning a patient, especially if recumbent.
Warmed fluid bags and 'hot hands' (gloves filled with warmed water) (Figure 14.44)	Are of limited use for patients that are mobile, as there is a high risk of puncture resulting in leakage of warmed water on to the patient. They can be useful for recumbent or anaesthetized patients when heated for a short period of time to make them warm; they can then be placed around a patient due to their flexible nature. Care should be taken not to make these items too hot, as they can cause thermal burns if placed too close to the patient. Towels or bubble wrap can be used as thermal protection. A food dye added to the fluid bag will be a visual aid that it is not to be infused. Fluid bags can be reheated multiple times, but 'hot hands' should be discarded when cooled.
Heat lamps	Should be used with caution. They must be used with extreme care if the animal is recumbent and unable to move away from the heat. Lamps can become very hot and there is a risk of overheating the patient, contact burns if the bulb is touched and shattering of the bulb if it comes into contact with water. Heat lamps should only be used in areas where constant supervision can be provided.
Circulating warmed air systems (Figure 14.45)	Are now commonly available for purchase or hire. These systems provide a safe, thermoregulated source of warmed air that is circulated through a special blanket, allowing the air to escape through small holes and circulate around the patient. Various sized blankets are available for different sizes of patient and can be positioned either under or over the patient. These systems are extremely effective.

14.41 Sources of supplementary warmth for small animals.

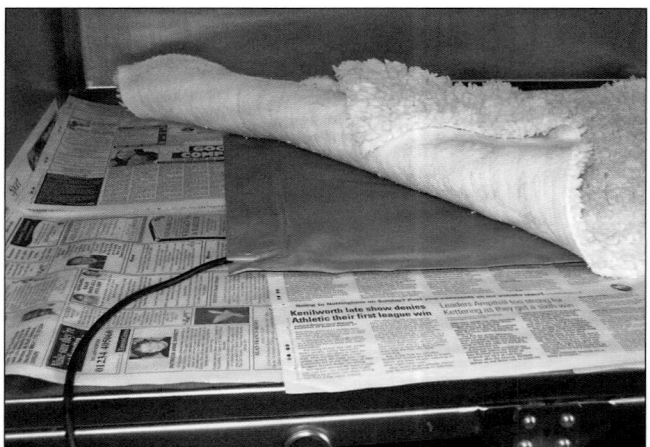

14.43   A heat pad placed under fleece bedding.

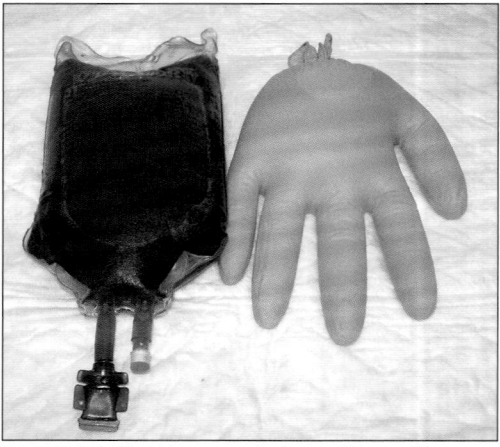

14.44   Fluid bags and gloves filled with warm water may be useful for short-term use in warming recumbent or anaesthetized patients.

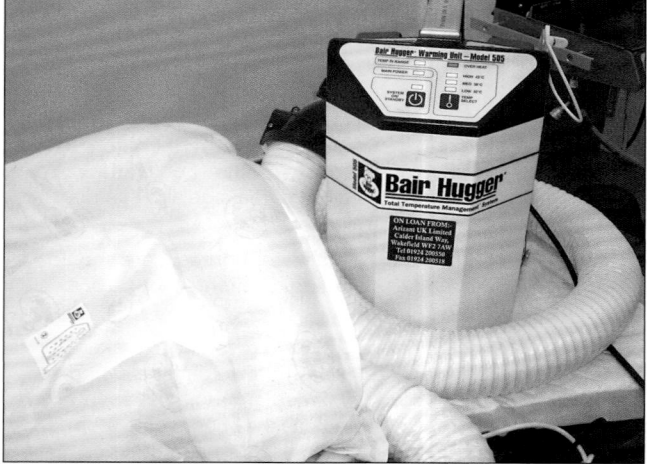

14.45   A circulating warmed air system is an efficient way to provide supplementary warmth.

Hygiene

Strict hygiene protocols and fundamental infection control procedures should be in place to support the nursing of animals in a hospital environment. Good hand hygiene should be implemented and gloves should be worn at all times when dealing with patients. Patients should be assessed on a regular basis and any abnormalities should be noted in their hospital record.

Urine and faecal soiling should be removed as soon as possible. Patients that are left in contact with soiled material or bedding may develop urinary or faecal scalds. In addition, some patients may become distressed as a result of soiling their kennel. The patient should be bathed, if appropriate, to prevent skin irritation and a barrier cream applied if necessary.

Vomit, regurgitation or excessive salivation should be removed with damp swabs. Patients with facial or oral fractures should have their faces wiped and groomed daily as they are unable to complete this task themselves. These patients often benefit from extensive TLC; one of the most important roles of the veterinary nurse.

Surgical wounds, abrasions, wound and chest drains, feeding tubes, indwelling urinary catheters and intravenous catheter sites should be examined twice daily for any signs of infection (see Chapter 23). Bandages and dressings that become wet must be replaced to prevent strikethrough; this is the process by which bacteria can wick through the wet material and into the wound. Discharges should be cleaned without disturbing the sutures or the wound. A water-resistant barrier cream can be useful to protect the skin against constant wound discharge. Other discharges noted (e.g. ocular) must not be cleaned until directed by the clinical team.

Patients that are not kept clean are at risk of developing a hospital-acquired infection (such as a wound or skin infection). Infection with meticillin-resistant *Staphylococcus aureus* (MRSA) or resistant *Pseudomonas* is a risk in these patients (see Chapter 7).

Provision of food

Every patient requires the appropriate nutrition for its species, breed, life-stage and health status (see Chapter 13). Good nutrition is required for basic metabolic function. Patients that are unwell, recovering from surgery or trauma, or have neoplasia may have additional requirements in order to provide the nutrition needed to repair and protect the body.

Monitoring food intake

Patients that are admitted to the practice for hospitalization should have a daily energy requirement calculated (see Chapter 13). Knowing the daily requirements for food intake will allow easier monitoring of whether or not these are being met (see 'Changes in appetite', above). Food charts can be a useful visual check of how much food a patient has consumed, what food was consumed and how much was left; this allows the patient's intake of food to be monitored over a period of time.

The amount of food consumed by exotic pets may be harder to assess than for dogs and cats; measuring/weighing of the food can assist this process. The provision of fresh food makes it easier to determine how much has been consumed. Dry diets are often scatter fed and some patients may store food, making it difficult to determine how much has been eaten. Rabbits can sometimes appear to be masticating (eating food), but close observation is required to determine whether the food has been eaten.

Observation of the type and amount of faecal matter passed will allow assessment of how efficient the digestive system of the animal is. It is very important to record the faecal passage of rabbits. Caecotroph pellets should not be visible; the rabbit should ingest these overnight. Caecotrophic animals must eat these pellets; if they do not, they are at risk of intestinal stasis. If caecotrophs are not being consumed, then nutritional supplementation and medication must be provided to encourage gut motility.

Choice of diet

Diets that are given to patients within the hospital may be chosen to meet the requirements of their specific illness; however, it should be noted that some animals may develop a behavioural link between the food and the practice. Thus, it may be advisable to introduce specific diets when the patient returns home. It is also important to gather information from owners about the patient's favourite foods and whether they have any allergies or dislikes when they are admitted (see Client questionnaires at the end of the chapter).

Other feeding considerations

Some animals are not affected by the hospital environment and continue to eat well throughout their stay. Other patients may require supportive measures for feeding. There are various nursing considerations that can be implemented to encourage voluntary food intake:

- Reduce stressors such as noise and other patients in the ward
- Ensure the animal has appropriate analgesia
- Offer the patient its normal diet or favourite foods
- Increase palatability by warming the foods
- Do not place food and water bowls by litter trays
- On admission determine what type of bowl the animal prefers to eat from (e.g. plastic or metal)
- Use wide shallow bowls for small mammals; being able to see over the bowl whilst eating can decrease their feeling of vulnerability
- Some dogs may prefer to eat their food outside the kennel
- Some cats may prefer hiding whilst eating; cover the kennel to give them some privacy
- Groom the animal prior to eating (if appropriate); this can sometimes work as an appetite stimulant
- Spend time with the animal provide TLC and handfeeding (Figure 14.46)
- Remove the food if it is obvious that the patient does not like it
- Offer small amounts of food but not many selections at a time
- Remove any uneaten food from dogs after a short time; feline patients may be more suited to grazing throughout the day.

Assisted feeding

This term generally refers to patients that have feeding tubes in place to ensure that their nutritional requirements are met (see Chapter 13). As the patient starts to eat voluntarily, tube feeding can be reduced or used to supplement the voluntary intake. If a patient continues to refuse voluntary feeding, then syringe feeding could be considered; however, this can be stressful for the patient and can increase the risk of aspiration pneumonia. In addition, it should be borne in mind that the technique of placing food on to a paw or directly into the mouth can reinforce the original aversion to food.

Appetite stimulants

Anorexia is not normally a primary condition and a thorough investigation of the cause of inappetence should be undertaken. However, even with treatment, the patient may still show no appetite. In these cases, drugs such as diazepam and mirtazapine can be used as appetite stimulants for a short period of time. Assisted feeding may prove more beneficial for these patients.

Provision of water

All patients within the hospital should have free access to water at all times, unless advised otherwise by the clinical team (e.g. when a water deprivation test is being performed or the patient is awaiting anaesthesia). It is important to ask the owner on admission how water is normally provided, as this may affect intake. For example, small mammals may be used to a bottle/bowl and some cats may prefer dripping water than a bowl. In these cases, a water fountain may be beneficial. Some patients may benefit from provision of an elevated water supply (Figure 14.47).

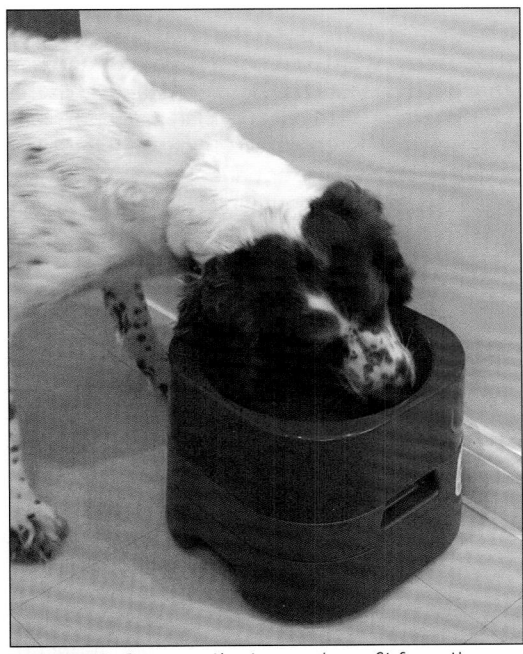

14.47 Some patients may benefit from the provision of an elevated water or food supply.

Exercise

Although unnecessary interaction with hospital patients should be avoided due to infection risks, time spent away from the kennel may further stimulate the patient. Outdoor or out of kennel exercise, fresh air and a change of scene, even for non-ambulatory animals, should be encouraged. Dogs should be given the chance to urinate and defecate at regular intervals throughout the day; many of these patients will have been trained not to soil in the house, so may become very stressed if soiling in the kennel environment. Some

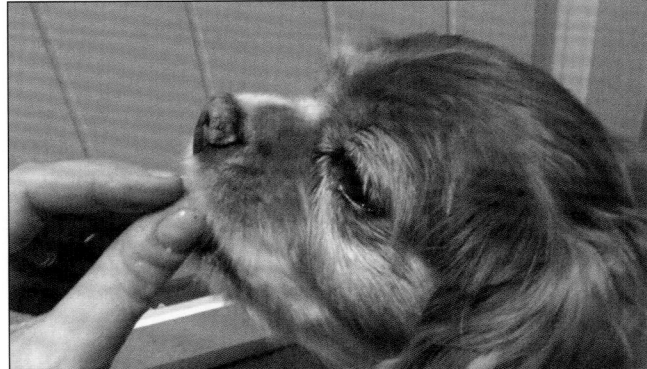

14.46 Handfeeding a dog that had been anorexic for 24 hours. Hand feeding can stimulate the animal to eat.

animals may become agitated or vocal when needing to go to the toilet. Patients suffering from polyuria (see above) will need more frequent opportunities to go outside.

Human interaction

Patient stimulation and interaction with people is important when the animal is hospitalized. If the animal is kept in a caged environment for long periods of time, boredom or self-trauma may occur.

All patients, but specifically those that are young, recumbent or intelligent (e.g. parrots), may benefit from human contact and the use of toys that promote behaviour. Educational toys, such as those that release food as a reward if moved around, and indestructible toys are useful. Consideration must be given to using toys brought in from home, and to the risk of infection from cross-contamination with toys and bedding.

Patients that are not responding well to the hospital environment and are subdued or anorexic may benefit from a visit from their owners. This can be beneficial to both parties and can encourage the animal to eat and provide mental stimulation for the animal.

Anorexic patients can be stimulated to eat in the presence of their owners; however, consideration must be given to the fact that these patients may become very withdrawn and subdued when the owners leave and thus whether a visit is suitable.

Rest

It is important that patients are given the chance to rest and have undisturbed sleep. Ward environments are often busy and noisy, with many hospitals having night staff within the wards. This can interfere with the normal day and night patterns that the animal is used to. Critical patients that require high levels of monitoring, or patients that are undergoing diagnostic tests (such as hourly blood glucose measurement), will all need a time that they can sleep. Many owners often report that their animals are exhausted when returning from the hospital.

Special considerations in older animals

Geriatric animals do not adapt as quickly to changes in routine and environment as younger animals. Many older patients that spend most of the day at home sleeping, can find it difficult to acclimatize to a hospital ward. Older patients should be treated and restrained more gently and may require additional assistance getting into and out of the kennel.

Older patients may also suffer with sensory loss and some animals may have altered sight and/or hearing. It is important for these animals that routines are followed and additional time should be allocated to provide the full support required. Any procedures should be carried out with care and the animal must be stimulated to ensure that they are aware that a procedure is about to take place. These patients should be approached and handled in a calm manner at all times.

See Chapter 15 for more information on nursing care of hospitalized geriatric patients.

Special considerations in neonates

Depending on their age and species, neonates will tend to have cycles of activity (Figure 14.48). Careful observation must be completed to ensure that a normal pattern is followed. Neonatal patients require extensive nursing skills and equipment (see Chapter 24).

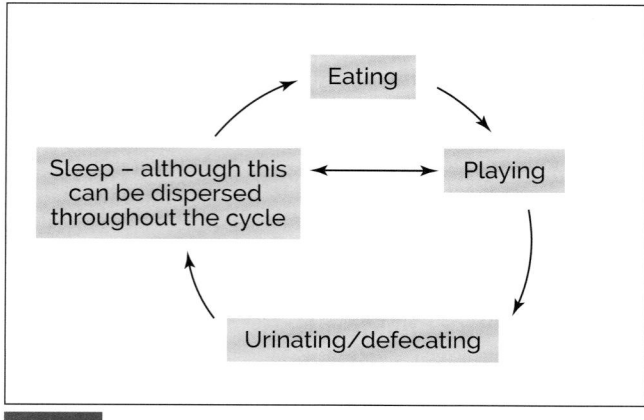

14.48 Activity cycle of young animals.

Daily routine and clinical records

It is important that there are a set of daily protocols (e.g. for feeding, medication, walking and rest of each patient) within the hospital environment. Suitable records, with an appropriate amount of clinical information, need to be kept to demonstrate that these protocols have been completed (see Figures 14.15 and 14.49).

The requirements for the type and frequency of records kept also differ between the different tiers of the RCVS PSS.

RCVS Practice Standards Scheme for daily patient care

Core practice

There must be a documented protocol for the frequency, type and combination of checks for individual patients.

General practice

All hospitalized animals (other than those admitted as day cases for short/routine surgical procedures) must have inpatient sheets that record basic husbandry parameters, with timed and initialled entries (see Figures 14.15 and 14.49 for examples). These parameters include:

- Temperature
- Pulse
- Respiration
- Treatments
- Food and water intake
- Urine and faeces output
- Clinical signs.

Hospital practice

Hospital practices must meet the above criteria plus:

- The practice must have the ability to provide 24-hour inpatient care, including intensive care
- A person directly responsible for the nursing care of inpatients must be within the curtilage of the site at all times
- There must be a minimum of a daily examination of all inpatients by a veterinary surgeon, which should be recorded on the patient records.

However, it is good practice to record a variety of tasks beyond those required by the RCVS PSS.

Inpatient sheet

Client	Mrs Hills	Date/day	09.11.19
Animal	Bramwell	Weight	9 kg
Condition	BSC 1–9 (6) Admit pos gastrointestinal infection	Breed/age	Cavalier King Charles (5 yrs) M(N)

ISOLATION

Checks

Time	HR/pulse	RR	Temp	CPRT	MM colour	Demeanour	Pain score 1–4
9.30	92	22	38.6C	<2 secs	Pink	Quiet, alert, responsive	1–2
12.30	82	18	38.4C	<2 secs	Pink	Quiet, alert, responsive	1

Medication (amount, frequency, route)

Time	SID 1ml Maropitant s/c	SID 10ml Omeprazole po	SID Co-amoxiclav s/c	Q6–8hrs Buprenorphine i/v
9.30	☑ VLB	☑ VLB	☑ VLB 0.45ml	☑ VLB 0.6ml

Comments

Time	E	D	U	F	V	Notes
09/11/19 9.30	NA	NA	✓	✓ D+	✓ +	Admit = Hx vomiting + diarrhoea. Slight dehydration. Provide water, iv fluids (Hartman n's 0.5l) 2ml/kg/hr rate
11.30	NA	NA	X	✓ D+	✓ +	Passed diarrhoea ++ and vomit within kennel. Kennel cleaned, iv site monitored, feathers cut on legs
12.30	NA	Small	X	X	X	Monitoring QAR, TPR taken, no vomit/diarrhoea, so given 50mls water in bowl, monitor 1 hour

Fluid therapy

Placed	℞ fore iv cannula
Type	Hartmann's
Rate (1st)	2ml/kg/hr
Rate (2nd)	

Bloods required	Taken
PCV 42%	09/11/19
Glu 5 mmol/l	09/11/19
TP 70 gl/l	09/11/19

Vet contact owner	am		pm	
Booked out	am	/	pm	/

14.49 An example of an inpatient monitoring form that should be completed for each patient.

Daily tasks that should be documented and recorded

- Record temperature, pulse and respiration – these are essential vital signs and it is best if the patient is calm prior to completing these assessments
- Record bodyweight on a weight chart – if a 10% weight loss is identified, consideration must be given to providing nutritional support
- Evaluate the mental state of the patient – is the animal BAR, QAR, progressing or deteriorating
- Provide the animal with the opportunity to go outside and exercise – 3–4 times a day is recommended for dogs
- Assess any wounds – the wound should be showing signs of healing. If there are any signs of infection, the clinical team should be informed. Dressings and bandages should be changed as required
- Monitor for signs of pain and discomfort – this should be performed continually throughout the day and analgesic protocols amended if necessary
- Administer any prescribed medications (see Chapter 8)
- Provide nutrition, unless the animal is nil by mouth. The correct amount of the right type of food should be calculated and fed to the patient. The quantity of food consumed by the animal should be recorded
- Care of intravenous cannulae – peripheral intravenous catheters should be flushed regularly and checked for patency (see Chapter 20). The insertion sites should be checked for any signs of infection. Cannulae should be removed and replaced if necessary
- Care of wound drains, cavity drains and feeding tubes – insertion sites should be checked at least twice daily and bandaged when required (see Chapter 15). Drained fluid should be measured and the volume recorded
- Physiotherapy should be performed on recumbent or inactive patients to ensure good circulation and lymphatic drainage (see Chapter 15) – this is usually undertaken 2–4 times a day (Figure 14.50)

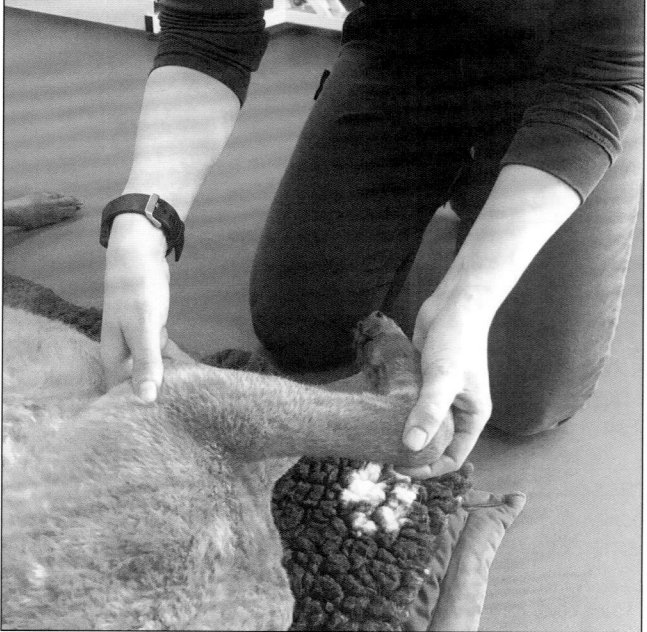

14.50 Physiotherapy should be provided on a daily basis for recumbent or inactive patients.

Grooming and bathing

Maintaining the cleanliness of the patient is essential to its clinical care and wellbeing. Such care may include bathing, grooming and clipping of the coat. Grooming should be performed on a regular basis, not only when soiling makes it necessary; self-grooming is often part of the animal's natural behaviour and suggests that they are comfortable in the environment. Patients that are stressed, anxious or extremely unwell may not groom themselves. Some species may have special grooming requirements; for example, chinchillas have fine, dense fur that can become matted and greasy when handled, so a sand bath should always be provided in their cage.

Reasons for grooming and bathing patients

The importance of grooming and bathing can be summarized by the acronym CHAIRS:

- Cleanliness
- Health
- Appearance
- Inspection
- Relationships
- Showing.

A hospitalized patient requires grooming to keep them free from debris and to provide mental stimulation and comfort. It can be completed in a systematic way, enabling a physical assessment of the patient to be carried out at the same time. Bathing (see Figure 14.53) may be useful for the management of specific skin conditions, especially in cases where medicated shampoos or topical treatments are required. Grooming and bathing may also be recommended before extensive surgical procedures are performed. Bathing and clipping areas will disturb the natural skin flora and should be completed at least 24–48 hours prior to the surgery.

Regular grooming throughout the patient's stay in hospital will ensure that the animal is in a presentable condition when they are discharged. Prior to being returned to their owner, the patient should be checked to ensure that they are clean and there are no areas of soiling or discharge. Owners are very conscious of the condition of their pet, so sending it home in a clean and tidy condition promotes the image of a caring professional environment.

The grooming and bathing of animals is a skilled job; veterinary nurses must be able to perform basic grooming and bathing tasks to maintain the cleanliness and hygienic condition of their patients. Clipping, stripping and de-matting of animals requires advanced knowledge and the correct use of grooming equipment.

Variations in coat types

There is a wide variation in coat types (Figure 14.51) between breeds and species; many breeds are recognizable by their coat and shape (see Appendix 1). The coat type of the patient will influence the amount of grooming and care required to keep it in good condition. Breeds with longer, thicker hair will require more intensive grooming techniques.

Cat coats are broadly divided into two types: long hair and short hair. These coats are made up of different types of hair:

- Guard hairs – these are long coarse hairs that make up the outer coat layer; they taper into a point to protect the undercoat. They are connected to the autonomic nervous system and respond to sensory information
- Awn hairs – these are intermediate length hairs (i.e. shorter than guard hairs but longer than down hairs). These hairs are the most visible of the coat, they help with insulation and protect the coat
- Down hairs – these are fine, soft fluffy hairs that are closest to the skin. They help to trap air and insulate the animal.

The amount and distribution of the hair depends on the breed; for example, the Sphynx cat is not considered to have any hair, however, they actually have a very fine covering of down hair, and the curly coat of the Devon Rex comprises curly awn hair and no guard hairs.

Changes in the animal's coat coincide with the natural seasonal changes and changes in daylight. Spring days initiate the production of the less dense summer coat and shedding of the winter coat. In the autumn, the reverse occurs; the thicker winter coat is produced and the lighter summer coat is shed. Seasonal coat changes are seen more often in animals that live outdoors; animals that live indoors are affected by environmental temperature (e.g. due to central heating) and tend to shed permanently. Endocrinological disorders such as Cushing's syndrome and hypothyroidism can cause coat changes in the dog. Animals that are fed an inadequate diet also have visible coat changes.

Useful advice for owners on grooming:

- Introduce at an early age
- Start with short sessions and slowly increase
- Start with the hand, then replace with a suitable brush
- Make the experience fun – use toys or titbits
- Include a physical examination at the same time
- Always reward good behaviour.

Grooming small animals

There is a wide range of grooming equipment available, but a selection of basic brushes and combs is suitable for the grooming needs of most small animal patients (Figure 14.52). Dedicated grooming areas and specialized equipment, such as grooming tables and walk in baths, are not normally found in most veterinary practices. Larger patients can be groomed in a quiet area of the ward; small recumbent patients can be groomed within their kennel. It should be remembered that some patients are unwell or uncomfortable, so gentle techniques must be used at all times. The patient's temperament and patience also needs careful consideration. The patient's coat type should be evaluated, along with areas that may need extra attention, such as sores or warts, in order to select the appropriate types of brushes and combs to be used. De-matting tools should only be used by staff that are confident and competent with their use.

Bathing patients

Bathing may be required to remove soiling from the coat of the animal, in order to maintain hygiene and cleanliness in the hospital environment (Figure 14.53). Bathing may also be required to apply topical medication to a patient's skin (e.g. treatment for demodectic or sarcoptic mange) or to use medicated shampoos for conditions such as *Malassezia* infection and skin hypersensitivities (see Chapter 18). Specialist equipment is required for those animals that have come

Coat	Type	Examples
Smooth coat	Short length and close to the body; minimal maintenance to keep clean	Boxer, Dachshund, Chihuahua, short-haired German Shepherd Dog, Corgi
Wire coat	Top coat is harsh and thick, softer undercoat; some breeds require hand-stripping to maintain the correct coat condition. With many breeds it proves easier to clip them to keep them clean and hygienic	Wire-haired terriers
Double coat	Long topcoat, thick, soft undercoat. Some of the breeds with this type of coat may be trimmed into a short style to aid coat care and cleanliness	Rough Collie and long-haired German Shepherd Dog
Silky coat	Varies in length from medium to long with a fine texture	Spaniels, setters, some retrievers, Afghan Hound, Bearded Collie
Woolly coat	Many breeds could be described as having a wool coat; these require special trimming	Poodle, Bedlington Terrier, Curly-coated Retriever, Irish Water Spaniel
Felt	Maintenance of the coat focusses on ensuring the felts are not too wide and maintaining skin condition with regular grooming and bathing. This is especially important in the first 3 years of life whilst the coat is developing	Bergamasco
Corded	There are various types of cord, from small rounded ones to a wider, flatter ribbon type. The cords need to be kept clean and dust free. Regular bathing will benefit both cords and skin	Hungarian Puli, Komondor

14.51 Most canine coat types can be divided into seven broad groups for the purposes of grooming.

Equipment	Features and use
Slicker brush 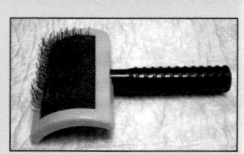	Can be used with all coat types except smooth coats. Fine directional bent pins remove loose hair. Correct use of the brush is required to avoid skin abrasion by the pins. Only light pressure should be applied to a brush that is positioned flatly against the coat in small sections to allow access to the undercoat. The pins on new brushes can be harsh and care should be taken not to damage the skin until the pins have 'relaxed'
Deep pin brush 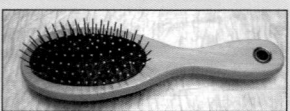	Long metal pins with rounded ends that protect the skin. Useful for thick double coats and long silky coats
Soft-bore bristle brush 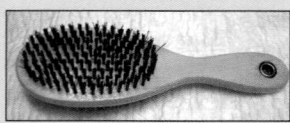	Often found on the reverse side of a deep pin brush. Firm bristles good for wire coats and removing dried dirt from short coats, less useful for thicker longer coats as bristles may be too dense to separate coat
Combs 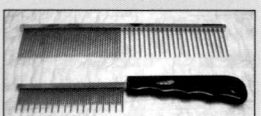	Variety of wire-toothed combs, with variation in tooth position and length. Suitable for all coats except smooth coats. Usually used after brushing to smooth coat and remove remaining knots, especially in longer coats
Rubber comb 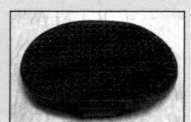	Used in smooth-coated breeds to remove undercoat and smooth the topcoat
Shedding blade 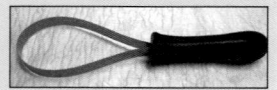	Used to remove dead hair and hairs on the verge of shedding. Useful on short- and longer-coated breeds. Smaller blades can be used for cats. Double-sided with different sized teeth. Excessive pressure should be avoided so as not to damage the skin
Undercoat rake 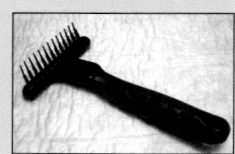	Used with thicker and double coats to remove dead undercoat and untangle small knots and matts. Light pressure should be used as the metal pins can be abrasive if pulled along the skin
Coat king 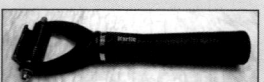	Used for thinning out coats. A selection of different sized blades is available with variable sized teeth. Mostly used by professional groomers as care is needed not to remove too much coat
Matt breaker 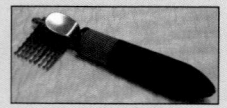	These tools break through knots and matts, they should not pull them out. Care is required as teeth and blades may cut the skin if used incorrectly
Stripping stone 	Light 'airy' pumice type stone that is used for hand stripping wire-coated breeds
Scissors 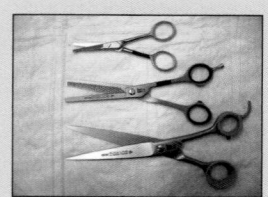	Wide variety of sizes and styles are available. From top to bottom: safety scissors, with rounded ends for trimming around delicate areas; thinning scissors, used with thicker coats; trimming scissors, used for finishing coats

14.52 Grooming equipment for small mammals.

continues ▶

Equipment	Features and use
Electric and battery clippers 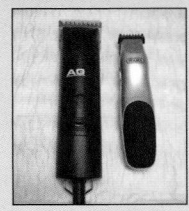	Can be used to trim fur and remove matts safely that are tight to the skin. Avoid using against the skin for extended periods of time as the clipper blade can become hot. Keep clean and well lubricated
Nail clippers 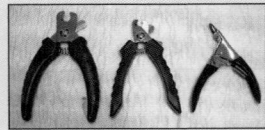	A wide variety of nail clippers is available. Heavy duty clippers may be required for larger breeds' nails. Sharp cutting types may be preferable to guillotine style cutters, which tend to squash the nail when it is cut

14.52 *continued* Grooming equipment for small mammals.

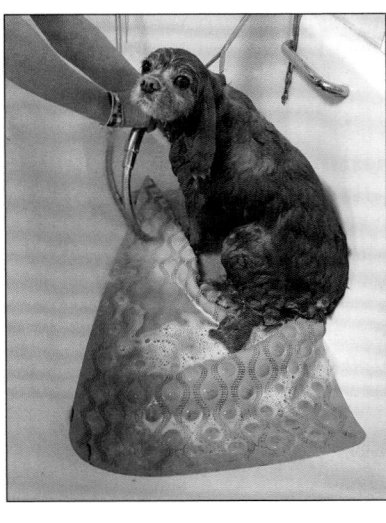

14.53 Bathing can be beneficial in dogs with allergic skin conditions or parasitic infestations, or to generally help maintain cleanliness.

into contact with contaminants such as engine oil, as these substances are difficult to remove. Care should be taken when removing potentially toxic substances, as the use of detergents may increase their absorption through the skin.

Some patients may require bathing of a specific area, such as the feet, perineal area (common in obese and geriatric rabbits) or skin fold areas around the mouth (to treat skin fold dermatitis which affects breeds with large jowl skin, e.g. St Bernard). Each patient should be assessed prior to bathing as this may be contraindicated in certain circumstances:

- Initial days after surgery to prevent contamination of the wound
- In patients with dressings or wounds (such as skin grafts); these require minimal disturbance and should be kept clean and dry
- In patients with unstable fractures
- In the initial days after extensive orthopaedic procedures; if the patient struggles or slips in the bath, damage can occur
- In weak or dyspnoeic patients where stress could exacerbate their condition.

In these special cases, cleanliness can be achieved by 'bed bathing' the patient using a bowl of warm water and cotton wool. Damp cotton wool swabs can also be used to clean ocular and nasal discharges; scabs should never be picked off unless directed by the clinical team. Animals with facial injuries that may be wearing an Elizabethan collar should be cleaned frequently; food and water can drip down the collar and collect around the neck area, causing significant sores.

Bathing small animal patients

Depending on the size of the patient and the equipment available in the veterinary practice, bathing can be performed in a sink or bath (see Figure 14.53) or using a 'tub table' where the patient is placed upon a metal grid supported above the bath. All items required, including towels, shampoo, sponges and jugs, should be prepared in the area of the bath. All baths should have non-slip bottoms to avoid accidental injury to the patient. PPE should be worn at all times, especially when medicated shampoo or topical treatment is being used. Water temperature should be monitored during the procedure to ensure that it is consistent and not too hot.

Bathing a dog

1. Restrain the dog using a slip lead. Patients unfamiliar with bathing should have the lead held by the groomer or an assistant in case they try to jump out, causing injury or possibly strangulation.
2. Wet the patient's coat thoroughly using a shower head or jugs of warm water.
3. Apply the shampoo and massage it into the coat, avoiding the face (medicated washes should be applied with a damp sponge around the facial area in order to prevent the substance from running into the patient's eyes, ears or mouth). Leave the shampoo or medicated wash on for the appropriate contact time (the manufacturer's recommendations should be followed). Gently holding the muzzle of the dog will prevent it from shaking and stop the possible introduction of shampoo into its or the handler's face.
4. Rinse the patient thoroughly, working from the upper body down to the undercarriage and legs; excess water can be squeezed from the coat.
5. Lift the patient out of the bath or move it on to a non-slip absorbent surface to be towel-dried. A hairdryer can be used to dry the patient if tolerated; care should be taken not to burn the patient by holding the hairdryer too close.
6. Once fully dry, the coat can be brushed through and the patient returned to a warm, draught-free environment.

Cleaning ears

The ears of inpatients should be checked regularly and cleaned when required.

1. Check for any aural discharge or inflammation.
2. If dirty, clean each ear with a separate piece of cotton wool and species-specific ear cleaner.
3. Apply a few drops of the cleaner and massage the ear canal.
4. Only clean the vertical ear canal. Never use cotton buds in the horizontal canal as this could cause damage to the inner ear.

Cleaning eyes

The eyes of inpatients should be checked regularly and cleaned when required.

1. Check for any ocular discharge or inflammation.
2. If the eyes require cleaning, warm or sterile water and separate pieces of cotton wool for each eye (to prevent cross-infection) should be used (Figure 14.54).

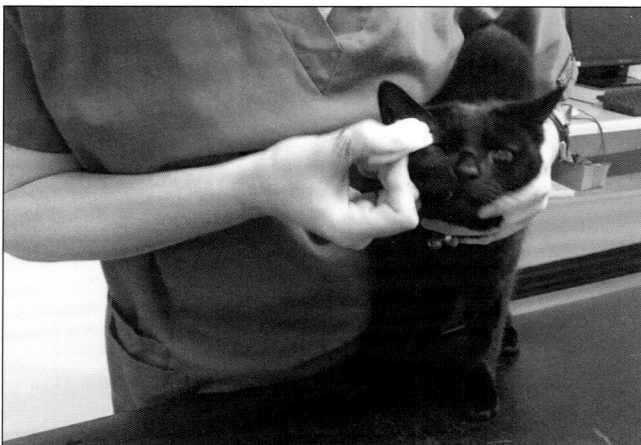

| 14.54 | A cat having its eyes cleaned. A separate piece of cotton wool should be used for each eye to prevent cross-infection. |

Nail clipping

The average healthy animal does not usually require attention to its claws (apart from the dewclaws). The reasons that an animal may require its nails clipping include:

- Animals not exercised on hard ground
- Animals whose normal behaviour or exercise is restricted by their housing or management
- Elderly animals that are unable to exercise normally
- Animals with immobilized fractured limbs
- Animals with injury or disease of the foot or nails
- Previous injury to the foot or leg causing an abnormal gait
- Animals causing damage to the owner's property (this is a controversial reason as training may be a better approach to the problem).

Equipment

The equipment needed for clipping nails includes:

- Nail clippers (the size is dependent on species and breed)
- Styptic (e.g. silver nitrate pencil)
- Restraint equipment (e.g. muzzles and towels).

Specialized nail clippers of various sizes are available, and an appropriate size and strength clipper should be selected for each patient; for example, the nails of a hamster require only small delicate clippers compared with the nails of a Labrador Retriever, which require significantly larger and stronger nail clippers.

To clip the nails, the patient should first be gently restrained; commonly an assistant is required. Small animals may benefit from being held firmly in a towel in order to prevent injury (Figure 14.55). The patient's digit should be firmly held and the nail examined to determine whether trimming is required. The hard part of the nail is an extension of the epidermis and varies in colour from transparent to pigmented. Beneath this layer is the dermis, which contains the blood and nerve supply to the nail and will be painful to the patient if cut. Transparent nails often allow visualization of the dermis, which aids in deciding how far to cut the nail. Clipping of pigmented nails should be performed with care; small trimmings at a time should be taken.

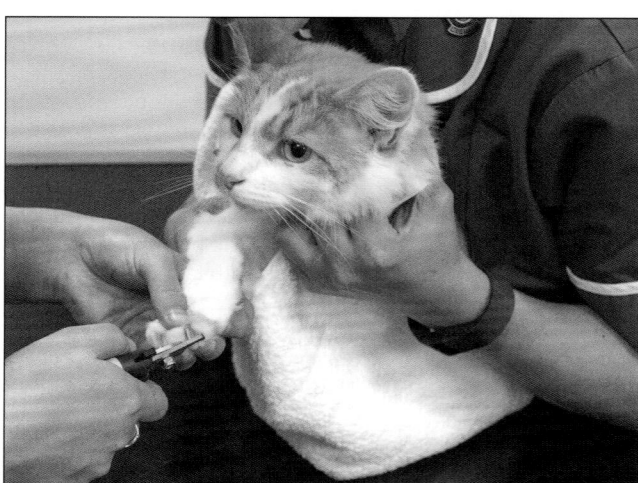

| 14.55 | A cat wrapped in a towel being restrained by a veterinary nurse for nail clipping. |

Examples of client questionnaires

Client Questionnaire – Canine Patients

It would be helpful if you could take a few minutes to tell us a little bit about your dog. Coming into hospital can be a stressful time, and some dogs will develop behaviours or signs that can affect our interpretation of their recovery from disease or surgery. By knowing more about your dog's general routines and personality, we will be able to care more for his/her individual needs during his/her stay with us.

Dog's name _____   **Your surname:** _____

Personality

How does your dog get on with people? _____

How does your dog get on with other dogs? _____

Is your dog shy at home? _____

Does your dog get stressed easily? _____

Other comments: _____

Toilet habits

Where does your dog prefer to urinate at home?   Anywhere ☐   Grass ☐   Gravel ☐   Bushes ☐

Will your dog go to the toilet when walked on lead?   Yes ☐   No ☐

Toilet command (if any) _____

Other comments: _____

Diet

What is your dog's normal diet? _____

What is your dog's favourite snack? _____

Would you be surprised if your dog chose not to eat while in hospital?   Yes ☐   No ☐

How often do you feed your dog? _____

Other comments: _____

Vaccinations

Are your dog's vaccinations current?   Yes ☐   No ☐

When did your dog last receive a kennel cough vaccine (given into the nose)? _____

*Note: If your dog has **not** received kennel cough vaccination within the last six months, it is our policy to administer this to all dogs that are in sufficiently good health and are likely to stay 3 nights or more. There is no charge for this vaccination. Although this will not eliminate the chance of your dog developing kennel cough, we have found it does reduce the incidence of outbreaks within our hospital. **If you would rather your dog did NOT receive this vaccination, please speak with your clinician during the consultation.***

Example of a client questionnaire for admission of canine patients. (Courtesy of Davies Veterinary Specialists)

Client Questionnaire – Feline Patients

Coming into hospital can be a stressful time, and some cats will develop behaviours or signs that can affect our interpretation of their recovery from disease or surgery. By knowing more about your cat's general routines and personality, we will be able to care more for his/her individual needs during his/her stay with us.

We try and provide our cat patients with an environment which attempts to reduce the stress they may experience while in hospital. They are kept in a ward away from dogs, and noise in the ward is kept to a minimum. Soft classical music is also played, as this has been shown to have a calming effect. Timid cats may have a box in their cage where they can hide away if they wish. Feline pheromone sprays and 'plug-ins' are used throughout the ward as these have also been shown to reduce anxiety.

It would be helpful if you could take a few minutes to tell us a little bit about your cat.

Cat's name ....   **Your surname:** ....

Personality

How does your cat get on with people? ....

What type of bedding does your cat prefer? ....

Does your cat like being groomed? ....

Other comments: ....

Toilet habits

Will your cat use a litter tray? ....   Yes ☐   No ☐

What type of cat litter does your cat prefer? ....   Soil ☐   Woodchip ☐   Gravel ☐

Other comments: ....

Diet

What does your cat normally eat? ....

Does your cat prefer to be offered single meals, or does he/she prefer to 'graze' through the day? ....

What is your cat's favourite treat? ....

Does your cat drink out of a water bowl? ....   Yes ☐   No ☐

Other comments: ....

Vaccinations

Are your cat's vaccinations current? ....   Yes ☐   No ☐

Example of a client questionnaire for admission of feline patients. (Courtesy of Davies Veterinary Specialists)

Client Questionnaire – Rabbit Patients

Coming into hospital can be a stressful time, and some rabbits will develop behaviours or signs that can affect our interpretation of their recovery from disease or surgery. By knowing more about your rabbit's general routines and personality, we will be able to care more for his/her individual needs during his/her stay with us.

We try and provide our rabbit patients with an environment which attempts to reduce the stress they may experience while in hospital. They are kept in a ward away from cats and dogs, and noise in the ward is kept to a minimum. We provide them with hiding places to provide comfort.

It would be helpful if you could take a few minutes to tell us a little bit about your rabbit.

Rabbit's name .... **Your surname:** ....

Personality

How does your rabbit get on with people? ....

What type of bedding does your rabbit prefer? ....

Does your rabbit like being groomed? ....

Other comments: ....

Toilet habits

Will your rabbit use a litter tray? .... Yes ☐ No ☐

What type of litter does your rabbit prefer? .... Soil ☐ Woodchip ☐ Gravel ☐

Other comments: ....

Diet

What does your rabbit normally eat? ....

What is your rabbit's favourite treat? ....

Does your rabbit drink out of a water bowl or bottle Bowl ☐ Bottle ☐

Other comments: ....

Vaccinations

Are your rabbit's vaccinations current? .... Yes ☐ No ☐

Example of a client questionnaire for admission of rabbit/lapine patients.

References and further reading

Asres A and Amha N (2014) Effects of stress on animal health: a review. *Journal of Biology, Agriculture and Healthcare* **4**, 116–121

Bassert J, Thomas J and McCurnin D (2014) *McCurnin's Clinical Textbook for Veterinary Technicians*. Saunders Elsevier, Missouri

Birchard S and Sherding R (2006) *Saunders Manual of Small Animal Practice*. Saunders Elsevier, Missouri

Blood D, Gay C and Studdert V (2012) *Saunders Comprehensive Veterinary Dictionary*. Saunders Elsevier, London

Bowes V (2015) Making sense of nursing care models. *Veterinary Practice Today* **3**, 20–22

Carter C (2014) Reducing patient stress: considerations for nurses. *Veterinary Nursing Journal* **29**, 362–364

Dugdale A (2011) *Veterinary Anaesthesia*. Wiley, New York

Goic JB, Reineke EL and Drobatz KJ (2014) Comparison of rectal and axillary temperatures in dogs and cats. *Journal of the American Veterinary Medical Association* **244**, 1170

Girling S (2013) *Veterinary Nursing of Exotic Pets*. Wiley, New York

Haskey E (2015a) *Nursing the critical patient: Part 1. Veterinary Nursing Journal* **30**, 16–21

Haskey E (2015b) Nursing the critical patient. Part 2: case history. *Veterinary Nursing Journal* **30**, 47–50

Hotston-Moore A and Rudd S (2008) *BSAVA Manual of Canine and Feline Advanced Veterinary Nursing*. BSAVA Publications, Gloucester

Hotston-Moore P and Hughes A (2007) *BSAVA Manual of Practical Animal Care*. BSAVA Publications, Gloucester

Keeble E and Meredith A (2009) *BSAVA Manual of Rodents and Ferrets*. BSAVA Publications, Gloucester

Lamb V and McBrearty AR (2013) Comparison of rectal, tympanic membrane and axillary temperature measurement methods in dogs. *Veterinary Record* **173**, 524

Lawrence K (2006) Canine mobility and physiotherapy. *Veterinary Nursing Journal* **21**, 24–26

Maughan J (2012) The essentials of patient care. In: *The Complete Textbook of Veterinary Nursing, 2nd edn.*, ed. V Aspinall, pp. 247–268. Elsevier, London

Meredith A and Johnson-Delaney C (2010) *BSAVA Manual of Exotic Pets, 5th edn.* BSAVA Publications, Gloucester

Meredith A and Lord B (2014) *BSAVA Manual of Rabbit Medicine.* BSAVA Publications, Gloucester

Millis DL and Levine D (2013) *Canine Rehabilitation and Physical Therapy, 2nd edn.* Saunders, Philadelphia

Opperman E (2004) The recumbent patient. *Veterinary Nursing Journal* **19(5)**, 164–166

Orpet H and Welsh P (2011) *Handbook of Veterinary Nursing*. Wiley, Chichester

Siracusa C, Manteca X and Cuenca R (2010) Effect of a synthetic appeasing pheromone on behavioural, neuroendocrine, immune and acute-phase perioperative stress responses in dogs. *Journal of the American Veterinary Medical Association* **237**, 673–681

Sirois M, Castle Boyer S and Sirois M (2013) *Workbook for Elsevier's Veterinary Assisting Textbook.* Elsevier Mosby, Missouri

Urquhart C (2001) Appreciating the needs of elderly in patients. *Veterinary Nursing Journal* **16(6)**, 206

Varga M, Lumbis R and Gott L (2012) *BSAVA Manual of Exotic Pet and Wildlife Nursing.* BSAVA Publications, Gloucester

Welsh L (2013) *Anaesthesia for Veterinary Nurses.* Wiley, New York

Useful websites

Animal Welfare Act 2006:
http://adlib.everysite.co.uk/adlib/defra/content.aspx?id=000HK277ZX.0FG51IZNV9M42

International Cat Care:
https://icatcare.org/isfm

Royal College of Veterinary Surgeons (RCVS) Code of Professional Conduct for Veterinary Nurses:
www.rcvs.org.uk/advice-and-guidance/code-of-professional-conduct-for-veterinary-nurses/

Royal College of Veterinary Surgeons (RCVS) Practice Standards Scheme:
www.rcvs.org.uk/practice-standards-scheme/

Self-assessment questions

1. Identify six measures that can be used to minimize stress during hospitalization of small animals, birds and exotics.
2. Why is it important to perform a complete examination of the patient on admission?
3. Produce a systematic list for a full clinical examination.
4. What is considered the normal colour of mucous membranes? List the abnormal colours and the disease states these could be indicative of.
5. List the different sites for assessing CRT. What information can CRT provide regarding the patient's health status?
6. Identify and describe five clinical parameters that can be used to help assess the degree of dehydration in the small animal patient.
7. Identify and describe four other nursing methods that can be used to provide comfort to animals in addition to using pain relief drugs.
8. Draw a picture of a dog; indicate the sites where you would take a pulse.
9. Define the following terms: pyrexia, hypothermia, tachycardia, tachypnoea, bradycardia and bradypnoea.
10. What methods of assessing cardiac function are included in a routine clinical examination?
11. Why is it important for patients to be identified within the veterinary hospital? What are the two key methods for identifying patients?
12. List the eight key methods that may be used to provide supplementary warmth to a hospitalized patient.
13. Discuss the potential problems that could be associated with a recumbent patient.
14. Identify six factors that could influence the voluntary food intake of a hospitalized patient.
15. Why is it important for clinical staff to have all behavioural details prior to the patient being admitted to the hospital ward? What mental support could be provided to an animal whilst hospitalized?
16. What are the four main reasons for grooming a patient during hospitalization?

Chapter 15

Nursing interventions in hospitalized animals

Stuart Ford-Fennah and Elizabeth Mullineaux with complementary therapies by Helen Mathie

Learning objectives

After studying this chapter, readers will have the knowledge to:

- **Apply the principles of bandaging including the reasons for bandaging, basic bandage selection, application and care**
- **Select appropriate dressing materials and apply standard bandaging techniques to the limbs, head, body and tail of small animals**
- **Describe the different types of drain available and their management**
- **Select equipment for, and carry out, enemas**
- **Describe the different types of catheter available for urinary catheterization and their uses**
- **Recognize the situations for which oxygen supplementation may be required and describe the different types of equipment that can be used to provide oxygen supplementation**
- **List the more commonly recognized complementary therapies and their uses**
- **Describe the general nursing requirements for a range of patients, including those that are geriatric, neonatal, vomiting, soiled, recumbent or critically ill**

Nursing interventions

Bandages and dressings

The ability to dress a wound correctly or place an effective bandage can make the difference between success and failure for any given surgical or non-surgical intervention where these are required. Bandages and dressings can *create* wounds, or make existing wounds worse, if applied incorrectly or without due care. To be able to apply appropriate dressings and bandages to wounds it is essential to have knowledge of the way in which wounds heal, as this will affect their management (see Chapter 23).

Veterinary nurses should be able to:

- Recognize the different types of wound
- Select correct materials appropriate to dress the wound
- For standard, uncomplicated applications, apply materials in the correct order and manner, resulting in an effective bandage
- Monitor for and recognize bandage-related problems
- Instruct owners on care and observation of the bandage
- Assist with application of specialized bandages.

Indications for bandaging

Bandaging is used to:

- Hold dressings in place
- Provide support for:
  - Fractures or dislocations
  - Sprains or strains
  - Healing wounds.
- Provide protection against:
  - Self-mutilation
  - Infection
  - The environment
  - Further injury.
- Provide even pressure to:
  - Arrest haemorrhage
  - Prevent or control swelling.
- Immobilize to:
  - Restrict joint movement
  - Restrict movement at fracture site
  - Provide comfort and pain relief.
- Protect indwelling devices (e.g. intravenous catheters).

Bandaging and dressing materials

Primary (contact) bandage layer

The primary or contact layer of a bandage is usually some form of dressing, which is applied directly to the wound before any other materials. Dressings prevent subsequent layers from sticking to, or contaminating, the wound area, as well as creating a suitable environment for wound healing. The choice of dressing depends upon the wound type (see Chapter 23); dressings may be adherent or non-adherent to the wound, and be absorbent or non-absorbent. Dressings are also described in terms of how 'occlusive' they are (occlusive, semi-occlusive, non-occlusive) to air (gas/vapour) and moisture. Dressings are invariably sterile and need to be handled in a sterile manner to avoid contamination, especially of the surface which will be in contact with the wound. There are many different dressings available, some examples of which are given in Figure 15.1. More information on the uses of different dressing types is given in Chapter 23.

Secondary bandage layer

The secondary layer of a bandage is there to hold the primary layer in place, provide padding and, where necessary, absorb exudate and/or apply even pressure to the wound to prevent swelling. Types of padding material are described in Figure 15.2. The padding layer is usually secured

Dressing type	Description	Uses/comments	Examples
Dry and adherent	Plain gauze swabs	Debridement of wounds Can be used 'dry-to-dry' or 'wet-to-dry' (saline-soaked)	Millswabs™ sterile (Millpledge)
Semi-occlusive	Usually with a layer of permeable non-stick material on one or both sides and a central absorbent core; may have an adhesive section around the edge to enable accurate, stable placement	Surgical wounds Wounds with mild to moderate discharges	Primapore™ (Smith and Nephew) OPSITE™ Post-Op (Smith and Nephew)
Absorbent	Made of various materials. Usually thicker than a semi-occlusive dressing and often with a coloured side that faces the wound; may have an adhesive section around the edge to enable accurate placement	Large wounds where there is a large amount of exudate; helps to remove fluid from wound area whilst preventing drying at the wound surface	Allevyn™ (Smith and Nephew) Biatain® (Coloplast)
Hydrogels	Gel-based dressing sheet, or gels alone, that need to be used in conjunction with other dressings	Where maintenance of moisture is essential (granulating wounds) Where there is a large deficit beneath the skin level that is difficult to dress in any other manner Used for wounds that are leaking little or no fluid Can be used on burns and necrotic wounds Designed to maximize patient comfort and reduce pain	Intrasite™ (Smith and Nephew) Manuka (Kruuse) Activon® Tulle (Advancis)
Impregnated	■ Petroleum gel ■ Antibiotic ■ Silver-impregnated ■ Iodine-impregnated	Superficial open wounds; have specific properties proven to help to prevent infections and encourage speed of healing	■ Jelonet™ (Smith and Nephew) ■ Bactigras™ (Smith and Nephew) ■ Acticoat™ (Smith and Nephew) ■ Iodoflex™ (Smith and Nephew)

15.1 Examples of types of primary wound dressings.

Type	Description	Uses/comments	Examples
Cotton wool	Natural or man-made absorbent material in rolls	Can be used as sole padding material in most bandages Can be difficult to apply compared with others	Millsoft™ (Millpledge)
Padding bandage	Natural absorbent material supplied in rolls of various sizes	Preferable to cotton wool in most cases due to ease of application Particularly good for limbs	Orthowool™ Vet (Millpledge)
Synthetic padding	Supplied in rolls of various sizes; thinner and lighter	Good where less bulk is needed (e.g. under casts, smaller patients) Can cause sweating and is not so absorbent	Soffban™ plus (BSN Medical)
Foam	Variety of thicknesses	Useful when external fixators are bandaged or under drains	Tegaderm™ Foam Adhesive Dressing (3M)
Cotton wool/gauze	Cotton wool sandwiched between gauze layers; supplied in rolls	Very useful for abdomens and thorax bandages; holes may be cut to accommodate legs and prepuce	Equi-Wool™ (Millpledge)

15.2 Examples of types of secondary bandage padding materials.

using a conforming stretch bandage that achieves the correct degree of compression and completes the secondary layer. Conforming materials (Figure 15.3) are supplied in two basic varieties: those with an elastic/latex component and those without. Each manufacturer uses a different design, construction and proportion of elastic/latex. It may be possible to use a cohesive conforming bandage to fulfil both secondary and tertiary (see below) bandage functions in one; however, caution is advised if this is used in a limb bandage as slippage may occur more readily. The use of a cohesive conforming bandage in this way is best restricted to a simple dressing (e.g. an intravenous catheter dressing).

Tertiary bandage layer

The tertiary bandage layer is to protect the underlying layers from dirt, soiling or trauma by the animal. Protective materials may be adhesive or cohesive (Figure 15.4).

Bandaging principles

When applying a bandage, materials must be selected carefully with consideration given to what is required from each layer:

- Is a primary (contact) layer required and if so, what are its functions?
- What is required of the secondary layer (support, absorption, pressure)?
- What level of protection is required from the tertiary layer?

General rules for bandaging:

- Avoid departing from the basic primary/secondary/tertiary layers wherever possible

- Always attempt to include enough padding to provide comfort
- Avoid sticking adhesive material to the skin to prevent bandage slippage; poorly applied previous layers will tend to 'slip' below the adhesive bandage, causing 'drag' on the skin, which may result in skin sores or more serious complications
- The bandage should be firm but never overly tight
- Never leave more than the tips of the toes out on limb bandages
- Ensure that the bandage is achieving its aims (e.g. immobilizing a joint) and that it is comfortable for the patient (i.e. no patient interference, patient able to move easily)
- Check bandages regularly and change if necessary (see 'Management of bandages', below).

Bandaging techniques
Limb bandages

Limb bandages are commonly required in general veterinary practice. They can be used for the distal portion of the limb only (e.g. for cut pads, dew claw removal) or for the entire limb (e.g. many surgical procedures or trauma).

Procedure for lower limb and foot bandages

1. Ensure the patient is suitably restrained.
2. Place cotton wool padding between the patient's toes, pads and dew claws to absorb sweat and prevent irritation (Figure 15.5a). →

Type	Description	Uses/comments	Examples
Loose open weave	Has no elastic component but loose weave aids conforming property	Can be used to hold padding to any area of the body	W.O.W Band™ (Millpledge)
Conforming	Has an elastic component	Designed to provide sustained compression; however, can be placed too tightly. Care needs to be taken during application, especially if not a lot of padding underneath; blood/fluid flow can be compromised, resulting in swelling or death of tissue	Knit-Fix™ (Millpledge)
Tubular	Bandage supplied in a tube construction	Under casts and on the abdomen and thorax; holes can be cut for legs/prepuce	Stretchnet™ (Millpledge)
Crepe	Washable cotton fibre material on a roll	Not commonly used but may be useful to hold small dressings in place on the thorax	Millcrepe™ (Millpledge)

15.3 Example of secondary bandage conforming materials.

Type	Description	Uses/comments	Examples
Adhesive	Thick cotton-based material with an adhesive side; supplied in rolls of various widths	Good for foot bandages (due to thickness); avoid applying direct to skin and hair	Tensoplast® (BSN Medical)
Cohesive	Latex-containing material that 'sticks' to itself but not to skin or hair; supplied in rolls of various widths, colours and designs	Most commonly used protective material; performs well and can be used in any bandaging. Care must be taken as the latex component has a 'memory' and will tighten once in place, especially if stretched too much during application	Co-Form™ (Millpledge) Vetrap™ (3M)

15.4 Description and uses of adhesive and cohesive tertiary bandage protective materials.

Procedure for lower limb and foot bandages *continued*

3. Apply a layer of cotton wool or soft dressing material around the foot. If using pre-rolled padding bandage, apply it longitudinally to the cranial and caudal surfaces of the limb (Figure 15.5b).
4. Twist the bandage to cover the medial and lateral aspects of the foot (Figure 15.5c).
5. Wind it around the foot in a figure-of-eight pattern (Figure 15.5d).
6. Continue up the limb.
7. Apply the conforming bandage, similarly, longitudinally to the cranial and caudal surface of the limb.
8. Wind the conforming bandage around the foot in a figure-of-eight pattern, ensuring even tension throughout (Figure 15.5e).
9. Continue up the limb.
10. Apply the protective layer in the same manner (Figure 15.6).

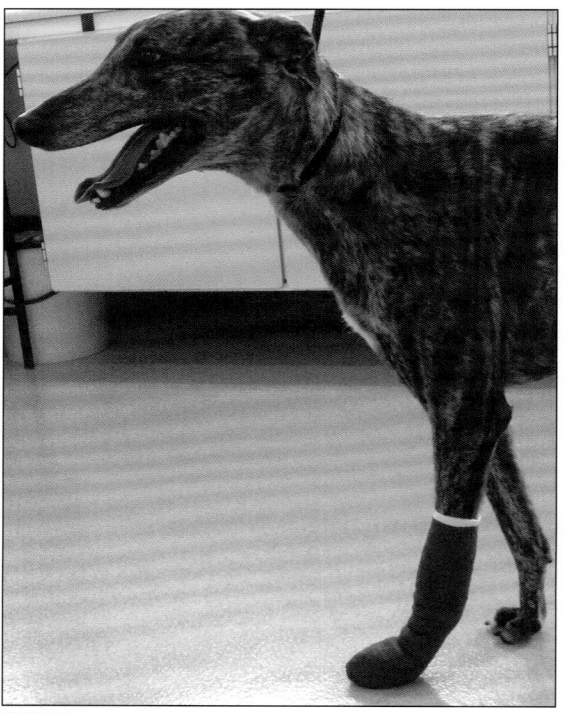

15.6 Completed foot and lower limb bandage.

If it is necessary to extend the limb bandage over the hock (tuber calcis) or elbow (olecranon), then adequate padding on these bony prominences must be used. Extension of the bandage to include the stifle can be especially prone to slippage and careful compression of the padding layers to produce a bandage that is firm but not tight is required.

This method of limb dressing encloses the digits. Alternatively, the very tips of the toes can be left out of the bandage to enable peripheral circulation to be monitored. In these cases, the bandage at each stage is simply started by passing the bandage around the foot excluding the toes. Either technique is acceptable and effective.

WARNING

If they are left out, only the very tips of the toes should be seen. Avoid leaving the whole foot out of a limb bandage; the foot invariably swells and such bandages are prone to significant slippage

Ear bandages

Ear bandages are used either to help stop haemorrhage (usually from the pinna) following trauma, or to keep ear dressings in place following surgery. Both ears may be bandaged; although it is usually only necessary to bandage one ear.

Any wounds should be covered with a sterile dressing before applying appropriate padding to the ear. A conforming bandage should then be placed over the padding. The position of the pinna beneath the bandage is usually indicated in ink on the conforming layer (see 'Procedure for bandaging a single ear' and Figure 15.7 below).

After application, the patient should be observed for a few minutes to ensure that the bandage is not too tight and does not interfere with swallowing or breathing. The aim is to

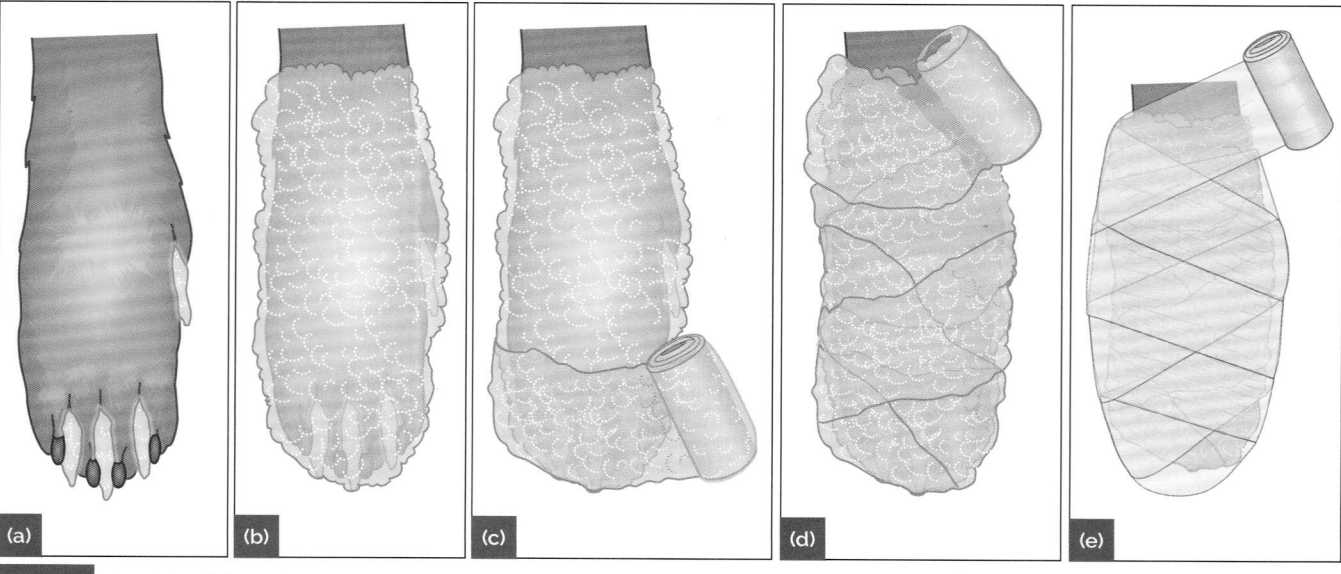

(a)   (b)   (c)   (d)   (e)

15.5 (a–e) Applying a foot and lower limb bandage (see 'Procedure for lower limb and foot bandages').

Procedure for bandaging a single ear

1. Apply appropriate sterile dressings to any wounds on the pinna (Figure 15.7a).
2. Place a pad of cotton wool on the top of the cranium, fold the dressed ear on to the pad and place further padding over the dressing (Figure 15.7b).
3. Wrap cotton wool roll around the head and ear in a figure-of-eight pattern.
4. Apply conforming bandage in a figure-of-eight pattern around the head, using the free ear for additional anchorage (Figure 15.7c), ensuring the padding stays level with or proud of the conforming layer to prevent constriction or rubbing.
5. Cover the bandage with adhesive tape or cohesive bandage using the same figure-of-eight pattern around the head and opposite ear (Figures 15.7d and 15.8).
6. Use marker pen to indicate on the outer layer the position of the pinna (see Figure 15.7e).

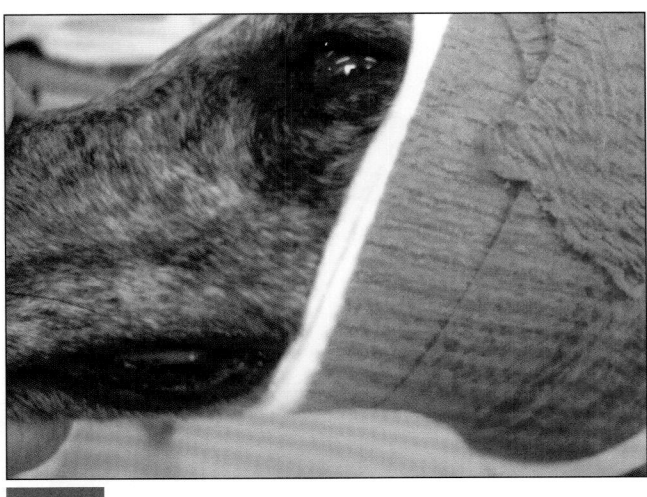

15.8 Completed ear bandage.

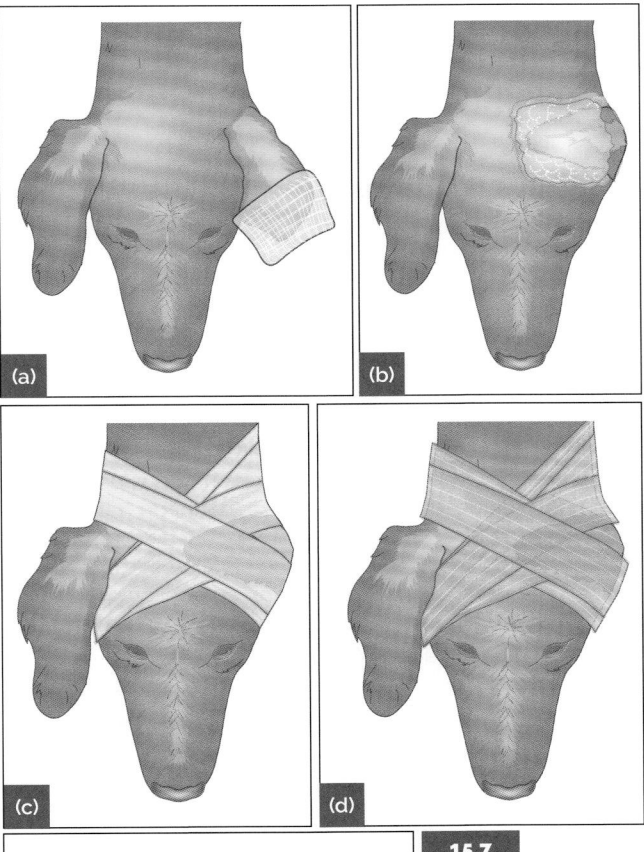

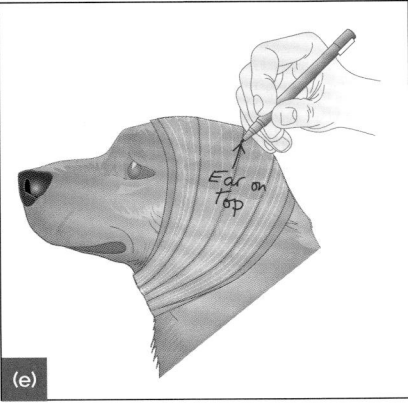

15.7

(a–e) Applying an ear and head bandage (see 'Procedure for bandaging a single ear').

have the bandage as far forward as possible (without interfering with sight), otherwise it will slip backwards (the most common complication) and its role will be compromised. Checking that two fingers can be passed under the edges of the bandage ensures it has not been applied too tightly.

Chest (thorax) bandages

Chest bandages may be applied to wounds of the chest wall or used to hold chest drains in place. The chest bandage is prevented from slipping by passing the bandaging materials between the front legs in a figure-of-eight fashion, resulting in a cross-over of bandages between the forelimbs on the ventral surface.

Procedure for chest (thorax) bandage

1. Apply appropriate sterile dressings to any wounds on the chest wall.
2. Starting dorsally mid thorax, apply a padding layer around the chest wall (Figure 15.9a).
3. Incorporate the forelimbs in a figure-of-eight pattern to help secure the bandage (Figure 15.9b).
4. Return back along the chest wall ending caudally to where the bandage started (Figure 15.9c).
5. Cover the padded layer with a conforming bandage using the same figure-of-eight pattern (Figure 15.9de), ensuring the padding stays level with or proud of the conforming layer to prevent constriction or rubbing.
6. The conforming layer can then be covered in a similar manner with a cohesive layer.

If cohesive bandage is used it must not be placed too tightly, as tightness may result in the patient having difficulty in breathing. Checking that two fingers can be passed under the edges of the bandage ensures it has not been applied too tightly. Adhesive material should be avoided as it tends to make the patient very hot and has minimal ability to expand and retract with respiration.

Commercially available 'vests' (Figure 15.10) may be used as an alternative to chest bandages to hold drains or dressings in place, or can be used over a chest dressing to provide extra bandage security.

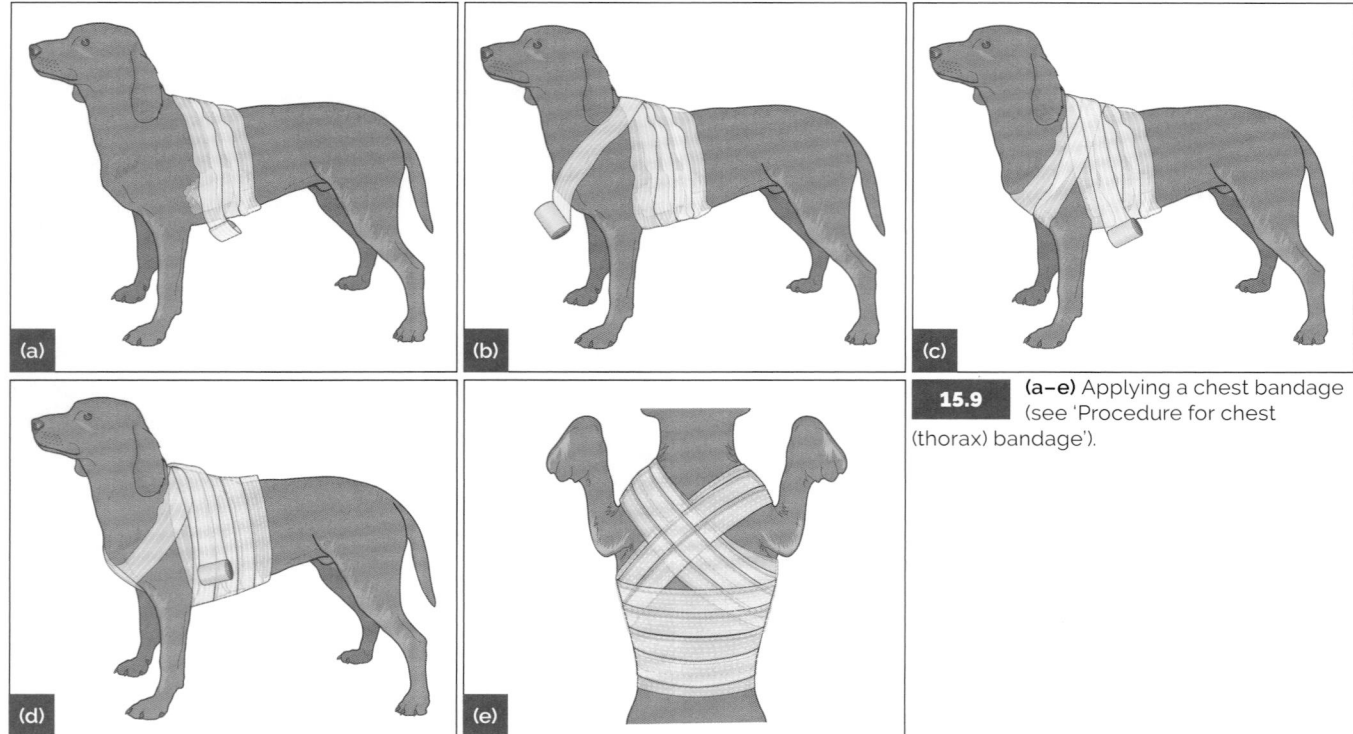

15.9 (a–e) Applying a chest bandage (see 'Procedure for chest (thorax) bandage').

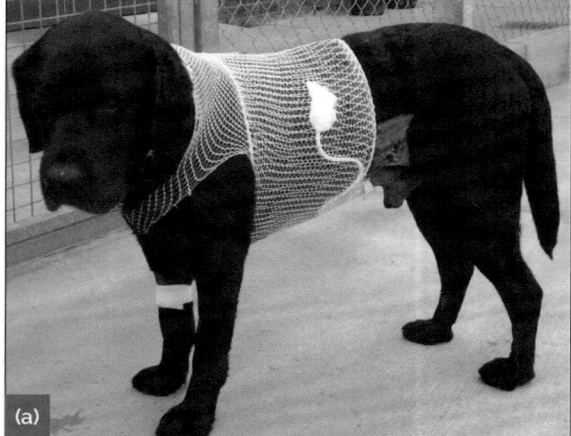

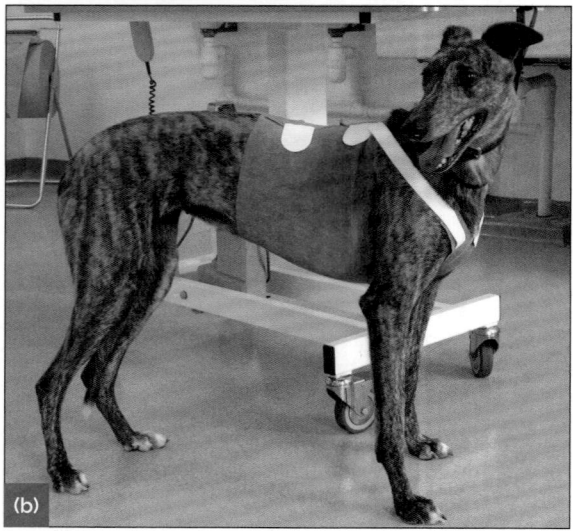

15.10 Vests may be used to hold chest dressings and drains in place. **(a)** Stockinette vest. **(b)** Commercial tapeless vest.

Abdominal bandages

Abdominal bandages may be applied to wounds of the abdominal wall or used to apply pressure in cases of intra-abdominal haemorrhage. The abdomen is difficult to bandage in dogs due to the relative narrowness of the area compared with the thorax, and the technique used will depend upon the species and breed. In some relatively immobile animals, padding layers can simply be laid around the abdomen and secured with conforming and protective layers. In more mobile animals, 'bunching' of bandaging material tends to occur in front of the hindlimbs. Attempts to prevent this situation from occurring include extending a chest bandage (see above) down over the abdomen (e.g. in round-chested breeds such as Dachshunds) or incorporating the hindlimbs (e.g. in deep-chested breeds such as Dobermanns; see below). The incorporation of the hindlimbs does, however, make the bandage more prone to soiling, necessitating regular changes.

Procedure for abdominal bandage incorporating the hindlimbs

1. Apply appropriate sterile dressings to any wounds on the chest wall.
2. Starting mid abdomen, apply a padding layer around the abdominal wall (Figure 15.11a).
3. Incorporate the hindlimbs in a figure-of-eight pattern to help secure the bandage (Figure 15.11b).
4. Return back along the abdominal wall ending cranially to where the bandage started (Figure 15.11c).
5. Cover the padded layer with a conforming bandage. Pay particular attention to anatomy of genitalia in both male and female animals: be careful not to cover vulva or prepuce (Figure 15.11de).
6. The conforming layer can then be covered in a similar manner with a cohesive layer.

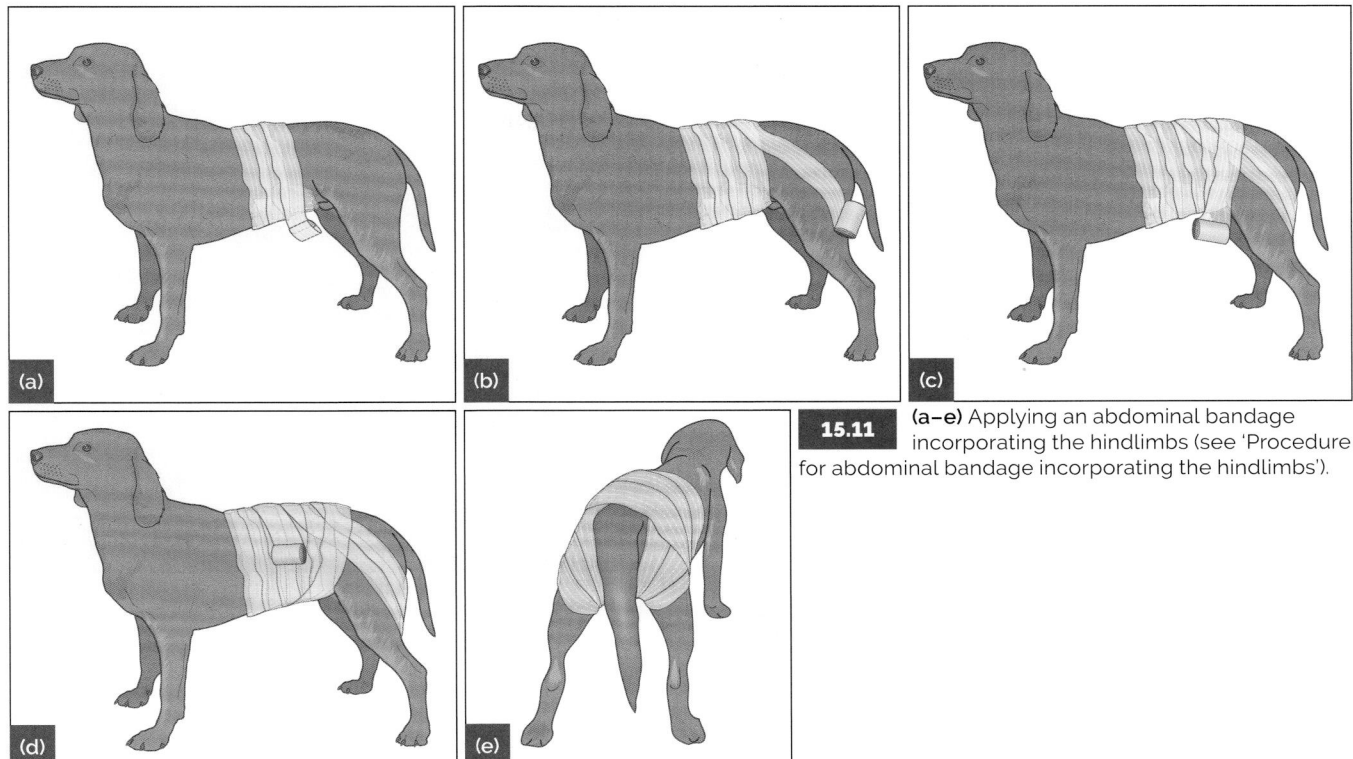

15.11 **(a–e)** Applying an abdominal bandage incorporating the hindlimbs (see 'Procedure for abdominal bandage incorporating the hindlimbs').

Tail bandages

The tail may need to be bandaged to stop haemorrhage (especially from the tail tip), to keep a dressing in place, to protect the tail tip from injury, to keep the tail clean following surgery or in cases of perineal soiling.

Procedure for a tail bandage

- Apply appropriate sterile dressings to any wounds (Figure 15.12a).
- Using a conforming bandage, roll from the base, along the dorsal aspect of the tail, to the tip of the tail. Go under the tip, along the ventral aspect of the tail and back to the base (Figure 15.12b).
- Fold the bandage back on itself and return along the ventral surface to the tip of the tail (Figure 15.12c).
- Spiral the bandage from the tip in a proximal direction towards the base, ensuring even pressure up to the base of the tail (Figure 15.12d).
- Apply a conforming layer using the same methodology; from tip to base (Figure 15.12e).
- Return from base to tip (Figure 15.12f).
- The conforming layer can then be covered in a similar manner with a cohesive layer.

Tail bandages are often difficult to keep in place. Options for helping keep the bandage in place include: flicking hair into some turns of the initial layer of bandage; using adhesive dressing and bandaging materials; covering the bandage with a plastic syringe case; and using plastic tail splints. Avoiding excessive weight in the bandage is always wise.

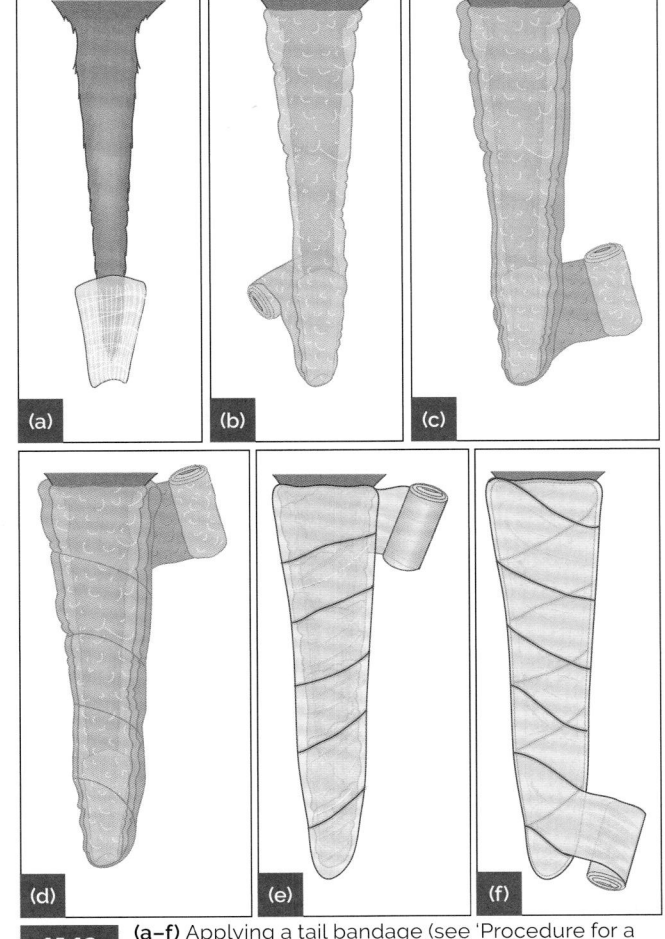

15.12 **(a–f)** Applying a tail bandage (see 'Procedure for a tail bandage').

Other bandaging techniques

The four most common special bandaging techniques are:

- Ehmer sling: to support the hindlimb following reduction of hip luxation (surgical or non-surgical)
- Velpeau sling: to support the shoulder joint following luxation or surgery
- Robert Jones bandage: to provide support and immobilization to fractured limbs in a first aid situation or following surgery
- Spica bandage: to immobilize the forelimb, in particular the elbow joint and associated bones.

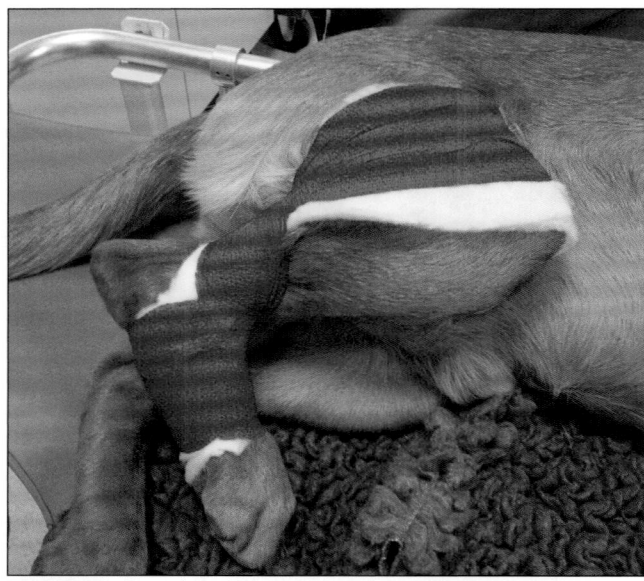

15.14 Completed Ehmer sling. (Reproduced from the *BSAVA Manual of Canine and Feline Musculoskeletal Disorders, 2nd edn*)

Procedure for an Ehmer sling

1. Apply light padding material to the metatarsus (Figure 15.13a); too much padding will cause the bandage to slip.
2. Apply conforming bandage (some people prefer adhesive tape) to the metatarsus from medial to lateral (Figure 15.13a).
3. Flex the leg and rotate the foot inwards; this will turn the hock outwards and the stifle inwards, engaging the hip joint into the acetabulum (Figure 15.13b).
4. Bring the bandage up under the medial aspect of the stifle. A small amount of padding may be applied to the cranial aspect of the stifle (Figure 15.13b).
5. Bring the bandage over the lateral aspect of the thigh and around the medial aspect of the hock, returning to the lateral aspect of the metatarsals (Figure 15.13c).
6. Apply several more layers until the leg is secure and the hip is supported (Figure 15.13d).
7. Repeat this for a cohesive dressing layer as required.
8. Tension of the bandage must be checked carefully on application: if too tight, it could result in ischaemic damage to the lower limb.
9. The completed dressing (Figure 15.14) is usually kept in place for 4–5 days.

Procedure for a Velpeau sling

1. Apply light padding material to the carpal area (Figure 15.15a).
2. Apply conforming bandage to the carpal area from lateral to medial (Figure 15.15b).
3. Bring the bandage from the medial carpus, up over the lateral aspect of the shoulder and around the opposite side of the chest behind the contralateral elbow (Figure 15.15c).
4. Ensure the carpus, elbow and shoulder are flexed and incorporate the carpus into the sling (Figure 15.15d).
5. Repeat this until the complete forelimb has been covered, producing a sling effect (Figure 15.15e).
6. The whole bandage can be covered with a cohesive layer, or a custom-made jacket can be used (Figure 15.16).
7. Tension of the bandage must be checked carefully on application: if too tight, it could result in ischaemic damage to the lower limb.

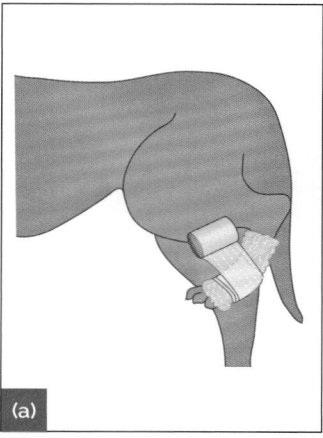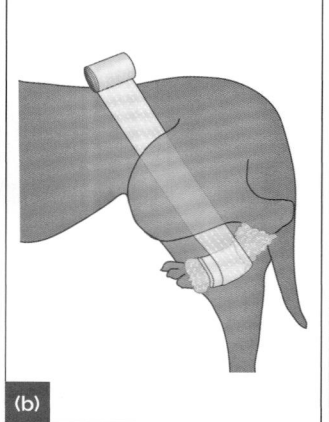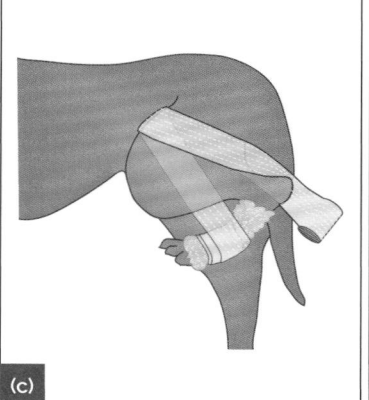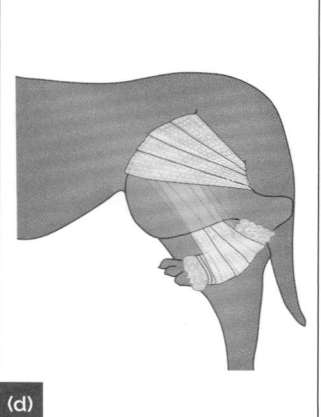

15.13 (a–d) Applying an Ehmer sling (see 'Procedure for an Ehmer sling').

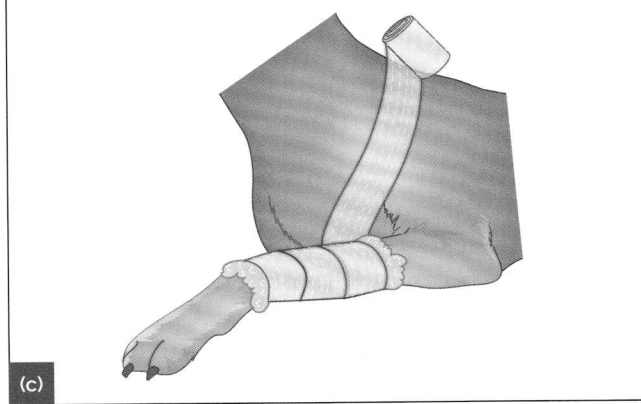

(a)

(b)

(c)

Procedure for a Robert Jones bandage

1. Place two lengths of zinc oxide tape to cover 15–20 cm up the leg and 10–13 cm overlap at the toes; place on each side of the leg to form 'stirrups' (see below; Figure 15.17a).
2. Place padding between the toes as necessary.
3. Place cotton wool layer: start halfway up nail and reverse roll cotton wool four or five times around the leg (Figure 15.17b).
4. Place conforming bandage: this should compress the cotton wool as firmly and as evenly as possible and should cover it entirely (Figure 15.17c).
5. Unstick two ends of zinc oxide tape and fold back to secure the bandage (Figure 15.17d).
6. Cover the bandage with cohesive bandage for protection and extra support (Figures 15.17ef).
7. Check that the bandage is not too tight: it should be possible to insert two fingers between the bandage and the animal. When flicked, the bandage should sound like a ripe melon.
8. The two middle toes should remain exposed (Figures 15.17g and 15.18).
9. The bandage may be kept in place for up to 2 weeks.

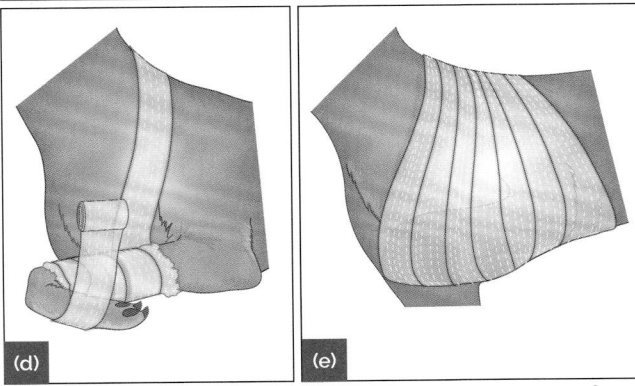

(d)

(e)

15.15 (a–e) Applying a Velpeau sling (see 'Procedure for a Velpeau sling').

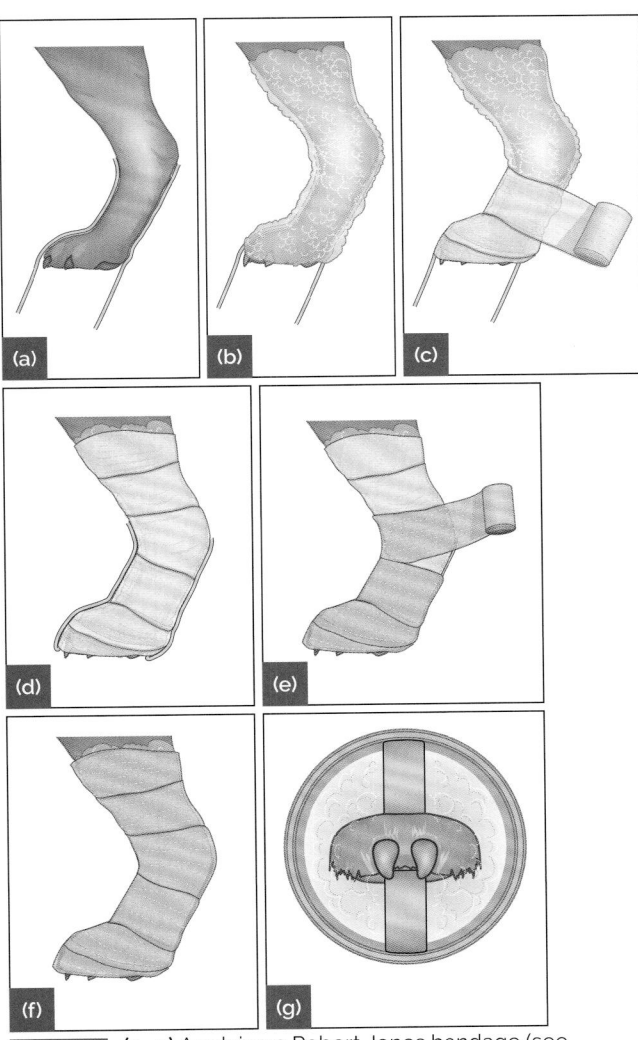

(a)

(b)

(c)

(d)

(e)

(f)

(g)

15.17 (a–g) Applying a Robert Jones bandage (see 'Procedure for a Robert Jones bandage').

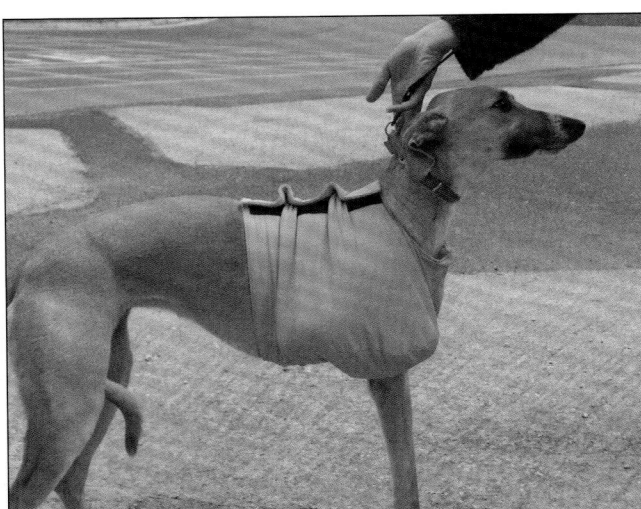

15.16 A custom-made jacket used as a Velpeau sling. (Reproduced from the *BSAVA Manual of Canine and Feline Musculoskeletal Disorders, 2nd edn*)

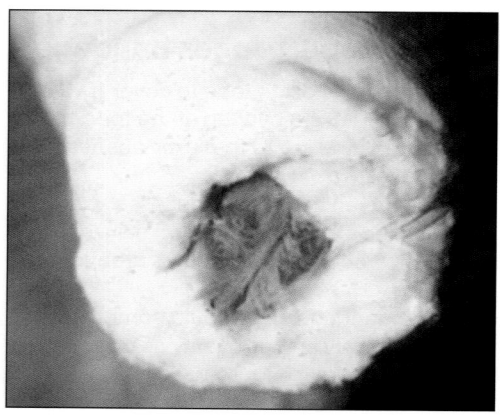

15.18

Completed Robert Jones bandage.

Note: the use of tape 'stirrups' in an attempt to stop bandage slippage can be helpful in some taper legged patients; however, a good technique and correct tension should negate the need for stirrups. Stirrups anchor adhesive tape on to the patient's fur/skin, which can cause irritation and pull if the bandage begins to slip. This irritation often leads to further patient interference and trauma under the dressing from the adhesive and fur/skin damage. Thus, stirrups should be used with caution.

Spica bandages

This specialized bandage is used to immobilize the elbow joint or associated bones (e.g. scapula, humerus, proximal radius and ulna). The antebrachium is padded with a Robert Jones bandage and there is some padding over the scapula. A flat lateral splint is placed over the midline at the tip of the scapula and all the way down to the foot. The splint can be made from a sheet of thermosetting cast material and pleated for resistance to bending. It is held in place with adhesive tape over the Robert Jones dressing and a body bandage around the thorax (Figure 15.19)

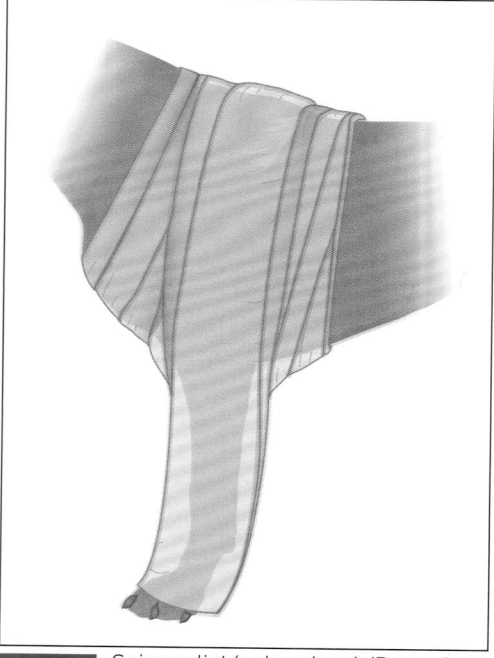

15.19 Spica splint (or bandage). (Reproduced from the *BSAVA Manual of Canine and Feline Emergency and Critical Care, 3rd edn*).

Management of bandages

Once the bandage has been applied, regular checks should be carried out until it is removed to ensure that it does not cause any discomfort or injury to the animal.

- The bandage should be checked to ensure that it is not uncomfortable, has not slipped or is too tight.
- Any evidence of odour, oedema, discharge, skin irritation or wetness due to the wound itself ('strike through' of discharges or blood) should be investigated – usually by changing the bandage.
- It is important that the dressing does not become soiled or wet from environmental factors (e.g. urine, water, mud). The dressing should be covered with a protective covering when the patient is taken outside; there are commercial 'booties' available, but empty, dried and adapted drip bags are durable and work well as a protective 'do-it-yourself' boot. Any covering should be removed indoors to prevent the bandage becoming wet with condensation. Ensure any protective covering is not too tight.

Patient interference with bandages

Constant chewing or licking at the bandage by the patient should be discouraged; however, it should be noted that patient interference can indicate that the bandage is uncomfortable, causing irritation or causing pain and should be investigated. Reasons for patient interference with the bandage include:

- Bandage being too tight
- Wounds may have become infected
- Pain from the bandaged site as a result of slippage or tightness causing rubbing
- The patient may be allergic to the adhesive in the tape being used
- The bandage may have become wet
- There may be a pressure sore developing or present
- The patient's personality – may not like dressings or bandages.

Interventions to prevent interference

In order to establish the cause of the interference, potential causes should be eliminated by carefully checking the bandage. If there is evidence of 'strike through', slippage and/or tension, then the dressing should be changed. A pain assessment should be carried out (see Chapter 21) and the patient's clinical variables (e.g. temperature, pulse, respiration (TPR); see Chapter 14) should be recorded as these may indicate infection. If there are signs of pain or infection, these should be brought to the attention of a veterinary surgeon.

If there are no obvious wound or dressing factors leading to the bandage interference, then patient personality factors should be considered and the following implemented:

- Increase mental stimulations:
  - Grooming
  - Toys
  - Food-based toys.
- Provide physical barriers:
  - Elizabethan collars (both rigid and soft options (Figure 15.20) can be effective)
  - Pet shirts/vests (see Figure 15.10).
- Anxiolytic medications.

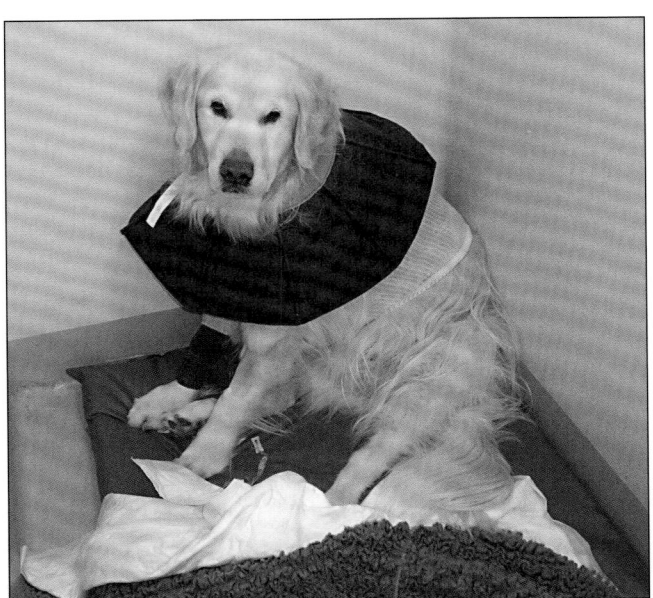

15.20 A soft cloth Elizabethan collar can be used to prevent self-trauma of wounds or inadvertent removal of bandages and indwelling catheters and/or drains. (Reproduced from the *BSAVA Manual of Canine and Feline Musculoskeletal Disorders, 2nd edn*)

Special bandaging considerations for exotic pets

The basic bandaging principles described above may be applied to small mammals, birds and other exotic pets, although a certain amount of creativity is often required to ensure that the aim of the bandage is achieved. All the dressing types mentioned above are appropriate for use in small patients, although they are often too large and must therefore be cut to size. Rolls of bandage can be cut in half with a sharp knife to provide a more suitable size for easier application. Adhesive tape to secure dressings and bandages may be more appropriate in small animals, compared with dogs and cats, provided fur and feather damage can be avoided. Imaginative use of non-veterinary products (e.g. the use of lollipop sticks as splints) is common and can be very successful.

Wing bandages in birds can be essential to prevent further damage to both fracture sites and feathers. For some simple fractures in birds, bandaging may be all that is needed to allow the fracture to repair (Figure 15.21). It must be remembered that joints in birds can rapidly fuse when immobile, so bandages must not be left in place for more than 2–3 days at a time. Further information is provided in the *BSAVA Manual of Wildlife Casualties*.

Management of drains

A variety of different passive and active drains are used within veterinary practice. Drains are used to remove possibly harmful material (e.g. pus, blood, exudate, air) from a site or to prevent the collection of fluid within a dead space (e.g. the cavity left behind after a large mass removal). Drains (e.g. chest drains) can also be used to administer local anaesthetic drugs to an area.

- Passive drains rely on gravity for the movement of fluids.
- Active drains rely on a vacuum drawing material away from the site.

Further information on the types of drain available and their placement is given in Chapter 23.

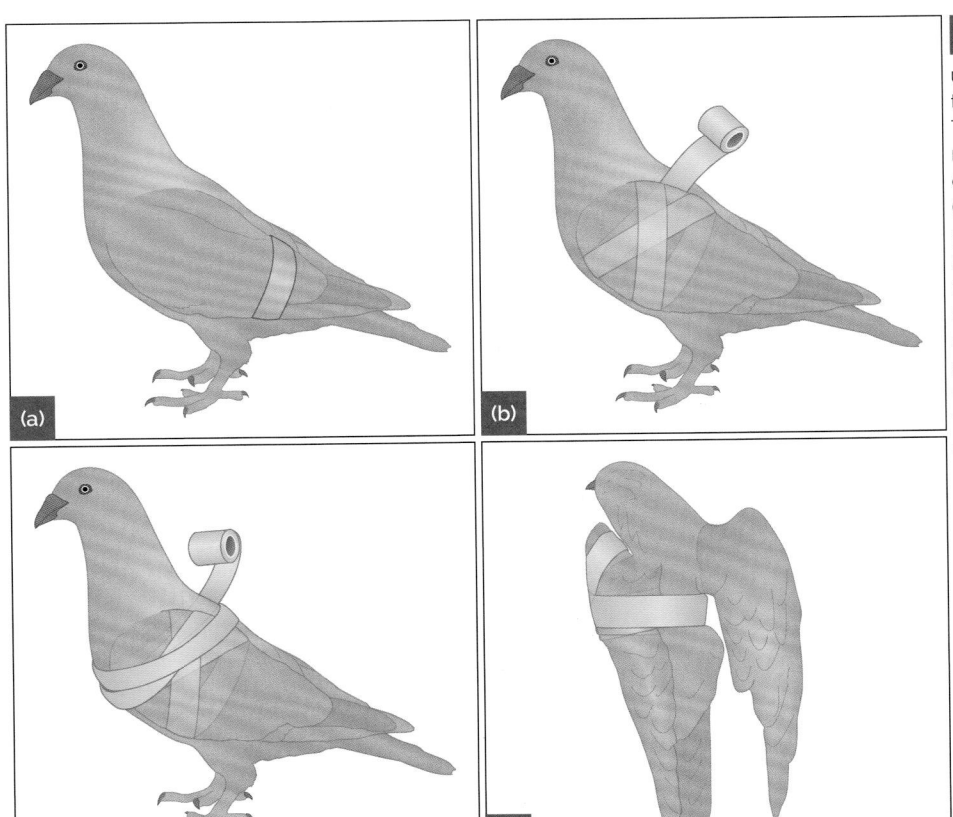

15.21 Wing bandaging technique. **(a)** Medical tape can be used to hold the primary feathers to the tertiary feathers in a closed wing. This is suitable for fractures of the manus or simple fractures of the radius or ulna alone.
(b) Conforming bandage can be used to produce a 'figure-of-eight' dressing to support fractures of the radius and ulna. The radius and ulna are held against the humerus, the carpal and elbow joints are held flexed but the shoulder maintains movement. The wing is not strapped to the body and the opposite wing remains free.
(c) Conforming bandage can also be used to produce a 'figure-of-eight' dressing to support the humerus. In this case the body of the bird is included in the dressing to restrict movement at the shoulder as well as the elbow and carpus. Care should be taken not to make the dressing too tight and so impede normal respiration.
(d) The opposite wing remains free. In all cases strapping should be removed and the wing reassessed after 2–3 days in order to help prevent the risk of joint stiffness.
(Reproduced from the *BSAVA Manual of Wildlife Casualties, 2nd edn*)

The key management point with these patients is prevention of interference with the drain, which can occur due to pain, discomfort or availability of access by the patient. The use of an Elizabethan collar (see Figure 15.20), or a similar device, is essential in these patients and this should be applied during the recovery period following surgery for placement of the drain (often a time when disoriented patients can cause inadvertent damage/trauma). Pain should be appropriately managed; the use of a local anaesthetic should be considered. The drain must be deactivated if local anaesthetic is being instilled down it as part of the analgesia plan, and it is essential this is done in an aseptic manner. If a patient is interfering with a drain, it is often due to discomfort.

It is important that the area around the drain is kept clean and monitored for any signs of infection. The use of products such as Surgifix®, patient jackets (see Figure 15.10) and Elizabethan collars (see Figure 15.20) can help keep the drain safe and secure, and can help to reduce the incidence of patient interference. All drains should be considered a possible source of infection, therefore, clean gloves should always be used during handling, and particular attention paid to the cleanliness of the bedding. Some drains have integral bacterial filters to help reduce the risk of infection.

Body temperature monitoring, at least twice daily, in these patients is also important for detecting the development of systemic infections.

Assessment of the material collected from the drain is important; the volume, viscosity and colour (Figure 15.22) should be noted during patient checks and recorded on the patient's hospital record. The protein concentration in the drain fluid can be measured using a refractometer.

Fluid type	Appearance	Protein concentration (g/dl)
Transudate	Clear	<2.5
Modified transudate	Hazy	2.5–4.5
Exudate	Turbid to opaque	>3.0

15.22 Monitoring of fluid collected from surgical drains.

Enemas

Enemas are defined as the placement of a liquid substance into the colon and rectum, which results in the stimulation of the patient's normal reflexes to expel the contents. It is important to remember to place a tail bandage (see above and Figure 15.12) prior to their administration.

Why administer enemas?

There are various reasons why an enema may be prescribed, including:

- Evacuation of rectal contents:
  - Due to impaction or constipation
  - Prior to lower gastrointestinal (GI) endoscopy (see Chapter 16)
  - To facilitate drug administration (see Chapter 8)
  - As part of a radiographic contrast study (see Chapter 16)
  - To facilitate abdominal and urinary tract radiographs (overlying rectal and colonic contents can impair the ability to accurately interpret caudal abdominal radiographic findings)

- Prior to some surgical interventions (e.g. rectal prolapse) – this is dependent on the veterinary surgeon, as some prefer manual evacuation and managing harder faeces rather than the more liquid content left behind after enema administration.
- Diagnostics – barium sulphate enemas can be used to silhouette the rectal and colonic walls (see Chapter 16)
- Administration of medications – the rectal route of drug administration can be very useful, both due to the ease of administration and the fact that some drugs are highly absorbed via this route (due to the large surface area and good blood supply). A good example of this is the administration of diazepam (Figure 15.23) in an emergency situation when it is not possible to gain intravenous access in a safe and timely fashion. It is also a very useful route for owner management prior to transportation of seizuring patients.

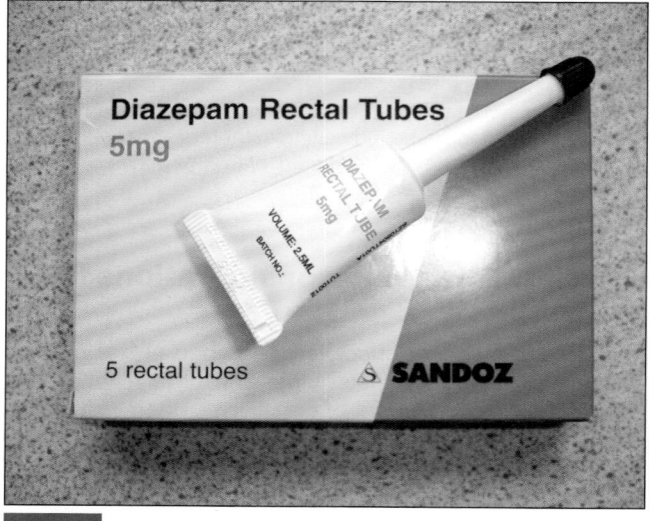

15.23 Diazepam rectal tubes.

Solutions available

There are a number of different enema solutions available (Figure 15.24), including:

- **Warm water** – the advantages of this technique is that it is readily available, non-toxic and non-irritant. It also does not create difficulties in cleaning the perianal area, which can be a problem with some products
- **Phosphate enemas** (Figure 15.25) – these often come in a sachet that is added to water prior to administration. They have a high osmolarity and draw water into the colon, which then stimulates defecation. These are not suitable for small patients (<15 kg) and those with gut motility issues (due to pooling and retention of the solution causing electrolyte imbalances), as they may result in toxicity. The use of phosphate enemas is also contraindicated in patients with renal disease
- **Liquid paraffin** – the advantages of this method is that it is both readily available and cheap. Liquid paraffin is useful in constipated patients due to its softening action, aiding evacuation of hard compacted faeces. The main disadvantage is that due to the oily nature of the solution, extensive bathing of the patient with warm soapy water is often required, which can be challenging in some patients. It can also be administered orally as a laxative (faecal softener)

Solution	Use	Volume used (ml/kg)	Frequency	Advantages	Disadvantages
Warm water	Enema	5–10	Every 20–30 minutes if necessary	Readily available; non-toxic; non-irritant; easy to clean	Non-lubricant; no stimulatory effects; relatively large volumes required
Phosphate enema (see Figure 15.25)	Enema	Not recommended	Not recommended	Low volume; stimulates defecation; rapid onset	May cause toxicity; not suitable for patients <15 kg; not suitable for patient with gut motility problems; contraindicated in patients with renal disease
Liquid paraffin	Enema or oral	2–3	Every 1–2 hours	Readily available; cheap; softens faeces; lubricates evacuation	Causes significant perineal contamination; can be hard to clean
Ready-to-use mini-enema (e.g. Micralax®; see Figure 15.25)	Enema (works as a fast-acting laxative)	5 ml single dose for all weights	May be repeated multiple times	Small volume; easy to use; well tolerated by most animals	May need to be repeated several times; may be ineffective in moderate to severe constipation
Barium sulphate	Enema or oral	5–10	Single administration	Used as an enema to silhouette the rectal and colonic walls; used orally to silhouette the upper digestive tract (see Chapter 16)	Not useful as a conventional enema
Gastrointestinal cleansing products (e.g. Klean Prep®)	Oral	20	Every 8–12 hours as required	Oral laxative; rapid onset	Not very palatable; may require repeat treatments
Lactulose	Oral laxative or enema (usually reserved for seizuring animals)	0.1–0.5 ml/kg	Every 4–12 hours	Relatively palatable; useful for chronic constipation; can be used to treat seizures in hepatic encephalopathy	May cause sustained loose stools

15.24 Common enema and laxative solutions and information for their use.

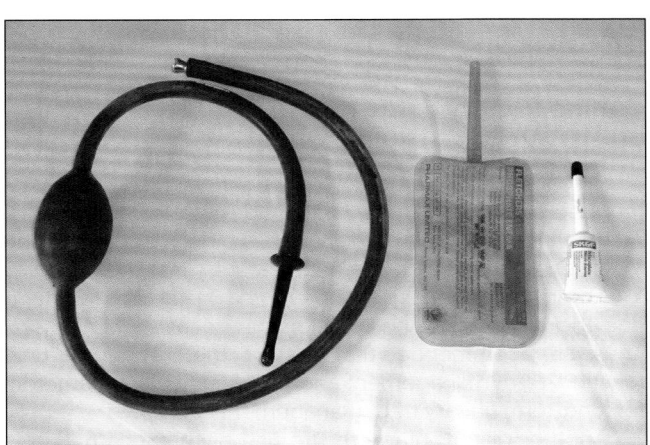

15.25 Example equipment for enemas: Higginson's syringe, phosphate enema and Micralax®.
(Reproduced from the *BSAVA Manual of Practical Veterinary Nursing*)

- **Ready-to-use mini-enemas** (e.g. Micralax®, Figure 15.25) – these are ready-to-use preparations contained within an applicator. Due to the small volume and the small applicator, ready-to-use enemas are usually very well tolerated, particularly by cats. These products are actually ultra-fast acting laxatives, rather than enemas

- **Lactulose** – used particularly in patients that are seizuring due hepatic encephalopathy associated with hepatic disease (e.g. portosystemic shunts), by drawing ammonia into the colon. Lactulose can also be administered orally as a laxative and is useful in cases of chronic constipation (e.g. in elderly cats)
- **Gastrointestinal cleansing products** (e.g. Klean Prep®) – these products are commonly used prior to lower gastrointestinal endoscopy. They are orally administered laxatives but have the same effect as an enema. Often they require administration a couple of times prior to the procedure (i.e. the evening prior and the morning of the endoscopy). The administration of gastrointestinal cleansing products often requires the use of a stomach tube; however, some dogs will drink the solution – this can be facilitated by using water that has been used to cook chicken in
- **Miscellaneous enema solutions** – the following solutions are not recommended and have been replaced:
  - Olive oil and water
  - Glycerine and water
  - Water-based medical lubricant
  - Soap and water solution.

Equipment

The general equipment required to administer an enema includes:

- Gloves
- Tail bandage material
- Lubricant
- Method of administration:
  - Higginson syringe (see Figure 15.25)
  - Bucket/can and tubing
  - Catheter (e.g. Foley).
- In dogs, if the patient is conscious, outside access and a lead and collar to take them outside immediately (if not available, perform the enema outside)
- Cats require a litter tray with an appropriate substrate for the individual (really important to reduce stress as far as possible).

Techniques

The general technique for any type of enema is essentially the same: a short tube is inserted per rectum and an enema is given. This can prove easier with some patients than others, and appropriate precautions should be taken to ensure the safety of the patient and the staff involved. Adequate restraint is essential and the patient's condition and temperament will dictate which method is best. Physical restraint of a conscious animal should be employed where possible and if patient temperament permits; however, chemical restraint in the form of sedation or anaesthesia should be considered when the patient is less compliant in order to reduce the risk of injury to the patient or staff. It is advised that the owner of a patient should not be involved in any clinical situation where procedures are being carried out.

Giving an enema to an amenable dog or cat

This method requires two people.

1. Prepare all equipment.
2. The assistant restrains the patient in a suitable area; this is preferably outdoors, where cleaning will be easier.
3. Lubricate the end of the tube or nozzle.
4. Elevate the patient's tail and place the tube into the anus. Rotate gently until access to the rectum is achieved (this is easy in the dog but occasionally more difficult in the cat).
5. Advance the tube into the rectum.
6. Stand to the side of the patient and allow fluid to run into the rectum by gravity, or gently pump/syringe in fluid.
7. Allow dogs free exercise to evacuate bowels and supply cats with litter trays (with appropriate litter) and an adequately sized cage.

Urinary catheterization

Urinary catheterization involves placement of a catheter (a hollow tube) into the urinary bladder, though which fluid/urine can be expelled from the body or fluid/air introduced.

Indications for urinary catheterization

The indications for catheterization include:

- Voiding of bladder contents prior to:
  - Pneumocystography
  - Surgery (manual expression is often adequate)
  - Urinary tract surgery
  - Long surgical procedures.
- Obtaining a sterile urine sample for culture and sensitivity testing or, alternatively, obtaining a urine sample for analysis in a patient where other methods of collection (e.g. free-catch) are not possible/challenging
- Introduction of a contrast agent for radiographic evaluation of the urinary tract (see Chapter 16)
- Retrograde flushing to dislodge urinary calculi in cases of urethral obstruction. Hydropulsion can be used as part of an emergency treatment protocol or prior to cystotomy surgery
- To maintain constant or controlled bladder management
- To prevent soiling in recumbent or incontinent patients
- Postoperative management
- Monitoring urine output (e.g. when the patient is under anaesthesia or in intensive care for conditions such as acute renal failure)
- Monitoring fluid balance
- Maintenance of a patent urethra
- To enable patient stabilization prior to surgery
- Treatment of male cats suffering from feline lower urinary tract disease (FLUTD) while management strategies are implemented.

Types of catheter

There are several different types of urinary catheters for dogs and cats (Figure 15.26). The majority of urinary catheters commercially available are supplied sterilized (usually gamma radiation has been used). The packaging may also contain an inner sleeve to aid aseptic placement. As with all sterile equipment, it is important to check the integrity of the packaging for any damage and the expiry date.

Canine urinary catheters
Plastic catheters

These catheters are made of fairly rigid plastic. They have a rounded tip with two holes in the side wall towards the tip. Along with their rigidity, which makes placement easier, the main advantage of these catheters is their cost.

The rigidity of these catheters is a major disadvantage due the discomfort and irritation they cause when *in situ*. Thus, it is recommended that plastic catheters are used only for short-term management and not as indwelling catheters for long-term urinary tract management.

Another disadvantage to the use of these catheters is that they do not have a balloon to both prevent flow around the catheter and keep the catheter *in situ*. These catheters require suturing in place. The recommended technique for this is to place adhesive tape 'wings' next to the Luer connector and to then secure this with sutures to the patient.

Foley catheters

Foley catheters are supplied in various diameters and lengths, with longer length catheters required for dogs and shorter length catheters used for bitches. They are made from either a soft silicone or latex. This does make placement more

Type	Photograph	Species	Sex	Material	Indwelling	Sizes (FG)	Length (cm)	Luer fitting
Plastic dog catheter		Dog	Male and female	Flexible grade of nylon (polyamide)	No but can be adapted to be indwelling	6–10	50–60	Yes
Foley		Dog	Female	Teflon-coated latex	Yes	8–16	30–40	No
Silicone Foley		Dog	Male and female	Flexible medical grade silicone	Yes	5–10	30 and 55	No
Tieman's		Dog	Female	PVC (polyvinyl chloride)	No	8–12	43	Yes
Plastic cat catheter		Cat	Male and female	Flexible grade of nylon	No	3 and 4	30.5	Yes
Jackson cat catheter		Cat	Male and female	Flexible grade of nylon	Yes	3 and 4	11	Yes
Silicone cat catheter		Cat	Male	Medical grade silicone	Yes	3.5	12	Yes
Slippery Sam™ catheter		Cat	Male	PTFE (Teflon™)	Yes	3–3.5	14 and 11	Yes

15.26 Types of urinary catheter.

challenging; however, they are often supplied with a stylet/guidewire. The stylet/guidewire is commonly passed down the inner lumen, but can be inserted directly into the tip of the catheter via the holes in the wall close to the tip (Figure 15.27). Often these stylets/guidewires are not particularly stiff (they are usually made of a more rigid catheter material). Commercially available J-wires (narrow gauge flexible wire with rounded tips) can be used to provide more rigidity to aid placement. Once correctly in place, the balloon should be inflated using saline/water (Figure 15.27). This balloon maintains the catheter's position and also helps to prevent flow around the catheter.

If using a latex Foley catheter, it is essential that a water-based, not petroleum-based, lubricant is used, as petroleum-based products cause degradation of the latex. If the catheter is intended for indwelling use, the silicone version is recommended as it is non-irritant.

The soft flexible nature of Foley catheters makes them the ideal choice for indwelling use. They are the preferred type of catheter for performing retrograde urethrograms in the bitch because their flexible nature allows a better seal to be achieved, and provides better air or contrast medium retention.

The absence of a Luer connector has historically caused collection/drainage problems; however, as the use of these catheters has increased, more solutions to this problem have become available to the veterinary market (e.g. spigots, catheter-tipped syringes (Figure 15.28; see also below), urine collection bags and the plunger from a 2.5 ml syringe can all be used).

Tieman's catheters

This type of catheter is rarely used in modern veterinary medicine. It was originally designed for use in the human male. It has a curved tip and this is why it was believed that it could be useful in the bitch. Tieman's catheters are extremely long and flexible, making placement extremely challenging.

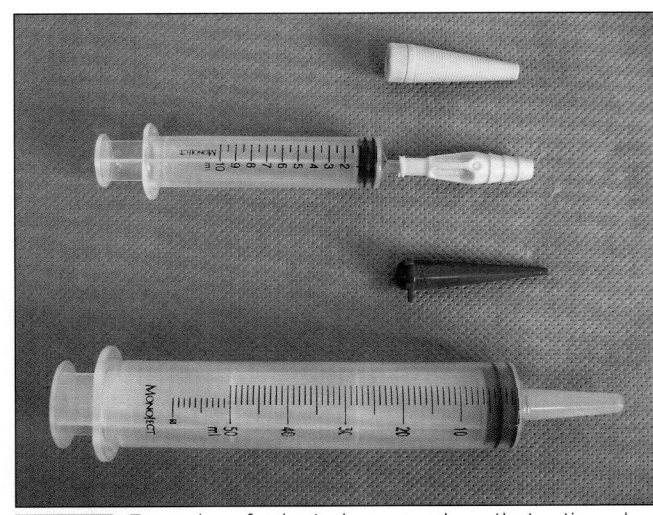

15.28 Examples of spigots, bungs and a catheter-tipped syringe (from top: catheter bung, spigot attached to 10 ml syringe, spigot, catheter-tipped 50 ml syringe).

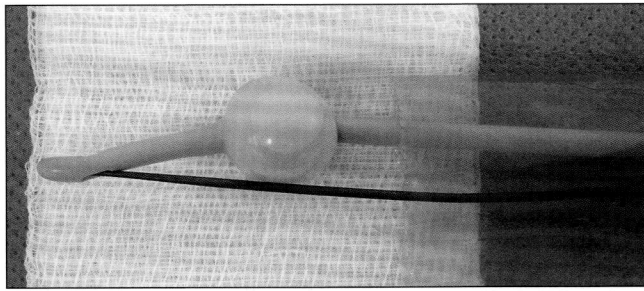

15.27 Tip of Foley catheter showing the balloon inflated and stylet in place.

Feline urinary catheters
Plastic catheters

These are similar to the canine plastic catheters, but are slightly smaller in gauge and length. These catheters are suitable for short-term use.

Jackson catheters

These catheters were primarily designed for use in male cats; however, they can also be used for female cats. They are short plastic catheters with a fine wire insert, which increases rigidity but also prevents/clears obstructions (e.g. protein/mucus plugs or calculi) during placement. This guidewire is removed once the catheter is *in situ*.

Due to their short length, Jackson catheters are designed to be fully inserted and have a plastic flange with appropriate holes located just in front of the Luer connector, allowing the catheter to be sutured in place.

These catheters are also available in silicone (**silicone tomcat catheter**) and Teflon™ (polytetrafluoroethylene (PTFE); e.g. Slippery Sam™ Tomcat Urethral catheter). The Teflon™ coating on the plastic of the catheter makes it extremely smooth and non-irritant, aiding insertion. They are the catheter of choice in cats for long-term indwelling urinary catheter management. The use of a rotating Luer attachment may help with the management of indwelling catheters when attached to a closed collection system.

Equipment to aid urinary catheter placement
Speculum and light source
Speculum

A speculum is used to assist catheterization of bitches by aiding good visualization of the urethral orifice and helping to hold back the tissue in the vestibule. Visual catheterization is usually much easier than digital catheterization (where the urethral opening is gently palpated), especially for those less familiar with the technique. All specula should be sterilized before use. There are several varieties, most of which are not specifically designed for urinary catheterization.

- **Nasal specula:** there are many slight variations, the adult size being the most appropriate. All have two flat blades that separate when the handles are closed together (Figure 15.29a). Some have a retaining device; others have to be held open. A light source may be attached to one of the blades to illuminate the vagina. If this is not available, a pen torch held by an assistant is an effective alternative.
- **Rectal specula:** these are used rarely, mainly due to expense. Rectal specula (Figure 15.29b) are conical in shape and, once in place, a section of the conical arm slides out to allow viewing of the urethral orifice. The main problem is to align the removable section with the urethral orifice; this is easy in theory, but difficult in practice.
- **Vaginal specula:** this is usually a normal auriscope handle and light, but the conventional aural attachment is replaced by a vaginal speculum with a section removed from its wall (Figure 15.29c).

Batteries and transformers

These should be electrically tested and working correctly. Spare batteries should always be in stock. Transformers do not come into contact with the vulva and so do not require sterilization.

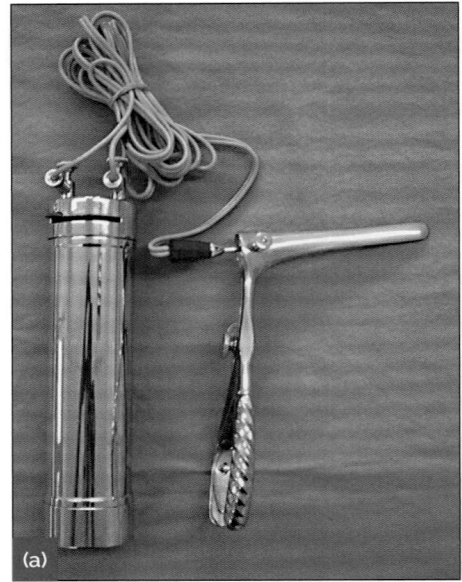

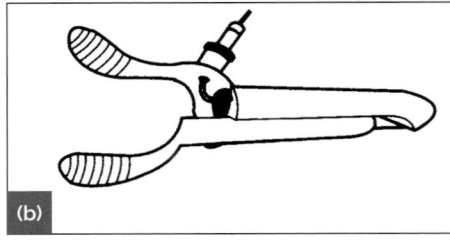

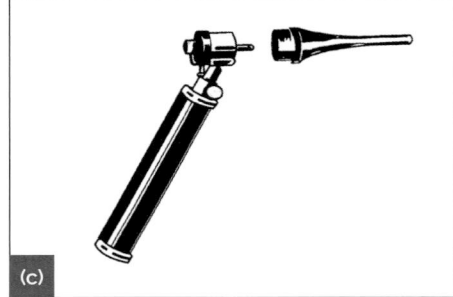

15.29 Specula used for urinary catheterization. **(a)** Nasal speculum, suitable for use as a bitch vaginal speculum. Pressing together the handles causes the blades to move apart and open the vestibule. **(b)** Rectal speculum, suitable for use as a bitch speculum. The lower sliding panel is removed after insertion into the vestibule to expose the urethral opening. The lighting attachment, which is connected to a battery, provides a self-contained light source. **(c)** Catheterization speculum for attachment to an auriscope; resembles an ear speculum except that a segment of its wall is absent.

Speculum light bulbs

These are best stored separately as they break easily. They cannot be sterilized in the autoclave and therefore need ethylene oxide or, more readily available, chemical sterilization.

Stylets

Stylets can be made or bought. They should be long enough for easy use; they must be at least two-thirds the length of the longest Foley catheter stocked. Stylets can be packed and autoclaved or chemically sterilized. Metal guidewires are supplied for use with silicone Foley catheters (see above). These are placed through the centre of the catheter and therefore need to be longer than the length of the Foley catheter. They can be autoclaved.

Ancillary equipment

Urine collection bags

Manufactured varieties are pre-packed and sterile; they are designed for single use. Previously used drip bags can be used with a giving set attached. The end of the giving set must be thoroughly cleaned and chemically sterilized before being attached to the urinary catheter. A screw attachment bung should be attached to the end of the giving set during storage to keep it clean from dust and dirt. Closed collection sets must be carefully attached to the urinary catheter to avoid tension and irritation of the prepuce (Figure 15.30).

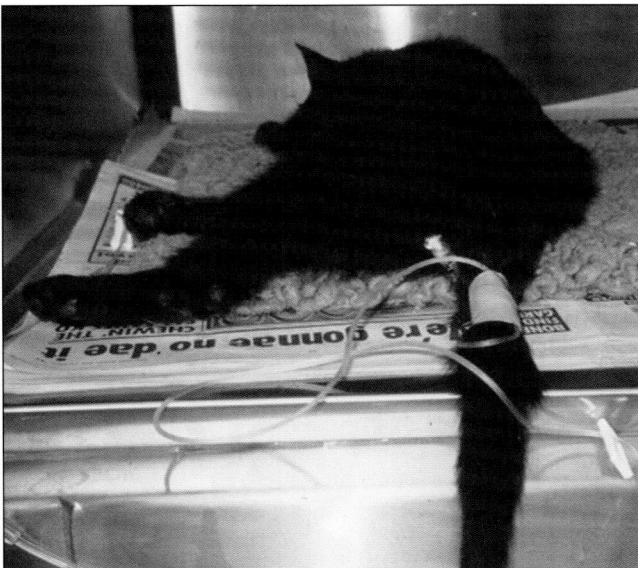

15.30 Urinary catheter *in situ* in a cat. A sterile extension set and closed-collection system has been attached and taped to the tail (without putting any tension on the prepuce). An Elizabethan collar should be placed on the cat. (Reproduced from the *BSAVA Manual of Feline Practice*)

Spigots and bungs

Plastic spigots and bungs (see Figure 15.28) are supplied in multi-packs requiring sterilization, or as individually packed sterile units. Chemical sterilization is the only practical method for these plastic items. Metal spigots can be autoclaved or placed in chemical sterilizing solution until needed but are rarely used in modern practice.

Three-way taps

These are invaluable when draining the bladder via a catheter. They avoid leakages by controlling urine flow whilst syringes are emptied.

Lubricants

All urinary catheters should be well lubricated to aid atraumatic placement. All catheters can be lubricated with water-based lubricants. A safe alternative to water-based lubricant is a medical grade silicone spray (Silkospray™). Petroleum-based lubricants are not recommended. The use of local anaesthetics (typically lidocaine due to the fast onset of action) can further aid catheterization.

Gloves

The use of gloves is recommended for the health and safety of personnel. In general, multiple packs of non-sterile gloves are adequate because the catheter will be fed from its package using a 'no touch' technique. Gloves are, therefore, used to prevent contamination of staff with urine, rather than protection of the patient from infection. Sterile gloves will be required when digital catheterization is performed, as the catheter tip is inevitably guided by the finger.

Techniques for urinary catheterization

Preparation

Regardless of the species or sex of the patient, some general principles should be followed in all cases:

- Analgesia is appropriate for all urinary catheterization procedures and may form part of a sedative protocol (see Chapter 21)
- Some patients, especially male dogs, will allow urinary catheterization under gentle physical restraint without resistance. If necessary, a muzzle may be used on a dog (see Chapter 11)
- In many patients, urinary catheterization will only be possible under appropriate sedation (see Chapter 21). General anaesthetic is sometimes required (e.g. in very traumatized patients) and/or urinary catheterization may take place whilst the patient is anaesthetized for other procedures
- All equipment, as above, should be prepared before restraining the patient
- An appropriate urinary catheter should be chosen and an approximation made of the length of catheter required before it is unpacked. This can be made by measuring against the patient, from roughly the urethral orifice along the urethra to the bladder
- The area around the prepuce or vulva should be cleaned with an antiseptic solution to remove any debris, discharges and surface dirt. It may be necessary to clip the hair around the area, especially in longhaired breeds
- The patient should be positioned at a comfortable working height for urinary catheterization to take place.

Catheterizing a male dog

Equipment

- Catheter
- Swabs for cleaning
- Sterile water-based lubricant (or silicone spray)
- Syringe to assist urine drainage
- Three-way tap (if required)
- Sample pot
- Gloves
- Urine bag or a bung
- Kidney dish

If the catheter is to be made indwelling, the following equipment is also required:

- Suture material
- Zinc oxide tape
- For silicone male Foley catheters, water sufficient to fill balloon
- Guide wire
- Syringe.

Restraint

Dogs may be restrained in a standing position or in lateral recumbency.   →

Catheterizing a male dog *continued*

Procedure

1. Wash your hands and put on gloves.
2. Clean the prepuce.
3. Extrude the penis; if not experienced, ask an assistant to do this.

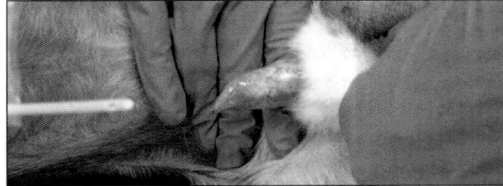

4. Clean the prepuce again.
5. Remove the catheter from the outer wrapping and cut a feeding sleeve from the inner sterile packaging. This allows easy feeding of the catheter from the packaging into the urethra using a 'no touch' technique. For silicone male Foley catheter placement, feed the guide wire up the centre of the catheter.

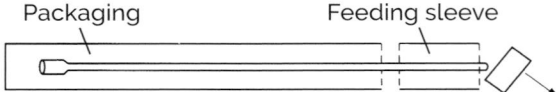

6. Lubricate the catheter and insert the tip into the urethra.
7. Advance the catheter up the urethra. Resistance may be met at the os penis, where there is a slight narrowing of the urethra, at the ischial arch and at the area of the prostate gland if enlarged. Steady but gentle pressure should overcome this resistance. If the catheter cannot be passed, re-evaluate catheter size.
8. Inflate the balloon once the tip of the catheter is in the bladder if using a silicone male Foley.
9. Proceed according to the reason for catheterization (e.g. drain bladder, collect sample, hydropropulsion).

To make an indwelling dog catheter from a polyamide catheter, either:

■ Place zinc tape around the catheter near to the prepuce

OR

■ Stitch or stick the catheter to the prepuce.

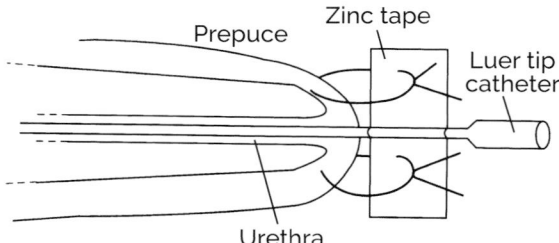

Neither of these options is ideal because dog catheters are not designed to be indwelling. It is best to use a silicone indwelling male Foley.

Catheterizing a bitch: Method 1. Urethra viewed in dorsal recumbency

Equipment

■ Speculum (with or without light source)
■ Alternative light source if required
■ Catheter
■ Sterile water-based lubricant (or silicone spray)
■ Swabs for cleaning
■ Gloves

If a Foley catheter is being placed, the following equipment is also needed:

■ Stylet
■ Sterile water/saline to inflate cuff
■ Urine bag
■ Syringe.

Restraint

Bitches should usually be sedated for this procedure. The bitch should be positioned in a straight dorsal recumbent position with the hindlimbs flexed and drawn forward. The tail must also be under control.

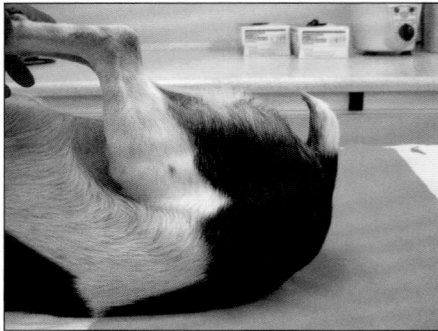

Procedure

1. Wash your hands and put on gloves.
2. Clean the vulva.
3. Remove the catheter from its outer wrapping and expose the tip only from the inner sleeve.
4. If a Foley catheter is being used, insert the stylet.
5. Place the lubricated speculum blades between the vulval lips as caudally as possible to avoid the clitoral fossa.

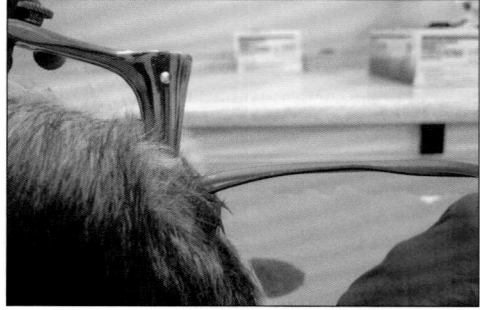

6. Insert vertically into the vestibule and turn the handles cranially.
7. Open the blades of the speculum. The urethral opening will be visible on the cranial side of the vertically oriented vestibule, approximately half way between the vulva and cervix.

Catheterizing a bitch: Method 1. Urethra viewed in dorsal recumbency *continued*

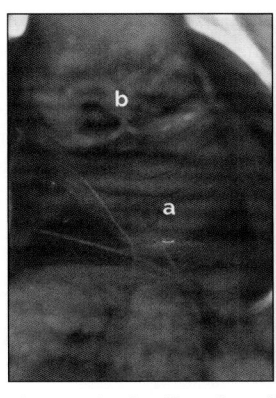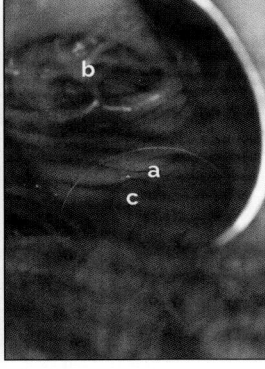

a = the urethral orifice; **b** = clitoral fossa; **c** = catheter in position.

8. Insert the tip of the catheter into the urethral orifice. Draw the hindlimbs caudally. This straightens the urethra, making it easier to push the catheter into the bladder.
9. Proceed depending on the reason for catheterization. If a Foley catheter is being used, inflate the balloon, withdraw the stylet, attach the urine collecting bag and place an Elizabethan collar.

Catheterizing a bitch: Method 2. Urethra viewed standing

Equipment
The equipment required is as for Method 1. Generally only one assistant is required.

Restraint
The bitch should generally be standing for this procedure, although positioned in a straight ventral recumbency with the hindlimbs forwards is also possible. Ensure the tail is well restrained.

Procedure
1. Wash your hands and put on gloves.
2. Clean the vulva.
3. Place the speculum between the vulval lips and advance at a slight angle towards the spine, then horizontally.

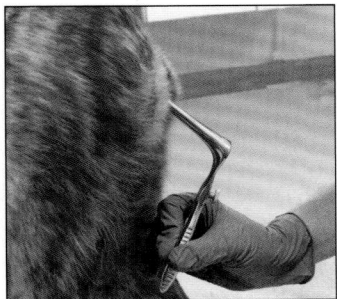

4. Open the blades and identify the urethral orifice. This will be on the ventral floor of the vestibule.
5. Insert the catheter at a slightly ventral angle so as to follow the direction of the urethra into the bladder.
6. Proceed as for Method 1.

Catheterizing a bitch: Method 3. Digital

Equipment
- Sterile gloves
- Catheter
- Sterile water-based lubricant (or silicone spray)
- Swabs for cleaning
- Collection pots

If a Foley catheter is being placed, the additional equipment required is as for Method 1.

Restraint
The bitch should generally be standing for this procedure, although lateral recumbency is also possible.

Procedure
1. Scrub your hands and put on sterile gloves in an aseptic manner.
2. Ask an assistant to clean the vulva.
3. The assistant removes the outer wrapping from the catheter and you (the scrubbed person) remove the inner package.
4. Holding the sterile part of the packaging, place the stylet if necessary.
5. Lubricate the first finger of your non-writing hand.
6. Place your finger into the vestibule and feel along the ventral surface for a raised pimple.
7. Place your finger just cranial to this raised area, which is the urethral orifice.

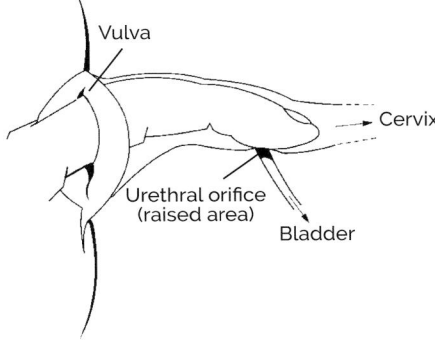

8. Raising your hand and finger dorsally, digitally guide the catheter, tipped slightly ventrally (as for Method 2) into the urethral orifice. The catheter will run past the fingertip if the orifice is missed.
9. Proceed as for Method 1.

The digital method may be difficult or even impossible in smaller breeds.

Catheterizing a tomcat

Equipment
As for dog catheterization.

Restraint
The cat should usually be sedated and positioned in lateral recumbency with the hindlimbs pulled slightly cranially. The tail should be held away from the perineal area.

Procedure
1. Wash your hands and put on gloves.
2. Prepare the feeding sleeve as for the dog catheter and lubricate the tip. →

Catheterizing a tomcat *continued*

3. With one hand, extrude the penis by applying gentle pressure each side of the prepuce with two fingers.
4. Introduce the catheter into the urethra gently.
5. Collect the sample or drain the bladder.
6. If a Jackson catheter is being placed for continuous drainage, stitch the flange to the prepuce.

Catheterizing a queen

Equipment
As for dog catheterization.

Restraint
The cat should usually be sedated and positioned in lateral recumbency with the hindlimbs pulled slightly cranially. The tail should be held away from the perineal area.

Procedure
1. Wash your hands and put on gloves.
2. Remove the outer wrapping and cut a feeding sleeve.
3. Lubricate the tip of the catheter.
4. Place the catheter between the vulval lips and 'blindly' introduce it into the urethra. Angle the catheter ventrally, placing gentle pressure until the catheter slips into the urethra.
5. The catheter is not designed to be indwelling.

Management of indwelling urinary catheters

Patients with urinary catheters *in situ* require close monitoring. All patients should have an Elizabethan collar (see Figure 15.20) or a similar device placed to prevent interference. If the patient is paying a lot of attention to the catheter site, this could indicate a problem (e.g. infection).

Patients with indwelling catheters should have their temperature taken at least twice daily to aid in the identification of urinary tract infections. Regular urinary dipstick tests (see Chapter 17) should also be undertaken to aid monitoring. If infection is suspected, culture and sensitivity testing of a urine sample may be indicated. If a urine collection system is being used, it should not be placed directly on the floor; a clean litter tray can be useful to contain it. Gloves should be used when handling any part of the urine collection system.

Urine output should be monitored. In normal animals, urine output is 1–2 ml/kg/h. If the rate of production drops below this value, further investigations/assessments should be carried out (e.g. hydration status, blood pressure measurement as hypotension can lead to reduced glomerular filtration rates).

Care and consideration should be taken to prevent any tension being placed on the catheter as this will increase discomfort and the risk of patient interference. The use of a cohesive bandage or adhesive tape to reduce tension on the catheter, for example by taping the catheter to the patient's tail (Figure 15.30), must be carried out carefully so as not to cause trauma to the tail.

Possible complications associated with urinary catheterization

Complications as a result of urinary catheterization can arise for a number of reasons; methods of prevention and actions to be taken should they arise are summarized in Figure 15.31.

Failure to catheterize the urethra
Failure to catheterize the urethra may occur in the bitch if the urethral orifice is passed and the catheter cannot be advanced because it meets the cervix. Catheterization of the cervix is a rare occurrence and is easily identified:

- By viewing the urethral orifice with a lighted speculum
- Because no urine flows through the catheter; although it should be noted that catheters can be placed correctly and still not produce urine, due to either an empty bladder or an obstruction to urine flow (e.g. excessive lubricant blocking the drainage holes).

Complication	Prevention	Action
Failure to catheterize the urethra in the bitch	■ The only prevention is to gain experience in bitch catheterization ■ The easiest way for the student nurse to appreciate the position of the urethral orifice is by use of a lighted speculum to provide viewed introduction of the catheter	■ If catheterization of the cervix occurs, remove the catheter and begin with a new one
Urethral damage	■ Never use force ■ Use adequate lubrication ■ If an obstruction or difficulty occurs, stop and inform a senior member of staff	■ If trauma caused by catheterization is suspected, a veterinary surgeon will have to decide what further action is to be taken ■ Minor trauma may require antibiotic treatment to prevent secondary bacterial infection
Infection	■ Use only new or re-sterilized catheters ■ Use sterile gloves to handle catheters or employ the 'no touch' technique described for dog catheterization ■ Use sterile lubricants ■ Clean penis or vulva thoroughly before catheterization; clip surrounding hair if necessary ■ Catheterization should be carried out in a clean environment, not in the patient's kennel ■ Investigate infection where suspected: culture and sensitivity testing of urine sample. Use appropriate antibiotics as necessary	■ If infection becomes evident, treatment will consist of culture and sensitivity testing of urine sample followed by use of appropriate systemic antibiotics

15.31 Possible complications associated with catheterization.

continues ▶

Complication	Prevention	Action
Cystitis after catheterization	■ Gentle introduction of the catheter – no force should be necessary ■ Use of lubricants is beneficial – they help to limit the epithelial damage to the urethral mucosa, thereby reducing inflammation ■ Trauma is less likely if an experienced person catheterizes debilitated patients	With indwelling catheters there is inevitably some degree of cystitis after removal of the catheter. If it is significant: ■ Encourage the patient to increase its fluid intake, either as water or by adding water to the food, or by using intravenous fluids ■ Walk the patient frequently to allow urination; observe the colour and volume of urine passed
Blockage of indwelling catheters	■ General hygiene and cleaning ■ Flush catheter as necessary 2–3 times daily with sterile saline or water ■ Encourage increased water intake or use intravenous fluid therapy (this helps to maintain a continuous flow of urine through the catheter) ■ If bags are attached, check regularly to ensure that urine is able to drain freely	■ Flush with sterile saline or water 2–3 times daily as necessary
Catheter removal by the patient	■ Adequate suturing in male animals ■ Use of an Elizabethan collar	■ Re-catheterize as necessary ■ Use preventative measures

15.31 *continued* Possible complications associated with catheterization.

Infection

A urinary tract infection (UTI) can easily be caused by catheterization if bacteria present in the urethra are pushed into the bladder by the catheter. In most circumstances the bacteria are rapidly eliminated and cause no further concern. The risk of infection is increased when:

■ The bladder is traumatized
■ A preputial or vaginal discharge is present
■ Indwelling catheters are used, or repeated catheterization is carried out
■ The patient is immunosuppressed (i.e. its immune system is compromised in some way and the body's natural defences are not operating normally).

Good catheter placement technique (see above) and post-placement management of indwelling catheters (see above) should help to prevent infection.

Feeding tubes

There are many different types of feeding tube, including:

■ Naso-oesophageal/nasogastric tubes
■ Oesophagostomy tubes
■ Gastrostomy tubes (e.g. percutaneous endoscopic gastrostomy tubes)
■ Jejunostomy tubes.

Feeding tubes are commonly placed to provide nutritional support to patients who, for a variety of medical or surgical reasons, may be unable to eat themselves. The choice of type of feeding tube depends upon patient factors, the capabilities of the veterinary team providing the treatment, and the social economic status of the owner. The determining factors are associated with not only the cost of the procedure but also the duration the tube will remain in place (e.g. an economical tube choice will be best suited to short-term use, whilst longer terms solutions cost more in procedure time and consumables, as well as equipment and skill required to place).

The selection, use and management of feeding tubes is discussed in detail in Chapter 13.

Oxygen supplementation

Oxygen supplementation is indicated in patients that have conditions which affect their ability to obtain an oxygen supply (e.g. upper airway obstruction), or have a problem with gaseous exchange, or with poor supply of oxygen to the tissues as a result of poor perfusion (e.g. patients in shock) or anaemia.

Patients with an airway obstruction

In patients that have a problem with obtaining an oxygen supply, physical methods of providing oxygen are central. An example of this situation that is becoming more commonly seen in veterinary practice is patients suffering from brachycephalic obstructive airway syndrome (BOAS; e.g. French bulldog, pug; Figure 15.32). If these patients are presented in crisis, they require emergency management (see Chapter 19). Primarily this involves trying to keep the patient as calm as

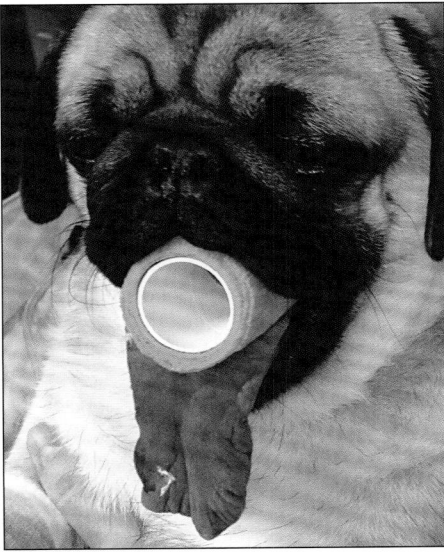

15.32 Pug recovering from anaesthesia after upper airway surgery. A bandage roll is placed in the mouth to keep the tongue pulled out and to maintain a patent airway. (Reproduced from the *BSAVA Manual of Canine and Feline Anaesthesia and Analgesia, 3rd edn*)

possible (sometimes this requires the use of mild sedatives, e.g. low-dose acepromazine; see Chapter 21), but patient positioning is also key.

The aim of restraint is not to put any additional pressure on the soft tissues of the upper airways and to extend the upper airways to reduce the obstruction. With this in mind, these patients should not be restrained in the typical manner of looping the arm around the neck; instead they should be held with a hand either side of the cranial neck/mandible, thereby avoiding pressure on the ventral neck. By using these bony prominences, the head can be effectively extended, stretching the soft tissues that are causing the obstruction.

If these patients are sedated, management of the tongue is vital. The tongue should be pulled/extended as far out of the mouth as possible (Figure 15.32), taking care not to be bitten. It is important to remember that any upper airway noise/snoring is due to obstruction. A roll of cohesive bandage can be used in a sedated patient to act as a soft gag (Figure 15.32). Care needs to be taken with BOAS patients as they have a higher incidence of regurgitation; patients should not be profoundly sedated without the head being raised and the equipment to convert to general anaesthesia (e.g. endotracheal tube and laryngoscope) should be readily available. These patients should be attached to a pulse oximeter to monitor oxygen saturation. The use of oxygen masks in these cases is indicated. Eyes should also always be lubricated to help prevent eye ulceration.

Patients with altered gaseous exchange

Patients may have problems at the point of gaseous exchange and long-term oxygen therapy may be required. There are a couple of considerations that need to be taken into account when administering this type of therapy:

■ Oxygen is a dry gas – oxygen delivered directly from a cylinder or pipeline is dry and will cause desiccation of the mucous membranes. This can be managed with the use of water humidifiers ('bubblers'; Figure 15.33), which pass the oxygen though water to increase the moisture content. The minimal flowrate that the patient can manage with should be used

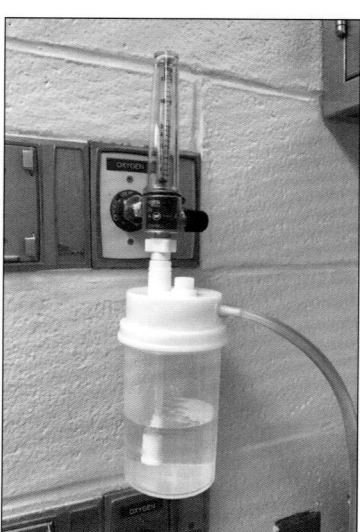

15.33 Commercial humidifier ('bubbler') attached to an oxygen supply. (Reproduced from the *BSAVA Manual of Canine and Feline Emergency and Critical Care, 3rd edn*)

■ The use of 100% oxygen long-term is toxic. However, it is unlikely that 100% oxygen would be delivered via the options available in veterinary practice. Venturi valves can be used to achieve a specific concentration; these are of particular use when using an oxygen cage/tent long term.

Patients with altered oxygen delivery to the tissues

The other subset of patients are those that have problems delivering oxygen to the peripheral tissues. This can be due to reduced oxygen-carrying capacity of the blood (e.g. anaemia) or due to circulatory problems (e.g. hypovolaemic shock, when oxygen cannot be delivered to the tissues). When monitoring anaemic patients, it is vital to remember that they can be hypoxaemic but still have a normal percentage (%) haemoglobin saturated with oxygen (SpO_2; see also Chapter 21); this is because of the overall reduced oxygen-carrying capacity of the blood. Oxygen therapy in these patients is only indicated to ensure that the maximum amount of oxygen is available to oxygenate the remaining haemoglobin. Treatment of these patients is a blood transfusion to increase the oxygen-carrying capacity (see Chapter 20).

Methods of providing oxygen therapy

With all methods of oxygen therapy, it is important to lubricate the eyes to prevent the formation of ulcers due to desiccation caused by the oxygen. It is also vital to remember that, although providing oxygen therapy is important, it may become counterproductive if patients become stressed. If this occurs, an alternative method for oxygen provision should be tried.

Mask

This involves simply placing a mask over the nose/muzzle of the patient (see Chapter 21). The use of a diaphragm on the mask can improve efficiency; however, a lot of patients will not tolerate this.

Flow-by

This involves either placing/holding a breathing system or oxygen tubing next to the patient. If using this technique, it is important to remember that oxygen is denser than room air, so it will sink. Thus, efficiency can be improved by holding the tubing just above the patient's nose so that the oxygen falls down in front of the nose and mouth.

Nasal oxygen prongs

These are commercially available; however, they are very patient-dependent. They rely on the prongs fitting the patient (Figure 15.34) and staying *in situ*. It can be helpful to use a small amount of tissue glue or skin staples to secure the tubing to the surrounding tissues. Patients can find this technique irritating. It is important to use humidified oxygen with this technique.

Nasal oxygen cannula/catheter

Soft catheters or nasogastric tubes can be used to provide oxygen further into the nares (see Chapter 19). The catheter is introduced nasally to the level of the medial canthus. The use of water based-lubricant is essential during placement. The use of local anaesthetic can also aid placement. It is essential to use humidified oxygen with this technique and to avoid high flow rates, as this may cause tissue damage.

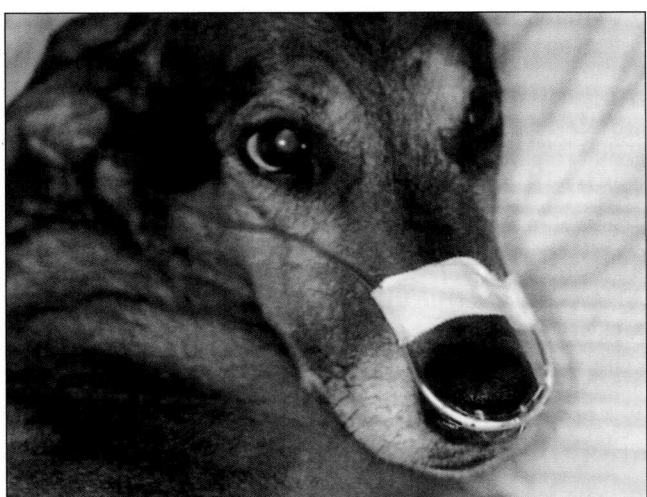

15.34 Supply of oxygen using nasal prongs. (Reproduced from the *BSAVA Manual of Canine and Feline Head, Neck and Thoracic Surgery, 2nd edn*)

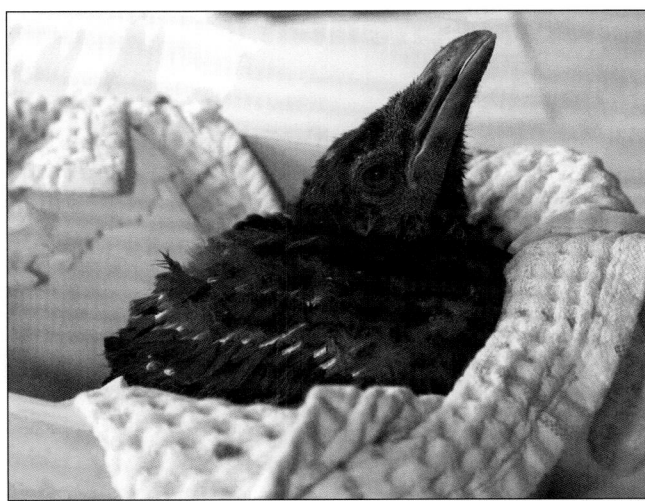

15.35 Bird in sternal recumbency in a 'doughnut nest'.

Oxygen cage/tent

These have become more commercially available in recent years. Oxygen cages (see Chapter 19) and tents can be very useful, especially for smaller patients (e.g. small dogs, small mammals and exotic pets), and are ideal for cats that require supplemental oxygen but become stressed with any hands-on techniques. It is very important to ensure that these cages/tents do not become too hot. It is also useful to have an oxygen concentration monitor to detect the concentration being delivered. It is important to avoid opening these cages/tents too frequently, as the oxygen will escape.

Further information on oxygen supplementation is given in Chapter 19.

Provision of oxygen to exotic pets

Most small exotic pets that are struggling to breathe (dyspnoeic) and have a reduced oxygen supply will be much less tolerant to handling than dogs and cats. The stress of handling will exacerbate the problems and should be avoided. This makes many of the methods of providing supplementary oxygen (above) unsuitable in these cases and alternatives must be found. Possible methods of supplying short-term oxygen to small pets include:

- Placing a clear face mask directly over the pet and on to a solid surface in order to enclose it within the mask space and provide high levels of oxygen quickly
- Place the pet into an anaesthetic chamber (see Chapter 21) and provide oxygen only
- Place the pet into a home-made oxygen cage produced by wrapping a small cage in cling film and piping oxygen into it
- Place the pet into a commercial incubator into which oxygen can be piped.

Oxygen supplementation to birds

Birds that require oxygen therapy present with clinical signs of open-beaked breathing and 'tail bobbing', and are often 'fluffed up'. In order to allow the air sacs and lungs (see Chapter 3) to function maximally, the bird should be placed in sternal recumbency (rather than in lateral). A 'doughnut nest' can be useful to help make this achievable (Figure 15.35). Excessive use of oxygen in birds can lead to 'oxygen

toxicosis' and careful reassessment of the need for oxygen supplementation should be made on a regular basis, with oxygen supplementation reduced as soon as improvement is seen.

Further information on first aid in exotic pets is provided in the *BSAVA Manual of Exotic Pet and Wildlife Nursing*.

Pain management and patient wellbeing

Pain recognition in hospitalized patients is key to ensuring patient wellbeing and welfare, and is important for staff safety. Pain is an emotional experience and, therefore, each individual animal responds in a unique manner. This makes both pain assessment and management challenging, but also rewarding.

Assessment of the patient's behaviour and changes in behaviour forms the backbone of pain assessment. Physiological signs are important to assess and occur due to stimulation of the sympathetic nervous system. It should be noted that behavioural assessments vary between different species (see Chapter 14). The use of pain scoring systems (see Chapter 21) can aid patient assessment and help to reduce variability between observers.

Opioids (e.g. methadone) are the mainstay for pain management. However, other classes of drugs, including non-steroidal analgesics (e.g. meloxicam), local anaesthetics (e.g. lidocaine) and adjunctive analgesics (e.g. ketamine) are also often used (see Chapter 21).

Due to the emotional aspect of pain, the importance of patient housing and nursing care cannot be underestimated (see Chapter 14). The more comfortable and relaxed a hospitalized patient is, the less they will preserve their pain and the more likely they are to rest. Thick, comfortable bedding can help enable the patient to manoeuvre themselves into the most comfortable position. It is important to question the owner regarding the patient's preferences and to incorporate these into the management plan where appropriate. Patient specific factors that might result in unnecessary patient distress should also be considered, particularly age, sex (entire male not housed next to entire bitch) and prey species (e.g. rabbits) being separated from predator species (see Chapter 14 for further information).

Pain management is covered in detail in Chapter 21.

Complementary therapies

Complementary therapies incorporate a range of treatment approaches designed to facilitate and promote healing alongside conventional veterinary medicine. There is growing evidence from the medical literature that they can aid recovery and promote restoration of health when used appropriately alongside conventional medications and following an accurate diagnosis. These techniques have since been extrapolated and applied with success to the field of veterinary medicine; however, further clinical trials are warranted to validate their effectiveness in animals. The complementary therapies discussed in this chapter include:

- Acupuncture
- Aromatherapy
- Homeopathy
- Chiropractic
- Osteopathy
- Physiotherapy (including hydrotherapy).

The Veterinary Surgeons Act 1966 currently restricts the practice of complementary therapies to registered members of the Royal College of Veterinary Surgeons (RCVS) with the exemptions of registered veterinary nurses and qualified physiotherapists (which includes osteopaths and chiropractors). Acupuncture may be performed by registered veterinary nurses under the direct supervision of a veterinary surgeon, but by no other individual, even though they may be qualified to use acupuncture in human medicine. In common with other medications, aromatherapy and homeopathy may only be prescribed to animals by a member of the RCVS who has those animals under their care. Animals may receive physiotherapy (encompassing also chiropractic treatment and osteopathy) once veterinary permission has been granted, usually in writing, by the referring veterinary surgeon. The roles of paraprofessionals working alongside the veterinary surgeon as part of a 'vet-led team', are currently being reviewed by the RCVS.

Acupuncture

Acupuncture has gained considerable popularity and credibility within the fields of human and veterinary medicine as a method of pain control. It is a treatment technique which originated in China and has been used in the Far East for the past 2000 years. It involves the insertion of fine metal needles at varying depths into the skin at localized points within the body to treat pain or disease.

The research suggests that the needles activate naturally occurring pain-relieving chemicals in the brain (endogenous opiates and endorphins) by sending messages via the spinal cord from the sensory nerves in the skin. The Chinese Medicine theory believes that acupuncture works by stimulating the body's natural energy known as 'Chi' via energy channels known as 'meridians'. However, the scientific literature to date has had difficulty proving the existence of these meridians as they cannot be objectively measured or quantified.

Nevertheless, acupuncture is a popular method of achieving natural pain relief in humans and has since been applied successfully by veterinary surgeons to animals. It can be a useful treatment adjunct for postoperative or chronic pain cases.

Acupuncture needle insertion may be slightly uncomfortable initially but seems to be tolerated well by most animals if performed correctly and sympathetically (Figure 15.36). The needles are left *in situ* for anything up to 30 minutes per treatment, during which they may be 'stimulated' by being gently rotated several times. The number of needles used during a treatment session varies depending on the condition being treated. Frequency of treatment also depends on the chronicity and nature of the presenting condition; an animal may start off with two treatments per week initially.

Under the Veterinary Surgeons Act (1966), acupuncture is classified as minor surgery and must therefore only be performed by a veterinary surgeon who has received specialist training, or by a registered veterinary nurse under their direct supervision.

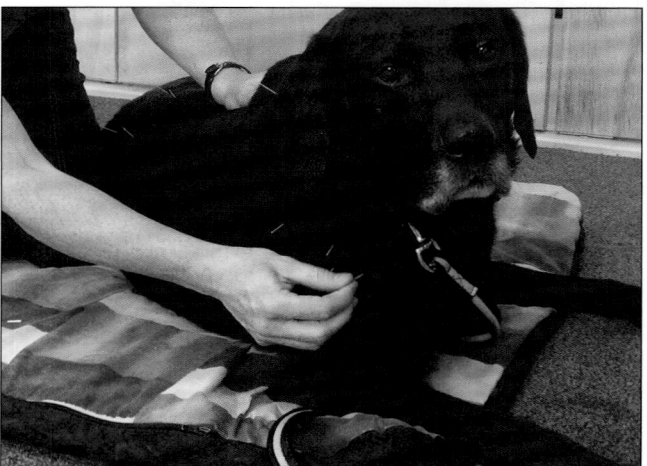

15.36 Dog receiving acupuncture.

Aromatherapy

Aromatherapy involves the use of aromatic plant extracts in oil form to promote health and wellbeing. Certain plant materials are believed to possess therapeutic properties, which may prevent illness and disease. The oils may be administered to the animal by massaging them into the skin or via direct inhalation. As with acupuncture, the Veterinary Surgeons Act (1966) restricts the treatment of animals (other than one's own) with aromatherapy to members of the RCVS.

Homeopathy

Homeopathy is the oral administration of diluted plant or mineral extracts designed to boost the body's natural energy and promote a state of health. The treatment can be given in tablet or liquid form and relies on the theory 'treat like with like', i.e. the substance given is meant to cause a similar effect to the clinical signs of dysfunction presented. The evidence to support this theory is debatable. As with acupuncture and aromatherapy, homeopathy can only be prescribed to animals by a member of the RCVS.

Chiropractic

Chiropractic treatment involves the identification and subsequent treatment of musculoskeletal dysfunction within the body. Particular emphasis and treatment is focused on the spine and its associated bony and soft tissue structures by performing a manipulation or 'adjustment' to correct areas of 'subluxation'. Chiropractors use the term 'subluxation' to describe a loss of function in an area of the spine and associated spinal nerves due to a reduction in normal movement or alignment. Chiropractors undergo specialized training before they can treat humans and animals and are regulated by the General Chiropractic Council in the UK. The chiropractic treatment of animals must be approved by a qualified veterinary surgeon in accordance with the Veterinary Surgeons Act (1966).

Osteopathy

Osteopathy involves the identification and subsequent treatment of imbalances and dysfunction within the skeleton, encompassing the bones, joints, muscles, ligaments, tendons and nerves. Osteopaths use a variety of treatment techniques, including joint manipulation, massage and stretches to create a state of balance within the body. They are required to undergo 4–5 years' specialist training at degree level in the human field prior to further postgraduate study which enables them to treat animals following veterinary permission. The osteopathic treatment of animals must be approved by a qualified veterinary surgeon in accordance with the Veterinary Surgeons Act (1966).

Physiotherapy

Physiotherapy or physical therapy is the treatment of illness and injury by physical means. It encompasses exercises, manual therapies (stretches, massage, joint mobilizations), hydrotherapy, thermal modalities (heat and cold), electrotherapeutic modalities (ultrasound, laser, TENS (transcutaneous electrical nerve stimulation), NMES (neuromuscular electrical stimulation)) and respiratory physiotherapy techniques.

Currently, in the UK there are three subgroups of physiotherapists treating animals:

■ ACPAT members (Association of Chartered Physiotherapists in Animal Therapy) – dually qualified healthcare professionals that train extensively in humans to degree level before embarking upon further postgraduate degree programmes (MSc/PGDip) to enable them to treat animals
■ IRVAP members (Institute of Registered Veterinary and Animal Physiotherapists) – train solely with animals
■ NAVP members (National Association of Veterinary Physiotherapists) – train solely with animals.

Physiotherapists can only treat an animal legally in the UK following permission from the referring veterinary surgeon in accordance with the Veterinary Surgeons Act (1966). Registered veterinary nurses can treat animals using physiotherapy techniques provided the referring veterinary surgeon feels they are competent to do so.

The most common treatment approaches and techniques used by physiotherapists in animals are discussed in an introductory format below. Further in-depth information on these topics can be found in the *BSAVA Manual of Canine and Feline Advanced Veterinary Nursing*.

Manual therapies

These include techniques such as massage, limb stretches and joint mobilizations, as well as specialized positioning methods used to treat respiratory patients, such as those requiring pleural drainage.

Massage

This involves the manipulation of the muscles and associated soft tissue structures by rhythmical motions of the therapist's hands. There are various different massage techniques designed to influence the tissues in different ways:

■ **Stroking** – this involves gentle sweeping movements across the muscles. It is generally used as a relaxation and preparatory phase of massage treatment prior to working the tissues using deeper techniques. Stroking allows the animal to become accustomed to the therapist's touch, thus enabling trust and patient compliance
■ **Effleurage** – this is similar to stroking but requires more pressure and is therefore only appropriate to use once the animal has become accustomed to the therapist and the muscles have been warmed up with stroking. The therapist should allow their hands to follow the contours of the animal's musculature, taking care not to put pressure over bony areas such as the spine
■ **Tapotement and petrissage** – these are more vigorous, stimulating techniques that need to be introduced gradually to prevent the animal becoming alarmed.
  • **Coupage** – this is a form of tapotement that can be used over most muscular areas, but the pressure must be kept light over more bony areas such as the scapula. Coupage if often used over the ribs to loosen secretions.

The research suggests that massage, when applied appropriately, can effectively promote blood and lymph circulation and is therefore an effective adjunct in oedema control. In addition, it helps to mobilize the tissues promoting collagen extensibility and elasticity, as well as providing relaxation and pain relief (due to stimulation of pressure receptors in the skin which interact with the nervous system involving the brain).

Animals seem to enjoy massage if performed in an appropriate, timely manner by a trained professional and research from human medicine suggests that it promotes psychological and emotional wellbeing. It must be noted that massage may be contraindicated in certain cases (e.g. around unstable fracture sites, around unstable joints, over bony prominences in general, and around neoplastic or infected tissue as it will promote blood supply). A thorough working knowledge of veterinary anatomy is an absolute pre-requisite before treating any animal with massage techniques to ensure appropriate application.

Limb stretches

Limb stretches involve gently taking a muscle to a lengthened position without causing pain. Again, a thorough working knowledge of animal anatomy is an absolute necessity prior to attempting these techniques in order to prevent damage to the soft tissue structures. When executed appropriately stretches can help maintain muscle/tendon length and health, thereby facilitating normal joint range of movement. This can help with restoration of movement and therefore, ultimately, function. Stretches can help prevent painful contractures and improve, as well as maintain, extensibility of collagen fibres within the connective tissue matrix, thus promoting flexibility and suppleness.

Joint mobilization

This technique involves gently moving the joints through their normal physiological range of motion. Joint mobilizations may be performed passively or actively.

- Passive joint mobilizations involve the therapist gently taking the animal's joints from flexion through to extension and back again. They are particularly useful in recumbent animals that are not actively able to move the joints themselves (e.g. paraplegics).
- Active joint mobilizations involve the animal taking the joints from flexion to extension and back again themselves (e.g. asking a dog to sit and then stand for a treat will result in hip, stifle and tarsus flexion followed by hip, stifle and tarsus extension).

Joint mobilizations, whether active or passive, are necessary for normal joint nutrition and ultimately cartilage health. Articular cartilage lines the surface of all synovial joints and obtains its nutrition via the synovial fluid present within the joint cavity. The synovial fluid is moved around the joint surface thus 'feeding' the articular cartilage with nutrients in response to flexion/extension movements of the limbs. Joints that have not been moved for some time or have only been moved in a restricted manner become stiff, dysfunctional and at more risk of degeneration. A thorough knowledge of anatomy, especially normal joint angle ranges, is essential before performing these techniques to ensure patient safety.

Electrotherapy

This involves treating soft tissue structures with specific machines that produce electrical energy in a variety of different wavelengths, which can help promote healing and repair at a cellular level. Electrotherapy includes modalities such as ultrasound, laser, pulsed magnetic fields and electrical stimulation (NMES, TENS, H-Wave® and microcurrent). These machines can cause significant damage if used at the wrong dosages and it is important that those administering such treatments have received appropriate training. In addition, there are specific precautions and contraindications to using these treatment modalities, which once again highlights the need for specialized training prior to use in animals. A thorough anatomical and physiological knowledge base is paramount for their safe use in animal treatments.

Ultrasound

Ultrasound machines generate vibrations similar to sound waves, creating energy that is then transmitted to the treated tissues (Figure 15.37). This waveform can produce both thermal and non-thermal effects within the tissues, depending on how much energy is absorbed by them. It is a useful modality for increasing tissue extensibility and promotes normal collagen fibril alignment. It is therefore advocated in managing contractures and scar tissue, as well as tendon and ligament injuries. A coupling medium, such as gel, is needed to transmit the ultrasound waves to the underlying tissues; alternatively, treatment can be delivered by submerging the body part (if appropriate) and treatment probe into a container of water.

Laser

This is defined as Light Amplification by Stimulated Emission of Radiation or, more simply, light energy. Lasers deliver light energy into the underlying structures, thus creating an optimum environment for healing to occur. Studies in animal and human models have found that laser therapy can help reduce inflammatory chemicals, which have an adverse effect on normal tissue homeostasis and function. Laser therapy is therefore beneficial for wound healing and, in addition, can help provide pain relief. Like all electrotherapy modalities, it is important that it is used only by trained personnel otherwise significant tissue damage may occur.

Pulsed electromagnetic field therapy (PEMF)

This involves stimulation of the body at a cellular level by exposure to a pulsed magnetic energy waveform. The literature published to date suggests that PEMF can help reduce pain and inflammation and facilitate healing. PEMF therapy can be delivered via a handheld device or a pad, which is subsequently applied to a limb or incorporated into a jacket.

Neuromuscular electrical nerve stimulation (NMES)

This involves stimulation of the nerve fibres on the skin surface by a series of gel covered electrodes, which are attached to a small handheld unit (Figure 15.38). TENS machines are one type of electrical stimulation unit. They can be used as a form of pain relief and work by stimulating the nervous system to release naturally produced pain-relieving chemicals from the brain. Depending on the electrical current frequency and intensity used, they can cause a muscle to contract by stimulating its motor unit. This can help promote blood and lymph circulation (thus reducing swelling), optimize muscle health and strength, and assist in healthy nerve functioning at a cellular level, depending on the machine type and frequency/intensity of the current used.

H-Wave®

This involves electrical stimulation via a waveform designed to mimic that found in nerve cells (Hoffman reflex). This treatment is thought to be beneficial in the relief of pain and is applied via electrode pads placed on the patient's skin, which are connected to a unit that delivers the waveform.

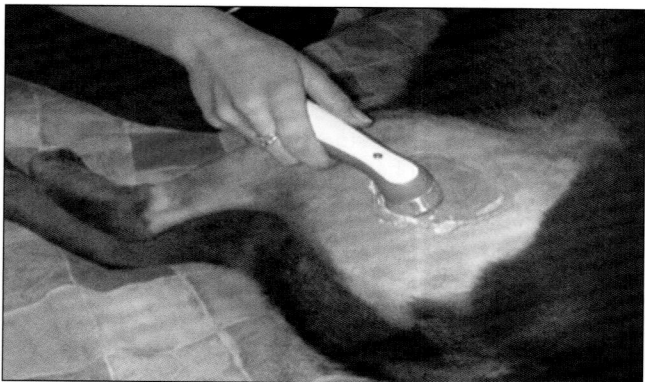

15.37 Dog receiving ultrasound treatment. Note the clipped area to enable more effective transmission of the ultrasound waves. (© Linhay Veterinary Rehabilitation Centre)

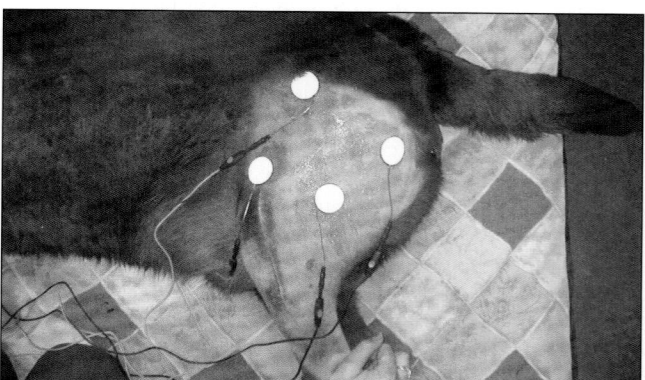

15.38 Dog receiving neuromuscular electrical stimulation. Note the clipped area to enable better electrode contact with the skin surface. (© Linhay Veterinary Rehabilitation Centre)

Microcurrent

This involves electrical stimulation via a waveform that is designed to mimic the naturally occurring bioelectrical field that exists within the cells and tissue, thus restoring a state of homeostasis. It has been postulated to have a variety of therapeutic effects, including pain relief and cellular and tissue repair, by increasing adenosine triphosphate (ATP) activity within the cells themselves. The waveform is delivered via a handheld unit that communicates with a series of electrode pads that are attached the patient's limbs and/or back.

Thermal modalities

These involve the application of cold (cryotherapy) or heat (thermotherapy) to the muscles and associated soft tissues of the body to promote pain relief and facilitate healing after injury.

Cryotherapy

The application of cold can help reduce swelling postoperatively or following trauma and provides a natural form of pain relief to the inflamed/injured structures. Initially, the application of cold causes the blood vessels to constrict (vasoconstriction), which reduces blood flow to the area. This is then followed by a period where the blood vessels expand again (vasodilatation), thereby enabling an increase in blood flow to the area. These changes in blood flow help control inflammation and are useful in the acute stage to limit further tissue damage. Cold can be applied by simply wrapping some ice in a damp towel or via special gel packs that can be kept in the freezer. Care must be taken not to expose the treated area to the cold for too long, otherwise an ice burn and further tissue damage may be caused (10–15 minutes is usually adequate per treatment).

Thermotherapy

This involves the application of heat to the tissues, which can help with pain relief, promotion of blood flow (causes vasodilatation) and tissue elasticity/extensibility. This can make it a useful treatment adjunct prior to massage or stretching in certain cases. Heat can be applied using special gel or wheat bag packs that can be warmed to a comfortable temperature in a microwave before direct application to the muscles. As with ice application, precautions must be taken to avoid skin burns to the animal. Hot packs can be left in place for 20–30 minutes as they tend to cool down during this time; however, the animal must be supervised at all times to ensure safety. It is important to note that neoplastic, infected or haemorrhaging tissue must not be exposed to thermotherapy treatments as heat causes increased blood flow to the underlying treated area.

Hydrotherapy

This involves swimming/walking in a body of water, such as a pool or water treadmill. Occasionally, open bodies of water such as lakes or ponds can be utilized; however, the water temperature is usually too cold and therefore will not have a thermal therapeutic effect on the joints and tissues. In addition, there is the issue of safety when swimming an animal in an open body of water due to external influences such as current, water depth and hidden reeds/weeds. Ideally, animals should receive hydrotherapy in a veterinary establishment (usually run in conjunction with a qualified physiotherapist) or in an establishment that has received approval from the Canine Hydrotherapy Association (CHA).

Hydrotherapy can help strengthen muscles (due to water resistance) without placing extra weight-bearing forces through the joints (due to the effect of buoyancy). It can also be used for cardiovascular/respiratory conditioning and oedema control, as well as psychological benefits by allowing the animal to exercise and expend energy in a controlled environment.

Care must be taken with geriatric animals and those with heart or lung conditions due to the extra pressure that the water will place on the heart and lungs when the animal is submerged. For this reason, each animal should be checked by a veterinary surgeon prior to undergoing any form of hydrotherapy. However, when used appropriately, the physiological effects of submerging an animal in water can be clinically advantageous.

General guidelines

Water temperature and quality should be strictly controlled to ensure patient safety and satisfy hygiene/infection control regulations. Water temperature should be between 26 and 30°C to enable a therapeutic effect on the musculoskeletal system. In addition, it is important that the animal is adequately dried following treatment to prevent chills, especially in colder weather.

Good control and handling of the animal in the pool/hydrotherapy treadmill is imperative to ensure appropriate, effective and safe treatment. A therapist must be present in the pool with the animal at all times and use appropriate buoyancy aids or harnesses to aid control, thereby ensuring animal/handler safety. Dogs on treadmills should be secured centrally on the treadmill belt via a harness and bungee system (see Figure 15.40) to facilitate a safe, therapeutic treatment and should be supervised at all times. In addition, all dogs must be introduced to the aquatic environment in a controlled, sympathetic manner, ideally via a shallow, non-slip ramp. In some cases, it may be appropriate to hoist the animal into the pool, but this needs to be undertaken by experienced personnel.

Therapeutic effects

Submerging an animal in water has a number of physiological effects that can help provide a therapeutic treatment if performed correctly by qualified physiotherapists or veterinary nurses who have received further specialist training. These therapeutic effects include the principles of buoyancy, hydrostatic pressure and viscosity.

- **Buoyancy** – this is based on Archimedes' principle that describes what happens when an object is submerged in water. When pushed under the surface, the object will experience an up-thrust equal to the weight of water it has displaced. From a clinical perspective, the effect of buoyancy means that weak patients or those with joint pain will be able to move more freely in water, with less pain, and therefore build muscle. By building up the relevant muscle groups and gently mobilizing the associated joints, the animal becomes stronger and therefore better able to cope with exercise on land.
- **Hydrostatic pressure** – this incorporates the principle that the deeper an object is immersed in water, the more pressure is exerted on it. Clinically, this means that submerging an animal's limbs in water can help control swelling, as the pressure exerted by the water will help pump the venous blood back to the heart. As a result, the limb may well be less swollen following hydrotherapy treatment, which will be more comfortable for the animal.

■ **Viscosity** – this is the resistance to movement created by water molecules and decreases as temperature increases. Clinically, this is advantageous as it will enable weak muscles to move bones and joints in water easier than on land. This is particularly useful in some orthopaedic postoperative or neurological cases. Treatment times need to be closely monitored and increased gradually, depending on the patient's problem. The skill lies in knowing when to challenge the musculoskeletal structures without causing a concomitant increase in pain and lameness.

Pool *versus* treadmill

Both of these forms of hydrotherapy can be useful rehabilitation tools if used sensibly, following a complete diagnosis and subsequent close liaison with the referring veterinary surgeon. However, it must be noted that in certain cases/conditions they can make the animal lame, increase pain and, in the case of postoperative orthopaedic patients, cause surgery to fail.

Swimming in a pool (Figure 15.39) often encourages the patient to take their joints through a large active range of motion, which may not always be appropriate immediately following surgery. For this reason, the hydrotherapy treadmill (Figure 15.40) may be a more suitable treatment option, but the water height and belt speed must be carefully controlled to prevent worsening of the condition. It is also easier to control the amount of work performed by the patient in a treadmill compared with a pool.

It is paramount that the physiotherapist/veterinary nurse collaborates with the referring veterinary/orthopaedic surgeon so as not to adversely affect treatment outcome. Thus, knowledge of normal healing timescales for both soft tissue and bone/fractures, alongside a thorough working knowledge of animal anatomy, are very important.

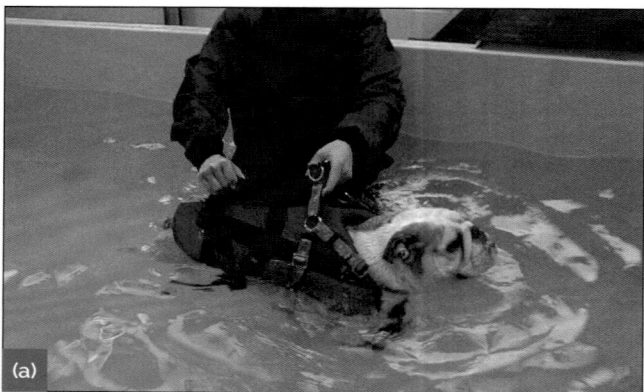

(a)

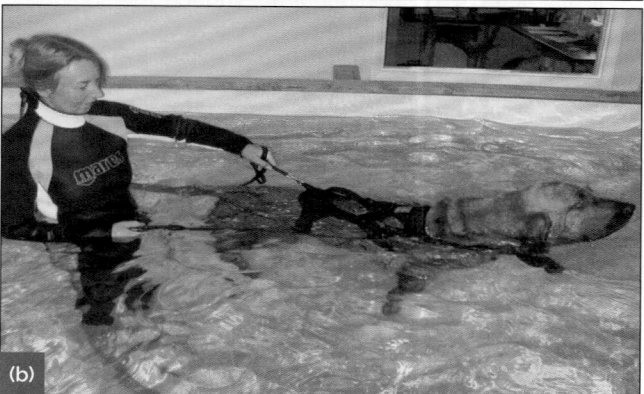

(b)

15.39 (a, b) Dogs undergoing treatment in a hydrotherapy pool. Note the harness control and use of a buoyancy aid. (b, © Linhay Veterinary Rehabilitation Centre)

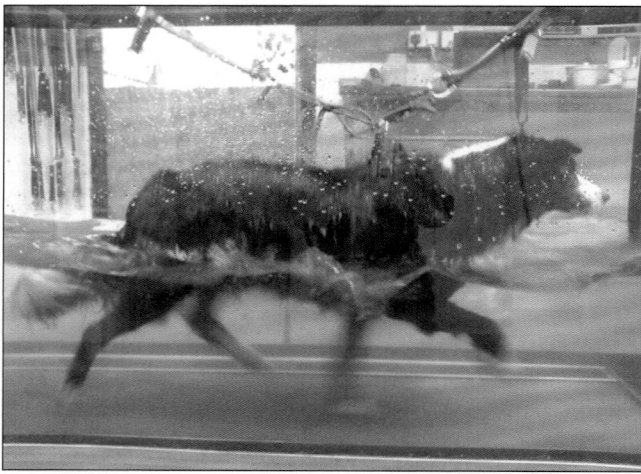

15.40 Dog undergoing treatment on a hydrotherapy treadmill. Note the harness and bungee control system. (© Linhay Veterinary Rehabilitation Centre)

Therapeutic exercises

Therapeutic exercises consist of a multitude of planned, repetitive series of events designed to facilitate muscle hypertrophy, activate joint range of motion and stimulate balance and coordination, as well as influence cardiovascular/respiratory endurance and fitness (Figure 15.41). They are intended to prepare condition and restore function to the neuromusculoskeletal, cardiovascular and respiratory systems following injury, surgery or disease. These exercises may include:

■ Harness-controlled lead walking up/down slopes/over different surfaces (e.g. sand, gravel, grass, through weave poles)
■ Using apparatus to challenge the animal's balance, proprioception and core stability (e.g. stepping over poles, facilitated balancing on wobble cushions, work over a 'physio-roll' and sit–stands exercises).

Such exercise programmes must be designed with clear goals in mind, which are ultimately influenced by the clinical diagnosis. They must be progressively incremental in design, thus allowing for training and subsequent recovery effect. The exercise programme should aim to deliver controlled stresses on the muscles, joints, ligaments, tendons and nervous system, which ultimately facilitate restoration of function without increasing pain or lameness. It should be noted that during the rehabilitation process, it is important for the animal to be provided with suitable analgesia. This will enable the patient to participate in the rehabilitation programme without causing unnecessary discomfort or suffering, and should be discussed with the referring veterinary surgeon.

Summary

The complementary therapies and treatment approaches discussed above are by no means an exhaustive list. It is beyond the scope of this chapter to include other alternative treatment approaches such as Shiatsu, Bowen therapy, Rolfing and Reiki, all of which need further research and evidence of their effectiveness in the treatment of animals. Furthermore, there is still a paucity of randomized, controlled clinical trials within the field of veterinary physiotherapy, since it is a fairly new, rapidly evolving specialist area. This warrants evidence-based research to help inform best practice for using these physiotherapy techniques in animals.

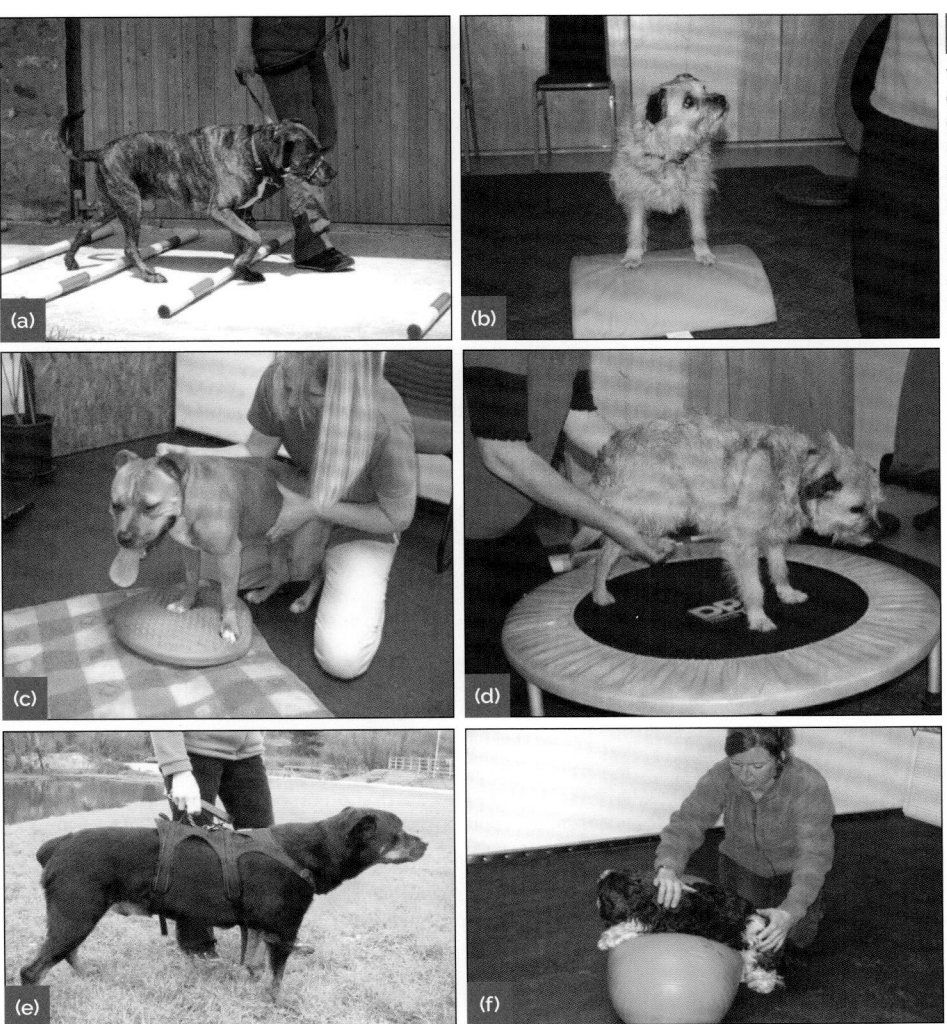

15.41 A variety of therapeutic exercises are used in veterinary practice.
(a) Walking over poles.
(b) Balancing on a wedge.
(c) Balancing on a wobble cushion.
(d) Limb lifts on a trampette.
(e) Harness control during outdoor exercise.
(f) Core stability/strengthening work over a 'physio-roll'.
(© Linhay Veterinary Rehabilitation Centre)

Nursing of common patient types

Nursing care often involves the sort of interventions that are described in this chapter (or elsewhere in this textbook) including: administration of prescribed medication (see Chapter 8); provision of appropriate nutrition (see Chapter 13); general patient care and comfort (see Chapter 14); fluid therapy (see Chapter 20); and appropriate analgesia (see Chapter 21). The combination of interventions required will vary between patients according to a variety of factors, including species, medical or surgical conditions and age. Some of these are discussed in more detail when medical nursing (see Chapter 18) and surgical nursing (see Chapter 23) are considered.

The common generic types of patients, often encountered in veterinary practice, and their requirements are discussed below. Nursing care planning for individual patients is considered in more detail in Chapter 12. For all patients, a full nursing history (see Chapters 12 and 14) must be taken, followed by a nursing assessment of real and potential problems (see Chapter 12) and likely nursing interventions.

The geriatric patient

The nursing of geriatric patients can be complex as these animals often have multiple conditions; however, they can also be amongst the most rewarding to treat. Physical changes as a result of natural ageing are often compounded by the effects of old injuries and concurrent medical problems. Changes due to disease must be carefully distinguished from those of old age, although disease can become more obvious or affect a patient more rapidly as they become older. Many conditions in elderly patients are subtle and multiple.

Common medical conditions associated with old age

- Neoplasia
- Chronic renal disease
- Cardiac disease
- Osteoarthritis (degenerative joint disease, DJD)
- Cataracts
- Dental disease
- Constipation
- Urinary and/or faecal incontinence
- Impaired cognitive function

Nursing assessment and possible interventions

A nursing assessment based upon a standardized approach, together with common nursing interventions for geriatric patients is summarized in Figure 15.42.

Parameter	Potential problems in these patients	Possible nursing interventions
Eating	■ May be fussier about foods than younger animals ■ May have dental disease or other medical conditions that make eating difficult	■ Tempt to eat: palatable diet, hand feed, warm food (see Chapter 14) ■ Adequate analgesia (see Chapter 21) ■ Appropriate dental care (see Chapter 25)
Drinking	■ May be polydipsic as a result of age-related medical conditions ■ May be prone to dehydration as a result of medical problems	■ Provide adequate fresh water, encourage drinking (e.g. water fountains for cats) ■ Use intravenous fluids as necessary (see Chapter 20)
Urinating	■ Urine production may be inadequate ■ May be polydipsic and polyuric ■ May be urinary incontinent	■ Use intravenous fluids as necessary (see Chapter 20) ■ Take out often for walks, provide clean litter trays ■ Provide appropriate bedding, including incontinence pads ■ Consider **urinary catheterization**
Defecating	■ May be prone to constipation	■ Provide **laxatives and enemas** as required
Breathing	■ May have pre-existing heart and/or lung conditions	■ Give any prescribed medication
Maintaining body temperature	■ May have reduced ability to maintain temperature	■ Monitor temperature ■ Provide appropriate bedding (see Chapter 14) ■ Encourage mobility
Grooming	■ Self-care may be poor ■ Nails may not wear adequately	■ Groom at least daily ■ Clip nails as necessary
Mobilizing	■ May be deaf and/or blind ■ May have osteoarthritis or other age-related medical problems affecting mobility	■ Offer physical and verbal support when walking ■ Give any prescribed medication ■ Exercise little and often. Provide appropriately supported exercise on non-slip floors
Sleeping/resting	■ May sleep more ■ May adjust poorly to changes in routine	■ Allow adequate time and conditions for sleep ■ Ask owners for information on normal routine. Try and maintain some routine
Expressing normal behaviour	■ May adjust poorly to changes in routine	■ Ask owners for information on normal routine. Try and maintain some routine. May benefit from owner visits

15.42 Nursing assessment, potential problems and possible nursing interventions in geriatric patients. Nursing interventions highlighted in **bold** are covered in more detail in this chapter.

Eating and drinking
Food

Geriatric patients without other medical complications require a diet that is relatively low calorie, but has adequate levels of protein, vitamins and minerals. The nutritional requirements of elderly dogs and cats are described in Chapter 13. Commercial 'senior' diets are appropriate for most cases. The patient's weight should be regularly monitored as many geriatric animals are overweight and this can affect their mobility. Geriatric animals with pre-existing medical conditions may conversely be underweight and prone to further weight loss in a hospital environment. Diets for specific medical problems may be used. Changes in bodyweight may require adjustments in the doses of any drugs being used.

In a hospital environment many geriatric patients will need extra encouragement to eat. Using palatable foods, warming food and hand feeding (see Chapter 14) may be necessary. Any changes in diet should be made slowly in order to encourage the new diet to be eaten and to avoid gastrointestinal upsets, which may be more common in elderly patients. Consideration should be given to the possibility of dental disease. Adequate analgesia should be provided if gums and/or teeth are painful, together with appropriate dental care (see Chapter 25).

Fluids

Some geriatric patients may be polydipsic as a result of underlying medical conditions. Other elderly pets may be poor at drinking and risk becoming dehydrated, this is especially the case in geriatric cats. Fresh water must be provided at all times and water intake measured to ensure that it is adequate. Adding water to food or using novel water sources (e.g. water fountains for cats) can assist with water intake. Where fluid intake is not adequate (or production of urine is inadequate), intravenous fluids may be required (see Chapter 20).

Urinating and defecating

Urine output should be measured to assess whether fluid intake is adequate. The elderly pet should be observed to ensure that urination is normal (e.g. no straining) and that the urine produced is normal (e.g. colour, concentration, volume, smell)

Inappropriate urination (e.g. in the house) in older dogs and cats is not always a result of urinary incontinence. Urinary incontinence arises from loss of bladder muscle or sphincter tone and may arise as part of the ageing process or for other medical reasons. Incontinent animals typically leak urine when relaxed or asleep. Older dogs and cats that consciously urinate in the house may do so as a result of increased urine output (polyuria), often associated with increased thirst (polydipsia), or as a result of loss of learned behaviour (training) that may be associated with senility.

Elderly dogs should be taken out for regular walks to encourage normal urination. Elderly cats and rabbits should be provided with clean and regularly changed litter trays. Water intake must not be restricted. Where animals are genuinely incontinent, appropriate bedding and the use of incontinence pads is necessary. Care must be taken to avoid urine scalding (see below) by clipping excess hair, keeping the patient clean, using barrier creams and, where appropriate, a tail bandage (see 'Bandaging', above).

Constipation is not uncommon in older animals due to loss of muscle tone. This situation can be made worse in a hospital environment where normal routine and familiar places to toilet have changed. Use of opioid drugs for analgesia may also result in constipation. Faecal output should be monitored carefully (frequency, volume and consistency). Laxative drugs and enemas (see 'Enemas', above) should be used appropriately where necessary.

Breathing

Older pets may have heart and lung conditions. It is important to ensure that any prescribed medication for these conditions is given. Diuretic drugs may result in an increase in thirst and subsequently increased urination. Recumbent geriatric pets may be at risk of hypostatic congestion (see 'The recumbent patient', below).

Maintaining body temperature

Geriatric pets may have a reduced ability to maintain their body temperature. Body temperature should be checked twice daily as routine and more often as necessary. The provision of good bedding and encouragement of mobility (see below) will help maintenance of body temperature.

Grooming

Geriatric patients may have problems with self-care including grooming (see Chapter 14) as a result of problems such as arthritis; this is especially the case in old cats. Grooming is particularly important in longer haired breeds of dog, cat and rabbit, where matting of the coat can be a source of dirt and subsequent bacterial growth. Grooming also helps to give the older pet a feeling of wellbeing, encourages surface blood circulation, provides an opportunity to check the coat and skin (e.g. for the development of sores and decubital ulcers, see below) and to clean discharges from eyes and nose. The human contact is in itself beneficial. Grooming should be reduced to a minimum in patients that find it stressful.

The nails of geriatric pets can become long as a result of inadequate wear or nail deformities related to age. In cats, a reduction in the ability to retract the front claws can result in these growing round and into the foot pads. Nails should be checked on admission and during hospitalization and trimmed (see Chapter 14) as required.

Mobilizing

Geriatric patients often suffer from visual and hearing impairments, so these patients should not be rushed, treated gently and nursed with compassion. It is important that patients suffering from visual impairment be prevented from walking into doors, cages etc.; this is of particular concern with the increased use of glass doors within veterinary practices.

Geriatric patients commonly have mobility problems due to osteoarthritis. Hospitalization can reduce the ability of the patient not only to move around as they are accustomed to, but also to rest properly (see below). Short but regular walks, along with massage (see 'Physiotherapy', above), can aid in maintaining mobility and reducing muscle stiffness.

If the patient is unstable or has particular difficulty in changing/shifting position, it is important that they do not fall or slip. The use of mats to prevent slipping on hard surfaces and slings to move less mobile patients can be beneficial.

All nursing interventions and supportive care should be undertaken gently, at appropriate time intervals, with minimal stress to the patient in order to reduce the risk of the patient hurting themselves. Confidence in these patients is key and can be very quickly lost if the animal hurts themselves or is hurt during handling.

Sleeping/resting

Generally, older pets tend to sleep more. Maintaining the pet's normal routine (see below) will help encourage normal sleeping patterns. Ensuring that lights are turned off appropriately for at least some of the night will also encourage normal sleep patterns. Adequate analgesia for mobility problems (see above) helps to ensure that the patient rests well.

Geriatric pets are often more recumbent that younger animals and this can be especially the case in a hospital environment. Adequate padded bedding (see Chapter 14) is required to help avoid any problems associated with recumbency (see 'The recumbent patient', below).

Expressing normal behaviour

Geriatric patients are usually very set in their routines and careful questioning of the owner is essential to know and try and replicate, where possible, that routine (see Chapter 14). Elderly patients are also more likely to become stressed when separated from their owner and gentle nursing and reassurance are required. The benefits/disadvantages of owner visits should be considered on an individual basis; for some pets they can be beneficial (e.g. the pet may eat for the owner), whilst other pets may not respond positively and become more depressed when the owner leaves.

Other nursing considerations
Medication

Geriatric patients are often on multiple medications. The patient's hospital sheets must be carefully completed to ensure that all medications are given at the correct times. These drugs should be continued on the same regime as at home, unless alternations need to be made. If a new drug regime is introduced in the hospital and needs to be continued in the home environment, it is important to communicate with the owner to ensure that the timings of drug administration are appropriate for their lifestyle. This will help improve long-term management and owner compliance.

The neonatal patient

Neonatal patients should, ideally, remain with the dam (mother) as much as possible. This allows the dam to compensate for the innate homeostatic mechanisms that are not yet present and/or fully functioning in the neonate, and also helps prevent maternal rejection. When the neonate is not with the dam, the veterinary nurse must take over this role. For further information on the care and management of neonatal patients, the reader is referred to Chapter 24.

Nursing assessment and possible interventions

A nursing assessment based upon a standardized approach, together with common nursing interventions for neonatal patients is given in Figure 15.43.

Parameter	Potential problems in these patients	Possible nursing interventions
Eating	■ Unweaned neonates, away from the dam, will require feeding every few hours	■ Feed with milk replacer
Drinking	■ May become dehydrated	■ Provide subcutaneous, intravenous or intraosseous fluids as required (see Chapter 20)
Urinating	■ Unweaned neonates are likely to require stimulation to urinate and defecate	■ 'Toileting' with damp cotton wool several times daily (see Chapter 24)
Defecating	■ Unweaned neonates are likely to require stimulation to urinate and defecate	■ 'Toileting' with damp cotton wool several times daily (see Chapter 24)
Breathing	■ May have reduced lung capacity	■ Provide **oxygen supplementation**
Maintaining body temperature	■ Neonates may be unable to maintain an adequate body temperature	■ Provide additional heat sources (e.g. an incubator; see Chapter 14)
Grooming	■ Self-care will be poor	■ Groom as necessary
Mobilizing	■ Limited movement	■ Provide appropriate mobilization
Sleeping/resting	■ Will sleep more than adults	■ Maintain a routine that allows adequate sleep
Expressing normal behaviour	■ Will require socialization, especially if single	■ Stimulate and TLC, especially if no litter mates

15.43 Nursing assessment, potential problems and possible nursing interventions in neonatal patients. The nursing intervention highlighted in **bold** is covered in more detail in this chapter.

Eating and drinking
Food
Unweaned neonates when with the dam feed ad libitum. When they are not with the dam, neonates are dependent upon the veterinary nurse for the provision of nutrition and/or glucose for energy. Due to their relatively high metabolic rates and reduced glycogen storage within the liver, neonates rapidly become hypoglycaemic if food is withheld. Frequent small feeds of an appropriate milk substitute product are required. The rate and volume of feeding will depend upon the age and species of neonate (see Chapter 24). Where the neonate is unwell or less responsive than normal, then blood glucose levels should be checked (see Chapter 17); supplementary glucose and repeated glucose monitoring may be required.

Fluids
Similar to the provision of nutrition/glucose, neonates normally have *ad libitum* access to milk to maintain adequate hydration when with the dam. When they are not with the dam, neonates are dependent upon the veterinary nurse for hydration. Due to a higher percentage of body water than adult animals, neonates are much more likely to become dehydrated if fluids are withheld. As above, frequent small feeds are required. Where the neonate presents or becomes dehydrated, intravenous, intraosseous or intraperitoneal fluid administration may be required (see Chapter 20).

Urinating and defecating
Neonates require stimulation from the dam to urinate and defecate. When they are not with the dam, neonates are dependent upon the veterinary nurse to perform this task. This can be carried out using damp cotton wool to stimulate 'toileting' by gently wiping the perineal area. This process should be carried out every 2 hours, usually around the time of feeding. The passage of urine and faeces should be carefully recorded.

Breathing
Neonates may have reduced lung capacity, especially if they are premature and the lungs are not fully developed.

Neonates that do not feed well or have congenital abnormalities, such as a cleft palate or harelip, may be prone to aspiration pneumonia. An oxygen tent or incubator can be used where necessary to provide supplementary oxygen (see 'Oxygen supplementation', above).

Maintaining body temperature
Due to their high body surface area to volume ratio and immature liver (important in the generation of heat), neonates need support to maintain their body temperature. An environmental temperature of 30–33°C for first 24 hours and then 26–30°C for 4–5 days should be maintained. This can be achieved with the use of warm bedding and warming devices, although a thermostatically controlled incubator is the best option. Care needs to be taken when using warming devices due to the risk of thermal burns and hyperthermia. Care should also be taken when feeding and toileting neonates to ensure that they do not become wet and cold.

Grooming
Neonates usually require minimal grooming. They do, however, need to be kept clean whilst at the same time avoiding getting them too wet and cold. Spilt milk should be cleaned off the coat immediately and care should be taken to avoid the risk of urine scalding by soaking up any urine passed with cotton wool.

Mobilizing
Movement in neonates will be intermittent with sleeping and eating in between. Appropriate soft bedding is required that keeps the animals warm but prevents the risk of injury to immature limbs if they become caught or tangled in it.

Sleeping/resting
Neonates will have long periods of sleeping. A feeding and toileting routine should allow undisturbed periods of rest.

Expressing normal behaviour
Neonates are best kept with their litter mates to allow normal socialization. They will require some stimulation and TLC ('tender loving care') if the dam is not with them.

Other nursing considerations

Caring for neonates can be very time-consuming. It is likely that they will require frequent (2–3 hourly) care with overnight feeds. Careful consideration must be given to practice resources and demands upon nursing staff if neonates are admitted for basic non-medical care that might be otherwise provided by the owner following careful discussion and training.

Medication

It is essential to ensure accurate dosing of drugs in neonates. Use of 1 ml or 100 IU syringes is advisable when drawing up small quantities of medication. Where appropriate, and directed by the prescribing veterinary surgeon, drugs may be diluted for use. This must be done with care; the drugs must be water-miscible and thoroughly mixed.

The vomiting patient

Vomiting or emesis is an active process whereby the contents of the stomach are forcefully ejected out of the mouth. The causes, diagnosis and treatment of vomiting patients is covered in Chapter 18.

Examples of medical conditions associated with vomiting

- Gastrointestinal disease (e.g. infectious conditions, foreign bodies)
- Endocrine disease (e.g. diabetes mellitus)
- Renal disease
- Hepatic disease
- Pancreatitis
- Some neoplastic conditions (e.g. lymphoma)

Nursing assessment and possible interventions

A nursing assessment based upon a standardized approach, together with common nursing interventions for vomiting patients is given in Figure 15.44.

Eating and drinking
Food

The nutritional management of vomiting patients can be challenging and is often dependent on the underlying cause. Even once the animal has ceased vomiting, it can be difficult to get them to start eating again. This can be due to ongoing nausea or food aversions. In these cases, medications (e.g. antiemetics and appetite stimulants) can be useful. The value of good basic nursing, developing a trusting relationship with the patient and providing TLC, cannot be underestimated.

It can be a tricky balance between tempting an animal to eat and providing an appropriate diet for the individual patient. The diet chosen will depend upon the cause of vomiting. In uncomplicated cases, a bland diet such as chicken and rice or a commercial gastrointestinal diet is usually indicated. If the patient will not eat, then syringe feeding may be considered; this must be carried out carefully to prevent the risk of regurgitation, aspiration and stress to the patient. Once a bland diet is being taken on a regular basis, it may be possible to return the pet to its normal food. Any diet change must be made slowly, ideally by mixing the bland diet with the pet's own food for several days.

Fluids

One of the main nursing considerations in the management of the vomiting patient, is the close monitoring of hydration status and the appropriate use of fluid therapy (oral or intravenous fluids; see Chapter 20). Electrolyte balance needs

Parameter	Potential problems in these patients	Possible nursing interventions
Eating	■ May vomit or be nauseous or food adverse ■ Will require a digestible diet	■ Tempt to eat: palatable diet, hand feed, warm food (see Chapter 14) ■ Provide medications as required ■ Feed an appropriate diet
Drinking	■ May become dehydrated and may vomit fluid	■ Intravenous fluids as required (see Chapter 20) ■ Monitor electrolytes and acid–base balance as required (see Chapter 17)
Urinating	■ May be reduced due to dehydration	■ Monitor urine output ■ Intravenous fluids as required (see Chapter 20)
Defecating	■ May develop diarrhoea	■ Provide medications as required ■ Feed an appropriate diet ■ Provide appropriate fluids
Breathing	■ Possible risk of aspiration of vomitus	■ Monitor carefully including chest auscultation
Maintaining body temperature	■ May become hyperthermic or hypothermic	■ Monitor temperature and treat accordingly
Grooming	■ May become soiled	■ Keep clean, especially around the mouth
Mobilizing	■ May be nauseous especially on movement	■ Move gently and carefully
Sleeping/resting	■ Maybe unsettled and sleep poorly	■ Keep clean ■ Provide medication etc. ■ Maintain a routine allowing for sleep as far as is possible
Expressing normal behaviour	■ Can become depressed	■ Provide TLC

15.44 Nursing assessment, potential problems and possible nursing interventions in vomiting patients.

to be closely monitored, along with acid–base status (see Chapter 17). Hypokalaemia (low potassium) is the most common derangement encountered, but other electrolyte abnormalities (e.g. sodium, chloride) and complex acid–base changes may also be seen. Patients suffering from vomiting often become head shy and in these cases, or in animals for which long-term intravenous access is required, it is important to consider the position of the catheter. Use of the saphenous vein can be helpful in these patients; this location for intravenous access also reduces contamination of the catheter site during vomiting.

Urinating and defecating

In vomiting patients, it is essential to ensure adequate urine output as this is an indication of adequate hydration. If urine production is low this may indicate dehydration and the need for intravenous fluids. Many vomiting patients will develop diarrhoea and this will need to be treated appropriately (diet modification, fluids, medication as necessary); see also 'The soiled patient', below.

Breathing

With all vomiting patients there is small but possible risk of aspiration of vomitus and the development of aspiration pneumonia. Careful observation and thoracic auscultation will enable this complication to be identified quickly.

Maintaining body temperature

The ability of a vomiting patient to maintain body temperature will depend upon the underlying cause; patients may be hypothermic, normothermic or hyperthermic. The patient's temperature must be taken routinely several times daily and more frequently if it is outside the normal range for that species. Vomiting animals may become wet and cold if not kept clean (see below).

Grooming

The vomiting patient needs to be kept clean with regular cleaning and grooming to avoid the risk of vomitus contaminating the coat. Gentle cleaning around the mouth is particularly important. Grooming should be carried out especially gently in these patients as excessive movement may make nausea worse and result in further vomiting.

Mobilizing

Vomiting patients should be handled gently when mobilizing them (e.g. walking dogs) to avoid further nausea and pain. Vomiting patients frequently develop diarrhoea, so taking dogs outside often can be of benefit and prevent additional soiling.

Sleeping/resting

Vomiting animals will have disturbed sleep as a result of the act of vomiting, which can be exhausting in itself, and the nursing interventions required to keep them clean and comfortable. The aim should be to treat the patient appropriately to stop the vomiting and have a care plan that allows for adequate rest.

Expressing normal behaviour

Vomiting patients are likely to become very depressed. They may also become reluctant to be handled if they begin to associate handling with nausea. Key to this is adequate medical management to stop the vomiting as soon as possible and appropriate nursing interventions to keep the patient clean and comfortable.

Other nursing considerations

Medication

The correct administration of prescribed medication (e.g. antiemetics, analgesics; see Chapter 8) is another key consideration in the vomiting patient. Medication should ideally be given by injection (parenterally) rather than orally, where possible. It is important that the underlying cause of the vomiting is identified and it is the role of the veterinary nurse to help prepare both the patient and the equipment required for any procedure deemed necessary (e.g. endoscopy).

Homecare information

It is important when vomiting patients are discharged back to their owners that they are given good information about how to feed their pet. This should include the type, volume and frequency of food to feed, and how and when to return to normal feeding.

The soiled patient

Hospitalized patients may become soiled at some time during their stay. Patients can be soiled by urine, faeces, vomit, blood, other bodily fluids and food. It is the responsibility of the veterinary nurse to ensure that all soiling is cleaned efficiently, effectively and quickly. Maintaining a high level of cleanliness can be both very challenging and time-consuming, and the use of disposable incontinence sheets can be invaluable.

> ## Common medical conditions associated with patient soiling
>
> - Vomiting (see 'The vomiting patient', above)
> - Diarrhoea as a result of medical problems (e.g. hepatic disease)
> - Increased urination as a result of medical problems (e.g. cystitis or renal disease)
> - Urinary incontinence (see 'The geriatric patient', above)
> - Faecal incontinence (e.g. associated with spinal disease)
> - Wounds that have not or cannot be adequately dressed
> - Problems eating (dysphagia, e.g. associated with dental problems) or drinking

Nursing assessment and possible interventions

A nursing assessment based upon a standardized approach, together with common nursing interventions for soiled patients is given in Figure 15.45.

Eating and drinking

Food

The willingness to eat and type of food provided will depend upon the cause of the soiling. The use of appropriate nutrition and tempting patients to eat is often key to the successful management of these cases. It may also form the mainstay of long-term treatment in chronic cases, therefore, owner education and compliance is vital. Early involvement and engagement of owners can help to achieve this goal.

Parameter	Potential problems in these patients	Possible nursing interventions
Eating	■ May require a special diet to treat underlying medical problems	■ Tempt to eat: hand feed as necessary
Drinking	■ May become dehydrated with electrolyte imbalances	■ Intravenous fluids as required (see Chapter 20) ■ Monitor electrolytes and acid–base balance as required (see Chapter 17)
Urinating	■ May be polyuric ■ May be urinary incontinent	■ Take dogs outside frequently ■ Provide clean litter trays for cats and rabbits ■ Provide appropriate bedding, including incontinence pads ■ Monitor carefully for **urine scalding**
Defecating	■ May have diarrhoea	■ Take dogs outside frequently ■ Provide clean litter trays for cats and rabbits ■ Feed an appropriate diet ■ Provide appropriate fluids ■ Provide appropriate bedding, including incontinence pads
Breathing	■ Possible risk of aspiration if vomiting	■ Monitor carefully, including chest auscultation
Maintaining body temperature	■ May not be able to maintain normal body temperature	■ Monitor temperature frequently ■ Avoid allowing to get wet and cold
Grooming	■ Coat may become soiled ■ May develop urine scalding	■ Groom frequently ■ Keep clean: clip hair as necessary; use barrier creams; **tail bandage** ■ Monitor for **urine scalding**
Mobilizing	■ May be reluctant or less able to move around	■ Take outside often ■ Encourage to move around
Sleeping/resting	■ Maybe unsettled and have disturbed sleep ■ Nursing interventions may disturb sleep	■ Provide care in a way that minimizes disturbance of sleep
Expressing normal behaviour	■ Can become very 'fed-up'	■ Provide encouragement and TLC

15.45 Nursing assessment, potential problems and possible nursing interventions in soiled patients. Nursing interventions highlighted in **bold** are covered in more detail in this chapter.

Fluids

Fluid balance needs to be monitored closely in these patients and appropriate oral or intravenous fluid therapy instituted as needed. Soiled patients can also experience acid–base changes and electrolyte derangements; appropriate monitoring of these (see Chapter 17) and associated management should be provided as needed.

Urinating and defecating

Animals may become soiled as a result of:

■ **Urinary incontinence:** the involuntary passing of urine. Leakage may be intermittent or continuous and occur when the animal is standing or recumbent
■ **Diarrhoea:** the increased passage of abnormally softer liquid faeces. It can be acute or chronic in nature.

The causes, diagnosis and treatment of both urinary incontinence and diarrhoea are covered in Chapter 18.

Animals at risk of urine or faecal soiling must be given the opportunity to urinate and defecate normally outside (in the case of dogs) or in a clean litter tray (in the case of cats and rabbits). For cats and rabbits, the use of a preferential litter, together with regular changes of litter trays is essential. Where soiling is taking place in the kennel, careful observation is required to ensure that the animal remains as clean as possible. Cleaning the animal and its environment frequently, together with the use of appropriate bedding including incontinence pads to draw fluid away from the patient, is essential. Urine scalding (see below) will occur if careful nursing care is not provided.

Breathing

Although soiling is unlikely to directly affect breathing, except in the case of vomiting (see above), the causes of soiling may result from diseases that also have a negative impact upon the respiratory system due to electrolyte imbalance. Careful monitoring of respiration is therefore required.

Maintaining body temperature

The ability of the soiled patient to maintain body temperature will depend upon underlying medical conditions. The patient's temperature must be taken routinely several times daily and more frequently if it is outside the normal range for that species. It is important to ensure that soiled patients do not get cold as a result of being wet. Care should be taken when cleaning and grooming these patients (see below) to ensure that they are dried adequately.

Grooming

The prevention of sores as a result of urine or faecal scalding is a key nursing consideration and is discussed further in 'The recumbent patient' (see below). The patient should be observed regularly and closely and any soiling removed quickly. The soiled area should be thoroughly washed using warm water and an appropriate shampoo where necessary. A barrier cream may be used around the perineal area and/ or a tail bandage applied (see 'Bandaging', above). It may be necessary to clip hair in long coated breeds. General grooming provides an opportunity to check carefully for any sore areas.

Where soiling around the mouth occurs (for example, as a result of dental disease in dogs, cats and small mammals),

417

this also needs to be carefully cleaned. The best time to clean this area is after feeding. Animals may become 'head shy' and a gentle approach is required.

Mobilizing

Regular walks outside for dogs can aid management of incontinence, reducing soiling and helping with their general wellbeing. Encouraging mobility in all patients helps avoid the complications of recumbency (see below).

Sleeping/resting

Patients that become soiled may have disturbed sleep as a result of the action of soiling or as a result of nursing interventions (cleaning, walking, medicating). Treating the underlying causes of the soiling and having a care plan that allows for adequate rest is essential.

Expressing normal behaviour

Understandably, these patients can become depressed and often 'fed-up' with the situation. Thus, it is important to approach them in a calm and considered manner and to bear in mind your safety and that of those around you.

Other nursing considerations

Other nursing considerations may be indicated as a result of underlying and/or concurrent problems.

The recumbent patient

An animal that is lying down and unable to rise by itself is described as recumbent. Patients may be recumbent for a number of reasons and it is essential that the cause is fully understood in order to be able to provide effective nursing care.

Common conditions associated with recumbency

- Fractures (e.g. pelvis, limbs)
- Spinal trauma (e.g. disc protrusion)
- Weakness due to medical disease
- Neurological injury or disease
- Heart failure
- Shock

Nursing assessment and possible interventions

A nursing assessment based upon a standardized approach, together with common nursing interventions for recumbent patients is given in Figure 15.46.

Parameter	Potential problems in these patients	Possible nursing interventions
Eating	■ May be unable to eat ■ May require a 'special' diet ■ May lose or gain weight inappropriately	■ Tempt to eat: provide palatable food, provide supportive feeding as required ■ Provide a food appropriate for any underlying medical conditions ■ Monitor weight regularly (daily)
Drinking	■ May be unable to drink or drink inadequately	■ Monitor water intake ■ Assess hydration (examination ± blood sample) ■ Provide intravenous fluids as necessary (see Chapter 20)
Urinating	■ May urinate in bedding ■ May be prone to urine scalding and decubital ulcers	■ Monitor urination carefully ■ Take dogs outside frequently, if possible ■ Provide appropriate bedding, including incontinence pads ■ **Urinary catheterization** as necessary ■ Monitor carefully for **urine scalding** and **decubital ulcers**
Defecating	■ May defecate in bedding ■ May become constipated ■ May develop diarrhoea ■ May be prone to urine scalding and decubital ulcers	■ Monitor defecation carefully ■ Take dogs outside frequently, if possible ■ Provide appropriate bedding, including incontinence pads ■ Provide treatments as necessary, including **enemas and laxatives** ■ Keep clean: clip hair as necessary; **tail bandage** ■ Monitor carefully for **urine scalding** and **decubital ulcers**
Breathing	■ May have underlying breathing problems ■ May be predisposed to and develop hypostatic pneumonia	■ Provide treatment for any existing problems, including analgesia ■ Prevent and monitor for **hypostatic congestion/pneumonia** – turn patients at least every 4h; use coupage 4–5 times daily; monitor, including auscultation and peripheral pulse palpation
Maintaining body temperature	■ May be hyperthermic, normothermic or hypothermic	■ Monitor temperature and provide appropriate nursing care, including heat provision as required (see Chapter 14)
Grooming	■ Unlikely to self-groom adequately; coat may become soiled ■ May be prone to urine scald and decubital ulcers	■ Groom frequently ■ Keep clean: clip hair as necessary; use barrier creams; **tail bandage** ■ Monitor for **urine scalding** and **decubital ulcers**
Mobilizing	■ Unlikely to mobilize normally ■ Prone to secondary problems (urine scalding, decubital ulcers, hypostatic pneumonia)	■ Turn patients at least every 4h ■ Provide good bedding (see Chapter 14) ■ Provide appropriate **physiotherapy**

15.46 Nursing assessment, potential problems and possible nursing interventions in recumbent patients. Nursing interventions highlighted in **bold** are covered in more detail in this chapter. *continues* ▶

Parameter	Potential problems in these patients	Possible nursing interventions
Sleeping/resting	■ May be unsettled and have disturbed sleep ■ May sleep during the day and have disturbed nights ■ Nursing interventions may disturb sleep	■ Provide stimulation and a regular routine ■ Provide nursing care in a way that minimizes disturbance of sleep
Expressing normal behaviour	■ Can become very bored	■ Provide encouragement and TLC ■ Take outside if possible: going outside will provide additional natural daylight stimulation supporting a normal circadian rhythm

15.46 *continued* Nursing assessment, potential problems and possible nursing interventions in recumbent patients. Nursing interventions highlighted in **bold** are covered in more detail in this chapter.

Eating and drinking

If the recumbent patient is able to eat and drink, food and water must be placed within easy reach or offered at regular intervals.

Food

The type of diet fed to recumbent patients will depend upon the underlying medical condition and the ability of the pet to eat normal amounts of food. Nursing care may be as simple as tempting the patient to eat (see Chapter 14), including hand feeding, or may be as complicated as providing total parenteral nutrition (TPN; see Chapter 13). If the recumbent patient fails to eat, advice should be sought from the owner regarding the animal's preferences and favourite foods. Feeding tubes (see Chapter 13) should be placed in animals that fail to eat despite appropriate medical and nursing interventions. The energy and feeding requirements for hospitalized patients are described in Chapter 13. Diets with an increased protein content, that are highly digestible and palatable are required. Highly digestible diets have the added advantage of generally producing less faecal material. Careful monitoring of the weight of these patients during hospitalization, and once they go home, is essential. Obesity may be a problem in some cases and a possible contributing cause of recumbency.

Fluids

Fluid intake and fluid balance need to be carefully monitored in recumbent patients. Hydration status should be assessed both on examination (see Chapter 14) and by blood tests (see Chapter 17). Patients that fail to drink sufficiently can have water added to their food, but in many instances appropriate intravenous fluid therapy is required (see Chapter 20).

Urinating and defecating

Recumbent dogs and cats should, where possible and medically indicated (following veterinary advice), be taken outside to be given the opportunity to urinate and defecate. Maintaining natural urination and defecation is always preferable to interventions (urinary catheterization and/or enemas), and movement, a standing position, a change of environment and fresh air may have a positive benefit on the mental attitude of many animals. Patients will require help standing and may need additional support to take them outside. Simple towel support is useful and appropriate in many cases (Figure 15.47), although other forms of support harnesses and frames (see Figure 15.49) are also available. When an animal is supported, if it does not urinate unassisted, gentle manual pressure may be applied to the bladder to encourage urination (Figure 15.48).

In patients that cannot be taken outside or moved into a standing position for natural or manual expression of the bladder, urinary catheterization (see 'Urinary catheterization',

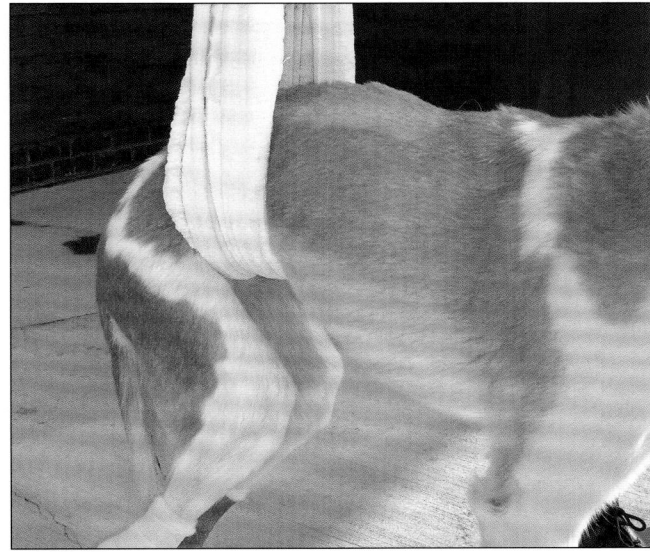

15.47 Assisted walking for the recumbent patient.

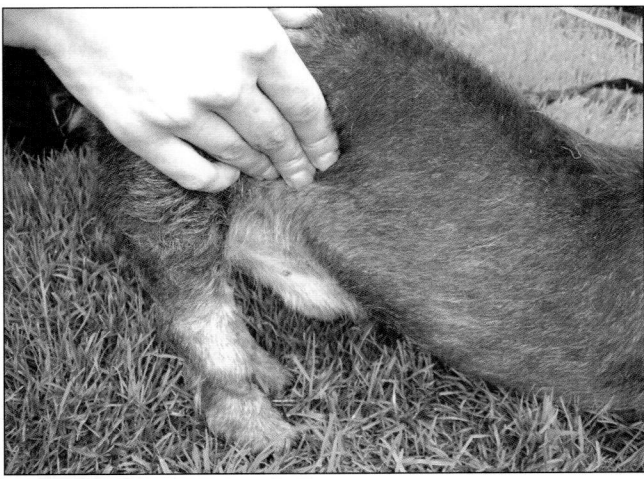

15.48 Manual bladder expression.

above) may make the patient both easier to nurse and more comfortable. A careful record of urination (volume, frequency, colour) should be kept for all recumbent patients.

Records should also be kept regarding defecation (frequency, volume, consistency, colour). Recumbent patients may become constipated as a result of inactivity, reduced intestinal movement and the side effects of opioid analgesics. Mild constipation will make animals uncomfortable and reluctant to eat, whilst severe constipation if not addressed can result in gut perforations leading to peritonitis. Where a patient's frequency of passing faeces is reduced, laxative medications (see Chapter 8) should be used under veterinary direction. Where significant constipation has already occurred, enemas may be needed (see 'Enemas', above).

Some recumbent patients may develop diarrhoea as a result of underlying medical conditions and/or dietary changes. Diarrhoea in recumbent patients increases their risk of sores (including decubital ulcers, see below), wound infections, myiasis ('fly-strike'), especially in the summer, and discomfort. If diarrhoea develops, the veterinary surgeon should be informed. As in the case of soiled patients (see above), regular bedding changes and good nursing are essential. Excess hair in the perianal/anal area of dogs and cats should be clipped and tail bandages (see 'Bandaging', above) appropriately applied.

Urine scalding

This may occur if patients are allowed to become soiled with urine and are not correctly nursed. Urine scalding initially appears as red inflamed areas of skin, but can progress rapidly into sores, which may become infected and/or develop into decubital ulcers (see below). Urine scalding should be prevented wherever possible through good nursing including:

- Giving patients as much opportunity as possible to urinate outside of their kennel
- Provision of appropriate bedding, including incontinence pads, to draw urine away from the patient
- Urinary catheterization where indicated
- Careful and regular patient examination and grooming to quickly recognize scalding when it occurs.

If urine scalding does occur, it should be treated by:

- Regular bathing of the affected areas with a mild antiseptic shampoo (e.g. dilute chlorhexidine gluconate), which should be rinsed off thoroughly
- Clipping the hair, tail bandaging as appropriate (see 'Bandaging', above) and applying an appropriate barrier cream
- Urinary catheterization, if necessary
- Use of analgesic drugs and other medication as indicated by a veterinary surgeon.

Breathing

Recumbent patients may suffer from breathing difficulties as a result of their underlying clinical conditions (e.g. fractured ribs in a dog that has been in a road accident) and these must be managed appropriately. Adequate analgesia is essential in all patients experiencing pain, as without it they are more likely to take shallow breaths, increasing the risk of the development of pneumonia. Recumbency itself may also predispose the patient to pneumonia secondary to hypostatic congestion.

Hypostatic pneumonia

This is caused by the pooling of blood, hypostatic congestion, and a consequent decrease in viability of the dependent lung, resulting in the development of pneumonia. It is more likely to occur in an old, sick and debilitated animal that has been in lateral recumbency for a long period of time and is a particular risk in large-breed dogs due to their size. ➔

Hypostatic pneumonia *continued*

Signs of hypostatic pneumonia include:

- Rapid shallow breathing
- Increased respiratory effort
- Moist noises when breathing, possibly even gurgling
- Depressed attitude.

Serious secondary chest infections may result if hypostatic pneumonia is allowed to develop and these can be life-threatening. If hypostatic pneumonia is suspected, a veterinary surgeon should be informed immediately. Auscultation of the lung field quadrants and radiography may be required to confirm the diagnosis. If hypostatic pneumonia is diagnosed, medication (including antibiotics) is likely to be prescribed. Good nursing, including methods to help prevent congestion, will be required.

Nursing interventions for the prevention of hypostatic congestion and pneumonia include:

- Turning the recumbent patient at least every 4 hours, 24 hours a day
- Placing the patient in sternal recumbency for some of the time; this can be assisted by using sandbags, water/sand-filled containers or radiography cradles. The patient's head must be supported
- Regular coupage (external impact massage of the thorax with cupped hands; see 'Physiotherapy', above) 4–5 times daily for 5 minutes will improve thoracic circulation. By promoting coughing, coupage also aids removal of secretions that build up in the bronchial tree. A veterinary surgeon should be consulted before coupage is undertaken, to ensure that there are no contraindications such as fractured ribs
- Chest auscultation (monitoring for the development of pneumonia)
- Peripheral pulse palpation (monitoring for the development of aortic thromboembolism and blood clots at other sites).

Maintaining body temperature

Temperature regulation in recumbent patients will be determined by any underlying disease processes. Body temperature should be monitored and recorded carefully. As recumbent patients are not moving around normally, in many cases they expend very little energy, heat production is lower than normal and they can become hypothermic. Normal body temperature, in some cases, may be maintained simply by having adequate bedding (e.g. covering canine and feline patients with warm blankets). In other cases, this may not be enough and additional external heat provision may be required (see Chapter 14).

Grooming

Grooming is essential in recumbent patients to ensure good hygiene and skin care (monitoring for areas of reddening, which could indicate the start of the development of pressure sores and/or decubital ulcers), as well as ensuring patient wellbeing.

Mobilizing

Mobilization of recumbent patients is essential to prevent the development of secondary problems, including decubital ulcers, hypostatic congestion and pneumonia, and urine scalding. The types and extent of mobilization possible will vary between individual patients, depend upon their underlying medical problems, and will need to be discussed in full with the responsible veterinary surgeon. Interventions should, where possible, include:

- **Positioning** – all patients should be turned at least every 4 hours, 24 hours a day. Positioning in sternal recumbency (see above) for part of the time will be beneficial
- **Bedding** – recumbent patients should be provided with padded/cushioned bedding (see Chapter 14). Mattresses are useful as they provide a more even surface and help avoid pressure points that can be created by creases and folds in multiple layers of bedding. Quilts can be useful to aid in patient positioning (i.e. propping them up in sternal recumbency)
- **Physiotherapy** – regular physiotherapy will help prevent muscle contracture, joint stiffness and associated discomfort. Coupage can also be used to prevent hypostatic congestion (see above and 'Physiotherapy', earlier in the chapter)
  - **Massage** – this is particularly useful for the limbs. The patient should be massaged from the toes/foot towards the body to encourage venous return to the heart
  - **Supported exercise** – for dogs and cats, towel walking is a common (and inexpensive) method (see Figure 15.47). Adequate staff must be available, as both the patient and the staff member can be injured if the patient is heavy and not supported adequately. Wheeled total support hoists for walking recumbent canine and feline patients assist mobility of heavier patients and enable effective active physical therapy with the patient in a normal walking position (Figure 15.49)
  - **Hydrotherapy** – swimming is very useful physiotherapy that can be used with dogs and cats. Small dogs can be swum in large sinks and baths in

the hospital; larger patients need pools. Swimming enables patients to move their limbs freely without weight-bearing forces. The temperature and the quality of the water must be checked before the patient enters. Constant support and observation are essential to prevent panic and possible drowning

- **Passive joint movement** – moving joints manually within their normal range of movement helps to prevent stiffness and improves circulation.

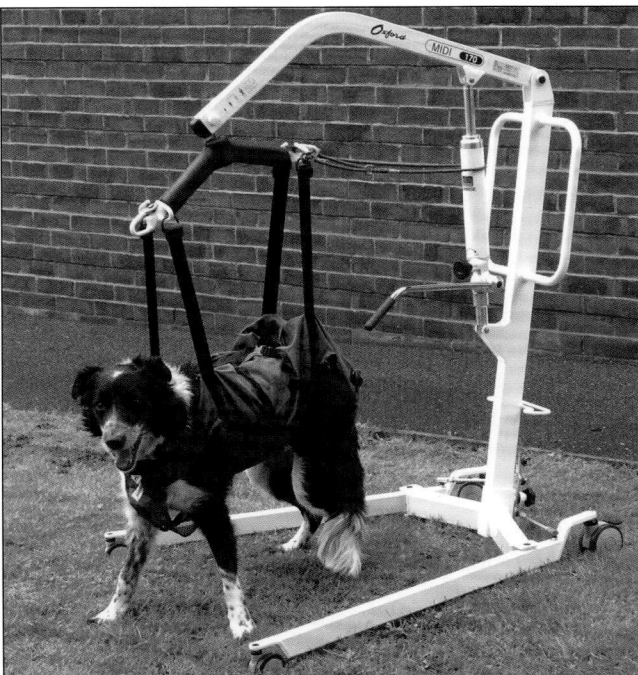

15.49 Wheeled 'total support' hoist for walking recumbent patients.

Decubital ulcers

Decubital ulcers ('pressure sores', 'bed sores') are wounds that develop, often at the site of bony areas (e.g. pelvis, hip, elbow, hock), as a result of consistent pressure on that area over a relatively short period of time. This type of pressure results in interruption to the local tissue blood supply and the skin and underlying tissues die (ischaemic necrosis), leaving open wounds (Figure 15.50). They are especially common in recumbent animals that are not managed correctly and/or have inadequate bedding. Urine scalding and faecal soiling further compromise the affected tissue. In common with urine scalding, it is better and easier to prevent decubital ulcers than it is to treat them.

Preventive measures against decubital ulcers

These include:

- The use of soft bedding with absorbable blankets
- Waterbeds may be useful for recumbent dogs and cats, but are rarely used in the UK
- Regular turning of the patient (at least every 4 hours)
- Bony prominences are most likely to suffer and these areas can be additionally padded with foam rings (e.g. those sometimes included in tablet pots; Figure 15.51)
- Regular supported exercise, where possible
- Slings to raise patients for longer periods (see Figure 15.49) are used in at some larger and referral veterinary hospitals
- Massage performed while the patient is recumbent or standing.

Decubital ulcers can be extremely difficult wounds to resolve, especially if their cause, ongoing recumbency, cannot be addressed. Further information on wound management is given in Chapter 23. Basic principles of decubital ulcer management are given below.

Management of decubital ulcers

Decubital ulcers are serious and can be extremely difficult to resolve. Treatment is as follows:

- Clip the area around the sore
- Clean with saline or a dilute antiseptic solution
- Dry thoroughly
- If possible, apply an appropriate permeable topical dressing (see 'Bandaging', above and Figure 15.1)
- If the decubital ulcer is on a lower limb, consider additional bandaging (see 'Bandaging', above)
- Ensure that all the methods described above to prevent decubital ulcers are employed.

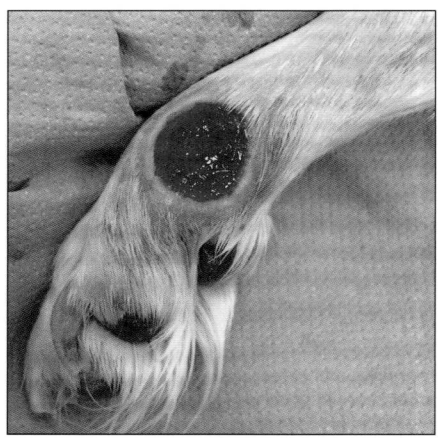

15.50

Decubital ulcer in a dog.

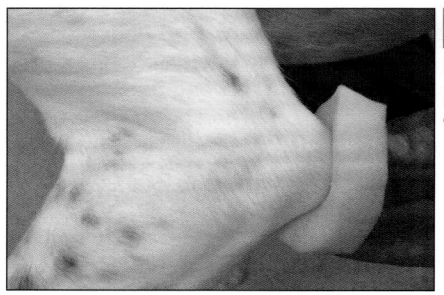

15.51

Padding of bony prominences on the elbow of a dog.

Sleeping/resting

Most recumbent patients benefit from being housed in an area of activity, provided that this is appropriate for their medical conditions. Some activity and interest can stimulate them and help relieve boredom. However, this should be considered on an individual basis, as some patients may require a very quiet environment in order to recover.

Trying to maintain a regular routine that allows for periods of rest is also necessary. Nursing tasks such as turning the patient, giving medication, changing dressings, etc. should, where possible, be carried out at the same time in order to give the patient a few hours of undisturbed rest.

Expressing normal behaviour

As described above, recumbent patients, especially those that are otherwise relatively clinically well, can become very bored. Being in a position in the hospital ward where they can see things going on can greatly improve wellbeing. Having some human contact and reassurance that is independent of any necessary, and possibly uncomfortable, nursing interventions also helps build patient confidence and contentment. If possible, regular trips outside for fresh air are beneficial; again this will depend upon the individual patient and the reasons for recumbency.

Other nursing considerations
Pain management

Appropriate and adequate analgesia provision is key to the management of recumbent patients. It should be noted that the patient's ability to display the common behavioural traits associated with pain will be altered. The use of pain scales that take this into account can be advantageous (e.g. the Glasgow Composite Pain Scale; see Chapter 21 for further details).

Pain management is important not only for the general welfare of the patient, but also for the prevention of hypostatic pneumonia (see above). There is also a health and safety aspect to ensuring that adequate analgesia is provided, as patients in pain are more likely to object to being moved or handled.

Monitoring

These patients require intensive care and thus close monitoring. The use of an appropriate hospital/intensive care record sheet (see Chapter 14) is essential to ensure that further complications do not develop.

Care at home

Recumbent patients are generally managed in a hospital environment, but some will be recumbent for a longer period of time and may need to be nursed at home. Most owners are quite capable of learning how to nurse their own pet, but tasks that come automatically to a veterinary nurse must be pointed out to an owner. It is helpful to write clear instructions to which owners can refer once they are home. Assistance with provision of suitable equipment for home nursing will also help. At least an initial home visit by the veterinary team is beneficial in order to ensure that the home environment is set up as well as possible. Assurance should be given to the owners that they can contact the practice at any time if they have any concerns. Weekly checks at the surgery, or home visits, should be arranged to monitor for signs of decubital ulcers, urine scalding or hypostatic pneumonia.

The critically ill patient

A patient may become critically ill from a broad spectrum of traumatic and disease conditions, each carrying its own challenges. Often several medical conditions are present concurrently. The age, species and breed of the patient may further complicate the nursing care that needs to be provided. All critical patients require a multimodal approach to their care and the holistic approach of the veterinary nurse is essential in complementing the disease-based care of the veterinary surgeon.

There must be adequate facilities for the care of critical patients. If these are not available, the patient should be moved to an alternative veterinary facility. As an absolute minimum, facilities must be:

- Quiet
- Well ventilated
- Well-lit with controllable lighting levels
- Able to provide oxygen if required
- Well served with electrical points for monitors.

There must also be adequate:

- Monitoring equipment for nursing staff to use effectively
- Veterinary staff members (for 24-hour care)
- On-site laboratory facilities.

Common critical medical conditions

- Hypercalcemia
- Pancreatitis
- Myasthenia gravis
- Acute renal failure
- Poisoning
- Acute anaemia
- Thrombocytopenia
- Leucopenia
- Raised intracranial pressure
- Diabetic ketoacidosis
- Acute heart failure
- Hepatic encephalopathy

Nursing assessment and possible interventions

A nursing assessment based upon a standardized approach, together with common nursing interventions for critical patients is given in Figure 15.52. Most critical patients are recumbent, and the nursing interventions described above are all relevant. Critical patients will, typically, be less independent and have a greater reliance upon veterinary staff, interventions and equipment for many normal functions.

Eating and drinking
Food

Intake of food and water by critical patients will depend upon:

- Whether the patient can physically eat and drink
- Whether the patient is allowed to eat and drink
- The position of food and water bowls
- Whether any adjustments to diet according to condition and impairment are required (e.g. supplements, probiotics and electrolytes)
- Whether feeding tubes are placed
- Whether TPN or fluid therapy is required.

There are implications for the level of nursing care required according to these factors. For the majority of critical patients, both feeding tubes (see Chapter 13) and intravenous fluid therapy (see Chapter 20) are standard requirements.

Critically ill patients should never be starved, as they have an increased basic energy requirement (see Chapter 13) as a consequence of inflammatory processes and tissue healing. Tube feeding or TPN must be started immediately if patients are unable to (or will not) eat for themselves (see Chapter 13). In many circumstances, fresh food should be offered to tube-fed patients regularly, as it is preferable for them to eat normally and for tube feeding to be stopped as soon as possible. In the seemingly unconscious or mentally 'dull' animal, the smell of food can sometimes produce a marked positive response, which can be a good indicator of overall improvement.

Fluids

Even if they are drinking themselves, most critical patients will require intravenous fluid therapy in order to stabilize and maintain hydration, electrolyte and acid–base requirements (see Chapter 20). Hydration status should be assessed on examination (see Chapter 14), including monitoring of blood pressure (see Chapter 21), and blood tests (see Chapter 17).

Parameter	Potential problems in these patients	Possible nursing interventions
Eating	■ May be unable to eat ■ May require tube feeding or total parenteral nutrition (TPN)	■ If appropriate, tempt to eat: provide palatable food and supportive feeding as required ■ Provide tube feeding or TPN as required (see Chapter 13)
Drinking	■ May be unable to drink ■ May be prone to dehydration, electrolyte and/or acid–base imbalances	■ Monitor hydration, electrolyte and acid–base status (examination and blood samples; see Chapter 17) ■ Provide intravenous fluids (see Chapter 20) ■ **Manage intravenous catheters** correctly
Urinating	■ May urinate in bedding ■ May be prone to urine scalding and decubital ulcers	■ Monitor urination carefully ■ Provide appropriate bedding, including incontinence pads ■ **Urinary catheterization** often necessary ■ Monitor carefully for **urine scalding** and **decubital ulcers**
Defecating	■ May defecate in bedding ■ May become constipated ■ May develop diarrhoea ■ May be prone to urine scalding and decubital ulcers	■ Monitor defecation carefully ■ Provide appropriate bedding, including incontinence pads ■ Provide treatments as necessary, including **enemas and laxatives** ■ Keep clean: clip hair as necessary; **tail bandage** ■ Monitor carefully for **urine scalding** and **decubital ulcers**
Breathing	■ May have compromised breathing ■ Predisposed to and may develop hypostatic pneumonia	■ Provide treatment for any existing problems, including analgesia ■ Maintain a patent airway ■ Provide **oxygenation** as necessary ■ Maintain chest drains correctly (see Chapter 23) ■ Prevent and monitor for **hypostatic congestion/pneumonia**: turn patients at least every 4 h; use coupage 4–5 times daily; monitor, including auscultation and peripheral pulse palpation
Maintaining body temperature	■ Unlikely to maintain normal body temperature	■ Monitor temperature frequently and provide additional heat as required (see Chapter 14)
Grooming	■ Will not self-groom adequately ■ Coat may become soiled ■ May be prone to urine scald and decubital ulcers	■ Groom frequently ■ Keep clean: clip hair; use barrier creams; **tail bandage** ■ Monitor for **urine scalding** and **decubital ulcers**
Mobilizing	■ Unlikely to mobilize normally ■ Prone to secondary problems (urine scalding, decubital ulcers, hypostatic pneumonia)	■ Turn patients at least every 4 h (take care with tubes and drains) ■ Provide good bedding (see Chapter 14) ■ Provide appropriate **physiotherapy**
Sleeping/resting	■ May have disturbed sleep ■ Nursing interventions may disturb sleep	■ Provide care in a way that minimizes disturbance of sleep
Expressing normal behaviour	■ Unlikely to behave normally ■ May have an altered mental state	■ Provide reassurance and TLC ■ Coma score as required

15.52 Nursing assessment, potential problems and possible nursing interventions in critically ill patients. Nursing interventions highlighted in **bold** are covered in more detail in this chapter.

Intravenous catheter management

Intravenous catheter management must be exemplary, as many critically ill patients are immunosuppressed and likely to contract infections easily. Hands must be washed before handling catheters and gloves worn. Any spilt blood around the catheter should be gently cleaned with dilute antiseptic solution, and checks should be made to ensure that all tapes securing catheters and dressings are clean. The use of impregnated dressings may be helpful in immunocompromised patients.

Catheter patency is maintained by flushing with saline (0.9% saline) every 4–6 hours. Regular changing of peripheral catheters (usually every 3–5 days) should be carried out as directed by the case veterinary surgeon. Jugular catheters are not normally changed if they are functioning well. The skin insertion site of jugular catheters requires particular care and should be inspected at least daily, preferably twice daily, with gloved hands. The sterile dressing at the site should be replaced at each dressing change. For more information on intravenous fluid therapy of small animals see Chapter 20.

Urinating and defecating

Many of the considerations for critical patients are the same as for recumbent patients (see above). Critical patients are much more likely to have indwelling urinary catheters than other recumbent patients.

Urinary catheter placement and management

Placement of urinary catheters poses a high risk of urinary tract infection (UTI), especially in critical patients that may be immunocompromised. Careful attention to catheter placement and management (see 'Urinary catheterization', above) is essential to reduce the risk of complications.

Breathing

Many critical patients will have compromised breathing as a result of medical conditions (e.g. heart or lung disease) or trauma (e.g. fractured ribs, lung contusions). Secondary problems such pneumostatic pneumonia as a result of recumbency may be additional complicating factors. Critical patients may have chest drains in place following treatment or surgery. The types of nursing interventions required will be patient-dependent, but may include:

- Maintaining a patent airway – the tongue should be pulled forward in unconscious patients and endotracheal intubation should be considered. In conscious patients, ensure that the head is extended
- Cleaning any secretions from the oral cavity – in unconscious patients suction or swabs should be used and the head lowered (e.g. over a foam or towel roll) to encourage drainage by gravity
- Ensuring adequate oxygenation (oxygen should be provided as necessary; see 'Oxygen supplementation', above). Oxygenation should be monitored appropriately, including via pulse oximetry (see Chapter 21). Even if oxygenation is not required, ensure that the patient is hospitalized close to an available oxygen supply
- Managing chest drains carefully and correctly (see below and Chapter 23)
- Ensuring medication is given in the correct manner and at the correct time
- Alerting the veterinary surgeon to any concerns.

Maintaining body temperature

These patients are unlikely to have adequate temperature control. Regular monitoring of the patient's temperature is paramount. Core temperature should be monitored every 30–120 minutes, depending on the underlying condition(s). External heat provision is often required in these patients (see Chapter 14). Warming patients gradually usually prevents inadvertent overheating.

Grooming

As with recumbent patients, grooming is essential for critically ill animals. Good hygiene and skin care, especially around orifices, is required at all times. Hair should be clipped as necessary and tail bandages used as appropriate (see 'Bandaging', above). There must be careful monitoring for urine scalding and decubital ulcers (see above).

Mobilizing

The basic requirements for mobilizing critical patients are the same as those described for recumbent patients above. Additional care and assistance from colleagues may be required during mobilization where patients have a number of tubes and drains in place, to ensure that these are not dislodged or contaminated.

Sleeping/resting

Critical patients will normally be placed in an 'intensive care' area of the veterinary practice, where adequate lighting, oxygen and other essential facilities are close at hand. Even though these patients require regular and often very intensive hands-on care, consideration should be given to the need for some peace, quiet and rest.

Expressing normal behaviour

The extent to which critical patients are able to express normal behaviour varies, depending upon the individuals and the medical conditions involved. It is important for veterinary nurses to remember that intensive care patients are still pet animals, with their own personalities and needs, and not just a series of tubes and drains and tasks to be carried out. Taking a little time for some basic TLC is important in these cases and is greatly appreciated by the owners.

Patient mental state

Critically ill patients often respond to stimuli in a very delayed fashion or may be unconscious. Levels of consciousness, motor activity and reflexes should be assessed using a coma scale, such as the Modified Glasgow Coma Scale (https://bvns.net/wp-content/uploads/2016/09/Neurotransmitter-2.0-MGCS-final.pdf). Even when animals are conscious, they may appear unresponsive to normal stimuli. This does not necessarily mean that they are unaware, and care must be taken when handling the patient, as well as with other stimuli such as noise and smell, to reduce stress. If care is not taken, aggression, panic and abnormal neurological activity (e.g. seizures) may occur, all of which will actively delay recovery times. In some cases, having a radio in the background may help to calm patients and taking time simply to sit and stroke or talk to the patient is good nursing care for these individuals.

Other nursing considerations
Regular monitoring

Regular monitoring of critical patients is essential. Findings must be recorded on an appropriate intensive care sheet (Figure 15.53) or in a series of separate documents (e.g. feeding charts, fluid charts, glucose curve sheets) depending upon patient requirements and practice policy. Care plans (see Chapter 12) should also be completed for these patients.

Title:

Last name:

Animal Name:

Age:

Species:

Gender:

Reason for admission:

Date:	Day no.	Case vet:

Admit weight: | Daily weight:

Character: | Vet check

I own:

Owner contact
AM ☐ PM ☐

Estimate:

Nutritional requirements

Diet required/chosen:

RER =   kcal/day

Amount of food per 24 hours =

Frequency of feeding: **SID/BID/TID/QID** (please circle)

Amount of food per feed =

Observation	00	01	02	03	04	05	06	07	08	09	10	11	12	13	14	15	16	17	18	19	20	21	22	23
Demeanour																								
Temperature																								
Pulse/ HR																								
Pulse quality																								
RR + effort																								
MMs																								
CRT																								
Hydration status																								
Pain score																								
Initial																								
Exercise/ Litter tray check																								
Urine																								
Faeces (faecal score – see chart)																								
Bed check/changed																								
Food offered																								
Food eaten																								
Water offered (quantity)																								
Water drank (quantity)																								
Vomit/regurge																								
Wound check																								
Bandage check																								
Physio																								

Medication/strength	Dose	Route	Freq.	00	01	02	03	04	05	06	07	08	09	10	11	12	13	14	15	16	17	18	19	20	21	22	23

| Catheter 1 –position/size/date placed: | | Flushed | | | | | | Dressed |
| Catheter 2 –position/size/date placed: | | Flushed | | | | | | Dressed |

Fluid bag	Bag 1	Bag 2
Type:	New bag: Booked: ☐	New bag: Booked: ☐
Additives		
ml/kg		
ml/hr		
Rate change/plan:		

15.53 Example of an intensive care sheet. (Courtesy of Quantock Veterinary Hospital)

Monitoring should take place at regular (30–120 minute) intervals, as appropriate to the individual case and medical conditions. Information recorded should, at a minimum, include:

- Temperature, pulse rate and quality, respiratory rate and rhythm, mucous membrane colour and capillary refill time
- Consciousness (using as appropriate a scale, e.g. the Modified Glasgow Coma Scale)
- Pain (using an appropriate scoring scheme, e.g. the Glasgow Composite Pain Scale for dogs and cats, grimace scales for rabbits and rodents) (see Chapter 21 for further details)
- Urine output (30-minute intervals if a catheter is in place)
- Intravenous fluid rates
- When turned and on to which side
- Other nursing interventions and outcomes (e.g. changes in dressings, enemas)
- Drug administration – doses, frequency and rates (continuous infusions).

Medication

Critical patients are often on a large number of medications. It is essential that these are given and recorded at the correct times. Most medications are likely to be parenteral in these cases (see Chapter 8) and must be given in a sterile manner; this is especially important for intravenous medications. When medication is given by continuous infusion, care should be taken to ensure that drip pumps and syringe drivers are correctly calibrated and in working order (see Chapter 20).

Management of tubes and drains

These may be chest drainage tubes, active drainage tubes from wounds, feeding tubes or nasal oxygen provision tubes (see also Chapters 13, 21 and 23). The same basic rules apply to all:

- Wash hands and wear gloves before handling tubes and drains
- Check insertion sites at an appropriate frequency (for some hourly; others daily)
- Dress sites that involve breaches in the skin with sterile dressings; change the dressings as appropriate, but at least daily
- Bandage (see 'Bandaging', above) so that the tubes are protected, but also in a manner that provides patient comfort; ensure that no clamps, etc., rub or press into the skin surface
- Prevent patient trauma using Elizabethan collars and/or protective vests
- Ensure that feeding tubes are flushed thoroughly to prevent blockage.

Acknowledgement

Sharon Chandler is thanked for her contribution to an earlier edition of this chapter.

References and further reading

Arthurs G, Brown G and Pettitt R (2018) *BSAVA Manual of Canine and Feline Musculoskeletal Disorders, 2nd edn.* BSAVA Publications, Gloucester

Bockstahler B, Wittek K, Levine D, Maierl J and Millis D (2019) *Essential Facts of Physical Medicine, Rehabilitation and Sports Medicine in Companion Animals.* VBS VetVerlag, Buchhandel und Seminar GmbH, Babenhausen

Brockman D, Holt D and ter Haar G (2018) *BSAVA Manual of Canine and Feline Head, Neck and Thoracic Surgery, 2nd edn.* BSAVA Publications, Gloucester

Carver D (2015) *Practical Physiotherapy for Veterinary Nurses.* Wiley Blackwell, Oxford

Chauvet A, Laclaire J, Elliot DA and German AJ (2011) Incorporation of exercise, using an underwater treadmill, and active client education into a weight management programme for obese dogs. *Canine Veterinary Journal* **52**, 491–496

Drum MG, Marcellin-Little DJ and Davis M (2015) Principles and applications of therapeutic exercises for small animals. *Veterinary Clinics of North America: Small Animal Practice* **45**, 73–90

Duke-Novakovski T, de Vries M and Seymour C (2016) *BSAVA Manual of Canine and Feline Anaesthesia and Analgesia, 3rd edn.* BSAVA Publications, Gloucester

Elliott J, Grauer GF and Westropp JL (2017) *BSAVA Manual of Canine and Feline Nephrology and Urology, 3rd edn.* BSAVA Publications, Gloucester

Harvey A and Tasker S (2013) *BSAVA Manual of Feline Practice.* BSAVA Publications, Gloucester

King LG and Boag A (2018) *BSAVA Manual of Canine and Feline Emergency and Critical Care, 3rd edn.* BSAVA Publications, Gloucester

Klide AM and Kung SH (2002) *Veterinary Acupuncture.* University of Pennsylvania Press, Philadelphia

McGowan C, Goff L and Stubbs N (2016) *Animal Physiotherapy – Assessment, Treatment and Rehabilitation of Animals.* Wiley Blackwell, Oxford

Millis DL and Levin D (2013) *Canine Rehabilitation and Physical Therapy, 2nd edn.* Elsevier, Philadelphia

Mullineaux E and Jones M (2007) *BSAVA Manual of Practical Veterinary Nursing.* BSAVA Publications, Gloucester

Mullineaux E and Keeble E (2016) *BSAVA Manual of Wildlife Casualties, 2nd edn.* BSAVA Publications, Gloucester

Nelson D and Welsh P (2015) Using the ability model to design and implement a patient care. *The Veterinary Nurse* **6(3)**, 141–149

Prydie D and Hewitt I (2015) *Practical Physiotherapy for Small Animal Practice.* Wiley Blackwell, Oxford

Ramey DW and Rollin BE (2004) *Complementary and Alternative Veterinary Medicine Considered.* Iowa State Press, Ames

Rew K (2007) Rehabilitation offers effective way to restore form and function. Veterinary Times October 22nd pp. 16–18

Rew K, Davies L and Sharples R (2009) Don't drown the dog: practical and safe approaches to rehabilitation. *Veterinary Times* February 2nd pp. 16–19

Sharp BJ (2008) Physiotherapy and rehabilitation. In: *BSAVA Manual of Canine and Feline Advanced Veterinary Nursing, 2nd edn,* ed. A Hotson Moore and S Rudd, pp. 72–102. BSAVA Publications, Gloucester

Watson P and Lindley S (2010) *BSAVA Manual of Canine and Feline Rehabilitation, Supportive and Palliative Care: Case Studies in Patient Management.* BSAVA Publications, Gloucester

Varga M, Lumbis R and Gott L (2012) *BSAVA Manual of Exotic Pet and Wildlife Nursing.* BSAVA Publications, Gloucester

Vitger AD, Stallknecht BM, Nielsen DH and Bjornvad CR (2016) Integration of a physical training program in a weight loss plan for overweight pet dogs. *Journal of the American Veterinary Medicine Association* **248(2)**, 174–182

Useful websites

Association of British Veterinary Acupuncturists:
www.abva.co.uk

Association of Chartered Physiotherapists in Animal Therapy (ACPAT):
www.acpat.org

Modified Glasgow Coma Scale:
https://bvns.net/wp-content/uploads/2016/09/Neurotransmitter-2.0-MGCS-final.pdf

National Association of Veterinary Physiotherapists:
www.navp.co.uk

Self-assessment questions

1. List six reasons for bandaging in dogs and cats.
2. For the following dressings state the type of dressing and a reason for its use:
    *   Hydrogel
    *   Synthetic padding
    *   Conforming.
3. State one reason why you would apply each of the following bandages and describe (and/or demonstrate) how you would apply the bandage:
    *   A food bandage in a cat
    *   An ear bandage in a dog
    *   A chest bandage in a dog
    *   A Robert Jones bandage in a dog
    *   An Ehmer sling in a cat
4. Identify one advantage and one disadvantage of using: a) a phosphate enema and b) a ready-to-use mini enema in a dog.
5. Describe how you would give a warm water enema to a dog.
6. Provide three indications for urinary catheterization and describe how you would catheterize a male cat and a female dog.
7. Identify three methods of oxygen supplementation in dogs.
8. When might the following therapies by used and why:
    *   Effleurage
    *   Petrissage
    *   Cryotherapy
    *   Hydrotherapy.
9. How can ultrasound benefit an injured tendon?
10. What role do the following professionals carry out when working alongside the veterinary team in providing alternative treatments to promote health:
    *   The chiropractor
    *   The osteopath
    *   The acupuncturist
    *   The physiotherapist.
11. What are the important considerations when nursing:
    *   A vomiting cat
    *   A critically ill dog.
12. What can be done to help prevent:
    *   Urine scalding
    *   Decubital ulcers
    *   Hypostatic pneumonia.

Chapter 16

Diagnostic imaging

Julie Sales, Abby Caine, Ruth Dennis and Philip Lhermette with exotic pets by Simon Girling

Learning objectives

After studying this chapter, readers will have the knowledge to:

- Apply the physical principles of diagnostic radiography, using both conventional film/screen systems and digital radiography
- Adopt a sound working knowledge of radiographic equipment, procedures and safety
- Demonstrate how to perform basic radiographic procedures in dogs, cats and exotic pets, and how to prepare for and assist in more complex investigations
- Identify faults in radiography and how to correct them
- Apply the principles of diagnostic ultrasonography and assist in ultrasound examinations in dogs, cats and exotic pets
- Appreciate the basic principles of magnetic resonance imaging (MRI), computed tomography (CT), scintigraphy and endoscopy
- Apply specific considerations for imaging exotic pets

Introduction

Diagnostic imaging techniques are a fundamental part of veterinary practice and are procedures in which most veterinary nurses become actively involved. The production of radiographic images requires skill in the use of radiographic equipment and in patient positioning. At the same time, the procedure must be carried out safely, without hazard to the handlers or patient. Increasingly, veterinary nurses are also involved in other diagnostic techniques, including ultrasonography, endoscopy, magnetic resonance imaging (MRI) and computed tomography (CT) with responsibilities for patient preparation, image processing, equipment maintenance and safety.

Basic principles of radiography

X-rays are produced by X-ray machines when mains electricity is transformed into a high-voltage current, converting some of the energy in the current to X-ray energy. X-rays are produced when rapidly moving electrons are decelerated or completely stopped following interaction with atoms of the target in an X-ray tube. The intensity and penetrating power of the emergent X-ray beam varies with the size and complexity of the apparatus and the exposure settings used; portable X-ray machines are capable of only a relatively low output, whereas larger machines are far more powerful.

X-rays travel in straight lines and can be focused into an area called the primary beam, which is directed at the patient. Some of the X-rays are absorbed within the patient's tissues; the remainder pass through and are detected either by a digital recording system or, now less commonly, by photographic X-ray film, producing in both cases a hidden (latent) image. More than 99% of the electron energy is converted into heat and less than 1% of energy is converted into X-rays. With digital radiography, the image is produced electronically and can be viewed on a computer screen. When X-ray film is processed chemically, a permanent image is produced and this can be viewed on a light box viewer.

Production and properties of X-rays

X-rays form part of the electromagnetic spectrum, a group of types of radiation that have some similar properties but which differ from each other in their wavelength and frequency (Figure 16.1).

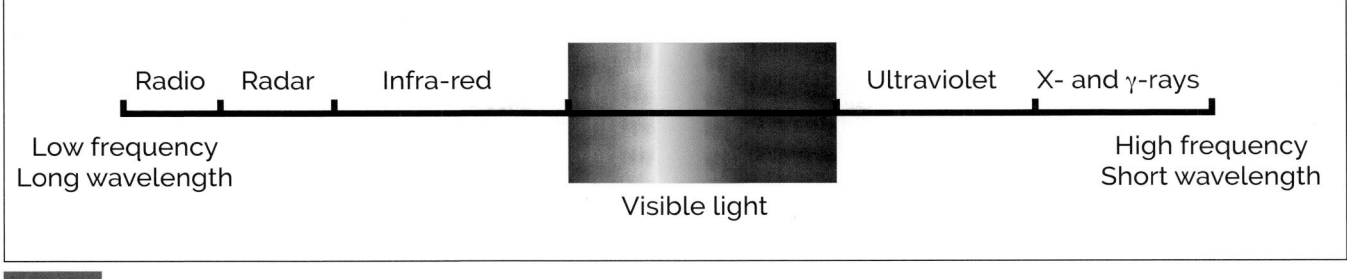

The electromagnetic spectrum.

The energy in a given type of radiation is directly proportional to the frequency of the radiation and inversely proportional to its wavelength. X-rays and gamma-rays are similar types of electromagnetic radiation that have high frequency, short wavelength and therefore high energy. X-rays are produced by X-ray machines and gamma-rays by the decay of radioactive materials.

All parts of the electromagnetic spectrum have the following common features:

- They do not require a medium for transmission and can pass through a vacuum
- They travel in straight lines
- They travel at the same speed: 3×10^8 m/s in a vacuum
- They interact with matter by being absorbed or scattered.

X-rays have some additional properties that mean they can be used to produce images of the internal structures of people and animals. They are also used in engineering for detecting flaws in pipes and construction materials.

- **Penetration:** Due to their high energy, X-rays can penetrate substances that are opaque to visible ('white') light. The X-ray photons are absorbed to varying degrees, depending on the nature of the substance penetrated and the energy of the photons themselves, and some may pass straight through the patient, emerging at the other side. The shorter its wavelength, the higher the energy of the X-ray photon and the greater the penetrating ability.
- **Effect on photographic film:** X-rays have the ability to produce a hidden or latent image on photographic film, which can be rendered visible by processing (film in cameras is damaged by exposure to X-radiation).
- **Fluorescence:** X-rays cause crystals of certain substances to fluoresce (emit visible light) and this property is utilized in the composition of intensifying screens, which are used in the recording of the image.
- **Energy storage:** With digital radiography systems, the energy of the emergent photons is captured and converted electronically to a digital image in several different ways, depending on the type of digital system used.

X-rays also produce biological changes in living tissues by altering the structure of atoms or molecules or by causing chemical reactions. Some of these effects can be used beneficially (e.g. the use of radiotherapy to treat tumours), but they are harmful to normal tissues and constitute a safety hazard. Aspects of radiation safety are considered later in the chapter.

Production of X-rays

X-ray photons, or quanta, are tiny packets of energy that are released whenever rapidly moving electrons are slowed down or stopped. Electrons are present in the atoms of all elements and, in order to grasp the fundamentals of simple radiation physics, it is necessary to understand the structure of an atom (Figure 16.2). Atoms contain the following particles:

- **Protons** – positively charged particles contained in the centre or nucleus of the atom
- **Neutrons** – particles of similar size to protons that are also found in the nucleus but carry no electrical charge
- **Electrons** – smaller, negatively charged particles that orbit around the nucleus in different planes or 'shells'.

The number of electrons normally equals the number of protons and so the atom as a whole is electrically neutral. The number of protons and electrons is unique to the atoms of each element and is called the atomic number. If an atom loses one or more electrons it becomes positively charged and may be written as X+ (where X is the symbol for that element). If an atom gains electrons it becomes negatively charged (X-). Atoms with charges are called ions or are said to be ionized; a positively charged ion is a cation and a negatively charged ion is an anion. Compounds are combinations of two or more elements and usually consist of positive ions of one element in combination with negative ions of another; for example, silver bromide (in X-ray film emulsion) consists of silver (Ag+) and bromide (Br−) ions.

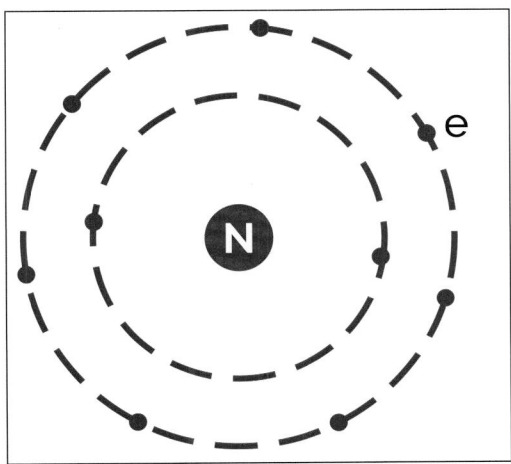

16.2 Structure of an atom. e = electron (dotted lines represent electron 'shells'); N = nucleus (protons and neutrons).

In an X-ray tube head, X-ray photons are produced by collisions between fast-moving electrons and the atoms of a 'target' element. Electrons that are completely halted by the target atoms give up all of their energy to form an X-ray photon, whereas those that are merely decelerated give up smaller and variable amounts of energy, producing lower-energy X-ray photons. The X-ray beam produced therefore contains photons of a range of energies and is said to be polychromatic. If the number of incident electrons is increased, more X-ray photons are produced and the intensity of the X-ray beam increases. If the incident electrons are faster-moving, they have more energy to lose and so the X-ray photons produced are more energetic; the quality of the X-ray beam is therefore increased and it has greater penetrating power. The intensity and quality of an X-ray beam can be altered by adjusting the settings on the machine, and the practical effect of this will be discussed in greater detail later.

The X-ray tube head

The X-ray tube head is the part of the machine where the X-ray photons are generated. A diagram of the simplest type of X-ray tube, a stationary or fixed anode tube, is shown in Figure 16.3.

The X-ray tube head contains two electrodes: the negatively charged cathode and the positively charged anode. Electrons are produced at the cathode, which is a coiled wire filament. When a small electrical current is passed through the filament it becomes hot and releases a cloud of electrons by a process called thermionic emission. Tungsten is used as the filament material because:

- It has a high atomic number, 74, and therefore has many electrons
- It has a very high melting point, 3380°C, and so can safely be heated
- It has helpful mechanical properties which mean that fine, coiled filaments can be made.

The electric current required to heat the filament is small and so the mains current to the filament is reduced by a step-down or filament transformer, which is wired into the X-ray machine (a transformer is a device for increasing or decreasing an electric current). Next, the cloud of electrons must be made to travel at high speed across the short distance to the target. This is done by applying a high electrical potential difference between the filament and the target so that the filament becomes negative (and therefore repels the electrons) and the target becomes positive (and attracts them). The filament therefore becomes a cathode and the target an anode.

The filament sits in a nickel or molybdenum focusing cup, which is also at a negative potential and so repels the electrons, causing them to form a narrow beam. The electron beam constitutes a weak electric current across the tube, which is measured in milliamperes or 'milliamps' (mA). Multiplying the mA by the duration (in seconds) of the exposure reflects the total quantity of X-ray photons emitted in milliampere seconds or mAs.

The potential difference applied between the filament and the target needs to be very high and many times the voltage of the mains supply of 240 volts. In fact, it is measured in thousands of volts, or kilovolts (kV), and is created from the mains in a second electrical circuit using a step-up or high-tension transformer, which is also part of the electrical circuitry of the X-ray machine. The stream of electrons strikes the target, or anode, at very high speed. Tungsten or rhenium–tungsten alloy is used as the target material because its high atomic number renders it a relatively efficient producer of X-rays. Unfortunately, the process is still very inefficient and >99% of the energy lost by the electrons is converted to heat, so the anode must be able to withstand very high temperatures without melting or cracking. Tungsten's high melting point is therefore useful in the target as well as in the filament.

In a simple type of X-ray tube (see Figure 16.3) the target is a small rectangle of tungsten about 3 mm thick set in a copper block. Copper is a good conductor of heat and so the heat is removed from the target by conduction along the copper stem to cooling fins radiating into the surrounding oil bath, which can absorb much heat.

The target is set at an angle of about 20 degrees to the vertical (Figure 16.4). This is so that the area of the target which the electrons strike (and therefore the area over which heat is produced) is as large as possible. This area is called the actual focal spot. At the same time, the angulation of the target means that the X-ray beam appears to originate from a much smaller area and this is called the effective focal spot. The importance of having a small effective focal spot – ideally a point source – is discussed later in the chapter with regard to image definition. The design of the target to maximize actual focal spot size whilst minimizing the effective focal spot is known as the line focus principle.

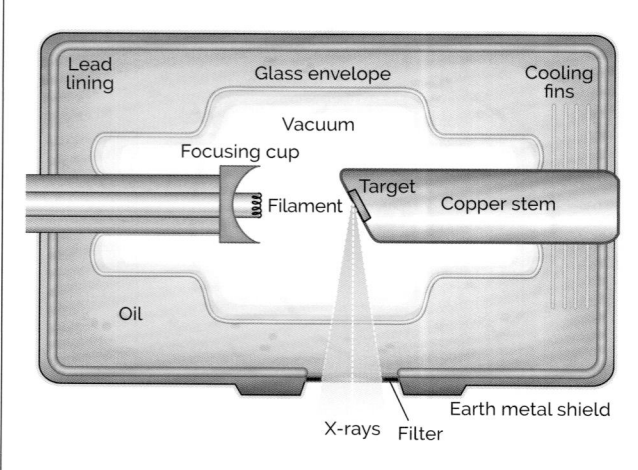

16.3 Stationary anode X-ray tubes are the simplest form of X-ray tube head.

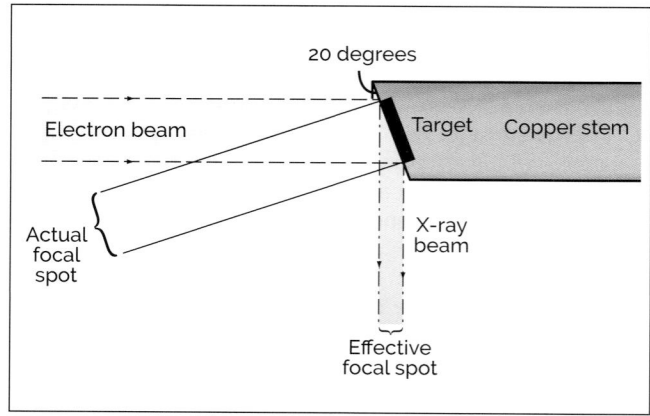

16.4 The line focus principle: how angulation of the target produces a large actual focal spot and a small effective focal spot.

Some X-ray machines allow a choice of focal spot size using two different-sized filaments at the cathode:

■ The smaller filament produces an electron beam with a smaller cross-sectional area and hence smaller effective and actual focal spots. This is known as fine focus. The emergent X-ray beam arises from a tiny area and will produce very fine radiographic definition. However, the heat generated is concentrated over a very small area of the target and so the exposure factors that can be used are limited

■ The larger filament produces a wider electron beam with larger effective and actual focal spot sizes – the coarse or broad focus. Higher exposures can be used but the image definition will be slightly less sharp due to the penumbra effect, a blurring of margins related to the geometry of the beam (Figure 16.5). X-ray photons produced at different points on the focal spot will travel along slightly different pathways and therefore hit the film in slightly different locations, even though they outline the same anatomical feature. 'Penumbra' is derived from Latin and means 'partial shadow'.

In practice, fine focus is selected for small parts where fine definition is required (e.g. the limbs), and coarse focus when thicker areas are to be radiographed (e.g. the chest and abdomen); the thicker areas require higher exposure factors and so the heat generated at the target is higher.

The cathode, anode and part of the copper stem are enclosed in a glass envelope (see Figure 16.3). Within the envelope is a vacuum, which prevents the moving electrons from colliding with air molecules and losing speed. The glass envelope is bathed in oil, which acts both as a heat sink and as an electrical insulator, and the whole is encased in an earthed, lead-lined metal casing. X-rays are produced in all directions by the target but only one narrow beam of X-rays is required. This emerges through a window in the casing, placed beneath the angled target, and is used for making a radiographic image. It is called the primary beam. X-rays produced in other directions are absorbed by the casing.

Within the X-ray beam are some low-energy or 'soft' X-ray photons, which are not powerful enough to pass through the patient but may be absorbed or scattered by the patient and therefore represent a safety hazard. They are removed from the beam by an aluminium filter placed across the tube window; these filters are legally required as a safety precaution and must not be removed.

In stationary anode X-ray tubes, the X-ray output is limited by the amount of heat generated at the target. Over-heating the target would produce melting and surface irregularity, which would reduce the efficiency of the tube; in modern machines, automatic overload devices prevent such high exposures from being used. Stationary anode X-ray tubes are found in low-powered, portable X-ray machines. These have limited ability to produce short exposure times for thoracic radiography or high output for large patients. More powerful machines require a more efficient way of removing the heat and this is accomplished using a rotating anode (Figure 16.6). In such tubes the target area is the bevelled rim of a metal disc of about 10 cm diameter whose rim is set at about 20 degrees, as in a stationary anode X-ray tube. The target area is again tungsten or rhenium–tungsten. During the exposure, the disc rotates rapidly so that the target area upon which the electrons impinge is constantly changing. The actual focal spot is therefore the whole circumference of the disc and so is many times greater than in a stationary anode X-ray tube. The heat generated is spread over a much bigger area, allowing larger exposures to be made, whilst the effective focal spot remains the same. The disc is mounted on a molybdenum rod and is rotated at speeds of up to 10,000 rpm by an induction motor at the other end of the rod. Molybdenum is used because it is a poor conductor of heat and therefore prevents the motor from overheating. Heat generated in the anode is lost by radiation through the vacuum and the glass envelope into the oil bath.

The size of the emerging X-ray beam must be controlled for safety reasons otherwise it will spread out over a very large area. This is achieved using a collimation device, preferably a light beam diaphragm. Methods of collimation are described later.

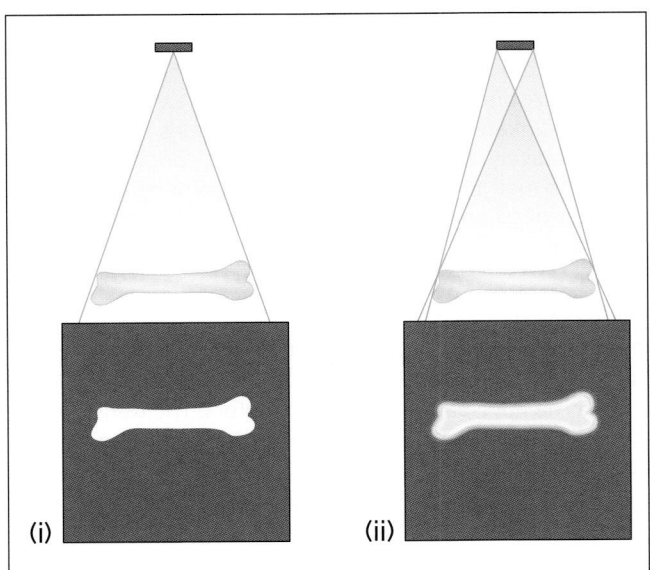

16.5 Effect of focal spot size. **(i)** The spot is a pinpoint and the projected image is sharp. **(ii)** The rays form a focal spot of larger dimensions cause a penumbra effect, which blurs the projected image.

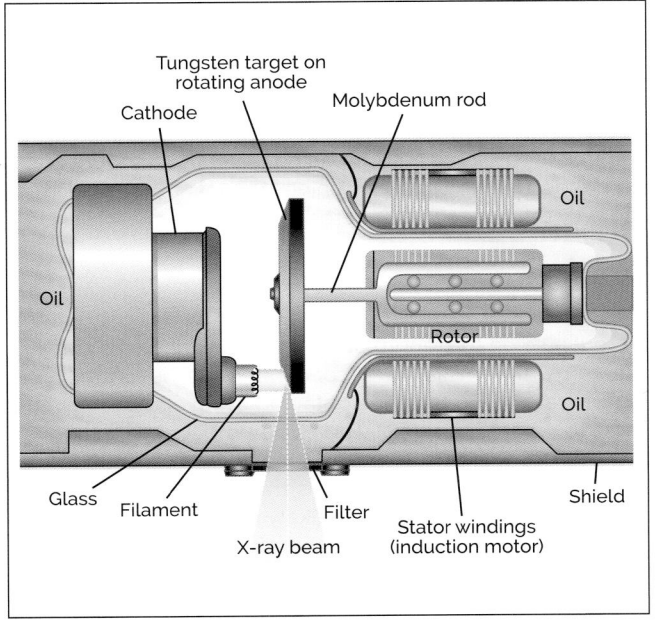

16.6 A rotating anode X-ray tube.

The X-ray control panel

X-ray machine control panels vary in their complexity; the majority having light-emitting diode (LED) displays, either touch screen or push buttons. Some or all of the following controls will be present.

On/off switch

As well as switching the machine on at the mains socket, there will be an on/off switch or key on the control panel. When the machine is switched on, a warning light on the control panel will indicate that it is ready to produce X-rays or, in the case of panels with digital displays, the displays will be illuminated. With larger fixed systems there must also be a link to a warning sign outside the X-ray room, which is illuminated whenever the X-ray machine is switched on. X-ray machines must always be switched off when not in use, so that accidental exposure cannot occur when unprotected people are in the room.

Kilovoltage (kV) control

The kV control selects the kV (potential difference) that is applied across the tube during the instant of exposure. It determines the speed and energy with which the electrons bombard the target and hence the quality or penetrating power of the X-ray beam produced. Depending on the power and sophistication of the X-ray machine, the kV is controlled in various ways. Ideally, it is controlled independently of the mA, often in increments of 1 kV, and the kV meter is usually a digital display, but in older machines dials may still be used.

Milliamperage control

The mA is a measure of the quantity of electrons crossing the tube during the exposure (the 'tube current') and is directly related to the quantity of X-rays produced. Moving electrons constitute an electrical current, which is measured in amperes (amps), but the tube current is very small and is measured in 1/1000 amperes or milliamps (mA). Adjusting the mA control alters the degree of heating of the filament and hence the number of electrons released by thermionic emission, the tube current and the intensity of the X-ray beam.

In smaller machines the kV is linked to the mA, so that if a higher mA is selected only lower kVs can be used. With older units there is often a single control for both kV and mA and as the kV is increased the mA available drops. This is not ideal since, for larger patients, a high kV and high mA may be required at the same time, meaning that long exposure times are needed. In very basic machines the kV and mA are fixed, and only the time can be altered.

Timer

The quantity of X-rays produced depends not only on the mA but also on the length of the exposure, and so a composite term, the milliamp seconds or mAs, is often used. A given rate of mAs may be obtained using a high mA with a short time, or vice versa. The two numbers are multiplied together, for example 30 mAs = 300 mA for 0.1 s or 30 mA for 1.0 s. The effect on the image is the same except that the longer the exposure, the more likely it is that movement blur will occur. One should always, therefore, use the largest mA allowed by the machine for that kV setting, in order to minimize the exposure time. It should now be clear why machines in which kV and mA are automatically inversely linked are less than ideal.

The timer is electronic and is commonly another display on the control panel, giving the choice of a wide range of exposure times up to several seconds long. Release of the exposure button terminates the exposure, even when long times have been selected. In larger machines, an automatic display of the resulting mAs is also present. Some machines have a single control for mAs, which automatically selects the shortest exposure time for the selected mAs.

Exposure button

The exposure button must be at the end of a cable that can stretch to >2 m, to enable radiographers to distance themselves from the primary beam during the exposure. Alternatively, the button may be on the control panel itself, provided that the panel is at least 2 m from the tube head or is separated from it by a lead screen. Most exposure buttons are two-stage devices: depression of the button to a halfway stage ('prepping') heats the filament and rotates the anode if a rotating anode is present; after a brief pause, further depression of the button causes application of the kV to the tube and an instantaneous exposure to be made. In some machines only a single-stage exposure button is present; in this case there is a slight delay between depression of the button and exposure, during which time the patient may move.

Types of X-ray machine

X-ray machines can be divided into three broad types: portable, mobile and fixed.

Portable machines

These are the commonest type of machine found in general practice. As their name suggests, they are relatively easy to move from site to site for large animal radiography and many come with a special carrying case. The largest weigh about 20 kg. The electrical transformers are located in the tube head, which is usually supported on a wheeled metal stand (Figure 16.7), though some may be wall-mounted. The tube head must never be held for radiography, as this is very hazardous to the person holding it. The controls may be either on a separate panel or on the head itself. Portable machines are low powered, usually producing only about 20–60 mA and often less. In most, the kV and mA are inversely linked. Although portable machines are still used, their relatively low output means that longer exposure times are needed, and chest and abdomen radiographs of larger dogs are often degraded by the effects of movement blur.

Mobile machines

These are larger and more powerful than portable machines but can still be moved from room to room on wheels (Figure 16.8); some have battery-operated motors. The transformers are bulkier and encased in a large box, which is an integral part of the tube stand.

Mobile machines usually have outputs of up to 300 mA and are likely to produce good radiographs of most small animal patients. Although they are more expensive to buy new, they can sometimes be obtained second-hand from human hospitals, where they will have had relatively little use yet been well cared for, having been used mainly for bed ridden patients.

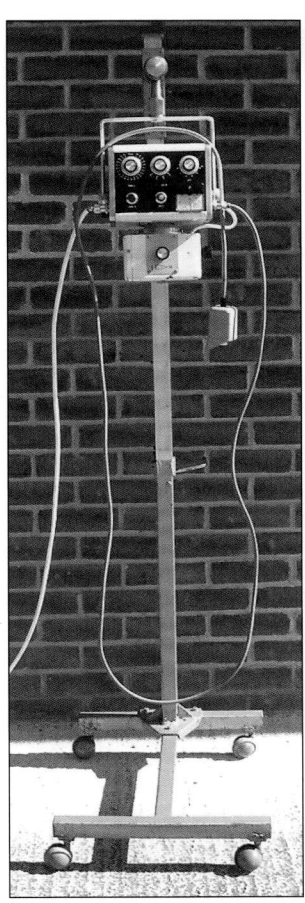

16.7 Portable X-ray machine.

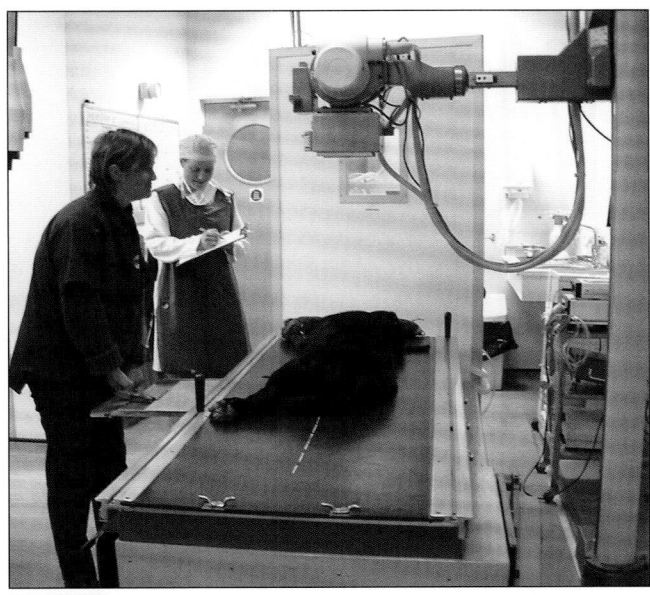

16.9 Fixed X-ray machine.

The largest fixed machines can produce up to 1250 mA and generate excellent radiographs of all patients but, because of the high cost of purchase, installation and maintenance, they are rarely found outside veterinary institutions. However, several companies are now producing smaller, fixed X-ray machines especially for the veterinary market, which are much more affordable. Fixed X-ray machines are often linked electronically to a floating table top and moving grid.

High-frequency machines

Many older X-ray machines, in particular portable machines, generate X-rays from a pulsating voltage supply. Most modern machines, including modern portable machines, use high-frequency generators to produce a stable high voltage supply to the X-ray tube. They do this by increasing the frequency of the waveform of the standard mains supply from 50 cycles per second (Hz) up to thousands of cycles per second (kHz). The advantage of this is that machines are capable of shorter exposure times, higher exposures, and improved efficiency.

Maintenance of X-ray machines

X-ray machines require little maintenance, but should be serviced annually by a qualified X-ray engineer, who will check both safety issues and calibration of the control buttons.

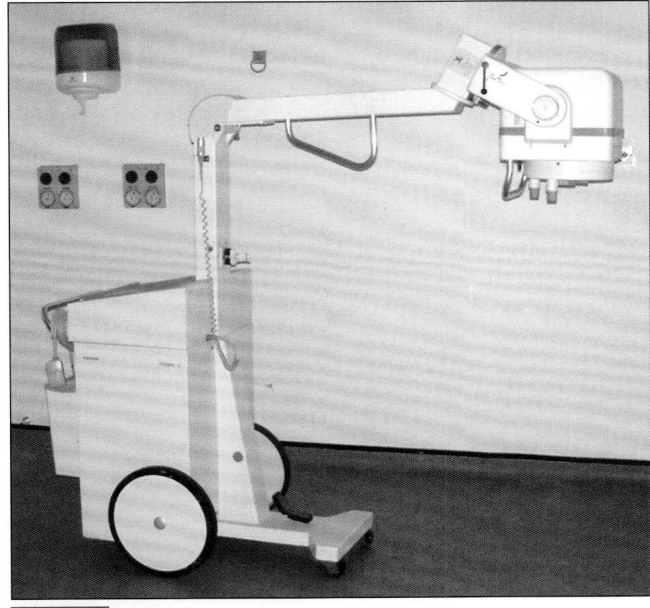

16.8 Mobile X-ray machine.

Fixed machines

The most powerful X-ray machines are built into the X-ray room and are either screwed to the floor or mounted on rails or overhead gantries (Figure 16.9). The tube head is usually quite mobile on its mounting and can be moved in several directions. The transformers are situated in cabinets some distance from the machine itself, and connected to it by high-tension cables.

Formation of the X-ray image

The X-ray image is essentially a 'shadowgraph', or a picture in black, white and varying shades of grey, caused by differences in the amount of absorption of the beam by different tissues and hence in differences in the amount of radiation reaching the digital detector system or X-ray film (Figure 16.10).

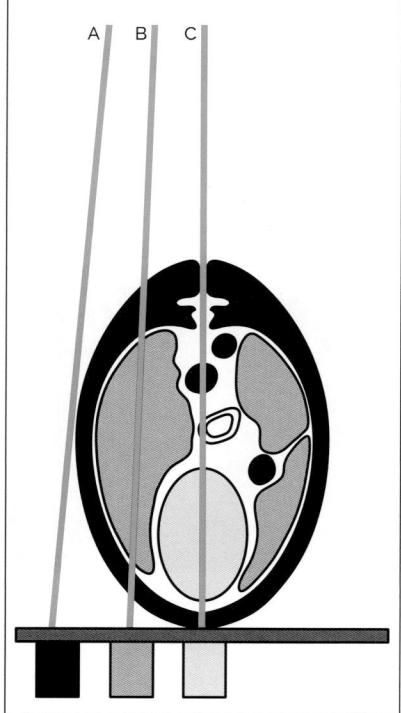

16.10 Cross-section through a thorax to illustrate formation of an X-ray 'shadowgraph'. X-ray photons passing along path C are largely absorbed, resulting in white areas on the radiograph. X-ray photons passing along path B are partly absorbed, producing intermediate shades of grey on the radiograph. X-ray photons passing along path A are outside the patient and so are not absorbed, producing black areas on the radiograph.

The degree of absorption by a given tissue depends on three factors:

- The atomic number (Z) of the tissue, or the average of the different atomic numbers present (the 'effective' atomic number)
- The specific gravity of the tissue
- The thickness of the tissue.

Bone has a higher effective atomic number than soft tissue and so absorbs more X-ray photons, producing paler areas on the radiograph. Similarly, soft tissue has a higher effective atomic number than fat.

Specific gravity is the density, or mass per unit volume. Bone has a high specific gravity, soft tissue a medium specific gravity and gas a very low specific gravity; hence gas-filled areas absorb few X-rays and appear nearly black on the radiograph.

The combination of effective atomic number and specific gravity produces five characteristic shades to be seen on a radiograph:

- Gas – very dark
- Fat – dark grey
- Soft tissue or fluid – mid grey
- Bone – nearly white
- Metal – white (as all X-rays are absorbed).

It should be noted that solid soft tissue and fluid produce the same radiographic appearance; therefore, fluid within a soft tissue viscus (e.g. urine in the bladder or blood in the heart) cannot be differentiated from the tissue that surrounds it. Fat is less radiopaque (darker) than soft tissue and fluid, so fat in the abdomen is helpful in surrounding and outlining the various organs. Overlap in the ranges of grey shades on the radiograph occurs due to the fact that thicker areas of tissue absorb more X-ray photons than thinner areas; hence a very thick area of soft tissue may actually appear more radiopaque (whiter) than a thin area of bone.

Selection of exposure factors

The following section provides information on the physics that underlies radiography using combinations of film and intensifying screens, used in medical and veterinary imaging. In many situations, digital imaging has replaced traditional film techniques and further comments about the selection of exposure factors for digital radiographs are given in the section on digital imaging. It is recognized, however, that there are still many veterinary practices that rely on film and intensifying screens.

Kilovoltage

The kilovoltage controls the quality or penetrating power of the X-ray beam. A higher kV is required for tissues that have a higher atomic number or specific gravity, or are very thick. Both the nature and depth of the tissue being X-rayed must therefore be taken into consideration when selecting the appropriate kV setting. A range of about 40–100 kV is generally used in veterinary radiography. The kV affects both the scale of contrast on the image (the number of grey shades) and the radiographic density (the degree of blackening of the film).

Increasing the kV will cause greater penetration of all tissues and hence a darker film. Too high a kV will overpenetrate tissues, resulting in a dark film with few different shades; this is called a 'flat' film or is said to be 'lacking in contrast'. Too low a kV will underpenetrate tissue (especially bone), which will appear white, on a black or dark grey background. This type of appearance is sometimes called 'soot and whitewash'; its contrast is too high. Figure 16.11 shows the effect of alterations in the kV.

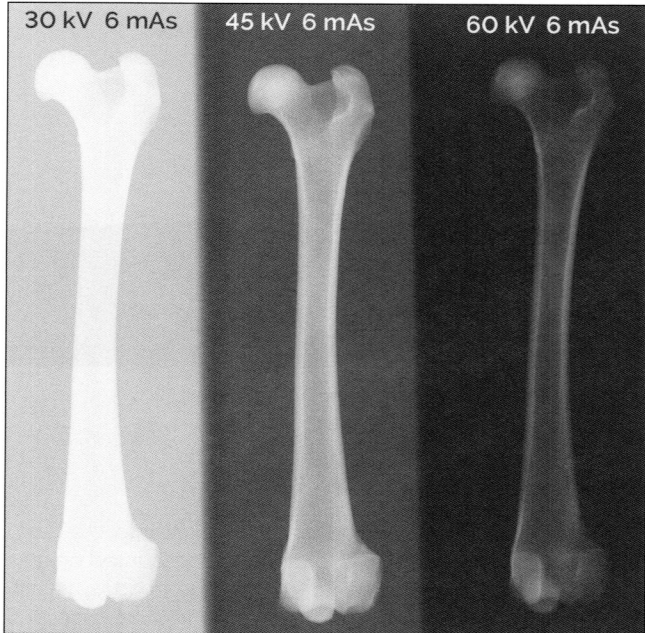

16.11 Effect on subject penetration of altering the kV but keeping the mAs constant. With low kV there is little penetration of the subject; with high kV there is too much.

Milliamperage and time

The mA setting determines the tube current and therefore the quantity of X-rays per second in the emergent beam, also known as its intensity. Altering the mA will not affect the penetrating power of the beam (i.e. the contrast of the image) but will change the degree of blackening of the film under the areas that are penetrated (the radiographic density).

The product of mA and length of the exposure produces the mAs factor or total quantity of X-rays used for that particular exposure. Normally the maximum mA and shortest time possible are used for the chest, in order to reduce the effects of movement blur (times of <0.05 s are preferred). Increasing the mAs will produce more X-ray photons to blacken the film, though they have no more penetrating ability. The contrast between adjacent tissues (the difference in shades of grey) will not change, but the overall picture will be darker. Figure 16.12 shows the effect of alterations in the mAs.

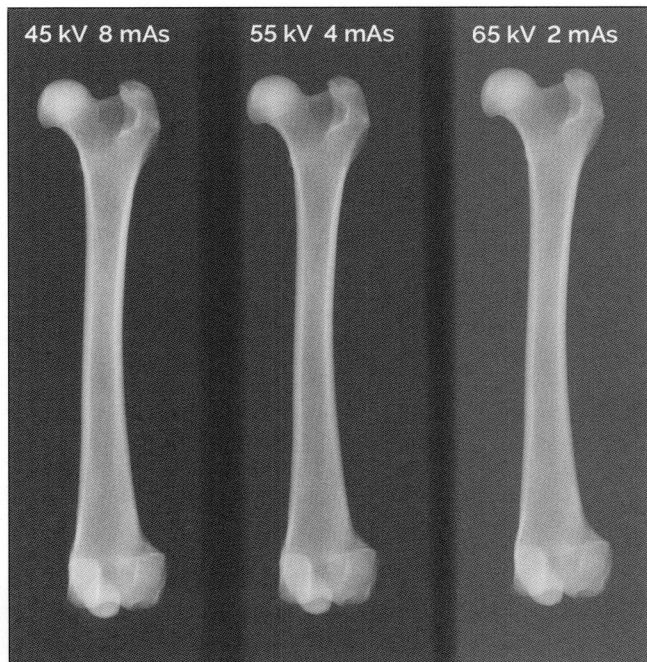

45 kV 8 mAs   55 kV 4 mAs   65 kV 2 mAs

16.13 Interplay between kV and mAs. If the kV is increased by 10 and the mAs is halved, the effect on the film is almost identical.

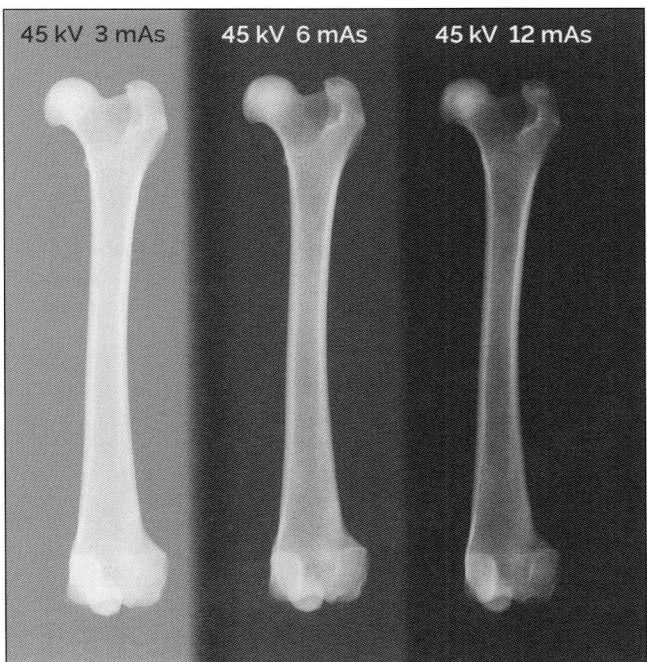

45 kV 3 mAs   45 kV 6 mAs   45 kV 12 mAs

16.12 Effect on film blackening of altering the mAs but keeping the kV constant. The patient penetration (internal detail) is similar in each case but the image is darker with higher mAs.

Although kV and mAs can be seen to govern different parameters of the X-ray beam, in the diagnostic range of exposures they are linked, in that images that appear similar can be produced by raising the kV and at the same time lowering the mAs, or vice versa. A useful and simple rule is that for every 10 kV increase, the mAs can be halved (Figure 16.13). Conversely, if the mAs is doubled, the kV must be reduced by 10. In practice, the time factor is usually paramount and so it is normal to work with as high a kV as possible, allowing the mAs to be kept low and therefore the time short.

Focal–film distance

The focal–film distance (FFD) is the total distance between the focal spot and the image receptor. It is important because, although the quality of the X-ray beam remains constant as it travels from the tube head, the intensity falls with increasing distance as the beam spreads out over a larger area. Figure 16.14 shows that if the FFD is doubled, the intensity of the beam over a given area is reduced to one-quarter and radiographic film will appear underexposed unless the mAs is raised. Conversely, if the FFD is reduced radiographic film will appear overexposed. (Note that digital receptors respond slightly differently and are less sensitive

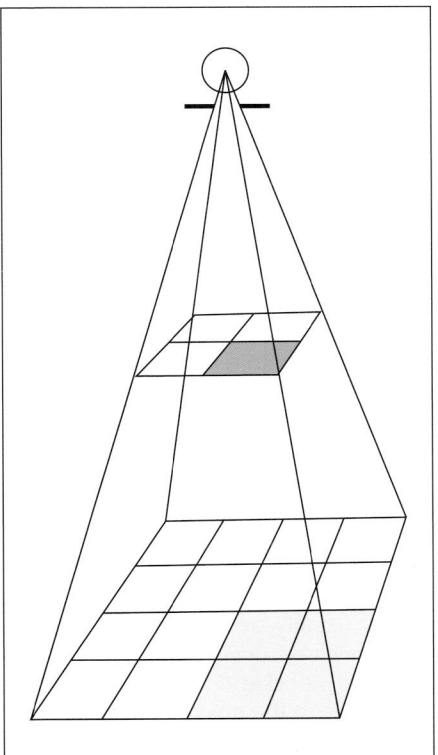

16.14 Inverse square law. The intensity of the beam falling on a given area is reduced to one-quarter by doubling the distance from the source.

to small changes in FFD.) The rule governing this effect is called the inverse square law, which states that the intensity of the primary beam projected on to an image receptor is reduced to one-quarter by doubling the distance from the X-ray film. Thus, a long FFD requires a higher mAs than a short FFD and the exact figure can be calculated mathematically from the equation:

$$\text{New mAs} = \text{Old mAs} \times \frac{\text{New distance}^2}{\text{Old distance}^2}$$

Although longer FFDs require a higher mAs to be used, image definition will be improved due to a reduction in the penumbra effect as the X-ray photons are travelling more nearly parallel to each other (see Figure 16.5). It is normal practice to work always at the same FFD for a given X-ray machine; a suitable distance for a portable X-ray machine is 75 cm, whilst 100 cm is normally used for more powerful X-ray machines that produce a higher mA.

Exposure charts

In order to avoid having to repeat radiographs, it is necessary to build up an exposure chart for each machine. An exposure chart is a list of the kV and mAs required for radiography of various areas of different-sized patients. For the exposure chart to be accurate, all other parameters must be kept constant (e.g. line voltage, quality of processing, FFD) and other changeable factors should also be given on the chart (i.e. digital receptor speed or film–screen combination and use of a grid). The chart may be compiled for patients of different types (e.g. cats and small, medium, large and giant dogs) or may be made more accurate still by measuring the thickness of the part to be X-rayed using callipers. The exposure chart can be built up over a period of time by recording all exposures made in the X-ray day book, with comments. Exposure charts are not usually interchangeable between types of machine and may not even be accurate for other machines of the same make and model, because of the varying factors listed above.

Exposure factors and digital radiography

Digital radiography systems are more tolerant of errors in selection of exposure factor, since the digital image can be computer-manipulated to optimize contrast and density. This means that there is less need to repeat exposures due to incorrect settings, saving time and money. The appearance of an underexposed digital image is different to that seen with a conventional X-ray film/screen system; instead of appearing pale it will have a grainy appearance as too few X-ray photons give rise to 'quantum mottle'. However, it is important not to allow the routine use of unnecessarily high exposure factors for obvious safety reasons. An additional advantage of digital radiography is that tissues of different density and thickness will usually be clearly seen using a single exposure, whereas with a conventional system two separate exposures may be needed. For example, in the thorax both the soft tissues and the spine can be demonstrated equally well with a single exposure, and an entire forelimb or hindlimb may be radiographed with one exposure, even when the difference in thickness of tissue from the proximal end to the distal is significant.

Scattered radiation

Although most of the X-ray photons entering the patient during the exposure are either completely absorbed or pass straight through, a certain proportion undergo a process known as scattering. Scattering occurs when incident photons interact with the tissues, losing some of their energy and 'bouncing' off in random directions as photons of lower energy (Figure 16.15). At lower kVs and when thin areas of tissue are being radiographed, the production of scattered or secondary radiation is small and most is re-absorbed within the patient. Scatter is therefore not a problem when cats, small dogs and the skull and limbs of larger dogs are being radiographed. However, when higher kVs are required in order to penetrate thicker or denser tissues, the amount and energy of the scattered radiation increases and substantial amounts may exit from the patient's body. The problems associated with this scattered radiation are two-fold:

- Scatter is a potential hazard to the radiographers, as it travels in all directions and may also ricochet back off the tabletop or the floor or walls of the room. In small animal practice, animals should not usually be manually restrained, allowing the radiographer to stand further away from the tube head, and the risks of scatter to be minimized (see 'Radiation protection', below)
- Scattered radiation will cause a uniform blackening of the X-ray film unrelated to the radiographic image, and will detract from the film's contrast and definition. The blurring that results is called fogging.

Scatter production increases with higher kV, thicker or denser tissues, and larger field sizes of the primary beam. Digital systems are especially sensitive to the effects of scatter. The amount of scattered radiation produced may be reduced in several ways.

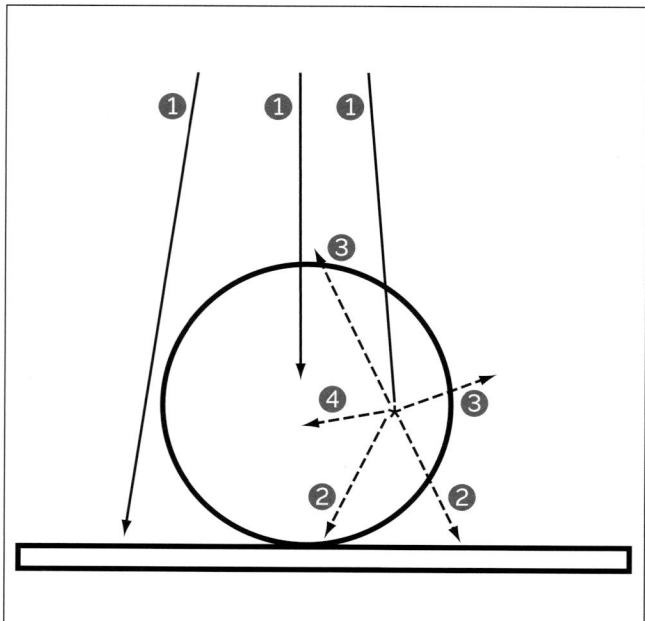

16.15 Formation of scattered radiation. 1 = Photons of the primary beam. 2 = Scatter in a forwards direction causing film fogging. 3 = Scatter in a backwards direction, which is a safety hazard. 4 = Some scatter is absorbed by the patient.

Reducing scattered radiation

- Reduction of the kV will reduce scattered radiation, so the lowest practicable kV should be selected. This is not always feasible, as in lower-powered X-ray machines the priority is usually to keep exposure time down using a low mAs factor and hence a large kV
- Collimation of the primary beam (i.e. restriction in the size of the primary beam, using a device such as a light beam diaphragm) has a very large effect on the production of scatter. The primary beam should therefore cover only the area of interest, and tight collimation on to very small lesions (such as areas of bone pathology) will greatly improve the quality of the finished radiograph
- Reduction of back-scatter from the tabletop can be achieved by covering it with a 1 mm thick lead sheet
- Compression of a large abdomen using a broad, radiolucent compression band will reduce the thickness of tissue being radiographed and will also reduce the amount of scattered radiation produced. Compression band devices may be attached to X-ray tables but should be used with caution in animals with abdominal pathology such as uterine or bladder distension. Compression techniques are no longer widely used in veterinary practice

Grids

Even when the above precautions are taken, scattered radiation is still often a significant problem. The amount of scatter reaching the film can be greatly reduced by using a device known as a grid, which is a flat plate placed between the patient and the cassette. A grid consists of a series of thin strips of lead, alternating with strips of a material that allows X-rays through, such as plastic or aluminium, all encased in a protective aluminium cover. X-ray photons that have passed undeflected through a patient will pass through the radiolucent plastic or aluminium strips ('interspaces') but obliquely moving scattered radiation will largely be absorbed by the lead strips (Figure 16.16). Thus, there will be a reduction in the degree of film fogging and an improvement in the image quality, though with coarse grids the grid lines will be visible. Significant amounts of scattered radiation are produced from depths of solid tissue >10 cm (or a 15 cm depth of chest, which contains much air) and so the use of a grid is usually recommended for areas thicker than this. Various types of grid are available, and there are two broad groups: stationary grids and moving grids.

Stationary grids

Stationary grids are either separate pieces of equipment or built into the front of special cassettes. Various sizes are available, but it is advisable to buy a grid large enough to cover the biggest cassette used in the practice. Grids are expensive and fragile and should be treated with care, as the strips may be broken if the grid is dropped.

Parallel grids

A parallel grid is the simplest and cheapest type of grid. The strips are vertical, and parallel to each other (Figure 16.17). This means that, since the X-ray beam is diverging from its

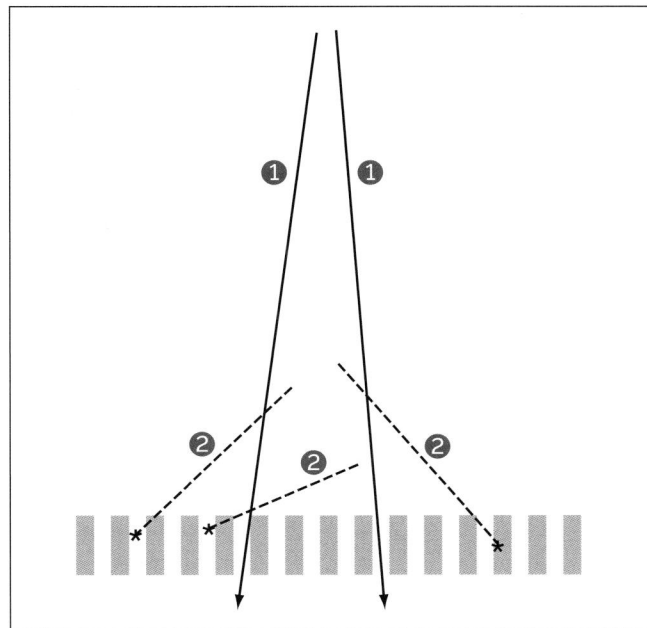

16.16 Effect of a grid. **1** = Most primary beam X-ray photons pass through the grid. **2** = Obliquely moving scattered radiation is absorbed by the strips of the grid.

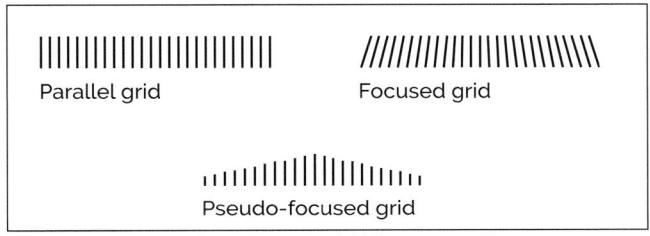

16.17 Types of stationary grid (diagrammatic cross-sections).

very small source, the X-ray photons at the edge of the primary beam may also be absorbed by the lead strips, as well as scatter. There may therefore be some reduction in the quality of the film around the edges; this is called grid cut-off.

Focused grids

A focused grid should prevent grid cut-off, as the central strips are vertical but those on either side slope gradually, to take into account the divergence of the primary beam (Figure 16.17). A focused grid must be used at its correct FFD and should not be used upside down. The X-ray beam must be centred correctly over the grid, at right angles to it.

Pseudo-focused grids

A pseudo-focused grid is intermediate between a parallel and a focused grid in efficiency and price. The strips are vertical but get progressively shorter towards the edges, so reducing the amount of primary beam absorbed (Figure 16.17). Pseudo-focused grids should also be used at the correct FFD and should not be used upside down.

Crossed grids

Most grids contain strips aligned only in one direction and therefore scattered radiation travelling in line with the strips will not be absorbed. Crossed grids contain strips running in both directions and so remove much more scattered radiation. The strips may be either parallel or focused. Crossed grids are expensive and are only used in establishments routinely radiographing equine spines, chests and pelvises.

Moving grids

The use of a stationary grid results in the presence of visible parallel lines on the radiograph. These lines may be eliminated by the use of a grid that oscillates slightly during the exposure. This requires an electronic connection between the X-ray machine and the moving grid or 'Potter–Bucky diaphragm', which is built into the X-ray table. Moving grids are used in larger veterinary clinics, and moving grid tables may sometimes be available for purchase second-hand from human hospitals.

Grid parameters

Grid factor

The use of a grid means that, as well as scattered radiation, the grid will absorb some of the useful, primary beam. The mAs factor must therefore be increased when using a grid (to increase the number of X-ray photons in the beam) by an amount known as the grid factor. This is usually 2.5–3 times, but will be specified for each grid. In most cases a longer exposure time will be required, as it is likely that the X-ray machine will already be set at its maximum mA output. The increase in time may increase the risk of movement blur on the film, and the radiographer will have to decide whether or not this is outweighed by the advantages of using a grid.

Lines per centimetre

The greater the number of lines per centimetre, the finer the grid lines on the film and the less the disruption to the image (coarse grid lines may be very distracting). The usual number is approximately 24 lines/cm for grids used in general practice. Grids with finer lines are more expensive.

Grid ratio

The grid ratio is the ratio of the height of the strips to the width of the radiolucent interspace. The higher the grid ratio, the more efficient it is at absorbing scatter, but the more expensive the grid and the larger the grid factor. Practice grids usually have a ratio of between 5:1 and 10:1. Grids used with more powerful machines may have a ratio of 16:1.

Recording the X-ray image

Once the X-ray beam has passed through the subject and undergone differential absorption by the tissues, it must be recorded in order to produce a visible and permanent image. For many years, the conventional way of doing this was by using X-ray film, which has some properties in common with photographic film, including its sensitivity to white (visible) light. It must therefore be enclosed in a light-proof container, either a metal or plastic cassette or a thick paper envelope, and handled only in conditions of special subdued 'safe-lighting' until after processing. However, this method is fast becoming replaced by digital imaging using computed or digital radiography equipment (this is considered separately, see 'Digital radiography', below).

Structure of X-ray film

The part of the film responsible for producing the image is the emulsion, which usually coats the film base on both sides in a thin, uniform layer. The emulsion gives unexposed film an apple green, fawn or mauve colour when examined in daylight (obviously an unexposed film examined in this way will then be ruined for X-ray purposes). The emulsion consists of gelatine, in which tiny grains of silver bromide are suspended. The silver bromide molecules are sensitive to X-ray photons and visible light, both of which change their chemical structure slightly. During a radiographic exposure, X-ray photons passing through the patient will cause this invisible chemical change in the underlying film emulsion, but the picture is not visible to the naked eye and the film will still be spoilt by blackening ('fogging') if exposed to white light. The picture is therefore a hidden or latent image and must be rendered visible to the eye by chemical processing or development. When the film is developed, the chemical change in the emulsion continues until those silver bromide grains that were exposed lose their bromide ions and become grains of pure silver, appearing black when the film is viewed.

The emulsion layers are attached to the transparent polyester film base by a sticky 'subbing' layer and the outer surfaces are protected from damage by a supercoat (Figure 16.18).

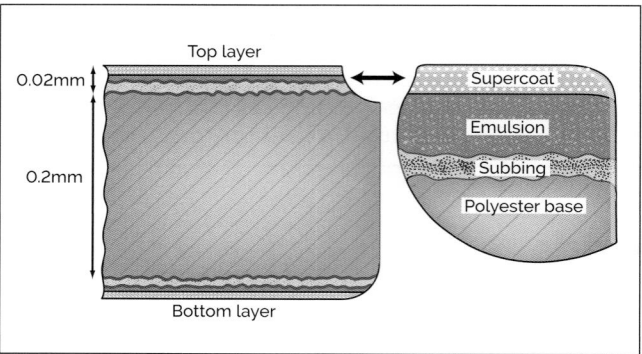

16.18 Section of X-ray film, showing emulsion coats bound to the base by subbing layers and protected by supercoats.

Intensifying screens and cassettes

Unfortunately, X-ray film used alone requires a very large exposure to produce an image and the use of film in this way is unacceptable in most circumstances. However, it was discovered many years ago that the exposure time could be greatly reduced for the same degree of blackening if some of the X-ray photons emerging from the patient were converted into visible light photons. This is achieved by coating flat sheets with crystals of phosphorescent material and holding these sheets against the X-ray film. These devices are known as intensifying screens (because they intensify the effect of the X-rays on the film) and for many years the most common phosphor used in the construction of intensifying screens was calcium tungstate, which emits blue light when stimulated by X-rays. In the 1970s a new group of phosphors was first used in intensifying screens; these were the so-called rare-earth phosphors, which produce blue, green or ultraviolet light. It is important that the X-ray film used is primarily sensitive to the right colour of light and for this reason some film–screen combinations are incompatible. One advantage of rare-earth screens is that they are more efficient at converting X-radiation into light than are calcium tungstate screens and so exposure factors can be markedly reduced, producing less scattered radiation and images with less movement blur. Additionally, they produce finer image definition. Often the trade name of the screen is embossed along its edge and can be seen on the edge of films exposed in that cassette.

The main benefits of intensifying screens are therefore that they:

- Allow much lower mAs settings to be used and so reduce movement blur, scatter production and patient exposure
- Prolong the life of the X-ray tube
- Increase radiographic contrast.

Screens consist of a stiff plastic base covered with a white reflecting surface and then a layer of the phosphor. Over the top is a protective supercoat layer. The screens are usually used in pairs and are enclosed in a light-proof metal, plastic or carbon fibre box known as a cassette (Figure 16.19) with the film sandwiched between. Occasionally a single screen is used together with single-sided emulsion film used for human mammography; such a combination produces images of higher definition but requires slightly longer exposures. For good detail, the film and screens must be in close contact; the cassette therefore contains a thick felt or foam pad between the back plate and the back screen. Poor screen–film contact causes blurring in that part of the film as the light from the intensifying screens spreads out slightly before impacting on the film. The top of the cassette must be radiolucent (allow X-rays through), and the bottom may be lead-lined to absorb remaining X-rays and prevent back-scatter, though this is uncommon with modern cassettes as it makes them very heavy. The cassette must be fully light-proof with secure fastenings and should be robust. Small flexible plastic cassettes containing one or two screens may be used for small animal intraoral radiography, since the larger sizes of non-screen film previously used are no longer manufactured and only small, dental non-screen film is available (see Chapter 25).

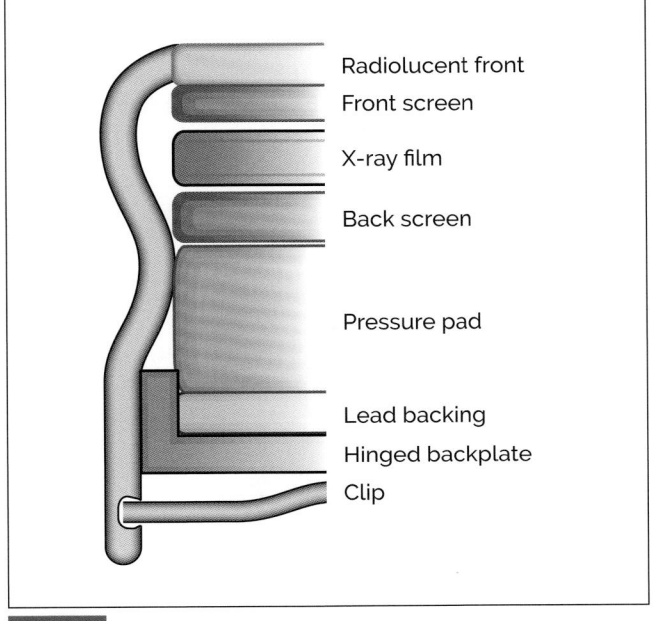

	Radiolucent front
	Front screen
	X-ray film
	Back screen
	Pressure pad
	Lead backing
	Hinged backplate
	Clip

16.19 Cross-section through an X-ray cassette.

Care of intensifying screens and cassettes

Intensifying screens are expensive and fairly delicate and should be treated gently. Scratches or abrasions will damage the phosphor layer permanently, resulting in white (unexposed) marks on all subsequent radiographs produced in that cassette. Screens should not be splashed with chemicals or touched with dirty or greasy fingers. Any dust particles or hairs falling on the screens when the cassette is open in the darkroom will prevent light from reaching the film and will produce fine white specks or lines on the image (even minute particles will prevent the visible light from the intensifying screens from blackening the film in that area, though they will not, of course, interfere with the passage of X-rays). Screens should therefore be cleaned periodically by wiping them gently with lint in a circular motion using a proprietary antistatic screen-cleaning liquid. The cassettes are then propped open in a dust-free environment in a vertical position to allow the screens to dry naturally. If they are reloaded whilst the screens are still damp, the film will stick to the screens and damage them.

Cassettes should be handled carefully and never dropped. They should be kept clean, as stains on the front may produce artefactual shadows on the radiograph and fluids seeping in will mark the screens. The catches must not be strained by closing the cassette when a film is trapped along the edges.

Types of X-ray film

Non-screen film

Non-screen film is film designed for use without intensifying screens, i.e. the image is solely due to X-rays. This requires very large mAs (usually a long exposure time) but produces extremely fine image definition. The film comes wrapped in thick, light-proof paper rather than being used in a cassette. Non-screen film is now only available as small dental film, which is used for dental radiography and other intraoral views in cats and small dogs. The patient will be anaesthetized for this type of study and so the very high exposure required is not a problem, as the radiographer can retire to a safe distance, and movement blur should not occur. The 13 x 18 cm film that was previously popular for intraoral radiography of dogs and for radiography of small exotic species is no longer manufactured; it has been replaced by flexible plastic cassettes of the same size containing one or two high-detail screens that can be inserted into the mouth of an animal for intraoral radiography. Image quality is inferior to that which is obtained with non-screen film. The flexible nature of these 'cassettes' means that image blurring due to poor screen–film contact will occur if the device is bent in the mouth, but they can be reinforced by taping thick cardboard to them. Care should be taken that the patient's teeth do not damage the device and so an appropriate level of anaesthesia is needed.

Screen film

Screen film is designed for use in cassettes and is used for all other studies. The detail produced is less than with non-screen film, as the visible light produced by the phosphor crystals spreads out in all directions and will result in blackening of a larger number of silver halide grains than the initial X-ray photon would have done – an effect called screen unsharpness (Figure 16.20). Monochromatic or blue-sensitive film is for use with calcium tungstate or blue light-emitting

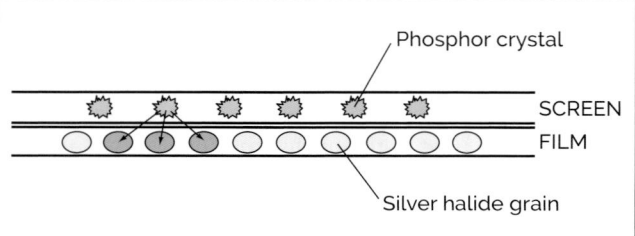

16.20 Screen unsharpness. The arrows show how visible light emitted from each phosphor crystal may affect several silver halide grains, resulting in some loss of definition of the image.

rare-earth screens; it is sensitive only to visible light in the blue part of the spectrum. For use with green light-emitting rare-earth screens, the sensitivity of the film emulsion is extended to include green as well as blue light; this is called orthochromatic film. It can therefore be appreciated that whilst green-sensitive film can be used with blue light-emitting screens as well (since it is sensitive to both colours), blue-sensitive film can only be used with blue light-emitting screens. One manufacturer produces ultraviolet light-emitting screens, which should therefore be used only with the same brand of film.

Most types of film are duplitized or double-sided, i.e. there is a layer of emulsion on both sides of the base, which doubles the efficiency of the film and the contrast and density of the image. However, this does result in some loss of definition, due to the superimposition of two slightly different images, and so single-sided emulsion film has become quite popular. Human mammography film is used when very finely detailed images with good soft tissue and bone detail are required; it is used in a cassette containing a single green light-emitting screen. The main disadvantages are that the system requires about five times more exposure and the film cannot be processed in glutaraldehyde-free developer.

Film and screen speed

The speed of a film, a screen or a film–screen combination describes the exposure required for a given degree of blackening of the film. The speed is due to the size of the silver bromide grains in the film emulsion and the shape of the phosphor crystals in the screens, as well as to the thickness of the layers. Fast film–screen combinations require less exposure but produce poorer image definition (the image is more blurred) whereas slow film–screen combinations produce finer detail and are often called 'high definition'. In practice, a medium-speed system is usually the best compromise for keeping exposure times down and still getting reasonable quality images. Rare-earth systems give better definition at the same speed. Different manufacturers describe their various films and screens with different terms, which makes it difficult to make direct comparisons, but most produce several speeds of film and screen, e.g. slow (high detail), medium and fast. If a choice of speeds of film–screen combinations is available in the practice, then a slow high-definition combination may be used where exposure times are not a problem (e.g. for bone detail in limbs and skulls) but a faster combination should be used where it is important to keep exposure times short in order to reduce movement blur (e.g. for the chest and abdomen), especially if a grid is used.

Films, screens and cassettes come in a range of sizes from 13 x 18 cm to 35 x 43 cm. It is wise to have several different sizes available so as not to waste film by radiographing small areas on large cassettes, though multiple exposures can be made on the same film. Hangers of corresponding size must be available if the films are processed manually. Some table-top automatic processors will not accept larger sizes of film.

Storage of X-ray film

As has already been mentioned, unexposed X-ray film is sensitive to light and so must be stored in a light-proof container. This may be either the original film box or a light-proof hopper. Film boxes and loaded cassettes should be kept away from the X-ray area in case they are fogged by scattered radiation; they should be kept in lead-lined cupboards if stored near a source of radiation.

Films are also sensitive to certain chemical fumes and of course to chemical splashes, so good darkroom technique is essential. They may be damaged by pressure or folding and so should be stored upright and handled carefully without being bent or scratched. In hot climates, high temperature or humidity may be a problem and so film should be refrigerated. This is not usually necessary in the UK. Film has a finite shelf-life that varies with the type of film. It is therefore wise to date the film boxes on arrival and use them in sequence, within the expiry date shown on the box.

Darkroom design and maintenance

Requirements

The darkroom is an important part of the radiography set-up within each practice (Figure 16.21). The following factors should be considered in its construction.

Size

Ideally it should be of a reasonable size to allow for satisfactory working conditions, and should not be used for any other purpose.

Light-proofing

The darkroom must be completely light-proof, and this must be checked by standing inside the darkroom for about 5 minutes until the eyes becomes dark-adapted, as small chinks of light entering may otherwise go unnoticed. The room must be lockable from the inside to prevent the door being opened inadvertently whilst films are being processed.

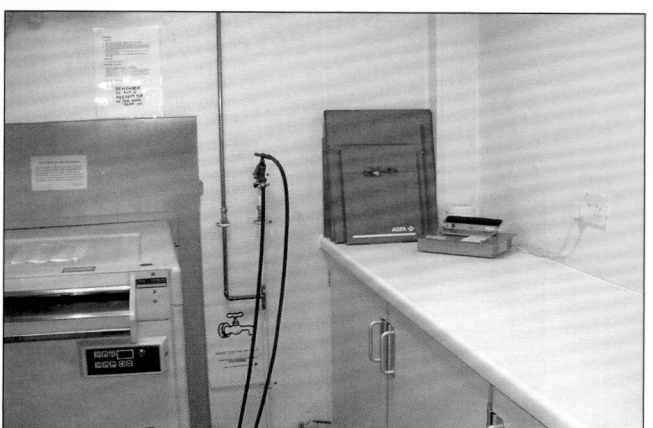

16.21 A darkroom for an automatic processor.

Services

There needs to be a supply of electricity and mains water and a drain. Access to a sink for cleaning the processor also needs to be considered when designing the room.

Ventilation

Due to the presence of chemical fumes, some form of light-proofed ventilation is essential.

Walls, floor and ceiling

The walls and ceiling should be painted white or cream (not black) so as to reflect the subdued lighting and make it easier for those working inside. The walls and floor should be washable and resistant to chemical splashes.

Safe-lighting

Since X-ray film is sensitive to white light until the fixing stage, illumination must be achieved using light of low intensity and a specific colour from safe-lights, which are boxes containing low-wattage bulbs behind brown or dark red filters. The colour of light produced must be safe for the type of film being processed, as green-sensitive films require different filters to blue-sensitive films. If the wrong filter is used, the films will become uniformly fogged whilst being handled in the darkroom. Safe-light filters must be checked carefully for flaws and damage as even small pinpricks will allow light leakage.

The efficiency of the safe-lights may be checked by laying a pair of scissors or a bunch of keys on an unexposed film on the work bench for periods of up to 2 minutes and then processing it. If significant fogging is occurring, the metal object will be visible on the film. It should be noted that no safe-light is completely safe if the films are exposed for too long or if the safe-light is too close to the handling area. Film manufacturers will advise on the correct filter colour needed for particular types of film.

Two types of safe-light are available: direct safe-lights shine directly over the working area and indirect safe-lights produce light upwards which is reflected from the ceiling. The number of safe-lights required varies with the size of the room but should be sufficient to allow efficient film handling without fumbling.

Dry and wet areas

If manual processing is used, the darkroom should be divided into two working areas: the dry area and the wet area. If the room is large enough, these areas may be separated by being on opposite sides of the room, but where this is not possible they must be separated by a partition to prevent splashes from the wet area reaching the dry bench and damaging the films or contaminating the intensifying screens.

- In the dry area, the films are stored in boxes (preferably in cupboards) or in film hoppers, loaded into and out of cassettes and placed in the film hangers prior to processing. Sometimes films are also labelled at this stage. Dry film hangers should be stored on a rack above the dry bench and there may also be a storage area for cassettes.
- In the wet area, the processing chemicals are kept and used. There should be a viewing box with a drip tray for initial examination of the films, a wall rack for wet hangers and some arrangement for allowing films to dry without dripping over the floor or other working areas.

Usually, the processing solutions are contained in tanks. The developer tank should have a well-fitting lid to slow down the rate of deterioration of the developer due to oxidation by the atmosphere. Ideally, the intermediate rinse water is held in a separate tank situated between the developer and the fixer so as to prevent splashes of developer falling into the fixer. The rinse water should be changed frequently. The final wash tank should contain running water if possible and should be at least four times the size of the developer tank.

In a busy radiography unit, the tanks should be housed together in a larger container filled with water and maintained at a constant temperature (usually 20°C). This water bath ensures that the chemicals are always at the correct, uniform temperature for processing and saves time, as well as helping to avoid underdevelopment of films. It is not essential to heat the fixer but inclusion in the water bath will prevent fixing from slowing down in very cold weather. Water bath arrangements may be purchased as special units or may be constructed, using an immersion heater and a thermostat.

If a water bath is not available, the tanks should sit in a shallow sink to prevent wetting the floor. In this case, the developer must be heated prior to use using an immersion heater with a thermostat or a thermometer. The solution must not be allowed to overheat and must be thoroughly mixed before the film is placed in the tank, as an uneven temperature in the solution will result in patchy development and a mottled appearance to the film.

If few radiographs are processed, the chemicals may be kept in dark, stoppered bottles and poured into shallow dishes when needed (as in photography). It may also be necessary to employ this technique should the automatic processor break down or for small dental films that cannot be put through an automatic processor. Unused cat litter trays make ideal processing dishes for radiographs and dental film can be processed in small plastic drinking cups. The correct development temperature is achieved by either heating the solution prior to use or by placing the dish on an electric heating pad. The solutions are usually discarded after use as the developer oxidizes rapidly.

Other darkroom equipment

Film hangers are required for manual processing and are available in two types: channel hangers and clip hangers. Each type has its advantages and disadvantages. Channel hangers are easier to load but may result in poor development of the edges of the film. Films must be removed for drying and attached to the drying line using clips. The hangers should be washed after the films are removed, as chemicals may otherwise build up in the channels, causing staining of subsequent films. Very large films may not be held securely in channel hangers. Clip hangers avoid these disadvantages but are more fragile and more cumbersome to use and they may tear the films if not used correctly. A timer is needed in the darkroom; ideally it should be capable of being pre-set to a given time.

General care of the darkroom

Most film faults arise during processing and often radiographs that have been carefully taken are spoilt by careless darkroom technique. Competent handling of the films during this stage is therefore vital to the success of radiography within the practice and it is a duty usually delegated to the veterinary nurse. Film faults can also arise during automatic processing.

The darkroom should be kept tidy, clean and uncluttered, with all the equipment in its correct place. Cleanliness is particularly important, as undeveloped films handled with fingers that are dirty or contaminated with developer, fixer or water will show permanent fingerprints. Splashes of liquid falling on to undeveloped films result in black (developer), grey (water) or white (fixer) patches on the film after processing. Splashes of liquid falling on to screens result in pale areas on all subsequent films placed in that cassette, due to interference with light emission. Dust and dirt falling into open cassettes will result in small white screen marks on the radiographs.

With manual processing, attention must also be paid to the maintenance of the processing solutions, as underdevelopment is a common film fault. The tanks should be topped up when the fluid levels fall and the chemicals should be changed regularly, with a record being kept of the date on which they are changed. Developer should be renewed every 90 days or when it has been replenished by the same volume as the original solution, whichever is sooner. Whether using manual or automatic processing, separate mixing rods should be used for making up developer and fixer and should be cleaned after use. The chemical solutions may damage clothing and so aprons should be worn while they are being mixed. The temperature of the solutions for manual processing should be checked regularly and the heater or thermostat adjusted if necessary.

Other important points are to ensure that the cassettes are always reloaded ready for use when the previous film is removed and to check that a sufficient number of film hangers are always clean and dry.

Radiographic processing

The invisible or latent image on the exposed X-ray film is rendered visible and permanent by a series of chemical reactions known as processing. As with photographic film, this must be carried out under conditions of relative darkness, as the X-ray film is sensitive to blackening by white light (fogging) until processing is complete. Although digital imaging is now the most widely used method of image production, an understanding of the principles of manual and automatic processing is still necessary since there are many practices that continue to use conventional imaging techniques. Manual processing is considered first, as the principles of this technique can then be used to understand the automatic process.

Manual processing

There are five stages in the procedure of manual film processing: development, intermediate rinsing, fixing, washing and drying.

Development

The main active ingredient in the developing solution is either phenidone-hydroquinone or metol-hydroquinone. These chemicals convert the exposed crystals of silver bromide into minute grains of black metallic silver, whilst the bromide ions are released into the solution. This process is known as reduction and the developer acts as a reducing

agent, (being itself oxidized). The length of time for which the film is immersed in the developer (usually 3–5 minutes) is critical, since longer development times will allow some of the unexposed silver bromide crystals to be converted to black metallic silver as well, causing uniform darkening of the film (chemical or development fog: see 'Film faults', below). The developer must also be used at a constant and uniform temperature (usually 20°C) and ways of achieving this are considered below (see 'Darkroom design and maintenance'). Precise times and temperatures for developing films are given in the manufacturer's instructions along with some indication of how the development time may be altered to compensate for unavoidable changes in the temperature of the solution.

Other chemicals present in the developing solution include an accelerator and a buffer, to produce and maintain the alkalinity of the solution necessary for efficient development, and a restrainer to reduce the amount of development fog (development of unexposed silver bromide crystals by fresh developer). X-ray developing solutions are purchased as concentrated liquids. Skin irritation may be observed after handling processing solutions; this may be due to an allergic reaction or due to the alkaline nature of the developer. Gloves should be worn when the chemicals are handled. If the problem is marked, a doctor should be consulted and informed of the chemicals involved.

During the development of each film a certain quantity of the developer will be absorbed into the film emulsion and so the level in the developer tank will gradually fall. On no account should the solution be topped up with water, as this will cause dilution and subsequent underdevelopment of films. The original developer solution is also unsuitable for topping up, as the proportions of the different chemical constituents of the developer change with each film that is developed and the solution becomes imbalanced. Instead, special developer replenisher solutions should be used, which take into account, and compensate for, this imbalance. Eventually, the developer will become exhausted as the active ingredients are used up and the solution becomes saturated with bromide ions.

Developer will also deteriorate with time by the process of oxidation, which will again result in underdevelopment of films. This process can be slowed by keeping the developer tank covered; in larger replenishment tanks there may also be a floating lid on the surface of the solution. Whether or not the developer is used, it is unlikely to be fit for use after 3 months and so the general rule is to change the developer completely either every 3 months or when an equal volume of replenisher has been used, whichever is the sooner.

Rinsing

After the appropriate development time the film and hanger are removed from the solution and quickly transferred to the rinse water tank. Surplus developer should not be allowed to drain back into the developer tank, because it will be saturated with bromide ions and will contribute to developer exhaustion. The film should be rinsed for about 10 seconds to remove excess developer solution and prevent carryover into the fixer tank. Ideally the rinse tank will be situated between the developer and the fixer to prevent splashes of developer falling into the fixer.

Fixing

Following immersion in the developer, development is halted and the image is rendered permanent by a process known as fixing. The fixer is acidic and this neutralizes the developer, preventing further development of the emulsion. The fixer also removes the unexposed silver halide crystals, leaving a metallic silver image that can be viewed in normal light, a process known as clearing. The fixer contains sodium or ammonium thiosulphate, which dissolves the unexposed silver halide, causing the emulsion to take on a milky-white appearance until the process is complete. The time taken for the removal of all of the unexposed halide is called the 'clearing time' and depends on the thickness of the film emulsion, the temperature and concentration of the solution and the degree of exhaustion of the fixer. The fixer becomes exhausted as the amount of dissolved silver halide builds up within it, and exhaustion of fixer will occur more quickly than exhaustion of developer.

Fixer temperature is not critical but warm fixer will clear a film faster than cold fixer. However, staining may occur above 21°C and so the fixer should not be overheated. Fixing can also be speeded up by agitating the film slightly in the fixer. After 30 seconds immersion in the fixer it is safe to switch on the darkroom light, and the film may be viewed once the milky appearance has cleared. The total fixing time should be at least twice the clearing time, a total of about 10 minutes.

A third function of the fixer bath is to harden the film emulsion (a process known as tanning) to prevent the film from being scratched when handled.

As well as the fixing agent (thiosulphate) and the hardener, the fixer solution contains a weak acid (to neutralize any remaining developer), a buffer (to maintain the acidity), and a preservative.

Fixing solutions are normally made up from concentrated liquids by the addition of water, according to manufacturer's instructions, as are developing solutions. They should be changed when the clearing time has doubled compared with that of the original fixer solution.

Washing

Following development and fixing, the film must be washed thoroughly to remove residual chemicals which would cause fading and yellow-brown staining of the film. Washing is best achieved by immersion of the film and hanger in a tank with a constant circulation of water, using at least 3 litres per minute so that the film is properly rinsed; static water tanks are much less satisfactory. Washing time should be 15–30 minutes.

Drying

Following adequate washing the films should be removed from their hangers for drying. Films left in hangers of the channel type will not dry adequately around the edges. The usual method is to clip the films to a taut line over a sink, taking care that they do not touch each other. The atmosphere should be dust-free with a good air circulation. Drying frames and warm-air drying cabinets are also available and are useful if film throughput is high.

Manual processing procedure

In order to ensure that no mistakes are made a strict protocol should be adhered to and all those involved in film processing must be familiar with it. The following steps should be carried out.

Preparation

1. Check that the developer and fixer are at the correct level. Check that the developer is at the required temperature and is adequately stirred.
2. Ensure that hands are clean and dry.
3. Select a suitable film hanger and check that new films for reloading the cassette are available.
4. Lock the door, switch on the safe-light (see 'Safe-lighting', above) and switch off the main light.

Unloading the cassette

Open the cassette and take hold of the film gently by one corner between finger and thumb, taking care not to damage the screen or the film emulsion; shaking the cassette slightly first may help to dislodge the film. Remove the film and close the cassette to prevent dirt falling into it.

Identifying the film

If labelling has not been performed during radiography, label the film using a light marker if available. These simple devices allow patient details written or typed on a thin piece of paper to be imprinted on to the corner of the film before processing, using a small flash of light. Often, cassettes contain small lead blockers in one corner to prevent that part of the film being exposed to X-rays and preserving it for the light-marking identification. The paper slips can be overprinted with the name of the practice, which adds a professional touch.

Loading the hanger

Load the film into the hanger, handling it as little as possible and touching it only at the edges.

Processing the film

The processing stages are illustrated in Figure 16.22.

1. Remove the developer tank lid, insert the film and hanger and agitate gently to remove air bubbles from the surface of the film.
2. Close the lid and commence timing. The lid is kept on for two reasons: first, it reduces the amount of oxidation of the developer by the atmosphere; secondly, the developing film is still sensitive to fogging by prolonged exposure to the safe-light.
3. The film may be agitated periodically during development to bring fresh developer into contact with the film surface and prevent streaking.
4. At the end of the development period, remove the film and transfer quickly to the rinse tank.
5. Immerse and agitate the film in the rinse water for about 10 seconds.
6. Transfer the film to the fixing tank. After 30 seconds the light may be switched on or the door opened. The film may be examined briefly once the milky appearance has cleared but it should be fixed for at least 10 minutes to allow hardening to take place.

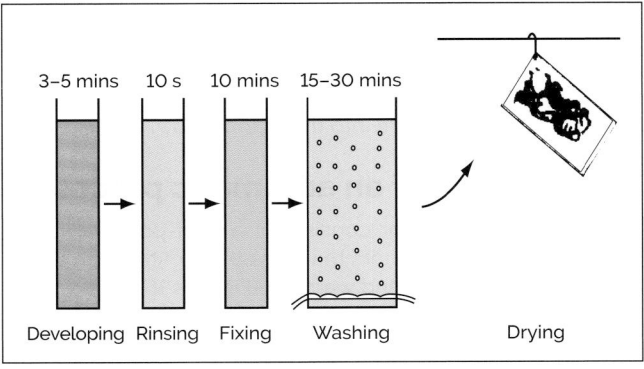

3–5 mins   10 s   10 mins   15–30 mins

Developing   Rinsing   Fixing   Washing   Drying

16.22   Manual processing routine.

7. Wash in running water for half an hour. (If running water is not available in the darkroom, the film may be washed elsewhere.)
8. Dry the film by hanging it on a taut wire in a dust-free atmosphere. Films in channel hangers must be removed first and hung by clips. Films must not touch each other during drying.

Reloading the cassette

This stage may be performed whilst the film is developing.

1. Ensure hands are clean and dry.
2. Open the cassette.
3. Remove a new film from the film box or hopper. Handle carefully without excessive pressure or bending, as unprocessed films are susceptible to damage by pressure.
4. Lay the film in the cassette and, with a fingertip, ensure that it is seated correctly and will not be trapped when the cassette is closed.

Manual processing of non-screen film

As the emulsion of non-screen film is thicker than that of screen film, it takes longer for the developing and fixing chemicals to penetrate the emulsion and act on the silver halide crystals. Development time should normally be increased by about 1 minute and clearing time in the fixer will be several minutes longer. Since the only non-screen film currently available is the very small dental film, it is more practical to process these in small plastic cups or trays.

Automatic processing

Automatic film processing has several advantages over systems of manual film development, as it saves considerable time and effort and produces a dry radiograph that is ready to interpret in a very short time (as little as 90 seconds with some machines). In addition, the films should be processed to a consistently high standard if the processor is operated and maintained correctly. However, with poor use of the automatic processor, film faults may still arise (see 'Assessing radiographic quality', below). Automatic processors are now widely used in general practice. A darkroom is still required to unload and reload the cassettes, but only a dry bench is necessary. The processor may be entirely within the darkroom, or the feed tray may pass through the darkroom wall to a processor that is located outside.

An alternative is a daylight processor; this automatically unloads and processes the exposed film and then reloads the cassette. Daylight processors do not require a darkroom but do require special cassettes and need regular servicing. A daylight processor found in some practices is a small automatic processor with light-proof sleeves into which the forearms are inserted, manipulating the cassette inside a dark area and feeding the film into the machine by feel.

Construction of an automatic processor

An automatic processor consists of a light-proof container enclosing a series of rollers that pass the film through developer, fixer, wash water and warm air (Figures 16.23 and 16.24). The intermediate rinse is omitted as excess developer is removed from the films by squeegee rollers. The chemicals are used at a higher temperature (about 28°C) to speed up the process, and the solutions are pumped in afresh for each

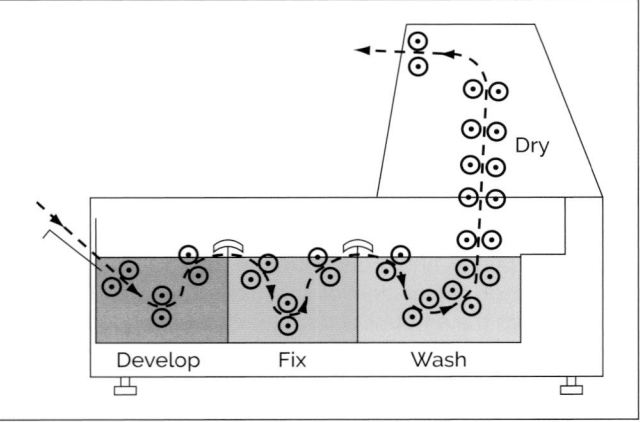

16.23 Essential features of an automatic processor.

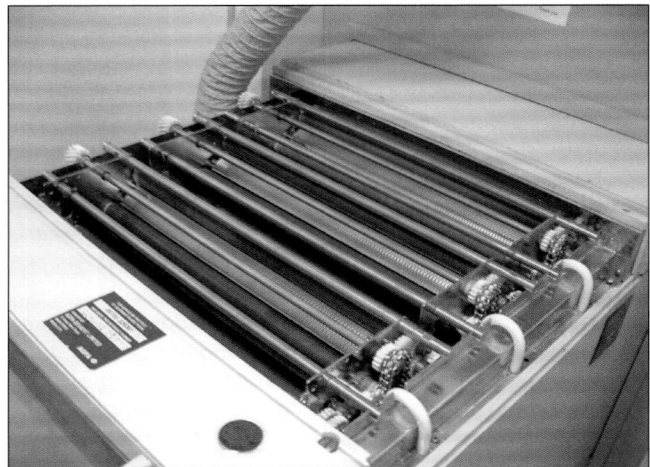

16.24 Automatic processor with lid removed, showing rollers and tanks.

film at a predetermined rate; there is therefore no risk of poor processing due to the use of exhausted chemicals. A considerable amount of water needs to flow through the unit for the final rinse and so there must be an adequate water supply and adequate drainage. Finally, the films are dried by a flow of warm air. If the film throughput is high, a silver recovery unit may be attached to the processor to retrieve silver from waste chemicals.

Maintenance of the automatic processor

Automatic processors usually require a warm-up period of 10–20 minutes prior to use (longer in cold weather). Films processed before the machine has reached its operating temperature will be underdeveloped, although some machines will not accept film until they have reached the correct operating temperature. After the warm-up period a piece of unexposed film should be passed through to check the correct functioning of the processor and to remove any dried-on chemicals from the rollers by adherence to the unhardened emulsion. At least 10 films per day should be put through the processor to ensure adequate replenishment of the chemicals in the tanks. If necessary these may be old films; although new, unfixed films work better at cleaning the rollers but this is more wasteful and expensive. At the end of the working day the machine should be switched off and the superficial rollers wiped or rinsed to remove any chemical scum.

Once a week the machine may be given a more thorough clean according to the manufacturer's instructions. This requires a deep sink so that the whole roller assembly for each of the three tanks can be removed and thoroughly cleaned. An old toothbrush is useful for cleaning around the cogs, especially in hard water areas in which lime scale will develop. The tanks also need to be cleaned once the chemicals have been drained out. An algicide solution, such as Milton® can be added to the wash tank to help to remove algae from the tank walls and roller assembly, and a lime scale treatment may also be required. Care should be taken when handling chemical solutions as they contain substances that are classified as irritant and can also lead to sensitization from cumulative exposure. Cleaning and mixing tasks should therefore always be undertaken using appropriate eye protection and protective clothing. Splashes of developer reaching work surfaces, walls and floors will quickly oxidize and become brown; this may cause a permanent stain and so any splashes should be wiped off quickly.

The chemicals required are produced specifically for automatic processors and are not usually interchangeable with solutions for manual processing as they are formulated for use at higher temperatures. Since fresh chemicals are pumped in for each film and then discarded, there is no need for developer replenisher solution. The chemicals are made up by mixing concentrated solutions thoroughly with water; in the case of the developer there are three concentrates, one acting as a 'starter' solution; for the fixer there are two. The constituents must be mixed in the correct order and with the correct amount of water. The developer and fixer solutions are mixed and then stored in tanks ready to be pumped into the processor.

An alternative means of mixing chemicals for automatic processors is by automatic mixer unit. This method provides a safer and more convenient way of mixing and storing chemical solutions. Chemical concentrates for automatic processors are packaged in bottles with plastic seals and screw caps. Mixing is achieved by removing the screw cap and placing the upturned bottle on to the seal opener of the mixing unit; the seal is automatically broken and the contents flow into the tank below, where the correct amount of water is then added. The prepared chemicals can be pumped directly from the mixer unit tanks into the processor.

The automatic processor and automatic mixer unit (if used) should be serviced regularly to reduce the chance of breakdown.

Film quality with automatic processing

Although automatic processing will produce films of a consistently good standard, there is always a slight loss of contrast compared with the best that can be achieved by perfect hand processing. The latter is not often achieved and so the automatic processor is usually of great benefit to a practice with a reasonable throughput of radiographic cases.

Automatic processing of non-screen film

Non-screen film may be put through the automatic processor but will usually require subsequent manual fixing and further washing and drying to finish the clearing process in the thicker emulsion layers. A small amount of the fixer solution placed in a small plastic box is adequate for this. Depending on the nature of the processor, dental non-screen film may be too small to pass through the roller system and will need complete manual development.

Film faults

Radiographic quality is often degraded by faults arising during exposure or processing of the film. It is important to be able to recognize the cause of film faults in order to correct them. Sometimes there may be several possible causes for a given fault. Common film faults, their causes and remedies are discussed in detail in the section 'Assessing radiographic quality', below.

Disposal of waste chemicals

Spent chemical solutions should not be poured into the normal drainage system as they are environmentally damaging. Solutions should be collected and disposed of by a licensed waste disposal company. It is now a legal requirement to notify the Environment Agency when hazardous waste, such as spent developer and fixer, is produced or removed from any premises. Records of types and quantities of hazardous waste must then be kept for at least 3 years. Certain types of premises, including veterinary practices, are exempt from having to notify the Environment Agency provided that <200 kg of hazardous waste is produced per year.

Fixer solution can be collected and re-used several times in automatic processors, using dipsticks to test for activity and to show when it is exhausted. To retrieve the silver content of waste fixer it can then be passed through a silver recovery system, though the cost-effectiveness of this depends upon the world price of silver.

Viewing the radiograph

Although the radiograph may be examined whilst it is still wet (for technical quality, a provisional diagnosis or the need for a contrast study), the image will be somewhat blurred due to swelling of the two layers of wet emulsion. Full examination must be delayed until the film has dried, when the emulsion will have shrunk and the image is clearer. Radiographs should be examined on clean viewing boxes (not held up to a window) in a dim area to allow the eyes to pick out detail on the film without distracting glare from elsewhere. If the film is small, the rest of the viewer may be masked off with black card or other opaque objects – a simple procedure that will allow much more detail to be appreciated. Relatively overexposed areas should be examined with a special bright light, and a magnifying glass is useful to look for fine detail.

Assessing radiographic quality

Radiographs must be of high technical quality if a radiographic examination is to produce maximum information about the patient. Errors can arise both during radiography and in the darkroom and the veterinary nurse should be able to assess the film for its quality, recognize any faults and know how to correct them (Figure 16.25). Before film faults can be recognized, it is necessary to understand the terms density, contrast and definition.

Density

Radiographic density is the degree of blackening of the film and is determined by two factors: the exposure used and the processing technique.

Fault	Cause	Remedy
Film too dark	Overexposure	Reduce exposure factors; check thickness of patient; check correct film/screen combination used
	Overdevelopment	Check developer temperature; time development accurately; check automatic processor cycle and thermostat
	FFD too short	Increase FFD
	Fogging	See 'fogging' below for causes and remedies
Film too pale	Underexposure (background black but image too light)	Increase exposure factors; check thickness of patient; check correct film/screen combination used
	Underdevelopment (background pale only)	Check developer temperature; time development accurately; check automatic processor cycle and thermostat
	FFD too long	See 'Exposure' below, for causes and remedies
Patchy film density	Developer not stirred; film not agitated in developer	Correct the development technique
Contrast too high ('soot and whitewash film')	kV too low	Increase kV
Contrast too low ('flat film')	Overexposure	Reduce exposure factors
	Underdevelopment	Correct the development technique
	Overdevelopment	Correct the development technique
	Fogging	See below for causes and remedies
Fogging	Scattered radiation from patient	Collimate the beam; use a grid
	Scattered radiation from elsewhere	Change storage area for films and cassettes
	Exposure to white light before fixing stage	Check darkroom and safe-lights, film hoppers, lids on film boxes, keep lid on developer whilst in film tank
	Storage fog	Use films before expiry date
	Chemical or development fog	Avoid overdevelopment
Image blurring	Patient movement Tube head movement Cassette movement Scattered radiation Fogging Poor film-screen contact Large object-film distance Double exposure	Depends on the cause
Extraneous marks:		
Small, bright marks	Dirt on the intensifying screens	Clean the screens
Black patches	Developer splashes on film	Careful processing
White patches	Fixer splashes on film	Careful processing
Grey patches	Water splashes on film	Careful processing
	Chemical splashes on intensifying screens	Clean the screens
Scratches	Careless handling of unprocessed film	Handle unprocessed film carefully
	Guideshoes of automatic processor misaligned	Handle unprocessed film carefully
Crescentic black crimp marks	Bending of unprocessed film	Handle unprocessed film carefully
Fingerprints	Handling of unprocessed film with dirty hands	Wash and dry hands before processing
Branching black marks	Static electricity	Handle unprocessed film carefully; use antistatic screen cleaner
Parallel marks on film	Roller marks	Check seating and cleanliness of rollers
Scum on surface	Scale or algae in processor	Clean processor; use water softener or anti-algal agents
Chemical stains:		
Yellowing/browning on storage	Insufficient fixing or washing	Correct fixing/washing
Areas of film supposed to be clear are grey and opaque	Insufficient fixing	Increase time; change fixer
Borders around films	Dirty channel hangers	Clean the hangers
Grid lines too coarse	X-ray beam not perpendicular to grid; focused or pseudo-focused grid used upside down	Correct alignment of beam and grid
Damp films for automatic processor	Thermostat malfunction	Call service engineer
	Dryer temperature too low	Call service engineer
	Insufficient fixing	Change fixer

16.25 Common faults and their remedies. FFD = focal–film distance; kV = kilovolts.

Exposure

Film blackening is affected by the quantity of X-rays passing through the patient and reaching the film. It is influenced by the kV, the mAs and the FFD. If the patient's image is generally too dark, then the film is overexposed and the exposure factors should be reduced or the FFD increased; conversely, if it is too light, then it is underexposed and the exposure factors should be increased or the FFD reduced. Usually, corrections are made to the exposure factors; the FFD should remain constant unless it has been inadvertently altered.

Processing

Radiographic density can also be affected by processing. Underdevelopment, due to the use of diluted, exhausted or cold developer or development for too short a time, will cause all areas of the film to be too light, including the background outside the area covered by the primary beam. Development can be tested by performing the finger test, i.e. putting a finger between the film and the light viewer in an area where the film was not covered by the patient and which should therefore be completely black. If the finger is visible, the film is underdeveloped. Underdevelopment is the most common film fault arising with manual processing, and should be corrected by topping up the developer with replenisher (not water), by changing the solution regularly and by ensuring that it is used at the correct temperature and for the correct length of time. Underdevelopment may also occur with automatic processing, if the machine is not working at the correct temperature. Overdevelopment may occur if the developer is too hot or if the film is inadvertently left in the solution for too long. In this case, some of the unexposed silver halide crystals will be converted to black metallic silver, leading to uniform darkening of the film or 'development fog'.

Overexposure and overdevelopment may be hard to differentiate, as both will cause an increased radiographic density. However, areas covered by metal markers during the exposure will remain white if the fault is overexposure but will darken if the film is overdeveloped.

Underexposure and underdevelopment can usually be easily differentiated. Underdevelopment will produce a grey background using the finger test; with underexposure the background should still be black but the area covered by the patient will be too pale as the tissues have not been adequately penetrated by the X-ray beam.

In general, films that are too dark are to be preferred to those that are too light, as they may still yield adequate information when examined under a bright light.

Contrast

Contrast is the difference between various radiographic densities (shades of grey) seen on the radiograph. A medium contrast film with a reasonable number of grey shades as well as white and black on the image is desirable, as it will yield most information. A film that shows a white image on a black background with few intermediate grey shades has too high a contrast ('soot and whitewash') and is due to the use of too low a kV with insufficient penetrating power. A film without extremes of density, showing mainly grey shades, has a very low contrast and is called a 'flat' film. Poor contrast is usually due to underdevelopment, in which case the background will be grey (use the finger test). Overexposure, overdevelopment and various types of fogging including scattered radiation will also produce a flat film but in this case the background density will be black and the remainder of the film will also be very dark.

Definition

Definition refers to the sharpness and clarity of the structures visible on a radiograph. Good definition is usually essential if the film is to be diagnostic. Definition may be affected by a number of factors, as follows:

Movement blur

This is the most common cause of poor definition on chest and abdomen radiographs and is usually due to respiratory movement or struggling by the patient. It may also occur if the tube stand is unstable or if the cassette moves during the exposure. Patient movement is minimized by the use of sedation or general anaesthesia and by adequate artificial restraint using sandbags, etc. The exposure time should be kept as low as possible as this will minimize the effect of motion.

Scattered radiation

Scattered radiation produced when thick or dense areas of tissue are X-rayed will produce random darkening of the film, resulting in loss of both definition and contrast. Its effects may be reduced significantly by collimating the beam and by using a grid.

Fog

Fogging is darkening of the film unrelated to the image and has a number of causes. These include the following: scattered radiation, accidental exposure of the film to radiation or white light prior to or during processing, poor light-proofing of the darkroom, the use of an unsuitable safelight filter, prolonged or incorrect storage of film and overdevelopment. The result is a loss of definition and contrast.

Poor film–screen contact

Poor contact between the intensifying screen and the film within the cassette due to shrinkage of the felt or foam pad will cause blurring of the image in the affected area as light produced by the intensifying screens spreads out slightly before contacting the film. It will be present in the same place on all films taken in that cassette. Poor film–screen contact may also occur if the edge of the film is trapped in the side of the cassette, preventing it from closing snugly.

Film and screen speed

Fast film–screen combinations require a lower exposure for a given degree of film blackening than do slower combinations, but the definition of the image is poorer due to the larger size of the phosphor crystals in the intensifying screens and to the characteristics of the film emulsion.

Focal spot size

Some machines allow a choice of focal spot size. Fine focus produces finer radiographic detail but the exposure factors available are limited. Coarse focus allows higher exposure factors but, since the effective focal spot is larger, some detail is lost by the penumbra effect (see Figure 16.5). The penumbra effect is reduced in two ways: first, by keeping the object–film distance as small as possible to reduce the amount of divergence between the photons; secondly, by using a reasonably long focus–film distance, which means that the photons are travelling more nearly parallel to each other.

Magnification and object–film distance (OFD)

As the X-ray beam diverges from the focal spot, the geometry of the X-ray beam results in some degree of magnification of the image. Magnified images will usually also be blurred, because the penumbra effect increases with increasing OFD. In order to reduce this effect, the part being radiographed should always be positioned as close as possible to the film, with the FFD as long as is practicable for that machine (Figure 16.26).

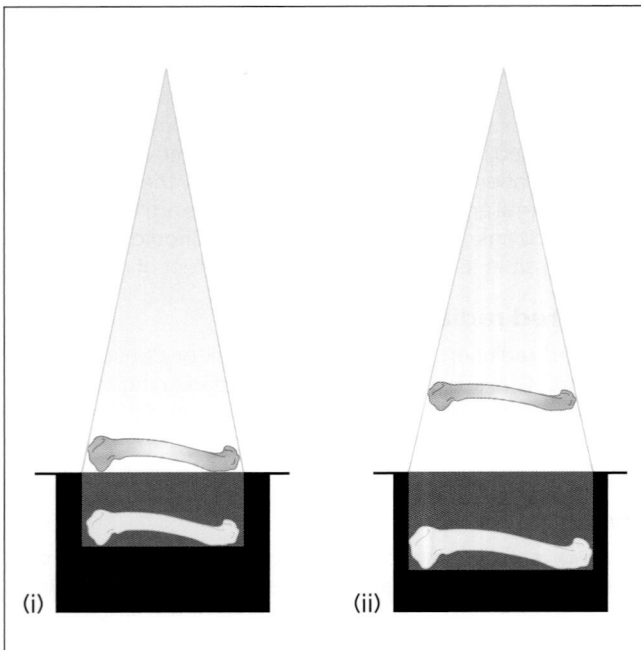

16.26 Magnification and object–film distance (OFD). **(i)** Object close to film, so reproduced accurately on radiograph. **(ii)** Object not close to film, so image is magnified.

Labelling, storage and filing of radiographic films

Labelling

All radiographic films should be permanently labelled with the case identification (name or number), the date, a right or left marker if appropriate and any other relevant details (e.g. time after administration of a contrast medium). Labelling of the paper sleeve or film envelope only is inadequate and liable to cause mix-ups, especially on busy days. Films can be labelled at one of three stages: during exposure, in the darkroom or on dry film after processing.

Labelling during exposure

Films can be identified during radiography by placing lead letters on the cassette or by writing details on special graphite tape, which is then stuck to the cassette. Care should be taken to ensure that the whole of the information appears on the film after processing and is neither lost on the edge of the film nor overexposed. Right or left markers should be used at this stage (and not substituted by the use of personal codes such as scissors or keys).

Labelling in the darkroom

Films may also be identified by labelling in the darkroom prior to processing. The most efficient method is to use a light marker, which is a small device that prints information, written or typed on paper, on to the corner of the film, using white light. A small rectangular area in the corner of the film must therefore be protected from exposure to X-rays by the incorporation of a piece of lead in the cassette to act as a blocker and leave a space on the film on which these details may be printed. There are also special cassettes available with a movable window, which can be inserted into a light-marking camera for imprinting the details; this can be done in daylight outside the darkroom.

Labelling of the dry film

Information may be written on the film after processing using a white 'Chinagraph' pencil, white ink or a black felt-tip pen. Such identification may not be acceptable for films used in legal cases, so labelling after processing is not good practice.

Identification of radiographs for the BVA/KC scoring schemes

The following information must be included on digital images, or in the case of radiographic film either superimposed on to the film at the time of exposure or added by light marker before processing, for the British Veterinary Association (BVA)/Kennel Club (KC) Hip and Elbow Dysplasia Scoring Schemes:

- The Kennel Club Registration Number (from the top right-hand corner of the KC Registration Certificate) for dogs registered with the KC. (Note that no other form of identification for KC registered dogs is acceptable.) For dogs not registered with the KC, identification as used by the veterinary practice, other registering body or breed club may be used
- Microchip or tattoo number
- The date the radiograph was taken
- Left and/or right marker(s).

Labelling after processing and computer-generated labelling with digital systems are not acceptable.

Storing and filing radiographic films

Radiographs may be required for retrospective study or as legal documents and so radiographs on film ('hard copies', as opposed to digital images) should be clearly labelled and carefully filed. Many films can accumulate within a short space of time in a busy practice and the filing system must be simple and foolproof.

Films processed manually must be completely dry before filing, otherwise they will be damaged by sticking to paper. Films may be stored in their original paper folders or in special X-ray envelopes, with case details (e.g. owner's name, patient information and date) marked clearly on the outside. These may then be kept in film boxes, filing cabinets or on shelving depending on the number of films involved. Films may be stored either chronologically or in alphabetical order of owner's surname, with films from each year usually being kept separately. Films of special interest and good examples of normal anatomy should be noted for future reference.

Digital radiography

With modern technological advances, new methods of acquiring and viewing radiographic images have become available. These methods are based on digital acquisition of the image, i.e. the image is created and stored electronically and viewed on a computer monitor rather than on radiographic film (Figure 16.27). Digital radiography systems convert the pattern of photons reaching the detector into stored energy; this is then electronically measured and converted into an image (digitized). The method of obtaining the image (generation of the X-ray beam, interaction of the X-ray beam with the patient and radiographic technique) is the same as for film–screen radiography; it is simply that the recording system is different. All images generated in this manner are referred to as 'digital radiographs', but there are two distinct processes associated with the production of such images: computed radiography (CR) and direct digital radiography (DDR).

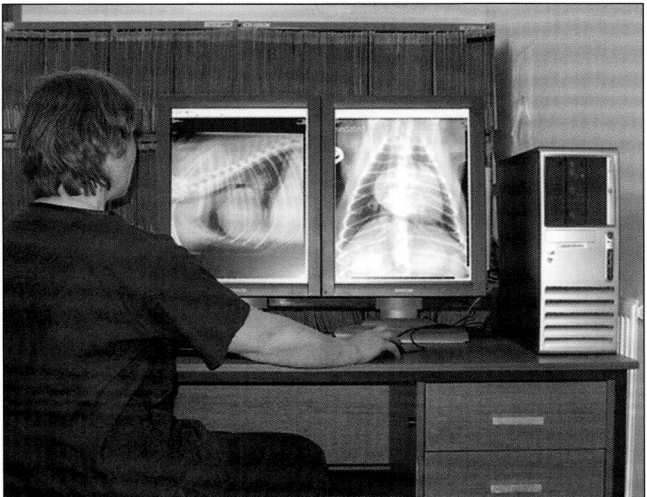

16.27 Digital radiographs are viewed on a computer screen.

The advantages of digital radiography include:

- Reduced exposure to radiation as the number of repeat exposures required is reduced; this is because exposure factors are less critical and tissues of different densities can be seen on the same image
- The radiographic examination is quicker (as little as seconds in some cases)
- Greater tolerance to suboptimal exposure factors, reducing the need for repeat exposures
- The ability to see a wide range of tissues on the same image
- The ability to computer-manipulate images
- There is no requirement for a darkroom, X-ray viewer or film archiving space; therefore, savings are made in processing costs and storage space, and there are associated environmental benefits (i.e. no use of harmful developing or fixer chemicals). Hard copies can still be made if required, using a type of film similar in appearance to X-ray film
- Important radiographs should never go missing provided a logical system of storing digital images is developed and used

- Images can be viewed anywhere in the practice where there is an appropriate workstation and can be transmitted offsite for rapid interpretation or referral
- Different types of digital image can be stored on the same network and viewed together (e.g. radiographs, ultrasonograms, computed tomography (CT) scans and magnetic resonance (MR) scans)
- Digital images can easily be inserted into letters, publications, lecture notes and presentations.

Computed radiography

Computed radiography replaces the conventional film and intensifying screens with an imaging plate (IP) made of a material (a photostimulable phosphor, usually a europium-activated barium fluorohalide compound) that can be excited by X-rays and light photons. These imaging plates are similar in appearance to conventional intensifying screens and they are contained within cassettes (similar to those used with conventional radiography and available in the same sizes). They are used with X-ray machines in the same way as film–screen cassettes (i.e. above or below the X-ray table top, with or without a grid). They may be exposed elsewhere (e.g. in an operating theatre or off-site) but should be processed within a couple of hours of exposure because the image will begin to degrade after this time. In an analogous way to conventional screens, the thickness, phosphor type and its structure will determine the efficacy and resolution of the phosphor.

During exposure, the photostimulable phosphors (storage phosphors) store energy from the incident X-ray photons in semi-stable areas of the crystal lattice called electron traps, creating a latent image. Following exposure, the cassette is labelled electronically with the patient's information and image details before being inserted into an image reader device (digitizer) (Figure 16.28). The imaging plate is usually

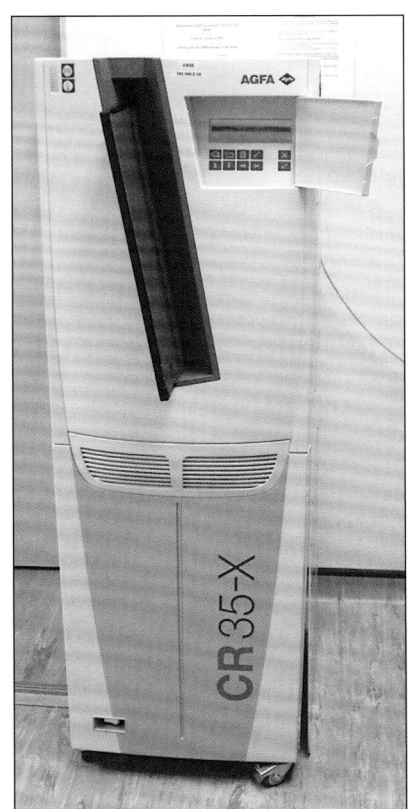

16.28 Digitizer for computed radiography. The cassette is inserted into the vertical slot, the image is 'read' by the laser, and the cassette cleared and ejected ready for its next use.

automatically removed from the cassette and passed through the reader assembly of the digitizer by means of a series of rollers. However, in some older systems, the imaging plate has to be manually unloaded from the cassette and then loaded into the reader. This is not ideal as it can increase the risk of artefacts being introduced into the final image or can lead to 'fading' of the latent image due to exposure of the plate to light.

The imaging plate is read by a helium–neon laser, which provides a small amount of energy to the electrons in the electron traps, allowing them to move back to their resting or equilibrium state and in doing so, releasing energy in the form of visible light. The visible light released has a different wavelength to that of the laser used to read the imaging plate. A device called a light guide collects the emitted light, which is then converted to an analogue electrical signal before being amplified by a photomultiplier tube and digitized by an analogue-to-digital converter (ADC). The intensity of the light emitted is proportional to the number of X-ray photons received by the imaging phosphor.

The residual image stored on the imaging plate after it has been read must be erased before it can be used again, otherwise a faint 'ghost' image will remain visible on subsequent exposures. The residual image is completely erased by automatic exposure to high intensity white light at the end of the 'read' cycle. The final stage of the process is reloading of the 'clean' imaging plate back into the cassette followed by automatic ejection of both from the digitizer.

In most CR digitizers, the phosphor is read using a point mechanism, whereby the laser repeatedly scans across the phosphor measuring the signal from each pixel location. Processing the entire image usually takes in the order of 1–2 minutes from insertion of the cassette into the digitizer to ejection of the cassette containing the 'cleaned' imaging plate free of any residual image. With more modern CR readers with dual-sided read out and line scan technology, the whole process is much faster with the laser being able to scan the imaging plate in 10 seconds or less. There are also automatic CR systems available that are integrated into Bucky systems and require no manual handling of cassettes.

Imaging plates are more sensitive to scattered radiation than are conventional intensifying screens and should be erased prior to use if they have not been used for a few days to avoid the build-up of artefacts. They should be used in rotation and periodically cleaned with the appropriate CR system manufacturer's imaging plate cleaner.

CR systems allow greater flexibility with exposures than conventional film–screen radiography, but the optimum quality image is still achieved with the correct exposure and radiographic technique, including accurate collimation. Most systems have an exposure range (exposure index) displayed, which indicates whether an image is under- or overexposed. The way that the exposure range is indicated varies between manufacturers (Figure 16.29). Under- and overexposure appear differently on digital images to the same faults on conventional images: an underexposed CR image may have a higher degree of 'noise', creating a grainy appearance; whereas, an overexposed image is less easily detected and may appear lacking in density. As an overexposed image can be adjusted on the workstation and a repeat texposure avoided (unless the image is extremely overexposed), it is important that the system exposure range is checked frequently to ensure that the minimum radiation dose to achieve an optimum quality image is used consistently.

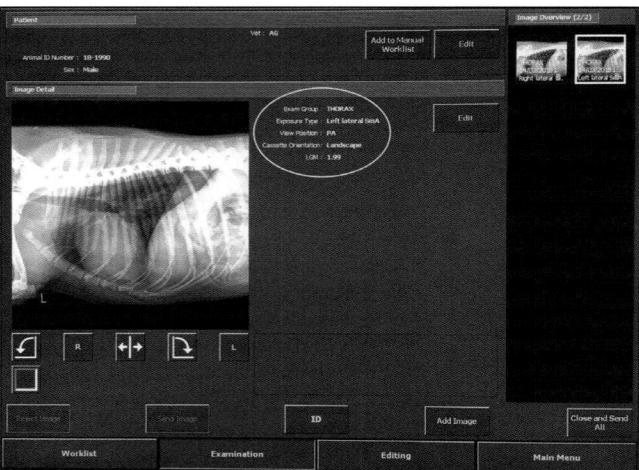

16.29 CR workstation in the 'examination' window. There is an image overview on the right-hand side of the screen with the highlighted view appearing in the image window on the left. Immediately to the right of this image is a description of the view (circled). The fifth row refers to LGM (log of the median value); in this case it is 1.99. This is the exposure index for the system. It should be between 1.8 and 2.2 for this particular system if the exposure technique is optimal.

Direct digital radiography

Direct digital radiography involves technology that produces an almost instantaneous image on the display screen of the controlling computer without the need for an intermediate 'processing' stage. Some systems convert X-ray energy directly into digitized electrical energy (direct flat panel detector systems), whilst others produce the electrical signal via an intermediate light phase (indirect flat panel detector systems). DDR provides major time-savings compared with CR and film–screen radiography. However, the equipment can be much more expensive than that for CR.

It is often marketed as an entire package, including the X-ray machine and table, although it is possible to retrofit the detectors to an existing system. DDR flat panel detectors contain a thin film transistor array, with the transistors arranged in a matrix and coupled to a scintillator. The image detectors are often hardwired to the acquisition computer; however, wireless detectors are becoming increasingly more widely used (Figure 16.30). The advantage of wireless systems is greater flexibility without the problems of long cables potentially becoming entangled with other equipment or even accidently damaged by movement of the X-ray tube column. Portable digital systems are now widely used. The advantage of these systems is the short image acquisition (and display) time without the need to return to the practice to process images.

There are three main types of direct digital radiography system:

- Flat panel detector with direct conversion of the X-ray photon into an electrical charge using a semiconductor, usually amorphous selenium, which is very efficient at absorbing the oncoming X-ray photons. There is direct conversion of the X-ray photon into an electrical charge, hence the term 'direct flat panel detector'. This charge is detected and read by a thin film transistor, electronically processed and then converted into an electronic file
- Flat panel detector with indirect conversion of the X-ray photon into an electrical signal. A scintillator (usually caesium iodide or gadolinium oxysulphide and similar in

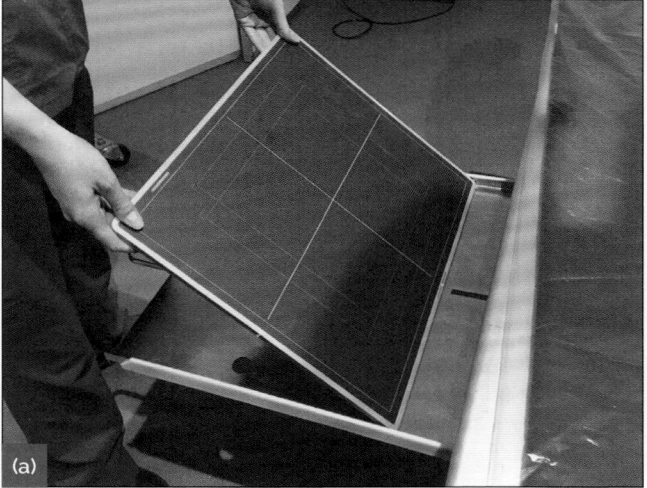

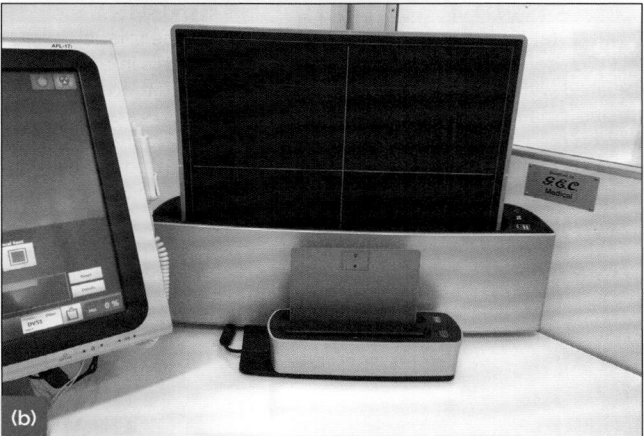

16.30 **(a)** Wireless flat panel detector with caesium iodide scintillator. **(b)** Wireless flat panel detector sitting in its docking station to recharge.

function to a conventional intensifying screen) is built into the flat panel detector, which emits light when struck by X-ray photons. A photodiode coupled with the thin film transistor array is then used to generate the electrical signal, which in turn creates the image. In this case, the production of light photons is an additional step, hence the term 'indirect flat panel detector'

- A charged-couple device (CCD) is a fixed image receptor located at the point at which the X-ray photons emerge from the patient after interaction (components usually found in the table assembly). It consists of a phosphor-type material that produces light when struck by the emerging X-ray photons. Light sensitive electrodes then convert the light patterns to a digital signal. They are very small devices and are often used for dental radiography. Compared with flat panel detectors, there is loss of efficiency and with some systems the image quality is poorer.

After the data are acquired, they are processed before being displayed by the computer. If there were no post-processing, the image would be useless with virtually no contrast. The type of post-processing has an effect on the appearance of the final image and specific algorithms are used for different body areas and systems. Post-processing may result in enhancement of edges and reduction in noise of the image. The resultant radiograph from the DDR system is displayed on the workstation screen almost immediately (within 2–10 seconds).

Production of digital images

There are three stages involved in the production of a digital image: acquisition of the image, processing the image and displaying the image. During the acquisition phase of the process, the image receptor used differs depending on whether a CR system or a DDR system is being used. Once the X-ray photons emerging from the patient have been converted to digital data, image processing and image display are essentially the same, irrespective of whether a CR or DDR system is being used.

The fundamental software component of the digital image is a computer file. This computer file contains information relating to the signal that has been measured and is called a DICOM (Digital Imaging and Communications in Medicine) format. It has some similarities to JPEG and TIFF file types, but as well as the image it contains a set of instructions (standards) that are tagged to the image. This information relates to patient identification, the specific equipment used (e.g. radiography, ultrasonography, CT, MRI, scintigraphy, endoscopy) and the protocols used for handling, storage, printing and transmission of the image. Typically, DICOM files are very large. The fundamental hardware components enabling the production of a digital image are a cassette containing a flexible plate in the case of CR, and a rigid flat panel detector in DDR.

Labelling digital images

Prior to radiography, the patient's details are entered on to the workstation computer of the digital system being used (CR or DDR) (Figure 16.31). At this point, the examination type is selected along with the views that are required (e.g. thorax, abdomen, spine; lateral, dorsoventral, ventrodorsal) (Figure 16.32). This allows the system to apply the correct image reconstruction technique ('algorithm') for the body part being imaged, providing optimal definition and contrast for that area.

It is important to ensure that the patient's details are entered correctly, as it can be very difficult to alter them once the images have been obtained. This obviously increases the risk of the images being placed in an incorrect patient's file and leads to the inability to retrieve all studies for a particular patient. These errors are minimized if registration details are computerized, although this facility is often only found in large referral centres dealing with a large number of cases.

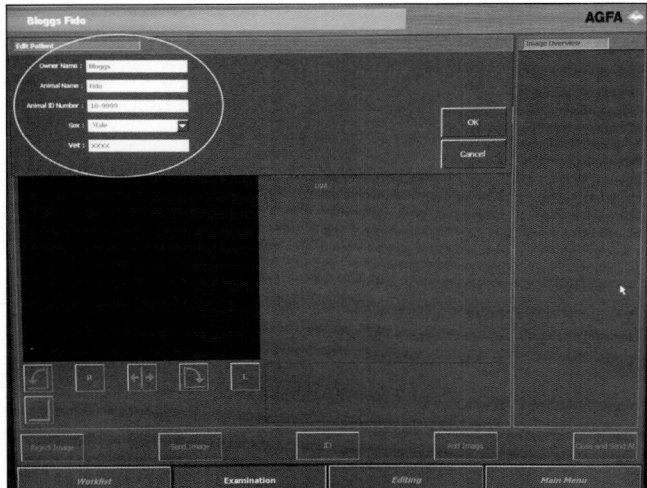

16.31 Example of the window on a CR system workstation where patient details are entered on the top left (circled).

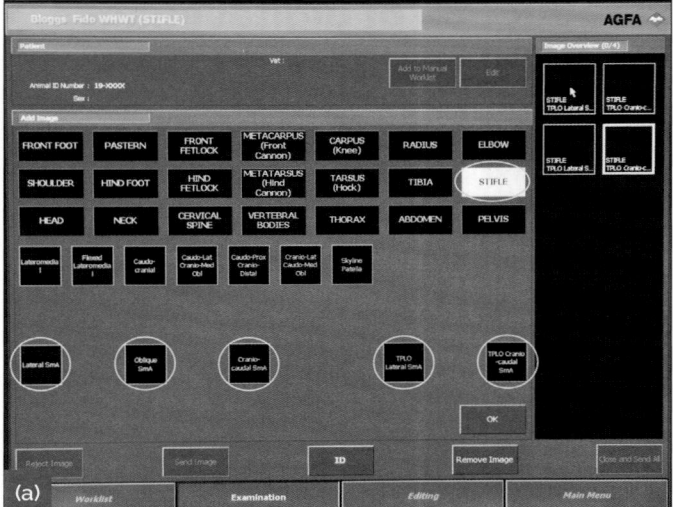

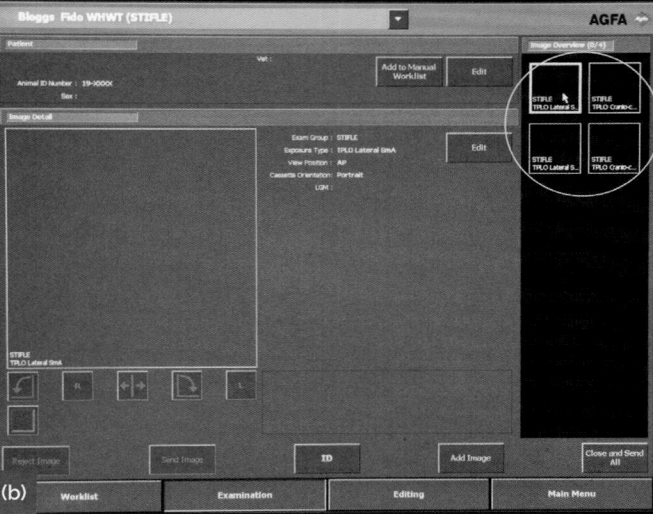

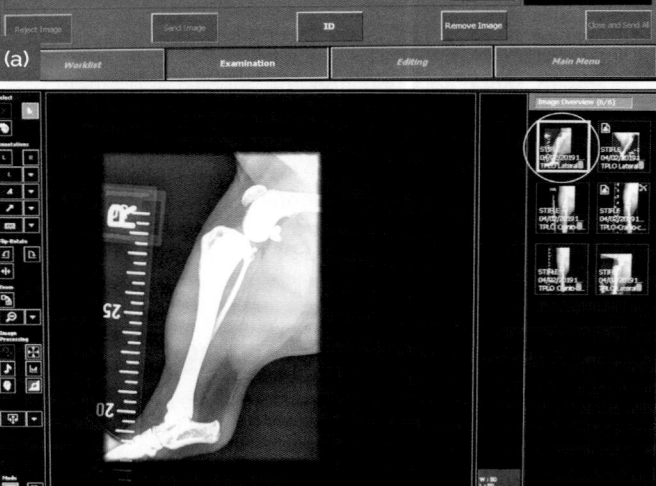

16.32 (a) Example of a CR workstation screen showing selection of anatomical area (stifle) and views associated with the chosen area (this screen shows the views for large and small animals; the small animal stifle views are those shown on the bottom row (circled)). **(b)** Examination screen showing selected views for chosen anatomical area before imaging plates are scanned and processed (thumbnail images on the right-hand side of the screen (circled)). **(c)** Editing screen showing lateral tibial plateau levelling osteotomy view of the right stifle (highlighted thumbnail image on the right-hand side of the screen (circled)).

Commonly, digital systems can be customized and set up with large animal, equine, small animal or a combination of examination algorithms, depending on the particular need of the practice. Additional views can be added easily during the study if required. Once available, the images of a given patient are shown in a list that identifies each view.

The digital image

Processing algorithms

Irrespective of the type of digital radiography system used, the electronic data files must be processed before the final image is displayed (see above). Without any image processing, the digital radiograph would lack contrast and be non-diagnostic. With both CR and DDR systems, the aim of image processing is to maximize contrast in the area of interest and discard information outside the collimated area. During image processing, the boundary of the collimated area is automatically detected. The pixel values for the area within the collimation are analysed, are assigned a shade of grey (using look-up tables in the processing software which contain data detailing how bright the pixel should be on the monitor for that amount of phosphor excitation) and then undergo data processing to optimize contrast and sharpness, which varies with anatomical area. The post-processed pixel values are then applied for the image display.

A variety of computer algorithms and techniques are used for post-processing and vary between manufacturers.

Many systems have packaged the appropriate look-up tables with other automatic image processing tools (such as edge enhancement), so that the technique for 'stifle' can be selected and should be optimized for thoracic radiographs (see Figure 16.32). The type of image processing has a huge impact on the appearance of digital images and it is important that appropriate algorithms are selected for each body area. Incorrectly set up algorithms or incorrectly chosen algorithms for a specific body area can lead to an inaccurate diagnosis (e.g. apparent lysis around surgical implants or the false impression of a trabecular pattern in bone where none exists).

Image quality

Image quality with digital systems may not be inherently better than with high standard conventional film–screen radiographs, although post-processing manipulation may permit more subtle lesions to be seen. The image quality with some cheaper digital systems is often poorer than that obtained with good conventional radiographs. The method of obtaining the image is the same as for film–screen radiography in terms of generation of the X-ray beam, interaction of the beam with the patient and the technique used. The best images are obtained using correct radiographic technique, and failure to do so may result in poor or even non-diagnostic digital images. Image quality also depends on the quality of the acquisition equipment and viewing monitors, as well as the software packages used for image manipulation.

Resolution and contrast

The digital radiographic image is created from a number of small rectangular picture elements (pixels) arranged in a matrix (Figure 16.33). The more pixels in an image, the bigger the matrix and the bigger the image file. The spatial resolution of the image is determined by the size of the pixels used to make the image. The smaller the pixel, the higher the spatial resolution; typical resolution is approximately 5–10 pixels per millimetre. It is worth noting that the spatial resolution of conventional film–screen radiographs is often higher than digital radiographs, but due to the poorer image contrast, the ability to detect small lesions on conventional radiographs may be no better than lower resolution digital images.

For each pixel, there is a limited but large number (approximately 4000) of potential shades of grey. Unlike conventional film–screen radiographs where the greyscale is limited by the human eye and brain, which can (on average) differentiate approximately 60 shades of grey, the digital image can be manipulated to use all these potential shades of grey. However, the spatial resolution of an image cannot be altered once it has been acquired; it is the perceived spatial resolution that can be manipulated by post-processing edge enhancement or smoothing.

With conventional radiographs, the relationship between radiographic exposure (number of photons) and optical density (blackness) of the film is known as the characteristic curve and is sigmoidal (S-shaped). If there are too few photons (underexposure) or too many (overexposure), the information that results from the distribution of photons is lost (Figure 16.34a). Within the straight part of the characteristic curve, there is a linear relationship between the number of photons and the resulting density on the film. When the exposure factors are set using a conventional film–screen system, the aim is to set the exposure such that the resulting density falls within the straight part of the characteristic curve. The human eye can only discern differences in density that lie within the straight part of the characteristic curve.

With digital systems, the relationship between the signal and the exposure remains linear throughout (Figure 16.34b). This means that there are no 'toe' or 'shoulder' regions at the top and bottom of the graph where information is lost, as is the case with conventional radiographs. In addition, once conventional film is black (or when the density has reached such a point as to render the eye unable to discern differences in it), extra photons (increase in exposure) do not provide any further useful information. In a digital system, the extra photons do carry useful information. The digital image can be manipulated after acquisition to alter the contrast and the brightness. This means that it is possible to view areas on the radiograph with marked differences in tissue thickness or to examine the soft tissues and bones without having to take separate images, simply by adjusting the brightness and contrast ('windowing') of the processed image (Figure 16.35).

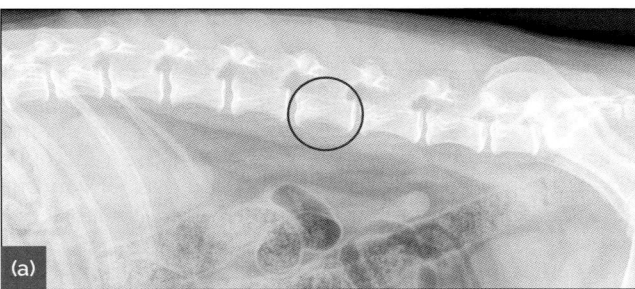

16.33   Digital radiography. **(a)** Lateral radiograph showing the lateral lumbar spine in a dog. **(b)** Magnified view of the area circled in (a). **(c)** The same circled area in (a) magnified further, allowing individual pixel elements constituting the matrix, as well as the greyscale, to be visualized.

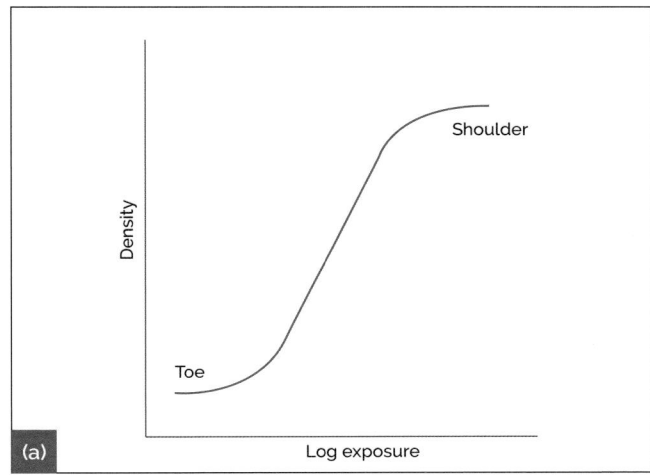

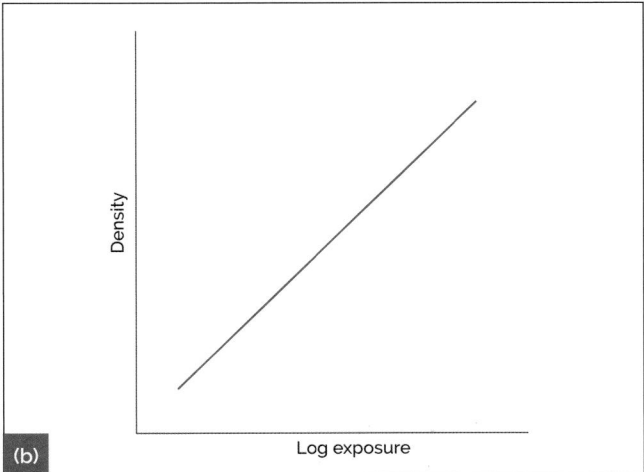

16.34   **(a)** Characteristic curve of radiographic film. The sigmoidal curve reflects the relationship between the relative exposure and optical density of the film. Contrast is highest along the linear part of the curve. The toe and shoulder areas of the curve are regions of low contrast. For radiographic film, the linear response extends over a narrow range of exposures. **(b)** Digital images have a linear response over a much greater range of radiation exposures. Therefore, structures with a large range of attenuation values can all be viewed on the same exposure.

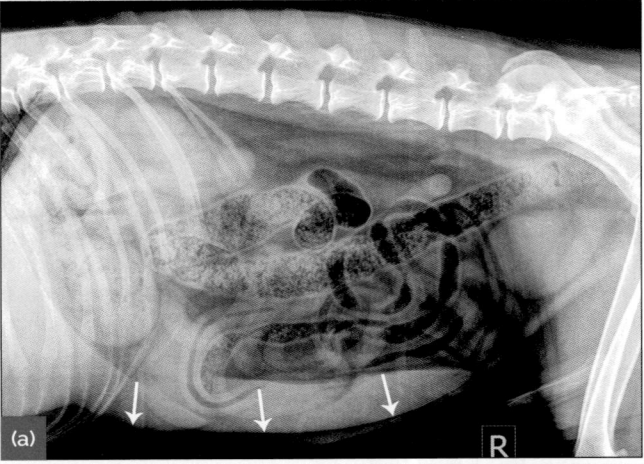

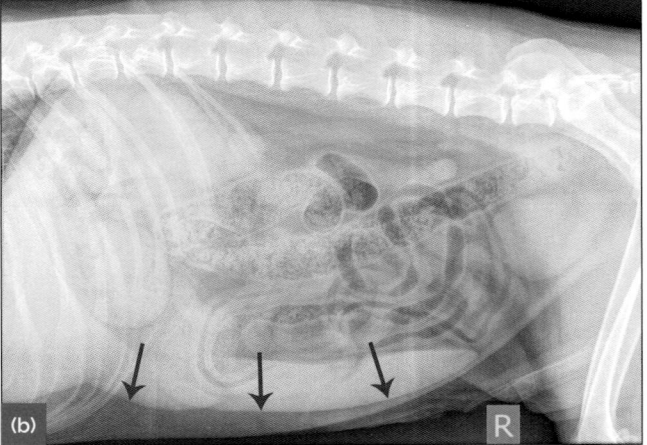

16.35 Lateral abdominal radiographs demonstrating the wide latitude of digital images. **(a)** The bones and thicker soft tissues are visible but the thinner soft tissues and fat along the ventral abdominal wall are overexposed (arrowed). **(b)** Adjustment of the brightness and contrast (window levelling) allows these soft tissues to be seen (arrowed).

Contrast

An important consideration of a digital image is its superior contrast resolution (sometimes referred to as contrast optimization) when compared with a conventional film–screen image. This is significant when visualizing small objects with similar densities (shades of grey) and the ability to see the recorded detail. Put in another way, it is the ability of a system to display in one image and therefore with one exposure, regions of high and low atomic number and regions of varying thickness. As stated above, the more shades of grey that can be displayed on a digital image, the better the contrast resolution. The kV is just as important in digital imaging as it is in conventional radiography and is the exposure factor to be considered in relation to penetration of a particular anatomical area and, more importantly, to produce the optimum level of contrast in that area.

Detector contrast refers to the ability of the detector to convert the X-ray beam exiting the patient into density on conventional X-ray film or into signal differences in digital systems. However, the effect of detector contrast is less important with digital systems. The very wide dynamic range of the detector in a digital system means that the detector contrast has relatively little effect →

Contrast *continued*

on the final image contrast, which is mostly determined by post-processing of the signal. The construction of the detector and its electronics (number of pixels), determines the grey shades that can be displayed. Display contrast refers to window and levelling (displaying pixels according to the values generated by look-up tables, which are part of the processing software). It allows all structures within an object with a wide range of attenuation values to be displayed.

Exposure factors

An exposure chart (see 'Exposure charts', above) is still required for digital systems as underexposure is common and results in reduced image quality. Overexposure is less common but also reduces image quality, as well as increases the radiation dose to the animal. As the direct relationship between film blackening and exposure factors is lost in digital systems, the degree of exposure is often given by a numerical value (exposure index) on the viewing console. Each equipment manufacturer has their own method of displaying exposure information and usually provides guidelines as to the range of recommended values.

The measurement of the number of X-ray photons on image quality is often expressed as signal to noise ratio (SNR). Images with a low SNR have a grainy mottled appearance, which may prevent visualization of finer detail. The effect of kV on image quality with digital systems is complex and difficult to measure, as the relationship between kV and image contrast is less apparent and is affected by multiple factors (e.g. image processing). The sensitivity of the X-ray detector to scattered photons and the effect of X-ray photon energy on detector efficiency varies with the type of detector, and advice should be sought from the equipment supplier regarding their recommendations for use of a grid and the choice of exposure factors. The rule varying the kV to optimize the image contrast should be followed as for conventional film. Increasing the kV may reduce the SNR by increasing noise but not signal.

When assessing quality, the images should be reviewed on a diagnostic workstation with an appropriate monitor, as subtle changes such as underexposure with poor SNR may not be apparent on the low-resolution monitor of the digital radiography console. In summary, optimum exposures should always be selected; although the digital imaging system can compensate for incorrect selection of exposure factors, increased patient dose or suboptimal image quality can result.

Exposure latitude

Exposure latitude is the ability of a digital imaging system, in particular the imaging detector, to compensate for exposures that would produce underexposure or overexposure in a conventional film–screen system. It is the range of exposures that can be successfully used to produce the image. There is a problem associated with a wide exposure latitude: there is a tendency to use higher exposures than necessary to produce an image. It is commonly referred to as *dose creep* and leads to unnecessary patient exposure to radiation. This situation does not arise in film–screen radiography because overexposure or excessive film blackening is easily recognized. Most manufacturers include an exposure index in the system, indicating whether an exposure is optimum for the chosen algorithm, is too high or too low (see 'Computed radiography', above).

Viewing digital images

Following the acquisition and processing stages of the digital process, the image is ready to be viewed and this is facilitated using dedicated DICOM software (see below). This represents the post-processing stage. Images acquired using CR or DDR systems are normally viewed on the associated LCD monitor (see Figure 16.27) and can be manipulated using the various viewing tools available (Figure 16.36). The computer image can be manipulated in several ways:

- Rotation
- Flipping
- Magnification
- Inversion of black and white
- Annotation (e.g. adding a L/R marker or time after contrast study)
- Measurement of line distance or angles.

Images can also be enhanced by adjusting the contrast and brightness ('window levelling'). This optimizes the distribution of greyscales so that the tissue of interest is best seen.

It is usually possible to compare different images from the same study on the same screen on the CR/DDR monitor. LCD monitors can vary in size and resolution and if the CR/DDR monitor is the only screen where images are to be viewed, it is important that this monitor is of a high specification.

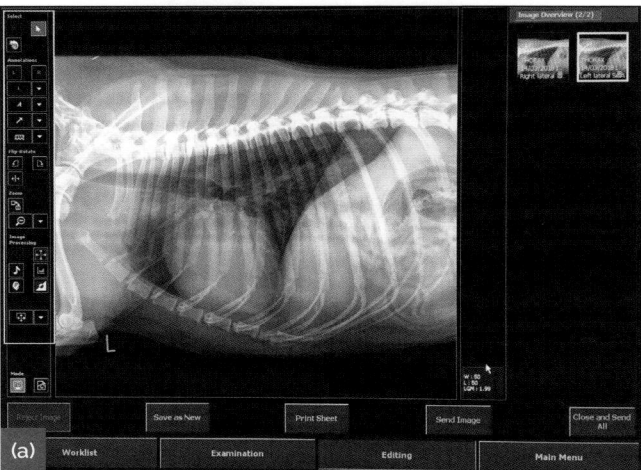

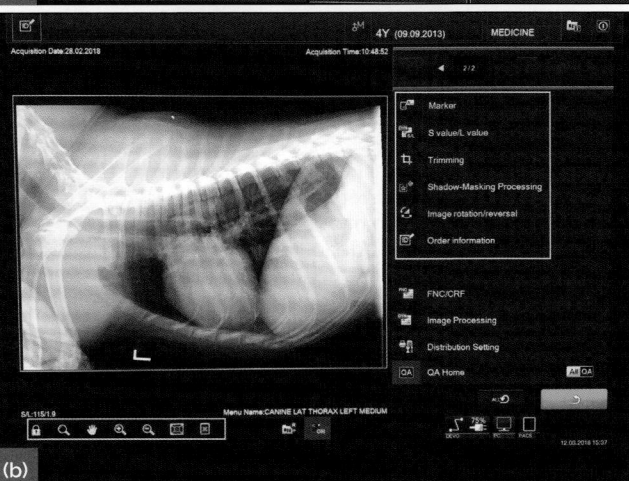

16.36 **(a)** A CR acquisition workstation displaying a left lateral view of the thorax. The various viewing tools are shown on the left of the image (highlighted with a yellow square). **(b)** A DDR acquisition workstation showing viewing tools on the right and along the bottom of the image (highlighted with yellow squares).

The larger veterinary establishments may have a dry laser printer, which allows the images to be printed on to thermal film from the CR/DDR system (having a similar appearance to a conventional radiograph) if required, although these are becoming redundant with the improvement and increased accessibility of PACS (Picture Archiving and Communication System, see below). Images may also be printed on photographic or standard paper, although this should be avoided as it results in very inferior reproduction.

Magnification

Manipulation of digital images after acquisition allows the image to be magnified or reduced in size, but it is important to be able to recognize the original size of the image. Most DICOM viewers automatically display the image so that it fits in its entirety on the viewing screen. This means that most images are automatically zoomed or reduced in size. Some DICOM viewers allow images to be displayed at 'True Size' or '100%', but this may require the calibration of the viewer settings as the monitor pixel size can affect the True Size display. A True Size or 100% display only shows the image plate/phosphor and does not mean that the image genuinely reflects the true size of the anatomical area being imaged, since geometric factors still apply with digital images. If accurate measurements are required, a marker of known length should always be included within the collimated area at the level of the anatomical structure of interest; the radiograph can then be digitally calibrated to this marker.

Digital Imaging and Communications in Medicine (DICOM)

DICOM was developed to prevent problems that can occur when different manufacturers use different protocols in their systems. The list of information required to make the image 'readable' can be very long; for example, in the many factors that make up each individual magnetic resonance (MR) image. It is very important that the information is easily and readily available so that the image can be processed on a workstation for viewing either at the time of acquisition or later after transmission.

DICOM allows a basic reference so that one system is able to communicate accurately with any other system set up to receive the information. DICOM is used worldwide to store, exchange and transmit veterinary images, and adheres to the General Data Protection Regulations (GDPR) in the EU. Each different piece of information sits in an area called a field. Each centre will have a unique identifier that can be found in one particular field and each imaging modality (e.g. radiography, ultrasonography, CT, MRI and radiation therapy) will have another unique identifier sitting in another field. In addition, there will be fields that are specifically for identification details (e.g. surname, name and date of birth).

In 2005, a veterinary DICOM working group was established to develop the specifications required in veterinary medicine. These specifications include patient information, owner, species, breed, area imaged and view. DICOM images are embedded with information that is unique to each image and which is very nearly impossible to alter. This has obvious implications with regard to security and fraud (for example, in the submission of images for hip dysplasia assessment to the BVA; see 'Labelling', above).

Exposure faults and artefacts in digital imaging

Exposure faults

Digital radiography copes much better with a wide range of exposures than conventional radiography. Under- and over-exposure do occur with digital systems, but have quite a different appearance to similar problems that occur with conventional radiography (Figure 16.37).

- Underexposure results in a grainy or 'noisy' appearance called quantum mottle. This is due to insufficient signal (photons) reaching the detectors, which means the system is unable to differentiate between background electronic noise and low signals created by the X-ray photons. This results in a non-uniform appearance, even in organs that should appear quite uniform (Figure 16.37a). Any attempt to improve the image quality by changing the contrast and density simply amplifies the quantum mottle and the graininess remains. Underexposed grainy radiographs also have reduced radiographic contrast.
- Digital radiography withstands overexposure quite well. These images have low quantum mottle and remain diagnostic due to the ability of digital systems to rescale the high signals within the visible greyscale range. With extreme overexposure there will still be detail visible, but areas with the lowest radiographic density may be displayed as completely black without any discernible anatomy (Figure 16.37c). This is because during pre-processing, certain pixel values are assigned to monitor brightness and pixel ranges beyond the chosen range are all shown as black. This results in what is known as 'clipping' of the image, with areas of low attenuation (e.g. thin soft tissues and the lungs) all displayed as black. No amount of post-processing with recover these areas and because only parts of the image are overexposed, and not the entire image as would be the case in film–screen radiography, the overexposed region can easily be interpreted as an area of abnormality or as a lesion.

Underexposure and overexposure may be indicated by the exposure index being outside the recommended range. Increasing or decreasing the kV by 10–15% is a good starting point to correct underexposure and over-exposure, respectively.

Digital imaging artefacts

To ensure a good image is obtained, the digital imaging device must be properly calibrated, configured, maintained and operated. Correct system calibration is essential to main-tain uniformity and systems must be correctly configured with the most up-to-date software, hardware and durable goods. Regular cleaning and servicing are also necessary to avoid artefacts.

Due to the differences in image creation, artefacts asso-ciated with image detection and formation are different for CR and DDR systems.

Computed radiography
Dirt on the phosphor or within the reader

This is a common artefact within CR systems and results in white marks on the image, which are visible on multiple

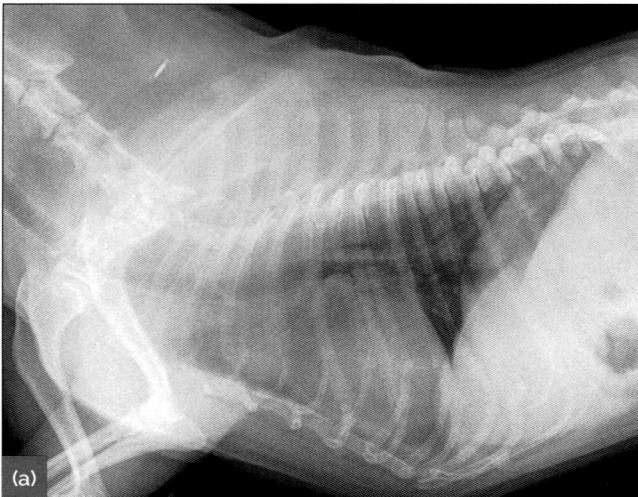
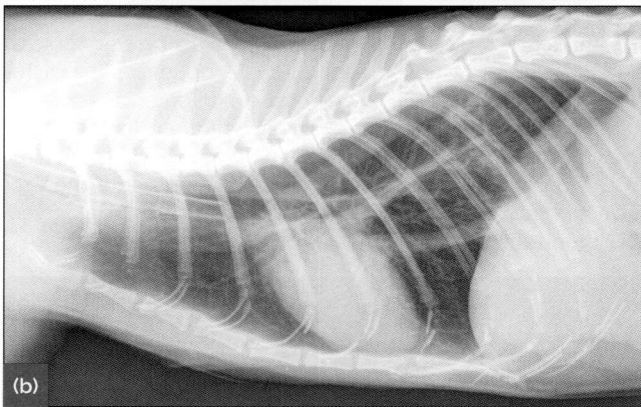
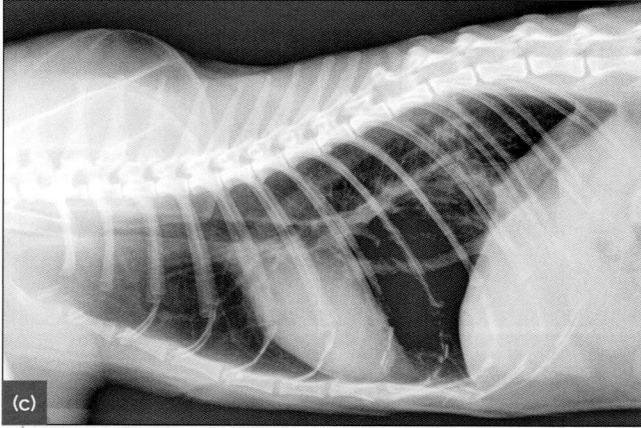

16.37 **(a)** Underexposed digital radiograph of the thorax. Underexposure results in a grainy or noisy appearance of the image and is called quantum mottle. It is particularly obvious in the region of the neck and shoulders where the exposure given has not been sufficient to demonstrate these areas adequately. Attempts to improve the appearance by changing the contrast and density only amplify the noise. **(b)** Correctly exposed digital thoracic radiograph demonstrating good detail of the lung fields and major vessels. **(c)** Digital image of the same thorax as in (b). This image demonstrates gross overexposure; detail is still visible but regions of low radiographic density are displayed as black areas without any discernible anatomy. It is referred to as clipping. No amount of windowing and levelling will retrieve this lost data.

exposures. The dirt prevents the light emitted from the phosphor from reaching the photodetector in the CR reader, in a similar way to the same artefact arising with conventional radiographic screens.

- Dirt on the phosphor results in small white marks on the image (in a similar way to conventional radiography screens). This can often be identified by inspecting the surface of the imaging plate.
- Dirt on the rollers or light guide in the digitizer results in thin linear white marks. Dirt within the CR reader requires a cleaning process as recommended by the manufacturer. Occasionally, this cleaning process is not adequate and an engineer will then need to remove the dirt (Figure 16.38).

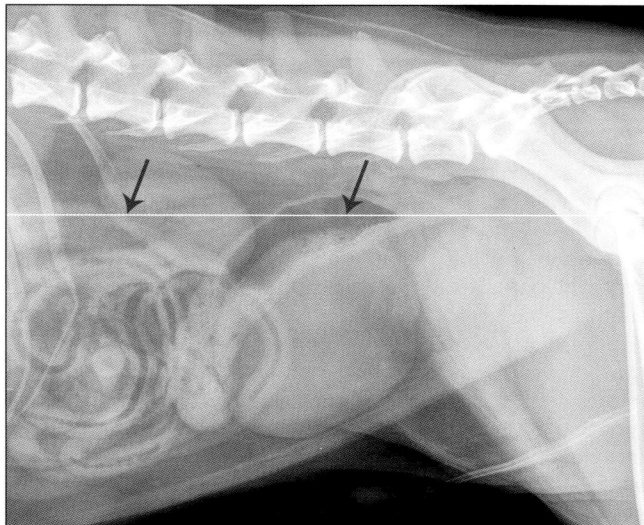

16.38 Digital abdominal radiograph demonstrating a thin, horizontal, linear white line just ventral to the spine (arrowed), which represents dirt on the light guide of the CR digitizer.

Delayed scanning of the cassettes

A long delay (>24 hours) between exposing and processing the imaging plate results in fading of the stored image on the phosphor. This may also occur due to exposure of the phosphor to light in CR systems where the phosphor is manually removed from the cassette for processing.

Direct digital radiography

Artefacts that appear solely with DDR systems include detector calibration artefacts and artefacts caused by problems with the readout circuit.

Common CR and DDR artefacts
Look-up table errors

- During image processing, the look-up table is necessary to allow the raw data on the imaging plate/detector to be converted into an image that can be viewed. The look-up table contains data detailing how bright the pixel should be on the monitor for the amount of phosphor that has been excited. This often comes as a package with other processing tools (such as edge enhancement), so that when, for example, the thorax is selected, the processed images should be optimized for thoracic radiographs. Therefore, it is very important to select the correct examination algorithm for the body area to be examined.
- Inadequate or no collimation in the region of interest can result in an artefact where parts of the image are not displayed or are blacked out. This occurs because the software attempts to apply automatic collimation to the straight lines identified on the image and

occasionally inadvertently collimates to straight lines in the patient (e.g. the spine). Reapplying the collimation during post-processing allows the software to 'find' the margins and the correct image to be displayed.

Überschwinger and Moiré artefacts

- Überschwinger artefacts result from an image processing error, which allows significant portions of the image with large differences in radiopacity between adjacent pixels to be excessively enhanced. This most often occurs with orthopaedic implants where the edge enhancement causes a radiolucent-like appearance or halo around the implant. This can be mistaken for loosening of the implant or low-grade infection (Figure 16.39).
- Moiré artefacts (alternating light and dark bands across the image) are seen on the computer monitor if a stationary grid has been used for CR or DDR, or if the grid is aligned with the readout of the CR cassette. Moiré artefacts occur due to interference of the grid lines and the monitor display and are more common with low-resolution monitors and coarse grids (Figure 16.40). They can be corrected by using a Potter-Bucky moving grid or by using a stationary grid with a higher number of lead strips per centimetre.

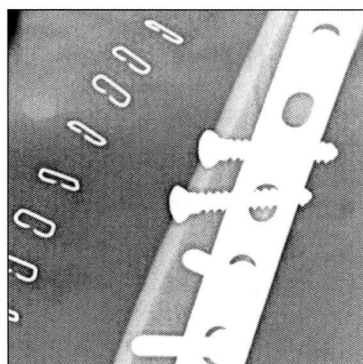

16.39 Überschwinger artefact. There is a radiolucent-like appearance or halo around the screws and around the central hole of the metal plate. It results from excessive edge enhancement of adjacent pixels with large differences in radiopacity.

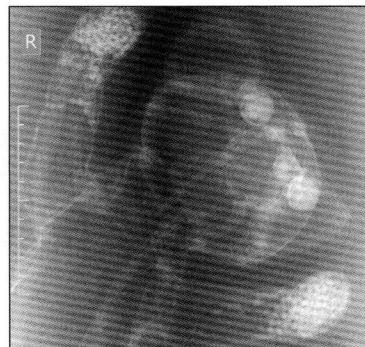

16.40 Moiré artefact. A digital radiograph of a soft toy taken with a stationary grid. Alternating light and dark bands can be seen across the image. The artefact is due to interference of the grid lines and the monitor display.

Storage and distribution of digital images

Storage

There is normally limited storage on CR/DDR systems without an internal disc back-up, so it is important that an additional storage method is used. The storage of digital images acquired from CR/DDR systems can be either offline or online. Offline storage can be on a CD/DVD, whereas online storage will typically be on a central archive.

Offline storage

For offline storage, images can be copied to a CD/DVD in a DICOM or JPEG format. Images copied in a DICOM format will normally include a DICOM viewer, which allows the CD/DVD to be read on a normal PC with the DICOM viewing tools available (as described above). DICOM 3.0 is an industry standard for the viewing and storage of X-ray images, which secures the patient's details, and the image is stored in full resolution on the CD/DVD. The CD/DVD may be used to store images at a practice, given to a referral veterinary surgeon or sent away for second opinion. Images copied into a JPEG format are compressed, of lower resolution, and may not contain the patient's details. They are used where emailing images is required or for lecture presentations. They should not be used for radiological interpretation or for teleradiology purposes (see 'Teleradiology', below).

Online storage

Online storage is typically on a central archive. An online archive system is known as a Picture Archiving and Communication System (PACS). It allows the automatic saving of images from CR/DDR or other digital imaging systems (e.g. CT, MRI, ultrasonography and scintigraphy) to a secure location without the manual task of copying to CD/DVD, as well as allowing retrieval and distribution for viewing.

A PACS consists of the imaging modality, an archive server and appropriate routing software and viewing workstations. It requires a network with a reasonable speed, since the images to be transmitted are very large. Veterinary-specific PACS for different sized establishments have been developed with the limitation on the number of images stored being due only to the amount of digital storage available. The central archive may connect to a single modality or to several imaging modalities with DICOM output; the initial archive system can be expanded with each procurement of a new imaging modality. A branch practice may install a CR/DDR system, but storage at the main practice archive server may be preferred. In these cases, a routing device can be added which encrypts and compresses the images and sends them to the main practice archive server for storage and distribution across all practice sites.

For referred patients, it may be possible to import DICOM or JPEG images or digital photographs acquired elsewhere into the archive from a CD, DVD or USB device, or via internet file transfer, for example, images imported from a mobile MRI scanner. Offsite back-up storage is helpful in case of local computer failure.

Distribution

Images can be viewed on the archive server, but even in a small veterinary practice it is very useful to be able to access images in consulting rooms, theatres and offices. An image archive can be supplied with a web browser to enable computers and dedicated workstations within the practice to access the archive server. The number of users able to access the web browser simultaneously can be predetermined, depending on the needs of the practice.

Staff can search for images using the patient's or the owner's name, the animal's identification (ID) number or the date of the examination, and can view and manipulate images in the full resolution DICOM format. Images from different dates and imaging modalities can be compared on the same screen for diagnosis or discussion with clients (Figure 16.41). In human medicine, the PACS is usually integrated with the hospital information system and radiology information system, allowing all patient data to be stored together and avoiding transcription errors in patient name and details. This is an ideal situation, but it is not yet widely available in veterinary medicine, although the image archive system may be integrated with the practice management system (PMS), enabling users to retrieve X-ray images from the PMS software.

Although DICOM images can be viewed in full resolution throughout the practice, PC monitors may not be of ideal resolution. If the dedicated CR/DDR monitor is not being used, one practice PC could be upgraded to a DICOM-calibrated monitor (available in a selection of sizes and resolutions). For more in-depth radiology reporting of CR/DDR, ultrasound, MR and CT images, a dedicated PACS workstation with DICOM-calibrated or diagnostic monitors is recommended. However, monitor resolution is reflected in the price.

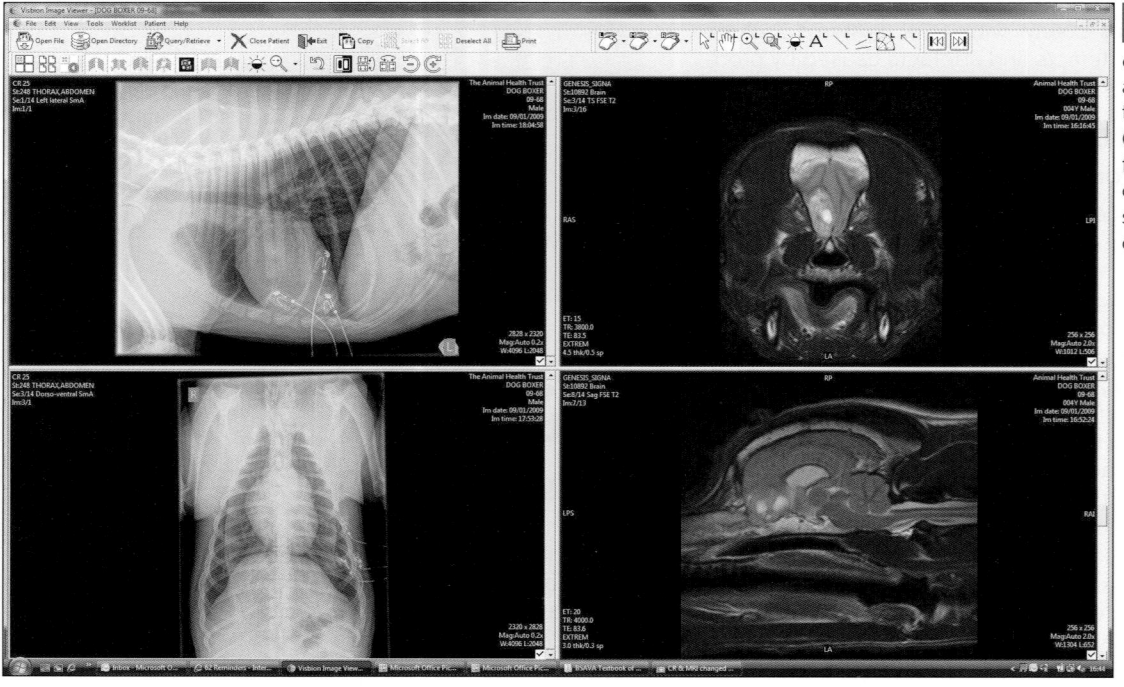

16.41 MRI scans (right) of a dog's brain showing a brain tumour, and thoracic radiographs (left) obtained to look for lung metastases, demonstrating simultaneous use of digital technology.

Teleradiology

Teleradiology is the transmission of digital imaging files for remote viewing, interpretation and reporting by a veterinary (or medical) radiologist. Images are sent electronically from one location to another (e.g. from a referring practice to a radiologist), either using a broadband internet connection or by being downloaded from a secure internet site or file-sharing service. It is a much more efficient system than sending the images on a CD or DVD. A report is subsequently transmitted back to the practice, meaning that expert advice may be obtained 24 hours a day, if necessary, from offsite professionals who may be working on different continents and in different time zones.

Radiation protection

Dangers associated with radiography

Exposure of the human or animal body to radiation is not without hazard, because of the biological effects that X-rays have on living tissues via cellular chemical reactions. X-rays have four properties that mean that the danger from them may be seriously underestimated:

- They are invisible
- They are painless
- The effects are latent, i.e. they are not evident immediately and may not manifest until some time later – even several decades in some cases
- Their effects are cumulative and so repeated very low doses may be as hazardous as a single large exposure.

Large doses are unlikely to occur in human or veterinary radiography but may be seen after nuclear accidents. It is the danger arising from repeated exposure to small amounts of radiation that concerns people working with radiation. Despite these hazards, it is possible to perform radiography in veterinary practice with no significant risk to any of the people involved, provided that adequate precautions are taken.

The adverse effects of radiation on the body may be divided into three groups: somatic, carcinogenic and genetic. They may also be classified as stochastic and non-stochastic or deterministic. Stochastic effects are those which occur by chance and have no threshold, so could be caused by any dose, irrespective of its magnitude (e.g. neoplasia and genetic mutations). Deterministic, or non-stochastic, effects have a dose-specific threshold beyond which acute radiation burns can occur.

Somatic effects

These are direct changes in body tissues that usually occur soon after exposure. They include skin reddening and cracking, blood disorders, hair loss, cataract formation and digestive upsets. Gastrointestinal side effects cause severe dehydration, which is the usual cause of death following nuclear accidents or bombs. Different tissues vary in their susceptibility to this type of damage, with the developing fetus being particularly susceptible. The somatic effect is used to advantage in the radiotherapy of tumours, since tumour cells are often more sensitive to radiation damage than are normal cells.

Carcinogenic effects

These concern the induction of cancer in tissues that have been exposed to radiation. There may be a considerable time lag before tumours arise; this may be as long as 20–30 years in the case of leukaemia.

Genetic effects

These occur when the gonads (ovaries and testes) are irradiated and mutations are induced in the chromosomes of germ cells. These mutations may give rise to inherited abnormalities in the offspring.

Sources of radiation hazard

During an exposure, there are three potential sources of X-rays that may be hazardous to anyone who needs to be present: the tube head, the primary beam, and secondary or scattered radiation (Figure 16.42).

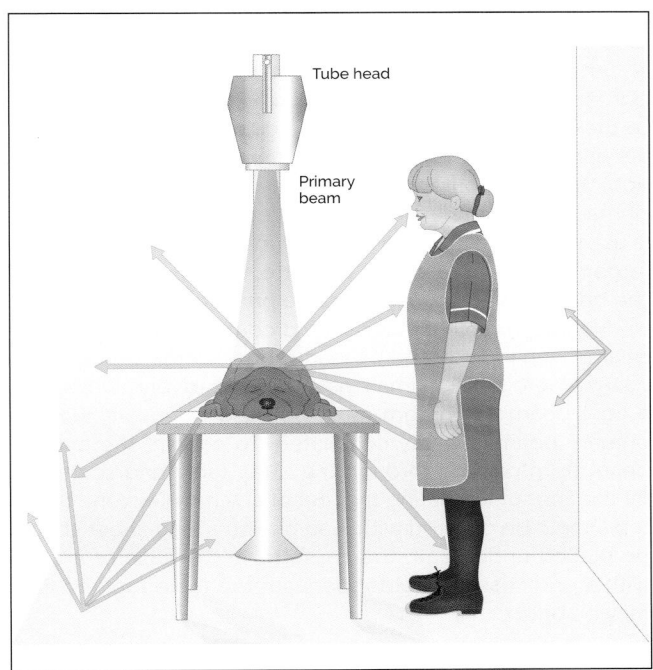

Tube head

Primary beam

16.42 Spread of scattered radiation. The radiographer is too close to the X-ray beam and should ideally be 2 m away from it and behind a lead screen.

Tube head

Although the tube head is lead-lined (except at the window where the primary beam emerges), older machines may have suffered cracks in the casing that allow X-rays to escape in other directions. For this reason, the tube head should never be held or touched during an exposure. Checks on the integrity of the casing can be made by taping a thermoluminescent dosimeter (TLD) to the tube head, leaving it for a few exposures and then processing it. Any cracks in the casing will cause a reading to be obtained on the TLD. The integrity of the tube head should be checked by an engineer during the machine's annual service, as well as testing for electrical safety. The tube window must be covered by an aluminium filter, which removes low-energy X-ray photons from the primary beam. These photons do not contribute to the useful X-ray beam but are still a radiation hazard.

Primary beam

The beam of X-rays produced at the anode is directed out of the tube head through the window. This primary beam constitutes the greatest safety hazard, since it consists of high-energy X-rays. It may be delineated using a light beam diaphragm, a device attached to the tube head that produces visible light over the area covered by the X-ray beam (Figure 16.43). The light beam diaphragm usually contains crossed wires that produce a shadow in the illuminated area, showing the position of the centre of the beam (the central ray).

Movable metal plates or diaphragms operated by knobs allow the area covered to be adjusted to the size required, a procedure known as collimation.

Collimation should always be to as small an area as possible and the accuracy of the light beam diaphragm should be checked periodically. This can be done by arranging pairs of coins along each margin of the light beam with their edges touching, so that one of each pair lies inside and the other outside the light beam, and making an exposure. After processing, the image should show four coins inside the black area and the other four coins outside, if the light beam diaphragm is accurate.

An alternative, but now uncommon, method of collimation is to use conical or cylindrical devices or cones attached to the tube window to produce a circular primary beam of varying diameter. Cones are much less satisfactory than light beam diaphragms, since the area covered by the primary beam is not seen. Whichever method of collimation is used, the area covered by the primary beam should be no larger than the size of the cassette, and so the borders of the beam should be visible on the processed radiograph.

No part of any handler should come within the primary beam, even if protected by lead rubber clothing. In the rare cases where small animals have to be held for radiography, a light beam diaphragm must be used to ensure that the primary beam is safely collimated. To prevent the primary beam from passing through the X-ray table and scattering off the floor or irradiating the feet of any handlers, the tabletop should be covered with lead or else a lead sheet should be placed underneath the cassette; in the case of a table with a grid cassette holder beneath the table top, the lead may be below this.

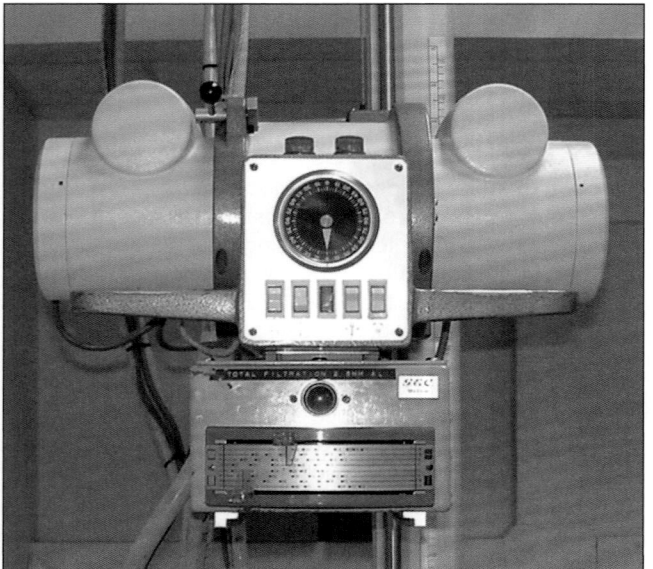

16.43 A light beam diaphragm attached to an X-ray tube head.

The use of a horizontal X-ray beam is especially hazardous, as the primary beam will pass, with little attenuation, through doors, windows and thin walls. This procedure should only be performed with great care, with the primary beam directed only towards a thick wall. The procedure for the use of horizontal beam radiography should be described in the practice's Local Rules (see 'Local Rules and written arrangements', below). Although the use of a horizontal beam is mainly employed for large animal radiography, there are occasions when it may be necessary for small animals; for example, when animals are too dyspnoeic to lie in lateral recumbency.

Secondary or scattered radiation

Scattered radiation is produced in all directions when the primary beam strikes a solid object (see Figure 16.42), and so it arises from the patient and the cassette. It is produced by the table or floor if the tabletop is not lead-lined; it can also bounce off walls and ceilings and travel in random directions. It is, however, of much lower energy than the primary beam and is absorbed by lead rubber protective clothing. Its intensity falls off rapidly with distance from the source, as described by the inverse square law. The best protection against scatter is to stand as far from the X-ray machine and patient as possible – a minimum of 2 m, and better still behind a lead-lined screen.

Ways of reducing the amount of scatter produced (see above) include close collimation of the primary beam, compression of large areas of soft tissue, reduction in the kV where possible, and the use of a lead-topped table or lead-backed cassettes. Protection against scatter is also afforded by radiographic protective clothing.

Legislation

In 1985 the law governing the use of radiation and radioactive materials was revised and updated with the publication of The Ionising Radiations Regulations (IRR) 1985; these were subsequently updated as The Ionising Radiations Regulations 1999 (IRR99). The Health & Safety Executive (HSE) consulted on changes to IRR99 in 2017 and these changes came into effect on 1st January 2018, replacing IRR99 with IRR17. The main changes were; a lower dose limit to the lens of the eye and changes to the way in which any work with ionizing radiation is notified to the HSE. Consequently, as of February 2018, all veterinary practices working with ionizing radiation are required to register with the HSE. IRR17 is a legal document that covers all uses of radiation and radioactive materials, including veterinary radiography.

As IRR17 is written in legal terms, and is somewhat lengthy, a second booklet called 'Work with ionising radiation. Ionising Radiations Regulations 2017. Approved Code of Practice and Guidance' was produced to explain the Regulations (www.hse.gov.uk/pubns/books/l121.htm). The 'Approved Code of Practice and Guidance' contains some specific references to veterinary radiography, but is also rather long and complex and so the British Veterinary Association (BVA) has produced guidance notes explaining the law as it applies to veterinary radiography; Guidance Notes for the Safe Use of Ionising Radiations in Veterinary Practice, Ionising Radiations Regulation 2017. A summary of the legislation is given in the following paragraphs.

Principles of radiation protection

Protection follows three basic principles:

- Radiography should only be undertaken if there is definite clinical justification for the use of the procedure
- Any exposure of personnel should be kept to a minimum. The three words to remember are: time, distance, shielding (i.e. reduce the need for repeat exposures, stand well back, and wear protective clothing or stand behind a lead screen)
- No dose limit should be exceeded.

The aim is to avoid exposure at all times, but failing this a high standard of protection will exist if the advice contained in the Guidance Notes is followed.

Local Rules and written arrangements

The Local Rules are a set of instructions drawn up by the practice's Radiation Protection Adviser (RPA), which set down details of equipment, procedures and restriction of access to the controlled area for that practice. The written arrangements are part of the Local Rules and include the sequence of actions to be followed for each exposure, including the method of restraint of patients for radiography and the precautions to be taken should manual restraint be necessary. A copy of the Local Rules should be given to anyone involved in radiography (veterinary surgeons and veterinary nurses) and should also be displayed in the X-ray room.

Radiation Protection Supervisor (RPS)

An RPS must be appointed within the practice and will usually be the principal or a senior partner, although may be the Head Nurse in some practices. The RPS is responsible for ensuring that radiography is carried out safely and in accordance with the Regulations, and that the Local Rules are followed. It is not necessary for the RPS to be present at every radiographic examination.

Radiation Protection Adviser (RPA)

Most practices will also need to appoint an external RPA. RPAs must hold a certificate of competence issued by an appropriate body, stating that they have the knowledge, experience and competence required to act as a veterinary RPA. They are usually medical physicists, although holders of the RCVS Diploma in Veterinary Radiology who have undertaken appropriate further training may also be eligible. The RPA will give advice on all aspects of radiation protection and the demarcation of the controlled area, and will advise on drawing up the Local Rules and instructions for safe working.

The controlled area

A specific room should be identified for small animal radiography and should have walls of sufficient thickness that no part of the controlled area extends outside the room (single brick is usually adequate; thin walls may be reinforced with lead ply or barium plaster). The room should be large enough to allow people remaining in the room to stand at least 2 m from the primary beam. If this is not possible, a protective lead screen should be provided, unless the radiographer can routinely step outside the room and stand behind a brick wall during the exposure. Unshielded doors and windows

may be acceptable if the workload is low and the room is large enough. Special recommendations are made for flooring in cases where there may be an occupied area below or above the radiography room.

Technically, the controlled area is the area around the primary beam within which the average dose rate of exposure exceeds a given limit (laid down in the Regulations). The controlled area for a typical practice is within a 2 m radius from the beam but usually needs to be defined by the RPA. Since the controlled area must be physically demarcated and clearly labelled, it is usually simpler to designate the whole X-ray room as a controlled area and to place warning notices on its doors to exclude people not involved in radiography. When the radiographic examination is completed, the X-ray machine must be disconnected from the power supply; the room then ceases to be a controlled area and may be entered freely.

A warning sign should be placed at the entrance to the X-ray room, consisting of the radiation warning symbol and a simple legend (see Chapter 2). For permanently installed equipment there should also be an automatic signal at the room entrance indicating when the X-ray machine is in a state of readiness to produce X-rays. This signal usually takes the form of a red light or an illuminated sign. Whilst not a legal requirement for portable and mobile X-ray machines (which comprise the majority of practice X-ray machines), many practices have installed red lights outside their radiography rooms to warn when radiography is in progress and prevent accidental entry, and this is to be recommended.

In addition, all X-ray machines should have lights visible from the control panel indicating (a) when they are switched on at the mains and (b) when exposure is taking place; sometimes exposure is indicated by a noise such as a beep or buzz. Illuminated signs outside the X-ray room may also have two different legends, for example one showing in yellow light when the X-ray machine is switched on and the other in red light when an exposure is taking place (Figure 16.44).

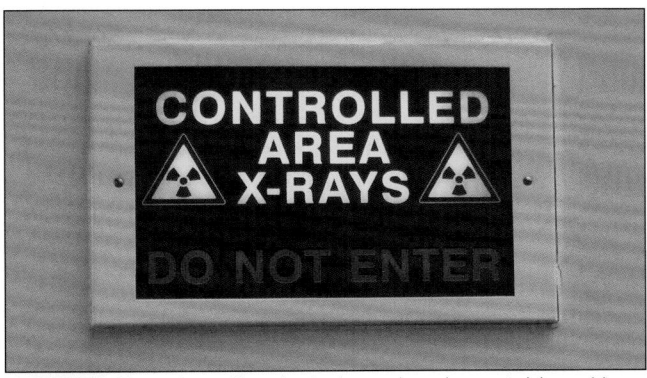

16.44 Two-stage illuminated warning sign outside an X-ray room.

X-ray equipment

Radiation safety features of the X-ray machine should be checked annually by a qualified engineer.

- Leakage of radiation from the tube housing must not exceed a certain level and the beam filtration must be equivalent to at least 2.5 mm aluminium.
- All machines must be fitted with a collimation device, preferably a light beam diaphragm.
- The exposure button must allow the radiographer to stand at least 2 m from the primary beam, which means

either that it must be at the end of a sufficiently long cable or else that it should be on the control panel, which is placed well away from the tube head.

■ The timer should be electronic (most X-ray machines) rather than clockwork, as exposures cannot be aborted with clockwork timers should the patient move.

Suppliers of X-ray machines have a responsibility to ensure that they are safe and functioning correctly, and they should provide a report to this effect when installing the equipment. Servicing of X-ray machines is a legal requirement and should be carried out at least once a year; all documentation pertaining to that service should be kept.

The X-ray table must be lead-lined or, alternatively, a sheet of lead 1 mm thick and larger than the maximum size of the beam should be placed on or below the table to absorb the residual primary beam and reduce scatter. Many practices now use purpose-built X-ray tables that are not only lead-lined but are also fitted with hooks to aid patient positioning using ties.

Film and film processing

The Regulations recommend the use of fast film–screen combinations in order to reduce exposure times. They stress the importance of correct processing techniques in order to minimize the number of non-diagnostic films and avoid the need for repeat exposures. Digital radiography has important safety benefits as the number of repeat exposures required is reduced, since exposure factors chosen are less critical, and since bone and soft tissues can be seen on the same exposure of a given area.

Recording exposures

It is necessary to record each radiographic exposure made and this is done using a daybook for radiography, including the following details for each exposure: date; patient identity and description; exposure factors used; quality of image; and means of restraint. If the animal has had to be held during radiography, the name(s) of the person(s) doing so must be recorded. As radiography is a potentially hazardous procedure, the HSE has the power to make unannounced inspections, so it is extremely important that these records, as well as those relating to X-ray generating equipment servicing and dosimetry (see 'Dosimetry', below), are kept.

Protective clothing

Protective clothing consists of aprons, gloves, sleeves and neck (thyroid) protectors and is usually made of rubber impregnated with lead. The thickness and efficiency of the garment is described in millimetres of lead equivalent (LE), i.e. the thickness of pure lead that would afford the same protection. It is important to remember that protective clothing is only effective against scatter and does not protect against the primary beam. Fixed or mobile lead screens with lead glass windows are also useful as the radiographer can stand behind them during the exposure and still see the patient. Unfortunately, they are very expensive.

Lead rubber aprons should be worn by any person who needs to be present in the X-ray room during the exposure unless they are behind a protective lead screen. They are designed to cover the trunk (especially the gonads) and should reach at least to mid-thigh level. Their thickness should be at least 0.25 mm LE; many are 0.35 or even 0.5 mm

LE, though the latter are rather heavy to wear. Single-sided aprons covering the front of the body but with straps at the back are cheaper but provide less protection than double-sided aprons covering both front and back, and are also less comfortable to wear for long periods. Aprons are expensive items and should be handled carefully; when not in use they should be stored on coat hangers or on rails (Figure 16.45). They must never be folded as this can lead to undetected cracking of the material.

Lead rubber gloves, open-palm mitts and hand shields must be available for use in those cases where manual restraint of the patient is unavoidable. Lead sleeves are tubes of lead rubber into which the hands and forearms may be inserted as an alternative to gloves. Single sheets of lead rubber draped over the hands are not adequate, as they do not protect against back-scatter.

Gloves, hand shields and sleeves should be at least 0.35 mm LE and must never appear in the primary beam, since they offer inadequate protection against high-energy primary beam X-rays. It is important to remember that, although a lead glove may appear completely opaque on a radiograph, the film is being protected by two layers of lead rubber but the hand by only one (Figure 16.46). Lead rubber neck guards for protection of the thyroid gland may also be used and are held in place using Velcro®. Their use should be defined in the Local Rules.

All items of protective clothing should be checked frequently for signs of cracking. A small defect may not allow many X-rays through but will always be over the same area of skin. If in doubt, the garment may be X-rayed or examined with fluoroscopy and image intensification (a moving X-ray image obtained with low energy photons, which is electronically enhanced) to check for cracks (Figure 16.47).

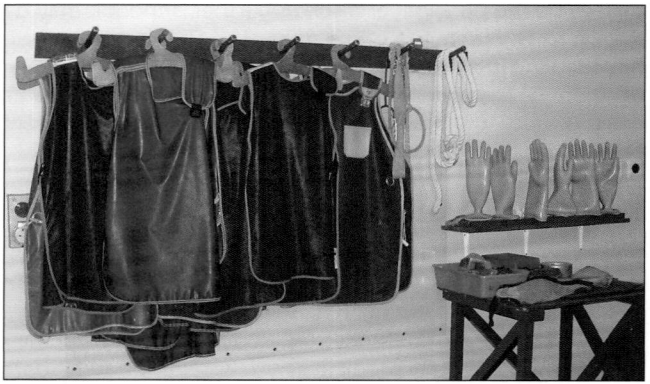

16.45 Correct storage of lead aprons and gloves.

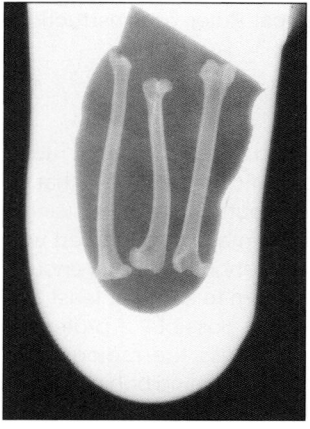

16.46 Radiograph of bones covered by a single thickness of lead rubber: compare with the edge, where there are two layers of lead rubber and all of the primary beam appears to have been absorbed.

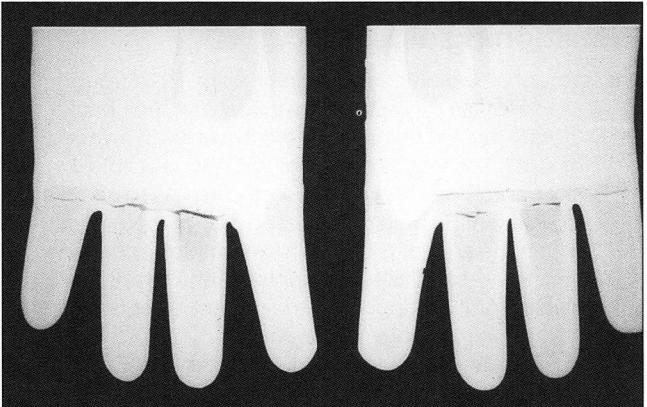

16.47 Radiograph of gloves showing cracking of the lead rubber at the usual site – the base of the fingers. These gloves should now be discarded.

Dosimetry

All persons who are involved in radiography should wear small monitoring devices or dosemeters to record any radiation to which they are exposed. Dosemeters can be obtained from dosimetry services, such as those offered by Public Health England (PHE), or from larger hospitals. The length of time that dosemeters can be worn before being sent back to the provider for reading is 1–3 months, depending on the radiographic caseload.

The main dosemeter should be worn on the trunk beneath the lead apron, but an extra dosemeter may be worn on the collar or sleeve to monitor the levels of radiation received by unprotected parts of the body. Extremity ring or fingerstall dosemeters are available for wearing on the hands beneath lead gloves and are used for large animal radiography and for work with radioactive materials (e.g. during scintigraphy). Each dosemeter should be worn only by the person to whom it is issued and it must neither be left in the X-ray room whilst not being worn nor exposed to heat or sunlight. Dosemeters should only be worn on the veterinary premises as it is important that they reflect accurately any radiation dose acquired at work and not false readings due to other factors.

Two types of dosemeter are available:

- Film badges contain small pieces of X-ray film and are usually blue. They contain small metal filters that allow assessment of the type of radiation to which the badge has been exposed. (It should be noted that this type of dosemeter is no longer widely used due to the ever-decreasing demand for conventional film)
- Thermoluminescent dosemeters (TLDs) contain radiation-sensitive lithium fluoride crystals. On exposure to radiation the electrons in the crystals are rearranged, thus storing energy. During the reading process the crystals are heated and give off light in proportion to the amount of energy that they have stored; this provides a quantitative reading.

Dosemeters may also be used to monitor radiation levels in the X-ray room or in adjacent rooms by mounting them on the wall. They can be used to check the adequacy of protection offered by internal walls and doors. The exact arrangement for dosimetry in the practice will be made in consultation with the RPA, and the records must be filed for easy retrieval or available for future employers if a staff member leaves. Anyone whose badge reveals a reading should be informed, so that the cause can be identified if possible and working practices adjusted accordingly.

Dose limits

Dose limits are amounts of radiation that are thought not to constitute a greater risk to health than those encountered in everyday life. Legal limits have been laid down for various categories of person and for different parts of the body. Maximum permitted doses (MPDs) are laid down for the whole body, for individual organs, for the lens of the eye and for pregnancy. 'Classified' persons are those working with radiation who are likely to receive >30% of any relevant MPD. However, in veterinary practice these levels should not be reached and so veterinary workers rarely need to be designated as classified persons, provided they are working under formal written arrangements drawn up by the practice's RPA.

Staff involved in radiography

The Local Rules will include a list of names of designated persons authorized to carry out exposures. It should be remembered that nurses and other lay staff aged 16 or 17 have a lower MPD than do adults aged 18 or over, and therefore their involvement in radiography should be limited. Young people under 16 years of age should not be present during radiography under any circumstances. Owners should not routinely be present as they are members of the general public and are neither trained in radiography nor wearing dosemeters. The Local Rules should ensure that doses to pregnant women are well within the legal limit, but nevertheless it is wise to avoid the involvement of pregnant women in radiography whenever possible.

The general rule is that the minimum number of people should be present during radiography. When, as is usual, the patient is artificially restrained, only the person making the exposure need be present and this should be the case in the majority of radiographic studies. Usually the radiographer will be able to stand behind a protective screen or outside the room during the exposure.

Radiographic procedures and restraint

Whenever possible, the beam should be directed vertically downwards on to an X-ray table. The minimum number of people should remain in the room and they should either stand behind lead screens or wear protective clothing. All those present must obey the instructions given by the person operating the X-ray machine. The beam must be collimated to the smallest size practicable and must be entirely within the borders of the film. Grids should only be used when the part being X-rayed is >10 cm thick, as their use necessitates an increase in the exposure.

The method of restraint of the patient is of paramount importance. The Approved Code of Practice states that 'only in exceptional circumstances should a patient or animal undergoing a diagnostic examination be supported or manipulated by hand'. These exceptional circumstances may include severely ill or injured animals for whom a diagnosis requires radiography but for whom sedation, anaesthesia or restraint with sandbags is dangerous (e.g. very young puppies and kittens, congestive heart failure, ruptured diaphragm or other severe traumatic injuries). In these cases, the animal may be held, provided that those restraining it are fully protected and provided that no part of their hands (even in gloves) enters the primary beam. A light beam diaphragm is essential for manual restraint. The majority of patients may be positioned and restrained artificially using positioning aids under varying degrees of sedation or general anaesthesia, and sometimes with no chemical restraint at all.

Radiographic positioning

In order to produce radiographs of maximum diagnostic value it is necessary to position the patient carefully and to centre and collimate the beam accurately. Poor positioning, with rotation or obliquity of the area being radiographed, will result in a film that is hard to interpret or misleading or that fails to demonstrate lesions adequately. There are several general rules that should be adhered to when positioning the patient.

Patient positioning

- Use a large enough cassette to cover the whole area of interest, such as the chest or abdomen in a large dog – it is very difficult to interpret images that are made up of a mosaic of smaller radiographs
- Place the area of interest as close to the film as possible in order to minimize magnification and blurring and to produce an accurate image
- Centre over the area of interest, especially if it is a joint or a disc space in the spine
- Ensure that the central ray of the primary beam is perpendicular to the film; otherwise distortion and non-uniform exposure of the structures will result. If a grid is being used, accurate alignment of the primary beam is essential to prevent grid faults
- Collimate the beam to as small an area as possible, to reduce the amount of scattered radiation produced
- Since a radiograph is a two-dimensional image of a three-dimensional structure, it is usually necessary to take two radiographs at right angles to each other (orthogonal views) in order to visualize the area fully. Oblique views may then be taken to highlight lesions seen on initial radiographs, if appropriate

---

Restraint

Small animals should be held for radiography only in exceptional circumstances (see 'Radiographic procedures and restraint', above), when a radiograph is essential for a diagnosis but where the condition of the animal renders other means of restraint unsafe. In practice, patients rarely need to be held and most views may be achieved using a combination of chemical restraint and positioning aids.

Simple lateral views of the chest, abdomen and limbs may be possible in placid animals without any form of sedation. Other views require varying degrees of sedation or general anaesthesia; the positioning requirements and the temperament of the patient must be taken into consideration when assessing the depth of sedation required. It is also important to handle patients gently, calmly and firmly during radiography, and to reassure them with touch and voice. The room should be quiet, and subdued lighting will not only help to settle the patient but is also necessary for optimum use of the light beam diaphragm.

Positioning aids

With skilful use of positioning aids and the correct degree of chemical restraint, almost any radiographic view may be achieved without the need to hold the animal. The following positioning aids should be present in the practice.

Positioning aids

- Troughs: Radiolucent plastic or foam-filled troughs are essential for restraining animals on their backs (dorsal recumbency). They are available in a variety of sizes. The edges of the trough will be visible on radiographs as straight lines, so care has to be taken to position the area of interest either completely within the area of the trough or completely outside of it. Bean-bags filled with polystyrene beads are also helpful in supporting the patient, although they may be very slightly radiopaque
- Foam pads: When lateral views are required, wedge-shaped pads may be placed under the chest, skull or spine to prevent rotation and to ensure that a true lateral view is achieved. They are also useful for accurate limb positioning. They are radiolucent and may therefore be used in the primary beam. It is useful to have several, in different shapes and sizes, and to cover them with plastic for easy cleaning
- Sandbags: Long, thin sandbags of various sizes may be wrapped around limbs or placed over the neck for restraint. They should only be loosely filled with sand, so that they can be bent and twisted. As they are radiopaque they should not be used in the primary beam. They should be plastic-covered for easy cleaning
- Tapes: Cotton tapes are looped around limbs and may then be tied to hooks on the edge of the table or wrapped around sandbags, for positioning of the limbs. Medical sticky tape may also be useful at times. Ties should only be attached to hooks in anaesthetized patients, in case of unexpected patient movement, which might lead to injury
- Velcro® bands: Fabric bands with Velcro® fastenings are especially useful for ventrodorsal (VD) hip radiographs, as they can be placed around the stifles to align the femora correctly. Non-stick elasticated bandage can also be used
- Wooden blocks: These are used to raise the cassette to the area of interest for certain views (e.g. dorsoventral (DV) skull). They are radiopaque and so should not be placed between the patient and the film

---

Nomenclature

Each radiographic view is named with a composite term describing the first the point of entry and then the point of exit of the beam. For example, a DV view of the chest involves the X-ray beam entering through the spine (dorsally) and emerging through the sternum (ventrally). An exception is the lateromedial (LM) or mediolateral (ML) view, which is commonly just called the lateral view. A standardized nomenclature has been devised for veterinary radiology (the naming of the various body regions is illustrated in Chapter 3). The correct terminology will be used throughout this section.

Note that the terms anterior and posterior are no longer used in veterinary radiography as they are not appropriate to four-legged creatures. Instead, anteroposterior (AP) and posteroanterior (PA) views of the limbs are called:

- Craniocaudal (CrCd) or caudocranial (CdCr) above the radiocarpal and tibiotarsal joints

- Dorsopalmar (DPa)/palmarodorsal (PaD) below the radiocarpal joint in the forelimb and dorsoplantar (DPl)/plantarodorsal (PlD) below the tibiotarsal joint in the hindlimb.

Dorsal recumbency (supine) describes an animal lying on its back and sternal recumbency (prone) describes the crouching position.

Positioning for common views in dogs and cats

The following notes describe in brief the positioning for the more common views performed in veterinary practice in small animals. The resultant images of various views can be found in BSAVA Manuals on diagnostic imaging.

Thorax

The right lateral recumbent position is usually preferred to the left lateral for a single screening film, as the heart outline is more consistent in shape. However, when assessing the lungs it is useful to perform the left lateral recumbent view too, as the uppermost lung field is better aerated in lateral recumbency and is therefore more likely to show pathology. Therefore, when investigating known or suspected lung disease (such as a search for metastases) both right and left lateral radiographs with or without a DV or VD view should always be obtained. For cardiac examination, a right lateral and DV view are recommended for consistency of cardiac shape.

If performing radiography under general anaesthesia, the animal should be radiographed as soon as possible after induction, as collapse of the dependent lung area occurs quickly and can mimic pathology. Ideally, the patient should be kept in sternal recumbency until the lateral radiograph is to be taken. Manual inflation of the chest (taking all necessary safety precautions for the person doing this) will be of great benefit in aerating the lungs and improving the image. The kV should be reduced slightly, by about 2–5 kV, for manually inflated lungs.

Lateral view

1. Place the patient in right or left lateral recumbency.
2. Place a radiolucent foam wedge under the sternum to raise it to the same height above the tabletop as the spine (Figure 16.48), thus ensuring that there is no lateral rotation of the chest.
3. Place a sandbag carefully over the neck for restraint if the patient is not anaesthetized.
4. Draw the forelimbs forwards and fix them in place with tapes or sandbags to prevent them from overlying the cranial thorax.
5. Restrain the hindlimbs with a sandbag, extending them slightly caudally.
6. Centre by palpation on the middle of the fifth rib and level with the caudal border of the scapula (slightly caudal to this if manual lung inflation is to be used).
7. Collimate to include lung fields and expose on inspiration for maximum aeration of the lungs.

The trachea, heart, aorta, caudal vena cava, diaphragm, bronchovascular lung markings and skeletal structures can be identified on a lateral view. The oesophagus is not normally visible on plain radiographs.

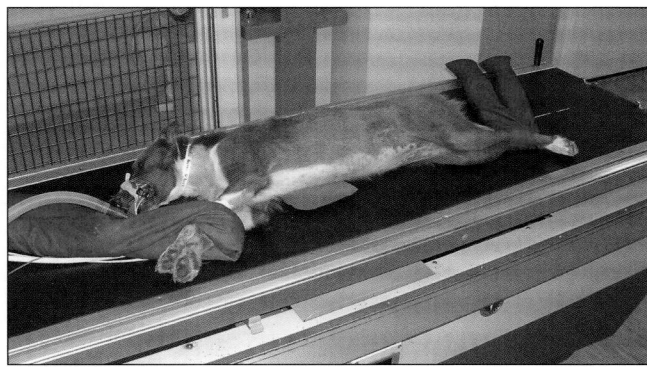

16.48 Positioning for lateral view of the thorax/abdomen.

In a very dyspnoeic patient, a lateral view may be obtained with the patient standing or crouching and using a horizontal X-ray beam. This is safer for the patient than being placed in lateral recumbency. Cats and small dogs may be restrained in narrow cardboard boxes instead of being held; larger dogs can usually be held on the end of a lead with the handler standing well back. Care should be taken with the direction of the primary beam, which should only be directed towards a substantial wall. Although the resulting image will be poor, with the elbow area overlying and obscuring the cranioventral thorax, in such dyspnoeic patients there is usually major thoracic pathology which is still easily visible.

Dorsoventral view

The DV and not the VD view must be used for assessment of the heart, because in the latter position the heart may tip to one side and appear distorted. Animals that are dyspnoeic or may have significant thoracic pathology must not be placed on their backs, and so the DV and not the VD view is required.

1. Position the patient in sternal recumbency, crouching symmetrically (Figure 16.49). This may be difficult in conscious animals that have arthritis of the elbows, hips or stifles.
2. Push the elbows laterally to 'prop' up the dog or cat symmetrically.
3. Drape a sandbag carefully over the neck to keep the head down, shaking the sand into either end to produce a sparsely filled area in the middle of the sandbag. It may be useful to rest the patient's chin on a foam pad or wooden block.
4. Centre in the midline between the tips of the scapulae.
5. Collimate to include the lung fields and expose on inspiration.

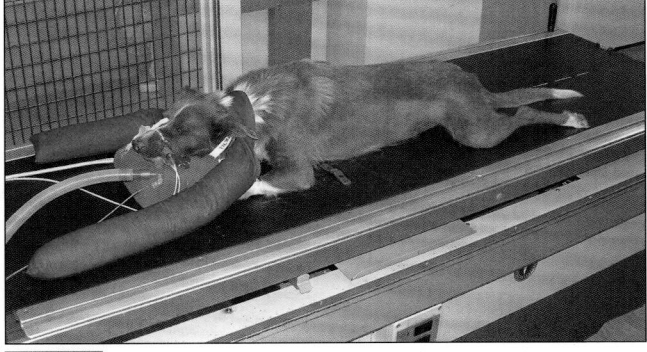

16.49 Positioning for dorsoventral view of the thorax.

The trachea, heart, aorta, caudal vena cava, diaphragm, bronchovascular lung markings and skeletal structures can be identified on a DV view. The oesophagus is not normally visible on plain films.

Ventrodorsal view

1. Position the patient in dorsal recumbency using a radiolucent trough or sandbags around the hind end (Figure 16.50). The hindlimbs may be flexed or 'frog-legged' and supported on foam wedges or sandbags.
2. Ensure that the patient is lying straight and not tipped to one side.
3. Draw the forelimbs forwards with tapes or by placing a sandbag gently over them. Secure the hindlimbs too if necessary.
4. Centre on the mid-point of the sternum, collimate to the lung field and expose on inspiration.

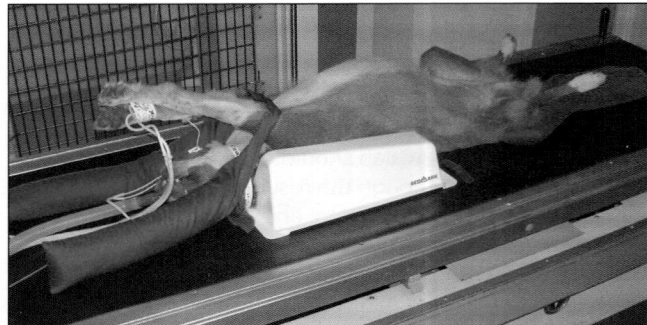

16.50 Positioning for ventrodorsal view of the thorax/abdomen.

The trachea, heart, aorta, caudal vena cava, diaphragm, bronchovascular lung markings and skeletal structures can be identified on a VD view. The oesophagus is not normally visible on plain films.

> **WARNING**
>
> Patients must never be placed on their backs if pleural fluid, pneumothorax or a ruptured diaphragm is suspected, as this may cause respiratory embarrassment

Abdomen
Lateral view

Positioning is similar to that for the thorax.

1. Position the patient in lateral recumbency and pad up the sternum if necessary (see Figure 16.49).
2. Place a sandbag carefully over the neck if the patient is not anaesthetized.
3. Restrain the fore- and hindlimbs with sandbags or ties, ensuring that the hindlimbs are pulled back so that they do not obscure the caudal abdomen.
4. Centre over the area of interest and collimate as necessary. In large dogs, two radiographs may be required to cover the entire abdomen, one for the cranial area and one for the caudal area.
5. Expose on expiration to give a more 'spread out' view of the abdominal viscera.

The liver, spleen, kidneys, bladder, stomach, small and large intestine, and skeletal structures can usually be identified on a lateral view.

Ventrodorsal view

Positioning is similar to that for the thorax.

1. Position in dorsal recumbency using a trough, or by placing sandbags on either side of the chest (see Figure 16.50).
2. Sandbag or tie the fore- and hindlimbs if necessary.
3. Centre and collimate as required and expose on expiration.

The liver, spleen, kidneys, bladder, stomach, small and large intestine, and skeletal structures can usually be identified on a VD view.

DV views of the abdomen are rarely taken, as the viscera are usually compressed and distorted, but they may be all that is possible if the patient is dyspnoeic, or very large and conscious, and cannot be placed on its back.

Skull

Skull views generally require general anaesthesia as accurate positioning cannot otherwise be achieved.

Lateral view

1. Position the animal in lateral recumbency, using small foam wedges under the nose and mandible to ensure that the line between the eyes (interpupillary line, IPL) is vertical and that the midline (median sagittal plane, MSP) is horizontal and parallel to the table (Figure 16.51). The degree of padding depends on the shape of the patient's skull.
2. It may also be necessary to place a pad under the middle of the neck and under the sternum.
3. Centre and collimate as required, according to the shape of the head and the area of interest.

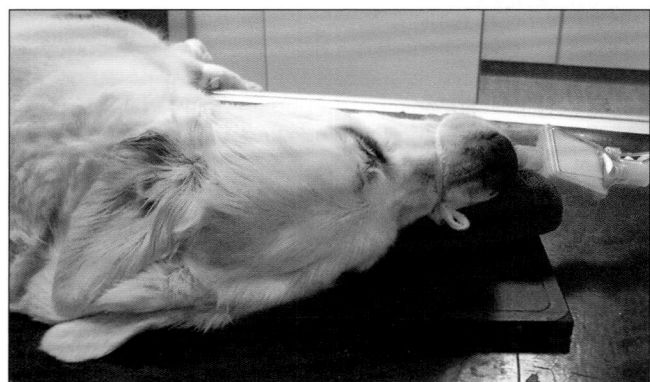

16.51 Positioning for lateral view of the skull.

The cranium, frontal sinuses, nasal cavity, teeth, maxillae, mandibles, temporomandibular joints and tympanic bullae can be identified on a lateral view.

Dorsoventral view

- Place the animal in a symmetrical crouching position, with the chin resting on a wooden or foam block, on which is placed the cassette (Figure 16.52).
- Secure the head with a sandbag draped loosely over the neck if necessary. Ensure that the line between the eyes (interpupillary line, IPL) is horizontal.
- Centre and collimate as required.
- If an endotracheal tube is being used, it may require removal before exposure so as not to obscure any structures in the midline.

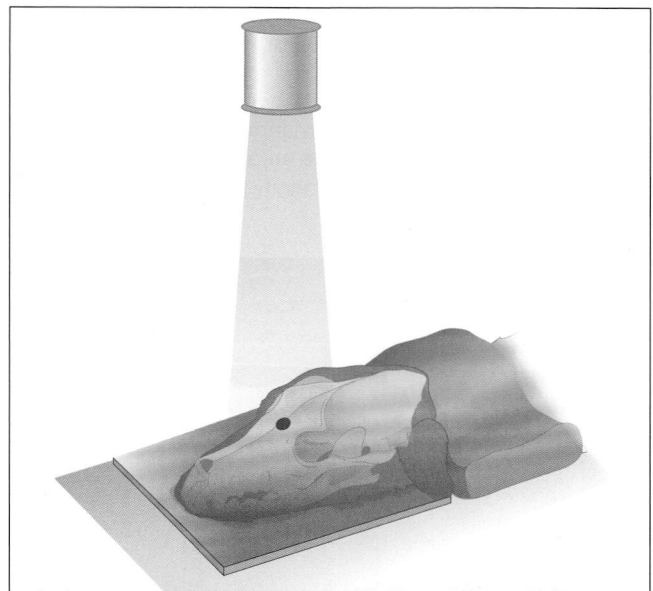

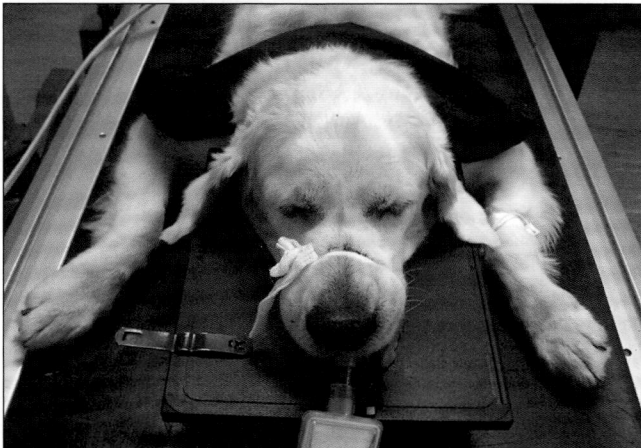

16.52 Positioning for dorsoventral view of the skull. (Illustration reproduced from the *BSAVA Guide to Radiographic Positioning*)

Ventrodorsal view

Symmetrical positioning is more difficult than for the DV view, as facial landmarks are not visible. The DV view is therefore usually preferred, and there is little benefit to a VD.

1. Place the animal in dorsal recumbency in a trough, with the head and neck extended (Figure 16.53).
2. Put foam pads under the neck and nose.
3. Fix the nose down using a tape placed over the chin, or using sticky tape.

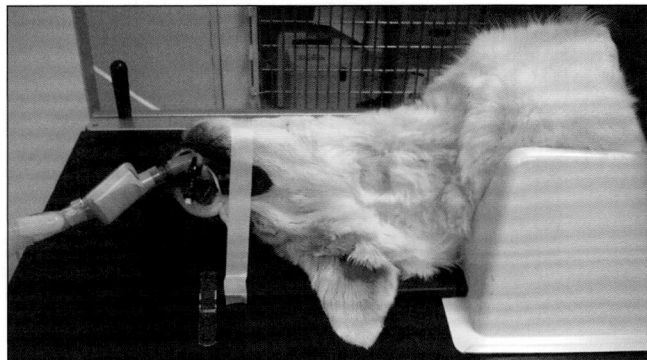

16.53 Positioning for ventrodorsal view of the skull.

Lateral oblique view for tympanic bullae

1. Place the animal in lateral recumbency with the side to be radiographed down.
2. Using foam pads, rotate the skull about 20 degrees around its long axis, towards the VD position (this will skyline the tympanic bulla nearer the table) (Figure 16.54).
3. Centre and collimate by palpation of the bulla, which will now lie ventral to the main part of the skull.
4. It is usually necessary to repeat the procedure for the other bulla, either to give a normal for comparison or to check whether it is also affected. Care should be taken to ensure that the positioning is the same for the two sides.

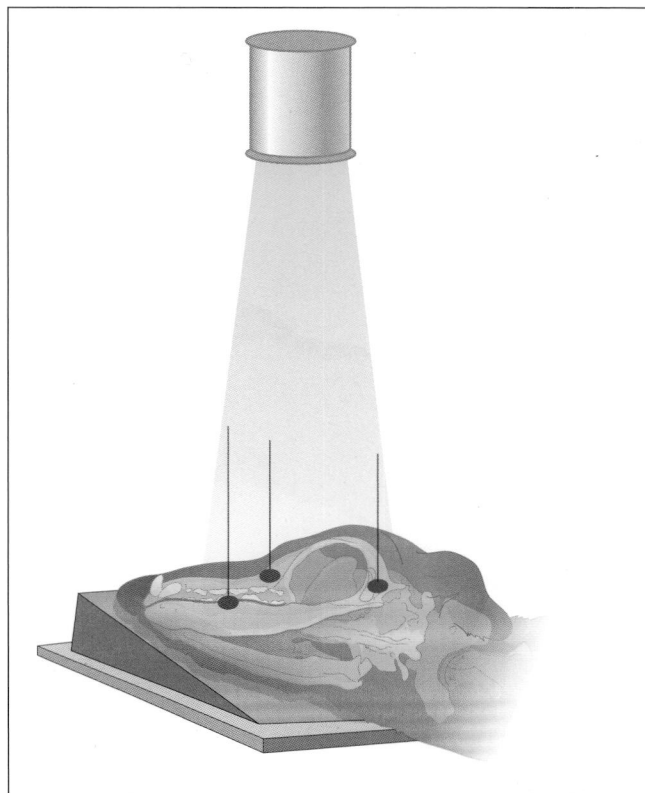

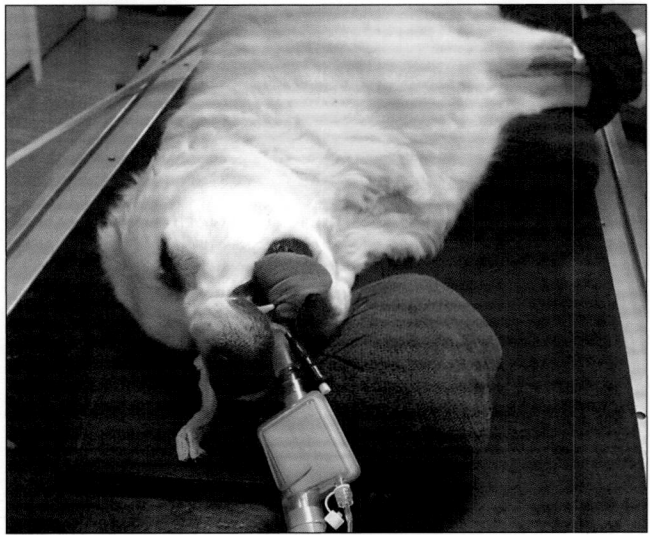

16.54 Positioning for oblique tympanic bullae view. (Illustration reproduced from the *BSAVA Guide to Radiographic Positioning*)

Intraoral DV (occlusal) view for nasal chambers

This view always requires general anaesthesia.

1. Place the animal in sternal recumbency with the chin resting on a wooden or foam block.
2. Insert a small dental non-screen film (cats and small dogs) or a thin, flexible plastic imaging plate holder for use with CR (medium and larger dogs) into the mouth above the tongue, placing it corner first so as to get it as far back in the mouth as possible (Figure 16.55). Dedicated receptors are available for direct digital dental systems.
3. Ensure that the head is level and not laterally tilted by looking for facial landmarks such as the eyes.
4. Centre and collimate over the nasal cavity, bearing in mind the size of the film (or imaging plate if using CR).

placing it corner first so as to get it as far back in the mouth as possible (Figure 16.56). The tongue can be moved so as not to obscure the main area of interest.
3. Ensure that the head is level and not laterally tilted by looking for symmetry of the mandibles.
4. Centre and collimate over the area of interest, bearing in mind the size of the film or imaging plate.

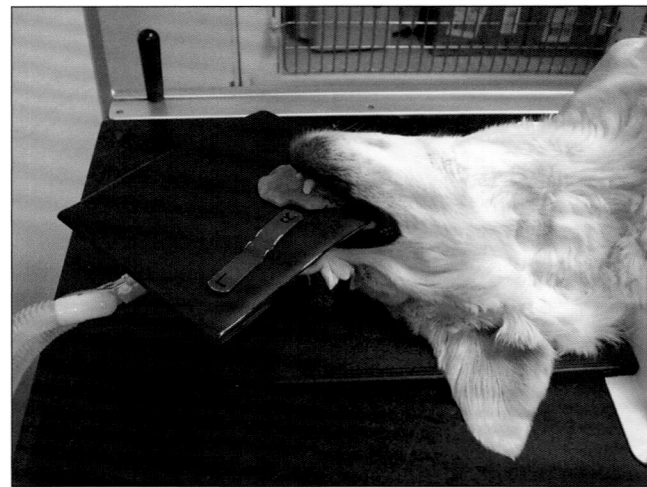

16.56 Positioning for ventrodorsal intraoral view of the mandible.

Other views

A number of other views of the skull are possible but their detailed description is beyond the scope of this chapter. They include special obliques for temporomandibular joints (Figure 16.57), obliques for dental arcades (Figure 16.58) and the frontal sinuses, skyline views of the frontal sinuses (Figure 16.59) and cranium and the rostrocaudal view for tympanic bullae (Figure 16.60) (see 'References and further reading').

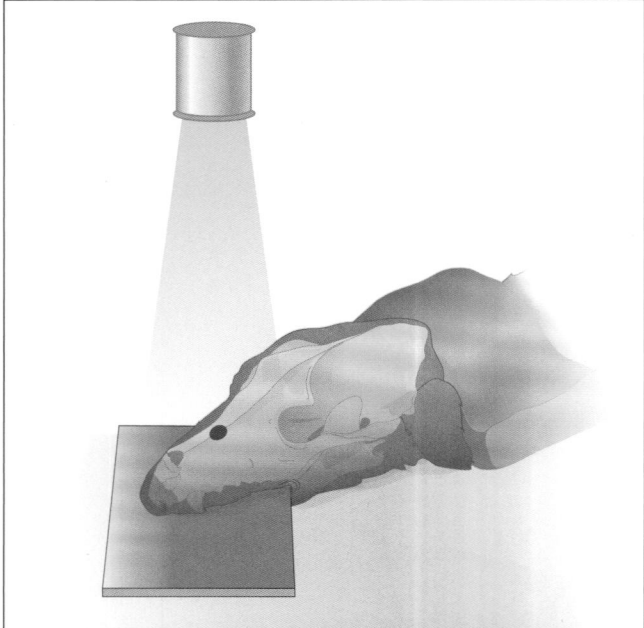

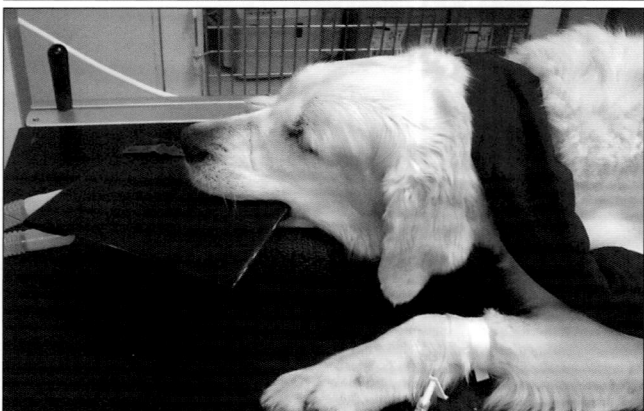

16.55 Positioning for dorsoventral intraoral view of the nasal cavity. (Illustration reproduced from the *BSAVA Guide to Radiographic Positioning*)

Intraoral VD (occlusal) view of the mandible

This view always requires general anaesthesia.

1. Place the animal in dorsal recumbency in a trough.
2. Insert a small dental non-screen film (cats and small dogs) or a thin, flexible plastic imaging plate holder for use with CR (medium and larger dogs) into the mouth,

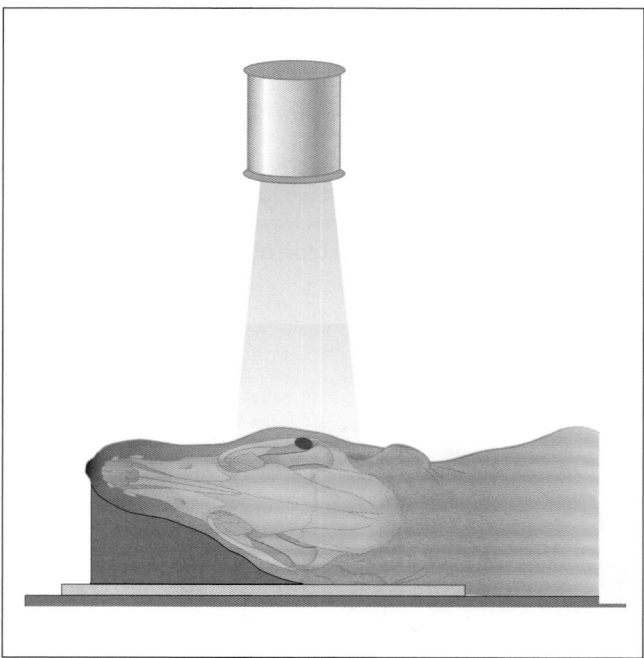

16.57 Positioning for sagittal oblique view of the temporomandibular joint. (Reproduced from the *BSAVA Guide to Radiographic Positioning*)

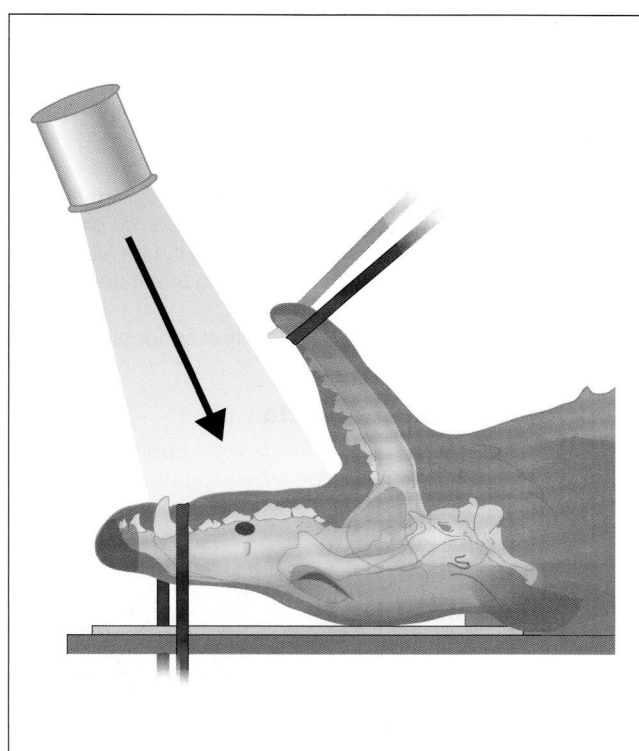

16.58 Positioning for open-mouth oblique view of the upper dental arcade. (Reproduced from the *BSAVA Guide to Radiographic Positioning*)

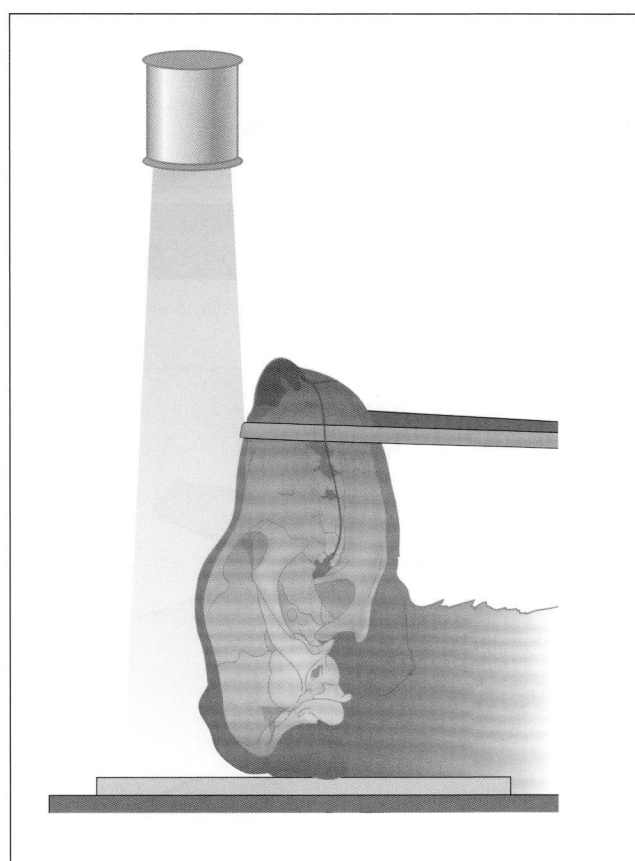

16.59 Positioning for rostrocaudal view of the frontal sinuses. (Reproduced from the *BSAVA Guide to Radiographic Positioning*)

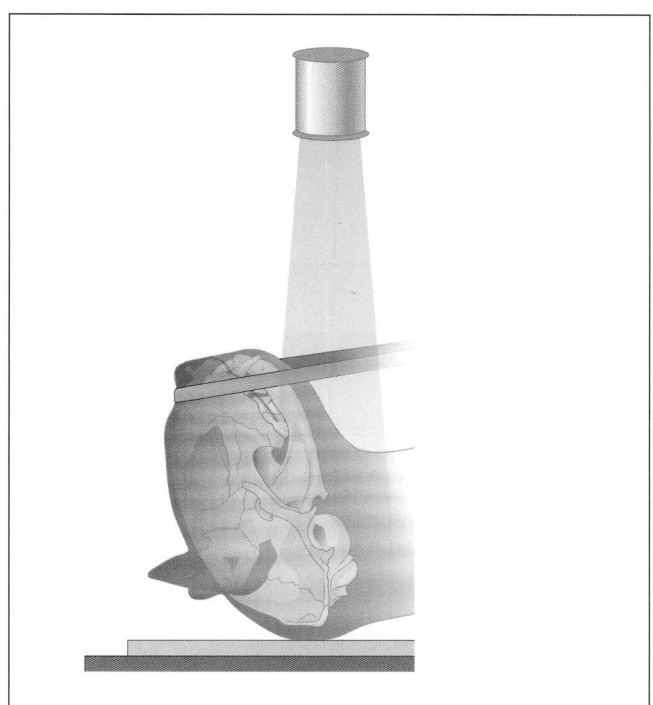

16.60 Positioning for a rostrocaudal view of the tympanic bullae. (Reproduced from the *BSAVA Guide to Radiographic Positioning*)

Spine

Spinal pathology is often undramatic using radiography and therefore requires particularly careful positioning, especially if disc spaces are under scrutiny. General anaesthesia is usually required in order to obtain diagnostic radiographs. Great care should be taken with patients that may have spinal fractures or dislocations in case positioning for radiography causes displacement of the fragments; in such cases, the use of a horizontal beam for VD views could be considered as this will remove the need to roll the patient on to its back.

It is not possible to get an accurate picture of the entire spine on one film, since the X-ray beam is diverging and will not pass equally through all disc spaces, and so it is usually necessary to take several radiographs of smaller areas. In medium and large dogs, up to six films may be required for a spinal survey, as follows: cervical C1–C6; cervicothoracic C6–T3; thoracic T3–T11; thoracolumbar T11–L3; lumbar L1–L7; sacral and caudal (coccygeal) L6–Cd4. Once a lesion is suspected, tightly collimated views taken over the area of interest should be made. For disc disease, only the few disc spaces in the centre of the film are fully assessable (Figure 16.61). It is important to note that many spinal diseases produce minimal or no radiographic changes, and that some apparent radiographic lesions, such as lumbosacral spondylosis, are clinically silent. MRI (see 'Magnetic resonance imaging' below) is a far superior technique for spinal imaging.

Lateral view

Judicious use of foam pads is required to prevent the spine sagging or rotating (Figure 16.62) and to ensure that it forms a straight line parallel to the tabletop. Otherwise, the positioning is similar to that for lateral chest and abdomen views (see Figure 16.48). It is necessary to centre and collimate to the area of interest by the palpation of relevant bony landmarks (in obese animals the spine may be some distance below the skin surface).

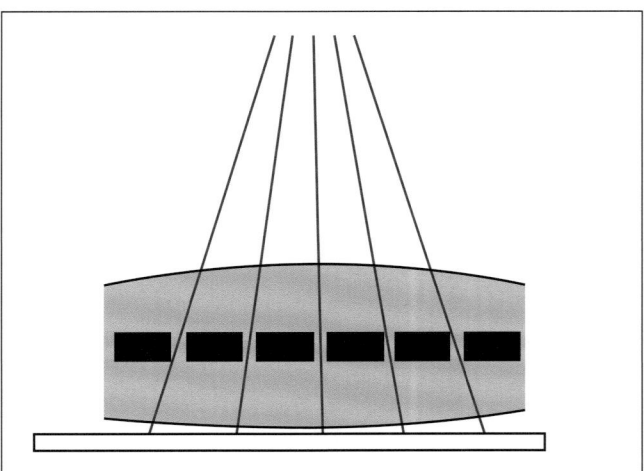

16.61 Radiography of disc spaces. Multiple images of the spine will be required as only the few disc spaces in the centre of the film are fully assessable.

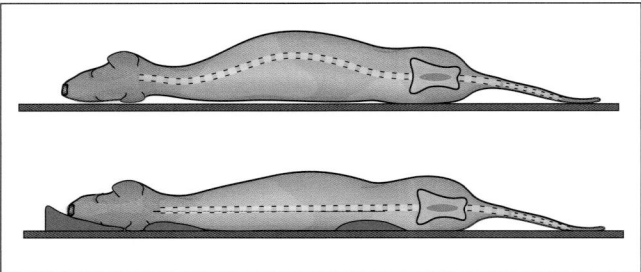

16.62 Use of foam pads for spinal radiography.

Ventrodorsal view

1. Place the animal in symmetrical dorsal recumbency, using a trough or sandbags (similar to positioning for VD chest and abdomen radiographs, see Figure 16.50).
2. Secure the limbs as appropriate.
3. Centre and collimate over the area of interest.
4. For VD views of the caudal cervical spine and cervicothoracic junction, the X-ray beam must be angled 15–20 degrees towards the patient's head in order to pass through the disc spaces, which lie obliquely at this level.

The DV view of the spine is rarely obtained, as the un-avoidably large OFD results in magnification and blurring of the image.

Forelimbs

Although many diagnoses may be possible from a single view (usually the mediolateral), it is often necessary to obtain the orthogonal view as well (i.e. the view at right-angles to this), and sometimes flexed views or obliques are also required. For investigation of suspected joint disease, centre over the joint of interest. Some joint diseases, such as osteochondrosis (OCD), are commonly bilateral and so the opposite limb should be radiographed as well. For long bones, the beam should be centred over the middle of the bone but including the joints above and below, with the long bone parallel to the film. If there is doubt about the significance of a lesion or if the normal length of a bone must be known for a fracture repair, then the opposite limb may be used as a useful control. Note that, except for the scapula and shoulder in giant dogs, a grid is not necessary for forelimb radiography.

Mediolateral (ML) scapula

The scapula is a difficult bone to radiograph, as it is very thin. The distal part of the scapula can be seen on shoulder radiographs, but the following special ML and CdCr views may occasionally be required for the proximal scapula.

1. With the animal lying on the side to be radiographed, pull the lower limb caudally and the upper limb cranially, flexing it towards the head and securing it with a tape. It may also be pushed slightly dorsally so that it lies above the level of the spine.
2. Centre and collimate to the dependent scapula by palpation.

Caudocranial (CdCr) scapula

1. Place the animal on its back in a trough, tipping it slightly over to the side that is not under investigation.
2. Draw the limb cranially and secure in maximum extension with a tape.
3. Centre and collimate to the scapula by palpation.

Mediolateral shoulder

1. With the animal lying on the side to be radiographed, draw the lower limb cranially and secure it with a tie or sandbag (Figures 16.63 and 16.64); pull the upper limb so that it is well back out of the way and secured.
2. Extend the head and neck to reduce the amount of soft tissue overlying the shoulder of interest.
3. Centre and collimate to the dependent shoulder joint by palpation.

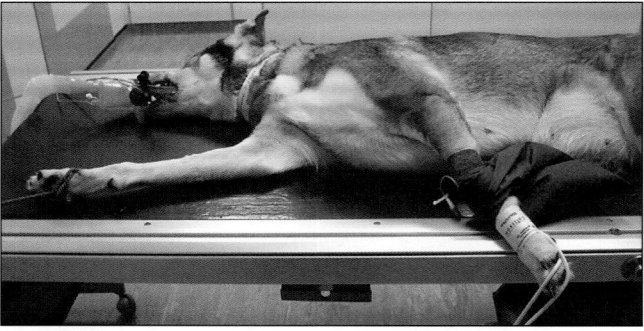

16.63 Positioning for mediolateral forelimb view.

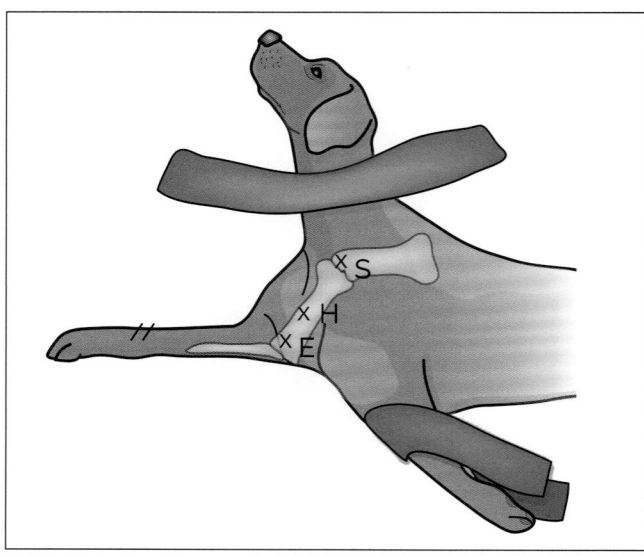

16.64 Centring points (X) for mediolateral forelimb views. E = elbow; H = humerus; S = shoulder.

Caudocranial shoulder

As for caudocranial scapula but centred on the shoulder joint (Figure 16.65).

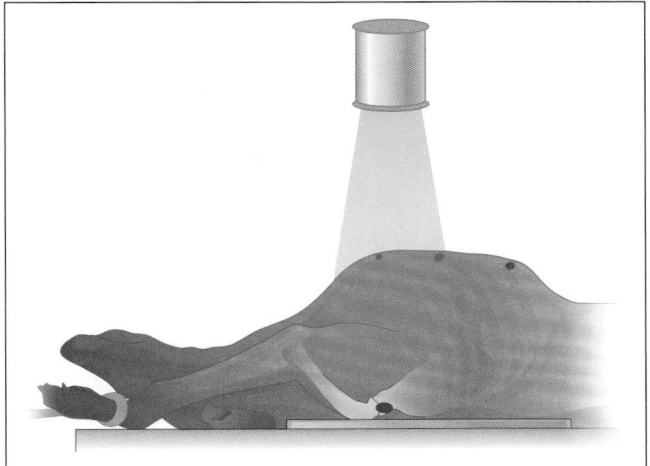

16.65 Positioning for caudocranial view of the shoulder. (Reproduced from the *BSAVA Guide to Radiographic Positioning*)

Cranioproximal-craniodistal (CrPr-CrDi) shoulder

This special oblique view is used to skyline the bicipital groove of the humerus in cases of suspected shoulder teno-synovitis, and is obtained with the shoulder flexed.

1. Place the patient in sternal recumbency (as for a DV chest) and flex the forelimb to be radiographed at the shoulder and elbow, the opposite side of the body being raised on a sandbag and the head displaced away from the shoulder under investigation.
2. Support the cassette above the forearm but beneath the shoulder joint, pushed back to contact the front of the elbow.
3. Centre and collimate to the humeral head by palpation.

Mediolateral humerus

As for the lateral shoulder (see Figures 16.63 and 16.64) but centred on the mid-humerus. Collimate to include both the elbow and shoulder joints.

Caudocranial humerus

As for the caudocranial scapula but centred on the mid-humerus. Collimate to include both the elbow and shoulder.

Craniocaudal humerus

An alternative view. The animal is placed on its back and the limb to be radiographed is pulled caudally, securing with a tape. The humerus should lie parallel to the film. It may not be possible to use a trough for this view.

Mediolateral elbow

Extended view

As for mediolateral shoulder (see Figures 16.63 and 16.64) but centred on the elbow by palpation and collimated to include the distal humerus and proximal radius and ulna.

Flexed view (more useful for assessing degenerative joint diseases)

As for mediolateral shoulder but with the lower limb flexed at the elbow so that the paw comes up towards the patient's chin.

1. Place the animal on its side with the elbow to be radiographed closest to the table.
2. Retract the upper limb caudally and dorsally and secure with a tie, so that it does not overlay the joint to be radiographed.
3. Flex the lower limb so that the angle between the humerus and the antebrachium is 45 degrees and secure with a tape or sandbag (Figure 16.66). Overflexion should be avoided, as this may cause rotation of the limb and distortion of the image.
4. Centre on the condyle of the humerus and collimate the X-ray beam to include approximately the distal third of the humerus and the proximal third of the antebrachium.

For the BVA/KC Elbow Dysplasia Scheme both an extended mediolateral and a flexed mediolateral view are required (see relevant Procedure Notes published by the BVA). Details of image labelling are given below.

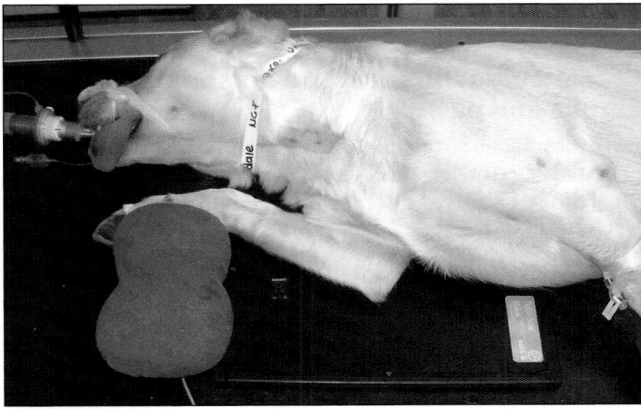

16.66 Positioning for flexed mediolateral elbow view.

Craniocaudal elbow

Position the animal in sternal recumbency with the forelimb to be radiographed extended and pulled cranially, and secured with a sandbag and/or tie. The other forelimb may be allowed to remain more flexed.

Turn the head and neck to the side that is not being radiographed and restrain by draping a sandbag over the neck. Take care that the elbow to be radiographed does not slide sideways (further sandbags and ties may be required) (Figure 16.67).

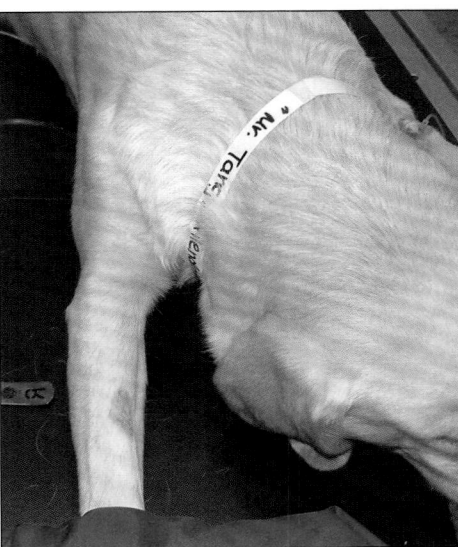

16.67 Positioning for craniocaudal elbow view.

Centre on the elbow joint by palpation, angling the beam about 10 degrees towards the patient's tail in order to demonstrate the joint space. Collimate to include the distal humerus and proximal radius and ulna.

Caudocranial elbow

An alternative view: as for caudocranial shoulder but centred on the elbow joint. However, the large OFD results in some magnification and blurring of the image.

Mediolateral forearm (radius and ulna), carpus and paw

1. With the animal lying on the side to be radiographed, draw the lower limb cranially and the upper limb caudally out of the way (see Figures 16.63 and 16.64).
2. Ensure that a lateral position is achieved, using foam pads or sticky tape.
3. Centre and collimate to the appropriate area.
4. For individual toes, it may be useful to separate them by drawing the affected one forwards and the others backwards with tapes.

Craniocaudal forearm and dorsopalmar (DPa) carpus and paw

As for craniocaudal elbow (see Figure 16.67), but centred and collimated to the appropriate area and using a vertical beam. The limb may be extended using a tie rather than a sandbag, as the latter is radiopaque.

Hindlimbs

Lateral pelvis and hips

The animal is positioned on its side, using foam pads under the spine and sternum to achieve a true lateral position. The beam is centred on the hip joints by palpation of the greater trochanter of the uppermost femur. For medium and large dogs, a grid is required, although no grid is required for more distal parts of the limb.

VD pelvis and hips: extended hip position

This position is described in some detail as it is required for official assessment of hip dysplasia in dogs under the BVA/KC Hip Dysplasia Scheme (see also the relevant Procedure Notes published by the BVA). This position requires general anaesthesia or a reasonable degree of sedation, and perfect positioning may be achieved without the need for manual restraint. For medium and large dogs, a grid is required.

1. Place the animal on its back in a trough, ensuring that the thorax is perfectly upright and not tipped to either side.
2. Extend the forelimbs cranially and secure them with tapes; a sandbag may also be draped over the sternum, taking care not to impair respiration.
3. Extend the hindlimbs caudally, using tapes looped just above the hocks and tied to hooks on the edge of the table. The femora should be parallel to each other and to the tabletop, and the stifles should be rotated inwards by means of a further tape, Velcro® band or bandage tied firmly around them so that they are also parallel (Figure 16.68).
4. Centre on the pubic symphysis at the level of the greater trochanter of the femur, by palpation of these bony landmarks. Generally, the whole pelvis is included in the image but note that it is not necessary to include the stifles in the radiograph; this is a common misconception, but in order to centre over the hips and still include the stifles an unacceptably large area would need to be irradiated.

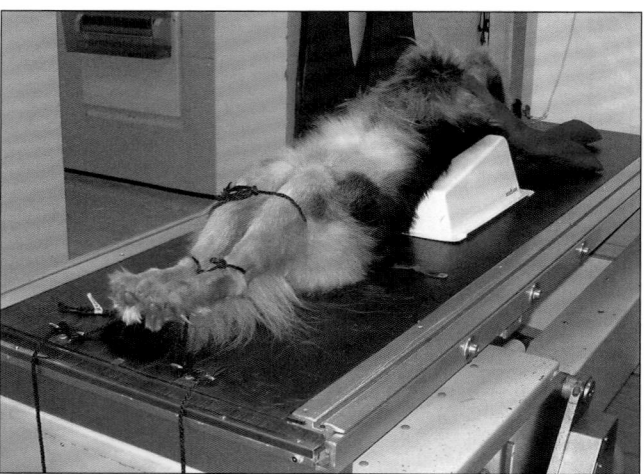

16.68 Positioning for assessment of hip dysplasia: extended ventrodorsal pelvic view.

For submission to the BVA/KC Hip Dysplasia Scoring Scheme, the images must be identified with the patient's Kennel Club number (or other identification if the dog is unregistered), microchip number, the date and a right or left marker. The owner's name must not be included. It should be noted that as from 2018, only DICOM images are accepted for these schemes.

The various anatomical areas of the hip joint assessed under the scoring scheme should all be identifiable; if the image is under- or overexposed certain important features may not be seen and the radiograph may be rejected. Lateral tilting of the pelvis results in the hip joint that has moved up and away from the table appearing falsely deeper (better) than it really is and the hip joint that has moved towards the table appearing shallower (poorer); therefore, the hip score will not accurately reflect the true hip status. This may also result in rejection of the radiograph, especially if the hips are very good and the scrutineers feel that the score on the tilted radiograph will be artificially high (i.e. poor). If the hips are dysplastic, lateral tilting is less important as the score is unlikely to be significantly affected.

PennHIP images

The Pennsylvania Hip Improvement Programme (PennHIP) is a programme designed to assess the hip joints of dogs, with the primary objective of reducing the prevalence of hip dysplasia. Three radiographs are taken from different angles whilst the dog is under anaesthesia. These views – a hip extended view, a compression view and a distraction view – are used to assess hip laxity and to predict the onset of osteoarthritis. Images may be submitted for assessment from animals as young as 16 weeks of age and are used to predict the risk of osteoarthritis in later life

---

VD pelvis and hips: flexed or frog-legged view

This view allows some assessment of the hips but is not as satisfactory as the extended view for assessment of subluxation or mild degrees of arthrosis. The hindlimbs are flexed and allowed to fall to either side. Sandbags may be used to steady the hindpaws (Figure 16.69).

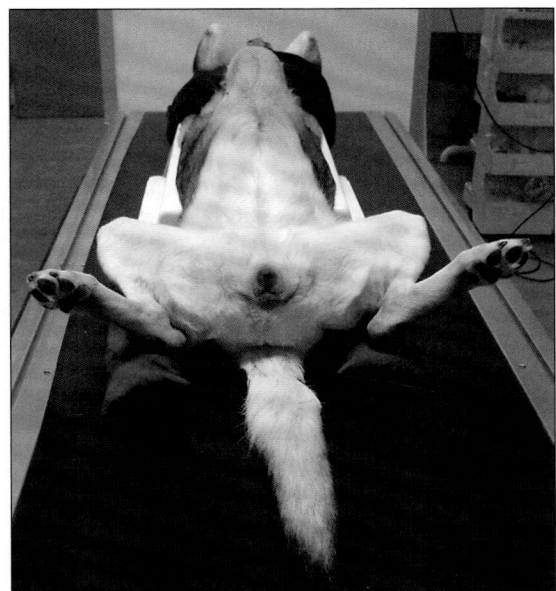

16.69 Positioning for flexed ventrodorsal pelvic view.

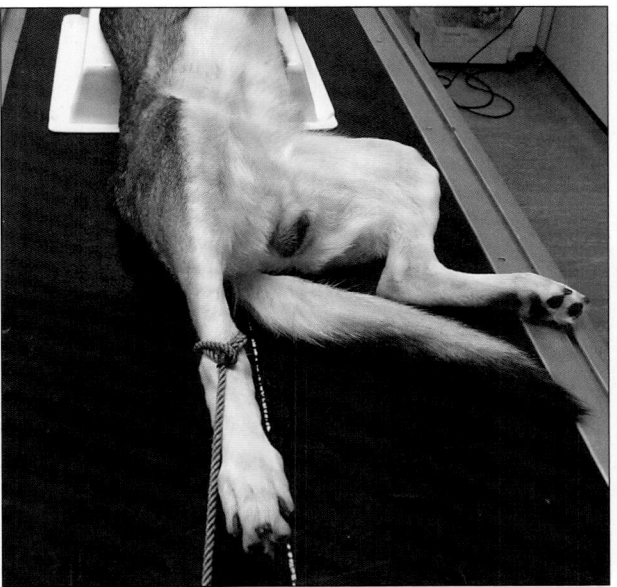

16.70 Positioning for craniocaudal hindlimb views.

VD pelvis and hips: dorsal acetabular rim (DAR) view

This is used to provide measurements prior to triple pelvic osteotomy surgery. The exposure needs to be increased by about 5–10 kV from that used for the extended VD view.

1. Position the dog in sternal recumbency with a trough under its chest.
2. Pull the hindlimbs forwards so that the pelvis is rotated towards a more vertical position and raise the hocks on sandbags.
3. Palpate the pelvis to ensure that it is symmetrical and extend the tail caudally.
4. Centre at the base of the tail.

Mediolateral femur

Two methods are used, both requiring the animal to lie on the side to be radiographed. In the first method the uppermost limb is pulled upwards so that it is roughly vertical, and is secured with tapes or sandbags. It may be difficult to prevent superimposition of part of this limb over the femur under investigation and so an alternative is to pull the lower hind-limb cranially and the upper hindlimb back. In this case the lower femur is radiographed through the soft tissues of the abdomen.

Craniocaudal femur

1. Position the animal in dorsal recumbency in a trough and extend and restrain the limb that is to be radiographed (Figure 16.70).
2. The other hindlimb may be left free.
3. It may be useful to tilt the animal slightly away from the side that is being radiographed to ensure a true craniocaudal view.
4. Centre on the mid-femur by palpation, and collimate to include the hip and stifle.

Mediolateral stifle

1. Position the animal so it is lying on the side to be radiographed (Figure 16.71).
2. Move the other hindlimb upwards or caudally so that it is not superimposed over the lower stifle.

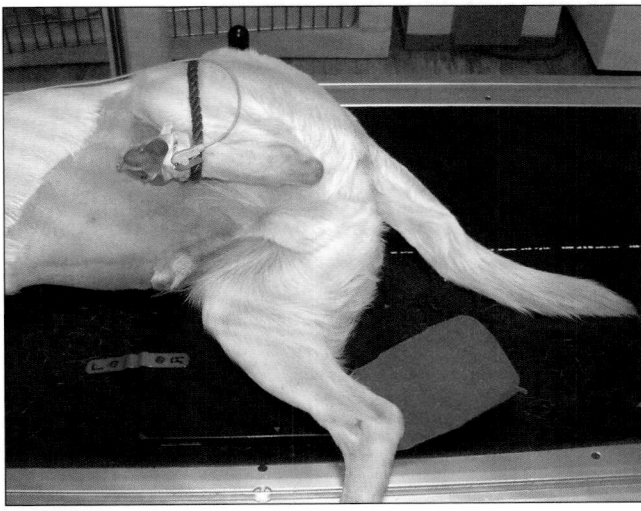

16.71 Positioning for mediolateral stifle view.

3. Ensure that a true lateral view is obtained by placing a small pad under the hock.
4. In obese animals, the mammary tissue or sheath may obscure the stifle joint; this may be prevented by tying a tape around the caudal abdomen to act like a corset.
5. Centre on the stifle by palpation, and collimate to include the distal femur and proximal tibia.

Craniocaudal stifle

This is identical to the extended CrCd femur view (see Figure 16.70), but centring and collimating to the stifle by palpation.

Caudocranial stifle

An alternative view (Figure 16.72), with the animal positioned in sternal recumbency and with the affected limb extended caudally. The opposite side of the animal may need to be raised on sandbags to obtain a true CdCr position. This position results in less magnification and sharper definition of the stifle than with the CrCd view as the stifle is closer to the film, but the joint space may be slightly distorted.

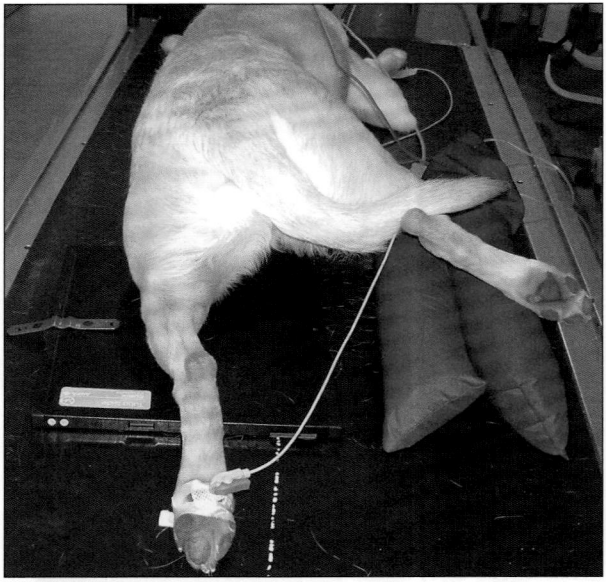

16.72 Positioning for caudocranial stifle view.

Mediolateral tibia, hock and paw

1. The patient lies on the side to be radiographed; the uppermost limb is drawn cranially or caudally to prevent superimposition.
2. Use foam wedges to achieve a true lateral position if necessary.
3. Centre and collimate to the required area by palpation.

Craniocaudal tibia and dorsoplantar hock

As for CrCd stifle, but centred and collimated to the appropriate area (see Figure 16.70). For the hock, the tape is looped around the paw. To reduce the object–film distance for the hock view, it may be necessary to raise the cassette from the table with a wooden block or rectangular foam wedge. The X-ray tube head should be raised by the same amount in order to keep the focal–film distance the same.

Dorsoplantar paw

Two methods are available. The patient may be positioned as above, but with the paw held down to the cassette with strong radiolucent tape. Alternatively, the animal may crouch, with the affected paw pulled slightly outwards and resting on the cassette; this results in a slightly oblique view.

Radiographic contrast studies

Although much information about soft tissues can be gained from good-quality radiographs, certain structures may be unclear either because they are of the same radiographic opacity as surrounding tissue or because they are masked by other structures. In addition, the inner lining (the mucosal surface) of hollow, fluid-filled organs cannot be assessed, because it is of the same radiographic density as the fluid contained within the organ. A good example is the urinary bladder, which appears simply as a homogeneous pear-shaped structure of soft tissue/fluid density on a plain (non-contrast) radiograph.

Contrast studies aim to render these structures and organs more visible and to outline the mucosal surface where appropriate, either by changing the radiopacity of the structure itself or by altering that of the surrounding tissue. Both methods increase the contrast (difference in grey shade) between the structure of interest and the surrounding tissues, allowing assessment of its position, size, shape and internal architecture. If serial films are taken over a period, it may also be possible to gain some idea of the function of the organ, for example the rate of stomach emptying or small intestinal transit time.

Many contrast techniques are possible, but only those of most relevance to veterinary radiography will be discussed.

Types of contrast media

Two broad groups of contrast media exist: positive and negative.

Positive contrast agents

Positive contrast agents contain elements of high atomic number that absorb a large proportion of the X-ray beam and are therefore relatively radiopaque, appearing whiter on radiographs than do normal tissues. They are said to provide positive contrast with soft tissues. The agents most commonly used are compounds of barium (atomic number 56) and iodine (atomic number 53).

Barium sulphate preparations

Barium sulphate is a white, chalky material, which may be mixed with water to produce a fine, colloidal suspension. It is available as a liquid, a paste or a powder that is made up to the desired consistency by the addition of water. It is used for gastrointestinal studies and is not suitable for injection into blood vessels. Being inert, it is non-toxic and well tolerated by the patient and it produces excellent contrast with clear delineation of the lumen of the gut. Its inert nature means that it does not become diluted by body fluids and so it maintains its contrast along the length of the gut. Its main disadvantages are that if it is inadvertently aspirated it may cause pneumonia and if it leaks through a perforated area of gut into the thoracic or abdominal cavities it may provoke the formation of granulomas or adhesions by causing a foreign body reaction. Barium should not be given to constipated patients as it may exacerbate the condition. It should also not be used if surgery is anticipated (e.g. for foreign body removal).

Water-soluble iodine preparations

The iodine compounds are water-soluble and may therefore be injected into the bloodstream. However, anaphylaxis is a possibility (although it is extremely rare) and so an emergency protocol for such an eventuality should be in place. Most of the iodine compounds are excreted by the kidney and they therefore outline the upper urinary tract (kidneys and ureters). They are also safe to use in many other parts of the body, for example the bladder, gut and sinus tracts. Despite being radiopaque, they appear as clear solutions to the eye (unlike barium). Iodine compounds fall into two categories: ionic media, which dissociate in solution; and non-ionic media, which remain as single molecules in solution. The ionic media have a higher osmotic pressure, several times that of normal body fluids. Intravascular injection of ionic media may cause nausea and retching and so the patient must be heavily sedated or anaesthetized. Ionic media must not be used for myelography as they can cause seizures and even death. The non-ionic media were developed in the 1970s for myelography, as their lower osmotic pressure means that they have much less effect on sensitive nervous tissues. They are also suitable for use in all the studies for which the ionic media can be used, although they are more expensive.

Being water-soluble, the iodine preparations are absorbed by the body and so should be used in the gut in preference to barium if there is a possibility of perforation. However, due to their high osmotic pressure, the ionic media absorb fluid during their passage through the gut, with the result that they become progressively diluted and so the pictures they produce have much less contrast than those obtained using barium; there is also a risk of collapse in a dehydrated patient. They are therefore not routinely used for gut studies. Non-ionic iodinated media can be used for gastrointestinal studies and produce an image quality intermediate between that of barium and the ionic iodinated media; non-ionic media should be used if gut perforation is a possibility. Many different water-soluble iodine preparations are available but most ionic media contain diatrizoate, metrizoate or iothalamate as the active ingredients. Non-ionic iodinated media include iohexol and iopamidol.

Negative contrast agents

These are gases, which because of their low density appear relatively radiolucent or black on radiographs, providing negative contrast with soft tissues. Room air is usually used in veterinary radiography although nitrous oxide (N_2O), carbon dioxide (CO_2) or oxygen (O_2) from cylinders may also be used.

Double-contrast studies

Studies on hollow organs may utilize both a positive and a negative agent in a double-contrast study. In these cases, a small amount of positive contrast agent is used to coat the inner lining of the organ, which is then distended with gas. This provides excellent mucosal detail and prevents the obscuring of small filling defects, such as calculi, by large volumes of positive contrast. Examples of commonly performed studies are double-contrast cystography (bladder) and double-contrast gastrography (stomach).

Patient preparation

Adequate patient preparation is essential before many of the contrast studies, which are usually performed as elective procedures. Prior to a barium study of the stomach or small intestine, the animal must be fasted for at least 24 hours to empty the gut of residual ingesta. If food remains in the gut it will mix with the barium, mimicking pathology. Patients should also be fasted prior to studies on the kidneys, as a full stomach may obscure the renal shadows. However, most patients are anaesthetized for these studies and so will have been fasted anyway.

The presence of faeces in the colon will also obscure much abdominal detail and so an enema is often required prior to the contrast study. This is particularly important before investigations of the urinary tract as faeces may obscure or distort the kidneys, ureters, bladder or urethra. The colon must be completely empty of faeces if a barium enema is to be performed as even a small amount of faecal material will produce filling defects, giving the appearance of severe pathology. The patient should therefore be fasted for 24 hours and the colon must be thoroughly washed out with tepid saline or water.

Plain radiographs must always be taken and examined before the contrast study commences. They are assessed for the following factors:

- Any pathology previously overlooked
- Correct exposure factors, to avoid the need to repeat films after the contrast study has begun
- Adequacy of patient preparation
- Assessment of the amount of contrast medium required
- Comparison with subsequent radiographs (to show whether any shadows on the images are due to contrast media or were already present).

Techniques for contrast radiography in dogs and cats

Oesophagus (barium swallow)

Indications

Regurgitation, retching and dysphagia (difficulty in swallowing).

Preparation

No patient preparation required; plain radiographs must be obtained first.

Equipment

- Barium paste is usually preferred as it is sticky and adheres to the oesophageal mucosa for several minutes.
- Barium liquid may be used if paste is not available (5–50 ml, depending on patient size).
- Oral water-soluble iodine preparations should be used if a perforation is suspected.
- Liquid barium mixed with tinned pet food should be used if a megaoesophagus is suspected clinically or on plain radiographs, as paste or liquid alone may fail to fill a dilated oesophagus.

Restraint

Moderate sedation sufficient to allow non-manual restraint is required. Heavy sedation or general anaesthesia is contraindicated because of the possibility of regurgitation and aspiration; in addition, both procedures may induce a transient megaoesophagus.

Technique

Barium paste is deposited on the back of the tongue. Barium or iodine liquids should be given slowly by syringe into the buccal pouch, allowing the patient to swallow a small amount at a time to avoid aspiration. Barium/tinned pet food mixture is often eaten voluntarily, as animals with megaoesophagus tend to be hungry; if not, then the patient may be hand-fed.

Radiographs are taken immediately after administration of the contrast medium. Lateral views are usually sufficient but VD views may also occasionally be indicated. In medium and large dogs two separate radiographs may be needed to cover the cervical and thoracic areas of the oesophagus due to the differences in exposure factors required and the length of the area of interest.

Stomach (gastrogram)

Three techniques are used: air alone (pneumogastrogram), barium alone (positive gastrogram), or barium and air (double-contrast gastrogram). The latter gives better mucosal detail. Gastrography is less often performed now due to the increasing use of endoscopy.

Indications

Persistent vomiting, haematemesis, displacement of stomach and assessment of liver size.

Preparation

Fasting for 24 hours; enema (if necessary); plain radiographs.

Equipment

- Barium liquid (20–100 ml, depending on patient size) unless the study is a simple pneumogastrogram. Note: barium paste and barium/tinned pet food mixtures are not suitable, and oral water-soluble iodine preparations should be used if a perforation is suspected.
- Syringe or stomach tube plus three-way tap.
- Barium impregnated polyethylene spheres (BIPS) are available in capsules and contain a powder that is a mixture of plastic and barium sulphate. They are used to estimate the gastric emptying rate and intestinal transit of food, which is useful when a gastrointestinal obstruction is suspected or when screening patients with chronic vomiting.

Restraint

Moderate sedation (to allow positioning and non-manual restraint); acepromazine has least effect on gut.

Techniques
Pneumogastrogram

This technique may be used to show position and distensibility of the stomach and large gastric masses or foreign bodies, but will not show mucosal detail.

1. Administer the required dose of room air by stomach tube.
2. Take four radiographs: DV, VD, left and right lateral recumbency; each will highlight a different area of the stomach.

Barium gastrogram

This technique will show position of the stomach and the thickness of its wall and may be followed by a small intestinal examination. However, smaller foreign bodies may be 'drowned' by the barium, and mucosal detail will not be shown.

1. Administer the required dose of barium liquid by syringe or stomach tube.
2. Roll the patient to coat the gastric mucosa.
3. Take four radiographs: DV, VD, left and right lateral recumbency; each will highlight a different area of the stomach with barium lying in the lowest part of the stomach and any gas which was present rising to the highest area.
4. Take further radiographs as indicated, e.g. to follow stomach emptying.

Double-contrast gastrogram (DCG)

This technique will give better distension of the stomach than a barium gastrogram, and will show mucosal detail. Small, radiolucent foreign bodies are more likely to be visible as 'filling defects' in the barium or else coated with residual barium after stomach emptying. A DCG is preferred if a definite gastric lesion is suspected, but follow-up radiographs of the small intestine may be hard to interpret because of the presence of the air creating bubbles in the barium.

1. Stomach tube the patient.
2. Give liquid barium, using the syringe and three-way tap, roll the patient (with the stomach tube still in place) and then distend the stomach with room air.
3. Remove the stomach tube and immediately take four views of the stomach as above.

Small intestine (barium series)
Indications

Persistent vomiting, haematemesis, abdominal masses, weight loss, malabsorption and intestinal dilatation (usually unrewarding in cases of chronic diarrhoea).

Preparation, equipment and restraint

As for stomach.

Technique

Liquid barium is administered by syringe or stomach tube. Serial lateral and VD radiographs are taken to follow the passage of barium through the small intestine (usually at intervals of 15–60 minutes, plus a 24-hour radiograph) depending on rate of transit and any pathology seen.

Large intestine

Three techniques are used: air only (pneumocolon), barium only (barium enema), and barium and air (double-contrast enema). A pneumocolon will outline soft tissue masses within the colon and the use of barium alone will demonstrate displacement or compression of the colon, but for most purposes a double-contrast enema is indicated, as it yields maximum information about the colonic mucosa. Large intestinal contrast studies are less often performed now due to the increasing use of endoscopy.

Indications

Tenesmus, melaena, colitis and identification of certain abdominal masses.

Preparation

Fasting for 24 hours; thorough enema (see Chapter 15), using tepid water or saline until no faecal matter returns; plain radiographs.

Equipment

- Cuffed rectal catheter or Foley catheter.
- For pneumocolon: three-way tap and large syringe.
- For barium and double-contrast enemas: gravity feed can and hose or a proprietary barium enema bag; barium sulphate liquid diluted 1:1 with warm water.

Restraint

Moderate to deep sedation or general anaesthesia is required, to allow positioning with non-manual restraint. With anaesthesia a purse-string suture may be used to hold the rectal catheter in place.

Techniques
Pneumocolon

The rectal catheter is positioned and the colon is inflated with room air, using the syringe and three-way tap, until air leaks out around the catheter. Lateral and VD radiographs are taken without removing the catheter.

Barium enema

The rectal catheter is positioned and barium allowed to flow into the colon under gravity, until it just begins to leak out around the catheter (usually 10–20 ml/kg is required). Lateral and VD radiographs are taken without removing the catheter.

Double-contrast enema (DCE)

The barium technique is followed for initial radiographs. Then, excess barium is allowed to drain out and the colon is re-inflated with air. This can be a very messy procedure unless a special barium enema bag is used; when the bag is lowered to the floor the barium drains back down the tube from the colon into the bag. If the bag is then compressed, the air within it will inflate the colon (Figure 16.73).

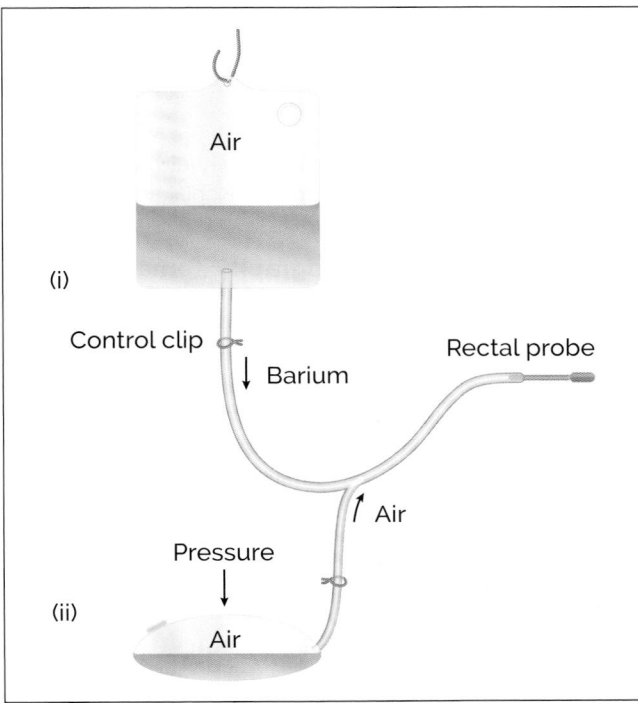

16.73 Barium enema bag. **(i)** In this position, barium flows down into the colon due to gravity. **(ii)** In this position, barium empties from the colon into the bag. Applying pressure to the bag will distend the colon with air to produce the double-contrast effect.

Kidneys and ureters: intravenous urography (IVU) and excretion urography

Contrast radiography of the upper urinary tract involves the intravenous injection of a water-soluble iodine preparation, which is subsequently excreted by, and opacifies, the kidneys and ureters. Two methods are used: rapid injection of a small volume of a very concentrated solution (bolus intravenous urogram) and a slow infusion of a large volume of a weaker solution (infusion intravenous urogram). The bolus IVU produces excellent opacification of the kidneys. The infusion IVU is preferred for investigation of the ureters, as it produces more ureteric distension by inducing a greater degree of osmotic diuresis.

Indications

Identification of kidney size, shape and position, haematuria and urinary incontinence.

Preparation

Fasting for 24 hours; enema; plain radiographs.

Equipment

- Intravenous catheter (perivascular leakage of contrast medium is irritant).
- For bolus IVU: syringe and three-way tap; concentrated contrast medium (300–400 mg iodine/ml) at a dose of up to 850 mg iodine/kg bodyweight, i.e. about 50 ml for a 25 kg dog (if there is poor renal function, the dose may be increased by up to 50% more).
- For infusion IVU: drip giving set; less concentrated contrast medium (150–200 mg iodine/ml) at a dose rate of up to 1200 mg iodine/kg bodyweight, i.e. about 200 ml for a 25 kg dog. Concentrated solutions may be diluted with saline for this study if necessary.

Restraint

General anaesthesia is required to prevent patient nausea and to allow positioning with non-manual restraint.

Techniques
Bolus IVU

1. Warm the contrast medium to body temperature to reduce its viscosity and make it easier to inject.
2. Inject the whole amount as quickly as possible.
3. Take VD and lateral radiographs immediately and at 2, 5, 10 minutes and so on as indicated by the initial images. The VD view is generally more helpful, as the two kidneys are seen without superimposition.

Infusion IVU

If the patient has urinary incontinence and the position of the ureteric endings is being assessed, a pneumocystogram should be performed first to produce a radiolucent background against which the location of the ureters can be seen.

1. Infuse the total dose over 10–15 minutes.
2. Take VD and lateral radiographs once most of the contrast medium has run in.
3. Oblique radiographs are also useful for ureteric endings.

Bladder (cystography)

Direct or retrograde cystography may be performed in three ways: using negative contrast alone (pneumocystogram), positive contrast alone (positive contrast cystogram) or a combination of the two (double-contrast cystogram). Non-ionic iodine media are preferred for the positive and double-contrast studies, as they are less irritant to inflamed bladder mucosa than the ionic media. Pneumocystography is quick and easy but gives poor mucosal detail and will fail to demonstrate small bladder tears, as air leaking out will resemble intestinal gas. Positive contrast cystography is ideal for the detection of bladder ruptures but will mask small lesions and calculi. Double-contrast cystography is usually the method of choice, as it produces excellent mucosal detail and will demonstrate all types of calculi as filling defects in the 'contrast puddle'. A positive contrast cystogram will also be seen following an IVU, if the patient cannot be catheterized for any reason. Excreted contrast should be mixed with urine already present in the bladder by rolling the animal. This type of cystogram is not ideal, as adequate bladder distension cannot be ensured.

Indications

Haematuria, dysuria, urinary incontinence, urinary retention, suspected bladder rupture, identification of the bladder if not visible on the plain radiograph and assessment of prostatic size.

Preparation

Enema (see Chapter 15), if faeces are present; plain radiographs.

Equipment

- Appropriate urinary catheter.
- Syringe and three-way tap.
- Dilute water-soluble iodine contrast medium for positive and double-contrast cystogram.

Restraint

Sedation or general anaesthesia is required to allow catheterization and positioning using non-manual restraint.

Techniques

The bladder is first catheterized (see Chapter 15) and drained completely of urine, obtaining a sterile urine sample if required.

Pneumocystogram

The drained bladder is inflated slowly with room air, using a syringe and three-way tap. The bladder should be inflated until it is felt to be moderately firm by abdominal palpation (usually requires 30–300 ml air, depending on patient size). It is important to avoid overdistension, especially if the bladder may be fragile or in cats with cystitis in which mucosal sloughing may occur.

Positive contrast cystogram

Procedure as for pneumocystogram but using diluted iodine contrast medium instead of air. However, for detection of bladder rupture, a much smaller quantity is required.

Double-contrast cystogram (DCC)

1. Inject 2–15 ml iodine contrast medium (depending on patient size) at a concentration of approximately 150 mg iodine/ml into the empty bladder via the catheter.
2. Palpate the abdomen or roll the patient to coat the bladder mucosa.
3. Inflate with air until the bladder feels turgid.
4. The bladder wall will be lightly coated with positive contrast, and residual contrast will pool in the centre of the bladder shadow, highlighting calculi and other filling defects.

Lateral radiographs are usually more informative, but VD and oblique views may be taken if required.

Urethra: retrograde urethrography (males) and retrograde vagino-urethrography (females)

These studies are less frequently performed in cats than in dogs, but may be carried out using simple cat catheters.

Indications

Haematuria, dysuria, urinary incontinence, urinary retention, prostatic disease and vaginal disease.

Preparation

Enema (see Chapter 15), if faeces are likely to obscure the urethra on either view; plain radiographs.

Equipment

- Appropriate urinary catheter.
- Syringe.

- Dilute iodine contrast medium (150 mg iodine/ml) (may be mixed with an equal amount of K-Y jelly for studies on male dogs, to increase urethral distension).
- Gentle bowel clamp (for bitches).

Restraint

Sedation (dogs) or general anaesthesia (bitches, cats).

Techniques
Retrograde urethrography (males)

1. Insert the urinary catheter into the penile urethra.
2. Occlude the urethral opening manually, to prevent leakage of contrast.
3. Inject 1 ml/kg bodyweight contrast or contrast/K-Y jelly mixture slowly.
4. Release the urethral occlusion and stand back prior to exposure (or make the injection via an extension tube wearing lead mittens and an apron, and ensuring tight collimation to exclude the hands).

Lateral views are most useful and should be taken with the hindlimbs pulled forwards for the ischial arch and backwards for the penile urethra.

Retrograde vaginourethrography (females)

1. Snip off the tip of a Foley catheter, distal to the bulb.
2. Insert the catheter just inside the vulval lips, inflate the bulb and clamp the vulval lips together with the bowel clamp to hold the catheter in place. In cats a non-cuffed catheter is used.
3. Carefully inject up to 1 ml iodine contrast medium/kg bodyweight (vaginal rupture has been reported).

Lateral views are most informative and demonstrate filling of the vagina and urethra.

Spine (myelography)

A narrow gap surrounds the spinal cord as it runs along the vertebral column; this is called the subarachnoid space and it contains cerebrospinal fluid (CSF). It may be opacified by the injection of positive contrast medium and will then demonstrate the spinal cord, showing areas of cord swelling (e.g. tumours) or cord compression (e.g. prolapsed intervertebral discs) not evident on plain radiographs. This technique, which is called myelography, requires the use of non-ionic water-soluble iodine preparations, which have lower osmotic pressures than do the ionic iodine media and which are therefore less irritant to nervous tissue. The two low osmolar contrast media currently used in veterinary myelography are iohexol and iopamidol.

Two approaches may be made to the subarachnoid space. The one most commonly used in veterinary radiology is the cisternal puncture, where the needle is inserted into the cisterna magna – the wide cranial end of the subarachnoid space just behind the skull. Myelography may also be performed by injection in the lumbar area via a lumbar puncture, which is more commonly used in humans. Lumbar myelography involves passing the needle through the cauda equina (the termination of the spinal cord) and injecting into the ventral subarachnoid space. Both techniques involve practice and skill and the patient must be anaesthetized to prevent movement during needle placement or injection.

Myelography is sometimes used in conjunction with CT; however, it has been largely replaced by MRI, as the latter is safer and gives much more information about the different spinal tissues.

Indications

Spinal pain, spinal neurological signs (ataxia, paresis or paralysis) and identification of location of prolapsed intervertebral discs prior to surgery.

Preparation

Clip relevant area, i.e. caudal to skull or over lumbar spine.

Equipment

- Spinal needle of suitable length, depending on patient size.
- Contrast medium, warmed to body temperature to reduce viscosity and ease injection (dose rate 0.25–0.45 ml/kg of 200–350 mg iodine/ml solution – dose administered depends on size of patient and expected site of lesion but no more than a maximum of 15 ml).
- Syringe.
- Sample bottles for CSF if required for analysis.
- Some means of elevating the head end of the table for cisternal punctures, to aid flow of contrast along the spine.

Restraint

General anaesthesia is essential.

Techniques
Cisternal puncture

1. Elevate the table to about 10 degrees of tilt, with the animal's head at the raised end.
2. Clip and surgically cleanse the injection site.
3. The veterinary surgeon will flex the head to an angle of 90 degrees to the neck. It is then held by an assistant, e.g. the veterinary nurse.
4. The veterinary surgeon will insert the needle carefully between the skull and atlas vertebra (Figure 16.74; see also Chapter 17), advancing the needle slowly until CSF drips out of the hub when the needle is in the cisterna magna.
5. Several millilitres of CSF will be collected. The veterinary surgeon will then slowly inject warmed contrast medium. The syringe plunger should be withdrawn very slightly at intervals to check that CSF flows back into the syringe, confirming that the tip of the needle is still in the correct place.
6. The needle is removed by the veterinary surgeon and the head is extended again.
7. Several lateral radiographs are taken, either until contrast medium reaches the lesion or until the whole spine is shown well. VD and oblique views may also be

taken, especially if a lesion is found. Improved filling of the subarachnoid space in the lower neck area can be ensured by obtaining DV rather than VD views of this area. When the animal is on its back for the VD view, this area is furthest from the table and contrast medium runs cranially and caudally away from the area of interest; with the dog in sternal recumbency, this area is closest to the table and therefore contrast medium pools here.

Lumbar puncture

1. Clip and surgically cleanse the injection site in the caudal lumbar area.
2. Flex the vertebral column by pulling the hindlimbs forwards; the animal may be in lateral or sternal recumbency depending on preference.
3. The veterinary surgeon will insert the needle carefully (usually at L5–6 for dogs and L6–7 for cats); as it passes through the cauda equina, the animal's hindlimbs and anus will usually twitch slightly. Little or no CSF may appear from this site and if this is the case a small test injection is required to check needle placement.
4. The veterinary surgeon injects contrast medium.
5. The needle is removed and the spine is extended again.
6. Radiographs are taken as above.

> **WARNING**
>
> It is important that the veterinary nurse keeps the animal's head raised during the recovery period after cisternal or lumbar myelography, since contrast medium entering the brain may precipitate fits

Other contrast techniques

Some other contrast techniques occasionally performed in small animals are described briefly.

Portal venography

Portal venography is used to diagnose certain types of liver disease (e.g. congenital portosystemic shunts, cirrhosis and acquired shunts) by demonstration of the vascular system within the liver parenchyma. Under general anaesthesia, a laparotomy is performed and a splenic or mesenteric vein is catheterized. A small quantity of concentrated iodine contrast medium is injected as a bolus and a single radiograph, either lateral or VD depending on preference, is taken at the end of the injection. The contrast medium enters the liver via the hepatic portal vein and in the normal animal shows branching and tapering portal vessels throughout the liver. In the case of a congenital shunt the liver is bypassed by an anomalous vessel, which connects to the caudal vena cava or azygos vein; with acquired shunts numerous small and tortuous vessels are seen between the hepatic portal vein and the caudal vena cava.

Arthrography

Arthrography is the demonstration of a joint space using negative contrast (air), positive contrast (iodine) or double-contrast techniques injected under sterile conditions. The joints most amenable to arthrography in small animals are the shoulder and stifle. General anaesthesia is required as the procedure is uncomfortable. Arthrography will demonstrate joint capsule distension or rupture, and defects in the articular cartilage, which is normally radiolucent. A sample of synovial fluid may also be collected for analysis.

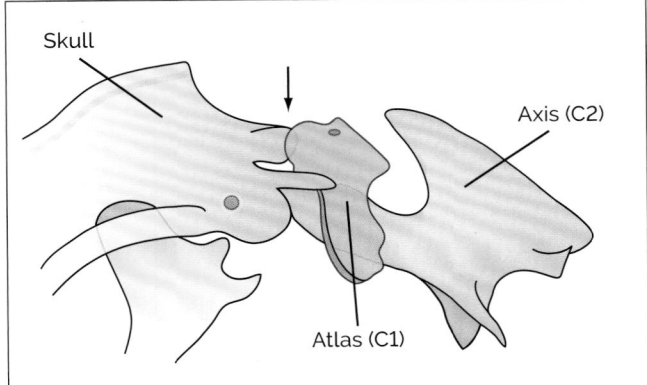

Skull

Axis (C2)

Atlas (C1)

16.74 Myelography: site for cisternal puncture (arrowed).

Dacryocystorhinography

Dacryocystorhinography uses opacification of the naso-lacrimal duct in order to demonstrate strictures, rupture, foreign material and communication with cystic maxillary structures. Under general anaesthesia, one of the nasolacrimal puncta in the eyelids is cannulated and a small quantity of warmed, non-ionic iodine contrast medium is instilled. Lateral views are usually most helpful.

Fistulography/sinography

Fistulography and sinography use the opacification of fistulae and sinus tracts by water-soluble iodine contrast media injected via cuffed catheters. They demonstrate the extent and course of these lesions and may outline radiolucent foreign bodies such as pieces of wood. These techniques have largely been superseded by MRI, which gives much more information about the soft tissues.

Angiography

Angiography comprises the opacification of blood vessels by injected iodine contrast medium and a rapid series of radiographic exposures made immediately after injection. It demonstrates the location and size of arteries (arteriography) or veins (venography), depending on the site of deposition of the contrast medium. Although still used in humans for the investigation of cerebral aneurysms and varicose veins, its applications in veterinary patients are extremely limited, with the exception of portal venography (described above). It has been largely superseded in both medical and veterinary diagnosis by ultrasonography, CT and MRI.

Radiography of exotic species

Most of the exotic species seen in general practice are smaller than the more commonly seen cats and dogs. The smaller size of the species means lower voltages (kV) are generally used, particularly in small mammals and birds. In chelonians, however, the kV may need to be disproportionately greater per kilogram of bodyweight, due to the density of the bony shell. Grids are rarely, if ever, used in commonly seen exotic species as few patients are >10 cm in depth. Due to the smaller size of these patients, non-screen films may be more helpful in demonstrating the finer details of their anatomy. In general, these types of film require a higher amperage (mAs). Alternatively, rare-earth intensifying screens and so-called 'detail' films (high-definition, fine-grain films) can be used.

For most small exotic pets, particularly birds, mammals, snakes and lizards, a radiography unit capable of a range of 40–70 kV with a rapid exposure time of 0.008–0.016 seconds is helpful. The rapid exposure time is important, as many small mammals in particular have rapid respiration rates and therefore longer exposures can lead to blurring of the image produced.

It may also be useful to have a radiography unit that has the facility to alter the focal–film distance, as reducing the distance can allow some magnification of the image produced, which may be of help when imaging very small patients.

Smaller radiographic units, such as human dental machines, are beneficial. They generally operate on a fixed voltage and amperage, the only variable being the exposure time, which may be varied from 0.1 to 3 seconds on modern digital machines. This will allow the fine detail imaging of distal limbs and the head, and, if combined with non-screen dental film, can provide superior imaging to standard veterinary radiography. Because of longer exposure times patients generally have to be restrained chemically to avoid motion blurring of the image.

Positioning and restraint

Small mammals

The usual two views (a lateral and a VD or DV view; Figure 16.75ab) for small mammals are advisable in order to build up a three-dimensional picture. In addition, further specialist views may be useful. For example, in rabbits and chinchillas particularly, where dental disease is a common problem, oblique lateral views (Figure 16.75c) with contrast medium injected into the lacrimal ducts may help to highlight dental and nasolacrimal disease (see Chapter 25).

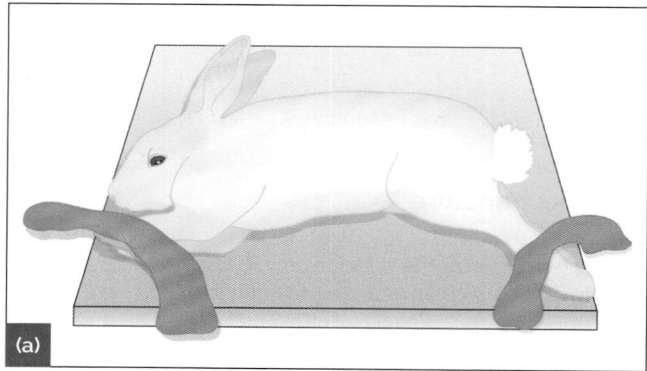

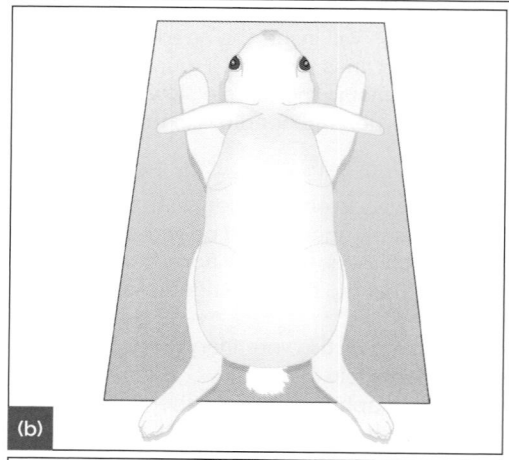

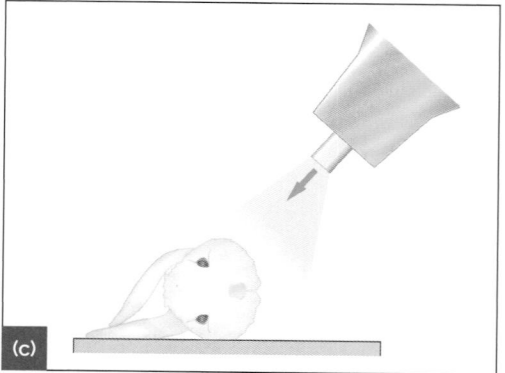

16.75 Positioning a rabbit for radiography. **(a)** Right lateral view: the limbs are drawn away from the body. **(b)** Standard dorsoventral whole body view. **(c)** Oblique lateral dental arcade and head view. (Reproduced from the *BSAVA Manual of Rabbit Medicine and Surgery, 2nd edn*)

Rabbits also commonly suffer from otitis media, and DV views specifically focusing on the auditory bullae are necessary to confirm the presence of disease. Skyline views of the frontal sinuses and craniocaudal views of the skull may also be used where disease is suspected in sinuses or in the temporomandibular joints. Advanced imaging techniques (CT and MRI) may be used instead or as well as radiography in these cases.

Dental disease is also common in ferrets, and bisecting angle radiographs as used in cat and dog dental radiography are helpful to obtain an accurate image of the roots of affected teeth.

Birds

As with small mammals, two views are essential and these usually comprise a lateral (generally a right lateral) and a VD view (Figure 16.76). For the lateral view the wings are pulled dorsally away from the body to prevent superimposition. It is advisable to anaesthetize the patient to prevent struggling and minimize stress.

These two views are suitable for imaging the body cavity, but they actually result in exactly the same view for the wings, i.e. a VD view. To obtain a caudocranial view of the wing, it is necessary to position the patient vertically. This is achieved by positioning the anaesthetized and intubated bird's head downwards and extending the wing over the radiographic cassette, which can be challenging.

It may also be necessary from time to time to perform skyline views of the skull when examining the sinuses for signs of disease.

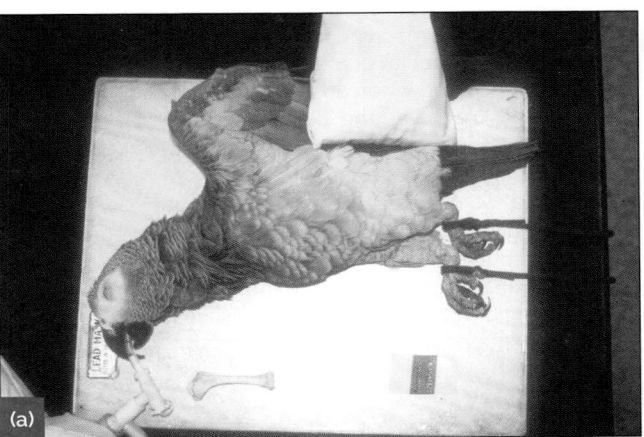

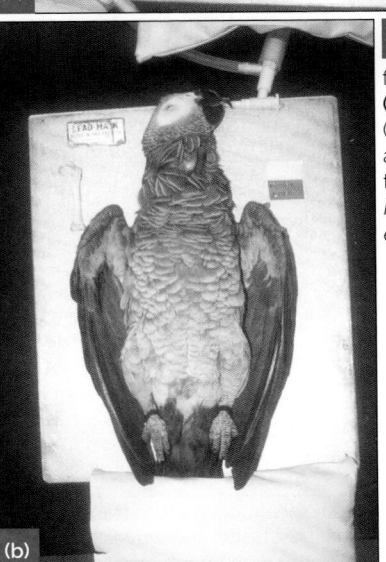

16.76 A Grey Parrot positioned for **(a)** lateral and **(b)** ventrodorsal views. (© Nigel Harcourt-Brown and reproduced from the *BSAVA Manual of Psittacine Birds, 2nd edition*)

Reptiles

Chelonians may be immobilized by propping up the centre of the plastron, for example with tin cans or upturned feeding bowls, so that the legs cannot reach the ground (Figure 16.77). Snakes can be encouraged to enter a clear plastic tube to restrain them for such procedures, but the tube itself will reduce the clarity of the image produced. Lizards, and some snakes, may be placed into a hypotonic immobility by using the vagovagal response. This is where pressure applied gently to the eyes stimulates the vagal nerve and results in a slowing of respiration, heart rates and a semi-sedated state. Pressure may be maintained by placing cotton-wool balls over the closed eyes and wrapping them in place with bandage material. Chemical restraint should be used for fractious animals or dangerous species.

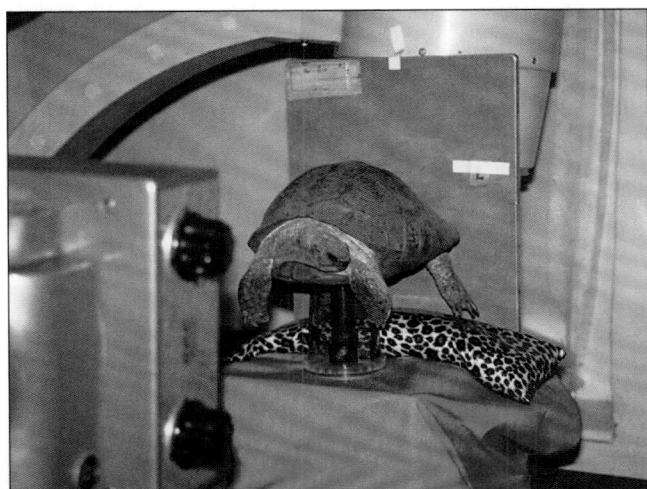

16.77 Tortoises can be propped up by the plastron to keep them immobile during radiography. (Courtesy of Mike Jessop)

Due to the absence of a diaphragm in reptiles, the lungs are fully collapsible (unlike birds, where the lungs are relatively rigid in structure). It is therefore advisable to use horizontal beam radiography when performing lateral radiography, to avoid the viscera obscuring the lung fields. This allows the assessment of the lung fields and viscera in their normal positions without superimposition.

A DV view is also necessary to provide a three-dimensional picture, and in chelonians a third view, the craniocaudal view (again using horizontal beam radiography), is helpful. This is because the chelonian lungs sit in the most dorsal part of the carapace. Lateral horizontal beam radiographs will allow the lungs to be examined, but the right and left lung fields are superimposed on each other. The DV view in chelonians provides little information on the lungs due to their superimposition on the ventrally situated viscera. Therefore, to compare left and right lung fields a craniocaudal horizontal beam radiograph (with the X-ray beam centred on the nuchal scute just behind the head) can be performed.

In snakes, it is not advisable to allow the snake to coil up on the cassette, as this distorts the anatomy and makes interpretation difficult. The snake should instead be stretched out; if necessary, sequential sections of body can be radiographed. It is helpful to place radiodense markers on the dorsal body wall when performing lateral radiographs, and on the lateral body wall when performing DV radiographs to help with the accurate localization of any abnormalities found.

Ultrasonography

Diagnostic ultrasonography is common in small animal practice as a complementary imaging tool to radiography. Ultrasound imaging can be performed on the conscious patient using manual restraint without the need for sedation or anaesthesia (Figure 16.78), although nervous or tense animals may be more easily scanned under some form of chemical restraint, especially for abdominal ultrasonography when a better image is usually obtained in a more relaxed patient. Ultrasonography requires clipping of the hair, unless the coat is sparse or can be parted; the owner should be warned of this before the procedure is undertaken.

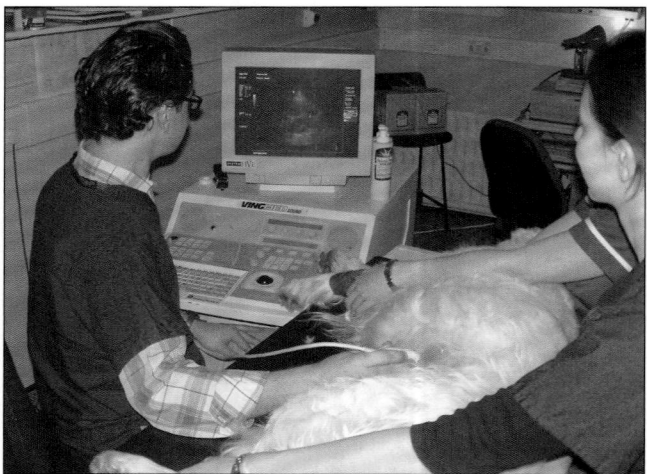

16.78 Ultrasonography of a conscious patient.

Ultrasonography can differentiate soft tissue from fluid, which radiography cannot, and shows the internal architecture of soft tissues that appear homogeneous on radiography. Unlike a conventional radiograph, the ultrasound image is a 'real-time' or moving picture, which is invaluable in the assessment of cardiac function and of peristalsis, and it therefore gives information about the function of certain organs. The applications of ultrasonography are continually advancing, and very small structures such as the adrenal glands, pancreas and lymph nodes, which were once thought to be beyond detection with ultrasonography, are now routinely examined. Furthermore, ultrasonography allows guided biopsy or fine-needle aspiration of very small lesions deep within the patient, and often avoids the need for a more invasive diagnostic procedure.

The main disadvantage is that ultrasound does not penetrate bone or air so it cannot usually be used for investigations of the skeletal system or lungs, with the exception of examination of superficial lesions. Bone reflects all of the incident ultrasound, resulting in 'acoustic shadows' or radiating black streaks in deeper tissues (Figure 16.79), whereas air in normal aerated lungs creates reverberations.

Ultrasonography is a difficult technique to master, since experience is required both to obtain and to interpret the images. Unlike radiographs, MR and CT images, ultrasound scans are not suitable for remote interpretation, since frozen images lose much of their value and much of the interpretation depends on hand–eye coordination of the operator. However, some simple interpretations, such as pregnancy, pericardial effusion, large abdominal masses or ascites, may be made even by relatively inexperienced operators. A range of normal and abnormal ultrasound images are presented in the *BSAVA Manual of Canine and Feline Ultrasonography*.

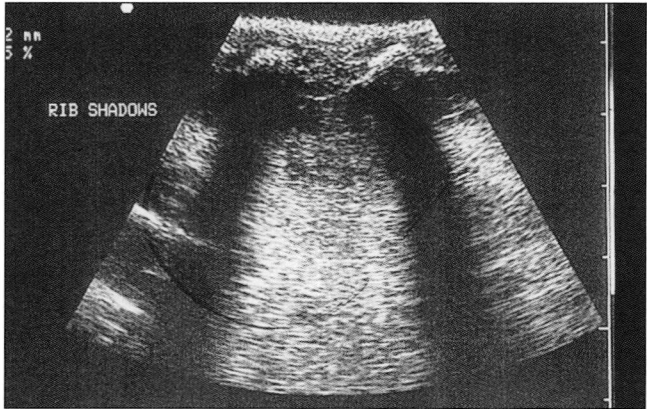

16.79 Acoustic shadows created by ribs.

Principles of ultrasonography

Ultrasound is sound energy at a higher frequency than can be detected by the human ear. In the diagnostic range, the frequencies used range from about 2.5 to 15 megahertz (MHz). Ultrasound of higher frequency produces better image resolution but cannot penetrate as far into the body as lower frequencies, and so the highest frequency compatible with the type of study and the patient is selected. For abdominal ultrasonography of larger dogs, a 5 MHz transducer is used. For rabbits, cats and smaller dogs, 7.5 MHz may be preferred; and for very superficial examinations, such as of the eye or tendons, transducers of 10 MHz or higher are needed.

In an ultrasound machine the sound waves are created by the vibrations of special crystals in the probe or transducer that alter their shape when an electrical current is applied to them. This is known as the piezoelectric effect. When the transducer is applied to the patient's skin, the sound waves are passed through the patient's soft tissues as pressure waves, and at interfaces between tissues or between clusters of different cells within an organ a certain percentage of the sound waves are reflected and may return to the transducer (Figure 16.80). Returning sound waves in turn

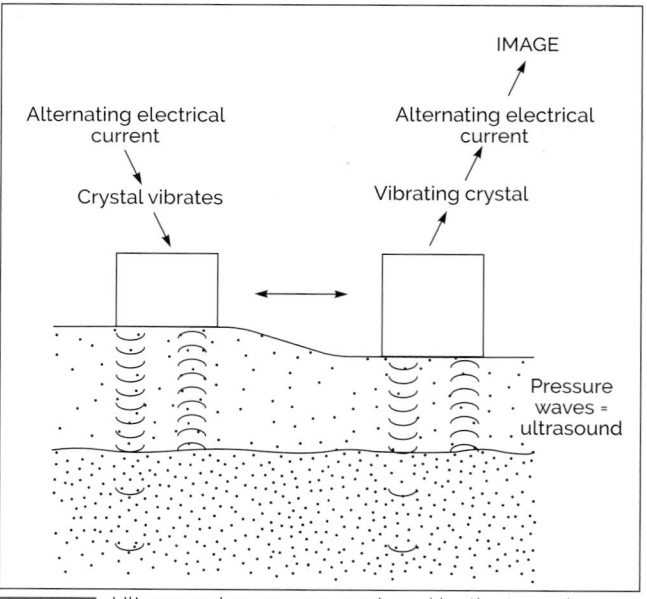

16.80 Ultrasound waves are produced by the transducer and pass into the tissues. Reflected waves are detected by the same transducer and an image created.

create a vibration of the tissues and of the crystals in the probe and this is converted back into electrical impulses, which are almost instantly converted by a computer into an image. The image is basically built up from many tiny dots of different brightness, depending on the strength of the returning pulses of ultrasound and the location in the body from which they have been reflected. It is a cross-sectional picture of the internal architecture of the tissues under investigation.

Equipment

Ultrasound equipment consists of one or more transducers, a TV monitor and a control panel (Figure 16.81). There is also likely to be some sort of printer for recording the images and a computer to record the studies.

Ultrasound transducers are of two main types: linear array and sector scanner (Figure 16.82). In linear array transducers, the piezoelectric crystals are arranged in a line and the image is rectangular. Although a wide image of the tissues close to the transducer is obtained, linear array transducers need a long contact area with the patient, which is hard to achieve in small animals (note: ultrasound does not pass through air). Linear array transducers are mainly used for rectal investigations in large animals. Sector scanning transducers are much more suitable for small animal work,

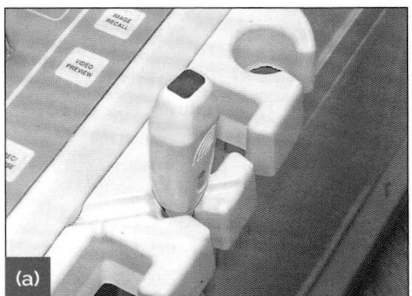

(a)

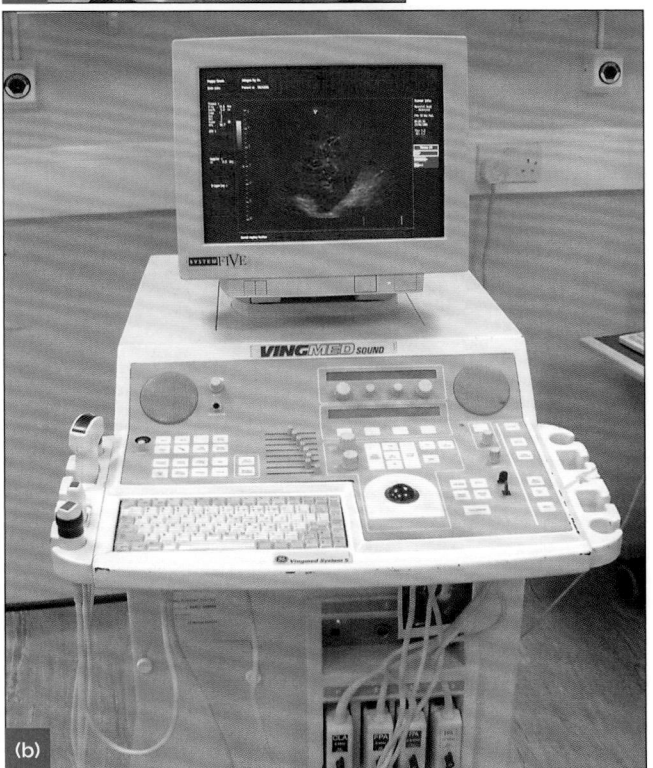

(b)

16.81 (a) Ultrasound transducer. (b) TV monitor and control panel.

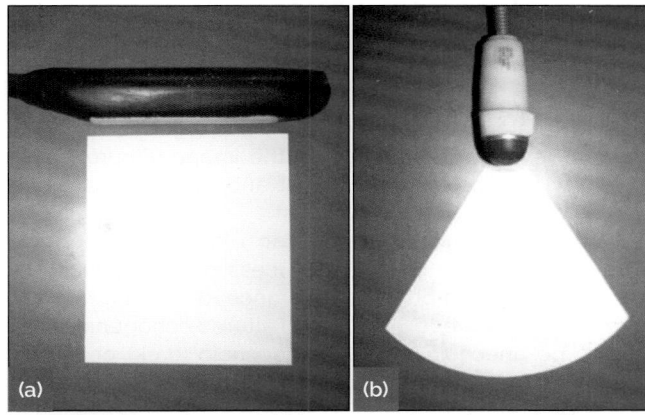

(a) (b)

16.82 Transducers. (a) Linear array transducer and image field. (b) Sector scanner transducer and image field.

since the crystals are arranged close together so that only a small area of contact with the patient is required. The ultrasound beam fans out to produce a triangular image that shows as much of the deeper tissues as possible. The image can be altered in depth, size, brightness and contrast, using the ultrasound machine's controls, and measurements and annotations can be made on a frozen image.

Care of the ultrasound machine

- Schedule regular machine maintenance visits by a service engineer
- Check the ultrasound equipment regularly
- Make sure that all connections are plugged in properly
- Check the integrity of the wiring, cables and transducers
- Wipe down the transducers and cables that monitor the heart rate after each patient examination, using a special cleaner
- Follow any recommended cleaning protocols, such as sterilization for certain types of transducers used for specific procedures
- Wipe down the machine thoroughly at the end of each use
- Report any problems to the service representative

Technique

Usually for dogs, cats and small mammals, the fur must be clipped to allow good contact between the transducer and the skin, as small air bubbles trapped in hair will greatly degrade the image. A special coupling gel is then applied to improve contact further. In long-haired animals it may be possible simply to part the hair and hold it aside using gel, but this means that only a small area can be examined.

Most ultrasound examinations are performed with the animal in lateral or dorsal recumbency, scanning from the ventral surface of the body or through the uppermost body wall. However, echocardiography (ultrasonography of the heart) is best performed from beneath, through a cut-out in a special tabletop. In lateral recumbency, the heart sinks towards the dependent chest wall, compressing the lung between it and the chest wall, and therefore the best 'acoustic window' (the least intervening lung) is on the underside.

Most ultrasonography performed uses B-mode ('brightness' mode ultrasound, described above) to create a two-dimensional image of the tissues. Small sound reflections within tissues create a fine granular pattern for parenchymatous organs, with different organs producing different levels of brightness on the image (Figure 16.83). Layers within the gastrointestinal and bladder walls can also be detected.

Pathology within an organ can often be recognized as a change in the overall brightness or echogenicity of the organ, or a mottled appearance disrupting normal architecture (Figure 16.84). Areas of altered echogenicity are said to be anechoic (black), hypoechoic (dark) or hyperechoic (bright). An area of mixed echogenicity is described as complex.

Fluid is usually seen as an anechoic area, because it gives rise to very few ultrasound reflections. Thus, free abdominal fluid can be seen as a black background surrounding abdominal organs (Figure 16.85). One of the main advantages of ultrasonography is that it allows examination of the abdominal structures when free fluid renders radiography unhelpful by obscuring the organs.

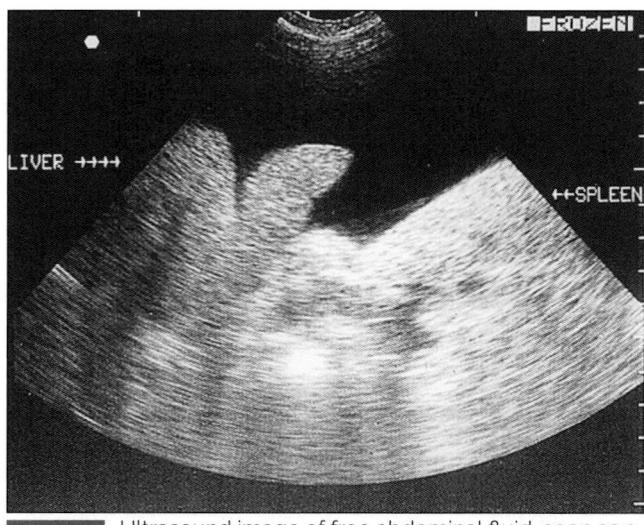

16.85 Ultrasound image of free abdominal fluid, seen as a black area outlining abdominal organs.

Special applications

Biopsy and fine-needle aspiration

Ultrasonography is increasingly used to assist biopsy or fine-needle aspiration (see also Chapter 17) of small diseased areas within organs, provided that a suitable and safe route to the area of interest exists via an appropriate acoustic window. Since the internal organ architecture and the needle tip can both be seen, the needle can be guided into the affected area without damaging other structures (Figure 16.86). Fine-needle aspiration can often be performed with the patient conscious; ultrasound-guided tissue biopsy is more likely to require general anaesthesia but avoids the need for surgery. Following sampling, the area should be scanned for several more minutes to ensure that there is no after-effect such as haemorrhage.

Ultrasound-guided cystocentesis is a very useful and quick procedure when the bladder is small and cannot be palpated for cystocentesis (see Chapter 17).

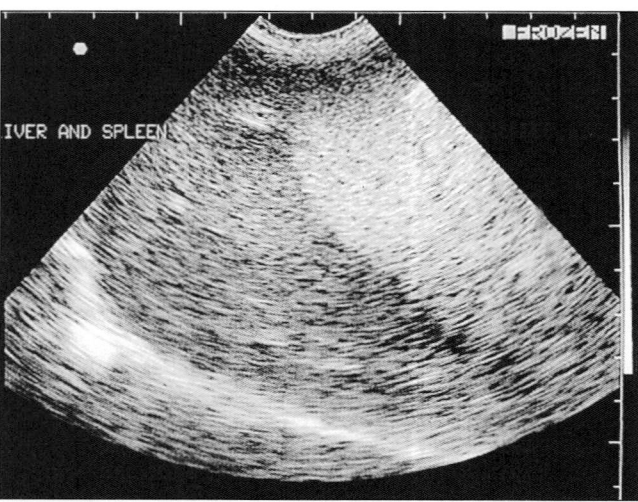

16.83 Ultrasound image of normal liver and spleen.

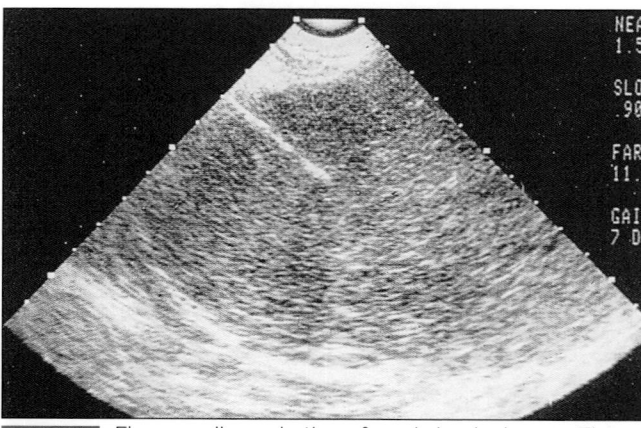

16.86 Fine-needle aspiration of an abdominal mass. The needle is seen as a bright line entering the mass.

Heart motion

A further refinement of ultrasonography is the use of M-mode ('movement' mode) to quantify heart motion. First, a B-mode image is obtained and a cursor (line of dots) is placed on it and moved right or left until it passes through

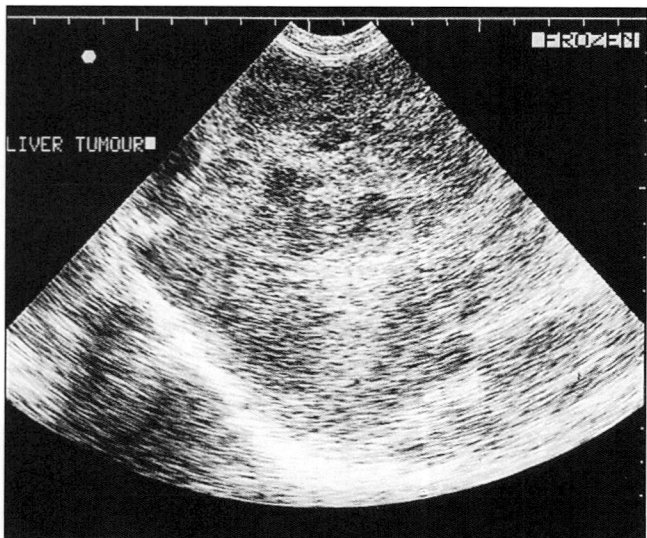

16.84 Ultrasound image of a liver tumour in a dog, giving rise to a mottled, irregular pattern to the liver.

the heart in the required position. At the touch of a button, the ultrasound beam produced by the transducer is converted into a thin line that produces a vertical band of dots, indicating reflections at tissue interfaces along that fixed line. This is rapidly updated with the movement of the heart and the image is scrolled along a horizontal axis with time. The resultant image shows the degree of heart motion and can be frozen to allow measurements of the heart chambers and walls in systole and diastole. Figure 16.87 shows a combined B-mode and M-mode image of a heart.

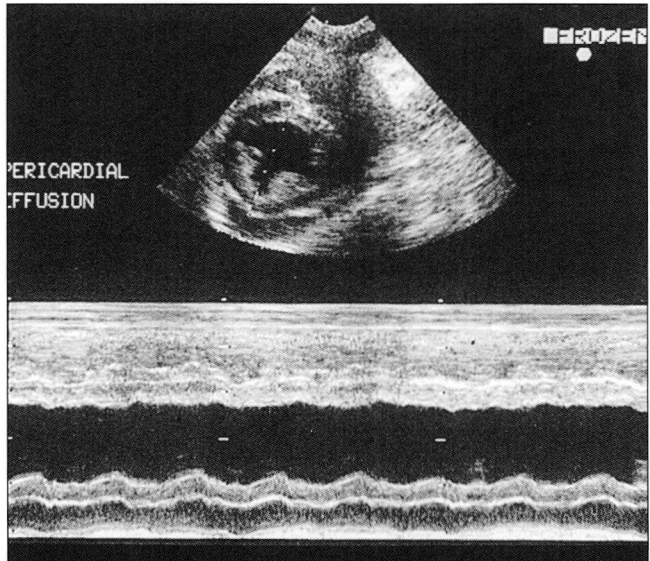

16.87 Ultrasound image from a dog with a pericardial effusion. Top: B-mode image of the heart; the line of dots indicates the position of the linear ultrasound beam. Bottom: M-mode image, with time along the horizontal axis. Blood in the left ventricle and the pericardial fluid are seen as black areas on both images.

Doppler ultrasonography

Doppler ultrasonography is the use of ultrasound waves to detect movement, usually blood flow. It is based on the principle that echoes returning from moving reflective surfaces will be of shorter wavelength if the movement is towards the transducer and longer wavelength if it is away. Spectral Doppler displays flow quantitatively and graphically against a baseline, whilst colour-flow Doppler assigns a colour according to speed and direction of flow and this colour mapping is superimposed over a B-mode or M-mode image. Doppler ultrasonography is used mostly in cardiac investigations (echocardiography) but can also be used to show the vascularity of structures, which is helpful prior to biopsy and to detect portosystemic shunts.

Contrast ultrasonography

There is increasing interest in contrast ultrasonography, in which small quantities of microbubbles of sulphur hexafluoride gas within phospholipid capsules suspended in liquid are injected into the blood stream. The microbubbles reflect ultrasound, producing increased echogenicity of the tissues in proportion to their vascularity. This allows vascular and non-vascular structures to be differentiated (e.g. tumour masses from blood clots), and the time scale of 'wash in' and 'wash out' of the contrast medium may suggest whether a lesion is benign or malignant, especially in the liver.

Computed tomography (CT scanning)

Principles and equipment

CT involves using X-rays to produce a highly detailed cross-sectional radiograph of the patient's tissues. Tissue contrast is much greater than with conventional radiography, and so fluid and solid tissue can be distinguished and some information about the internal architecture of soft tissues is given.

The CT scanner is a large piece of apparatus shaped like a ring doughnut with a central aperture within which is the patient table (Figure 16.88). The X-ray tube head moves rapidly around the circumference of the ring during the exposure, and radiation emerging from the patient is detected electronically and digitized, producing image information that can be manipulated by computer. The table moves forward slowly or in very small increments, and this movement results in the production of many cross-sectional, slice-like images of the area under investigation.

Differences in mathematical reconstruction of the emerging radiation, or 'algorithms', are used to emphasize different types of tissue and the grey scale of the final image can be altered further according to the tissue of interest. Thus, settings such as 'bone', 'lung' and 'soft tissue' can be selected. The grey scale of CT is described in terms of 'Hounsfield units' (HU), named after the engineer who invented CT, Sir Godfrey Hounsfield. The Hounsfield scale extends from approximately +3000 to –1000, with water being 0, bone being up to nearly 3000 and air being –1000 HU. Within the grey scale of the image, a range of Hounsfield units can be selected for viewing; all values higher and lower than these are displayed as white and black, respectively, and the values between are spread out over a range of grey shades that are discernible by the human eye. The centre of the range of Hounsfield units selected for viewing is known as the window level and the range is the window width. For examination of bone a window level of about +200 to +600 and window width of about +1000 to +2000 are used; for lung, the values are about –500 to –800 and +1000 to +2000, respectively.

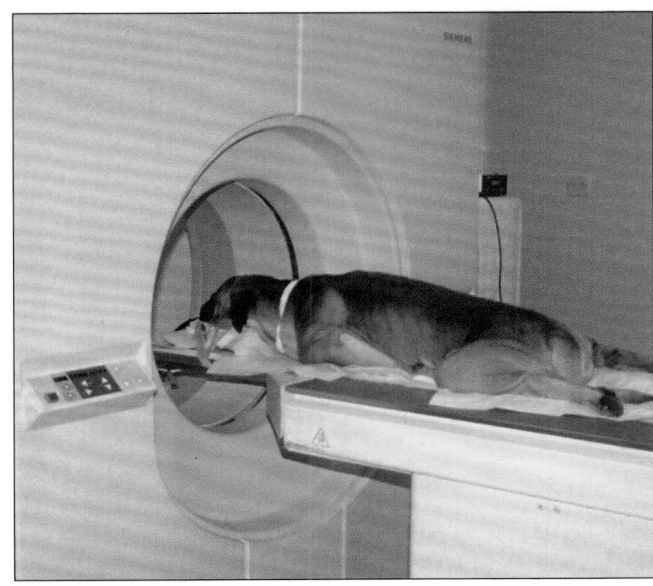

16.88 CT scanner and patient.

Technique

Veterinary patients must be anaesthetized or heavily sedated for CT scanning because the very high doses of radiation involved preclude manual restraint, but conventional anaesthetic and monitoring equipment can be used. Each exposure takes between a few seconds and one minute, depending on the study.

With older CT machines, images are always obtained transverse to the patient as it passes through the gantry. Images in other planes must be reformatted, which results in considerable loss of detail. The newer 'spiral' or 'helical' CT scanners are capable of producing images in any plane in very short scan times. Images can also be displayed in three dimensions and with different layers of tissue 'stripped away', allowing surgical planning. Advanced applications such as angiography and 'virtual endoscopy' are also possible.

Applications

Although this is essentially a radiographic technique, CT images have much more tissue definition than radiography and can differentiate between different types of soft tissue and between fluid and soft tissue. CT is especially valuable for imaging the skeletal system, as it is very sensitive to areas of osteolysis and new bone formation, and can therefore detect bony lesions that are invisible on radiography (Figure 16.89).

CT is also useful for imaging thoracic and abdominal masses, as it is less susceptible to movement artefacts than is MRI (see below). CT is especially valuable for imaging the lung, due to the very fine definition produced (Figure 16.90), and is the technique of choice for detection of lung metastases.

CT can be used for the brain, although the images are greatly inferior to those obtained with MRI. For the spine, excellent bone detail is obtained but changes in the spinal cord are not likely to be visible. Iodine radiographic contrast media can be given intravenously or into the spinal subarachnoid space to enhance the images further, demonstrating the vascularity of a lesion or damage to the blood–brain barrier and permitting myelography to be performed. CT-guided biopsy may be performed with the needle trajectory planned by computer from the CT images.

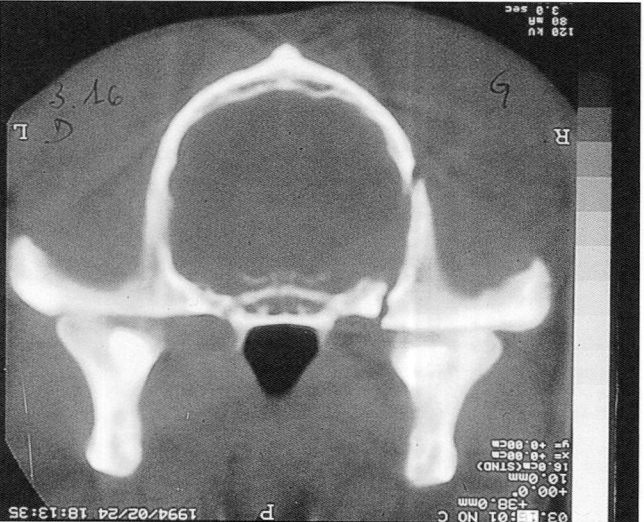

16.89 CT image of a skull fracture: bone appears white, as in radiography. This image has been 'windowed' by the computer to 'flatten' the soft tissues into a single grey shade to give better emphasis to bone.

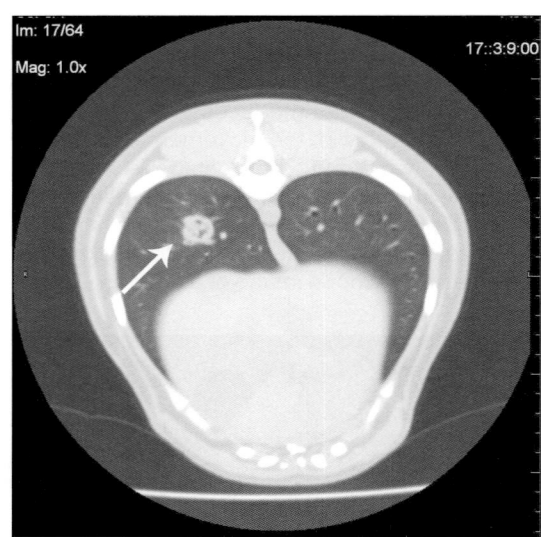

16.90 CT image of a bronchial foreign body, seen as a white (hyperdense) area (arrowed) within a thickened bronchus.

Magnetic resonance imaging (MRI scanning)
Principles and equipment

MRI involves completely different physical principles to radiography and CT, combining magnetism and radio waves. The scanner itself is a very powerful magnet, which may be cylindrical in the case of medium- and high-field magnets (Figure 16.91) or open in the case of low-field (weaker) systems. The tissues within the magnetic field become magnetized, which has the effect of aligning the protons of the hydrogen atoms in the body. The patient is then subjected to a series of radio waves emitted by a radiofrequency aerial, or RF coil, each lasting for several minutes; these disorientate the protons so that they emit tiny radio signals themselves. The emitted signals are detected by the same

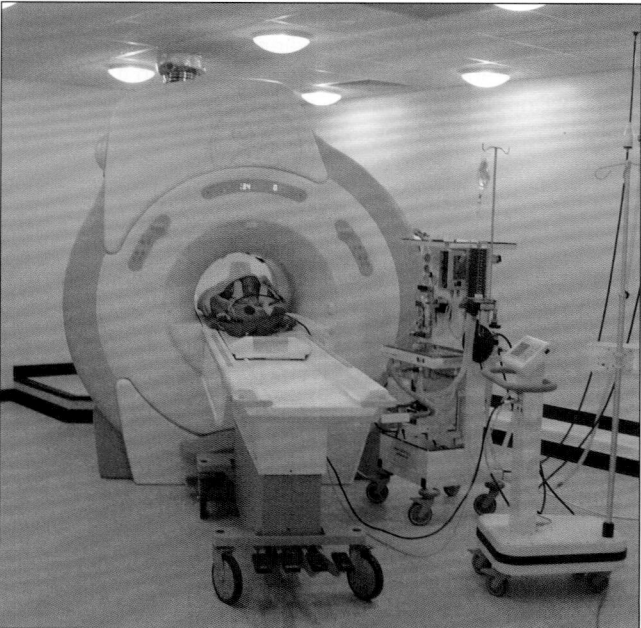

16.91 MRI scanner and anaesthetized patient.

RF coil and are converted to an image by a computer using very complex mathematical procedures.

As MRI does not use ionizing radiation, unlike radiography and CT, it is thought to be completely safe, but veterinary patients must be anaesthetized to keep them still during the scanning time, as any movement will render the images non-diagnostic. This may sometimes be for up to an hour or more in complex cases or when using low-field systems, in which scan times are longer. The main danger to patients and handlers lies in the fact that ferrous metal objects taken near the magnet may become dangerous missiles, and serious injuries and even deaths have occurred in medical MRI as a result. Fortunately, however, pet microchips remain un-affected by the powerful magnetic field and retain their data.

The presence of a strong magnetic field means that conventional anaesthetic and monitoring equipment cannot be used. In the case of low-field magnets, placing the anaes-thetic machine at a distance from the magnet and using a long circuit may be sufficient to overcome this problem. With higher-field systems, dedicated non-ferrous machines may be required and this of course adds to the expense of MRI. Although total intravenous anaesthesia may be possible, patients with severe disease, especially of the CNS, are often at high risk from anaesthesia, especially if they cannot be monitored adequately.

Technique

During scanning, the patient lies on the table in the magnetic field with the part to be imaged in an RF coil. The RF coils are of varying size and shape depending on the part of the body for which they are designed. There are now some MRI scanners and RF coils that are manufactured especially for veterinary patients, but most are designed for human patients; nevertheless, the equipment is well suited to scan-ning veterinary patients.

Unlike CT, in which there is a single image acquisition, with MRI many different types of scan can be performed to show tissues in different ways. For example, using a so-called T1-weighted scan, fluid such as CSF and ascites is dark, whereas with a T2-weighted scan it is bright. Other types of scan or 'pulse sequences' such as fat suppression can be employed to detect the nature of a tissue or lesion. As with CT, the images are in the form of cross-sectional 'slices' of the patient, but unlike CT they can be acquired in any plane. Studies usually comprise transverse, sagittal and dorsal plane images, although sometimes oblique slices are help-ful, for example for the orbital structures. Since many more studies are possible than with CT and since each set of image acquisitions takes a number of minutes, overall scan times are much longer than with CT.

Applications

The soft tissue information produced by MRI is much better than with CT, provided the tissue is still during scanning. Moving areas, such as the heart and lungs, require more complex 'gating' techniques during which the applica-tion of the RF pulses is synchronized with heartbeat or res-piration. Although slightly less sensitive for bony structures and calcification than CT, MRI provides excellent orthopaedic images by showing articular cartilage, joint fluid, subchondral bone and so on.

In veterinary work, MRI is used particularly in the diagno-sis of brain (Figure 16.92) and spinal (Figure 16.93) conditions in small animals in which it is by far the technique of choice.

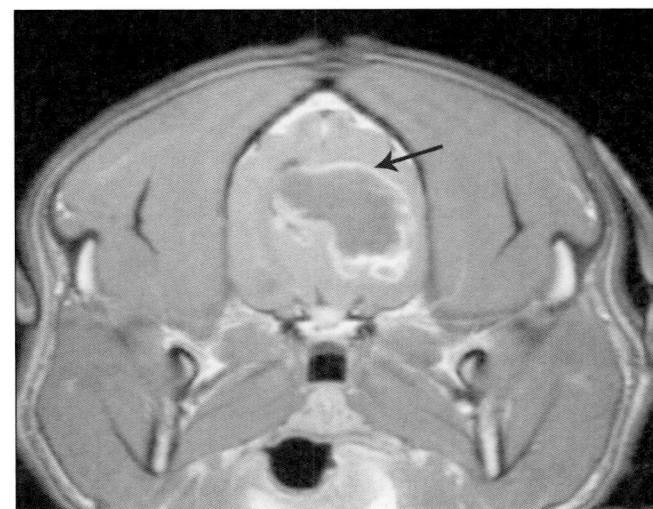

16.92 MRI scan of a brain tumour (arrowed) in a dog. On this contrast-enhanced, T1-weighted transverse brain image, the vascularized part of the brain tumour appears white and the necrotic part is dark.

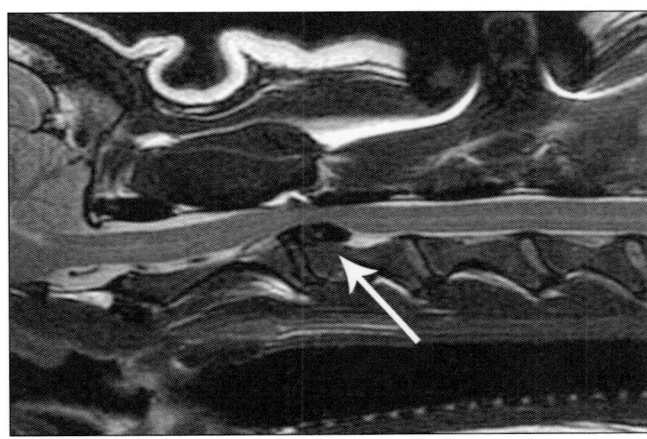

16.93 MRI scan of a calcified prolapsed disc (arrowed) causing spinal cord compression. Calcified material is black on MRI.

Conditions such as brain and spinal cord tumours, Chiari-like malformation and syringomyelia (see Chapter 4), inflamma-tory CNS disease, congenital deformities, disc disease and trauma can all be readily diagnosed, improving the diagnosis and treatment of the patients and allowing a more accurate prognosis to be given.

MRI can also be used to investigate many other disease processes, such as neoplasia, soft tissue foreign bodies and other space-occupying lesions, and inflammation. Intra-venous MRI contrast medium is given in many cases. MRI contrast media are complex molecules that usually contain the element gadolinium, which has 'paramagnetic' proper-ties. Use of contrast medium will show damage to the blood–brain barrier and vascularity of lesions, due to 'enhancement' of the tissues absorbing the contrast medium. As with CT, angiography can be performed to show blood vessels in three-dimensional detail.

The use of MRI, and to a lesser extent CT, has meant that surgery and radiotherapy of brain tumours in cats and dogs can now be performed successfully. The two techniques are also very helpful in planning surgery or radiotherapy for diseases elsewhere in the body, as the full extent of a disease process is often not evident on radiographs. MRI and CT are becoming increasingly used in veterinary diagnostic imaging as referral centres gain access to human scanners or mobile MRI systems or even obtain their own machines, and as owner expectations and the number of insured animals continue to rise. MRI and CT are, however, open to misuse. As with other imaging techniques, appropriate patient selection is required, together with expert acquisition and interpretation of images.

Nuclear medicine (scintigraphy)

Scintigraphic studies involve the use of radioactive isotopes which are defined as 'open sources'. Use of these isotopes is governed by the Radioactive Substances Act 1993. Licences must be obtained from the Environment Agency for activities involving radioactive isotopes. One is for keeping and using isotopes (the Registration), and the second governs the accumulation and disposal of radioactive waste (the Authorization). As with radiography, safe working procedures should be defined in the Local Rules.

Use in small animals

Scintigraphy is occasionally used in small animals. Figure 16.94 shows a sedated cat positioned on a gamma camera for scintigraphy of the thyroid gland. Radioactive iodine is injected intravenously and is taken up by the thyroid gland. The activity of the thyroid is compared with that of the zygomatic salivary glands in the head, and the relative activity of the two areas will show whether hyperthyroidism is present, in which gland (or both) the abnormality is, and whether or not there is any ectopic thyroid tissue elsewhere. Figure 16.95 shows the location of abnormal thyroid tissue in a hyperthyroid cat, allowing surgical planning if thyroidectomy is to be performed. Scintigraphy is occasionally used for other purposes such as detection of a portosystemic shunt and comparison of ventilation and perfusion in the lungs. However, this is a very specialized technique, which is performed in relatively few veterinary institutes. Following scintigraphy, small animals must be isolated, usually for 24 hours.

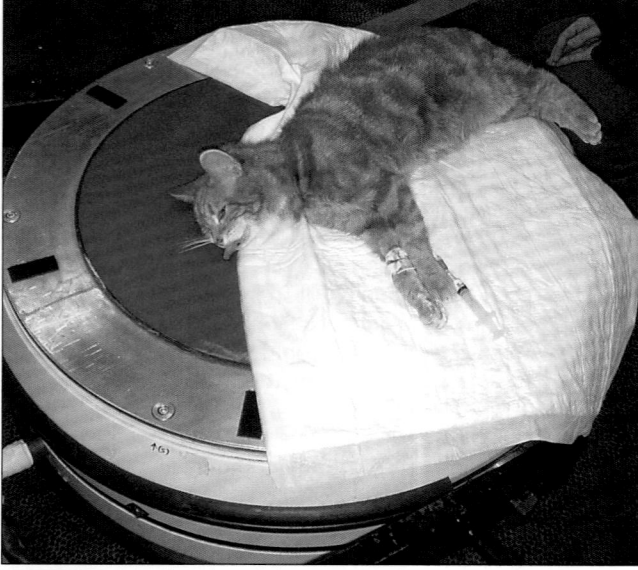

16.94 A sedated cat lying on a gamma camera during scintigraphy.

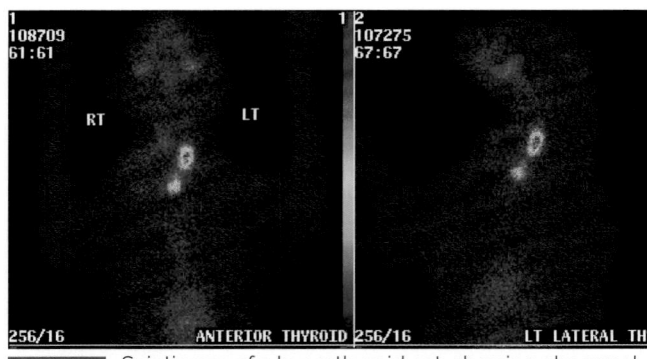

16.95 Scintigram of a hyperthyroid cat, showing abnormal tissue in the caudal neck.

Endoscopy

Principles and equipment

Endoscopy is the use of optical devices that give visual access to the inside of the body and provide high-quality magnified images of tissues and organ systems (Figure 16.96). With flexible endoscopes, foreign bodies can be removed and tissue samples taken from the digestive and respiratory tracts, often without the need for open surgery (Figure 16.97). Where surgery is required, rigid endoscopy provides a clear magnified image that allows greater precision and access to otherwise inaccessible places. Procedures are carried out through natural orifices or tiny incisions (keyhole surgery), resulting in less tissue trauma, reduced intraoperative and postoperative pain, quicker recovery and reduced infection

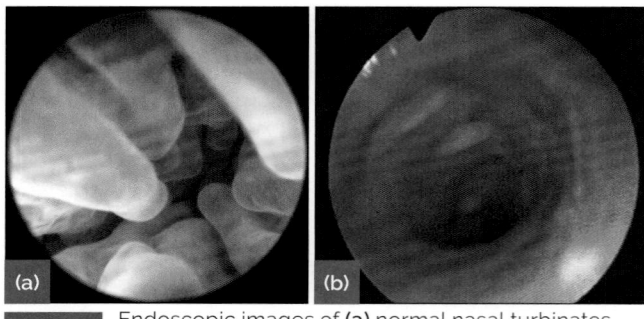

16.96 Endoscopic images of **(a)** normal nasal turbinates and **(b)** normal duodenum in a dog.

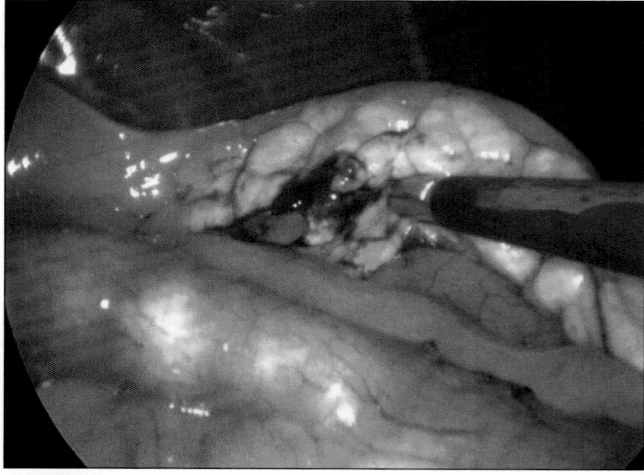

16.97 Laparoscopic biopsy of the pancreas.

rates. For these reasons, endoscopic procedures are termed minimally invasive. An increasing number of routine procedures, including exploratory laparoscopy, organ biopsies, bitch spays and cryptorchid testicle removal, are being carried out using these techniques (see Chapter 24), and this trend is continuing as it has in human surgery. Endoscopy can be divided into two broad categories: flexible endoscopy and rigid endoscopy.

Flexible endoscopy

Flexible endoscopes comprise an umbilical cord connected to a light source and suction/irrigation pump, a handpiece and a long flexible insertion tube, the tip of which can be manipulated in two directions (bronchoscopes) or four directions (e.g. gastroscopes). These endoscopes are used for examination of the respiratory tract and gastrointestinal tract, respectively, where they can be directed deep within the body to remove foreign bodies, visualize lesions and take fluid or tissue samples. Images are observed either through the eyepiece or preferably on a television monitor by means of an attached camera or dedicated video-endoscope. Patients are examined under general anaesthesia and a suitable mouth gag must always be used to prevent inadvertent reflex biting and damage to the endoscope. Flexible endoscopes should be pressure tested for at least 1 minute before each use, as any leak in the instrument channel or insertion tube may render the instrument irreparable.

Instrumentation

Instruments used in flexible endoscopy must be chosen to suit the diameter and length of the endoscope's instrument channel. Biopsy forceps (oval cupped with serrated edges are preferred) and a variety of grasping forceps are routinely used. Instruments are necessarily small and fragile and limit the size of biopsy specimen that can be obtained. Guarded brushes can also be obtained for retrieving samples for cytology and culture from the bronchial or intestinal mucosa. Sterile sample tubing may also be used through the instrument channel when performing bronchoalveolar lavage (BAL), although with smaller bronchoscopes samples are usually taken directly through the sterile instrument channel.

Routine positioning for flexible endoscopy

- Upper GI tract (gastroduodenoscopy) – left lateral recumbency.
- Lower GI tract (colonoscopy) – left lateral recumbency.
- Lungs (tracheobronchoscopy) – sternal recumbency.
- Nose/pharynx (rhinoscopy) – sternal recumbency.
- Urethra (especially male dogs) (urethroscopy) – lateral recumbency.

Special considerations

- Insufflation (filling with air) of the stomach in upper GI tract endoscopy may reduce diaphragmatic excursion and venous return. Air should always be removed by suction at the end of the procedure.
- Any fluid (acid reflux) in the oesophagus should also be suctioned to prevent oesophagitis and possible stricture formation.
- Airways will be partially occluded during bronchoscopy. Careful attention to the pulse oximeter/capnograph is essential. Examinations should be limited to 30–50 seconds to limit hypoxia. Patients should be maintained on oxygen for 10 minutes before and after the procedure.

Rigid endoscopy

Rigid endoscopes are relatively simple steel tubes containing rod lenses, with an eyepiece at one end, and a connection for a light guide cable. They are extremely delicate and require careful handling and care during cleaning. These endoscopes are used for a wide variety of diagnostic and surgical procedures, including:

- Otoscopy (examination of the ear)
- Fistuloscopy (examination of fistulae and stick injuries)
- Rhinoscopy (examination of the nose)
- Tracheoscopy (examination of the trachea)
- Colonoscopy (examination of the colon)
- Vaginoscopy and urethrocystoscopy (examination of the vagina and urogenital tract/bladder)
- Laparoscopy (examination of the abdomen)
- Coelioscopy (examination of the coelom in reptiles and birds)
- Thoracoscopy (examination of the thorax)
- Arthroscopy (examination of the joints).

Instrumentation

Smaller endoscopes (≤2.7 mm diameter) are always placed in a specially designed rigid sheath, often with instrument and irrigation channels to allow biopsy samples to be taken in restricted spaces (such as the nose and the bladder), and to protect the endoscope from torsion and damage. Grasping forceps or laser fibres can also be passed down the channel for foreign body removal or surgical resection, respectively. Arthroscopic sheaths are used to protect the endoscope in joints. These have no instrument channels, but have a tap with a luer fitting for instillation of saline under pressure from a pump or pressure bag to expand the joint space and flush away debris and haemorrhage. Instruments are introduced through separate cannulae.

Larger endoscopes, usually 5 mm diameter, are used in the abdomen or thorax through specially designed cannulae, which have gas-tight valves and are inserted through the body wall. A variety of endoscopic instruments may be passed through separate cannulae to perform surgical procedures or take tissue samples. Most instrumentation used in veterinary laparoscopy and thoracoscopy is of 5 mm diameter for use in 6 mm laparoscopic cannulae, although smaller instrumentation is available for cats and small dogs. A wide variety of instrumentation is available but most commonly used are biopsy forceps, Babcock's forceps, curved scissors, Maryland forceps and a palpation probe – a blunt metal rod used for manipulating tissues. A detachable camera clipped to the eyepiece enables procedures to be observed on a television monitor.

In addition to the basic instrumentation, a light source is required. Where possible, this is shared with a flexible endoscope using a suitable adapter for the light guide cable. A xenon, metal halide or LED light source is suitable.

For laparoscopy an electronic carbon dioxide (CO_2) insufflator is used and connected to the tap on a cannula via a filter and some sterile insufflation tubing. This maintains intra-abdominal pressure at a pre-set level, providing a space in which the surgeon can work.

Electrosurgery is the preferred method of haemostasis for routine minimally invasive procedures, and a radiosurgery generator is therefore essential. Many instruments are electrically shielded and have electrodes for attachment of monopolar leads. Bipolar instruments are also widely used, especially for operative surgery. Specialized vessel sealer/dividers are also commonly used and may require a bespoke generator. It should be noted that for monopolar electrosurgery, the generator should always be set on the 'cutting' current, even when coagulating vessels, as this has a lower voltage and is less likely to cause sparking to other instruments and cannulae, resulting in tissue damage. The tissue effect depends on the amount of tissue grasped, and anything other than a point electrode with minimal contact will result in slower tissue heating and therefore coagulation.

Routine positioning and preparation for rigid endoscopy

Vaginoscopy and otoscopy may sometimes be carried out on conscious patients, but all other procedures require general anaesthesia. Positioning will depend on the site being examined, and the procedure being undertaken.

- Rhinoscopy and urethrocystoscopy – sternal recumbency (some prefer lateral), with nose or abdomen propped up on a rolled-up towel. Dorsal recumbency may also be used for urethrocystoscopy.
- Laparoscopy – dorsal recumbency (sometimes dorsolateral or lateral).
- Thoracoscopy – dorsal recumbency (sometimes lateral).
- Arthroscopy – usually lateral but depends on the joint being examined.

Rhinoscopy and urethrocystoscopy are best carried out on a tub table as they require considerable amounts of saline irrigation. Alternatively, a deep tray covered with a wire grid may suffice.

Special considerations

Copious saline flushing of the nose or bladder may also result in the induction of hypothermia, especially in small patients. Careful monitoring of core body temperature is advisable and small patients should be maintained on heat mats or warm air circulation blankets.

It should be noted that laparoscopy requires insufflation of the abdomen with an inert gas (usually carbon dioxide). This reduces venous return and increases abdominal pressure on the diaphragm and can restrict respiration and cardiac output. In the healthy patient, homeostatic mechanisms readily compensate for these changes but careful monitoring during anaesthesia is essential.

Thoracoscopy is an open chest procedure, resulting in collapse of the lungs. All patients will require positive pressure ventilation throughout the operation and careful monitoring using pulse oximetry and capnography, if available. In most cases, a chest tube will be placed at the end of the procedure to allow drainage of exudate and re-inflation of the lungs through intermittent or continuous suction. It is not unusual for the surgeon to change the position of the patient during laparoscopy or thoracoscopy in order to allow gravity to move viscera out of the surgical field. For this reason, rigid ties should not be used, and movable cradles may be substituted. Alternatively, an adjustable operating table that can tilt in four directions is helpful.

Patients should be clipped wide enough to allow optimal positioning of cannulae and also to enable conversion to an open procedure if it should become necessary. A suitable surgical kit should always be immediately available for laparotomy or thoracotomy.

Care and cleaning of endoscopic equipment

All endoscopes require meticulous care and attention to cleaning protocols if they are not to suffer irreversible damage. Delay may make cleaning very difficult or impossible. Most endoscope suppliers will provide in-house training in care and maintenance, and it is advisable to ensure all cleaning is done by trained personnel.

Both rigid and flexible endoscopes and cameras may be gas-sterilized or soaked in a suitable cold sterilizer solution. Some rigid endoscopes are autoclaveable, although this is not recommended as the majority of veterinary autoclaves cycle too quickly and may shorten the life of the instrument. Most instruments, cannulae and trocars can be cleaned in an ultrasonic bath. Never attempt to clean an endoscope, camera or light guide cable in an ultrasonic bath as this will cause irreparable damage. Cannulae and most reusable instruments can also be autoclaved. Always check with the manufacturer first before cleaning endoscopic instruments.

- Rinse immediately after use to remove gross contamination.
- Flexible endoscopes should always be pressurized with a pressure tester before immersion. Check that there is no pressure drop over 1 minute before removing the leakage tester.
- Remove buttons and the instrument channel seal. Flush all channels using a 60 ml syringe and appropriate tubing attached to the button channels and soak everything in an approved enzymatic cleaner for up to 30 minutes.
- Dismantle all rigid instruments as far as possible and brush thoroughly.
- Brush all channels in flexible endoscopes and rigid cannulae.
- Rinse in clean water and flush channels.
- Flush all channels with an approved cold sterilizer and soak for a further 15 minutes.
- Never soak any endoscope for longer than one hour as this may result in damage to the seals.
- Rinse in deionized water and dry carefully.
- Clean lenses with 70% alcohol.
- Reconnect the leakage tester and release the pressure.
- Hang flexible endoscopes vertically with the umbilicus and insertion tube straight and all taps removed to allow drainage.
- Store rigid endoscopes in a protective sheath in a suitable container or drawer.

Single-use bipolar instruments, such as the Ligasure® (Coviden), Enseal® or Harmonic® Ace (Ethicon) or Powerblade® (LiNA Medical), designed for human surgery may be re-used if carefully cleaned and re-sterilized. These instruments cannot be autoclaved or cold-sterilized. Care must be taken not to allow fluids to run up the shaft towards the handle, which houses the electronic circuitry. The tip of the instrument is cleaned carefully with enzymatic cleaner, rinsed and dried. The instrument can then be gas-sterilized.

Endoscopy is typically very safe; however, the procedure does have a few potential complications. These include:

- Perforation (tear) of the gastrointestinal wall
- Bleeding
- Infection
- Reaction to sedation, anaesthetic and/or contrast medium.

It is therefore important to monitor the patient carefully following endoscopy.

References and further reading

Baines E (2005) Practical contrast radiography 3. Urogenital studies. *In Practice* **27**, 466–473

Barr F and Gaschen L (2011) *BSAVA Manual of Canine and Feline Ultrasonography*. BSAVA Publications, Gloucester

Barrett E (2007) Practice radiography: time to go digital? *In Practice* **29**, 616–619

Bradley K (2005) Practical contrast radiography 2. Gastrointestinal studies. *In Practice* **27**, 412–417

Bradley K (2006) Digital radiography – considerations for general practice. *UK Vet* **11**, 81–84

BSAVA (2018) *BSAVA Guide to Radiographic Positioning*. BSAVA Publications, Gloucester

BVA (2017) Guidance Notes for the Safe Use of Ionising Radiations in Veterinary Practice, Ionising Radiations Regulation 2017. (Available from: www.bva.co.uk/resources-support/practice-management/ionising-radiations-guide/)

Caine A (2009) Practical approach to digital radiography. *In Practice* **31**, 334–339

Crane L and Barrett E (2008) Advanced imaging. In: *BSAVA Manual of Canine and Feline Advanced Veterinary Nursing, 2nd edn*, ed. A Hotston Moore and S Rudd, pp. 220–249. BSAVA Publications, Gloucester

Dennis R, Kirberger RM, Barr FJ and Wrigley RH (2010) *Handbook of Small Animal Radiology and Ultrasound: Techniques and Differential Diagnoses, 2nd edn*. Elsevier, Oxford

Fauber TL (2016) *Radiographic Imaging and Exposure, 5th edn*. Elsevier, Missouri

Harcourt-Brown F and Chitty J (2013) *BSAVA Manual of Rabbit Surgery, Dentistry and Imaging*. BSAVA Publications, Gloucester

Harcourt-Brown N and Chitty J (2005) *BSAVA Manual of Psittacine Birds, 2nd edn*. BSAVA Publications, Gloucester

Holloway A and McConnell F (2013) *BSAVA Manual of Canine and Feline Radiography and Radiology: A Foundation Manual*. BSAVA Publications, Gloucester

Kirberger R and McEvoy F (2016) *BSAVA Manual of Canine and Feline Musculoskeletal Imaging, 2nd edn*. BSAVA Publications, Gloucester

Latham C (2005) Practical contrast radiography 1. Contrast agents. *In Practice* **27**, 348–352

Lhermette P and Sobel D (2009) *BSAVA Manual of Canine and Feline Endoscopy and Endosurgery*. BSAVA Publications, Gloucester

Llabres Diaz F (2005) Practical contrast radiography 4. Myelography. *In Practice* **27**, 502–510

Llabres Diaz F (2006) Practical contrast radiography 5. Other techniques. *In Practice* **28**, 32–40

Meredith A and Flecknell P (2006) *BSAVA Manual of Rabbit Medicine and Surgery, 2nd edn*. BSAVA Publications, Gloucester

O'Brien R and Barr F (2009) *BSAVA Manual of Canine and Feline Abdominal Imaging*. BSAVA Publications, Gloucester

Rudorf H, Taeymans O and Johnson V (2008) Basics of thoracic radiography and radiology. In: *BSAVA Manual of Canine and Feline Thoracic Imaging*, ed. T Schwarz and V Johnson, pp. 1–19. BSAVA Publications, Gloucester

Tams T and Rawlings C (2011) *Small Animal Endoscopy, 3rd edn*. Mosby, Philadelphia

Thrall D (2018) *Textbook of Veterinary Diagnostic Radiology, 7th edn*. Elsevier, Missouri

Wallack ST (2003) *The Handbook of Veterinary Contrast Radiography*. San Diego Veterinary Imaging Inc.

Ward A and Prior J (2007) Diagnostic imaging techniques. In: *BSAVA Manual of Practical Veterinary Nursing*, ed. E Mullineaux and M Jones, pp. 229–267. BSAVA Publications, Gloucester

Useful websites

British Veterinary Association (BVA) Canine Health Schemes:
- Chiari Malformation/Syringomyelia (CM/SM) www.bva.co.uk/Canine-Health-Schemes/CM-SM-Scheme/
- Elbow Dysplasia www.bva.co.uk/Canine-Health-Schemes/Elbow-Scheme/
- Hip Dysplasia https://www.bva.co.uk/Canine-Health-Schemes/hip-scheme

Self-assessment questions

1. How can the quality of an X-ray image be improved? What is scattered radiation and how is it produced? What steps may be taken to minimize the effect of scatter on radiographs?
2. Describe the stages of processing a radiographic film by the manual method. How does automatic processing differ?
3. Define the terms 'density', 'contrast' and 'definition', as applied to radiographic images.
4. What sources of radiation hazard exist in veterinary radiography? How may the potential risk to personnel involved be minimized?
5. Describe the restraint, positioning and views required for submission of hip and elbow radiographs to the BVA/KC Hip and Elbow Dysplasia Schemes.
6. What is the difference between linear array and sector scanning ultrasound transducers?
7. Define 'Hounsfield unit', 'window level' and 'window width', as applied to CT scan images.
8. What are the advantages and disadvantages of MRI scanning compared with CT?
9. Describe the cleaning and care of endoscopic equipment following its use. How should flexible and rigid endoscopes be stored?
10. What system is now in place for the communication and sharing of digital images?
11. What is PennHIP and when might it be used?
12. What patient preparation is required for a dog requiring double-contrast studies of the bladder?

Chapter 17

Veterinary laboratory equipment and techniques

Elizabeth Mullineaux

Learning objectives

After studying this chapter, readers will have the knowledge to:

- **Describe the requirements of an in-house veterinary laboratory, including safe working practices and the use of a range of laboratory equipment**
- **Collect, preserve and analyse diagnostic samples from animals, including blood, urine, faeces, skin and hair, other tissue samples and samples for culture of infectious organisms**
- **Safely and correctly package and transport samples to external laboratories**
- **Record and report laboratory findings**
- **Recognize the limitations of laboratory test results, identify inconsistencies and inaccuracies and recognize the significance of spurious results**

The importance of laboratory diagnostic aids

Laboratory tests are often an essential part of the diagnosis of clinical disease in animals. However, in common with all diagnostic tests, laboratory tests should be used in addition to good history-taking and clinical examination, with the clinical judgement of the veterinary surgeon guiding which tests are most appropriate.

Most veterinary practices have at least some basic in-house laboratory facilities and it is often the role of the veterinary nurse to carry out laboratory tests, as well as maintain equipment and the laboratory itself. Therefore, an understanding of the equipment, how it works, and how it should be maintained, is essential. In some instances, even with an extensive in-house laboratory, some samples will need to be sent to external laboratories for specialist procedures and/or the interpretation of results by a specialist clinical pathologist. Where an external laboratory is used, the veterinary nurse will often be required to correctly package and dispatch samples safely.

Regardless of where the sample is to be tested, some common veterinary nursing skills are required to ensure that the laboratory test results obtained are as reliable as possible:

- **Communication:** with the client, veterinary team and, where appropriate, external laboratory staff
- **Preparation:** through discussion with the veterinary surgeon, consideration of patient records, appropriate admission/consent (see Chapter 9), patient preparation (e.g. overnight withholding of food) and preparation of equipment (including appropriate calibration and quality control testing)
- **Sampling:** correct sampling methods, storage, preservation, procedure for sample rejection and, where necessary, transportation
- **Record keeping:** both clinical and client records
- **Communication of results:** to both the client and the veterinary team
- **Understanding the findings:** the limitations of the tests carried out, their relevance, recognition of spurious values
- **Health and safety considerations:** for the veterinary nurse, other veterinary staff, laboratory staff and clients (see also Chapter 2).

In all cases, before a diagnostic test is performed:

- Check with the veterinary surgeon to confirm which test is to be carried out
- Check the patient identification (ID) and clinical history
- Check that all equipment required is present and in full working order

- Check that a safe area is available in which to perform the test
- Check that another person is available in order to assist with sample collection if required.

The following samples are commonly collected for veterinary laboratory tests:

- Blood
- Urine
- Faeces
- Skin and hair samples
- Tissue and body fluid samples for cytology
- Samples for bacteriology, fungal or viral culture
- Samples for toxicology.

Details of each of these are given later in this chapter. In all cases, after the diagnostic test has been performed:

- Label all samples with the patient ID, date and sample type
- Record the date and type of diagnostic tests that have been carried out in patient's clinical records
- If the samples are to be sent to an external laboratory, they must be packaged and dispatched correctly (see 'Package and dispatch of samples', below)
- Record the results of the test(s) and date(s) received as soon as they are available (see 'Laboratory results', below)
- Inform other members of the veterinary team of the results and inform the clients as appropriate.

Laboratory health and safety

Collecting samples from animals, handling samples and carrying out procedures in the veterinary practice laboratory, are subject to legislative controls in order to minimize potential risks to people, animals and the environment. These include measures for the prevention of injury, to deal with injury, for the safe use of chemicals, and the disposal of waste. Further information is provided in Chapter 2.

Relevant legislation in England and Wales includes:

- Control of Substances Hazardous to Health Regulations 2002 (COSHH)
- Electrical Equipment (Safety) Regulations 2016
- Environmental Protection Act 1990
- Hazardous Waste (England and Wales) Regulations 2005 (amended 2016)
- Health and Safety at Work etc. Act 1974
- Health and Safety (First Aid) Regulations 1981
- Reporting of Injuries, Diseases and Dangerous Occurrences Regulations 2013 (RIDDOR)
- Scientific Procedures Act 1986 (amended 1993)
- Waste (England and Wales) Regulations 2011 (amended 2014).

In order to fulfil the legislative requirements, ensure personal protection and the protection of others, safe working practice in the laboratory is essential. 'Risks' and 'hazards' (see Chapter 2) must be identified and standard operating procedures (SOPs) developed and regularly reviewed. Some chemicals may be labelled with standard 'Chemical hazard'

symbols (Figure 17.1) and it is important to understand the meaning of these. Potential hazards and risks in the laboratory include:

- Chemicals that may have toxic, corrosive or flammable effects, resulting in harm to people or the environment (Figure 17.1)
- Equipment, including electrical equipment
- Infectious biological agents, including zoonoses (see Chapters 5, 6 and 7)
- Waste, including sharps
- Fumes and aerosols
- Fire/explosion (Figure 17.1)
- Slips/trips/falls.

Personal protective equipment (PPE), such as aprons, gloves and eye shields, should be provided in the laboratory and worn by staff as required. Staff who may be pregnant or who are immunosuppressed may be at greater risk in the laboratory; appropriate measures must be taken to minimize risks, which may include those that are especially vulnerable not carrying out certain procedures. A general code of conduct should be followed when working within the laboratory; further information is given in Chapter 2.

Example laboratory code of conduct

- All staff must have read and understood the practice health and safety policy, as well as specific task and risk assessments including SOPs for the laboratory area
- Entry must be restricted to authorized persons only
- Authorized members of staff should be fully trained and supervised wherever necessary
- Jewellery must be removed and long hair tied back
- Mobile phones should not be taken into the laboratory (or must be switched off)
- PPE (e.g. apron or laboratory coat) must be worn whilst in the laboratory. Additional PPE should be available and worn wherever necessary (e.g. gloves, mask, goggles)
- No eating, smoking or drinking should take place within the laboratory
- The laboratory must be kept well organized, tidy and clean
- All hazardous items should be clearly labelled and stored securely
- Cupboards should not be above eye level
- A sink should be provided in the laboratory
- Containers, chemicals and other material should all be fully labelled and datasheets available
- All waste should be disposed of correctly (see below)
- A well-stocked and in-date first aid box must be available, including eye wash. A trained First Aider must be available within the practice
- Firefighting equipment must be available and appropriate for the area. Staff should be appropriately trained to use such equipment
- Records of diagnostic tests carried out on patients should be kept within the laboratory (electronic or paper)
- Care should be taken to avoid cross-contamination of samples
- Any accidents or spillages (see below) must be reported to a senior member of staff immediately
- All staff should be aware of potential zoonotic risks, such as from faeces, urine, blood and bacterial samples

---

Pictogram and classification	Precautions
Acute toxicity	Toxic material which may cause life threatening effects even in small amounts and with short exposure. ■ Do not swallow the material, allow it to come into contact with skin or inhale it
Explosive	May explode if exposed to fire, heat, shock, friction. ■ Avoid ignition sources (sparks, flames, heat) ■ Keep your distance ■ Wear protective clothing
Highly flammable	Flammable if exposed to ignition sources, sparks, heat. Some substances with this symbol may give off flammable gases in contact with water. ■ Avoid ignition sources (sparks, flames, heat) ■ Keep your distance ■ Wear protective clothing
Oxidizing	Can burn even without air, or can intensify fire in combustible materials. ■ Avoid ignition sources (sparks, flames, heat) ■ Keep your distance ■ Wear protective clothing
Corrosive	Corrosive material which may cause skin burns and permanent eye damage. May corrode metals. ■ Avoid contact with skin and eyes ■ Do not breathe vapours or sprays ■ Wear protective clothing ■ Keep away from metals
Gas under pressure	Contains gas under pressure. Gas released may be very cold. Gas container may explode if heated. ■ Store correctly ■ Do not heat container ■ Avoid contact with skin or eyes
Health hazard/ hazardous to the ozone layer	May cause irritation (redness, rash) or less serious toxicity. ■ Keep away from skin and eyes ■ Avoid release to the environment May damage the ozone layer. ■ Avoid release to the environment
Hazardous to the environment	Toxic to aquatic organisms and may cause long lasting effects in the environment. ■ Avoid release to the environment
Serious health hazard	May cause serious and prolonged health effects on short or long-term exposure. ■ Do not swallow the material, allow it to come into contact with skin or breathe it

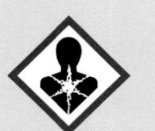

17.1 Classification, labelling and packaging (CLP) hazard pictograms that may be found associated with laboratory work.

Spillages

All spills should be made safe as soon as possible after the spillage is discovered. Clearing blood or body fluid spillages may expose an individual to infectious microorganisms, so care must be taken to ensure the member of staff is protected by the appropriate use of protective clothing. Local codes of practice should specify procedures (e.g. spill kits) and the disinfectants to be used for dealing with spillage and other forms of contamination (see Chapter 2).

The following principles should apply, regardless of the scale of the spill:

- Gloves should be worn throughout and should be discarded safely after use
- If there is broken glass present, it is essential that the fragments are not gathered up by hand either before or after treatment with disinfectant. Bunches of paper towels or newspaper, pieces of card or a plastic dustpan should be used to remove the fragments to a sharps container without risk of sharps injury
- Gloves should be worn and lesions on exposed skin covered with waterproof dressings
- Contamination should be wiped up with a paper towel soaked in disinfectant
- Towels and gloves should be placed in a clinical waste bag for incineration and hands washed
- If the spillage is extensive, disposable plastic overshoes or rubber boots may be necessary
- If splashing is likely to occur while cleaning up, other protective clothing should be worn, e.g. to protect the eyes, clothing
- Liquid spills should be covered with dichloroisocyanurate granules and left for at least 2 minutes before clearing up with paper towels and/or a plastic dustpan.

Disposal of laboratory waste

The disposal of waste within the laboratory is regulated by the legislation listed above and discussed in detail in Chapter 2. It is important that correct segregation, labelling, storage, removal and destruction of laboratory waste are carried out in accordance with these regulations and in line with the practice's waste collection service:

- Much of the waste in the laboratory is likely to be potentially contaminated with microorganisms and is therefore usually considered to be 'Hazardous waste' (which includes 'infectious clinical waste') (see Chapter 2)
- Sharps, syringes and other contaminated items must be placed in the appropriate containers (see Chapter 2)
- Culture plates should be autoclaved and then disposed of appropriately (see Chapters 2 and 5)
- Untrained staff and students should not handle hazardous waste until they have received training on the use of PPE and the Safety Data Sheets (SDS).

Laboratory equipment

A wide range of equipment may be used within the veterinary practice laboratory. In order that equipment is used safely, reliably and accurately, correct management is required. Faults should be identified and rectified quickly; damaged or faulty equipment should be labelled as such and not used. Procedures should be in place to control infection and avoid possible cross-contamination of samples. These procedures should be followed carefully.

Microscopes

A microscope is one of the most commonly used pieces of equipment within a laboratory. A binocular microscope with a built-in light source (Figure 17.2) is the most suitable for veterinary practice laboratory use. Figure 17.3 explains the functions of the various components. Microscopes are valuable pieces of laboratory equipment and must be carefully stored and maintained (see below).

Microscope lenses

The first magnifying lens on a microscope is the eyepiece, which typically magnifies X10. In addition, most binocular microscopes are usually equipped with four **objective lenses** (some have only three) that magnify at X4, X10, X40 and X100 (oil immersion).

- Scanning lens (X4): a very low power lens used for scanning the slide, usually to look for areas of interest. This lens may be absent on some microscopes.
- Low power objective (X10): a low power lens used for locating areas of interest on a slide.
- High power objective (X40): a higher power lens used for more detailed focusing on an area of interest.
- Oil immersion (X100): a high power lens used for very detailed examination of an area of interest. This lens uses light that is refracted through a thin layer of oil rather than through air.

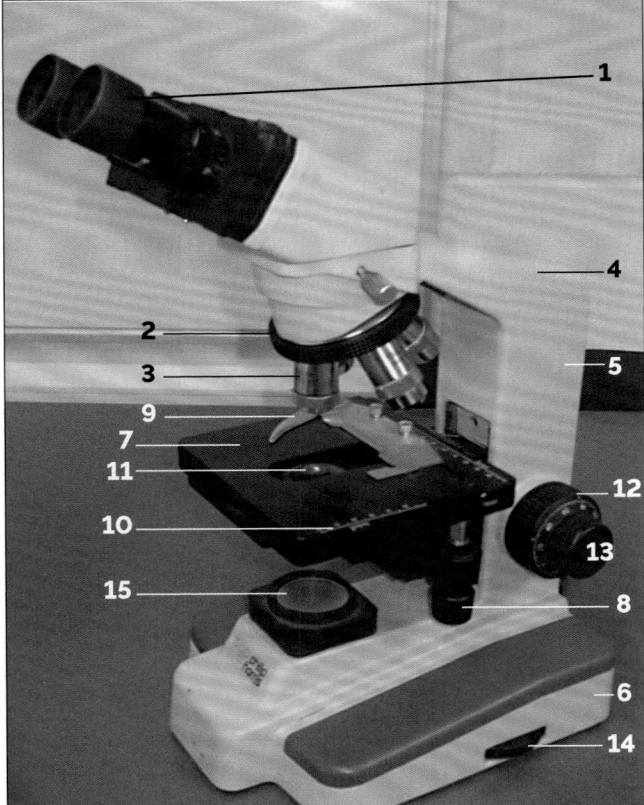

17.2 Binocular microscope with a built-in light source (see Figure 17.3 for additional information). **(1)** Eyepiece containing ocular lenses. **(2)** Rotating nosepiece. **(3)** Objective lens. **(4)** Limb. **(5)** Body. **(6)** Base. **(7)** Stage. **(8)** Mechanical stage control. **(9)** Clips. **(10)** Vernier scale. **(11)** Substage condenser and iris diaphragm. **(12)** Coarse focus knob. **(13)** Fine focus knob. **(14)** Rheostat. **(15)** Light source.

Component	Function
Eyepiece **(1)**	The eyepiece, through which the operator views the specimen, contains ocular lenses that magnify the primary image formed by the objective lens. Typically X10
Nosepiece **(2)**	The rotating nosepiece holds the objective lens
Objective lenses **(3)**	There are normally four objective lenses, each with a different magnification. Typically X4, X10, X40 and X100 (oil immersion)
Limb **(4)**, body **(5)** and base **(6)**	The microscope should be carried by its limb **(4)** with the base **(6)** supported. When using the microscope, the base **(6)** should always be placed on a flat surface.
Stage **(7)**	A flat platform that holds the microscope slide using clips **(9)**. The hole in the centre of the platform allows light to illuminate the specimen. The stage can then be moved up and down using the focus control knobs **(12** and **13)**. The stage houses the mechanical stage with a control **(8)** that allows the slide to be moved left, right, horizontally and vertically
Vernier scale **(10)**	A horizontal and vertical Vernier scale allows the location of specific points of the specimen to be recorded and relocated
Substage condenser **(11)**	Condenses light from the light source on to the specimen. The position of the substage condenser and the amount of light passing through it can be adjusted using the iris diaphragm
Iris diaphragm **(11)**	By adjusting the iris diaphragm, the amount of light passing through the condenser can be increased or decreased. It is useful to close the diaphragm when looking at things such as parasites, this reduces detail but increases the contrast making the parasites more obvious. For more detailed work such as cytology the diaphragm should be opened which reduces the contrast but gives the most detailed image
Focus knobs **(12** and **13)**	Coarse (larger knob, **12**) and fine focus (smaller knob, **13**) raise and lower the stage to allow the image to be focused
Rheostat **(14)**	Alters the level of light produced by the light source **(15)**

17.3 The main components of a microscope (numbering relates to labelled parts of Figure 17.2).

Microscope slides

Microscope slides are usually thin flat pieces of glass, typically 75 x 26 mm and 1 mm thick. Slides are used to hold samples for examination under a microscope in a manner that avoids contamination of the microscope and lenses. The most common type of slide is a 'plain slide' that can be used either way up. Some plain slides may be frosted on one side at one end, allowing labelling; with these slides the frosted section should be uppermost. Other specialized slides include 'concavity slides' that have an indentation on one side, 'graticule slides' that have gridlines etched on them to allow counting (an example of this is the McMasters slide used for microscopic examination of faecal samples for endoparasites; see 'Faecal samples', below) and 'coated slides' to assist with sample adhesion to the slide.

Cover slips

Cover slips should be used to view most slides and certainly all 'wet' slides. Cover slips help protect the microscope lenses, as well as improve the image and help viewing by giving a defined area to scan. When making tape strips for dermato-logical examinations (see 'Adhesive tape impressions', below), the tape itself acts as a cover slip.

Using a binocular light microscope

1. Use PPE if necessary.
2. Remove the dust cover and ensure the microscope is plugged into an electrical socket.
3. Check the rheostat to ensure that it is turned down to its lowest setting to avoid damaging the bulb.
4. Turn the microscope on.
5. Move the stage down to its lowest point.
6. Move the lowest objective lens (X4 or X10 depending on the microscope) into position, ensuring it clicks firmly in place.
7. Place the microscope slide on to the stage (the correct way up), using clips to hold it in position if required.
8. Without looking down the eyepiece (look at the stage directly), move the stage up until it almost touches the objective lens. Ensure that the lens does not touch the slide.
9. Look down the eyepieces and adjust the distance between them as necessary so that the two fields can be viewed as one.
10. Adjust the rheostat to a medium light setting.
11. Adjust the substage condenser so that it is a few millimetres below the stage.
12. Slowly move the stage downwards using the coarse focus control, whilst looking down the eyepiece, until the image comes into view.
13. Once an image can be seen, use the fine focus control to sharpen the image.
14. In order to move from the X4 lens to the X10 objective lens, take your eyes away from the eyepiece and slowly move the X10 objective into place, checking that it does not come into contact with the slide. Use the fine focus control to focus the image.
15. In order to move to the X40 objective lens, take your eyes away from the eyepiece and slowly move the X40 objective lens into place, checking that it does not come into contact with the slide. Use the fine focus control to focus the image.
16. Record the Vernier scale coordinates so that you can relocate a particular organism or artefact on the slide (see below).

Using oil immersion

The oil immersion lens should always be used last, in order to avoid getting oil on any of the other lenses. First, carry out steps 1 to 15 above, then:

1. Fully open the iris diaphragm.
2. Move the stage down and place a drop of oil on the specimen. (Note, remove the coverslip first if one is in place.)
3. Rotate the oil immersion lens (X100) into place.
4. Without looking down the eyepiece, move the stage upwards slowly until the objective lens comes into contact with the oil on the slide.
5. Look down the eyepiece and slowly focus the image using the fine focus control.

Viewing the slide

Once a focused image is in view, the slide must be viewed in a methodical manner. Use the 'battlement technique' to scan the slide (Figure 17.4).

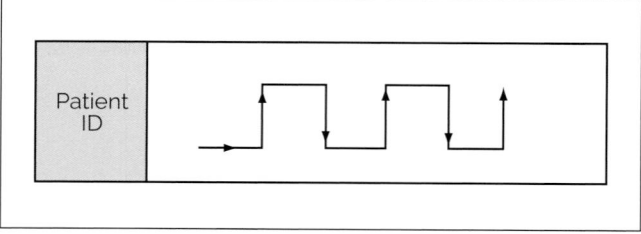

17.4 Diagrammatic representation of scanning a slide using the battlement technique: when viewing a slide, start on the left hand side. Move two fields to the right and view again; then move two fields vertically (i.e. away from you) and view again; then move two fields to the right and view again; then two fields downwards (i.e. towards you) and view again. This is continued across the slide, forming a 'battlement' pattern.

Vernier scales

The Vernier scales can be used to record the location of a particular part of an image or specimen (e.g. an ectoparasite on a skin scraping or a blood cell in a blood smear), so that it can be relocated easily on a subsequent viewing. There are two scales: the horizontal Vernier scale (X axis running from left to right) and the vertical Vernier scale (Y axis running from top to bottom). Both must be read and recorded, stating horizontal and vertical values (X, Y).

Using a Vernier scale

- The stage can be lowered if needed to enable the scale to be read accurately but should not be touched again
- For each direction, there is a main scale (marked on the stage) and a smaller Vernier scale located next to the main scale
- For the main scale reading, read the last whole increment before the Vernier scale zero (0), i.e. 28 in the diagram below
- For the Vernier scale reading, read the point on the Vernier scale at which a line on that scale best matches one on the main scale, i.e. 4 in the diagram below
- This will give the complete reading as 28.4 mm

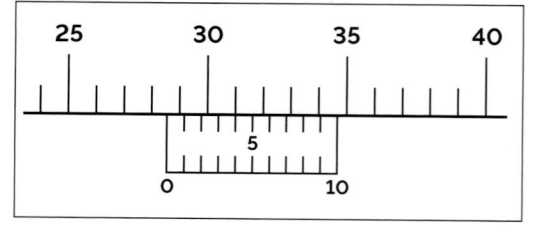

After viewing a slide under the microscope

- Work out the magnification factor of the image by multiplying the eyepiece lens magnification (usually X10) by the objective lens magnification (e.g. X40, so magnification factor = X10 x X40 = X400).

- Turn down the light using the rheostat.
- Lower the stage completely.
- Remove the slide.
- Rotate the nosepiece to the lowest objective lens.
- Move the stage up but do not touch any of the lenses.
- Switch off the light.
- Remove the plug from the electrical socket.
- Clean the microscope, including the lenses.
- Replace the dust cover.

Microscope care and cleaning

- The microscope must be stored in a safe position away from water, moisture, dust, vibrations (e.g. centrifuge) and excessive heat
- When not in use the microscope should be covered with a dust cover
- The microscope should be lifted by the 'limb' (see Figure 17.2) with the base supported
- The microscope must never be pulled or pushed along a surface; it should instead be lifted and placed where required
- The microscope must be cleaned regularly, using a suitable disinfectant
- The stage must be kept clean by wiping the underside of slides, using cover slips (see above) and avoiding excessive amounts of fluid on the slide
- Lenses should be wiped with lens cleaner using fine tissue or lens cloth
- Moving parts should be oiled as necessary
- Safety checks must be carried out regularly including electrical testing
- The light must be switched off when not in use and never be left on for long periods of time, in order to prolong the life of the bulb
- If the bulb needs changing it should first be allowed to cool. The microscope should be switched off and unplugged before the old bulb is removed and a new one put in

Centrifuges

A centrifuge uses centrifugal force to separate substances of varying densities. Dense particles, such as solids, will settle to the bottom of the samples; this is known as the sediment. The less dense liquid portion will remain at the surface; this is known as the supernatant. There are three types of centrifuge:

- **Angle-head:** this is the most common type of centrifuge. Tubes are held in a fixed position, usually 40 degrees from vertical (Figures 17.5a and 17.6). Care must be taken when removing the sample from the fixed angle position
- **Swing-out head:** the sample starts in a vertical position. As the rotor turns the head, the buckets swing out (Figure 17.5b). Once the centrifuge slows and eventually stops, the buckets revert to a vertical position
- **Microhaematocrit:** this centrifuge has a special type of rotor consisting of individual slots on a horizontal surface for holding blood capillary tubes (Figure 17.6).

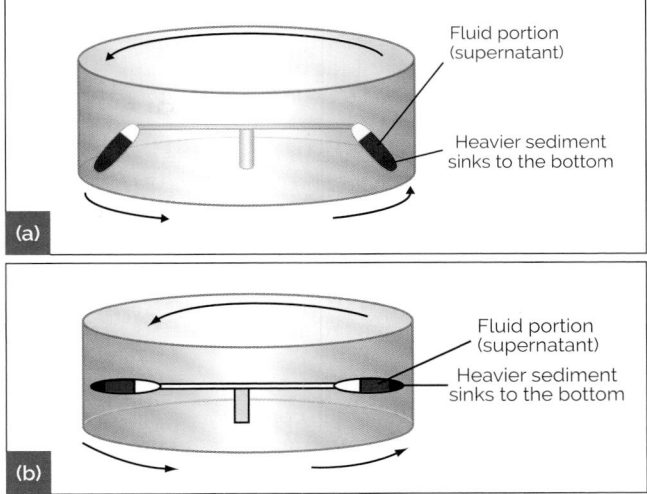

17.5 Diagrammatic representation of two centrifuge types. **(a)** Angle-head. **(b)** Swing-out head.

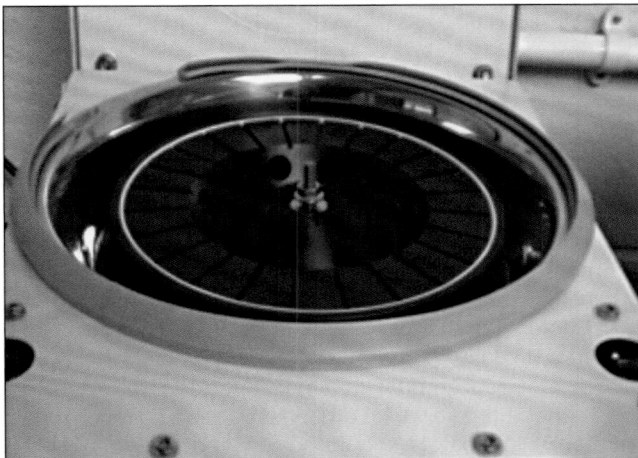

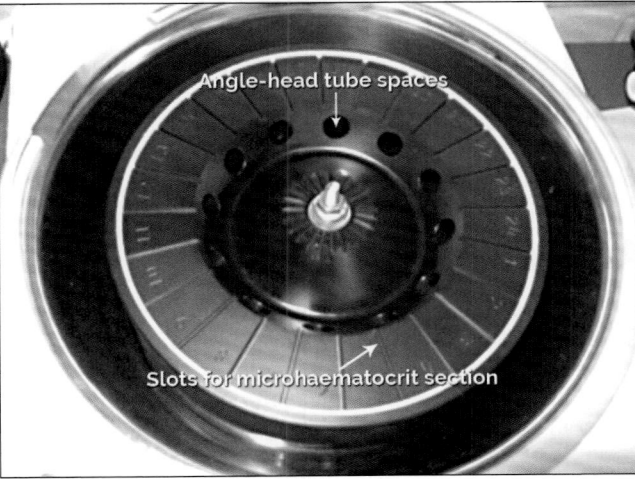

17.6 Angle-head centrifuge, with a section for microhaematocrit tubes, within a solid metal inner bowl. The safety plate lid has been removed.

Centrifuges have the potential to be dangerous, as the contents (which often include glass) are spinning at high speeds. As a result, they have built-in safety modifications, including a solid metal inner bowl (Figure 17.6) with a safety plate lid. The lid usually locks in place and cannot be opened until the rotor stops moving. In addition, if the machine is not correctly loaded, it will not start to rotate.

Using a centrifuge

- Always use the centrifuge on a flat surface
- Make sure the safety plate in the lid is secure before turning on
- Always balance the samples around the machine (e.g. two samples should be placed at 180 degrees to each other)
- Select the most appropriate speed for the sample and the centrifuge. As a guide:
  - Urine: 1500–2000 rpm for 5 minutes
  - Blood including microhaematocrit: 10,000 rpm for 5 minutes
  - Faeces: 1000–1500 rpm for 3 minutes
- Never lift the lid whilst the centrifuge is still rotating (this is usually not possible as the lid is locked in place; see above)
- Clean the whole centrifuge after each use; wipe and disinfect the interior and lid
- The centrifuge must be serviced regularly according to the manufacturer's recommendations

All analysers should:

- Be kept in a safe and secure position
- Be kept at the appropriate room temperature, which should be monitored
- Be used in accordance with manufacturer's instructions by trained personnel
- Be serviced regularly by the provider, including electrical testing
- Have quality control performed regularly for reliable results (see below).

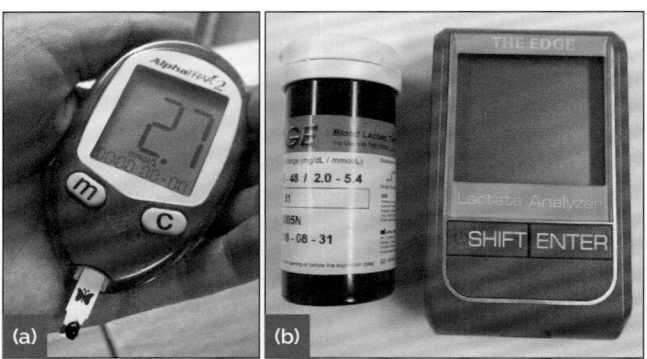

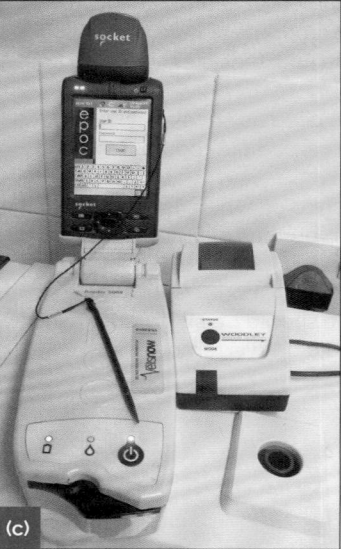

17.7 Handheld analysers are now more commonly available for veterinary practice. Examples include; **(a)** AlphaTRACK® pet glucometer; **(b)** The EDGE™ lactate analyser; **(c)** epoc® portable blood gas, electrolyte and critical care analyser.

Incubators

Laboratory incubators are heated cabinets usually used for culturing bacteria or fungi (see 'Bacteriology', below). Most incubators are run at 'body temperature' (37°C). Incubators commonly have an inner glass door to allow the contents to be checked without opening the main door and losing heat. Bacterial or fungal culture plates are placed inside the incubator, usually with the lid downwards, and incubated for the required amount of time (this depends upon the culture medium and which organisms are being grown) (see Chapter 5). Incubators should be cleaned after use with a disinfectant at a dilution and contact time appropriate to kill the organisms that it has been used to grow. Incubators must also be serviced at regular intervals according to the manufacturer's recommendations. It is important to ensure that the incubator has at least 3 inches of space around the cabinet to allow venting of heat and provide access to cords and hook ups.

Analysers

An analyser is any instrument or device that performs chemical or other analyses on samples. Biochemistry, haematology, electrolyte and hormone analysers are the types most commonly found in veterinary practice laboratories. In-house analysers can provide quick and reliable results and avoid the delay of sending samples to external laboratories; this is particularly important in urgent cases. Analysers vary from small hand-held machines (Figure 17.7) measuring only a limited number of parameters (e.g. a glucometer to measure blood glucose levels; Figure 17.7a) to large worktop machines measuring a wide range of different parameters. Many modern machines require only very small sample sizes. Commercial machines vary in how they operate and most manufacturers provide specific training for staff.

Regardless of the make and function of practice analysers, some basic rules should be applied.

Quality control and quality assurance

Quality control (QC) and quality assurance (QA) procedures must be carried out on any analyser used within the in-house laboratory. Both QC and QA are ways of avoiding errors in laboratory findings and their interpretation, and this subject is discussed further at the end of the chapter (see 'Inconsistencies and inaccuracies in laboratory results', below).

Quality control

QC includes all the steps taken to determine the validity of a specific test procedure. QC checks are usually performed internally by veterinary practice staff. Manufacturers produce QC products for each of their analysers. These consist of samples with known values, e.g. biochemical ranges, which can then be compared with the results formulated by the in-house analyser. Any inconsistencies in the results produced by the machine should be reported to the manufacturer. Analyser QC should ideally be carried out:

- At the beginning of each shift or day
- After an analyser is serviced
- When reagent lots are changed
- After calibration
- When patient results seem inappropriate
- As indicated by the manufacturer.

Quality assurance

QA is the broader programme of controls that ensures that the final results reported are correct. QA includes things like ensuring that the right test is carried out on the right specimen, and that the right result and right interpretation are delivered to the right person at the right time (see 'Inconsistencies and inaccuracies in laboratory results', below). QA also usually includes some sort of external monitoring of standards. QA through referral of internal samples to external laboratories, or internal analysis of external samples, should be routinely undertaken and the results documented. The frequency of external QA testing should be related to the number of tests undertaken, but is likely to be at least quarterly.

Biochemistry analysers

These measure levels of biochemical substances (e.g. calcium, glucose, lactate; see Figure 17.7) contained within a patient's blood. Some biochemical analysers have additional functions such as hormone analysis (e.g. T4 (thyroxine) levels). There are two types of machine.

- **Dry chemistry analysers:** These use slides impregnated with chemicals. The machine drops the sample on to the slides and then reads and interprets the colour change. The colour change reflects the level of the biochemical substance in the patient sample.
- **Wet chemistry analysers:** These use containers of wet fluids. The machine uses chemical reactions creating colour changes to determine the biochemical levels in the patient sample.

Analysers usually measure a colour change in order to determine the result. This measurement may be made using a **colorimeter** (a device which measures absorbance of specific colours of light), or using a **spectrophotometer** (a device that measures transmittance or reflectance of light as a function of wavelength).

Electrolyte analysers

These can vary from large in-house laboratory analysers to hand-held portable analysers. They are able to give rapid results on the levels of electrolytes (e.g. Na$^+$, K$^+$, Cl$^-$) in a sample. Some machines can be used for additional tests, such as measuring blood gas levels (see Figure 17.7c), which can be extremely important in emergency and critical care patients (see Chapter 19), in fluid therapy (see Chapter 20) and during general anaesthesia (see Chapter 21).

Haematology analysers

These are used to perform tests on the cellular components of the blood such as cell counts, coagulation tests and erythrocyte sedimentation rates. Most commonly, veterinary practice haematology equipment is used to determine the quantities of each type of red and white blood cell within a blood sample, providing a **differential count** of each cell type. Haematology analysers work on either a Coulter Principle (electrical impedance) or flow cytometry (including fluorescent flow cytometry); both involve the cells rapidly passing through a small aperture or a laser beam where they are differentiated and counted. Most veterinary practice haematology machines are calibrated for specific species of animal and it is important that the correct species is inputted into the machine at the start of the test, or the results will not be valid.

Glassware

Glassware, such as flasks and beakers, should be thoroughly cleaned before use to avoid contamination.

Cleaning and care of laboratory glassware

1. Wear suitable PPE including gloves.
2. Remove organic material/contaminants from the glassware. Appropriate soaking in detergent may be required in order to remove dried substances. A soft-bristled brush or ultrasonic cleaner may be used to assist with cleaning.
3. Wash the glassware in detergent to remove remaining organic material, grease, etc. Rinse well.
4. Disinfect using an approved solution at the correct dilution for the required contact time for the organisms involved (see Chapter 14).
5. Rinse 2–3 times in distilled or deionized water.
6. Allow to drain.
7. Dry in a drying cabinet or oven.
8. Ensure the glassware is thoroughly clean, free from cracks/chips and suitable for use before storage. Any mark in the uniform surface of glassware is a potential breakpoint, especially when the piece is heated.
9. Store in a clean, dry and dust-free environment.

Bunsen burner

Bunsen burners are used for heating and sterilizing equipment. They are usually only used in practice laboratories where in-house bacteriology is carried out (see 'Bacteriology', below). Bunsen burners can be dangerous, so some precautions should be taken when using them.

Precautions for using a Bunsen burner

- Ensure that long hair is tied back
- Ensure that nothing flammable is close to the Bunsen burner; for example, paper laboratory notices or flammable liquids
- Ensure that the Bunsen burner is placed on a flat surface with no obstructions around it (e.g. it should not be placed under a shelf)
- Switch on the gas supply
- Close the air hole and then light the Bunsen burner, which should show a golden flame
- Open the air hole to show a blue flame for direct heating of equipment
- Close the air hole to return to a more visible gold flame when not being used
- Always turn off the Bunsen when not in use. NEVER leave a lit Bunsen unattended
- Turn off gas supply once all procedures have finished

Blood samples

As with all clinical sampling, basic rules of communication, consent and record keeping must be adhered to when blood samples are collected (see 'The importance of laboratory diagnostic aids', above). In addition, special consideration will need to be given to patient preparation as well as ensuring that the sample is collected, handled and stored correctly. Poor patient preparation and/or mishandling of blood samples can mean that the results of any tests are invalid (see 'Inconsistencies and inaccuracies in laboratory results' below). Blood samples must always be handled gently and with respect.

Patient preparation

Some test results can be affected by physiological factors and/or the timing of drug administration.

- Exercise, excitement and fear can result in an increase in white blood cell counts (neutrophils and sometimes lymphocytes) and in blood glucose levels. Patients should consequently be kept as calm as possible when taking blood samples and consideration given to the possibility of spurious results if this is not the case.
- Recent food consumption can affect biochemistry test results, especially cholesterol, triglycerides, glucose and urea, as well as make the sample lipaemic (fatty; see also Figure 17.12) and unsuitable for some other tests (albumin, total protein and electrolytes). For these reasons, unless post-feeding samples are specifically required (e.g. for bile acid test) or there are medical reasons for avoiding withholding food, all animals should be starved for 8–12 h (usually by withholding food overnight).
- The collection of samples for drug monitoring (e.g. for thyroxine in hypothyroidism or trilostane in hyperadrenocorticism) must be timed appropriately after the administration of medication. The time of drug administration and of sample collection should be carefully recorded. Consideration should also be given to any possible delay in sample analysis after collection; this is especially the case if postage to an external laboratory is required. Samples for glucose, ammonia and coagulation factors need to be either analysed quickly and/or collected in appropriate tubes (see 'Sample preservation', below and Figure 17.10).

Sample collection

Preparation and equipment

Before the patient is restrained for blood sample collection (venepuncture) all equipment should be prepared.

Selection and preparation of equipment for blood sample collection

- Gloves
- Clippers to remove hair
- Clipper blade of an appropriate size
- Attach blade to clippers and check they are working correctly →

Selection and preparation of equipment for blood sample collection *continued*

- Skin antiseptic preparation (chlorhexidine and surgical spirit) and swab(s)
- Dry swab for pressure after sample collection
- Needle of appropriate size (largest gauge possible to avoid rupturing red blood cells) and syringe of appropriate size (smallest size possible to reduce the pressure and avoid rupturing red blood cells)
- Put together the syringe and needle in a sterile manner and pre-loosen the syringe plunger
- Select appropriate tube/receptacle (e.g. blood tube, vacutainer; see Figure 17.10 for cap colours)
- Label tube

Venepuncture

Restraint of the patient is described in Chapter 11 and the sites for venepuncture are given in Figure 17.8.

Species/group	Example veins used for blood sample collection
Dog	Cephalic, jugular, lateral saphenous
Cat	Jugular, cephalic, lateral saphenous
Rabbit	Jugular, cephalic, lateral saphenous, marginal ear
Birds	Right jugular, superficial ulnar, medial metatarsal
Tortoises	Subcarapacial, jugular, dorsal coccygeal
Lizards	Jugular, ventral coccygeal (only in larger species)
Snakes	Jugular, ventral coccygeal, palatine (in non-venomous species)

17.8 Common sites for venepuncture in a range of species.

Technique for needle venepuncture

1. Assemble the equipment required (see 'Selection and preparation of equipment for blood sample collection', above). Ensure the equipment such as the needle and syringe are sterile and assembled aseptically. Ensure the plunger is pre-released on the syringe. It is also useful to pre-label blood collection tubes.
2. Ensure correct identification of the patient.
3. Confirm the tests/samples required from the patient.
4. Request assistance from a colleague to restrain the patient. The restraint technique will vary depending on the species and site used for venepuncture (Figure 17.9).
5. Put gloves on.
6. Prepare the venepuncture site aseptically. This may involve clipping in mammalian species.
7. Depending on the venepuncture site, ask the assistant to occlude the vein if required.
8. Once the vein is visible, insert the needle into the vein at a slight angle from the skin surface. →

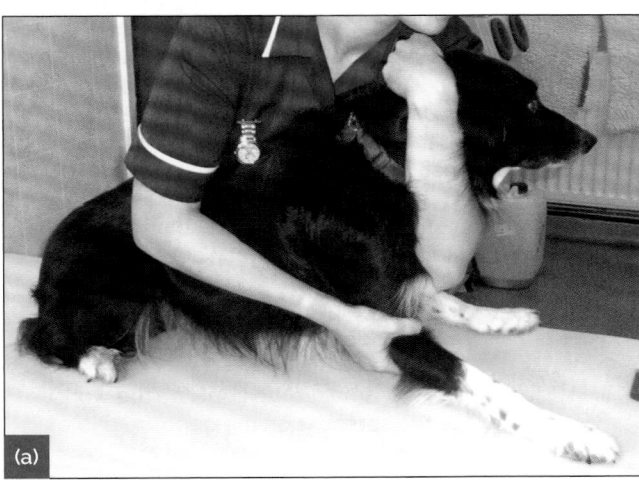

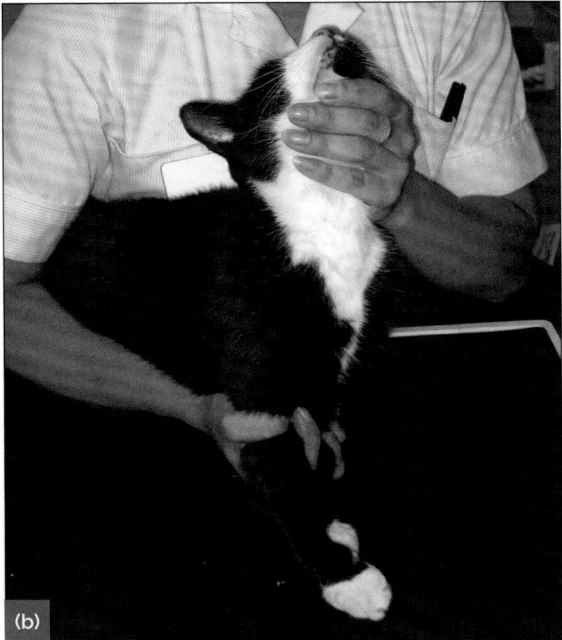

17.9 (a) Restraint of a dog for cephalic venepuncture. (b) Restraint of a cat for jugular venepuncture.

Volume collected

The volume of blood needed for diagnostic tests in dogs and cats is usually quite small relative to their size. For smaller species, care needs to be taken with the amount collected so as to avoid excessive blood loss. As a general rule, no more than 1% of the animal's blood volume should be collected in healthy patients and less than that in those that are debilitated.

Sample preservation

The preservation method chosen is dependent upon the required diagnostic test. In order to preserve a sample, the following can be used:

- A receptacle containing an anticoagulant
- A receptacle containing no anticoagulant, allowing the sample to clot so that the serum can be removed
- Preparation of a blood smear, possibly including the use of stains, so that it can be viewed with a microscope.

Anticoagulants

Anticoagulants prevent blood clotting (Figure 17.10). A collection tube with the appropriate anticoagulant for the diagnostic test to be carried out must be selected, as incorrect selection can result in invalid results.

- For routine haematology EDTA (ethylenediamine tetra-acetic acid) is used. The benefit of this anticoagulant is that it causes minimal changes in the morphology of the blood cells, thus making it useful for blood smears and cell counts.
- Samples for glucose estimation are collected into a tube containing fluoride/oxalate or into a vacutainer that inhibits the oxidation of glucose.
- Heparin salts may be used for blood samples that are to undergo biochemical tests where plasma is required. Heparin salts (sodium, ammonium and lithium) bind and inhibit thrombin, thus preventing the formation of clots. Samples with heparin may also be used for various hormone tests.

In all cases, the sample must be quickly and gently placed into the appropriate container via the syringe not the needle. The sample should then be mixed, which is best achieved by gently rolling the tube between the fingers. Poor mixing (as well as poor sampling and a delay in mixing) may result in the blood, at least in part, clotting and make any results invalid.

Serum samples

Serum is obtained from a clotted sample (i.e. there is no anticoagulant within the tube; Figure 17.11). Serum samples are used for serology and for some biochemical tests (see below). Serum does not contain clotting factors, such as fibrinogen, as they have been used in forming the blood clot. Serum may be extracted from a naturally clotted sample and analysed in-house or sent to an external laboratory. Alternatively, the serum can be separated from the clotted blood using a serum-separating tube (serum gel tube), which contains a special gel that creates an impermeable barrier between the serum and the clot; some tubes also contain 'clot activators' which speed up the rate of clot formation. Care should be taken when using serum gel tubes for drug and hormone assays as they are not always appropriate for these tests. Separated serum can be

Anticoagulant	Tube cap colour	Vacutainer cap colour	Used for
Lithium heparin	orange	green	Biochemistry
Ethylenediamine tetra-acetic acid (EDTA)	pink	mauve	Haematology
Fluoride/oxalate	yellow	grey	Glucose
Sodium/lithium citrate	blue	blue	Coagulation profiles
No anticoagulant	white brown	red	Serum collection

17.10   Common anticoagulants used in blood collection containers.

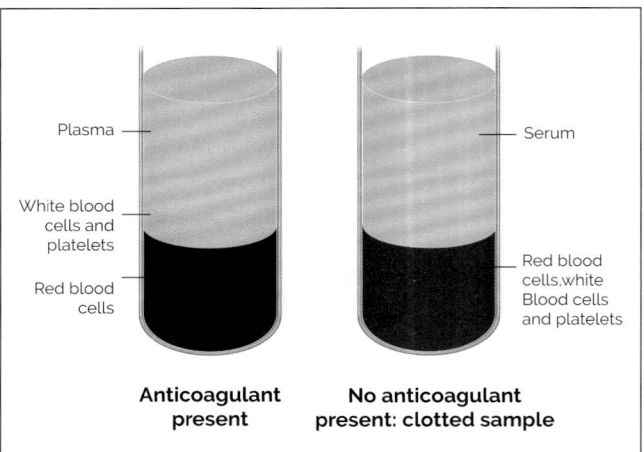

Anticoagulant present   **No anticoagulant present: clotted sample**

17.11   Diagrammatic representation of the individual components of a blood sample once it has been centrifuged. Plasma is obtained from samples collected into tubes containing anticoagulant. Serum is obtained from a clotted sample (no anticoagulant).

stored in a refrigerator for a few days or, for some tests, the serum may be frozen and then thawed to room temperature before use. The appearance of serum and plasma may vary for a number of reasons (Figure 17.12).

Abnormal serum colour	Reason for change
Pink/red	Haemolysed sample – red blood cells have been damaged due to incorrect sampling or preservation
Yellow	Icteric sample – the colour change is caused by the presence of bilirubin, which may indicate haemolytic disease, liver disease or biliary obstruction
Milky white	Lipaemic sample – due to the presence of fat in unstarved animals or evidence of liver disease

17.12   Serum or plasma sample may have an abnormal colour for a variety of reasons.

Blood smears

A blood smear, or blood film as it is sometimes known, is a thin layer of blood spread across a glass slide. The method is used to produce a sample that may be sent to an external laboratory, or used in house, to be examined for a differential white blood cell count or cellular abnormalities. Some form of staining (see below) is usually used to help differentiate cell types. Blood smears are an important tool, even in practices with haematology analysers, as they can detect cell abnormalities and inclusions not detected by an automatic analyser.

Preparation of a blood smear

1. Put on gloves.
2. Select a microscope slide and clean it using ethanol or absolute alcohol (methanol) and dry with lint-free tissue.
3. Select a blood sample containing EDTA.
4. Gently mix the sample.
5. Select a plain capillary tube.
6. Insert the capillary tube into the blood sample and draw up a small amount of blood into the tube.
7. Place a finger over the top of the tube or keep the tube horizontal to prevent leakage of blood.
8. Remove the tube and place a small dot of blood near one end of the slide.
9. Discard the capillary tube as hazardous waste.
10. Select a spreader slide; ensure that it is clean and dry.
11. Holding the blood sample slide firmly on the work surface, place the spreader on the opposite end of the slide to the blood.

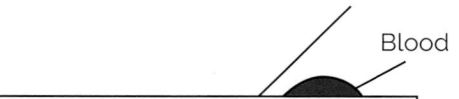
Blood

12. Draw the spreader back into the drop of blood at an angle of 45 degrees and allow blood to spread along the edge of the spreader.

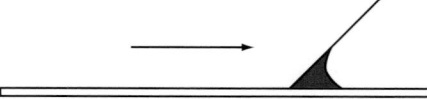

13. Push the spreader away from the blood drop using a single, smooth motion.

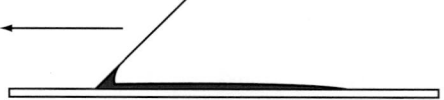

14. Rapidly air-dry the slide.
15. Label the slide.
16. Check and comment on the quality of the smear.
17. Place in a slide transport container.

The final blood smear should look like a thumbprint with a 'feathered edge'. The slide should be examined in the 'monolayer' close to the feathered edge (Figure 17.13). Common faults in blood smears include 'hesitation bands', grease spots, thick/thin smears and uneven smears. Faults can be avoided through correct preparation and technique.

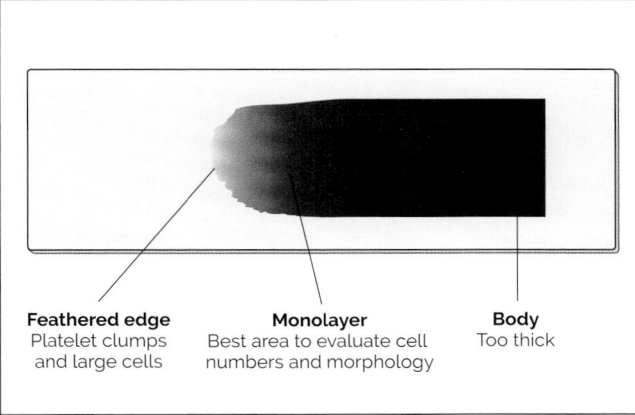

Feathered edge
Platelet clumps
and large cells

Monolayer
Best area to evaluate cell
numbers and morphology

Body
Too thick

17.13 Diagrammatic representation of the correct appearance of a blood smear.

Staining

Smears are usually stained prior to examination to distinguish individual cells and to identify cellular abnormalities. There are two common types of stain used for blood smears in veterinary practice:

- **Romanowsky stain** – e.g. Leishman's, Giemsa, Diff-Quik®. These stains can be used when performing a differential white blood cell count. They will also detect the presence of blood parasites such as *Babesia*
- **Supravital stain** – e.g. methylene blue. Supravital stains can be used for smears that are to be used to perform a reticulocyte count. They will also detect Heinz bodies.

Staining procedures for blood smears
Leishman's stain

1. Put on gloves.
2. Place slide on staining rack with smear uppermost.
3. Cover with Leishman's stain and leave for 2 minutes.
4. Add twice the stain's volume of buffered distilled water pH 6.8 and gently mix using a Pasteur pipette.
5. Leave for 10–15 minutes.
6. Wash the slide with buffered distilled water pH 6.8.
7. Allow slide to dry.

Giemsa stain

1. Put on gloves.
2. Fix the slide by dipping in methanol for 1 minute.
3. Flood the slide with diluted Giemsa stain and leave for 30 minutes.
4. Rinse the slide with distilled water.
5. Allow slide to airdry.

Staining procedures for blood smears *continued*
Diff-Quik® stain

1. Put on gloves.
2. Dip slide into the fixative (methanol) solution (pale blue) five times for 1 second each time. Allow excess fluid to drip back into the jar.
3. Dip slide into stain (eosin) solution 1 (red) five times for 1 second each time. Allow excess fluid to drip back into the jar.
4. Dip slide into stain (methylene blue) solution 2 (purple) five times for 1 second each time. Allow excess fluid to drip back into the jar.
5. Rinse slide with distilled water.
6. Place slide vertically and leave to dry.

Once the slide has been correctly stained and is dry, examination can be carried out. The smear should be examined under a microscope at low power (X10), high power (X40) and oil immersion (X100) objectives.

Blood smear examination

Blood cell morphology

Qualitative examination of the blood smear should be carried out first. This involves examination of the red blood cells (RBCs, erythrocytes), white blood cells (WBCs, leucocytes) and thrombocytes (platelets) in the monolayer (see Figure 17.13) for morphological abnormalities. Normal blood cell morphology in dogs and cats is shown in Figure 17.14 and in Chapter 3. Blood cell morphology differs in many 'exotic' species and is discussed further in Chapter 3. Erythrocyte abnormalities in dogs and cats are described and illustrated in Figures 17.15 to 17.17.

Common abnormalities in white blood cells include:

- Toxic neutrophils: Blue/pink cytoplasm with blue cell inclusions
- Left shift: Increase in the number of immature neutrophils. Indicates the presence of an inflammatory condition.

White blood cell counts

A differential white blood cell count is performed to determine the relative proportions of the different cell types (see Figure 17.14 for reference ranges). For the most accurate estimation counts should be made on both the edge and the middle of the body of the blood smear using a battlement technique (see Figure 17.4). The procedure is time-consuming but can be a crucial aid to diagnosis in practices that do not have a haematology analyser.

- The main body of the smear is examined under oil immersion.
- Cells are counted and recorded using a standard manual laboratory 'clicker' type counter or using an electronic tabulator. If these are not available a tally chart can be used.
- Usually 100 cells are counted, so that the number of each cell counted can be expressed as a percentage.

Once the quantitative analysis of the smear has been carried out, the results must be correctly recorded and passed to the veterinary surgeon who will interpret the results (Figure 17.18).

Cell type	Normal appearance	Description	Role/significance	Reference ranges (number of cells per litre of blood or percentage of white blood cells)	
				Cat	Dog
Erythrocyte		Pink, biconcave disc with no nucleus	Transport of blood gases	$5–10 \times 10^{12}/l$	$5.5–8.5 \times 10^{12}/l$
Mature neutrophil		Multi-lobed nucleus, pale granules in cytoplasm	Phagocytosis	60%	70%
Immature neutrophil		Horseshoe-shaped nucleus	Phagocytosis	Variable	Variable
Eosinophil		Pink granules with bilobed or segmented nucleus	Increased in parasitic conditions	4%	$0.1–1.25 \times 10^{9}/l$
Basophil		Irregular nucleus with blue granular cytoplasm	Increased in allergic reactions	Rare	Rare
Lymphocyte		Larger cells, nucleus occupies majority of cell	Immune response: B cells and T cells	30%	20%
Monocyte		Horse-shaped nucleus. Larger cells. No granules in cytoplasm	Phagocytosis	3%	5%
Thrombocyte		Very small cells	Clotting	$200 \times 10^{9}/l$	$200 \times 10^{9}/l$

17.14 Normal blood cell morphology and reference ranges in dogs and cats. (Modified Wright's stain, original magnification X100). (Courtesy of Axiom Laboratories)

Abnormality		Description
Size	Macrocyte	Larger than normal
	Microcyte	Smaller than normal
	Anisocytosis	Great variation in size of cells
Shape	Crenation (crenellation)	Distortion giving a spiky appearance (Figure 17.16a). Caused by damage to the cell. Seen in patients with autoimmune haemolytic anaemia
	Schistocyte	Red blood cell fragment (Figure 17.16b)
	Spherocyte	Spherical (Figure 17.16c)
	Rouleaux	Individual cells are of normal shape but cells are stacked and formed into chains (Figure 17.16d)
Colour	Hypochromasia	Reduced cellular haemoglobin, giving paler appearance
	Polychromasia	Larger bluer cells (Romanowsky stain). Often seen in regenerative anaemia
Inclusions	Heinz bodies	Blue (Supravital stain) and granular appearance; formed from denatured haemoglobin
	Howell-Jolly bodies	Basophilic nuclear remnants seen in young blood cells (Figure 17.17a). Seen in regenerative anaemia and after splenectomy
	Babesia	Parasite transmitted by ticks. Detected using Romanowsky staining techniques
	Mycoplasma haemofelis	Parasite causing feline infectious anaemia
Immaturity	Reticulocyte	Immature red blood cells (anuclear) with sustainable cytoplasmic RNA (blue cytoplasm, Supravital stain) (Figure 17.17b)

17.15 Common abnormalities of red blood cells (erythrocytes).

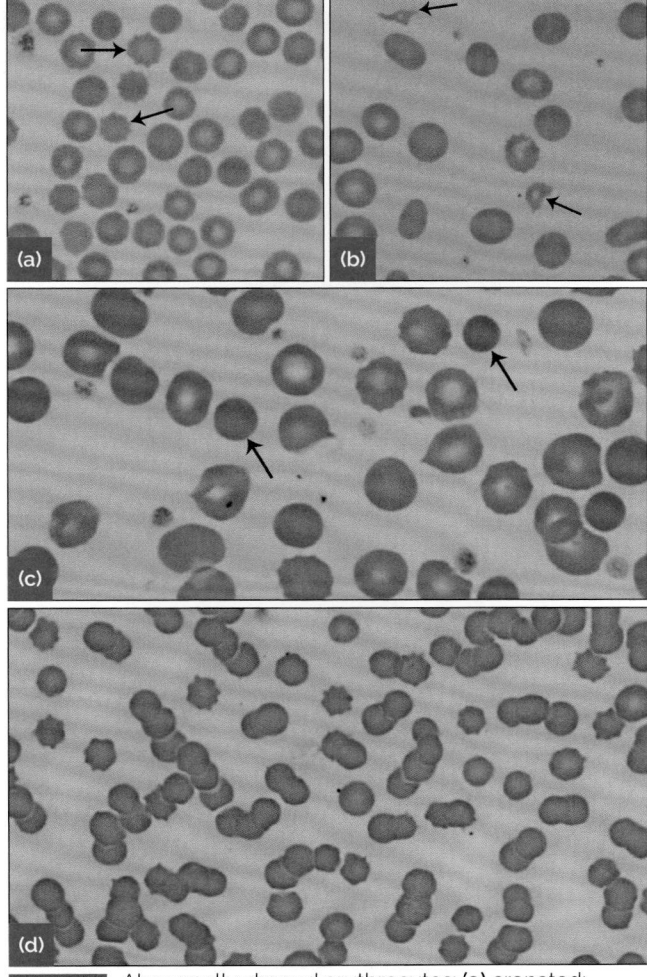

17.16 Abnormally shaped erythrocytes: **(a)** crenated; **(b)** schistocytes; **(c)** spherocytes; **(d)** rouleaux. (Modified Wright's stain; **a**, **b** and **c**, Original magnification X100; **d**, Original magnification X50). (Courtesy of Axiom Laboratories)

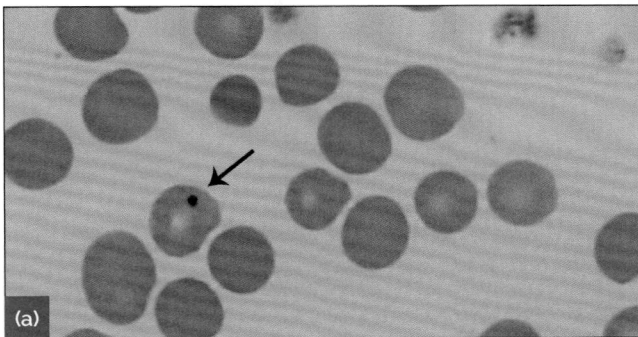

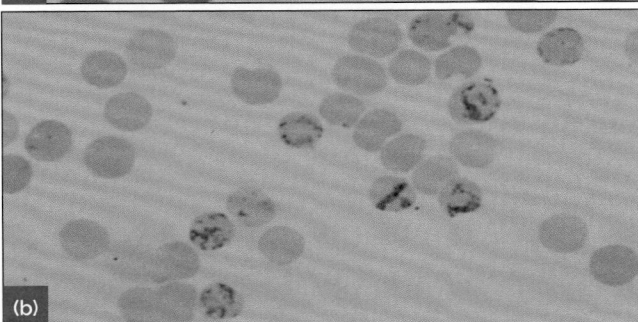

17.17 Erythrocytes with inclusions: **(a)** Howell–Jolly body (Wright's stain); **(b)** canine reticulocytes (new methylene blue). (Original magnifications X100). (Courtesy of Axiom Laboratories)

Cells counted	Increase and possible causes	Decrease and possible causes
All white blood cells	**Leucocytosis:** Presence of infection, neoplasia, haemorrhage	**Leucopenia:** Severe bacterial infection/ sepsis, some viral disease, Cushing's disease, bone marrow suppression
Neutrophils	**Neutrophilia:** Bacterial infection, inflammation, stress, neoplasia	**Neutropenia:** Severe bacterial infections, some viral infections, cytotoxic medications, bone marrow disorders
Eosinophils	**Eosinophilia:** Allergic reactions, parasitism	**Eosinopenia:** Cushing's disease, corticosteroid therapy
Basophils	**Basophilia:** Rare, sometimes seen with allergy, parasitism or neoplasia	**Basopenia:** Basophils rare in all common domestic animals. Therefore basopenia difficult to document and of no diagnostic significance
Lymphocytes	**Lymphocytosis:** Chronic disease, exercise/excitement, stress, lympho-proliferative disease	**Lymphopenia:** Cushing's disease, corticosteroid therapy, acute viral or bacterial infection
Monocytes	**Monocytosis:** Infection/ inflammation, steroids/stress, immune-mediated conditions	**Monopenia:** Rare

17.18 Interpretation of quantitative analysis of white blood cells (leucocytes).

Packed cell volume

Packed cell volume (PCV) (also known as the **haematocrit**) is the percentage of the total blood volume that is occupied by red blood cells. This quick and easy test rapidly gives information on hydration status, level of blood loss in haemorrhaging patients, or degree of anaemia.

Preparing a PCV sample

1. Put on gloves.
2. Select a blood sample with EDTA.
3. Mix the sample gently.
4. Remove plain microhaematocrit capillary tubes from their container (1 or 2).
5. Insert a microhaematocrit tube into the sample (holding the sample tube at an angle) and fill the tube to at least three-quarters full by capillary action.
6. Place a finger over the top end of the tube or keep the tube horizontal to prevent leakage of blood.
7. Remove the tube from the sample.
8. Wipe the outside of the tube with a tissue.
9. Plug one end of the tube with soft clay sealant.
10. Place the tube into the microhaematocrit centrifuge with the clay plug against the rim.
11. Balance the centrifuge with a second tube.
12. Screw the inner safety lid down over the samples. ➔

Preparing a PCV sample *continued*

13. Close and lock the main lid.
14. Set at 10,000 rpm (or fast setting, depending on make of centrifuge) for 5 minutes.
15. Dispose of any used capillary tubes and other used materials as hazardous waste.

Once the microhaematocrit tube has been centrifuged the blood will have separated into three layers: red cells, buffy coat and plasma (Figure 17.19).

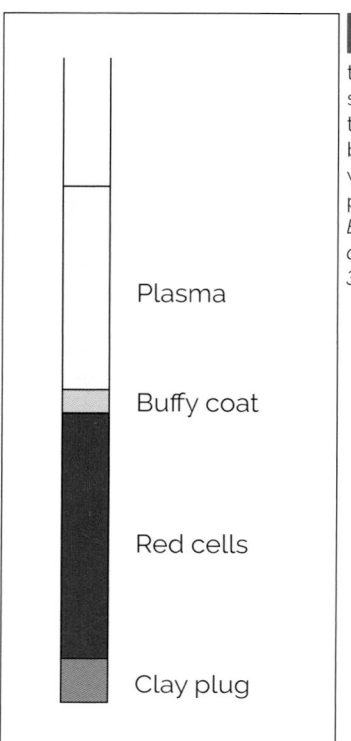

17.19 Diagrammatic representation of the layers of a centrifuged sample in a microhaematocrit tube for PCV evaluation. The buffy coat layer contains the white blood cells and platelets. (Reproduced from *BSAVA Manual of Canine and Feline Clinical Pathology, 3rd edn*)

Plasma

Buffy coat

Red cells

Clay plug

Ideally, the PCV should be read using a Hawksley micro-haematocrit reader (see below). If one is not available a ruler can be used along with the following calculation:

PCV (%) = (height of red blood cells/total column height) x 100

For example, if the height of the red blood cells is 2.2 cm and the total column height is 5.0 cm, then the PCV is 2.2/5.0 x 100 = 44%.

Reference ranges for PCV in dogs and cats are included in Figure 17.20. For common exotic pets they are given in Figure 17.21.

It is important to note that in all species, PCV readings vary significantly with breed, age and fitness; for example, Greyhounds have significantly higher numbers of red blood cells than other breeds of dog, which is one reason why they are often popular as blood donors.

Using a Hawksley PCV reader

1. Place the tube into the slot in the reader, with the sealed end downwards.
2. Align the top of the seal, i.e. the bottom of the red blood cell layer, with the zero line on the reader.

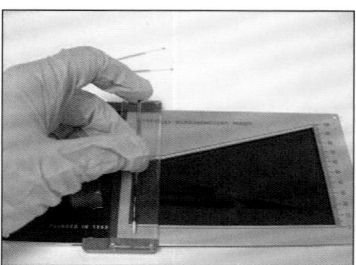

3. Move the tube holder across until the top of the plasma is lined up with the 100% line on the reader.

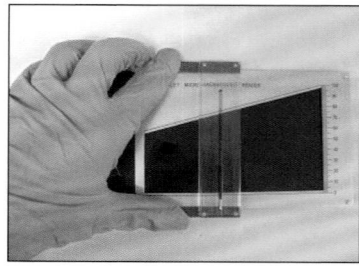

4. Move the adjustable PCV reading line to intersect the top of the RBC layer.

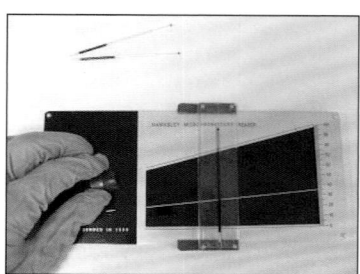

5. Record the PCV reading correctly as a percentage.

Species	Packed cell volume (PCV)
Rabbit[a]	30–40%
Mouse[b]	35–40%
Rat[b]	37.6–50.6%
Hamster[b]	45–50%
Guinea pig[b]	35–45%
Birds[c]	35–55%
Reptiles[d]	18–38%

17.21 Reference ranges for PCV in common exotic pets ([a]*BSAVA Manual of Rabbit Medicine*; [b]*BSAVA Manual of Rodents and Ferrets*; [c]*BSAVA Manual of Avian Practice*; [d]*BSAVA Manual of Reptiles, 3rd edn*).

Species	RBC count (10¹²/l)	WBC count (10⁹/l)	PCV (%)	Hb (g/dl)	MCV (fl)	MCHC (g/dl)
Dog	5.5–8.5	6–17	37–55	12—18	60–70	32—36
Cat	5–10	5.5–19.5	24–45	9—17	39–55	30—36

17.20 Reference ranges of haematological values for dogs and cats. For values in exotic pets please refer to Figure 17.21 and the relevant BSAVA Manuals.

An *increase* in PCV may indicate dehydration due to reduced plasma levels, but an increase is also present in other conditions such as endotoxic shock and splenic contraction. A decrease in PCV may indicate anaemia or haemorrhage, due to a decrease in the number of red blood cells. Use of other parameters, such as total protein or total solids, urine specific gravity and a blood smear, alongside PCV, helps to differentiate between clinical conditions (Figure 17.22; see also Chapter 20).

Blood PCV	Blood total protein/ total solids	Urine specific gravity	Possible cause
Increased	Increased	Increased	Dehydration
Normal (or decreased)	Normal	Decreased	Renal failure
Increased	Normal	Normal	Polycythaemia, normal in some dog breeds (e.g. greyhounds)
Normal	Increased	Normal	Hyperglobulinaemia
Normal	Decreased	Normal	Hypoalbuminaemia
Decreased	Normal	Normal	Chronic anaemia
Decreased	Decreased	Normal	Haemorrhage

17.22 Interpretation of PCV alongside blood total protein/ total solids and urine specific gravity.

Total solids

Once the PCV has been recorded, the same blood haematocrit tube can be used to measure total solids (TS) using a refractometer in the plasma fraction of the tube (Figure 17.19). Although the TS value is made up of the plasma protein plus other non-protein solids (e.g. triglycerides, cholesterol) in most patients it provides a clinically useful approximation of the plasma total protein (see below). This is, however, not the case if the non-protein solids are increased, for example if the animal is lipaemic or jaundiced (icteric) (see Chapter 18), or if larger molecules such as colloids or mannitol have been administered to the patient (see Chapter 20).

Reference ranges for TS are: 60–75 g/l in dogs and 60–75 g/l in cats. TS values can be used alongside PCV to help differentiate between clinical conditions (Figure 17.22).

Measuring total solids using a refractometer

1. Prepare and measure PCV on a microhaematocrit tube as above (see 'Preparing a PCV sample', above).
2. Ensure that the refractometer is calibrated (see 'Using a refractometer', below).
3. Carefully break the capillary tube near the bottom of the plasma fraction. This will give two fragments, one containing the plasma and the other the packed cells.

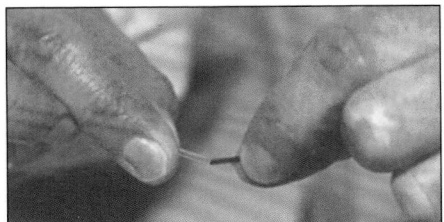

Reproduced from the *BSAVA Manual of Canine and Feline Clinical Pathology, 3rd edn* →

Measuring total solids using a refractometer *continued*

4. Discard the packed cells fragment into a sharps bin.
5. Dab the unbroken end of the fragment containing the plasma on to the refractometer surface. Be careful not to cut yourself on the sharp edges of the glass.

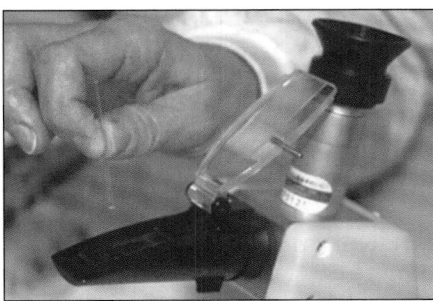

Reproduced from the *BSAVA Manual of Canine and Feline Clinical Pathology, 3rd edn*

6. Read the appropriate scale on the refractometer to determine the plasma protein; this is usually the left hand scale and may be labelled 'Serum P'.

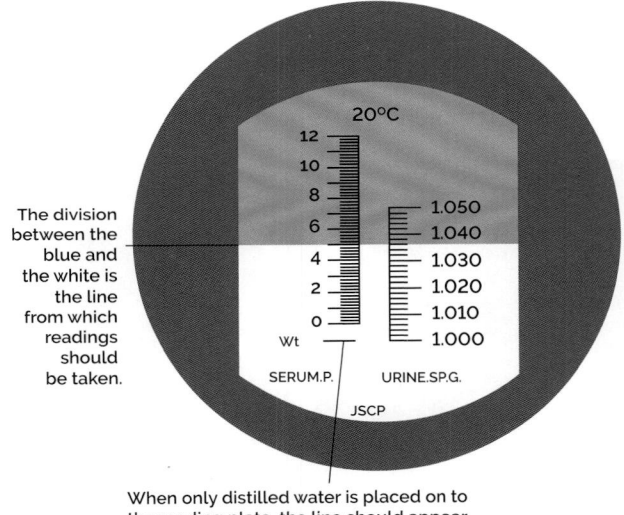

The division between the blue and the white is the line from which readings should be taken.

When only distilled water is placed on to the reading plate, the line should appear at this point if properly calibrated.

7. The measurement will be g/100 ml so needs to be multiplied by 10 to give g/litre (e.g. 50 g/litre above).
8. Dispose of the remaining glass into a sharps bin.

Additional haematological parameters

Additional parameters may be provided by automated haematology analysers. These include:

- **Mean corpuscular volume (MCV)**, which indicates the average size of the red blood cells
- **Mean corpuscular haemoglobin concentration (MCHC)**, which indicates the average haemoglobin concentration per red blood cell
- **Haemoglobin (Hb)** estimations, which indicate the level of haemoglobin found in the red blood cells.

Reference ranges for these parameters in dogs and cats are shown in Figure 17.20.

Blood clotting (coagulation) tests

Thrombocytes assist in haemostasis through the coagulation of blood. Blood clotting analysis (coagulation times) can be vital in the diagnosis and treatment of many conditions, such as von Willebrand's disease and warfarin poisoning, as well as liver disease (see below and Chapter 18). The normal clotting time of blood is usually 1–2 minutes. Buccal mucosal bleeding time, activated clotting time and thrombocyte counts can all be used to determine the animal's coagulation profile.

- **Buccal mucosal bleeding time** (BMBT; Figure 17.23): A commercially available kit can be used to create a small incision in the mucosa – normally in the patient's inner lip. Blotting paper or tissue is held against the incision and a timer used to calculate the length of time taken for it to stop bleeding.
- **Activated clotting time** (ACT): This is measured by placing 1 ml of whole blood into a small glass tube or ACT tube. The tube should be kept at 37°C. The time is recorded from aspiration to the formation of the first clot.
- **Thrombocyte counts** are performed manually on blood smears (see above) or using automated haematology analysers.
- Coagulation tests such as **prothrombin time** (PT), **activated partial thromboplastin time** (aPTT) and thrombin time (TT) can also be used to assess blood clotting function in patients (see Chapter 18). Citrated plasma samples are required (see Figure 17.10). These samples may be run in-house (Figure 17.24) or sent to an external laboratory.

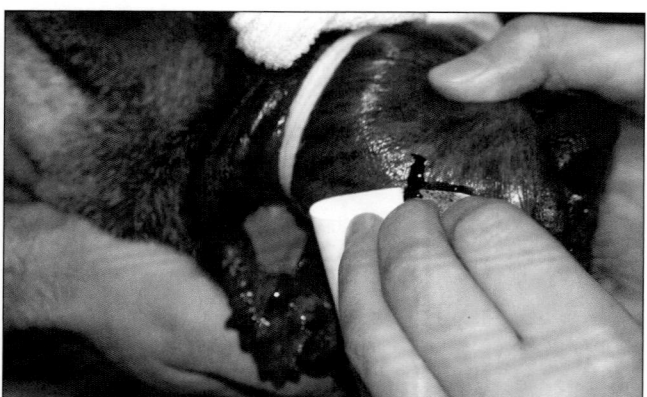

17.23 A veterinary nurse performing a buccal mucosal bleeding time test. Note the upper lip is everted by a bandage; Filter paper is used to absorb excess blood without disturbing the primary clot. (Reproduced from *BSAVA Manual of Advanced Veterinary Nursing*, 2nd edn)

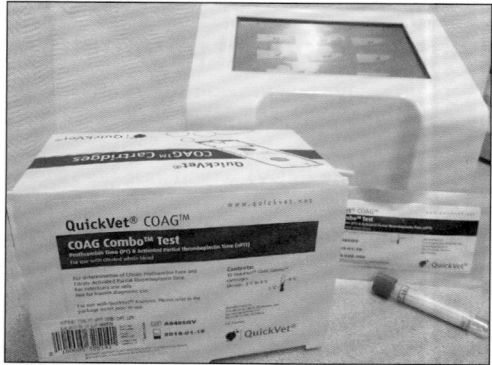

17.24 In-house blood coagulation factor analyser that can analyse prothrombin (PT) and activated partial thromboplastin time (aPPT). Note the use of a citrate blood tube.

Blood biochemistry

Biochemical parameters are used in the diagnosis of many medical conditions through the interpretation of values that fall outside the reference ranges (see Figure 17.25, Chapter 18 and below). Exact reference ranges for biochemical parameters vary for each laboratory. A variety of methods can be used to measure biochemical parameters, including:

- Desktop in-house biochemistry analysers
- Commercial test strips
- Hand-held analysers
- External laboratories.

Samples for biochemistry must be collected into the correct anticoagulation tube (see Figure 17.10). Regular quality assurance tests (QC and QA) must be carried out on biochemistry analysers to ensure that reliable results are produced (see 'Quality control and quality assurance', above). Figure 17.25 provides some common biochemical ranges for the cat and dog and summarizes possible reasons for the variations outside of these reference ranges.

Ammonia

This is the result of metabolism of protein and should be excreted. Elevated levels in blood may be associated with portosystemic shunts. High concentrations of ammonium can cause neurological problems.

Blood urea nitrogen (BUN)

This is a waste product formed by the liver and excreted by the kidneys as a result of amino acid metabolism. Elevated BUN is most commonly seen as a result of dehydration, urethral obstruction, renal failure and a ruptured bladder, but may also be found in cases of infection, metabolic disease, high-protein diet, chronic heart failure and corticosteroid therapy. Decreases in BUN can occur as a result of low-protein diet, anabolic steroids, liver failure or portosystemic shunts.

Calcium

The majority of calcium is found in bone and it is also involved in the maintenance of neuromuscular function. Calcium concentrations are usually related to phosphorus concentrations. Increased levels of calcium may occur in parathyroid gland disease, renal disease and some types of neoplasia. It is important to note that EDTA or citrate anticoagulants will affect the calcium result produced by analysers making the findings invalid.

Cholesterol

Cholesterol is a plasma lipoprotein that is produced primarily in the liver, but is also obtained from food. An increase in cholesterol may be seen in patients with diabetes mellitus, hypothyroidism, hyperadrenocorticism, liver disease and renal disease and also in post-feeding samples. Decreases may be seen in patients with maldigestion, malabsorption and severe hepatic insufficiency.

Creatine kinase (CK) (creatine phosphokinase, CPK)

The highest levels of CK are found in skeletal and cardiac muscle and brain tissue. When muscle cells become damaged CK is excreted into the blood. The most common cause of a rise in blood CK in small animals are muscle disorders such as exertional hyperthermia. Hypothyroidism, heart disease, recent exercise prior to a blood test, selenium/vitamin E deficiencies and trauma to the muscles may also contribute to a rise in the CK value.

Biochemical parameter	Reference ranges (adult)		Possible causes of an increased value outside the reference range	Possible causes of a decreased value outside the reference range
	Dogs	Cats		
Ammonia (µmol/l)	0–98	0–95	Portosystemic shunts	
Albumin (g/l)	23–40	22–40	Dehydration	Liver disease, intestinal disease, kidney disease
Alanine aminotransferase (ALT) (IU/l)	10–125	12–130	Liver cell damage (primary and secondary), heart disease, kidney failure, muscle damage	
Alkaline phosphatase (ALP) (IU/l)	23–212	14–111	Liver disease, bone disease, hyperadrenocorticism, corticosteroid and anticonvulsant medication	
Aspartate aminotransferase (AST) (IU/l)	0–50	0–48	Skeletal muscle damage, cardiac disease, liver disease, haemolysis	
Blood urea nitrogen (mmol/l)	2.5–9.6	5.7–12.9	Dehydration, renal infection, urethral obstruction, renal failure, ruptured bladder, high-protein diet, chronic heart failure, pancreatic disease, corticosteroid therapy	Low-protein diet, anabolic steroids, liver failure, portosystemic shunts.
Calcium (mmol/l)	1.98–3.00	1.95–2.83	Hyperparathyroidism, renal disease, some types of neoplasia	Pregnancy, lactation, parathyroid abnormalities
Cholesterol (mmol/l)	2.84–8.27	1.68–5.81	Diabetes mellitus, hypothyroidism, hyperadrenocorticism, liver disease, renal disease, post-feeding blood samples	Maldigestion, malabsorption, severe hepatic insufficiency
Creatine kinase (CK) (IU/l)	10–200	0–314	Muscle disorders, muscle trauma, exertional hyperthermia, hypothyroidism, heart disease, selenium/vitamin E deficiencies	
Creatinine (µmol/l)	44–159	71–212	Dehydration, renal infection, urethral obstruction, renal failure, pancreatic disease	
Fructosamine (µmol/l)	177–314	191–349	Diabetes mellitus	
Globulin (g/l)	25–45	28–51	Infection, immune-mediated disease	Immune compromise, intestinal disease, liver disease
Glucose (mmol/l)	4.11–7.94	4.11–8.83	Diabetes mellitus, hyperadrenocorticism, pancreatitis, corticosteroid therapy, stress, post-feeding blood samples	Hepatic insufficiency, hypoadreno-corticism, neoplasia, malabsorption, starvation, insulin treatment
Lactate (mmol/l)	<2.5	<2.5	Dehydration, hypoperfusion (shock), hypoxia, anaemia, sepsis, gastric dilation–volvulus (GDV), significant muscle activity, seizures, prolonged restraint	
Lipase (IU/l)	200–1800	100–1400	Pancreatitis, kidney disease and corticosteroid drugs (dogs, not cats)	
Pancreatic amylase (IU/l)	500–1500	500–1500	Pancreatitis, intestinal disease (dogs, not cats)	
Phosphate (mmol/l)	0.81–2.19	1.00–2.42	Renal insufficiency, pancreatic disease	
Total bilirubin (µmol/l)	0–15	0–15	Haemolytic anaemia, liver disease, biliary obstruction	
Total protein (g/l)	52–82	57–89	Elevations in albumen and/or globulin; dehydration, immune-mediated disease, lactation, infection or neoplasia	Reductions in albumen and/or globulin; liver disease, intestinal disease, kidney disease

17.25 Reference ranges for common biochemical tests in dogs and cats, together with possible reasons for values outside of the reference range. (Ranges quoted are those for the Idexx Catalyst Chemistry Analyser, note that precise reference ranges vary from laboratory to laboratory).

Creatinine

Creatinine is formed from creatine, which is found in skeletal muscle. Creatinine diffuses out of the muscle cell and into most body fluids, including blood. In normal conditions the creatinine is filtered through the glomeruli in the kidney and is eliminated in urine. Creatinine is not an accurate indicator of early kidney function compromise because approximately 75% of the kidney tissue must be non-functional before elevated blood creatinine levels are seen.

Fructosamine

This is formed by the glycosylation (bonding of glucose) of circulating proteins and is a marker of mean blood glucose concentration, with fructosamine concentration being proportional to the blood glucose concentration. The concentration of fructosamine in the blood is, unlike glucose, not affected by stress, making it ideal for monitoring diabetic animals, particularly cats. A fructosamine measurement indicates the average glucose concentration over the previous 2–3 weeks. Fructosamine results must be evaluated in the context of the patient's total clinical findings. Falsely low fructosamine results may be seen with decreased blood total protein and/or albumin levels, with conditions associated with increased protein loss, or with changes in the type of protein produced by the body. In this case, a discrepancy between the results obtained from daily glucose monitoring and fructosamine testing may be noticed.

Glucose

This is the main source of energy for cells in the body and its concentration is controlled by the hormones insulin and glucagon. Elevated levels may be seen in diabetes mellitus, hyperadrenocorticism, corticosteroid therapy, stress and pancreatitis and in post-feeding samples. Decreased levels may be seen in hepatic insufficiency, hypoadrenocorticism, neoplasia, malabsorption, starvation or insulin treatment. Handheld analysers are available to measure glucose (see Figure 17.7a).

Lactate

This is produced in anaerobic respiration and its formation results in acidosis (see Chapter 20). Failure of the body to correct the acidosis, causing increased blood lactate levels, may result from dehydration, hypoperfusion (shock), hypoxia, anaemia, sepsis, gastric dilation–volvulus (GDV). Lactate levels may also be elevated through significant muscle activity (e.g. in seizuring animals) and restraint (e.g. in blood sample collection). Hand-held analysers are available to measure lactate (see Figure 17.7b).

Lipase

This is a water-soluble enzyme secreted by the pancreas. Its function is to break down fats in the intestinal tract. In acute pancreatitis (see Chapter 18), destruction of pancreatic tissue results in the escape of pancreatic enzymes into the pancreas and peritoneal cavity. The enzymes enter the blood by way of lymphatics or capillaries with subsequent elevation of serum levels. Increases lipase levels in the blood are not however, specific for pancreatitis. Lipase levels may also be increased by kidney disease and corticosteroid drugs. Lipase levels may be elevated in normal cats, so are not of diagnostic value in this species. In both dogs and cats, pancreatic immunoreactivity tests (see below) are preferred for the diagnosis of pancreatitis.

Pancreatic lipase

This is a specific lipase found only in pancreatic tissue and increases in the circulation when the pancreas is inflamed. Enzyme Linked Immunosorbent Assay (ELISA) tests (Canine/Feline Pancreatic Lipase Immunoreactivity; cPLI / fPLI) are available to test specifically for serum canine pancreatic lipase (cPL) or feline pancreatic lipase (fPL). These tests can be carried out in the practice laboratory or sent to an external laboratory. cPLI and fPLI are useful diagnostic tests for acute pancreatitis (see Chapter 18).

Pancreatic amylase

This is a water-soluble enzyme secreted by the pancreas. It is involved in starch digestion. In acute pancreatitis (see Chapter 18), destruction of pancreatic tissue results in the escape of pancreatic enzymes into the pancreas and peritoneal cavity. The enzymes enter the blood by way of lymphatics or capillaries with subsequent elevation of serum levels. Pancreatic amylase levels may also be increased in intestinal disease. Amylase levels may be elevated in normal cats, so are not of diagnostic value in this species.

Plasma proteins

Albumin

This is one of the most important proteins in plasma or serum, making up 35–50% of the total plasma protein in most animals. Hepatocytes synthesize albumin, and levels may therefore be influenced by liver disease. In addition, intestinal disease and kidney disease can lead to loss of albumin from the blood.

Globulins

These are high molecular weight proteins (higher than albumin) produced by the liver or the immune system. Globulin concentration is usually calculated by subtracting albumin from total protein. Measurement of specific immunoglobulins is useful in determining the immune status of the patient.

Total protein (TP)

Total plasma protein measurements include fibrinogen, whereas total serum protein levels do not as it is used in the clotting process. Elevated TP levels may occur as a result of dehydration, immune-mediated disease, lactation, infection or neoplasia. Decreased levels may occur as a result of renal disease, haemorrhage, malnutrition, malabsorption, hepatic insufficiency or pancreatic insufficiency. An approximation of TP levels may be made by measuring TS using a spun haematocrit tube and a refractometer (see above). TP (or TS) can be usefully interpreted alongside PCV and urine specific gravity (see Figure 17.22).

Phosphate

Levels of phosphate are very closely linked with calcium levels (see above). Increased levels are seen in renal insufficiency in cats and dogs.

Total bilirubin

Formed from the breakdown of haemoglobin, bilirubin is a component of bile. Elevated levels may be seen in haemolytic anaemia, liver disease and biliary obstruction. An animal with an elevated bilirubin level may appear icteric (jaundiced; see Chapter 18).

Liver enzymes and liver function tests

In dogs and cats, the enzymes ALP, ALT and AST are the most useful markers for liver disease.

- **Alanine aminotransferase (ALT)** is found within the cytoplasm of the hepatocyte, as well as in renal cells, cardiac muscle, skeletal muscle and pancreas. Damage to cells in these areas results in elevations in ALT as the enzyme escapes from the damaged cells. Alterations in ALT levels in dogs and cats are most commonly indicative of liver cell damage, although this can be primary liver damage or secondary to other disease.

- **Alkaline phosphatase (ALP or ALKP)** is widely distributed in the body, including liver, intestines and bone. Younger animals have naturally higher levels due to the growth and development of bone. Elevated levels of ALP may indicate liver disease or hyperadrenocorticism. Corticosteroids and anticonvulsant medication may also result in elevated levels.
- **Aspartate aminotransferase (AST)** is found in the liver, red blood cells, cardiac and skeletal muscle tissue. Increases in blood levels in dogs and cats can reflect muscle damage or liver disease.

Other enzymes are released from damaged liver cells and can be analysed but are more useful in other species (e.g. ruminants and horses) than they are in small animals.

- **Gamma-glutamyl transferase (GGT):** Alterations in levels may indicate liver disease/cholestasis.
- **Glutamate dehydrogenase (GLDH):** A liver-specific enzyme that can indicate acute liver damage.
- **Lactate dehydrogenase (LDH):** Not liver-specific, but can be useful when measured with other liver enzymes.

The biochemical assays described above may indicate liver cell damage and bile stasis (cholestasis) but they are not necessarily good measures of liver function. Albumin and ammonia levels (see above) may reflect abnormalities in liver function, as may measurement of blood clotting factors (see above). The most commonly used liver function test is the measurement of bile acids, often as part of a bile acid stimulation test (see below). Liver biopsy (see below and Chapter 18) is, however, often the only definitive way to diagnose liver disease.

Following a fatty meal, the normal gall bladder contracts and releases bile acids into the duodenum, to allow emulsification and absorption of fats. Bile acids are then reabsorbed from the small intestine, via the portal blood stream and into the hepatocytes. In healthy animals this process is very efficient, with only low levels of bile acids being present in the blood stream after a meal. Liver dysfunction or shunting of blood away from the liver can result in high post-feeding bile acid levels.

Bile acid stimulation test

1. Fast the animal for 12 hours.
2. Collect about 1–2 ml of blood into a plain (serum) tube.
3. Feed a fatty meal – puppy or kitten food is good. If the pet is not eating, give it vegetable oil carefully by syringe. →

Bile acid stimulation test *continued*

4. Take a second sample of blood into a plain (serum) tube 2 hours after eating.
5. The blood tests measure pre and post meal levels of bile acids. High levels may be indicative of liver or hepatic vasculature problems.

Electrolytes and acid–base balance

Electrolytes are the negative and positive ions found in body fluids. Electrolytes commonly measured are sodium (Na^+), potassium (K^+) and chloride (Cl^-). Their functions (Figure 17.26) include water balance in the body. Serious consequences can follow even relatively small changes in their absolute or relative levels (acid–base balance; see Chapters 18 and 20). Measurements of electrolyte concentrations are used in the diagnosis and management of many conditions, including renal, endocrine and metabolic disorders.

Electrolytes are measured by a process known as potentiometry. This measures the potential difference (voltage) that develops between the inner and outer surfaces of an electrode that is selectively permeable to the ion being measured. This is then compared to that of a reference electrode. Electrolyte tests can be performed on whole blood, plasma or serum. Hand-held (see Figure 17.7c), bench top and external laboratory analysers are available.

Sodium

This is required for many vital functions in the body, including the regulation of blood pressure and volume, and the transmission of nerve impulses. **Hypernatraemia** (increased levels of sodium in the blood) may be seen where there has been an abundant loss of water through the gastrointestinal tract along with sodium intake, perhaps caused by excessive sodium replacement in fluid therapy or low water intake (dehydration). **Hyponatraemia** (decreased levels) may arise as a result of excessive loss of sodium, which may be seen in renal failure, intestinal obstruction or urinary tract problems.

Chloride

This plays an important role in helping to maintain a normal balance of fluids. Significant increases (**hyperchloraemia**) may be associated with diarrhoea, kidney disease and overactivity of the parathyroid glands. Vomiting or excessive sweating may be associated with a decrease in chloride (**hypochloraemia**).

Electrolyte	Importance	Reference ranges (adult) (mmol/l)		Causes of increase	Causes of decrease
		Dogs	*Cats*		
Sodium (Na^+)	Water distribution; osmotic pressure maintenance; temperature control	144–160	150–165	Intestinal disease Kidney disease	Hypoadrenocorticism Intestinal disease
Potassium (K^+)	Muscular function; respiration; cardiac function; nerve impulse transmission; carbohydrate metabolism	3.5–5.8	3.5–5.8	Hypoadrenocorticism Renal disease Diabetes melitus	Intestinal disease
Chloride (Cl^-)	Water distribution; osmotic pressure; normal anion/cation ratio	109–122	112–129	Renal disease	Renal disease

17.26 Reference ranges and functions of electrolytes in dogs and cats. (Ranges quoted are those for the Idexx Catalyst Chemistry Analyser. Note that precise reference ranges vary from laboratory to laboratory.)

Potassium

This has a key role in maintaining the electrical potential of the cell membrane. Increases in potassium levels (**hyperkalaemia**) may be caused by diabetes mellitus, hypoadrenocorticism, renal failure, urinary tract obstruction or rupture, or massive tissue damage (e.g. trauma, neoplasia). Decrease in potassium (**hypokalaemia**) may be caused by; anorexia, gastrointestinal disease, losses through the urinary tract, myopathy in Burmese cats. Decrease in potassium can result in muscle weakness, commonly with ventroflexion of the neck.

Hormones

Thyroid hormones

Measurement of thyroxine (T4) is the most commonly used test to assess thyroid function (triiodothyronine, T3, is also sometimes measured). Increased T4 may be seen in hyperthyroidism (cats), oestrus, pregnancy and in the young animal. Decreased levels may be seen in hypothyroidism (dogs), hyperadrenocorticism, chronic illness, advanced age and iodine deficiency. Many factors, including illness and drug therapy, can affect levels of T4 in the blood and so testing can be unreliable. Additional tests (e.g. thyroid stimulating hormone, TSH) are used to confirm conditions such as hypothyroidism (see also Chapter 18).

Adrenal hormones

The most common conditions affecting the adrenal cortex are hyperadrenocorticism (Cushing's disease) and hypoadrenocorticism (Addison's disease), where levels of cortisol are affected (see Chapter 18). A basal cortisol test is unreliable in the diagnosis of these conditions and so adrenocorticotrophic hormone (ACTH) stimulation or dexamethasone suppression tests are performed. These tests are also used to monitor the response to treatment of adrenal disorders (see Chapter 18).

- **ACTH stimulation test:** Basal cortisol level is first measured in a sample of the patient's blood. The patient is then given an intravenous injection of synthetic ACTH, which will stimulate the release of cortisol. A second blood sample is taken 2 hours later (depending upon specific laboratory preferences) and the cortisol level is measured. Elevated post-injection levels of cortisol indicate Cushing's disease, whereas a reduced level indicates Addison's disease, although interpretation of the test results may be influenced by other clinical factors.
- **Low-dose dexamethasone suppression test:** Basal cortisol level is first measured in a sample of the patient's blood. The patient is then given an intravenous injection of a low dose of dexamethasone. A second blood sample is taken 8 hours later (depending upon specific laboratory preferences), to assess the response. Cortisol levels should normally decrease significantly, and a high post-injection cortisol level may be indicative of hyperadrenocorticism.
- **High-dose dexamethasone suppression test:** This is used to distinguish between pituitary-dependent and non-pituitary-dependent hyperadrenocorticism in dogs. Basal cortisol level is first measured in a sample of the patient's blood. The patient is then given an intravenous injection of a high dose of dexamethasone. A second sample is taken 3 hours later and a third at 8 hours (depending upon specific laboratory preferences), to

assess the response. Patients with pituitary-dependent Cushing's disease commonly have a post-injection cortisol level below the base level, whereas those with non-pituitary-dependent Cushing's will have a post-injection cortisol level above the base level.

Serology

Serology is the term used for tests carried out on blood serum (see 'Serum samples', above). Most commonly these are tests for antibodies generated in response to infectious disease. Sometimes serological tests are 'paired' on two occasions some time apart (typically weeks), in order to indicate recent exposure to infectious agents (see Chapter 7). There are several types of serology tests that can be used, depending on the antibodies being studied. These include ELISA, agglutination and fluorescent antibody tests. Some tests can be carried out in-house and may be combined with virus assays (see 'Virology', below).

Urine samples

Analysis of urine samples can be a relatively non-invasive, simple, quick and inexpensive method of investigating some aspects of the health status of a patient and can provide additional information to that provided by other investigations such as the analysis of blood samples. The veterinary surgeon can be assisted in the diagnosis of many conditions of the urinary system and other body systems using such tests.

Patient preparation

On average, a cat or dog will produce 1–2 ml/kg of urine per hour. Alterations to normal production may occur (see Chapter 18). Some indications of thirst can be assessed and measured by the owner, as can an indication of urine output; however, in order to assess water intake and urine output fully, a thorough 12-hour or 24-hour measurement is required, usually in the veterinary practice.

Preparation of the patient for urine collection depends on which tests are to be carried out. In most instances, withholding food overnight in order to avoid post-feeding (post-prandial) changes in the urine and collecting the sample first thing in the morning when the bladder has been allowed to fill and urine concentration is higher, is most appropriate. Water should not be withheld or restricted in any way unless directed by a veterinary surgeon. Collection of a sample first thing in the morning is often easy and convenient for owners too, if a 'mid-stream free-catch' sample is required (see 'Collection methods', below).

Sample collection

A variety of methods are available for collecting urine (see below). In all cases, care should be taken to avoid self-contamination as there are some significant zoonotic risks associated with urine (e.g. leptospirosis infection). PPE (gloves) should be worn and hands washed well after the sample has been collected. Owners should be provided with gloves and appropriate containers if they are requested to collect samples.

Ideally, a morning sample should be collected. Any urine sample should ideally be examined within 60 minutes of collection. If a urine sample is left at room temperature for extended periods of time, cells and casts may degenerate, crystals may dissolve or precipitate, levels of some chemicals (glucose, bilirubin and ketones) may reduce, bacteria may multiply and the pH may increase as a result of bacterial breakdown of urea to ammonia. Urine samples can be stored in a refrigerator until tested or sent to an external laboratory, but must be allowed to warm to room temperature before analysis. Some laboratories request that samples are preserved for bacteriology and cytology (see below).

Suitable containers

Depending on the method of collection, urine should ideally be collected straight into a sterile universal container. As mentioned above, owners asked to collect urine samples should be provided with suitable containers, as well as disposable gloves. If the client brings in a sample in an alternative container (e.g. jam jar, ice cream tub, kidney dish), this needs to have been thoroughly cleaned and dried before the sample was collected, otherwise the laboratory findings may be invalid.

All containers used for sample collection and/or storage must be adequately labelled with: patient identification; date, time and 'urine' to identify the type of sample collected; and the name and amount of any preservatives that may have been used. The preference for the use of preservatives for urine samples varies between laboratories and it is always best to check with the laboratory first. Preservatives generally increase the 'lifespan' of the urine before testing to 24–72 h.

Urine for microbial examination can be collected directly into a container with boric acid (red-topped container). Boric acid helps to preserve the existing bacteria and prevent the growth of further microorganisms. Thymol (1 mg/ml), 10% formalin (1 drop per 2.5 ml of urine) and toluene (volume sufficient to create a thin film on the top of the sample) are alternatives.

Collection methods

For all methods of collection, PPE, including gloves, should be worn. Collection methods include:

- Mid-stream free-catch collection
- Catheterization
- Cystocentesis.

Mid-stream free-catch collection

This method involves collecting the sample either during normal urination or by expressing the bladder. The first portion of the urine should, in most instances, not be collected as it is frequently contaminated; instead, a 'mid-stream' sample is usually ideal. Catching the urine during normal elimination is an ideal method of collection for owners to carry out at home and creates no discomfort for the pet. It can, however, be challenging, particularly in some species and some individual animals.

Commercial collection kits are available and consist of a funnel with a universal container attached (Figure 17.27a). Urine from cats can be collected using non-absorbable cat litter (Figure 17.27b), and can then be transferred to a universal container using a pipette. In the veterinary practice, it may be possible to obtain a mid-stream free-catch sample by manual expression of the bladder, although this can be uncomfortable for the pet unless it has a neurological problem that makes manual expression easy. Urine samples

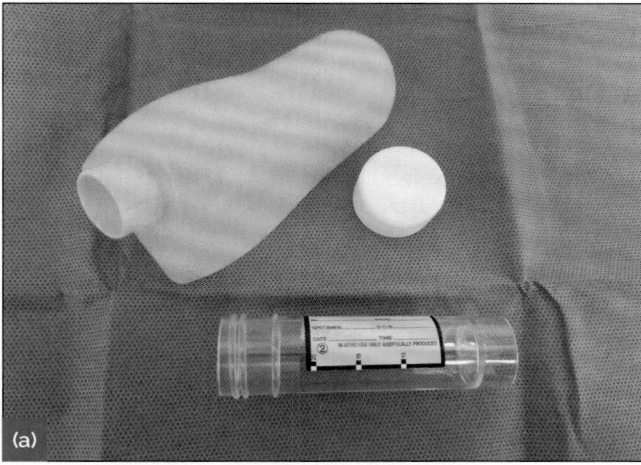

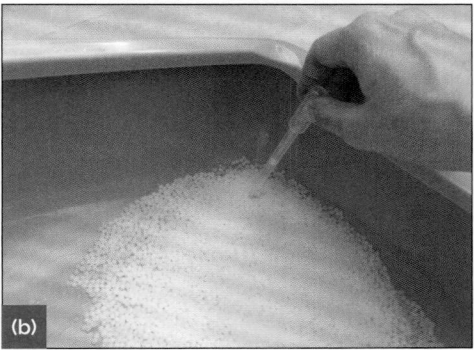

17.27 **(a)** Commercial urine collection funnel with container. **(b)** Non-absorbable cat litter can be used to collect free-catch samples in cats. (a, Courtesy of Louise Marshall; b, reproduced from the *BSAVA Manual of Canine and Feline Clinical Pathology, 3rd edn*)

collected using the mid-stream free-catch method are non-sterile and therefore not suitable for microbial examination.

Catheterization

This method involves passing a urinary catheter directly into the bladder via the urethra. (Details of catheterization techniques are given in Chapter 15.) Catheterization should only be used to collect a urine sample if the bladder is being catheterized for another reason (e.g. removal of a urethral obstruction, for contrast imaging or to monitor urine output and maintain urethral patency).

Catheterization is relatively easy to perform (see Chapter 15), but sedation or general anaesthesia may be required and there is a risk of infection and urethral tract trauma. Sterile equipment (catheter, collection container, gloves) should be used. However, it should be noted that even with the use of sterile equipment, the sample may be contaminated by bacteria in the lower urogenital tract, making it less suitable for bacteriology in most instances than a sample collected by cystocentesis; discarding the first portion of the sample helps to overcome these problems to some extent.

Cystocentesis

This method involves the passage of a sterile needle through the abdominal wall and into the bladder. It can be a relatively quick method of obtaining a sterile sample and is easily performed if the bladder is at least partially full. Ultrasound guidance can be useful. Strict asepsis is required and the sample collected is ideal for bacteriology. Cystocentesis can, however, result in blood contamination of the sample, which can be difficult to differentiate from existing haematuria. Care should be taken when carrying out cystocentesis in a very full bladder, as bladder rupture is possible; cystocentesis should not be used in cases with bladder distension as a result of urethral obstruction. Cystocentesis should also not be used in animals with known or suspected blood clotting disorders (see Chapter 18). The technique should not be used in patients with known or suspected bladder tumours, as seeding of the tumour may occur where the needle has been inserted.

Sample analysis

A range of terms are used to describe urine sample characteristics (see text box). Urinalysis can be split into several parts, which should generally be carried out in the following order:

1. Physical appearance.
2. Specific gravity.
3. Chemical tests.
4. Microscopic analysis.

Terms used in urine sampling

- **Anuria** – Lack of any urine production
- **Bilirubinuria** – Presence of bilirubin in the urine
- **Calculi** – Abnormal concretion usually composed of mineral salts
- **Cystitis** – Inflammation of the bladder
- **Dysuria** – Abnormal, painful or difficult urination
- **Glucosuria** – Presence of glucose in the urine
- **Haematuria** – Presence of blood in the urine
- **Haemoglobinuria** – Presence of haemoglobin in the urine
- **Hypouresis** – reduced flow of urine
- **Ketonuria** – presence of ketone bodies in the urine
- **Micturition** – the act of urination, passage of urine
- **Oliguria** – reduced urine production
- **Pollakiuria** – increased urination frequency
- **Polyuria** – increased volume of urine production
- **Proteinuria** – presence of increased protein in the urine
- **Urobilinuria** – presence of increased urobilinogen in the urine
- **Urolith** – a urinary calculus
- **Urolithiasis** – presence of calculi in the urinary system

---

Physical appearance

Before tests are performed on urine, the physical characteristics of the sample should be recorded. Normal urine has the following characteristics:

- **Colour:** Dog and cat urine should be pale yellow in colour indicating normal hydration. The pigment urochrome is responsible for this colour. The depth of colour may change according to the concentration of the urine; more concentrated samples appear darker and more orange. Normal rabbit urine can range in colour from yellow through orange to red or rust
- **Turbidity:** Dog and cat urine is usually clear; although, if the urine is left to stand, precipitation of phosphate can occur and cause turbidity. Rabbit urine can appear turbid due to the presence of naturally occurring calcium

carbonate crystals (see Figure 17.35). Urine from birds and reptiles is cloudy due to the presence of uric acid crystals
- **Odour:** Normal urine has a slight sour smell. The urine of entire male cats can have a distinct putrid smell, which contributes to scent marking.

Alterations and abnormalities in the physical appearance of the urine sample can be useful for diagnosis (Figure 17.28).

Specific gravity

Specific gravity (SG) is the relative density (mass per unit volume) of a known volume of fluid compared with an equal volume of distilled water. Distilled water has an SG of 1.000 and is used in the calibration of SG measuring devices, such as refractometers (see below). Normal urine SG values (depending on hydration status and water intake) are given, together with some possible causes of higher and lower values, in Figure 17.29. Urine SG can be higher in 'normal' rabbits due to the presence of crystals (see Figure 17.35). Urine specific gravity is a useful parameter to assess alongside blood PCV and total protein measurements (see Figure 17.22).

Chemical test strips (see below) provide an approximation of urine SG; a refractometer is required for an accurate measurement of this parameter.

Characteristic	Abnormality	Causes
Colour	Pale/clear	Polyuria/polydipsia
	Dark yellow/orange/brown	Dehydration
	Red, brown or black	Presence of blood Certain drugs
	Green/yellow	Biliverdin (oxidization of bilirubin)
	Blue/green tinged	Certain drugs
Turbidity	Cloudy	Contamination, e.g. pus, semen Presence of mucus Phosphate precipitation
Odour	Sweet/fruity	Presence of ketones (ketonuria), e.g. in diabetes mellitus
	Ammonia	Fresh samples – bacteria present Old samples – stale
	Foul	Excess protein

17.28 Abnormalities in the physical characteristics of canine urine.

Species	Reference range for urine specific gravity (SG)	Possible causes of urine SG above the reference ranges	Possible causes of urine SG below the reference ranges
Dog	1.015–1.045	Dehydration, acute renal failure, shock, diabetes mellitus, fluid loss, sediment such as crystals (Figures 17.34, 17.35)	Chronic renal failure, diabetes insipidus, polydipsia, fluid therapy, corticosteroid therapy.
Cat	1.035–1.060		
Rabbit	1.003–1.036		

17.29 Urine specific gravity references for dogs, cats and rabbits and common reasons for abnormal findings.

Using a refractometer

Calibrate the refractometer:

1. Place 2–3 drops of distilled water on the prism surface of the refractometer.
2. Hold the refractometer up to a light source and look down the eyepiece.
3. Calibrate the refractometer to 1.000 on the urine SG (or W) scale.
4. Lift the cover and dry the prism surface using a dry tissue.

Test the sample:

1. Put on gloves.
2. Invert the tube to mix the urine sample gently.
3. Pipette 1–2 drops of urine on to the prism surface.

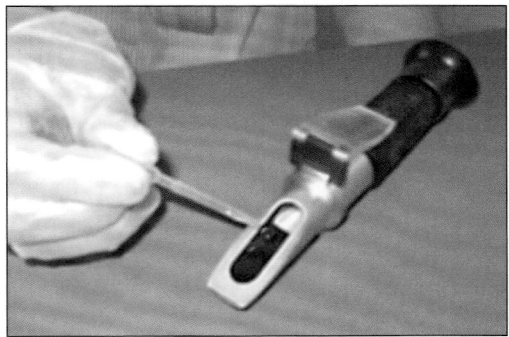

4. Close the cover.
5. Hold up to the light source and look down the eyepiece.

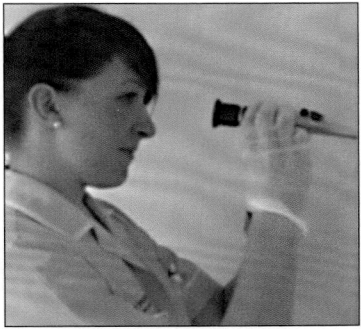

6. Read and record the actual urine SG reading.
7. Rinse the prism with water.
8. Dry the prism.
9. Dispose of used materials as hazardous waste.

Chemical tests

Commercial reagent strips are available for quick and inexpensive analysis of urine in house. Multistix® and Chemstrip® (Figure 17.30) are the most common type of 'dipstick' used in veterinary practice and cover a range of chemical parameters (other dipsticks such as Diastix®, Clinistix®, Clinitest® and Ketostix® are available for one or more parameters).

For accurate results, it is important to ensure that:

- The test strips come in an airtight container
- The test strips are in date before using
- The sticks are not damp or discoloured
- The lid is closed immediately after removing the strip
- Urine ideally less than 60 minutes old is used (see 'Sample collection', above)

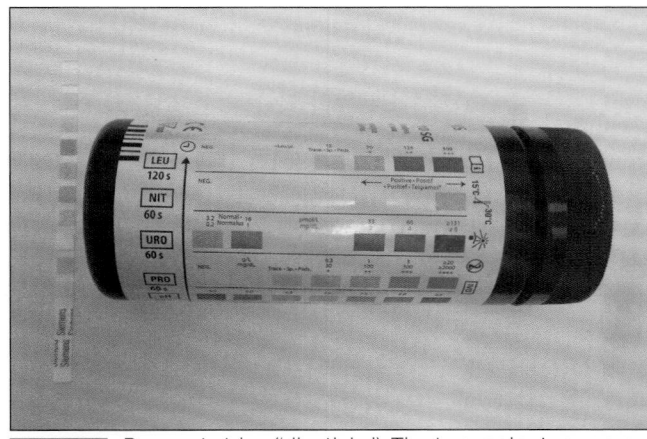

17.30 Reagent strips ('dipsticks'). The two major types are Multistix® and Chemstrip®.

- The urine has been kept at room temperature (or brought to room temperature if refrigerated), away from sunlight, in a closed container.

Dipstick analysis

1. List the chemicals on a piece of paper before starting, to enable results to be recorded efficiently.
2. Put on gloves.
3. Invert the fresh urine sample to mix.
4. Select urine dipstick test strips; remove one test strip and replace the lid immediately.
5. Cover the test strip pads with urine (ideally using a 1 ml syringe; alternatively, the test strip can be immersed in the urine sample).
6. Immediately note the time.
7. Wait for the appropriate length of time for each test component and then read and record the dipstick measurements correctly.
8. Dispose of used dipsticks as hazardous waste.

Dipsticks (such as Multistix®) measure pH, proteins, glucose, ketones, bilirubin, urobilinogen, nitrite, leucocytes and blood in urine. Although some dipsticks measure SG, these are not reliable, and SG should be measured using a refractometer (see above). Normal values and causes of abnormal dipstick findings are described in Figure 17.31.

Microscopic analysis

Microscopic examination of urine is inexpensive and can be carried out within the practice laboratory relatively quickly. Centrifugation (see 'Centrifuges' above) of the urine sample allows the sediment to be separated from the supernatant and produces a large enough sample to be examined microscopically. The sediment may be stained to facilitate examination. Sedi-Stain® (modified Sternheimer-Malbin urinary stain) is most commonly used, but Leishman's or Gram stains can also be utilized.

Normal urine may contain a small amount of sediment, consisting of:

- Epithelial cells
- Mucus
- Blood cells
- Bacteria.

515

Chemical test	Normal value	Possible causes of increase	Possible causes of decrease
pH	Dogs: 5–7 Cats: 7–9	Bacterial infection, cystitis, alkalosis, certain drugs	Fever, starvation, diabetes mellitus, chronic renal failure, acidosis
Proteins	Trace	Renal failure, haemorrhage, inflammatory disease	Rare
Glucose	None	Stress, excitement, diabetes mellitus, Cushing's disease, hyperthyroidism	Not applicable
Blood	None	Oestrus, cystitis, urolithiasis, acute nephritis	Not applicable
Ketones	None	Diabetes mellitus, starvation, liver damage	Not applicable
Bilirubin	Trace	Liver disease, haemolytic or obstructive jaundice	Rare
Nitrate	None	Bacterial infection	Not applicable
Urobilinogen	Trace/small amount	Liver dysfunction	Liver dysfunction

17.31 Chemical analysis of urine using dipsticks in dogs and cats.

Method for microscopic analysis of urine

1. Select a pipette, microscope slide and a plain centrifuge tube.
2. Put on gloves.
3. Mix the urine sample gently and pipette urine into the centrifuge tube.
4. Centrifuge the sample at 1500–2000 rpm for 5 minutes.
5. Remove most of the supernatant without disturbing the sediment; leave a few drops of supernatant in which to re-suspend the sediment.
6. Add a stain to the sediment if required (e.g. Sedi-Stain®).
7. Re-suspend the sediment (and mix the stain if used) by 'flicking' the base of the tube or very gently shaking it.

To make a wet preparation for examination of crystals and casts:

8. Pipette a drop of the suspension (supernatant and suspended sediment) on to a clean, labelled microscope slide.
9. Carefully place a coverslip on top of the sediment. Avoid creating air bubbles by lowering the coverslip at an angle of 45 degrees.
10. Label the slide.

To prepare a smear for examination of cells and bacteria:

11. Place a small drop of urine on the slide and smear using the same method as for blood (see 'Preparation of a blood smear', above).
12. Allow the smear to air dry and label the slide.
13. Dispose of the used pipette, urine and used materials as hazardous waste.
14. Examine the slide(s) using the battlement technique under low power, X10 then X40.
15. Record any findings. The Vernier scale reading can be used to relocate items.

- Squamous cells from the lower urethra, vagina and prepuce – these are large granular cells with nuclei
- Renal tubular cells – these are cuboidal to columnar cells; a large number would indicate active renal (kidney) tubule disease.
- Blood cells:
  - Erythrocytes – these indicate trauma, oestrus and infection/inflammation
  - Leucocytes (Figure 17.32) – these indicate inflammation and infection.
- Spermatozoa:
  - These may be seen in entire male dogs (less so in male cats).
- Yeast cells:
  - These are non-nucleated round or oval cells, and usually a result of contamination of the urine sample.
- Bacterial cells:
  - A small number of bacterial cells are always present
  - Further staining, culture and sensitivity may be required.

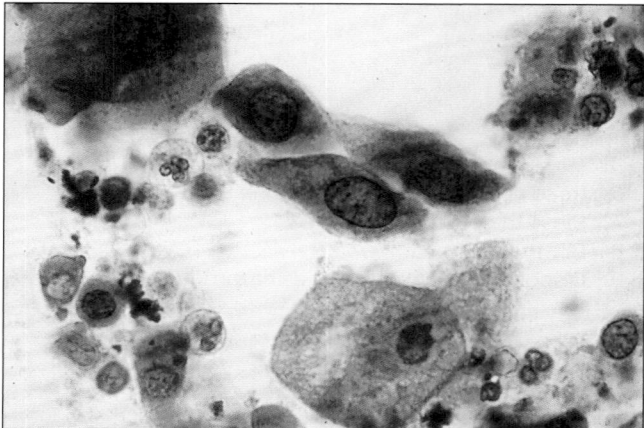

17.32 Mixed population of epithelial cells and leucocytes in canine urine sediment. (Sedi-Stain®; original magnification X400). (Reproduced from *BSAVA Manual of Canine and Feline Nephrology and Urology, 2nd edn*)

Sediment analysis: cells

The following cells may be found in a stained urine smear or wet preparation:

- Epithelial cells (Figure 17.32):
  - Transitional cells from the bladder – these are small round polyhedral cells and indicate cystitis or pyelonephritis

Sediment analysis: casts

Casts are formed in the distal convoluted tubules and collecting ducts of the kidney, where the concentration and acidity of urine are greatest. Secreted protein is precipitated in acidic conditions. Casts are composed of a matrix of protein and mucoprotein. Mucus threads can be differentiated from casts by their irregularly spaced, twisting sides and pointed, wispy ends.

- **Hyaline casts** (Figure 17.33a):
  - Clear, colourless, composed only of protein
  - More easily identified in stained samples
  - Present in patients with poor renal perfusion and fever, and those that have recently undertaken strenuous exercise.
- **Granular casts** (Figure 17.33b):
  - The most common cast type seen in animal urine
  - Appear granular due to the degeneration of other cells, such as red blood cells
  - Seen in patients with acute nephritis and chronic renal failure.
- **Cellular casts:**
  - **Epithelial casts** (Figure 17.33c):
    - Consist of epithelial cells from the renal tubules in a hyaline matrix
    - Seen in patients with acute nephritis.
  - **Leucocyte casts:**
    - Contain white blood cells (normally neutrophils)
    - Indicate inflammation in the renal tubules.
  - **Erythrocyte casts:**
    - Formed from red blood cells
    - Indicate renal haemorrhage.
- **Waxy casts** (Figure 17.33d):
  - Similar to hyaline casts but have a square end
  - Indicate extensive renal damage.
- **Fatty casts** (Figure 17.33e):
  - Contain small droplets of fat
  - Mainly seen in cats with renal disease and dogs with diabetes mellitus.

Sediment analysis: crystals

The presence of crystals in a urine sample may or may not be of clinical significance. Some crystals form through normal renal activity, others form as a result of metabolic disturbances or may be secondary to urinary tract problems, such as inflammation, infection or neoplasia. Crystals may aggregate to form large uroliths (also called calculi). The damage these cause to the urinary tract is known as urolithiasis (see Chapter 18). It is important to note that the microscopic appearance of crystals can vary greatly depending on their orientation within the sample being viewed and whether they are incomplete or complete.

- **Struvite (magnesium ammonium phosphate or triple phosphate) crystals** (Figure 17.34a):
  - Typically resemble the shape of coffin lids, although their shape may vary
  - Found in alkaline urine.
- **Cystine crystals** (Figure 17.34b):
  - Flat and thin with hexagonal outline
  - Found in acidic urine and associated with renal tubular dysfunction.
- **Calcium oxalate crystals** (Figure 17.34c):
  - Dihydrate crystals appear as small square crystals with an 'X' in the centre
  - Found in acidic or neutral urine
  - Commonly seen in urine from certain breeds that are genetically predisposed (e.g. Yorkshire Terrier, Miniature Poodle, Lhaso Apso, Miniature Schnauzer and Burmese, Himalayan and Persian cats)
  - Also found in animals that have ingested ethylene glycol (antifreeze).
- **Ammonium urate crystals** (Figure 17.34d):
  - Appear as spindles, thorn apple-shaped or rosettes
  - Found in acidic and neutral urine
  - Seen in clinically normal Dalmatians due to the way they metabolize and excrete protein
  - In other dog breeds and in cats their presence can indicate liver disease or portosystemic shunts.
- **Uric acid crystals** (Figure 17.34e):
  - Vary in shape but usually diamond-shaped or rhomboid
  - Occur in acidic urine, although they are rare.
- **Calcium phosphate crystals:**
  - Long and flat with a rectangular outline
  - Typically form in alkaline urine but are rare.
- **Calcium carbonate crystals** (Figure 17.35):
  - Commonly seen in urine from clinically normal rabbits
  - Causes urine to appear turbid and cloudy, which is normal in these species.

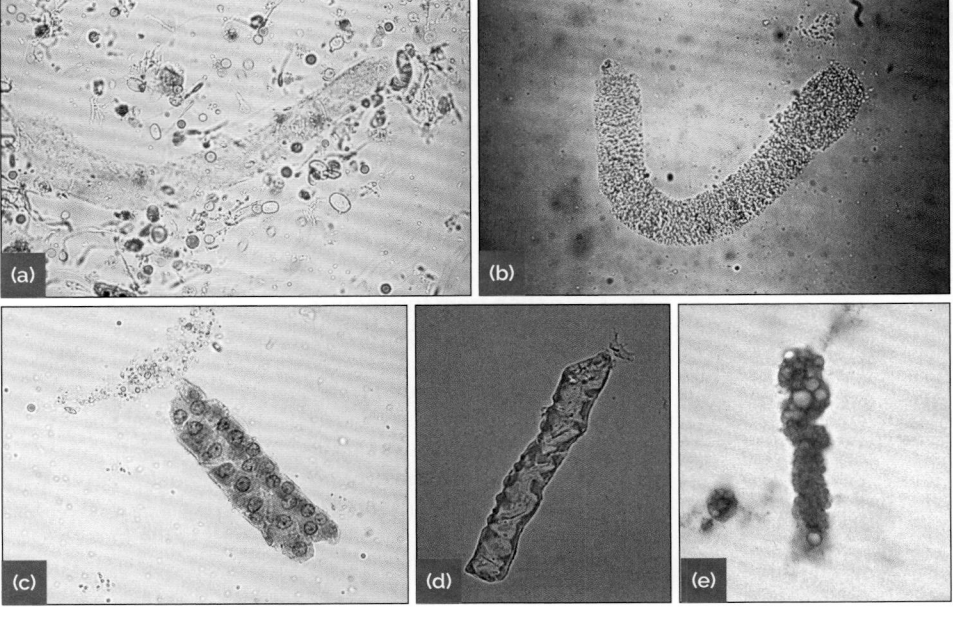

17.33 Casts found in urine. **(a)** Curved hyaline renal tubular cast. (Unstained; original magnification X400). **(b)** Granular cast. (Unstained; original magnification X400). **(c)** Epithelial cast from a dog with acute renal failure. (New methylene blue; original magnification X400). **(d)** Waxy cast with characteristic broken, blunt ends. (Unstained; original magnification X400). **(e)** Fatty cast in feline urine; note the lipid droplets. (New methylene blue; original magnification X100). (Reproduced from the *BSAVA Manual of Canine and Feline Nephrology and Urology, 2nd edn*)

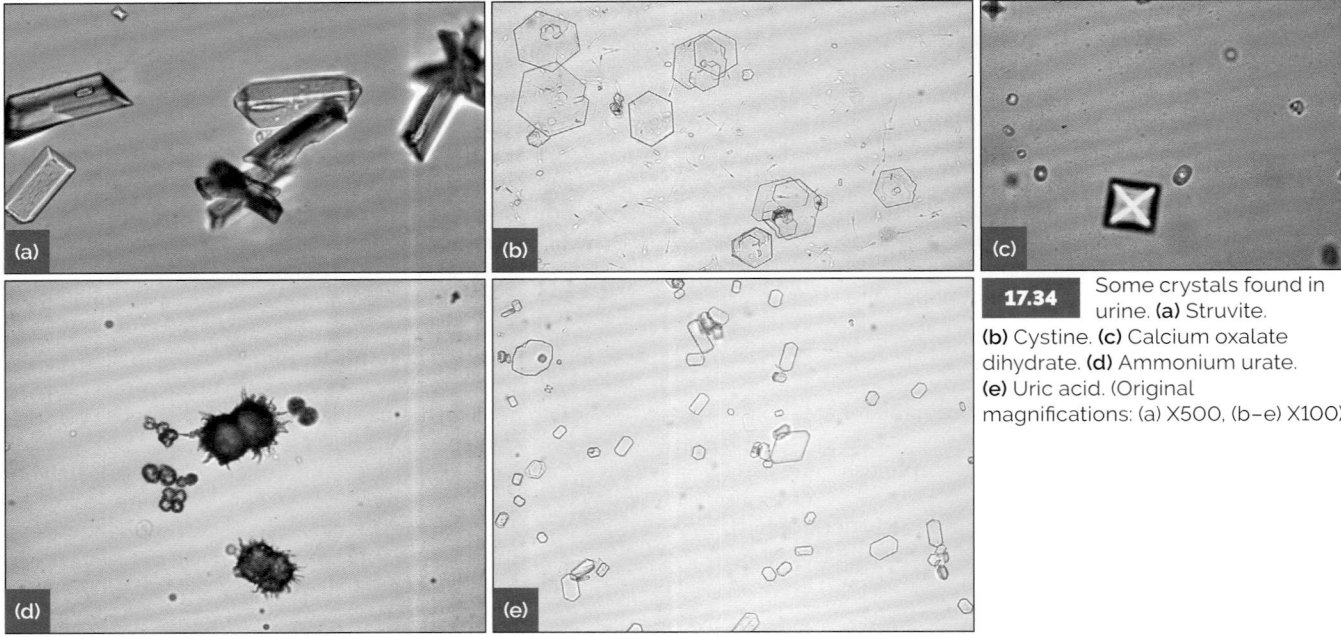

17.34 Some crystals found in urine. **(a)** Struvite. **(b)** Cystine. **(c)** Calcium oxalate dihydrate. **(d)** Ammonium urate. **(e)** Uric acid. (Original magnifications: (a) X500, (b–e) X100)

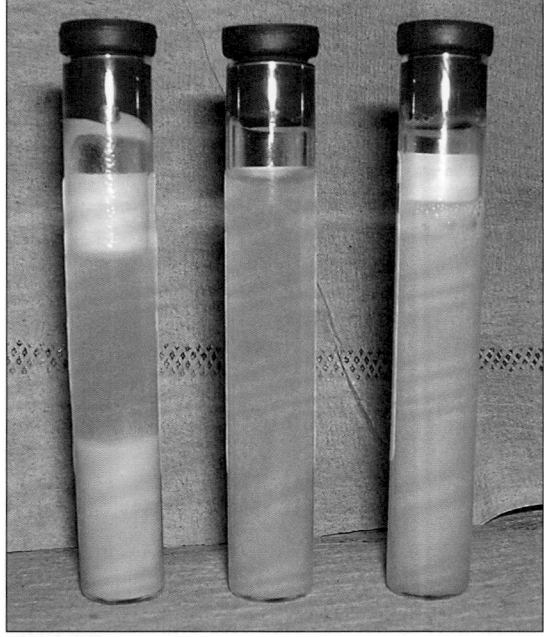

17.35 Normal rabbit urine may contain variable amounts of calcium carbonate crystals as shown in these three samples. (Reproduced from the *BSAVA Manual of Rabbit Medicine*)

Sediment analysis: other findings

Other findings may include:

- **Mucus:**
  - May be present associated with renal damage, recent surgery or retrograde ejaculation in male animals.
- **Faecal material:**
  - May be associated with contamination of the sample.
- **Helminth eggs:**
  - The eggs of the bladder worm (*Capillaria plica*) may rarely be found.

Faecal samples

Faecal samples can be very useful as an aid to the diagnosis of endoparasites (nematodes, cestodes, protozoa; see Chapter 6), viral, bacterial and yeast infections (see Chapter 5), and functional gastrointestinal diseases (see Chapter 18). Although the collection of faeces may be simple, it is important that strict hygiene is employed to avoid contamination and exposure to potential zoonoses (e.g. *Salmonella* spp., *Echinococcus* spp., *Toxoplasma* gondi). PPE (gloves, apron, facemask) must be worn and good hygiene (hand washing) is essential.

Patient preparation

Depending on the diagnostic test to be performed, it may be necessary to withdraw medication, such as antibiotics or antidiarrhoeal preparations, or to withhold red meat from the diet, for a period of time prior to sampling.

Sample collection

Samples can be collected directly from the rectum or from voided faeces. It is important to consider contamination if faeces have been collected from the animal's enclosure or from the ground, and also the date on which they were passed.

- **Collection from the rectum** can be carried out by gently using a gloved finger with sterile lubricant. The animal should be firmly but gently restrained and care must be taken not to damage the anorectal mucosa. Direct collection is particularly useful in animals that are generally housed with others.
- **Collection from the ground** involves transferring the faeces into a universal container using gloves, and a spatula if required. Ideally the top part of the faeces that has not been in contact with the ground should be collected.

Once the sample has been collected, it should be carefully transferred to a universal container with a screw cap in order to avoid contamination. Using an appropriate size of container and filling the container as far as possible will help avoid the sample drying out. The sample should be labelled with the pet and owner's names, date of collection and details of any preservative used (see below). Hands should be washed well after collection.

Sample preservation

Specimens that cannot be examined within a few hours can be refrigerated for up to 7 days. Samples should not be frozen. An equal part of 10% formalin may be used to preserve the sample, but it should be noted that this method of preservation will make the specimen unsuitable for bacteriological examinations such as culture and sensitivity testing.

Sample analysis

All faecal samples should be handled with care, as they may contain bacteria, viruses and parasites that may be potentially zoonotic or harmful to humans. Special attention must be paid to hygiene and personal protective clothing (e.g. gloves, apron, facemask), not only during collection but also during examination of the sample.

Normal contents of faeces of carnivorous animals include:

- Water (60–80%)
- Undigested food (small amounts only)
- Enzymes such as trypsin
- Bile products (biliverdin)
- Small amounts of mucus
- Bacteria
- Small numbers of epithelial cells
- Small amounts of blood from prey
- Small amounts of hair from prey.

Normal contents of faeces of herbivorous animals include large amounts of undigested fibre and seeds.

Gross/macroscopic examination

Appearance

This depends upon the species of animal, but in dogs and cats should usually be 'sausage-shaped' with pinched ends. The sample should be checked for gross evidence of parasites, which may be mobile (e.g. *Toxocara canis* round worms appear like spaghetti several inches long; tapeworm segments appear like flat grains of rice). Foreign material that has passed through the digestive tract (e.g. string, bone fragments, grass) should also be looked for.

Consistency

This will depend on the species of the animal. In most cases, the faeces should be formed and any variations such as hard dry faeces (**constipation**) or liquid faeces (**diarrhoea**) should be noted. Observations of **tenesmus** (straining) when the animal was passing the faeces should also be noted.

Colour

This will depend on the species of the animal and the food that it eats. Colour will also change as the age of the specimen increases, hence the need to examine fresh samples.

Blood may appear in faeces as fresh blood (bright red; **haematochezia**) originating in the lower part of the digestive tract (colon, rectum, anus) or digested blood (darker red/brown; **melena**) originating in the upper part of the digestive tract (stomach, small intestine). It is therefore important to note the colour, as this can help to identify the site of clinical problems. Variations in colour for canine faeces are described in Figure 17.36.

Colour	Possible causes
White	Increased fat in the diet Feeding of bones Digestive problems such as exocrine pancreatic insufficiency (EPI; see Chapter 18)
Yellow	Increased bile pigments due to liver disease
Pink	Hepatic dysfunction such as biliary obstruction
Bright red	Fresh blood (normally seen on top/coating the faeces) Haemorrhage from the lower part of the gastrointestinal tract
Dark red/brown/black	Older blood Diet high in red meat Haemorrhage from the upper part of the gastrointestinal tract

17.36 Colour abnormalities in canine faeces.

Odour

This will depend on the species, as well as the diet the animal receives. Animals on high-protein diets may have very strong smelling faeces. Increased fat levels in the diet can result in rancid smells. Some conditions cause distinct odours, e.g. with haematochezia (fresh blood; see Figure 17.36) in parvovirus infection.

Mucus

Any presence of mucus should be noted. In some cases, it can indicate the presence of digestive disorders (in particular colitis) and parasitic conditions.

Microscopic examination

A **direct smear** ('wet preparation') can be made by spreading a small amount of fresh faeces (collected from the rectum or off a rectal thermometer) on to a microscope slide. The faeces are gently mixed on the slide with saline or water, using a toothpick, and a coverslip applied. The smear should be examined using the low power (X10) and high power (X40) objectives. This is a quick method, requiring minimal equipment. The following abnormalities may be seen on a basic microscopic examination:

- Starch, fat or muscle fibres, which may be indicative of poor digestion
- Bacterial or yeast infection
- Helminth (worm) adult, larvae or eggs
- Protozoa, such as *Giardia* spp. or *Toxoplasma*
- Artefacts and foreign bodies, such as bone spicules, clothing fibres, grass and plant cells.

However, the small sample used in a direct smear may not be sufficient to detect low parasite burdens. Faecal samples can be 'concentrated', either by flotation (using sugar or salt solution) or by sedimentation, to more easily identify parasitic burdens. Two commonly used techniques are the **Modified McMaster technique** (for eggs) and the **Baermann technique** (for larvae).

Modified McMaster technique for eggs

1. Assemble the equipment required; beaker, stirrer, tea strainer, bowl, test tube(s), saturated salt solution, McMaster chamber.
2. Put on gloves.
3. Measure 3 g of faeces and place in a glass beaker.
4. Add 42 ml of water to the beaker and mix with the faeces (a mechanical stirrer is useful).
5. Pour the mixture through a tea strainer or sieve, collecting the filtrate in a separate bowl.
6. Discard the debris in the sieve as hazardous waste.
7. Add 15 ml of the filtrate to a test tube and centrifuge at 1000–1500 rpm for 5 minutes.
8. Remove the supernatant and discard.
9. Add a few millilitres of saturated salt solution to the sediment and resuspend. Once suspended, add further amounts of saturated salt solution until 15 ml of fluid is present.
10. Remove a small amount (0.15 ml) with a Pasteur pipette and fill one side of a McMaster chamber.
11. Repeat step 10, filling the other side of the McMaster slide.
12. Examine the McMaster slide under X40 magnification.
13. Using the grid on the McMaster slide examine each section, recording the eggs present. Repeat this technique using the grid on the other side of the slide.

To calculate the number of eggs per gram of faeces, add the numbers counted in each chamber together and multiply by 50 (this is because 3 g of faeces gave 45 ml suspension and 2 x 0.15 ml fluid in chamber (0.3 ml in total) are examined).

Baermann technique for larvae

1. Assemble the equipment required; Baermann apparatus (funnel, metal clamp stand, short section of rubber tube, clip), gauze/muslin, centrifuge tube, microscope slides, glass coverslips, Lugol's iodine.
2. Put on gloves.
3. Attach the rubber tubing to the end of the funnel. Place the clip over the end of the rubber tubing to seal.
4. Clamp the funnel in the metal clamp stand.
5. Fill the funnel with warm water, up to about 1 cm from the rim.
6. Place the gauze/muslin (twice the diameter of the funnel) on top of the funnel.
7. Place 5–15 g of faeces on to the gauze/muslin, ensuring it is covered with water.
8. Allow the apparatus to stand overnight.
9. In the morning unclip the clip from the tubing and fill a centrifuge tube with the filtrate.
10. Centrifuge the tube for 1 minute at 1500 rpm.
11. Remove the supernatant and place the sediment on a microscope slide using a pipette.
12. Add a drop of Lugol's iodine and examine under the microscope under X40 and x100 magnification.
13. Record any findings.

Skin and hair samples

The testing of skin and hair is invaluable in the diagnosis of ectoparasites and conditions such as ringworm (dermatophytosis). It is important that the correct technique is used for sample collection, and knowledge of the potential condition is also required.

Patient preparation

It is useful to record any recent skin treatments (e.g. shampoos, creams, anti-parasitic spot-on products) that may have been used prior to the investigation of skin disease. It may be advantageous to stop some treatments, such as antibacterial drugs and immune therapy, prior to investigation; the veterinary surgeon will make these decisions often on the advice of a pathologist. Many skin investigations can be easily carried out in the conscious patient without causing any distress. Where the skin is painful, as is often the case with ear disorders, sedation or anaesthesia may be required.

Sampling techniques

Various methods are used to collect skin and hair samples. The clinical signs, along with differential diagnoses, should be considered to ensure that the correct sampling technique and area of sampling are used. Whilst sampling, it is important to be aware of potential zoonoses (e.g. *Sarcoptes scabiei*, dermatophytes) and cross-contamination. PPE (long sleeved gloves, aprons) should be worn at all times, and the risk of contamination of other patients avoided. Many of the techniques included below are used for investigating parasitic skin infections; information is given in Chapter 6 on the identification of these parasites.

Skin scrapes

Skin scraping is one of the most common diagnostic procedures used for evaluating patients with dermatological conditions. The area selected is usually one that has clinical lesions or is the most likely to harbour the particular parasite (e.g. ear margins for *Sarcoptes scabiei*).

Skin scrape procedure

1. Assemble the equipment required: clippers and clipper blades (size 40), size 10 scalpel blade (blunt), liquid paraffin or 10% potassium hydroxide, microscope slide, glass coverslip, chinagraph pen/permanent marker and microscope.
2. Put on gloves.
3. Select the area to be scraped.
4. Clip the area (if necessary) using the clippers; this will allow more accurate scraping and will remove hair that may obscure findings. Clipping is not usually necessary where surface-dwelling parasites are suspected.
5. Dip the scalpel blade into liquid paraffin or potassium hydroxide, which will act as a mounting medium and moisten the surface of the skin. This will make the detection and identification of the ectoparasites easier.
6. Hold the blade between the thumb and forefinger. →

Skin scrape procedure *continued*

7. Stretch the skin to be scraped with the other hand and then gently scrape the area (usually a 3 cm by 3 cm area). The depth of scraping will vary according to the parasite in question, although most scraping should result in a small amount of capillary ooze.

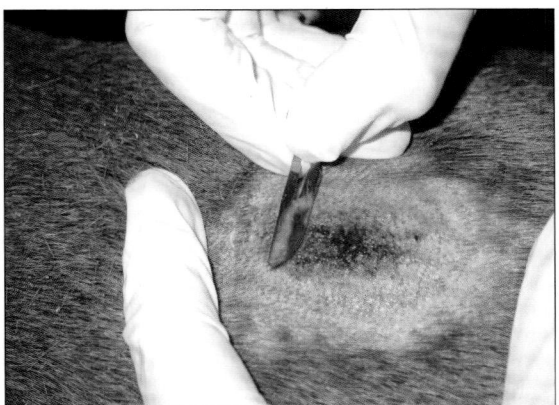

8. Transfer the collected material from the forward surface of the blade on to a glass slide. A drop of liquid paraffin or 10% potassium hydroxide can be added to the slide.
9. Place a coverslip over the top of the sample and label the slide.
10. Set up the microscope and examine the slide using the lowest power first. Vernier scale readings can be used to relocate parasites, although live parasites may move.
11. Slides should be viewed immediately after the sample has been collected to avoid parasites leaving the slide.
12. Once the slide has been examined and results recorded, dispose of in a sharps container.

Adhesive tape impressions

This method can be used to detect superficial parasites (e.g. *Cheyletiella*), as well as bacteria, fungi and yeasts (e.g. *Malassezia*). Clear adhesive tape is applied to the skin to collect epidermal debris. The adhesive side of the tape is then placed directly on a glass microscope slide, which is labelled with the patient's details. The slide is then viewed with a microscope, starting with the lowest power.

Hair plucks

Hair plucks may be used to identify the presence of fungal spores, superficial mites (including *Demodex*, which live in the hair follicles) and parasitic eggs such as those from *Cheyletiella*. A small number of hairs (including the roots) are plucked from the affected area using artery forceps. The hairs are placed on a glass slide with a drop of liquid paraffin. A glass coverslip is placed on top and the slide labelled. The slide can then be examined using a microscope, starting with the lowest power.

Hair brushings

Hair brushings can be used to identify superficial parasites and eggs. This method is also used to identify the faeces of fleas where the fleas cannot be seen on the coat by the naked eye. The animal or part of the animal being tested should be placed close to some white material (e.g. white paper). The coat is then brushed by hand or using a comb, over the white material and the debris collected. The debris can be examined on the white material; this allows flea faeces to be identified as they look like small bits of black soil but are actually digested blood. A 'wet paper test' can be performed to confirm this observation. If the material is dabbed with wet cotton wool, flea faeces will dissolve and appear as red/brown tinged marks. Some of the collected debris can also be transferred to a labelled microscope slide with liquid paraffin and a coverslip placed on top. This can then be examined using the microscope.

Impression smears

Impression smears can be used to detect bacterial, fungal or yeast skin conditions. The hair is first clipped and then a microscope slide pressed directly on to the skin. The slide can then be appropriately stained (see 'Bacteriology', below) and viewed with a microscope.

Swab samples

Skin swabs can be used to identify bacterial, fungal and yeast skin conditions. The swab is rolled over the surface of the affected area (e.g. skin, inside the ear canal). The swab can then be rolled/smeared on a microscope slide, stained (see 'Bacteriology', below) and viewed with a microscope. In cases where *Otodectes* ear mites are suspected, small amounts of wax can be collected from the ear canal and transferred to a microscope slide with liquid paraffin. A glass coverslip should be placed over the top before the slide is labelled and examined with a microscope. Alternatively, the swab can be labelled, correctly packaged (see 'Package and dispatch of laboratory samples', below) and sent to an external laboratory for bacteriology, fungal culture and cytology (see below), as appropriate. Charcoal swabs should be used for transportation of samples for bacterial and fungal culture.

Ear swab collection

1. Assemble the equipment required: gloves, appropriate swabs, pen for labelling.
2. Wear gloves.
3. Select appropriate swab (e.g. charcoal for bacteriology).
4. Ask for assistance and give instructions for the animal to be restrained.
5. Collect sufficient material for analysis by gently rotating the swab to cover all surfaces without traumatizing the ear or causing any discomfort; avoid any contamination.
6. Replace the swab into the cover tube without any further contamination and secure the lid.
7. Remove gloves and ensure correct disposal.
8. Label the swab with the location the sample was collected from (e.g. 'right ear').
9. Label the swab with the animal's name, owner's name and the date.
10. Package the swab following packaging guidelines (see 'Package and dispatch of laboratory samples', below).

Cytology

Cytology uses microscopic examination of tissue or fluid samples to differentiate normal from abnormal cells to aid diagnosis. The samples may be obtained from a variety of body areas; examples of which are listed below. Frequently samples are sent for microbiology at the same time as cytology. Various sampling techniques are used, according to the area of interest, and testing can be carried out in house or via an external laboratory.

> ## Samples for cytological examination may include:
>
> - Tracheal washes
> - Vaginal swabs (see Chapter 24)
> - Ear swabs
> - Semen (see Chapter 24)
> - Cerebrospinal fluid
> - Abdominal fluid
> - Synovial fluid
> - Thoracic fluid
> - Urine.

Patient preparation

The preparation of the patient depends upon the site of sample collection, as well as patient temperament and the clinical condition being investigated. Samples such as skin and ear canal swabs (see above) can usually be collected in a conscious patient, as can fine-needle aspirates and most centesis samples (see below). Other more invasive sampling techniques such as those used for cerebrospinal fluid collection (see below) and tissue biopsy (see below) require some form of anaesthesia. In these cases, the need for chemical restraint and therefore withholding of food need to be taken into consideration as part of the patient preparation. It may be beneficial to stop some drug treatments for a period of time before sampling and the veterinary surgeon will make this decision.

Sample collection

Swabs

Swabs are generally used to collect samples from mucous membranes such as those lining the nasal cavity, vagina (see Chapter 24) or eyes. The swab should be gently placed into the cavity and rolled/stroked on the lining. Once removed from the cavity, the swab should be gently stroked down the length of a clean microscope slide. The slide should be air-dried or heat-fixed. The slide can be stained (e.g. with Diff-Quik® (Romanowsky stain); see 'Bacteriology', below) before microscopic examination. The cells seen should be identified and recorded. Bacterial cells are identified using Gram staining (see 'Bacteriology', below). Swabs can also be used to collect samples from the skin and ear canal (as described above).

Direct smears

Inflammatory exudate from ulcerated surface lesions can be sampled by direct application of a microscope slide to the lesion. This may be of limited value, however, as deeper tissues are not included. Impression smears may also be made of biopsy specimens (see below) to give an immediate indication of the type of lesion before sending a sample

for histopathological interpretation. The cut surface of the sample is blotted to remove surface blood and serum. The dried surface is then applied to a clean dry slide, using gentle pressure. Several areas can be sampled on a single slide. The preparations are quickly air-dried and then stained as for a fluid sample.

Fine-needle aspiration

Specimens for cytology may be collected from organs, lymph nodes and masses. The most common method used in practice is fine-needle biopsy, commonly known as fine-needle aspiration (FNA). Ultrasound guidance may be helpful (see Chapter 16). The procedure will be carried out by a veterinary surgeon but may require assistance from a veterinary nurse.

> ## FNA collection
>
> 1. Equipment should be prepared, including microscope slides, syringes and needles.
> 2. The mass is stabilized using the hand and a fine sterile needle (21–27 G) inserted. The needle is redirected several times while still in the mass.
> 3. The needle is then removed from the mass.
> 4. A syringe is then filled with air and attached to the needle. Pushing down on the plunger gently forces the sample on to a clean microscope slide.
> 5. The sample is then spread on to the slide using either a 'squash technique' (Figure 17.37) or smeared like a blood smear (see 'Blood smear preparation', above) and then air-dried.
> 6. The process is usually repeated to collect several samples.
> 7. The samples may be stained and examined in house (Figure 17.38) or sent to an external laboratory.

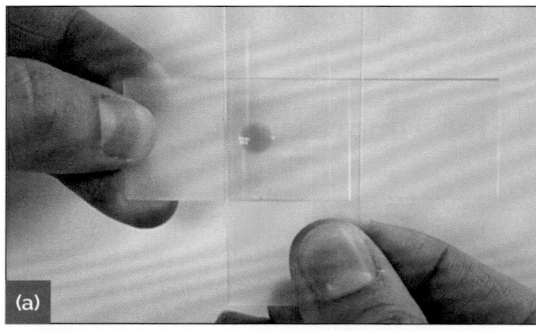
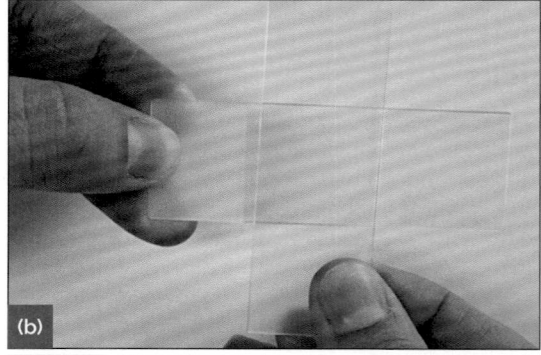

17.37 'Squash technique' for preparing a slide from tissue collected using a fine-needle aspiration. **(a)** A drop of specimen is placed on one edge of the bottom slide. **(b)** A second slide is gently applied on top and drawn across at right angles. (Reproduced from the *BSAVA Manual of Feline and Canine Clinical Pathology, 3rd edn*)

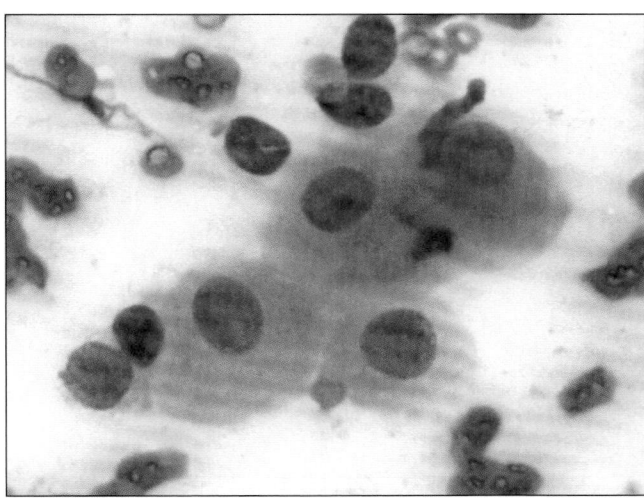

17.38 Fine-needle aspirate from a perianal mass on a dog, showing a cluster of epithelial cells with round nuclei and grainy cytoplasm. (Wright's stain; original magnification X1000) (Courtesy of Elizabeth Villiers; reproduced from the *BSAVA Manual of Canine and Feline Clinical Pathology, 2nd edn*)

The technique described above is sometimes referred to as 'needle off' (or needle only) FNA. Some veterinary surgeons prefer to use a 'needle on' (or suction) technique, in which negative pressure is created at Stage 1 by attaching an appropriately size syringe (2–20 ml) to the needle. The needle is inserted into the mass and the syringe plunger drawn back to about three-quarters its length. The plunger is released before the needle is withdrawn. The syringe and needle are detached before the process in continued from Stage 3.

FNA techniques have the advantages that they are cheap to carry out, minimally invasive and rarely require sedation or anaesthesia. The samples collected, however, are limited in their ability to diagnose a problem since the number of cells collected is small and those harvested may not be representative of the mass as a whole. A more representative sample may be collected through tissue biopsy (see below) or removal of the whole lesion or lymph node.

Tissue biopsy

Tissue biopsy can be used to obtain samples for cytological and histopathological examination. A biopsy can be performed on most organs and tissues for the investigation of conditions such as suspected tumours (neoplasia), cysts, abscesses, haematomas, foreign body reactions and allergic reactions. Depending on the location and accessibility of the organ in question, surgery may be aided by endoscopy or laparoscopy (see Chapter 16). Biopsy procedures usually require at least sedation and local anaesthesia and, frequently, general anaesthesia. Procedures will be carried out by a veterinary surgeon where entry into a body cavity is required.

The biopsy procedure may involve cutting into the affected organ or lesion. These are described as incisional biopsies and include:

- **Wedge biopsy:** Commonly performed using a surgical scalpel. Specific lesions can be included within the sample and a good cross-section of the mass/area can be obtained
- **Punch biopsy:** Normally much easier and quicker to perform than wedge biopsy. Specialized punch biopsy instruments are available (e.g. skin punches and Tru-Cut® needles).

Alternatively, the biopsy procedure may involve removal of the organ (or part of it) or the lesion. These are described as **excisional biopsies** and may be:

- **Intracapsular:** Removal of the mass without the capsule of surrounding tissue
- **Marginal:** Removal of the mass with its capsule only
- **Wide:** Removal of the mass with a margin of normal tissue around it
- **Radical:** Removal of the mass with the entire surrounding tissue compartment (muscle, fascia).

Sample preservation

All tissue samples should ideally be preserved in 10% neutral buffered formalin (3.7%–4.0% formaldehyde in phosphate-buffered saline) using 10 parts formalin solution to 1 part tissue; other preservatives are also available (Figure 17.39). Samples should be collected into large histology pots, with a wide-mouth and base, that are made of tough polypropylene with strong plastic leak-proof lids.

Preservative	Details
10% formalin	This contains 40% formaldehyde gas
10% formal saline	Most common solution used. It is made by diluting formalin with saline solution
10% neutral buffered formalin	This is a 10% solution of formalin with added buffers. The buffers prevent any changes in pH, which may affect cells
Alcohol	This may be used but causes unwanted shrinkage of tissue and hardness

17.39 Examples of tissue preservatives.

Preservation of tissue samples

- Be aware of health and safety (see Chapter 2). The sample is a pathological hazardous specimen and formalin is toxic and irritant. PPE should be worn at all times.
- Check with the laboratory for details on how they would like specific samples to be sent.
- A wide-necked container should be used so that samples can be removed easily after they have been fixed. Remember samples are likely to swell in the preservative and increase in size.
- Sample containers should be robust, leak-proof and tightly secured.
- Every container/microscope slide should be labelled.
- Tissue samples should be of a small size (ideally no more than 1 cm thick), to allow penetration of formalin for preservation of the cells. Slicing down into the tissue can help with penetration of the preservative.
- Enough fluid should be used for preserving. All tissue samples should be immersed in 10 times the volume of fixative to the tissue volume.
- Samples should not be frozen, as this damages the cells.
- Only representative samples should be collected and sent to external laboratories. Whole organs should not be sent. →

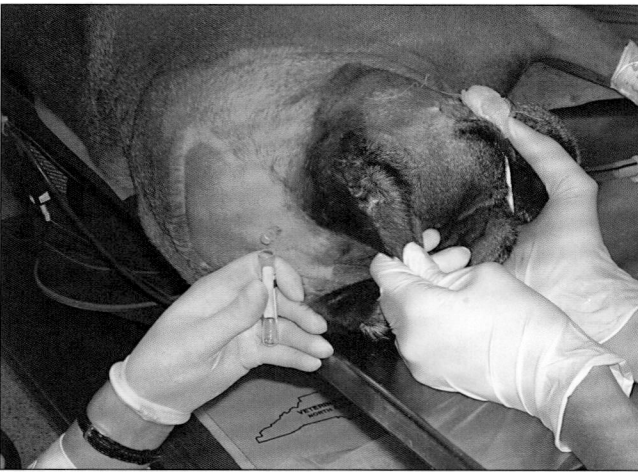

17.40 CSF collection from the cisterna magna via the atlanto-occipital joint in a dog. (Reproduced from the *BSAVA Manual of Canine and Feline Neurology, 4th edn*)

Preservation of tissue samples
continued

- Correct paperwork should accompany the tissue sample. This must include the details of the submitting veterinary surgery, the patient's details, and details of the area sampled (a diagram is useful), including the margins. Gross appearance including size and location of the lesion, previous treatment (if any) and if a zoonotic disease is suspected.

Tissue fluid collection

Collection of fluid from a body cavity or organ can be a useful aid to diagnosis. When fluid is removed from a body cavity, the term 'centesis' is used, for example, pericardiocentesis is removal of fluid from the pericardial sac, cystocenteis is removal of urine from the bladder (see 'Cystocentesis', above). Examples of other 'centesis' are included below and some are discussed in more detail in Chapter 18. The technique involves placing a needle into a body cavity or organ in order to remove fluid for diagnostic and other clinical reasons (see Chapter 18). Strict asepsis is required. This procedure will be carried out by a veterinary surgeon, but may require assistance from a veterinary nurse.

Cerebrospinal fluid (CSF)

Examination of CSF is often required in the diagnosis of neurological conditions such as meningitis. Fluid is collected from the subarachnoid space of the brain or spinal cord. The technique should only be carried out under general anaesthesia, by experienced personnel, using strict asepsis. CSF must be collected prior to injecting contrast media, otherwise the sample will be contaminated.

- In dogs and cats, the patient is anaesthetized and placed in lateral recumbency.
- The area for needle insertion must be aseptically prepared by clipping the hair and using skin disinfectants. The usual sites for collection of CSF are the cisterna magna via the atlanto-occipital joint (Figure 17.40) and lumbar vertebral space L5–L6 in the dog or lumbar vertebral space L6–L7 in the cat.
- All personnel must adhere to aseptic techniques by wearing sterile surgical gloves and using sterile equipment and consumables.
- The head and neck are flexed and held securely in position. Care must be taken not to compress the endotracheal tube.
- The veterinary surgeon inserts a 20–22 G spinal needle carefully into the subarachnoid space.
- The CSF is collected by allowing the fluid to drip into the collecting tubes (Figure 17.40). A maximum of 1 ml per 5 kg of bodyweight should be collected, using EDTA and plain tubes.
- The veterinary surgeon then slowly removes the needle.
- The point of insertion is covered with a sterile adhesive dressing.

Normal CSF should be clear, colourless and slightly viscous. Alterations in the visual appearance should be noted. Cytological analysis must be performed on CSF in order to assess the fluid accurately, and should be carried out as soon as possible after collecting the sample. The sample is examined for the presence of red blood cells and nucleated white blood cells. Other tests performed on CSF include: protein analysis; bacteriology; antibody titres; and electrolyte concentrations.

Thoracic fluid

Thoracocentesis can be undertaken in order to obtain fluid from the thoracic cavity. The procedure is described in Chapter 18. Fluid should be collected into EDTA and plain collection tubes, and the amount aspirated should be measured. Visual inspection of the fluid should also be carried out, and any differences in colour and turbidity such as pus (pyothorax), blood (haemothorax) or chyle (chylothorax) noted (see Chapter 18). Cytology and microbiology can then be carried out.

Abdominal fluid

Abdominocentesis is collection or drainage of fluid from the abdominal cavity. Small amounts of fluid may be collected in the conscious animal; however, sedation (plus local anaesthesia) or even general anaesthesia may be required for larger volumes of fluid. The usual site for abdominocentesis is a few centimetres to one side of the midline, midway between the umbilicus and bladder. Ultrasound guidance may be helpful. A 1–2 inch needle (18–19 G) or butterfly catheter (14–16 G), with a three-way tap connected to a 10–20 ml syringe, is ideal for sample collection. It may be necessary to reposition the needle during the procedure as it can become blocked with omentum.

Fluid should be collected into EDTA and plain collection tubes and the amount aspirated should be measured.

Visual inspection should also be carried out, noting differences in colour and turbidity, which can assist with sample interpretation (Figure 17.41). Additional testing for protein levels, specific gravity, cytology and bacteriology can also be carried out, which may be useful in confirming a clinical diagnosis.

Synovial fluid

Synovial fluid is collected from a joint via arthrocentesis. This can be very useful in assisting the diagnosis of inflammatory or infectious joint conditions. The most common sites for arthrocentesis in small animals are the stifle joint, shoulder and elbow. The procedure is usually carried out under general anaesthesia. Small amounts of fluid should be

Fluid colour and appearance	Likely fluid type	Possible causes
Clear (specific gravity <1.012, does not clot, low cell content)	True transudate	Hypoalbuminaemia; chronic liver disease, renal disease, gastrointestinal disease
Pink/yellow	Modified transudate	Hypertension; portal hypertension, obstruction of venous flow (e.g. neoplasia), cardiac disease (right-sided heart failure)
Yellow/red and turbid (specific gravity >1.012, may clot, high cell content)	Exudate	Sepsis; peritonitis, feline infectious peritonitis (FIP) Sterile; secondary to bile or urine leakage (see below)
Red	Blood	Bleeding; trauma, splenic rupture, neoplasia (haemangiosarcoma), clotting disorders (e.g. rodenticide toxicity)
White and turbid	Chyle	Damage to lymphatic vessels; trauma, neoplasia
Brown	Gut contents	Perforation of gut; trauma (e.g. foreign body), ulceration, neoplasia
Yellow	Urine	Urinary tract (kidney, bladder, ureter) rupture; trauma, urine outflow obstruction (e.g. urolithiasis)
Green	Bile	Gall bladder rupture; trauma, neoplasia

17.41 Interpretation of fluid types that may be collected by abdominocentesis.

collected into plain and EDTA tubes. Analysis usually includes visual assessment, total protein assay, cytology and bacteriology. Normal synovial fluid is clear to straw yellow in colour and non-turbid. Turbidity can indicate the presence of cells, protein or cartilage.

Airway washes

Tracheal wash or bronchoalveolar lavage (BAL) can be particularly useful for the diagnosis of respiratory disease. An endoscope is used to visualize the area to be investigated. Saline is then flushed into the area via the port on the endoscope and drawn back up with a syringe or suction device on the endoscope. The collected fluid should be placed in sterile containers (EDTA and plain), which are typically sent to an external laboratory for cytology and bacteriology.

Bone marrow sampling

The bone marrow may need to be sampled in animals with non-regenerative anaemia as a result of neoplasia or immune disease. The bone marrow may be sampled by either collecting a bone marrow aspirate or by core biopsy; the two sample types may be taken at the same time. Several sites may be used; the iliac crest, trochanteric fossa of the femur, tibial crest and proximal humerus. Bone marrow sample collection is usually carried out under general anaesthesia, although it can be carried out in some sites (e.g. iliac crest) under appropriate sedation and local anaesthesia. The preferred biopsy site is the proximal humerus and general anaesthesia is used for this procedure. Bone marrow sampling is a sterile procedure. The dog should be placed in lateral recumbancy and the site prepared (clipped and scrubbed) as for surgery. A small incision is made in skin over the greater tubercle of the humerus. A bone marrow needle (usually Jamshidi type) with a central stylet is inserted until it hits bone and the needle is then 'screwed' through cortex of bone into marrow cavity. The stylet of the needle is removed and a syringe is attached to take the sample. The sample is quickly transferred to a series of microscope slides and allowed to run down them, leaving marrow spicules behind on the slide. Squash preparation of these spicules (see Figure 17.37) are then made and can be stained (usually with Diff-Quik®) and examined under a microscope or sent to an external pathologist.

Bacteriology

When bacterial infection is suspected bacteriological samples may be investigated. Through bacteriology, a bacterial infection may be confirmed, the type of bacteria (see Chapter 5) can be identified and further testing, such as drug sensitivity testing (see below and Chapters 5 and 7), can be undertaken to aid treatment of the condition. A range of samples (e.g. blood, skin, CSF, faeces) may be collected for bacteriology using a variety of sampling techniques. In all cases, some basic principles for bacteriological sample collection should be adhered to.

Considerations for bacteriological samples

- Speak to the laboratory first if there is any uncertainty about what/how to sample, or when dealing with unusual clinical situations
- A generous sample, or multiple samples, should be submitted
- Samples should be taken from living or recently deceased animals
- Samples should be taken from recent or new lesions
- The edge of a lesion should be sampled
- Ideally, sampling should be carried out prior to treatment with antibacterials or antibacterial drugs stopped for a period of time before sampling. Any antibacterials used should be listed on the submission form
- Samples should be collected using aseptic techniques and sterile equipment (see 'Ear swab technique', above as an example)
- Samples should be collected and transported in appropriate media and containers
- The collection/transport container should be sealed as soon as possible to avoid contamination
- All containers should be clearly labelled on the outside of the container, to avoid confusion
- Samples should be examined as soon as possible after collection
- Samples should be refrigerated (at 2–4°C) if there is any delay in examination
- Samples should be delivered as soon as possible to the laboratory, if sending externally. Special delivery post or a courier should be used

Bacterial culture

Bacteria are specialized microorganisms that will only grow in a suitable environment. The correct environment for growth usually includes:

- Water
- Essential nutrients
- Correct pH
- Correct temperature (most bacteria are normothermic and therefore require body temperatures of 37–40°C)
- Correct gaseous environment.

Culture media

Bacteria are grown on or within a culture medium. Culture media provide the essential nutrients the bacteria require in order to reproduce. There are two types of medium; liquid (also known as broth) and solid media. For bacteriology, culture media may be purchased as dehydrated powder or as prepared agar plates in Petri dishes or liquid media jars. Solidifying agents used in solid media include gelatine and agar (dried extract of sea algae). Unused agar plates should be kept refrigerated at 5°C.

Simple media

Simple agar or nutrient agar media provide the basic nutrients for undemanding species such as *Escherichia coli*.

Enriched media

These media are used to culture bacteria that require additional nutrients. Examples include:

- **Blood agar:** This contains 5–10% blood, and is used to support the growth of most mammalian pathogens. It may also be used to detect haemolysis
- **Chocolate agar:** This contains blood that has been heated to 80°C. By heating the blood, the red blood cells rupture and release haemoglobin, which adds nutrition to the agar.

Enrichment broths are also used. This liquid medium is selective for a particular bacterium. Enrichment broth has no inhibitory agent preventing growth of other organisms. It allows the growth of the target species and allows it to outgrow other species that may be present. An example of an enrichment broth includes selenite broth used for the growth of *Salmonella*.

Selective media

This type of medium allows a particular bacterium or group of bacteria to grow whilst inhibiting the growth of unwanted species. Some of these media change colour with microbial growth; these are known as indicator media. Examples include:

- **MacConkey's agar:** This contains crystal violet (which suppresses the growth of Gram-positive bacteria) and bile salts (selective for lactose-fermenting enteric bacteria and other bile salt-tolerant Gram-negative bacteria)
- **Deoxycholate–citrate agar:** This inhibits non-enteric bacteria and is used for growing *Salmonella*.

Transport agar

This is used for the temporary storage and transport of a specimen, by acting as a maintenance agar. It merely supports survival of the organism rather than aiding growth.

Producing a bacterial culture

In order to culture bacteria, a sample is transferred to an appropriate culture medium. The aim is to obtain single bacterial colonies in order to observe colonial morphology, antibiotic sensitivity and biochemical identification. The quadrant streak method is the preferred method of inoculating an agar plate.

The quadrant streak method

1. Put on PPE.
2. Label the Petri dish.
3. Heat a wire inoculation loop by passing it through the flame of a Bunsen burner (see 'Bunsen burner' above for information on use). Cool the loop in the air for a few seconds or by touching it gently on to the surface of the agar at the edge of the plate.
4. Dip the loop into the sample.
5. Pick up the Petri dish and smear the loop over one-quarter of the agar surface. Be sure to keep the loop almost parallel to the agar surface to avoid digging into it.

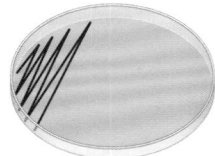

6. Pass the inoculating loop through the Bunsen burner flame again and allow it to cool.
7. Place the inoculating loop on the edge of the first set of streaks and create further streaks at right angles to them.

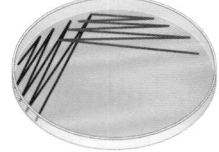

8. Pass the inoculating loop through the Bunsen burner flame again and allow it to cool.
9. Place the inoculating loop on the edge of the second set of streaks and create further streaks at right angles.

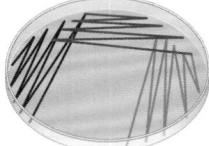

10. Pass the inoculating loop through the Bunsen burner flame again and allow it to cool.
11. Place the inoculating loop on the edge of the third set of streaks and create a final set, again at right angles.

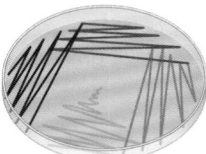

12. Place the lid on the dish and place in the incubator at 37°C.
13. Remove the plate after 18–24 hours and examine for colony growth. Re-incubate if necessary.

Examining the colony

Appropriate health and safety precautions should be taken when examining bacterial plates; gloves, an apron, goggles and a facemask should be worn. An experienced microbiologist can recognize several bacteria on gross examination of cultured colonies. When looking at the colonies, the following examination and recordings should take place:

- Size (either measured or described as pinpoint, medium, large)
- Pigment/colour
- Density (opaque, transparent)
- Elevation (raised, flat, convex, drop-like)
- Shape (circular, irregular)
- Texture (smooth, sticky)
- Odour, if appropriate (sweet, pungent)
- Haemolysis.

Once gross examination has occurred, individual colonies can be isolated and grown on if required. An inoculation loop is used to remove an individual part of the bacterial culture and a new agar plate inoculated as described above. Culture samples may be transferred to a microscope slide, stained and examined with a microscope.

Bacterial smear preparation

1. Put on PPE.
2. Clean a microscope slide with ethanol and lint-free tissue and label it.
3. Pass the slide through a Bunsen burner flame (see 'Bunsen burner', above for information on use).
4. Place one drop of water on to the slide using a sterile inoculating loop.
5. Using the sterile inoculating loop, remove a portion of the bacterial culture and place it on to the slide.
6. Mix the sample on the slide and spread evenly.
7. Allow the smear to dry thoroughly.
8. Fix the slide by passing through the Bunsen burner flame three times.

Staining

Once the smear is prepared and fixed, a stain may be used to aid identification. Taking into consideration the colour, size, shape and arrangement, common types of bacteria may be identified.

There are three types of stain that can be used:

- **Simple stains:** These colour the cell or the background so that the size, shape and arrangement of the cells can be seen (e.g. methylene blue)
- **Differential stains:** These stains use a combination of two dyes to differentiate between cell types (e.g. Gram stain)
- **Structural stains:** These stains only dye part of the cell structure.

Methylene blue

This is a simple stain, which can be used to identify size, shape and arrangement. Methylene blue is relatively cheap and easy to use.

Methylene blue staining

1. Put on PPE.
2. Place the microscope slide on a staining rack.
3. Flood the slide with 1% methylene blue stain.
4. Leave for 2 minutes.
5. Wash off with distilled water.
6. Stand vertically and allow to dry.
7. Examine under the microscope, using X100 with oil immersion.

Gram stain

The Gram stain is the most common differential stain used, as it divides bacteria into two groups: Gram-positive and Gram-negative (see Chapter 5).

Gram staining procedure

1. Put on PPE.
2. Place the microscope slide on a staining rack.
3. Flood the slide with crystal violet for 30 seconds.
4. Gently rinse in tap water.
5. Flood slide with Gram's iodine for 30 seconds.
6. Gently rinse in tap water.
7. Wash slide with decolorizer (acetone) for 5 seconds.
8. Gently rinse in tap water.
9. Flood slide with carbol fuchsin or safranin for 30 seconds.
10. Gently rinse in tap water.
11. Air-dry smear or gently blot with paper towel.
12. Examine under the microscope, using X100 and oil immersion.

Results
- Bacteria that stain **purple** are termed **Gram-positive**
- Bacteria that stain **pink** are termed **Gram-negative**

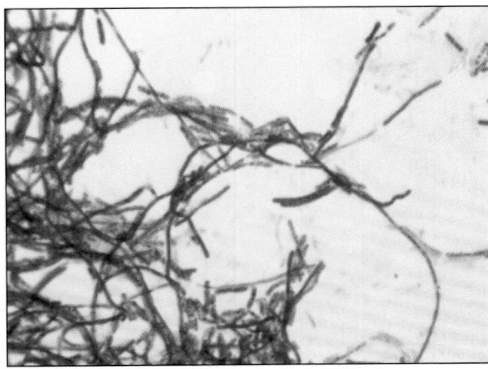

Gram-positive bacilli

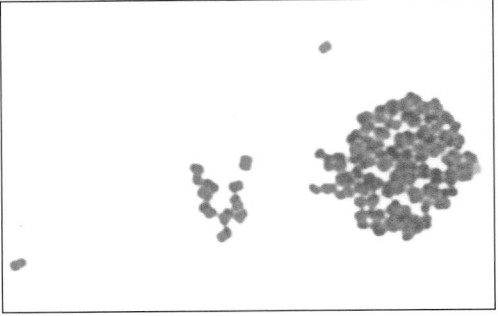

Gram-negative cocci

Ziehl–Neelsen/acid-fast staining

This stain is used to identify acid-fast bacteria such as *Mycobacterium* spp.

> ## Ziehl–Neelsen staining procedure
>
> 1. Put on PPE.
> 2. Place the microscope slide on a staining rack.
> 3. Flood the slide with Ziehl–Neelsen carbol fuchsin solution and apply gentle heat until steam rises.
> 4. Leave for 5 minutes.
> 5. Rinse gently with tap water.
> 6. Decolorize with acid alcohol for at least 1 minute.
> 7. Rinse gently in tap water and repeat decolorization until the smear is pale pink.
> 8. Flood with Loeffler's alkaline methylene blue.
> 9. Leave for 2–3 minutes.
> 10. Rinse gently with tap water.
> 11. Blot dry with paper towel and examine.
>
> **Results**
> - **Acid-fast** bacteria stain **bright red**
> - **Non-acid-fast** bacteria stain **blue**

Antimicrobial sensitivity testing

In order to establish the best treatment for a bacterial infection, antimicrobial sensitivity testing (see Chapters 5 and 7) can be carried out using agar Petri dish cultures. Specialized discs impregnated with antibiotics are placed on the surface of the agar, which has been previously inoculated with a pure bacterial culture. After incubation of 18–24 hours the plate is removed and examined. Where bacteria are sensitive to a particular antibiotic, there will be a clear zone of growth inhibition around that disc (Figure 17.42).

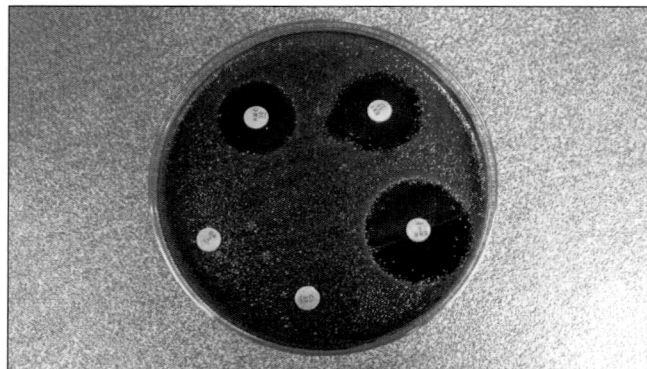

17.42 Antibacterial sensitivity plate: the organism was sensitive to three of the antibiotics (no growth zone around the disc) but resistant to the other two (no zone of inhibition).

Fungal culture

Using similar methods as for bacteriology, clinical samples can be collected and cultured for fungal infections (for example, fungal culture is used in the diagnosis of dermatophytosis (ringworm); see Chapter 5). Special selective media is required for fungal culture. Sabouraud's agar has a high glucose content and low pH, which is ideal for fungal growth. It is used as an indicator medium, changing from yellow to red in the presence of fungal growth (Figure 17.43).

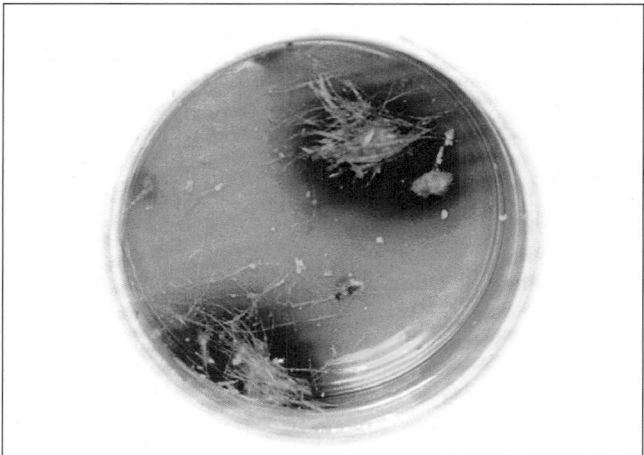

17.43 Sabouraud's agar changes from yellow to red in the presence of fungal growth.

Virology

Testing for some viruses (see Chapter 5) can be carried out in the practice using simple in-house testing kits (see above). These test kits often use ELISA, which is one of the most sensitive and reproducible diagnostic technologies available. Kits are available for the detection of viral diseases in small animals, as well as in other species. A commonly used kit combines a test for feline leukaemia virus with one for feline immunodeficiency antibodies (see 'Serology', above). For testing for other viruses, samples will need to be sent for testing to external laboratories.

Toxicology

Toxicological testing, to detect poisonous substances affecting an animal, is carried out by specialist laboratories. Veterinary practices should check with the laboratory which are the most appropriate samples and/or tests available before sampling. Samples can be collected from both living and deceased animals and include blood, tissue samples from organs, stomach contents and vomit. Strict attention should be paid to PPE when dealing with suspected poisoning cases, as the majority of toxins affecting animals can also potentially be toxic to humans.

Package and dispatch of samples

It is very likely that, at some point, it will be necessary to send samples from the veterinary practice to a specialized external laboratory. It is very important that samples sent to an external laboratory are correctly packaged, in order to ensure that they arrive in excellent condition and that all legal packaging requirements are complied with.

Legal packaging requirements

Packaging regulations are in place in order to protect postal workers, transportation and laboratory staff, as well as to ensure that samples arrive in good condition. It is the responsibility of the sender to ensure samples are packaged correctly.

The World Health Organization provides guidance for the transportation of pathological samples. Since air transport regulations are the most restrictive, packaging and shipping that complies with the International Air Transport Association (IATA) regulations should be used. Almost all samples sent from veterinary practices to laboratories are classed as 'diagnostic substances' and these fall under classification UN3373 (Category B infectious substances). Samples that fall under classification UN3373 must be packed for transport according to a set of guidelines known as P650 or Packing Instruction 650. This is a list of requirements covering the quality and construction of the packaging used for transport. These regulations state that the packaging must have the following components (Figure 17.44):

- A primary receptacle containing the specimen
- A secondary container or receptacle
- Outer packaging with suitable cushioning or sturdy protective material for the sample being sent.

The packaging must also:

- Be capable of withstanding a 1.2 m drop test
- Be able to withstand internal pressure of 95 kPA
- Be leak proof
- Have enough absorbent material to absorb leakages
- Clearly show 'Diagnostic specimen Licence no. UN3373' with diamond shaped mark (Figures 17.44 and 17.45).

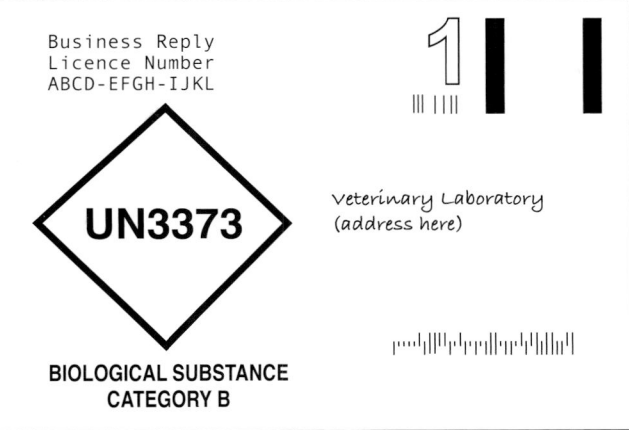

17.45 Example of address label on packaging for UN3373 (Category B infectious substances).

External laboratories often provide veterinary practices with their own supplies, containers and packaging to be used for submitting laboratory samples. These may include:

- Containers, including blood collection tubes and universal containers (as described above)
- Forms/paperwork (see below)
- Absorbent material
- Secondary layer (e.g. plastic biohazard bag, polystyrene box) (Figure 17.44)
- Tertiary layer (e.g. padded bag-type envelope, cardboard box) (Figure 17.44)
- Labels for the tertiary layer, including 'UN3373 Category B Infectious Material' together with the UN3373 symbol, laboratory address and space for the practice address (see Figures 17.44 and 17.45).

Samples should be packaged carefully, in a clean environment.

Further details on the correct packaging and posting of samples are available from the Royal Mail and/or courier services.

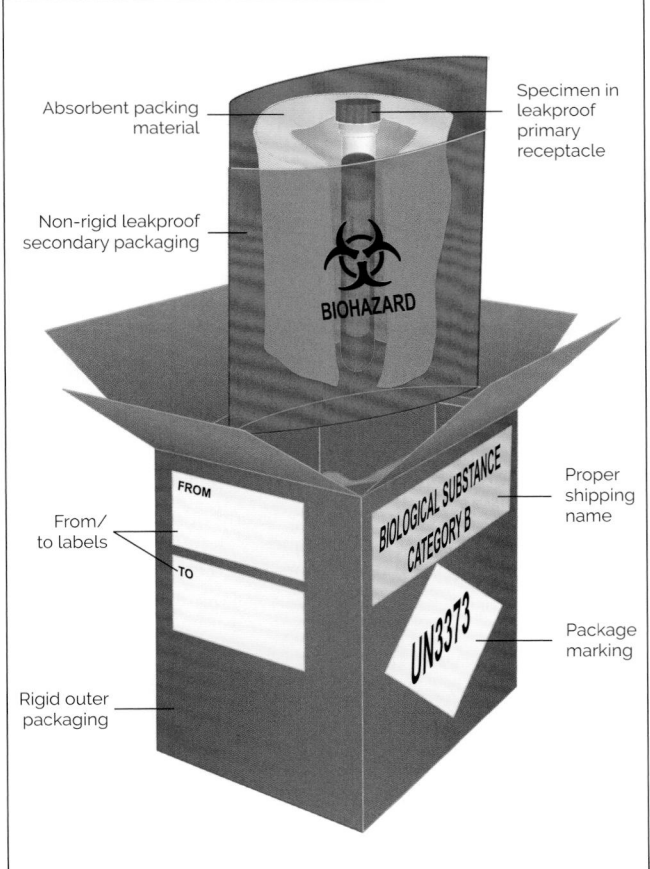

17.44 Example of packing and marking for Category B infectious substances.

Packing and posting samples

1. Put on PPE, to avoid contamination and potential zoonoses.
2. Check that the sample is preserved correctly (e.g. is there adequate formalin?).
3. Ensure the container is labelled with the animal's name, species, breed, age, sex, owner's name and date.
4. Ensure the container is airtight, moisture-proof and robust.
5. Ensure the total volume/mass of the sample in one package does not exceed 50 ml or 50 g.
6. Wrap the container in sufficient absorbent material to absorb the total volume of fluid in the sample, should the container leak or break.
7. As an additional precaution, it is good practice to also wrap the container in bubble wrap.
8. Place the sample in a secondary layer (e.g. plastic biohazard bag), expel any excess air from the bag and seal it securely.
9. Ensure that the laboratory paperwork/form has been completed and place this in a plastic bag separate from the sample. Ideally use a waterproof marker for labelling specimen bags and containers →

Packing and posting samples *continued*

10. Place all the items into the tertiary layer (e.g. a prepaid padded bag supplied by the laboratory) and ensure that this is sealed securely.
11. Ensure the outer packaging contains the sender's name and address.
12. Ensure the outer packaging states the nature of the sample and any special instructions (e.g. handle with care, fragile, pathological specimen).
13. Ensure the sample is sent by first class post or via a courier.

Paperwork for laboratory samples

Most external laboratories provide paperwork for completion and dispatch with any samples being sent to the laboratory. Often the paperwork is specific to a certain type of test (e.g. bacteriology, histopathology, virology). Forms should include:

- Practice details and veterinary surgeon's name
- Owner's name and address
- Animal's name
- Species, age and sex of animal
- Test required
- Date sample collected
- Date sample dispatched
- Sample type
- Sample site
- Relevant history, clinical findings and therapy.

It is good practice to keep internal records of all samples processed 'in-house' or sent to an external laboratory. These may be computerized or written in a laboratory book. Information to record might include:

- Name of owner and animal
- Types of sample(s)
- Quality of samples

- Tests requested or carried out
- If sent externally, to which laboratory
- Date and time of posting
- Name of person packaging and posting sample
- When results were received.

Laboratory results
Recording and reporting laboratory findings

Laboratory test results must be recorded carefully on the animal's clinical record. It is important that results are updated promptly so that they can be used, where necessary, to review or change a clinical diagnosis or treatment plan. Results should also be communicated accurately, as soon as possible, to the appropriate clinician. Trainee and newly qualified veterinary nurses may need to seek the assistance of a more experienced veterinary nurse prior to reporting to the veterinary surgeon. Where indicated, usually upon the request of the veterinary clinician, results may also be communicated to the client.

Inconsistencies and inaccuracies in laboratory results

As explained earlier in the chapter, laboratory tests form a part of the data on which a veterinary surgeon makes a clinical diagnosis. The history, clinical examination and other ancillary tests such as diagnostic imaging (see Chapter 16) should all be interpreted together. When laboratory test results are evaluated, their clinical significance should be taken into account and any possible errors considered. All laboratory tests are subject to potential errors. Errors may be pre-analytic, analytic or post-analytic. The types of error that may occur and ways of avoiding them are summarized in Figure 17.46 (many of these have been discussed throughout the chapter).

Stage of error	Possible causes	Methods of avoiding errors (further information is given in the main text)
Pre-analytic	Inappropriate choice of test	■ Check clinical records ■ Ensure that laboratory tests are part of a package of investigations including careful history-taking and clinical examination ■ Contact a clinical pathologist in an external laboratory if in doubt
	Incorrect preparation of the patient	■ Avoid exercise, stress, excitement and fear prior to and during sampling ■ Starve the patient appropriately prior to sampling ■ Ensure that tests for monitoring drug therapy are timed correctly
	Poor sample collection and handling	■ Collect samples carefully, using the correct sized needle and syringe to avoid haemolysis ■ Handle samples gently to avoid haemolysis ■ Mix anticoagulant tubes quickly, carefully and gently ■ Do not over- or under-fill anticoagulant tubes ■ Avoid any sample contamination
	Incorrect sample/patient identification	■ Take care in labelling of the sample with patient/client details ■ Take care in completion of information on the laboratory submission form
Analytic	Errors in the actual test and its findings	■ Have in place internal quality control (QC) procedures ■ Have in place external quality assurance (QA) procedures

17.46 Examples of types of error that may occur in laboratory sampling and ways of avoiding them.

continues ▶

Stage of error	Possible causes	Methods of avoiding errors (further information is given in the main text)
Post-analytic	Incorrect recording of the findings	■ Check clinical records, owner and patient details
	Incorrect interpretation of the results	■ Compare with appropriate known reference ranges for that species ■ Ensure that both results and reference ranges are in the same units of measurement ■ Remember individual variation outside reference ranges may be influenced by, for example, breed and age
	Delay in reporting	■ Record results on the patient's file promptly ■ Report findings to the veterinary surgeon promptly ■ Recognize delays in reporting (e.g. when samples are sent to an external laboratory) and follow up on delayed results

17.46 *continued* Examples of types of error that may occur in laboratory sampling and ways of avoiding them. (continues)

Acknowledgement

The author would like to acknowledge the contribution of Gemma Irwin-Porter to an earlier version of this chapter.

References and further reading

Bexfield N and Lee K (2014) *BSAVA Guide to Procedures in Small Animal Practice, 2nd edn.* BSAVA Publications, Gloucester

British Veterinary Association (2011) *Good practice guide to handling veterinary waste in England and Wales.* BVA Publications, London.

Chitty J and Monks D (2018) *BSAVA Manual of Avian Practice: A Foundation Manual.* BSAVA Publications, Gloucester

Girling SJ and Raiti P (2018) *BSAVA Manual of Reptiles, 3rd edn.* BSAVA Publications, Gloucester

Keeble E and Meredith A (2009) *BSAVA Manual of Rodents and Ferrets.* BSAVA Publications, Gloucester

Knottenbelt C (2007) Practical laboratory techniques. In: *BSAVA Manual of Practical Veterinary Nursing,* ed. E Mullineaux and M Jones, pp. 205–228. BSAVA Publications, Gloucester

Meredith A and Lord B (2014) *BSAVA Manual of Rabbit Medicine,* BSAVA Publications, Gloucester

Sirois M (2014) *Laboratory Procedures for Veterinary Technicians, 6th edn.* Elsevier, Mississippi

Villiers E and Blackwood L (2011) *BSAVA Manual of Canine and Feline Clinical Pathology, 2nd edn.* BSAVA Publications, Gloucester

Villiers E and Ristić J (2016) *BSAVA Manual of Canine and Feline Clinical Pathology, 3rd edn.* BSAVA Publications, Gloucester

Useful websites

Health and Safety Executive (HSE) – Hazard pictograms:
www.hse.gov.uk/chemical-classification/labelling-packaging/hazard-symbols-hazard-pictograms.htm

Self-assessment questions

1. What magnification does the eyepiece of a microscope usually have?
2. What is the difference between plasma and serum?
3. Identify two possible sites for blood collection in a bird.
4. Which anticoagulant is usually used for coagulation profiles and what is the colour of the sample tube top that contains that anticoagulant?
5. Name three possible stains for blood smears and identify when they might be used.
6. State three methods of urine collection from a dog and the advantages and disadvantages of each.
7. Which tests concentrate faecal samples for examination for a) parasite eggs b) parasite larvae?
8. Which skin pathogens might be identified on an adhesive tape impression from a dog?
9. On a Gram-stained slide what is the significance of purple-staining bacteria?
10. What are the components of legal packaging for pathological samples?

Chapter 18

Medical disorders of dogs and cats and their nursing

Robyn Gear

Learning objectives

After studying this chapter, readers will have the knowledge to:

- **List common medical disorders of dogs and cats**
- **Identify how disease affects the normal function of the animal – pathophysiology and resulting clinical signs**
- **Explain how to plan and deliver care for animals with a range of commonly encountered conditions**
- **Provide safe, effective and efficient nursing care to patients in the medical setting**
- **Explain the purpose and rationale for various interventions including procedures, diagnostic tests and medications**
- **Develop written plans of care for animals utilizing the nursing process**
- **Describe how to facilitate effective home and follow-up care for animals with long-term illness**

Introduction

Veterinary nurses play a vital role in the care of pets and are important members of the veterinary team. They carry out a range of duties, under the direction of the veterinary surgeon, including performing diagnostic tests and providing nursing care for a range of medical conditions. Information on managing the hospital ward and basic patient care is provided in Chapter 14, whilst nursing interventions in hospitalized patients is covered in Chapter 15. The reader is referred to Chapter 12 for information on the nursing process and care plans.

Upper respiratory tract disease

The upper respiratory tract comprises the nasal cavity, pharynx, larynx and trachea.

Definitions

- Acute – of short duration
- Chronic – of long duration
- Sinusitis – inflammation of one or more sinuses
- Rhinitis – inflammation of the nasal lining
- Epistaxis – bleeding from the nose
- Laryngitis – inflammation of the larynx
- Tracheitis – inflammation of the trachea

Nasal disease

Clinical signs

- Sneezing.
- Snorting.
- Facial swelling.
- Facial rubbing.
- Dyspnoea (cats).
- Nasal discharge.

Nasal discharge

Nasal discharge can be either bilateral or unilateral, depending on whether one or both nasal passages are affected, and this can help differentiate the causal factor. A good indicator as to the causal factor can be the type of discharge:

- Serous
- Mucoid
- Mucopurulent (Figure 18.1)
- Bloody.

Causes of nasal discharge (Figure 18.2) include viral, bacterial and fungal infections, allergies, neoplasia and foreign bodies. Trauma, tumours, coagulopathies and fungal infections can cause epistaxis (Figure 18.3).

Diagnostics

- History and clinical examination.
- Blood tests – complete blood count, biochemistry, clotting profile and serology if pathogens are suspected.

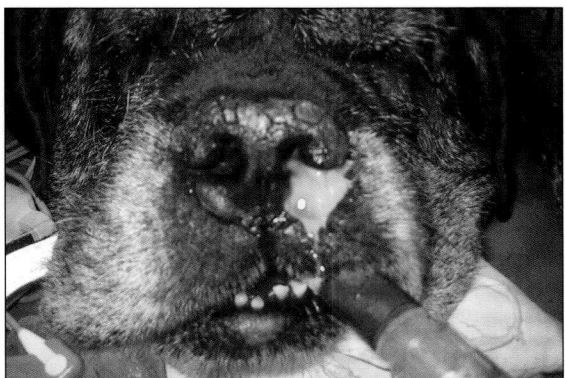

18.1 Mucopurulent nasal discharge from a dog with a nasal tumour.

Dogs
■ Distemper virus infection
■ Kennel cough complex
■ *Aspergillus* spp. infection
■ Foreign bodies (e.g. grass seeds)
■ Neoplasia

Cats
■ Feline upper respiratory tract disease (highly infectious viral and/or bacterial disease)
■ *Chlamydia* infection
■ Foreign bodies (e.g. blades of grass)
■ Neoplasia
■ Trauma

18.2 Common causes of nasal discharge and respiratory disease in dogs and cats (note that this list is not exhaustive).

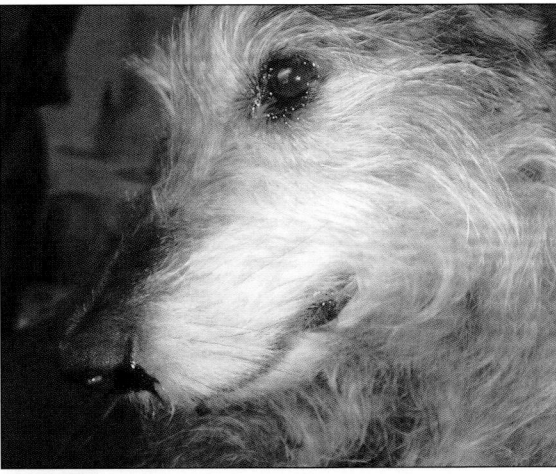

18.3 Epistaxis in a dog with a nasal tumour.

■ Radiography of the nasal chambers and thorax.
■ Rhinoscopy.
■ Magnetic resonance imaging (MRI) and computed tomography (CT).
■ Bacterial (often secondary to other causes and may be of limited value) and fungal culture.
■ Nasal flush for cytology examination (may be of limited value).
■ Nasal biopsy and histopathology.

Treatment

The correct treatment depends on the causal factor (e.g. supportive treatment for viral infections; antibiotics for primary and secondary infections; antifungal treatment for aspergillosis; removal of foreign bodies; surgery or radiotherapy for neoplasia).

Nursing care

The nursing considerations for nasal disease are detailed in Figure 18.4 and these can be incorporated into a care plan (see Chapter 12). A similar approach may be taken with other medical conditions.

Laryngeal disease

This can include conditions such as laryngitis, laryngeal paralysis, oedema and trauma. Causes of laryngitis include persistent barking in dogs and respiratory tract infections in dogs and cats.

Clinical signs

■ Panting.
■ Noisy respiration.
■ Change in character of the bark or meow (dysphonia).
■ Coughing or gagging when attempting to bark.
■ Problems associated with swallowing food and/or water.
■ Reduced tolerance to increased temperature (less able to pant).
■ Exercise intolerance.
■ Polyneuropathy syndrome resulting in decreased or absent reflexes.

Diagnostics

■ History and clinical examination.
■ Examination of the larynx under a light plane of anaesthesia for paralysis diagnosis.
■ Smears, fine-needle aspirates and biopsy samples may be taken in chronic cases.
■ Ultrasonography.
■ Electromyogram (EMG).

Treatment

Treatment depends on the cause:

■ Severe laryngeal paralysis – surgery often indicated (unilateral arytenoid lateralization)
■ Laryngitis – supportive treatment. Anti-inflammatory medication should be considered. Antibiotics should be considered for bacterial infections.

Nursing care

The nursing considerations for laryngeal disease are detailed in Figure 18.5.

Tracheal disease

This can include conditions such as tracheitis (kennel cough or inflammation), tracheal collapse and trauma.

Clinical signs

■ Honking noise (tracheal collapse) – middle-aged obese small dogs, especially Yorkshire Terriers.
■ Dry hacking cough or a 'goose honking' cough.
■ Exercise intolerance or dyspnoea in tracheal collapse.

Diagnostics

■ History and clinical examination.
■ Radiography, tracheoscopy and tracheal wash (submitted for cytology, culture and sensitivity testing).

Parameter	Problem	Nursing considerations	Monitoring
Breathing	■ Potential problem if patient insists on breathing through nose ■ Potential breathing problems after invasive procedures (e.g. nasal biopsy)	■ Prepare oxygen supplementation ■ On recovery from sedation and anaesthesia, dedicate one nurse to patient – have the ability to open the mouth or allow patient to breathe through the mouth (e.g. syringe case) ■ Keep nose clean	■ Monitor respiratory rate and pattern
Bleeding	■ Potential after biopsy or due to underlying disease	■ Apply pressure ■ Cold compresses ■ Sedation ■ Intranasal medication as directed by the veterinary surgeon ■ Fluids	■ Monitor bleeding ■ Monitor mucous membrane colour ■ Monitor heart rate ■ Monitor blood pressure ■ Monitor PCV/TS if bleeding excessive
Pain	■ Destructive nasal disease could be painful ■ Biopsy painful	■ Analgesia ■ Local block: infraorbital	■ Pain assessment scoring
Drinking	■ Normal	■ Provide fresh water	■ Monitor hydration
Eating	■ Inappetence or anorexia	■ Hand-feed palatable, strong smelling and warm food as necessary	■ Monitor and record food intake ■ Monitor weight
Urinating	■ Normal	■ Provide regular opportunities to urinate	■ Monitor urine output
Defecating	■ Normal	■ Provide regular opportunities to defecate	■ Monitor faecal output
Grooming	■ May not be grooming ■ Nasal discharge	■ Keep clean and groom ■ Bathe away discharge with warm saline ■ Prevent excoriation around orifices with the use of petroleum jelly ■ Humidify air to loosen discharges	■ Monitor for excoriation
Housing	■ Animal potentially infectious	■ Keep in isolation and barrier nurse as required	■ Good disinfection ■ Good ventilation
Mobilizing	■ Normal	■ Good hygiene and maintenance of barrier nursing whilst exercising	■ Disinfect areas that the animal comes into contact with

18.4 Nursing considerations for patients with nasal disease. PCV = packed cell volume; TS = total solids.

Parameter	Problem	Nursing considerations	Monitoring
Breathing	■ Potential respiratory distress ■ Potential for developing aspiration pneumonia	■ Provide oxygen as required ■ May require anaesthesia and intubation ■ Minimize stress	■ Monitor respiratory rate and mucous membrane colour for cyanosis ■ Pulse oximetry ■ Auscultate lungs ■ Monitor heart rate ■ Monitor temperature
Pain	■ Unlikely to be painful	■ Provide analgesia if required	■ Monitor for signs of pain
Drinking	■ Normal	■ Provide fresh water	■ Monitor hydration
Eating	■ Normal ■ Risk of aspiration	■ Use balls of food or dry food to try to avoid aspiration. Avoid dusty food	■ Monitor food intake
Urinating	■ Normal	■ Take out to toilet regularly	■ Monitor urine output
Defecating	■ Normal	■ Take out to toilet regularly	■ Monitor faecal output
Grooming	■ May not be grooming	■ Keep clean and comfortable	■ Good hygiene
Housing	■ Stress impacts oxygen requirement	■ Minimize noise and stress ■ Cool environment	■ Monitor animal's behaviour ■ Monitor stress
Mobilizing	■ Reduced exercise tolerance	■ Cage rest ■ Gentle walks to toilet ■ Use harness	■ Monitor exercise tolerance

18.5 Nursing considerations for patients with laryngeal disease.

Treatment

■ Treat the underlying cause.
■ Use of cough suppressants, bronchodilators, corticosteroids (to control inflammation) and antibiotics.
■ Weight loss for obese patients.

■ Surgery.
■ In severe cases, tracheal stent placement may be considered.

Nursing care

The nursing considerations for tracheal disease are detailed in Figure 18.6.

Parameter	Problem	Nursing considerations	Monitoring
Breathing	■ Potential respiratory distress	■ Provide oxygen as required ■ Minimize stress and excitement	■ Monitor respiratory rate and mucous membrane colour for cyanosis ■ Pulse oximetry ■ Auscultate lungs ■ Monitor heart rate ■ Monitor temperature
Pain	■ Unlikely to be painful	■ Provide analgesia as necessary	■ Monitor carefully
Drinking	■ Normal	■ Maintain hydration	■ Monitor fluid intake
Eating	■ Normal ■ May be overweight	■ Weight-reducing diet if appropriate	■ Monitor weight
Urinating	■ Normal	■ Take out to toilet regularly	■ Monitor urine output
Defecating	■ Normal	■ Take out to toilet regularly	■ Monitor faecal output
Grooming	■ May not be grooming	■ Keep clean and comfortable	■ Avoid hair balls
Housing	■ Stress impacts oxygen requirement ■ Irritants can exacerbate problem	■ Minimize excitement ■ Avoid dry, dusty and smoky environments	■ Maintain ambient temperature
Mobilizing	■ Potential reduced exercise tolerance	■ Restrict exercise ■ Use harness	■ Monitor controlled exercise and weight

18.6 Nursing considerations for patients with tracheal disease.

Lower respiratory tract disease

The lower respiratory tract comprises the bronchi, bronchioles and alveoli.

Definitions

- Dyspnoea – difficulty in breathing
- Apnoea – cessation of breathing
- Tachypnoea – increased breathing rate
- Orthopnoea – dyspnoea in lateral recumbency (usually improved in sternal recumbency)
- Hypoxia – reduced oxygen availability
- Hypercapnia – excess carbon dioxide in the blood
- Cyanosis – bluish appearance of the tongue and mucous membranes as a result of insufficient oxygen reaching the tissues

---

Acute respiratory disease

Acute respiratory disease will occur when any part of normal respiration is interrupted or fails to function adequately. This will lead to the failure of oxygen being transferred to the circulation and of carbon dioxide being eliminated, resulting in hypoxia and hypercapnia. Causes can include the following:

- Diseases of the pleural space:
  - Ruptured diaphragm
  - Pneumothorax, haemothorax, pyothorax and chylothorax.
- Diseases of the upper airways:
  - Airway obstruction (e.g. foreign body, tracheal collapse, laryngeal paralysis).

- Diseases of the pulmonary parenchyma (lower airways):
  - Infection – pneumonia (e.g. canine aspiration pneumonia)
  - Pulmonary oedema (e.g. in heart failure)
  - Pulmonary haemorrhage (e.g. due to trauma).
- Neoplasia (e.g. nose, paranasal, larynx, trachea and primary lung tumours)
- Paraquat poisoning.

Clinical signs

- Tachypnoea, orthopnoea and dyspnoea.
- Mouth breathing.
- Cyanosis.
- Tachycardia.
- Collapse.

Nursing care

The nursing considerations for acute respiratory disease are detailed in Figure 18.7.

Equipment should be prepared in case the patient deteriorates further and requires intervention to support respiration. This equipment might include:

- Various sizes of endotracheal tube (local anaesthetic spray for cats) and bandage for securing the tube in place
- Oxygen supply and suitable anaesthetic circuit to provide intermittent positive pressure ventilation (IPPV)
- Laryngoscope
- Tracheostomy tube and surgical kit or large-gauge needle
- Thoracocentesis equipment
- Emergency equipment box
- Intravenous antibiotics and fluids
- Isolation and biosecurity measures if infectious disease is suspected.

Parameter	Problem	Nursing considerations	Monitoring
Breathing	■ Respiratory distress - triage patient on arrival ■ Lung exudate	■ Provide oxygen therapy (e.g. nasal catheter, nasal prongs, tracheal catheter, Buster collar oxygen hood, flow by oxygen, oxygen tent with oxygen provided at 1 l/min) ■ Humidification if oxygen is to be administered for >1 h ■ Nebulization ■ Minimize stress with minimal restraint ■ Loosen tight fitting collars and leads ■ Sternal recumbency ■ Cooling fans ■ Coupage (see Chapter 15)	■ Monitor respiratory rate and mucous membrane colour for cyanosis ■ Pulse oximetry ■ Regular auscultation of the chest to determine changes to breathing ■ Monitor heart rate ■ Monitor temperature ■ Inform veterinary surgeon of any changes
Pain	■ Unlikely to be painful	■ Provide analgesia as necessary	■ Monitor for signs of pain
Drinking	■ Normal to reduced	■ Intravenous access: place catheter with minimal stress ■ Intravenous fluid treatment if required	■ Monitor hydration and for overhydration if on intravenous fluids
Eating	■ Will depend on underlying condition ■ Infection: inappetent/anorexia ■ Respiratory distress: unlikely to eat	■ Wait until breathing improved ■ Provide palatable food as necessary	■ Monitor and record food offered and eaten
Urinating	■ Normal to reduced, if unable to mobilize	■ If possible, take out to toilet ■ Minimize stress ■ Keep bedding clean	■ Monitor bladder size and urine output ■ Monitor bedding for soiling
Defecating	■ Normal	■ If possible, take out to toilet	■ Monitor faecal output
Grooming	■ May not be grooming	■ Keep clean and comfortable	■ Good hygiene
Housing	■ Stress impacts oxygen requirement	■ Minimize noise and stress ■ Cool environment	■ Important to monitor if patient is receiving supplemental oxygen in an enclosed space
Mobilizing	■ Poor exercise tolerance	■ Cage rest ■ Gentle walks to toilet/or assist to grass ■ Use harness	■ Monitor level and tolerance of exercise

18.7 Nursing considerations for patients with acute respiratory disease.

Chronic pulmonary disease

Causes of chronic pulmonary disease (CPD) include:

■ Bronchitis
■ Pulmonary oedema (e.g. in cardiac failure)
■ Feline asthma
■ Lungworm (*Angiostrongylus vasorum*)
■ Neoplasia (e.g. alveolar parenchyma).

Clinical signs
■ Coughing.
■ Wheezing.
■ Tachypnoea.
■ Exercise intolerance and lethargy.

Diagnostics
■ History and clinical examination.
■ Blood tests – complete blood count, biochemistry and DNA testing for lungworm.
■ Thoracic radiographs.
■ Bronchoscopy.
■ Faecal analysis for lungworm larvae.
■ Bronchoalveolar lavage to obtain a sample for culture and cytology.

Treatment
Treatment is aimed at the underlying cause, but may include:

■ Anti-inflammatory medication – to reduce inflammation
■ Bronchodilators – to treat narrowing of the airways (e.g. in the case of feline asthma)
■ Mucolytics – to reduce mucus viscosity to aid removal
■ Expectorants – to aid removal of secretions
■ Antibiotics – for primary or secondary bacterial infections
■ Anthelmintics – for lungworm infections
■ Antitussives – to suppress coughing if indicated, when coughing is persistent and unproductive
■ Diuretics – for pulmonary oedema.

Nursing care
The nursing considerations for chronic pulmonary disease are detailed in Figure 18.8.

Extrapulmonary disease
Clinical signs
The lungs are unable to inflate adequately as a result of air, fluid, abdominal organs or neoplasia in the thoracic cavity (Figure 18.9). The clinical signs are directly attributable to this. The signs depend on the severity of the underlying condition but may include:

■ Severe respiratory distress – tachypnoea, shallow respiration, orthopnoea, dyspnoea and cyanosis
■ Shock
■ Collapse.

Parameter	Problem	Nursing considerations	Monitoring
Breathing	■ Potential respiratory distress ■ May require long-term inhalational medication	■ Provide oxygen as required ■ Nebulization/inhalation of isotonic saline for patients with thick tenacious secretions ■ Coupage/percussion (see Chapter 15) for those patients that do not have chest injuries ■ Minimize stress ■ Teach owners how to administer inhalational medication to the patient (long-term treatment)	■ Monitor respiratory rate and mucous membrane colour for cyanosis ■ Pulse oximetry ■ Auscultate lungs ■ Monitor heart rate ■ Monitor temperature
Pain	■ Unlikely to be painful	■ Provide analgesia as necessary	■ Monitor for signs of pain
Drinking	■ Normal	■ Maintain hydration	■ Monitor fluid intake. May be increased if patient on steroids or diuretics
Eating	■ Normal	■ Warm food if necessary	■ Monitor weight
Urinating	■ Normal	■ Take out to toilet regularly	■ Monitor urine output. May be increased if patient on steroids or diuretics
Defecating	■ Normal	■ Take out to toilet regularly	■ Monitor faecal output
Grooming	■ May not be grooming	■ Keep clean and comfortable	■ Good hygiene
Housing	■ Stress impacts oxygen requirement	■ Minimize noise and stress ■ Cool environment	■ Monitor stress levels
Mobilizing	■ Often normal	■ Cage rest, if required ■ Short walks to prevent atelectasis and to allow patient to toilet ■ Use harness	■ Monitor exercise tolerance

18.8 Nursing considerations for patients with chronic pulmonary disease.

Condition	Description	Cause	Other information
Diaphragmatic rupture	Abdominal organs in the thoracic cavity	Rupture of the diaphragm due to blunt trauma (e.g. road traffic accident, being kicked)	Heart can sound muffled, depending on extent of condition Size of rupture can determine how many of the abdominal organs are present in the chest cavity Patient should be handled carefully as viscera can move around, making the condition worse
Pneumothorax	Accumulation of air in the thoracic cavity	Trauma to the chest wall either blunt or penetrating (e.g. often seen following road traffic accidents)	Can be classified as open (e.g. when thoracic wall is penetrated, air is sucked into thorax from outside) or closed (e.g. following rupture to lungs, allowing air to leak from lungs into thoracic cavity) Chest percussion will produce increased resonance
Haemothorax	Accumulation of blood in the thoracic cavity	Trauma or disease affecting pulmonary veins, arteries or other blood vessels in the chest cavity Coagulopathy Neoplasia	Heart can sound muffled depending on the extent of the condition Chest percussion will show decreased resonance in ventral thorax when patient in sternal recumbency
Hydrothorax	Accumulation of fluid (pure or modified transudate) in thoracic cavity	Hypoproteinaemia causing fluid to leak from blood vessels (pure transudate) Congestive heart failure or neoplasia (modified transudate) Fluid overload	Appearance of fluid (pure = clear and colourless; modified = straw coloured, pink, slightly opaque) Laboratory test will reveal: nucleated cell count <7 (1×10^9/l), specific gravity ≤1.018 with pure transudate, protein content <35 g/l Chest percussion as above
Exudate	Accumulation of pus (or exudates) in thoracic cavity	Bacterial infection (pyothorax) Feline infectious peritonitis (wet) Neoplasia	Appearance of fluid – often thick, yellow-brown and foul smelling Laboratory test will reveal: nucleated cell count 5–300 (1×10^9/l), specific gravity >1.018, protein content >30g/l Chest percussion as above These patients are often pyrexic

18.9 Extrapulmonary disease.

continues ▶

Condition	Description	Cause	Other information
Chylothorax	Accumulation of chyle in thoracic cavity	Trauma or rupture of thoracic duct Idiopathic abnormalities of thoracic duct Feline heart failure	Appearance of fluid – milky, fails to clear when centrifuged Triglyceride levels of the fluid should be tested to confirm that it is chyle Chest percussion as above
Neoplasia	Development of neoplasia involving thymus, mediastinal and sternal lymph nodes	Lymphosarcoma – common in ferrets Mediastinal lymphoma Thymoma	Neoplasia if large enough will interfere with normal lung expansion, but usually it is the pleural effusion generated that produces the clinical signs A non-compressable cranial mediastinum may be present with dull heart and lung sounds on auscultation

18.9 *continued* Extrapulmonary disease.

Diagnostics

- Clinical examination.
- Blood tests (e.g. white blood cell count; leucocytosis likely).
- Thoracic radiographs.
- Thoracic ultrasonography.
- Thoracocentesis – submit sample for cytology, culture and sensitivity testing.

Treatment

- Thoracocentesis (see 'Nursing assistance with a thoracocentesis procedure' below).
- Indwelling chest drain (indicated for pyothorax and chylothorax) (see Chapter 15).
- Specific treatment depending on the cause of the condition (e.g. surgery to repair ruptured diaphragm) (see Chapters 15 and 23).
- Supportive treatment (e.g. appropriate intravenous fluid therapy).

Nursing care

The nursing considerations for patients with extrapulmonary disease are as for acute respiratory distress (see Figure 18.7).

Nursing assistance with a thoracocentesis procedure

Equipment
- Clippers
- Cotton wool swabs and skin disinfectant
- Local anaesthetic
- Sterile gloves
- Intravenous catheter or butterfly catheter (veterinary surgeon's preference) – suitable size for patient, extension set and three-way tap, and suitable size syringe
- Bowl for collection of any fluid
- Sterile sample pots (plain and EDTA)

Procedure
1. Place patient in sternal recumbency.
2. Clip thorax over the 7th/8th intercostal space.
3. Veterinary surgeon will inject local anaesthetic and wait for it to take effect.
4. Surgically prepare the thoracocentesis site.
5. Veterinary surgeon will put on sterile gloves.
6. Hand equipment (catheter, extension set, three-way tap and syringe) to surgeon in a sterile manner. ➜

Nursing assistance with a thoracocentesis procedure *continued*

7. Veterinary surgeon will insert catheter into thoracic cavity and connect the extension set, three-way tap and syringe.
8. Veterinary surgeon will hand syringe to nurse.
9. The veterinary nurse will then turn the three-way tap to open.
10. Gently withdraw plunger.
11. Once syringe is full, turn the three-way tap and empty of fluid or air.
12. Repeat procedure until no further air or fluid can be aspirated.
13. Repeat on other side of chest if required.
14. Fill sample pots and send for analysis (from the initial fluid removed).

Circulatory system disease

Definitions
- Endocarditis – inflammation of the endocardium (endothelial membrane lining the cavities of the heart), most commonly involving a heart valve
- Endocardiosis – chronic fibrosis and thickening of the atrioventricular (AV) valves
- Tachycardia – rapid heart rate
- Bradycardia – slow heart rate
- Pericarditis – inflammation of the pericardium (sac around the heart)
- Cardiomyopathy – primary disease of the heart muscle. Dilated cardiomyopathy (DCM) is a disease of the heart muscle characterized by poor contractility. Hypertrophic cardiomyopathy (HCM) is characterized by a thickening of the walls of the heart, which leads to an inadequate amount of blood being pumped around the body when the heart contracts
- Cardiac tamponade – compression of the heart due to fluid accumulation in the pericardial sac
- Diastole – time within the heart contraction cycle when the heart chambers are relaxed and able to fill with blood
- Systole – time within the heart contraction cycle that the heart contracts and forces blood into the circulation

Congenital heart disease

Congenital heart disease is present at birth. Many breeds have a predisposition to a specific defect or defects. Often it is detected at the first vaccination, when a heart murmur is detected on auscultation. Clinical signs depend on the severity of the defect and include poor growth, collapse and signs of heart failure: exercise intolerance, lethargy, dyspnoea and increased respiratory rate. The diagnosis is made from the signalment of the patient, history, clinical examination and echocardiography. Thoracic radiographs (including contrast studies) may be used in a referral setting and an electrocardiogram (ECG) may be taken if an arrhythmia is auscultated. Congenital conditions include: patent ductus arteriosus, valvular defects, septal defects and persistent right aortic arch. Some congenital heart defects can be corrected with surgery or interventional radiology (e.g. patent ductus arteriosus, persistent right aortic arch) or improved with interventions (e.g. pulmonic stenosis), but others can only be managed by treating the clinical signs that occur due to heart failure (see 'Heart failure' below) or collapse.

Acquired heart disease

Endocardial disease: endocardiosis and endocarditis

Disease of the heart valves is most commonly due to chronic fibrosis (scarring) and is called endocardiosis. Endocardiosis is the most frequently encountered heart disease in older small-breed dogs, but is very rare in cats. The mitral (left AV) valve is most commonly affected, although the tricuspid (right AV) valve can be affected. It is a progressive condition. Endocardiosis prevents the valves from functioning correctly. During the cardiac cycle, the valves close, followed by contraction of the heart pumping the blood into the arteries. In the case of endocardiosis, the valves cannot close completely, and so as the heart contracts some of the blood flows (leaks) backwards (described as regurgitation) from the ventricles into the atria. This increases the workload of the heart, ultimately, resulting in poor forward flow of blood, congestion and heart failure. Infection of the heart valves (endocarditis) is less common.

Clinical signs

The clinical signs of mitral valve endocardiosis include a murmur, which may be an incidental finding on clinical examination. Other signs are those of left-sided heart failure (see 'Heart failure' below). Clinical signs of tricuspid valve endocardiosis are those of right-sided heart failure (see 'Heart failure' below).

Endocarditis is inflammation of the inside lining of the heart chambers and heart valves (endocardium), most commonly caused by bacteria. Clinical signs of endocarditis include:

- Pyrexia
- Lethargy
- Anorexia
- Heart murmur
- Coughing
- Exercise intolerance.

Diagnostics

A presumptive diagnosis can be made on history and clinical examination:

- Echocardiography (ultrasonography of the heart)
- Thoracic radiographs – right lateral and dorsoventral views
- ECG
- Blood culture – to culture bacteria if endocarditis is suspected.

Treatment

- Patients with endocardiosis are treated when heart failure has developed (see 'Heart failure' below). Treatment with pimobendan prior to developing heart failure may be considered.
- Endocarditis is initially treated with broad-spectrum antibiotics, which may be changed after receiving the blood culture results.

Recording an electrocardiogram

This should be carried out with minimal stress to the patient and without sedation.

- The animal is placed in right lateral recumbency and gently restrained.
- ECG pads can be placed on the main pads of the paws. Alligator forceps can be traumatic and painful and should, if possible, be reserved for emergency situations; they can be attached on the upper part of the leg, where there is some loose skin.
- Good contact is made by using ECG gel or spirit. The latter should not be used if there is a chance that the animal may need to be defibrillated.
- The electrodes are attached as follows (the colour of the leads can vary between countries):
  - Red – right forelimb
  - Yellow – left forelimb
  - Green – left hindlimb
  - Black – right hindlimb.
- A standard six-lead ECG is recorded (leads I, II, III, aVL, aVR, aVF), usually at settings of 10 mV and 25 mm/s.
- The ECG should be labelled with the animal's details, date, settings and leads used.
- Ensure that it is of diagnostic quality, with minimal interference.

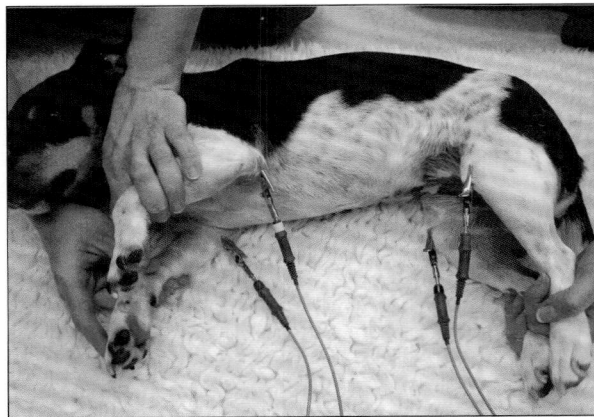

The electrode placement can be remembered as 'Red = Right' (both begin with R) and then work in an anticlockwise direction (when viewing from the dorsal aspect of the patient) in the order of traffic lights – yellow, green. Black is placed on the remaining limb, i.e. right hindlimb.

Myocardial disease

Cardiomyopathies are diseases of the myocardium (heart muscle) that result in cardiac dysfunction. Cardiomyopathy is the most frequently recognized cardiac condition in cats (commonly hypertrophic cardiomyopathy). It is also seen in large and giant breeds of dog (commonly dilated cardiomyopathy).

Hypertrophic cardiomyopathy

The normal functioning heart has a period within its cycle when it relaxes to create space within the ventricles to fill up with blood. As the heart contracts this blood is then pumped forward. Thickening of the heart muscle interferes with this relaxation, space is not created, and the ventricles cannot fill normally with blood. Therefore, there is only a small amount of blood available to pump forward. This is described as poor diastolic function and results in decreased cardiac output and heart failure. In cats, the condition is not uncommon and may be secondary to hyperthyroidism. It is heritable in some breeds (e.g. Maine Coon).

Clinical signs

Many cases in cats are clinically 'silent', but if congestive heart failure is present signs include:

- Dyspnoea and tachypnoea
- Tachycardia and a gallop rhythm
- Heart murmur.

A common complication in cats is feline aortic thromboembolism (FATE, sometimes called a saddle thrombus), where a thrombus (blood clot) leaves the heart and lodges in the caudal aorta (most commonly), obstructing blood flow to the hindlimbs. Clinical signs include:

- Acute painful onset of unilateral/bilateral paresis/paralysis of the hindlimbs
- Lack of arterial pulse in the affected leg(s)
- Hindlimb(s) cool to the touch
- Acute dyspnoea and tachypnoea.

Diagnostics

- Echocardiography.
- Thoracic radiographs – right lateral and dorsoventral views.
- ECG.
- Blood pressure measurement.
- Blood tests – T4 (for hyperthyroidism) and renal function.
- Additional tests if a clot is suspected include blood tests (complete blood count and biochemistry) and abdominal ultrasonography.

Treatment

Beta-blockers may be used (e.g. atenolol). Treatment may also be indicated to reduce the risk of blood clots occurring (e.g. clopidogrel). Once blood clots occur, the patient is treated supportively with pain relief; euthanasia should be considered as the prognosis for FATE can be poor.

Dilated cardiomyopathy

This is characterized by dilatation (enlargement) of the heart chambers. The heart muscle is unable to contract effectively and in essence the 'pump' fails. This is described as poor systolic function. The heart is unable to pump blood forward effectively, resulting in congestion and heart failure. In dogs,

dilated cardiomyopathies are seen most frequently in large breeds and there is a familial predisposition in Dobermanns, Irish Wolfhounds, Great Danes, Newfoundlands and Boxers, as well as other breeds. More recently, dilated cardiomyopathy has also been diagnosed in some dogs fed grain-free diets. In cats, the cause may be idiopathic, or due to taurine deficiency, although the latter is now rare because of good commercial diets containing adequate taurine levels.

Clinical signs

- Anorexia, weight loss, reduced exercise tolerance and lethargy.
- Usually present with signs of left-sided heart failure (dyspnoea, tachypnoea, soft cough) and sometimes concomitant right-sided heart failure.
- Ascites.
- Slow capillary refill.
- Heart murmur and tachycardia. Pulse quality should be checked.
- Arrhythmias.
- Sudden death.

Diagnostics

- Echocardiography.
- Thoracic radiographs – right lateral and dorsoventral views.
- ECG.

Treatment

Each patient is assessed and treated based on the severity of the disease. Treatment (e.g. pimobendan) is aimed at improving contractility of the heart. Heart failure is managed as below.

Arrhythmias

Arrhythmias occur as a result of a disturbance of the electrical activity in the heart. This can be due to primary heart disease, or secondary to another systemic disease (for example, electrolyte disturbances). Arrhythmias can be broadly categorized into bradycardic (slow) arrhythmias and tachycardic (fast) arrhythmias (Figure 18.10). They are further categorized according to where the arrhythmia arises, either in the ventricles (ventricular) or above the ventricles (supraventricular). This distinction is important to determine the right treatment for the patient.

Clinical signs

- May be asymptomatic.
- Collapse.
- Exercise intolerance and weakness.
- Sudden death.

Diagnostics

- Blood tests – including electrolytes.
- ECG to document type of arrhythmia (Figure 18.10).
- Holter monitor (24-hour ECG) for intermittent arrhythmias.
- Thoracic radiographs, echocardiography and abdominal ultrasonography to identify underlying cause.

Treatment

This is based on the type of arrhythmia and whether or not the patient is symptomatic. If possible, the underlying cause should be treated. Tachycardia is treated with antiarrhythmic drugs. Bradycardia can be treated with a pacemaker.

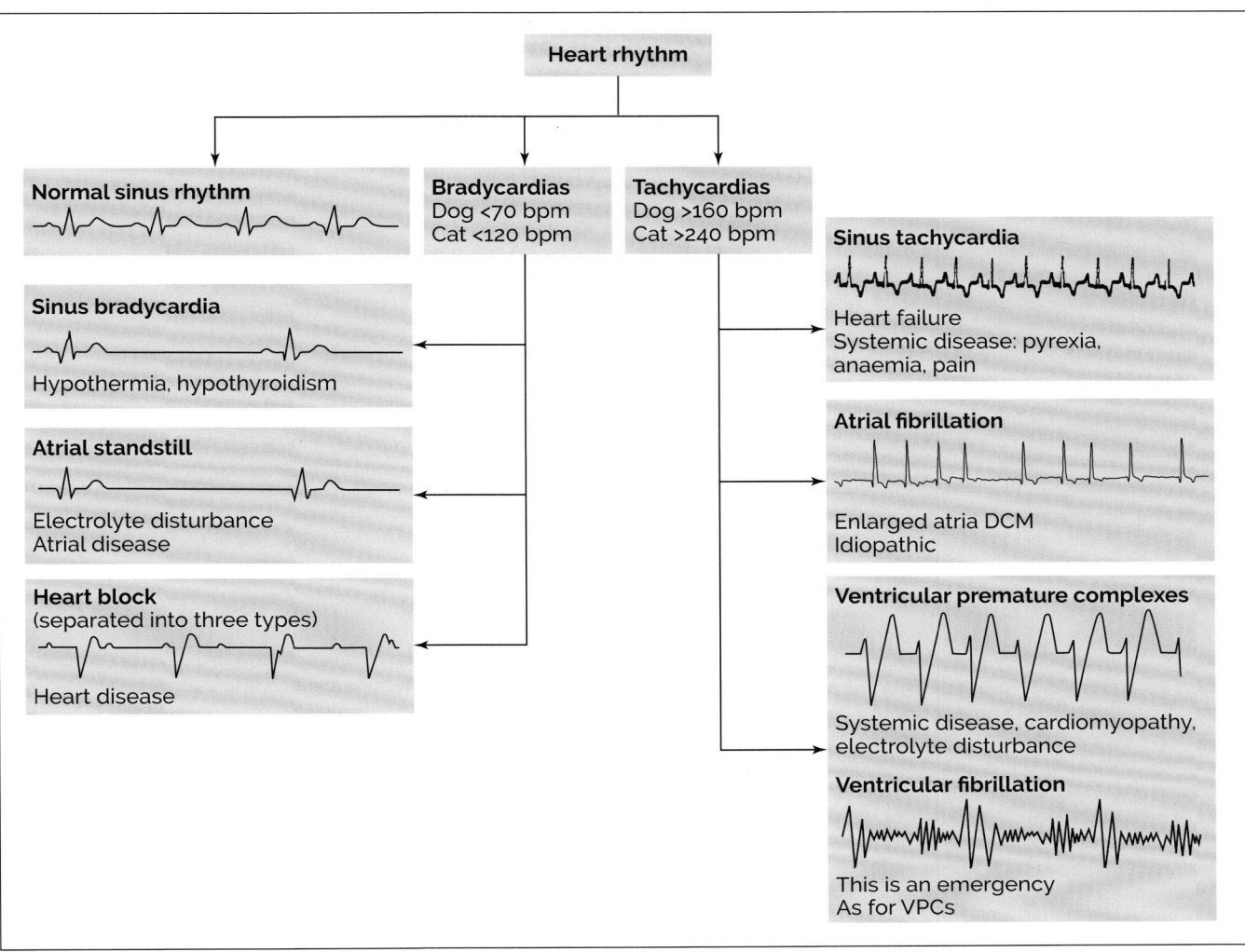

18.10 Arrhythmias and their common causes in dogs and cats.

Pericardial disease

An effusion (fluid) accumulates within the pericardial sac and restricts filling of the right side of the heart with blood, leading to congestion and right-sided heart failure. A pericardial effusion is usually either idiopathic (unknown cause) or secondary to a tumour of the heart. Cardiac tamponade is the result of compression of the heart due to fluid accumulation in the pericardial sac.

Clinical signs

- Collapse.
- Exercise intolerance.
- Pale mucous membranes.
- Muffled heart sounds and tachycardia.
- Distended abdomen.
- Variable pulse quality.
- Changes in ECG characteristics.

Diagnostics

- Echocardiography.
- Thoracic radiographs – right lateral and dorsoventral views.
- ECG.
- Pericardial fluid analysis.

Treatment

This involves relieving the pressure around the heart and removing the fluid via pericardiocentesis; samples should be sent for analysis (cytology). Subsequent management depends on the underlying cause, but if pericardial effusion recurs, surgical removal of the pericardium (pericardectomy) is indicated. Administration of oxygen and/or an oxygen cage to assist those with respiratory distress.

Nursing assistance with a pericardiocentesis procedure

The following is one of various pericardiocentesis techniques.

Equipment

- 60 ml syringe
- Three-way stopcock
- Intravenous fluid extension line
- 16 G 3¼ inch or 5 inch over-the-needle catheter
- Sterile gloves
- Lidocaine for local anaesthesia
- Scalpel blade

Technique

This is a sterile procedure. It is usually performed with the patient in sternal or left lateral recumbency.
If sedation is required, it should be administered according to the veterinary surgeon's instructions.
The patient should be constantly monitored throughout the procedure. The patient should be monitored with ECG.

→

Nursing assistance with a pericardiocentesis procedure *continued*

1. Surgically clip the ventral third of the right hemithorax from the 3rd to the 8th intercostal space.
2. The veterinary surgeon will infiltrate the area with lidocaine.
3. Surgically prepare the clipped area.
4. Pass the equipment to the surgically scrubbed and gloved veterinary surgeon in a sterile manner.
5. The veterinary surgeon will pass the syringe, three-way stopcock and one end of the extension set to the veterinary nurse. Connect the syringe to the three-way stopcock and intravenous extension tubing.
6. The veterinary surgeon will make a small cutaneous incision with the scalpel blade and advance the catheter into the pericardial space. The veterinary surgeon's end of the intravenous extension is then attached to the catheter.
7. The veterinary nurse will then be instructed to aspirate the fluid slowly. A small volume is removed first to check it does not clot. If it does, this may indicate incorrect placement of the needle within a vessel or the heart.
8. During the procedure the catheter may become blocked and the veterinary surgeon will need to reposition it.
9. Ventricular premature complexes may be seen during the procedure. These usually resolve once the procedure is completed. The ECG should be monitored intermittently for abnormal rhythms once the procedure is complete.
10. The fluid is usually very bloody. Collect a sterile sample, label it and submit for cytological examination and culture.
11. Measure the packed cell volume (PCV) of the fluid and compare with venous PCV.
12. Monitor the patient's vital signs once the procedure is completed.

Heart failure

Heart failure may be defined as circulatory failure where the heart is unable to maintain an adequate circulation for the needs of the body. It may arise as a result of several causes of cardiac abnormality or disease as have been described above. The heart has some capacity to compensate for disease by increasing heart rate and retaining fluid to maintain blood pressure. Ultimately, however, this results in the excessive accumulation of fluid, congestion and congestive heart failure. Right-sided heart failure is the failure of the right side of the heart. Blood enters the right side of the heart from the venae cavae and congestion results in excess fluid within the systemic venous circulation and ascites can develop (peritoneal/abdominal effusion). Left-sided heart failure is failure of the left side of the heart. Blood enters the left side of the heart from the pulmonary vein. If the left side fails, congestion occurs in the lungs and generally manifests as pulmonary oedema in dogs and a pleural effusion in cats.

Clinical signs

Some cases will be recognized early on with mild clinical signs, whilst others will present with acute decompensation, have severe clinical signs and acute congestive heart failure. These cases require emergency treatment.

Acute congestive heart failure

- Collapse.
- Pale mucous membranes.
- Slow capillary refill time.
- Weak pulse.
- Tachycardia.
- Tachypnoea.

This is an emergency and requires immediate treatment (see Chapter 19).

Left-sided congestive heart failure

- Tachypnoea and dyspnoea.
- Pulmonary oedema – increased lung sounds on auscultation.
- Tachycardia and weak pulses.
- Pleural effusion (cats) – reduced lung sounds on auscultation.
- Murmurs and arrhythmias (in many cases).
- Exercise intolerance, fatigue and lethargy.
- Cyanosis in severe cases.
- May have a soft cough.

Right-sided heart failure

- Ascites and abdominal distension.
- Exercise intolerance, fatigue and lethargy.
- Pale mucous membranes, tachycardia and weak pulses.
- Dyspnoea, tachypnoea and cyanosis.
- Murmurs and arrhythmias (in many cases).

Diagnostics

Heart murmurs can be identified on clinical examination prior to the development of heart failure. Owners can be taught to monitor the sleeping respiratory rate of their pet (i.e. the number of breaths the animal takes during 1 minute). An increase in rate to over 30 breaths per minute can indicate the onset of pulmonary oedema and further investigation is indicated.

- Thoracic radiographs – right lateral and dorsoventral views.
- Echocardiography.
- ECG.
- Blood tests – biochemistry, especially urea, creatinine and electrolytes.
- Urine specific gravity.

The blood tests and urinalysis are to obtain baseline values for renal parameters. These are monitored after treatment is commenced to ensure renal function does not deteriorate.

Treatment

The reader is referred to Chapter 19 for additional information on cardiovascular emergencies.

Acute congestive heart failure

- Diuretics (e.g. furosemide).
- Strict cage rest.
- Oxygen supplementation.
- Vasodilators (e.g. glyceryl trinitrate) (applied topically to inside of ear; wear gloves).

Chronic congestive heart failure (left-sided, right-sided, congestive)

- Reduce exercise.
- Reduce obesity if present.
- Low salt diet (see Figure 18.12).

- Diuretics – furosemide to relieve congestion (i.e. pulmonary oedema, pleural effusion or ascites). Pleural effusions are generally managed with thoracocentesis to improve respiration. Peritoneal drainage may be required if there is poor response to the diuretic treatment and to relieve discomfort.
- Cardiac drugs – angiotensin-converting enzyme (ACE) inhibitors (decrease upregulation of fluid retention) and positive inotropes (pimobendan) (improves contractility).
- Antiarrhythmic drugs if required.

Nursing care

The reader is referred to Chapter 19 for additional information on cardiovascular emergencies.

Acute heart failure

The nursing considerations for acute heart failure are detailed in Figure 18.11.

Chronic congestive heart failure

The nursing considerations for chronic congestive heart failure are detailed in Figure 18.12.

Parameter	Problem	Nursing considerations	Monitoring
Breathing	■ Cardiac insufficiency	■ Provide oxygen therapy ■ Important to minimize stress to reduce oxygen requirement	■ Monitor respiratory rate and effort (sleeping respiratory rate should be <40 breaths per minute or halved from admission) ■ Monitor heart rate
Maintaining body temperature	■ Hypothermia as a result of poor perfusion	■ Administer medication	■ Only occasionally take temperature in order to minimize stress
Drinking	■ Dehydration is a potential problem due to diuretic treatment ■ May be a desired effect to reduce congestion	■ Provide *ad libitum* water ■ Consider intravenous fluids	■ Monitor hydration
Eating	■ Anorexia/inappetence	■ Tempt with warmed, palatable food ■ Avoid invasive feeding method to minimize stress and therefore oxygen demand	■ Monitor and record food offered and eaten
Urinating	■ Polyuria due to diuretics (increased urination)	■ Regularly take out to toilet with the minimum of exertion	■ Monitor urine output ■ Monitor weight: fluid loss (desired)
Mobilizing	■ Exercise intolerance	■ Restrict exercise to reduce oxygen demand	■ Monitor respiratory rate
Other nursing considerations			
■ Blood tests to monitor renal function and electrolyte concentrations ■ Catheter placement for intravenous medication			

18.11 Nursing considerations for patients with acute heart failure.

Parameter	Problem	Nursing considerations	Monitoring
Breathing	■ Cardiac insufficiency Pulmonary oedema	■ Diuretics ■ Cardiac medication	■ Teach owners to monitor sleeping respiratory rate: should be <30 breaths per minute
Eating	■ Anorexia/inappetence	■ Cardiac diet: reduced salt ■ Reduced salt treats ■ Important to eat, therefore, offer palatable warmed food if patient inappetent	■ Monitor and record food offered and eaten ■ Monitor weight
Urinating	■ Polyuria due to diuretics (increased urination)	■ Regularly take out to toilet ■ May need to go out during the night ■ Discuss with owner	■ Monitor weight ■ Monitor hydration
Mobilizing	■ Exercise intolerance	■ Minimize exercise	■ Monitor exercise tolerance and do not overexert
Other nursing considerations			
■ Regular bodyweight checks if the animal is over- or underweight with dietary adjustments as needed ■ Clinical examination and blood tests (biochemistry and electrolyte concentrations) to identify and monitor potential fluid and electrolyte imbalances ■ Blood tests 5–7 days after the start of treatment to monitor renal function and electrolyte concentrations			

18.12 Nursing considerations for patients with chronic congestive heart failure.

Haemopoietic system disease

Definitions

- Anaemia – reduced number of red blood cells or reduced quantity of haemoglobin
- Erythrocytosis – increased number of red blood cells
- Leucocytosis – increased number of white blood cells
- Leucopenia – reduced number of white blood cells
- Thrombocytopenia – reduced number of platelets
- Lymphocytosis – increased number of lymphocytes
- Neutropenia – reduced number of neutrophils
- Neutrophilia – increased number of neutrophils
- Leukaemias – distorted proliferation and development of leucocytes and their precursors in the blood and bone marrow

Anaemia

Anaemia is a clinical sign rather than a diagnosis. There are many causes of anaemia (Figure 18.13). To aid diagnosis anaemias are defined as either regenerative or non-regenerative.

- Regenerative anaemias – the stimulation and production of red blood cells is normal. In response to anaemia, erythropoietin (EPO) is released from the kidney. In turn, the EPO stimulates the bone marrow to produce more red blood cells, as well as to release immature red blood cells (reticulocytes) to boost the number of red blood cells in the circulation. Regenerative anaemias are distinguished by the presence of these reticulocytes in the blood. This can take a couple of days to occur after an animal has become anaemic.
- Non-regenerative anaemias – either there is no EPO produced or the bone marrow is incapable of responding to it. Therefore, there is no increase in red blood cell production in the anaemic patient. Reticulocytes are not present in circulation.

Clinical signs

Patients with acute anaemia can have severe clinical signs and require emergency treatment. Conversely, patients with mild and chronic anaemia can have very few apparent clinical signs.

- Collapse, weakness and exercise intolerance.
- Lethargy.
- Inappetence.
- Pale or jaundiced mucous membranes.
- Tachypnoea and dyspnoea.
- Tachycardia sometimes with an anaemia-induced (haemic) murmur.

Diagnostics

- Blood tests – haematology (complete blood count and fresh blood smear, reticulocyte count (this differentiates regenerative from non-regenerative anaemias); the morphology of the cells can help identify the cause of anaemia).
- Biochemistry (disease in other organs may result in secondary anaemia, e.g. tumours of the kidneys, bladder or spleen).
- In-saline agglutination (slide agglutination test) for autoimmune haemolytic anaemia.
- Serology, especially if travel history. Heavy infestations of blood-sucking parasites (fleas, ticks and hookworms).
- Feline leukaemia virus (FeLV) and feline immunodeficiency virus (FIV) tests in cats.
- *Mycoplasma* infection – polymerase chain reaction (PCR; see 'Feline infectious anaemia', below).
- Faecal occult blood (feed a red-meat-free diet for 3 days).
- Non-regenerative anaemias – bone marrow aspiration (see Chapter 17).

Other tests that may be indicated include:

- Coagulation profile (see Chapter 17)
- Imaging:
  - Radiography – thorax, abdomen (e.g. evidence of bleeding or neoplasia)
  - Ultrasonography – thorax, abdomen (e.g. evidence of bleeding or neoplasia)
  - CT scan.

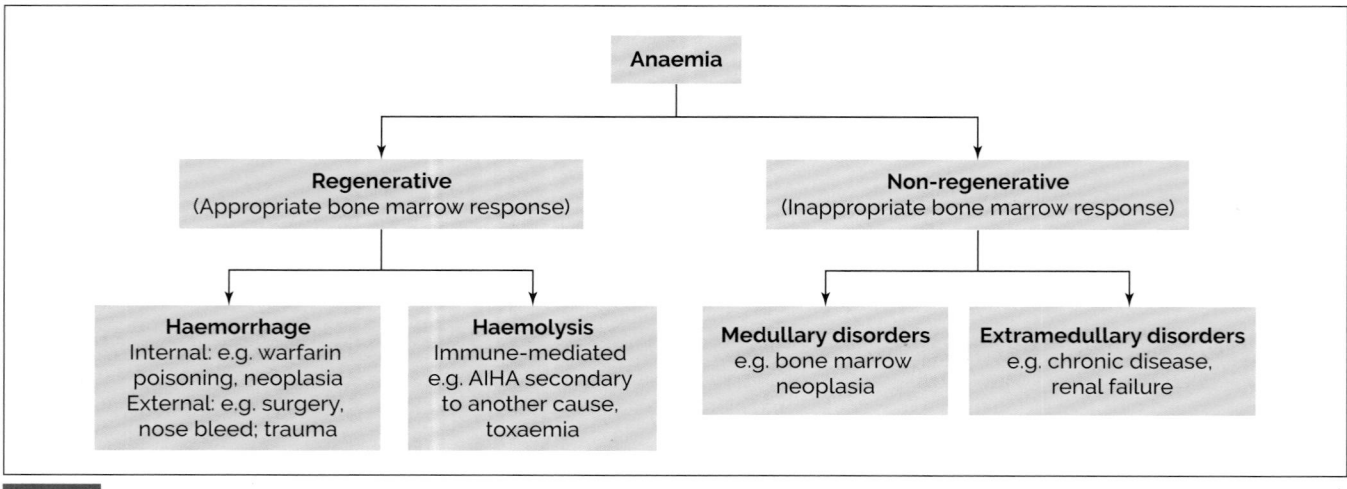

18.13 Types and causes of anaemia. AIHA = autoimmune haemolytic anaemia.

Treatment

The patient may need a blood transfusion (Figure 18.14) if the anaemia is severe or if the clinical signs are severe. Treatment is targeted at the underlying cause (e.g. immuno-suppression for immune-mediated disease; chemotherapy for neoplasia; tetracyclines for *Mycoplasma*).

Nursing care

The nursing considerations for anaemia are detailed in Figure 18.15.

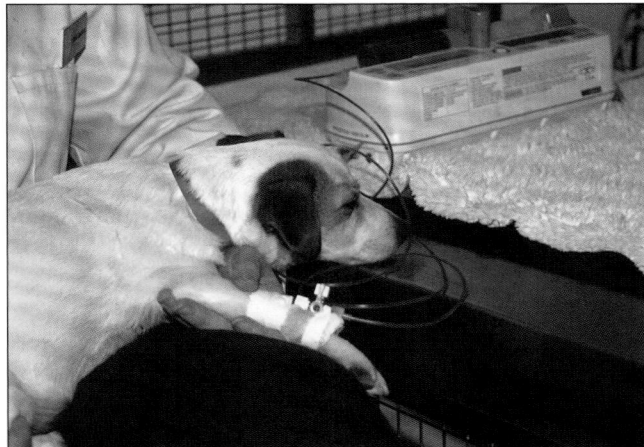

| **18.14** | Blood transfusion in an anaemic dog. |

Clotting disorders

The normal blood clotting mechanism (haemostasis) is described in Chapter 3. Clotting defects can result in haemorrhage and thus give rise to anaemia. Clotting disorders may result from primary or secondary defects:

- Primary haemostatic defect:
  - Blood vessel defect
  - Platelets (decreased number, platelet dysfunction or increased consumption)
  - von Willebrand factor deficiency (rarely seen in cats but commonly seen in certain breeds of dog, e.g. Dobermann). Often presents with excessive bleeding following an event after which the patient should normally be able to produce a clot and stop bleeding (e.g. a cut, bitch in oestrus, or surgery)
  - Signs may include nose bleeds, vaginal or penile bleeding and petechiae.
- Secondary haemostatic defect:
  - Decreased levels of clotting factors
    - Decreased production (e.g. liver disease, warfarin toxicity)
    - Increased consumption (e.g. disseminated intravascular coagulation, DIC).

Clinical signs

A primary abnormality in haemostasis usually leads to haemorrhages in the skin or mucous membranes. These are referred to as petechial (pinpoint) or ecchymotic (Figure 18.16) haemorrhages. An abnormality in clotting factors can lead to bleeding into body cavities such as the pleural or peritoneal space. If the blood loss is severe, the patient will have clinical signs of anaemia. Other clinical signs will be related to the underlying cause and to the physical effect of accumulation of blood (e.g. dyspnoea if there is bleeding into the pleural space).

Diagnostics

Caution is required when nursing these patients as they are at risk of bleeding. It is important to have a confident and careful approach to taking blood and to ensure that there is adequate pressure applied to the venepuncture site afterwards to prevent haemorrhage. To avoid excessive bleeding, blood should be taken from a peripheral vein and not the jugular vein as this is difficult to apply pressure to. For coagulation factors, fresh blood should be collected

Parameter	Problem	Nursing considerations	Monitoring
Breathing	■ Reduced red blood cells for oxygen transport		■ Monitor vital signs
Pain	■ Potentially if due to trauma or neoplasia	■ Analgesia	■ Pain assessment scoring
Drinking	■ May be increased with medication	■ Water available at all times	■ Monitor hydration
Eating	■ May be decreased	■ Tempt to eat	■ Monitor and record food offered and eaten
Urinating	■ May be increased with medication	■ Gentle walks to toilet regularly	■ Monitor and record urine output
Defecating	■ Can be normal ■ Potential melaena (indicates bleeding in the upper gastrointestinal tract) or diarrhoea due to medication	■ Take out to toilet ■ Keep clean ■ Wrap tail and apply barrier cream as required	■ Monitor faecal output
Grooming	■ May not be grooming	■ Keep clean and groom	■ Monitor for fleas, ticks and lice
Housing	■ Minimize stress	■ Soft bedding ■ Turn if recumbent ■ Quiet, calm environment	■ Keep environment clean and free from ectoparasites
Mobilizing	■ Exercise intolerance	■ Restrict exercise, gentle walks to toilet	■ Monitor exercise tolerance
Other nursing considerations			
■ Monitor for side effects if the animal has been treated with potentially immunosuppressive drugs			

| **18.15** | Nursing considerations for patients with anaemia. |

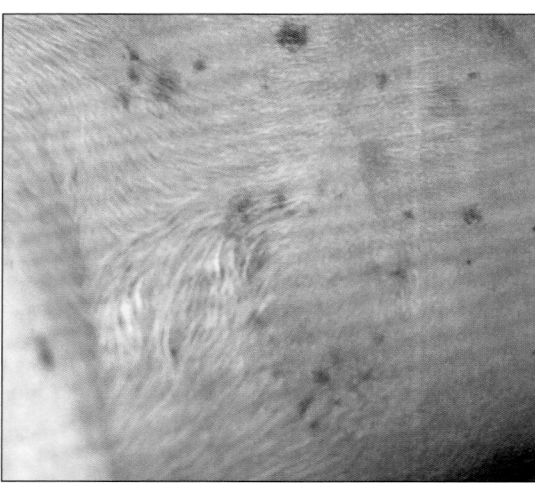

18.16 Ecchymotic haemorrhages in the skin as a result of a primary haemostatic disorder.

into a tube containing sodium citrate anticoagulant and tested within 2 hours. Further information on diagnostic tests is given in Chapter 17.

- Complete blood count (including blood smear) and biochemistry.
- Clotting profile – prothrombin time and activated partial thromboplastin time.
- Activated clotting time.
- von Willebrand factor.
- Coagulation factor assays.
- Platelet function tests.
- Buccal mucosal bleeding time (this is performed if the platelets and clotting tests are normal; it assesses primary haemostasis).

Treatment

Treatment is targeted at the underlying cause (e.g. immuno-suppression for immune-mediated disease; vitamin K for warfarin poisoning). If the bleeding is severe, the patient may require whole blood or plasma to replace clotting factors. Desmopressin can be used to increase von Willebrand factor and can be used prior to surgery in affected animals.

Nursing care

The nursing considerations for clotting disorders are detailed in Figure 18.17.

Parameter	Problem	Nursing considerations	Monitoring
Breathing	■ May be increased if bleeding into the lungs or chest	■ Oxygen therapy	■ Monitor vital signs
Bleeding	■ Bleeding following blood sample collection ■ Bleeding following injection	■ Take blood samples from peripheral veins ■ Apply pressure after the procedure ■ Avoid intramuscular injections	■ Monitor vital signs ■ Monitor for signs of petechiae
Pain	■ Bleeding into tissues may be painful	■ Pain relief considered: may need to avoid injections due to bleeding	■ Pain assessment scoring
Drinking	■ Likely to be normal	■ Maintain hydration	■ Monitor fluid intake, particularly if the patient is on steroids and hydration is altered
Eating	■ Likely to be normal	■ Provide well balanced diet	■ Monitor weight
Urinating	■ Likely to be normal but may bleed into bladder	■ Take out to toilet regularly	■ Monitor urine output
Defecating	■ Melaena or fresh blood may be present in the faeces	■ Take out to toilet regularly	■ Monitor faecal output
Grooming	■ May not be grooming	■ Groom as necessary	■ Good hygiene
Housing	■ Bleeding patient requires gentle handling	■ Soft bedding ■ Maintain regular routines	■ Good hygiene
Mobilizing	■ May be painful if bleeding into joints	■ Gentle walks	■ Monitor exercise tolerance

18.17 Nursing considerations for patients with clotting disorders.

Lymphoma

This is a cancer of the lymphoid tissue.

Clinical signs

- Enlarged lymph nodes (see Figure 18.48).
- Weight loss.
- Anorexia and inappetence.
- Vomiting and diarrhoea.
- Clinical signs associated with other organs affected (e.g. mediastinal lymphoma may result in difficulty breathing; cutaneous lymphoma may cause dry flaky skin) or other abnormalities associated with the lymphoma (e.g. hypercalcaemia).

Diagnostics

- Haematology (e.g. complete blood count).
- Biochemistry (e.g. high levels of calcium are seen with T-cell lymphoma; high levels of thymidine kinase (TK) indicates activity of tumour cells).
- Fine-needle aspiration (FNA) of an enlarged peripheral lymph node (ideally not associated with the head).
- Biopsy of the lymph node if FNA cytology non-diagnostic.
- Thoracic and abdominal radiography.
- Abdominal ultrasonography.
- CT.
- Bone marrow aspiration.

Treatment

- Chemotherapy (e.g. oral prednisolone and cyclophosphamide or intravenous vincristine, cyclophosphamide and doxorubicin).
- Surgery (e.g. bone marrow transplant).
- Radiotherapy.
- Intravenous fluids.
- Steroids (e.g. prednisone and dexamethasone).
- Canine lymphoma blood test (cLBT) to check for disease remission and recurrence.

Nursing care

The nursing considerations for lymphoma are detailed in Figure 18.18 (see also Chapters 2 and 8).

Parameter	Problem	Nursing considerations	Monitoring
Breathing	• May be compromised due to a mass in the chest	• Oxygen therapy	• Monitor vital signs • Monitor respiratory rate and character • Monitor mucous membranes for pallor (extreme or unnatural paleness), icterus (jaundice), petechiae and ulceration
Pain	• Unlikely to be painful	• Provide analgesia if needed	• Pain assessment scoring
Drinking	• May be increased (due to hypercalcaemia)	• Water freely available • Intravenous fluids if required	• Monitor hydration and water intake
Eating	• May be inappetent or anorexic	• Tempt to eat	• Monitor food intake
Urinating	• May be increased	• Take out to toilet frequently • Check bedding for soiling • Care should be taken when handling waste if patient is on chemotherapy	• Record urine output
Defecating	• May have diarrhoea	• Take out to toilet frequently • Care should be taken when handling waste if patient is on chemotherapy	• Monitor faecal output
Housing	• Normal	• Keep accommodation clean	• Good hygiene
Mobilizing	• May have exercise intolerance	• Gentle exercise	• Monitor exercise tolerance

Other nursing considerations

For patients on chemotherapy:

- Care should be taken when administering chemotherapeutic drugs
- Care should be taken when disposing of cytotoxic bodily waste
- Monitor for side effects relating to the chemotherapy treatment (e.g. vomiting, diarrhoea, lethargy and weakness)
- Instruct owners in how to safely dispose of cytotoxic bodily waste and to monitor for side effects
- To avoid risk of exposure to cytotoxic drugs, which can result in organ damage, impaired fertility, fetal malformation and cancer, personal protective equipment (PPE) should be worn. This includes when preparing and administering chemotherapy drugs and also when handling patient excreta, cleaning up spills or disposing of materials and equipment that have been in contact with these drugs

18.18 Nursing considerations for patients with lymphoma.

Gastrointestinal tract disease

The gastrointestinal (GI) tract comprises the oesophagus, stomach, small intestine, colon and rectum. Dysfunction or disease affecting these organs can lead to regurgitation, vomiting and diarrhoea.

Definitions

- Dysphagia – difficulty in swallowing
- Coprophagia – eating of faeces
- Anorexia – absence of appetite
- Pica – depraved appetite (e.g. eating of unusual foodstuff)
- Inappetence – reduced appetite
- Polyphagia – increased appetite
- Megaoesophagus – flaccid dilatation of oesophagus
- Regurgitation – passive process of returning ingesta, usually from oesophagus
- Vomiting – active process of expelling stomach contents
- Diarrhoea – increased passage of abnormally softer liquid faeces
- Tenesmus – straining to pass faeces
- Dyschezia – pain on defecation
- Melaena – dark tar-like faeces containing digested blood
- Constipation – failure to pass faeces of normal frequency or consistency

---

Regurgitation

It is important to be able to differentiate regurgitation from vomiting. Regurgitation is a passive process: there is no contraction of the abdominal muscles; the head is lowered and undigested food is ejected from the mouth. The severity of the condition can vary from the regurgitation of all solid food to regurgitation of only some ingested matter and saliva. Malnutrition and aspiration pneumonia can develop if the condition is severe.

Causes of regurgitation can include:

- Megaoesophagus (this can have various causes)
- Oesophagitis (this can result if reflux occurs whilst the patient is anaesthetized, secondary to capsule retention in the oesophagus (e.g. doxycycline in cats), oesophageal foreign bodies and vomiting)
- Oesophageal foreign bodies
- Oesophageal strictures (as a consequence of oesophagitis)
- Persistent right aortic arch (congenital cardiac abnormality).

Diagnostics

- Blood samples for haematology and biochemistry; other specific tests may be requested if the patient is found to have megaoesophagus (myasthenia gravis – acetylcholine receptor antibodies; or hypoadrenocorticism (Addison's disease) – adrenocorticotrophic hormone (ACTH) stimulation test).
- Plain radiographs. Contrast radiographs may be considered; water-soluble contrast medium is preferred for these studies.
- Fluoroscopy.
- Oesophagoscopy.

Treatment

The treatment will vary depending on the underlying cause of the problem:

- Medical management to treat any underlying disease that causes megaeosophagus
- Analgesics, gastric acid reduction (omeprazole and histamine (H2) blockers) and polyaluminium sucrose sulfate for oesophagitis
- Endoscopic or surgical removal of oesophageal foreign bodies
- Endoscopic ballooning of oesophageal strictures
- Surgery for animals with persistent right aortic arch
- Fluids and electrolytes
- Dietary modification.

Nursing care

The nursing considerations for regurgitation are detailed in Figure 18.19.

Further management can include feeding animals from a height (see Chapters 13 and 14). Gravity-assisted feeding can help to control the clinical signs if the problem is not too severe. Keeping the patient's head and forelimbs elevated for 10 minutes after a meal will allow the food to enter the stomach. In other cases, liquid food can be fed to pass a stricture, or balls of food may be given for megaoesophagus if some peristaltic activity is present.

Parameter	Problem	Nursing considerations	Monitoring
Breathing	■ Potential aspiration pneumonia	■ Feed smaller meals ■ Slow speed of eating – avoid using deep dishes. In the case of cats, use a wide flat tray as this spreads out the food and encourages the cat to spend more time eating	■ Auscultate lungs ■ Monitor respiratory rate ■ Monitor for coughing ■ Monitor heart rate
Pain	■ Oesophagitis	■ Analgesia	■ Pain assessment scoring
Drinking	■ Dehydration; unable to drink adequately ■ Regurgitation of saliva	■ Fluids: intravenous or subcutaneous if oral intake inadequate ■ Gastric feeding tube can also be considered	■ Monitor for dehydration ■ (weight loss and urine output) ■ Monitor blood electrolyte concentrations

18.19 Nursing considerations for patients with regurgitation.

continues ▶

Parameter	Problem	Nursing considerations	Monitoring
Eating	■ Unable to swallow ■ Regurgitation	■ Use food of different consistencies to ascertain which is swallowed better ■ Feed from a height, maintain upright for 10 minutes after eating ■ Consider gastric feeding tube ■ Multiple small meals throughout the day ■ Feed high quality, calorific dense food to limit volume necessary to meet nutritional needs	■ Monitor weight ■ Monitor and record frequency and volume of regurgitation
Urinating	■ Dehydration	■ Take out to toilet regularly	■ Monitor urine output
Defecating	■ Poor food intake	■ Take out to toilet regularly	■ Monitor faecal output
Grooming	■ Saliva around the mouth, poor grooming	■ Clean around mouth, chin and neck as required	■ Monitor for excoriation
Mobilizing	■ Potential problem; some conditions can also affect other muscles and nerves	■ Take out to toilet using a harness	■ Monitor for difficulty mobilizing
Other nursing considerations			
■ Poor oesophageal function – provide medication (generally parenteral), as directed by the veterinary surgeon			

18.19 *continued* Nursing considerations for patients with regurgitation.

Vomiting

Vomiting is an active process, where the stomach contents are forcefully ejected out of the mouth by the contraction of the abdominal muscles. It is a common clinical sign of many conditions, as it is a protective mechanism that helps to eliminate toxic substances from the body. Receptors in the brain are triggered by the presence of certain toxins or when normal levels of substances found in the body are exceeded (e.g. urea). Causes of vomiting are shown in Figure 18.20.

Prior to vomiting the animal may show signs of restlessness, abdominal pain, salivating or licking of the lips. An episode of vomiting may occur many hours after the animal has eaten and the vomitus may contain partially digested food, bile or a mixture of both.

Vomiting can be classified as acute or chronic, depending on the speed of onset and its duration. Depending on the frequency of vomiting and the volumes involved, there can be a significant loss of water from the body and dehydration if the animal is unable to replace these losses. Electrolytes (sodium, chloride and potassium) are also lost, along with hydrogen ions, and this can result in electrolyte imbalances and metabolic alkalosis (see Chapter 20).

Diagnostics

It can sometimes be difficult to identify the cause of vomiting in a patient. Obtaining a detailed history is an important part of the diagnostic approach. It is equally important that close observations of a patient are made if an animal is hospitalized.

- History (see below).
- Clinical examination – abdominal palpation important.
- Blood samples for haematology and biochemistry to confirm or rule out systemic disease. (Other specific blood tests may be requested by the veterinary surgeon.)
- Abdominal radiography and/or ultrasonography.
- Barium meal (not used before endoscopy if this is carried out).
- Endoscopy.
- Gastroscopy or exploratory laparotomy – biopsy samples are taken routinely during these procedures.

Gastrointestinal disease
- Dietary indiscretion
- Infectious agents: viral (e.g. parvovirus); bacterial (e.g. *Salmonella*); parasitic (occasionally) (e.g. roundworms)
- Gastric foreign bodies
- Intestinal foreign bodies
- Intussusception
- Gastrointestinal ulceration
- Pyloric stenosis
- Gastrointestinal neoplasia

Systemic disease
- Uraemia – due to either renal disease or urinary tract obstruction
- Hepatic inflammation
- Pyometra
- Pancreatitis
- Peritonitis

Metabolic/endocrine disorders
- Diabetic ketoacidosis
- Hypercalcaemia
- Hypoadrenocorticism

Drugs/toxins
- Non-steroidal anti-inflammatory drugs (NSAIDs)
- Chemotherapy drugs
- Heavy metal toxicity
- Insecticide toxicity (e.g. organophosphates)
- Herbicide toxicity (e.g. chlorates)
- Molluscicide toxicity (e.g. metaldehyde)

18.20 Causes of vomiting (note that this list is not exhaustive).

Assessing the vomiting patient
- Demeanour – a depressed or lethargic patient is more likely to have systemic disease, dehydration or electrolyte imbalances
- Body condition – weight loss and general body condition can also provide important information about the cause of vomiting →

> ## Assessing the vomiting patient *continued*
> - Age – older animals are more likely to have neoplasia. Younger animals are more likely to have infections or have eaten foreign bodies or toxins
> - Environmental – indiscretion (e.g. table scraps, sudden diet change, rubbish bin ingestion, toxins, plants)
> - Other clinical signs – clinical signs such as polyuria and polydipsia can indicate the presence of systemic disease
> - Vaccination history – up-to-date vaccination status can help to rule out some infectious agents
> - Dietary changes – changes in feeding can help to confirm or rule out uncomplicated gastroenteritis. A history of scavenging (or opportunity to scavenge) should also be ascertained. The time that vomiting occurs in relation to eating is also helpful
> - Type and frequency of vomiting – can provide important information about the causal factor (e.g. projectile, chronic intermittent, cyclic or morning only). For example, infectious agents such as parvovirus or *Salmonella* are often associated with acute bouts of frequent vomiting
> - Content of the vomitus – vomit containing blood can indicate ulceration or severe inflammation of the GI tract. Vomiting undigested food long after a meal can suggest gastric motility problems including obstruction
> - Faeces – lack of faeces can indicate obstruction. Diarrhoea indicates intestinal involvement. Melaena (blackened by digested blood) indicates ulceration and bleeding from the upper GI tract. Fresh (undigested) blood indicates bleeding from the lower GI tract

Treatment

Uncomplicated acute vomiting is managed by starving the patient for 24 hours, whilst providing oral or intravenous fluid and electrolyte replacement. If the animal responds successfully, an investigation of the cause is often not undertaken. Further symptomatic treatment may also be required.

Treatment for chronic vomiting is aimed at treating the underlying disease, controlling the clinical signs and correcting dehydration, if necessary. Drug therapy may include:

- Specific drugs acting on the GI tract (see Chapter 8) including antiemetics
- Fluid therapy – important to correct dehydration, electrolyte and acid–base imbalances (see Chapter 20)
- Analgesia – to make the patient more comfortable (non-steroidal anti-inflammatory drugs (NSAIDs) should be avoided).

Surgery may be indicated for correction of pyloric stenosis, removal of foreign bodies, treatment of intussusception and removal of gastrointestinal tumours.

Nursing care

The nursing considerations for vomiting are detailed in Figure 18.21 (see also Chapter 15).

Parameter	Problem	Nursing considerations	Monitoring
Breathing	Low potential for compromise	Check vital signs	Monitor for aspiration
Pain	Potential for gastrointestinal tract pain	Analgesia if required	Pain assessment scoring; Assess with abdominal palpation q4–6h
Drinking	Dehydration; unable to drink adequately; Vomiting	Fluids: intravenous or subcutaneous if oral intake inadequate; Consider electrolytes in water	Monitor for dehydration (weight loss and urine output); Monitor blood electrolyte concentrations
Eating	Anorexia or vomiting	Palatable, easily digestible, bland single protein source; Offer food little and often; Medication: antiemetics as directed by the veterinary surgeon; Acute vomiting: withhold food for 24 hours; Chronic vomiting: hypoallergenic diet	Monitor weight; Monitor blood electrolyte concentrations
Urinating	Dehydration	Take out to toilet	Monitor for dehydration; Record urine output
Defecating	Potentially reduced due to poor intake or obstruction; Diarrhoea: gastroenteritis	Toilet frequently	Monitor and record faecal output
Grooming	May not be grooming	Groom as required	Good hygiene
Housing	Animal potentially infectious	Keep in isolation and barrier nurse as required	Good disinfection; Good ventilation
Mobilizing	Unlikely to be a problem unless severely debilitated	Provide regular opportunities to exercise	Monitor exercise tolerance

Other nursing considerations

- Prepare patient as required for diagnostic and/or surgical procedures
- Provision of medication, including antiemetics, as directed by the veterinary surgeon – generally parenteral administration in animals with gastrointestinal disease as they have poor absorption from the gastrointestinal tract. Ensure oral medication is not vomited

18.21 Nursing considerations for patients with vomiting.

Diarrhoea

Diarrhoea can be classified as either acute or chronic and can originate from the small intestine, the large intestine or both (Figure 18.22). It results in a loss of water from the body, leading to dehydration, electrolyte imbalances and metabolic acidosis.

Clinical sign	Origin: small intestine	Origin: large intestine
Vomiting	Commonly seen	Occasional
Weight	Loss common	Maintained
Appetite	Often increased	Normal
Faecal volume	Increased	Normal
Faecal type	Watery	Varies with cause
Faecal frequency	3–4 times daily	Up to 10 times daily
Faecal mucus	None	Often present
Blood in faeces	Melaena	Heamatochezia
Urgency to pass faeces	Not present	Present; straining on defecation
Flatulence	Minimal	Common

18.22 Clinical signs suggesting the origin of diarrhoea.

Causes

Acute diarrhoea

- Sudden change of diet or scavenging.
- Dietary intolerance or hypersensitivity (allergy).
- Viral infections (e.g. parvovirus).
- Bacterial infections (e.g. *Salmonella*, *Campylobacter*, *Escherichia coli*).
- Intestinal parasites (e.g. *Toxocara*, *Giardia*, *Cryptosporidium*).
- Intussusception.
- Neoplasia of the colon.
- Foreign bodies.
- Metabolic and endocrine diseases.
- Stress.

Chronic diarrhoea

- Chronic dietary intolerance or hypersensitivity.
- Chronic infections (e.g. *Giardia*, *Campylobacter*).
- Antibiotic-responsive diarrhoea.
- Inflammatory bowel disease.
- Malabsorption.
- Maldigestion (e.g. exocrine pancreatic insufficiency, EPI).
- Colitis.
- Intussusception.
- Neoplasia.
- Foreign bodies.
- Liver disease.
- Endocrine disease (e.g. hyperthyroidism, hypoadrenocorticism).

Clinical signs

- Acute diarrhoea can be mild or severe. In mild cases the animal appears bright and alert with no signs of dehydration. In severe cases the animal is dull, depressed and dehydrated, especially if accompanied by vomiting.
- Patients with chronic diarrhoea may suffer weight loss and loss of bodily condition, as a result of the animal receiving inadequate nutrition over a period of time. However, this is not always the case if the diarrhoea is due to large intestinal disease (colitis).

Diagnostics

A thorough history can provide important information as to the cause of the diarrhoea. Questioning the owner can also help differentiate whether the diarrhoea is arising from the small or large intestine. In addition, observation of the frequency and the consistency of the diarrhoea (e.g. steatorrhoea) can help identify whether the diarrhoea is small or large intestinal in origin.

- Clinical examination.
- Routine biochemistry and haematology to rule out systemic disease.
- Specific blood tests – trypsin-like immunoreactivity (TLI); to confirm or rule out EPI, cobalamin (vitamin B12) is checked as it can be low in gastrointestinal disease.
- Faecal analysis – for parasites, undigested food and culture; PCR for infectious disease and enzyme-linked immunosorbent assay (ELISA) for parvovirus antigen.
- Abdominal radiography and/or ultrasonography.
- Contrast radiography.
- Endoscopy of the upper and/or lower GI tract, exploratory laparotomy and biopsy.

Treatment

Acute diarrhoea

Traditionally, food was withheld from patients with acute diarrhoea; however, more recent research suggests that patients should continue to be fed during the episode with the addition of probiotics. If withholding food is indicated, fasting for 24–48 hours is usually sufficient as long as during this period of time the animal is not vomiting, and fluid and electrolytes are supplemented. In severe acute cases, intravenous fluid therapy is indicated to prevent dehydration and electrolyte imbalance. Fasting for longer periods should be avoided, as the intestine obtains a large proportion of its nutrition from the digested food that passes through it. Long periods of starvation can therefore result in reduced functioning capabilities of the intestine. Food during this period and recovery should be a bland, easy-to-digest, low-fat and single-source protein diet. This should be fed for a number of days before gradually reintroducing normal food. Treatment of any underlying cause is also important.

Chronic diarrhoea

In cases with chronic diarrhoea, investigation of the underlying cause is important for successful treatment. Treatments can include:

- In cases of hypersensitivity to diet, feeding a protein that the animal has never eaten before
- Anthelmintics and other antiparasitic drugs
- Antibacterials for antibiotic-responsive diarrhoea
- Corticosteroids and other immunosuppressives for inflammatory bowel disease
- Enzyme supplementation in cases with EPI
- Surgery for intussusception, neoplasia and foreign bodies
- Treatment of underlying systemic disease.

Nursing care

The nursing considerations for diarrhoea are detailed in Figure 18.23 (see also Chapter 15).

Parameter	Problem	Nursing considerations	Monitoring
Breathing	■ Unlikely to become compromised	■ Awareness of normal respiratory pattern	■ Monitor vital signs
Pain	■ Potential for gastrointestinal tract pain	■ Analgesia if required	■ Pain assessment scoring ■ Assess with abdominal palpation q4–6h
Drinking	■ May be reduced. May need to drink more	■ Fluids: intravenous or subcutaneous if oral intake inadequate ■ Consider electrolytes in water	■ Monitor for dehydration (weight loss and urine output) ■ Monitor blood electrolyte concentrations
Eating	■ Potential for anorexia/ inappetence or developing vomiting	■ Palatable, easily digestible, low-fat single protein source ■ Small frequent meals ■ Various approaches to the management of acute diarrhoea from withholding food to the new recommendations of feeding throughout the episode with the addition of probiotics	■ Monitor weight ■ Monitor blood electrolyte concentrations
Urinating	■ Dehydration	■ Take out to toilet	■ Monitor for dehydration ■ Record urine output
Defecating	■ Diarrhoea	■ Toilet frequently	■ Monitor and record faecal output
Grooming	■ Faecal soiling	■ Keep clean and dry ■ May need to wrap tail and/or clip hair ■ Barrier cream may need to be applied to prevent damage to skin around perineum	■ Monitor and record faecal soiling
Housing	■ Animal potentially infectious	■ Keep in isolation and barrier nurse as required	■ Good disinfection ■ Good ventilation
Mobilizing	■ Unlikely to be a problem unless severely debilitated	■ Provide regular opportunities to exercise	■ Monitor exercise tolerance ■ Good hygiene

Other nursing considerations

■ Prepare patient as required for diagnostic and/or surgical procedures
■ Provision of medication, as directed by the veterinary surgeon – animals with gastrointestinal disease have poor absorption from the gastrointestinal tract. Ensure desired response to medication indicating adequate absorption

18.23 Nursing considerations for patients with diarrhoea.

Constipation

Constipation is the failure to pass faeces either in normal quantity or at normal frequency, resulting in impaction of the colon and rectum with faecal material. There are many causes of constipation (Figure 18.24). It is seen more commonly in elderly patients. An enlarged prostate gland, bones in the diet, tumours and dehydration can all contribute to the development of constipation.

Clinical signs

■ Failure to pass faeces.
■ Tenesmus.
■ Passing of very hard faeces (often with fresh blood).
■ Vomiting.
■ Dyschezia (pain on passing faeces).

Diagnostics

■ Physical examination/rectal examination.
■ Radiography.
■ Ultrasonography.
■ Proctoscopy.

Treatment

It is important to find the underlying cause to provide the best treatment, but treatment may include:

■ Enemas – various types (use most suitable) (see Chapter 15)
■ Correct dehydration

Dietary

■ Fibre content of diet is too low
■ Eating bones

Colonic

■ Rectal strictures
■ Rectal foreign bodies
■ Rectal tumours
■ Perineal hernia
■ Megacolon (dysautonomia)
■ Anal sac disease

Orthopaedic

■ Pelvic fractures causing narrowing of pelvic canal

Other

■ Dehydration
■ Neurological dysfunction (Key–Gaskell syndrome; spinal damage)
■ Prostatic hyperplasia

18.24 Common causes of constipation (note that this list is not exhaustive).

■ Changes to diet
■ Stool-softening agents (e.g. lactulose, pumpkin)
■ Bulking agents
■ Surgical correction of obstruction
■ Increased exercise.

Nursing care

The nursing considerations for constipation are detailed in Figure 18.25.

Parameter	Problem	Nursing considerations	Monitoring
Breathing	■ Unlikely to be compromised	■ Awareness of normal respiratory pattern	■ Monitor vital signs
Pain	■ Potential for gastrointestinal tract pain	■ Analgesia if required (opiates can potentially cause constipation)	■ Pain assessment scoring
Drinking	■ Dehydration	■ Fluids: intravenous or subcutaneous if oral intake inadequate	■ Monitor for dehydration (weight loss and urine output) ■ Monitor blood electrolyte concentrations
Eating	■ Anorexia or vomiting	■ Appropriate diet: can include high-fibre diets ■ Stool softeners	■ Monitor weight ■ Monitor blood electrolyte concentrations
Urinating	■ Dehydration	■ Take out to toilet	■ Monitor for dehydration ■ Record urine output
Defecating	■ Constipation	■ Administer enemas ■ Toilet frequently	■ Monitor and record faecal output

18.25 Nursing considerations for patients with constipation.

Hepatic disease

Definitions

- Hepatitis – inflammation of the liver
- Cirrhosis – a degenerative change, causing fibrosis of the organ, resulting in a loss of functional cells and therefore loss of normal function
- Ascites – accumulation of fluid in the abdominal cavity.
- Jaundice – elevated levels of bilirubin in the tissues and circulation, resulting in a yellowing of the skin and mucous membranes

Causes

Liver disease may be congenital or acquired, and acute or chronic. There are many causes of hepatic disease but often the cause is not identified. Causes include:

- Acute:
  - Drug-induced (e.g. lomustine)
  - Toxins (e.g. bacterial endotoxin, blue-green algae)
  - Bacterial infection (e.g. *Leptospira*)
  - Viral infection (e.g. adenovirus I (ICH))
  - Surgical hypotension or hypoxia
  - Trauma (e.g. bruising or rupture).
- Chronic:
  - Drug-induced (e.g. phenobarbital)
  - Neoplasia
  - Metabolic (e.g. diabetes mellitus, hyperadrenocorticism)
  - Copper toxicity (in Bedlington Terrier and West Highland White Terrier)
  - Immune-mediated (inflammatory, e.g. cholangiohepatitis, chronic hepatitis)
  - Congenital (e.g. portosystemic shunts).

Portosystemic shunts

The hepatic portal system enables the products of digestion that are absorbed by the gut to be transported directly to the liver for storage or use (see Chapter 3). In a normal animal the blood flows:

- From the heart to the capillary beds of the stomach and intestines
- From here to the liver via the hepatic portal vein, where it enters the capillary bed of the liver (Figure 18.26)
- From the liver via the hepatic vein to the caudal vena cava.

With a portosystemic shunt the blood bypasses the liver and deposits blood directly back into the systemic circulation. Clinical signs are frequently seen post-feeding when blood ammonia levels are elevated. Shunts can be a developmental abnormality, or they can be due to advanced cirrhosis. Poor muscle development, behavioural abnormalities, polyuria, polydipsia, vomiting, diarrhoea and blindness may also be seen.

Ultrasonography is used to identify the location and extent of shunting and possible treatment options. Congenital shunts can be surgically ligated; it is also possible to manage the clinical signs medically. In cirrhosis multiple shunting vessels develop which cannot be ligated.

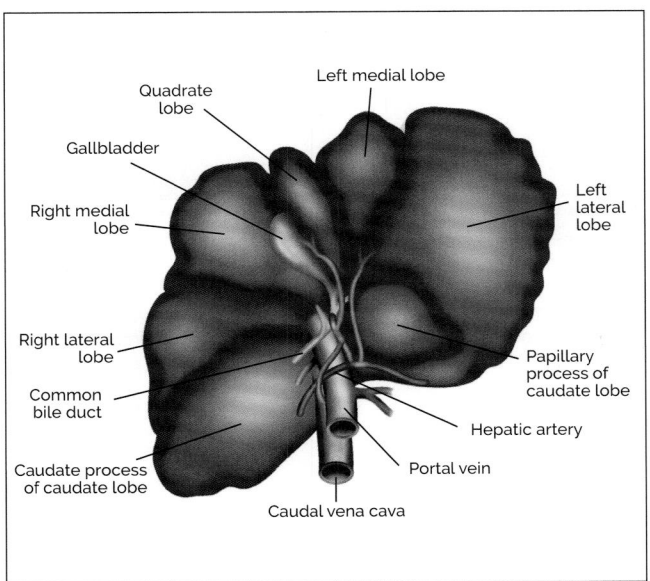

18.26 Anatomy of the liver. (Reproduced from the *BSAVA Manual of Canine and Feline Abdominal Surgery, 2nd edn*)

Clinical signs

The liver has enormous regenerative capabilities and chronic clinical signs will not be noticed until 70–80% of the liver cells have been lost due to damage.

Non-specific clinical signs may include:

- Vomiting
- Diarrhoea
- Weight loss
- Polydipsia
- Polyuria
- Anorexia or inappetence.

Specific signs include:

- Cranial abdominal pain
- Jaundice
- Ascites
- Hepatomegaly
- Neurological signs due to hepatoencephalopathy
- Dark urine – due to bilirubin
- Bleeding disorders – due to clotting factor deficiency (the clotting factors are made in the liver).

Jaundice (icterus)

Jaundice of the skin (Figure 18.27) and mucous membranes will occur if the capacity of the liver to excrete bilirubin in the bile becomes unbalanced:

- Prehepatic (e.g. excessive haemolysis)
- Intrahepatic (e.g. liver dysfunction)
- Posthepatic (e.g. bile flow obstruction).

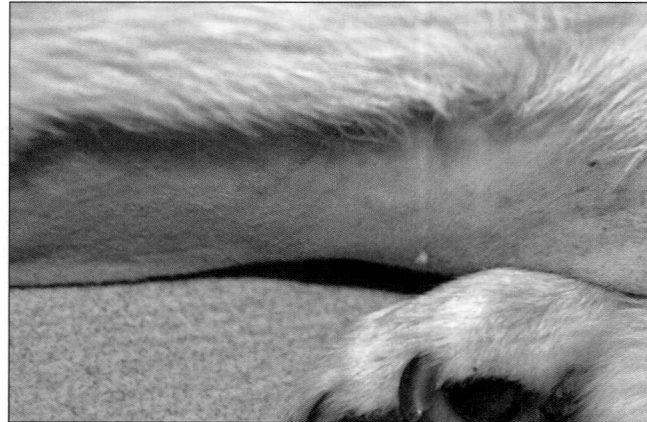

18.27 Jaundice as a result of haemolytic anaemia in a 6-year-old Labrador Retriever.

Hepatic encephalopathy

This occurs when >70% of hepatic tissue is lost and neurotoxic substances build up, causing toxaemias and neurological signs. The toxins are mainly from the gastrointestinal tract (e.g. ammonia is a by-product of protein breakdown).

Diagnostics

- Biochemistry:
  - Albumin
  - Globulin
  - Alanine aminotransferase (ALT) and alkaline phosphatase (ALP) are liver enzymes and indicate liver damage or cholestasis
  - Gamma glutamyltransferase (GGT) (cats)
  - The liver has multiple functions and other results on the biochemistry panel can also be abnormal when the patient has liver dysfunction.
- Bile acid stimulation test (liver function test).
- Haematology:
  - Full blood count
  - Coagulation screen.
- Radiography – can provide information about the size of the liver.
- Ultrasonography – can give a more useful indication of internal structure of the liver and can identify focal (discrete lesions) or diffuse (throughout) lesions.
- Fine-needle aspirate of the liver – can give indication as to the cause or nature of the disease.
- Liver biopsy – will most likely provide a definitive diagnosis. As the liver produces clotting factors, a coagulation screen should be requested first to minimize the risk of bleeding. Liver biopsy samples can be taken with ultrasound guidance or during an exploratory laparotomy.

Treatment

The treatment options depend on the underlying cause and whether or not hepatic dysfunction exists, but can include the following:

- Intravenous fluids (acute cases).
- Antibiotics (to reduce bacterial load).
- Anti-inflammatories.
- Water-soluble bile acids.
- Lactulose (helps to bind ammonia).
- Special diet and supplements (see Chapter 13).

Nursing care

The nursing considerations for hepatic disease are detailed in Figure 18.28.

Parameter	Problem	Nursing considerations	Monitoring
Breathing	■ Unlikely to be compromised	■ Awareness of normal respiratory pattern	■ Monitor vital signs
Pain	■ Acute disease may be painful	■ Pain relief: different doses and frequency may be required due to drug metabolism through the liver	■ Pain assessment scoring
Drinking	■ Polydipsia ■ May not be drinking adequately. Vomiting and diarrhoea could contribute to dehydration	■ Fluids: intravenous or subcutaneous if oral intake inadequate	■ Monitor for dehydration (weight loss and urine output) ■ Monitor blood electrolyte concentrations

18.28 Nursing considerations for patients with hepatic disease.

continues ▶

Parameter	Problem	Nursing considerations	Monitoring
Eating	■ Anorexia or vomiting	■ Tempt with palatable, easily digestible food. If hepatic dysfunction then feed low-protein diet or hepatic diet	■ Monitor weight ■ Monitor proteins long term if on a low-protein diet
Urinating	■ Polyuria ■ Dehydration	■ Take out to toilet	■ Monitor for dehydration ■ Record urine output
Defecating	■ May have diarrhoea ■ Malaena	■ Take out to toilet	■ Monitor and record faecal output
Grooming	■ May not groom adequately	■ Keep clean and groom	■ Good hygiene
Housing	■ Animal potentially infectious (e.g. zoonotic disease)	■ Keep in isolation and barrier nurse as required	■ Good hygiene
Mobilizing	■ Circling, ataxia	■ Remove objects that patients may injure themselves on	■ Monitor exercise tolerance

Other nursing considerations

■ Prepare patient as required for diagnostic procedures (e.g. blood tests, biopsy)
■ Monitor for adverse reactions to medication (e.g. antiemetics, antibiotics and lactulose administered as directed by the veterinary surgeon). Consider dose reductions for drugs metabolized by the liver
■ Monitor for bleeding

18.28 *continued* Nursing considerations for patients with hepatic disease.

Pancreatic disease

The pancreas is composed of two types of tissue:

■ Exocrine – produces digestive enzymes (trypsin, chymotrypsin, amylase and pancreatic lipase)
■ Endocrine – produces hormones (insulin, glucagon).

Diseases of the exocrine pancreas can be divided into:

■ Pancreatitis – acute and chronic
■ Exocrine pancreatic insufficiency
■ Exocrine tumours.

Pancreatitis

Pancreatitis, inflammation of the pancreas, is caused by self-digestion (autolysis) of the pancreas by the digestive enzymes that are stored inside specialized storage pockets. It can be acute or chronic.

Acute pancreatitis

This can be life-threatening, as complications such as peritonitis can develop. Usually the cause of pancreatitis is unknown. Some breeds have a predisposition to this condition. Other potential risk factors include:

■ Obesity
■ High-fat diet
■ Hypertriglyceridaemia
■ Pancreatic duct occlusion
■ Hypotension
■ Some medications.

Clinical signs

The severity of clinical signs ranges from mild to severe.

■ Vomiting (not seen as often in cats).
■ Pyrexia.
■ Anorexia.
■ Acute cranial abdominal pain.
■ Dehydration.

■ Shock.
■ Collapse.
■ Diarrhoea (occasional).

Diagnostics

■ Blood tests (biochemistry, complete blood count; elevated levels of canine-specific pancreatic lipase (cPLI) or feline-specific pancreatic lipase (fPLI)).
■ Radiography.
■ Abdominal ultrasonography.
■ CT.

Treatment

■ Supportive treatment:
  • Intravenous fluid therapy
  • Analgesics
  • Low-fat diet
  • Antiemetics.

Nursing care

The nursing considerations for acute pancreatitis are detailed in Figure 18.29.

Chronic pancreatitis

This is a low-grade but continual inflammation of the pancreas. In cats, inflammatory bowel disease and biliary tract disease may be risk factors.

Clinical signs

■ Recurrent vomiting or discomfort.
■ Weight loss.
■ Reduced appetite.
■ Abdominal pain.

Diagnostics

Diagnostic tests are as for acute pancreatitis, with the addition of testing for TLI and vitamin B12 levels.

Treatment

■ Long-term dietary management (low fat).
■ Fluid and electrolyte support.
■ Enzyme supplementation if EPI occurs.

Parameter	Problem	Nursing considerations	Monitoring
Breathing	■ Potential to deteriorate quickly	■ Regular checks of temperature, pulse and respiration	■ Monitor vital signs as they can deteriorate quickly
Pain	■ Can become very painful	■ Analgesia	■ Regular pain assessment scoring
Drinking	■ Dehydration	■ Fluids: intravenous or subcutaneous if oral intake inadequate	■ Monitor for dehydration (weight loss and urine output) ■ Monitor blood electrolyte concentrations
Eating	■ Anorexia or vomiting	■ Palatable low-fat diet ■ Parenteral or enteral nutrition	■ Monitor weight ■ Monitor blood electrolyte concentrations
Urinating	■ Dehydration	■ Take out to toilet	■ Monitor for dehydration ■ Record urine output
Defecating	■ Can be reduced or can have diarrhoea or colitis	■ Toilet frequently	■ Monitor and record faecal output
Housing	■ Normal	■ Provide comfortable bedding	■ Good hygiene

18.29 Nursing considerations for patients with acute pancreatitis.

Exocrine pancreatic insufficiency (EPI)

This condition is caused by insufficient production of pancreatic enzymes, resulting in maldigestion and malabsorption of food. Pancreatic atrophy occurs. It can be congenital and may be hereditary in German Shepherd Dogs. It can also occur following chronic pancreatitis if the cells of the pancreas are damaged. The condition is relatively common in dogs but rare in cats.

Clinical signs

- Diarrhoea.
- Steatorrhoea (fatty faeces).
- Ravenous appetite.
- Coprophagia (eating faeces) – due to presence of undigested food.
- Weight loss.

Diagnostics

- Blood tests – complete blood count and biochemistry, to include TLI, vitamin B12 and folate.
- Faecal analysis for undigested food.

Treatment

Supplementation of food with pancreatic enzymes such as amylase, lipase and protease; dietary management is still required.

Nursing care

The nursing considerations for exocrine pancreatic insufficiency are detailed in Figure 18.30.

Renal disease

Definitions
- Nephritis – inflammation of the kidney
- Glomerulonephritis – inflammation of the glomerulus
- Pyelonephritis – inflammation of the kidney and renal pelvis
- Interstitial nephritis – inflammation of the renal interstitium

Acute kidney injury

Acute kidney injury may occur as a consequence of:

- Decreased blood flow to the kidneys (e.g. hypovolaemic shock)
- Direct effect on the cells of the kidneys (e.g. toxins: ethylene glycol toxicity (antifreeze); grapes; infectious causes: leptospirosis)
- Post-renal obstruction (e.g. ureteral or urethral stone causing obstruction, blocked bladder or rupture of the urinary tract)
- Acute exacerbation of chronic renal failure.

Parameter	Problem	Nursing considerations	Monitoring
Breathing	■ Unlikely to be compromised	■ Awareness of normal respiratory pattern	■ Monitor for any changes from normal
Pain	■ Unlikely to be painful	■ Provide analgesia if necessary	■ Monitor for signs of pain
Drinking	■ Should be normal	■ Maintain hydration	■ Monitor fluid intake
Eating	■ Increased	■ Good quality, easily digestible food ■ Pancreatic enzyme supplementation required ■ Avoid feeding treats	■ Weekly monitoring of weight
Urinating	■ Should be normal	■ Take out to toilet regularly	■ Monitor urine output
Defecating	■ Cow pat	■ Pancreatic enzyme supplementation	■ Regular monitoring of faecal output

18.30 Nursing considerations for patients with exocrine pancreatic insufficiency.

Clinical signs

- Sudden-onset anorexia, lethargy and depression.
- Oliguria and anuria, followed by polyuria.
- Vomiting and diarrhoea.
- Polydipsia.
- Dehydration.
- Uraemic breath.
- Abdominal pain.

Diagnostics

- Blood tests – complete blood count and biochemistry (urea, creatinine, electrolytes – specifically potassium, phosphate).
- Urinalysis – specific gravity, dipstick and sediment examination, culture and sensitivity.
- Abdominal radiography – right lateral and ventrodorsal views.
- Abdominal ultrasonography.
- CT.
- Blood pressure may be increased (hypertension).

Treatment

Treatment involves, if possible, removing the inciting cause and treating the underlying cause. It is usually supportive.

- Intravenous fluid therapy is very important for several reasons: to decrease potassium (which is the initial life-threatening complication); to dilute the built-up waste products; and to rehydrate the animal. It is also the first line in establishing urine output.
- If oliguria persists, drugs such as furosemide may be administered to improve urine output.
- Antiemetics can be used to manage persistent vomiting.

- Peritoneal dialysis is used to remove nitrogenous waste products when urine output has failed to be re-established with the above treatment.
- Patients can also be referred for continuous renal replacement therapy (CRRT) at a specialist hospital.

The condition is often reversible if the patient comes through the acute crisis. However, there can be residual renal damage.

Nursing care

The nursing considerations for acute kidney injury are detailed in Figure 18.31.

Chronic renal failure

This slowly progressive loss of renal function over an unidentified period of time results in azotaemia (uraemia). The onset of the clinical signs is gradual and may only become noticeable when 75% of the nephrons have already been lost. It is most often seen in animals over 7 years of age (Figure 18.32) but this can depend on the causal factor, as younger animals can be affected. It is a common cause of illness in older cats.

Causes of chronic renal failure include:

- Idiopathic
- Can occur after acute kidney injury
- Nephrotoxins
- Pyelonephritis
- Glomerulonephritis
- Ischaemic damage
- Hypercalcaemia
- Congenital/hereditary disease (e.g. polycystic kidney disease).

Parameter	Problem	Nursing considerations	Monitoring
Breathing	- Potential volume overload with intravenous fluid	- Regular checks of temperature, pulse and respiration	- Auscultate lungs - Monitor sleeping respiratory rate
Pain	- Potentially painful	- Provide analgesia as needed	- Pain assessment scoring
Drinking	- Polydipsia	- Water freely available if not vomiting - Intravenous fluid therapy	- Monitor for vomiting and dehydration - Monitor potassium concentrations in the blood
Eating	- Anorexia, inappetence, vomiting	- Tempt with palatable food - Naso-oesophageal tube placement may be considered	- Monitor and record food intake
Urinating	- Anuria - Oliguria Polyuria	- Intravenous fluid therapy - Take out to toilet frequently	- Monitor and record hourly urine output (should be 1–2 ml/kg/h) - Placement of a urinary catheter should be considered for monitoring purposes - Monitor weight - Palpate bladder - Weigh bedding or litter tray
Defecating	- Potential diarrhoea	- Take out to toilet - Keep clean	- Monitor and record faecal output
Grooming	- Poor grooming	- Keep clean and comfortable	- Good hygiene
Housing	- Animal potentially infectious	- Keep in isolation and barrier nurse as required	- Good hygiene - Correct disposal of waste and bedding
Mobilizing	- May be lethargic	- Take out to toilet	- Monitor exercise tolerance
Other nursing considerations			

- Provision of medication as directed by the veterinary surgeon – monitor for response to treatment and for side effects. Check drugs and doses to ensure they are not nephrotoxic. Check pharmacokinetics of drugs to determine whether they are metabolized or eliminated by the kidneys and adjust the dose rate as required
- Monitor blood pressure

18.31 Nursing considerations for patients with acute kidney injury.

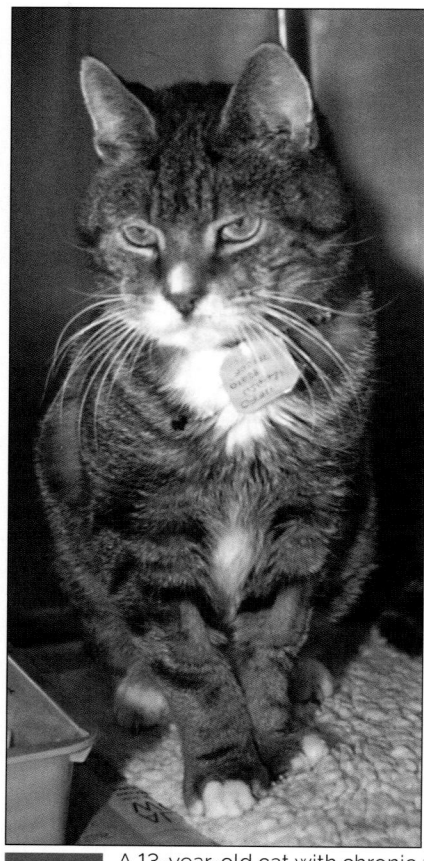

18.32 A 13-year-old cat with chronic renal failure showing poor body condition.

Clinical signs

- Polyuria/nocturia (as the kidney loses its ability to concentrate the urine).
- Polydipsia.
- Uraemia – anorexia, vomiting, lethargy and depression.
- Weight loss.
- Dehydration.
- Oral ulceration and halitosis.
- Non-regenerative anaemia (due to lack of erythropoietin production by the kidney).
- Hypertension.
- Rubber jaw (renal hyperparathyroidism) – kidneys fail to excrete phosphorus effectively causing phosphorus levels in blood to become elevated (hyperphosphataemia); parathyroid gland responds by triggering release of parathyroid hormone (PTH), resulting in demineralization of calcium from bones to correct imbalance in blood.
- Seizures – end-stage disease.

Diagnostics

- Biochemistry – high levels of symmetric dimethylarginine (SDMA), urea, creatinine and phosphorus.
- Hypokalaemia often evident.
- Complete blood count – non-regenerative anaemia.
- Urinalysis – isosthenuric urine specific gravity (1.008–1.012). May also be reduced concentrating ability in association with elevated SDMA, urea and creatinine. Sediment and urine protein:creatinine ratio assessment.
- Abdominal radiography and/or ultrasonography.
- Blood pressure frequently increased (hypertension).

International Renal Interest Society (IRIS) staging is undertaken following diagnosis of chronic kidney disease in order to facilitate appropriate treatment and monitoring of the patient. Staging is based, initially, on fasting blood creatinine concentration assessed on at least two occasions in the stable patient. The patient is then substaged based on proteinuria and blood pressure (www.iris-kidney.com).

Treatment

Chronic renal failure is not reversible. Treatment is aimed at preventing further damage and reducing the workload of the remaining nephrons.

- Treatment of any underlying cause.
- Intravenous fluid therapy if required (allow water to drink, unless vomiting). Subcutaneous fluid if the patient is treated as an outpatient.
- Antiemetics if vomiting.
- Electrolyte supplementation, if required, due to increased losses.
- Treatment of hyperphosphataemia.
- Dietary management (see Chapter 13).
- ACE inhibitors such as benazepril can be used to treat proteinuria. Urea and creatinine are monitored to ensure renal function does not deteriorate while the patient is on this medication.
- Treatment of hypertension.
- Vitamin B supplementation.
- Erythropoietin by injection may be considered.

Nursing care

The nursing considerations for chronic renal failure are detailed in Figure 18.33.

Parameter	Problem	Nursing considerations	Monitoring
Breathing	■ Unlikely to be a problem but potential for fluid volume overload	■ Regular checks of temperature, pulse and respiration	■ Monitor sleeping respiratory rate
Pain	■ Unlikely to be painful	■ Provide analgesia if needed	■ Monitor for signs of pain
Drinking	■ Polydipsia ■ May be dehydrated	■ Water freely available ■ Subcutaneous fluid therapy	■ Monitor for dehydration
Eating	■ Inappetence, anorexia, vomiting	■ Palatable food if inappetent ■ Renal diet if appetite adequate: introduce early in course of disease	■ Monitor appetite ■ Monitor weight
Urinating	■ Polyuria	■ Water freely available ■ Take out to toilet regularly ■ Change litter frequently	■ Monitor for dehydration

18.33 Nursing considerations for patients with chronic renal failure.

continues ▶

Parameter	Problem	Nursing considerations	Monitoring
Defecating	■ Potential for diarrhoea or developing constipation	■ Take out to toilet regularly	■ Monitor faecal output
Grooming	■ Reduced grooming	■ Keep clean and groom	■ Good hygiene
Other nursing considerations			
■ Prepare patient as required for diagnostic procedures (blood tests for urea, creatinine and electrolyte concentrations, urinalysis, culture and sensitivity testing)			
■ Provision of medication as directed by the veterinary surgeon – monitor for response to treatment and for side effects. Check doses to ensure they are not nephrotoxic			
■ Monitor blood pressure			

18.33 *continued* Nursing considerations for patients with chronic renal failure.

Lower urinary tract disease

The lower urinary tract comprises the ureters, bladder and urethra. Disease of these organs results from inflammation, obstruction or dysfunction.

Definitions
- Cystitis – inflammation of the urinary bladder
- Urinary incontinence – involuntary passing of urine
- Urinary tenesmus – straining to pass urine
- Haematuria – the presence of blood in the urine
- Polyuria – passing of increased volumes of urine
- Dysuria – difficulty and pain passing urine
- Oliguria – reduced urine production
- Anuria – absence of urine production
- Pollakiuria – abnormal frequency of urination passing very small amounts of urine
- Stranguria – painful urination characterized by slow drips of urine

Diagnostics

The following diagnostic tests should be performed for lower urinary tract disorders:

- Blood tests – biochemistry and complete blood count
- Urinalysis – specific gravity, dipsticks, sedimentation examination, culture and sensitivity (urine for this test must be obtained via cystocentesis)
- Abdominal ultrasonography
- Radiography – contrast studies such as pneumocystograms and double-contrast cystograms
- Intravenous excretory urography (IVU)
- Retrograde urethrography
- CT
- Histopathology.

Cystitis

Causes of cystitis include:

- Idiopathic
- Feline lower urinary tract disease (see 'Feline lower urinary tract disease (FLUTD)' below)
- Trauma
- Urolithiasis (see 'Urolithiasis (urinary calculi)' below)
- Neoplasia
- Primary bacterial infection – often ascending, common in female dogs
- Bacterial infection secondary to other diseases (e.g. diabetes mellitus, hyperadrenocorticism (Cushing's disease), immunosuppressive infection such as FIV and FeLV).

Clinical signs
- Pollakiuria.
- Urinary tenesmus.
- Haematuria.
- Stranguria.
- Incontinence.
- Dysuria.
- Inappropriate urination.
- Excessive grooming.

Treatment
- Identification and treatment of any underlying cause.
- Appropriate antibiotic therapy only if a bacterial infection has been diagnosed – bacteria such as *Escherichia coli*, *Staphylococcus*, *Streptococcus* and *Pseudomonas* have all been identified as causal agents.

Nursing care

The nursing considerations for cystitis are detailed in Figure 18.34.

Parameter	Problem	Nursing considerations	Monitoring
Breathing	■ Unlikely to be a problem	■ Regular checks of temperature, pulse and respiration	■ Monitor respiratory rate
Pain	■ Urinary tenesmus	■ Analgesics	■ Monitor for discomfort when urinating and excessive licking of the area
Drinking	■ Likely to be normal	■ Water freely available	■ Monitor fluid intake

18.34 Nursing considerations for patients with cystitis.

continues ▶

Parameter	Problem	Nursing considerations	Monitoring
Eating	■ Likely to be normal, but can be inappetent	■ Cats: prescription diets	■ Monitor food intake
Urination	■ Pollakiuria ■ Haematuria	■ Ensure opportunities to toilet outside ■ Cats: a litter tray should be provided for each cat plus one extra ■ Clean litter tray frequently ■ At home: use strategies to increase drinking (e.g. water fountains) ■ Use wide bowls (so cats do not knock their whiskers) ■ Bacterial culture and sensitivity testing ■ Administration of antibiotics as directed by the veterinary surgeon	■ Monitor urine output: ensure urethral obstruction does not develop ■ Record frequency, volume and haematuria
Defecation	■ Likely to be normal	■ Take out to toilet regularly	■ Monitor faecal output
Grooming	■ May groom excessively	■ Analgesics	■ Good hygiene
Housing	■ Stress	■ Maintain a stress-free environment	■ Monitor behaviour.

18.34 *continued* Nursing considerations for patients with cystitis.

Urolithiasis (urinary calculi)

Urinary calculi or uroliths (see Chapter 17) can form within the urinary tract in the renal pelvis, ureters, bladder or urethra. Causes include:

- Urinary tract infection
- High dietary intake of certain minerals
- Systemic disease (e.g. liver disease)
- Genetic predisposition (e.g. high incidence of urate calculi in Dalmatians).

See also 'Feline lower urinary tract disease (FLUTD)' below.

Clinical signs

- Pollakiuria.
- Urinary tenesmus.
- Haematuria.
- Dysuria.
- Distended bladder.

Treatment

Diet plays a major role in the control and management of some types of urinary calculi (i.e. struvite, urate and cystine) (see Chapter 13). Dietary dissolution of calculi is possible for certain uroliths, but surgical removal is required for others, such as those composed of calcium oxalate or calcium phosphate.

The main goal of treatment is to reduce the patient's urine specific gravity and increase urination. Diet can help prevent the recurrence of calculi after removal. These diets change the urinary pH, make the urine more dilute, and contain lower dietary levels of the minerals that contribute to calculi formation.

If urinary obstruction occurs, the same steps should be followed as for obstructed feline lower urinary tract disease (see 'Feline lower urinary tract disease (FLUTD)' below).

Nursing care

The nursing considerations for urolithiasis are detailed in Figure 18.35.

Parameter	Problem	Nursing considerations	Monitoring
Breathing	■ Unlikely to be a problem	■ Regular checks of temperature, pulse and respiration	■ Monitor breathing
Pain	■ Can have some discomfort	■ Analgesia	■ Monitor for signs of pain
Drinking	■ Normal	■ Encourage increased drinking (e.g. water fountains, ice, increased fluid in food)	■ Monitor hydration
Eating	■ Normal	■ Prescription diets for offending minerals ■ Increase moisture: use tinned or soaked food	■ Monitor urine specific gravity
Urinating	■ Dysuria ■ Haematuria ■ Anuria	■ Increase water intake ■ Take out to toilet regularly	■ Monitor urine output and specific gravity ■ Monitor for straining
Defecating	■ Likely to be normal	■ Take out to toilet regularly	■ Monitor faecal output
Grooming	■ May be excessive around the perineum	■ Analgesia	■ Monitor for trauma
Housing	■ Stress (cats)	■ Ensure the number of litter trays, beds, etc. exceeds the number of cats in the household to reduce stress	■ Monitor stress levels
Mobilizing	■ Likely to be normal	■ Provide regular opportunities to exercise	■ Monitor exercise tolerance

18.35 Nursing considerations for patients with urolithiasis.

Urinary incontinence

Urinary incontinence is the involuntary passing of urine. Leakage of urine may be continuous or intermittent and may occur when the animal is recumbent or standing. Causes include:

- Urethral sphincter mechanism incompetence (USMI)
- Ectopic ureters (congenital; more common in females; ureter often ends in vagina)
- Bladder-neck tumour (transitional cell carcinoma)
- Prostatic disease
- Neurological disease
- Cystitis.

Clinical signs

- Passing of urine when lying down or walking.
- Urine around perineum which can cause urine scalding.

Treatment

Treatment will be specific to the cause, but can include:

- Phenylpropanolamine or oestrogen for sphincter mechanism incompetence. Surgery considered in cases where medical treatment has failed
- Surgery for ectopic ureters
- Surgery with or without chemotherapy for tumours
- Castration or hormone treatments for prostatic hyperplasia
- Antibiotic therapy for bacterial cystitis.

Nursing care

The nursing considerations for urinary incontinence are detailed in Figure 18.36.

Feline lower urinary tract disease (FLUTD)

FLUTD may be obstructive (usually in male cats) or non-obstructive. In many cases the cause is unclear, but FLUTD is commonly seen in overweight, young to middle-aged cats with limited access to outdoors and in multi-cat households. It is likely that the cause of the syndrome is multifactorial. It is thought that these cats have a tendency to urinate less frequently than outdoor cats, resulting in stale urine remaining in the bladder for longer periods, which gives rise to increased precipitation of crystals. Stress is also thought to be a major contributing factor in feline idiopathic cystitis. Research has found that cats with cystitis have reduced levels of glycosaminoglycan (GAG), a component of the bladder membrane.

FLUTD affects both male and female cats, but male cats tend to be affected by obstructive disease due to the narrow size of the urethra in comparison with females. The distal end of the urethra becomes blocked with calculi or clumps of crystals and mucus (urethral plugs).

Causes of FLUTD include:

- Idiopathic (up to 65% of cases)
- Urethral plugs
- Uroliths
- Bacterial infection.

Clinical signs

Clinical signs for both non-obstructive and obstructive FLUTD are as for cystitis (see 'Cystitis', above). With obstructive FLUTD these signs may lead to:

- Distress – vocalizing and signs of abdominal pain
- Anuria
- Distended hard bladder
- Clinical signs of renal damage
- Anorexia and vomiting
- Lethargy and depression
- Dehydration
- Collapse and death if untreated.

Treatment of obstructive FLUTD

Urethral obstruction is a serious life-threatening condition, which requires urgent medical attention.

Parameter	Problem	Nursing considerations	Monitoring
Breathing	■ Unlikely to be a problem	■ Regular checks of temperature, pulse and respiration	■ Monitor for any changes
Pain	■ Unlikely to be painful	■ Provide analgesia if needed	■ Monitor for any changes
Drinking	■ Likely to be normal	■ Ensure water is freely available	■ Monitor hydration
Eating	■ Likely to be normal	■ Normal diet	
Urinating	■ Incontinence	■ Clean bedding regularly/use incontinence pads ■ Ensure urine scald does not develop ■ Use dog diapers	■ Monitor urine output ■ Monitor for cystitis: pollakiuria
Defecating	■ Likely to be normal unless neurological disease present; in which case faecal incontinence can develop	■ Taker out to toilet regularly	■ Monitor faecal output
Grooming	■ Urine scald ■ Urine smell	■ Clean perineum regularly and apply barrier cream if necessary	■ Monitor perineum for urine scald
Housing	■ Soiled bedding	■ Clean regularly	■ Good hygiene
Mobilizing	■ Likely to be normal unless incontinence due to neurological disease	■ Frequent short walks	■ Monitor exercise tolerance

18.36 Nursing considerations for patients with urinary incontinence.

- Blood tests should be performed to assess the patient's metabolic state (urea and creatinine often elevated due to postrenal azotaemia; potassium levels elevated: this can be life-threatening; analysis of blood gases if available).
- Cystocentesis should be performed to empty the bladder or at least alleviate the pressure. This should be done with great caution as the bladder may be friable and prone to tearing. A sample can be taken at this time for urinalysis and culture.
- Intravenous fluid therapy should be initiated to reduce the potassium, improve the azotaemia and rehydrate the patient (a fluid type that does not contain potassium).
- Once the cat is stable it should be sedated or anaesthetized.
- The blockage can then be dislodged; massage of the penis tip or retrograde flushing is often required to pass a urinary catheter, and the bladder should then be flushed with saline.
- The veterinary surgeon will decide whether an indwelling catheter should be left in place, as this can increase the urethral inflammation already present.
- If a urinary catheter is fitted, it should be sutured in place and either plugged or a closed collection system fitted, to prevent ascending bacterial infection. The patient should also be fitted with an Elizabethan collar to prevent interference.

- Antibacterial drugs can be considered after culturing the urine or the catheter once it has been removed.
- Analgesia must be provided.

Nursing care of obstructive FLUTD

The nursing considerations for obstructive FLUTD are detailed in Figure 18.37.

Treatment of non-obstructive FLUTD

- Prescription urinary diet. Some diets promote the acidity or alkalinity of the urine, which can reduce the risk of certain types of urinary calculi. Animal-based protein can help to promote acidic urine, whereas grains can promote a more alkaline urine.
- Increasing water intake will increase urination and dilute the urine, which may be helpful. This can be achieved with a wet food. Use other strategies to increase drinking as for urolithiasis.
- Environmental enrichment and stress reduction; feline pheromones may help in some cases or, in severe chronic cases, antidepressants may be beneficial.
- Analgesics during episodes.
- Dietary supplements.
- Weight reduction and increasing exercise.

Parameter	Problem	Nursing considerations	Monitoring
Breathing and cardiovascular system	■ Life-threatening complications ■ Bradycardia due to hyperkalaemia is possible	■ Intravenous fluid therapy to reduce potassium concentration as necessary	■ Monitor vital signs ■ Monitor blood potassium levels ■ Monitor electrocardiogram
Pain	■ Pain likely	■ Analgesics	■ Pain assessment scoring
Drinking	■ Reduced intake as a result of anaesthesia ■ Increased drinking after obstruction relieved	■ Intravenous fluid therapy Long-term management: ■ Water freely available ■ Use large shallow bowls (so the cat's whiskers do not touch the sides), water fountains. Place in multiple areas where the cat feels safe	■ Monitor blood pressure ■ Monitor hydration
Eating	■ Inappetence, anorexia, vomiting	■ May have an Elizabethan collar if catheterized. Remove this under supervision while offering palatable food Long-term management: ■ Diet: prescription urinary diet ■ Increase fluid intake – use tinned or moistened food ■ Weight reduction diet if overweight	■ Monitor weight
Urinating	■ Anuria	■ Placement of urinary catheter as required Long-term management: ■ Encourage elimination; provide several litter trays, cleaned regularly. Keep litter trays in quiet, safe areas of the house with privacy ■ Access to outside	■ Monitor and record frequency and volume of urine output
Defecating	■ Likely to be normal	■ Take out to toilet regularly	■ Monitor faecal output
Grooming	■ Poor	■ May have an Elizabethan collar. Remove under supervision ■ Keep clean and groom	■ Good hygiene
Housing	■ Stress	■ Minimize stress and changes to routine ■ Ensure the number of litter trays, beds, etc. exceeds the number of cats in the household to reduce stress ■ Avoid multi-cat households	■ Good hygiene ■ Monitor stress

18.37 Nursing considerations for patients with obstructive FLUTD.

Prostatic disease

The prostate can be affected by:

- Benign prostatic hyperplasia (BPH)
- Prostatitis
- Prostatic abscessation
- Prostatic cysts
- Prostatic neoplasia (rare).

Clinical signs

- Haematuria.
- Dysuria.
- Urinary incontinence.
- Urinary and faecal tenesmus.
- Constipation.

Diagnostics

- Ultrasonography.
- Radiography.
- Urinalysis (haematuria, leucocyturia and bacteriuria).
- Prostatic massage/flushing/biopsy.
- Blood tests – complete blood count and biochemistry.

Treatment

- BPH is treated by neutering (castration) or hormone treatment.
- Prostatitis is treated as for BPH plus antibiotics following culture and sensitivity.
- Surgical intervention is required for cysts and abcessation.
- Palliative treatment for neoplasia.

Nursing care

The nursing considerations for geriatric patients, including those with prostate disease, are covered in Chapter 15.

Reproductive system disease

Diseases of the reproductive system are discussed in detail in Chapter 24.

Endocrine and metabolic disorders

Hormones are made and secreted by various endocrine glands and the functions of those hormones are described in Chapter 3.

Diabetes mellitus

Diabetes mellitus is caused by the lack of insulin, or a relative lack of insulin. Insulin is required to regulate glucose in the body. In the absence of insulin, the animal will become hyperglycaemic. Clinical signs are attributable to this.

In the majority of dogs, the condition is caused by immune destruction of the insulin-producing cells in the pancreas (similar to type 1 diabetes in humans). Dogs generally require insulin therapy for treatment. In cats, diabetes is often a result of insulin resistance due to obesity (similar to type 2 diabetes in humans). These cats may produce insulin but the cells do not respond adequately. Cats are also treated with insulin. Cats may go into remission but generally develop diabetes again. Insulin resistance can also be seen in entire bitches, in hyperadrenocorticism (Cushing's disease) and pancreatitis. If diabetes is left untreated, fats are broken down, leading to a build-up of ketones. These patients quickly become dehydrated, are acidotic and have electrolyte abnormalities. This condition is called diabetic ketoacidosis (DKA).

Clinical signs

The majority of cases present with a history of:

- Polyuria/polydipsia
- Increased appetite (polyphagia) with weight loss.

More serious clinical signs that may indicate that the animal has developed DKA include:

- Vomiting
- Diarrhoea
- Anorexia
- Weight loss
- Depression
- Collapse.

Other clinical signs include:

- Cataracts in dogs
- Plantigrade posture in cats.

Diagnostics

- Blood – complete blood count and biochemistry (plus fructosamine levels).
- Urinalysis – dipstick, especially for the presence of glucose and ketones, culture and sensitivity testing.

Treatment

- Treatment involves the subcutaneous administration of insulin.
- Caninsulin® is the insulin of choice in dogs. It is a porcine lente insulin (40 IU/ml). Cats require longer-acting insulins and ProZinc® is the treatment of choice for cats in the UK. Insulin glargine may be used overseas. Generally, insulin is administered to dogs and cats twice daily. Note: volumes of insulin given are very small. Insulin syringes are used and the units are 'International Units (IU)'.
- Patients undergoing anaesthesia should have their glucose levels measured on the morning of the surgery and insulin given as directed by the veterinary surgeon. Blood glucose levels should be monitored during anaesthesia, and dextrose saline administered intravenously as necessary.
- If there is insulin resistance, the underlying cause must be treated in order to control the blood glucose levels (e.g. treat hyperadrenocorticism; neuter a diabetic bitch).
- Stabilization – the correct insulin dose is determined and a suitable daily routine for the pet and owner is established.
- Maintenance – the pet is monitored regularly to follow the progression of its diabetes and thus determine changes in insulin requirements.

The diabetic ketoacidotic patient

DKA is a life-threatening condition and needs intensive treatment.

- Fluid therapy to rehydrate the patient and correct acidosis and electrolyte imbalances.
- A short-acting human neutral (soluble) insulin is given intravenously or intramuscularly to lower blood glucose. This allows the glucose level to be lowered in a controlled manner.
- Glucose, electrolytes and phosphate are monitored frequently and treatment adjusted as directed by the veterinary surgeon. Potassium and phosphate can both become very low.

Further information on diabetic ketoacidosis is given in Chapter 19.

The 'well' diabetic dog

It is very important that patients follow a routine in their insulin administration, diet and exercise. The routine should be adapted to the owner's lifestyle and can be flexible, to a degree.

- Insulin therapy – type, dose rate and frequency (usually twice daily) will be decided by the veterinary surgeon. Note that insulin preparations authorized for veterinary use are usually 100 IU/ml or 40 IU/ml and it is important to use the correct syringe for the particular type of insulin being administered. Insulin 'pens', similar to those used in the management of diabetes in humans, are now available for dogs and cats (e.g. VetPen®).
- Diet – a high-fibre, medium-protein, low-fat diet should be provided.
  - If the patient is receiving once-daily insulin, feed the first meal when the insulin is administered and the second meal 6–8 hours later to coincide with lowest glucose point.
  - If the patient is receiving twice-daily insulin, meals are given at the time of insulin administration, usually every 12 hours.
- Exercise – same time and amount every day.

The 'well' diabetic cat

It is very important that patients follow a routine in their insulin administration, diet and exercise. The routine should be adapted to the owner's lifestyle and can be flexible, to a degree. Note that this is harder to achieve in cats compared with dogs.

- Insulin therapy:
  - ProZinc® (or other type of insulin) administered as per veterinary surgeon's instructions. Usually administered twice daily.
- Insulin therapy can be discontinued in some cats with non-insulin-dependent diabetes if they go into remission.
- Glucose is monitored closely for hypoglycaemia.
- Diet – high-protein or high fibre/low carbohydrate, *ad libitum* (see Chapter 13) or twice daily to coincide with insulin (as for dogs above).
- Exercise – as per usual.

Long-term monitoring

The diabetic patient is monitored by owner observations (appetite, water consumption, urine output, weight control, exercise routine) and blood tests. The insulin is adjusted on the basis of a combination of these findings.

- Serial blood glucose curves – these curves indicate how long the insulin is effective for and the time the lowest glucose level occurs. Blood is usually taken every 2 hours over a 24-hour period and the glucose level plotted on a graph (Figure 18.38). For example, the action of Caninsulin® on blood glucose concentrations, following subcutaneous administration, peaks in diabetic

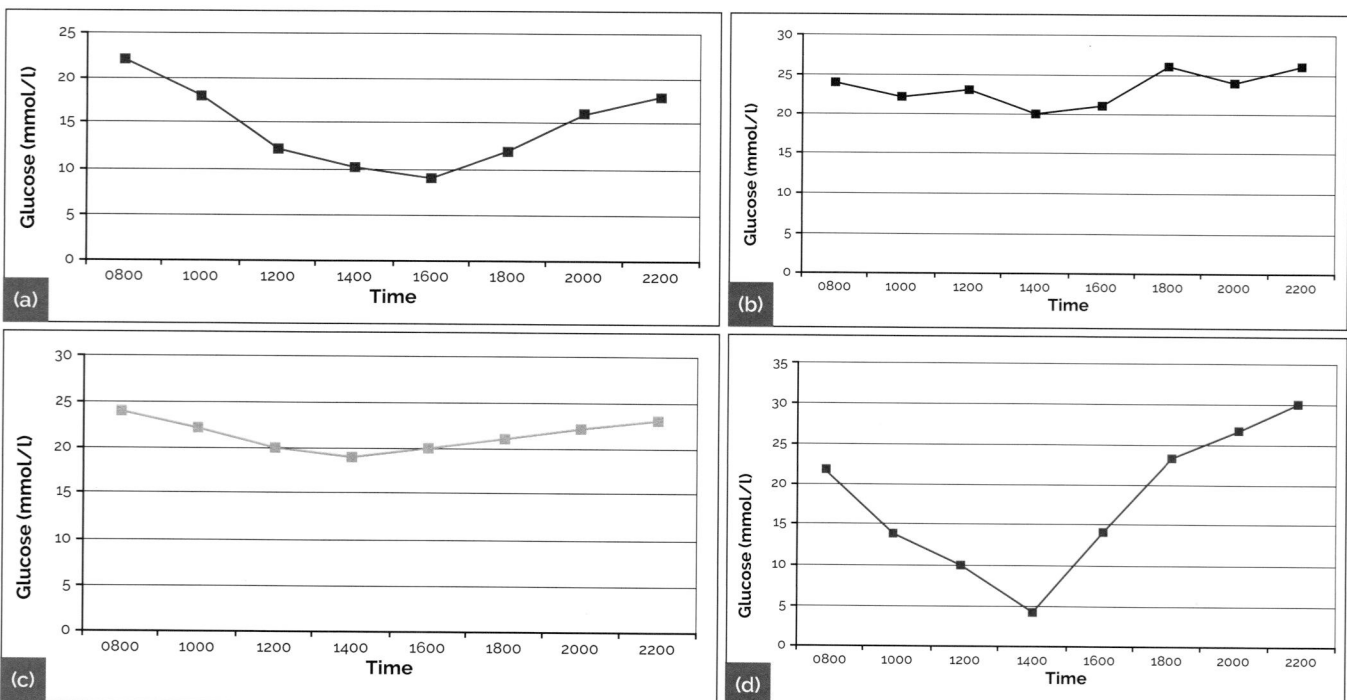

18.38 Blood glucose curves in diabetic cats. **(a)** Appropriate response to insulin. **(b)** Minimal response to insulin, insulin resistance or stress hyperglycaemia. **(c)** Inadequate response to insulin. **(d)** Rapid decline in glucose concentration in response to insulin with marked rebound (Somogyi overswing). (Reproduced from the *BSAVA Manual of Canine and Feline Endocrinology, 4th edn*)

dogs at approximately 6–8 hours following the injection and lasts for about 14–24 hours; in diabetic cats it peaks at approximately 4–6 hours following the injection and lasts for about 8–12 hours. Blood collection should follow as normal a routine as possible, with minimal stress to the patient, as stress causes hyperglycaemia (this is especially important in cats).

- Continuous blood glucose monitoring is becoming more commonly available.
- Urinalysis to monitor for ketones, glucose and developing urinary tract infections.
- Fructosamine: indication of blood glucose control over 2–3 weeks.

Urine glucose monitoring and subsequent adjustment of insulin by the owner is not recommended, as urine glucose can be misleading. The presence of glucose in the urine can be a result of underdosing with insulin but can also be as a result of overdosing in the case of insulin-induced hyperglycaemia (see below).

Hyperglycaemia

Hyperglycaemia in diabetic patients most commonly results from underdosing with insulin or poor control of diabetes due to other medical conditions (e.g. hyperadrenocorticism, infections). Hyperglycaemia can also confusingly arise as a result of overdosing with insulin. The reason for this is a compensatory mechanism called the Somogyi overswing (see Figure 18.38). This results from a normal physiological response to hypoglycaemia induced by excessive insulin. When the blood glucose level drops to below 3.3 mmol/l or falls very quickly (note: it is not only the level it falls to, but also the rate at which it falls), several important protective hormones are released (the 'diabetogenic' hormones). These are catecholamines, cortisol, growth hormone and glucagons. Glucose levels will often rise above normal levels subsequent to their release. The animal persists with diabetic signs because the majority of the 24-hour cycle is spent with high glucose levels. The typical clinical response (based on clinical signs alone without glucose curve

information) is to raise the insulin dose. This results in an even more severe drop, an even more vigorous endocrine response and an even higher overswing hyperglycaemia. The correct course of action to take in these cases is to reduce the dose of insulin. Thus, if a patient is found to have an unexpected increase in blood or urine glucose prior to the administration of the morning insulin, it may be an indication to perform a serial blood glucose curve or other diagnostic tests.

Hypoglycaemia

Hypoglycaemia is a complication that occurs as a result of an insulin overdose. Clinical signs include:

- Lethargy
- Ataxia
- Muscle twitching
- Severe seizures.

It is most likely to occur at the time of peak activity of the insulin. Immediate action must be taken, which may involve feeding, rubbing honey or glucose on the gums, or administering intravenous dextrose (as directed by veterinary surgeon). If left untreated, coma and death will ensue.

Nursing care

Uncomplicated diabetes mellitus

The nursing considerations for uncomplicated diabetes mellitus are detailed in Figure 18.39.

Diabetic ketoacidosis

The nursing considerations for diabetic ketoacidosis are detailed in Figure 18.40.

Nutrition

Successful management of a diabetic patient involves an appropriate dietary regime as well as insulin therapy (see Chapter 13).

Parameter	Problem	Nursing considerations	Monitoring
Breathing/ vital signs	■ Unlikely to be a problem in uncomplicated diabetes mellitus cases but the patient has potential to become complicated	■ Regular checks of temperature, pulse and respiration	■ Monitor respiratory rate ■ Monitor heart rate
Pain	■ Unlikely to be painful	■ Provide analgesia if needed	■ Monitor for signs of pain
Drinking	■ Polydipsia	■ Ensure water is available at all times	■ Monitor and record water intake; a decrease indicates better control ■ Monitor for dehydration
Eating	■ Polyphagia	■ Ensure diet is consistent: type, amount and feeding times ■ Dogs: usually fed twice daily with insulin ■ Cats: fed ad lib or as for dogs ■ See text for recommended diet	■ Monitor weight, appetite and for vomiting ■ Avoid obesity
Urinating	■ Polyuria	■ Ensure regular opportunities to urinate to prevent soiling bedding	■ Monitor urine output ■ Monitor urine for ketones
Defecating	■ Unlikely to be a problem	■ Take out to toilet	■ Monitor faecal output

18.39 Nursing considerations for patients with uncomplicated diabetes mellitus.

continues ▶

Parameter	Problem	Nursing considerations	Monitoring
Grooming	■ Unlikely to be a problem	■ Keep clean and groom	■ Good hygiene
Mobilizing	■ Weakness; plantigrade in cats ■ Lethargy	■ Exercise routine: same exercise each day	■ Monitor for excessive lethargy, which may indicate hypoglycaemia

Other nursing considerations

- Prepare patient as required for diagnostic procedures (blood glucose curve or continuous glucose monitoring; urinalysis to monitor ketone concentrations)
- Provision of insulin (twice daily) as directed by the veterinary surgeon – monitor for hypoglycaemia and ketonuria (see also Chapter 8)
- Owner support and instructions – caring for an animal with diabetes mellitus is often a scary prospect for owners
  - Spend time teaching the owners how to store and administer the insulin prior to discharge
  - Suggest owners keep a diary to monitor clinical signs such as drinking, urinating, eating, behaviour, weight and response to treatment
  - Advise owners on how to monitor for side effects, including lethargy and collapse due to hypoglycaemia
  - Advise owners to discuss neutering of bitches with the veterinary surgeon
  - Provide written discharge instructions
  - Follow up with regular phone calls

18.39 *continued* Nursing considerations for patients with uncomplicated diabetes mellitus.

Parameter	Problem	Nursing considerations	Monitoring
Breathing/vital signs	■ Increased respiratory rate as acidotic ■ Heart rate variable	■ Intravenous fluid therapy and electrolyte supplementation	■ Monitor respiratory rate ■ Monitor heart rate ■ Monitor blood electrolyte concentrations ■ Blood tests
Pain	■ Unlikely to be a problem	■ Provide analgesia if needed	■ Monitor for signs of pain
Drinking	■ Polydipsia ■ Dehydration	■ Ensure water is available at all times ■ Intravenous fluid therapy to correct acidosis and electrolyte abnormalities, reduce glucose and rehydrate. If the patient's glucose becomes too low, dextrose may need to be added to the fluids	■ Monitor and record water intake ■ Monitor dehydration ■ Monitor glucose and electrolyte concentrations
Eating	■ Vomiting	■ Tempt with palatable food. Once appetite has improved, transition on to long-term diet	■ Monitor weight, appetite and for vomiting
Urinating	■ Polyuria	■ Ensure regular opportunities to urinate to prevent soiling bedding	■ Monitor urine output ■ Monitor urine for ketones
Defecating	■ Diarrhoea	■ Take out to toilet	■ Monitor faecal output
Grooming	■ May not be grooming	■ Keep clean and groom	■ Good hygiene
Housing	■ Normal	■ Change litter trays frequently	■ Good hygiene
Mobilizing	■ Weakness; plantigrade in cats ■ Lethargy	■ Take out to toilet only	■ Monitor exercise tolerance

Other nursing considerations

- Prepare patient as required for diagnostic procedures (blood glucose, electrolyte and fructosamine (may not be important in DKA cases) concentrations; urinalysis to monitor ketone concentrations)
- Provision of medication, including insulin (note type, amount and frequency) and antiemetics as directed by the veterinary surgeon
- Monitor blood glucose and electrolyte concentrations – note that management is adjusted according to these results

18.40 Nursing considerations for patients with diabetic ketoacidosis.

Hyperadrenocorticism (HAC) (Cushing's disease)

Hyperadrenocorticism is common in the dog but rare in the cat. It occurs as a result of excessive cortisol in the body. This may be due to excessive administration of steroid medication or an overproduction of cortisol by the adrenal glands. The latter is a result of either a tumour in the pituitary gland (pituitary-dependent HAC), which overstimulates the adrenal glands to produce cortisol, or a tumour of the adrenal gland (adrenal-dependent HAC). Pituitary-dependent HAC is the most common form.

Clinical signs

- Polyuria/polydipsia.
- Polyphagia.
- Pot-belly (Figure 18.41).
- Panting.
- Bilateral alopecia and skin changes (thin inelastic skin).
- Muscle atrophy and weakness.

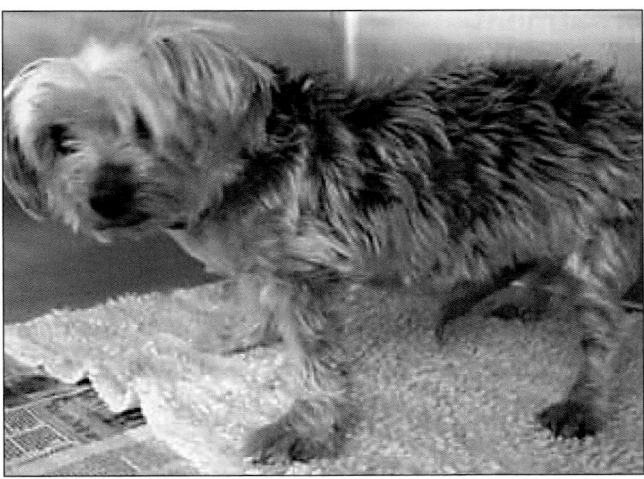

18.41 A dog with hyperadrenocorticism. Note the pot-bellied appearance.

Diagnostics

- Blood tests – complete blood count and biochemistry.
- Adrenocorticotrophic hormone (ACTH) stimulation test.
- Low-dose dexamethasone suppression test (LDDST).
- High-dose dexamethasone suppression test (HDDST).
- Endogenous ACTH assay.
- Abdominal ultrasonography.
- Abdominal radiography.
- MRI or CT (pituitary and adrenal areas).

The ACTH stimulation and LDDST are confirmatory tests. The HDDST and endogenous ACTH assay are used to differentiate between pituitary-dependent and adrenal-dependent HAC (see Chapter 17).

Treatment

Pituitary-dependent HAC is treated medically. Trilostane (veterinary licensed product) is the first-line medication. Mitotane (human-licensed product) may be administered if there are complications with trilostane. Adrenal tumours can be treated with drugs or by surgical removal.

Nursing care

The nursing considerations for hyperadrenocorticism are detailed in Figure 18.42.

Hypoadrenocorticism (Addison's disease)

Hypoadrenocorticism is a reduction in, or failure of, steroid production by the adrenals. This usually occurs as a result of immune destruction of the adrenal gland, but may also be a consequence of treating hyperadrenocorticism. Hypoadrenocorticism causes electrolyte imbalances, hypo-natraemia (low sodium), hyperkalaemia (high potassium) and dehydration. The hyperkalaemia can be life-threatening and must be treated promptly.

Clinical signs

Clinical signs are often initially vague and wax and wane; they include lethargy and inappetence. In the untreated patient this will progress to:

- Anorexia
- Vomiting
- Haemorrhagic diarrhoea

Parameter	Problem	Nursing considerations	Monitoring
Breathing	■ Rare for this to be a problem	■ Regular checks for temperature, pulse and respiration	■ Monitor respiratory rate
Pain	■ Unlikely to be a problem	■ Provide analgesia if needed	■ Monitor for signs of pain
Drinking	■ Polydipsia	■ Ensure water is available at all times	■ Monitor and record water intake; a decrease indicates better control
Eating	■ Polyphagia	■ Normal diet	■ Monitor weight ■ Reduced appetite is seen with response to treatment
Urinating	■ Polyuria	■ Ensure regular opportunities to urinate to prevent soiling bedding	■ Monitor urine output
Defecating	■ Unlikely to be a problem	■ Take out to toilet	■ Monitor faecal output
Grooming	■ Unlikely to be a problem	■ Keep clean and groom	■ Monitor for hair loss
Mobilizing	■ Exercise intolerance	■ Exercise according to the tolerance of the patient	■ Monitor for excessive panting and muscle weakness

Other nursing considerations

- Prepare patient as required for diagnostic procedures (blood tests). Minimize stress as this can interfere with results. Apply pressure to the venepuncture site and monitor for bruising
- Provision of medication as directed by the veterinary surgeon – monitor for vomiting, diarrhoea and poor appetite; contact veterinary surgeon if this occurs
- Monitor blood cortisol concentrations
- Owner support and instructions
  - Suggest owners keep a diary to monitor clinical signs such as drinking, urinating, eating, behaviour and weight
  - Advise owners on how to monitor for lethargy and gastrointestinal signs. It is important that the owner contacts the clinic if this occurs
  - Advise owners on how to monitor for side effects to medication, including collapse, vomiting and diarrhoea
  - Provide written discharge instructions
  - Follow up with regular phone calls

18.42 Nursing considerations for patients with hyperadrenocorticism.

- Hypotension
- Weakness
- Bradycardia (see Figure 18.43)
- Collapse.

Diagnostics

- Blood tests – complete blood count and biochemistry (sodium:potassium ratio reveals low levels of sodium and high levels of potassium).
- ACTH stimulation test (protocol as for hyperadrenocorticism).
- ECG (Figure 18.43).

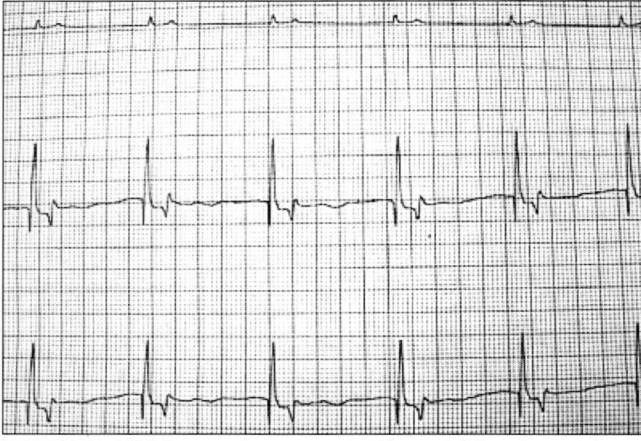

| 18.43 | ECG from a dog presented in an Addisonian crisis. There is bradycardia and no P waves are evident. |

Treatment

An acute crisis is an emergency. Treatment involves fluid therapy at shock rates to reduce the potassium level and rehydrate the hypovolaemic patient (see Chapter 20). Intravenous corticosteroids are administered. In the stable patient, glucocorticoids (prednisolone) and mineralocorticoids (desoxycortone pivalate, DOCP) are administered. Treatment is monitored by measuring the sodium:potassium ratio.

Nursing care

The nursing considerations for hypoadrenocorticism are detailed in Figure 18.44.

Hyperthyroidism

Patients with hyperthyroidism have an overactive thyroid gland usually as a result of benign hyperplasia (increased production of cells). There is overproduction of thyroxine (T4) that increases the metabolic rate. This is a common condition in the older cat but rare in dogs.

Clinical signs

- Polyphagia with weight loss.
- Emaciation.
- Aggression and hyperactivity.
- Heart murmur and tachycardia.
- Polyuria/polydipsia.
- Vomiting and diarrhoea.
- Depression.
- Weakness.

Parameter	Problem	Nursing considerations	Monitoring
Breathing/ vital signs	■ Potential for bradycardia ■ Shock	■ Intravenous fluid therapy to address hypovolaemia, hypotension, dehydration and hyperkalaemia. Saline (low potassium) is indicated	■ Monitor heart rate ■ Monitor electrocardiogram ■ Monitor blood pressure ■ Monitor blood electrolyte concentrations, particularly potassium
Pain	■ Unlikely to be painful	■ Provide analgesia if required	■ Monitor for signs of pain
Drinking	■ Reduced initially due to shock and vomiting	■ Intravenous fluid therapy ■ Water freely available once patient no longer collapsed	■ Monitor for dehydration
Eating	■ Reduced initially ■ Vomiting	■ Tempt to eat after the initial crisis. Appetite should improve quickly	■ Monitor and record appetite
Urinating	■ May be increased or reduced	■ Patient may be recumbent initially and will need to be monitored for soiled bedding	■ Monitor and record urine output
Defecating	■ May have diarrhoea	■ Patient may be recumbent initially and will need to be monitored for soiled bedding	■ Monitor and record faecal output
Grooming	■ May not be grooming	■ Keep clean and dry	■ Good hygiene
Housing	■ Intensive case	■ Intensive care: close monitoring required	■ Good hygiene
Mobilizing	■ Collapsed initially	■ Intravenous fluids will improve shock and animal should recover quickly	■ Monitor exercise tolerance

Other nursing considerations

- Monitor clinical signs and electrolyte concentrations
- Owner support and instructions
  - Important medication is administered for life
  - Advise owners to seek veterinary assistance if the animal's condition deteriorates
  - Advise owners that more medication may be required if there is a stressful event

| 18.44 | Nursing considerations for patients with hypoadrenocorticism. |

Diagnostics

- Blood tests – complete blood count, biochemistry and total T4.

Treatment

Treatment involves administration of thiamazole (methimazole) or carbimazole, a prescription diet, radioactive iodine or thyroidectomy. Treatment is monitored by measuring T4 levels.

Nursing care

The nursing considerations for hyperthyroidism are detailed in Figure 18.45.

Hypothyroidism

Patients with hypothyroidism have an underactive thyroid gland. There is decreased production of thyroxine (T4) as a result of atrophy or lymphocytic infiltration of the thyroid gland. This results in a decreased metabolic rate. It is most common in middle-aged dogs and rare in the cat. It is occasionally seen in cats after thyroidectomy.

Clinical signs

- Lethargy, exercise intolerance.
- Obesity.
- Bradycardia, hypothermia.
- Dermatological abnormalities – alopecia, seborrhoea, hyperpigmentation and pyoderma.

Diagnostics

- Blood tests – complete blood count and biochemistry.
- Total T4, free T4 and thyroid-stimulating hormone (TSH) assay.
- Treatment trial.

Treatment

Supplement thyroxine (levothyroxine). Treatment is monitored by measuring T4 levels and observing clinical signs.

Nursing care

The nursing considerations for hypothyroidism are detailed in Figure 18.46.

Parameter	Problem	Nursing considerations	Monitoring
Breathing/ vital signs	■ Tachycardia, potential heart failure	■ Treat underlying disease ■ Heart failure	■ Monitor sleeping respiratory rate ■ Monitor heart rate
Pain	■ Unlikely to be painful	■ Provide analgesia if required	■ Monitor for signs of pain
Drinking	■ Potentially increased	■ Free access to water	■ Monitor hydration
Eating	■ Increased	■ Normal diet unless treated with low iodine prescription diet	■ Monitor weight
Urinating	■ Potentially increased	■ Provide litter trays and clean regularly	■ Record urine output frequency
Defecating	■ Potentially diarrhoea	■ Provide litter trays	■ Monitor weight
Grooming	■ Poor coat	■ Clean and groom as necessary. Although may be fractious and patience likely required	■ Good hygiene

Other nursing considerations

- Prepare patient as required for diagnostic procedures (T4 and renal (urea and creatinine) blood tests)
- Provision of medication as directed by the veterinary surgeon – monitor for side effects and response to treatment (T4 and renal (urea and creatinine) blood tests)
- Implement surgical nursing protocols and monitor for hypocalcaemia
- Implement radioactive iodine nursing protocols
- Diet
- Owner support and instructions
  - Spend time teaching the owners how to administer medication
  - Advise owners how to monitor for adverse side effects
  - Advise owners that regular blood tests will be required

18.45 Nursing considerations for patients with hyperthyroidism.

Parameter	Problem	Nursing considerations	Monitoring
Breathing	■ Unlikely to be a problem	■ Regular checks of temperature, pulse and respiration	■ Monitor vital signs
Pain	■ Unlikely to be a problem	■ Provide analgesia if required	■ Monitor for signs of pain
Drinking	■ Unlikely to be a problem	■ Ensure that water is freely available	■ Monitor fluid intake
Eating	■ Unlikely to be a problem	■ Normal diet	■ Monitor weight; avoid obesity
Urinating	■ Unlikely to be a problem	■ Take out to toilet	■ Monitor urine output
Defecating	■ Unlikely to be a problem	■ Take out to toilet	■ Monitor faecal output

18.46 Nursing considerations for patients with hypothyroidism.

continues ▶

Parameter	Problem	Nursing considerations	Monitoring
Grooming	■ Poor coat and other dermatological problems	■ Clean and groom patient as necessary	■ Good hygiene
Housing	■ Unlikely to be a problem	■ Keep clean	■ Good hygiene
Mobilizing	■ Exercise intolerance	■ Gentle exercise	■ Monitor exercise tolerance
Other nursing considerations			
■ Provision of medication (i.e. thyroxine) as directed by the veterinary surgeon – monitor clinical signs and T4 concentrations via regular blood tests			

18.46 *continued* Nursing considerations for patients with hypothyroidism.

Hypercalcaemia

Calcium is required for many functions in the body. It is regulated in the body by vitamin D, which is ingested and metabolized in the kidneys, and parathyroid hormone (PTH) produced in the parathyroid gland (Figure 18.47). Increased vitamin D and PTH will increase the calcium in the body. There are other substances that are able to increase calcium in the body and they are released in certain disease states. In excess, calcium can cause renal failure and death.

Differential diagnoses

- Neoplasia (e.g. lymphoma see above, Figure 18.48).
- Primary hyperparathyroidism.
- Vitamin D toxicity (e.g. some toxic rat baits).
- Renal failure (see 'Chronic renal failure').

Clinical signs

- Polyuria and polydipsia.
- Anorexia, lethargy and weakness.
- Vomiting and diarrhoea.
- Tremors.

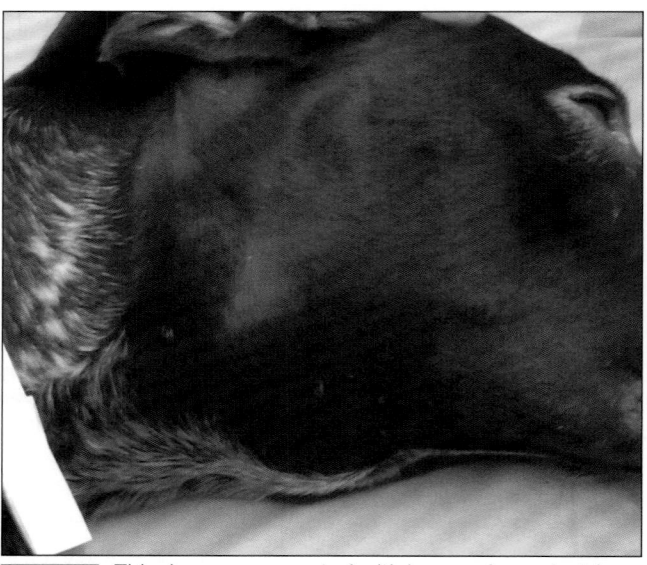

18.48 This dog was presented with hypercalcaemia. It has enlarged submandibular lymph nodes and was diagnosed with lymphoma.

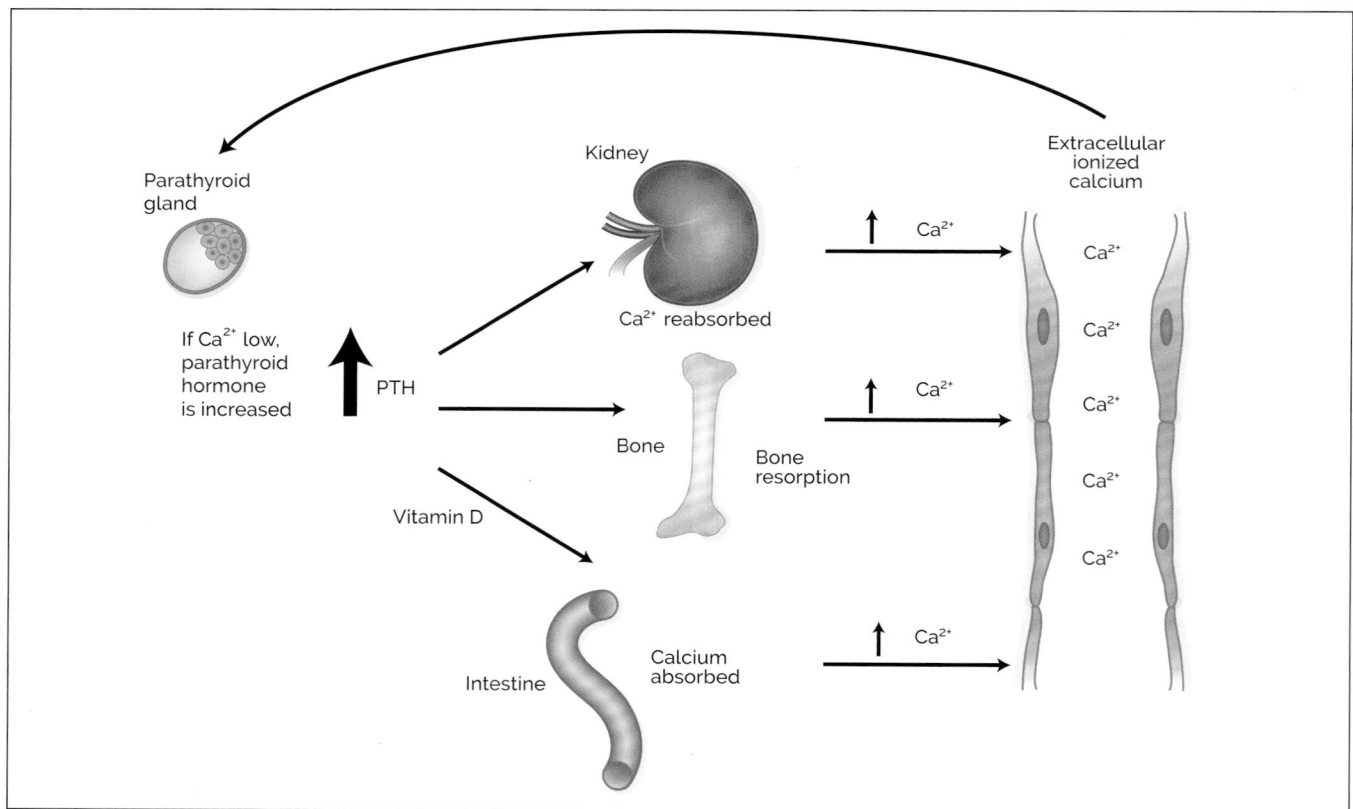

18.47 Calcium regulation in the body. Low calcium: PTH production rises; calcium absorbed by the intestine and kidney. High calcium: PTH production decreases; calcium lost in urine and taken up by bones.

Diagnostics

- Blood tests – complete blood count and biochemistry (total calcium and ionized calcium).
- Urinalysis – specific gravity, dipstick and sediment.
- Fine-needle aspiration of a lymph node to rule out lymphoma.
- Radiography.
- Ultrasonography.
- PTH assay and parathyroid-related protein assay to diagnose occult tumours.

Treatment

Hypercalcaemia should be treated promptly to decrease risk of permanent renal damage. Patients should be placed on intravenous fluids. Once a diagnosis has been made, the underlying cause should be treated (e.g. chemotherapy for lymphoma; parathyroidectomy for primary hyperparathyroidism). After surgery for primary hyperparathyroidism the patient should be monitored for hypocalcaemia. Clinical signs of hypocalcaemia include tremors, seizures and facial rubbing.

Nursing care

The nursing considerations for hypercalcaemia are detailed in Figure 18.49.

Diabetes insipidus

Diabetes insipidus (DI) disease is caused by an impairment in the production of ADH (antidiuretic hormone/vasopressin) or a failure in response. The animal produces large quantities of dilute urine with a compensatory polydipsia. The condition may be referred to as water diabetes. Animals are normally well in all other aspects.

There are two forms of diabetes insipidus:

- Central DI – a deficiency in ADH produced by the pituitary, thought to be either congenital or as a result of damage to the hypothalamus (e.g. tumours, head trauma)
- Nephrogenic DI – failure of the collecting tubules in the nephrons to respond to ADH. A primary problem is very rare.

Normally, ADH controls the water balance within the body by concentrating the urine. If the animal's water intake is decreased, the body will respond by producing more ADH and this will then stimulate the collecting tubules to retain water, preserving the body's water balance.

Clinical signs

- Marked polyuria.
- Marked polydipsia.
- Vomiting after drinking large amounts.
- Weight loss due to poor appetite, due to constant thirst.

Diagnostics

- Blood tests – complete blood count and biochemistry (normal).
- Urinalysis – specific gravity (<1.009).
- Water deprivation test (note: this test in becoming more controversial and some veterinary surgeons are moving away from performing it for the diagnosis of DI).
- Desmopressin test.

Protocols for water deprivation test and desmopressin test

Prior to starting this test, the patient should be well hydrated and have a normal blood urea level. The test should only be performed under close observation.

1. Empty the bladder and measure urine specific gravity.
2. Weigh animal and calculate 5% of its bodyweight.
3. Place animal in a kennel with no access to food or water.
4. Empty bladder every hour, check specific gravity and weigh the animal.
5. Once 5% of the animal's bodyweight has been lost, stop the test.
6. Normal result: specific gravity >1.025. If specific gravity is <1.020, suspect DI.

Once rehydrated, repeat as above but give desmopressin injection or drops.

- Increased urine specific gravity = central DI.
- No change in specific gravity = nephrogenic DI.

Treatment
Central DI

Desmopressin acetate (DDAVP) is a vasopressin analogue. Formulations available incluse intranasal, metered spray, injectable solution and tablets. It can be administered intravenously, intramuscularly, orally, intranasally or topically directly on to the conjunctiva.

Nursing care

The nursing considerations for diabetes insipidus are detailed in Figure 18.50.

Parameter	Problem	Nursing considerations	Monitoring
Breathing/vital signs	■ Unlikely to be a problem	■ Regular checks of temperature, pulse and respiration	■ Monitor vital signs
Pain	■ Unlikely to be a problem	■ Provide analgesia if needed	■ Monitor for signs of pain
Drinking	■ Polydipsia	■ Water freely available ■ Intravenous fluid therapy with saline for diuresis	■ Monitor blood concentrations of calcium, urea and creatinine
Eating	■ Inappetent ■ Vomiting	■ Offer palatable food ■ Antiemetics	■ Monitor food intake
Urinating	■ Polyuria	■ Take out to toilet regularly	■ Record urine output frequency
Defecating	■ Potentially diarrhoea	■ Take out to toilet regularly	■ Monitor faecal output
Grooming	■ Polyuria/polydipsia ■ Potential soiled bedding	■ Groom and clean as necessary	■ Good hygiene
Mobilizing	■ May have weakness	■ Assist on walks	■ Monitor exercise tolerance

18.49 Nursing considerations for patients with hypercalcaemia.

Parameter	Problem	Nursing considerations	Monitoring
Breathing	■ Unlikely to be a problem	■ Regular checks of temperature, pulse and respiration	■ Monitor for vital and clinical signs
Drinking	■ Polydipsia	■ Ensure that water is freely available (except during the water deprivation test)	■ Monitor for dehydration
Urinating	■ Polyuria ■ Decreased if dehydrated	■ Take out to toilet regularly	■ Monitor urine output
Defecating	■ Occasional house soiling	■ Take out to toilet regularly	■ Monitor faecal output
Grooming	■ Poor hair coat	■ Clean and groom patient as necessary	■ Good hygiene
Other nursing considerations			
■ Prepare patient as required for diagnostic procedures ■ Provision of medication as directed by the veterinary surgeon			

18.50 Nursing considerations for patients with diabetes insipidus.

Nervous system disease

Definitions

- Convulsions – a series of involuntary contractions of the muscles
- Seizures – clinical manifestation of a paroxysmal cerebral disorder resulting from a transitory disturbance of brain function due to abnormal electrical activity
- Epilepsy – an intracranial disorder that produces recurrent seizures
- Status epilepticus – life-threatening series of epileptic spasms without intervals of consciousness
- Paresis – weakness of one or more limbs
- Hemiplegia – paralysis of one side of the body
- Paraplegia – paralysis of the caudal limbs
- Tetraplegia – paralysis of all four limbs

Clinical signs of nervous system disease include:

- Cerebral:
  - Behaviour changes
  - Ataxia
  - Circling
  - Pacing
  - Seizures
  - Weakness.
- Cerebellar:
  - Ataxia
  - Tremors
  - Dysmetria
  - Hypermetria
  - Head tilt
  - Nystagmus.
- Spinal:
  - Abnormal spinal reflexes
  - Weakness
  - Paresis/paralysis
  - Faecal/urinary incontinence.

Seizures

Differential diagnoses

Seizures can result from abnormalities within or outside the brain. Causes within the brain include:

- Idiopathic epilepsy
- Brain tumours
- Head trauma
- Infections (e.g. canine distemper)
- Congenital abnormalities (e.g. hydrocephalus).

Causes outside the brain include:

- Metabolic (e.g. hypoglycaemia, hypocalcaemia, hepatic encephalopathy, uraemia)
- Toxins (e.g. chocolate, permethrin flea collars in cats).

Idiopathic epilepsy is more likely to occur in dogs under 3 years of age. Most brain tumours are more common in the older animal.

Clinical signs

Signs can vary from animal to animal, but usually take the form of three phases.

- Preictal – just before the fit the animal will usually be asleep or resting; it will then appear restless or anxious.
- Ictal – this period describes the actual fit, varying degrees of collapse, clonic and tonic activity. Unconsciousness, vocalization, jaw champing, hypersalivation, involuntary urination or defecation may also be present.
- Postictal – this is the period following the fit: the animal may be exhausted, disorientated or anxious.

Seizures may be single, multiple (cluster seizures) or continuous (status epilepticus). They also need to be differentiated from syncopal episodes (fainting).

Diagnosis

- History and neurological examination.
- Blood tests – complete blood count, biochemistry (including electrolytes) and bile acids (liver function tests). Other blood tests may also be requested.
- Cerebral spinal fluid (CSF) tap (EDTA and plain tube)
- MRI.
- CT.
- Electroencephalography (EEG).

Treatment

Any underlying cause should be treated. To control cluster seizures or status epilepticus, initial treatment involves:

- Diazepam initially, under the direction of the veterinary surgeon; can be repeated (intravenously or per rectum) if unsuccessful. This should be used with care in cats
- Phenobarbital or propofol infusion under the direction and supervision of the veterinary surgeon
- Status epilepticus should be dealt with as an emergency
- If idiopathic epilepsy is diagnosed, anticonvulsant therapy should be started.

Imepitoin or phenobarbital is usually the first-line oral medication to control seizures. If ineffective, additional anti-epileptic treatments (e.g. zonisamide or levetiracetam) can be added.

Nursing care

The nursing considerations for seizures are detailed in Figure 18.51. Additional information on nursing recumbent patients is given in Chapter 15.

Spinal injuries

Differential diagnoses

- Intervertebral disc disease.
- Fibrocartilaginous embolism.
- Discospondylitis.
- Wobbler syndrome.
- Cauda equina syndrome.
- Tumour.
- Fracture.

Clinical signs

- Ataxia.
- Paresis of one or more limbs.
- Paralysis of one or more limbs (paraplegia, tetraplegia, hemiplegia).
- Urinary or faecal incontinence.
- Lack of the panniculus reflex, which is used to help localize a spinal cord lesion. This reflex is evaluated by pinching the skin just lateral to the vertebral spines bilaterally. A positive response is seen by a skin twitch.
- Lack of tail function.
- Pain.

Parameter	Problem	Nursing considerations	Monitoring
Breathing/ vital signs	■ Seizures can cause difficulty with breathing Hyperthermia ■ Anaesthetized patient can become hypothermic	■ Keep airway clear ■ Oxygen if required ■ Cool patient: wet towels, fans ■ Warm if cold	■ Monitor oxygen saturation and breathing rate ■ Monitor temperature
Drinking	■ Could be reduced if sedated	■ Water freely available if patient conscious ■ Consider intravenous or subcutaneous fluid therapy	■ Monitor hydration and urine output
Eating	■ Could be reduced if sedated or seizuring ■ May be increased as a side effect of medication	■ Offer food regularly if conscious	■ Monitor appetite ■ Monitor weight
Urinating	■ May be increased with medication ■ May urinate when seizuring	■ If conscious: take out to toilet regularly ■ If recumbent: express bladder and consider urinary catheter ■ Keep clean	■ Record urine output frequency and volume
Defecating	■ Should be normal	■ Take out to toilet ■ If recumbent keep clean	■ Monitor faecal output
Grooming	■ Urine scald	■ Check bedding regularly ■ Keep clean and comfortable	■ Monitor skin
Housing	■ Trauma as a result of seizuring	■ Padded kennel best with walls/doors that will not cause trauma or allow the patient to get stuck amongst the bedding ■ Quiet and dimly lit	■ Good hygiene
Mobilizing	■ May be recumbent ■ May be ataxic when on treatment	■ If recumbent turn regularly ■ Care when taking out if ataxic. Support hindlimbs: under abdomen support	■ Monitor exercise tolerance

Other nursing considerations

- Prepare patient as required for diagnostic procedures (blood tests)
- Monitor and record seizures and monitor trends
- Provision of medication as directed by the veterinary surgeon – maintain patency of the intravenous catheter whilst the animal is hospitalized. The animal may also be anaesthetized whilst hospitalized; monitor for side effects of sedation
- Owner support and instructions
  - Spend time teaching owners how to administer medication at the correct frequency and emphasize to not stop treatment suddenly
  - Ongoing monitoring may required blood tests to check concentration of drugs in the blood
  - Advise owners how to monitor for side effects
  - Suggest owners keep a diary of seizure activity
  - Advise owners how to stop the animal from injuring itself
  - Advise owners how to reassure the animal following a seizure
  - Provide regular contact initially and discuss when veterinary advice should be sought

18.51 Nursing considerations for patients with seizures.

Diagnosis

Neurological assessment

- Full neurological examination.
- Localization of pain.
- Examination of gait.
- Detection of proprioceptive deficits.
- Assessment of cranial nerves.
- Assessment of muscle atrophy/tone.
- Assessment of limb, tail, anal and panniculus reflexes.
- Assessment of deep pain.
- Assessment of bladder function.

Other diagnostic tests

- Radiography.
- Myelography.
- MRI/CT.
- CSF analysis.

Treatment

Surgical correction of some conditions is possible. Other conditions cannot be corrected surgically, or surgical repair is precluded by financial constraints. These patients are then managed by medical treatment, which includes:

- Analgesia
- Restricted or supported exercise (depending on condition)
- Urinary and faecal management – expressing bladder or urinary catheter placement
- Physiotherapy (depending on condition).

Nursing care

The nursing considerations for spinal injuries are detailed in Figure 18.52. Additional information on nursing recumbent patients and physiotherapy is given in Chapter 15.

Parameter	Problem	Nursing considerations	Monitoring
Breathing/ hyperthermia	■ Patients with spinal injuries that are recoverable should not have breathing difficulties ■ Some other neurological problems can affect the respiratory nerves: poor ventilation ■ Potential pyrexia if infection occurs	■ Oxygen ■ May consider ventilation if short-term respiratory compromise	■ Monitor vital signs ■ Monitor breathing rate and character
Pain	■ Painful	■ Analgesia	■ Pain assessment scoring
Drinking	■ Likely to be normal but may have difficulty with mobility and drinking water	■ Offer water regularly	■ Monitor hydration ■ Monitor urine output ■ Monitor weight
Eating	■ Likely to be normal but may have difficulty with mobility and moving to the food	■ Offer food directly to patient; may need to tempt by hand/assisted feeding	■ Monitor and record food intake ■ Monitor weight
Urinating	■ Abnormal; difficulty urinating or incontinence	■ Express bladder regularly or place urinary catheter if difficult to express ■ Aseptic technique to reduce urinary tract infection ■ Check perineum regularly to ensure not soiled or developing urine scald: apply barrier cream	■ Monitor and record bladder size, ease of expression and volume of urine produced ■ Monitor for urinary tract infection ■ Monitor weight
Defecating	■ Could be abnormal	■ Monitor for defecation and clean away as necessary ■ Check not soiling	■ Monitor and record faecal output
Grooming	■ Urine scald and faecal soiling ■ May not be able to groom or groom excessively	■ Groom and keep patient clean	■ Monitor urination and defecation
Housing	■ Poor mobility, recumbent	■ Padded, orthopaedic mattress ■ Water and food bowls easily accessible or food offered directly to the patient	■ Good hygiene
Mobilizing	■ May be unwilling to move ■ Difficulty going up and down stairs ■ Paresis, paralysis ■ Recumbent	■ If possible, sling around abdomen to take out to toilet ■ Recumbent: turn regularly to prevent bed sores ■ Minimize movement if spinal fracture ■ Regular physiotherapy ■ Hydrotherapy	■ Monitor for improvement and deterioration

Other nursing considerations

- Owner support and instructions
  - Advise owners that there will be a prolonged recovery
  - Advise owners that the animal's movement should be restricted/cage rest
  - Educate owners about nursing the patient and providing physiotherapy
  - Maintain regular contact with the owners

18.52 Nursing considerations for patients with spinal injuries.

Musculoskeletal system disease

Definitions
- Myositis – inflammation of a voluntary muscle
- Tendonitis – inflammation of a tendon
- Arthritis – inflammation of a joint

Bone disease

Rickets

This disease is seen in young growing animals that are fed a diet deficient in vitamin D. Vitamin D is required for the absorption of calcium from the intestines (see Chapter 3). If insufficient calcium is absorbed from the intestines, this can lead to reduced bone mineralization around the growth plates. Clinical signs include lameness, bowing of limbs and swollen joints. Enlargement of growth plates is evident on radiographs. Treatment involves feeding an appropriate balanced diet for a young growing dog.

Secondary nutritional hyperparathyroidism

This is caused by a diet grossly deficient in calcium or containing an excess of phosphorus. It is most commonly associated with feeding all-meat diets. Calcium is resorbed from bone, giving rise to lameness, pain, reluctance to stand or walk, and pathological fractures of long bones. Treatment consists of feeding a balanced diet, cage rest to allow fractures to heal, and analgesics.

Metaphyseal osteopathy

This is also known as hypertrophic osteodystrophy. Metaphyseal osteopathy occurs in young growing dogs, particularly giant breeds. It is associated with abnormal metaphyseal bone formation, usually affecting long bones of the distal limbs. Clinical signs include swollen and painful growth plate regions on all limbs, severe lameness, pyrexia, depression and anorexia. The cause of metaphyseal osteopathy is unknown. Treatment consists of pain relief and feeding an appropriate diet for a young growing dog.

Hypertrophic osteopathy

This is also known as pulmonary osteopathy or Marie's disease. It is usually associated with a thoracic mass. There is periosteal proliferation, particularly of the metacarpals and metatarsals. There is no joint involvement. Clinical signs include lameness, bilateral soft tissue swelling of the lower limbs and pain (see Chapter 21 for information on pain scoring). These changes are usually seen before thoracic signs develop. Treatment depends on the underlying condition but the prognosis is usually poor unless the thoracic mass is operable.

Osteomyelitis

Osteomyelitis is inflammation, most commonly due to infection, of bone. Clinical signs include pain, swelling, lameness, loss of function, pyrexia, depression and inappetence. A draining sinus tract may develop. Causes include bacterial or fungal infection (the latter is uncommon in the UK) and corrosion of surgical implants. Radiography reveals destruction of existing bone and new bone formation. Treatment includes administration of antibiotics (based on culture and sensitivity results), antifungals and removal of surgical implants or necrotic bone fragments (sequestra) that may be associated with the osteomyelitis.

Nursing care

The nursing considerations for patients with bone disease are detailed in Figure 18.53.

Parameter	Problem	Nursing considerations	Monitoring
Breathing	■ Unlikely to be a problem	■ Regular checks of temperature, pulse and respiration	■ Monitor respiratory rate
Pain	■ Painful	■ Analgesics	■ Pain assessment scoring
Drinking	■ May be reduced with reduced mobility	■ Offer water regularly ■ If the patient is systemically unwell, may require intravenous fluid therapy	■ Monitor and record hydration, urine output and weight
Eating	■ May be reduced with reduced mobility ■ Poor nutrition ■ Inappetence	■ Offer palatable food ■ Hand feed if necessary ■ Feed an appropriate growth diet for puppies	■ Monitor and record appetite and weight
Urinating	■ Should be normal ■ May have difficulty with mobility	■ Assist to go out to toilet	■ Monitor and record urine output ■ Check no soiling
Defecating	■ Should be normal ■ May have difficulty with mobility	■ Assist to go out to toilet	■ Monitor and record faecal output ■ Check no soiling
Grooming	■ May not be grooming	■ Groom and keep clean	■ Good hygiene
Housing	■ Painful limbs	■ Padded orthopaedic bedding	■ Good hygiene
Mobilizing	■ Painful to walk ■ Potentially recumbent	■ Gentle exercise ■ Assist with walking if necessary ■ Recumbent: turn regularly to avoid bed sores ■ Soft bedding ■ Physiotherapy	■ Monitor exercise tolerance

18.53 Nursing considerations for patients with bone diseases.

continues ▶

18.53 *continued* Nursing considerations for patients with bone diseases.

Arthritis

Joint disease can be categorized as immune-mediated (e.g. idiopathic polyarthritis, systemic lupus erythematosus, rheumatoid arthritis), inflammatory (infectious or non-infectious) or degenerative (Figure 18.54). It should be noted that some conditions fall into more than one category; for example, immune-mediated arthritis is not only immune-mediated but also inflammatory.

Clinical signs

Patients with arthritis have a variable degree of lameness, pain in the affected joint or joints, and exercise intolerance. A specific clinical sign of degenerative joint disease is that the condition improves with exercise.

- Degenerative:
  - Gradual onset
  - Improvement with exercise
  - Crepitus on extension/flexion.
- Immune-mediated:
  - Pyrexia
  - Inappetence
  - Usually multiple joints involved
  - Other signs of systemic disease.
- Infectious:
  - Joint pain (usually one joint)
  - Pyrexia
  - Recent history of surgery or medication.

Cats

As cats are relatively sedentary, degenerative osteoarthritis is a little harder to recognize. Some signs that may be noted include reduced agility, a reluctance to jump and less time spent being active.

Diagnostics

- Blood tests for complete blood count and biochemistry.
- Radiography.
- Joint tap (arthrocentesis) for cytology and culture.

Treatment

Treatment is aimed at the underlying cause, or managing the pain associated with degenerative changes:

- Immune-mediated – immunosuppressive drugs
- Infectious – antibacterials and pain relief
- Degenerative – pain relief (NSAIDs), diet and glycosaminoglycans
- Physiotherapy (see Chapter 15).

Nursing care

The nursing considerations for arthritis are detailed in Figure 18.55.

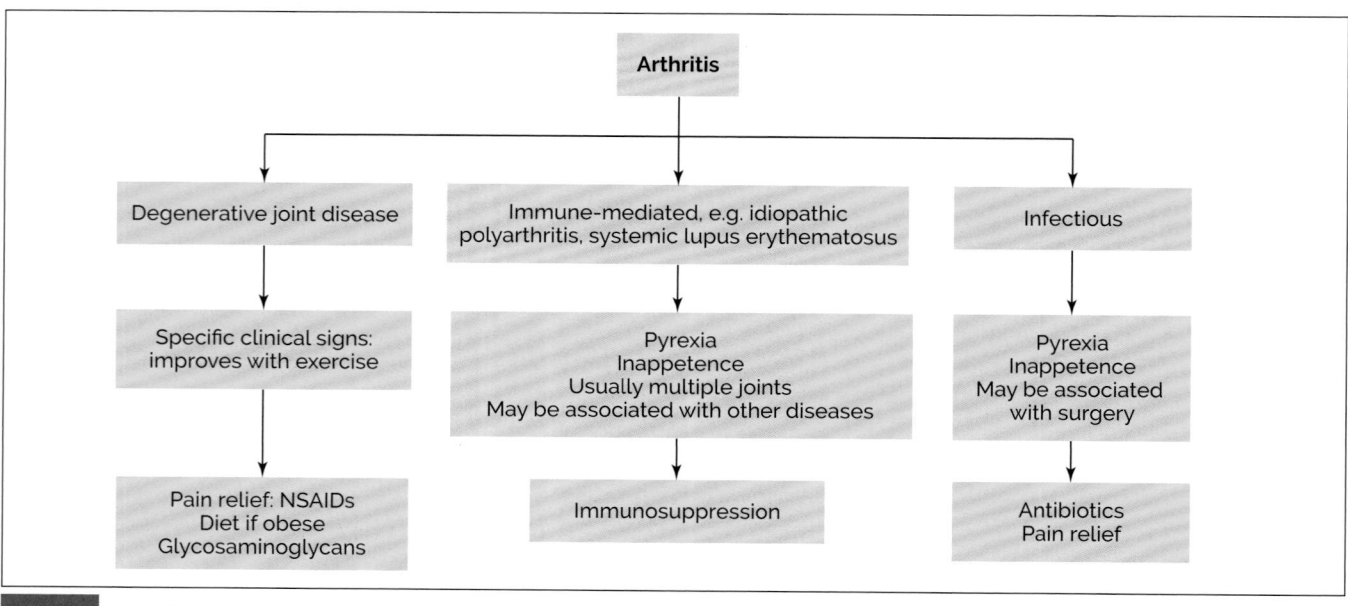

18.54 Classification, clinical signs and treatment of arthritis.

Parameter	Problem	Nursing consideration	Monitoring
Breathing	■ Normal	■ Regular checks of temperature, pulse and respiration	■ Monitor respiratory rate
Pain	■ Painful joints	■ Analgesia administration as directed by the veterinary surgeon	■ Pain assessment scoring
Drinking	■ May be reduced due to reduced mobility	■ Offer water to patient regularly	■ Monitor and record urine output, hydration and weight
Eating	■ May be reduced due to reduced mobility	■ Offer food to patient regularly ■ Weight reduction diet if overweight	■ Monitor and record food intake and weight; avoid obesity
Urinating	■ May have difficulty due to reduced mobility	■ Take out to toilet: assist if required	■ Monitor for soiling and scalding ■ Record and monitor urination
Defecating	■ May have difficulty due to reduced mobility	■ Take out to toilet: assist if required	■ Monitor for soiling ■ Record and monitor defecation
Grooming	■ May not be grooming	■ Keep clean and comfortable	■ Monitor for decubitus ulcers
Housing	■ Reduced mobility, pain	■ Padded, soft orthopaedic mattress	■ Good hygiene
Mobilizing	■ Reduced	■ Assist: sling and support weight, especially when rising (see Chapter 15) ■ Keep warm ■ Gentle short walks ■ Physiotherapy	■ Monitor exercise tolerance

Other nursing considerations

- Provision of medication as directed by the veterinary surgeon – monitor for side effects
- Provide acupuncture and cold laser treatments as directed by the veterinary surgeon
- Assist with weight reduction
- Implement surgical nursing protocols
- Owner support and instructions
  - Advise the owners that the animal should be regularly weighed
  - Advise the owners that the animal should be provided with nutritional supplementation if needed

18.55 Nursing considerations for patients with arthritis.

Muscle disease

Myopathies can be classified as inflammatory or non-inflammatory:

- Inflammatory:
  - Infectious (e.g. *Toxoplasma gondii*, *Neospora caninum*)
  - Immune-mediated.
- Non-inflammatory:
  - Endocrinopathies (e.g. hyperadrenocorticism, hypothyroidism)
  - Hereditary (e.g. 'floppy Labrador').

Clinical signs

- Exercise intolerance and lethargy.
- Muscle weakness and loss of function.
- Muscle atrophy.
- Muscular pain.
- Lameness.

- Pyrexia; anorexia if inflammatory.
- Regurgitation if the oesophageal muscle is affected.

Diagnostics

- Complete blood count, biochemistry and serology.
- Electromyography.
- Muscle biopsy.

Treatment

The underlying cause should be treated:

- Infectious – antibiotics
- Immune-mediated – immunosuppressive drugs
- Endocrinopathies – treat underlying disease
- Hereditary – usually no treatment available.

Nursing care

The nursing considerations for muscle disease are detailed in Figure 18.56.

Parameter	Problem	Nursing considerations	Monitoring
Breathing	■ Potential as muscular function is required for breathing	■ Oxygen supplementation as required ■ Ventilation	■ Monitor breathing rate and character ■ Monitor pulse oximetry
Pain	■ May or may not be painful	■ Analgesia	■ Pain assessment scoring regularly
Drinking	■ May not be able to drink adequately if oesophagus affected or poor mobility	■ Offer water directly to patient ■ Oral fluids ■ Gastric feeding tube ■ Intravenous fluid therapy ■ Subcutaneous fluid therapy	■ Monitor and record volume consumed ■ Monitor hydration, weight and urine output

18.56 Nursing considerations for patients with muscle disease.

continues ▶

Parameter	Problem	Nursing considerations	Monitoring
Eating	■ May not be able to eat adequately if oesophagus affected or poor mobility	■ Assisted feeding from a height ■ Try different consistencies of food to see what is kept down ■ Gastric feeding tube	■ Monitor and record amount consumed ■ Monitor weight
Urinating	■ May have difficulty with mobility	■ Take out to toilet: assist if required	■ Monitor urine output ■ Monitor for soiling and scalding ■ Monitor mobility
Defecating	■ May have difficulty with mobility and squatting	■ Take out to toilet: assist if required	■ Monitor faecal output ■ Monitor for soiling ■ Monitor mobility
Grooming	■ May not be grooming	■ Keep clean and dry	■ Monitor for decubitus ulcers
Housing	■ May be recumbent	■ Soft bedding and turn frequently	■ Good hygiene
Mobilizing	■ Recumbent	■ Soft bedding and turn frequently ■ Physiotherapy	■ Monitor mobility

18.56 *continued* Nursing considerations for patients with muscle disease.

Tumours of the musculoskeletal system

- Bone tumours – most commonly osteosarcoma (malignant); other tumours include fibrosarcoma, haemangiosarcoma and chrondrosarcoma.
- Soft tissue sarcomas (tumours) – fibrosarcoma and haemangiosarcoma.

Clinical signs

- Osteosarcomas most commonly affect the long bones of large-breed dogs. Patients may present with only a swelling (Figure 18.57) but they are usually very painful and the patient will be lame and often unable to bear its weight on the affected leg.
- Chondrosarcomas affect bones such as ribs and the nasal cavity.
- Fibrosarcomas usually affect the bones of the axial skeleton, including the skull and mandible.

Diagnostics

- Complete blood count and biochemistry.
- Radiography – local area and thorax (metastasis); ultrasonography – abdomen (metastasis); or CT of the body.
- Biopsy for histopathology.

Treatment

Treatment of osteosarcomas usually involves amputating the affected leg to relieve pain. The majority of osteosarcomas have metastasized (spread) by the time they are diagnosed. The best results are achieved by combining amputation with chemotherapy to slow the development of metastases. The primary tumour can also be treated with radiotherapy to provide pain relief. Soft tissue tumours are best treated by surgical excision.

Nursing care

The nursing considerations for musculoskeletal tumours are detailed in Figure 18.58.

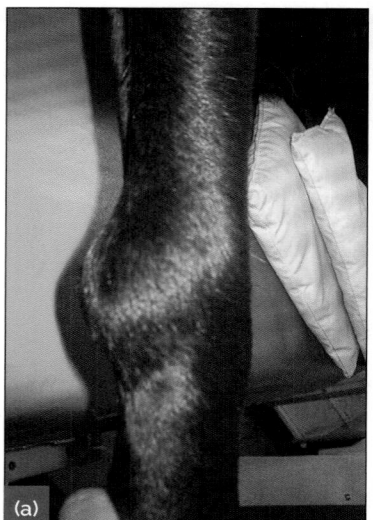

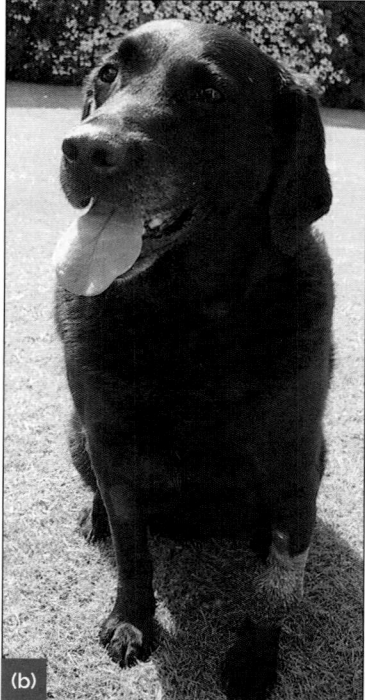

18.57 Bone tumour. **(a)** A swelling on the distal left forelimb of a dog, which was diagnosed as an osteosarcoma. **(b)** The dog underwent a course of radiotherapy, as evidenced by the white square of hair on the left forelimb.

Parameter	Problem	Nursing considerations	Monitoring
Breathing	■ Unlikely to be a problem unless very advanced disease and spread of the tumour	■ Oxygen as required	■ Monitor breathing rate
Pain	■ Painful	■ Analgesia	■ Pain assessment scoring
Drinking	■ May have difficulty with mobility	■ Offer water directly to patient	■ Monitor hydration
Eating	■ May have difficulty with mobility	■ Offer food directly to patient	■ Monitor appetite ■ Monitor weight
Urinating	■ May have difficulty with mobility	■ Sling and assist to toilet	■ Monitor urine output
Defecating	■ May have difficulty with mobility	■ Sling and assist to toilet	■ Monitor faecal output
Grooming	■ May not be grooming	■ Keep clean and dry	■ Monitor for decubitus ulcers
Housing	■ Animal may be in pain	■ Soft orthopaedic bedding	■ Good hygiene
Mobilizing	■ Limb amputation	■ Sling when walked	■ Monitor for exercise tolerance
Other nursing considerations			

- Chemotherapy – assist veterinary surgeon with treatment (wear gloves)
- Monitor for gastrointestinal clinical signs and lethargy
- Monitor haematology and biochemistry parameters
- To avoid risk of exposure to cytotoxic drugs, which can result in organ damage, impaired fertility, fetal malformation and cancer, personal protective equipment (PPE) should be worn. This includes when preparing and administering chemotherapy drugs and also when handling patient excreta, cleaning up spills or disposing of materials and equipment that have been in contact with these drugs.

18.58 Nursing considerations for patients with musculoskeletal tumours.

Diseases of the skin and coat

Definitions

- Alopecia – the absence of hair from areas of the skin where it is normally present; can be partial or complete, symmetrical or patchy, diffuse or focal
- Erythema – reddening of the skin
- Pyoderma – a pyogenic (pus-forming, e.g. infected) condition of the skin
- Pruritus – sensation within the skin that provokes the desire to scratch (animal may persistently lick, chew, or rub itself to alleviate the irritation; this can lead to self-trauma)
- Seborrhoea – excessive secretion of sebum by the sebaceous glands within the skin, giving the coat and skin an oily appearance

Parasitic and fungal skin disease

These conditions are discussed in Chapters 5 and 6.

Pyoderma

This condition is more common in the dog than the cat and there is usually an underlying cause for its development. The severity of the condition is determined by the depth of the tissue affected (Figure 18.59). *Staphylococcus pseudintermedius* is the most commonly involved bacterium, but other secondary opportunist bacteria such as *Pseudomonas* spp. may also be present.

Feline pyoderma is associated with cat bites. Bacteria such as *Pasteurella* spp., *Staphylococcus* spp. and *Fusiformis* spp., which are routinely found in the cat's mouth, cause cellulitis when bite wounds penetrate deep within the skin. Other clinical signs include pyrexia, anorexia, depression, pain and swelling at the site of the bite wound. This condition is usually successfully treated with drainage of pus from the site of infection with or without antibiotics.

Tissue depth	Condition	Presentation	Treatment
Surface	Acute moist dermatitis	Often occurs where skin has become damaged due to self-trauma Can occur anywhere but especially over face, feet and tail base Erythema often present and are is often moist or crusty due to serum exudates	Treatment of underlying cause (e.g. ear infection) Clip hair from site – patient may require sedation as area can be very painful Clean area with dilute chlorhexidine Elizabethan collar to prevent further self-trauma Topical treatments
	Skin fold dermatitis	Commonly found around lip folds, vulval folds and tail folds Common in breeds with excessive skin folds	Treat as above Surgical correction or cosmetic surgery may be required to correct anatomy of skin in severe cases that recur

18.59 Classification of pyoderma.

continues ▶

Tissue depth	Condition	Presentation	Treatment
Superficial	Impetigo	Often known as juvenile pustular dermatitis or puppy pyoderma Multiple pustules and yellow scabs commonly found along ventral abdomen	Antibacterial shampoo with additional systemic antibiotic and anti-inflammatory therapy if condition extensive
	Folliculitis	Formation of pustules with hair protruding Sometimes the lesions in ring-like formation, especially ventral abdomen As a result of underlying disease	Treatment of underlying disease Appropriate antibiotic selection
Deep	Interdigital pyoderma (pyodermatitis)	Often seen in short-haired dogs – paws become painful and swollen and may discharge pus Area of alopecia seen with ulceration and fistulas in severe cases	Surgical drainage of infected material Treatment of underlying cause Long-term antibiotic therapy
	Furunculosis	Often associated with underlying disease such as demodicosis, dermatophytosis or hypothyroidism Clinical signs include pustules, discharging pus, fistulas, alopecia, pain Lesions often found on muzzle, flanks and anal regions but can occur anywhere on body	Treatment of any underlying disease Long-term antibiotic therapy In severe cases, surgical resection of fistulas may be required if problem recurs

18.59 *continued* Classification of pyoderma.

Allergic skin disease

This is caused by an inappropriate immune response to an antigen, which in cases of allergic skin disease can include many factors. Figure 18.60 outlines the causes, presentation, diagnoses and treatments of various allergic skin diseases.

Hormonal alopecia

This is usually associated with one of the following:

- Hypothyroidism (see 'Hypothyroidism', above)
- Hyperadrenocorticism (Cushing's disease, see 'Hyperadrenocorticism', above)
- Sertoli cell tumour.

In conjunction with clinical signs of the underlying condition, it usually presents as a bilateral alopecia, often on the flanks. It is usually non-pruritic and the skin is not inflamed. Treatment is based on identifying and treating the underlying cause.

Nursing care

The nursing considerations for skin and coat diseases are detailed in Figure 18.61.

Condition	Cause	Presentation	Diagnosis	Treatment
Urticaria	Induced by drugs, vaccines and insect stings	Sudden development of multiple oedematous swellings or wheals on skin, with hair becoming erect; they are pruritic and can remain for hours or days	Based on clinical signs and accurate history	Removal of cause Treatment with corticosteroids Future avoidance of causal agent
Atopic dermatitis	Large numbers of unknown antigens, including house dust mites, pollens, danders	Usually affects dogs 1–3 years old Intense pruritus and alopecia, especially around eyes, feet, axillae and ventral abdomen Secondary infection common, due to self-trauma Otitis externa and ocular discharges may also be present Cats may present with miliary eczema and eosinophilic granuloma complex	Intradermal skin testing with multiple allergens to determine cause Serum testing for specific antigens	Allergies usually lifelong Depending on causal factors, changes to environment may be required Treatment may include oclacitinib, lokivetmab, corticosteroids, antihistamines, essential fatty acid supplementation, desensitizing injections
Food hypersensitivity	Causes individual to each animal but can include beef, milk, gluten	Pruritic skin disease and/or gastrointestinal symptoms	Clinical signs and exclusion diet food trial (see Chapter 13)	Avoidance of specific allergens identified by food trial Long-term feeding of novelty diet fed during exclusion trial

18.60 Causes, diagnosis and treatment of allergic skin diseases. *continues* ▶

Condition	Cause	Presentation	Diagnosis	Treatment
Contact dermatitis	Commonly caused by soaps, detergents or chemicals of any kind	Pruritic erythematous lesions mainly on feet, ventral abdomen, neck and face Often secondary bacterial infection due to self-trauma Intolerance generally develops 4-6 weeks after initial exposure	Patch testing: suspected allergen applied to clipped area of skin and kept in contact for 48 hours then examined for reaction Contact elimination: hospitalize animal from usual environment to see if clinical signs resolve; suspected items or substances then reintroduced and patient observed for reaction	Avoid contact with identified allergens

18.60 *continued* Causes, diagnosis and treatment of allergic skin diseases.

Parameter	Problem	Nursing considerations	Monitoring
Breathing	■ Normal	■ Regular checks of temperature, pulse and respiration	■ Monitor respiratory rate
Pain	■ Skin could be painful	■ Analgesia	■ Pain assessment scoring
Drinking	■ Polydipsia (hyperadrenocorticism) (may also be caused by corticosteroid therapy)	■ Provide fresh water	■ Monitor fluid intake
Eating	■ Weight gain with certain medications ■ Allergic reaction to corn, soya or wheat ■ Colourings and fillers ■ Appetite may increase (hyperadrenocorticism)	■ Appropriate hypoallergenic diets ■ Dietary supplements (essential fatty acids)	■ Monitor weight
Urinating	■ Normal ■ Polyuria (hyperadrenocorticism)	■ Urinalysis to identify cause	■ Monitor urine output
Defecating	■ Normal ■ Diarrhoea	■ Treat underlying cause	■ Monitor faecal output
Grooming	■ May not be grooming ■ Primary and secondary skin disorders ■ Ectoparasites ■ Bacterial or yeast infections as a result of another disorder ■ Loss of hair along the back	■ Keep the patient clean and groom regularly ■ Control ectoparasites ■ Keep fur short	■ Monitor for ectoparasites ■ Shampoos and grooming products may irritate the skin
Housing	■ Seasonal allergies	■ Pollen, weeds, dust, mites, mould, grass ■ Eliminate environmental allergies	■ Monitor behaviour ■ Toys/chews to limit boredom
Mobilizing	■ Self-mutilation	■ Regular walks to toilet ■ Prevent self-mutilation – consider use of a collar/Elizabethan collar or cone ■ Consistent routine	■ Encourage play to minimize stress and boredom

Other nursing considerations

- Prepare patient as required for diagnostic procedures (skin scrape/hair plucking, skin lesion biopsy, cytology, complete blood count and biochemistry, radiography and ultrasonography for testicular abnormalities, adrenocorticotrophic hormone test, gonadotrophin releasing hormone test, urinalysis, antibody test)
- Provision of treatment based on the results of the diagnostic procedures, as directed by the veterinary surgeon (oral antibiotics, antibacterial ointments or shampoos, ectoparasiticides, steroids, surgery)
- Control of allergic reactions/allergies – provision of medication, including antibiotics, steroids, antifungals, antihistamines, non-steroidal anti-inflammatory drugs, trilostane and corticosteroids, as directed by the veterinary surgeon. Regular veterinary checks to monitor response to treatment
- Owner support and instructions
  - Spend time teaching owners how to administer topical and/or oral medication to the patient
  - Advise the owners on care of patients with skin conditions and the use of topical applications
  - Advise the owners on treatment of the environment
  - Advise the owners on what personal protective equipment is required
  - Advise the owners that regular dermatology reviews are required

18.61 Nursing considerations for patients with skin and coat diseases.

Diseases of the eye

Definitions

- Blepharospasm – constant blinking
- Cataracts – cloudy appearance to the eyes, resulting in blurred vision
- Distichiasis – extra row of eyelashes behind the normal row
- Ectropion – eversion of the lower eyelid away from the eyeball with exposure of the conjunctiva
- Entropion – turning in of the upper or lower eyelid towards the eyeball
- Glaucoma – increased fluid pressure within the eye, leading to optic nerve damage
- Intraocular pressure – fluid pressure inside the eye
- Keratoconjunctivitis sicca – 'dry eye' (lack of tear production)
- Lens luxation – an inherited condition in which the lens dislocates causing damage to the optic nerve
- Progressive retinal atrophy (PRA) – an inherited condition that caused diminished peripheral vision or blindness
- Trichiasis – eyelashes growing in the wrong direction

Conditions that affect the eyelids

- Entropion – often hereditary.
- Ectropion – less common than entropion.
- Distichiasis – most common hereditary eye abnormality in the dog.

All of these abnormalities can result in irritation, inflammation, infection or damage to the cornea and conjunctiva, depending on the severity.

Clinical signs

As well as visible evidence of one of the above conditions, clinical signs may include:

- Blepharospasm (constant blinking)
- Squinting
- Increased lacrimation (tear production)
- Ocular discharge.

Treatment

- Anti-inflammatory eyedrops.
- Antibacterial eyedrops.
- Surgical correction of condition.

Conjunctivitis

Inflammation of the conjunctiva can be unilateral or bilateral, depending on the cause.

Causes include bacterial infections (sometimes primary but usually secondary), viral infections (e.g. distemper, herpesvirus) or allergies. It may also be associated with foreign bodies, environmental irritants, trauma and ectropion.

Clinical signs

- Blepharospasm.
- Increased lacrimation.

- Chemosis (oedema and swelling of the conjunctiva).
- Conjunctival hyperaemia.
- Ocular discharge ranging from serous to mucopurulent.

Treatment

This will vary depending on the causal factor, but may include:

- Surgical correction of eyelid deformities, removal of foreign bodies
- Antibiotic eyedrops
- Anti-inflammatory eyedrops
- Antiviral eyedrops.

Keratoconjunctivitis sicca

KCS ('dry eye') is due to a reduction in aqueous tear production from the lacrimal and third eyelid gland. This often results in an overproduction of mucus as an attempt to keep the cornea moist. Most commonly the condition is immune-mediated but it may also be caused by drug toxicity (e.g. sulfasalazine), trauma or surgery (e.g. following removal of the third eyelid gland in dogs with 'cherry eye'). There is considerable variation in the degree of severity.

Clinical signs

- Vascularization, ulceration and opacity of the cornea.
- Recurrent conjunctivitis.
- Mucoid or mucopurulent discharge on and around the surface of the eye.

Diagnostics

A Schirmer tear test (Figure 18.62) will show insufficient tear production. Readings of <10 mm in a minute will confirm the diagnosis, but the test should be repeated for monitoring purposes. Fluorescein is applied to the cornea to detect ulceration.

Treatment

- Ciclosporin to treat immune-mediated destruction of the lacrimal gland.
- Tear substitutes.
- Antibiotic drops if infected.
- Good ocular hygiene and frequent cleaning to remove discharge from around the eyes.

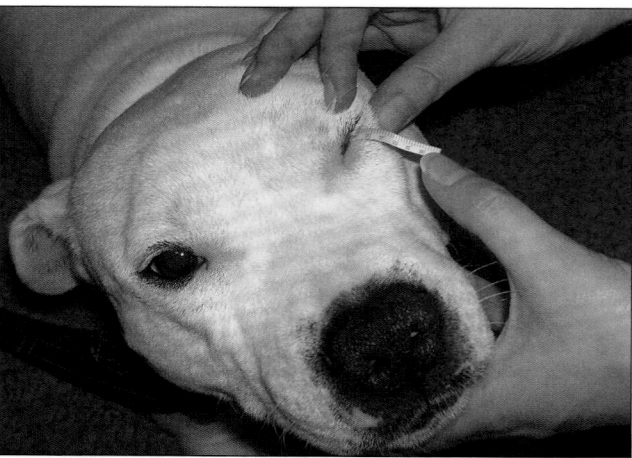

18.62   Schirmer tear test.

Corneal ulceration

This common condition can vary in severity depending on depth. Deep ulcers may result in corneal rupture. Causes include:

- Eyelash/eyelid disorders
- Trauma (e.g. cat scratch)
- Keratoconjunctivitis sicca
- Bacteria (primary trauma due to any of the above often allows bacterial overgrowth)
- Melting ulcers – these occur due to bacterial infections (e.g. *Pseudomonas*), resulting in enzymes being released to aid removal of devitalized cells and debris. These enzymes also contribute to the melting of the cornea.

Clinical signs

- Ocular pain.
- Ocular discharge.
- Blepharospasm.
- Increased lacrimation.

Diagnostics

- Visual inspection of the cornea.
- Fluorescein dye – this dye is taken up by any exposed stroma so that epithelial erosions can be detected.

Treatment

This will vary depending on the severity of the ulcer but may include:

- Remove the cause
- Antibiotic eyedrops
- Analgesia
- Complicated ulcers:
  - Surgical procedures (e.g. debridement of damaged cornea, grid keratotomy)
  - Contact lenses may be used to protect the eye in slow-healing ulcers. They protect the eyelids from rubbing the open area and may assist in holding water-soluble drops over the ulcerated lesion. They have no impact on the vision of the patient.

Uveitis

Uveitis is inflammation of the iris, ciliary body and/or choroid. It can be caused by trauma, neoplasia, infection or immune-mediated disease, lens-induced, or associated with corneal insult.

Clinical signs

Clinical signs vary according to duration of the condition, the cause of the inflammation and the extent of the uveal tract involvement. Bilateral uveitis usually indicates systemic involvement. Secondary complications include glaucoma and cataracts.

- Pain.
- Blepharospasm.
- Miotic pupil.
- Red eye.
- Photophobia.
- Lacrimation.
- Reduced intraocular pressure.

Diagnostics

Underlying cause must be determined.

- Haematology, biochemistry, specific diagnostic tests (e.g. FeLV, FIV, feline infectious peritonitis (FIP)).
- Serology.
- Ophthalmoscopy.
- Tonometry.
- Fluorescein staining.
- Diagnostic imaging.

Treatment

- Treat underlying cause.
- Topical atropine (contraindicated if glaucoma present).
- Topical corticosteroids (avoid in corneal ulceration, with caution in viral/fungal infections) or topical NSAIDs.
- Systemic corticosteroids.
- Systemic NSAIDs if systemic corticosteroids contraindicated.
- Evaluate response to treatment at regular intervals.

Glaucoma

This is a condition in which there is an elevation in intraocular pressure due to inadequate drainage of aqueous humour within the globe. This eventually affects the vision and health of the eye, and the condition can be very painful. In acute cases permanent blindness can result if untreated. The condition may be idiopathic: many breeds have a predisposition (including many terrier and spaniel breeds as well as the Great Dane and Flat-coated Retriever). There is a list of breeds that are tested for this condition on the KC/BVA eye testing scheme (see Chapter 4). Other causes include:

- Uveitis
- Cataracts
- Lens luxation
- Neoplasia.

Clinical signs

- Painful red eye(s).
- Corneal oedema.
- Swelling of the globe.
- Dilated pupil.
- Retinal damage.

Diagnostics

- Examination of the eye with an ophthalmoscope.
- Measuring the intraocular pressure with a tonometer (this is also monitored to check the response to treatment) (Figure 18.63).
- Gonioscopy to measure the iridocorneal drainage angle.

Treatment

- Emergency treatment: prostaglandin analogue; intravenous mannitol, to help to draw fluid from the aqueous and vitreous humours and therefore decrease intraocular pressure.
- Carbonic anhydrase inhibitors reduce formation of aqueous humour.
- Miotics to increase aqueous outflow.
- Analgesia.
- Surgical treatment in specialist centres.
- Enucleation.

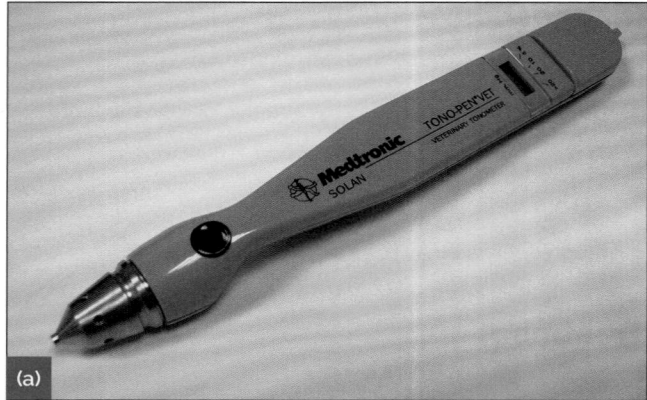

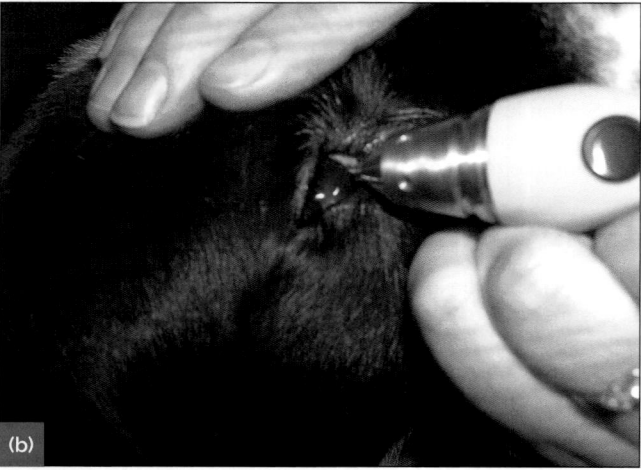

18.63 (a) Tonometer. (b) Using a tonometer to measure intraocular pressure.

Conditions affecting the lens

These include cataract formation and lens luxation, both of which require surgical correction (see Chapter 23). Cataract formation is a common finding in dogs with diabetes mellitus. Visual inspection of the eye reveals a clouding of the lens. Poor night vision leading to progressive blindness is the common progression of the disease.

Conditions affecting the retina

Collie eye anomaly

This is a disorder of the deep structures of the eye that affects collie breeds. It is a congenital disorder and can be detected with an ophthalmoscope in puppies. It can affect the eye in the following ways:

- Choroid hypoplasia – inadequate development of the choroids
- Coloboma – a cleft or defect in the optic disc
- Staphyloma – an area of thinning in the sclera, adjacent to the choroids
- Retinal detachment, with or without haemorrhage.

The severity of the condition varies. In its mildest form there is little effect on sight. In a severe form, total retinal detachment will cause blindness. Affected animals should not be used for breeding (see Chapter 4 for details of BVA/Kennel Club/International Sheep Dog Society Eye Scheme).

Progressive retinal atrophy (PRA)

This is a hereditary disease of the eye that causes blindness. The retina comprises two types of photoreceptor cells: rods and cones. The rods function in dim light and the cones function in bright light. A dog affected with PRA begins to have difficulty seeing in dim light and then gradually loses the ability to see in bright light, eventually becoming completely blind. Although most common in dogs, some forms can occur in cats. Age at onset and rate of progression vary. Generalized retinal thinning occurs, manifesting as tapetal hyper-reflectivity and attenuation of the superficial retinal vessels. There is no available treatment. Genetic testing is now available to identify carrier animals that are unaffected (see Chapter 4).

Nursing care

The nursing considerations for patients with inflamed or irritated eyes are given in Figure 18.64. The nursing considerations for patients with poor vision are given in Figure 18.65.

Parameter	Problem	Nursing considerations	Monitoring
Breathing	■ Normal	■ Regular checks of temperature, pulse and respiration	■ Monitor respiratory rate
Pain	■ Eyes could be painful	■ Analgesia	■ Pain assessment scoring
Drinking	■ Locate bowls in same place for those with vision problems	■ Provide fresh water in bowls that are unlikely to be knocked over	■ Monitor hydration
Eating	■ Locate bowls in same place for those with vision problems	■ Warm food	■ Monitor appetite
Urinating	■ Normal	■ Take out to toilet regularly	■ Monitor urine output
Defecating	■ Normal	■ Take out to toilet regularly	■ Monitor faecal output

18.64 Nursing considerations for patients with inflamed or irritated eyes.

continues ▶

Parameter	Problem	Nursing considerations	Monitoring
Grooming	■ May not be grooming	■ Keep the patient clean and groom ■ Bathe away any eye discharge with warm saline (0.9%) ■ Prevent excoriation around face with the use of petroleum jelly ■ Humidify air to loosen discharges	■ Monitor for excoriation
Housing	■ Prevent infection ■ Avoid bright lights ■ Avoid hazards	■ Clean environment ■ Avoid risk of cross-infection ■ Minimize stress and dry, dusty environment	■ Monitor animal's behaviour
Mobilizing	■ Normal	■ Gentle walks to toilet ■ Wear a harness for exercise ■ Remove objects that patients may injure themselves on	■ Monitor exercise tolerance

Other nursing considerations

- Prepare patient as required for diagnostic procedures based on the underlying cause (blepharospasm, squinting, increased tear production, ocular discharge, conjunctivitis, purulent discharge)
- Swab discharging eyes to enable identification of infective organisms and enable culture and sensitivity testing to be carried out
- Perform Schirmer tear test (>10 mm/min) and fluorescein test
- Provision of medication, including anti-inflammatory eye drops, antibacterial or antiviral eye drops/ointment, artificial tears and anti-immune treatments, as directed by the veterinary surgeon
- Implement surgical nursing protocols
- Owner support and instructions
  - Spend time teaching owners how to administer ophthalmic medication to the patient
  - Advise the owners how to store the medication (in the fridge, away from sunlight)
  - Advise the owners to wash hands thoroughly before applying the medication
  - Advise the owners to check the medicine prescription against the label on the eye medication prior to applying to the eyes
  - Advise the owners to check the expiry date
  - Advise the owners of any likely side effects
  - Advise the owners that all treatments given should be recorded
  - Advise the owners on how to prevent self-mutilation (use of a collar or cone)
  - Advise the owners that regular re-examination by the veterinary surgeon is required

18.64 *continued* Nursing considerations for patients with inflamed or irritated eyes.

Parameter	Problem	Nursing considerations	Monitoring
Breathing	■ Normal	■ Regular checks of temperature, pulse and respiration	■ Monitor respiratory rate
Pain	■ Eyes could be painful	■ Analgesia	■ Pain assessment scoring
Drinking	■ Locate bowls in same place for those with vision problems	■ Maintain oral health ■ Care of teeth ■ Use of a drinking fountain (dog can hear running water)	■ Monitor fluid intake ■ Monitor hydration
Eating	■ Locate bowls in same place for those with vision problems	■ Age appropriate diet	■ Monitor food intake
Urinating	■ Normal	■ Take out to toilet regularly	■ Monitor urine output
Defecating	■ Normal	■ Take out to toilet regularly	■ Monitor faecal output
Grooming	■ May not be grooming	■ Keep the patient clean and groom regularly ■ Bathe away any eye discharge with warm saline (0.9%)	■ Monitor for excoriation ■ Check nails (reduced exercise)
Housing	■ Provide a safe area ■ Avoid hazards ■ Let other people know that the animal cannot see or has reduced vision	■ Large soft bed	■ Monitor animal's behaviour
Mobilizing	■ Normal	■ Gentle walks to toilet ■ Little and often ■ Always on a lead ■ Consistent routine	■ Monitor exercise tolerance

Other nursing considerations

- Prepare patient as required for diagnostic procedures based on the underlying cause (poor sight/blindness, cataracts, injury)
- Provision of medication, including artificial tears and insulin (for patient with diabetes), as directed by the veterinary surgeon
- Implement surgical nursing procedures
- Owner support and instructions
  - Spend time teaching owners how to administer ophthalmic medication (e.g. artificial tears) to the patient
  - Advise the owners on how to care for patients with impaired vision
  - Advise the owners to regularly talk to the animal to reassure them of their presence
  - Advise the owners to keep all bowls, sleeping area and equipment in the same place; avoid moving furniture around; put corner protectors on sharp furniture; provide baby gates at the top of the stairs

18.65 Nursing considerations for patients with impaired vision.

Infectious diseases – canine

Information on common canine infectious diseases is summarized in Figure 18.66. Two important features in the care of patients with infectious diseases are barrier nursing and the provision of isolation facilities, which are described in Chapter 14.

> ## Vaccination
>
> Vaccination is important for the control of viral diseases in dogs and cats. Countries with good vaccination programmes have fewer cases of infectious diseases than those with poor overall population vaccination. Therefore, within the UK and other developed countries, the likelihood of seeing infectious diseases is much lower. The subject of vaccination is discussed in principle in Chapter 7

Canine distemper

Canine distemper is caused by canine distemper virus (CDV), a morbillivirus related to measles virus in humans. Both dogs and ferrets are susceptible. Transmission is mainly from dog to dog. It only persists in the environment for 1–2 days and is susceptible to routine disinfection.

The disease is most commonly seen in unvaccinated 3–6-month-old puppies. This time coincides with the waning of maternal antibodies (see Chapter 7). In susceptible populations a dog of any age may be affected. Outbreaks occur where there is a high density of dogs, such as rescue centres, housing estates and cities generally.

The virus is shed most commonly in respiratory exudates as well as in urine, faeces, saliva, vomitus and ocular discharges, up to 60–90 days post-infection. The incubation period is 7–21 days and infection is via inhalation. The aerosol droplets, when inhaled, come into contact with the upper respiratory epithelium of the susceptible animal and spread through the body from this point. The respiratory, gastrointestinal and central nervous systems, nose, footpads and conjunctiva can be affected. The severity of the disease depends on the efficacy of the immune response that is mounted and ranges from no clinical signs to death. Secondary bacterial infections can complicate the infection.

Clinical signs (generalized distemper)

- Depression.
- Pyrexia.
- Anorexia.
- Lymphadenopathy.
- Conjunctivitis giving ocular discharge (initially serous but rapidly becoming mucopurulent with secondary bacterial infection).

Disease/ infection	Type of infectious agent	Incubation period	Major organs affected	Main method of transmission	Zoonotic	Diagnostics	Major nursing needs	Control/ prevention
Canine distemper	Virus	7–21 days	Respiratory, gastrointestinal systems	Inhalation	No	History, clinical signs Blood analysis Post-mortem examination	Fluid therapy Symptomatic	Vaccination Client education
Infectious canine hepatitis	Virus	5–10 days	Liver	Inhalation/ ingestion	No	History, clinical signs Blood analysis	Pain management Fluid therapy	Vaccination Client education
Canine parvovirus	Virus	3–5 days	Gastrointestinal system, bone marrow, heart (rare)	Ingestion of faecally contaminated material	No	History, clinical signs CITE faecal test	Fluid therapy Symptomatic Antibiotics for secondary infections	Vaccination Isolation Avoid risk
Leptospirosis	Bacteria	5–7 days	Kidneys, liver	Through mucous membranes and skin abrasions	Yes	History, clinical signs Urinalysis Blood analysis	Antibiotics Fluid therapy	Vaccination Avoid risk
Kennel cough complex	Mixed – bacteria/ virus	5–7 days	Respiratory system	Inhalation	No	History, clinical signs	Antibiotics Symptomatic	Vaccination Isolation
Rabies	Virus	1 week to 6 months, normally 3–8 weeks	Nervous system	Saliva to skin wound	Yes – fatal	History, clinical signs Post-mortem examination	N/A	Stray dog control Vaccination Pet Travel Scheme
Salmonellosis	Bacteria	2–3 days following a stressful experience	Gastrointestinal system	Ingestion of faecally contaminated material	Yes	History, clinical signs Culture	Fluid therapy ± antibiotics	Hygiene, disinfection

18.66 Common canine infectious diseases (note that this list is not exhaustive).

- Rhinitis giving nasal discharge (initially serous but rapidly becoming mucopurulent with secondary bacterial infection).
- Cough (initially dry, may become moist and productive).
- Exudative pneumonia – complicated by a secondary bacterial infection – leading to tachypnoea and dyspnoea.
- Vomiting, diarrhoea, dehydration and loss of body condition.
- Hyperkeratosis of nose and footpads; footpads become thickened and fissures appear ('hard pad').
- Enamel hypoplasia – permanent damage to tooth enamel in puppies under 6 months old.
- Neurological signs (see below).
- Skin rash – pustules, thought to be associated with an immune response (animals that develop rashes often recover).

Neurological signs

Some animals, including those with subclinical infection, can develop neurological signs 2–3 weeks after infection. Clinical signs are usually acute in onset and progressive and are associated with a poor prognosis. Clinical signs depend on the part of the nervous system that is affected and include seizures, paresis/paralysis of one or more limbs, and optic neuritis. Involuntary twitching of muscles (myoclonus) may also occur and is said to be a classic sign.

Diagnostics

A presumptive diagnosis is usually based on the history and classical clinical signs in an at-risk patient.

- Blood tests: haematology and biochemistry.
- Thoracic radiographs: right lateral and ventrodorsal views.
- CSF sample.
- Specific tests (note: some tests can be affected by previous vaccination giving false results):
  - PCR
  - Epithelial cells with eosinophilic bodies
  - Antibody titre rising at least four-fold on subsequent sampling
  - Immunofluorescence for virus in lymphoid tissue
  - Detection of antibody in CSF.
- Post-mortem examination.

Treatment

Prevention is by vaccination. Specific treatment is not available and the patient is treated symptomatically:

- Isolation and barrier nursing – of particular importance (see Chapters 7 and 14)
- Intravenous fluids for dehydration and electrolyte losses (see Chapter 20)
- Broad-spectrum antibiotics for secondary bacterial infections
- Anticonvulsants for seizures
- Antiemetics for vomiting.

Infectious canine hepatitis

Infectious canine hepatitis (ICH) is caused by canine adenovirus type 1 (CAV-1), similar to the CAV-2 adenovirus that causes respiratory disease (see 'Kennel cough complex', below). It is a resistant virus and can survive for months on fomites in the environment. It survives disinfection with various chemicals but is inactivated at temperatures >50°C.

The incubation period is 5–10 days. During the initial infection, virus is shed in all bodily secretions. From around 10 days' post-infection, the virus is shed in the urine for at least 6 months. Animals become infected through the oronasal route. The virus localizes in the tonsils and regional lymph nodes before disseminating to other parts of the body and localizing in the liver and vascular endothelial cells. If an appropriate immune response is not made, acute or chronic hepatitis can occur. Immune complexes (antibody and viral antigen complexes) can lodge in the uveal tract and glomerulus and cause a severe uveitis and corneal oedema, or glomerulonephritis.

Dogs younger than 1 year are usually affected, but unvaccinated dogs of any age can be affected. Mortality rate can be high in unweaned puppies. Disease can progress rapidly and the puppies may die within a few hours of developing clinical signs. Infection in older animals is less severe.

Clinical signs

Clinical signs in acute infections may include:

- Pyrexia, depression and anorexia
- Lymphadenopathy
- Vomiting and diarrhoea
- Shock
- Hepatomegaly and anterior abdominal pain
- Jaundice (in a third of cases)
- Petechial haemorrhages
- Corneal oedema (blue eye)
- Neurological signs (in terminal stages)
- Severely affected dogs may die suddenly, without the owner noticing other clinical signs.

In subacute infections, clinical signs include depression, anorexia and mild pyrexia.

Diagnostics

- History and clinical signs.
- Blood tests: haematology, biochemistry (especially liver enzymes) and clotting profile.
- Serological tests – rising antibody titre (can be complicated by vaccination).
- Intranuclear inclusion bodies found within hepatocytes.
- Post-mortem examination.

Treatment

Prevention is by vaccination (CAV-2 cross-protective). ICH patients are treated symptomatically:

- Intravenous fluids to rehydrate the animal
- Analgesics to control abdominal pain
- Ocular topical steroids should only be used with caution under the guidance of the veterinary surgeon
- Antimicrobials should be considered to treat secondary bacterial infections.

The corneal changes may remain, leading to permanent visual impairment, but in the majority of cases these are temporary.

Canine parvovirus

Canine parvovirus (CPV) is the most important canine virus diagnosed in susceptible patients. It is very resistant and can survive in the environment for months to years. It is not killed by normal routine disinfection and a parvocidal disinfectant must be used.

It is a common infection and is highly contagious with a high mortality rate without appropriate treatment. Young puppies are most susceptible between the waning of maternal antibodies and the synthesis of their own antibodies in response to the vaccine. However, an unvaccinated dog of any age can potentially be affected.

Parvovirus is shed in the faeces. It is spread by direct or indirect contact with infected dogs or their faeces. Infection occurs through ingestion. The incubation period is 3–5 days; however, an incubation period of 7–14 days has been reported in experimental cases. The severity of the disease depends on the age, immune/antibody status of the animal, stress and concurrent infections. The virus targets rapidly dividing cells, i.e. the gastrointestinal tract and bone marrow. In the gastrointestinal tract there is generalized inflammation, causing the gastrointestinal signs. The virus causes flattening of the villi, which causes malabsorption. Destruction of the bone marrow causes immunosuppression and susceptibility to secondary bacterial infections. In puppies under 4 weeks of age, the myocardium is rapidly dividing and will also be targeted by parvovirus, causing heart failure. The infection is often complicated by secondary bacterial infections.

Clinical signs

- Anorexia, depression and lethargy.
- Vomiting and foul-smelling haemorrhagic diarrhoea.
- Pyrexia.
- Shock, dehydration and hypothermia.
- Sudden death.

Diagnostics

A presumptive diagnosis is based on history (general and vaccination) and clinical signs.

- Blood tests: haematology (leucopenia) and biochemistry.
- Faecal sample: antigen tests – CPV antigen ELISA test.
- Post-mortem examination – histopathology.

Treatment

Prevention is by vaccination and reducing the exposure of at-risk animals. Treatment involves:

- Isolation and barrier nursing (see Chapters 7 and 14)
- Supportive – intravenous fluid therapy to correct dehydration and electrolyte imbalance (see Chapter 20)
- Antiemetic and prokinetic medication if vomiting is intractable
- Nutrition (microenteral nutrition has been shown to decrease the time for which a patient is hospitalized)
- Antibiotics to treat secondary bacterial infections.

Microenteral nutrition delivered via a nasogastric tube provides nutrients to the lining of the gut wall and improves gut health. However, if this is not available or possible then, once the vomiting has ceased, water can be introduced. If this is kept down, small highly digestible low-fibre, low-fat meals can be offered to the patient. The amounts are gradually increased over the following few days. Sometimes parvovirus causes permanent damage to the gastrointestinal tract and malabsorption may then occur; these patients will need to be maintained on a special diet.

Leptospirosis

This is a zoonotic disease. It is important that effective precautions are taken when nursing these cases.

Leptospirosis is caused by the Gram-negative bacterium *Leptospira*. There are several serovars including *L. canicola* and *L. icterohaemorrhagiae*. Leptospires can survive in a suitable environment and contaminate water supplies. They are destroyed by desiccation, disinfection and ultraviolet light.

Transmission occurs through contact with infected urine and contaminated water sources, food, soil or bedding. Exposure to farm animals and rats also increases the risk. Recovered dogs can excrete organisms, through urine, intermittently for months. Some species of animal can be carriers without exhibiting signs. The organism penetrates through mucous membranes or damaged skin, spreads through the body and infects many tissues. The incubation period is approximately 7 days. The extent of damage to organs depends on the serovar. *L. icterohaemorrhagiae* predominantly causes hepatocellular damage, giving rise to hepatitis; whereas, *L. canicola* predominantly causes renal dysfunction, leading to an acute interstitial nephritis.

Young animals are usually more severely affected but there is a spectrum of disease from mildly affected (subclinical) cases to sudden death (peracute). Mortality rates can be high, with sudden death or rapid deterioration within a few hours.

Clinical signs

- Anorexia, pyrexia, depression and dehydration.
- Vomiting and diarrhoea.
- Anterior abdominal pain, jaundice, petechiae and bleeding from gum margins (*L. icterohaemorrhagiae*).
- Renal enlargement and pain, polyuria/polydipsia or oliguria (*L. canicola*).

Diagnostics

A presumptive diagnosis is usually made based on history and clinical signs.

- Blood tests: haematology, biochemistry (hepatic and renal abnormalities) and clotting profile.
- Urinalysis: specific gravity, dipstick, sediment and dark field microscopy and culture for leptospires.
- Serological testing: demonstration of a four-fold increase in antibody titre (note, vaccination can interfere with this).
- PCR (blood and urine).
- Post-mortem examination.

Treatment

Prevention is through pest control and vaccination. Antibiotics are used specifically to treat the infection. Penicillins are effective against the bacteraemic state but other antibiotics are required to eliminate the carrier state. Doxycycline is recommended to treat the renal carrier state (the kidney infection). Supportive treatment is aimed at restoring fluid and electrolyte balance. If acute kidney injury has occurred, the aim of treatment is to restore urine production. Blood transfusions may be required if the patient is anaemic.

It should be noted that leptospirosis is a zoonotic disease and care must be taken when nursing these patients. In addition, owners must be given appropriate advice for the management of their animal once they have been discharged.

Canine infectious respiratory disease ('kennel cough complex')

A complex of microorganisms can cause the clinical signs of kennel cough. The organisms include canine parainfluenza virus 5 (PI-5), canine herpesvirus, canine respiratory coronavirus, canine pneumovirus, canine adenovirus 2 (CAV-2), *Bordetella bronchiseptica* and *Mycoplasma*. *B. bronchiseptica* can cause the most severe form of kennel cough when involved in an outbreak. Parainfluenza virus does not last long away from the host. CAV-2, like CAV-1, is relatively resistant but is susceptible to heat. Quaternary ammonium disinfectants are effective against these viruses. *Bordetella* can be shed for months.

Kennel cough is highly infectious but mortality rate is low. Spread usually occurs in areas of high density by direct dog-to-dog contact, hence the name kennel cough. Transmission occurs through aerosol droplets that localize in the respiratory system and cause tracheobronchitis. The incubation period is 5–7 days and the clinical signs tend to resolve after 3–7 days. Damage to the respiratory epithelium can predispose to secondary bacterial infections.

Clinical signs

These are usually restricted to a goose-honking cough that is dry and unproductive, and may be associated with retching. Gentle pressure on the trachea will elicit this cough. The animal will remain bright and alert unless the condition is complicated by bronchopneumonia, in which case anorexia, pyrexia, depression, tachypnoea and dyspnoea will be present.

Diagnostics

A presumptive diagnosis is usually made on history and clinical signs.

Treatment and prevention

Vaccination is available against *B. bronchiseptica* (intranasal and subcutaneous vaccines), CAV-2 and PI-5. The disease is usually self-limiting, but antibiotics should be considered if clinical signs persist or there is evidence of bronchopneumonia. Antitussives can be used to reduce the persistent cough, but should not be used if a productive cough is present (see Chapters 7 and 14).

Nursing care

Nursing plans for patients with infectious diseases are based on the body system that the infectious agent targets (see above for specific body system nursing plans). For example, if a disease causes vomiting refer to Figure 18.21.

Figure 18.67 provides a general nursing plan for patients with infectious diseases.

Parameter	Problem	Nursing considerations	Monitoring
Breathing/vital signs	■ May be a problem depending on infection	■ Regular checks of temperature, pulse and respiration	■ Monitor vital signs
Pain	■ May be a problem depending on infection	■ Provide analgesia as required	■ Monitor for signs of pain
Drinking	■ May be a problem depending on infection	■ Provide fresh water	■ Monitor fluid intake
Eating	■ May be inappetent or anorexic	■ Palatable food. May require prescription diet if the infection has resulted in organ dysfunction ■ Use of convalescing diet and assisted feeding may be required	■ Monitor food intake
Urinating	■ May be affected or a source of infection	■ Care where patient toilets and cleaning this area ■ Barrier nurse	■ Monitor urine output
Defecating	■ May be affected or a source of infection	■ Care where patient toilets and cleaning this area ■ Barrier nurse	■ Monitor faecal output ■ Correct disposal of waste
Grooming	■ Nasal/ocular discharges	■ Groom but take care not to contaminate with bodily fluid ■ Clean discharges and apply petroleum jelly to prevent skin excoriation	■ Good hygiene
Housing	■ Often very contagious or zoonotic	■ Barrier nurse or isolation ■ Disinfect the environment	■ Good hygiene
Mobilizing	■ May be affected or the patient may be recumbent	■ Care where the patients are walked ■ Isolation	■ Monitor exercise tolerance

Other nursing considerations

■ Provision of medication as directed by the veterinary surgeon
■ Owner support and instructions
  • Discuss prevention and vaccination protocols with the owners

18.67 General nursing considerations for patients with infectious diseases.

Infectious diseases – feline

Common feline infectious diseases are summarized in Figure 18.68.

Feline panleucopenia

Feline panleucopenia (feline infectious enteritis, FIE) is caused by a feline parvovirus and infects domestic and wild cats. It is very similar to the canine parvovirus, with similar properties. It survives for long periods in the environment and is very resistant to heating and routine disinfectants. Parvocidal products are required for disinfection.

The disease is usually seen in unvaccinated kittens living in close proximity (e.g. in rescue shelters). Maternal antibodies protect the kittens in the first 3 months of life.

The virus is shed in faeces, vomit, saliva and urine up to 6 weeks after infection. Transmission occurs via the faecal–oral route or transplacentally. Fomites play an important role in transmitting the virus. The incubation period is 2–10 days.

As a parvovirus, feline panleucopenia targets rapidly dividing cells: the lymphoid tissue, bone marrow and intestinal mucosal crypts. Destruction of the lymphoid tissue and bone marrow results in immunosuppression. Damage to the gastrointestinal system leads to gastroenteritis. In the late prenatal and early neonatal stages, the lymphoid tissue, bone marrow and central nervous system can be affected. Early in utero infection can cause abortion and infertility.

Damage to the bone marrow (panleucopenia results in low white blood cell counts) and enteritis increase susceptibility to bacterial infections.

Clinical signs

Many cats will have mild or subclinical infection and the disease is unlikely to be recognized. In peracute cases there will be sudden death. In acute cases the clinical signs include:

- Pyrexia, depression and anorexia
- Vomiting
- Diarrhoea (less frequent)
- Dehydration and hypothermia
- CNS signs: ataxia, tremors and incoordination. Cerebellar hypoplasia if the fetus is infected in the second half of pregnancy
- Retinal lesions
- Queens: abortion and infertility.

Diagnostics

A presumptive diagnosis is usually made on history, clinical signs and demonstration of leucopenia on haematology.

- Blood tests: haematology and biochemistry.
- ELISA test: faecal sample.

Treatment

Prevention is by vaccination. Supportive treatment includes intravenous fluid therapy, antibiotics for secondary bacterial infections and antiemetics for intractable vomiting.

Disease/ infection	Type of infectious agent	Incubation period	Major organs affected	Transmission	Zoonotic	Diagnostic methods	Major nursing needs	Control/ prevention
Feline panleucopenia	Virus	2–10 days	Gastro-intestinal system Bone marrow	Body excretions	No	History, clinical signs Faecal analysis	Fluid therapy Symptomatic Antibiotics	Vaccination
Feline upper respiratory disease	Virus Bacteria	1–10 days	Upper respiratory tract	Saliva Ocular and nasal discharges	No	History, clinical signs Swabs	Symptomatic Antibiotics for secondary bacterial infections	Vaccination Isolation
Feline leukaemia	Virus	Months–years	Immune system Neoplasia	Saliva	No	Blood analysis	Symptomatic	Vaccination
Feline immuno-deficiency	Virus	Variable – may not show clinical signs for many years	Immune system	Cat bites – saliva	No	Blood analysis	Symptomatic	Restrict cat's movements
Feline infectious peritonitis	Virus	Variable	Severe inflammation of body tissues	Ingestion	No	Combination of history, clinical signs, blood tests, tissue biopsy	Symptomatic	Unknown
Feline infectious anaemia	Bacterium	–	Red blood cells	Unknown Fighting/ fleas?	No	Blood analysis	Antibiotics, immuno-suppressants Symptomatic	Flea control, cat fight control
Toxoplasmosis	Coccidia	3–10 days	Intestinal tract system	Ingestion faeces, meat	Yes	Tissue biopsy Serology	Antibiotics	Keep cat indoors

18.68 Common feline infectious diseases (note that this list is not exhaustive).

Feline upper respiratory disease

Feline upper respiratory disease (FURD, cat 'flu) is a common disease involving several primary infectious agents. It usually causes high morbidity but low mortality. The main infectious agents are:

- Viral:
  - Feline herpesvirus type 1 (FHV-1)
  - Feline calicivirus (FCV).
- Bacterial:
  - *Mycoplasma felis*
  - *Bordetella bronchiseptica*
  - *Chlamydia felis*.

FHV-1 and FCV account for 80% of cases. FURD is a highly infectious disease and the infectious organisms are shed in nasal and ocular discharges and saliva from cats exhibiting clinical signs or from asymptomatic carriers. Close contact, aerosolized droplets and contaminated fomites transmit the viruses to susceptible individuals. It should be noted that FHV-1 can only survive hours in the environment, whilst FCV can persist for as long as 4 weeks.

Cats of all ages are susceptible, but the disease may be more severe in kittens, elderly cats and immunocompromised cats.

After inhalation, the virus replicates in the local lymph nodes before targeting the epithelial cells of the respiratory tract and conjunctiva. Most cats will become carriers after the clinical signs are no longer evident.

Infectious agents and clinical signs

Feline herpesvirus type 1

FHV-1 survives in the environment for hours only and is killed by routine disinfection. The incubation period is 2–10 days and infection usually lasts for 10–14 days. After infection cats often become carriers, shedding the virus when stressed. They will remain carriers for life. Severe illness and fatalities can occur in young and old cats. Some cats develop chronic rhinitis or sinusitis ('chronic snufflers').

Clinical signs

- Depression.
- Inappetence/anorexia.
- Paroxysmal sneezing.
- Pyrexia.
- Conjunctivitis.
- Rhinitis (serous ocular/nasal discharges rapidly become mucopurulent with secondary bacterial infection).
- Salivation.
- Dyspnoea and cough if pneumonia develops.

Feline calicivirus

The incubation period is 1–7 days and infection usually lasts for 7–14 days. Disease is usually not as severe as with FHV-1. Carriers of FCV shed the virus continuously, some for a short period and some for years.

Clinical signs

- Mild ocular/nasal discharge (becoming mucopurulent with secondary bacterial infection).
- Sneezing.
- Inappetence.
- Depression.

- Pyrexia.
- Ulceration of hard and soft palates, tongue and cheeks.
- Chronic ulcerative stomatitis and gingivitis in some individuals.

Bordetella bronchiseptica

Infection with this bacterium causes mild upper respiratory tract disease in cats. Coughing is less prominent than in infected dogs. Bronchopneumonia may develop and can cause death, especially in kittens. Recovered cats may remain infectious for several months. Infections are more prevalent in multi-cat households, in rescue catteries and in cats in contact with dogs with respiratory disease, suggesting interspecies transmission.

Clinical signs

- Sneezing.
- Nasal discharge.
- Coughing.
- Submandibular lymphadenopathy.

Chlamydia felis

Chlamydia felis (formerly *Chlamydia psittaci* var. felis) is an intracellular parasite. Strains are species-specific. It is present on the ocular, respiratory, gastrointestinal and genitourinary mucosa of infected cats. The organism is very short lived off the host and transmission is likely to occur through direct contact with infected ocular and nasal discharges. All ages can be affected but kittens the most severely. The incubation period is 4–10 days. Infection may be unapparent to overt. The most common illnesses are acute, chronic and relapsing conjunctivitis. Improvement is normally seen after 2–3 weeks. The organism can also cause nasal and lower respiratory infections. Abortions or infertility may also be caused by *Chlamydia felis* but this remains to be proven clinically.

Clinical signs

- Conjunctivitis, hyperaemia and blepharospasm.
- Serous to mucopurulent ocular discharge.
- Mild upper respiratory tract disease (less common).

Diagnostics

A presumptive diagnosis is usually made on history and clinical signs.

- Oropharyngeal swab in viral transport medium for isolation of FHV-1 or FCV.
- PCR.
- Oropharyngeal or nasal swab in charcoal Amies transport medium for culture of *Bordetella* and PCR.
- Ocular swab for PCR detection of *Chlamydia* DNA.

Treatment

Prevention is by vaccination. Treatment is symptomatic and supportive. Nursing care is particularly important.

- Antibiotics if viral infection complicated by secondary bacterial infection.
- Chlamydosis: topical or systemic tetracyclines. In multi-cat households the whole cat population should be treated at the same time. Treatment should continue for 2 weeks after clinical signs have abated.
- Bordetellosis: antibiotics (tetracyclines).
- Intravenous fluid therapy if cat dehydrated and anorexic.

Preventive measures in a cattery

- Ensure that all animals are vaccinated before entering the premises.
- Good quality housing and management to ensure good air quality, to reduce fomite transmission, reduce stress and reduce overpopulation.
- Cats should not be able to gain access to other cats. Ideally runs should have Perspex walls to provide a sneeze barrier.
- Use of disposable feeding bowls to reduce fomite transmission.
- Maintain correct disinfection protocols.
- Isolate any cats showing clinical signs.

For more information, see the *BSAVA Manual of Canine and Feline Shelter Medicine: Principles of Health and Welfare in a Multi-animal Environment*.

Feline leukaemia

Feline leukaemia virus (FeLV) is a retrovirus. It is host species-specific and affects both domestic and wild cats around the world. It is associated with leukaemia and other lymphoproliferative diseases and non-neoplastic disease.

The virus is shed constantly in saliva; therefore, close contact and mutual grooming are required for spread. Cats in close contact or living in the same household are most likely to become infected. Vertical transmission from dam to off-spring via the placenta and milk also occurs. The main source of infection is the persistently viraemic cat that is either a healthy carrier or has FeLV-related disease. Kittens are more susceptible than adults and are more likely to become persistently viraemic.

Although the virus is shed in other bodily fluids (e.g. mucus and faeces), it is unlikely to be spread via this route; it is readily inactivated in the environment. Iatrogenic spread could occur through blood transfusions and contaminated needles or instruments.

After initial oronasal infection the animal may exhibit mild, vague clinical signs of lethargy and inappetence and a lymphadenopathy. At this point, cats can mount an appropriate immune response, recover and do not become carriers. In other cases, cats become permanently viraemic and are carriers. The most important factors that determine whether a cat recovers or is permanently infected are its age at infection and the dose of virus to which it is exposed. Cats with persistent viraemia have a high risk of developing FeLV-related disease.

The diseases caused by FeLV can be divided into two categories: neoplastic and non-neoplastic. Malignancy may be caused by the virus being inserted into the genome and causing changes in the expression of the oncogene, which results in abnormal 'growth' and control of some cell lines. The transformation is usually of lymphoid and myeloid cells, causing lymphoma, leukaemias and myelodysplastic disorders. Anaemias may occur as a result of interference with normal maturation of the red blood cell line in the bone marrow or due to anaemia of chronic disease. Thrombocytopenia and leucopenia are a result of decreased production caused by suppressed or infiltrated bone marrow. The virus also interferes with a normal immune response; therefore, these cats are more prone to infections. Circulating immune complexes may cause immune-mediated disease (e.g. glomerulonephritis, polyarthritis). Reproductive disorders include infertility and abortions.

Latent infections may revert to overt viraemia in times of stress, such as pregnancy and glucocorticoid treatment, but this is unusual and latent infection is most likely to be eliminated over time.

The prevalence of FeLV has declined over the years with effective routine testing of kittens in shelters and use of early vaccination.

Clinical signs
Neoplastic FeLV
Lymphoma can be categorized by the site of origin. FeLV may be associated with some sites, including mediastinal lymphoma. Clinical signs for the latter include:

- Tachypnoea
- Dyspnoea
- Regurgitation
- Horner's syndrome
- Non-specific signs of disease.

Alimentary lymphoma (intestinal lymphoma) is usually FeLV-negative even though other lymphomas can be associated with FeLV.

Clinical signs for leukaemia include:

- Lethargy
- Bleeding
- Sepsis
- Splenomegaly.

Non-neoplastic FeLV
- Anaemia (see 'Anaemia', above).
- Platelet abnormalities:
  - Bleeding tendencies (see 'Clotting disorders', above).
- Leucocyte abnormalities:
  - Increased incidence of bacterial infections
  - Gingivitis.
- Immunosuppression:
  - Increased incidence of infections (e.g. toxoplasmosis, cat 'flu, gingivitis).
- Reproductive disorders:
  - Infertility
  - Abortions.

If kittens are infected *in utero* they often die at an early age of 'fading kitten' syndrome (see Chapter 24). They fail to nurse and become dehydrated and hypothermic within the first 2 weeks of life.

Diagnostics
If an apparently healthy cat has a positive FeLV ELISA test, a confirmatory test is recommended. The result should be interpreted in light of the clinical signs of the patient. As the cat may still be able control the infection, a repeat test at a later time is recommended.

- Specific blood tests: ELISA for FeLV.
- Other blood tests: haematology for haemopoietic cell lines.
- FIV test as may occur concurrently.
- Bone marrow cytology.
- Fine-needle aspiration/biopsy of lymph nodes.
- Radiography and/or ultrasonography.

Treatment

Prevention is by vaccination of at-risk cats. Treatment is supportive: although the underlying virus cannot be treated, the secondary disease should be treated as for an FeLV-negative cat.

Good routine management of disease needs to be maintained to avoid stress to the immune system. For example, good flea and worm control and routine vaccinations should be continued.

FeLV-positive cats should be removed from multi-cat households if the other cats are found to be negative, using 'test and remove' schemes.

Feline immunodeficiency

Feline immunodeficiency virus (FIV) is a retrovirus. It is related to human immunodeficiency virus (HIV) but is host species-specific, i.e. it only infects cats, both wild and domestic. It is labile and does not survive in the environment.

The virus is transmitted predominantly via bite wounds. The virus is found in large quantities in the saliva. Transmission to other cats in a multi-cat household is infrequent. Intact male cats are at increased risk as they are most likely to roam and fight. The average age of infected cats is around 6 years.

After infection, replication of the virus occurs in the salivary glands and lymphoid tissue. At this point there may be mild and vague clinical signs or infection may be subclinical. An immune response can be mounted that decreases the circulating virus and the cats generally become asymptomatic for a period of time. The virus, however, continues to replicate and over time there is destruction of the cat's immune system. This leaves the cat susceptible to infections and developing various tumours. The brain and kidneys can also be affected, leading to neurological signs and renal failure, respectively.

Clinical signs

Clinical signs are non-specific. After the initial infection the cats may have mild lethargy, inappetence and pyrexia. In the later stage of infection, clinical signs are associated with opportunistic infections, neoplasia or other syndromes, such as wasting, and include:

- Weight loss and emaciation
- Lethargy
- Inappetence
- Lymphadenopathy
- Pyrexia
- Gingivitis/stomatitis
- Chronic diarrhoea
- Chronic nasal discharge
- Chronic ocular discharge
- Anterior uveitis (directly FIV-related or as a result of toxoplasmosis)
- Chronic respiratory infection
- Abscesses
- Neurological signs (behavioural changes, seizures, paresis).

Diagnostics

- Blood tests: haematology and biochemistry.
- FIV-specific ELISA for antibodies (false results may be seen in cats vaccinated for FIV and in cats with maternal antibody still present).
- Confirmatory tests: serology or PCR (for cats vaccinated against FIV).
- FeLV test as can be concurrent.

ELISA-based tests

It can take a couple of months for cats to produce antibodies against FIV. Therefore, if a cat has been recently exposed to FIV and tests negative, then the test should be repeated after 8–12 weeks (anti-FIV antibodies may not develop until 8 weeks after infection).

Queens transfer antibodies to their newborn kittens via milk. These maternally derived antibodies (MDA) are then detected when the kittens are tested. FIV is usually only passed on to about one-third of the litter, but all the kittens will have MDA at the time of sampling as they may remain in the kitten's immune system for up to 4 months. Kittens that have been infected with the virus do not usually produce their own antibodies to the virus for a further 2 months. Therefore, to avoid false-positive results, kittens born to FIV-positive queens should not be tested until 6 months old or should be tested repeatedly until at least 6 months old.

Treatment

At this time there is no specific treatment with proven long-term efficacy, although antiviral drugs may be used. Treatment is aimed at the complications of FIV infection, i.e. opportunistic infections and neoplasia. Infections should be treated with appropriate antimicrobials. Dental hygiene is important to reduce stomatitis.

Routine inactivated vaccines can be given to asymptomatic FIV-positive cats living in a high-risk population to reduce the effects of stress that these diseases could have on the cat. Other measures include:

- Routine flea and worming prevention
- Neutering
- Removal of kittens from FIV-positive queens from birth
- Keeping FIV-positive cats indoors and away from FIV-negative cats.

Feline infectious peritonitis

Feline infectious peritonitis (FIP) is caused by a coronavirus. Although the incidence is low, the disease is usually fatal. It is a disease of multi-cat households and there is an increased risk in pedigree households. Clinical disease is seen most frequently in cats under 2 years of age, stressed or with concurrent disease.

The virus is shed via the faeces. Cats are usually infected via the oronasal route by direct contact with infected individuals or indirectly through contaminated fomites. Although the virus may survive in the environment, it is readily destroyed by routine disinfection.

Coronavirus infection is common. In the majority of cases the cats are asymptomatic or develop mild signs of diarrhoea and eliminate the virus. Less commonly the virus causes FIP. The reason why these cats develop FIP is not fully understood. One school of thought is that the virus mutates to a more pathogenic form and can multiply within macrophages, which are then dispersed around the body via the circulation, targeting the vascular beds of the peritoneum, pleura, eyes, meninges or kidneys. Antibodies produced against the coronavirus form complexes with the antigen that lodge in the vasculature and cause a vasculitis.

- If this occurs in the peritoneum or pleura, it causes protein-rich fluid leakage and accumulation in the cavities. This is referred to as wet effusive FIP and is generally seen in cats under 2 years old.
- The dry form of FIP is seen in older cats, often after stress. There is inflammation and development of pyogranulomatous lesions throughout the body, without fluid accumulation.

Both forms are difficult to treat and the disease is invariably fatal. Therefore, the prognosis is poor.

Clinical signs

FIP cats have clinical signs of systemic disease – anorexia, lethargy and depression. The signs may be variable depending on the affected organs.

Wet effusive FIP
- Pleural effusion: dyspnoea and tachypnoea.
- Ascites: pot-bellied appearance.
- Weight loss.

Dry FIP
Common presenting signs include:

- Weight loss
- Inappetence.

Other signs depend on the organs affected:

- Neurological signs
- Ocular disease
- Gastrointestinal disease
- Renal disease.

Diagnostics

Diagnosis can be difficult, as the majority of cats are seropositive for coronavirus but do not have FIP. A combination of criteria is therefore used to make a diagnosis of FIP:

- History and clinical signs
- Blood tests: haematology and biochemistry (especially looking for increased globulins)
- FeLV and FIV test as may occur concurrently
- Fluid analysis: exudates with increased proteins
- Biopsy of enlarged organs
- Post-mortem examination.

Treatment

The prognosis is poor and treatment is palliative. Corticosteroids may target the inflammation and slow the deterioration of the cat's condition, but may also result in immunosupression. Supportive treatment involves thoracocentesis to relieve dyspnoea associated with a pleural effusion.

Prevention is aimed at managing the multi-cat households by reducing faecal contamination, keeping cat numbers low, and isolation and early weaning of the kittens.

Feline infectious anaemia

The organism causing feline infectious anaemia (FIA) was previously known as *Haemobartonella felis* but has been reclassified as *Mycoplasma haemofelis* and *Candidatus Mycoplasma haemominutum*. They are parasites of feline red blood cells and live on the cell surface.

The route of transmission is not completely understood. It is potentially spread by cat bites, fleas and blood transfusions. There is an increased incidence in cats that are FIV or FeLV-positive, unvaccinated, roaming or involved in frequent cat fights.

Usually the severe anaemias attributable to mycoplasmas are caused by *Mycoplasma haemofelis*. The organism causes damage to the red blood cell surface. This is recognized by the immune system and the red blood cells are destroyed. This results in anaemia, which can be severe, especially if there is a concurrent FeLV infection.

The severity and length of infection varies between cats. Some cats have a cyclical parasitaemia, resulting in cyclical anaemia. Whether cats remain carriers may differ depending on the species of *Mycoplasma* causing the infection.

Clinical signs

Clinical signs are usually a result of anaemia (see 'Anaemia', above) and pyrexia.

- Collapse, lethargy and anorexia.
- Dyspnoea, tachypnoea and tachycardia.
- Pale mucous membranes.
- Splenic enlargement.
- Enlarged lymph nodes.
- Pyrexia.

Diagnostics

The diagnostic plan for anaemia is followed:

- Blood tests: haematology (including reticulocytes: the anaemia is regenerative) and biochemistry
- Fresh blood smears to stain for *Mycoplasma* (Wright–Giemsa stain). The parasites are visible on the surface of the red blood cells. Due to the cyclical nature, multiple smears over time may need to be examined
- PCR for *M. haemofelis* and *Candidatus M. haemominutum* FeLV and FIV testing (see above).

Treatment

The infection is treated with doxycycline for 2–3 weeks. As there is an immune component to the red blood cell destruction, the patient is often given immunosuppressive drugs. Supportive care includes blood transfusions for severe anaemia.

Toxoplasmosis

This is an important zoonotic disease, especially for pregnant women. *Toxoplasma gondii* is an intracellular protozoan parasite (see Chapter 6). It infects all warm-blooded animals, but cats are the only species in which the parasite can complete its life cycle (the definitive host) and the only species that sheds oocysts (in their faeces). The other species act as intermediate hosts. The organism has a predilection for placental tissue, especially in ewes and in women. It is a multisystemic infection. Neurological signs are seen in 10% of affected animals.

Clinical signs

Most infections are subclinical. Most adult cats are immune to infection as a result of previous exposure. If infection occurs in a previously uninfected queen during pregnancy, the parasite can multiply in the placenta and spread to the fetuses. Affected kittens may be stillborn or may die before weaning.

Clinical signs depend on the organs affected:

- Pyrexia
- Anorexia
- Lethargy
- Weight loss
- Ophthalmitis (especially uveitis)
- Pneumonia
- Hepatitis
- Myositis
- Pancreatitis
- Myocarditis
- Skin lesions (rare)
- Diarrhoea
- Vomiting
- Muscle hyperaesthesia
- Lameness
- Ascites
- Neurological signs
- Sudden death.

Diagnostics

- Blood tests: haematology and biochemistry.
- FeLV and FIV testing as may occur concurrently.
- CSF sample if neurological signs are present.
- Faecal examination.
- Serology.
- Biopsy.

Treatment

Systemic disease should be treated with clindamycin. Corticosteroids are contraindicated.

Advice for clients on avoiding toxoplasmosis

- Prepare animal food in a separate area, using separate utensils and feeding bowls
- Do not allow pets to lick bowls, utensils or cooking items that will be used by people
- Empty cat litter trays daily and clean with boiling water and disinfectant
- Regular and prompt cleaning of litter trays will prevent oocysts from sporulating and becoming infectious
- Pregnant women should avoid cleaning litter trays and should wear waterproof protective gloves when gardening to avoid contact with buried or decomposed cat faeces, as the oocysts in the environment will have sporulated and become infectious. Hands should be washed thoroughly prior to contact with cups, food, etc
- Wash all vegetables thoroughly for the same reason
- Cook meat thoroughly
- Cover children's sand pits to prevent cats using as litter trays

---

Nursing care

A general nursing plan for patients with infectious diseases is given in Figure 18.67. For specific body system nursing plans, relevant to the body system that the infectious agent targets, see text above. For example, if a disease causes diarrhoea, refer to Figure 18.23.

Infectious diseases – canine/feline

Rabies

This is a zoonotic disease.

Rabies is caused by a lyssavirus. It is quite labile and does not survive in the environment. Rabies is an important fatal zoonotic disease and is widely spread through the rest of the world except Australasia and Antarctica. The UK is currently free of terrestrial rabies; however, European bat lyssaviruses (EBLV-1 in a Serotine bat and EBLV-2 in Daubenton's bats) have been identified and can be responsible for causing 'bat rabies' in humans. Control of stray dogs and rabies vaccinations have been important in reducing the number of rabies cases in pet dog and human populations. Dogs that travel abroad as part of the Pet Travel Scheme are required to be vaccinated against rabies (see Chapter 7).

Rabies is transmitted directly via saliva in bite wounds or abrasions from infected animals. All warm-blooded animals are variably susceptible to infection. Wild animals can act as a reservoir of infection.

The incubation period can be prolonged, with an average of around 2 months. The length of time to clinical signs is related to the infective dose and the distance the virus has to travel to the central nervous system: after the animal is bitten, the virus replicates locally before spreading up the nerves to the central nervous system. It replicates in the central nervous system before spreading along nerves to other parts of the body and into the salivary glands, where it is secreted in the saliva and capable of infecting another animal. Clinical signs of abnormal behaviour and paralysis are caused by direct damage to the central nervous system. The disease is considered fatal.

Clinical signs

The clinical signs of rabies have classically been divided into two major types: excitative ('furious') and paralytic ('dumb'). However, atypical signs are commonly seen. From the onset of clinical signs in pets, death usually occurs within 2–7 days.

Excitative

These animals become irritable, restless and vicious. They usually develop other neurological signs of incoordination, disorientation and generalized grand mal seizures. Wild animals may be less fearful of humans.

Paralytic

Incoordination is one of the first signs of the paralytic form. The motor neurons are damaged, resulting in hindlimb ataxia progressing to paralysis. Progressive laryngeal and pharyngeal paralysis occurs, giving difficulty in swallowing and profuse salivation and drooling. Facial expression is affected, resulting in drooping eyelids, sagging jaw and squinting. Progressive paralysis ensues, leading to respiratory arrest and death.

The distinction between the two forms is often not clear-cut and both forms progress toward paralysis, coma and death. The paralytic form is very uncommon in cats.

Diagnostics

There are no reliable ante-mortem tests for the diagnosis of rabies; therefore, a presumptive diagnosis needs to be based on history and clinical signs. As rabies is a fatal zoonotic disease, suspected cases are euthanased and the diagnosis is made on post-mortem examination of the brain. Rabies is a notifiable disease. Suspect cases should be isolated and Department for Environment, Food and Rural Affairs (Defra) contacted immediately.

Any animal that has potentially been exposed should be handled with great care. Transmission routes should be borne in mind and any abrasions, especially to the hands and face, should be covered. Masks with visors should be worn to avoid infection via mucous membranes.

Treatment

- Dogs are vaccinated in areas where there is a risk of rabies and in those taking part in the Pet Travel Scheme (see Defra website and Chapters 7 and 10).
- Humans are vaccinated if they are deemed at risk (e.g. staff working in quarantine kennels or handling certain wildlife species such as bats).
- Dogs with clinical signs should be placed in strict isolation and Defra contacted immediately. These cases are not treated.
- If bitten, the wound should be washed immediately with detergent and then 40–70% alcohol. Medical attention should be sought urgently.

Salmonellosis

This is a zoonotic disease. Salmonellosis is caused by *Salmonella*, of which there are many serotypes. The bacterium is not host species-specific and occurs commonly in the intestinal tract of healthy mammals, birds and reptiles. Under certain circumstances it can cause systemic disease. It can survive for relatively long periods in the environment.

It is shed in the faeces, and transmission occurs through ingestion of faecally contaminated food, water or fomites. The bacteria multiply rapidly in foodstuffs stored at room temperature and in food that is inadequately cooked. Shedding can be intermittent and is usually increased when the animal is stressed. Younger animals are more susceptible to infection and illness. Overcrowding, stress and immunosuppression increase the risk of salmonellosis in dogs and cats.

After ingestion, the bacteria localize in the intestinal epithelium. Acute gastroenteritis is the most common clinical manifestation, but septicaemia can occur and the infection may become established in other tissues (placenta, conjunctiva, joints, meninges). Carrier animals may exhibit GI signs when subject to stress.

Clinical signs

- Anorexia and depression.
- Diarrhoea – haemorrhagic in severe cases.
- Vomiting and abdominal pain.
- Dehydration.
- Weight loss.
- Pyrexia.
- If severely affected and has a bacteraemia, will present in shock.
- *In utero* infections result in abortions, stillbirths and the birth of weak puppies.

Diagnostics

The diagnosis may be suspected from history and clinical signs.

- Blood tests: haematology/biochemistry are non-specific.
- Faecal culture: may be supportive but bear in mind that *Salmonella* can be isolated from healthy individuals.

Treatment

- Barrier nursing and isolation.
- Antibiotics are only used if the disease is systemic, as they (except fluoroquinolones) may increase risk of shedding once the animal has recovered. The disease is usually self-limiting.
- Fluid therapy and other supportive care for acute diarrhoea.

Campylobacteriosis

This is a zoonotic disease. The bacterium *Campylobacter* is an opportunistic organism whose role as a primary pathogen is not fully known. *Campylobacter* species probably act synergistically with other infections. Spread is through ingestion of undercooked raw food, contaminated water or faeces from infected animals, or via food/water bowls. Clinical infection is more common in animals under 6 months of age.

Clinical signs

- Watery or mucoid diarrhoea.
- Faecal tenesmus.
- Dullness and inappetence.

Diagnostics

- Culture of organisms from fresh (<24h old) faeces, using selective media.
- Detection of *Campylobacter* – it should be borne in mind that this is not always diagnostic on its own because of the carrier state.

Treatment

- The disease is self-limiting.
- Antibiotics may be given to reduce duration and severity of diarrhoea, minimizing risk of infection to humans and other animals.
- Fluid therapy.

Nursing care

A general nursing plan for patients with infectious diseases is given in Figure 18.67. For specific body system nursing plans, relevant to the body system that the infectious agent targets, see text above. For example, if a disease causes vomiting, refer to Figure 18.21.

References and further reading

Arthurs G, Brown G and Pettitt R (2018) *BSAVA Manual of Canine and Feline Musculoskeletal Disorders, 2nd edn.* BSAVA Publications, Gloucester

Dean R, Roberts M and Stavisky J (2018) *BSAVA Manual of Canine and Feline Shelter Medicine – Principles of Health and Welfare in a Multi-animal Environment.* BSAVA Publications, Gloucester

Dobson JM and Lascelles DX (2011) *BSAVA Manual of Canine and Feline Oncology, 3rd edn.* BSAVA Publications, Gloucester

Elliott J, Grauer GF and Westropp JL (2017) *BSAVA Manual of Canine and Feline Nephrology and Urology, 3rd edn.* BSAVA Publications, Gloucester

Fuentes VL, Johnson LR and Dennis S (2010) *BSAVA Manual of Canine and Feline Cardiorespiratory Medicine, 2nd edn.* BSAVA Publications, Gloucester

Hall EH, Simpson JW and Williams DA (2005) *BSAVA Manual of Canine and Feline Gastroenterology, 2nd edn.* BSAVA Publications, Gloucester

Harvey A and Tasker S (2013) *BSAVA Manual of Feline Practice.* BSAVA Publications, Gloucester

Hutchinson T and Robinson K (2015) *BSAVA Manual of Canine Practice.* BSAVA Publications, Gloucester

Mooney CT and Peterson ME (2012) *BSAVA Manual of Canine and Feline Endocrinology, 4th edn.* BSAVA Publications, Gloucester

Nelson C and Couto CG (2019) *Small Animal Internal Medicine, 6th edn.* Elsevier, Missouri

Williams JM and Niles JD (2015) *BSAVA Manual of Canine and Feline Abdominal Surgery, 2nd edn.* BSAVA Publications, Gloucester

Self-assessment questions

1. Describe the clinical signs of acute heart failure and identify the key features when nursing patients with heart failure.
2. What are the clinical signs of pancreatitis in the dog? How does the treatment and nursing care differ between the cat and dog with pancreatitis?
3. What are the clinical signs of acute and chronic renal failure? How are patients with chronic renal failure nursed?
4. What are the clinical signs of diabetes mellitus? How is diabetes mellitus managed? What short term nursing protocols would you put in place for managing ketoacidosis?
5. What are the causes of arthritis? How is arthritis treated and nursed?
6. How is parvovirus shed? What age group is most susceptible to infection? Describe how to nurse these patients.
7. Describe how to nurse a patient with cat 'flu.
8. Advise a client on how to avoid contracting toxoplasmosis.
9. What is the difference between regurgitation and vomiting? How would nursing differ between the two conditions?
10. What are the clinical signs of a bleeding disorder and how is it diagnosed and nursed?

Chapter 19

Small animal first aid and emergencies

Amanda Boag and Racheal Marshall

Learning objectives

After studying this chapter, readers will have the knowledge to:

- **Define a veterinary emergency and provide advice on emergency care over the telephone**
- **Recognize the severity of an emergency and perform appropriate triage**
- **Describe the approach to the assessment of the emergency patient**
- **List the major body systems and understand their importance in the evaluation of the emergency patient**
- **Describe the procedure to follow if a patient undergoes cardiopulmonary arrest**
- **Explain the veterinary nurse's role when evaluating emergency patients and understand professional limitations**
- **List common veterinary emergencies, their presenting signs and their initial stabilization and treatment**

Introduction

Veterinary emergency medicine is a rapidly developing area of the profession. In general, an emergency is classified as any illness or injury where the animal's owner or guardian perceives that urgent veterinary attention is needed. Once the animal has been examined by a trained veterinary professional (veterinary surgeon or veterinary nurse), emergencies may be further categorized as those that are unstable where immediate/urgent diagnostics and treatment are required and those that are stable where further diagnostics and treatment may be delayed safely.

The Royal College of Veterinary Surgeons (RCVS) requires that all veterinary surgeons in practice take steps to provide 24-hour emergency first aid and pain relief to animals, according to their skills and the specific situation. The RCVS has confirmed that the responsibility for the welfare of an animal rests primarily with the owner, keeper or carer of that animal. When the owner, keeper or carer is concerned that the animal is suffering or requires attention and contacts a veterinary surgeon, they then place the onus of decision-making on to the veterinary surgeon. With the benefit of prior knowledge of the animal, or relevant enquiry of the client, the veterinary surgeon must decide whether attention is required immediately, or whether it can be reasonably delayed. Full details on the professional responsibilities of veterinary surgeons and nurses when dealing with emergencies can be found in the relevant professional code of conduct (www.rcvs.org.uk/advice-and-guidance/code-of-professional-conduct-for-veterinary-surgeons/ and www.rcvs.org.uk/advice-and-guidance/code-of-professional-conduct-for-veterinary-nurses/).

While veterinary surgeons and nurses are able to develop a special interest in this field, it is vital that all members of nursing staff are confident and competent in dealing with emergencies. These can present at any time, including during routine daily clinics, and some practices (especially in rural areas) will continue to provide their own out-of-hours cover. Although practices may focus on treating only certain species, on an emergency basis 'a veterinary surgeon on duty should not unreasonably refuse to facilitate the provision of first aid and pain relief for all other species until such time as a more appropriate emergency veterinary service accepts responsibility for the animal'.

This chapter will outline the general approach to the veterinary emergency patient and the role of the nurse, and will summarize some of the common clinical conditions seen in an emergency practice. Emergency work is always a team effort and the emergency nurse is a vital part of the veterinary team.

A successful outcome for the patient depends on:

- Early recognition of the severity and nature of the problem
- Good communication with the owner and with other members of the team
- Implementation of appropriate treatment
- Careful and diligent monitoring.

BSAVA Textbook of Veterinary Nursing, sixth edition. Edited by Barbara Cooper, Elizabeth Mullineaux and Lynn Turner.

Although a veterinary surgeon will ultimately examine every patient, the experienced emergency nurse should be able to assess the severity of illness of each animal. This allows cases to be prioritized on the basis of clinical need and determines the optimal order in which they should be treated. The goal is to ensure a successful outcome for as many patients as possible, recognizing that the decision to euthanase an individual patient will sometimes need to be made.

Rules for emergency practice

- Remain calm
- Be prepared
- Do not put yourself, the owner or other staff members at risk
- Ensure that the animal is at no further risk
- Assess severity of injury/illness
- Administer appropriate first aid where necessary
- Contact the veterinary surgeon as soon as possible

Types of emergency

Veterinary emergencies comprise a wide range of clinical problems, ranging from those that are imminently life-threatening to minor injuries and ailments.

Triage is the process of rapidly classifying patients on the basis of their clinical priority, allowing identification of those patients that need urgent life-saving help and ensuring that this occurs immediately and before patients with less severe problems are dealt with.

In emergency practice, one of the nurse's major roles is to perform triage so that the veterinary surgeon can focus their attention on the patients that need them the most. The process of triage involves assessing information from the patient's history and initial clinical examination, in particular an assessment of their major body systems (i.e. the cardiovascular, respiratory and neurological systems).

- Severe life-threatening emergencies are those that involve significant disturbances in the major body systems, where there is the potential for rapid deterioration and death.
- The list of minor emergencies is long but includes problems such as minor wounds, mild vomiting or diarrhoea, polydipsia, skin lesions/scratching and lameness. Although these animals may be dealt with on an emergency basis, their full evaluation and treatment can be delayed until after the needs of those patients with life-threatening emergencies have been addressed.

Telephone calls

This form of communication is often the first contact the practice will have with a client and their pet during an emergency. Understandably, clients may be very distressed and concerned at this time. It is vital that the veterinary nurse or receptionist remains sympathetic, calm and patient, and shows that they are aware that the client is distressed. Owners may not understand why certain questions are being asked and may become upset. They need to be reassured that the questions are being asked in order to ensure that the best advice and help are provided.

The immediate aim of the telephone conversation is to establish whether the pet has a life-threatening problem. If this is the case, the owner should be advised that the pet should be brought to the practice as soon as possible. Further questioning at this point will only delay the pet's arrival at the practice and may have a negative impact on its chances of survival.

Emergencies for which examination at a veterinary practice should be advised without delay

- Respiratory distress
- Severe bleeding, either from wounds or from body orifices
- Collapse or unconsciousness
- Rapid and progressive abdominal distension
- Inability to urinate
- Sudden onset of severe neurological abnormalities
- Protracted vomiting, especially if animal is also depressed
- Severe diarrhoea, especially if haemorrhagic
- Witnessed ingestion of toxin
- Severe weakness or inability to stand
- Extreme pain
- Fracture with bone ends visible or wounds in close proximity to fracture site
- Dystocia

In other situations, further questioning may be needed to determine whether the animal needs to be seen immediately or whether an appointment can be made. Examples of this include:

- Mild to moderate vomiting
- Non-haemorrhagic diarrhoea
- Small wounds with minimal blood loss
- Discomfort on urinating but urine is being passed
- Polyuria/polydipsia
- Weight-bearing lameness.

Questions to be asked if the emergency is not life-threatening

- What is the breed, age and sex of the pet?
- Is it on any medication? If so, what medication is this and when was it last given?
- What is the exact nature of the problem?
- When did the problem start and has it been progressive?
- Has the animal ever had this problem before? If so, when? Was it treated?
- Does the animal seem depressed or lethargic?
- Does the animal have any other signs?

It is advisable to take the client and pet's name plus a contact telephone number at the beginning of the call. This allows the client and pet to be referred to by name, which can help to calm the situation, and should the call be disconnected enables the client to be called back. Following this, the focus should be on the current problem. It can be frustrating for a distressed owner to be asked questions about the longer term medical history (e.g. vaccination history) before being asked about their pet's problem. To gain maximum information, questions should be specific and concise. To avoid misunderstanding, it is preferable to speak directly to the owner rather than to a third party.

Occasionally telephone advice is sought when the pet seems relatively normal but a serious incident has occurred recently. It is recommended that the following advice is given.

- Recent trauma (e.g. glancing blow from a car, fall from a height) has occurred and the animal appears to have recovered.
  - In this situation a full clinical examination by a veterinary surgeon should be recommended. It is possible that the animal has internal injuries. A veterinary surgeon may be able to identify these injuries, allowing early treatment. If the owners are unwilling to bring the pet to the practice, they should be asked to observe the pet closely and call back immediately if any unusual signs (especially respiratory distress, weakness and pale mucous membranes) are observed.
- The animal has suffered a seizure but it has stopped by the time the owner contacts the veterinary practice.
  - It is recommended that the animal be seen promptly. Although many seizures are single incidents, an underlying medical problem predisposing to further seizures may be identified.

Owners will often ask if there is any treatment or first aid they can give at home. Any advice should be given with caution. Very few owners have medical training and their interpretation of clinical signs may be misleading. If in doubt, it is always advisable to recommend that a pet is seen at the practice in order that it may be examined by a trained professional.

In some situations, first aid provided by the owner before reaching the practice may be helpful:

- With haemorrhage, owners should be advised to apply pressure directly over an area of profuse bleeding, using a clean towel or cloth, whilst the animal is transported to the clinic
- In rare cases where a foreign object is present in the wound, the owner should be instructed not to remove it but to transport the animal to the practice with the object in place. It may be possible to apply pressure around the foreign object. Removing the object can potentially make any bleeding much worse
- On rare occasions, either as a result of trauma or if a surgical wound has broken down, owners may report being able to see internal organs (often fat or intestines) protruding through the wound. The owners should be advised to cover the pet's abdomen lightly (not tightly) with a clean towel for transportation and prevent the animal from licking the area
- With thermal burns, owners should be advised to run the affected area under cool water for 5–10 minutes, otherwise the area will continue to burn whilst the patient is being transported and result in further tissue damage
- For patients with heat stroke, owners should be instructed to dowse their pet with tepid water and take measures to cool the car prior to transportation to ensure the animal's temperature does not continue to increase on the journey to the practice.

The owner's personal safety is paramount and it may not be possible for first aid measures to be carried out on animals with painful wounds.

Rules for telephone conversations

- Always answer the phone by introducing yourself and your practice. A panicking owner needs to know that they have contacted a vet
- Always be polite and calm
- Ascertain as quickly as possible whether the problem is life-threatening
- Ensure the client knows where they need to attend and be able to provide clear directions to the practice
- Be able to offer alternative means of transport (local pet ambulances, taxi firms) in case the owner has transport difficulties
- Give the owner advice on how to safely transport their pet
- Obtain an estimated time of arrival
- Obtain the owner's contact details, including a mobile telephone number if possible. Repeat this information back to the caller to ensure that it is correct
- Give the owner a financial quote for an emergency consultation
- Check whether the pet regularly attends a veterinary surgery and, if so, which one

---

Practices should consider having a telephone logbook where details of emergency telephone calls can be recorded. They should also have a list of local pet ambulances or taxis that will transport pets to give out to clients who have no transport or are unable to drive. Clients should be offered advice on how to transport their pet to prevent making the condition worse and to reduce the risk of owners being bitten.

When an emergency call is taken, the veterinary nurse or receptionist should inform the rest of the team about the nature of the emergency and its expected arrival time. The surgery should be prepared to receive the patient. This may include preparing equipment for oxygen administration, intravenous fluid administration or wound dressings.

Handling and transport of emergency patients

Emergency patients generally have the same considerations regarding handling and transportation as other patients (see Chapter 11). Importantly, emergency patients may be shocked and in pain. Dogs and cats that are normally considered to be friendly and placid may become aggressive when injured and in pain. Veterinary staff should be cautious when approaching these animals and should use a muzzle or other restraint if concerned. Analgesia, under veterinary direction, should be given at the earliest possible opportunity; this will facilitate further handling. Owners should also be reminded that they should be cautious even when handling their own pet.

The dyspnoeic patient, especially the dyspnoeic cat, warrants special consideration. These patients may already be stressed due to their underlying disease and the journey to the practice. Further handling of these patients on arrival, especially if they struggle, may precipitate cardiopulmonary arrest. Dyspnoeic animals should be placed in an oxygen-enriched environment and given time to settle after arrival before a full examination or further procedures (e.g. catheter placement, thoracocentesis, further diagnostic tests) are carried out.

Consideration should also be given to location when handling small mammal and exotic emergencies; many of these species are natural prey species and can find the presence and even odour of dogs and cats very distressing.

Arrival at the surgery

The key to treating emergencies successfully is to be prepared. As much paperwork as possible, including a consent form, should be prepared in advance. All practices, including both general practices and those that predominantly carry out emergency or out-of-hours work, should have a designated area for dealing with emergency patients. This emergency area or room should be easily accessible from as many other areas of the building as possible, including the client entry area/consulting rooms and areas with diagnostic equipment such as the laboratory and radiography room. Oxygen and anaesthetic equipment should be readily available. In most practices, the preparation area or induction room is best suited, as it is usually fitted with most of the emergency equipment required. Figure 19.1 gives a suggested list of equipment and drugs that should be readily available.

All staff (veterinary surgeons, veterinary nurses, other patient care staff and reception staff) should know that this area is where emergencies should be taken. The area should be well lit and spacious, with items and equipment stored tidily.

There should be a mobile crash box or trolley that is fully stocked and ready for use at all times (Figure 19.2). It should be the responsibility of one person in the practice (usually a veterinary nurse) to ensure that it is checked after every use and at least once weekly.

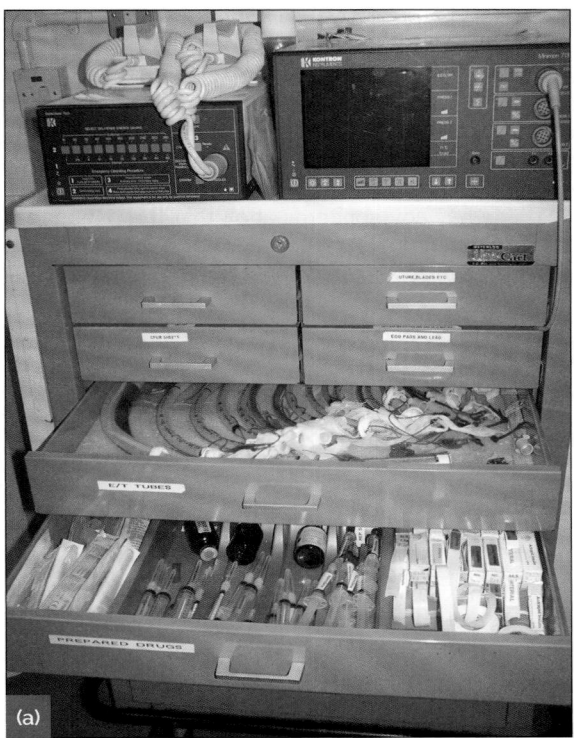
(a)

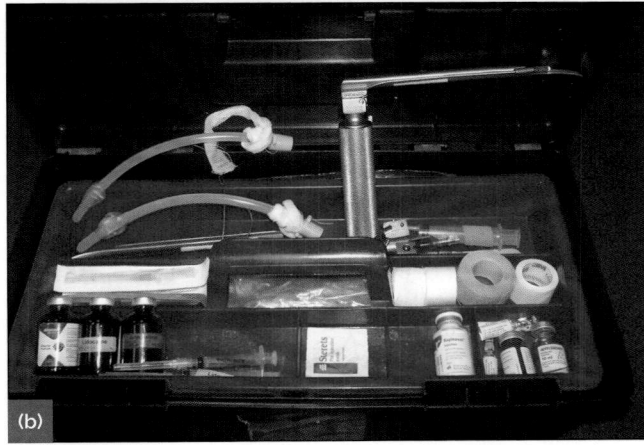
(b)

19.2 Example of **(a)** a crash trolley from a large veterinary hospital and **(b)** a crash box from a smaller practice. A variety of endotracheal tubes, intravenous catheters, drugs and monitoring equipment is present.

Any patient with a potentially life-threatening condition should be taken immediately to the designated emergency area on arrival at the practice for a primary survey.

Primary survey

This starts with an assessment of whether the animal has just undergone, or is likely to undergo, imminent cardiopulmonary arrest. The mnemonic ABC should be followed:

- Airway – does the patient have a patent airway?
- Breathing – is the patient making useful breathing efforts?
- Circulation – does the patient have evidence of spontaneous circulation (heartbeat, pulses)?

Emergency equipment

- Endotracheal (ET) tubes (varying sizes)
- Laryngoscope
- Oxygen supply
- Anaesthetic circuits
- Intravenous catheters (varying sizes)
- Tape for tying in ET tube
- Tape for securing intravenous (IV) catheters
- Multi-parameter monitor including electrocardiogram (ECG)
- Assortment of syringes and needles
- Suction machine/bulb syringe
- Dog urinary catheter (for difficult intubations)
- Good light source
- Drug dosage chart
- Fluid administration equipment
- Scalpel blades/suture material

Emergency drugs

- Adrenaline (epinephrine)
- Atropine
- Lidocaine
- Diazepam
- Calcium gluconate (10%)
- Dextrose solution (50%)
- Furosemide
- Dexamethasone
- Propofol
- Opioid analgesics
- IV fluid – hypertonic saline
- Mannitol

19.1 Emergency equipment and drugs that should be readily available in the designated emergency area.

It should also be determined whether the patient is conscious or unconscious.

The primary survey should take approximately 30 seconds to perform. Once this assessment has been carried out and it is established that the patient is unlikely to undergo cardiorespiratory arrest, the triage nurse should carry out a major body systems assessment.

If the nurse has any concerns at all that the patient has arrested, cardiopulmonary resuscitation should be started and a veterinary surgeon called immediately.

Major body system assessment

The three major body systems are considered to be:

- Cardiovascular
- Respiratory
- Neurological.

When triaging a patient, these systems should always be examined first, regardless of any other injuries. Dysfunction in any of these systems is potentially life-threatening. If a patient dies, it is always the result of failure of one of these systems.

Although other injuries may be more obvious, they are unlikely to kill the patient unless they have a secondary effect on one of the major body systems. For example, in a dog that has been hit by a car and has a fracture of the femur with a large open wound, although that injury may appear dramatic it will not on its own lead to the dog's death. However, the haemorrhage from the fracture site may lead to hypovolaemic shock, cardiovascular system compromise and death. Shock is detected by examination of the cardiovascular system.

The major body system assessment provides a means of assessing whether the patient's injuries are life-threatening. All parameters should be recorded at the time they are measured. It is helpful to have a triage sheet that includes a scoring system; this allows accurate recording of parameters and helps to identify those patients who need urgent intervention.

Parameters that should be recorded during a major body systems assessment

- Heart rate
- Pulse quality
- Mucous membrane colour
- Capillary refill time
- Respiratory rate
- Respiratory effort
- Gait
- Mentation
- Temperature

Cardiovascular system

Information from the cardiovascular system examination is the best way the veterinary team has of quickly assessing the degree and type of shock. Repeat cardiovascular system examination, as the animal receives treatment for shock, is the simplest and most cost-effective way of monitoring the animal's response to treatment. The information provided by the nurse has a vitally important role in the outcome of the case.

The cardiovascular system examination involves assessment of a patient's heart rate, pulse quality, mucous membrane colour and capillary refill time.

Heart rate

Heart rate should be measured while auscultating the patient's heart with a stethoscope (see Chapter 14) and should be compared with the patient's pulse rate. The heart and pulse rates should be the same. If they are not, the veterinary surgeon should be alerted.

Pulse

The easiest pulse to feel is the femoral pulse. It is felt by sliding the fingers gently into the inguinal region (see Chapter 14). In some patients (e.g. those with femoral or pelvic fractures, heavily muscled or obese animals) this pulse can be difficult to feel and palpation of a metatarsal pulse on the dorsomedial aspect of the metatarsus may be easier (Figure 19.3).

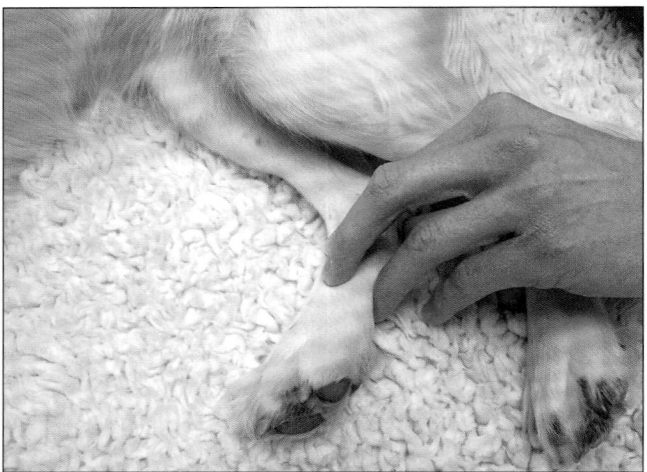

19.3 Locating the metatarsal pulse. Palpation of this pulse is especially useful in patients with pelvic or femoral fractures.

With practice, pulse quality can be assessed. Pulse quality can be classified as: normal; tall and narrow (bounding or hyper-kinetic); or weak (thready). Information on the quality of the pulse should be recorded each time it is felt.

A pulse deficit occurs when a heartbeat is heard but there is no corresponding pulse. Thus, the pulse rate measured will be lower than the heart rate. Pulse deficits are a sign of arrhythmia.

Mucous membrane colour

The normal colour is pale pink (paler in cats than dogs), though it should be remembered that some breeds (e.g. Chow-Chow) have pigmented dark mucous membranes. Some disease states cause abnormalities in mucous membrane colour; for example, pale or white in hypovolaemic shock or anaemia, bright red in distributive shock, or blue with hypoxia.

The capillary refill time (CRT) is checked by applying firm pressure with the thumb on the gingival mucosa to blanche the mucous membranes and timing how quickly the colour returns. If it is not possible to check the gingival mucosa, the vaginal or preputial mucosa can be used (see Chapter 14). A normal refill time is 1–2 seconds. The CRT may be rapid (<1 second) in early shock or slow (>2.5 seconds) in late shock.

Respiratory system

Respiratory system assessment involves evaluation of the animal's respiratory rate and effort. It is useful to record whether there are any audible noises associated with the respiratory effort and, if possible, whether the greater effort is associated with inspiration (breathing in) or expiration (breathing out). This information can assist the veterinary surgeon in diagnosing the cause of the breathing difficulty.

Findings that suggest severe respiratory distress

- Cyanotic (blue) mucous membranes; however, it is important to note that patients can be hypoxic without being cyanotic
- Open-mouth breathing (especially in cats)
- Abducted elbows
- Extended neck
- Paradoxical abdominal movement (abdomen moves in while chest moves out)
- Dilated pupils
- Anxious facial expression

Oxygen should always be supplied while a dyspnoeic animal is being examined (Figures 19.4, 19.5 and 19.6). Care should be taken that the method of oxygen supplementation does not distress the patient further. It is advisable to avoid face masks, especially in dyspnoeic cats. Flow-by oxygen is generally tolerated by dogs, especially if the oxygen flow is directed across the nose rather than directly into the face; with cats it may be necessary to place them in an oxygen cage/tent to allow them to settle and perform the examination in stages, placing them back into the oxygen cage/tent between the stages.

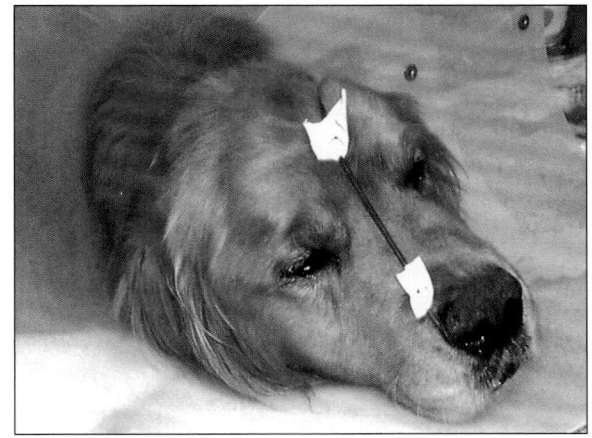

19.5 Nasal oxygen catheter in place.

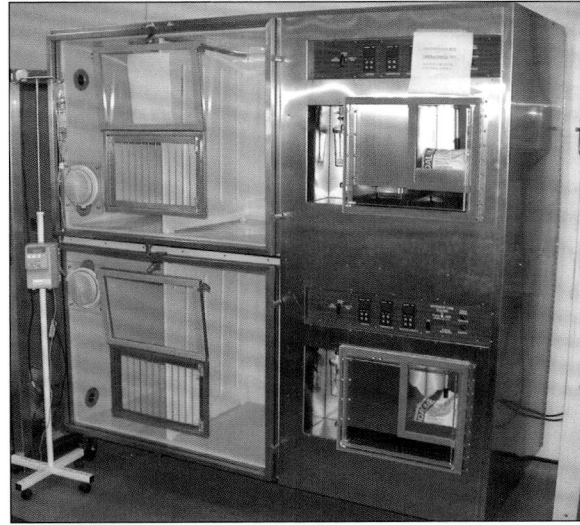

19.6 Oxygen cage allowing supplementation of up to 90% oxygen, with temperature and humidity control.

Method of oxygen supplementation	Advantages	Disadvantages
Flow-by (hold oxygen source close to patient's nose or mouth)	■ Cheap ■ Easy ■ Well tolerated	■ Does not allow high inspired concentration of oxygen
Mask	■ Cheap ■ Easy	■ Not tolerated by some patients ■ Does not allow high inspired concentration of oxygen
Nasal prongs	■ Cheap	■ Not tolerated by some patients ■ Tend to fall out frequently (designed for human noses) ■ May cause sneezing; use with care in head trauma
Nasal catheter (Figure 19.5)	■ Cheap ■ Catheter easy to place with practice	■ May require sedation for placement of catheter ■ Catheter irritates some patients ■ May cause sneezing; use with care in head trauma
Transtracheal catheter	■ May be useful in patients with upper airway problems	■ Difficult to maintain and use in conscious patient ■ Not tolerated by some patients
Improvised oxygen cage (e.g. Elizabethan collar with cling-film)	■ Cheap ■ Widely available	■ Patients rapidly become hot ■ Can get CO_2 build-up
Oxygen cage/ incubator (Figure 19.6)	■ Allows delivery of up to 90% oxygen ■ Minimal stress ■ May allow temperature and humidity control	■ Not widely available ■ Expensive
Intubation and ventilation	■ Allows 100% oxygen delivery ■ Allows control of breathing	■ Requires anaesthesia ■ Not possible long term except in specialist institutions

19.4 Methods of oxygen supplementation.

Nervous system

Initial evaluation of the nervous system involves an assessment of the patient's gait and mentation.

Gait

During assessment of gait, the following terms are used:

- Paresis – weakness
- Plegia – paralysis (unable to move)
- Quadriplegia – paralysis of all four limbs
- Paraplegia – paralysis of any two limbs
- Hemiplegia – paralysis of one side of the body
- Hypermetria – exaggerated limb movements.

In a paralysed animal it is important to note whether the animal can feel its limbs (e.g. turns its head toward the handler when its toes are squeezed) even though it may be unable to move them.

Mentation

The animal's mentation may be classified as:

- Alert
- Obtunded (mentally dull)
- Stuporous (semi-conscious, able to be roused only by a painful stimulus)
- Coma (unconscious and unable to be roused).

Other neurological features to note include:

- Pupil size and symmetry
- Presence or absence of pupillary light reflexes
- Presence or absence of palpebral reflex
- Facial asymmetry and any head tilt
- Nystagmus (abnormal flicking eye movements)
- Presence of gag reflex (in stuporous or comatose patients only)
- Anal tone (may be assessed when taking the temperature).

Body temperature

Once the major body system assessment has been completed, the animal's temperature can be taken and recorded. These points should be noted:

- Any faecal staining of the perineum
- Any blood or melaena on the thermometer
- Whether normal anal tone was present.

After the primary survey has been completed, any major body system conditions can be prioritized, and stabilization started as soon as possible.

Secondary survey

A secondary survey to establish other abnormalities can be performed once the primary survey is complete and treatment for any major body system abnormalities has been started. A head-to-tail approach is recommended to ensure that a systematic examination is performed.

Nose

Note any discharge (serous, purulent, haemorrhagic) and whether it is unilateral or bilateral. Note any swellings or asymmetry that may suggest nasal fractures or tumours.

Mouth

Note the colour of the mucous membranes. Initial examination of mucous membrane colour and capillary refill time (CRT) should have been performed as part of the major body systems assessment (see above). Normal mucous membranes are pale to medium pink in colour.

Abnormal mucous membrane colours

- Pale – suggestive of anaemia or hypovolaemic shock
- Red – suggestive of distributive shock or localized inflammation (gingivitis)
- Cyanotic (blue) – suggestive of severe hypoxia
- Jaundiced (yellow) – suggestive of liver disease or haemolytic anaemia
- Cherry red – suggestive of carbon monoxide poisoning. (This is rare. Red mucous membranes are much more likely to be seen with distributive shock)
- Brown – suggestive of methaemoglobinaemia, which can be seen with paracetamol toxicity

---

The oral cavity should be examined for any signs of haemorrhage, including both gross haemorrhage and petechial (pinprick) haemorrhages in the mucosa. The moistness of the mucous membranes can be assessed. Dry mucous membranes are suggestive of dehydration. Any ulcers on either the mucosa or the tongue should be noted. The hard palate should be assessed to see if it is split (a common injury in cats with head trauma). The mouth should be closed and an assessment made of whether the jaw closes properly or whether there is any asymmetry that may suggest a fracture. Excessive salivation should be noted.

Eyes

The eyes should be assessed for any discharge (serous or purulent) and whether it is unilateral or bilateral. The symmetry of the eyes should be assessed and any blepharospasm (indicative of ocular pain) noted. If there is no obvious ocular injury, the conjunctival mucous membranes should be assessed for their colour and the presence of haemorrhage. The position of the eyeball should be noted. An abnormal position is known as strabismus ('squint') and the direction of the strabismus should be noted. Abnormal ocular movements (nystagmus) should be noted and the direction of the fast component of the movement should be recorded. The pupil size and symmetry should be noted. The presence of asymmetrical pupils is known as anisocoria and it should be noted which pupil is larger. The palpebral reflex and pupillary light response should be checked.

Ears

Both ears should be checked for any discharge and the nature of the discharge noted. The pinnae should be observed for any petechial haemorrhages and for signs of haematoma caused by damage to the pinna. It presents as a swelling of the pinna due to pooling of blood between the skin and the cartilage. It is often painful and warm to the touch.

Limbs

Any obvious wounds should be noted. The limbs should be gently palpated and any swellings, pain or crepitus (abnormal cracking or grinding sound or sensation) should be recorded. If a limb is clearly being held at an abnormal angle and a fracture is suspected, this limb should not be palpated but the veterinary surgeon should be alerted. The animal should be prevented from using this limb until the veterinary surgeon has examined it. If the animal is ambulatory, it should be noted if it is lame and if so on which limb(s) it is lame and how severe the lameness is.

It is important to note whether the neurological function of each limb is intact. If the animal is moving the limb voluntarily, there must be some functioning nerve supply. If there are concerns that an animal cannot move or feel a limb, the toes on that foot should be pinched. Withdrawal of the limb implies that local nerve reflexes are intact but does not necessarily mean that the spinal cord is functioning normally. The animal should be closely observed to see whether there is pain sensation accompanying the pinching. This may involve vocalizing, turning its head towards the limb or attempting to bite. Loss of conscious pain perception in a limb indicates a poor prognosis.

Thorax

Any external wounds or swellings should be noted. If there is any evidence of a penetrating chest wound (e.g. a piece of skin sucked in and out as the animal breathes, sometimes accompanied by a gentle hissing sound) the wound should be covered with a sterile adherent dressing until it can be examined by the veterinary surgeon.

Thoracic auscultation is a useful skill for the emergency nurse to develop. When auscultating the chest, the nurse should listen to whether the lung sounds are abnormally quiet or loud. The distribution (e.g. left *versus* right, dorsal *versus* ventral) of any abnormal sounds should be recorded.

Abdomen

The hands should be run gently over the abdomen. Any wounds, swellings or bruising should be noted. Deep abdominal palpation is a skill that can take years to develop. The ability to palpate the bladder in the caudal abdomen is a useful skill for the emergency nurse to master. An obstructed bladder or urethra is a common emergency. Obstructed bladders feel firm, hard and enlarged. If this condition is suspected, the nurse should not attempt to express the bladder as there is a chance it may rupture.

External genitalia

In both sexes, the external genitalia should be checked for any discharge and for discoloration of the mucous membranes. Any evidence of urine scalding should be noted, as this could be suggestive of a more chronic urinary problem.

Tail

Any wounds should be noted. It should also be noted whether the animal can move its tail. Neurological injuries to the tail are common in cats following trauma and may be accompanied by neurological injury to the bladder and anus.

Capsule history

A 'capsule history' should be obtained from the owners of all emergency patients. This history focuses on the essential information that could alter the early management of the patient. A more detailed history may be taken once the patient is more stable.

Important questions to ask for a capsule history

- What is the age, sex and neutering status of the animal?
- If an entire female, when was her last season or litter?
- Is the animal on any medications? If so, when was the last dose given?
- Has the animal been diagnosed with any long-term medical problems?
- Does the animal have any known allergies?
- Has the animal had access to any known toxins?
- When was the last time the animal ate and drank?
- When was the last time the animal passed faeces and urinated, and was it normal?
- How long has the animal been showing signs of its current problem?
- Has this problem got better, worse or stayed the same since it was first noticed?

Intravenous access

Vascular access is required in most emergency and critically ill patients, and the placement of intravenous catheters (see Chapter 21) is a key skill for nurses working in emergency and critical care to master. Intravenous access is required for the administration of fluid and drug therapy and can provide a means of atraumatic serial blood sampling. Vascular access should be obtained early in the management of many emergency patients and sometimes before the secondary survey is complete.

In dogs and cats, the most common vein used is the cephalic vein; patients can generally be restrained in sternal recumbency during placement and the vein is easily identified with practice. If the cephalic vein cannot be used (e.g. injuries to both forelimbs), the saphenous vein is a useful alternative. In very collapsed or very small patients, the peripheral veins may be difficult to identify. In this situation, options include placement of a catheter directly into the jugular vein or placement of an intraosseous catheter into the bone marrow. Intraosseous access is usually obtained via the femur, although the tibia, humerus and ilium may all be used.

In rabbits, the ear vein is the most easily catheterized vessel, although the cephalic vein can be used. Obtaining vascular access in smaller mammals is challenging, and jugular or intraosseous access is usually required.

In avian emergencies, options for venous access include the right jugular vein (larger than the left in all avian species), the ulnar vein running on the ventral aspect of the wing or the medial metatarsal vein. Intraosseous access can also be used in avian species, although bones that contain air sacs must be avoided. Suitable bones include the distal ulna and proximal tibiotarsus.

Regardless of the site used, the catheter chosen should be the largest that will fit into the vessel; this facilitates rapid fluid administration and reduces the risk of thrombophlebitis. In large dogs, it may be necessary to place two catheters to allow sufficient volumes of fluid to be administered over a short timeframe. Aseptic technique should always be used during catheter placement, and the catheter should be carefully secured immediately following placement.

General nursing care

The stabilization of life-threatening medical conditions must take priority but, having addressed these, the patient's general physical comfort and level of psychological stress should be considered (see Chapter 14).

Mental welfare

Many emergency patients are distressed, in pain or confused. Being in the unfamiliar environment of the veterinary practice surrounded by strangers can serve to make this worse.

- Be kind and gentle with the patient. Talk softly and use the patient's name as much as possible.
- Be aware if the patient has any physical disabilities, such as being blind, deaf or recumbent, that may make the situation more unsettling.
- Always approach the patient slowly and perform any procedures with the minimum handling necessary. Some patients may benefit from a period in a kennel or basket without being handled whilst they become accustomed to the environment.
- Emergency patients should never be covered from view.
- Be aware that some patients (especially prey species, e.g. rabbits) may find the presence of other animals stressful; organize kennelling to reduce this if possible.

Physical comfort

The patient should be given a warm and comfortable bed. If the patient is recumbent, it should be turned regularly and at least every 4 hours. A well-padded kennel should be provided for patients that may be at risk of self-trauma through seizuring, vestibular disease or visual impairment. Environmental temperature should allow maintenance of a normal body temperature. Hypothermia is a common problem in small critically ill patients (cats and other small mammals).

If the patient is able to stand and walk, then it should be allowed to do this. Critically ill patients should not walk long distances, however the benefit of standing and walking around the room should not be underestimated, especially in older patients who may have concurrent chronic orthopaedic disease (e.g. arthritis). Patients that are able to walk outside will benefit from the fresh air and sunshine.

Toileting needs

The necessity for the patient to urinate and defecate should be considered. Although it may not be possible or advisable for critically sick dogs to be walked outside, they should be allowed to leave their kennel regularly for toileting purposes. If they are recumbent, a urinary catheter should be considered.

If a patient soils itself or its bedding, it should be cleaned immediately. In patients with diarrhoea, clipping the perineal and caudal thigh region should be considered and a barrier cream applied. A tail bandage may be beneficial, and should be replaced regularly. Cats should be provided with a litter tray, containing a familiar type of litter if possible.

Dressings, catheter sites and tube sites

All dressings and catheter or tube insertion sites should be checked regularly. Any dressings that become soiled or displaced should be changed as soon as possible. All catheter sites should be unwrapped and checked at least once daily, and more frequently if the site appears to cause discomfort. Other tubes (e.g. oesophagostomy tubes, gastrostomy tubes) should be checked and rewrapped on the advice of the veterinary surgeon.

A record should be made each time dressings are replaced; the necessity for frequent dressing changes, especially if this represents an increase on previous needs, may indicate a problem, e.g. local infection.

Oral food and water

The decision to offer food and water should be made by the veterinary surgeon and is dependent on the underlying disease process. The nurse should be proactive in ascertaining when food and water can be offered. If food can be offered, small amounts of fresh food should be placed in the patient's kennel. If the patient does not want to eat, the food should be removed after 1 hour and more fresh food offered at a later time. The presence of stale food in the patient's kennel may act as an adverse stimulus and decrease the patient's appetite. Some patients may have trouble moving to their water or food bowl and may benefit from hand-feeding.

Monitoring

The nurse is responsible for monitoring the patient. Although many advanced monitoring techniques are now available in veterinary practice, the most important monitoring tool is the serial clinical examination.

The following parameters should be recorded at regular intervals (up to every 15 minutes in unstable patients; every 6–8 hours in stable patients).

Regular monitoring

- Pulse rate
- Pulse quality
- Mucous membrane colour
- Capillary refill time
- Respiratory rate
- Respiratory effort
- Temperature
- Pain score
- Demeanour
- Bodyweight (every 12 hours)

Other monitoring techniques that can be considered include:

- Urine output
- Urine specific gravity
- Blood pressure

- Pulse oximetry
- Electrocardiogram (ECG)
- Central venous pressure
- Serial bloodwork, including glucose, lactate, packed cell volume (PCV), total solids (TS), electrolytes and blood gas parameters (see Chapter 17).

It is vital that any parameter monitored is recorded accurately. Successful management of emergency patients often involves several members of staff and it is essential that the patient's status is communicated accurately between staff members. Emergency patients often require a great deal of effort but can be some of the most rewarding patients to nurse.

Pain scoring

It is vital to assess pain levels at regular intervals; failure to identify and adequately control pain can lead to increased morbidity and mortality in patients. A pain scoring system can be used objectively to quantify the patient's level of pain, allow the response to analgesia to be monitored and indicate when further analgesia is required. There are several pain scoring models available; however, they will only be effective if staff are trained in their use and confident at interpreting signs of pain in patients. Models that are commonly used in emergency medicine include the University of Glasgow Short Form Composite Pain Scale (www.newmetrica.com/acute-pain-measurement/) and the Colorado State University Acute Pain Scale (http://csu-cvmbs.colostate.edu/vth/diagnostic-and-support/anesthesia-pain-management/Pages/pain-management.aspx); both have canine and feline versions (see Chapter 21).

Cardiopulmonary arrest, resuscitation and death

The information in this section is based on the guidelines produced by the Reassessment Campaign On Veterinary Resuscitation (RECOVER) initiative. This was a collaborative project that carried out a systematic review of the experimental and clinical evidence in cardiopulmonary resuscitation (CPR) research and devised a series of evidence-based, consensus CPR guidelines for cats and dogs. Full details of the project and the guidelines can be found on their website (https://recoverinitiative.org/). Early recognition of cardiopulmonary arrest (CPA) is vital; the longer it takes to recognize CPA and start CPR the worse the outcome is likely to be.

Signs of impending or actual cardiac arrest

- Agonal (gasping) breathing pattern or absence of useful respiratory movements
- Absence of a heartbeat and pulse, or weak and rapid pulses that will usually slow rapidly and dramatically shortly prior to arrest
- If the patient is having their end-tidal carbon dioxide (ETCO$_2$) level monitored, it will drop to below 20 mmHg prior to arrest
- Loss of consciousness
- Fixed dilated pupils and lack of a palpebral and corneal reflex

---

Patients that go into CPA prior to arrival need to be quickly identified and CPR should be started immediately. Within 4 minutes of CPA ischaemic tissue damage occurs and within 10 minutes this damage is irreversible.

Evaluation of the patient should take less than 15 seconds, with the focus being to check whether the patient is breathing and the airway is clear. Current CPR guidelines do not recommend pulse palpation prior to starting CPR, as several human studies have shown that pulse palpation is an insensitive and time-consuming test for the diagnosis of CPA.

In patients that are unresponsive and not breathing, CPR should be started immediately. It may be necessary to initiate CPR before the veterinary surgeon arrives and prior to speaking to the owner. When diagnosing CPA, it should be noted that the mucous membranes may remain pink with a normal capillary refill time for several minutes after cessation of effective circulation; for patients being monitored by ECG, this may also remain normal for many minutes following cessation of cardiac contractions. It should also be noted that breathing efforts must be useful; agonal gasping is not a useful breathing effort.

Cardiopulmonary resuscitation

The aim of CPR is to temporarily support the patient's ventilation and circulation (basic life support) until spontaneous circulation and breathing are restored and sustained.

- Basic life support is the administration of external chest compressions and manual artificial ventilation.
- Advanced life support refers to the administration of drugs or other treatments to restart and maintain spontaneous circulation.

Cardiopulmonary resuscitation procedure

Successful CPR requires a team approach. Ideally, there should be 3–5 team members, however, it can be performed with a minimum of two people. All members of staff, including student nurses, animal care assistants, kennel hands and receptionists should be trained in basic CPR, and regular drills and refreshers should be completed to keep skills current. One person should be nominated to 'run' the crash team; this will usually be a veterinary surgeon, however, an experienced nurse may need to fulfil this role until a veterinary surgeon arrives.

Depending on the size of the team, the following roles should be assigned:

- Leader – overseas and directs the team
- Compressor – provides chest compressions
- Ventilator – provides adequate ventilation
- Monitor – checks pulses, attaches multi-parameter monitor/ECG if available
- Drug handler/recorder – draws up drugs and records the medication administered, along with any interventions.

It is usual for team members to carry out multiple tasks during a resuscitation attempt.

Effective communication during CPR plays a vital role in patient outcome. Closed loop communication should be used to help avoid mistakes and to ensure that instructions have been understood and carried out.

Following recognition that a patient has gone into CPA, the following tasks should be carried out as quickly and smoothly as possible:

- Start cardiac compressions
- Call for assistance if team members are not already present
- Provision of ventilation
- Placement and securing of an intravenous catheter
- Placement of ECG or multi-parameter monitor to assist the veterinary surgeon in making decisions with regard to appropriate medication and assist with monitoring the effectiveness of CPR.

After any CPR attempt or drill, a debriefing session should be held to allow all staff to feedback on what went well and what could be improved, to encourage and facilitate ongoing improvements.

Basic life support

Compressions

Current CPR guidelines recommend that chest compressions are started immediately; they should not be delayed whilst an airway is established (see Chapter 21).

In all cats and the majority of dog breeds, chest compressions are best performed with the patient in lateral recumbency. In flat-chested breeds, such as Bulldogs, where the width of the chest is greater than the depth, compressions may be performed with the patient in dorsal recumbency.

In cats, small dogs and keel-chested breeds such as Greyhounds, where the depth of the chest is greater than the width, pressure should be applied using the heel of the hand directly over the heart (Figure 19.7). Use of a one-handed technique should be considered in cats and small dogs. In round-chested dogs, where the width of the chest is equal to the depth, pressure should be applied using the heel of the hand at the widest part of the chest (Figure 19.8). In flat-chested breeds, pressure is applied over the centre of the sternum using the heel of the hands (Figure 19.9).

Chest compressions should be delivered at a rate of approximately 100–120 per minute. Compression depth should be one-half to one-third the width of the chest. It is important to allow the chest to fully recoil after every compression, so that the heart can refill with blood.

Compressions should be performed in cycles of 2 minutes without interruption to allow the blood pressure to reach

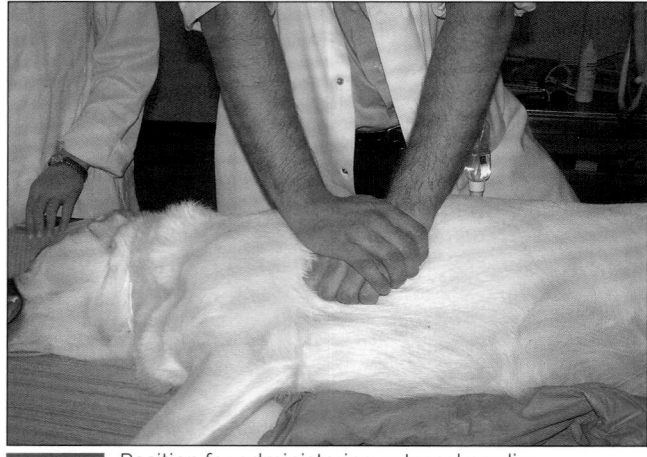

19.8 Position for administering external cardiac compression to a medium-large round chested dog.

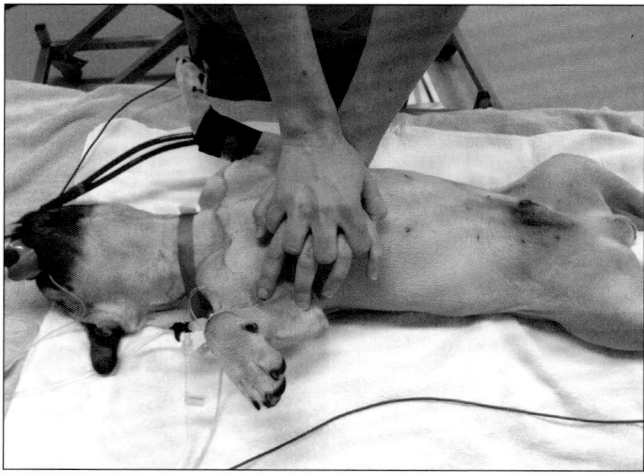

19.9 Hand position in a flat-chested dog. The animal is positioned in dorsal recumbency with chest compressions occurring over the sternum.

a level which provides perfusion to the heart and tissues. After each 2-minute cycle, the compressor should change to prevent fatigue, which leads to less effective compressions.

Ventilation

Early endotracheal intubation is recommended in canine and feline CPR. The tube should be placed and tied in whilst compressions are being delivered.

On rare occasions, an animal will have gone into CPA because of an obstructed airway. If airway obstruction is suspected, a variety of endotracheal tubes should be available, including some much smaller than would normally be chosen for the size of patient. A stiff male dog urinary catheter is also useful, as it can be placed through the larynx and passed beyond the obstruction. It can then be used to deliver oxygen whilst the obstruction is addressed.

Very rarely, an endotracheal tube cannot be placed and an emergency tracheotomy must be carried out. The patient should be rolled into dorsal recumbency and the neck hyperextended. An area over the trachea in the mid-cervical region should be rapidly clipped and a brief surgical preparation performed. The veterinary surgeon will rapidly make an incision through the subcutaneous tissues of the neck and then between the tracheal rings. Ideally, a specially designed tracheostomy tube (see Chapter 23) is placed through the tracheal incision into the airway, but if this is not available a standard endotracheal tube can be used.

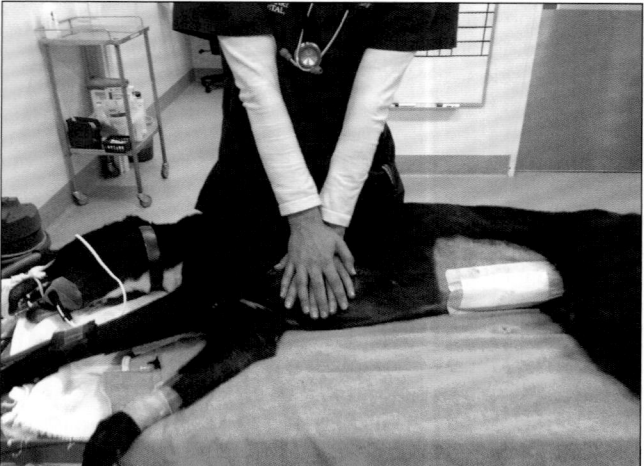

19.7 Hand position in a keel-chested dog. Chest compressions occur over the heart.

Following intubation, ventilation should be provided by connection to an anaesthetic circuit (preferably a Bain) or an Ambu bag. Breaths should be delivered simultaneously with the compressions, at a rate of one breath every 6 seconds (10 breaths per minute). The volume of air per breath should be judged so that the chest wall can be seen to rise only a small amount, and the inspiratory time should be 1 second. It is essential to maintain a respiratory rate of 10 breaths/minute and a short inspiratory time, as hyperventilation or hypoventilation during CPR are both detrimental as they lead to reduced venous return to the heart and therefore reduced cardiac output.

Advanced life support

Once ECG monitoring has started, the veterinary surgeon may wish to administer drugs to return the heart to a normal rhythm. Although a veterinary nurse does not need to understand fully the mechanism of action of each drug, having an understanding of which drug is appropriate and why can make both the veterinary nurse's and the veterinary surgeon's job quicker and easier. An experienced nurse can start to prepare drugs that are likely to be necessary, so that they can be administered as soon as they are requested.

The three common cardiac arrest rhythms in dogs and cats (Figure 19.10) are:

- Pulseless electrical activity (PEA)
- Asystole
- Ventricular fibrillation.

The three drugs used most commonly during resuscitation are:

- Adrenaline (epinephrine), a peripheral vasoconstrictor that acts to increase blood flow to the heart and brain. It is used in asystole and PEA
- Atropine, an anticholinergic drug used to reduce vagal tone. It is used to control severe bradycardia, which may lead to asystole or PEA
- Lidocaine, an antiarrhythmic drug. It is used for the treatment of ventricular arrhythmias such as fast ventricular tachycardia. It may be used as a chemical defibrillator but is rarely successful in this situation.

Drugs are generally administered via an intravenous catheter; however, rarely, it may not be possible to achieve venous access in a rapid timeframe. On these occasions, all three drugs may be administered by the intratracheal route by placing a urinary catheter down the endotracheal tube. A dose double the intravenous dose is used and the urinary catheter is flushed with saline following administration. A large breath is given following drug administration to facilitate dispersion of the drug to the alveoli, where it can be rapidly absorbed and reach the heart.

Electrical defibrillation

Electrical defibrillation is occasionally used to shock the heart from chaotic non-pulse-producing electrical activity (commonly ventricular fibrillation) to normal sinus rhythm. A large electrical charge is passed through the heart, with the aim of causing the cardiac cells to depolarize and then repolarize synchronously.

Defibrillation is only useful in cases where arrest has been caused by ventricular fibrillation or rapid ventricular tachycardia. The most common arrhythmia in human cardiopulmonary arrest is ventricular fibrillation and this is why defibrillators are so readily available and commonly used in human medicine. It is, however, a rare cause of arrest in dogs and cats. The earlier a heart is defibrillated, the better chance the patient will have of survival. The energy necessary for external defibrillation is approximately 5 joules/kg. Excessive energy levels and repeated defibrillation can cause myocardial damage; therefore, it is advisable to start at the lower energy levels and increase as needed.

Extreme caution must be exercised whenever a defibrillator is being used. One person who is trained to operate the machine should be in charge and should instruct all other personnel to 'Clear!' before discharging the defibrillator. To prevent risk of serious injury, all personnel must be clear of the patient and the table on which the patient is lying before the defibrillator is discharged. Defibrillators should never be used by untrained personnel. Alcohol-based solvents should never be used in the proximity of the defibrillator.

Collapse and unconsciousness

Many emergency patients will present because of collapse. The term collapse is used when an animal is unable or unwilling to stand and walk but remains aware of its surroundings. During the initial major body systems assessment, it should be ascertained whether an animal is:

- An alert collapsed animal with normal mentation
- A depressed collapsed animal that is quiet but will respond to stimuli such as calling its name or clapping hands behind its head
- An obtunded collapsed animal with a decreased level of consciousness that will only respond to painful stimuli such as squeezing hard on its toes or touching a painful area
- An unconscious (comatose) collapsed animal that does not respond to stimuli but has a palpable pulse and heart rate.

If the animal does not respond to stimuli and has no heart beat on thoracic auscultation, then it is considered to be dead. However, if it is still making breathing movements, death may only just have occurred and resuscitation efforts should be started.

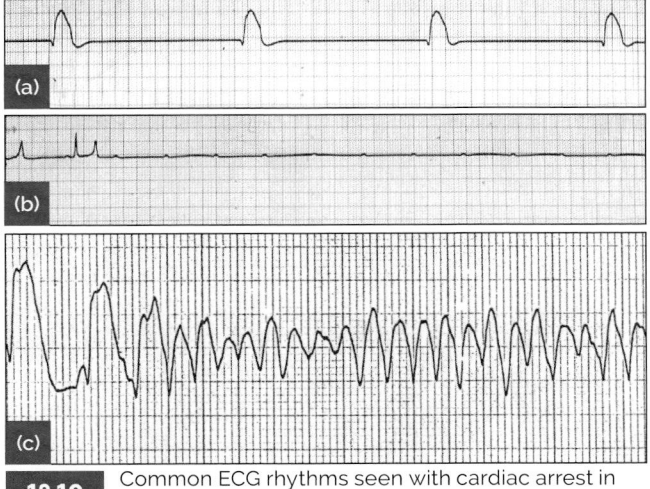

19.10 Common ECG rhythms seen with cardiac arrest in dogs and cats: **(a)** pulseless electrical activity, **(b)** asystole, **(c)** ventricular fibrillation. (Courtesy of V Luis Fuentes)

In an unconscious collapsed patient the airway may become blocked or narrowed due to the position of the neck and the tongue. The patient's muscles will tend to relax and can occlude the pharyngeal region, especially in breeds with a large amount of soft tissue in this area, such as Bulldogs. If this occurs, it can lead to respiratory and then cardiac arrest. It is vital that the airway is clear and open to allow adequate ventilation and oxygen delivery to the lungs.

Unconscious patients should be placed in lateral recumbency with their heads tilted dorsally (up), their mouths held gently open and the tongue gently pulled out. The airway should be examined to ensure that it is clear, but caution should be exercised and the safety of veterinary personnel must not be compromised.

There are many potential causes of collapse. The most common groups are summarized in Figure 19.11.

Presentation	Possible causes of collapse
Alert collapsed animal	Orthopaedic disease Peripheral neurological disease
Depressed collapsed animal	Mild to moderate shock Pain
Obtunded collapsed animal	Moderate to severe shock Neurological disease Metabolic disease
Unconscious collapsed animal with very fast or slow heart rate	Severe shock – cardiopulmonary arrest imminent
Unconscious collapsed animal with normal heart rate	Neurological disease Metabolic disease (e.g. hypoglycaemia)

19.11 Groups of differential diagnoses to be considered in a collapsed animal.

Shock

Shock is defined as a state of acute circulatory collapse where the circulation is unable to transport sufficient oxygen to meet the tissues' needs. The consequences of untreated shock are severe, as a lack of oxygen supply to the tissues will have significant effects on all organs, especially the brain, heart and kidneys. If the state of shock is prolonged, it may lead to organ failure and death.

The lack of tissue oxygen supply may be secondary to a number of circulatory system problems. Four major types of shock are recognized and are described in Figure 19.12. The distinction between the types of shock is important, as the treatment strategy varies. In most situations, the different types of shock can be distinguished by a careful and thorough physical examination focusing on the cardiovascular system and, most importantly, the perfusion parameters (heart rate, pulse quality, mucous membrane colour and capillary refill time).

Types of shock

Hypovolaemic shock

Physical examination findings of severe hypovolaemic shock

- Tachycardia (up to 220 beats per minute (bpm) in dogs and 250 bpm in cats)
- Prolonged capillary refill time
- Pale mucous membranes
- Poor pulse quality
- Low blood pressure

Hypovolaemic shock is the most common form of shock seen in veterinary patients. It occurs secondary to significant loss of circulating fluid volume that may happen following haemorrhage or rapid fluid loss through other sites, such as the gastrointestinal tract, urinary system or into third spaces, e.g. peritoneal cavity.

Fluid replacement

As hypovolaemic shock occurs due to reduced circulating blood volume, treatment revolves around replacing the fluid deficit. The fluid used to restore the deficit is dependent on the type of fluid loss (e.g. haemorrhage, vomiting, diarrhoea). The commonest fluids used are isotonic replacement crystalloid fluids, such as Hartmann's solution, but occasionally it is necessary to use other fluids, such as blood products.

When treating shock, the fluid is given intravenously (or, rarely, via the intraosseous route). Initially the fluid is given at a fast rate over a relatively short period. The dose (or bolus) of fluid used varies; a full shock dose of crystalloid is considered to be 60–90 ml/kg bodyweight in the dog and 40–60 ml/kg in the cat although this is very rarely used. More commonly in patients with moderate-severe shock a 10–40ml/kg dose is given initially with monitoring of response and for any side effects such as development of oedema or increased respiratory rate. As cats are particularly susceptible to volume overload, it is recommended that boluses are given in 5–10 ml/kg increments. Depending on the severity of the shock, this dose may be given over a period as short as

Type of shock	Description	Common causes
Hypovolaemic	Decreased circulating blood volume	Haemorrhage Severe vomiting and diarrhoea Third spacing (loss of fluid into body cavities, e.g. abdomen)
Distributive (includes anaphylactic, toxic and septic shock)	Abnormal distribution of body fluids secondary to body-wide dilation of all blood vessels	Sepsis Systemic inflammatory response syndrome (e.g. severe pancreatitis) Severe allergic reaction
Cardiogenic	Failure of the heart to act as an effective pump	Dilated cardiomyopathy Severe arrhythmias
Obstructive	Physical obstruction to blood flow within the vascular system	Pulmonary thromboembolism Pericardial effusion

19.12 Different forms of shock.

30 minutes (see Chapter 20). The principles of treating hypovolaemic shock with a large fluid bolus delivered over a short time frame should also be used when treating small mammals and exotic species.

Arrest of haemorrhage

Haemorrhage is one possible cause of hypovolaemic shock. The haemorrhage may be external or internal. When dealing with very small patients, it should be remembered that shock can result from only small blood losses; for example, a budgerigar can show signs of shock with the loss of only 20 drops of blood. If there is an obvious site of haemorrhage, efforts should be made to arrest it. However, external haemorrhage is a rare cause of severe hypovolaemic shock in dogs and cats.

Methods of arresting haemorrhage

- Direct digital pressure – ensure that gloves are worn and apply pressure for at least 5 minutes
- Artery forceps (haemostats) – if a bleeding vessel can be seen it may be possible to clamp it directly with artery forceps
- Pressure dressing – apply direct pressure over the bleeding area using an absorbent pad and cohesive bandage. If blood seeps through, apply another layer. Do not remove the initial layer as a clot may be dislodged. If a pressure dressing is used on a limb, the toes should be monitored carefully for both swelling and colour; if the toes become markedly swollen or lose their pink colour the pressure being applied should be carefully reduced

---

Haemorrhage into the peritoneal cavity is a common cause of hypovolaemic shock in dogs. If this is suspected, the veterinary surgeon may suggest placement of an abdominal pressure (belly) wrap (Figure 19.13). The aim is to increase pressure within the abdominal cavity to promote the formation of a clot at the site of bleeding. As this increase in pressure can lead to decreases in blood flow to intra-abdominal organs, the wrap should only be left in place for relatively short periods of time and certainly no longer than 12 hours.

Distributive shock

This type of shock occurs when the body suffers an insult (often severe infection or inflammation) that causes the generalized release of inflammatory mediators (cytokines) that promote peripheral vasodilation. The body can no longer

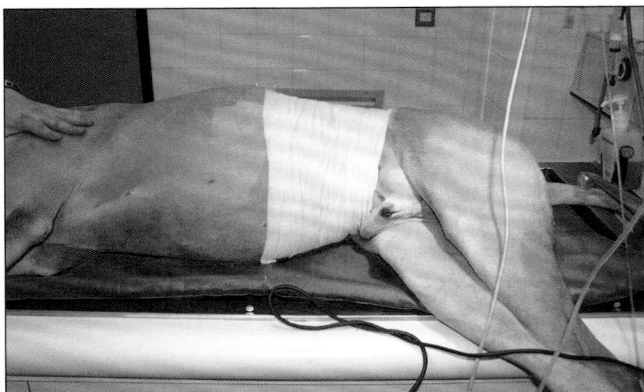

19.13 Abdominal pressure wrap for a patient with haemoabdomen. (Courtesy of D Hughes)

properly control where the blood volume is distributed. The peripheral tissues may have an increased blood supply to the detriment of the more important internal organs. Anaphylactic, toxic and septic are all forms of distributive shock.

Physical examination findings of distributive shock

- Tachycardia
- Poor pulse quality
- Red mucous membranes
- Capillary refill time initially rapid, progressing to slow

As the body is unable to constrict its blood vessels normally, the mucous membranes appear abnormally red. It is the presence of these inappropriately red mucous membranes that should alert the nurse to the presence of distributive shock.

The successful treatment of distributive shock involves rapidly identifying and treating the underlying cause. This may involve medical therapy (e.g. anaphylactic shock, pneumonia) or surgical therapy (e.g. ruptured pyometra). Fluid therapy is important but complications of fluid therapy (development of oedema or effusions) are more common in these patients, as they frequently have inflamed and leaky blood vessels. Drugs to support blood pressure, such as noradrenaline (norepinephrine) or dopamine, may be needed. Peripheral oedema is common if a large volume of crystalloid fluid is used.

In anaphylactic shock (e.g. insect stings) the patient can be treated with adrenaline, corticosteroids, antihistamines and fluid therapy if seen soon after exposure to the allergen.

Cardiogenic shock

This is seen in conditions where the heart can no longer pump effectively. It is most commonly seen in degenerative conditions of the heart muscle, such as dilated cardiomyopathy, or in severe arrhythmias. The findings on physical examination depend on the nature of the heart disease but may include heart murmurs, irregular pulses (especially if pulse deficits are present) and either very fast (>240 bpm) or very slow heart rates. Treatment depends on the underlying heart disease and is covered in the cardiovascular emergencies section. Fluid therapy is generally contraindicated in this form of shock.

Obstructive shock

This is the rarest form of shock in veterinary medicine. It may be seen in pericardial effusion and pulmonary thromboembolism. These conditions are covered under the cardiovascular and respiratory emergencies sections, respectively.

General treatments for shock

Patients with shock are likely to benefit from oxygen supplementation and being hospitalized in a comfortable stress-free environment. They may have a reduced body temperature and should be rewarmed slowly, but only after fluid therapy has started. Patients with shock require careful and close monitoring, especially in the first few hours after presentation.

Other markers of shock

Blood pressure

A drop in blood pressure is a late change in shock, as the body has a number of mechanisms to maintain blood pressure. A mean arterial blood pressure of <60 mmHg is of serious concern, as there may be damage to vital organs such as the brain, heart and kidneys.

Urine output

When monitoring a patient in shock, measurement of urine output (in ml per kg bodyweight per hour) is useful as it is a non-invasive method of evaluating blood supply (perfusion) to the kidneys. If the animal is producing plenty of urine (>2 ml/kg/h) the kidneys are likely to be well perfused. Normal urine production is 1–2 ml/kg/h. Serial measurements of urine output are a useful and cheap monitoring tool that can be used in most practice situations.

Lactate

Lactate is generated secondary to anaerobic respiration in the tissues and is the best objective marker of shock. Until recently it could not easily be measured in veterinary patients but there are now several machines available to veterinary practices allowing in-house measurement of lactate (see Chapter 17). Normal lactate values are <2.5 mmol/l and values >6 mmol/l imply severe shock. Lactate values should return rapidly to normal if the shock is treated successfully.

Cardiovascular emergencies

Many emergency patients present with cardiovascular system abnormalities on examination (e.g. tachycardia, poor pulse quality). In many cases these abnormalities represent the cardiovascular response to shock and are not indicative of primary cardiovascular system disease. This section focuses on those emergencies that are primarily cardiovascular in nature.

Acute congestive heart failure

Congestive heart failure (CHF) may occur secondary to a number of heart conditions. The most common are:

- Chronic mitral valve disease in small-breed dogs
- Dilated cardiomyopathy (weakness of the heart muscle) in large-breed dogs and older rabbits
- Hypertrophic cardiomyopathy (thickening and stiffening of the heart muscle) in cats.

CHF is usually seen in older patients but can occur in younger animals. Whatever the underlying cause, the clinical signs and emergency stabilization procedures are the same.

Clinical signs

- Cough, especially at night.
- Dyspnoea/tachypnoea.
- Reluctance to exercise.

- Tachycardia.
- Poor pulse quality.
- Pale mucous membranes.
- Cyanosis.
- Heart murmur or gallop rhythm on cardiac auscultation.

Diagnostic aids

If the patient is stable:

- Thoracic free fluid ultrasound scan
- Thoracic radiography (Figure 19.14)
- ECG
- Echocardiography (ultrasonography of the heart).

Treatment

- Do not stress.
- Oxygen therapy.
- Medical intervention, including:
  - Thoracocentesis if pleural effusion (commoner in cats)
  - Loop diuretic, e.g. furosemide intravenously or intramuscularly
  - Glyceryl trinitrate paste has been used topically (on skin in ear or groin) in these patients. Use non-latex gloves to apply.
- Once stabilized, medical therapy including one or more of: ACE (angiotensin-converting enzyme) inhibitors, diuretics, pimobendan, digoxin, calcium-channel blockers may be used depending on the nature of the underlying disease.

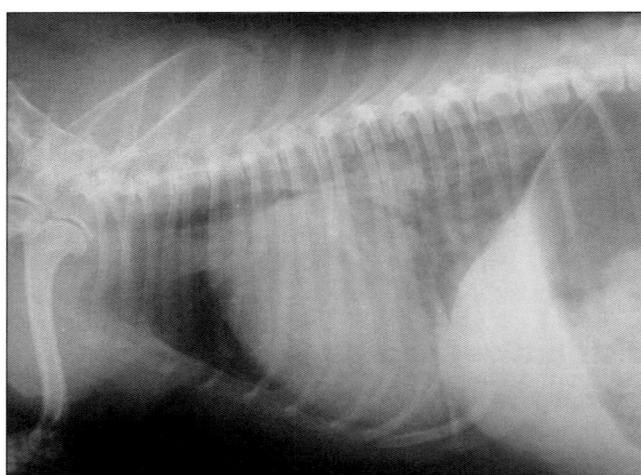

19.14 Right lateral radiograph of a Yorkshire Terrier with congestive heart failure. Note the enlarged cardiac silhouette and the increased opacity in the perihilar and caudal lung fields.

Pericardial effusion

This condition is principally seen in older large-breed dogs where the pericardial sac becomes full of fluid. This puts pressure on the heart so that it cannot fill properly and leads to signs of right-sided congestive heart failure.

Clinical signs

- Exercise intolerance.
- Dyspnoea/tachypnoea.
- Ascites (fluid in the abdomen).

- Muffled heart sounds on cardiac auscultation.
- Tachycardia.
- Poor pulse quality.

Diagnostic aids

- Echocardiography (ultrasonography of the heart).
- Thoracic radiography.
- ECG – electrical alternans (height of QRS complex alters from beat to beat) due to fluid in the pericardial sac.

Treatment

- Pericardiocentesis (a needle is used to drain the fluid from the pericardial sac) (Figure 19.15).
- Placement of intravenous catheter in case emergency treatment with lidocaine is necessary due to arrhythmias during pericardiocentesis.
- In recurrent cases, surgery to remove the pericardial sac may be necessary.
- Medical therapy is not effective.

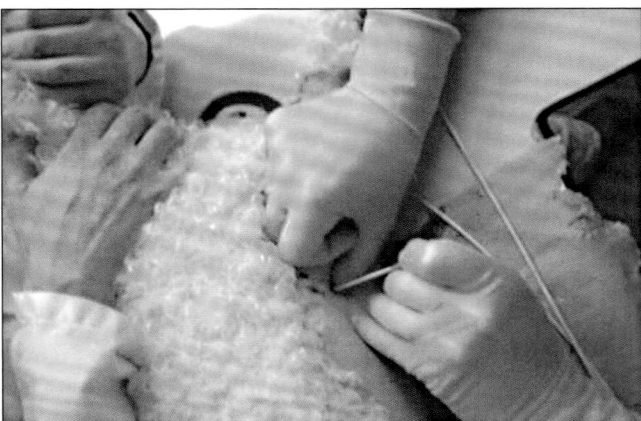

19.15 Placement of a large-bore intravenous catheter into the pericardial sac during pericardiocentesis in a Bichon Frise. Note the ECG leads running to the patient's feet, allowing essential monitoring of the patient.

Aortic thromboembolism

This is a relatively common condition in cats but a rare condition in dogs. A thrombus (clot) blocks the aorta, disrupting blood flow to the hindlimbs. In cats it usually occurs secondary to underlying heart disease, whereas in dogs it usually occurs secondary to abnormal blood clotting. Rarely, thrombi can occur at other sites.

Clinical signs

- Unilateral or bilateral paresis or paralysis of the hindlimb(s); forelimbs can be affected, but much less commonly.
- Cold hindlimb(s) with non-palpable pulse(s).
- Extreme pain (vocalizing) – less common in dogs.
- In the cat, dyspnoea or tachypnoea (signs of underlying cardiomyopathy).
- History of heart disease.

Diagnostic aids

Diagnosis is usually based on a physical examination; supportive tests may be useful, especially in dogs, where an underlying medical disease is often the precipitating factor:

- Haematology and biochemistry
- Urinalysis
- Abdominal ultrasonography
- Echocardiography
- Thoracic radiography
- Blood pressure
- Endocrine testing.

Treatment

- Prognosis poor.
- Oxygen therapy.
- Analgesia.
- Environmental comfort.
- Treatment of underlying disease.
- Thrombolytic drugs – for example tissue plasminogen activator. There is limited experience of their use in veterinary medicine. They are very expensive and associated with a number of side effects. If used, they are likely to be more effective within hours of the clot first forming.
- Antithrombotic drugs (e.g. aspirin, heparin) – these may help to reduce the risk of further clots forming but will not break down clots that are already present.

Arrhythmia – tachycardia

Animals present with an abnormal heart rhythm that is so fast that the heart does not have time to fill properly with blood between beats. This is a rare emergency but needs to be identified quickly or heart failure can follow.

Clinical signs

- Collapse or syncope.
- Exercise intolerance.
- Severe tachycardia (>240 bpm).
- Poor or intermittent pulses.

Diagnostic aids

- ECG (Figure 19.16).

Treatment

- Medical therapy with antiarrhythmic drugs.
- Therapy is challenging as the drugs used have side effects, including the potential to worsen the arrhythmia.

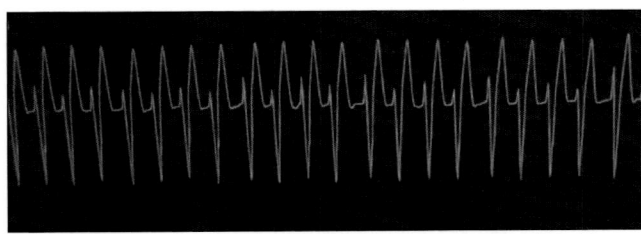

19.16 Ventricular tachycardia in a German Shepherd Dog that presented with gastric dilatation–volvulus.

Arrhythmia – bradycardia

Animals present with an abnormally slow heart rate, leading to collapse. This is rare. Medical causes such as hyperkalaemia should be ruled out at an early stage.

Clinical signs

- Collapse or syncope.
- Exercise intolerance.
- Marked bradycardia (usually <60 bpm).

Diagnostic aids

- ECG (Figure 19.17).
- Serum potassium level.
- Other medical tests dependent on potassium level.

Treatment

- If serum potassium level high, this should be treated urgently (see 'Metabolic emergencies').
- Cage rest.
- Medical therapy unlikely to be effective unless patient is hyperkalaemic.
- Pacemaker implantation may be necessary.

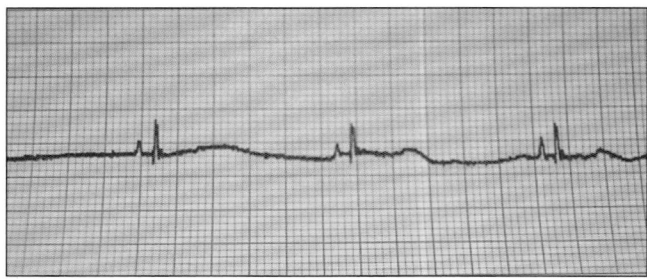

19.17 Sinus bradycardia in a Miniature Poodle that presented with severe head trauma and raised intracranial pressure.

Respiratory emergencies

Respiratory emergencies are very common and can be challenging to treat successfully. Several treatment strategies can be used irrespective of the cause of the dyspnoea, notably:

- Oxygen therapy
- Stress-free cool (but not cold) environment
- Maintain in sternal recumbency.

Upper airway disease

Upper airway problems generally present as dyspnoea associated with an audible noise (stridor or stertor). The emergency treatment of upper airway disease involves oxygen therapy and calming and cooling the patient. If the patient is in severe distress, it may be necessary to bypass the upper airway temporarily by anaesthetizing and intubating the patient. Emergency tracheotomies need to be performed rarely.

Common causes of upper airway dyspnoea are discussed in more detail below. Rarer causes include laryngeal masses, severe trauma to the upper airway and airway foreign bodies.

Laryngeal paralysis

This is a common cause of dyspnoea in older large-breed dogs. The muscles that hold the larynx open during inspiration become paralysed and the larynx collapses as the dog tries to breathe in.

Clinical signs

- Marked dyspnoea, often with paradoxical abdominal movement.
- Stridor (audible whistling noise) on inspiration.
- Exercise intolerance.
- History of change in bark.
- Cyanosis.
- Hyperthermia.

Diagnostic aids

The diagnosis is often suspected on the basis of the history and physical examination.

- Laryngoscopy under a light plane of anaesthesia is confirmatory.

Treatment

- Oxygen therapy.
- Sedation (commonly low doses of acepromazine) to reduce stress and inspiratory effort.
- Cooling.
- If severe, the patient may need to be anaesthetized and intubated. The patient can then be cooled and allowed to recover slowly from the anaesthetic. Rarely, a tracheostomy needs to be performed.
- Long-term treatment requires surgery (usually a 'tie-back' procedure) but this is not commonly done on an emergency basis.

Brachycephalic obstructive airway syndrome (BOAS)

This is a common disease in brachycephalic breeds such as Bulldogs and Pugs. It can be seen in brachycephalic cats such as Persians, but is typically less severe in this species. The dyspnoea is caused by airway obstruction secondary to the abnormal anatomy of these breeds. It is considered to include several components:

- Stenotic nares
- Long soft palate
- Everted laryngeal saccules
- Hypoplastic (narrow) trachea.

Clinical signs

- Dyspnoea.
- Exercise intolerance.
- Stertorous (snoring) breathing sounds.
- Collapse/syncope.
- Cyanosis.

Diagnostic aids

Diagnosis is usually made on the basis of compatible clinical signs, breed and physical examination. Anaesthesia and examination of the upper airway confirms the diagnosis.

Treatment

- Oxygen therapy.
- Sedation (commonly acepromazine).
- Cooling.
- If severe, the patient may need to be anaesthetized and intubated. The patient can then be cooled and allowed to recover slowly from the anaesthetic. Rarely, a tracheostomy needs to be performed.

- If severe, surgery may be needed to correct the anatomical abnormality, but this surgery is not commonly done on an emergency basis.

Tracheal collapse

This condition typically occurs in small-breed dogs where the cartilaginous tracheal rings are abnormal or degenerate and the trachea collapses as the animal breathes in and out.

Clinical signs

- Cough (goose-honk) and dyspnoea commonly occur with stress or excitement.
- Cyanosis.
- Collapse/syncope.

Diagnostic aids

Diagnosis is usually made on history, clinical signs and examination. Thoracic radiography and/or tracheal endoscopy may be used to confirm the diagnosis.

Treatment

- Oxygen therapy.
- Stress-free environment and strict rest.
- Sedation if necessary.
- If severe, the patient may need to be anaesthetized and intubated. This should be avoided if possible as the endotracheal tube will cause further irritation to the trachea and the patient may be worse following an anaesthetic.
- Long-term medical management includes weight loss and drug therapy but is rarely curative.
- Invasive treatment options are available (e.g. placement of a tracheal stent, surgery) but these have a variable success rate and are only available at specialist institutions.

Pleural space disease

Animals with dyspnoea secondary to pleural space disease commonly present with short shallow respiration and dull lung sounds on thoracic auscultation.

Pleural effusion

This occurs when fluid accumulates in the pleural space. There are a number of types of fluid but the emergency treatment is the same.

Types of fluid

- Transudate – secondary to severe hypoalbuminaemia (low blood protein)
- Modified transudate – secondary to heart failure
- Neoplastic exudate – secondary to neoplasia within the chest, commonly lymphoma in cats
- Pyothorax – infected purulent fluid in the chest
- Haemothorax – blood in the chest secondary to trauma or a clotting disorder
- Chylothorax – a milky fluid that builds up due to problems with lymphatic drainage in the chest or rupture of the thoracic duct

Clinical signs

- Dyspnoea and tachypnoea.
- Dull lung sounds on auscultation.
- Inappetence.
- Weight loss.

Diagnostic aids

- Thoracocentesis – this is therapeutic as well as diagnostic. The fluid obtained should be analysed.
- Thoracic free fluid ultrasound scan.
- Thoracic radiography.
- In dyspnoeic patients, radiographs should not be taken until after thoracocentesis has been performed.
- In non-traumatic cases, advanced imaging (computed tomography, CT) may be useful.

Treatment

- Oxygen therapy.
- Thoracocentesis.
- Treatment of the underlying cause – this may be medical or surgical.
- Occasionally it is necessary to place thoracostomy (chest) tubes to allow frequent drainage.

Pneumothorax

This occurs when air accumulates in the pleural space. Causes include:

- Trauma – most common cause
- Inhaled foreign body
- Idiopathic (especially in large-breed dogs)
- External penetrating wound (open pneumothorax).

Clinical signs

- Dyspnoea with short shallow respirations.
- Dull lung sounds on auscultation.
- External wound (open pneumothorax).
- Cyanosis.

Diagnostic aids

- Oxygen therapy.
- Thoracocentesis – this is therapeutic as well as diagnostic.
- Thoracic ultrasound scan.
- Thoracic radiography.
- In non-traumatic cases, advanced imaging (computed tomography, CT) may be useful.

Treatment

- Thoracocentesis – in most cases of traumatic pneumothorax, thoracocentesis is the only treatment required as the leak will heal itself.
- In non-traumatic cases, surgical exploration of the chest may be necessary.
- Thoracostomy tubes may need to be placed if large volumes of air are produced quickly.
- Open pneumothorax requires surgical treatment; a sterile adherent dressing should be placed over the wound until the patient is stable for surgery.

Feline asthma

This is the only lower airway disease of importance in veterinary emergency patients.

Clinical signs

- Dyspnoea principally on expiration.
- Wheezes on auscultation.
- Abdominal effort on expiration.

Diagnostic aids

- Physical examination.
- Thoracic radiography.
- Cytology on wash samples taken from the airways.

Treatment

- Oxygen therapy.
- Medical treatment:
  - Corticosteroids
  - Bronchodilators
  - Inhaled medications (Figure 19.18).

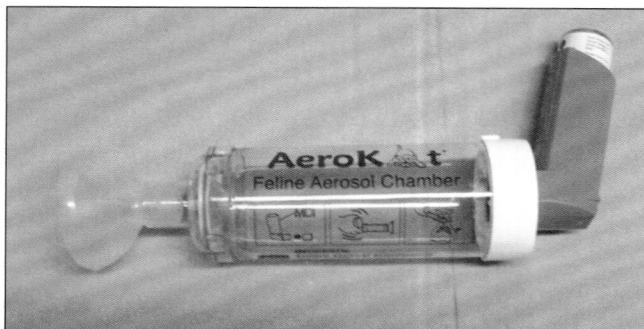

19.18 An inhaler with spacer and face mask used for administration of inhaled medications.

Parenchymal disease

Parenchymal disease develops when the alveoli become filled with either fluid or tissue.
Common causes include:

- Heart failure (pulmonary oedema)
- Pneumonia (bacterial or parasitic) (Figure 19.19)
- Neoplasia
- Non-cardiogenic oedema (e.g. secondary to head trauma, airway obstructions, severe systemic illness)
- Pulmonary contusions (bleeding into lung following trauma)
- Pulmonary thromboembolism.

Clinical signs

- Dyspnoea.
- Cyanosis.
- Crackles on auscultation of the lungs.
- Inappetence.

Diagnostic aids

- Thoracic radiography.
- Thoracic ultrasonography for the identification of fluid within the lungs is a relatively new technique, but may be useful.

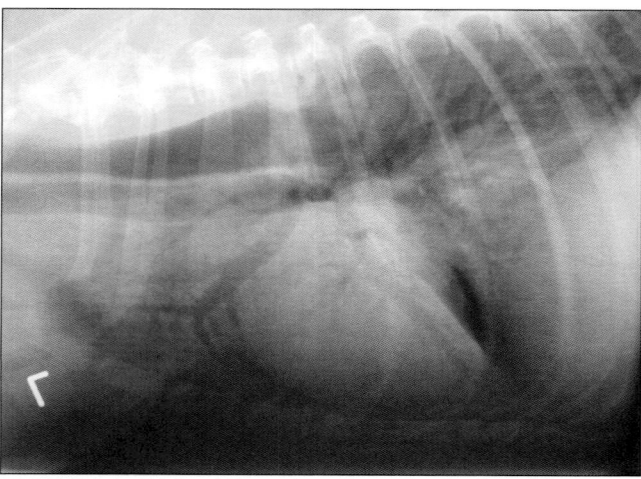

19.19 Left lateral thoracic radiograph of a dog with megaoesophagus and aspiration pneumonia. Note the branching air bronchogram in the cranial lung field.

- Haematology and biochemistry.
- Urinalysis.
- Bronchoscopy with airway washes in some patients.
- Echocardiography (heart ultrasonography).

Treatment

- Oxygen therapy.
- Medical treatment of the underlying disease may include:
  - Diuretics (e.g. furosemide)
  - Antibiotics
  - Anthelmintics.

Neurological emergencies

Head trauma

Head trauma is a common emergency in both dogs and cats. It can occur secondary to road traffic accidents, falling from a height or being attacked by other animals (bitten by a dog or cat, kicked by a large animal). Head trauma may or may not be associated with traumatic brain injury. Clinical signs are variable, depending on whether the brain has been damaged and, if so, which part.

Clinical signs

- Depression.*
- Anisocoria (variation in pupil size).*
- Nystagmus.*
- Strabismus.*
- Cranial nerve deficits.*
- Epistaxis.
- Bruising or swelling of face.
- Asymmetry of face or jaw.
- Inability to close mouth properly (mandibular or maxillary fractures).
- Ocular haemorrhage (scleral or within eye).
- Bradycardia.*
- Abnormal breathing pattern.*

- Seizures.*
- Coma.*
- Signs of trauma in other body areas (especially thorax or limb fractures).

(Those marked * indicate brain injury.)

Diagnostic aids

- Frequent neurological examination – these should be recorded using a standard system such as the modified Glasgow Coma Scale. This scale is an objective way of recording the severity of neurological injury by assigning a point value (1–6) to the patient's level of consciousness, motor activity and brainstem reflexes. A low score indicates more severe injury.
- Haematology and biochemistry.
- Blood pressure – an increasing blood pressure associated with a decreasing heart rate can indicate that intracranial pressure is rising.
- Skull radiographs.
- Advanced imaging techniques (CT, MRI).

Treatment

- Ensuring patent airway.
- Supplementing oxygen (take care that this does not cause stress).
- Intravenous fluid therapy to maintain blood pressure.
- Head elevated at 30 degrees to reduce intracranial pressure.
- Avoidance of any techniques that may increase intracranial pressure, such as jugular venepuncture or intranasal oxygen catheterization.
- Monitoring and maintaining body temperature.
- If recumbent, turning every 4 hours.
- Monitoring bladder size and catheterization or expression if necessary.
- Medical therapies to reduce intracranial pressure (e.g. hypertonic saline, mannitol).
- Analgesia.
- Treat concurrent injuries.
- Corticosteroids are now considered to be contraindicated in patients with head trauma.

Seizures

Seizures occur relatively commonly in dogs and rarely in cats. They represent an acute and usually brief disturbance of normal electrical activity in the brain and can be very distressing for both the patient and the owner. Most seizures are short (<2 minutes) and owners often only manage to telephone for veterinary advice once the seizure is over. As seizures can sometimes occur close together, it is always best to advise that the animal is examined by a veterinary surgeon as soon as practical even if the seizure has stopped. This is particularly important in very young (<6 months old) and older animals where there is more likely to be a medical cause for the seizures.

Seizures are often described as having a pre-ictal, ictal and post-ictal phase. During the pre-ictal phase, the animal may show mild behaviour changes, though these are not always recognized by owners. The ictal phase represents the seizure itself and the post-ictal phase a period after the seizure where the animal displays abnormal neurological signs.

Status epilepticus is a condition where seizures are prolonged (>5 minutes) or where there are multiple seizures in a short space of time (e.g. 30 minutes) and the animal does not recover completely between them. Animals with status epilepticus should be seen immediately, as prolonged or very frequent seizures may cause permanent brain damage.

Clinical signs

Ictal phase

- Loss of motor coordination with paddling of the limbs.
- Rigid collapse.
- Loss of consciousness.
- Hypersalivation and abnormal chewing movements.
- Defecation.
- Urination.
- Signs are usually generalized but, rarely, partial seizures are seen where the animal does not lose consciousness totally but becomes less aware, with focal twitching of the face or a single limb.

Post-ictal phase

- Confusion.
- Depression/listlessness.
- Ataxia.
- Visual disturbances, including blindness.

The post-ictal phase may last for several hours after a seizure episode.

Causes

- Idiopathic epilepsy.
- Brain tumour (neoplasia).
- Trauma.
- Infection.
- Inflammation.
- Toxin.
- Metabolic problems (hypoglycaemia, hepatic encephalopathy).

Diagnostic aids

- Blood glucose level (especially in young animals).
- Haematology and biochemistry.
- Full neurological examination.
- Cerebrospinal fluid (CSF) tap.
- Brain imaging (CT, MRI) if available.

Treatment

If the animal is having a seizure when it arrives at the practice, or starts to do so whilst hospitalized, medications should be given to control the seizure. Although most seizures are short, longer seizures (especially if lasting >5 minutes) can lead to further brain damage. Drugs used to treat seizures include:

- Diazepam (valium) – intravenous or per rectum
- Phenobarbital – intravenous or oral
- Potassium bromide – oral or per rectum
- Levetiracetam – intravenous or oral.

The drug of choice for acute control of seizures is diazepam given by the intravenous route, but the rectal route can be used if intravenous access cannot be obtained. If diazepam does not work for the acute control of seizures, other intravenous drug therapy such as propofol infusions may need to be considered. Phenobarbital, levetiracetam and potassium bromide are more commonly used as oral medications for the longer-term control of seizures, although are sometimes also used for acute control.

If a seizuring animal develops respiratory distress or cyanosis, it is important to secure an airway. However, drugs (sedative or anaesthetic) must be given to allow this to happen safely. Never put your hand in the mouth of a seizuring animal.

Nursing care

- Monitor body temperature and cool if hyperthermic. Conversely, patients that are sedated to control seizures may become hypothermic and require warming to maintain body temperature.
- Monitor heart rate and respiratory rate.
- Ensure patent intravenous access in case further seizures occur.
- Turn patient every 4 hours.
- Monitor bladder size and catheterize or express if necessary.
- Lubricate eyes.
- Maintain a calm environment. However, it is not necessary to maintain a dark room and this can in fact be detrimental, as it can compromise the ability to monitor the patient.

Spinal cord disease

Causes

- Intervertebral disc disease.
- Direct trauma (e.g. road traffic accident, inadequate restraint (rabbit)).
- Anatomical abnormalities (e.g. 'wobbler' dogs).
- Vascular disease (e.g. fibrocartilaginous emboli).
- Spinal cord haemorrhage.
- Spinal cord neoplasia.
- Infection.
- Degenerative spinal cord disease (e.g. degenerative myelopathy).

Clinical signs

These will be variable depending on the site and severity of the spinal cord injury. In general, cervical spinal cord disease has signs involving all four limbs, whereas thoracolumbar spinal cord disease has signs involving the hindlimbs only. It is very important to assess whether the animal can feel pain in each of its legs, which is usually done by squeezing firmly on one of the animal's toes. It should be remembered that the animal simply withdrawing its leg when the toe is squeezed is a local reflex arc and does not necessarily mean that the animal is aware and feeling the sensation. Signs that the animal can feel the sensation include vocalization, turning the head to look at the leg or pupillary dilation at the time the toe is squeezed. If deep pain sensation is lost, the animal's prognosis, in terms of the likelihood of it walking again, is much worse.

Clinical signs may include:

- Limb weakness (paresis) and proprioceptive deficits (mild disease)
- Ataxia (mild disease)
- Paralysis (severe disease)
- Recumbency/inability to walk (severe disease)
- Pain on palpation of spine
- Urinary incontinence
- Lack of anal tone
- Loss of deep pain sensation (severe disease)

- Change (either decrease or increase dependent on location of lesion) of the strength of the local reflexes (e.g. patellar reflex)
- Normal mentation and cranial nerve examination.

Rarely, severe thoracolumbar spinal cord disease will cause the Schiff–Sherrington phenomenon, where the forelimbs are rigid and the hindlimbs flaccid. This is most often seen following trauma and has a poor prognosis.

Treatment

- Analgesia.
- Cage rest.
- Monitoring bladder size and expression or catheterization if necessary.
- Maintaining warm and comfortable environment.
- Turning regularly (every 4 hours) if recumbent.
- Surgical treatment required for most causes of acute spinal cord disease.
- Use of corticosteroids (e.g. methylprednisolone, dexamethasone) is no longer recommended.
- Intravenous fluids only required if the animal shows concurrent signs of hypovolaemia or dehydration, or if the animal is not eating and drinking.

If a spinal fracture is suspected, great care must be taken when moving the patient. If possible, the animal should be strapped to something rigid during transport to the practice. A specially designed animal stretcher is ideal but other rigid objects may be used in an emergency.

Vestibular disease

The vestibular system controls balance and the animal's awareness of its body position in space. Vestibular disease may occur at the level of the inner ear, where the sense organs of balance are located (known as peripheral vestibular disease), or within the brain (known as central vestibular disease). Vestibular signs are not uncommon in rabbits where infection with *Pasteurella* spp. or *Encephalitozoon cuniculi* are common causes.

Causes

- Infection (e.g. otitis media).
- Inflammation.
- Neoplasia.
- Benign polyps (especially in young cats).
- Idiopathic ('old dog' vestibular disease).
- Trauma.
- Toxic (including drugs, e.g. high doses of metronidazole).
- Postsurgical (e.g. following ear surgery).

Clinical signs

- Nystagmus (abnormal eye movements).
- Strabismus.
- Ataxia.
- Mental depression.
- Other neurological signs.
- Horner's syndrome (constricted pupil, flaccid eyelids, enophthalmos, third eyelid protrusion).
- Nausea.
- Signs of external ear disease.

Figure 19.20 summarizes the clinical signs that can help to distinguish peripheral from central vestibular disease.

Clinical sign	Peripheral	Central
Nystagmus	Usually horizontal	Can be vertical or rotatory
Horner's syndrome	May be present	Absent
Mentation	Normal	May be depressed
Hemiparesis	Absent	Possible

19.20 Clinical findings that can help to differentiate between peripheral and central vestibular disease.

Treatment

- Treatment of underlying cause (medical or surgical).
- Maintaining in a comfortable padded environment.
- May need intravenous fluids and/or nutritional support as may be unable to eat or drink.
- Time.

Reproductive emergencies

Dystocia

Dystocia refers to problems during the parturition (birthing) process (see also Chapter 24). There are a large number of causes of dystocia but some of the more common ones are:

- Primary uterine inertia (i.e. failure of uterus to contract)
- Secondary uterine inertia after prolonged straining
- Fetal malpresentation
- Maternal–fetal disproportion (common in breeds such as Bulldogs)
- Maternal pelvic abnormalities (e.g. previous fractured pelvis)
- Fetal death.

Clinical signs

If the bitch is showing any of the following signs, veterinary advice should be urgently sought:

- She has been straining unproductively for more than 1 hour from the onset of stage II labour without producing a puppy
- She has been straining unproductively for more than 30 minutes without producing subsequent puppies
- She has a green/black vulval discharge or fetal fluids are seen and 2 hours have elapsed without producing a puppy
- She rests for more than 2 hours between puppies without straining
- She appears unwell or depressed
- A puppy can be seen stuck in the birth canal.

For queens, the interval between kittens may be much longer and the entire parturition process may take up to 24 hours. If concerned, it is better to err on the side of caution and recommend that the pet is examined for signs of fetal or maternal distress.

The occurrence of dystocia in exotic pets is very variable between the species. Egg binding in birds and reptiles may also occur. Reasons for dystocia in small mammals may

include those factors listed above. Other factors may be related to husbandry, such as lack of suitable substrate or nesting material, or to hormonal or metabolic imbalances. A clinical history should therefore include how the pet is managed and all relevant husbandry information. Veterinary advice should be sought if there is unproductive straining or an abnormal vulval or cloacal discharge. The reader is referred to exotic pet texts for specific information on individual species.

Diagnostic aids

- Digital vaginal examination.
- Abdominal radiography.
- Abdominal ultrasonography.
- Bloodwork to check glucose and ionized calcium levels.

Treatment

- Keep the bitch/queen in a warm and comfortable environment.
- If a puppy/kitten is visible in the birth canal, manually assisted delivery may be attempted.
- Medical therapy (e.g. oxytocin).
- Surgical delivery (Caesarean operation).
- If the bitch is weak or unwell, stabilization such as intravenous fluids may be required.

Nursing care for Caesarean operation

For a successful outcome, the time taken for the anaesthesia and surgical procedure should be minimized. The bitch should receive oxygen supplementation for at least 5 minutes and may be clipped and an initial surgical preparation carried out prior to anaesthesia. All instruments for the surgery and for neonatal resuscitation and care should be prepared before the procedure

Neonatal resuscitation

Equipment that should be prepared prior to delivery includes:

- A warm environment (incubator) or box with heat lamp
- Plenty of soft, dry, warm towels
- Haemostats for clamping the umbilical cord
- Suture material
- Suction bulb syringe for clearing oral secretions
- Emergency drugs (adrenaline, naloxone).

The following procedures should start once the neonate has been handed over to the nurse:

- Clean the fetal membranes from the puppy's mouth and gently suction the oral cavity (check for cleft palate when doing this)
- Clamp and cut the umbilical cord approximately 3 cm from the puppy's abdomen
- Stimulate and dry the neonate by rubbing with a warm towel
- Check that the puppy is breathing and has a heartbeat (using digital palpation).

If a puppy is not breathing or does not have a heartbeat, supply oxygen via a tight-fitting face mask or endotracheal tube and continue vigorously rubbing the puppy to stimulate respiration. 'Swinging' puppies is no longer recommended, due to the potential for causing harm. The use of doxapram is also no longer recommended due to a lack of evidence for its efficacy. If there is no heartbeat, start gentle external compressions and administer adrenaline.

Pyometra

This is an infection of the uterus that is common in older entire female dogs and occasionally cats. It occurs secondary to hormonally induced changes and is commonest about 5–6 weeks after a season.

Clinical signs

- Vomiting.
- Polyuria/polydipsia.
- Weakness and lethargy.
- Purulent vaginal discharge (not always present).
- Abdominal pain.
- Shock.

Diagnostic aids

- Haematology and biochemistry.
- Urinalysis.
- Vaginal swab.
- Abdominal radiography.
- Abdominal ultrasonography.

Treatment

- Intravenous fluid therapy.
- Antibiotic therapy.
- Surgery to remove the infected uterus.

Eclampsia

This is hypocalcaemia secondary to pregnancy or more commonly lactation. It is most often seen in small-breed dogs within 2 weeks of parturition.

Clinical signs

- Restlessness and anxiety.
- Panting.
- Hypersalivation.
- Twitching/muscle spasms.
- Hyperthermia.
- Tachycardia.
- Collapse.

Diagnostic aids

- Blood calcium level.

Treatment

- Slow intravenous infusion of 10% calcium gluconate (monitor heart rate and ideally ECG while doing this).
- Oral calcium supplementation.
- Wean the puppies.

Paraphimosis

This is an inability to retract the penis into the prepuce. It commonly occurs in entire male small-breed dogs following an episode of sexual excitement.

Clinical signs

- Engorged protruding penis, often dry and may be necrotic.
- Dysuria.
- Pain and excessive licking associated with penile region.

Treatment

- Analgesia.
- Gentle cleaning of penis with warm water or saline solution.
- Topical hyperosmolar solution to reduce swelling.
- Manual replacement of penis within prepuce (commonly requires heavy sedation or anaesthesia).
- Surgical correction, especially if situation recurs.

Paediatric emergencies

Young puppies, kittens and neonates of other species may present in a collapsed state. It is often challenging to achieve a specific diagnosis but the two most common problems are:

- Hypoglycaemia
- Hypothermia.

Clinical signs

- Weakness or collapse.
- Persistent crying.
- Decreased feeding.
- Decreased movement.

Treatment

Due to patient size, diagnostic tests and treatment are challenging but the following guidelines should be used:

- Monitor body temperature and warm if hypothermic
- Measure blood glucose (NB if a blood sample to measure glucose cannot be obtained, it is recommended that treatment with glucose is started, as hypoglycaemia is common)
- Supplement glucose:
  - Intravenous – a standard intravenous catheter may be used in the jugular vein in paediatric patients
  - Intraosseous – easy to place in paediatric patients and can be life saving
  - Oral – much less effective.
- Supplement fluids
- Once normothermic, initiate oral feeding regime
- Appropriate empirical antimicrobial therapy may also be used as bacterial infection is a possible underlying cause.

Nursing the paediatric patient

- Ensure warm and comfortable environment.
- Feed regularly by bottle or stomach tube:
  - Every 2 hours in puppies and kittens up to 5 days old
  - Every 4 hours in puppies and kittens >5 days old.
- Use a commercial hand-rearing formula to supply the patient's needs.
- After feeding, stimulate the patient to defecate by gently rubbing the perineum with a damp cotton bud (this function is usually undertaken by the mother).

For further information on neonatal care, see Chapter 24.

Urological emergencies

Urethral obstruction

This occurs when there is a blockage in the urethra and therefore the animal cannot pass urine. As urine cannot be voided from the body, waste products (especially potassium, hydrogen ions, urea and creatinine) build up rapidly in the bloodstream and can cause life-threatening signs within 24 hours of the obstruction occurring. It occurs most commonly in overweight male neutered cats, but some dog breeds (e.g. Dalmatians) and rabbits are also predisposed. It is very rare in female animals, as they have a much shorter wider urethra.

Causes

- Urethral calculi (stones).
- Urethral plug (consists of crystals and a mucoid material).
- Urethral neoplasia (cancer) (rare).
- Urethral stricture (may occur secondary to previous obstruction with stones or a plug).

Clinical signs

- Stranguria (straining to urinate without passing any urine). It should be noted that clients frequently confuse stranguria with constipation.
- Frequent visits to litter tray with no urine produced.
- Vocalization (pain) when attempting to urinate.
- Licking at urethra.
- Depression (dependent on duration of blockage, but most animals are markedly depressed by 24–36 hours after the blockage occurs).
- Anorexia.
- Bradycardia (secondary to potassium build-up in bloodstream).
- Distended painful bladder on palpation of the abdomen.
- Vomiting.
- Collapse.

Urethral blockage must be distinguished from cystitis, where the bladder is inflamed but not blocked. Animals with cystitis may also strain to urinate, urinate frequently and show pain when urinating, but they will pass small amounts of urine. Cystitis is more common in female animals. Cystitis is an uncomfortable condition but, as the animal can still void urine, it is not life-threatening.

Diagnostic aids

- Palpation and gentle attempts at expression of the bladder.
- Blood tests, especially blood potassium level.
- ECG – can help to identify signs of hyperkalaemia (high blood potassium).

Once the patient has had the obstruction relieved (been 'unblocked'), the following tests can be carried out:

- Urinalysis and culture
- Ultrasonography of the bladder
- Radiography, including retrograde urethrography.

Treatment

- Fluid therapy.
- Treatment for hyperkalaemia if present (see 'Metabolic emergencies').

- Urinary catheterization – commonly requires sedation and should be carried out once the animal has been stabilized with fluid therapy.
- Urinary catheter should be left in place for 24–72 hours after initial decompression of the bladder. Urine production should be monitored during this time ideally by connecting the urinary catheter to a closed collection system. Patients may develop post-obstructive diuresis, where they have a high urine output for up to 24 hours. During this period, it is important to match the intravenous fluid therapy rate to the urine output.
- Analgesia/anti-inflammatories.
- If bladder stones are present surgery may be required to remove them. Longer-term medical treatment may be used to dissolve or prevent recurrence of calculi.

Uroabdomen

This condition occurs when urine leaks into the abdominal cavity, often secondary to a tear in the bladder wall (ruptured bladder). As in urethral obstruction, urine is not voided from the patient and high levels of potassium, hydrogen ions, urea and creatinine can build up in the blood, leading to severe clinical signs.

Causes

- Trauma.
- Following cystocentesis (this is most often a concern when a cystocentesis is performed while the urethra is blocked).
- Bladder neoplasia (cancer).

Clinical signs

- Distended and/or painful abdomen.
- Depression.
- Anorexia.
- Vomiting.
- Bradycardia.
- Lack of urination (as urine is leaking into abdomen). If the tear in the bladder wall is small, it is possible that the animal may still be able to void small amounts of urine via the urethra.

Diagnostic aids

- Blood tests (especially potassium, urea and creatinine levels).
- Abdominal ultrasonography.
- Analysis of fluid collected from the abdominal cavity by abdominocentesis.
- Radiography, including contrast studies.

Treatment

- Intravenous fluid therapy.
- Treatment for hyperkalaemia if present (see 'Metabolic emergencies').
- Surgical repair of the rupture.

Acute kidney injury

This can happen if the kidneys suddenly fail. It is much less common than chronic renal failure in veterinary patients.

Causes

- Shock with significant reduction of blood supply to the kidneys (most commonly prolonged hypovolaemic shock).

- Infection (e.g. leptospirosis, bacterial pyelonephritis).
- Toxic damage (e.g. ethylene glycol).
- Metabolic (e.g. prolonged hypercalcaemia).
- Drug therapy (e.g. non-steroidal anti-inflammatory drugs, especially if given while the patient is in shock).
- Blood clots in the arteries supplying the kidneys (rare).
- Progression of chronic renal failure.

Clinical signs

- Depression.
- Anorexia.
- Vomiting.
- Uraemia (may be smelled on animal's breath).
- Abnormality in urine production, most commonly reduced (anuria/oliguria) but occasionally massively increased (polyuria).

Diagnostic aids

- Blood gas and electrolyte analysis.
- Haematology and biochemistry.
- Urinalysis, including urine culture.
- Abdominal ultrasonography.
- Abdominal radiography.
- Serology (blood tests for infectious agents such as leptospirosis).

Treatment

- Intravenous fluid therapy.
- Treatment for underlying cause, if known (e.g. antibiotics for infection, specific treatment for hypercalcaemia).
- Drugs to encourage urine production (furosemide, mannitol).
- Peritoneal dialysis. Haemodialysis may be used, but is only available in a small number of institutions and is very expensive.
- Monitor urine production and blood tests.

Metabolic emergencies
Hypoglycaemia

This is a low level of blood glucose (sugar). It is the commonest reversible cause of collapse in neonatal/paediatric patients but can occur in older animals. It may also be seen in the smaller exotic species where metabolic rates are high.

Causes

- Young patient, especially toy breeds of dog.
- Insulin overdose in diabetic patients.
- Insulinoma (functional cancer of pancreas).
- Other types of neoplasia.
- Hypoadrenocorticism (Addison's disease).
- Liver failure.
- Sepsis or severe infection.
- Toxicity (xylitol – artificial sweetener used in human foodstuffs).

Clinical signs

- Weakness.
- Exercise intolerance.
- Collapse.
- Seizures.
- Coma.

Diagnostic aids

- Blood glucose level (glucometer).
- Haematology and biochemistry.

Treatment

- Intravenous (or intraosseous) glucose supplementation.
- Food offered as soon as able to eat.
- Rub glucose syrup on oral mucous membranes – unlikely to be effective if animal is severely hypoglycaemic, but may be attempted whilst intravenous access is obtained.

Hyperkalaemia

This is an increased blood potassium level. The normal level of potassium in blood is approximately 3.5–5.5 mmol/l. Levels >8.0 mmol/l may be fatal. Death occurs as the high potassium level leads to disturbances in electrical conduction within the heart initially causing bradycardia but ultimately asystole and death.

Causes

- Urethral obstruction.
- Acute kidney injury.
- Uroabdomen.
- Hypoadrenocorticism (Addison's disease).
- Reperfusion injury.

Clinical signs

- Bradycardia (slow heart rate).
- Poor pulse quality.
- ECG changes.
- Other signs dependent on cause of hyperkalaemia.

Diagnostic aids

- Serum potassium level.
- ECG.
- Other tests dependent on underlying cause.

Treatment

Ultimately, successful treatment depends on identifying and treating the underlying cause of the hyperkalaemia. However, as it may be immediately life-threatening, the following therapies may be used to stabilize the animal, whatever the cause of the hyperkalaemia:

- Intravenous calcium gluconate
- Intravenous insulin and dextrose supplementation
- Intravenous fluid therapy.

Hypercalcaemia

This is an increased level of blood calcium.

Causes

- Neoplasia (cancer), especially lymphoma and anal sac carcinoma.
- Toxicity (e.g. human psoriasis cream, some rat poisons).
- Primary hyperparathyroidism (hormonal disease).
- Hypoadrenocorticism (Addison's disease).
- Granulomatous infections (e.g. lungworm, fungal disease).

Clinical signs

- Inappetence/anorexia.
- Polyuria/polydipsia.
- Depression.
- Vomiting.
- Tremors.
- Renal failure if prolonged.

Diagnostic aids

- Measurement of ionized calcium; the total calcium level on a biochemistry panel may be within the reference range, even though the animal has clinically significant hypercalcaemia, therefore, ionized calcium should be measured wherever possible.
- Haematology and biochemistry.
- Urinalysis.
- Imaging studies (radiography, ultrasonography).

Treatment

As with hyperkalaemia, successful treatment requires identification and treatment of the underlying disease. However, while diagnostic tests are being carried out to allow this, the following medical treatments can be used to lower the calcium level and reduce the risk of renal damage:

- Intravenous fluid therapy with 0.9% saline
- Furosemide
- Bisphosphonates
- Calcitonin.

Hypoadrenocorticism (Addison's disease)

This is a disease where there is impaired secretion of hormones from the adrenal cortex. The animal becomes deficient in a number of hormones, most importantly aldosterone (a mineralocorticoid) and cortisol (a glucocorticoid). Aldosterone is a hormone that helps the body to maintain electrolyte balance (especially potassium), and cortisol is a hormone that helps the animal to maintain normal blood pressure and gastrointestinal tract function and to cope with stress. It is most commonly diagnosed in young to middle-aged female dogs and is very rare in cats.

Clinical signs

- Collapse.
- Weakness.
- Depression/lethargy.
- Polyuria/polydipsia.
- Intermittent gastrointestinal signs (vomiting, diarrhoea, inappetence).
- Bradycardia.
- Poor pulse quality.
- Pale mucous membranes with a prolonged capillary refill time.

Diagnostic aids

- Acid–base and electrolyte panel.
- Haematology and biochemistry.
- Urinalysis.
- ACTH stimulation test (this is the only way to make a certain diagnosis).
- ECG.

Treatment

- Intravenous fluid therapy.
- Treatment of hyperkalaemia if severe (see section above on hyperkalaemia).
- Hormone replacement therapy (both mineralocorticoid and glucocorticoid).

Diabetic ketoacidosis

This is a complication of diabetes mellitus where the body starts to produce ketones as an energy source. As these ketones are organic acids, if produced in large quantities they can cause the blood to become acidic, with severe systemic effects. Diabetic ketoacidosis may occur both in previously undiagnosed diabetics and in diabetic animals that have been on insulin treatment for some time. In addition, there is almost always a concurrent disease such as a bacterial infection or pancreatitis that acts as a trigger.

Clinical signs

- Collapse.
- Inappetence/anorexia.
- Vomiting.
- Polyuria/polydipsia.
- Dehydration.
- Signs of shock (tachycardia, poor pulses).
- Tachypnoea (increased breathing rate).
- Ketones may be smelled on the breath (pear drop smell).

Diagnostic aids

- Haematology and biochemistry.
- Blood gas analysis (allows quantification of how acidic the blood is).
- Urinalysis and culture.
- Abdominal ultrasonography.
- Other tests as necessary (such as canine pancreatic lipase immunoreactivity (cPLI)) to identify concurrent disease.

Treatment

- Intravenous fluid therapy.
- Insulin therapy – generally using a short-acting insulin by intravenous or intramuscular route for initial stabilization. A longer-term protocol of subcutaneous insulin for use at home can be introduced once the patient is stable.
- Antiemetics.
- Antibiotics.
- Careful monitoring of electrolytes with supplementation if necessary. Potassium, phosphorus and magnesium may all need supplementing.

Disseminated intravascular coagulation

During disseminated intravascular coagulation (DIC), the clotting system of the body becomes overactivated. This leads to consumption of the patient's clotting factors and the development of a generalized bleeding tendency. DIC always occurs secondary to a severe underlying problem such as septic shock, pancreatitis or heat stroke. It is a serious complication but can be reversible.

Clinical signs

- Petechiation/ecchymoses.
- Excesssive bleeding from catheter or venepuncture sites.
- Haemorrhage at mucosal surfaces.
- Presence of a severe underlying disease.

Diagnosis

- Platelet count (will be low with DIC).
- Clotting times (will be prolonged with DIC).
- Other clotting parameters such as D-dimers or fibrinogen degradation products.

Treatment

- Treatment of underlying disease.
- Fluid therapy to maintain tissue blood flow.
- Fresh frozen plasma transfusions.
- Medical treatment such as with heparin may be used dependent on the stage and severity of DIC.

Gastrointestinal and abdominal emergencies

Pharyngeal or oesophageal fish hook

Dogs or, less commonly, cats may ingest fish hooks either directly or by eating fish or bait attached to them. The fish hook commonly lodges in the pharynx or proximal oesophagus but occasionally more distally. If there is still a line attached to the hook, the owners should be instructed neither to pull it, as this may cause further damage, nor to cut the line, as it may help the veterinary surgeon locate the hook.

Clinical signs

- Drooling, possibly with blood-tinged saliva.
- Dysphagia (difficulty eating).
- Facial/pharyngeal discomfort (pawing at face).
- It is possible that the animal may display no clinical signs but may simply have been observed to have eaten the hook.

Diagnostic aids

- Radiography.

Treatment

- Removal of hook, usually under general anaesthesia.

The ease with which the hook can be removed depends both on its location (e.g. hooks lodged in the pharynx are easier to remove than oesophageal ones) and the number of barbs the hook has. Hooks with multiple barbs embedded in the wall of the oesophagus may require careful manipulation to remove. Most hooks can be removed under either direct or endoscopic visualization. Occasionally surgical removal is necessary.

Oesophageal foreign body

This occurs most commonly in terrier breeds, especially West Highland White Terriers. The foreign body is most commonly a bone.

Clinical signs

- Witnessed ingestion of a foreign object (often fed to the dog by the owners).
- Regurgitation.
- Retching/coughing.
- Hypersalivation.
- Inappetence.
- Depression.
- Pain or discomfort on eating.

Diagnostic aids

- Radiography.
- Endoscopy.

Treatment

- Removal of foreign object via mouth, aided by endoscopy.
- Removal of foreign object via mouth, aided by fluoroscopy.
- Pushing foreign object into stomach and either removal by laparotomy and gastrotomy or left to be destroyed by gastric acid.
- Rarely, surgical removal of the object via thoracotomy and oesophagotomy.

Complications

- Aspiration pneumonia.
- Oesophageal rupture.
- Oesophageal stricture (may occur up to several weeks later).

Megaoesophagus

This is a condition where the oesophageal muscle cannot contract normally and loses its tone, meaning that food is no longer pushed normally from the mouth to the stomach following swallowing. It can be congenital but is more commonly an acquired condition in older dogs and less commonly cats. Its main clinical sign is regurgitation, which is the passive process whereby food that remains in the oesophagus is brought back. Although a chronic condition, these patients commonly present as an emergency either as the disease worsens or if the patient develops pneumonia.

Clinical signs

- Regurgitation (may occur for up to several hours after eating).
- Weight loss.
- Commonly a good appetite is maintained.
- Coughing/dyspnoea due to secondary aspiration pneumonia.

Diagnostic aids

- Radiography.
- Haematology, biochemistry and other blood tests to try to identify an underlying cause.

Treatment

- Treatment of underlying cause if one is identified.
- Nutrition – often necessary to feed directly into the stomach via gastrotomy tube.
- Treatment of concurrent aspiration pneumonia with antibiotics.

Vomiting

This is the active expulsion of gastric contents (as opposed to passive regurgitation). There are many causes of vomiting but they can be subdivided according to whether the origin of the problem is within the gastrointestinal (GI) tract or outside it.

Causes of vomiting

Primary gastrointestinal causes:

- GI infection (viral, bacterial, parasitic)
- Dietary indiscretion
- GI foreign body
- Intussusception (telescoping of the bowel)
- GI neoplasia.

Secondary causes:

- Pancreatitis
- Renal disease
- Liver disease
- Infection (e.g. pyometra)
- Endocrine disease (e.g. hypoadrenocorticism)
- Neurological disease
- Drug therapy.

Vomiting is commonly (but not always) accompanied by diarrhoea. Vomiting and diarrhoea vary considerably in their severity: some patients with vomiting require emergency evaluation and treatment, whereas other patients have much milder signs, where emergency treatment is not necessary. When dealing with an owner whose pet is vomiting, the following questions should be asked and can be used to make an assessment of the severity of the problem and whether the animal should be seen on an emergency basis.

- How many times has the pet vomited in the last 12 hours?
- Is there any blood in the vomit? How much?
- Is the pet still keen to eat and drink? Are they able to keep down anything they eat?
- Is the pet significantly depressed? If the pet is significantly depressed it should be seen as an emergency regardless of the answers to the other questions.
- Does the pet have any other signs of abdominal pain (e.g. vocalization, abnormal position)?
- Has the pet been witnessed to eat any toxins or drugs or any objects of a size that might have become stuck in the GI tract?
- Is the pet a known scavenger?

Diagnostic aids

- Thorough history, including vaccination status and worming history.
- Physical examination.
- Haematology and biochemistry, including in-house blood smear evaluation to assess for neutropenia (low

white blood cell count seen with severe GI infections, especially parvovirus).
- Acid–base and electrolyte analysis.
- Urinalysis.
- Faecal analysis (both for parasites and culture).
- Abdominal radiography.
- Abdominal ultrasonography.
- Serological testing of both blood and faeces for infectious disease.

Treatment

- Intravenous fluid therapy.
- Treatment of underlying cause (may be medical or surgical).
- Nil by mouth until diagnosis made.
- Antiemetic therapy unless GI obstruction suspected.
- Good nursing care – warm comfortable environment.

Diarrhoea

Diarrhoea refers to the voiding of abnormal liquid faeces. Patients with diarrhoea may present as an emergency if the diarrhoea is severe (with significant fluid loss), if there is a large amount of blood in the faeces or if it is accompanied by marked vomiting and depression. Diarrhoea is commonly divided into:

- Small-bowel – large volumes of watery faeces passed with a relatively low frequency
- Large-bowel – small volumes of semi-solid faeces passed frequently with straining. A small amount of fresh blood may be present.

When dealing with an owner whose pet has diarrhoea, the following questions should be asked and can be used to make an assessment of the severity of the problem and whether the animal should be seen on an emergency basis.

- How many times has the pet had diarrhoea in the last 24–48 hours?
- Is there any fresh blood in the diarrhoea? If so, how much?
- Is the diarrhoea black, very dark or tarry (suggestive of presence of digested blood)?
- Is the diarrhoea associated with straining?
- Is there a large or small volume of diarrhoea produced each time the animal passes something?
- Is the diarrhoea watery or semi-solid?
- Is the pet still keen to eat and drink?
- Is the pet significantly depressed? If the pet is significantly depressed it should be seen as an emergency regardless of the answers to the other questions.
- Does the pet have any other signs of abdominal pain (e.g. vocalization, abnormal position)?
- Has the pet been witnessed eating any toxins or drugs or any objects of a size that might have become stuck in the GI tract?

Small-bowel diarrhoea is more commonly an emergency than large-bowel diarrhoea, especially if melaena (digested blood presenting as black, sticky or tarry faeces) is present.

Diagnostic aids

- Thorough history, including vaccination status and worming history.
- Physical examination.

- Haematology and biochemistry, including in-house blood smear evaluation to assess for neutropenia (low white blood cell count seen with severe GI infections, especially parvovirus).
- Urinalysis.
- Faecal analysis (both for parasites and culture).
- Abdominal radiography.
- Abdominal ultrasonography.
- Serological testing of both blood and faeces for infectious disease.

Treatment

- Intravenous fluid therapy.
- Treatment of underlying cause (may be medical or surgical treatment).
- Nil by mouth until diagnosis made.
- Good nursing care – ensure perineal area does not become sore or inflamed. This may require frequent bathing and clipping of hair in this region, or a tail bandage.

Gastrointestinal obstruction

Patients with GI obstruction most often present with vomiting and sometimes diarrhoea. They also commonly show signs of both hypovolaemic shock and dehydration. The obstruction may be complete or partial. Animals with complete obstructions have more severe and rapidly progressive signs than those with partial obstructions.

Obstructions may occur secondary to:

- Foreign body ingestion
- Intussusception
- GI neoplasia
- Incarceration.

Clinical signs

- Vomiting, sometimes with blood.
- Anorexia.
- Depression.
- Abdominal pain.
- Palpable abdominal mass (classically intussusceptions are sausage shaped).
- Hypovolaemic shock.
- Dehydration.
- Weight loss – especially with partial obstructions.
- Diarrhoea/melaena (digested blood in stool), especially with partial obstructions.

Diagnostic aids

- Abdominal radiography, possibly including a barium study.
- Abdominal ultrasonography.
- Haematology and biochemistry.
- Electrolyte and blood gas analysis.
- Urinalysis.
- Faecal analysis.

Treatment

- Intravenous fluid therapy for stabilization.
- Surgical removal of the obstruction – this may require resection of a portion of the bowel.
- Endoscopic removal may be attempted for gastric foreign bodies.

Postoperative monitoring and nursing care

This is crucial for a successful outcome. Patients should initially be maintained on intravenous fluids, with gradual reintroduction of water and then food over the 12–48 hours after surgery. Breakdown (dehiscence) of the incision in the bowel can occur for several days after surgery. Postoperative monitoring should include:

- Perfusion parameters (heart rate, pulse quality, mucous membrane colour and capillary refill time)
- Urine output
- Pain score
- Any vomiting or regurgitation
- Any faeces passed
- Bodyweight
- Hydration status
- Repeat electrolytes and acid–base status.

Gastric dilatation–volvulus

Gastric dilatation–volvulus (GDV) is a condition of principally large-breed deep-chested dogs. The stomach becomes dilated with gas and then twists along its long axis. It typically causes a sudden onset of severe clinical signs.

Clinical signs

- Collapse.
- Severe hypovolaemic shock.
- Unproductive retching.
- Distended tympanic abdomen (though this can be hard to see in some of the most deep-chested dogs where the distended stomach is hidden under the ribcage).
- Tachycardia, possibly with arrhythmia.
- Pale mucous membranes with prolonged capillary refill time.
- Restlessness in early stages.
- Hypersalivation.
- Tachypnoea.

Diagnostic aids

- Abdominal radiography – right lateral view is most important.
- Haematology and biochemistry.
- Electrolyte and blood gas including lactate level.
- ECG (see Figure 19.16).

Treatment

- Intravenous fluid therapy for stabilization – this should be tailored to the clinical signs of shock the animal is showing, but large boluses of fluid via a large-bore catheter are often required.
- Gastric decompression via a stomach tube – this is not always possible and a stomach tube should never be forced in, as this may result in tearing of the oesophagus at the oesophageal gastric junction (cardia).
- Gastric decompression via percutaneous trocharization – a needle or catheter is inserted through the abdominal body wall in the area where tympany is detected, with the aim of entering the stomach and allowing gas to escape.
- Surgery – this is the definitive treatment and is typically performed as soon as the patient has been stabilized for anaesthesia with fluid therapy. Clipping and initial surgical

preparation can be carried out whilst the patient is being stabilized, and oxygen should be given for at least 5 minutes prior to induction of anaesthesia. At surgery, the stomach is derotated and then emptied (usually by passing a stomach tube following derotation). A gastropexy should then be performed. This involves anchoring the stomach in the correct position by suturing the stomach to the body wall. There is an increased risk of aspiration during surgery; consideration should be given to patient positioning and suction should be prepared.

■ Good postoperative care is essential – the monitoring is as for the patient with GI obstruction.

Pancreatitis

This is a generalized inflammation of the pancreas. In most cases, it is unknown why it happens but it may be associated with obesity, a high-fat diet and certain diseases such as hyperadrenocorticism. One of the functions of the pancreas is to make the digestive enzymes. When the pancreas becomes inflamed, these enzymes are released into the circulation and can cause severe systemic signs, including shock and death.

Clinical signs

■ Vomiting – may be severe.
■ Anorexia.
■ Collapse.
■ Tachycardia.
■ Severe abdominal pain – dogs may show the 'praying position'.
■ Dehydration.
■ Diarrhoea.

Diagnostic aids

■ Haematology and biochemistry.
■ Specific pancreatic blood tests, such as trypsinogen-like (TLI) and canine pancreatic lipase (cPLI) immunoreactivity.
■ Abdominal ultrasonography.
■ Abdominal fluid analysis (if present).
■ Abdominal radiographs.

Treatment

■ Intravenous fluid therapy.
■ Antiemetics.
■ Analgesia.
■ Nil per mouth while vomiting is severe; small amounts of low-fat food can be introduced once vomiting has been controlled.
■ Antibiotics.

Haemoabdomen

This occurs when an abdominal organ ruptures and the animal bleeds into its abdominal cavity. The spleen is the most common organ to rupture, often because there is a splenic tumour.

Clinical signs

■ Collapse.
■ Tachycardia.
■ Poor pulse quality.
■ Pale mucous membranes.
■ Abdominal distension with a fluid thrill.

Diagnostic aids

■ Haematology and biochemistry.
■ Clotting profile.
■ Abdominal ultrasonography.
■ Abdominal fluid analysis.
■ Thoracic radiographs to look for signs of metastasis (spread of cancer) to the chest.
■ Abdominal radiographs.

Treatment

■ Intravenous fluid therapy.
■ Blood transfusion.
■ Abdominal pressure wrap (see Figure 19.13).
■ Surgery to identify and remove the bleeding organ. Surgery should be performed once the patient has been stabilized with fluid therapy.

Septic peritonitis

This is a condition where a septic (infected) fluid builds up in the abdominal cavity. The infection most commonly gains entry to the abdominal cavity from a ruptured GI tract, but other sources (e.g. ruptured urogenital or biliary tract) are possible.

Clinical signs

■ Collapse.
■ Tachycardia.
■ Poor pulse quality.
■ Red mucous membranes.
■ Abdominal pain.
■ Abdominal distension.
■ Vomiting.
■ Diarrhoea.
■ Anorexia.

Diagnostic aids

■ Acid–base and electrolyte analysis.
■ Haematology and biochemistry.
■ Clotting profile.
■ Abdominal ultrasonography.
■ Abdominal fluid analysis (cytology, biochemistry and culture).
■ Abdominal radiography.
■ Urinalysis.

Treatment

■ Intravenous fluid therapy.
■ Intravenous antibiotic therapy.
■ Analgesia.
■ Exploratory surgery to lavage (flush) the abdomen and identify and treat the source of infection.

Nursing care

Postoperative nursing care is vital to a successful outcome. Parameters to be monitored should include:

■ Heart rate
■ Pulse quality
■ Mucous membrane colour
■ Blood pressure
■ Urine output
■ Pain score
■ Electrolytes and acid–base.

These parameters can be used to guide postoperative fluid and analgesia requirements.

Hepatic failure

Animals with liver disease may present as an emergency, either because they have developed acute liver failure or have chronic liver disease with acute deterioration.

Causes

- Infection (e.g. leptospirosis).
- Toxin.
- Inflammation.
- Neoplasia.
- Acute deterioration of chronic disease.

Clinical signs

- Weakness.
- Inappetence.
- Vomiting, including haematemesis.
- Neurological signs (seizures, unusual behaviour, blindness).
- Jaundiced mucous membranes.
- Increased tendency to bleed.
- If underlying chronic disease, the animal may have weight loss, polyuria/polydipsia and/or abdominal distension.

Diagnostic aids

- Haematology and biochemistry.
- Clotting profile.
- Liver function tests (bile acid stimulation tests, ammonia level).
- Abdominal ultrasonography.
- Aspirate or biopsy of the liver.
- Urinalysis.

Treatment

- Intravenous fluid therapy.
- Antibiotics.
- Glucose supplementation.
- Lactulose to treat neurological signs (hepatic encephalopathy).
- Blood or plasma transfusion.
- Treatment of primary cause.

Ocular emergencies

Ocular emergencies are relatively common. Although they are rarely life-threatening, prompt action may need to be taken to prevent loss of sight in the eye. They are also often particularly distressing to owners, as they can look very dramatic, and it is recommended that the animal is admitted to the practice as soon as possible. As even minor ocular problems have the potential to deteriorate rapidly, with the possibility of loss of vision, all animals showing a sudden onset of signs related to the eye should be seen urgently.

With all ocular emergencies the following rules can be applied:

- Assess condition of the patient – abnormalities in the major body systems should always be addressed first, no matter how severe the injury to the eye
- Assess extent of ocular injury

- Prevent self-trauma (place Elizabethan collar)
- Give analgesia
- Keep the eye moist with a false-tear solution
- Keep the patient in a quiet dimly lit environment.

Traumatic proptosis

This represents the forward displacement of the entire globe, with entrapment of the eyelids behind the equator of the globe. It is most commonly seen following trauma and in breeds with shallow orbits, such as the Pekingese.

Clinical signs

- Anteriorly displaced globe.
- Swelling around the orbit.
- Signs of other head injuries (e.g. bleeding, bruising).

Treatment

The globe should be replaced into its correct position as quickly as possible if the animal is to regain vision in that eye; however, any concurrent injuries must be considered when deciding whether immediate replacement of the globe is the correct course of action.

- Sterile saline-soaked swab over the proptosed globe to keep eye moist – the saline may be slightly cooled to help to reduce periorbital swelling.
- Prevention of self-trauma.
- Analgesia.
- Sedation/anaesthesia with replacement of globe. Following replacement, the eyelids are commonly sutured closed for a period of time.

Ocular foreign body

Clinical signs

- Foreign body visible (Figure 19.21) or may be trapped under eyelids or third eyelid.
- Blepharospasm.
- Rubbing eye or face.
- Epiphora (excess tear production).
- Chemosis (conjunctival swelling).
- Photophobia.

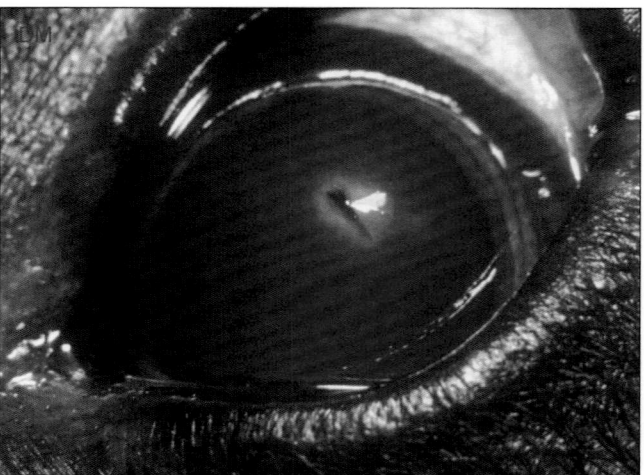

19.21 Corneal foreign body. (Courtesy of D Moore)

Treatment

- Prevention of self-trauma (Elizabethan collar).
- Topical local anaesthesia.
- Flushing eye with large volume of sterile saline.
- Sedation or anaesthesia if foreign object lodged (especially under third eyelid).
- If foreign object does not appear to have penetrated the cornea, it should be gently grasped and removed.
- If foreign object has clearly penetrated the cornea, it should be left in place and advice sought from a specialist veterinary ophthalmologist.
- Topical antibiotics.

Corneal scratch/laceration

This is where the surface of the cornea is damaged. It occurs most commonly secondary to scratches from other animals or damage from vegetation.

Clinical signs

- Ocular pain.
- Blepharospasm.
- Photophobia.
- Epiphora.
- Squinting.
- Rubbing eye or face.
- Visible disruption of the corneal surface.
- Corneal oedema (blue discoloration of cornea) (Figure 19.22).
- If the cornea is penetrated, there may be anterior uveitis (see below) or prolapse of the iris into or through the corneal wound.

Diagnostic aids

- Fluorescein stain of the eye – areas where the corneal epithelium is damaged will take up the stain.

Treatment

- Prevention of self-trauma.
- Topical local anaesthesia for analgesia and to allow a full examination.
- Topical medical treatment (antibiotics, treatment for uveitis if present).
- Deep scratches, especially if the cornea is penetrated, may require surgery and advice from a specialist veterinary ophthalmologist should be sought.

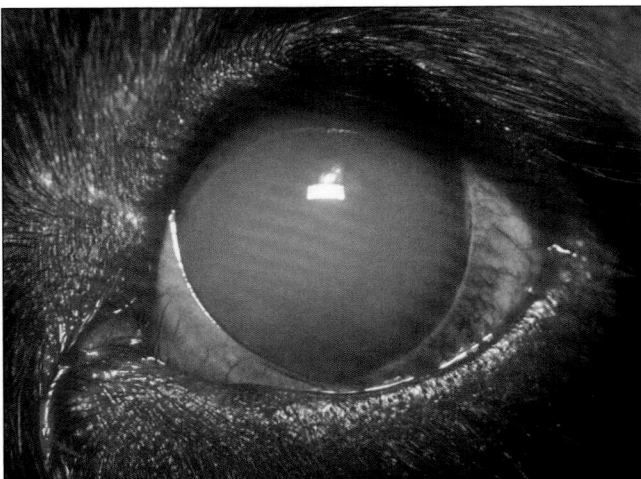

19.22 Blue discoloration of cornea indicative of corneal oedema. (Courtesy of D Moore)

Corneal ulcer

Causes

- Corneal trauma.
- Anatomical (e.g. exophthalmos, abnormal eyelashes).
- Breed-related (e.g. Boxer).
- Infectious.
- Lack of tear production.
- Chemical injury.

Clinical signs

- Ocular pain.
- Blepharospasm.
- Photophobia.
- Epiphora.
- Squinting.
- Rubbing eye or face.
- Purulent ocular discharge.
- Corneal oedema (blue discoloration of cornea) (see Figure 19.22).
- Secondary uveitis.

Diagnostic aids

- Full ophthalmological examination.
- Fluorescein staining – ulcerated areas will take up the fluorescein stain, unless the ulcer is very deep, with exposure of Descemet's membrane.

Treatment

- Prevention of self-trauma.
- Topical medical treatment (not corticosteroid).
- Treatment of underlying cause.
- Severe rapidly progressive ulcers (known as melting ulcers) may require surgical therapy.

Uveitis

This refers to inflammation of the uveal tract, which includes the iris, ciliary body and choroid layer. It may occur as a localized ocular problem or may be seen with a wide range of systemic infectious or inflammatory diseases.

Causes

- Ocular trauma.
- Infection.
- Inflammation.
- Neoplasia.
- Secondary to problems with the lens.

Clinical signs

- Ocular pain.
- Blepharospasm.
- Photophobia.
- Rubbing eye or face.
- Squinting.
- Miotic (constricted) pupil.
- Aqueous flare (cloudiness to anterior chamber).
- Secondary corneal oedema (blue discoloration of cornea) (see Figure 19.22).

Diagnostic aids

- Full ophthalmological examination.
- Careful full physical examination for signs of systemic disease.
- Haematology and biochemistry.
- Urinalysis.

Treatment

- Treatment of underlying cause.
- Analgesia (topical and/or systemic).
- Prevention of self-trauma.
- Topical anti-inflammatory.
- Topical mydriatic (agent that causes the pupil to dilate e.g. atropine)

Glaucoma

This represents an increased intraocular pressure (i.e. pressure within the eyeball). It can be very painful and if not treated quickly can lead to permanent blindness in that eye. It is an inherited condition in some breeds (e.g. Cocker Spaniel, Springer Spaniel) due to anatomical abnormalities that predispose to poor outflow of the aqueous humour. This is known as primary glaucoma. Secondary glaucoma may occur in any breed, secondary to a number of other ocular problems (e.g. lens luxation).

Clinical signs

- Often unilateral, sudden onset, severe ocular pain.
- Reduced or absent vision.
- Episcleral vascular congestion.
- Corneal oedema (blue discoloration of cornea) (see Figure 19.22).
- Dilated unresponsive pupil.
- Elevated intraocular pressure.

Diagnostic aids

- Full ophthalmological examination.
- Measurement of intraocular pressure using:
  - Indentation tonometry (Schiøtz tonometer)
  - Applanation tonometry (Tonopen).

Treatment

- Prevention of self-trauma.
- Analgesia (topical or systemic).
- Topical treatment to:
  - Reduce production of aqueous humour
  - Improve outflow of aqueous humour.
- Systemic treatment to reduce pressure within globe (e.g. mannitol).
- Surgical intervention by a specialist ophthalmologist may be necessary.
- If the eye remains non-visual but painful, enucleation can be considered.

Hyphaema

This refers to bleeding within the anterior chamber.

Causes

- Trauma.
- Coagulation disorder.
- Hypertension.
- Neoplasia.
- Inflammation.

Clinical signs

- Blood visible in anterior chamber (Figure 19.23).
- Disturbed vision.
- Secondary uveitis.

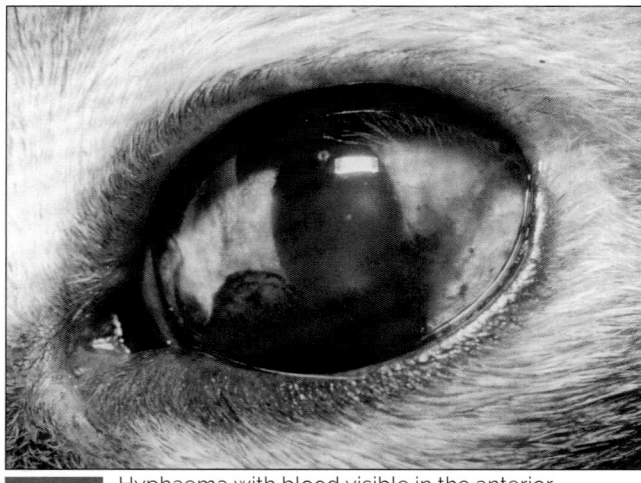

19.23 Hyphaema with blood visible in the anterior chamber. (Courtesy of D Moore)

Diagnostic aids

- Full clinical examination.
- Full ophthalmological examination.
- Haematology and biochemistry.
- Clotting profile.
- Blood pressure measurement.

Treatment

- Treatment of underlying cause.
- Treatment of uveitis symptomatically if present.

Sudden-onset blindness

Animals that suddenly become blind may appear disoriented or confused or may become depressed and withdrawn. If the eyes appear outwardly normal, owners may not immediately realize their pet has become blind.

Causes

- Chorioretinitis (inflammation of the choroid and retina).
- Retinal detachment secondary to:
  - Hypertension (especially in cats)
  - Trauma.
- Retinal degeneration (e.g. sudden acquired retinal degeneration syndrome (SARDS) in dogs).
- Optic neuritis (inflammation of the optic nerve).
- Intracranial disease (e.g. pituitary tumour).
- Glaucoma (although eye is usually painful).

Clinical signs

- Blindness.
- Bumping into things, especially in a new environment.
- Depression and unwillingness to move (especially cats).
- Inappetence/anorexia.
- Dilated non-responsive pupils.

Diagnostic aids

- Full ophthalmological examination.
- Full neurological examination.
- Blood pressure measurement (especially cats).
- Haematology and biochemistry.
- Urinalysis.

Treatment

- Treatment of underlying cause.

The animal may be very anxious, especially in a strange environment. To reduce its anxiety:

- Always use the animal's name whenever handling it
- Maintain a familiar smell if possible
- Reassure the animal verbally with a calm tone of voice as much as possible
- Move slowly and gently when handling the animal.

Nasal emergencies

Epistaxis

This refers to bleeding from the nostrils. It may be bilateral or unilateral. Although the volume of blood produced may seem to be large, it is rare for dogs or cats to become significantly anaemic or hypovolaemic following nasal bleeding. In small pets, however, even what appears to be a small blood loss may be more significant.

Causes

- Trauma.
- Nasal tumour.
- Infection, especially aspergillosis.
- Nasal foreign body.
- Coagulation disorder.
- Hypertension.

Clinical signs

- Nasal bleeding – always note if it is unilateral or bilateral.
- Stertorous breathing.
- Open-mouth breathing.
- Sneezing.
- Melaena (if blood is being swallowed).

Diagnostic aids

- Haematology and biochemistry.
- Clotting profile.
- Blood pressure.
- Nasal radiography.
- Nasal endoscopy plus biopsy.

Treatment

- Maintain a calm environment.
- Sedation.
- Cold compress externally.
- Topical application of adrenaline (either squirted into nostril or soaked on to a swab and placed in nostril).
- Absorbent dressing within nostril (e.g. tampon). It is vital to keep a record of the number of swabs/tampons used so it can be ensured that all are retrieved.
- Monitor for signs of hypovolaemia, which may occur if epistaxis is severe and/or prolonged. Treat with fluid therapy if it occurs.
- Treat underlying disease.

Nasal foreign body

The commonest nasal foreign bodies are grass seeds, blades of grass and small pieces of wood.

Clinical signs

- Sneezing, may be paroxysmal.
- Nasal discharge, usually unilateral, occasionally blood tinged.
- Rubbing or pawing at nose.

Treatment

Removal of foreign body by:

- Endoscopy
- Flushing.

Nasal foreign bodies can be particularly hard to identify. They are rarely seen on radiographs. Endoscopy may be useful but the size of the endoscope often precludes a thorough and complete search of the entire nasal chamber, especially in small patients. If a foreign body cannot be seen and retrieved under direct visualization, nasal flushing should be performed.

If foreign material is not found, it is possible that it had already been sneezed out before the animal reached the practice. However, it is also possible that it may remain *in situ*. This is unlikely to be dangerous for the animal, but a chronic nasal discharge may develop if any foreign material has been left behind. Owners should be warned of this possibility.

Nasal flush procedure

1. Ensure that a cuffed endotracheal tube is in place, with cuff inflated.
2. Pack the pharynx with swabs – count swabs and record. It is vital to double check that all swabs are removed before the animal is recovered from anaesthesia.
3. Place the animal in sternal recumbency with the rostral end of nose tipped downward.
4. Fill 60 ml syringe with saline (20 ml for a cat).
5. Place the nozzle of syringe up nostril that is most likely to be affected and squeeze both nostrils shut around it.
6. Empty the syringe with moderate force into nostril.
7. Hold an empty bowl beneath the nostril to catch any fluid.
8. Repeat multiple times and with both nostrils (recommend using at least 1 litre saline for a 20 kg dog).
9. Ensure that all swabs are retrieved from the pharynx before the patient is recovered from anaesthesia – the foreign material may sometimes be found on these swabs when they are removed.

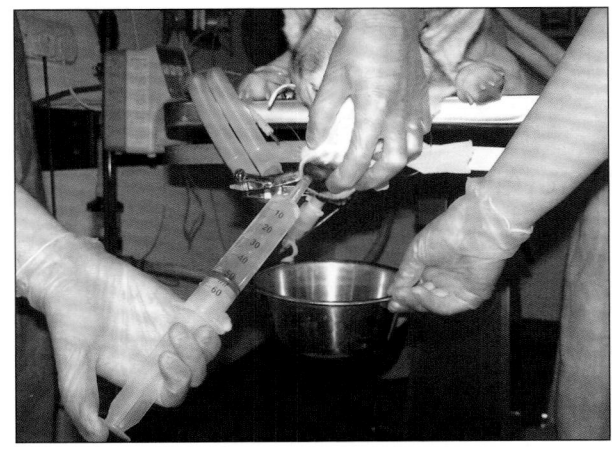

Aural emergencies

Although emergencies involving the ear are very rarely life-threatening, they can cause some distress to both the patient and the owner.

Aural foreign body

Clinical signs

- Head shaking.
- Rubbing or scratching ear.
- Pain on touching of head or aural region.
- Visualization of foreign body on auroscopic examination.

Treatment

- Removal of foreign body – invariably requires sedation.

Otitis externa and media

This is an infection of the external ear canal (otitis externa) or middle ear (otitis media).

Clinical signs

- Head shaking.
- Rubbing of head or scratching of ear.
- Self-trauma of aural region
- Vestibular signs (with otitis media – see 'Neurological emergencies' above).
- Aural discharge – may be waxy or foul smelling.
- Auroscopic examination confirms aural inflammation.

Treatment

- Emergency treatment rarely necessary unless neurological signs develop.
- Antibiotics (topical and systemic).
- Analgesia.
- Aural flush under anaesthesia.

Aural haematoma

This is a haematoma of the pinna. Although these swellings are never life-threatening, patients may present as an emergency as they can develop quite rapidly and be quite large.

Causes

- Head shaking.
- Self-trauma.

Clinical signs

- Soft non-painful swelling of the pinna.
- Scratching of the ear.
- History of head shaking or aural trauma.

Treatment

- Drainage of the haematoma.
- Bandaging of the ear following drainage has been recommended but is very difficult to achieve.
- Injection of corticosteroids following drainage (sometimes used but is discouraged as it delays healing).
- Surgical techniques to maintain pressure across pinna whilst healing occurs.
- Reassurance to owners that it is not a life-threatening problem.

Environmental emergencies

Hyperthermia (heatstroke)

The normal body temperature of both the dog and cat is approximately 38.5°C. Dogs and cats are homeotherms and maintain this body temperature unless they suffer from hyperthermia or pyrexia. If a mammal is placed in a hot environment it will activate cooling mechanisms (e.g. panting, drinking cold water, moving to a cooler place, sweating in some species) that act to keep the body temperature close to this normal value. If these cooling mechanisms fail, then the animal's body temperature increases and can reach dangerously high levels (>41°C) and cause heatstroke.

Heatstroke must be distinguished from the other major cause of an elevated body temperature, which is pyrexia. In pyrexia, the animal's elevated body temperature is an appropriate response to an infection or inflammatory process and is actually a useful part of the animal's response to their underlying disease.

- In hyperthermia, cooling the animal is a vitally important part of treatment.
- In pyrexia, cooling the animal can place the patient under additional physiological stress.

Whenever an increased body temperature is found on examination, it must be decided whether it is elevated due to hyperthermia (in which case external cooling measures are appropriate) or pyrexia (in which case external cooling measures are inappropriate). Heatstroke is very rare in cats.

Causes

- Overexposure to a hot environment that the animal cannot remove itself from (e.g. locked in a car on a hot day, tied up outside in direct sunlight).
- Excessive exercise.
- Seizures (uncontrollable excessive muscle activity).
- Upper airway obstruction (inability to hyperventilate and thus loss of one of the dog's major cooling mechanisms).

Clinical signs

- Restlessness.
- Panting (or attempts to pant).
- Tachypnoea.
- Tachycardia.
- Poor pulse quality.
- Red mucous membranes.
- Markedly elevated body temperature (>41°C).
- Vomiting and diarrhoea.
- Ataxia.
- Collapse, coma, death.

Treatment

- Rapid-rate intravenous fluid therapy with fluids either at room temperature or slightly chilled.
- Active external cooling:
  - Wet animal's haircoat (running water will cool more efficiently than still water). Placing wet towels over the patient is not recommended due to the potential to increase the temperature by trapping warm air against the body

- • Clip animal's haircoat
- • Fan.
- ■ Cold-water enema.
- ■ Peritoneal lavage with cooled (not cold) fluids.

Aggressive cooling measures should be discontinued when the patient's body temperature reaches 40.5°C to avoid overcooling and the development of hypothermia. Frequent and regular (every 10 minutes) monitoring of body temperature should then be performed in conjunction with less aggressive cooling measures until body temperature reaches 39.5°C.

A number of very serious complications can result from heatstroke, especially if the rise in body temperature has been prolonged. Once cooled, animals should be closely monitored for the development of:

- ■ Disseminated intravascular coagulation
- ■ Hypoglycaemia
- ■ 'Shock gut' – with sloughing of the GI tract mucosa and development of haemorrhagic vomiting and diarrhoea
- ■ Acute kidney injury
- ■ Cardiac dysrhythmias
- ■ Pulmonary dysfunction.

If these develop, they should be treated symptomatically. With pyrexia, the underlying infection or inflammation should be identified and treated. Non-steroidal anti-inflammatory drugs may be used to reduce the fever whilst this investigation and treatment is ongoing.

Hypothermia

This refers to a subnormal body temperature in mammals. Severe hypothermia is considered to be a body temperature below 28°C and is rare. Mild to moderate hypothermia is common. Smaller animals are more prone to becoming hypothermic, due to their high ratio of surface area to weight. Younger animals are also prone to hypothermia, as they are not yet able to generate body heat in the same way as adults.

Causes

- ■ Severe disease/shock – especially common in cats.
- ■ Sedation/anaesthesia.
- ■ Prolonged exposure to low environmental temperatures.

Clinical signs

- ■ Shivering.
- ■ Depression.
- ■ Slow breathing rate.
- ■ Cardiac arrhythmias.
- ■ Coma.
- ■ Death.

Treatment

- ■ Warmed intravenous fluids.
- ■ Rewarming should only start once cardiovascular support (intravenous fluids) has been initiated.
- ■ Passive rewarming – maintain warm ambient environment.
- ■ Surface rewarming with circulating warm water or air blankets (Figure 19.24).
- ■ If temperature less than 30°C, consider active core rewarming with warm peritoneal dialysis.

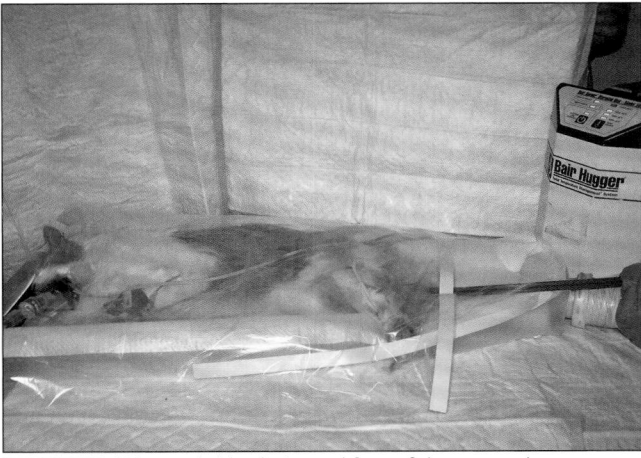

19.24 Warm-air blanket used for safely rewarming patients.

- ■ Electric heating pads and heating lamps not recommended, due to potential for causing burns.
- ■ Care should be taken not to warm the patient too rapidly, especially if they are also in shock. Rapid rewarming can worsen the signs of shock.

Burns

Burns result when intense heat (or, rarely, cold) damages the skin and subcutaneous tissues. Serum leaking from the damaged areas may lead to blister formation. Most burns seen in veterinary patients are iatrogenic (i.e. caused by veterinary intervention) – notably heat pads.

Burns can be classified by:

- ■ Cause (Figure 19.25)
- ■ Depth
  - • Superficial – affecting only outermost layer of skin
  - • Partial thickness – affecting slightly deeper layers of skin; blistering common
  - • Full thickness – affecting all layers of skin
- ■ Percentage of body surface affected.

Type of burn	Potential causes
Dry	Hot objects, flames, friction, heat pads
Scald	Hot liquid, steam
Cold	Very cold objects, especially metals
Electrical	Chewing on electric cables
Radiation	Sun
Chemical	Caustic soda, paint stripper

19.25 Burns and potential causes.

Clinical signs

- ■ Red, moist skin.
- ■ Charred, leathery skin (seen with full-thickness burns).
- ■ Pain (full-thickness burns are less painful, as nerve endings are destroyed).
- ■ Heat.
- ■ Signs of shock.

Treatment

- ■ Removing of the source of the problem, or moving the patient away from the source (taking care there is no risk to humans).

- Dousing the area in cold water for a minimum of 10 minutes (care should be taken not to overcool the patient and cause hypothermia).
- Very gently clipping the fur over a large area around the burn (burns can often be much larger than first thought).
- Covering the area, once cooled, with sterile non-adherent dressing or cling film.
- Analgesia.
- Elizabethan collar to prevent further self-trauma.
- Intravenous fluid therapy to treat concurrent shock.

WARNING

With electrical burns or electrocution, ensure that the electrical source is turned off before approaching patient. Do not put yourself at risk of being electrocuted – remember that both metal and water are good conductors of electricity

---

Smoke inhalation

Animals are occasionally seen for evaluation and treatment of smoke inhalation after being trapped in fires.

Clinical signs

- Cough.
- Dyspnoea.
- Nasal discharge.
- Singed whiskers/evidence of burns.
- Brick-red mucous membranes if carbon monoxide has been inhaled.
- Neurological signs – may occur up to several days after smoke inhalation.

Diagnostic aids

- Arterial blood gas analysis.
- Co-oximetry.
- Thoracic radiographs.
- Pulse oximetry less useful.

Treatment

- Oxygen therapy.
- Supportive care.

Toxicological emergencies

A large number of substances may poison animals. Owners of animals with an acute onset of clinical signs often query whether their animal could have been poisoned. Although this may occur, malicious poisoning is rare.

Due to the large number of potential toxins and the wide variety of clinical signs exhibited, poisoning is a differential diagnosis for many emergency patients.

All substances have the potential to be toxic if given in the wrong amount or at the wrong time. Figure 19.26 summarizes the types of toxins that may be encountered. Toxins are most commonly ingested but may also be inhaled (e.g. carbon monoxide) or absorbed through the skin (e.g. permethrin toxicity in cats).

Type of toxin	Examples
Veterinary prescription drugs	Insulin, NSAIDs, phenobarbital
Human prescription drugs	NSAIDs, human chemotherapy drugs, warfarin, human heart or asthma medication
Human recreational drugs	Cannabis, MDMA (ecstasy), cocaine
Human foodstuffs	Chocolate, onions, raisins, xylitol, mouldy food stuffs e.g. bread
Household chemicals	Bleach, oven cleaner, antifreeze, paint
Garden chemicals	Herbicides, pesticides, molluscicides, rodenticides
Plants	*Lilium* spp. including Tiger, Easter and Stargazer lilies, foxglove

19.26 Categories of common toxicities, with examples. NSAIDs = non-steroidal anti-inflammatory drugs.

History taking for the suspected poisoned patient

Poisoning is more likely to be seen in certain groups of patients:

- Young dogs (due to their tendency to eat indiscriminately)
- Cats (many chemicals and drugs are not adequately detoxified by the feline liver)
- Animals that are free-ranging on farmland or wasteland where chemicals are stored or used.

Sensitive questioning is required as some owners may not wish to reveal what substances their pet has had access to or may not even know that a substance was toxic to their pet. If poisoning is suspected, the following questions should be asked.

Questions for suspected poisonings

- Is the pet on any medication? If so, when did it receive its last dose? How much did it receive?
- Has the pet been given any human medications? If so, what and how much?
- Has the pet had access to any human medications? If so, what?
- Has the pet eaten any human foodstuffs recently? If so, what?
- What chemical products are kept in the home? Garage? Garden? Is there any way the pet could have had access to them?
- Does the pet have access to any farmland, parkland or industrial land? Can it be checked whether any chemicals are stored or used regularly there?
- Has the pet had any access to illegal substances? (Reassure the owner that this information is given in confidence)
- Has there been any building work or decorating at home with any unusual substances left around?
- Has the pet eaten anything unusual recently?
- Has there been anything on the pet's coat recently that it may have ingested while grooming?
- Have any flea products been administered to the pet or any other pets in the household?
- Are there any flowers in the house? If so, do they include lilies?

If an owner has witnessed a pet eating a potential toxin, they should be asked to bring as much information as possible about the toxin to the practice. This could include any packaging and an idea of how much of the substance might have been ingested. Further information on toxic doses and treatment options can be accessed in a number of ways, including online. In the UK, there is also a 24-hour poisons helpline (Veterinary Poisons Information Service or VPIS) that can be accessed by practices that subscribe to the service and also directly by clients. Some drugs used to treat toxicities are not stocked by most practices but may be available in an emergency through the VPIS/Vets NowTox Box initiative.

Clinical signs

Toxicities can lead to a huge variety of different clinical presentations, but common clinical signs of poisoning include:

- Gastrointestinal signs
- Profuse salivation
- Vomiting
- Diarrhoea
- Neurological signs
- Behavioural change
- Ataxia
- Seizures
- Collapse and coma
- Bleeding
- Unconsciousness and death.

The clinical signs and suggested treatments for some of the more common toxicities seen in the UK are summarized in Figure 19.27.

Toxin	Toxic dose (if known)	Principal clinical signs	Suggested treatment
Paracetamol	Cats 10 mg/kg. Dogs from 50 mg/kg but signs more commonly seen from 100 mg/kg	Cyanosis (muddy mucous membranes), respiratory distress, facial swelling (cat), liver failure (especially dog)	Induction of emesis. N-acetylcysteine orally or i.v. Ascorbic acid orally. Cimetidine i.v.
Ibuprofen	Dogs: GI signs from 25 mg/kg. Renal signs >175 mg/kg. CNS signs >400 mg/kg. Cats considered to be at least twice as sensitive	Gastric ulceration, vomiting, renal failure	Induction of emesis. Activated charcoal. Intravenous fluid therapy. Gastroprotectant drugs (e.g. H_2-blockers, omeprazole)
Anticoagulant rodenticides	Variable, depending on product	Haemorrhage – commonly starts 5–7 days following ingestion of toxin	Induction of emesis. Activated charcoal. Vitamin K (s.c. or orally). Whole blood or plasma transfusion
Metaldehyde (slug bait)	Median lethal dose (LD_{50}): Dog 100–300 mg/kg. Cat 207 mg/kg. Treatment recommended at 10 mg/kg	Severe seizures, depression, vomiting and diarrhoea, hyperthermia, metabolic acidosis	Gastric lavage. Activated charcoal. Control seizures. Cool
Xylitol	Hypoglycaemia from 0.05–0.1 g/kg. Acute hepatic necrosis from 0.25 g/kg	Collapse due to hypoglycaemia; may progress to liver failure with vomiting and icterus	Induction of emesis if patient is neurologically appropriate. Intravenous glucose for hypoglycaemia. Supportive care and hepatoprotectants for acute hepatic necrosis
Organophosphates/ carbamate insecticides	Variable, depending on product	Salivation, lacrimation, urination, vomiting and diarrhoea, muscle tetany (twitching), depression	Activated charcoal. Prevent further grooming. Bathe (if topical exposure). Atropine. Pralidoxime (2-PAM)
Ethylene glycol (antifreeze)	Cat 1.4 ml/kg. Dog 4.4 ml/kg	Vomiting, depression, ataxia, dehydration, oliguric renal failure	Induction of emesis. Intravenous fluid therapy. Administration of ethanol (alcohol). 4-methylpyrazole (specific antidote for use in dogs)
Theobromine (chocolate)	Dog 250–500 mg/kg (NB 64 g (2.25 oz) cooking chocolate or 560 g (20 oz) of milk chocolate may be toxic in a 10 kg dog)	Restlessness, panting, vomiting, tachycardia, cardiac arrhythmias	Induction of emesis. Activated charcoal. Arrhythmia treatment
Paraquat (weedkiller)	LD_{50} 25–50 mg/kg	Vomiting, renal and hepatic signs, dyspnoea (pulmonary fibrosis)	No specific treatment. Supportive care
Lilium spp. and *Hemerocallis* including Tiger, Easter and Stargazer lilies	Unknown – toxic to cats	Acute kidney injury	Supportive care
Permethrin (found in some over-the-counter flea treatments)	Toxic to cats – even small amounts topically can cause clinical signs	Twitching, muscular tremors, seizures	Wash area with warm water and detergent. Consider intralipid therapy. Heavy sedation/anaesthesia to control seizures may be required. Supportive care

19.27 Toxic dose, clinical signs and suggested treatment for some of the commoner toxicities seen in small animals in the UK.

Diagnostic aids

- Haematology and biochemistry.
- Urinalysis (especially sediment examination).
- Clotting profile (for suspected rodenticide).
- Any vomit, faeces and urine produced should be kept and frozen in case it is required for future toxicological investigation.

Stabilization and treatment

The key aims in initial stabilization of any poisoned patient are to:

- Identify the poison, the amount ingested and the time of ingestion as accurately as possible
- Prevent further absorption of the poison
- Treat any signs that develop symptomatically
- Administer any antidote or specific treatment (under the direction of a veterinary surgeon).

Preventing further absorption

Emetics

If an owner suspects that their animal has been poisoned, they should be asked to bring it to the practice immediately so that vomiting can be induced in a safe environment. Some owners may wish to try and induce vomiting at home but this is not recommended. Vomiting can be induced using a number of different emetics (Figure 19.28) under the direction of a veterinary surgeon.

Agent	Species	Dose	Route
Apomorphine	Dog	0.2 mg/kg is licensed dose in UK although 0.04–0.08 mg/kg may be effective	In conjunctival sac, s.c., i.m. or i.v.
Xylazine	Cat	1.1 mg/kg	i.m.
Washing soda crystals	Dog	1 crystal in small dog; 2 crystals in medium to large dog	Oral

19.28 Recommended compounds for induction of emesis.

Contraindications to emetics

Situations where vomiting should not be induced include:

- Where the toxin is a caustic or acidic substance or a volatile petroleum product that could cause further damage to tissues when it is vomited
- Where the patient is depressed or seizuring when there is a high risk of aspiration
- In species unable to vomit (e.g. rat).

When the administration of an emetic is contraindicated, gastric lavage may be employed. The animal is anaesthetized and the airway protected with a cuffed endotracheal tube.

Activated charcoal

Activated charcoal is administered in many patients following induction of emesis, as it adsorbs many toxins within the gastrointestinal tract and prevents further absorption of any remaining toxin. Some dogs will willingly eat activated charcoal mixed with food; in other patients the activated charcoal may have to be delivered by stomach tube. With some toxins, it is recommended that a dose of activated charcoal is repeated every 6 hours for 2–3 days.

Intravenous lipid emulsion therapy

Intravenous lipid emulsion (ILE) therapy is increasingly being used as a treatment option in toxicity cases. It is used for toxins that are lipophilic or cardiotoxic, and has most commonly been reported to be effective in baclofen, permethrin and ivermectin toxicities; however, it has also been used to treat other drug overdoses.

The exact mechanism of action is uncertain and there are two main theories:

- Lipid sink – it is thought that a lipid compartment is formed within the vascular space that acts as a 'sink' into which the lipophilic compound is drawn
- Energy source – with compounds that are cardiotoxic, it is thought that lipids provide an energy source for myocardial cells, reducing the toxic effects.

Topical toxins

In patients where the toxin is on the skin (e.g. flea products, paint, creosote), the following steps should be followed:

- Inform the veterinary surgeon (drug treatments may be available for the toxicity seen with some flea products)
- Fit the patient with an Elizabethan collar to prevent any grooming and possible ingestion of the toxin
- Treat any systemic signs symptomatically
- Wear gloves
- Remove the contamination with a combination of grooming, clipping and bathing. Use warm water for bathing, as water that is either too hot or cold can increase absorption of some toxins, such as permethrin. Rinse the patient with copious amounts of warmed water. Specialist cleansers such as Swarfega® are required for the removal of oily compounds such as creosote.

Symptomatic treatment

Most patients are treated symptomatically. The patient's cardiovascular, respiratory and neurological status and body temperature should be carefully monitored. Key treatments include:

- Intravenous fluid therapy to maintain intravascular volume and prevent dehydration
- Maintenance of normal body temperature
- Sedative or anti-seizure medication if neurological signs present.

Specific treatment

Specific treatments (antidotes) are available for only a small number of toxins. Some examples are given in Figure 19.27. It is only recommended that they are used if it is known that the toxin has been ingested. Antidotes may be expensive and may not be easily available in veterinary general practice.

Adder bites

The European Adder (*Viperis berus*) is the only native venomous snake present within the UK. Depending on geographical location, adder bites are not uncommon in dogs, especially in the warmer summer weather. Most bites occur on the limbs or muzzle. The incident is rarely witnessed by the owners as adders are very shy. The bites are rarely fatal.

Clinical signs

- Rapid swelling of bitten area.
- Fang marks may be present but are often difficult to identify.
- Depression.
- Rarely, distributive (anaphylactic) shock may occur.

Treatment

- Wound management – the adder bite should be treated as any other puncture wound.
- Fluid therapy if signs of shock are present.
- Medical treatment such as antihistamines.
- Cage rest.
- Antivenom if available.
- Techniques such as tourniquets, cutting the wound or attempting to suck the venom out are not recommended.

Insect stings (including bee and wasp)

Insect stings are a relatively common emergency. Although not life-threatening, they can be intensely irritating to the pet and distressing for the owner. They occur most commonly on the limbs or in the oral region. Rarely, if an animal is stung deep within the oropharynx, the associated swelling causes a degree of respiratory tract obstruction that may require emergency intervention.

Clinical signs

- Swelling and redness of bitten area.
- Pain.
- Pawing at mouth or chewing at limb.
- Development of distributive (anaphylactic) shock:
  - Tachycardia
  - Collapse
  - Dyspnoea
  - Vomiting
  - Seizures.

Treatment

- Local application of ice to reduce swelling.
- Antihistamines.
- Corticosteroids.
- Intravenous fluid therapy if signs of shock are present.

Toad poisoning

Toad poisoning that may be fatal occurs in the southern USA. In the UK, dogs will occasionally pick up and chew toads but, whilst this may result in local oral irritation and hypersalivation, it is not a life-threatening toxicity and is self-limiting. If the patient will allow, the mouth may be flushed with saline to speed resolution of signs.

Traumatic emergencies
Haemorrhage

Haemorrhage is defined as a loss of blood from the vessels. If haemorrhage is severe it leads to hypovolaemic shock and death. It is difficult to judge the severity of the haemorrhage simply from observing the amount of blood lost. The severity of the situation is best assessed by examining the animal's cardiovascular system parameters and assessing the patient for signs of shock. The principles of assessment and management of haemorrhage can be applied to all species.

Haemorrhage may be classified both by its location and by the type of vessel damaged:

- External haemorrhage occurs from wounds and is easily visible
- Internal haemorrhage may not be immediately obvious. Internal haemorrhage can occur in the thoracic or abdominal cavities, the gastrointestinal or urinary tract or in the muscle around a fracture site. Internal haemorrhage may be seen with:
  - Trauma
  - Clotting problems
  - Abnormalities of the internal organs, especially tumours.

Haemorrhage may occur from arteries, veins and/or capillaries:

- Arterial bleeding consists of bright red blood that spurts from the wound. It requires prompt recognition and urgent action to prevent significant blood loss. Haemorrhage from a major artery is seen uncommonly but can result in rapid blood loss and death
- Venous and capillary bleeding both consist of darker red blood that oozes rather than spurts from the wound. Differentiating between venous and capillary bleeding is often not possible and is rarely a clinically useful distinction.

In practice, most haemorrhage is a mixture of bleeding from different types of vessels. As the volume of blood lost can rarely be measured accurately, it is vital to assess the animal's perfusion parameters regularly. This gives an indication of the volume and rate of blood loss by the effect that it is having on the cardiovascular system (presence and severity of hypovolaemic shock). It also guides treatment (fluid therapy, see Chapter 20). Another useful assessment is the serial measurement of packed cell volume (PCV) and total solids/total protein.

Clinical signs

- Visible external blood loss.
- Bruising.
- Swelling of abdomen (if haemorrhage is into peritoneal cavity).
- Dyspnoea (if haemorrhage is into or around lungs).
- Melaena/haematemesis (if haemorrhage is into GI tract).
- Signs of shock dependent on severity of haemorrhage.

Treatment

- Control of haemorrhage.
- Intravenous fluids.
- Blood transfusion.

Control of haemorrhage

Although external arterial haemorrhage is uncommon, prompt action is required when it is seen. The following methods may be used to control arterial haemorrhage:

- **Direct digital pressure** – ensure gloves are worn and apply pressure for at least 5 minutes
- **Artery forceps (haemostats)** – if the bleeding vessel can be seen it may be possible to clamp it directly with artery forceps
- **Pressure points** – firm pressure can be applied directly over an artery. With enough pressure, flow through the artery will temporarily stop and bleeding distal to this point will be reduced. Three potential pressure points are described although they are used rarely:
  - Brachial artery on medial aspect of proximal humerus
  - Femoral artery on medial aspect of femur
  - Coccygeal artery on ventral aspect of tail
- **Tourniquets** – with severe arterial haemorrhage in a limb it may be necessary to apply a tourniquet temporarily while the bleeding artery is located and ligated by the veterinary surgeon. Tourniquets can be applied anywhere on the limb proximal to the site of bleeding. Patients with tourniquets must be continually monitored and the tourniquet removed as soon as possible. If left in place, there is a risk the limb may suffer significant compromise. A Penrose drain may be used as a tourniquet if a custom-made one is not available.

Venous and capillary bleeding is less likely to be imminently life-threatening; however, if severe, the following measures may be used to control the haemorrhage:

- **Pressure dressing** – apply direct pressure over the bleeding area using an absorbent pad and cohesive bandage
- **Abdominal pressure wrap** – if the patient is bleeding into the peritoneal cavity, an abdominal pressure wrap ('belly wrap') can be placed (see Figure 19.13). The increase in intra-abdominal pressure can aid haemostasis.

Wounds

Wounds are common emergencies. Most wounds are minor and do not put the animal at significant risk. However, some wounds can be life-threatening, especially if they are associated with significant blood loss or if they occur to the chest or abdomen and cause significant damage to underlying structures. The seriousness of a wound can be difficult to judge from its external appearance. An assessment of the animal's cardiovascular and respiratory systems gives a better indication of how life-threatening a wound is. Wounds can be described as shown in Figure 19.29 (see also Chapter 23).

Clinical signs

- Visible disruption of skin.
- Pain.
- Swelling.
- Haemorrhage.
- Shock.

Treatment

- Always treat shock or any other major body system condition first.
- Cover wound with sterile dressing to prevent further contamination whilst patient is being stabilized.
- Control haemorrhage.
- Analgesia.
- Once patient is stable:
  - Clip wide area around wound (especially bite wounds)
  - Remove any contaminating material
  - Flush wound with copious amounts of warmed fluids; for large heavily contaminated wounds, tap water can be safely used as the initial flush fluid to remove gross contamination
  - Wounds should be irrigated with sterile saline or lactated Ringer's solution at a pressure of 8–12 psi; this can be achieved using a 20–30 ml syringe with a 20–21 G needle
  - Dress or suture wound (depending on nature of wound).
- Antibiosis.

Classification	Description	Notes
Incised	Clean cut caused by sharp object (e.g. glass, scalpel blade)	Bleeding may be profuse, especially if wound is large or deep
Lacerated	Wound causing tearing of tissue and uneven edges (e.g. barbed wire)	Bleeding likely to be less severe than with incised wound but more likely to be contaminated
Abrasion (graze)	Superficial wound where full skin thickness is not penetrated	Embedded dirt or foreign bodies may be present
Contusion (bruise)	Blunt blow that has ruptured capillaries below surface	May be associated with deeper injuries (e.g. fracture)
Puncture	Small external wound but often associated with significant deeper damage	Often caused by dog or cat bites
Gunshot	Nature of wound depends on type of gun	Entry wound may be small but associated with possible significant internal damage

19.29 Wound classifications.

If any large foreign bodies are present in the wound, or if there is a chance the wound penetrates the thoracic or abdominal cavity, the patient will require anaesthesia to explore the wound safely and so that all possible complications can be dealt with if they arise. Bite wounds also require surgical exploration with extensive flushing. Even if a bite wound looks small, the tooth may have caused minimal skin damage but surprisingly extensive damage to underlying tissues. There will also have been inoculation of bacteria from the attacking animal's mouth into the deeper tissues with a high risk of infection if extensive flushing is not performed. The animal should be stabilized before surgical exploration.

Fractures

A fracture occurs when there is a break in the continuity of the bone. It most often occurs after trauma, but pathological fractures may be seen. Pathological fractures are fractures that occur with minimal trauma, due to an underlying weakness in the bone. They are most often seen with bone tumours and metabolic bone disease.

For classification of fractures, fracture healing and fracture management see Chapter 23.

Clinical signs

- Lameness (usually non-weight-bearing).
- Swelling.
- Pain.
- Bruising over fracture site.
- Wound (if open fracture).
- Abnormal orientation to limb.
- Crepitus.

Diagnostic aids

Radiographs are necessary to classify the fracture and decide on a definitive treatment plan. It is rarely necessary to take radiographs on an emergency basis; rather the patient should be stabilized and the radiographs taken under the direction of the veterinary surgeon who will be performing the fracture repair.

Treatment

Fractures most commonly occur following trauma but are rarely life-threatening. Concurrent injuries to the patient affecting the major body systems should always be addressed before specific treatment for the fracture is considered.

As the pain caused by the fracture is related to movement of the broken ends of the bone, the emergency management includes:

- Analgesia
- Immobilization of fracture site
  - Cage rest
  - Dressing – this should be applied as soon as possible to limit pain and further damage. The dressing must include the joint both above and below the fracture site. If it is not possible to place this dressing with the animal conscious or lightly sedated, strict cage rest should be employed until the patient can be anaesthetized to allow safe placement of the dressing or fracture repair. Further information on dressings can be found in Chapters 15 and 23

- Preventing further patient interference with fracture site
- Ensuring patient comfort
  - If limited mobility, consider placement of a urinary catheter.

Luxations

A luxation or dislocation occurs when the normal anatomy of a joint is disrupted so that the articular surfaces are no longer aligned normally. They generally occur secondary to trauma. Any joint can be affected but luxations of the hip, elbow, carpus and tarsus are most commonly seen.

For classification of luxations, treatment and complications, see Chapter 23.

Clinical signs

- Pain.
- Swelling of joint.
- Lameness.
- Abnormal angulation of the limb.

Treatment

- Provide analgesia.
- Limit patient movement.
- Do not attempt to reduce with patient conscious.
- Inform the veterinary surgeon as soon as possible. Patients usually require general anaesthesia for reduction of the luxation, but reduction may be easier if the procedure is attempted soon after the injury.

References and further reading

Aldridge P and O'Dwyer L (2013) *Practical Emergency and Critical Care Veterinary Nursing*, Wiley-Blackwell, Oxford

Battaglia AM and Steele AM (2016) *Small Animal Emergency and Critical Care for Veterinary Technicians, 3rd edn*. WB Saunders, Philadelphia

BSAVA/VPIS (2012) *Guide to Common Canine and Feline Poisons*. BSAVA Publications, Gloucester

Epstein ME, Rodan I, Griffenhagen G *et al*. (2015) AAHA/AAFP Pain Management Guidelines for Dogs and Cats. *Journal of Feline Medicine and Surgery* **17(3)**, 251–272

Hackett TB and Mazzaferro EM (2012) *Veterinary Emergency and Critical Care Procedures, 2nd edn*. Wiley-Blackwell, Ames, Iowa

King L and Boag A (2018) *BSAVA Manual of Canine and Feline Emergency and Critical Care, 3rd edn*. BSAVA Publications, Gloucester

Macintire DK, Drobatz KJ, Haskins SC and Saxon WD (2012) *Manual of Small Animal Emergency and Critical Care Medicine, 2nd edn*. Wiley-Blackwell, Ames, Iowa

Peterson ME and Talcott PA (2012) *Small Animal Toxicology 3rd edn*. WB Saunders, Philadelphia

Silverstein D and Hopper K (2014) *Small Animal Critical Care, 2nd edn*, Saunders, Philadelphia

Useful websites

BSAVA Poisons Database:
Available for BSAVA members at www.bsava.com

Colorado State University Acute Pain Scale:
- **Canine:** http://csu-cvmbs.colostate.edu/Documents/ anesthesia-pain-management-pain-score-canine.pdf
- **Feline:** http://csu-cvmbs.colostate.edu/Documents/ anesthesia-pain-management-pain-score-feline.pdf

RCVS Codes of Professional Conduct:
- **Veterinary surgeons:** www.rcvs.org.uk/advice-and-guidance/code-of-professional-conduct-for-veterinary-surgeons/
- **Veterinary nurses:** www.rcvs.org.uk/advice-and-guidance/code-of-professional-conduct-for-veterinary-nurses/

Reassessment Campaign On Veterinary Resuscitation (RECOVER) initiative: https://recoverinitiative.org/

University of Glasgow Short Form Composite Pain Scale: www.newmetrica.com/acute-pain-measurement/

Veterinary Poisons Information Service: https://vpisglobal.com/

Self-assessment questions

1. List the three major body systems and explain why these should be evaluated before other systems in an emergency patient.
2. What is the commonest cause of shock in veterinary emergency patients?
3. A cat presents with dyspnoea and the veterinary surgeon tells you it has dull lung sounds. List four possible causes for this. What is the emergency treatment likely to be and what should you prepare?
4. A patient has just undergone cardiorespiratory arrest. There is not a veterinary surgeon present although you have called for help. Whilst waiting for the veterinary surgeon, what are the most important tasks you should perform?
5. What clinical signs are commonly seen with pyometra in the bitch?
6. A male cat presents with a history of straining to urinate and has a large firm bladder. His heart rate is only 80 bpm. Why is his heart rate so slow? Is this a worrying finding and if so why?
7. An owner calls your practice as they are concerned that their dog is vomiting. What questions should you ask to help decide if the pet needs to be seen as an emergency?
8. A dog presents with a temperature of 42.5°C and the veterinary surgeon diagnoses heat stroke. How would you cool this patient and at what temperature would you stop active cooling? Why is it not recommended to place wet towels over the dog?
9. When treating shock with fluid therapy boluses, what side effects should you monitor for?
10. A cat presents with a large skin wound on its distal right hindlimb? What are the priorities for managing this patient? How and when would you start decontamination of the wound?

Chapter 20

Small animal fluid therapy

Louise O'Dwyer† with exotic pets by Simon Girling

Learning objectives

After studying this chapter, readers will have the knowledge to:

- **Define the terms used to describe the distribution and composition of body fluids**
- **Describe the distribution of water within the body, explain fluid losses and gains, and how fluid is regulated**
- **Identify the difference between hypovolaemia and dehydration, and how they are assessed clinically**
- **Identify the common parenteral fluid types and when they are indicated**
- **Describe how to create fluid therapy plans and how the correction of hypovolaemia and dehydration differ**
- **Calculate fluid requirements for a dehydrated patient**
- **Identify the different routes of fluid administration and their relative advantages and disadvantages**
- **Describe the different techniques for the placement of intravenous catheters**
- **Identify the complications with fluid therapy**
- **Describe the different products available for blood transfusion and their indications**

Introduction

Restoring and maintaining fluid balance in animals can be a challenging aspect of patient management. Consideration needs to be given to the individual patient's fluid requirements and veterinary nurses need to have a thorough understanding of the different composition of fluids available. There are a wide range of crystalloids, colloids and blood products available, and it can be difficult to determine both the most appropriate fluids to keep in stock and to use for a specific condition. It is therefore essential that veterinary nurses have a good knowledge and understanding of water and solute movement between fluid compartments in healthy patients (see Chapter 3), as well as those with hydration and perfusion deficits. Figure 20.1 contains definitions related to fluid therapy.

Term	Definition
Solvent	A substance, usually a liquid, capable of dissolving another substance (the solute). Water is the main solvent in the body
Solution	A mixture in which a solute is dissolved and evenly distributed in a solvent
Diffusion	The movement of particles from a region of higher concentration to one of lower concentration so that they become evenly distributed
Osmosis	Movement of water through a semi-permeable membrane from an area of low solute concentration to one of high solute concentration
Colloid osmotic pressure	The pressure that must be applied to a solution to prevent the inward flow of water across a semi-permeable membrane; this is related to the number (not size) of solute particles in the solution
Crystalloid solution	An aqueous solution of electrolytes, mineral salts or other water-soluble molecules that can pass through a semi-permeable membrane into all body fluid compartments

20.1 Definitions of terms related to fluid therapy.

continues ▶

Term	Definition
Colloid solution	A solution in which small particles are permanently suspended and cannot pass through a semi-permeable membrane
Hypotonic fluid	A solution (administered fluid) that contains a lower concentration of impermeable solutes than the solution (extravascular fluid) on the other side of the semi-permeable membrane
Isotonic fluid	Two solutions (in this case administered fluid and extravascular fluid) that contain an equal concentration of solutes
Hypertonic fluid	A solution (administered fluid) that contains a greater concentration of impermeable solutes than the solution (extravascular fluid) on the other side of the semi-permeable membrane
Tonicity	A measure of the osmotic pressure of two solutions separated by a semi-permeable membrane, the two solutions may, for example, be fluid administered intravenously and the body's extravascular fluid separated by the capillary membrane
Anion	A negatively charged ion (e.g. Cl^-, HCO_3^-)
Cation	A positively charged ion (e.g. Na^+, K^+)
Electrolyte	A substance that breaks down into negative and positive ions when dissolved in water
Cl^-	Chloride ion
H^+	Hydrogen ion
HCO_3^-	Bicarbonate ion
K^+	Potassium ion
Mg^{2+}	Magnesium ion
Na^+	Sodium ion
NaCl	Sodium chloride

20.1 *continued* Definitions of terms related to fluid therapy.

Distribution and composition of body fluid

The distribution of body water is shown in Figure 20.2 and the approximate compositions in Figure 20.3. The average water content of an adult animal is 60% of their bodyweight. The water content of a healthy animal varies with age (young animals may be 70–80% water, older animals may be 50–55% water) and body condition (fatty tissue contains less water than other soft tissue and therefore fat animals have lower percentage of water than thinner animals). Of the total body water:

- Two-thirds is inside the cells of the body: intracellular fluid (40% of the bodyweight)
- One-third is outside of the cell membranes: extracellular fluid (20% of the bodyweight)
  - Approximately three-quarters of the extracellular fluid is found around cells: interstitial fluid (15% of the bodyweight)
  - Approximately one-quarter of the extracellular fluid is intravascular: in the plasma (4% of the bodyweight)
  - The remaining extracellular fluid is transcellular: e.g. cerebrospinal fluid, synovial fluid, lymphatic fluid and gastrointestinal tract secretions (1% of the bodyweight).

Intravascular volume comprises a relatively small proportion of total body fluid and any loss of fluid from this compartment (hypovolaemia) has much more severe physiological effects than global loss of fluid (dehydration). The body water content will depend on the balance between the volume of water that is acquired by the body and the volume that is lost (see Chapter 3).

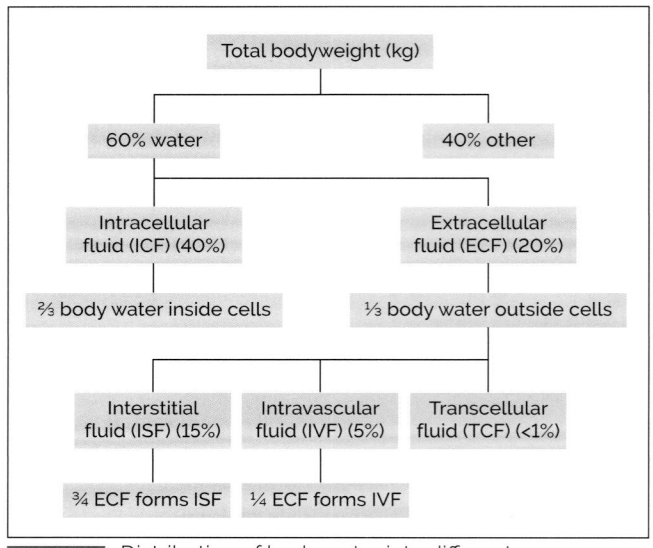

20.2 Distribution of body water into different compartments.

Extracellular fluid (mmol/l)	Substance	Intracellular fluid (mmol/l)
145	Na^+	12
110	Cl^-	4
24	HCO_3^-	12
4	K^+	140
1	Mg^{2+}	17
1.2	Ca^{2+}	2
15 in plasma	Protein	50

20.3 Approximate composition of different body fluid compartments.

Normal water intake and fluid loss

Normal water intake:

- Drinking
- Eating – moist diets may be 70–80% water
- Metabolism – oxidation of fat, carbohydrate and protein produces water
- Therapeutic (e.g. medications).

Normal fluid loss:

- Urination – regulated by healthy kidneys; fluid and electrolytes (24–48 ml/kg/day)
- Defecation – small volume; fluid and electrolytes (10–20 ml/kg/day)
- Respiration – evaporation; water only (20 ml/kg/day)
- Sweating – negligible volume in cats and dogs; fluid and electrolytes.

In some situations, or illnesses, the animal's ability to maintain fluid balance will be impaired.

Abnormal water intake and fluid loss

Causes of abnormal water intake include:

- Metabolic disorders
- Anaesthesia (preoperative, general anaesthesia, recovery)
- Systemic illness
- Dysphagia and/or physical difficulty
- Water deprivation.

Causes of abnormal fluid loss include:

- Vomiting (approximately 4 ml/kg per vomit)
- Diarrhoea (approximately 4 ml/kg per episode, up to 200 ml/kg/day)
- Increased respiratory evaporation (panting, dyspnoea)
- Pathological fluid losses (transudate, exudate, pyometra, burns, peritonitis)
- Haemorrhage
- Surgery (evaporation from the surgical site, haemorrhage).

Water will move via osmosis through a semi-permeable membrane until the concentration of impermeable solutes on either side of the membrane is equal (see Chapter 3). In health, both the cell membrane and the capillary wall function as semi-permeable membranes and concentrations of solutes are equal in all body fluid compartments. This can, however, change rapidly with disease. In some diseases, for example gastrointestinal tract disease, solutes may be lost leading to water movement by osmosis from areas of lower to higher solute concentration. In other diseases, such as pyometra or peritonitis, the capillary wall becomes leaky and no longer functions as a semi-permeable membrane meaning water and solutes may move out of the circulation. This kind of fluid movement is known as 'third spacing' and can result in excess fluid in the interstitium (oedema) or body cavities (e.g. ascites).

Body water balance

When considering administering fluid therapy to correct a fluid deficit, it is essential to think carefully about where the deficit exists. This should be straightforward based on the history of the patient and in conjunction with the clinical examination.

The history of the animal will give an indication of the type of fluid lost:

- Hypotonic fluid
- Isotonic fluid
- Hypertonic fluid.

Primary water depletion

With a primary water depletion, which occurs due to dehydration (e.g. lack of water availability, prolonged inability to drink, excessive panting, fever, diabetes insipidus), hypotonic fluid is lost initially from the extracellular fluid, and the extracellular fluid becomes hypertonic. Water moves from the intracellular fluid to equilibrate and the extracellular volume is supported, and therefore intravascular volume is maintained. This leads to a reduction of both intracellular and extracellular (interstitial and intravascular) fluid. Fluid loss is distributed across all of the fluid compartments, so although total body water content is reduced, the reduction in intravascular volume is small.

Mixed water and electrolyte depletion

Isotonic fluid loss represents loss of water and electrolytes and leads to no change in osmolality of the extracellular fluid, so therefore no movement of water from the intracellular fluid to compensate. This loss of extracellular fluid can be the result of internal or external haemorrhage, vomiting or diarrhoea. The resulting loss of intravascular volume is termed **hypovolaemia** and may lead to a perfusion deficit.

With hypertonic fluid loss, the extracellular fluid becomes hypotonic relative to the intracellular space and water moves out of the circulation and into the cells. This worsens the situation, causing **profound hypovolaemia** (e.g. as a result of haemorrhagic enteritis or secretory diarrhoea, where electrolyte absorption is impaired and leads to acute, severe haemoconcentration and hypovolaemia).

Dehydration and hypovolaemia

Dehydration and hypovolaemia are not interchangeable terms.

- Dehydration refers to a hydration deficit, where water is lost from the whole of the body, but predominantly from the intracellular and interstitial fluids.
- Hypovolaemia refers to a reduction in intravascular volume, which therefore reduces perfusion of the tissues, leading to a perfusion deficit.

Both hydration and perfusion parameters are initially assessed via physical examination (see Chapter 14). Hydration status is assessed by looking at parameters such as moisture of mucous membranes, skin turgor and the presence of retraction of the globe, which are affected by interstitial and intracellular fluid levels. Perfusion status is assessed by physical parameters that are affected by intravascular volume and perfusion, including: heart rate, pulse quality, mucous membrane colour, capillary refill time and urine output. The two conditions cause distinctly different clinical signs and must be managed in different ways, with different fluids at different rates of administration. Thus, appreciating the difference and recognizing the clinical signs, is essential in formulating a treatment plan.

Indications for fluid therapy

There are numerous indications for fluid therapy, including correction of dehydration, expansion and support of intravascular volume, and correction of some electrolyte disturbances. The history and physical examination of the patient will indicate which type of fluid deficit exists (i.e. dehydration *versus* perfusion deficit) and should include the duration of illness, frequency of vomiting or diarrhoea, water intake, food intake, blood loss, etc., to allow an assessment of fluid losses and therefore provide appropriate fluid types and volumes.

Dehydration

Hydration is a measure of the fluid content of the whole body. As the intravascular fluid compartment is only a small percentage of the overall body fluid (Figure 20.2), a patient can be dehydrated without appreciable signs of hypovolaemia, and life-threatening hypovolaemia can occur in the face of normal or even increased levels of hydration.

The body consists of approximately 60% water: significant increases or decreases in this volume result in clinical signs of over hydration or dehydration, respectively. Unfortunately, the clinical assessment of fluid gain or loss is only ever an approximation, as there is no single reliable test of hydration status. The clinical assessment of an individual's hydration status is important for the creation of a fluid therapy plan, as well as for the ongoing monitoring of fluid therapy.

Clinical assessment

The clinical assessment of hydration status requires evaluation of the patient history, physical examination findings and clinical judgment. In terms of the physical examination, the hydration status of an animal is usually assessed by measuring parameters that are affected by the reduction of fluid in the interstitial and extracellular compartments. This assessment includes:

- Moistness of gums or cornea – it should be remembered that conditions such as nausea can cause hypersalivation and make the membranes appear moist, even if the patient is dehydrated, and that panting can cause dry mucous membranes in a normally hydrated patient (Figure 20.4)

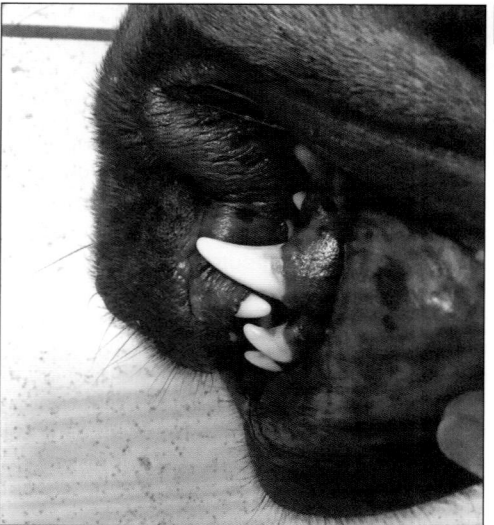

20.4 Dry mucous membranes in a dehydrated patient.

- Skin turgor or tenting – dehydration causes the skin to remain tented for several seconds
- Retraction of the globe (sunken eyes) – the retrobulbar fat pad, like the subcutaneous fat, will change in nature with hydration status
- Cardiovascular status
- Urine output
- Packed cell volume (PCV) and total protein (TP) or total solids (TS) (see Chapter 17).

Estimated degree of dehydration

Severity of dehydration estimated as a percentage of bodyweight	Clinical signs
<5%	- No detectable clinical signs - Increased urine concentration
5–6%	- Subtle loss of skin elasticity (tenting)
6–8%	- Marked loss of skin elasticity - Slightly sunken eyes - Dry mucous membranes
10–12%	- Tented skin stays in place - Sunken eyes, protruded third eyelid - Dry mucous membranes - Progressive signs of shock

Skin turgor and tenting

Skin turgor is an evaluation of the elasticity of the skin and is very much dependent on the volume of fat and water in the subcutaneous tissues. Increased amounts of fat will increase skin turgor, as will an increased water content. Reduced amounts of fat and/or water content are associated with decreased skin turgor.

The most common method of evaluating skin turgor is by observing the speed at which a pinch of skin that is 'tented' away from the body returns to its original position. Reduced skin turgor is indicated by a delay in the return of the skin to its original position, and may also reflect a loss of skin elasticity. For consistency, it is recommended that skin tenting is always performed in the same location on an animal; the skin between the shoulder blades is commonly used.

Since fat increases skin turgor, overweight animals may maintain 'normal' skin turgor despite dehydration, resulting in this clinical sign being less reliable in these patients. Conversely, very thin animals almost always appear dehydrated on skin tenting, so this clinical sign should be interpreted with caution in this group of patients. Young animals also tend to have very elastic skin and may require higher levels of dehydration before a decrease in skin turgor is detected. Normal skin turgor in these patients does not rule out dehydration and when reduced turgor is detected, this may indicate significant dehydration. With age, the inherent elasticity of the skin is lost and tented skin may lose its tendency to regain its original shape; in addition, elderly animals are often underweight and this combination can lead to dramatic decreases in skin turgor, making it a less reliable indicator of hydration in this group of patients.

Bodyweight

Fluctuations in bodyweight may be the most accurate method of measuring alterations in fluid balance. Acute changes in bodyweight relate to gain or loss of fluid, with 1 g = 1 ml. Ideally, all animals should be accurately weighed on presentation and then again as soon as their condition has stabilized. Patients should be re-weighed two to three times a day; this will provide valuable information to allow the clinician to amend the fluid therapy plan.

Laboratory testing

Serial measurements of PCV, TP (or TS) and urine specific gravity (USG) can provide information regarding a patient's hydration status. When a patient is significantly dehydrated, an increase in both PCV and USG is likely to be seen; whilst as hydration improves, a reduction in these parameters will be observed. It should always be remembered that there are numerous factors that may influence PCV and USG, so these results should be interpreted giving due consideration to all the patient information available. For example, an increase in USG is consistent with dehydration in patients with normal renal function, whereas a patient with compromised renal function will be unable to properly concentrate its urine and will have inappropriately diluted urine even in the face of dehydration. Dehydration causes a relative increase in PCV and TP (or TS) because of a total body water deficit; however, a normal PCV and TP (or TS) will be seen in an anaemic, dehydrated patient. Although a decrease in PCV and TP (or TS) is consistent with blood loss, an increased or normal PCV, with a decreased TP (or TS), can also be consistent with acute blood loss due to splenic contraction, which occurs in response to acute haemorrhage (see Chapter 17).

Central venous pressure

Central venous pressure (CVP) is a reflection of intravascular volume and can help guide volumes and rates of fluid therapy. It does not measure hydration but can be used as an assessment of hypovolaemia (see Chapter 21).

Hypovolaemia and shock

The term 'shock' is used where oxygen delivery to the tissues is poor due to tissue hypoperfusion. This leads to cell damage and, if not corrected, to organ dysfunction, organ failure and death. Cell damage and cell death will lead to the release of inflammatory mediators, which can result in systemic inflammatory response syndrome (SIRS).

Tissue hypoperfusion may be due to:

- Decreased circulating blood volume (hypovolaemic shock)
- Decreased ability of the heart to pump blood (cardiogenic shock)
- Decreased ability of vascular system to maintain vasomotor tone (distributive shock)
- Obstruction of blood flow from or to the heart (obstructive shock).

See Chapter 19 for further information on shock.

Hypovolaemic shock

Hypovolaemic shock is the most common form of shock seen in veterinary medicine, where tissue hypoperfusion is due to loss of circulating blood volume. This loss of volume may be due to blood loss (internal or external), loss of fluid from the gastrointestinal tract (vomiting, diarrhoea) or the kidneys, or due to the presence of an effusion and/or transudate in the peritoneal or pleural space.

If the circulating blood volume falls, blood flow is diverted away from capillary beds that are less essential (e.g. skin, gastrointestinal tract), so that the circulating volume can be sent to the more 'vital' organs such as the brain, heart and kidneys. This is a normal physiological response, and saves lives, but the volume needs to be restored before irreversible cell damage occurs.

Clinical assessment

A diagnosis of hypovolaemic shock is made by careful physical examination and the recognition of signs of poor tissue perfusion (Figure 20.5):

- Heart rate – increases in heart rate can be seen as an early indicator of volume loss; the increase in rate attempts to increase cardiac output. In dogs, regardless of size, these increases are fairly uniform. However, caution is advised in cats, as hypovolaemic animals can often have slower than normal heart rates
- Pulse quality – subjective impression of the fullness or width of a pulse. Vasoconstriction and a small stroke volume lead to poor pulse quality
- Mucous membrane colour – severe vasoconstriction means less haemoglobin and oxygen in the mucous membranes, so they appear pale or white
- Capillary refill time – a measure of peripheral vasomotor tone. Capillary refill time will be increased in hypovolaemic shock
- Mentation/level of consciousness – the brain has a high metabolic rate and low energy reserves, so is dependent on a constant supply of oxygen and glucose
- Extremity *versus* rectal temperature – due to

Clinical parameter	Mild hypovolaemia	Moderate hypovolaemia	Severe hypovolaemia
Heart rate (dog)	120–140	140–170	170–220
Mucous membranes	Normal/pinker	Pale pink	Pale/white/grey
Capillary refill time	Brisk (<1 second)	Normal (1–2 seconds)	Slow/absent
Pulse amplitude	Increased	Decreased	Very decreased
Pulse duration	Mildly reduced	Reduced	Very reduced
Peripheral pulse	Easily palpable	Faintly palpable	Non-palpable
Plasma lactate	3–5 mmol/l	5–8 mmol/l	>8 mmol/l

20.5 Clinical parameters used to assess the degree of hypovolaemia.

vasoconstriction, blood flow to the extremities decreases and so they become colder. The toe web temperature in hypovolaemic patients is usually 4°C lower than the core temperature of the animal.

The extent of the alteration in the perfusion parameters should give the clinician an accurate idea of the severity of the hypovolaemic shock present.

Physical examination is the main basis on which hypovolaemic shock is recognized, but laboratory samples can be of some use. Lactate is produced when cells metabolize anaerobically (i.e. without oxygen). If tissues are poorly perfused, oxygen delivery is reduced and lactate production increases. Due to poor perfusion, lactate clearance is also decreased. Thus, increased levels of lactate (>2 mmol/l) in the blood are an indicator of poor perfusion and, in some cases, can be used as a prognostic indicator (see Chapter 17).

Cardiogenic shock

Cardiogenic shock arises due to the heart's inability to efficiently create forward flow. This could be related, for example, to valvular disease, arterial thromboembolism or chamber enlargement. Cardiogenic shock is frequently accompanied by increases in pulmonary vascular pressures and hence fluid leakage into the alveoli causing pulmonary oedema and breathing difficulty. Cardiogenic shock may also be caused by severely abnormal heart rhythms. If there is a severe arrhythmia and the heart is no longer beating in a coordinated way this can lead to a severe reduction in cardiac output and hypoperfusion. This is identified by an irregular heart rhythm and pulse deficits on physical examination and confirmed by an electrocardiogram (ECG). In this scenario, the animal's breathing is usually normal as there are no changes to pulmonary vascular pressures.

Distributive shock

In distributive shock, poor perfusion of tissues exists due to loss of vasomotor tone and therefore inappropriate vasodilation. This leads to the intravascular fluid being distributed across the body in an abnormal way, as the body has effectively lost control of the regulation of perfusion. Clinical signs of distributive shock include rapid capillary refill time (CRT), red mucous membranes and tachycardia. Causes of distributive shock are anaphylaxis or SIRS. SIRS is a clinical state where localized pathology leads to widespread systemic inflammation, associated with dilatation and increased permeability of blood vessels. Initiating causes may be infectious (sepsis) or non-infectious (pyometra, pancreatitis, severe tissue injury, burns, neoplasia).

Obstructive shock

Obstructive shock occurs when there is a physical impediment to blood flow in the large vessels, predominantly the veins. This physical blockage to venous return results in blood being trapped distal to the obstruction, resulting in decreased stroke volume, decreased cardiac output and decreased blood being delivered to the tissues. A classic example of obstructive shock is the patient with gastric dilatation and volvulus (GDV). Another common cause is pericardial effusion, where the pressure of the fluid on the right side of the heart means blood cannot flow back into the heart and hence is an effective obstruction.

Types of parenteral fluid
Crystalloids

Crystalloids are water-based solutions that can easily leave the intravascular fluid and enter all body fluid compartments (Figure 20.6). They contain small molecules, electrolytes and other solutes that are osmotically active within body fluids, and are able to cross the capillary membrane. The varying concentrations and relative amounts of these electrolytes and solutes determine the indications for the different crystalloid fluids. The volume of crystalloid that remains within the blood vessels following its administration is dependent on Starling's forces (Frank Starling's Law is the intrinsic ability of the heart to adapt to increasing volumes of blood. The greater the myocardium is stretched during filling, the greater is the force of contraction) and the distribution of total body water. The sodium concentration of the fluid provides the greatest contribution to crystalloid osmolality.

Crystalloids can be divided into isotonic, hypertonic and hypotonic solutions:

- Isotonic fluids have an osmolality very similar to that of plasma/extracellular fluid; as such when administered they distribute to the intravascular and interstitial space but do not change the intracellular volume
- Hypertonic fluids have an osmolality greater than that of plasma; as such when administered intravenously they will tend to 'pull' additional water from the interstitial and intracellular space into the intravascular space
- Hypotonic fluids have an osmolality less than plasma; as such when administered intravenously a large volume of the fluid will move into the interstitial and intracellular spaces.

Isotonic crystalloids

Isotonic replacement crystalloids are the most commonly used fluid type in small animal medicine. They are versatile and can be used to treat hypovolaemia, dehydration and to replace ongoing losses. Where fluid and electrolyte loss has occurred (e.g. vomiting, diarrhoea, effusions, haemorrhage), a perfusion deficit will be likely. Isotonic crystalloids have a similar tonicity to plasma and are used mainly to replace perfusion deficits. Large volumes can be given rapidly where necessary, without much risk of dramatic electrolyte imbalances. When used for expansion of the intravascular fluid, crystalloids will equilibrate with the interstitial fluid, meaning that <25% of the fluid will be left in the intravascular space after an hour (Aldridge and O'Dwyer, 2013).

Examples of isotonic crystalloids include 0.9% saline (Figure 20.7a), Ringer's solution and Hartmann's solution (Figure 20.7b). Hartmann's solution is a balanced buffered isotonic replacement crystalloid, in that it contains electrolytes and a buffer (lactate) that regulates pH. As such, it is usually the preferred replacement crystalloid. Saline 0.9% may be preferred in cases of hypercalcaemia, hyperkalaemia or where the liver is unable to metabolize the lactate.

Isotonic crystalloids are often referred to as replacement crystalloids; the electrolytes are similar in composition to extracellular fluid (i.e. relatively high sodium and low (or no) potassium). When used long-term, there is a tendency towards hypokalaemia if the patient is not eating. Supplementation with potassium should be considered once the volume deficits have been replaced. Maintenance isotonic crystalloids with relatively high potassium levels (e.g. Plasma-Lyte® M) are available, but can only be given slowly, and their use is limited.

Crystalloid solution	Na⁺ (mmol/l)	K⁺ (mmol/l)	Cl⁻ (mmol/l)	Ca²⁺ mmol/l	Tonicity relative to ECF
Replacement					
Hartmann's solution	131	5	111	2	Isotonic
Lactated Ringer's solution	130	4	109	1.5	Isotonic
0.9% NaCl ('normal' saline)	154	0	154	0	Isotonic
Maintenance					
0.45% NaCl + 2.5% dextrose (glucose)	77	0	77	0	Hypotonic
Normosol-M + 5% dextrose (glucose)	40	13	40	0	Mildly hypotonic
Others					
0.45% NaCl (half strength saline)	77	0	77	0	Hypotonic
0.9% NACl + 5% glucose	154	0	154	0	Hypertonic
7.2% NaCl (hypertonic saline)	1232	0	1232	0	Hypertonic
Duphalyte®	N/A?	2.6	3.5	1.0	Unknown

20.6 Composition of the various types of crystalloid parenteral fluids available in practice.

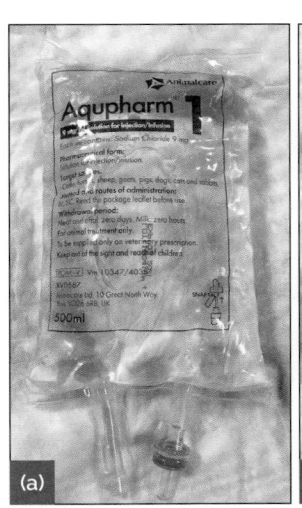
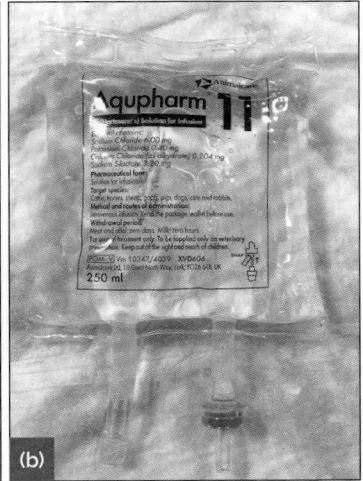

20.7 Isotonic crystalloids. **(a)** 0.9% saline. **(b)** Hartmann's solution.

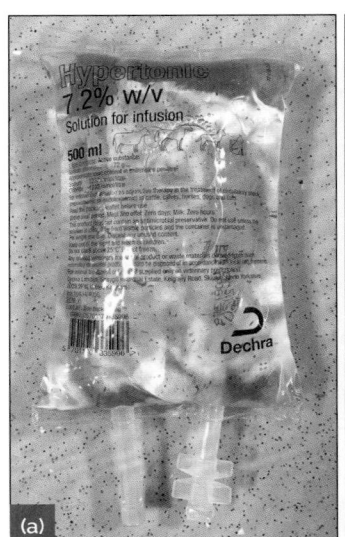
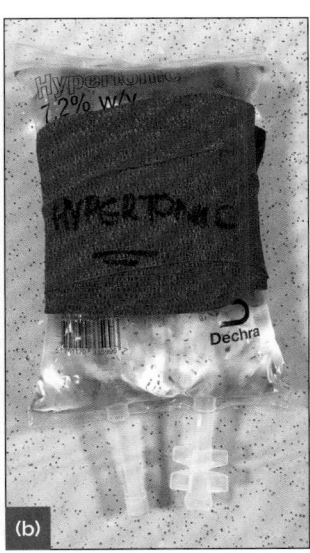

20.8 Hypertonic crystalloids. **(a)** 7.2% saline (hypertonic saline). **(b)** Hypertonic saline should be carefully labelled to avoid accidental administration.

Hypertonic crystalloids

Hypertonic crystalloids have roughly eight times the osmolality of plasma. By administering hypertonic fluids into the intravascular space, an osmotic gradient is created that draws fluid from the interstitial space into the circulation. An example of a hypertonic crystalloid is 7.2% saline (Figure 20.8). This is a very effective rapid means of increasing intravascular volume, as long as there is fluid in the interstitium to be drawn in. Therefore, hypertonic saline should not be used in patients with concurrent dehydration. The saline will redistribute, so its effect is temporary and needs to be followed by other fluids. A dose of 4–7 ml/kg in the dog or 2–4 ml/kg in the cat is given over 2–5 minutes, and produces a response similar to that seen with an isotonic crystalloid dose of 60–90 ml/kg. This is useful in large-breed dogs where an isotonic crystalloid bolus would take a long time to administer. It is also useful for the resuscitation of patients with a head injury that are at risk of intracranial pressure increase. The use of hypertonic solutions should be avoided in severe dehydration because of the oncotic pull.

Hypotonic crystalloids

Where primary water loss and dehydration only are suspected, with no evidence of hypoperfusion, then the loss may be hypotonic or isotonic. Electrolytes (especially sodium) must be measured to tell the difference; isotonic fluid loss is associated with normal sodium and hypotonic fluid loss is associated with high sodium (hypernatraemia). Hypotonic fluids have an osmolality less than that of the intracellular fluid. These crystalloids are poor volume expanders and dilute serum electrolytes, so are unsuited for the replacement of intravascular volume in perfusion deficits. Examples of hypotonic crystalloids are 5% dextrose and 4% dextrose in 0.18% sodium chloride. The dextrose in these solutions is immediately metabolized once it is in the bloodstream, effectively leaving water behind. The water is distributed according to the osmotic gradients that determine the distribution of total body water. The dextrose in the bag is present to ensure the fluid is isotonic at the point of administration, preventing lysis of erythrocytes and damage to the capillary endothelium close to the catheter. The level of glucose is not enough to provide meaningful calories. These fluids may be referred to as maintenance crystalloids; they provide the body's water requirement but not ongoing electrolyte requirements.

Colloids

Colloids are large molecules that increase the oncotic pressure of plasma, they hold fluid in the intravascular space and increase volume. Because they remain in the intravascular space, and do not equilibrate with the interstitial fluid like crystalloids, colloids are more effective at maintaining volume. Blood products, including whole blood, packed red blood cells and plasma, technically fall within this category as natural colloids, along with albumin, as they contain proteins. Synthetic colloids, such as hydroxyethyl starches (e.g. hetastarch) and gelatins (e.g. Geloplasma®), are also available. Recent studies have suggested an association of synthetic colloid administration with renal injury and coagulopathies, which have been reported in the human literature. Studies involving veterinary patients are currently ongoing to determine whether the same associations are seen (Fenger-Eriksen *et al.*, 2009; Zarychanski *et al.*, 2013).

Provided vascular permeability is normal, colloids maintain the oncotic gradient between the intravascular and interstitial spaces, reducing fluid movement from the vasculature. They will have the desired effect until they are broken down or degraded by the body, or until they leak from the vessels. The rate at which their effect diminishes depends on the molecules involved. Artificial colloids contain a mixture of molecules of differing weights. Initial volume expansion will depend on the number of molecules, not the molecule size. The duration of the effect will be dependent on the molecule size; larger molecules will persist longer and take longer to degrade.

Synthetic colloids

There are three common types of artificial colloid:

- Gelatins – produced from mammalian collagen (e.g. Geloplasma®). These products tend to have a shorter duration of action than any other colloid because of their small molecule size. Following infusion over 90 minutes, intravascular volume expansion is only 24% of the volume infused (similar to an isotonic crystalloid, where 20–25% of the volume infused remains in the intravascular space after an hour)
- Dextrans – prepared from polysaccharides (e.g. Dextran 40 or 70); not commonly used in veterinary medicine. It should be noted that there are no licensed dextrans products available for veterinary use
- Hydroxyethyl starches – derived from amylopectin, a branched form of plant starch (e.g. hetastarch, pentastarch, tetrastarch). Hydroxyethyl molecules are substituted on to the amylopectin to prevent intravascular hydrolysis. Estimates of initial volume expansion vary from 70% to 170% of the infused volume. At the current time, in Europe, there are no veterinary licensed hydroxyethyl starch products available.

Natural colloids

Blood products are administered when albumin, antithrombin, coagulation factors, platelets or red blood cells are required. The blood product should ideally be typed and cross-matched with the recipient when whole blood or packed red blood cell (PRBC) transfusions are needed. If blood typing or cross-matching is not available, then a DEA 1 negative transfusion is generally selected. A cross-match is always recommended in the cat. See 'Blood transfusion and products', below.

Albumin, the most abundant natural colloid molecule found in plasma, can be administered in the form of a plasma transfusion or concentrated human albumin. Frozen plasma, fresh frozen plasma and whole blood contain approximately 2.5% albumin, and concentrated human albumin solutions contain 25% recombinant albumin. Plasma transfusions have an albumin concentration equal to plasma and may not be an effective colloid when used alone.

Due to its high concentration of albumin and colloid osmotic pressure (COP) of 200 mmHg, 25% human albumin has the greatest capability of increasing plasma COP. When capillary permeability is normal, 25% human albumin can be a very effective colloid when administered to the hypovolaemic, oedematous patient. However, when increased capillary permeability prevents plasma albumin retention, it will leak into the interstitium, and the COP effect of any albumin infusion will be temporary. This can eventually lead to an increase in interstitial COP and oedema, as well as hypovolaemia.

Clinical application: the fluid plan

The five 'R's'

Veterinary professionals are encouraged to consider the five 'R's' of intravenous fluid therapy, which are terms referred to when drawing up fluid plans:

- Resuscitation – correcting shock and life-threatening deficits
- Routine maintenance – providing fluids to support and maintain homeostasis
- Replacement – replacement of dehydration deficits
- Redistribution – this is where fluid and electrolyte balance may result in shifts or lack of shifts of fluids between different body compartments (e.g. in cardiac disease)
- Reassessment – regular monitoring of intravenous fluid therapy.

Fluid therapy plans depend entirely on where the patient's fluid deficit is (i.e. whether the patient is hypovolaemic or dehydrated). Chronic fluid plans are suitable for patients with normal perfusion parameters (i.e. those patients that have hydration deficits only, or patients whose perfusion deficits have been corrected and are now moving to a longer term plan). If no hypovolaemia exists, then hydration, electrolyte and acid–base abnormalities can be corrected over 24–48 hours.

Fluid plan for the hypovolaemic patient

Three components need to be taken into consideration when determining a fluid therapy plan:

- Replacement of losses
- Maintenance requirements
- Ongoing losses.

Replacement of losses

The volume required to replace fluid losses is based on bodyweight and an estimation of dehydration.

Deficit (ml) = bodyweight (kg) x % dehydration x 10

For example: for a 20 kg Border Collie, estimated to be 8% dehydrated, the fluid deficit is calculated as:

Deficit (ml) = 20 x 8 x 10 = 1600 ml

Fluid plan for the hypovolaemic patient *continued*

Maintenance requirements

This is the normal fluid requirement of the animal over a 24-hour period. This is estimated at 50 ml/kg/day.

For example: for a 20 kg Border Collie, the maintenance requirements are calculated as:

Daily requirement (ml/day) = 50 x 20 = 1000 ml/day

Ongoing losses

Ongoing losses (e.g. due to diarrhoea, vomiting) need to be estimated. However, occasionally, they can be measured (e.g. chest drain output, weighing dressings to assess exudates).

For example: for a 20 kg Border Collie with diarrhoea and vomiting, the ongoing losses per day can be estimated as:

- Diarrhoea: 5 episodes at 4ml/kg = 400 ml/day
- Vomiting: 5 episodes at 4ml/kg = 400 ml/day
- Total ongoing losses (day) = 400 + 400 = 800 ml/day

Total fluid requirement

The aim is to replace any fluid deficits over 24 hours, so the total daily requirement is:

Replacement of losses + Maintenance requirements + Ongoing losses

For example: for a 20 kg Border Collie with diarrhoea and vomiting that is estimated to be 8% dehydrated, the total daily fluid requirement can be calculated as:

Total fluid requirement (ml/day) = 1600 ml + 1000 ml + 800 ml = 3400 ml/day
Hourly fluid requirement = 3400 ml/24 h = 142 ml/h

Fluid requirements given in millilitres per hour will need to be converted into drips per minute if an infusion pump is not available. Always double check how many drips are in a millilitre for the giving set to be used. The majority of 'adult' giving sets have a rate of 20 drops/ml, but some are manufactured at 15 drops/ml. Paediatric giving sets and burettes are normally calibrated at 60 drops/ml, but again the packaging should be checked.

Hourly fluid requirement = 142 ml/hour

The giving set to be used has a rate of 20 drops/ml, so the hourly rate can be calculated as:

142 ml x 20 drops/ml = 2840 drops/h
Minute fluid requirement = 2840 drops/ h ÷ 60 = 47 drops/minute

Treatment of hypovolaemic shock

The aim of treatment for hypovolaemic shock is to rapidly replace the intravascular volume. The effectiveness of treatment can be monitored by using the same perfusion parameters as mentioned above. The goal or endpoint of the resuscitation is normal perfusion parameters; measurements of lactate and urine output can also be used.

Observation of these parameters should be made every 15 minutes and fluid therapy tailored depending on the response. After assessing the degree of hypovolaemia present, a bolus dose is selected and administered with a view to correcting the intravascular volume and therefore normalizing the perfusion parameters (Figure 20.9). The bolus should be given over 15–60 minutes, depending on the severity of the hypoperfusion. After the dose has been administered, perfusion parameters should be re-assessed. If they have returned to normal, the ongoing fluid plan should now concentrate on replacing ongoing losses at a much slower rate. If the parameters are still abnormal, a further acute dose should be administered.

Degree of hypovolaemia	Bolus dose: dogs	Bolus dose: cats
Mild	5–10 ml/kg	3–5 ml/kg
Moderate	10–20 ml/kg	5–10 ml/kg
Severe	20–40 ml/kg (may need repeating)	10–15 ml/kg (may need repeating)

20.9 Bolus doses of fluids for hypovolaemic patients.

These fluids need to be administered rapidly into the intravascular space, so an intravenous or intraosseous route is required. Wide bore catheters are indicated to optimize flow rates (Figure 20.10). Before initiating aggressive fluid therapy, it should be remembered there are some contra-indications, including cardiac disease, respiratory disease and brain injuries. Patients with anuric renal failure require careful fluid therapy to prevent fluid overload, but fluid is required to confirm the diagnosis. Cats have a smaller fluid volume compared with dogs and tolerate volume overload poorly, so rates and volumes need to be reduced by one-third to one-half. Whilst a full dose of isotonic crystalloid for shock is considered to be 60–90 ml/kg in the dog and 40–60 ml/kg in the cat, in practice this size dose is very rarely given as a single bolus. An incremental approach is recommended with smaller doses (see Figure 20.9) and frequent reassessment with the dose being repeated if necessary. Occasionally, in suspected cases of uncontrolled ongoing internal haemorrhage (e.g. splenic rupture, hepatic laceration), a more limited resuscitation may be indicated.

Weight of patient	Catheter gauge
Replacement and maintenance fluid therapy	
<5 kg	27–22
5–15 kg	22–18
>15 kg	20–16
Shock rate fluid therapy	
<5 kg	24–20
5–15 kg	20–16
>15 kg	18–14

20.10 A selection of peripheral (over-the-needle) catheter sizes for use in replacement and maintenance fluid therapy and shock fluid therapy.

Fluid choice

Isotonic replacement crystalloids are often the first choice for fluid resuscitation of hypovolaemic animals (Hartmann's solution being commonly used), but colloids, hypertonic saline and blood products all have their place. Colloids provide a profound and persistent effect on intravascular volume, and a smaller volume is required compared with crystalloids (e.g. a 20 ml/kg dose of colloid would have similar effect to a 60–90 ml/kg dose of isotonic crystalloid).

It is common to use a combination of a crystalloid and a colloid to give intravascular expansion, with a longer duration.

Hypertonic saline should be considered where large patients in severe hypovolaemic shock are presented. In these cases, it may not be possible to administer isotonic crystalloids fast enough. A hypertonic saline (7.2% NaCl) bolus can be administered, followed by isotonic crystalloids. Hypertonic saline also has a role in the resuscitation of patients that have concurrent haemorrhage within an enclosed space (e.g. intracranial haemorrhage). In these cases, the intravascular volume can be expanded without the large volumes of isotonic crystalloid that would extravasate and contribute to haemorrhage and swelling.

Routes of fluid administration

Oral

If the animal is willing to drink, and is not vomiting, then oral fluids are suitable for cases of mild dehydration. In a clinical context this would only really apply to animals that have accidentally been deprived of water. Patients with a clinical condition that has led to water loss in excess of intake are obviously already unable to keep up with their requirements. Naso-oesophageal tubes, or oesophagostomy tubes, can be used for maintenance of fluid and food requirements where there is trauma or anorexia preventing the animal from eating and drinking.

Intravenous

The vast majority of patients admitted for medical or surgical procedures, or treatment of conditions, are likely to have an intravenous catheter placed at some point during their hospitalization period. In emergency or critical cases, the rapid placement of an intravenous catheter is a vital part of the treatment protocol, but the placement of catheters in this group of patients can be challenging due to factors such as patient size or hypovolaemia. In cases where intravenous catheter placement is difficult, then alternative routes of administering fluids and medications may be required. Additional factors that may influence catheter placement include patient temperament, the type of medications or fluids that are likely to be administered via the catheter, concurrent disease and trauma sustained.

Peripheral veins

Numerous veins can be used for vascular access, with the cephalic vein being most commonly used in dogs and cats. However, the medial and lateral saphenous veins, medial branch of the cephalic vein, the auricular vein and the dorsal common digital vein can also be used.

For the majority of patients, a peripherally placed intravenous catheter is usually appropriate and is considered one of the first stages in the treatment and stabilization of emergency patients (Figure 20.11). In patients where fluid administration is likely to be required for longer periods of time (e.g. more than 3–5 days), then it may be more appropriate to place a central catheter or 'line', which has its tip in the cranial or caudal vena cava.

1. Hair is clipped over the proposed site and the skin aseptically prepared. Gloves should be worn and aseptic technique observed.
2. An assistant applies pressure to 'raise' the vein.
3. The skin should be held taut to stabilize the underlying vein. An over-the-needle catheter is inserted through the skin at an angle of 45 degrees and into the vein.
4. If the vein is penetrated, blood will be seen in the hub of the catheter.

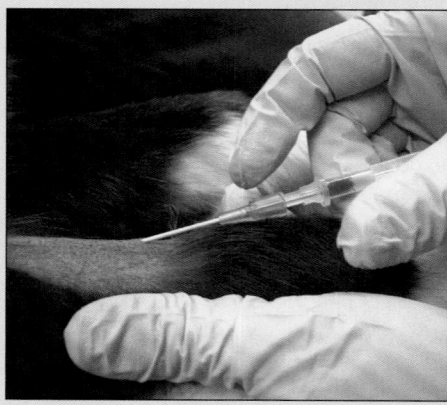

5. The angle of the catheter to the skin is reduced and the catheter advanced further into the vein.
6. The stylet is now held still, while the outer cannula is advanced into the lumen.

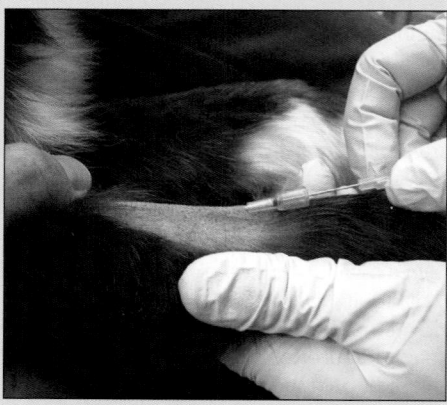

7. The assistant can now occlude the vein over the catheter tip to prevent haemorrhage.
8. An injection port, or fluid administration set, is now connected and the catheter secured in place with adhesive tape.

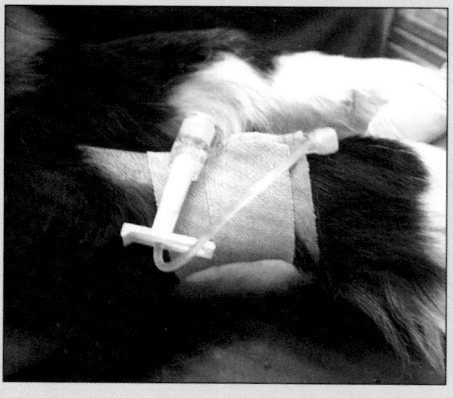

20.11 Procedure for peripheral catheter placement. (Reproduced from the *BSAVA Manual of Practical Veterinary Nursing*)

Central veins

Catheter selection

The placement of a central venous catheter requires some technical skill and specialized catheters.

- The catheters come in different sizes, lengths and number of lumens. The selection of the catheter size and desired number of lumens depends on the intended use of the catheter.
- A triple lumen catheter allows more flexibility for the use of the catheter, but will have narrower individual lumens than a double lumen catheter. This should be taken into consideration when selecting catheter size, especially if fluids may need to be rapidly administered.
- The placement of a jugular catheter in the cranial vena cava is preferable for the measurement of central venous pressure (see Chapter 21). The length of the catheter should be pre-measured from jugular insertion site to the 2nd rib space.

Catheter placement techniques

Central venous catheters (CVCs) are long catheters that are introduced through an accessible vein (ideally the distal tip of the catheter should be situated within the thoracic cavity to be classified as a central venous catheter). CVCs are generally placed in the cranial or caudal vena cava, which are accessed via the jugular or femoral veins (Figure 20.12).

1. The area is clipped, aseptically prepared and then draped.
2. A facilitative skin incision is made and a needle or introducer catheter is inserted into the vein.

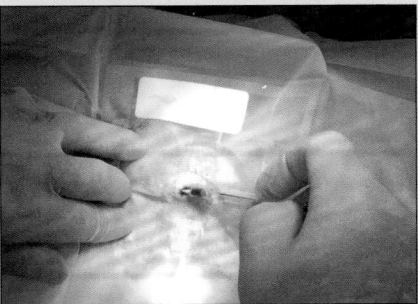

3. The guidewire is inserted into the vein via the introducer catheter. The introducer catheter is then removed, leaving the wire within the vein.

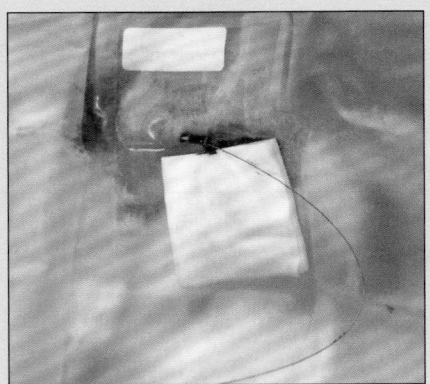

20.12 Procedure for central line placement into the jugular vein using the Seldinger technique.

continues ▶

4. A dilator is passed over the wire into the vein. This dilates the subcutaneous tunnel and the hole in the vein wall.

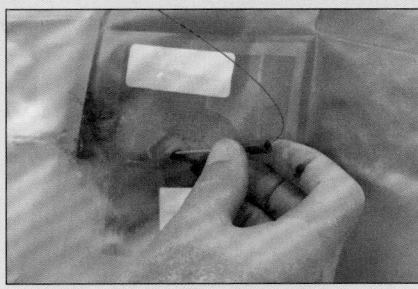

5. The catheter is advanced over the wire a premeasured distance into the vein, so that the tip lies within the central compartment.

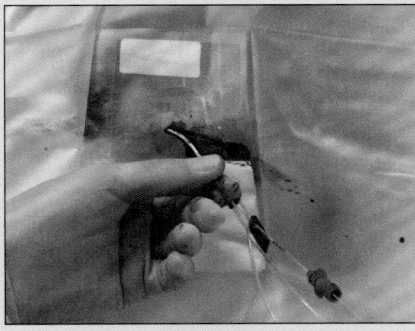

The wire is removed, all ports are aspirated and flushed using saline or heparinized saline, and the catheter is then sutured in place. The insertion site is covered with a sterile dressing and a neck bandage is applied.

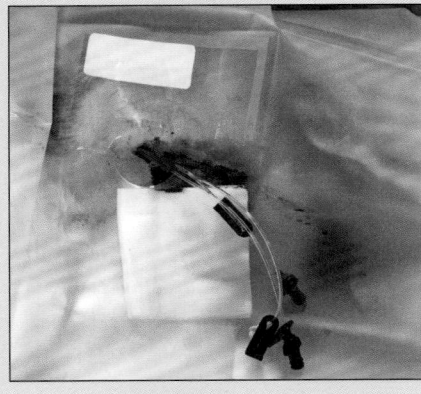

20.12 *continued* Procedure for central line placement into the jugular vein using the Seldinger technique.

Peripheral indwelling central catheters (PICCs) are introduced via a smaller peripheral vein (e.g. the lateral saphenous vein; see Figure 20.13) and so they need to be much longer and smaller in diameter; these catheters are generally utilized more for long-term venous access.

It is important that veterinary nurses are aware of the three most commonly used types of central venous placement:

- Seldinger technique: venous access is gained with a regular intravenous catheter. A guidewire is passed through the catheter into the vessel. The catheter is removed whilst taking care not to let go of the wire. A dilator is fed over the wire and pushed through the skin to create a tunnel. The dilator is removed and the CVC is fed over the wire. The guidewire is finally removed and the CVC is flushed and sutured in place (Figure 20.12)

1. The area is clipped, aseptically prepared and then draped.
2. Wearing sterile gloves, the cannula is inserted into the vessel (e.g. the lateral saphenous vein) and the stylet is removed.

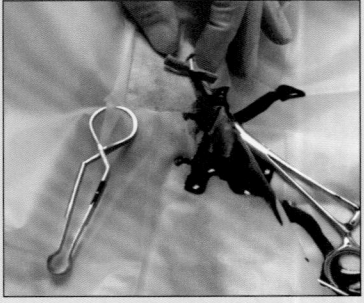

3. The long central catheter is fed through the cannula to the premeasured point.
4. Once *in situ*, the 'wings' on the cannula are broken, peeled apart and removed, leaving the catheter in place.

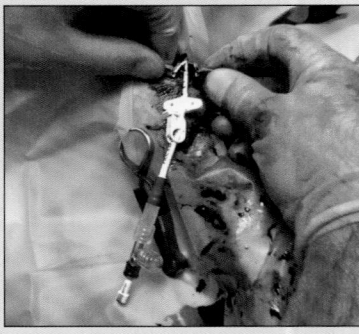

5. The catheter is aspirated and flushed with saline or heparinized saline and then sutured in place.

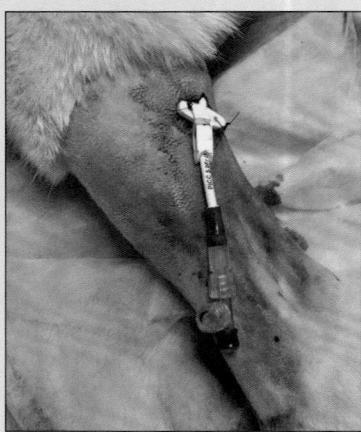

The catheter insertion site is covered with a sterile dressing and then bandaged in place.

20.13 Procedure for placement of a peel-away central line into the lateral saphenous vein. This is also referred to as a peripherally inserted central catheter (PICC).

- Peel-away technique: venous access is gained with the peel-away catheter with two tabs at the proximal end. The stylet is removed and the CVC is fed through the peel-away catheter. Once *in situ* the catheter is peeled away using the tabs. The CVC is positioned, flushed and sutured in place (Figure 20.13)
- Through-the-needle placement: this is the same principle as the peel-away method, however, the needle is simply removed by backing it out once the CVC is *in situ*.

Central venous catheters can be very beneficial, particularly in the critical care setting.

Indications for central venous catheterization

- It is likely that the patient will require long-term fluid therapy
- Administration of intravenous hyperosmolar or hypotonic fluids
- Administration of intravenous medications
- Administration of total parenteral nutrition
- Measurement of central venous pressure is to be performed
- Complications are present that cause peripheral catheter placement to be problematic (e.g. peripheral oedema, fractures, burns/wounds)
- Multiple blood samples are likely to be required (e.g. in diabetic ketoacidosis (DKA) and septic patients)

Potential contraindications for central venous catheterization

- Blood disorders (e.g. von Willebrand's disease)
- Coagulopathy disorders
- Thrombocytopenia
- Hypercoagulable states (e.g. disseminated intravascular coagulation, DIC)
- Increased intracranial pressure (e.g. head trauma)
- Respiratory disease (e.g. patients may not tolerate handling for catheter placement)
- Skin disease (e.g. infection/inflammation at the insertion site)
- Vasculitis

Catheter care

Once the catheter is placed, its ongoing monitoring and maintenance are essential. The area should be checked several times a day for any swelling, pain, leakage, heat or reddening of the skin. Ensure that the dressing is not too tight, as this may result in the swelling of the foot, or head/face in the case of jugular catheters. Check for swelling proximal to the catheter, which may indicate extravasation of fluid. Dressings should be replaced daily. Discharge, reddening or thickening of the vein may be signs of phlebitis. If present, the catheter should be removed and, ideally, the tip sent for culture. If the peripheral catheter site looks problem-free then the catheter should be left in as long as it remains that way. Repeated connection and disconnection of Luer junctions should be avoided, as this is a common source of contamination

---

Intraosseous

The placement of intraosseous catheters is not a commonly performed procedure in dogs and cats, but is a useful technique in cases where intravenous access cannot be established and rapid volume resuscitation is required. Intraosseous catheter placement is particularly useful in collapsed puppies and kittens, as their softer bones make placement easier (Figure 20.14).

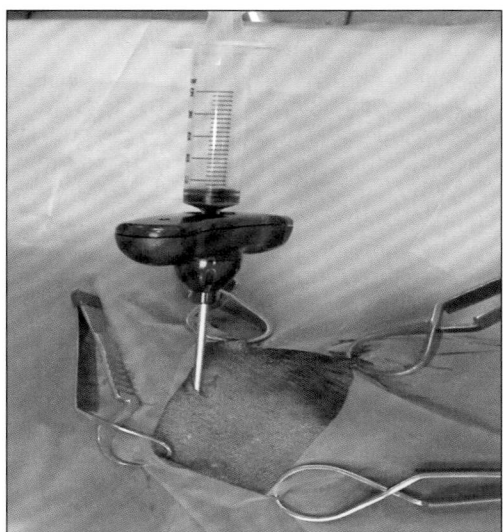

20.14 Intraosseous catheter placement.

Indications for intraosseous catheterization

- Severe burns
- Extensive subcutaneous oedema
- Shock
- Cardiac arrest
- Intravenous access difficult due to size of the patient

Catheter selection

There are commercially available intraosseous needles, but bone marrow biopsy needles or spinal needles can also be used. Both these devices contain a stylet, which prevents the needle clogging with bone during placement.

Catheter placement

Intraosseous catheters may be placed into any bone with a good marrow cavity; however the most common site is the medial aspect of the trochanteric fossa of the femur. The ilium, humerus and tibia may all be used. The site is prepared in a similar way as for intravenous placement with clipping and antiseptic preparation.

Subcutaneous

Subcutaneous fluids are totally unsuitable for patients with perfusion deficits as they will not bring about rapid resuscitation and will be poorly absorbed due to peripheral vasoconstriction. In mildly dehydrated animals, subcutaneous fluids will slowly rehydrate the patient; absorption can take 4–8 hours. Only small volumes should be injected in any one site (10–20 ml/kg) of an isotonic fluid. This route is sometimes used for maintenance of water intake in cats with chronic renal failure.

Intraperitoneal

Injecting fluids into the peritoneal cavity gives similar results to subcutaneous administration, but with risk of damage to the abdominal organs. This route is used by some clinicians in small animals or neonates.

Fluid administration equipment

The vast majority of veterinary patients will have their intravenous fluids administered via a giving or fluid administration set. In most patients, an 'adult' giving set is likely to be used; these sets deliver fluids at a rate of 20 drops/ml, although some may deliver fluids at 15 drops/ml. Paediatric administration sets are also available, which are calibrated to deliver fluids at 60 drops/ml. Burettes, which deliver a set volume of fluid via a chamber, also tend to have a rate of 60 drops/ml. With all fluid administration sets, the packaging should be checked before use to ensure that fluids are not under- or over-administered.

Fluid infusion pumps and syringe pumps (or syringe drivers) are useful to deliver fluids and medications at a set rate (Burkitt-Creedon and Davis, 2014) (Figure 20.15). This may be essential in some situations; for example, for the administration of continuous rate infusions of some medications.

Additional equipment includes drip stands or poles, which are used to hold fluid bags at an appropriate height above the patient. Fluid and syringe pumps can also be

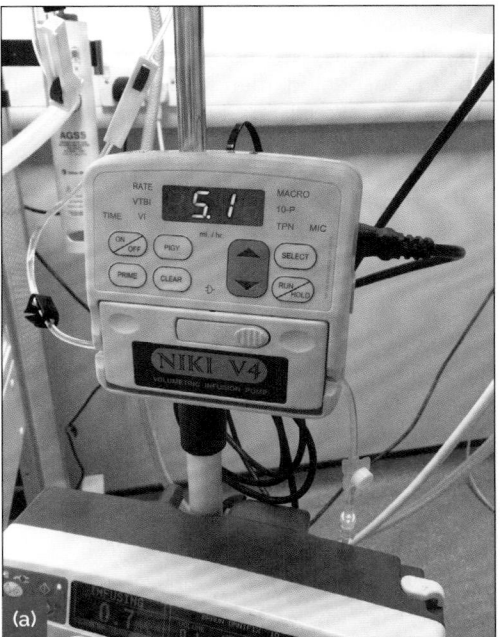

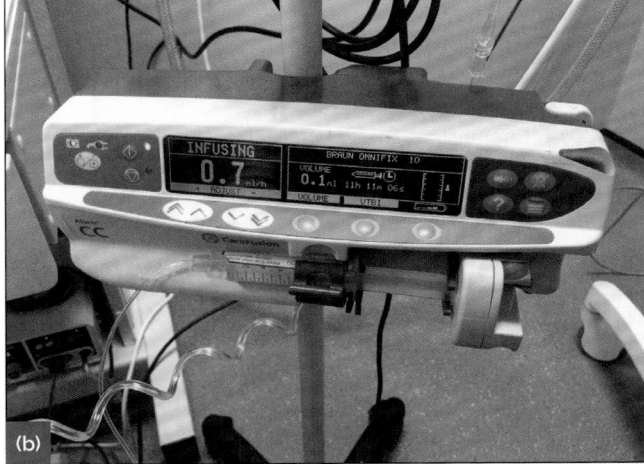

20.15 Example of **(a)** an infusion pump and **(b)** a syringe driver used for fluid therapy administration.

attached to these stands, meaning that they can easily be transported around with the patient.

Fluid pressure bags are useful for the rapid administration of intravenous fluids. These bags are basically a 'sleeve' that inflates around a fluid bag; they apply pressure and act as if someone is 'squeezing' the fluid bag, resulting in the rapid administration of large volumes of fluids.

Complications and monitoring

The most important complication is fluid overload. If too much fluid is administered, the body, especially the interstitial space, can become overloaded. Excessive fluid in the interstitial space may appear as:

- Pulmonary oedema
- Peripheral oedema (feet, legs, axillae, face)
- Serous nasal discharge
- Chemosis (oedema of the conjunctiva) (Figure 20.16)
- Cerebral oedema.

Other complications can include catheter-associated infection, catheter embolism, air embolism, fluid extravasation, blood loss and thrombus formation.

If fluid overload is suspected, then fluid therapy should be stopped and diuretics administered if appropriate, along with ongoing monitoring of the patient.

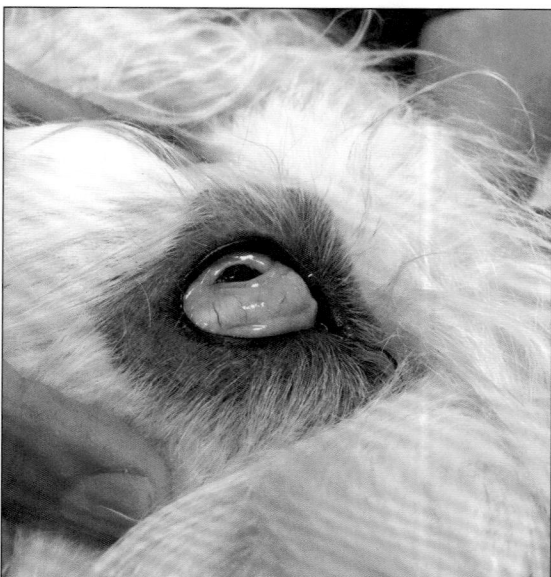

20.16 Chemosis in an Old English Sheepdog following overhydration.

Fluid balance measurement

When administering maintenance fluids to hospital in-patients, the best way to monitor volume status is by keeping an accurate record of the volume of fluid going into the patient versus the volume of fluid leaving the patient. Fluids 'in' are easily measured and recorded; this includes the volume of intravenous fluids administered, the volume of water consumed and amount/type of food eaten by the patient.

Fluids 'out' are less easy to measure. Urine output is easily measured if a urinary catheter is in place, otherwise soiled bedding should be weighed, non-absorbent cat litter should be used or urine should be caught in a kidney dish. When weighing cage liners, it is assumed that 1 g is equal to 1 ml of fluid. The volume of any vomit or diarrhoea must also be estimated.

The fluid balance of the patient should be measured every 6 hours. The volume of fluids 'in' should be approximately 10% more than the fluids 'out' (in addition some fluid is lost by sweating or evaporation from the respiratory tract). If the volume of fluids 'out' is greater than the volume of fluids 'in', then the fluid rate needs to be increased. If the volume of fluids 'in' is much greater than the volume of fluids 'out', this needs further investigation. If the patient is still dehydrated, this would be normal; the patient should therefore be examined for signs of dehydration. If not, other causes for the increase in water absorption (e.g. exudates, oliguric renal failure, overhydration) should be investigated.

Overhydration can occur if too much fluid is administered; it is the process by which the body becomes overloaded by fluid, especially the interstitial space. Excessive fluid in the interstitial space may present as peripheral oedema of the feet, legs, axilla and face, chemosis (swelling of the third eyelid), serous nasal discharge, pulmonary oedema and cerebral oedema. Signs of overhydration should be assessed via patient monitoring, including thoracic auscultation, potentially central venous pressure measurement and measurement of fluids 'in' versus fluids 'out'.

Special considerations

Patients where a modified approach to fluid therapy may be required include:

- Patients with respiratory disease/trauma
- Cardiac patients
- Renal patients
- Head trauma patients
- Paediatric patients.

Respiratory disease and trauma

Lung diseases that necessitate a modified fluid therapy plan are mostly pulmonary parenchymal diseases such as pneumonia and pulmonary haemorrhage secondary to trauma. Due to the additional fluid losses and systemic inflammation, pleural space diseases such as pyothorax also alter the fluid plan. Minor influences on the fluid plan occur with upper airway diseases such as laryngeal paralysis and tracheal collapse.

Patients suffering from pneumonia are challenging in regard to fluid therapy. Pneumonia causes multiple disorders of fluid homeostasis. Inflammation of the local endothelium, as well as the glycocalyx layer (a component of the endothelial surface layer lining blood vessels), ultimately leads to fluid and protein extravasation into the interstitium and alveoli. Hyperthermia, the extravasation of fluids and systemic inflammation, as well as the increased respiratory rate and decreased food and water intake, may lead to hypovolaemic shock, distributive shock, dehydration and ongoing fluid losses. The fluid plan need to address all of these factors.

In polytrauma patients, pulmonary involvement (e.g. pulmonary contusions or haemorrhage) is common. These patients often suffer from hypovolaemic shock. By increasing blood pressure with aggressive fluid therapy, haemorrhage is more likely to continue or restart. In addition, large fluid boluses decrease the concentration of coagulation factors in the plasma by dilution. Thus, in this group of patients, fluid volumes are often more restrictive, in order to maintain the balance between optimizing perfusion and preventing complications such as pulmonary oedema (Serrano and Boag, 2014).

Patients with severe systemic inflammation may have increased capillary permeability, leading to hypovolaemia in conjunction with interstitial overhydration.

Cardiac disease

Patients with congestive heart disease can have local increases in pulmonary vascular volume, leading to pulmonary oedema, whilst at the same time having a reduced total circulating volume due to chronic treatment with diuretics and afterload reducers.

Renal disease

With renal disease, care must be taken not to overload the patient with fluids. The primary reason for fluid overload is failure to adjust the administration rate in the face of decreased urine production. The oliguric or anuric patient is incapable of effectively excreting an excessive fluid load, so bodyweight and indices of hydration should be monitored closely.

Head trauma

In head trauma patients, the initial use of large volumes of crystalloids, which will extravasate within an hour and may make cerebral oedema worse, is contraindicated. Hypertonic saline is often used for the initial treatment of patients with concurrent hypovolaemia.

Neonatal and paediatric patients

The neonate is particularly susceptible to dehydration as water makes up 82% of its bodyweight and water turnover is about twice that of an adult. The higher percentage of body water (caused mostly by extracellular water), the greater surface area:bodyweight ratio, the lower percentage of body fat and the higher urine production are the main contributing factors. Maintenance rates in paediatrics usually range from 100 to 180 ml/kg/day. Evaluating the hydration status of the animal can be difficult using physical examination parameters (normally mucous membranes are wet even if the puppy or kitten is severely dehydrated, and skin tenting is present in well hydrated animals due to the lack of fat) or clinical pathology. Due to the same developmental limitations, paediatric patients are more susceptible to overhydration. Puppies or kittens should be weighed at least twice a day using an accurate paediatric gram scale.

Understanding electrolyte balance

Some of the most important electrolytes in the body are sodium, potassium, calcium, phosphorus and chloride. There are a wide variety of diseases associated with electrolyte abnormalities.

Sodium

Sodium is primarily an extracellular cation with less than 10% of total body sodium found intracellularly. An increase or decrease in serum sodium concentration will almost always be a reflection of the water balance of the patient, rather than an absolute increase or decrease in the amount of total body sodium. For this reason, it is important to evaluate a patient's circulating volume and hydration status whenever a serum sodium concentration is assessed. When the plasma concentration of sodium is decreased or increased, it alters the osmolality of the blood, which will trigger either the thirst mechanism or antidiuretic hormone (vasopressin) release, respectively. Hence, water is added or excreted, bringing the body's sodium concentration back to normal.

Hyponatraemia

Normal serum sodium is approximately 145–155 mmol/l in the dog and 149–160 mmol/l in the cat. Clinical signs from hyponatraemia are, however, unlikely unless solium is <125 mmol/l in the dog or <135 mmol/l in the cat.

Causes
The causes of hyponatraemia include:

- Gastroenteritis
- Kidney disease
- Diuretics
- Polydipsia
- Inappropriate antidiuretic hormone (ADH) release
- Congestive heart failure
- Hypothyroidism
- Burns, tissue trauma
- Third space losses
- Post-obstructive polyuria
- Iatrogenic administration of hypotonic fluids.

Clinical signs
The clinical signs associated with hyponatraemia include:

- Hypotension/shock
- Weakness
- Vomiting, anorexia, abdominal pain
- Ileus
- Altered level of consciousness
- Seizures.

Hypernatraemia

Clinical signs from hypernatraemia are unlikely unless sodium is >170 mmol/l in the dog or >180 mmol/l in the cat (see normal values above).

Causes and clinical signs
The causes of hypernatraemia and their associated clinical signs include:

- Hypovolaemic hypernatraemia – Vomiting, diarrhoea, adipsia, hypodipsia, hyperventilation, urinary obstruction, diuresis, renal disease and third space losses
- Normovolaemic hypernatraemia – Diabetes insipidus, iatrogenic hypernatraemia and hypodipsia/adipsia
- Hypervolaemic hypernatraemia – Hyperaldosteronism, hyperadrenocorticism, iatrogenic (hypertonic sodium administration and sodium bicarbonate administration).

Chloride

Chloride is one of the most important anions in the body, representing approximately two-thirds of the anions in the blood. Fluids and drugs containing chloride, such as 0.9% saline, hypertonic saline and potassium chloride, can increase patient's chloride levels. Chloride retention in the renal system can occur secondary to renal failure, renal tubular acidosis, diabetes mellitus and chronic respiratory alkalosis. Loop diuretics and thiazide diuretics can cause an increased loss of chloride relative to sodium. Hypochloraemia can occur with gastric vomiting and as an adaptive mechanism with chronic respiratory acidosis. Pseudohyperchloraemia can occur when patients are being treated with potassium bromide. Most chloride abnormalities are associated with acid–base abnormalities and clinical signs relate primarily to the acid–base disturbance rather than the alteration in chloride. Hyperchloraemia is typically associated with acidosis and hypochloraemia with an alkalosis (see Chapter 17 for reference ranges).

Hypochloraemia

Hypochloraemia is associated with metabolic alkalosis because chloride concentration varies inversely with bicarbonate concentration.

Causes

The causes of hypochloraemia include:

- Gastric vomiting
- Pyloric outflow obstruction
- Duodenal foreign body
- Severe pancreatitis
- Administration of diuretics.

Hyperchloraemia

Causes

The causes of hyperchloraemia include:

- Severe diarrhoea
- Renal retention of chloride
- Long-term administration of 0.9% NaCl.

Potassium

Hypokalaemia

Hypokalaemia is common in critically ill patients. It can result from excessive loss (renal disease, polyuria, diuretics, vomiting or diarrhoea), decreased intake (anorexia, potassium deficient fluids) or translocation from extracellular to intracellular fluid (insulin and glucose administration, bicarbonate, alkalosis).

Causes

The causes of hypokalaemia include:

- Vomiting and diarrhoea
- Anorexia
- Renal disease
- Burns
- Diuretic administration
- Polyuria
- Insulin therapy
- Acidosis.

Clinical signs

The clinical signs associated with hypokalaemia include:

- Muscular weakness (ventroflexion of neck in cats)
- Lethargy
- Vomiting
- Anorexia
- Arrhythmias
- Dyspnoea – respiratory paralysis in severe hypokalaemia
- Flaccid hemiplegia
- Ileus.

Guide to potassium supplementation

Serum K+ (mmol/l)	Amount K+ to add/250 ml 0.9% NaCl (mmol/l)	Max infusion rate (ml/kg/h)
<2	20	6
2.0–2.5	15	8
2.5–3.0	10	12
3.0–3.5	7	16
3.0–3.5 (anorexic patients)	5	16

Hyperkalaemia

In general terms, hyperkalaemia can be the result of increased intake with movement of potassium extracellularly and inadequate excretion in the kidneys secondary to renal or post-renal causes. Massive tissue damage such as that which occurs with crush injuries, as well as rapid reperfusion (e.g. following aortic thromboembolism treatment) can result in hyperkalaemia. Iatrogenic causes include fluid therapy, administration of spironolactone and angiotensin-converting enzyme inhibitors, loop and thiazide diuretics. Clinical signs of hyperkalaemia relate to weakness of skeletal, cardiac and gastrointestinal muscles due to hyperpolarization of the membranes. Cardiotoxic effects can become evident when potassium concentrations exceed 7.5 mmol/l.

There are distinct electrocardiographic findings associated with hyperkalaemia, although the order in which they appear in cats seems to be less consistent than in dogs. The electrocardiographic abnormalities appear to be less apparent in acute cases of hyperkalaemia (e.g. feline lower urinary tract obstruction). The abnormalities, in the order they typically appear, include tall or peaked T waves, a prolonged PR interval, an absent P wave, a prolonged QRS complex, bradycardia, atrial standstill, sine wave complexes, ventricular fibrillation and complete standstill.

Causes

The causes of hyperkalaemia include:

- Renal failure
- Urethral obstruction

- Addision's disease
- Tissue trauma, bladder or urethral rupture
- Ingestion of potassium salts
- Acidosis.

Clinical signs

The clinical signs associated with hyperkalaemia include:

- Arrhythmias (particularly bradycardia)
- Muscular weakness
- Reduction in tissue perfusion.

Calcium

Serum calcium levels should be checked in any patient with unexplained weakness, stiffness, polyuria, enlarged lymph nodes, seizures or periparturient illness.

Hypocalcaemia

Hypocalcaemia is commonly seen in small-breed bitches within 21 days post-whelping (see Chapter 24). Hypocalcaemia may also occur post-thyroidectomy in cats if the parathyroid glands have accidentally been removed or damaged.

Causes

The causes of hypocalcaemia include:

- Hypoalbuminaemia
- Vitamin D deficiency (gastrointestinal malabsorption)
- Hypoparathyroidism
- Eclampsia
- Acute pancreatitis
- Ethylene glycol toxicity
- Phosphate enemas
- Citrate toxicity
- Low calcium/high phosphorus diet
- Renal failure.

Clinical signs

The clinical signs associated with hypocalcaemia include:

- Seizures
- Tetany
- Weakness
- Ataxia
- Anorexia
- Vomiting
- Arrhythmias
- Panting
- Muscle tremors.

Hypercalcaemia

The causes and clinical signs of hypercalcaemia are listed below. It should be noted that haemolysis and hyperlipaemia may falsely raise calcium concentration.

Causes

The causes of hypercalcaemia include:

- Neoplasia (especially lymphosarcoma)
- Anal sac adenocarcinoma
- Multiple myeloma
- Metastatic bone tumours
- Primary hyperparathyroidism

- Acute kidney injury or chronic renal failure
- Hypoadrenocorticism
- Vitamin D rodenticide toxicity.

Clinical signs

The clinical signs associated with hypercalcaemia include:

- Renal, neuromuscular and cardiovascular system abnormalities
- Anorexia
- Lethargy
- Polyuria/polydipsia (PU/PD)
- Vomiting
- Muscle weakness
- Cardiac arrhythmias
- Seizures.

Blood gas analysis

Blood gas analysis provides information about both respiratory function and acid–base status (see also Chapter 21) and is essential in order to make a diagnosis, provide treatment and monitor the progress of patients with either respiratory or metabolic abnormalities. Acid–base status can be evaluated on arterial blood gas (ABG) or venous blood gas (VBG) samples. In order to evaluate oxygenation, however, an arterial sample is required. Four key pieces of information are provided from the ABG: partial pressures of both oxygen (PaO_2) and carbon dioxide ($PaCO_2$), blood pH and bicarbonate concentration (HCO_3^-). It is vital to know the normal values in order to evaluate samples accurately.

Assessing oxygenation and ventilation

P_aO_2 (measured in mmHg or kPa) is an accurate reflection of the ability of the lungs to transfer oxygen to the blood. A low P_aO_2 represents hypoxaemia and can initiate hyperventilation. The oxygen saturation of haemoglobin, S_aO_2 (as measured by the pulse oximeter) measures the percentage of haemoglobin actually carrying oxygen, which is why 95–100% is normal.

P_aCO_2 (in mmHg or kPa) indicates the efficiency of alveolar ventilation. Alveolar ventilation determines P_aCO_2. Hyperventilation results in a decreased P_aCO_2 (hypocapnia), whereas hypoventilation increases P_aCO_2 (hypercapnia). Changes in ventilation may occur in patients with primary pulmonary disease, central nervous system (CNS) impairment, or may occur as a compensatory change in patients with metabolic disturbances.

Metabolic assessment

Serum bicarbonate levels provide information about the metabolic aspect of acid–base balance. HCO_3^- is controlled by renal retention and excretion; this can be accurately measured in either venous or arterial samples. An increase in HCO_3^- results in a metabolic alkalosis, whilst an abnormally low HCO_3^- results in a primary metabolic acidosis. Primary metabolic acid–base disorders are predominantly corrected by treating the underlying disease. The kidneys respond to metabolic acid–base disturbances by retaining or excreting increased amounts of HCO_3^-. This compensatory response occurs far more slowly than respiratory changes.

Step by step approach to blood gas analysis

As previously stated, the body functions best at a pH of 7.4. Any physiological event that causes a change in blood pH is called a primary disorder. A **primary disorder** will stimulate a compensatory response in an attempt to restore the pH to normal.

1. Examine the P_aO_2 and determine whether the patient is hypoxaemic – administer oxygen if necessary.
2. Examine the pH. If the pH is <7.35, an acidaemia exists; if the pH is >7.45, an alkalaemia exists.
3. Is there a respiratory component? Examine the P_aCO_2. If it is high or low, a respiratory component exists (could be primary or secondary/compensatory); if it is normal, no respiratory component is present.
4. Is there a metabolic component? Examine the HCO_3^-, if it is high or low, a metabolic component exists (could be primary or secondary/compensatory); if it is normal, no metabolic component is detected. If the HCO_3^- is high, a metabolic alkalosis exists; if low, a metabolic acidosis exists.
5. Determine which component is the primary disorder. In simple acid–base disturbances, the primary disorder is the component that has changed in the same manner as the pH. If an acidaemia exists, the primary disorder will be the component that corresponds to an acidosis. For example, if the pH and the HCO_3^- are low, the primary disorder is metabolic (a metabolic acidosis). Conversely, if the pH is low, and the pCO_2 is elevated (respiratory acidosis), the primary disorder is respiratory. If both the metabolic and respiratory components have changed in the manner of the pH, then a mixed acid–base disturbance exists.
6. Determine whether there is a compensatory response. Compensatory responses will cause the component to move in an opposite manner from the pH. That is, if an acidaemia exists, the compensatory response to an acidaemia would be an alkalosis. Thus, a compensatory response to an acidaemia would be an elevated HCO_3^-, or a decreased pCO_2; a compensatory response to an alkalaemia would be a decreased HCO_3^- or increased pCO_2. For example, if the pH, HCO_3^- and pCO_2 are low, then a primary metabolic acidosis with respiratory compensation exists. If the pH is low, and the HCO_3^- and pCO_2 are high, a primary respiratory acidosis, with metabolic compensation, exists.

Treating acid–base disorders

Acid–base disorders are best treated by addressing and correcting the underlying problem. Occasionally, however, intervention to directly adjust pH must be initiated, usually if the pH becomes life-threatening.

Other indications for fluid therapy

Fluid administration recommendations for anaesthetized patients and patients with fluid disturbances were created by the American Animal Hospital Association (AAHA) and the American Association of Feline Practitioners (AAFP) in 2013 (Davis et al., 2013; www.aaha.org/globalassets/02-guidelines/fluid-therapy/fluidtherapy_guidlines_toolkit.pdf). These guidelines highlight that the previously recommended high fluid rates could potentially lead to worsened outcomes for patients, including increased bodyweight, reduced pulmonary function, coagulation problems, decreased gut motility and reduced tissue oxygenation. In addition, a decrease in packed cell volume, total protein concentration and body temperature have all been associated with use of high fluid rates.

The 2013 AAHA/AAFP guidelines recommend the use of 3 ml/kg/h in cats and 5 ml/kg/h in dogs as a starting point, and that any pre-existing fluid deficits should be addressed prior to the induction of anaesthesia. For further information on fluid therapy during anaesthesia, see Chapter 21.

Blood transfusions and blood products

Patients that have lost a large volume of blood due to some form of internal or external haemorrhage should, ideally, receive a whole blood transfusion, or a combined packed red blood cell (PRBC) and plasma transfusion. Patients that are anaemic due to a lack of production, or destruction, of red blood cells should be transfused with packed red blood cells, or if PRBCs are not available, whole blood may be administered cautiously, bearing in mind that these patients may have a normal circulating volume.

The decision regarding when to transfuse a patient is an ongoing debate; consideration needs to be given to the patient's volume status, the degree of anaemia and the species, when determining the specific PCV at which an animal should be transfused. For example, a normovolaemic anaemic patient (such as a dog with immune-mediated haemolytic anaemia) is likely to have compensated for its ongoing anaemia and, therefore, may not require a transfusion until the PCV decreases to around 12–18%. Cats appear to be able to tolerate anaemia to a greater degree compared with dogs and often only demonstrate clinical signs when the PCV decreases to 10–15%.

Generally, when anaemic patients begin to show early clinical signs (e.g. weakness), in combination with a decrease in PCV to below 20% in dogs and 15% in cats, a transfusion is indicated.

Anticoagulant/preservative in blood bags

Commercial blood bags all contain an anticoagulant/preservative solution. The most common ones are citrate-phosphate-dextrose (CPD) and citrate-phosphate-dextrose-adenine (CPDA-1) although acid-citrate-dextrose (ACD) may also be used. The duration of time for which the blood product can be stored varies depending on the anticoagulant/preservative solution, and the guidelines produced by blood bag manufacturers should be observed. CPD and CPDA-1 are typically used in a ratio of 1 ml anticoagulant to 7 ml of blood and ACD is used at a ratio of 1 ml of anticoagulant to 7–9 ml of blood

Canine blood groups

Dog erythrocyte antigens (DEAs) are glycoproteins and glycolipids that occur on the surface of the red blood cells, and the presence or absence of these determine a dog's blood type. At least 13 blood groups have been identified so far in dogs, and this is an ongoing area of research as new antigens continue to be discovered.

There are currently seven recognized antigen types within the DEA system: these antigen sites are known as DEA 1, 3, 4, 5, 6, 7 and 8. DEA 6 and DEA 8 are two examples of antigens that have been identified, but for which typing sera is unavailable at this time.

The DEA 1 group is considered to be the most antigenic. The antigen can be expressed in varying degrees, classified as 'weak', 'moderate' or 'intermediate', 'strong', or negative.

Canine erythrocytes were previously considered to be either positive or negative for certain blood types (e.g. DEA 4+ or DEA 4–); however, new research has shown that in the DEA 1 system, dogs can be DEA 1 negative or weakly, moderately or strongly DEA 1 positive. In 2007, a new common blood type, named Dal, was identified. Whilst it was initially thought that it was only Dalmatians that lacked this antigen (and therefore would be the only breed at risk of delayed and acute haemolytic transfusion reactions), the Dal antigen has subsequently been found to be absent in some Dobermanns, Beagles and other breeds, including the Lhasa Apso. In addition to Dal, two new red cell antigens were found in a dog in South Korea, after which they are named: Kai 1 and Kai 2.

Historically, it was thought that dogs did not have any naturally occurring antibodies to other red blood cell antigens, which is the reason why dogs were previously given blood transfusions without blood typing first. However, naturally occurring antibodies against DEA 3, 5 and 7 have been identified. When blood from a dog positive for DEA 3, 5 or 7 is transfused into animals that are negative for these antigens, there is no immediate transfusion reaction, but there is permanent red blood cell sequestration and loss of the red blood cells within 3–5 days. In addition, although usually DEA 4 antigen–antibody interactions have no influence on red blood cell survival, there have been clinical case reports of rare individuals who have had an acute haemolytic reaction.

The DEA 1 canine blood group is the one of most clinical significance. Dogs do not possess naturally occurring antibodies against the DEA 1 system; thus, a dog that is negative for DEA 1 that is given a transfusion from a dog that is positive will not have an immediate reaction. However, antibodies will be induced and all transfusions after this will carry the potential to be extremely dangerous. DEA 1 antibody interactions result in severe acute haemolysis of transfused donor red blood cells within 12 hours. This can be a life-threatening situation.

Dogs negative for Kai 1 and Kai 2, as well as DEA 1 dogs, do not have any naturally occurring alloantibodies in their plasma. Although acute haemolytic transfusion reactions have been documented in previously transfused dogs due to DEA 1, DEA4 and Dal incompatibilities, there is no published evidence of alloantibody production and acute haemolytic reactions due to mismatched Kai transfusions.

Universal Donors

The only 'universal donor' is a dog that is negative for DEA 1, 3, 5, and 7, and positive for DEA 4.

Blood typing cards

Blood typing cards that are based on serological identification of agglutination reactions have been available with modifications since the mid-1990s as a simple method to classify dogs as either DEA 1 negative or DEA 1 positive. A standardized simple immunochromatographic technique became available in the mid-2000s

Feline blood groups

Cats have three blood types belonging to a single recognized blood group: A, B and AB. Unlike dogs, cats do have naturally occurring (at birth) antibodies against other blood types. Type A cats can have a low titre of anti-B antibodies: type A cats receiving type B blood can have transfusion reactions that result in the removal of red blood cells within 2-4 days. However, type B cats have a very high titre of naturally occurring anti-A antibodies. When a type A cat is transfused with type B blood, it may have a slight reaction. However, transfusing as little as 1 ml of type A blood into a type B cat can result in acute haemolysis and death. Type AB, the third feline blood type, is extremely rare. There are no universal donor cats.

Type A is the most common blood type; however, the distribution of type A and type B amongst purebred cats varies markedly, as does the frequency of type A and type B in Domestic Shorthaired cats worldwide. British Shorthair, Cornish Rex, Devon Rex, Abyssinian, Himalayan, Birman and Scottish Fold cats all have a markedly increased frequency (5–50%) increase in blood B type frequency.

A new antigen was reported in 2007 after a haemolytic transfusion reaction was seen in a previously non-transfused cat that had been administered a matched AB unit of blood. The Mik antigen was identified but its relevance is not entirely understood at this time. The Mik antigen has been shown to be absent in about 6% of cats tested so far; the possibility exists in cats without Mik to develop an acute haemolytic reaction after transfusion with the appropriately matched AB blood. As feline antibodies are naturally occurring and typing serum for Mik is not available at this time, cross-matching even type-matched cats is a prudent decision.

Cross-matching

A cross-match is a test performed to determine whether there are antibodies in the patient's plasma against the red blood cells of the donor and *vice versa*. When a dog has received a prior transfusion, even with a compatible blood type, it is essential to cross-match the blood between the donor and recipient if the patient is receiving the transfusion 3–4 days after another transfusion. It is also important to perform a cross-match if a dog has an unknown history that may include a prior transfusion.

The traditional tube cross-matching procedure is performed with washed EDTA-anticoagulated blood from the recipient and the potential donor being mixed together to see if agglutination occurs. Cross-matching detects whether antibodies strongly react to red blood cell antigens and, therefore, decreases the chance of an acute haemolytic transfusion occurring. Cross-matching does not, however, eliminate the chance of an immediate or delayed reaction altogether, as it does not detect antibodies that may arise only following the transfusion. Nor does it detect antibodies to white blood cells or platelets, and it cannot detect the potential for acute hypersensitivity reactions or reactions based on non-immune causes.

Blood products and component therapy

Blood is composed of a variety of cells and components that each has their own role within the patient. Whole blood comprises red blood cells (RBCs), platelets, white blood cells (WBCs) and plasma. Plasma also contains coagulation factors, plasma proteins, antibodies and immunoglobulins.

Component therapy is the use of products that have been created from a single blood donation, each of which can be used for specific patient needs.

Fresh whole blood

Fresh whole blood is blood that is collected directly from the donor into a closed collection system and then administered directly to the recipient. Whole blood contains RBCs, functional platelets, coagulation factors and plasma proteins. Fresh whole blood is administered for a number of different reasons, including replacement therapy in patients with reduced oxygen-carrying capacity, generally as a result of haemorrhage or sometimes due to anaemia. Whole blood is often chosen in preference to blood components because it is the only product available to the patient at the time of transfusion. Fresh whole blood should be used within 4–6 hours of collection.

Stored whole blood

Stored whole blood is similar to fresh whole blood, except that these units are stored under refrigeration at 1–6°C until use. Platelets almost immediately begin to lose viability and function when refrigerated, with a 50% decrease occurring within the first 12–18 hours. Approximately 72 hours after refrigeration, there are no longer any viable platelets found within the stored unit (Abrams-Ogg, 2000). Labile clotting factors, such as factors V, VIII and von Willebrand factor (vWf), also lose function under refrigeration. There is very little loss of the non-labile clotting factors and antithrombin, which are thought to remain viable throughout the entire storage process (Abrams-Ogg, 2000). The administration of stored whole blood is similar to that of fresh whole blood, but obviously the platelets will not be viable.

Packed red blood cells

Packed red blood cells (PRBCs) are produced when a unit of fresh whole blood is centrifuged. PRBC units provide mainly RBCs and contain little plasma components. Packed red cell units should be stored in a specialized blood bank fridge, a designated blood product fridge, or in a laboratory fridge that has a separate area for the storage of blood products (Figure 20.17).

The main indication for the use of PRBCs is anaemia, but packed red cell units can also be administered to patients requiring a fresh whole blood transfusion, where no donor is available and the patient requires an immediate source of red cells.

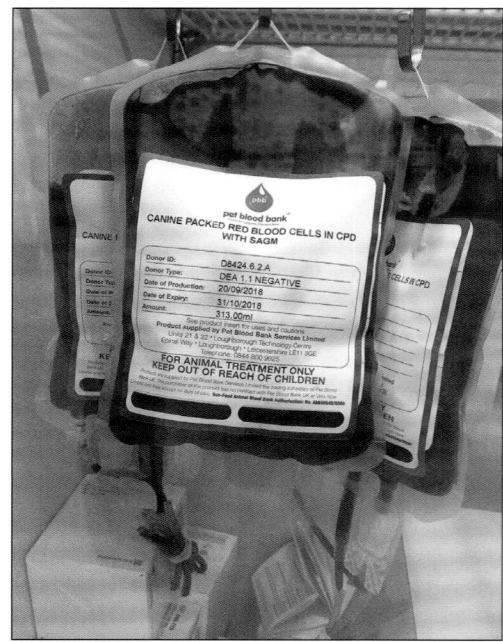

20.17 Packed red blood cells correctly suspended in a blood refrigerator.

Plasma products

Fresh frozen plasma (FFP)

This is defined as the plasma portion separated from the red cells via centrifugation and subsequently frozen to –18°C within 24 hours of collection (Figure 20.18). FFP expires within 1 year of preparation and collection. Once stored for 1 year, the unit should be relabelled as frozen plasma (FP) and can be stored for an additional 4 years. FFP contains coagulation factors (factors II, VII, IX, X), albumin and immunoglobulins.

Frozen plasma

This includes plasma that is unable to be frozen within 24 hours of collection or FFP that has been stored for 1 year and subsequently relabelled as frozen plasma (with a 4-year

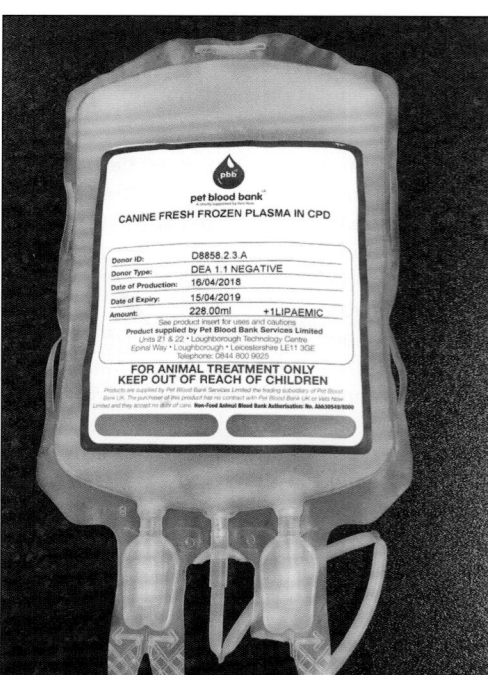

20.18

Unit of fresh frozen plasma.

shelf-life). Frozen plasma does not contain labile clotting factors (factors V, VIII, IX, vWf), but does contain non-labile clotting factors (factors II, VII, X) and plasma proteins such as albumin and globulin.

Cryoprecipitate

Cryoprecipitate is made by slowly thawing a unit of FFP at a steady temperature (4°C) until the unit has a slush-like frothy appearance. The unit is then centrifuged at 5000 x g for 5–7 minutes. The supernatant is removed and the small amount of precipitate remaining is the cryoprecipitate. This contains 50% factor VIII/vWf from the original unit, 20–40% fibinogen and some factor XIII. Cryoprecipitate is the treatment of choice for haemophilia A, von Willebrand disease and hypo-fibrinogenaemia.

Cryoprecipitate poor plasma (cryopoor plasma or cryosupernatant)

This is the supernatant that was removed during the production of cryoprecipitate. Following thawing and centrifugation, it is refrozen at less than –18°C within 24 hours. Cryoprecipitate poor plasma contains the remaining clotting factors, including the vitamin K dependent clotting factors (factors II, VII, IX, X), plus albumin and immunoglobulins. Cryoprecipitate poor plasma can be administered for vitamin K dependent coagulopathies (e.g. rodenticide toxicities) and immunoglobulin transfer.

Volume of blood products required

Once an animal has been typed and an appropriate component identified, the next step is to determine the volume of blood product to transfuse. This is determined by a set of factors, including the recipient's medical status, combined with the following calculation:

Donor blood (ml) (in anticoagulant) =

$$80 \text{ (dog) or } 60 \text{ (cat)} \times \text{BW (kg)} \times \left(\frac{\text{Desired PCV} - \text{recipient PCV}}{\text{PCV of the blood to be transfused}} \right)$$

How to set up and administer blood transfusions
Filters and transfusion sets

Whole blood and blood products should always be administered via an appropriate blood filter to eliminate the possibility of clots and other tissue components in the blood creating a potential embolus. Filters used in companion animals range from 170–230 μm. When transfusing a small volume into a cat or small dog (i.e. <60 ml), a haemonate filter is indicated (Figure 20.19). These filters incorporate less dead space than transfusion sets (which leave a significant volume of blood in the line) and keep out platelets and fibrin that pass through a standard filter. A standard transfusion set contains a 170 μm filter; these catch most of the macro-aggregates but fewer of the microaggregates than haemonate filters.

Fluid and blood administration pumps

The debate regarding the use of fluid/blood administration pumps is ongoing. Some clinicians are convinced that only

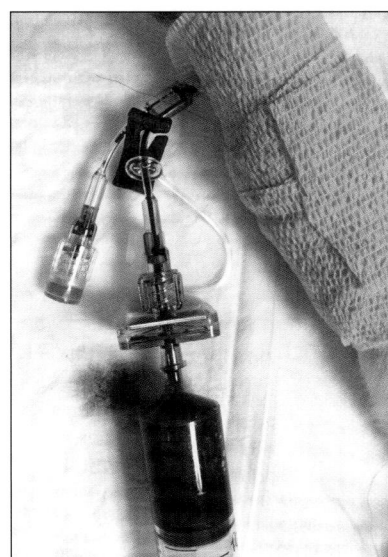

20.19 Inline haemonate blood filter.

by using an infusion pump can the volume and the rate of administration of RBC products be controlled, whilst others opposed to their use point to the damage sustained by RBCs caused by the pumps.

Recent studies

Two recent studies evaluated this issue:
- The study by McDevitt et al. (2011) reported the following findings:
  - 100% chance of PRBC survival to 49 days post-transfusion with gravity delivery (no pump)
  - 50% chance of PRBC survival to 49 days with a volumetric pump (peristaltic intravenous pump)
  - 0% chance of PBRC survival beyond 24 hours with a syringe pump.

  It is important to note that the syringe pumps pushed the blood through an 18 μm pore size filter instead of a 170–260 μm filter, which was used with the administration set; this was noted as a potentially significant contributing factor to the low PRBC survival rate.
- The study by Heikes and Ruaux (2014) on cat blood found that there was no difference in PRBC survival time up to 42 days' post-transfusion between gravity delivery and syringe pump infusions, despite the difference in filter pore size.

While gravity flow with close monitoring of rate and volume may seem to be indicated by one study, more research needs to be undertaken before a broad statement recommendation for blood transfusion via 'pump versus no pump' can be made (at least in dogs).

If infusion via a pump is elected, blood should be administered through a pump that will do minimal to no damage to the RBCs. To determine which pumps are 'safe' to administer red blood cell products, the manufacturer should be contacted directly to discuss whether their pumps have been evaluated for red blood cell transfusion. Most infusion pumps are intended to administer crystalloids and they may incorporate rollers or wheel mechanisms that crush the red blood cells. Whilst research in dogs has shown that pumps approved for transfusing human blood are also typically 'okay' for transfusing canine blood, dog RBCs are slightly more fragile than human RBCs. Some practices administer all red blood cell products using a filter, 3-way tap and a syringe to run blood through the syringe pump; this set-up is acceptable as the force is exerted from behind the syringe and does not compress the actual fluid line.

Blood temperature

When large volumes need to be rapidly administered (especially into small patients), blood products should be carefully warmed to no more than 37°C (and should not exceed 42°C) prior to administration to the patient in order to minimize heat loss and prevent hypothermia, as well as to reduce vasoconstriction. However, for typical administration rates, the blood being administered will reach room temperature before entering the patient and thus will not create a hypothermic reaction. Active warming efforts should be directed at raising the core temperature of hypothermic patients, rather than at increasing the temperature of the blood being transfused, as this is more effective and less damaging to the red blood cells.

Frozen plasma can be placed into two sealed plastic bags and placed into a water bath for warming. Plasma should not be thawed in boiling water as this will coagulate the plasma proteins. In emergency situations (i.e. massive haemorrhage as a result of a road traffic accident), a bag of blood can be removed from the refrigerator and given at a rapid rate, as long as the blood in the intravenous line is warmed by passing through some form of warm water bath.

Administration rate

In normovolaemic patients, blood should be administered at a rate of 5–10 ml/kg/h; this rate can be increased to 20 ml/kg/h in severely hypovolaemic animals. In patients at risk of intravascular volume overload (i.e. animals with cardiac or renal impairment), the rate can be decreased to 2 ml/kg/h. Blood is administered at a slower rate for the first 30 minutes of transfusion (0.25 ml/kg over the first 30 min) with the remainder delivered over 1–4 hours, depending on the volume to be given and the medical condition of the patient.

In emergency situations (e.g. severe haemorrhage), blood can be administered as rapidly as deemed necessary. Whole blood or blood components should not be infused over a period longer than 4 hours as this greatly increases the risk of bacterial contamination. Blood products should not be administered concurrently with fluids that contain calcium (i.e. Hartmann's solution, lactated Ringer's solution) as this can cause chelation, or with hypotonic fluids (i.e. 5% dextrose in water) as these substances can cause RBCs to lyse.

Plasma transfusions are typically administered at an initial rate of <5 ml/kg/h for the first 15–30 minutes, which is then increased to 5–10 ml/kg/h if no signs of complications are seen. Rates can be reduced to 1–2 ml/kg/h for patients at risk of circulatory overload.

Transfusion reactions

Whilst blood typing and cross-matching donors and their potential recipients significantly reduces the chances of acute haemolytic transfusion reactions, they do not eliminate the possibility of transfusion reactions altogether. This is because they do not detect antibodies to white blood cells or platelets, do not detect weakly binding antibodies and cannot detect the potential for acute hypersensitivity reactions or reactions based on non-immune causes. Blood contains many components, including red blood cells, white blood cells, proteins, platelets and potentially infectious agents, all of which are capable of causing a reaction in a patient receiving a blood transfusion. Considering the risk of a transfusion reaction cannot be eliminated, risk is further reduced by monitoring patients closely during the procedure.

Not all transfusion reactions are alike and they are classified according to their aetiology and the timeframe in which they occur: immune versus non-immune reactions; and immediate versus delayed reactions. Each type of transfusion reaction is important but treated differently.

Immediate transfusion reactions

Immune-mediated

- **Haemolytic transfusion reactions** may be considered the most serious. This type of reaction involves antibodies present in the recipient's plasma destroying the donor's red blood cells, resulting in intravascular haemolysis. Clinical signs include pyrexia, tachycardia or bradycardia, hypotension, dyspnoea (more commonly observed in cats), cyanosis, vomiting, diarrhoea, weakness, seizures, collapse, haemoglobinaemia, haemoglobinuria and, potentially, cardiac arrest. Treatment involves stopping the transfusion immediately and aggressive supportive care. Intensive monitoring, including blood pressure measurement and urine output should be performed.
- **Febrile reactions.** These usually occur due to an antibody reaction against donor leucocytes or platelet antigens. Clinical signs involve an increase in body temperature by 1–2°C within 1–2 hours of the transfusion being administered. These types of transfusion reactions are often self-limiting and treatment commonly involves slowing or stopping the transfusion and the administration of antihistamines.
- **Urticarial reactions** occur due to binding of the antigen from the donor's blood products to preformed antibodies bound to the recipient's mast cells and basophils, which subsequently degranulate. Clinical signs include pruritus, erythema and urticaria. Acute allergic reactions potentially manifest as signs of anaphylactic shock, including vomiting, dyspnoea and non-cardiogenic pulmonary oedema. Treatment involves slowing or stopping the transfusion, the administration of antihistamines and (potentially) corticosteroids if the clinical signs do not improve.
- **Non-cardiogenic pulmonary oedema/transfusion-related acute lung injury.** This is thought to involve leucocyte (white blood cell) antigen reactions with leucocyte aggregates trapped in the pulmonary circulation. Clinical signs include respiratory distress without other signs of volume overload or acute hypersensitivity. Treatment involves the administration of intravenous fluids and oxygen therapy.

Non-immune-mediated

These transfusion reactions generally arise due to problems during blood collection, administration and/or storage of donor blood.

- **Sepsis** can occur due to bacterial contamination of the blood product. Clinical signs of a septic reaction include pyrexia, hypotension, hypoglycaemia and DIC. Treatment includes culture of the blood administered, antibiotics and supportive care.

- **Circulatory overload** can occur due to the administration of a large volume of blood, or very rapid administration. Clinical signs of circulatory overload may include respiratory compromise, including increased respiratory rate and effort, and a cough.
- **Citrate toxicity** can occur due to the rapid infusion of products with citrate anticoagulants, which cause hypocalcaemia. This condition is more likely to occur in patients with hepatic impairment as they have a reduced capacity to deal with citrate. Clinical signs include vomiting, tremors, muscle spasms and cardiac arrest. Treatment involves stopping the transfusion and, if the condition does not improve, the slow administration of intravenous calcium gluconate, whilst monitoring the ECG and heart rate.
- **Haemolysis** can arise due to excessive warming, cooling or damage to the RBCs during administration. Clinical signs include haemoglobinaemia and haemoglobinuria without the concurrent signs present in an immune-mediated haemolytic reaction. Treatment is not required, but it should be noted that the blood transfusion will not be effective.
- **Hyperammonaemia** can result from the excessive accumulation of ammonia during the storage of blood products. This is more commonly seen in patients with liver disease. Central nervous system signs resembling hepatic encephalopathy may also be seen. Supportive treatment is required and care should be taken to administer 'fresh' blood products in patients with liver disease.

Delayed transfusion reactions

Delayed transfusion reactions arise due to the development of antibodies to the antigen in the transfused blood products. This reaction can occur any time from 3 days to 2 weeks following a transfusion, with antibodies developing and adhering to the transfused cells. These cells are removed from the recipient's circulation and extravascular haemolysis occurs. No clinical signs are observed other than a drop in PCV.

Infectious disease transmission can occur due to the administration of transfusions; hence, it is important that potential donors are screened appropriately.

Fluid therapy in exotic pets

Small mammals

Small mammals lose very little water as sweat, due to a lack of sweat glands, but because they have an increased metabolic rate and a large lung and renal filtration surface area in relation to volume, they do lose large volumes of fluid via respiration and glomerular filtration. This means that small mammals have significantly higher maintenance fluid requirements (almost twice that of dogs and cats) (Girling, 2013). In addition, a patient that presents with diarrhoea, respiratory disease or skin infections, can have significantly increased fluid requirements.

Fluid selection

Common fluid types used in exotic pets include lactated Ringer's and Hartmann's solutions, which are often used for rehydration and maintenance fluid requirements, as well as for fluid therapy during routine surgical procedures. The lactate makes these crystalloid solutions very useful for small mammals with metabolic acidosis as a result of chronic gastrointestinal problems, as it acts as a buffer for the acid.

Glucose and saline solutions (e.g. 0.45% NaCl + 5% dextrose) are useful in small mammals that have been anorexic for a length of time prior to presentation, in order to treat or prevent hypoglycaemia. These fluids may also be more suitable for guinea pigs who are prone to ketosis, but should preferably be given intravenously or intraosseously to avoid tissue irritation due to the glucose.

Hypertonic saline can be administered in small mammals that are acutely hypovolaemic and works in a similar manner in these groups of patients as it does in dogs and cats. Boluses of hypertonic saline may be given intravenously or intraosseously at a rate of 1–3 ml/kg bodyweight whilst measuring peripheral blood pressure in species such as rabbits and guinea pigs. Blood pressure is measured in a similar manner to cats and dogs (see Chapter 21); a Doppler probe is attached to the caudal aspect of the lower limb proximal to the foot with an inflatable cuff applied just below the elbow or hock, depending on whether the forelimb or hindlimb is used.

The greatest challenge is finding a cuff small enough to be effective (the width of the cuff needs to be around 40% of the circumference of the limb). Systolic blood pressure for most small mammals is similar to cats and dogs, at 120–130 mmHg.

Amino acid and vitamin supplements (e.g. Duphalyte®) are commonly used as additional nutritional support in small mammals, generally at a rate of 1 ml/kg/day (Girling, 2013). They are particularly useful in animals that are malnourished, those with a protein-losing enteropathy or nephropathy, and patients with hepatic disease or certain skin diseases (Girling, 2013). Amino acid and vitamin supplements are contraindicated in dehydration, hepatic encephalopathy, severe azotaemia, shock, congestive heart failure and significant electrolyte imbalances.

Colloids are also appropriate for use in small mammals; they are generally administered as a bolus following blood loss. In extreme cases, blood transfusion may be considered (particularly when the PCV decreases to 20% or less). Blood transfusion must be species-to-species, with blood collections typically being around 1% of the donor's bodyweight (Girling, 2013). Blood is generally collected using heparin or citrate acid dextrose as the anticoagulant. The blood collected should be immediately transferred to the recipient as a bolus, administering 1 ml over 5–6 minutes.

Calculating fluid requirements

Maintenance requirements

Maintenance fluid rates for small mammals are estimated to be 80–100 ml/kg/day; this is twice that required by dogs and cats and is due to the smaller surface area and higher metabolism in small mammals.

Fluid deficits

Estimation of fluid deficits in small mammals is very similar to that in larger mammals. It is generally assumed that 1% dehydration will require the administration of 10 ml/kg fluid to replace the deficit; this should be added to the ongoing maintenance requirements.

Estimated degree of dehydration in small mammals

Severity of dehydration estimated as a percentage of bodyweight	Clinical signs
3–5%	■ Slight lethargy ■ Tacky mucous membranes ■ Increased thirst
7–10%	■ Depression/dullness ■ Skin tenting ■ Dry mucous membranes ■ Dull corneas ■ Increased thirst ■ Anorexia
10–15%	■ Dull to comatose ■ Persistent skin tenting ■ Very dry mucous membranes

In patients with large fluid deficits, it may be necessary to restrict the administration of fluids to avoid fluid overload and pulmonary oedema. In these cases, the following protocol can be utilized:

- Day 1 – maintenance fluid levels + 50% of calculated dehydration deficit replacement volume
- Day 2 – maintenance fluid levels + 50% of calculated dehydration deficit replacement volume
- Day 3 – maintenance fluid levels.

In severely dehydrated patients, it may be necessary to replace the fluid deficit over 72 hours rather than 48 hours.

Routes of fluid administration

Oral

Oral fluid administration may be appropriate for mildly dehydrated patients, but in severe dehydration or hypovolaemia, this route is unlikely to be sufficient. Volumes of oral fluids are generally restricted to a maximum dose of 10 ml/kg at any one administration. For most debilitated patients, the use of oral fluids will require placement of a nasogastric or naso-oesophageal feeding tube.

Subcutaneous

The scruff region or lateral thorax are good locations for the administration of subcutaneous fluids. It is a technique often used for intraoperative or postoperative fluids, as well as maintenance fluids. A maximum fluid volume of 10 ml/kg should be used and this should be divided over several sites. Fluid administration into the scruff of guinea pigs can be painful as this area is highly innervated and so is best avoided in this species.

Intraperitoneal

This technique is useful when intravenous or intraosseous fluid administration is not possible. For the administration of fluids, the animal should be tilted head downwards whilst in dorsal recumbency, thereby allowing the gastrointestinal tract contents to move away from the area where the injection is to be placed. This technique is, therefore, not used regularly in the conscious patient, as it can be aversive. After insertion of the needle in the animal's right lower quadrant at a 30 degree angle, aspiration should be performed before injecting, with any blood or other fluid indicating improper placement. If this occurs, the syringe should be removed and a replacement used. The volume of fluid to be administered varies from 20–30 ml in rabbits, 15–20 ml in guinea pigs and chinchillas, and 1–4 ml in rats, gerbils, hamsters and other small mammals.

Intravenous

Intravenous access can be achieved in many small mammal species, including rabbits, guinea pigs and ferrets. Irrespective of the species and the vein selected, ideally EMLA™ cream (a combination of lidocaine and prilocaine) should be applied to the site 30–40 minutes prior to catheter placement, or sedation/general anaesthesia may be required. Numerous sites can be used, depending on the species, but commonly include the marginal (lateral) ear vein in rabbits (Figure 20.20), the lateral saphenous vein in rabbits (Figure 20.21), guinea pigs and chinchillas, the cephalic vein in rabbits, guinea pigs and chinchillas and the lateral tail vein in rats and mice. Cricetidae (gerbils and hamsters) are extremely difficult to administer intravenous injections to and so if central venous access is required, consideration should be given to using the intraosseous route.

Intraosseous

Intraosseous catheter placement requires anaesthesia and aseptic preparation of the catheter placement site, but can be a life-saving procedure where it is not possible to catheterize a vein and rapid support of blood pressure is required. The majority of fluids and medications that can be administered intravenously may be administered via this route. Common sites for placement include the proximal femur, proximal tibia and proximal humerus.

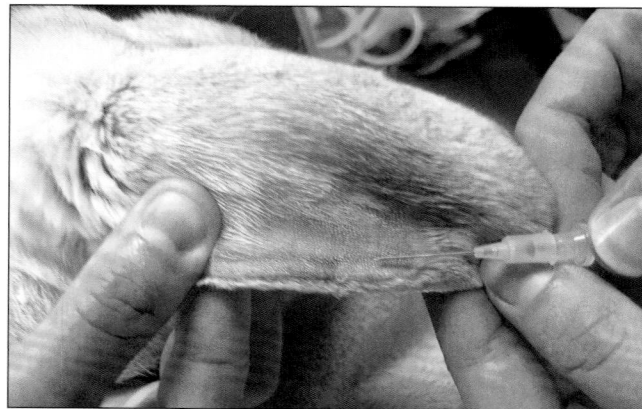

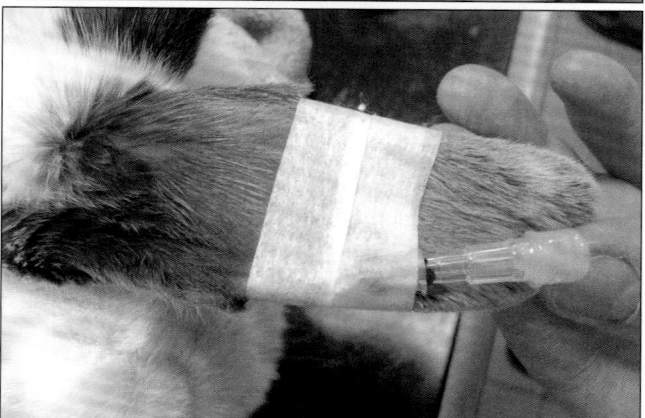

20.20 Venepuncture of the marginal ear vein in a rabbit. (Reproduced from the *BSAVA Manual of Rabbit Medicine and Surgery, 2nd edn*)

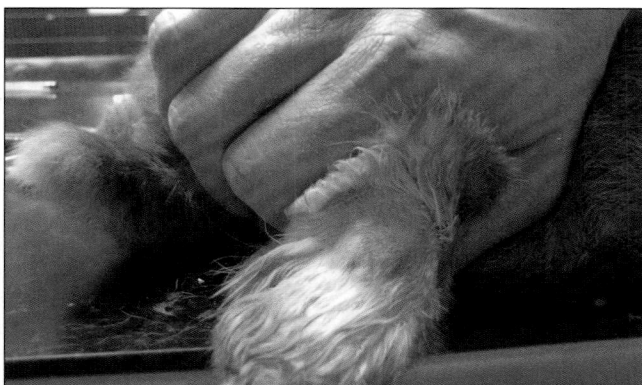
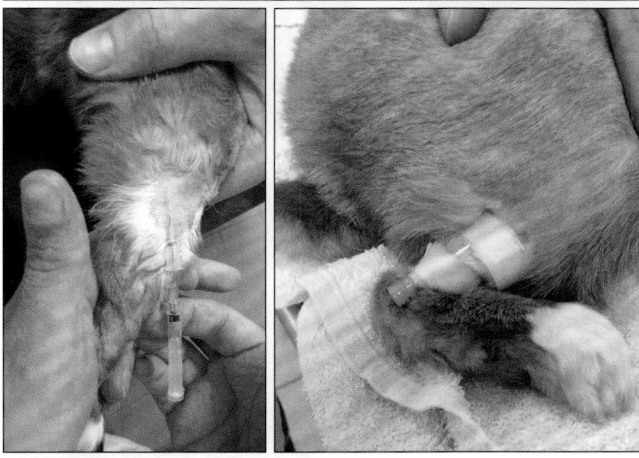

20.21 Venepuncture of the lateral saphenous vein in a rabbit. (Reproduced from the *BSAVA Manual of Rabbit Medicine and Surgery, 2nd edn*)

Hypovolaemic shock

In hypovolaemic shock, fluids are generally administered at body temperature at a rate of 10–15 ml/kg or, in severe cases, hypertonic saline may be administered at 3–4 ml/kg intravenously or intraosseously. Hypertonic saline works in a similar way is these patients as it does in dogs and cats. Colloids may also be administered (e.g. Geloplasma®) at a rate of 5 ml/kg intravenously over 5–10 minutes. A repeat dose of a crystalloid can be administered after 15–20 minutes if the desired response to the initial fluid bolus is not seen. Patients should also be warmed whilst being treated for hypovolaemia as the adrenergic receptors do not tend to respond to fluid therapy and catecholamines if the body temperature is less than 36.6°C.

Birds

Fluid selection

Lactated Ringer's and/or Hartmann's solutions are useful for rehydration, ongoing maintenance and surgical fluids (both for maintenance as well as the potential replacement of fluid losses). In birds, fluids are commonly delivered by the intravenous or intraosseous route. In anorexic birds, glucose/saline fluids can be useful to prevent hypoglycaemia; in dehydrated patients, a 5% glucose/saline or lactated Ringer's/Hartmann's solution can be administered.

As with small mammals, amino acid/vitamin supplements (such as Duphalyte®) may be used in malnourished patients or those suffering from protein-losing conditions, and can be administered at a rate of 1 ml/kg/day. However, it should be noted that toxicity issues have been reported in some species of bird, such as raptors and pigeons, when using compounds that contain vitamin B6 (pyridoxine). Thus, Duphalyte® and other vitamin B6 containing compounds should be avoided in these groups of birds (Samour *et al.*, 2016). Colloids can be used in birds, most commonly following haemorrhage, but also in hypoproteinaemic patients to help support colloid oncotic pressure.

In patients where haemorrhage is significant, a blood transfusion may be indicated (normally if the PCV drops below 15%). Transfusions should be performed within species (e.g. cockatiel to cockatiel) and the blood sample can be placed into citrate acid dextrose anticoagulant or, in extreme cases, heparin may be used. Alternatively, hypertonic saline (7.2–7.5%) can be used to attempt to maintain blood pressure at doses of 1–3 ml/kg bodyweight.

Systolic blood pressure monitoring should be performed, where possible, by placing a cuff on the distal humerus or femur and the Doppler probe on the medial surface of the proximal ulna (proximal ulnar artery) or tibiotarsus (medial metatarsal artery). Cuff widths should be 40% of the circumference of the humerus or distal femur, which means that for small avian patients the commercial cuffs available are too large. Systolic blood pressure monitoring using an indirect method correlates better with directly measured blood pressure in birds than it does in mammals (Lichtenberger and Ko 2007). A blood pressure below 90 mmHg is considered hypovolaemic for birds (and above 200 mmHg is considered hypervolaemic).

Calculating fluid requirements

Maintenance requirements

Maintenance fluid levels in birds are similar to those in dogs and cats at 50 ml/kg/day.

Fluid deficits

Critically ill birds are generally assumed to be at least 5–10% dehydrated, with 1% dehydration requiring 1 ml/kg bodyweight of fluid to correct it. Once calculated, the deficit should be added to the ongoing maintenance requirements.

Estimated degree of dehydration in birds

Severity of dehydration estimated as a percentage of bodyweight	Clinical signs
3–5%	■ Slight lethargy ■ Tacky mucous membranes ■ Increased thirst ■ Increased heart rate
7–10%	■ Depression/dullness ■ Skin tenting ■ Slower return of skin over the eyelid or foot ■ Increased thirst ■ Dry mucous membranes ■ Dull corneas ■ Wrinkled skin in chicks
12–18%	■ Dull to comatose ■ Skin tenting remains ■ Sunken eyes ■ Desiccated mucous membranes

When fluid deficits are significant, these may need to be replaced over a longer period of time to avoid fluid overload. One suggested protocol by Girling (2013) is as follows:

- Day 1 – maintenance fluid levels + 50% of calculated dehydration deficit replacement volume
- Day 2 – maintenance fluid levels + 50% of calculated dehydration deficit replacement volume
- Day 3 – maintenance fluid levels.

Routes of fluid administration

As a general rule, isotonic crystalloids can be administered at a rate of 10–15 ml/kg per bolus, but when needed large volumes of up to 30 ml/kg can administered without causing problems, provided this is performed slowly over 10–15 minutes. Fluid administration in birds needs to be carried out accurately. The use of syringe drivers and fluid pumps is ideal as they allow the accurate administration of small volumes of fluid under general anaesthesia. Drip sets are not well tolerated in the conscious bird and so the daily fluid rate is often split into several (4–6) individual boluses administered across the day.

Oral

Oral fluid administration is carried out via a crop tube. This method is also used for supplying nutrition. Maximal volumes of fluid or food that can be administered as one 'bolus' range from 0.5 ml in a budgerigar to 15 ml in large macaws (Girling 2013) (Figure 20.22).

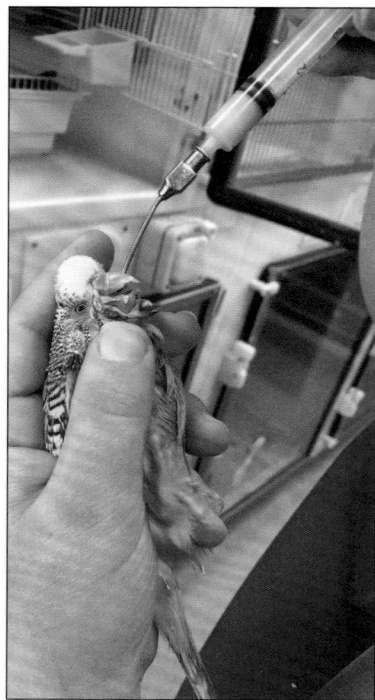

20.22 Crop feeding a budgerigar.

Intravenous

Avian vessels are extremely fragile and small; it may be possible to place small catheters (25 to 27 G) in budgerigars or small parrots, and slightly larger catheters (23 to 25 G) in larger parrots or waterfowl. Butterfly catheters should not be used as these are likely to damage the vessel. Veins that can be used include: the right jugular vein in most species; the basilic vein (brachial vein) and ulnar vein in larger birds; and the median metatarsal vein in waterfowl and poultry.

Intraosseous

Spinal needles are useful for the administration of intraosseous fluids; they have a central stylet that prevents clogging of the lumen of the needle on insertion. Hypodermic needles can also be used for intraosseous 'catheter' placement and for the administration of subcutaneous fluids. For most birds, 21–25 G needles are appropriate. Common sites for intraosseous catheter placement are the distal or proximal ulna and the proximal tibiotarsus (Figure 20.23). The femur and humerus should not be used as they connect to the air sacs and fluid administration via this route will lead to drowning of the bird.

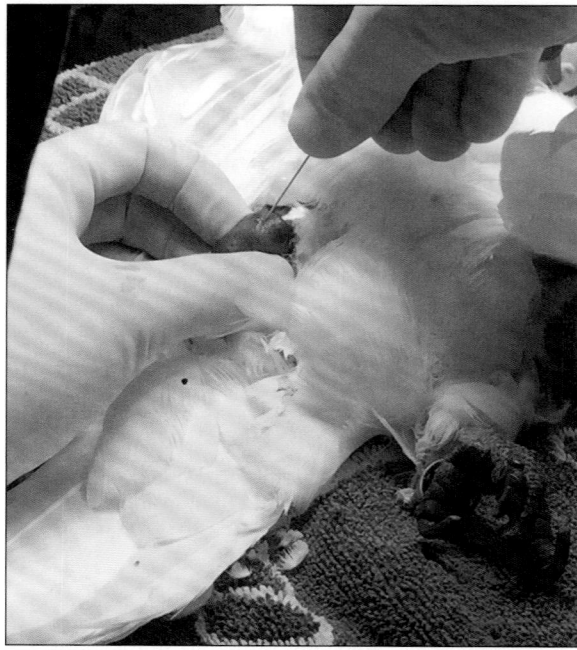

20.23 Placement of an intraosseous catheter into the tibiotarsus of an Umbrella Cockatoo.

Reptiles and amphibians

Reptiles are generally good at conserving water, with most reptile species being uricotelic (i.e. they excrete uric acid rather than urea as their main form of urinary protein waste product) (Girling, 2013). Since uric acid requires very little water to be excreted along with it, their maintenance requirements are much lower than other taxa (e.g. mammals). Some of the aquatic and semi-aquatic species of reptile (e.g. Crocodylia) excrete predominantly ammonia and sometimes urea, as well as small amounts of uric acid. Aquatic amphibians excrete ammonia and terrestrial amphibians generally excrete urea.

There is wide variation in terms of conservation of fluids, and therefore maintenance fluid requirements in different reptile species; much depends on their normal habitat and the route by which the species normally consumes water. Herbivorous reptiles (e.g. *Testudo* spp. of tortoises) obtain most of their daily fluid requirements via their diet. An additional consideration is that many reptiles do not drink from water bowls but will lick water droplets from leaves (e.g. chameleons, green iguanas, etc.) and so the way water is presented is important to avoid dehydration. Temperature is another factor to consider. Reptiles need to be kept at the appropriate temperature, their 'preferred optimum temperature zone' (POTZ). If this does not happen, then they are unable to achieve the correct (preferred) body temperature and inefficient body functions, including water usage, will occur (Girling, 2013).

Fluid selection

Lactated Ringer's and/or Hartmann's solutions are commonly used for rehydration, ongoing maintenance and surgical fluids. Hypertonic saline can be used in hypovolaemic patients, but most reptiles and amphibians have low blood pressure normally (often a systolic pressure of 40–50 mmHg) and so care should be taken with these fluids to avoid cardiac overload. Following periods of anorexia, glucose/saline fluids can be useful to prevent hypoglycaemia. Historic publications suggested that the isotonicity of extracellular fluid in reptiles is lower than that of mammals (0.8% for reptiles *versus* 0.9% mammals); however, more recent studies in lizards such as bearded dragons and chelonians have suggested that the isotonicity in many commonly kept reptiles is similar to that of mammals (0.9%), and so mammalian isotonic fluids are generally considered appropriate.

As with small mammals, amino acid/vitamin supplements (such as Duphalyte®) can be used in malnourished patients or those suffering from protein-losing conditions, and are generally administered at 1 ml/kg/day. Colloids can also be used in reptiles, most commonly following haemorrhage, but also in hypoproteinaemic patients to help support colloid osmotic pressure.

Blood transfusions are generally indicated when the PCV has dropped below 5–10%; reptiles (dependent on species) have much lower PCVs compared with birds and mammals, typically around 20–40% (Girling, 2013). Blood transfusions can be administered by either the intravenous or intraosseous routes. As with other species, same species transfusion should be performed (e.g. green iguana to green iguana). Up to 2% bodyweight of blood may be taken from healthy species, ideally into a pre-heparinized or citrate phosphate anticoagulant-coated syringe, and following collection should be immediately transfused into the recipient.

Calculating fluid requirements

Fluid rates of 10–50 ml/kg/day have been suggested for the rehydration of reptiles and amphibians, with many authors assuming reptile daily maintenance is approximately 25 ml/kg/day. As with other species, in reptiles it is assumed that 1% dehydration (or a 1% increase in PCV) is equivalent to a 10 ml/kg fluid requirement.

Estimated degree of dehydration in reptiles and amphibians

Severity of dehydration estimated as a percentage of bodyweight	Clinical signs
3%	■ Decreased urates ■ Increased thirst ■ Slight lethargy
7%	■ Dullness ■ Skin tenting ■ Dull corneas ■ Increased thirst ■ Anorexia
10%	■ No urates/urine output ■ Dull to comatose ■ Persistent skin tenting ■ Desiccated mucous membranes

Overall, a 30 ml/kg/day fluid rate intravenously or intraosseously should not be routinely exceeded, irrespective of the level of dehydration present. This is due to the normal low blood pressure of reptiles, which if increased can lead to cardiac and renal overload; this means it may take weeks to rehydrate severely dehydrated patients.

Routes of fluid administration

As with other species, the main routes of administration of fluids include oral, subcutaneous, intracoelomic, intravenous and intraosseous routes. One major problem with the administration of fluids to most reptiles and amphibians is that the intravenous and intraosseous routes are often limited and therefore the intracoelomic route is commonly used in dehydrated reptiles. The intracoelomic route, however, has its limitations as both reptiles and amphibians do not possess a diaphragm (i.e. the thorax and abdomen are connected), meaning that when intraperitoneal fluids are administered, the fluid can result in compression of the lungs and lead to respiratory dysfunction (Girling, 2013). The intracoloemic route should not be used for administering glucose-containing fluids as it increases the risk of coelomitis. As with other species, a range of catheters, needles and syringe drivers can be used in reptiles and amphibians.

Oral

Stomach tubing of snakes is straightforward. Canine urinary catheters or cat and dog feeding tubes may be premeasured from the snout to the end of the first third of the length of the snake (approximate stomach position). The snake is held vertically and the lubricated tube gently inserted using a tongue depressor or plastic syringe as a mouth gag. Lizards are more difficult, but again a tube may be premeasured from the snout to the caudal end of the sternum (approximate stomach position). In chelonians, the tube length is measured from the snout with the head extended to the mid-abdominal plastral scute; removing the head from the shell can be the most challenging part of the procedure. However, if an oesophagostomy tube has been placed, which is common practice in debilitated chelonians, the oral route can be easily used for fluid as well as nutrition and medication administration.

Subcutaneous

In snakes, the lateral aspect of the dorsum in the caudal third of the body is a suitable location for subcutaneous fluid administration. In lizards, the lateral thoracic area can be used for the administration of small volumes of fluid, but the volume needs to be restricted (usually less than 1–2 ml per site), and frequently the development of a dark, pigmented area around the injection site may make it a less suitable technique. In chelonians, the administration of fluids in the area cranial to the hindlimbs, or in the skin folds lateral to the neck, can be performed easily in mildly dehydrated patients and these sites permit the administration of relatively large volumes of fluid.

Intracoelomic

The intracoelomic route is appropriate in more severely dehydrated animals, as the vasculature in this region allows for better fluid absorption. This procedure is relatively simple to perform in snakes. The needle insertion site in snakes is between the ribs, just through the body wall in the caudal third of the body, cranial to the vent, two rows of scales dorsal to the ventral scutes. In lizards, the patient positioning required for the administration of fluids may make the procedure too stressful, as the animal needs to be placed in dorsal recumbency with its head downwards. This technique can be used in chelonians, using the fossa cranial to each hindlimb, but the volume of fluid administered needs to be restricted to 20–25 ml/kg/day otherwise, due to the rigid shell, the fluid administered will place too much pressure on the lung fields.

Intravenous

In snakes, there are no major vessels that are suitable for catheterization and the administration of fluids; if intravenous fluids are required in snakes, the ventral tail vein, palatine vein, jugular vein and intracardiac site can be used with a hypodermic needle. In small lizards, the intravenous route can be difficult, or even impossible, in conscious patients, but there are a few sites which can be used, particularly in larger reptiles, including the cephalic vein, jugular vein and ventral tail vein, however, catheter placement is difficult. The intravenous route is suitable in chelonians via the jugular vein for catheterization or dorsal tail vein for a one-off bolus of intravenous fluids. In larger amphibians, particularly anurans (frogs or toads), the ventral midline abdominal vein may be used.

Intraosseous

This route of fluid administration is impossible in snakes but is useful in lizards, particularly smaller species where the intravenous route is not possible. Suitable sites for intraosseous fluids include the distal femur and proximal tibia. Intraosseous fluid administration is possible in chelonians via the plastrocarapacial junction/pillar or the proximal tibia, although the former is difficult in adult tortoises due to the thickness of the shell and the latter site may require placing a cotton wool ball into the fossa in front of the hindlimb to prevent retraction of the limb in to the shell and so damage to the catheter. The distal femur may be used in large anurans.

Cutaneous

Amphibians are unique in that the cutaneous route can be used, due to their semi-permeable skin, as absorption occurs across the skin membrane. Water is directly absorbed especially via the cloaca. When an amphibian is placed in water this also encourages drinking, appetite and defecation. This route is only suitable in mildly dehydrated animals and should involve the use of oxygenated, dechlorinated, plain water warmed to the patient's preferred body temperature.

Acknowledgement

The editors would like to acknowledge the contribution of Amanda Boag to this chapter.

References and further reading

Abrams-Ogg A (2000) Practical blood transfusion. In: *BSAVA Manual of Canine and Feline Haematology and Transfusion Medicine*, ed. M Day *et al.*, pp. 263–302. BSAVA Publications, Gloucester

Aldridge P and O'Dwyer L (2013) *Practical Emergency and Critical Care Nursing*. Wiley Blackwell, Oxford

Burkitt-Creedon JM and Davis H (2012) *Advanced Monitoring and Procedures for Small Animal Emergency and Critical Care*. Wiley Blackwell, Oxford

Davis H, Jensen T, Johnson A *et al.* (2013) AAHA/AAFP fluid therapy guidelines for dogs and cats. *Journal of the American Animal Hospital Association* **49**, 149–159

Fenger-Eriksen C, Tonnwawn E, Ingersley J and Sorensen B (2009) Mechanisms of hydroxyethyl starch-induced dilutional coagulopathy. *Journal of Thrombosis and Haemostasis* **7**, 1009–1105

Girling S (2013) *Veterinary Nursing of Exotic Pets*. Wiley Blackwell, Oxford

Heikes BW and Ruaux CG (2014) Effect of syringe and aggregate filter administration on survival of transfused autologous fresh feline red blood cells. *Journal of Veterinary Emergency and Critical Care* **24**, 162–167

Lichtenberger M and Ko J (2007) Critical care monitoring *Veterinary Clinics of North America: Exotic Animal Practice* **10(2)**, 317–344

McDevitt RI, Ruaux CG and Baltzer WI (2011) Influence of transfusion technique on survival of autologous red blood cells in the dog. *Journal of Veterinary Emergency and Critical Care* **21**, 209–216

National Institute for Health and Care Excellence (2017) Intravenous fluid therapy in adults in hospital. (Available at: https://www.nice.org.uk/guidance/CG174)

Roberts C (2013) The VN's role in jugular catheter care and patient management. *Veterinary Nursing Journal* **28**, 356–360

Samour J, Perlman J, Kinne J, Baskar V, Wernery U and Dorrestein G (2016) Vitamin B6 (pyridoxine hydrochloride) toxicosis in falcons. *Journal of Zoo & Wildlife Medicine* **47(2)**, 601–608

Serrano S and Boag AK (2014) Pulmonary contusions and haemorrhage. In: *Small Animal Critical Care Medicine, 2nd edn*, ed. DC Silverstein and K Hopper, pp. 138–144. Elsevier, Oxford.

Weil AB and Ko J (2006) Intravenous indwelling catheters: use and care. *NAVC Clinician's Brief*

Whitlock E (2012) Fluid therapy and intravenous access in exotic mammals. *Proceedings of the 9th ECC UK Annual Congress*

Zarychanski R, Abou-Setta AM, Turgeon AF *et al.* (2013) Association of hydroxyethyl starch administration with mortality and acute kidney injury in critically ill patients. *Journal of the American Medical Association* **309**, 678–688

Self-assessment questions

1. Identify five causes of abnormal fluid loss.
2. State from which compartment hypotonic fluid is lost in cases of primary water depletion.
3. List four possible routes of fluid administration.
4. On physical examination, state the techniques used to identify reduced tissue perfusion.
5. What laboratory sample is useful in the assessment of reduced tissue perfusion?
6. List the main types of crystalloid fluid.
7. List the three types of artificial colloids.
8. State the indications for intraosseous catheter placement.
9. List the bones most appropriate for intraosseous catheter placement in reptiles.

Chapter 21

Anaesthesia and analgesia

Jo Murrell and Vicky Ford-Fennah

Learning objectives

After studying this chapter, readers will have the knowledge to:

■ **Apply the principles of anaesthesia and recognize the physiological effects of anaesthetic drugs on body systems**
■ **Appreciate the physiology and assessment of pain in animals**
■ **Recognize the principles of premedication, induction and maintenance of anaesthesia**
■ **Explain the use of local anaesthetic techniques**
■ **Describe the steps necessary to evaluate and prepare an animal for anaesthesia**
■ **Prepare and use various types of anaesthetic equipment, including endotracheal tubes, equipment for administering inhalation anaesthetics, non-rebreathing and rebreathing circuits**
■ **Explain the principles and risks of monitoring an anaesthetized animal, including the techniques and equipment required**
■ **Assist the veterinary surgeon in preparing, operating and maintaining anaesthetic equipment used in dogs, cats and exotic pets**
■ **Assist with anaesthetic preparation, premedication and induction of anaesthesia in dogs, cats and exotic pets**
■ **Monitor small animal anaesthesia and recovery**
■ **Recognize and respond to anaesthetic emergencies**

Introduction

General anaesthesia is routinely carried out in small animal practice and most cats and dogs will receive at least one general anaesthetic during their lifetime, often for the purposes of neutering. Many of the principles of anaesthesia in dogs and cats also apply to exotic pets, however some aspects of exotic pet anaesthesia differ and information on anaesthesia in these species is given at the end of this chapter.

Veterinary nurses play a critical role in the management of anaesthetized patients, commonly with responsibility for:

■ The administration of premedication drugs
■ Establishing intravenous access before induction of anaesthesia
■ Maintenance and setting up of the anaesthetic machine and monitoring equipment
■ Monitoring the patient during the anaesthesia and recovery period.

Veterinary nurses are also critical in pain assessment during the perioperative period. It is therefore imperative that they have a good understanding of the principles of anaesthesia, including the pharmacology and the use of anaesthesia equipment for both maintenance and monitoring of anaesthesia.

Who may carry out anaesthesia in animals?

The Royal College of Veterinary Surgeons (RCVS) has clearly defined the procedures that are permitted to be carried out by a qualified Registered Veterinary Nurse (RVN) and by Student Veterinary Nurses (SVN) enrolled with the RCVS with regard to anaesthesia:

■ Inducing anaesthesia by administration of a specific quantity of medicine directed by a veterinary surgeon may be carried out by a RVN or, under supervision by a veterinary surgeon, a SVN ➜

What is anaesthesia?

There are many different definitions of anaesthesia available in the literature.

Definition

For the purposes of this chapter, general anaesthesia is defined as a reversible immobile state that induces amnesia (loss of memory)

Both immobility and amnesia have useful clinical connections: the surgeon requires immobility, and the patients (certainly in the field of human anaesthesia) desire amnesia. The triad of anaesthesia has three components that contribute to the anaesthetized state:

- Muscle relaxation
- Unconsciousness
- Pain relief (analgesia/antinociception).

It is useful to think about the triad of anaesthesia when considering provision of a balanced anaesthesia protocol.

The principle of balanced anaesthesia

The underlying principle behind modern anaesthesia techniques is balanced anaesthesia. This can be defined as the use of multiple anaesthetic drugs in combination, in order to provide general anaesthesia. Instead of using a single anaesthetic agent for induction and maintenance of anaesthesia (e.g. the volatile anaesthetic agent isoflurane), for which high concentrations will be required to achieve the components of the anaesthesia triad, combinations of drugs are used. The side effects of most anaesthetic drugs are dose-dependent and the mechanisms by which these side effects occur vary for different classes of analgesic agent. Using combinations of drugs allows the dose of each individual agent to be reduced. Therefore, adoption of the principle of balanced anaesthesia usually allows for provision of better quality general anaesthesia associated with a reduction in cardiovascular and respiratory side effects.

Balanced anaesthesia may involve:

- Premedication with a sedative and analgesic drug
- Induction with an intravenous agent
- Maintenance with an inhalant agent
- Further analgesic drugs, if required (e.g. a constant rate infusion (CRI) of a short-acting opioid).

Effects of anaesthesia on major organ systems

Due to the profound effects of anaesthesia on most body organ systems, good preoperative assessment and the careful monitoring of animals during anaesthesia is vital in order to try and minimize physiological disturbances.

Brain

The mechanism by which most anaesthetic agents produce a state of anaesthesia is unknown, although it is suggested that agents act through a combination of effects on specific receptors in the central nervous system (CNS) and through an effect on the cell membrane of neuronal cells. Anaesthesia causes a reversible depression of CNS function, resulting in loss of consciousness.

Cardiovascular system

Depression of cardiovascular function is common during anaesthesia and may result from the central depressant effects of the drug (e.g. depression of the cardiovascular control centre in the brain) or through peripheral effects. This depression is usually manifest as a reduction in cardiac output and therefore blood flow to central and peripheral organs, with the potential to produce inadequate oxygenation of the tissues. Changes in the tone of blood vessels may also occur (peripheral vasodilation or vasoconstriction depending on the specific effects of the drugs that have been administered).

Respiratory system

Central depression of the respiratory centre in the brain is common during anaesthesia, leading to a reduced sensitivity to blood carbon dioxide (CO_2) concentration and reduced respiratory drive. This can result in:

- Hypercapnia (a higher concentration of CO_2 in the blood than normal)
- Hypoxia (when tissues receive an inadequate supply of oxygen, O_2).

Hypoxia occurs less frequently than hypercapnia because animals commonly receive >30% inspired O_2 during anaesthesia, which is higher than the O_2 concentration of room air. Reduced thoracic muscle tone can also reduce the effectiveness of ventilation, with the potential to cause hypercapnia.

Liver

The blood supply to the liver is via two routes: the hepatic artery and the portal vein. These two blood supplies work in tandem in order to maintain total liver blood flow within narrow limits. If portal blood supply decreases, the resistance in the hepatic artery is reduced in order to increase the blood supply via this route. All inhalant agents have the potential to reduce total liver blood flow through a reduction in cardiac output and through disturbing the reciprocal mechanism in the hepatic artery and portal vein.

Kidneys

The kidneys normally receive approximately 20% of total cardiac output, and adequate renal blood flow is essential to maintain normal renal function. General anaesthesia usually decreases renal blood flow, glomerular filtration rate, urine output and electrolyte excretion. These parameters usually return to normal a few hours after anaesthesia in healthy animals when the duration of anaesthesia is short.

Preparation for anaesthesia

Informed owner consent

Consent for carrying out an anaesthetic and the accompanying procedure must always be obtained (see Chapters 1 and 9). The purpose of the consent form is to record the client's agreement to treatment based on knowledge of what is involved and the likely consequences. The client may be the owner of the animal, someone acting with the authority of the owner or someone with other appropriate authority.

Before being asked to sign an anaesthesia consent form the person should be able to understand and retain the information provided and use it to come to a decision. Clients should be provided with the opportunity to read the form and ask questions before being asked to consent to the procedure or treatment. It is important to remember that children under the age of 16 should not be asked to sign a consent form.

Clinical history

It is important that, when possible, a full clinical history is obtained from the owner of every patient prior to anaesthesia. This will provide information on previous disease and anaesthetic history and will alert the anaesthetist to potential health problems at the time of presentation, which can be used to guide the clinical examination and the requirement for further evaluation before anaesthesia. Questions should be asked to obtain information on:

- The status of diagnosed chronic disease in the patient, including current medications such as non-steroidal anti-inflammatory drugs (NSAIDs), steroids, insulin, diuretics and cardiac medications
  - Generally, it is recommended that current medications are continued around the time of anaesthesia to avoid abrupt changes in drug regime; however, this must be determined on an individual animal and drug basis
  - It is important to question the owner carefully about concurrent NSAID administration (as this will influence administration of NSAIDs in the perioperative period) and steroids (as this will be a contraindication to the administration of NSAIDs in the perioperative period)

- Previous anaesthetic history
- Recent changes in bodyweight (may signal underlying undiagnosed disease)
- Recent changes in water consumption (increased drinking is a common sign of renal and endocrine disease)
- Recent changes in food consumption (may also be an indication of endocrine disease)
- Exercise intolerance (in dogs) – reduced willingness to exercise can be an indicator of underlying cardiovascular disease
- The temperament of the patient (useful to guide management of the patient while hospitalized)
- Vaccination status.

Clinical examination

A clinical examination (see Chapter 14) should be carried out before anaesthesia, with particular attention being paid to the systems affected by anaesthesia. It will also allow the temperament of the patient in response to handling to be assessed in a new environment, which may guide decisions about choice of premedication protocol and the requirement for sedation. Appropriate handling and safety measures should be observed at this time (see Chapters 2 and 11).

Pre-anaesthetic examination

The physical examination should concentrate on the body systems most affected by anaesthesia.

- Central nervous system:
  - Check that the animal has normal mentation (behaviour and level of consciousness), with no evidence of CNS depression.
- Cardiovascular system:
  - Palpate the peripheral pulses, assessing pulse quality and regularity
  - Auscultate the heart and listen for murmurs; concurrent auscultation and palpation of the pulse will allow any pulse deficit to be detected
  - Check mucous membrane colour and capillary refill time
  - Carrying out an exercise test by walking the animal a short distance on the lead can be used to aid detection of marked cardiovascular abnormalities (dogs)
  - Signs of dyspnoea, reluctance to move or collapse all signal that the animal will be at significant risk under anaesthesia and further investigation of the cardiovascular system is warranted.
- Respiratory system:
  - Observe the respiratory rate and pattern when the animal is at rest, looking for signs of laboured breathing or abnormal respiratory rate
  - Auscultate the chest to detect abnormal lung sounds that may indicate respiratory disease.

Additional pre-anaesthetic tests

Routine blood tests before anaesthesia should usually only be carried out on the basis of abnormalities detected on clinical examination or the clinical history. There is currently no evidence base to support routine pre-anaesthetic blood testing in healthy animals. In geriatric animals, where there is likely to be a higher incidence of concurrent disease, routine pre-anaesthetic blood testing may be more justifiable. Further information on specific blood tests is given in Chapter 17.

Anaemia may be detected by measuring haemoglobin concentration or packed cell volume (PCV). A blood coagulation profile is warranted in animals with a suspected blood clotting disorder.

Biochemical testing can be used to assess liver disease (through measurement of liver enzymes and bile acid concentration); and serum urea and creatinine concentrations are used as a marker of renal function. Measurement of plasma total protein (TP) concentration will detect hypoproteinaemia. Measurement of serum electrolyte concentrations (sodium, potassium and chloride) is indicated in some animals with systemic disease.

If marked disturbances in fluid therapy or blood volume are expected during anaesthesia and surgery, it is useful to take a baseline blood sample to measure PCV and TP. Changes in these parameters can then be used to guide fluid administration in response to disturbances in fluid balance during anaesthesia (see Chapter 20).

The cardiovascular and respiratory systems may require further evaluation using radiography, ultrasonography and electrocardiography.

Significance of clinical findings

Central nervous system disease

Systemic disease resulting in depression of the CNS can significantly reduce the amounts of anaesthetic agents required to induce and maintain anaesthesia: lower doses should be used and the agents given slowly and to effect, to reduce the likelihood of overdose. Seizures are common in animals with CNS disease and animals should be carefully monitored during the peri-anaesthetic period so that seizures can be managed promptly should they occur. Raised intracranial pressure, resulting from space-occupying lesions in the cranium, is associated with a number of specific anaesthetic considerations and knowledge of these is required before undertaking anaesthesia of this group of patients.

Cardiovascular disease

Cardiovascular disease is common in both cats and dogs and should not be considered a contraindication to anaesthesia. However, most cardiovascular diseases are likely to increase the risk of reduced cardiac output and hypotension during anaesthesia, increasing the likelihood of tissue hypoxia. Where possible, stabilization of the patient before anaesthesia is indicated, and the cardiovascular system should be monitored carefully so that derangements in cardiovascular function can be treated promptly.

Respiratory disease

Respiratory disease increases the risk of hypoxaemia and hypercapnia during anaesthesia. Supplementation with 100% O_2 is usually indicated immediately prior to induction of anaesthesia in patients with respiratory disease, in order to reduce the risk of hypoxaemia. Ventilation may require support with intermittent positive pressure ventilation (IPPV).

Hypovolaemia and dehydration

Reduced circulating blood volume predisposes the animal to reduced cardiac output and hypotension during anaesthesia.

Correction of disturbances in fluid balance is indicated before induction of anaesthesia, using appropriate fluid therapy given intravenously (see Chapter 20).

Coagulation disorders

Abnormalities in blood coagulation promote blood loss during surgery. Correction of the coagulation disorder before surgery, by the administration of blood products (see Chapter 20) or appropriate drug therapy, is indicated.

Liver and renal disease

Most anaesthetic drugs are metabolized in the liver, and therefore liver disease can prolong the duration of action of anaesthetic agents, leading to drug accumulation and a prolonged recovery time. Use of short-acting agents, given to effect, is recommended. Renal disease can be worsened by anaesthesia, particularly if adequate renal blood flow is not maintained, leading to renal ischaemia. Careful management of fluid therapy is required to prevent worsening of renal function.

Unstable blood glucose concentration

Common conditions leading to an unstable blood glucose concentration are diabetes mellitus and severe liver disease. Very young animals (<3 months of age) are also less able to regulate blood glucose concentration. Hypoglycaemia is a risk during anaesthesia, particularly as it cannot be detected by changes in mentation. Monitoring of blood glucose concentration during anaesthesia is recommended and an intravenous glucose solution should be administered if the blood glucose concentration is low (<3.3 mmol/l).

Electrolyte abnormalities

Disturbances in serum electrolyte concentrations are relatively common in animals suffering from systemic disease, particularly renal disease or some endocrine disorders (see Chapters 18 and 20). Hyperkalaemia (an elevated concentration of potassium in the blood) has particularly serious consequences during anaesthesia, as it results in heart conduction abnormalities and bradycardia. Normalization of blood potassium concentration is always indicated before induction of anaesthesia.

Anaemia

Oxygen is mainly carried in the blood bound to haemoglobin; therefore, severe anaemia will affect the oxygen-carrying capacity of the blood and may predispose the patient to hypoxia. Depending on the chronicity and severity of the anaemia, a blood transfusion may be indicated before anaesthesia.

Hypoproteinaemia

Most anaesthetic drugs are carried in the blood, bound to plasma proteins. It is only the unbound fraction of the drug that is active and able to cross the blood–brain barrier, in order to exert an anaesthetic effect. Drug doses should be reduced in hypoproteinaemic animals and drugs should be given slowly and to effect.

Pyrexia

Increased body temperature is a common finding in animals with acute illness, and detection during clinical examination should prompt further evaluation of the patient to establish the underlying cause. If pyrexia is severe (>40°C) it can result in increased heart rate and reduced myocardial contractility, decreasing cardiac output. If possible, body temperature should be normalized before the induction of anaesthesia.

American Society of Anesthesiologists (ASA) classification of anaesthetic risk

The information gathered from the patient history, clinical examination and auxiliary tests can be used to assign an ASA status to the patient. This system classifies the anaesthetic risk of the patient on a 5-point scale and can be used to guide selection of the anaesthesia protocol and the complexity of intraoperative monitoring.

ASA scale of anaesthetic risk

I.   A normal healthy patient – e.g. a young dog presented for elective ovariohysterectomy

II. A patient with mild systemic disease – e.g. a dog with a low-grade heart murmur that is not showing any clinical signs of cardiac disease

III. A patient with severe systemic disease – e.g. a dog with a heart murmur that has resulted in reduced exercise tolerance

IV. A patient with severe systemic disease that is a constant threat to life – e.g. a dog with a cardiac arrhythmia that is causing severe circulatory compromise

V.   A moribund patient that is not expected to survive without the operation – e.g. a dog with gastric dilatation and volvulus

E.   Denotes that the procedure is an emergency

Additional preparations

Fasting

It is currently recommended that cats and dogs are starved for a minimum of 6 hours prior to induction of anaesthesia or sedation. Puppies and kittens <12 weeks of age may be at risk of hypoglycaemia during preoperative starvation and therefore should have food withdrawn for 3 hours only and should be observed for signs of hypoglycaemia during this period. It is good practice to confirm normoglycaemia with monitoring of blood glucose concentration during the period of starvation and throughout anaesthesia. Provision of glucose intravenously (via fluid therapy) should be considered in very young animals with limited glucose reserves. Some endocrine diseases can also predispose to hypoglycaemia during periods of starvation (e.g. insulinoma) and at-risk animals should be carefully monitored during starvation, and glucose support considered.

Withdrawal of water

Water should not be withdrawn until the time of premedication, in order to prevent dehydration prior to induction of anaesthesia. It is very important to withdraw the water bowl from the cage when the animal is premedicated, in order to prevent the possibility that they could become sedated with the head in the water bowl and drown.

Weighing

All animals should be weighed before anaesthesia in order to calculate drug doses accurately.

Placement of intravenous catheters

Ideally, all animals should have some form of intravenous access established prior to anaesthesia, to allow administration of agents for induction, fluid therapy, additional drugs and in case of emergency. Placement of intravenous catheters is described in Chapter 20.

In conscious cats and dogs, the easiest vessels to catheterize are the cephalic (Figure 21.1a) and the saphenous (Figures 21.1b and 21.2) veins. If these vessels are unavailable (e.g. due to previous catheter placement or the site of surgery) an intravenous catheter can be placed into the auricular vein that runs along the edge of the ear (Figure 21.1c). When using this site, it is vital to palpate the area and ensure that there is no pulse to avoid placing the catheter in the artery. This site is invaluable in Basset Hounds and Dachshunds (as the shape of their legs makes other sites less suitable).

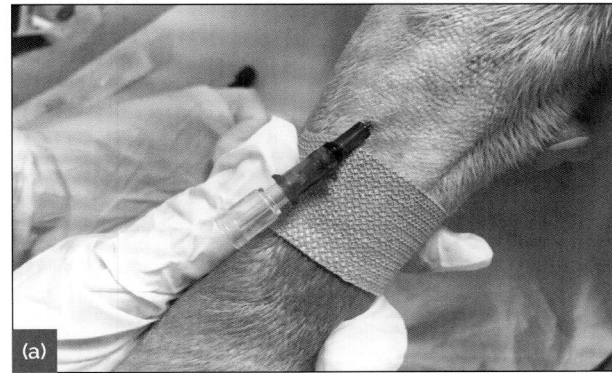

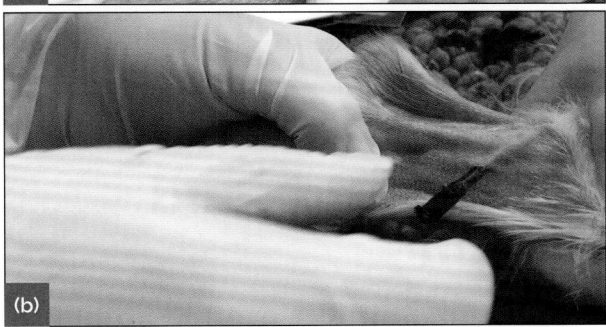

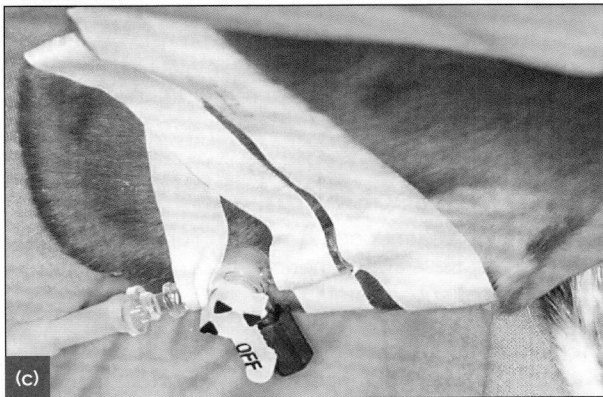

21.1 Intravenous catheterization sites in the dog. **(a)** Placement of a 22 G catheter into the cephalic vein of a dog. **(b)** Placement of a 22 G catheter into the saphenous vein of a dog. **(c)** Catheter in the auricular vein and connected to a three-way tap.

When choosing a catheter of an appropriate size, it is important to consider the nature of the procedure to be carried out and the potential risks associated with the surgery, e.g. a 20 G catheter is suitable for a healthy 15 kg dog being castrated; however, if the same dog were having an exploratory laparotomy, an 18 G catheter would be more appropriate because of the higher risks associated with the procedure and the possible need to provide rapid intravenous fluid therapy.

Once the catheter is placed, it must be fixed securely in order to prevent displacement when the patient is moved (Figure 21.2). Techniques vary depending on the species, site of placement and individual preference. If the patient is going to receive intravenous fluid therapy perioperatively (which is recommended), the catheter is usually connected to a short extension set (Figure 21.2) or T-port to allow fluids to be administered easily.

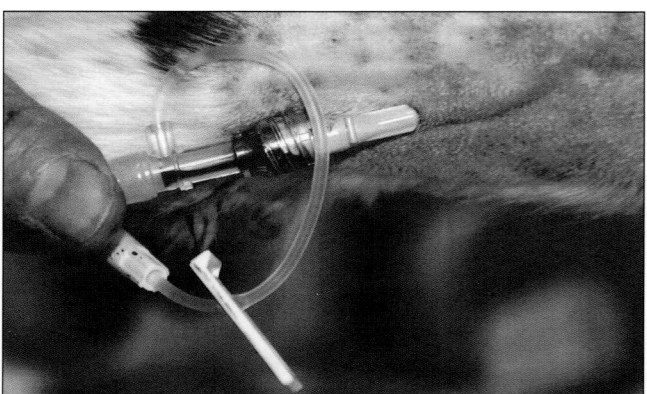

21.2 Intravenous catheter taped securely in the saphenous vein. A short extension set allows the catheter to be connected to a fluid administration set.

Rest and exercise

Where possible, dogs should be walked prior to anaesthesia, to allow them to pass urine and faeces. Cats should be provided with a litter tray.

Premedication and sedation

Premedication is an integral part of the total anaesthesia protocol. The choice of premedicant drugs will determine the characteristics of the ensuing anaesthesia. Therefore, when monitoring anaesthesia during the maintenance phase, vital parameters should be considered in light of the premedicant drugs administered.

Aims of premedication:

- To calm the patient prior to induction of anaesthesia
- To reduce stress during induction of anaesthesia for both the patient and staff
- To reduce the dose of anaesthetic drugs required for induction and maintenance of anaesthesia
- To contribute to a balanced anaesthesia technique
- To provide analgesia
- To counter adverse effects of other anaesthetic drugs
- To smooth recovery from anaesthesia through residual sedation and pain relief.

Sedation

Depending on the species and temperament of the patient, some procedures can be carried out under sedation rather than general anaesthesia. The drugs used for sedation are similar to those used for premedication, although higher doses are commonly used for sedation in order to achieve adequate chemical restraint. The principles of drug selection and monitoring are similar for sedation and premedication.

When deciding whether to sedate or anaesthetize an individual patient for a particular procedure, it is important to consider that sedation is not necessarily safer than general anaesthesia. Generally, less cardiovascular and respiratory support can be given to a sedated than to an anaesthetized patient, particularly with respect to control of the airway. Therefore, in high-risk patients it is often better to elect for general anaesthesia rather than sedation, even though it might be possible to carry out the procedure under sedation alone.

Routes of premedication and sedative drug administration

Premedication and sedative drugs may be administered via several routes:

- Intravenous: Rapid onset of action but requires restraint of the patient and intravenous access to be established
- Intramuscular: Slower onset of action than the intravenous route but requires minimal restraint for injection. Large volumes injected intramuscularly can be painful. Site of injection does not appear to affect onset or depth of sedation
- Subcutaneous: Onset of sedation is slowest, but associated with least pain on injection.

Drugs used for premedication of small animals

Several classes of drug are commonly used for premedication in small animals, each with advantages and disadvantages (Figure 21.3). Most premedication protocols involve administration of a drug with sedative properties combined with an opioid analgesic drug. This usually increases the quality of sedation that is achieved, due to synergism between opioids and drugs with sedative properties. Synergism means that the sedation is greater than can be achieved by simply summing the individual effects of the drugs. This protocol also ensures that analgesia is provided. Administration of NSAIDs prior to induction of anaesthesia can be helpful to provide improved intraoperative analgesia, but there are contraindications to this technique in some patients (see 'Analgesia', below).

It can be very useful to consider the ASA status of the patient (see above) when determining the premedication regimen (Figure 21.4). This takes the health status of the patient into consideration and allows some standardization of premedication protocols, which can be helpful within a busy practice situation. However, the individual requirements of each patient, such as the procedure to be carried out, must always be taken into consideration.

Class or drug	Advantages	Disadvantages
Phenothiazines, e.g. acepromazine	Synergism with opioids increases sedation (neuroleptanaesthesia). Provides reasonable sedation. Relatively wide margin of cardiovascular safety. Anti-arrhythmic action (mediated through an antagonistic action at alpha-1 receptors). Long duration of action (6 hours); can smooth recovery from anaesthesia. Can be given i.v., i.m. or s.c.	Relatively slow onset of action (30–45 min). Sedation not as profound as that provided by alpha-2 agonists; improved if environment is quiet and animal is left undisturbed. Long duration of action (may prolong recovery from anaesthesia). No antagonist available. Causes peripheral vasodilation through antagonism of alpha-1 receptors. **Do not use** in animals that are shocked or have significant cardiovascular disease. Peripheral vasodilation promotes heat loss and hypothermia
Alpha-2 agonists, e.g. medetomidine, dexmedetomidine	Profound sedation, synergism with opioids further increases sedation, allows a lower dose of the alpha-2 agonist to be used. Good muscle relaxation due to potency of hypnotic effect. Analgesia: contributes to a multimodal analgesia technique. Profound drug-sparing effect: contributes to a balanced anaesthesia technique. Peripheral vasoconstriction reduces heat loss and minimizes hypothermia. Rapid, smooth recoveries from anaesthesia. Can be given i.v., i.m. or s.c. Antagonist available (atipamezole).	Significant cardiovascular system effects: causes an intense initial vasoconstriction associated with a reduction in heart rate. Heart rate remains low due to central sympatholytic effects. Cardiac output is reduced. **Do not use** in animals with some types of cardiovascular disease. Reduces liver blood flow: **do not use** in animals with significant liver disease. Can cause vomiting: **do not use** in animals where vomiting is undesirable, e.g. raised intraocular pressure or linear foreign body. Analgesia is of short duration (45–60 min) reversed by administration of atipamezole
Ketamine	Good sedation/anaesthesia when given in combination with another sedative drug: dependent on dose. Minimal effects on the cardiovascular system. Provides analgesia. Profound drug-sparing effect. Useful in cats where profound sedation is required, given in combination with a benzodiazepine. Can be given i.v. or i.m.	Causes excitation and muscle rigidity unless combined with another sedative drug, commonly a benzodiazepine. Poor quality of sedation in dogs, even when given in combination with another agent. Animals can be 'spacey' in recovery due to the hallucinogenic effects
Benzodiazepines, e.g. diazepam, midazolam	Sedation is enhanced by combination with an opioid. Good sedation in sick or young animals. Minimal effects on the cardiovascular system: useful in patients with cardiovascular disease. Midazolam can be given i.v., i.m. or s.c.	Sedation is minimal in healthy animals; combination with an opioid is required. Can cause excitement in healthy animals. Muscle relaxation may reduce ventilatory effort. Diazepam solubilized in propylene glycol causes pain on i.m. injection and thrombophlebitis i.v; use midazolam if possible
Opioids, e.g. buprenorphine, methadone (see also 'Opioid analgesics', later in chapter)	Enhance sedation when combined with acepromazine, alpha-2 agonists and benzodiazepines. Provide analgesia: choice of opioid depends on severity of pain expected from the procedure. Can be given i.v. (not pethidine), i.m. or s.c.	Morphine can cause vomiting when administered to animals that are not in pain. High doses of potent opioids may cause a reduction in heart rate; bradycardia can be managed by the administration of an anticholinergic if severe. Administration of a partial mu opioid agonist (e.g. buprenorphine) prior to induction of anaesthesia may reduce the effectiveness of full opioid agonists administered during anaesthesia
Anticholinergics; parasympatholytics, e.g. atropine, glycopyrrolate	Will counter bradycardia produced by potent opioids. Will counter bradycardia caused by stimulation of the parasympathetic nervous system during surgery, e.g. oculocardiac reflex, exploratory neck surgery. Can be given i.v., i.m. or s.c.	Rarely required as premedicant in modern anaesthesia protocols. Usually advisable to give in response to bradycardia rather than pre-emptively

21.3 Advantages and disadvantages of drugs used for premedication and sedation in small animals.

ASA status	Dogs	Cats
i. Normal, healthy patient	Acepromazine plus opioid Medetomidine/dexmedetomidine plus opioid	Acepromazine plus opioid Medetomidine/dexmedetomidine plus opioid
ii. Patient with mild systemic disease	Acepromazine plus opioid Medetomidine/dexmedetomidine plus opioid (if no evidence of CVS disease)	Acepromazine plus opioid Medetomidine/dexmedetomidine plus opioid (if no evidence of CVS disease)
iii. Patient with severe systemic disease	Acepromazine plus opioid Midazolam plus opioid	Acepromazine plus opioid Ketamine plus midazolam
iv. Patient with severe systemic disease that is a constant threat to life	Midazolam plus opioid	Ketamine plus midazolam Midazolam plus opioid
v. Moribund patient not expected to survive without the operation	Midazolam plus opioid, or either drug alone	Midazolam plus opioid, or either drug alone

21.4 Examples of premedication protocols for dogs and cats with differing ASA status. CVS = cardiovascular system.

Alpha-2 adrenergic agonists

Alpha-2 adrenergic agonists, such as medetomidine and dexmedetomidine, are commonly used for premedication in cats and dogs in combination with an opioid. Combining an alpha-2 agonist with an opioid provides synergistic sedation and analgesia, which is advantageous and may allow lower doses of each individual agent to be used.

Medetomidine is a racemic mixture of levomedetomidine and dexmedetomidine; the active component of the drug is dexmedetomidine, which is now available as a single agent. This class of drug can provide profound sedation and analgesia, which is advantageous, particularly in excitable or fractious animals. However, these drugs also have marked effects on physiology that can limit their use, particularly in animals with concurrent cardiovascular disease.

The typical cardiovascular profile of medetomidine and dexmedetomidine comprises an initial hypertension immediately following administration associated with peripheral vasoconstriction and a consequent reduction in heart rate (bradycardia). Subsequently, the vasoconstriction wanes and blood pressure returns to normal or slightly below normal while heart rate remains low due to loss of sympathetic nervous system tone.

These changes in cardiovascular physiology are also associated with a profound reduction in cardiac output to approximately one-third of pre-administration levels. Thus, alpha-2 adrenergic agonists are generally not recommended in animals with significant cardiovascular disease.

Acepromazine

Acepromazine is probably the most widely used sedative for premedication in the UK. It is generally administered in combination with an opioid to provide synergistic sedation (neuroleptanaesthesia) and allow a lower dose of acepromazine to be used while still retaining adequate sedative properties. Acepromazine does not have any analgesic properties. The degree of sedation that can be achieved with acepromazine is generally lower than that which can be achieved with an alpha-2 adrenergic agonist. This can influence drug selection, particularly in fractious patients where a high degree of sedation is needed, especially if intravenous access is not possible in the patient when fully awake.

The major cardiovascular side effect of acepromazine is peripheral vasodilation produced by blockade of alpha-1 adrenoreceptors in the peripheral vasculature. This can result in severe hypotension in animals with some types of cardiovascular disease, particularly animals that present with cardiovascular collapse. Acepromazine also causes splenic sequestration of red blood cells and therefore should be avoided in animals with significant anaemia.

Benzodiazepines

Typically, when administered alone to healthy patients, the benzodiazepines midazolam and diazepam produce excitation due to loss of learned inhibitory behaviour; although in very sick or very young patients it may be possible to achieve some sedation from a benzodiazepine administered alone. However, benzodiazepines can provide good sedation in healthy animals when combined with an opioid (dogs) or with ketamine (cats). In contrast to acepromazine and the alpha-2 agonists, benzodiazepines have minimal effects on the cardiovascular system, which renders them suitable for use in patients with concurrent cardiovascular disease.

Ketamine

Ketamine is commonly used for premedication in cats in combination with a benzodiazepine; it should not be administered alone due to the risk of excitation and associated poor muscle relaxation. However, the combination of ketamine and a benzodiazepine is relatively cardiovascularly stable because ketamine, by stimulating the sympathetic nervous system, tends to preserve cardiovascular function, which is advantageous. One disadvantage of ketamine is that cats can often be 'spacey' in recovery and show clinical signs such as head bobbing and mild excitatory behaviour. It is important that cats are hospitalized and this behaviour is allowed to wane before discharge of the cat to their owner.

Alfaxalone

Although not licensed for intramuscular administration in the UK, alfaxalone administered intramuscularly can be a useful sedative drug for cats and small dogs in which administration of other sedatives are contraindicated and profound sedation is required. The volume of alfaxalone required to produce sedation precludes its use in larger dogs (e.g. dogs >10 kg) because of the pain associated with intramuscular administration of large volumes of injectate.

Monitoring premedicated patients

Drugs used for premedication can have profound effects on body systems, and careful monitoring of patients is therefore required. This should include:

- Monitoring the degree of sedation:
    - Marked sedation can result in airway obstruction in brachycephalic dogs and cats
    - Stretching out the head and neck and pulling the tongue forward can reduce respiratory obstruction in sedated patients
    - Acute respiratory obstruction is an indication to proceed directly to induction of anaesthesia and placement of an endotracheal tube.
- Monitoring of body temperature:
    - Support body temperature to prevent onset of hypothermia, particularly in animals of low bodyweight and after acepromazine.
- More invasive monitoring of high-risk patients after premedication, e.g. electrocardiography, pulse oximetry, oxygen supplementation.

Premedication tips

Premedication can be made safer and easier by remembering the following:

- Weigh all animals so that drug dosing is accurate. Dose recommendations for very potent drugs such as the alpha-2 agonists (dexmedetomidine) may be given based on body surface area rather than bodyweight (conversion charts are available)
- Give the premedication agents at the correct time relative to the expected onset of peak sedation and induction of anaesthesia
- Record the time of drug administration and the drugs given on the anaesthetic record on the front of the kennel
- A quiet environment with minimal stimulation will promote good sedation following premedication.

Analgesia

Nurses play a huge role in both recognizing pain in animals and delivering analgesia protocols. It is therefore imperative that veterinary nurses have a good theoretical grounding in analgesic drug pharmacology as well as a sound practical knowledge of analgesia techniques.

Pathophysiology of pain

The neuroanatomy and pathophysiology of pain pathways are complex. Nevertheless, a basic understanding of these pathways is essential in order to understand the underlying principles of analgesic strategies and the mechanism of action of analgesic drugs. Informed decisions about different analgesic drug combinations and the timing of analgesic interventions can contribute to improved analgesia provision in veterinary practice. This section will focus on changes that occur in the pain pathway in response to noxious input, particularly the clinical relevance of these changes and how they might influence analgesia protocols.

What is pain?

The International Association for the Study of Pain defines pain in humans as 'a sensory or emotional experience associated with actual or potential tissue damage'. The absence of the ability to communicate does not negate the possibility that a person is experiencing pain or requires pain-relieving treatment. Recently this definition has been adopted for animals. It acknowledges that animals can also suffer as a result of pain. However, it is important to consider that pain is a conscious sensation or experience; therefore, when an animal is adequately anaesthetized and is unconscious, by definition it cannot experience pain.

What is a noxious stimulus?

A noxious stimulus is one that is damaging to tissues, for example a thermal, mechanical or chemical stimulus that is of sufficient magnitude to cause tissue damage. Nociception is activity in nociceptive pathways, caused by a noxious stimulus, which is transmitted to the CNS. Nociception usually results in pain perception in conscious animals; however, in an adequately anaesthetized animal nociception will not result in pain until recovery from anaesthesia.

Activation of the pain pathway

Large changes in pain sensitivity are recognized to occur after peripheral tissue injury. The resultant pain is not merely localized and short term at the site of the injury but surrounding tissues may also become painful following activation of the pain pathway. Repeated activation of the nociceptive pathway results in a heightened sensitivity to pain. Understanding these changes is important in order to manage clinical pain effectively.

Types of pain

It is now recognized that pain is not homogeneous (i.e. it is not a single entity); rather it comprises three categories – physiological, inflammatory and neuropathic pain.

Physiological pain

Physiological pain is an essential early warning device that alerts an animal to the presence of potentially damaging stimuli in the environment. An example of physiological pain is the response to a needle prick. The pain is 'appropriate' to the degree of stimulation, i.e. a stimulus–response relationship is maintained. If the force of the needle prick increases, the pain also increases in a linear manner. The pain stops when stimulation stops and the pain is localized; only the area that is stimulated causes pain. Physiological pain results from 'normal' activation of the pain pathways and is considered to serve a protective function.

Inflammatory pain

This type of clinical pain is initiated by tissue damage and inflammation and is the inevitable consequence of surgery or trauma to a patient. It differs from physiological pain in that it is associated with changes in the pain pathways that result in heightened pain sensitivity.

Neuropathic pain

This type of clinical pain is initiated by damage to the nervous system itself, such as damage to a peripheral nerve. An example of neuropathic pain in humans is 'phantom limb' pain, which commonly occurs following amputation of a leg or arm. Despite the large number of amputations carried out in a variety of veterinary species, the clinical significance of neuropathic pain in animals following amputation is not yet established and clinical management of chronic neuropathic pain following amputation can be extremely challenging.

How does clinical pain differ from physiological pain?

When clinical pain arises, there is hypersensitivity to pain at the site of tissue damage and in adjacent normal tissue. Pain may arise spontaneously. Stimuli that would not normally produce pain, such as touch, begin to do so (this is known as allodynia) and noxious stimuli evoke greater and more prolonged pain than in a healthy animal (hyperalgesia). Inflammatory pain hypersensitivity will usually return to normal if the disease process resulting in pain is controlled.

Why does pain sensitivity change?

Peripheral sensitization

Understanding peripheral sensitization is important because it is the mechanism by which noxious stimuli at the site of tissue injury produce a more intense and prolonged pain response once clinical pain is established. This is termed primary hyperalgesia.

Nociceptors are the free nerve endings of primary afferent nociceptive fibres, predominantly A and C fibres. These sensory fibres relay information from the periphery to the spinal cord (see Chapter 3); this is the first step in the relay of nociceptive information from the site of tissue damage in the periphery to the brain. The peripheral terminals of nociceptors (heat, mechanical, chemical and polymodal receptors that are activated in response to noxious stimuli) become more excitable following tissue damage, so that further noxious stimuli applied to the area are more likely to cause nociceptor activation and trigger activity in nociceptive pathways (which will usually ultimately result in pain). This modulation occurs following exposure of the nociceptor to sensitizing agents such as inflammatory mediators released during tissue damage. Administration of NSAIDs can be an effective strategy for reducing primary peripheral hyperalgesia because NSAIDs reduce the release of inflammatory mediators at the site of tissue damage, thereby decreasing nociceptor sensitization.

Central sensitization

Understanding central sensitization is important because it is a major mechanism by which increased pain sensitivity occurs following tissue damage and the onset of clinical pain. It results in secondary hyperalgesia, allodynia and spontaneous pain.

The spinal cord is the first site at which modulation of nociceptive information relayed from the periphery via A and C fibres occurs and, as such, is an important target site of many analgesic drugs. A and C fibres synapse with sensory neurons in the dorsal horn of the spinal cord and it is at this communication between primary afferent A and C fibres and spinal cord neurons that many of the changes associated with central sensitization occur. Modulation in central pain pathways is triggered by peripheral afferent sensory fibre input and results in enhanced responsiveness of pain transmission neurons.

The NMDA receptor

Neurotransmitters, including excitatory amino acids and peptides, ensure that an action potential arriving at the dorsal horn of the spinal cord via A and C fibres is transmitted to higher brain centres. The neurotransmitters released at the synapse between A and C fibres and the dorsal horn neuron are different in animals with physiological pain compared to those with clinical pain. The N-methyl-D-aspartate (NMDA) receptor plays a key role in clinical pain but is not normally activated during transmission of 'physiological pain'. Activation of the NMDA receptor is central to the development of central sensitization leading to enhanced pain sensitivity.

The conditions needed for activation of the NMDA receptor are complex, but essentially this receptor contributes to the transmission of noxious input from the periphery to the CNS following repeated input to the spinal cord by A and C fibres of noxious information caused by tissue injury and inflammation. Once the NMDA receptor is activated, there is a sudden augmentation of the amount of noxious input to the spinal cord that is relayed to the brain, where it is perceived as pain. This amplification of the response initiated by activation of the NMDA receptor seems to underlie central sensitization.

Pre-emptive analgesia

Pre-emptive analgesia can be defined as an analgesic treatment initiated before the start of surgery or tissue trauma. The underpinning theory behind this concept is that once peripheral and central sensitization have occurred, pain management becomes much more difficult because of the increased sensitivity to pain that results from the consequences of the activation of the nociceptive pathways. Administration of analgesic drugs 'pre-emptively' aims to prevent the development of sensitization and therefore make provision of effective analgesia easier to achieve after surgery.

An overwhelming amount of experimental data has demonstrated that various antinociceptive techniques applied before injury are more effective at reducing the post-injury central sensitization phenomenon than administration after injury. However, there is little evidence that this translates effectively to the clinical arena. Human clinical research studies over the last two decades have overwhelmingly demonstrated that pre-emptive administration of analgesics to surgical patients does not confer major benefits in terms of immediate postoperative pain relief or the need for supplementary analgesics. A number of caveats must, however, be considered: measuring postoperative pain in human patients is problematic; the requirement for analgesics after surgery is influenced by many psychological and physical factors, not only the degree of pain experienced by the individual; and pre-emptive analgesia in a clinical setting may not be adequate to prevent central and peripheral sensitization.

A few studies have investigated the effects of pre-emptive administration of analgesic drugs to dogs (see 'References and further reading'). Pre-emptive administration of opioids to bitches undergoing ovariohysterectomy has been shown to reduce secondary hyperalgesia, suggesting a positive benefit. However, caveats applied to the human studies are also applicable to studies in animals.

Despite the lack of clinical scientific evidence supporting pre-emptive analgesia, the general consensus amongst veterinary and medical professionals is that early administration of analgesics is good practice for the following reasons:

- No major deleterious effects from pre-emptive analgesic techniques have been identified
- Intraoperative analgesic administration will blunt the surgical stress response
- Intraoperative analgesics will reduce the requirement for other anaesthetic agents (balanced anaesthetic protocol)
- Pre-emptive analgesia may confer clinical benefits that cannot be detected by current study designs.

Preventive analgesia

Due to the lack of evidence associated with pre-emptive analgesia techniques, the concept of pre-emptive analgesia has now been replaced by a broader principle for analgesic administration termed preventive analgesia. This is an analgesic strategy designed to reduce short- and long-term post-surgical pain by preventing the onset of peripheral and central sensitization. It involves giving analgesics early enough in the disease and/or trauma process, and for long enough after peripheral tissue injury, to prevent upregulation of the pain pathways.

Multimodal analgesia

Multimodal or balanced analgesia is the principle of using different classes of analgesic drugs in combination. Because of the complexity of pain pathways, it is unrealistic to expect to achieve adequate analgesia by using single agents. Using drugs in combination causes pharmacological modulation of the pain pathway at different levels and sites, and is more effective at preventing pain sensation. There may also be synergistic benefits, as with premedication (see earlier). Drug combinations will usually allow the dose of individual agents to be reduced, which may reduce the incidence of side effects.

Recognition and quantification (scoring) of pain

Recognizing that an animal is in pain is probably one of the most challenging and important aspects of a veterinary nurse's role. Pain management in human medicine is challenging because the experience of pain is an emotion and is therefore difficult to measure and quantify and affected by many factors. Similarly, in veterinary patients it is vitally important to remember that pain is an emotional experience and varies greatly between individuals. The mainstay of pain recognition is observation of the patient's behaviour. To assess this appropriately it is important to have a full appreciation of the full range of behaviours exhibited by different species and knowledge of what is normal behaviour for an individual patient.

Pain-related behaviour

Variations in pain behaviour between different species are considered to be linked to whether they are a predator (e.g. cats, dogs) or prey (e.g. rabbit) species in nature, and reflect the mechanism they employ for coping with dangerous situations. For example, dogs tend to fight whereas many rabbits 'freeze'. Further, within each species different breeds also have different behavioural traits: Labrador Retrievers have a reputation for being stoical, while Whippets tend to be more sensitive and vocalize. It is essential to appreciate that all patients are individuals and have different perceptions as to how severe a pain is. Each patient should therefore be given analgesic drugs according to its own individual requirements for analgesia.

Typical behaviours that may be exhibited by dogs in pain:

- Sudden development of aggression – a previously friendly dog becomes aggressive or nervous, or a naturally aggressive or nervous dog becomes more aggressive or nervous
- Attention-seeking behaviour
- Guarding the site of injury or tissue damage
- Biting or scratching that may progress to extreme mutilation
- A patient licking a wound could indicate that it is in pain (remember this postoperatively and consider additional analgesia rather than just applying an Elizabethan collar)
- Changes in sleep pattern and restlessness
- Posture: hunching; or the stereotypical 'praying' position typical of patients with abdominal pain (Figure 21.5)
- Anorexia or inappetence
- Vocalization, whimpering and whining, barking or growling
- Abnormal gait or movement – either non-weight-bearing or lameness on an affected leg or an abnormal gait when not wanting to stretch the abdomen or thorax
- Facial expression, including ear and eye position
- Weak or limp tail-wagging.

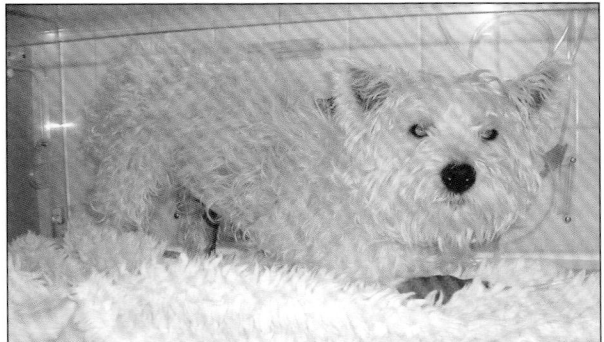

21.5 A dog in an incubator showing the 'praying' posture typically associated with cranial abdominal pain.

Specific behaviours more likely to be exhibited by cats in pain:

- Posture, hunched in sternal recumbency rather than curled up and relaxed in lateral recumbency
- Immobility
- Anorexia
- Sudden development of aggression
- Cats in pain quite often bite themselves during their recovery from anaesthesia
- Lack of grooming
- Facial expression, ears rotated and flattened with 'frowning' expression
- Shying away from attention, sitting at the back of the kennel and hiding under bedding (although some cats will do this anyway as they find it reassuring)
- Spontaneous vocalization and hissing.

Other factors influencing the expression of pain behaviour

There are many factors that can alter both the expression of pain behaviour in a species and the experience of pain by individuals, making recognition of pain even more challenging, particularly in a hospital environment or following surgery. These include:

- Age: Younger patients may be more sensitive to painful stimuli. With the exception of neonates, this cannot be explained by differences in the pathophysiology of pain and nociceptive processing; it is more likely to relate to the perception or expression of pain by younger animals
- Sex: Females tend to be more sensitive to pain than males, except when pregnant. This is due to the effect of sex hormones on pain processing
- The source of the pain
- Pain history: Presence of CNS sensitization or a prior pain experience
- Temperament: A nervous patient may experience more pain and anxiety, increasing stress and fear
- Presence or absence of additional stressors (e.g. being away from their owner)
- The patient's potential inability to perform the pain behaviour due to concurrent illness
- Drugs: Opioids and alpha-2 agonists often produce sedation, which can mask or prevent pain-related behaviour
- Presence of a predator species in the vicinity of a prey species (e.g. housing cats next to dogs).

Physiological effects of pain

Pain may also result in physiological changes, primarily as a result of stimulation of the sympathetic nervous system. Physiological changes can be induced by many factors, however, including stress. It is therefore important not to rely on physiological changes alone as indicators of pain, but to combine these with behavioural assessment. Physiological signs can also be significantly affected by drug administration.

Physiological changes induced by pain include:

- Tachycardia
- Increased blood pressure
- Tachypnoea

Physiological changes induced by pain include *continued*:

- Changes in respiratory pattern, e.g. rapid shallow breathing caused by thoracic pain
- Panting
- Pyrexia
- Salivation
- Pupillary dilation
- Shaking and shivering.

Recommended protocol for pain assessment

Assessing a patient for pain is a dynamic process, requiring interaction between the patient and the assessor. The best person to carry out pain assessment is the person who knows the patient best, having spent the most time with them during hospitalization. This person is often the veterinary nurse.

Pain assessment should involve identification of the behaviours described above and should follow a set protocol.

Pain assessment protocol

1. Assessment/observation of behaviour and demeanour within the pen without any interference by the observer.
2. Observation of how the patient interacts with people when approached in the pen.
3. Assessment of patient movement outside of the pen (if appropriate).
4. Response to gentle palpation/manipulation of the site of injury and surrounding tissue.

Clinical use of pain scoring systems

Pain scoring systems are used for many reasons, the main one being to improve perioperative pain management. All patients are individuals and thus have different requirements for analgesia. A pain scoring system ensures a reflective approach, helping to improve standards, identify problem areas and optimize patient care. Patients that are in pain can pose a danger to personnel as they are more likely to be aggressive; improving their experiences within the veterinary environment should make them easier to manage on future occasions. A pain scoring system helps to assess the appropriate type, dose and frequency of required analgesic drug administration. It also standardizes care by reducing the inter-observer variability of pain level. There are several different types of pain scoring systems.

Simple descriptive scale

In a simple descriptive scale (SDS), after pain assessment the observer rates the pain as follows:

- No pain
- Mild pain
- Moderate pain
- Severe pain.

Usually descriptors to aid classification are provided. Although this system is fairly crude, it is simple to use and can work well in a clinical environment.

Simple numerical rating scale

In a simple numerical rating scale (NRS) the observer assesses how much pain they think the patient is experiencing and then assigns a number appropriate to the degree of pain; usually this number is between 0 and 10. The system has been shown to be reasonably sensitive and appropriate for use by multiple observers; it is also simple to use.

Visual analogue scale

A visual analogue scale (VAS) is a simple method of recording pain (Figure 21.6). After pain assessment, the observer scores pain by marking a line that is 10 cm in length at a point corresponding to the degree of pain that the observer thinks the patient is experiencing. The line is anchored at two points: 0 cm (no pain) and 10 cm (worst possible pain for that procedure).

Advantages of this system are that the scoring system is continuous rather than having discrete categories (as in the NRS or SDS) and the result can be quantified numerically by measuring the distance of the mark along the line from the 0 mm anchor. The VAS is more sensitive than the NRS, but this is a disadvantage when used by more than one assessor. Therefore, the VAS is often used for research studies carried out by a single observer but is not so helpful in a clinical environment.

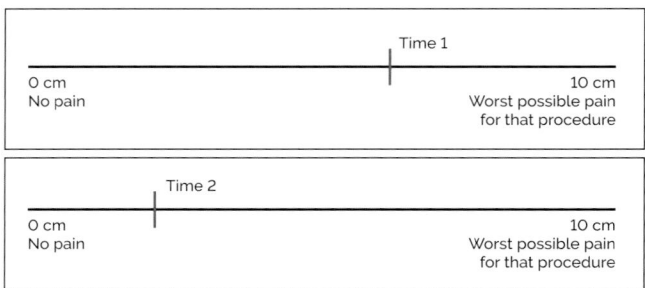

21.6 Example of a visual analogue scale for quantification of pain. A mark is made on the line by the observer according to their perception of the magnitude of pain experienced by the animal. At Time 2, following the administration of analgesia, this patient is perceived to be in less pain than at Time 1.

Multidimensional or composite pain scales

Multidimensional or composite pain scales are more complex than the unidimensional scales described above, and try to take into account both the emotional effects of pain and its intensity. They comprise a number of separate assessments of different aspects of behaviour that can be associated with pain (e.g. posture, demeanour, attention to the wound). The Glasgow Composite Pain Scale (GCPS) Short Form is a composite pain scale that has been validated in dogs and is probably the most widely used scoring system in the UK. The scale can be downloaded from: www.newmetrica.com/acute-pain-measurement/. There are validated translations of the scale into French, Spanish, German, Italian, Norwegian and Swedish.

Recently, two composite pain scales have been developed for cats: the UNESP-Botucatu Multidimensional Composite Pain Scale for assessing postoperative pain in cats (www.animalpain.com.br/assets/upload/escala-en-us.pdf); and the Glasgow Composite Pain Scale – Feline (www.newmetrica.com/acute-pain-measurement/). The Botucatu scale is only validated for pain associated with cats undergoing ovariohysterectomy, although it seems to translate well to post-surgical pain in cats in general. However, it is quite a complex scale to use and is time-consuming to complete, which is a disadvantage. In contrast, the GCPS for cats is simple to use and similar in layout and design to the scale for dogs. Thus, if you are used to using the canine scale it is easy to apply the feline scale in a hospital setting.

Although composite scales are more time-consuming to complete than unidimensional scales, they provide more information about the pain experience of the animal and their use is encouraged in clinical practice.

Facial expression of pain

In recent years there has been increasing recognition of the value of using facial expression as an indicator of acute pain. The work started in the field of rodent pain, where researchers first developed a mouse grimace scale that characterized changes in the eyes, ears, nose and whiskers of mice associated with severe pain. This work has now expanded and grimace scales, using facial expression changes to identify pain, have been developed for mice, rats, rabbits (see later in this chapter) and horses. It is notable that the Glasgow Composite Pain Scale – Feline also incorporates two questions that relate to changes in facial expression of the cat being assessed.

Opioid analgesics

The opioid group of drugs is diverse, and the drugs within it differ with respect to their analgesic efficacy, duration of action and potential for side effects. Opioids are generally a very safe and versatile group of drugs to use. It is important to understand the differences in order to choose the most appropriate drug for a given situation. Opioids can be classified by which opioid receptor they bind to and according to whether they have agonist, partial agonist or antagonist effects (Figure 21.7). Most opioids are Controlled Drugs (see Chapter 8).

Pharmacological effects of opioids

- Analgesia: Depending on the opioid chosen, different intensities of analgesia can be obtained. Opioids are a key element of perioperative pain control; mu (µ) agonists are the most effective analgesics. Generally, the more efficacious the opioid (e.g. fentanyl), the greater the likelihood of clinically significant side effects.
- Sedation: The sedative effect of opioids is usually dose- and drug-dependent. Sedation from phenothiazines and alpha-2 agonists is enhanced when they are combined with opioids (see above).
- Respiratory system: Opioids such as methadone and buprenorphine do not cause clinically significant respiratory depression in animals at clinical dose rates. Fentanyl and alfentanil given intravenously during anaesthesia are likely to cause clinically significant respiratory depression, and animals may require support of ventilation.
- Cardiovascular system: Opioids have few negative effects on haemodynamics. They can cause a reduction in heart rate through stimulation of the vagal nerve, which can be managed by co-administration of an anticholinergic. The effect on heart rate is most apparent when the drugs are given intravenously or in high doses.
- Gastrointestinal system: Morphine directly stimulates the vomiting centre, and animals sedated or premedicated with morphine often vomit shortly after administration. This effect is less apparent (or not evident at all) when morphine is used postoperatively for management of perioperative pain. Opioids stimulate the sphincters of the gastrointestinal tract, causing an overall action that is constipating; increased intestinal peristalsis tends to combat this effect.

Drug	Market Authorization in the UK	Opioid receptor effects	Duration of action	Routes of administration	Controlled Drug status
Morphine	No	Mu receptor agonist	2–4 hours	i.v. (dilute with saline and give slowly i.v.), bolus or CRI i.m., s.c. Epidural (use a preservative free solution)	Schedule 2
Methadone	Yes (in dogs and cats)	Mu receptor agonist	3–4 hours	i.v., i.m., s.c. Not routinely given by CRI or epidurally	Schedule 2
Pethidine	Licensed product (dogs and cats) no longer available in UK	Mu receptor agonist	1–1.5 hours	Do not give i.v. i.m., s.c.	Schedule 2
Fentanyl	Yes (in dogs)	Mu receptor agonist	10–20 minutes unless given by continuous rate infusion	i.v. (CRI or bolus)	Schedule 2
Alfentanil	No	Mu receptor agonist	10–20 minutes	i.v. (CRI)	Schedule 2
Buprenorphine	Yes (in dogs and cats)	Mu receptor partial agonist	6 hours	i.v., i.m., s.c. (not recommended) Oral transmucosal (in cats)	Schedule 3
Butorphanol	Yes (in dogs and cats)	Kappa receptor agonist	1–1.5 hours	i.v., i.m., s.c.	Not subject to Controlled Drug regulations
Naloxone	No	Mu receptor agonist	30–40 minutes	i.v.	Not subject to Controlled Drug regulations

21.7 Characteristics of the commonly used opioid drugs. CRI = constant rate infusion.

Choice of opioid

The choice of opioid drug depends on a number of drug- and animal-related factors. Figure 21.7 shows the duration of action and relative efficacy of different opioid drugs. It is also important to consider the Marketing Authorization (SPC, Summary of Product Characteristics) of the different opioid drugs available and choose drugs that are licensed where possible and follow the Prescribing Cascade.

Severity of pain

A full opioid agonist (methadone) should be given to animals that are likely to experience moderate or severe pain. Methadone has a relatively long duration of action and can be given repeatedly if analgesia is inadequate. Use of multimodal techniques may allow the dose of methadone to be reduced, or allow a partial agonist such as buprenorphine to be used instead. Fentanyl is an excellent analgesic drug but needs to be given continuously to provide effective analgesia postoperatively. Low doses given by constant rate infusion (CRI) postoperatively can provide good analgesia without significant respiratory depression or bradycardia. When given intraoperatively, respiratory depression is more likely because of the concurrent anaesthesia.

Expected ongoing plan for pain management

Clinical evidence suggests that administration of a partial opioid agonist (e.g. buprenorphine) with a full opioid agonist (e.g. methadone) does not produce additive analgesia. Therefore, if it is planned to use full opioid agonists intraoperatively or postoperatively, it is not ideal to premedicate with a partial opioid agonist.

Time of administration (premedication, intraoperative, postoperative)

Opioids given for premedication usually need to be longer acting. A choice is made between buprenorphine, butorphanol, and methadone depending on the severity of pain and the overall analgesia plan. Sedation from buprenorphine is usually less than from the other drugs; therefore, if an animal is very excitable or aggressive, a higher dose of methadone should be given. Buprenorphine combined with alpha-2 agonists is a good combination for premedication. The analgesia and sedation provided by the alpha-2 agonist means that a full opioid agonist is often unnecessary.

When giving opioids intraoperatively to provide additional analgesia, good analgesia is required. It is therefore sensible to choose a full agonist (e.g. methadone, fentanyl). Fentanyl is ideally given by CRI; however, if only a short duration of additional analgesia is required (e.g. during ovary removal in a spay procedure) then a single bolus dose is effective. Fentanyl CRI will also significantly reduce the amount of inhalant agent required to maintain anaesthesia, contributing to a balanced anaesthesia technique.

Ability to re-dose

If animals are not checked frequently overnight, then administration of a longer-acting opioid (e.g. buprenorphine) is desirable in order to achieve the longest duration of analgesia. This is also true for animals going home after surgery, when there is only a single chance to administer an injectable opioid.

Routes of administration

Fentanyl can be given by CRI, but animals should be monitored at regular intervals. Buprenorphine can be given by the orotransmucosal route in cats, which removes the need for repeated injections.

Non-steroidal anti-inflammatory drugs

NSAIDs are an important component of polymodal therapies aimed at providing perioperative analgesia in dogs and cats and are also used in the management of chronic pain, particularly osteoarthritis. Evidence suggests that the analgesic efficacy of most veterinary NSAIDs is comparable, so the most important factor in choice of NSAID is safety. Differences in the relative risk of side effects from different NSAIDs are apparent, particularly when used during the perioperative period.

NSAIDs inhibit the production of prostaglandins through inhibition of the cyclooxygenase (COX) enzyme system. Tissue damage causes the release of cell membrane lipids and prostaglandins are generated by the action of COX enzymes on products derived from those lipids. There are two isoforms of the enzyme: COX-1 and COX-2. Prostaglandins produced by the COX-1 pathway function largely (though not exclusively) in the gastrointestinal system, genital tract and brain. Many side effects of prostaglandins arise through inhibition of the production of such 'housekeeping' prostaglandins. Prostaglandins produced by the COX-2 pathway are largely (though not exclusively) generated following tissue damage and are termed inducible prostaglandins. It is these prostaglandins that are most important in mediating inflammation.

Side effects

The most important adverse effects of NSAIDs are: impairment of renal function and gastrointestinal irritation and ulceration. Although all NSAIDs can have antithrombotic effects by inhibiting the production of thromboxane A2, at therapeutic doses most NSAIDs (with the exception of aspirin) do not impair clotting mechanisms or impair bleeding time.

In the kidney locally produced prostaglandins are continually active in maintaining afferent arteriolar dilatation, and during periods of hypotension (such as may occur during anaesthesia) these prostaglandins assume an important role in the maintenance of normal renal haemodynamics. If the production of these prostaglandins is inhibited through the administration of an NSAID, renal hypoperfusion may occur with the potential to cause renal failure.

In the stomach and gastrointestinal system, prostaglandins promote the secretion of protective mucus, maintain mucosal blood flow and play a role in the modulation of gastric acid secretion. An NSAID-mediated decrease in prostaglandin production through inhibition of COX-1 can result in gastrointestinal ulceration (see Chapter 8).

Probably the most significant variation in NSAIDs lies in the safety of their administration during the perioperative period. The use of NSAIDs perioperatively has been shown to provide effective analgesia following a variety of orthopaedic and soft tissue procedures in both dogs and cats. Meloxicam, carprofen and robenacoxib (injectable form) are specifically authorized in the UK for perioperative administration to cats and dogs. Firocoxib and cimicoxib are also authorized for preoperative administration to dogs, but are not available as injectable preparations. Administration of all other commercially available NSAIDs (e.g. ketoprofen) should be delayed until the animal is fully recovered from anaesthesia and normotensive. It is strongly advisable to avoid the perioperative administration of all NSAIDs in animals with impaired renal function. Gastrointestinal side effects are a particular problem during the chronic use of NSAIDs, for example in the management of osteoarthritis.

Clinical recommendations for perioperative NSAIDs

- Only administer NSAIDs that are authorized for preoperative administration in the perioperative period
- Only administer an NSAID preoperatively to healthy animals undergoing routine procedures when hypotension during anaesthesia is not anticipated. Renal compromise is possible if an animal becomes hypotensive during anaesthesia when any NSAID has been given. If in doubt, delay NSAID administration until the animal is fully recovered from anaesthesia
- Do not give NSAIDs to trauma or shock patients until they are normotensive and cardiovascularly stable
- Do not give NSAIDs to animals with pre-existing renal disease
- Do not give NSAIDs to animals with disorders of haemostasis
- NSAIDs are liver metabolized, so liver dysfunction may alter the half-life of NSAIDs and lead to inadvertent drug overdose. Use carefully in animals with pre-existing liver disease and monitor the animal for altered liver function (blood biochemistry testing)
- Do not combine different NSAIDs or give NSAIDs and corticosteroids together
- Check ongoing medications before perioperative drugs are administered

Other drugs used for analgesia

Ketamine

Ketamine has been available for many years and is widely used in veterinary medicine for sedation and injectable anaesthesia. Use of ketamine in human patients had dwindled due to problems on recovery, such as hallucinations. However, interest in ketamine has recently resurged due to recognition of its profound analgesic properties, which are present at sub-anaesthetic doses. The use of low doses of ketamine to provide analgesia has been adopted into small animal analgesic protocols. Ketamine is a Schedule 2 Controlled Drug with regulations affecting its storage and dispensing (see Chapter 8).

The principal analgesic action of ketamine is attributed to its NMDA receptor antagonist effects. Ketamine should be used as an adjunctive analgesic in combination with opioids, NSAIDs or other analgesics. It is not a drug that should be used alone to provide analgesia. It can be used safely in low doses to provide analgesia during surgery and during the postoperative period. At sub-anaesthetic doses, ketamine is not generally associated with CNS excitatory effects and concurrent sedation is minimal. CRI is advantageous to provide a stable background level of analgesia. Although a fluid infusion pump or syringe driver is not a prerequisite for this, it will allow more accurate and controlled administration. Ketamine by CRI is often used for 24–48 hours in dogs and cats, despite limited data describing the pharmacokinetics of ketamine after prolonged infusions. Ketamine is metabolized to norketamine, which may contribute to the pharmacological effect.

Alpha-2 adrenergic agonists

Alpha-2 adrenergic agonists (alpha-2 agonists) are potent sedative, hypnotic and analgesic agents; these properties make them useful adjuncts for anaesthesia in small animal practice. Alpha-2 agonists have a potent antinociceptive action in experimental and clinical studies in animals and humans. The mechanism of alpha-2 agonist-mediated antinociception is not entirely understood; both supraspinal (brain) and spinal sites of action are involved. Extensive laboratory animal studies investigating the mechanism of alpha-2 agonist antinociception are confounded by the effects of sedation on behavioural evaluation of analgesia. Sedation complicates conclusions, particularly those involving supraspinally organized pain-related behaviours, upon which some experimental tests are based.

Medetomidine and dexmedetomidine are most commonly used for sedation or premedication (see above) but their additional analgesic effects should not be forgotten. Incorporation of an alpha-2 agonist into a premedication protocol will contribute to intraoperative analgesia, particularly if the alpha-2 agonist is re-dosed during anaesthesia. Dexmedetomidine has been recently evaluated as a postoperative analgesic in a clinical study in dogs; given by CRI it was found to be equally efficacious as morphine CRI. Sedation provided by the two drugs was also not different. Therefore, although dexmedetomidine by CRI is not a first-line drug for perioperative analgesia, it can be a useful adjunct where adequate analgesia is problematic. Due to the relatively short duration of analgesia from a single dose compared with the duration of sedation, a CRI is required. It should be remembered that administration of atipamezole will reverse both sedative and analgesic effects.

Lidocaine

Systemically administered lidocaine has been shown to be effective in the treatment of acute postoperative pain and experimentally induced pin-prick pain and hyperalgesia in human studies. There are few robust clinical studies that have evaluated the use of systemic lidocaine for perioperative analgesia in animals.

The mechanism of analgesia following systemic lidocaine is not fully elucidated. Following peripheral nerve injury, sodium channel expression becomes modulated so that there is upregulation of sodium channel subtypes. This is associated with the presence of random and spontaneous ectopic discharges from injured nerves that occur in the absence of input from peripheral nociceptors. This abnormal activity causes abnormal input to the CNS and higher brain centres, which is interpreted as pain. Lidocaine is most effective at blocking sodium channels in a frequency-dependent manner. It is postulated that lidocaine may preferentially block the upregulated sodium channel subtypes, resulting in a reduction in perceived pain without any effect on normal conduction. Evidence suggests that the postoperative analgesic effect of an intraoperative lidocaine infusion cannot be simply attributed to residual plasma drug concentrations, suggesting the systemic lidocaine may have a pre-emptive analgesic effect.

Low-dose lidocaine by CRI is not associated with cardiovascular side effects, and heart rate and blood pressure have been shown to be well maintained in dogs; there are limited data describing the use of lidocaine by CRI in awake cats. More information on lidocaine is given under 'Local anaesthesia/analgesia', below.

Morphine/lidocaine/ketamine combination

A combination of morphine, lidocaine and ketamine (MLK) is relatively widely used for the provision of perioperative analgesia in cats and dogs. The drugs are usually mixed together in a single fluid bag and given simultaneously at a single rate that does not allow the rate of administration of the individual drugs in the mix to be adjusted. The underpinning rationale is that the combination is the ultimate multimodal analgesia protocol. There are, however, limited clinical data to support the use of this protocol.

Should a combination of drugs be required by intravenous infusion, it is optimal to give the drugs separately via separate infusion apparatus. This allows flexibility in dosing of the individual agents and also allows the animals to be weaned off the different drugs individually, rather than having to adopt an 'all or nothing' approach.

Gabapentin

Gabapentin, available as an oral preparation, has been proven to be effective for the treatment of neuropathic pain resulting from diabetic neuropathy and post-herpetic neuralgia in humans. Although its exact mode of action is not known, it appears to have a unique effect on voltage-dependent calcium ion channels at the post-synaptic dorsal horn. Other suggested mechanisms include enhanced inhibitory input of GABA-mediated pathways and antagonism of NMDA receptors.

Animal studies have shown that gabapentin does not alter acute nociception but suppresses experimentally induced hyperalgesia. There is strong experimental evidence that gabapentin prevents the development of neuronal sensitization and reverses established neuronal sensitization. This suggests that gabapentin may prove effective in acute pain disorders involving neuronal sensitization, such as postoperative pain.

There are no published clinical studies describing the use of gabapentin in cats or dogs for acute or chronic pain management. Anecdotal evidence suggests that it is widely used in specialist clinics in the management of osteoarthritis pain and cancer pain refractory to conventional analgesic strategies. In this setting it is used as an adjunctive agent with therapies such as NSAIDs, fentanyl patches and tramadol. The quoted dose range for gabapentin in cats and dogs is wide; it is advisable to start at the low end of the dose range and then increase the dose gradually until an effect is achieved. Gabapentin is metabolized by the liver and excreted via the kidneys, so that liver and kidney dysfunction may result in drug accumulation unless the dose is adjusted. Side effects include lethargy, sedation and ataxia, and sometimes nausea. The pharmacokinetics of gabapentin in cats and dogs have been described, but optimal dosing regimens to provide analgesia and the effects of prolonged gabapentin administration have not been investigated.

Tramadol

Although tramadol has been available as an analgesic drug for a number of years, it is only recently that the mechanism of action has been fully understood. Tramadol is a unique analgesic with opioid and non-opioid properties. Its action on mu opioid receptors is weak, and naloxone antagonizes only 30% of its analgesic activity. Alpha-2 antagonists significantly reverse tramadol analgesia, and therefore much of its analgesic action is thought likely to be via inhibition of reuptake of neurotransmitters such as noradrenaline. It is now accepted that in addition to a mu opioid agonist effect, tramadol enhances the function of the spinal descending inhibitory pathway by inhibition of reuptake of both 5HT (5-hydroxytryptamine, serotonin) and noradrenaline, together with presynaptic stimulation of 5HT release.

Similarly to gabapentin, tramadol is widely used as an adjunctive analgesic for chronic pain, yet there are limited published studies describing clinical use in cats or dogs. In contrast to gabapentin, tramadol is also used for perioperative pain management. It is available in the UK in licensed tablet and injectable formulations for dogs. The tablets are very bitter and cats especially find them distasteful. It is a Schedule 3 Controlled Drug and the RCVS recommends that all Schedule 3 drugs are kept in a locked cabinet. Metabolism is principally via hepatic biotransformation, with a small amount excreted unchanged by the kidneys. Side effects, though rare, may include gastrointestinal upset and sedation. Because of tramadol's monoamine reuptake inhibition, it should not be given to animals taking tricyclic antidepressants, serotonin reuptake inhibitors or monoamine oxidase inhibitors.

Routes of analgesic drug administration

In common with other drugs (see Chapter 8), the route of administration of analgesics is affected by authorization, pharmacological effects and onset of activity (see Figure 21.7).

- **Intravenous injection:** Best when analgesia is required quickly. Efficacious opioids such as fentanyl and alfentanil, when administered in the aqueous form, should only be given by slow intravenous injection. Pethidine cannot be given intravenously due to histamine release. Morphine must also be diluted and given slowly to prevent histamine release.
- **Intramuscular injection:** Care must be taken with the volume of drugs given and when choosing the injection site, as repeated injection at the same site will cause soreness. This is especially true for animals with low bodyweight where a limited muscle mass increases the pain of repeated injection.
- **Subcutaneous injection:** Few pharmacokinetic data are available about the onset of action following subcutaneous injection of most drugs, although uptake is generally slower than with intramuscular or intravenous administration. The route is not recommended for buprenorphine, as current evidence suggests that uptake is slow, delaying the onset of action and ultimate efficacy.
- **Transmucosal** (Figure 21.8)**:** Shown to be effective in cats for the administration of buprenorphine. The newer multidose formulation of buprenorphine appears to be unpalatable to cats when given transmucosally, and 1 ml vial preparations are preferred.

Transdermal administration

Both fentanyl and buprenorphine transdermal patches are available and can provide a valuable non-invasive source of long-term analgesia. Data surrounding the clinical use of buprenorphine patches are limited and their effectiveness is currently unknown in dogs and cats. There is more research knowledge surrounding the use of fentanyl patches.

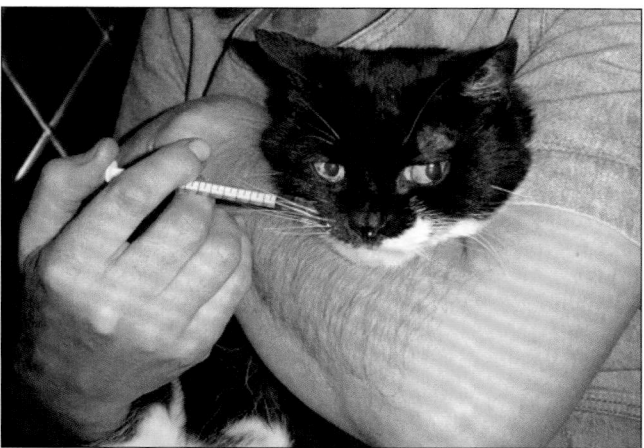

21.8 Oral transmucosal administration of buprenorphine.

Most patches comprise a reservoir of the drug covered with a membrane that limits the rate of absorption, surrounded by an adhesive dressing with which to attach the patch to the patient's skin. Matrix patches, where the drug is embedded in the adhesive plaster, are also available. The patches are designed for human skin, and transdermal bioavailability of fentanyl is much lower in feline (34%) or canine skin (64%). The site of patch placement is also likely to be important, as the characteristics of the skin (such as thickness and vascularity) over different sites of the body are likely to affect the rate of drug absorption, although this has not been formally evaluated in a controlled clinical study.

Commonly used sites of patch placement are the lateral thorax, medial aspect of the thigh, and tail. The contact between the patch and the skin must be optimal to promote drug absorption. It is important that the patient is not able to gain access to the patch and ingest it. The site of application of the patch should be gently clipped, the skin cleaned using a detergent and allowed to air dry. Although patches have an adhesive strip this is not robust enough for veterinary patients, and a dressing should be applied over the patch (Figure 21.9) to promote adhesion; use of tissue glue can also be helpful.

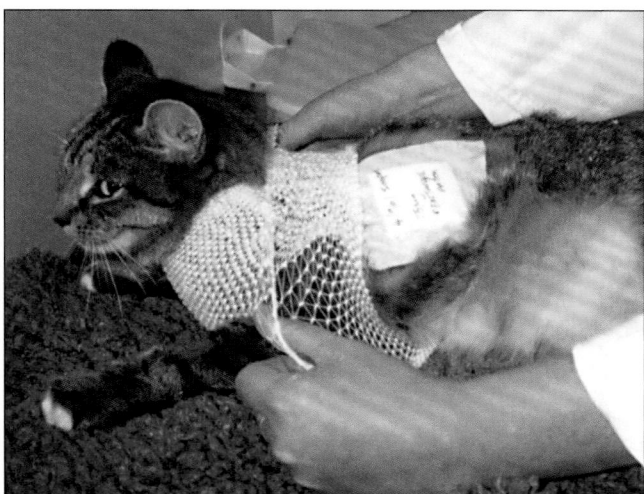

21.9 A fentanyl patch can be placed on clipped skin and covered with a flexible dressing to prevent the edges curling and excessive interference from the cat. It takes several hours to provide peak plasma fentanyl concentrations so it should be placed well in advance of surgery, and additional analgesia provided for the first few hours. (Courtesy of Polly Taylor)

Care should be taken when patches are used perioperatively as the patient's temperature and the temperature around the patch can affect the rate of drug absorption. If a patient is placed on to a warming device (e.g. a heat mat), the amount of drug released by the patch will increase. This can lead to severe respiratory depression in the case of fentanyl patches.

It takes approximately 24 hours in dogs and 12 hours in cats for the plasma concentration of fentanyl to reach therapeutic levels, so up until this time additional analgesia must be provided. There are many variables affecting the absorption of drugs via the transdermal route and using them as the sole method of analgesia is consequently unwise.

Constant rate infusions

The use of CRIs has increased in popularity over the last few years, in both the peri- and postoperative periods. The main advantage compared with repeated injections is that peaks and troughs in plasma concentration, and therefore fluctuations in the level of analgesia provision, can be avoided. This reduces the risk of breakthrough pain and consequently minimizes stimulation of the pain pathways, potentially reducing further central and peripheral sensitization. Another advantage is that the patient does not need to have repeated injections, particularly intramuscular ones.

When using a CRI, a 'loading' dose must first be administered to rapidly achieve plasma concentrations levels close to therapeutic levels. The infusion is started simultaneously to ensure that the therapeutic plasma concentration is maintained. The rate of infusion depends on the plasma concentration required as well as the rate at which the drug is redistributed and metabolized. The theory behind CRI is that as the drug is lost out of the circulation it is replaced, maintaining a constant plasma concentration.

CRI is mainly used for the intravenous administration of analgesics but is also useful for local anaesthetics, such as via epidural or wound catheters. When administering a drug by CRI, accuracy is vitally important. Although 'recipes' using only a standard giving set and a drip rate are available, they are not recommended, and use of either infusion pumps or syringe drivers is preferable (see Chapter 20). Selection of infusion apparatus with a high degree of accuracy for drug administration is important.

> ## Considerations for preparing drugs for CRI
>
> ■ The required rate of administration of potent analgesic drugs is often low, so diluting the drug with normal saline or lactated Ringer's (Hartmann's) solution will increase the accuracy of drug dosing. However, it is important to remember to adjust the volume in the bag or syringe before adding the drug. For example, for a 50 ml syringe, take up 45 ml of saline and then 5 ml of drug. If using a 500 ml bag of fluids and adding 5 ml of drug, remove 5 ml of the fluids from the bag first and then add the drug
> ■ Ensure that the drug solution is labelled with the patient details so that the infusion solution is uniquely linked with the patient for which it is intended
> ■ Ensure that the drug solution is clearly labelled with the date, drug name and concentration and intended infusion rate. It may be useful to add maximum and minimum infusion rates to guide administration ➜

Considerations for preparing drugs for CRI *continued*

- Ensure that the extension set or giving set is long enough to prevent the lines from becoming disconnected and that they are long enough to allow the patient to move around in the kennel
- Do not use needles to deliver the drug via an injection port but ensure that infusion lines are firmly connected using three-way taps or via a T-port
- Connect the infusion line delivering the drug as close as possible to the site of intravenous access in the patient. This reduces the time delay when the infusion is initially started.
- Ensure that connections and infusion lines are secured above ground level to prevent contamination of the infusion apparatus

Nursing considerations for CRI

- As CRI relies on the patency of the intravenous catheter, good catheter management is vital (see Chapter 20)
- If CRI is being used in a non-anaesthetized patient it is important to remember that the drugs commonly given by CRI usually cause some degree of sedation and, consequently, recumbency. It is important to nurse these patients like any other recumbent animal (see Chapter 15)
- It is vital to ensure that no joints in the fluid line (e.g. where two extension sets join) or three-way taps are on the floor, as this could be a source of contamination and could lead to a catheter infection.
- Remember to include the volume of fluids being used to administer the CRI in any fluid therapy calculation for the patient

Local anaesthesia/ analgesia

Local analgesia/anaesthesia techniques are widely used in human medicine. Use of a local technique can often reduce the dose of other anaesthetic drugs required for maintenance of anaesthesia and can contribute to a multi-modal analgesic technique. Use of specific nerve blocks to prevent the relay of nociceptive information from the site of injury to the spinal cord can also provide pre-emptive analgesia, and prevent or reduce the development of central sensitization.

Local anaesthetic agents

Mechanism of action

Local anaesthetics reversibly block the conduction of action potentials in neurons by causing changes in the neuron membrane that prevent depolarization and thus block the propagation of an action potential; this is termed membrane stabilization.

An action potential can be described as a brief fluctuation in membrane potential caused by the rapid opening and closing of voltage-gated sodium ion channels. In resting mode nerve fibres are polarized, with higher concentrations of sodium ions outside than inside the nerve, with the reverse true for potassium ions. The sodium and potassium channels are closed. Depolarization is caused by the sodium channels opening, which allows an influx of sodium ions into the nerve fibre. Local anaesthetics prevent the sodium channels from opening so that depolarization and therefore action potential transmission is prevented. Sensory neurons are more sensitive to the effects of local anaesthetics than are motor neurons and are therefore blocked by lower concentrations of local anaesthetics. However, although it would be highly desirable to produce a blockade of sensory nerve fibres without any concurrent effects on motor nerves and therefore movement, achieving a sensory block without concurrent motor effects is rarely possible.

Systemic toxicity

These agents are lipid-soluble, have low molecular weight and readily cross the blood–brain barrier. At sub-toxic doses, local anaesthetics can act as anticonvulsants, sedatives and analgesics. At higher concentrations they can cause convulsions, and generalized CNS depression occurs. Due to a combination of slowing of conduction in the myocardium, myocardial depression and peripheral vasodilatation, hypotension, bradycardia and cardiac arrest can occur.

Systemic toxicity depends on:

- Site of injection: vascular sites lead to rapid absorption. Intercostal injections give much higher plasma concentrations than subcutaneous injections
- Drug used
- Speed of injection: only important when given intravenously
- Addition of adrenaline: causes local vasoconstriction, resulting in slow absorption with reduction in peak concentration of up to 20–50%.

Cats are considered to be more susceptible than dogs to local anaesthetic toxicity, but problems are uncommon if appropriate doses are given. Safe maximum doses of lidocaine and lidocaine plus adrenaline are 4 mg/kg and 7 mg/kg respectively in both dogs and cats. The safe maximum doses of bupivacaine and ropivacaine are 2 mg/kg. When performing intercostal or intrapleural injections, the dose should be reduced by 25% because of the vascularity of the area that is being injected into.

Local anaesthesia techniques

Topical anaesthesia

The application of local anaesthetics to mucous membranes (transmucosal) produces analgesia rapidly (within 5 minutes). Common areas for topical administration include the cornea (for ocular examinations), the nasal passages (for placement of a nasal oxygen cannula) and the larynx (during intubation). The depth of analgesia produced in tissues is usually superficial (1–2 mm).

Absorption of local anaesthetic through the skin (stratum corneum) is poor. EMLA cream (APP Pharmaceuticals; contains lidocaine and prilocaine) is capable of producing anaesthesia if applied to the skin and covered with a non-permeable dressing for 30–60 minutes.

Infiltration anaesthesia

The infiltration of local anaesthetics is commonly performed in veterinary practice; it is safe, reliable and does not require extensive experience. Sterile sharp needles should be used. If subsequent injections are made at the periphery of each wheal, then only one needle prick is felt.

- Local anaesthetic should be diluted with 0.9% sodium chloride and not sterile water.
- Adrenaline at a concentration of 1:200,000 may be used to delay the absorption of local anaesthetics and increase the duration of effect.
- Adrenaline should not be used where an end-arterial supply exists, as skin necrosis may result (ears, tails).

Regional anaesthesia

The principle underlying regional anaesthesia is that the nerve supply to a specific region or area is blocked where the nerves are easily accessible from the skin. The nerves must be readily palpable and follow a fixed course next to easily identifiable anatomical structures (usually bones) or be known to be found at fixed positions. Use of a nerve stimulator (Figure 21.10) to locate the peripheral nerve can significantly increase the accuracy of drug deposition and therefore effectiveness of the block. This can also allow a lower total volume of the local anaesthetic drug to be used, reducing motor side effects and the risk of toxicity due to absorption of local anaesthetic agents into the systemic circulation.

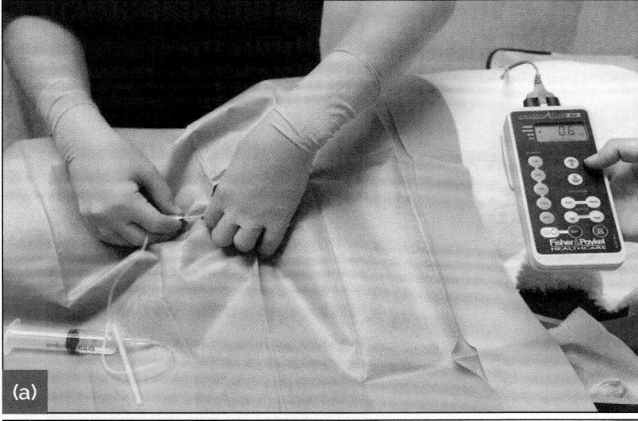

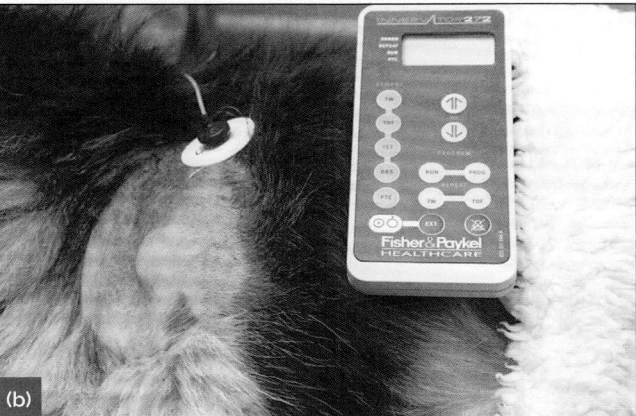

21.10 (a) Using a peripheral nerve stimulator to facilitate a brachial plexus block. The stimulating needle is being placed while an assistant holds the stimulator device. (b) The reference electrode is placed remote from the site of stimulation on a clipped area of skin.

The use of ultrasonography to guide placement of nerve blocks is becoming increasingly common; although, it requires the technical skill of knowing how to locate peripheral nerves using ultrasound guidance. In human medicine, it has been shown that blocks performed using ultrasound guidance were more likely to be successful, took less time to perform and had a faster onset time and longer duration of action than blocks performed using a peripheral nerve stimulator technique.

Brachial plexus block

This block provides analgesia distal to the elbow and is therefore useful during distal forelimb surgical procedures.

Preparation of the patient

The patient is positioned in lateral recumbency. The site of injection is just proximal to the point of the shoulder (Figure 21.11); therefore, a wide area should be clipped (approximately 6 cm x 6 cm) at this site, with the point of the shoulder at the centre. The skin should be prepared as if for surgery.

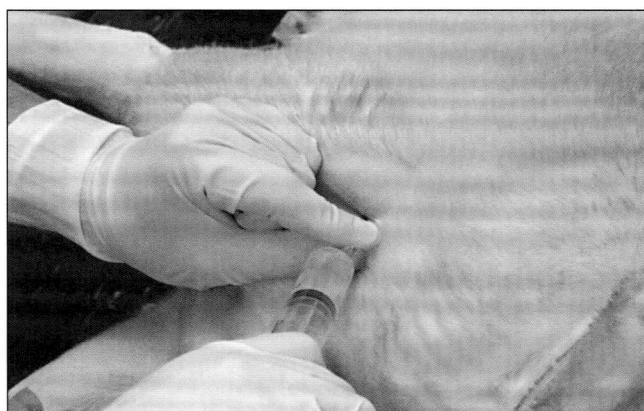

21.11 Brachial plexus block in a dog. The needle has been placed without using a peripheral nerve stimulator (see Figure 21.10) and bupivacaine is being injected.

Clinical notes

The two most important complications following brachial plexus blocks are pneumothorax due to puncture of the cupulae (the apex of each pleural cavity lying at the thoracic inlet) and haemorrhage as a result of puncture of the axillary artery and vein. The needle should be aspirated prior to injection of the local anaesthetic block to prevent inadvertent intravenous injection of the local anaesthetic. This will also allow identification of needle placement in the cupulae. Some resistance should be felt during injection. Damage to the brachial plexus nerves themselves is also possible if the needle penetrates the nerve bundle. This is uncommon, particularly if a nerve stimulator or ultrasonography are used to allow accurate location of the individual nerves that comprise the brachial plexus.

Femoral and sciatic nerve block

This block provides analgesia distal to the mid-shaft of the femur and is therefore particularly useful for providing intra- and postoperative analgesia for surgery of the stifle.

Preparation of the patient

The patient is positioned in lateral recumbency with the limb to be blocked uppermost. There are a number of potential injection sites for a femoral nerve block in dogs and cats. The authors favour a lumbar plexus approach to the femoral nerve using a peripheral nerve locator. The skin area corresponding to the lumbar (L) vertebrae L4–L6 is aseptically prepared after clipping the hair, and the needle is inserted parallel to the sagittal plane 1–2 cm lateral to the spinal process of L5. An alternative approach to block the femoral nerve is to use a medial approach, locating the nerve by its proximity to the femoral artery. The sciatic nerve is most easily approached between the greater trochanter of the femur and the ischiatic tuberosity.

Clinical notes

Similarly to the brachial plexus block, it is important to aspirate to confirm that the needle has not been inadvertently placed in a peripheral vein or artery before injection. The main advantage of a femoral and sciatic nerve block compared with epidural anaesthesia for stifle surgery is that only unilateral motor paralysis is produced, facilitating a rapid return to ambulation after surgery. Although bupivacaine has a duration of action of approximately 6 hours, studies have shown equivalent analgesia for the first 24 hours postoperatively in dogs undergoing unilateral stifle surgery that received either a femoral and sciatic nerve block with bupivacaine or epidural analgesia with morphine and bupivacaine. The incidence of urinary retention and intraoperative complications was also reduced in the group receiving a femoral and sciatic nerve block compared with epidural anaesthesia.

Epidural anaesthesia

Lumbosacral epidural anaesthesia may be used to provide analgesia for all procedures caudal to the thoracolumbar junction. It is especially useful for orthopaedic procedures in the hindquarters. Use of a combination of preservative-free morphine and bupivacaine is optimal. Morphine has a prolonged duration of action (18–24 hours) and therefore provides significant postoperative analgesia. Veterinary nurses are not permitted to carry out epidural administration of drugs, as placement of catheters or needles for epidural anaesthesia involves entering a body space, which may only be carried out by a veterinary surgeon. It is important, however, that veterinary nurses have knowledge of the technique and the effects of drugs injected into the epidural space.

Preparation of the patient

Careful preparation of the patient to ensure that the epidural injection can be made aseptically is important. Epidural injection is usually carried out with the animal in sternal recumbency with the hindlimbs directed forward, although some people prefer to have the animal in lateral recumbency. The epidural space between L7 and S1 is identified in order to ensure that the site of clipping is correct. The dorsal spinous process of L7 is more pronounced than the preceding dorsal processes and immediately caudal to it a dip can be felt. A large window (approximately 6 cm x 6 cm) is clipped around the L7–S1 space and the skin prepared aseptically in a similar way to that for surgery. Drugs for administration into the epidural space should be drawn up and administered aseptically using sterile gloves, needles and syringes.

Technique

A spinal needle (22 G) (Figure 21.12) or Tuohy needle (17 G or 18 G) (Figure 21.13), is placed perpendicular to the skin surface and slowly advanced through the skin by the veterinary surgeon.

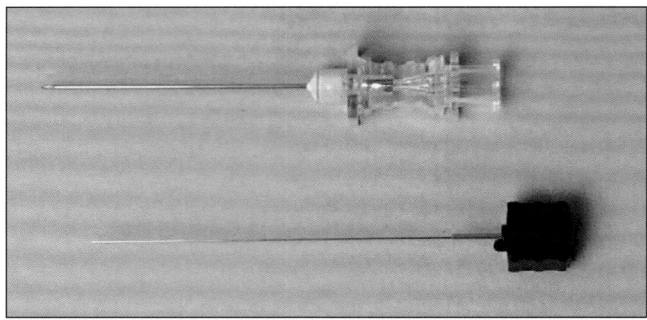

21.12 A 22 G short spinal needle suitable for use in a cat or dog. The stylet has been removed from the needle.

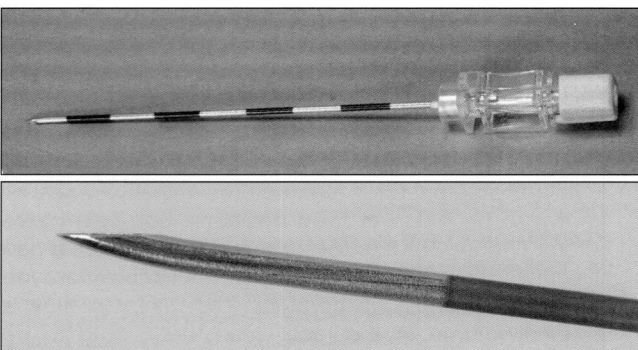

21.13 Tuohy needle, showing detail of curved distal end.

Initially the stylet is left *in situ* in the needle, but as the point of the needle nears the anticipated site of the epidural space the stylet is removed. A popping sensation is felt as the needle penetrates the ligamentum flavum. Correct placement of the needle is checked in two ways:

- Loss of resistance: Correct placement of the needle is confirmed by a lack of resistance to the injection of either air or saline into the epidural space. Air may be associated with a patchy block as the air tends to localize around the nerve roots, resulting in an ineffective block
- Hanging drop: Once the epidural needle and stylet have been advanced through the superficial tissue, the stylet is removed and a drop of saline placed on the hub of the needle (Figure 21.14). The needle is then gradually advanced; entry of the tip of the needle into the epidural space is associated with the rapid movement of the drop of saline into the epidural space so that it can no longer be seen.

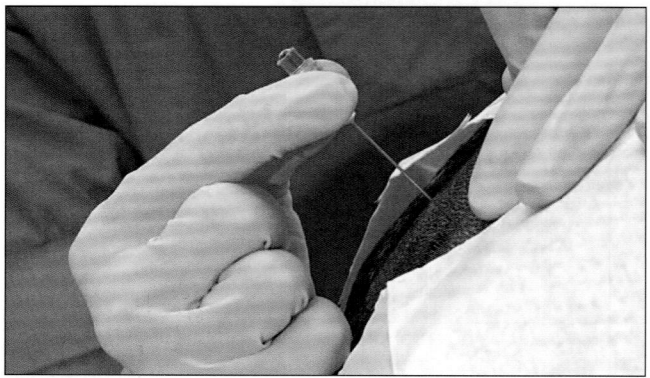

21.14 Epidural analgesia in a dog. The stylet has been removed from the spinal needle and a hanging drop is being used to locate the epidural space.

The presence of blood in the hub of the needle indicates that the needle has penetrated a blood vessel (usually the spinal ventral sinus), which typically occurs if the needle is not inserted in the midline. The needle should be withdrawn and placement started again once the position of the animal has been checked and the location of L7–S1 confirmed.

If cerebrospinal fluid (CSF) is present in the needle, the dose of local anaesthetic should be reduced by 50% or the needle replaced in a new space. Injection of local anaesthetic into the CSF is known as spinal anaesthesia, which has a more rapid onset than epidural anaesthesia.

Clinical notes

Epidural anaesthesia with local anaesthetic agents can induce vasodilation of the mesenteric blood vessels due to blockade of sympathetic nervous system tone to the splanchnic vessels. Caution should be exercised in hypovolaemic patients, although fluid administration readily resolves the hypotension. Hypoventilation and paralysis may occur if the local anaesthetic spreads too far cranially (e.g. too large a volume has been injected). Artificial ventilation is instigated until the local anaesthetic block resolves and no adverse effects are seen. Epidural anaesthesia should not be carried out in patients with septicaemia or when the needle would have to traverse an area of infected skin. Coagulation disorders are also a contraindication to epidural anaesthesia due to the risk of continued bleeding around the spinal cord if a blood vessel is damaged during needle placement.

Morphine injected epidurally can be associated with urinary retention; therefore, urination should be monitored in all animals for approximately 24 hours following epidural administration of morphine. If urinary retention occurs, placement of a urinary catheter to facilitate urination is likely to be indicated.

Local anaesthetics injected epidurally will cause motor effects and hindlimb paralysis for their duration of action (typically 6–8 hours for bupivacaine). This should be considered when walking dogs that have received epidural local anaesthetics, and hindlimb support should be provided.

Hair regrowth at the site of epidural injection is more prolonged than for other body areas; it can therefore be prudent to warn owners that regrowth may take up to 6 months after clipping.

Epidural catheters

Placement of an epidural catheter can be useful in patients that will benefit from a longer period of epidural analgesia, avoiding the need for repeat epidural injection. Kits are commercially available that contain all the equipment required for placement of an epidural catheter by the veterinary surgeon.

The first stage is the placement of a Tuohy needle in the epidural space. Tuohy needles have a rounded blunt-ended curved tip (see Figure 21.13), so that there is no risk of damaging or cutting the catheter as it is threaded through the needle. The tip of the catheter is usually inserted up to the level of L3–L4, although more caudal placement may be required if the site of injury is distal to this. To prevent motor effects during catheter placement, usually morphine alone is injected into the epidural space for pain management. However, the catheters can become irritating after 12–24 hours, and injection of a low dose of lidocaine or bupivacaine before the injection of morphine can be helpful.

A bacterial filter is placed between the end of the catheter and the injection port to reduce the risk of infection being introduced into the epidural space. It is imperative that epidural catheters are managed aseptically and clearly labelled, so that other drugs are not inadvertently injected through the injection port.

Intercostal nerve block

Intercostal nerve blocks are useful for relieving pain following thoracic surgery and trauma. Following thoracotomy, the surgeon can easily place these blocks prior to closing the chest, using direct visualization of the intercostal nerve, artery and vein bundle. Bupivacaine is usually chosen because of its longer duration of action.

Intrapleural anaesthesia

Intrapleural application of local anaesthetics is a very effective technique for providing analgesia following thoracotomy or rib trauma. The local anaesthetic can be administered either through an over-the-needle catheter or through an indwelling chest drain (Figure 21.15). The site of injection is the cranial edge of a rib. The animal should be placed with the injured side downwards for the block to be maximally effective. Local anaesthetics are acidic and this route of administration is very painful in conscious animals. Diluting the dose of local anaesthetic with 0.9% saline (up to 40 ml total volume in a large dog) can reduce pain. Alternatively, sodium bicarbonate can be added to the local anaesthetic, though it is difficult to achieve physiological pH without generating precipitation. Bupivacaine produces analgesia of approximately 8 hours' duration.

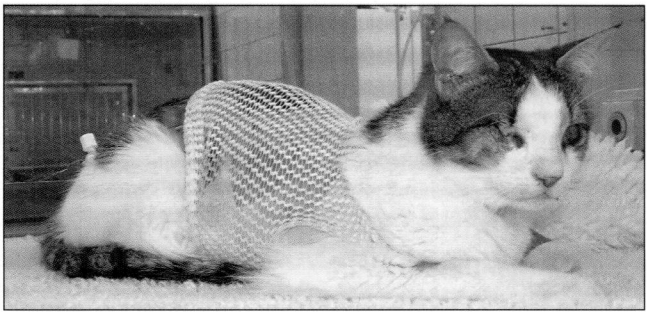

21.15 Cat with a chest drain placed after surgery. Intrapleural analgesia can be provided by injection of bupivacaine down the chest drain every 8 hours.

Maxillary and mandibular nerve blocks

These are extremely useful for analgesia for dental procedures or jaw surgery. The maxillary (Figure 21.16) and mandibular (Figure 21.17) nerves can be blocked as they exit from the infraorbital and mental foramina, respectively, or can be blocked more proximally, to provide a wider area of analgesia.

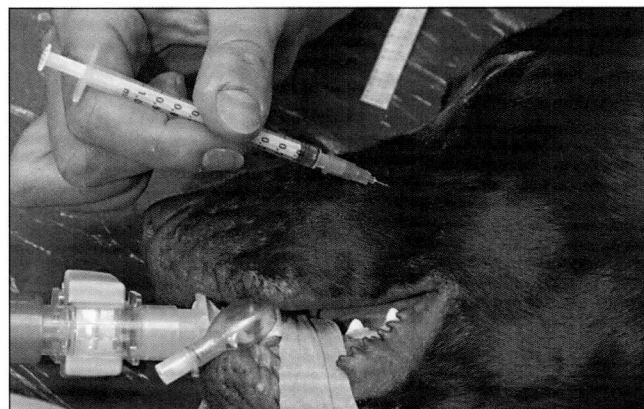

21.16 Site of injection for a distal maxillary nerve block, with the needle placed in the infraorbital foramen. Injection of local anaesthetic to block the infraorbital nerve will desensitize the ipsilateral soft tissues and upper incisor, premolar and canine teeth.

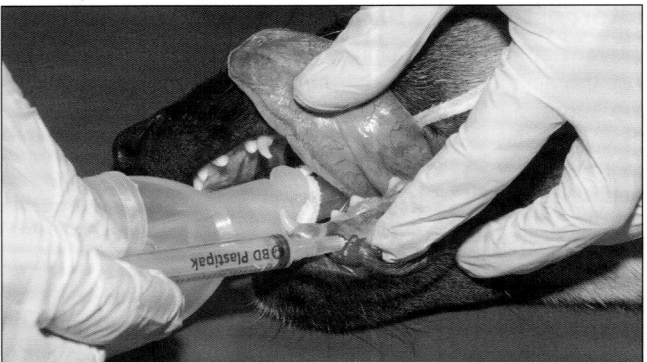

21.17 Distal mandibular nerve block. Local anaesthetic is being injected into the mental foramen. This will desensitize the ipsilateral lower incisors, premolar and canine teeth.

The use of dental nerve blocks will lower the concentration of inhalant agent required for surgery and provide postoperative analgesia. Using a combination of lidocaine and bupivacaine for the block has the advantage of a short-onset of action and a prolonged duration of action, facilitating postoperative analgesia. Small gauge needles (25 G, 5/8 inch) are suitable for carrying out dental blocks, as they reduce the risk of trauma to the dental tissues and only small volumes of injectate are required (typically 0.25 to 0.5 ml of local anaesthetic per block). When carrying out multiple blocks, it is important to calculate the safe maximum dose of local anaesthetic for the patient and ensure that this dose is not exceeded. Care must be taken when performing a maxillary nerve block in cats because of the proximity of the injection site to the globe of the eye; penetration of the globe has been reported as an adverse event following maxillary nerve block in the cat.

Intrasynovial analgesia

Injection of local anaesthetics and morphine is being increasingly employed to provide analgesia in small animals following joint surgery or arthroscopy. Generally, it is recommended that these drugs are infused at the end of surgery so they are not flushed out of the joint prior to closure. The injection is usually made by the surgeon using sterile needles and syringes as aseptic technique is important. Intrasynovial analgesia has not undergone rigorous evaluation in the clinical arena, however, and information regarding clinical efficacy is lacking; it should therefore only be adopted as part of a multimodal analgesia protocol. The optimal doses of local anaesthetic and morphine have not been determined.

Wound catheters

Soaker or wound catheters are commonly used in human anaesthesia to provide postoperative analgesia following surgery. The catheters are placed by the surgeon at the end of the surgical procedure and sutured loosely in place (Figure 21.18). Postoperatively, local anaesthetic agents such as bupivacaine can be injected down the catheter to provide topical analgesia. The catheters come in different lengths and have holes along the distal third of the catheter to allow the injected local anaesthetic to spread into the area of surgical trauma. This technique usually allows the dose of systemic analgesics to be reduced, contributing to a multimodal protocol. A good example of a surgical procedure for which wound catheters can be very helpful is limb amputation. The catheter can be left in place for 24–36 hours after surgery and bupivacaine instilled every 8 hours to provide pain relief. It is important that the catheter is secured in place and covered to prevent removal by the patient.

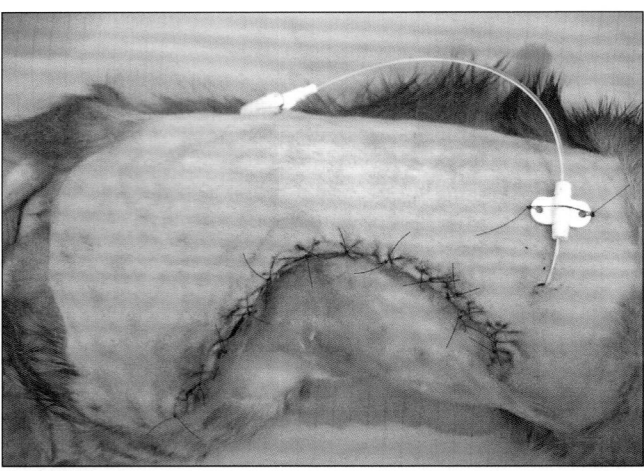

21.18 Wound catheter placed following reconstructive surgery in the flank of a cat. Bupivacaine administered through the wound catheter every 6–8 hours was used to provide analgesia.

Induction of general anaesthesia

Induction of anaesthesia may be carried out using one of the following techniques:

- Injectable anaesthetic agent or combination of agents (usually short-acting) given intravenously
- Injectable anaesthetic agent or combination of agents given intramuscularly
- Inhalant agent given via mask or an induction chamber.

Placement of an intravenous catheter should be mandatory before induction of anaesthesia whichever technique is used.

Choice of induction technique depends upon several factors:

- Species: In some animals, such as feral cats, intravenous access may not be easily achieved
- Temperament of the patient: In some animals it may not be possible to administer an injectable agent. If gaseous anaesthesia is used for induction, temperament may influence the use of a mask or an induction chamber
- Anaesthesia protocol: The anaesthetist may choose to use a total injectable anaesthetic technique or maintenance with an inhalant agent (see below)
- Age of the patient: It may be preferable to avoid injectable agents in very young animals where liver metabolism of injected drugs will be slower, thereby prolonging recovery.

Drugs commonly used to induce anaesthesia

Injectable agents

Figure 21.19 gives the key pharmacological properties of commonly used injectable induction agents, together with the advantages and disadvantages associated with them. Further information is given on these agents in the section on 'Maintenance of anaesthesia'.

Drug	Routes of administration	Cardiovascular system effects	Respiratory system effects	Drug formulation and preparation	Other notes
Propofol	i.v.: does not cause thrombophlebitis if injected outside of the vein	Myocardial depression, vasodilation & bradycardia	Respiratory depression, may cause apnoea after injection	Two preparations of propofol are available. In both preparations the propofol is solubilised in egg phosphatide and soya bean oil. One preparation contains a preservative allowing a 28 day shelf life once the vial is broached; the other preparation does not contain a preservative and the remainder of the vial should be discarded immediately after use	Propofol is relatively non-accumulative in dogs and can be used to maintain anaesthesia by incremental injection or CRI. Cats are less able to metabolise phenols than dogs and accumulation with repeated dosing or administration by CRI is likely, leading to a prolonged recovery. The preparation containing a preservative should not be used by CRI because of the risk of benzyl alcohol (preservative) toxicity
Alfaxalone	i.v. i.m. (unlicenced)	Myocardial depression associated with a compensatory increase in heart rate	Respiratory depression, may cause apnoea after injection	Alfaxalone is solubilised in a cyclodextrin that does not cause histamine release, can be used in cats and dogs	Recoveries can be stormy if given to unpremedicated animals. Can be used to maintain anaesthesia by incremental injection or CRI. Preparation does not contain a preservative, should be discarded or used immediately once the bottle is opened. A new multi-dose preparation is now available that contains a preservative and has a shelf life of 28 days once the bottle is broached. Alfaxalone administered i.m. can be a useful technique to sedated cats and small dogs. Be aware that this route of administration is unlicensed. Research indicates that puppy vitality is well maintained when alfaxalone is used for induction of anaesthesia prior to caesarean section
Ketamine	i.v. i.m.	Stimulates the sympathetic nervous system, increases heart rate, minimal effects on cardiac output	Minimal effects on the respiratory system, may cause an apneustic breathing pattern	Preparation contains a preservative	Can cause pain on i.m. injection. Only use in premedicated animals, commonly combined with a benzodiazepine when used for induction of anaesthesia. Low doses are used for induction of anaesthesia, higher doses are required to produce a period of anaesthesia as part of a total injectable technique. Recoveries after ketamine can be "spacey" or stormy, particularly in dogs. Analgesic
Etomidate (unlicensed in cats and dogs)	i.v.	Minimal effects on heart rate or inotropy	Minimal effects on the respiratory system	Two formulations are available; in one formulation the etomidate is solubilised in propylene glycol which can be associated with hydrolysis, pain on injection and thrombophlebitis. The other form of etomidate is solubilised in a hyperlipid emulsion (similar to propofol)	Etomidate is suitable to induce animals with severe cardiovascular compromise. Stormy inductions of anaesthesia and recovery from anaesthesia are likely in poorly premedicated patients. The product suppresses endogenous adrenocortical function for up to three hours after administration. Not suitable for administration by CRI

21.19 Key pharmacology of injectable drugs used for induction of anaesthesia.

Inhalant agents

Two methods are used to deliver an inhalational agent for induction of anaesthesia. The advantages and disadvantages of chamber *versus* mask induction techniques are described in Figure 21.20.

Chamber induction technique

It is better to use a chamber that is as small as possible without compromising and squashing the animal. Use of a clear plastic chamber allows constant observation of the animal during induction, which is advantageous. An entry and an exit port are built into the chamber. The entry port (usually 15 mm in diameter) allows connection of an anaesthetic breathing circuit to the chamber for the delivery of inhalant agent and oxygen via an anaesthetic machine. The exit port (usually 22 mm in diameter) allows the connection of a scavenging system to the chamber to remove the inhalant agent.

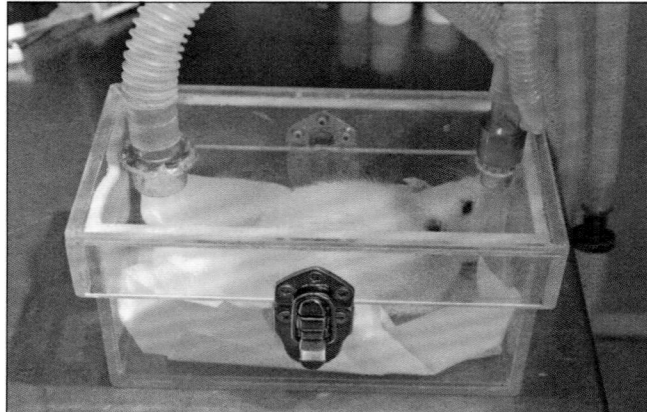

21.21 Rat placed in a clear chamber for induction of anaesthesia using an inhalant agent. The green tube is delivering inhalant anaesthetic vaporized in oxygen into the chamber; the clear plastic tube is scavenging.

1. First fill the chamber with oxygen.
2. Place the patient inside the closed chamber.
3. The inhalant agent is delivered via an anaesthetic machine (Figure 21.21). It is necessary to use a high percentage of volatile anaesthetic carried within high fresh gas flow in order to achieve anaesthesia in a timely fashion (e.g. 3–4% isoflurane or 7–8% sevoflurane).
4. Once the patient has lost the righting reflex (i.e. it does not try and correct its position when the chamber is tipped slightly), flush the chamber with oxygen to remove excess inhalant agent via the scavenging pipeline.
5. Open the chamber and remove the patient quickly before re-sealing the chamber.
6. Use a face mask to deliver further inhalant agent to maintain anaesthesia until a suitable plane has been obtained and the patient can be intubated. It is also possible to maintain anaesthesia via inhalant agent delivery by face mask, but this has health and safety implications for staff working in the area.

Mask induction technique

The animal is restrained and anaesthetic gases are delivered via a face mask and anaesthetic breathing circuit. There are two commonly used types of mask: clear ridged polycarbonate masks with a rubber diaphragm to provide a good fit of the mask over the nose and face of the animal (Figure 21.22); and flexible black rubber masks. Flexible rubber masks help reduce the potential for trauma during induction

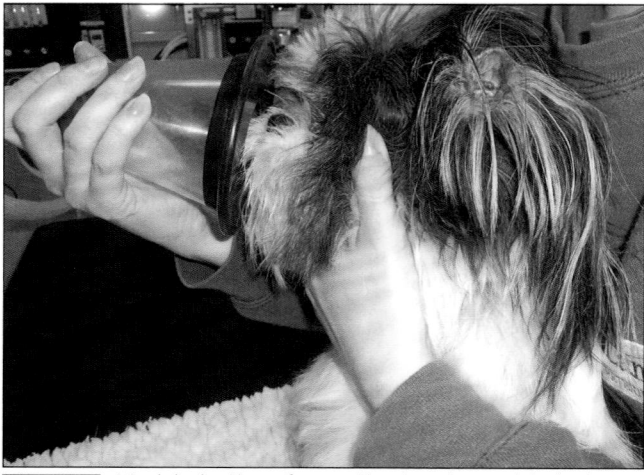

21.22 Mask induction of anaesthesia using an inhalant anaesthetic agent in a dog.

of anaesthesia. This type of mask, however, tends to lack a rubber diaphragm where the mask fits over the face of the animal, making them inappropriate for use with inhalant agents due to the atmospheric pollution caused by not having a tight seal around the patient's nose and face. They are also not transparent, and so visual observation of the patient is impaired.

Technique	Advantages	Disadvantages
Chamber induction	Does not require restraint of the patient	Depending on the size of the chamber it can take a relatively long period of time to build up a high concentration of inhalant agent inside the chamber; induction can be prolonged. Most animals find the technique aversive; injury may occur if the animal becomes excited and can move freely in the chamber. Movement can be limited by using a chamber size that is appropriate for the size of the animal. Significant environmental contamination occurs when the chamber is opened to remove the animal
Mask induction	Does not require any additional equipment, although suitably sized face masks must be available for delivery of the anaesthetic agent to the patient. Easy to deliver a high concentration of inhalant agent rapidly. The animal is restrained and cannot injure itself	Most animals find the technique aversive. Use of sevoflurane provides a faster induction than other agents. Difficult to restrain aggressive or unsedated patients. Use of 'cat bags' can be useful to improve control of the patient. Leaking of inhalational agent around the face mask results in environmental contamination

21.20 Advantages and disadvantages of chamber and mask induction using inhalant agents.

Monitoring during induction

As the induction agent is being administered by the veterinary surgeon it is important to observe respiration and measure pulse rate by palpation (see later).

Preparation of equipment

It is important to ensure prior to inducing anaesthesia that all equipment required for the procedure (including emergency equipment and drugs) is available and has been checked. The equipment typically needed includes:

- Intravenous catheterization equipment
- Larygnoscope and appropriately sized blade (usually a straight Miller blade)
- Tube tie (e.g. white open weave bandage)
- Swab to hold the tongue during intubation
- Endotracheal tubes – appropriate selection (see below for further information regarding endotracheal tubes)
- Cuff inflation syringe
- Eye lubricant – eyes should be lubricated after the induction of anaesthesia; this should be repeated at least hourly during anaesthetic
- Saline flush
- Intravenous fluids (if appropriate)
- Drugs as instructed by veterinary surgeon
- Additional monitoring equipment:
  - ECG pads
  - Blood pressure cuff
  - Capnograph connector.

The anaesthetic machine and appropriate breathing system should also be checked at this point to ensure they are in safe working order. Further details on this procedure are covered below.

Safety checklists

The use of safety checklists has become increasingly more popular over recent years. They originate from the aviation industry, where safety is paramount. The aim of these checklists is not only to prompt everyone involved in the process of anaesthetizing a patient to check that all equipment is present and correct, but also to improve dialogue amongst the whole team to ensure that everyone is aware of all possible considerations and problems with the individual patient. This was highlighted by the World Health Organization's Safe Surgery Saves Lives initiative, in its attempt to reduce the number of surgical deaths worldwide. This initiative was first published in 2008 and has now been widely adopted.

Bearing this in mind, the Association of Veterinary Anaesthetists (AVA) has produced a checklist and an implementation manual to assist practices in the process of introducing this initiative to the veterinary environment (https://ava.eu.com/wp-content/uploads/2015/11/AVA-Checklist-Booklet-FINAL-Web-copy.pdf and https://ava.eu.com/wp-content/uploads/2015/11/AVA-Anaesthetic-Safety-Checklist-FINAL-UK-WEB-copy-2.pdf) (Figure 21.23). Each of the steps involved in the checklist has been included to reduce the risk of significant harm to the patient; it is not designed to be a comprehensive list of actions involved with anaesthetizing a patient. These checklists emphasize that all members of the team are responsible for patient safety – it is not only the responsibility of the veterinary surgeon in charge of the case. The idea is that it is not just a box ticking exercise, rather, it is the performance of the associated actions and the communication and information sharing that it promotes which is important.

Safety checklists should form part of the wider anaesthetic record for the patient and be saved in paper form or scanned electronically onto the patient's records. The requirements for patient records are discussed in Chapter 9.

In human medicine, the poor transfer of information has been identified to be a major risk factor associated with medical errors, as well as poor patient outcomes, decreased patient satisfaction and increased length of hospital stay. The checklist is performed at three specific time points during the procedures, prior to the commencement of the following:

- Pre-induction
- Pre-procedure
- Recovery.

Pre-induction checklist

The pre-induction checklist includes confirmation of:

- Patient name, owner consent and procedure
- Intravenous cannula in place and patent
- Airway equipment available and checked to be functioning (including additional equipment, i.e. dog urinary catheter, if difficult airway suspected)
- Endotracheal tube cuffs checked
- Anaesthetic machine checked
- Adequate oxygen supply for the procedure
- Breathing system connected, checked and the adjustable pressure limiting (APL) valve open
- Dedicated person assigned to monitor the patient
- Risks identified and communicated to all members of the team
- Emergency interventions available.

Pre-procedure checklist

The pre-procedure checklist includes confirmation of:

- Patient name and procedure
- Appropriate depth of anaesthesia
- Safety concerns communicated – this is another point at which any concerns regarding the patient should be aired to the whole team; an intervention plan should be made, if necessary, at this point.

Recovery checklist

The recovery checklist includes confirmation of:

- Safety concerns:
  - Airway
  - Breathing
  - Fluid balance
  - Body temperature
  - Pain.
- Assessment and intervention plan
- Analgesia plan
- Person assigned to monitor patient.

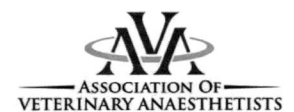

Anaesthetic Safety Checklist

ASSOCIATION OF VETERINARY ANAESTHETISTS

Pre-Induction

- ☐ Patient NAME, owner CONSENT & PROCEDURE confirmed
- ☐ IV CANNULA placed & patent
- ☐ AIRWAY EQUIPMENT available & functioning
- ☐ Endotracheal tube CUFFS checked
- ☐ ANAESTHETIC MACHINE checked today
- ☐ Adequate OXYGEN for proposed procedure
- ☐ BREATHING SYSTEM connected, leak free & APL VALVE OPEN
- ☐ Person assigned to MONITOR patient
- ☐ RISKS identified & COMMUNICATED
- ☐ EMERGENCY INTERVENTIONS available

Pre-Procedure — Time Out

- ☐ Patient NAME & PROCEDURE confirmed
- ☐ DEPTH of anaesthesia appropriate
- ☐ SAFETY CONCERNS COMMUNICATED

Recovery

- ☐ SAFETY CONCERNS COMMUNICATED
  Airway, Breathing, Circulation (fluid balance), Body Temperature, Pain
- ☐ ASSESSMENT & INTERVENTION PLAN confirmed
- ☐ ANALGESIC PLAN confirmed
- ☐ Person assigned to MONITOR patient

This checklist was written by the AVA with design and distribution support from **jurox**

21.23 Anaesthetic safety checklist. (© Association of Veterinary Anaesthetists)

Endotracheal intubation

Most patients should be intubated during anaesthesia, regardless of the technique being used to maintain anaesthesia, for the following reasons:

- To protect the airway during anaesthesia
- To maintain a patent airway
- To prevent soft tissue from obstructing the airway
- To prevent secretions (e.g. salivation and regurgitated material) from causing airway obstruction.

WARNING

Remember that an intubated airway can still become obstructed, as tubes can become kinked (especially red rubber-type tubes) or be blocked by plugs of secretions or lubricant. It is important to observe the patient's breathing pattern and tidal volume during anaesthesia to assess airway patency

The intubation of very small patients with a narrow airway can result in trauma to the larynx and trachea; the costs and benefits of intubation must therefore be considered when attempting intubation of puppies and kittens. As a general rule, intubation of patients with a bodyweight of <2 kg may be problematic and the placement of a very small endotracheal tube may increase respiratory resistance (due to the small tube diameter) compared with allowing the animal to breathe naturally through the mouth.

Endotracheal tubes

There are a number of different types of endotracheal (ET) tube, each with differing advantages and disadvantages (Figure 21.24). They can be made of red rubber, polyvinyl chloride (PVC) or silicone and be cuffed or uncuffed; examples of each are shown in Figure 21.25.

Tube type	Advantages	Disadvantages
Red rubber (see Figure 21.25a)	Re-useable. Wide range of sizes available. Can be autoclaved. Easy to intubate, as pre-moulded	Fairly expensive (especially larger sizes). Perish with time. Not malleable. Kink easily (extreme care should be taken to ensure airway patency is maintained when the head is kinked, e.g. during cervical CSF taps). Irritant to the airway. Impossible to detect contamination without looking directly down the lumen. No self-sealing valve. Only available with low-volume, high-pressure cuff
PVC (see Figure 21.25b)	Cheap. Although designed to be disposable, can be re-used. Malleable when warmed. Fairly kink-resistant. Non-irritant. Easy to place. High-pressure, low-volume and low-pressure, high-volume cuffs available. Easy to see any contamination, e.g. plugs within the lumen. Cuffs are valved	Designed to be disposable. Cannot be repaired. Limited sizes available (no large sizes >11 mm internal diameter). Cannot be autoclaved. Connections can become loose once the PVC becomes warm
Silicone (see Figure 21.25c)	Can be repaired (long life). Can be autoclaved. Malleable when warmed. Fairly kink-resistant. Non-irritant. Cuffs are valved. Wide range of sizes available. Possible to see contamination when examined carefully	Expensive to purchase. May require a stylet to facilitate intubation because the tubes do not have a moulded curve. Only available with low-volume, high-pressure cuff

21.24 Advantages and disadvantages of endotracheal tubes made from different materials.

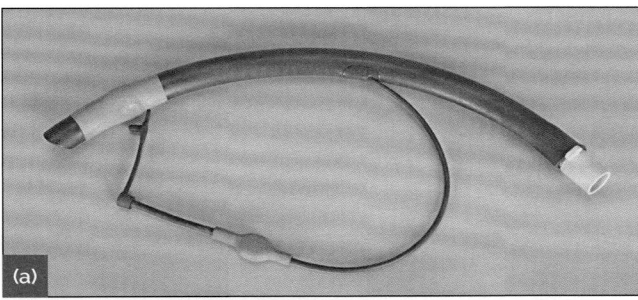

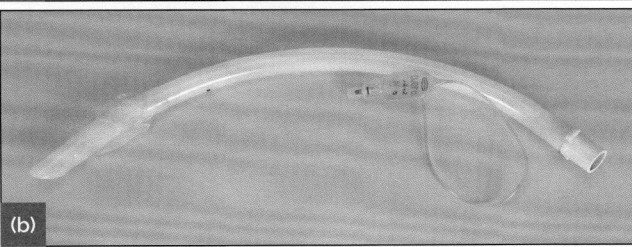

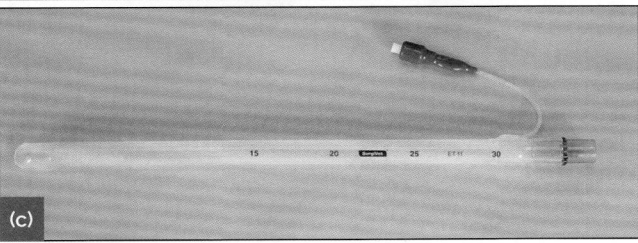

21.25 Endotracheal tubes. **(a)** Red rubber. The pilot balloon and cuff on the tube are maintained inflated using the cap on the pilot balloon. The cuff is a high-pressure, low-volume type. **(b)** PVC. This cuff is a low-pressure, high-volume type. The pilot balloon has a valve on it to maintain cuff inflation. **(c)** Silicone. This tube is much straighter than the other two types.

Cuffs may be of a high-volume, low-pressure or low-volume, high-pressure type:

- A low-pressure, high-volume cuff is safer in terms of the health of the tracheal mucosa, as the pressure of the inflated cuff is spread over a larger area; however, it does not provide such good protection of the airway as fluids can traverse folds in the cuff and enter the lungs

- A high-pressure, low-volume cuff provides more secure protection of the airway; however, there is a higher risk of tracheal necrosis due to the pressure of the cuff being exerted on a small band of tissue.

Armoured or guarded ET tubes are usually made from PVC with a thick wall in which a wire coil is placed. They are designed to prevent kinking when the patient's neck is flexed, for example, during a cisternal puncture to collect CSF. These tubes can become permanently occluded if over-flexed (unlikely to be possible with new designs) or if they are bitten by the patient.

A 'Murphy eye' may be present in some silicone and PVC tubes; this is an oval hole in the tube wall opposite to the bevel. The hole allows gases to enter and exit the tube if the end becomes occluded by sitting against the wall of the trachea or by secretions.

Choice of endotracheal tube

When selecting the size of ET tube for the patient it is important to consider both its diameter and length. The tube should be as wide as comfortably fits down the trachea, to minimize the amount of air needed in the cuff (if a cuffed tube is being used) to provide a tracheal seal.

- Most adult cats can take a 4.5 or 5 mm uncuffed tube.
- In dogs, a rough guide for tube sizes are 8 mm for a 10 kg dog, 10 mm for a 20 kg dog and 12 mm for a 30 kg dog. However, it is important to consider tube size in terms of lean bodyweight and breed. Brachycephalic breeds often have a relatively narrow laryngeal diameter and trachea compared to their bodyweight.

Tube length is also important, tubes that are too short displace easily, while overly long tubes carry a risk of one lung intubation due to the tube being placed down one bronchus. The tube end should be level with the front incisors and not sitting out proud of the mouth as this increases the equipment dead space (the volume of gas contained within equipment that is rebreathed without any changes in composition). To ensure tube length is optimal, the tube should be measured against the side of the patient, using the jaw and the thoracic inlet as marker points.

In cats, uncuffed tubes are generally preferred, except when it is known that a good tracheal seal will be needed (e.g. during IPPV) or if the patient is at a high risk of regurgitation (e.g. during dental procedures or cranial abdominal surgery). If a cuffed tube is used it is vital that the cuff is inflated carefully and not over-pressurized, because cats are at a high risk of tracheal necrosis. An alternative to using a cuffed tube in situations where the risk of regurgitation is high is placement of a throat pack (or rolled up swab attached to a piece of suture to allow easy retrieval) in order to prevent regurgitated material from entering the pharynx and the trachea. The throat pack must provide a good seal at the back of the mouth and must be removed at the end of anaesthesia. The use of cuffed red rubber ET tubes in cats is not recommend by the authors.

Before using an ET tube:

- Visually inspect for any gross contamination and damage to the tube (e.g. bite marks)
- Check the lumen for contamination by holding the tube up to the light and looking down the lumen. Patency should never be checked by blowing down the tube, for reasons of health and safety
- Check the cuff. The cuff should be fully inflated and left for a few minutes to ensure that it stays inflated. If using a lubricant on the tube to aid intubation it is best applied at this time. Ideally, use a silicone spray designed specifically for this purpose. A water-based lubricant can be used; however, these can dry out and become sticky and may plug the tube if care is not taken during application. Fully deflate the cuff before intubation.

Cleaning ET tubes

- ET tubes should never be cleaned or come into contact with chlorhexidine-containing products as these cause tracheal irritation. ET tubes should be cleaned using a solution of washing-up liquid and water with a pipe cleaner brush to clean the lumen and a cloth to clean the exterior. The cuff should be inflated to enable thorough cleaning. They should then be thoroughly rinsed with copious amounts of water, including flushing down the lumen. The tubes should be then placed into a sterilizing solution, made up to the manufacturer's recommended concentration, and left to soak for a minimum of 15 minutes (for Milton solution; for other sterilizing solutions soak according to manufacturers instructions). It is recommended that the tubes are not soaked for a prolonged period of time (i.e. greater than 30 minutes)
- ET tubes used for patients suffering from contagious diseases should either be disposed of or be sterilized (e.g. using an autoclave or ethylene oxide as per manufacturer's guidelines)

Technique

Following induction, once a suitable plane of anaesthesia to allow intubation has been achieved, cats and dogs should be positioned for intubation in the following way:

- Hold the upper jaw by the lateral aspect of the mucous membrane (gums) under the lips. It is also acceptable to use a length of bandage positioned behind the canine teeth to hold the mouth open
- Straighten and extend the neck to open the airway and facilitate intubation. Be aware that in some circumstances neck extension is contraindicated (e.g. cervical disc disease)
- Do not distort the soft tissues of the neck by pulling the scruff. Place the hand behind the base of the skull (feel for the bony prominence) and lift and extend the neck to place the head and neck in a straight line.

WARNING

To avoid the risk of being bitten, do not place your fingers in the patient's mouth

---

Intubation is a procedure that veterinary nurses are permitted to perform and it is important that they are both proficient and confident in the technique. Intubation can be carried out either with (Figures 21.26 and 21.27) or without the use of a laryngoscope. Laryngoscopes facilitate laryngeal visualization and thus aid quick intubation and reduce the risk of laryngeal trauma. When using a laryngoscope, pull the tongue firmly out of the mouth between the canine teeth and place the blade of the laryngoscope at the base of the tongue (just in front of the larynx, not on the epiglottis); depress the blade downwards to improve laryngeal visualization. Two types of laryngoscope blade are commonly used in veterinary practice: Miller (straight blade) and Macintosh (curved) blade (Figure 21.28).

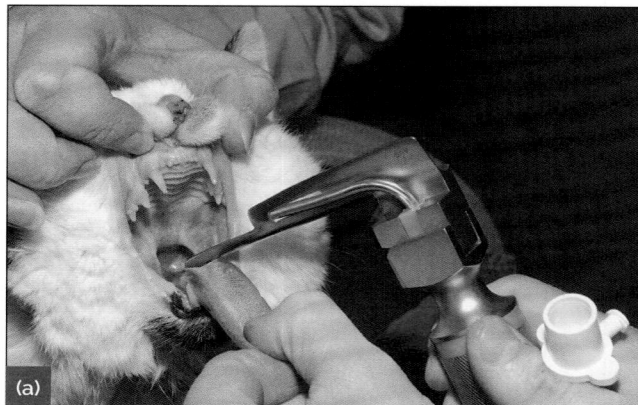

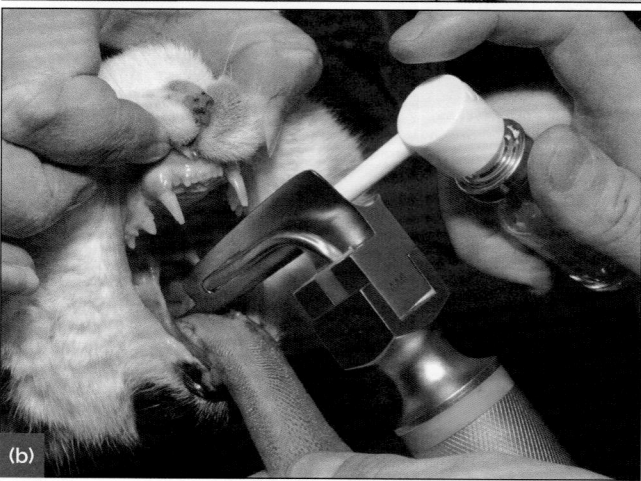

21.26 Endotracheal intubation of a cat. **(a)** Positioning the cat. **(b)** Using a laryngoscope to facilitate visualization of the larynx. Local anaesthetic spray is used to desensitize the larynx prior to intubation. *continues* ▶

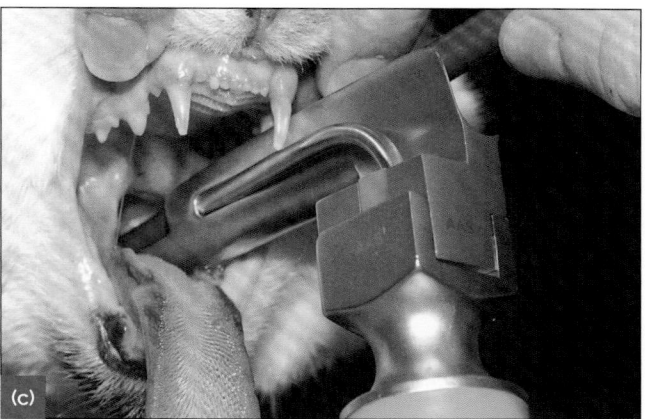

21.26 *continued* Endotracheal intubation of a cat.
(c) Placement of the endotracheal tube.

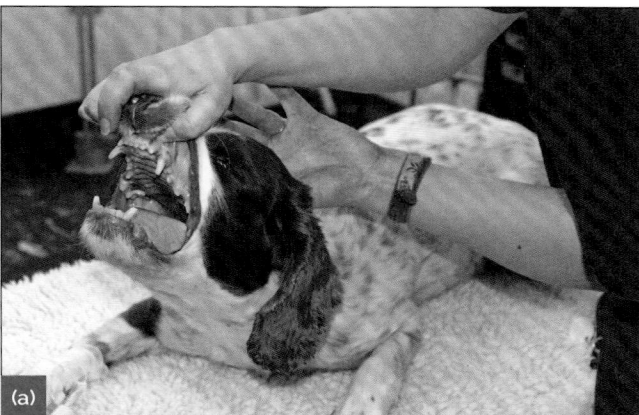

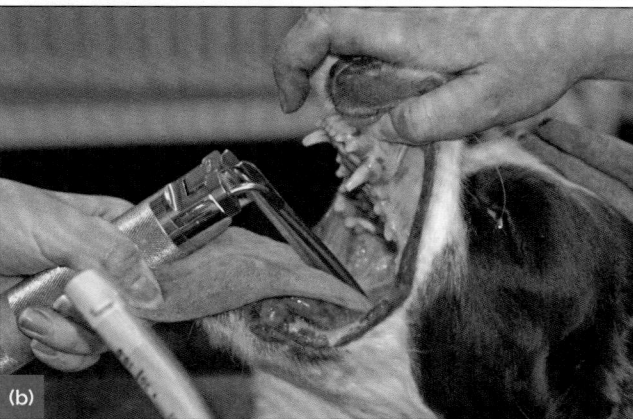

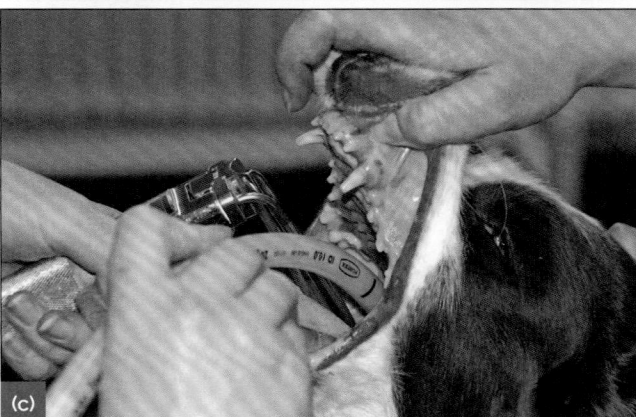

21.27 Endotracheal intubation of a dog. **(a)** Positioning the dog. **(b)** Using a laryngoscope to facilitate visualization of the larynx. **(c)** Placement of the endotracheal tube.

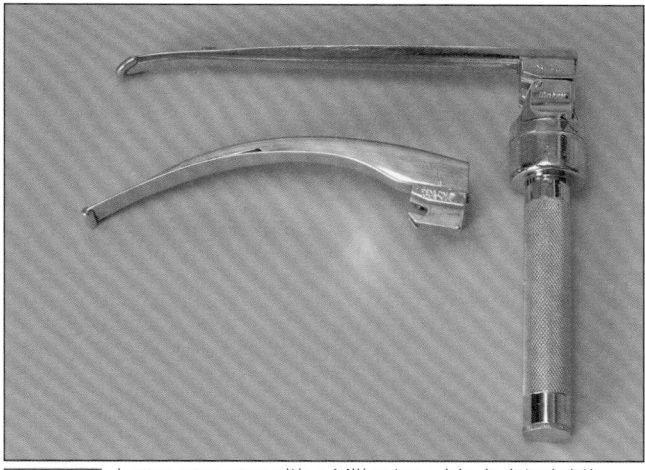

21.28 Laryngoscope with a Miller type blade (straight) attached. A Macintosh type blade (curved) is also shown.

Stylets can also aid intubation by stiffening the ET tube or acting as a guidewire. To stiffen the ET tube, the tube is threaded over the top of the stylet. A stylet can also guide placement of the tube by gently intubating the patient with the stylet and then threading the ET tube over it until the tube is introduced into the trachea. A polyurethane dog urinary catheter can be used as a stylet if plastic stylets are not available.

In cats, it is vital to spray the larynx with topical local anaesthetic (see Figure 21.26b). This prevents laryngeal spasm during intubation. It is necessary to wait 1 minute after application of the local anaesthetic to allow mucosal absorption before attempting intubation. Laryngeal spasm is an emergency as the patient is unable to open the larynx and breathe. Care should be taken not to overdose the patient with topical local anaesthetics; positioning and priming of the spray prior to administration is key. The most commonly used proprietary preparation to desensitize the larynx in cats is Intubeaze® (Dechra Veterinary Products), which delivers 2–4 mg of lidocaine in a single spray. Therefore, when using Intubeaze® only deliver a single spray to the larynx to avoid overdose.

Management of ET tubes during anaesthesia

In most species, securing the ET tube in place is vital to ensure maintenance of the tube during anaesthesia. This can be achieved using gauze fixed to the tube and tied behind the patient's ears. Care should be taken to avoid nasal congestion if the tube is tied around the muzzle (in dogs) as this is not only uncomfortable for the patient but can result in respiratory distress during the recovery period.

Procedure immediately after intubation

1. Secure the ET tube in place.
2. Attach the ET tube to an appropriately sized breathing circuit and switch on the oxygen flow.
3. Attach the cuff inflation syringe to the pilot balloon.
4. Give the patient a breath via the bag on the breathing system and listen by the patient's mouth for any leaks around the tube. Inflate the cuff gradually until no leaks can be heard. The minimum amount of ➔

air needed to create a seal around the tube should be used during cuff inflation, to reduce the risk of tracheal necrosis.
5. Assess patient depth.
6. Start administration of the inhalant agent (if applicable).

Periodically re-check for leaks around the tube, as the trachea can relax slightly and small movements in the tube can create spaces around it. It is important to remember that if gas can escape around the tube, regurgitated material can also pass by the cuff, increasing the risk of aspiration if regurgitation does occur.

> **WARNING**
>
> If the patient has a history of regurgitation or has a condition that could increase the risk of regurgitation (e.g. myasthenia gravis or advanced pregnancy) the cuff should be inflated immediately after intubation, before the head and neck are lowered. The animal's head should also be kept raised throughout pre-medication, induction and intubation to reduce the risk of aspiration

If regurgitation does occur, it is important first to drop the head of the patient down below the height of the thoracic outlet to facilitate drainage. The seal around the ET tube should be checked at the earliest opportunity and material sucked out of the patient's mouth and airway. This can be performed using a footpump-operated suction unit, a hand-held suction device (widely available from medical equipment suppliers), or a surgical suction unit (care should be taken not to traumatize the soft tissues); alternatively, if these are not available, a 20 ml syringe attached to a three-way tap and a 6 French dog urinary catheter may be used. These patients should be extubated as late as possible (i.e. when a strong gag reflex is present) during recovery.

Heat moisture exchangers (HMEs)

HMEs (Figure 21.29) contain a porous material that absorbs the heat and moisture from exhaled air and then warms and moistens inspired gases as they pass through the chamber, thereby reducing tracheal drying and heat loss via the respiratory system. A HME is placed between the ET tube and the breathing system. Care should be taken when using HMEs in small patients as they increase dead space and resistance. They are designed for use in human medicine and different sizes are manufactured for different bodyweights. Animals of lower bodyweight have a relatively smaller tidal volume and choosing an HME with appropriate dead space is important. When using a HME the patient should be monitored for signs of increased respiratory effort that could indicate that the HME has become obstructed with secretions or become very wet, which can increase the resistance imposed by the device. HMEs are designed for single use only.

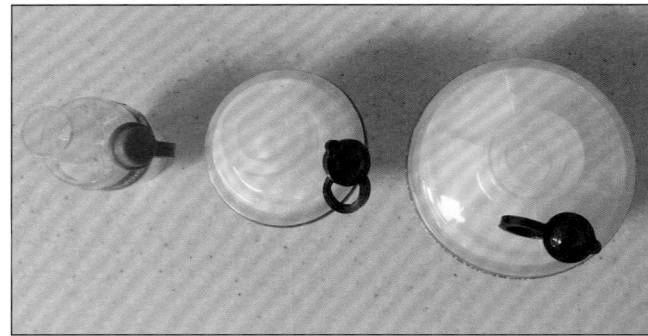

21.29 Heat moisture exchangers (HMEs) with different sized chambers and therefore dead space. The capped ports are the sites of attachment for a gas sampling line for capnography (gas analysis).

Maintenance of anaesthesia

Anaesthesia can be maintained using a variety of different techniques and anaesthetic agents:

- Inhalant agents alone
- Total intravenous anaesthesia (TIVA) – injectable agents given intravenously in incremental doses or by CRI
- Partial intravenous anaesthesia (PIVA) – using a combination of intravenous injectable agents (e.g. propofol) and inhalant anaesthetics (e.g. isoflurane)
- Injectable agents given intramuscularly.

The advantages and disadvantages of total injectable *versus* total inhalant anaesthesia are shown in Figure 21.30. The advantages and disadvantages of TIVA *versus* PIVA are shown in Figure 21.31. ET intubation and provision of supplementary oxygen is recommended, where possible, for all types of anaesthetic maintenance.

Inhalant agents

The inhalant agents, with the exception of nitrous oxide (N_2O), are all liquids at room temperature and are vaporized for use and mixed with carrier gas(es). Oxygen is the predominant carrier gas, but may be combined with nitrous oxide or medical air.

The vapour and carrier gas mixture are delivered to the patient via a breathing system into the respiratory tract and lungs. Absorption of the agent across the alveolar membrane allows the agent to be transported via the blood to the brain, where anaesthesia is induced or maintained.

Available inhalant agents differ in terms of their:

- Potency
- Volatility
- Solubility in tissues
- Flammability
- Chemical stability
- Effect on organ function
- Metabolism
- Analgesic properties.

The pharmacology of the common inhalant agents is summarized in Figure 21.32.

Technique	Advantages	Disadvantages
Total injectable anaesthesia	No expensive equipment required Drugs may be given i.v. or i.m. (depending on agent) Induction usually rapid and stress-free Easy to induce and maintain: requires little technical expertise Although recommended, ET intubation and oxygen not mandatory No scavenging required	Difficult to regulate depth of anaesthesia if agents given i.m. I.V. access may be required Plasma concentration of drugs cannot be measured in real time Drugs must be metabolized before recovery can occur Duration of recovery depends on duration of anaesthesia if agents not rapidly metabolized
Total inhalational anaesthesia	Patient usually intubated and inhalant agent vaporized in oxygen: ensures airway is protected and oxygen supplementation provided Depth of anaesthesia easy to control by altering vaporizer dials Delivered concentration of agent can be easily measured by sampling airway gases Recovery not dependent on drug metabolism (inhalants largely excreted by exhalation) Long duration of anaesthesia does not necessarily mean a prolonged recovery time Useful for rats, mice and guinea pigs, when rapid recovery desired.	Requires anaesthetic machine and oxygen supply; equipment can be expensive Understanding of how anaesthetic machine works is required to use equipment safely Induction is relatively slow (compared to i.v. injection); can be stressful for patient and staff restraining them Waste anaesthetic gases must be removed from the immediate environment of the patient and staff Scavenging of waste gases is difficult during recovery period, leading to environmental contamination Inhalant agents are greenhouse gases and contribute to degradation of the ozone layer, as well as having potential health and safety risks for staff

21.30 Advantages and disadvantages of total injectable *versus* inhalant anaesthesia techniques.

Technique	Advantages	Disadvantages
Total intravenous anaesthesia	Does not require anaesthetic machine and oxygen supply (although oxygen recommended) Useful when maintenance with inhalant agents problematic, e.g. during bronchoscopy Drugs with specific actions can be given to provide triad anaesthesia, e.g. propofol plus analgesic	Long duration of drug administration can result in drug accumulation and prolonged recovery time Plasma concentration of agent difficult to predict and likely to increase over time, even when given by CRI Unless given by CRI, peaks and troughs in depth of anaesthesia occur with redosing CRI requires controlled administration through syringe driver
Partial intravenous anaesthesia	Administration of selected injected agents usually provides analgesia and reduces concentration of inhalant required to maintain anaesthesia Balanced anaesthesia technique, often with improved cardiovascular stability	Injectable agents usually potent and require controlled administration through syringe driver More complex protocol necessitates experience Injectable agents can accumulate and prolong recovery time

21.31 Advantages and disadvantages of total *versus* partial intravenous anaesthesia.

Agent	MAC[a]	Blood/gas coefficient[b]	Pharmacological characteristics
Isoflurane	1.15%	1.4	Pungent smell and irritant to airways: animals may resent induction. Dose-dependent respiratory and cardiovascular system depression. Reduces systemic vascular resistance, leading to vasodilation and compensatory increase in heart rate. Little liver metabolism; most excreted via respiratory system at end of anaesthesia. Minimal effect on liver blood flow
Sevoflurane	2.05%	0.6	Odourless, non-irritant. Lower solubility in blood than isoflurane. Agent of choice for induction. Dose-dependent reduction in myocardial contractility and mean arterial blood pressure. Very little liver metabolism; rapidly excreted via lungs. Unstable in presence of moist soda lime, producing small amounts of compound A, which is nephrotoxic in rats but not considered to be clinically significant in dogs and cats
Desflurane	5–10%	0.42	High saturated vapour pressure; vaporizes very rapidly at room temperature. Delivery requires special vaporizer that heats liquid desflurane to a constant temperature, enabling agent to be available at constant vapour pressure and negating effects that fluctuating ambient temperatures would otherwise have on concentration imparted into fresh gas flow of anaesthetic machine. Pungent smell; despite low blood solubility, rarely used for induction. Dose-dependent myocardial and respiratory system depression. Heart rate may increase due to stimulation of sympathetic nervous system. Very little liver metabolism; rapidly excreted via lungs

21.32 Key pharmacology of the common inhalant agents. MAC = minimum alveolar concentration. [a] Values in humans given as examples; similar to MAC across veterinary species. [b] Solubility in blood: a higher coefficient indicates greater solubility.

Minimum alveolar concentration (MAC)

> ## Definition of MAC
>
> The minimum alveolar concentration of the inhalant agent at equilibrium at 1 atmosphere pressure that is required to suppress movement in response to a supramaximal noxious stimulus in 50% of patients

MAC is used as a measure of anaesthetic potency; inhalant agents that are more potent have a lower MAC value, i.e. a lower concentration of the agent is required to suppress movement. The mechanism of immobility caused by inhalant agents is considered to be at the level of the spinal cord, therefore potency as measured by MAC is a spinal cord rather than a brain phenomenon.

Solubility in blood

The solubility of an inhalant agent in blood (blood/gas partition coefficient) determines the speed of induction and recovery. The greater the solubility, the slower the onset of effect and the more slowly the patient goes to sleep. At the end of anaesthesia, agents that are highly soluble will have accumulated a large reservoir in the blood, fat and other tissues, and therefore blood levels of the agent fall slowly and recovery from anaesthesia is relatively slower. The newer anaesthetic agents (e.g. isoflurane, sevoflurane) are less soluble in blood than is halothane; therefore, induction and recovery are more rapid, which is advantageous. Sevoflurane is the inhalant agent of choice for mask or chamber induction of anaesthesia because it is non-irritant and odourless and will produce the most rapid induction.

Health and safety considerations

Maximum workplace exposure limits for nitrous oxide, isoflurane and sevoflurane have been established by nationalized agencies in many industrialized countries. It is a legislative requirement in the UK that practices carry out monitoring of anaesthetic pollutants in operating areas and maintain written records of this. It is also a legislative requirement that veterinary practices provide facilities for the scavenging of anaesthetic gases – passive, active (pump and air brake system) or charcoal absorbers (see Chapter 2).

The dangers to veterinary staff are difficult to quantify because most studies have failed to identify an association between waste anaesthetic gases and an increased incidence of adverse effects. Studies that have been carried out have focused on healthcare workers rather than members of the veterinary profession, so any findings of these studies can only be extrapolated to the veterinary workplace. A number of confounding variables usually affects these studies, including the effects of work stresses and long working hours.

The principal occupational health hazards associated with exposure of health workers to nitrous oxide include the potential for effects on the bone marrow caused by depression of vitamin B12 function, diminished reproductive health and abusive self-administration. High concentrations of nitrous oxide have also been shown to be teratogenic in experimental animals. Some studies have demonstrated that chronic exposure to inhalant anaesthetic agents is associated with physiological changes in healthcare staff, including an inhibition of neutrophil apoptosis, depressed central neurorespiratory activity and a higher incidence of DNA single strand breaks compared to controls. These findings should be balanced, however, against the findings of a systematic review of the subject that was unable to demonstrate an association between exposure and health risks. This study, however, still highlighted the importance of minimizing exposure to eliminate potential risks.

Nitrous oxide

Nitrous oxide (N_2O) is a vapour at room temperature and atmospheric pressure. It is not a potent enough anaesthetic agent to cause anaesthesia when administered alone, but is often used as a carrier gas. There are several reasons for including N_2O in the carrier gas mix:

- N_2O is a CNS depressant and is analgesic at concentrations >20%. Use of N_2O will reduce the concentration of inhalant agent required to maintain anaesthesia, contributing to a balanced anaesthesia technique
- N_2O has relatively minor effects on the cardiovascular and respiratory systems
- The second gas effect: N_2O is very insoluble in blood (blood/gas partition coefficient 0.47); its rapid absorption from the alveoli causes an abrupt increase in alveolar concentration of the administered inhalant agent, thereby also increasing the rate of uptake of that agent into the blood and increasing the speed of induction of anaesthesia or attainment of the desired brain concentration of the agent.

N_2O should not be administered at concentrations >70% in the inspired gas mixture (delivery of a minimum of 30% inspired O_2 concentration) in order to prevent hypoxia during anaesthesia.

When administration of N_2O is stopped, due to its very low solubility in blood, the volume of N_2O entering the alveolus from the blood is greater than the volume of nitrogen entering the pulmonary capillary. The N_2O effectively dilutes the alveolar air and if the animal is breathing room air at this point hypoxia can result due to dilution of the available O_2; this is termed diffusion hypoxia. To avoid this 100% O_2 should be administered for approximately 5–10 minutes after N_2O is discontinued.

> ## Contraindications for nitrous oxide use
>
> - N_2O is 40 times more soluble than nitrogen in blood and therefore expands air-filled cavities because it passes from the blood into the cavity faster than nitrogen can diffuse out. This can double the size of a pneumothorax in 10 minutes when delivered at a concentration of 70%. N_2O should therefore not be used in patients with a gas-filled cavity, such as in cases of:
>   - Pneumothorax
>   - Bowel obstruction
>   - Gas-filled eye (e.g. following intraocular surgery)
> - Administration of N_2O should be avoided in animals with significant cardiovascular or respiratory disease and at high risk of hypoxaemia
> - N_2O should be avoided in patients with raised intracranial pressure because it causes cerebral vasodilation and a further increase in intracranial pressure

Injectable agents

Propofol

Propofol is used in TIVA in small animals, given as a constant rate infusion (CRI, see above) or by incremental injection. Low-dose CRI results in sedation (see above). Propofol is relatively non-accumulative in dogs and therefore can be used to maintain anaesthesia without a long duration of recovery. Cats metabolize propofol poorly and therefore prolonged administration may lead to a long recovery time. Propofol is not analgesic and is a poor reflex suppressant. A better quality of anaesthesia, as well as provision of analgesia, can be ensured by combining it with an analgesic agent such as ketamine or a potent opioid.

Alfaxalone

Alfaxalone is used in TIVA, given by CRI or incremental injection. Low-dose CRI of alfaxalone results in sedation (see above). The drug is authorized for use in dogs and cats. It is rapidly metabolized by the liver; therefore, repeated administration does not cause a prolonged recovery from anaesthesia.

Lidocaine

Lidocaine may be used in PIVA, given by CRI using a syringe driver. Systemic lidocaine provides analgesia and contributes to hypnosis; therefore, administration is designed to provide analgesia and reduce the concentration of inhalational agent required to maintain anaesthesia, particularly in cardiovascularly unstable patients. Lidocaine may be continued postoperatively to provide analgesia.

> **WARNING**
>
> Lidocaine is not recommended for PIVA in cats, due to negative effects on the cardiovascular system when administered in combination with inhalant agents

Potent opioids

Potent opioids are used in PIVA, given by CRI or incremental injection. The drugs used are usually short-acting mu agonists, such as fentanyl and alfentanil. Remifentanil is an ultra-short-acting mu opioid that is metabolized extremely rapidly, regardless of the duration of administration. Opioids are commonly used to provide analgesia during inhalant anaesthesia, allowing the dose of inhalant agent to be reduced and contributing to a balanced anaesthesia technique. Administration by CRI will reduce drug accumulation and the potential for a prolonged recovery. Accumulation is less likely with alfentanil or remifentanil than with fentanyl. Potent mu opioids cause respiratory depression; therefore, support of ventilation (IPPV, see later) may be required. Considerations for storage and record keeping of opioids are discussed in Chapter 8.

Ketamine

Low doses of ketamine given by CRI are used in PIVA, and higher doses can be used to maintain anaesthesia as part of TIVA. Ketamine is analgesic at subanaesthetic doses; therefore, inclusion in the anaesthesia protocol will contribute to provision of perioperative analgesia. Low-dose ketamine infusion may be continued postoperatively to provide analgesia. Ketamine, given at low doses, does not cause excitation in cats or dogs. Considerations for storage and record keeping are discussed earlier in this chapter and in Chapter 8.

Management of the patient during the maintenance phase

Positioning

Care should be taken when positioning the patient on the surgery table:

- Overstretching limbs and tying them in a fixed position can lead to pain on recovery, particularly in patients with osteoarthritis
- Leg ties should be positioned carefully. On the hindlimbs they should be placed just above the stopper pad and not around the Achilles tendon. For the forelimbs, care should be taken when tying a leg back over the patient's thorax for some surgeries carried out in lateral recumbency. This is to prevent restriction of thoracic movement, which may impair spontaneous respiration
- Putting excessive pressure on superficial peripheral nerves can lead to nerve damage and neuropathy on recovery. Superficial nerves should not be placed against the hard edges of the table and ties should not be too tight around limbs
- Myopathy can occur in animals that are recumbent for a long period of time on an unsupported hard surface. Tables and table edges should therefore be padded
- Positioning for perineal surgery, where the hindlimbs hang over the end of the table and the patient is positioned with head down and the perineal area elevated, should be carried out very carefully. Adequate padding of the medial thighs is required to prevent damage to the superficial nerves in this region (Figure 21.33)
- Animals positioned in dorsal recumbency often have impaired ventilation due to the pressure of abdominal contents on the diaphragm. This is particularly the case in obese animals. The requirement for IPPV (see later) should be assessed rapidly after placement in dorsal recumbency
- The potential for skin burns in animals placed on heat pads or other contact warming devices should also be recognized.

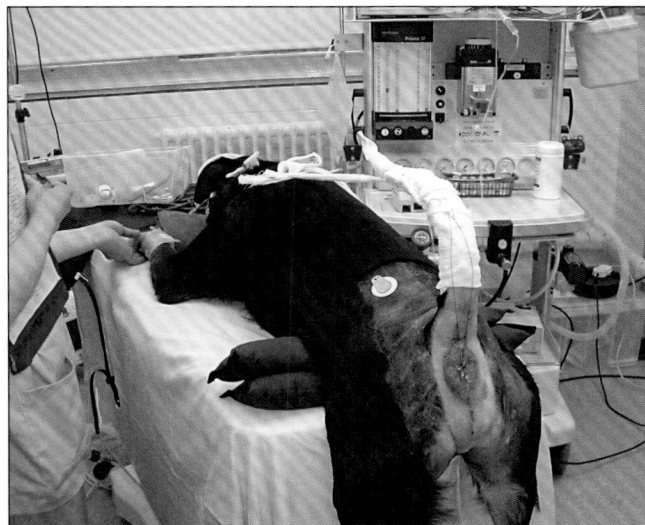

21.33 A dog positioned for perineal surgery showing how padding has been placed between the medial aspect of the thigh and the operating table. The perineal area of the dog is slightly elevated relative to the head and the tail elevated and fixed to allow visualization of the perineal area. A purse-string suture has been placed in the anus to prevent contamination of the surgical field with faeces.

Muscle relaxation and neuromuscular blockade

Adequate muscle relaxation during surgery is vital. Reduced muscle tone decreases the requirement for traction on tissue during surgery, reducing pain and inflammation on recovery from anaesthesia. Prevention of movement may also be mandatory when sudden movement may be catastrophic, e.g. during intraocular (eye) surgery.

Muscle relaxation can be produced in four ways:

- General anaesthesia: High concentrations of anaesthetic agents are usually required to produce marked muscle relaxation and cannot guarantee prevention of sudden movement during anaesthesia
- Administration of a local anaesthetic drug around a peripheral nerve: Block conduction in motor neurons (see earlier)
- Administration of local anaesthetic drug into the intrathecal or epidural space (see earlier)
- Use of a neuromuscular blocking agent (NMBA): This technique can be used to provide good muscle relaxation and prevent movement, while avoiding the need for a high concentration of inhalant agent which can have marked cardiovascular and respiratory system effects. It provides whole body muscle relaxation in contrast to techniques involving local anaesthetic agents.

Movement is the cardinal sign of inadequate anaesthesia; very careful attention should therefore be paid to monitoring depth of anaesthesia following administration of an NMBA in order to prevent inadequate anaesthesia and awareness in a patient that is unable to respond.

> **WARNING**
>
> - NMBAs must always be administered in combination with adequate general anaesthesia
> - Administration of an NMBA will stop respiration due to blockade of activity in respiratory muscles. The facility to support ventilation with IPPV must be available

Indications for neuromuscular blockade

- Intraocular surgery: To prevent downward rotation of the eye and unpredictable body movement that might be catastrophic during surgery. The eye must be in a central position in order to allow surgical access
- Facilitate IPPV: Respiration can be controlled without use of NMBAs, but in some animals their use is helpful to over-ride voluntary respiratory movements
- Laparotomy: It can be helpful to reduce abdominal muscle wall tone and therefore reduce the traction required during exploration of the abdomen
- Cardiovascularly unstable patients: NMBAs will contribute to a balanced anaesthesia technique and reduce the concentration of other drugs required to maintain anaesthesia, thereby reducing the negative cardiovascular consequence of anaesthesia. However, care must be taken to ensure that depth of anaesthesia is adequate

Action of NMBAs

Muscle contraction is initiated by a nerve impulse or action potential in a motor nerve. The motor nerve connects with the muscle at the neuromuscular junction (NMJ) (Figure 21.34). Action potentials in the motor nerve arriving at the NMJ cause the release of acetylcholine (ACh) into the synaptic cleft. When activated by ACh, receptors on the post-synaptic membrane of the NMJ allow an ion channel to open which allows sodium ions to enter the muscle fibre. Sodium enters the muscle, resulting in depolarization of the post-synaptic membrane, generating a small action potential in the motor endplate and muscle fibre membrane, termed a motor endplate potential (Figure 21.34b). When sufficient summation of motor endplate potentials occurs this results in muscle contraction. Neuromuscular blocking agents act at the NMJ to prevent action potential depolarization of the muscle fibre and muscle contraction.

Two classes of drug are used for neuromuscular blockade:

- Depolarizing agents (e.g. suxamethonium) bind reversibly to the ACh receptor to cause opening of the ion channel. This results in initial muscle contraction

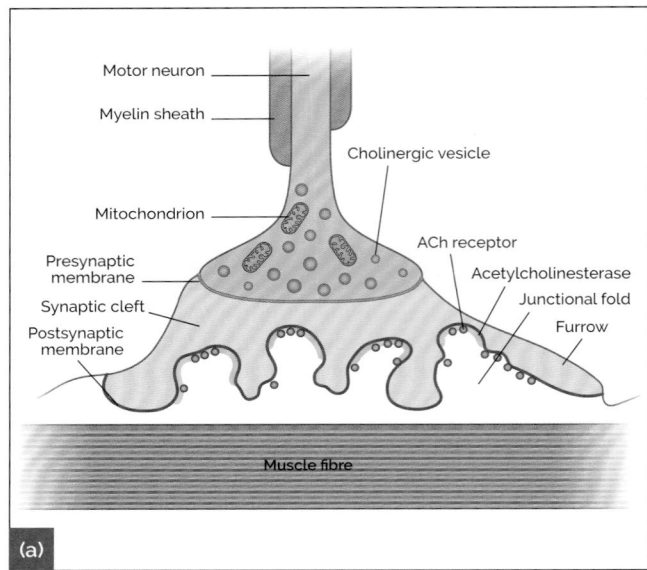

(a)

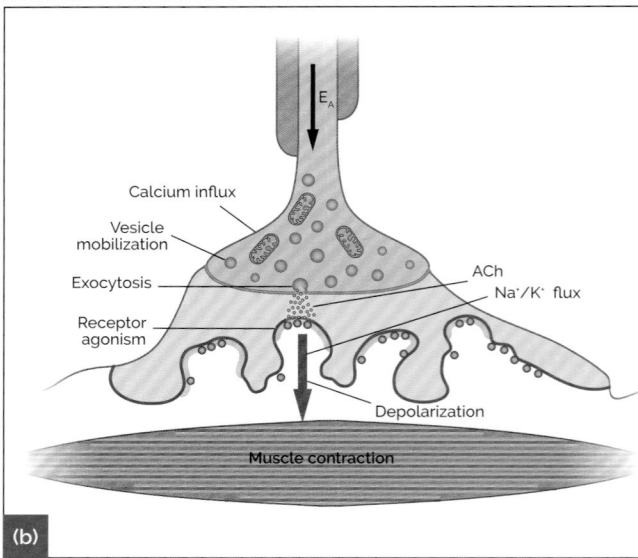

(b)

21.34 (a) Anatomy and (b) physiology of the neuromuscular junction. E_A = action potential. (Redrawn after Clutton, 2007)

followed by muscle relaxation; further muscle contraction is prevented due to occupation of the receptor by the drug. Suxamethonium is rarely used clinically in veterinary practice
■ Non-depolarizing agents (e.g. atracurium, vecuronium) bind reversibly to the ACh receptor (but do not cause the ion channel to open and initiate muscle contraction) and prevent ACh from binding to the receptor. This prevents muscle contraction. Non-depolarizing agents are used clinically in veterinary practice.

Monitoring neuromuscular blockade

Monitoring is important because it allows the re-dosing interval to be determined and helps to ensure that return of respiratory activity is sufficient before ventilatory support is withdrawn. Neuromuscular blockade is monitored by electrically stimulating a superficial peripheral nerve and measuring the response in terms of resulting muscle contraction. This can be assessed by observation or palpation of a muscle twitch or by measuring movement resulting from the muscle contraction, e.g. by using an accelerometer placed on the body part that will move when the muscle contracts.

Peripheral nerve stimulators (Figure 21.35) can be purchased to monitor neuromuscular blockade. It is important that the electrodes used to stimulate the nerve are placed before the administration of the NMBA. This allows correct placement to be confirmed (by observation of the appropriate muscle contraction) before the onset of the blockade.

Superficial nerves commonly stimulated to assess neuromuscular blockade include:

■ The facial nerve – to cause contraction of the dilator nasolabialis muscle and flare of the nostrils

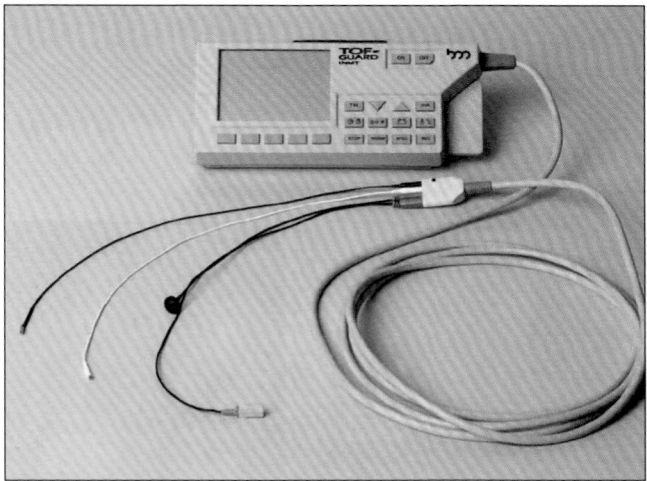

21.35 Peripheral nerve stimulator for monitoring neuromuscular blockade. The black and white leads with a 2 mm plug connector at their ends (on the far left of the picture) connect, respectively, to the negative and positive needle electrodes; these electrodes are placed subcutaneously over the peripheral nerve to be stimulated. At the end of another black lead is a small rectangular grey accelerometer that can be placed on the body part that will be moved as a result of stimulation of the muscle. A third black lead, between the white lead and the lead with the accelerometer, ends in a small round disc that is a temperature sensor. The accelerometer and temperature sensor are not essential.

■ The ulnar nerve – to cause contraction of the muscles that flex the carpus; the site of placement of the electrodes for stimulation of the ulnar nerve are shown in Figure 21.36
■ The deep peroneal nerve – to cause contraction of the digital extensors of the hindlimb.

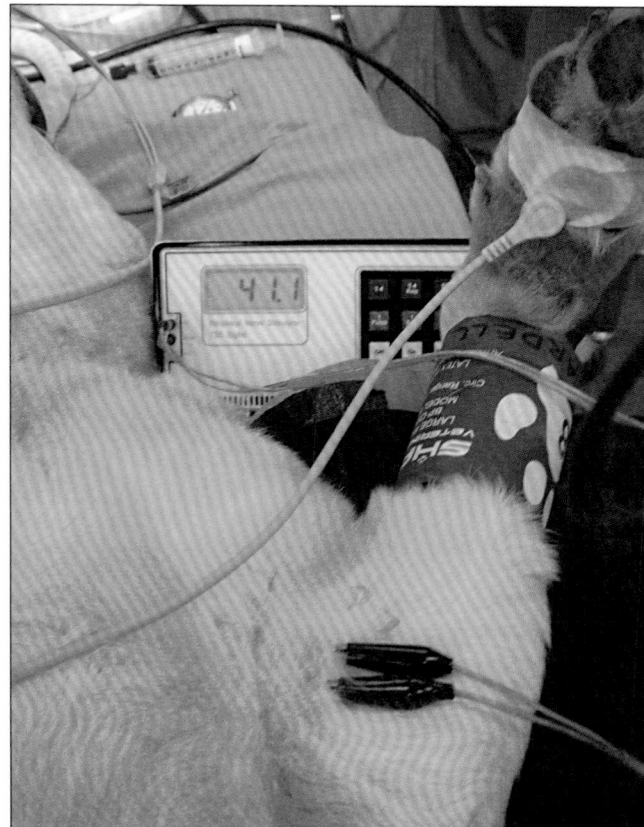

21.36 Site of subcutaneous placement of stimulating electrodes (needles) to stimulate the ulnar nerve to monitor neuromuscular blockade. The nerve runs medial to the olecranon and causes contraction of the carpal flexor muscles and flexion of the carpus. The electrodes are two 25 gauge ⅝ inch needles placed approximately 3 cm apart from each other. The black (negative) electrode is located distally to the red (positive) electrode. The electrodes are connected to a nerve stimulator. The display on the nerve stimulator shows the stimulating current in mA. A cuff for non-invasive measurement of blood pressure using the oscillometric technique is placed on the left forelimb. An ECG electrode and lead are also connected to the left forelimb footpad.

Reversal of neuromuscular blockade

Muscle contraction is normally terminated by the action of acetylcholinesterase. This enzyme breaks down ACh so that the ACh receptor is no longer occupied; the ion channels close and repolarization of the post-synaptic membrane occurs, resulting in muscle relaxation. Modern non-depolarizing agents are relatively short-acting (e.g. atracurium 45 min, vecuronium 20 min), and for many procedures duration is shorter than the anaesthesia period required. Duration of neuromuscular blockade is, however, unpredictable in some animals and reversal can be beneficial. Reversal also ensures that ventilatory function is returned to normal by the end of anaesthesia, so that the animal can safely recover from anaesthesia without respiratory compromise. Human data indicate that visual assessment of adequate respiratory activity following neuromuscular blockade is ineffective and that NMBAs should always be reversed at the end of anaesthesia combined with monitoring of muscular function.

Reversal of non-depolarizing NMBAs can be achieved by administration of an anti-acetylcholinesterase such as neostigmine or edrophonium. These drugs block the activity of the enzyme so that the concentration of ACh in the synaptic cleft rises. ACh is then able to compete effectively with the NMBA for the ACh receptors, and muscle contraction can occur. In order to prevent unwanted systemic effects, an anticholinergic drug is administered concurrently (e.g. atropine or glycopyrrolate). This specifically prevents the bradycardia that would otherwise occur due to a prolonged activity of ACh on myocardial ACh receptors, causing increased parasympathetic nervous system effects. The anticholinergic drug should have a similar onset of action time to the anti-acetylcholinesterase. Due to differing onset of action times of edrophonium and neostigmine, atropine should be used with edrophonium whilst either atropine or glycopyrrolate are appropriate with neostigmine.

Rocuronium is a relatively new NMBA, closely related to vecuronium, with a very rapid onset of action (the shortest onset of action time of all currently available NMBAs). Sugammadex is a C-cyclodextrin used to reverse aminosteroidal neuromuscular blocking agents such as rocuronium and vecuronium. It was originally designed to selectively bind rocuronium by encapsulation. Encapsulation occurs in the blood and can be used to reverse profound neuromuscular blockade in less than 2 minutes. The interaction is tight and long lasting; the complex formed is biologically inert and excreted from the plasma via the kidneys. Sugammadex has none of the severe limitations associated with the use of other NMBA reversal agents (anti-acetylcholinesterases) such as limited effectiveness when reversing profound to deep neuromuscular block or cardiovascular side effects.

Equipment for maintaining anaesthesia

The anaesthetic machine

A basic understanding of how an anaesthetic machine works is vital if the veterinary nurse is to assist in the safe administration of anaesthesia. Anaesthetic machines consist of several parts (Figure 21.37).

Gas supply

The gas supply can be from a cylinder, a pipeline or both.

Colour coding

The gas supply is colour coded for safety (Figure 21.38):

- Black cylinders with a white head and white pipelines for oxygen
- Blue cylinders and pipelines for nitrous oxide
- White necked cylinders with grey body and black pipeline for medical air (check that there is a 4 bar supply before connecting to any anaesthetic machines).

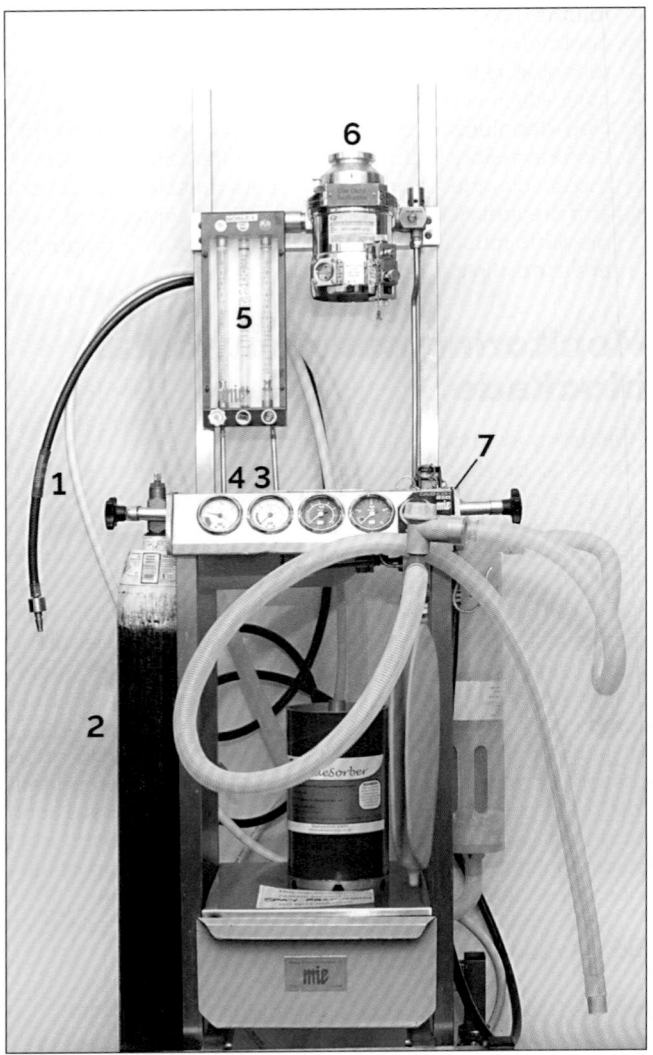

21.37 A simple anaesthetic machine. 1 = oxygen pipeline (white), nitrous oxide pipeline (blue); 2 = oxygen cylinder; 3 = pressure gauge for pipeline oxygen supply; 4 = pressure gauge for cylinder oxygen supply; 5 = oxygen and nitrous oxide flowmeters; 6 = isoflurane vaporizer; 7 = oxygen flush.

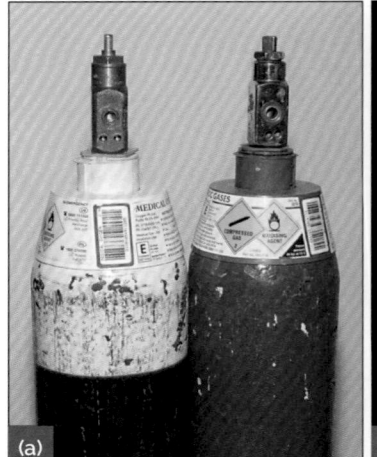
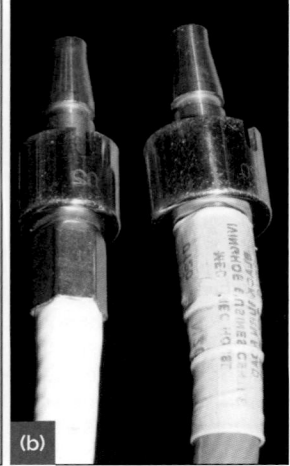

21.38 Colour coding. **(a)** In the UK, oxygen cylinders have a white neck, whereas nitrous oxide cylinders are blue. **(b)** Oxygen pipelines are white, whereas nitrous oxide pipelines are blue.

Another safety feature is the pin index system. This is the configuration of the pin holes on the cylinder and pins on the yoke (where the cylinder is attached to either the anaesthetic machine or the cylinder manifold on the pipeline supply). This prevents an oxygen cylinder being attached to an N_2O yoke or vice versa. Schrader probes (Figure 21.39a) and pipeline gas outlets also only fit the correct probe or outlet. On the yoke there is a Bodok seal (Figure 21.39b) that maintains a gas-tight seal between the cylinder and the yoke. These often need changing.

> **WARNING**
>
> It is vital that no carbon-based oils and greases are used around the valves on cylinders and anaesthetic machines due to the risk of explosion

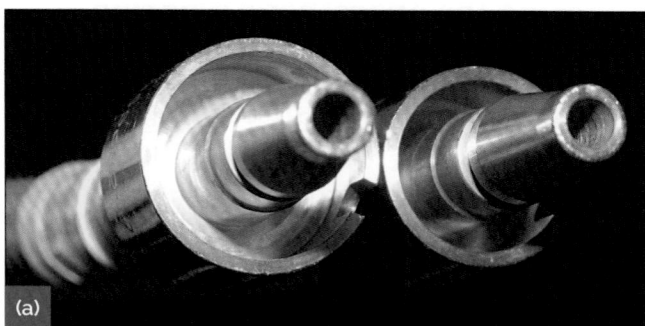

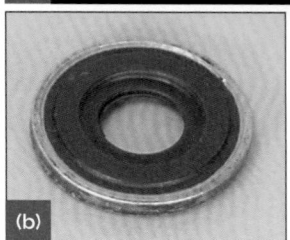

21.39 (a) Connection between oxygen and nitrous oxide pipelines to Schrader outlets; different gases have different sized connectors to prevent inadvertent misconnection of gas pipelines to the incorrect outlet. **(b)** A Bodok seal.

Pressure gauge

The pressure gauge provides information about the amount of gas left in the cylinder or pipeline gas supply (Figure 21.40). It should be remembered that pressure gauges do not give reliable information about the amount of gas remaining in N_2O cylinders or pipelines because N_2O is in liquid form; the cylinder must therefore be weighed to find out the content.

Pressure-reducing valve (regulators)

Regulators (pressure-reducing valves) (Figure 21.41) reduce the pressure of the gas coming from the cylinder and maintain a constant pressure to prevent any surges in the pressure

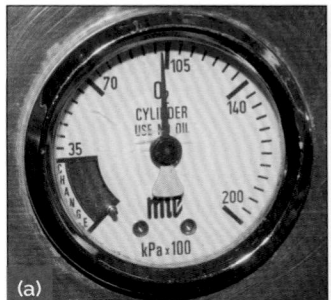
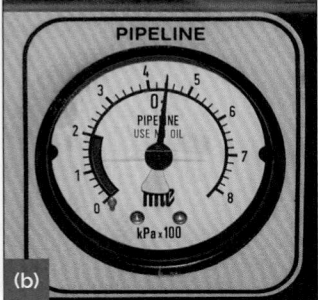

21.40 (a) Pressure gauge for a cylinder of oxygen. (b) Pressure gauge for pipeline oxygen supply.

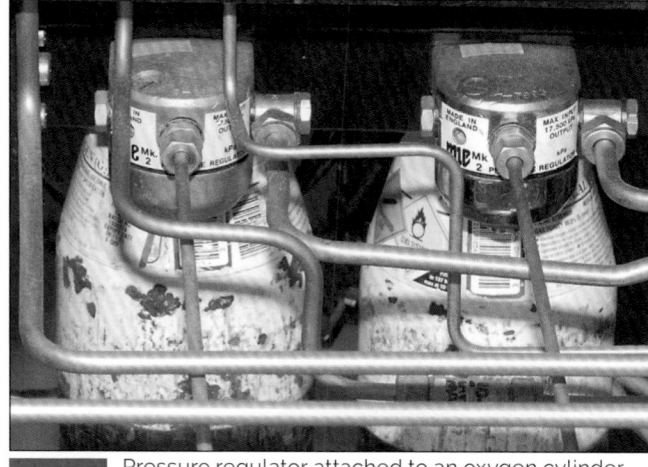

21.41 Pressure regulator attached to an oxygen cylinder on an anaesthetic machine.

of the gas being relayed to the patient. They are only present in anaesthetic machines that have cylinders. When a pipeline is used as the gas source, the pressure-reducing valve is present at the source of the gas.

Flowmeters

Flowmeters (rotameters) provide the final stage in the reduction of the pressure of the gas and allow manual adjustment of the volume of gas (O_2, medical air, N_2O) delivered to the patient (Figure 21.42). The flowmeter comprises a tube of tapered glass or plastic (narrower at the bottom and getting wider towards the top). Contained within the tube is a lightweight ball or bobbin that is moved within the tube by the gas passing around it (the movement of the gas is both laminar and turbulent, thus the flowmeter needs to be calibrated

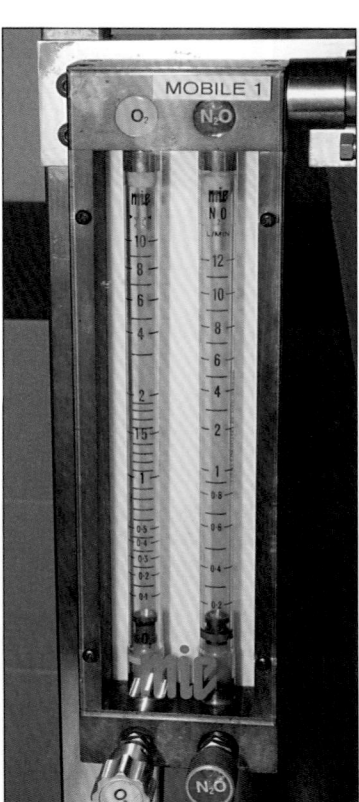

21.42 Oxygen and nitrous oxide flowmeters on an anaesthetic machine.

specifically for each gas). When setting the flow rate for a patient, the top of the bobbin or the middle of the ball should be used according to which is present on the anaesthetic machine in use.

Back bar

The back bar supports the flowmeters and it is here that the vaporizers are mounted. Most anaesthetic machines in the UK use the 'Ohmeda selectatec' system. When using this system, it is important that the vaporizer is 'locked' into place on to the back bar in order to ensure a seal and allow the vaporizer to work. Modern back bars that can mount more than one vaporizer have mechanisms to prevent more than one vaporizer being switched on at once, which would allow the potential for anaesthetic overdose.

Common gas outlet

The common gas outlet is the point at which the gases come out of the anaesthetic machine.

Additional features

Additional features that may be present on anaesthetic machines are:

- **Mini-Schrader sockets:** gas sockets that provide O_2 or air to power ventilators (Figure 21.43). They are usually found underneath the anaesthetic machine
- **Emergency oxygen flush** (Figure 21.44)**:** provides O_2 directly from the cylinder or pipeline, bypassing the vaporizer. Care should be taken when using this function as the oxygen is delivered at high flow rates that could produce barotrauma
- **Oxygen failure alarm:** sounds if there is a drop in the pressure of the O_2 supply. This is a very important safety feature

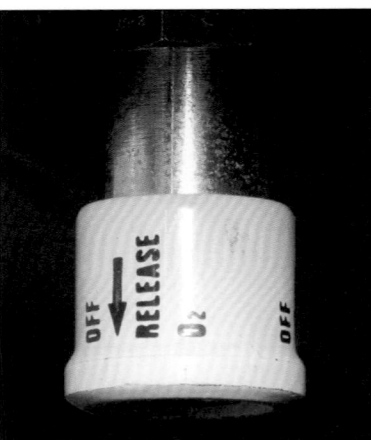

21.43 Mini-Schrader outlet used to attach a ventilator driven by oxygen to the machine oxygen supply.

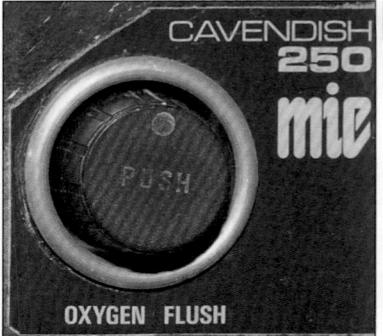

21.44 Oxygen flush on the front of an anaesthetic machine.

- **Nitrous oxide cut-off:** if the oxygen fails and N_2O is also being used, administration of N_2O is terminated
- **Hypoxic guard:** the anaesthetic machine will not allow the delivery of N_2O without the concurrent delivery of O_2. It prevents accidental delivery of a hypoxic mixture by ensuring that there is always a minimum percentage of oxygen present in the delivered mixture
- **Pressure relief valve:** opens if the pressure at the common gas outlet is too high, i.e. if the common gas outlet is blocked. This is designed to prevent the pressure within the anaesthetic machine becoming too high and thus damaging the machine. It does provide a degree of protection to the patient; however, the pressure that needs to be reached before the valve is activated would cause substantial damage to the lungs of the patient.

Checking the anaesthetic machine before use

A check should be performed at the start of each day before the anaesthetic machine is used. The following steps comprise a check of anaesthetic machine function:

- Attach the scavenging pipe to the common gas outlet and switch on the active scavenging system (if available)
- Perform a visual check of the anaesthetic machine and associated pipelines and cylinders; ensure cylinders are seated within the yoke correctly and firmly
- Open cylinders and check content; change if necessary (see text above for details on checking N_2O cylinder content)
- Turn on O_2 flow; check the bobbin moves slowly from low to high flows with the bobbin/ball spinning continuously. Turn the flow to 4 l/min. Repeat for N_2O if present
- Turn off O_2 cylinder and press oxygen flush; as the flow drops, the O_2 supply failure alarm will sound and N_2O should cut off (if a hypoxic guard is present on machine)
- If a pipeline is available, connect. If not, switch the O_2 cylinder back on. Flow should resume to 4 l/min
- Check pipeline pressure (most run at around 4.2 bar). Press O_2 flush; the pressure should only drop slightly (contact engineer if the drop is greater than 0.5 bar)
- Switch off N_2O
- With the O_2 flow at 4 l/min, occlude the common gas outlet with your thumb; watch that the bobbin drops and listen for the pressure relief valve to open (sounds like a small hiss/squeak); release the occlusion (not all anaesthetic machines have a pressure relief valve on the back bar).

Vaporizers

The majority of vaporizers used in the UK are temperature-compensated (TEC) vaporizers. This means that they automatically compensate if the temperature changes, to ensure maintenance of a constant concentration of inhalant agent in the delivered gas mixture. Vaporizers work by splitting the gas into two channels: one channel passes through the vaporizing chamber and becomes saturated with anaesthetic vapour (with isoflurane this equates to a concentration of 32%); while the other channel bypasses the vaporizing chamber. The two channels are then combined before exiting the vaporizer. When the concentration of anaesthetic gas required is dialled up on the vaporizer, the amount of gas that is split off into the vaporizing channel is adjusted to achieve the required concentration. It is important not to tip vaporizers, to prevent contamination of the bypass chamber with inhalant agent that would make the output of the vaporizer unreliable and be potentially dangerous. It is important to follow the manufacturer's guidelines on servicing. Many vaporizers should not be used with fresh gas flow rates <0.75 l/min, as the output of the vaporizer may become inaccurate. Again, it is important to follow the manufacturer's guidelines.

Filling vaporizers

Due to the different physical properties of the agents it is important that each vaporizer is calibrated and designed to deliver a single gas. For example, using an isoflurane-specific vaporizer to deliver sevoflurane would result in concentrations different to those predicted. In order to prevent filling with the wrong agent, modern vaporizers have a keyed filling system. An agent-specific filler tube is used: one end slots into a fitting on the vaporizer and the other end slots on to a collar on the bottle of anaesthetic (Figure 21.45). Both the fitting on the vaporizer and the collar on the bottle are specific for one agent. This closed system, unlike older funnel fill systems, also minimizes environmental contamination. Nevertheless, vaporizers should still be filled at the end of the working day and with all ventilation systems for the room switched on, so that any waste gases are dissipated before the working area is used again.

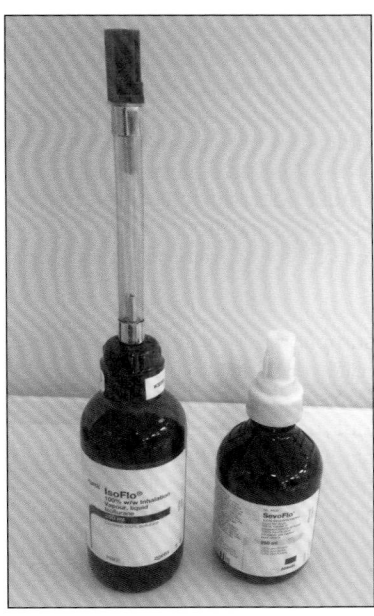

21.45 Bottles of isoflurane and sevoflurane with appropriate filler attachments (sevoflurane filler is integral to bottle).

Checking the vaporizer before use

The vaporizer should be checked at the start of each day before use:

- Check vaporizer content (vaporizers should be filled at end of the day to reduce exposure to personnel); if using the selectatec system, ensure that the vaporizer is seated on the back bar correctly and locked into place
- Check the dial rotates smoothly
- With the vaporizer switched on but set to zero, occlude the common gas outlet with your thumb; ensure that the bobbin drops (release pressure as soon as a drop is observed). This is performed to check there is no leak present on the interface between the anaesthetic machine and vaporizer.

Anaesthetic breathing systems

Anaesthetic breathing systems have several functions:

- Transfer of gases from the anaesthetic machine to the ET tube or face mask
- Removal of CO_2 breathed out by the patient, preventing rebreathing of CO_2
- Delivery of artificial breaths to the patient (IPPV, see later)
- Measurement of airway pressures, gas volumes and gas composition
- Scavenging of waste gases.

Important definitions

- Tidal volume (TV): The volume of gas exhaled by the patient in one breath
- Minute volume (MV): The volume of gas exhaled by the patient in 1 minute
- Rebreathing: Inhalation of previously breathed gases that have taken part in gas exchange
- Reservoir bag (rebreathing/breathing bag): An open-ended or closed bag that is attached to a breathing system
- Limbs of the anaesthetic breathing circuit (breathing tubes): The tubing of the breathing system within which the gases are carried. These can be inspiratory or expiratory
- Unidirectional valves (one-way valves): Ensure that the gases only flow in one direction
- APL (adjustable pressure limiting) valve (pressure relief valve, pop-off valve, scavenging valve): Controls the amount of gas contained within the reservoir bag and how much gas escapes from the breathing system via the scavenging system. This valve commonly contains a plastic disc suspended on a spring that is depressed when a set pressure is exerted on it, causing the valve to open, thus allowing gases to escape. This acts as a safety feature, although the pressure that must be reached before the valve opens is quite high for some models, by which time barotrauma is likely to have occurred
- Fresh gas inlet: The point where the gas enters the breathing system from the common gas outlet of the anaesthetic machine
- Anatomical dead space: The gas inhaled by the patient that does not undergo any gas exchange (i.e. the air within the upper airway and trachea)
- Apparatus dead space (equipment dead space): The volume of gas contained within the breathing system that is rebreathed by the patient and has not participated in gaseous exchange
- Non-rebreathing systems
  - Open breathing systems: These systems have no reservoir bag, unidirectional valves or CO_2 absorbent
  - Semi-open systems: These systems contain a reservoir bag and APL valve. They do not contain a CO_2 absorbent or unidirectional valve
- Rebreathing systems
  - Closed systems: Contain a reservoir bag, unidirectional valves, CO_2 absorbent and APL valve →

Important definitions *continued*

- Semi-closed systems: Same as a closed system except the circuit is used with the valve open or partially open
- Mapleson configuration: A method of classifying non-rebreathing systems developed in 1954
- Coaxial system: The inspiratory and expiratory limbs are contained one within the other. There is a possible advantage over parallel tubing in that the fresh gases are warmed; however, damage/disconnection of the inner tube is not easily visible and this can make the circuit potentially hazardous to use
- Parallel system: The inspiratory and expiratory limbs run side by side
- Compliance: How well the lungs stretch to accommodate a change in volume in relation to the pressure applied

Anaesthetic breathing systems are now described as either rebreathing or non-rebreathing (Figure 21.46) and there has been a move away from classifying them as open or semi-open, etc. (see text box). The easiest way to distinguish between these is to identify whether there is any CO_2 absorbent present in the system. This absorbs the CO_2 that the patient breathes out, enabling this gas to be reused by the patient. In non-rebreathing systems the CO_2 is flushed out by the continued flow of fresh gas into the circuit. Non-rebreathing systems can be further classified as coaxial or parallel; there are advantages and disadvantages to each type (Figure 21.47).

Rebreathing
- Circle
- To-and-fro
- Humphrey ADE–circle system

Non-rebreathing
- T-piece
- Bain (parallel or coaxial)
- Lack (parallel or coaxial)
- Magill
- Humphrey ADE

21.46 Breathing systems used in veterinary practice.

Rebreathing systems

These systems allow the gases that have been exhaled by the patient to be re-used after the absorption of CO_2. They are economical when used in a 'closed' manner because the only gas that needs to be added is oxygen to compensate for the relatively small amount of oxygen used by cells of the body during metabolism (metabolic oxygen consumption).

Circle system

The circle system (Figure 21.48) is the most commonly used rebreathing system. There are many different circle systems available, but they all work using the same principle. The main variation between models is the size of the soda lime canister and the tubing design. These factors determine the level of resistance to gas flow in the circuit and thus the size of patient the system can be used for. Most small circle systems are suitable for patients >10 kg. Circle systems contain unidirectional valves that ensure unidirectional gas flow. The gases that the patient breathes out pass through the canister containing the CO_2 absorbent before they are breathed again.

Practical considerations

When the patient is first anaesthetized and placed on to the circle system, high levels of nitrogen are exhaled due to the gas composition of room air breathed before induction. A higher gas flow, with the valve in an open or semi-open position, must be used for the first 15–20 minutes to allow denitrogenation, which prevents the development of a hypoxaemic mixture within the circle system. After 15–20 minutes the fresh gas flow can be reduced, either to the metabolic oxygen consumption rate (2–7 ml/kg), with the APL valve closed (closed circle), or to a rate of 1 litre/min (for patients <10 kg), with the APL valve semi-open (semi-closed system). The valve must be sufficiently open to prevent the bag from becoming over distended.

Use of a truly 'closed' circle is not recommended for a number of reasons:

- Metabolic oxygen consumption is very variable, not only between individuals of different age, sex and breed but also due to changes in temperature and drug administration throughout the anaesthetic period. Maintaining the reservoir of gas at the correct oxygen concentration is therefore extremely difficult
- Most anaesthetic machines used in veterinary practice do not have flowmeters that allow accurate delivery of very low gas flow rates

System type	Advantages	Disadvantages
Rebreathing	Require low gas flow rates reducing cost associated with anaesthetic agent delivery and environmental contamination with waste gases. Reduced heat loss, as gases require less warming by the patient than in non-rebreathing circuits	Altering the concentration of volatile agent within the circuit takes time, depending on gas flow rate and volume of circuit. CO_2 absorbent and valves create resistance. Require an understanding of how the circuit works. Require maintenance associated with changing CO_2 absorbent. Can be expensive to purchase
Non-rebreathing	Concentration of inhalant agent can be adjusted rapidly. Minimal circuit resistance. Easy to use. Cheap to purchase	High gas flow rates increase costs associated with gases and inhalant agents and increase environmental contamination. Potential for rebreathing if patient breathes rapidly; gas flow rate must be increased. Significant heat loss through respiratory tract due to warming of inspired gases

21.47 Advantages and disadvantages of rebreathing and non-rebreathing systems.

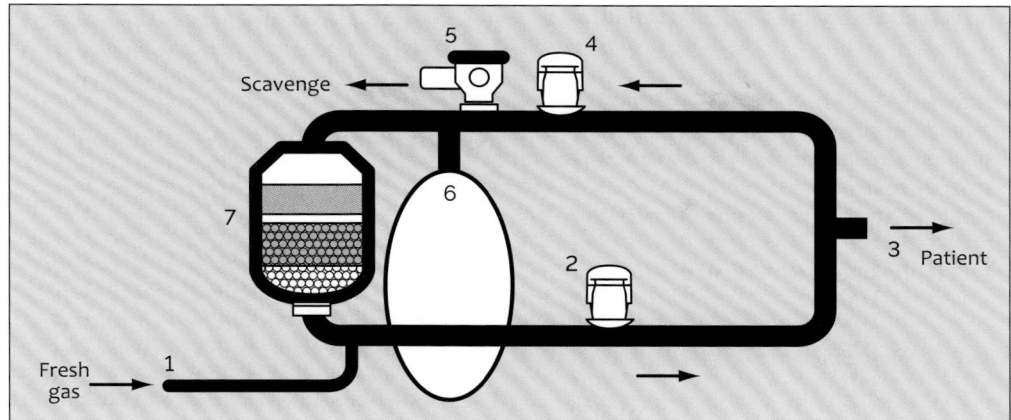

- ■ **1. Fresh gas inflow.** This pipe connects the circuit with the common-gas outlet on the anaesthetic machine.
- ■ **2 and 4. Unidirectional valves.** These are light transparent discs resting on knife-edge valve seats, enclosed within a transparent dome. Units should be easy to disassemble for drying and cleaning.
- ■ **3. 'Y' connector.** This connects inspiratory and expiratory limbs with endotracheal tube connectors or masks.
- ■ **5. Adjustable pressure limiting (APL) valve.** This is opened to release surplus gas from 'low-flow' systems, during denitrogenation, and closed when lung inflation is imposed. APL valves should be shrouded for attachment to scavenging hoses.
- ■ **6. Reservoir bag.** This allows IPPV; its volume should be 3–6 times the animal's tidal volume. Large bags increase circuit volume, make respiratory movement less obvious and are harder to squeeze. Inadequately sized bags collapse during large breaths and overdistend during expiration.
- ■ **7. Absorbent canister.** Canisters for circle systems may have two compartments. When absorbent in one becomes exhausted, it is discarded; after refilling, the canister is replaced in the reverse direction. This allows optimal use of absorbent.
- ■ **Hoses.** These are corrugated to prevent kinking.

21.48　Circle breathing system.

- ■ Most vaporizers used in veterinary practice are not calibrated to be accurate at very low flow rates
- ■ Analysis of exhaled (end tidal) gases is needed to work out the concentration of inhalational agent that is being delivered to the patient, along with capnography (see below) to ensure that no rebreathing of CO_2 occurs
- ■ Closed circle systems rely heavily on the CO_2 absorbent not being exhausted.

Advantages of circle systems

- ■ Low fresh gas flow requirements, reducing medical gas costs.
- ■ Decreased use of expensive volatile agents.
- ■ Less environmental contamination.
- ■ Reduced heat loss from the patient. The gases coming from the anaesthetic machine are cold but recirculation of gases though the soda lime (where an exothermic reaction takes place) warms the gases. The low flow rates also reduce the cold air being added to the system.
- ■ Inspired gases are moistened as they pass through the soda lime because the reaction within the CO_2 absorbent produces water. Less new fresh gas and hence dry air is also added to the system.
- ■ Ideal for IPPV.

Disadvantages of circle systems

- ■ The canister needs to be filled with a CO_2 absorbent in accordance with the manufacturer's guidelines.
- ■ Some canisters are fiddly to fill.
- ■ Some canisters are difficult to clean.
- ■ Canisters are often a source of gas leaks.

- ■ Maintenance takes time and skill (it is vital to check the circle system before every use) and there is a cost associated with purchase of CO_2 absorbent.
- ■ The CO_2 absorbent creates resistance.
- ■ Relatively expensive to purchase.
- ■ Water may collect in tubing and within the circle (must be allowed to dry out frequently).
- ■ May be unsuitable for anaesthesia of hyperthermic patients or large-breed dogs as excessive heat may be generated, exacerbating or creating hyperthermia (although this effect can be reduced by using higher gas flow rates).

Carbon dioxide absorption

The CO_2 absorbent is integral to rebreathing systems. The individual designs vary between manufacturers, but the basic components are the same:

- ■ Calcium hydroxide
- ■ Sodium hydroxide
- ■ Water
- ■ pH indicator
- ■ Silica
- ■ Zeolite
- ■ Calcium sulphate
- ■ Calcium chloride.

The most important components are calcium hydroxide, sodium hydroxide and water.

The CO_2 absorbent may have granular or spherical particles that give a high surface area to volume ratio to maximize the surface exposed to the gas. The preparation must not be too dusty. Dust in the CO_2 absorbent has several effects:

- It increases resistance
- It damages the breathing system – the dust can settle within valves, making them inefficient, and can gather in seals, making leaks more likely
- It may reach the patient and cause caustic burns to the airway
- It may be an irritant to the operator refilling or emptying the canister.

The reaction with CO_2 takes place in two stages:

Stage 1

H_2O + CO_2 $\leftrightarrows$ H_2CO_3
Water + Carbon dioxide $\leftrightarrows$ Carbonic acid

Stage 2

$2H_2CO_3 + 2NaOH + Ca(OH)_2 \leftrightarrows CaCO_3 + Na_2CO_3 + 4H_2O + heat$

Carbonic acid + Sodium hydroxide + Calcium hydroxide $\leftrightarrows$ Calcium carbonate + Sodium carbonate + Water + Heat

Carbon dioxide absorption results in a pH change, signalled by a colour change in the pH indicator. It is important to refer to the manufacturer's guidelines in order to be aware of the colour change that occurs with a particular absorbent. The most commonly seen colour changes are from pink to white, and from white to purple. The colour change indicates that the absorbent has been exhausted and so must be changed.

Other indicators of exhaustion include:

- Increased end-tidal CO_2 (hypercapnia) as measured by a capnometer (clinical signs are increased heart and respiratory rates and blood pressure, brick red mucous membranes and bounding pulses)
- Increased inspired CO_2 (there should be no CO_2 present in the inspired gases)
- The canister of absorbent is cool to the touch (the reaction between the absorbent and CO_2 generates heat).

WARNING

A CO_2 absorbent that is left overnight after it has become exhausted will return to its original colour, and so the following day will appear as if it has not been exhausted. This occurs because the reaction between the CO_2 and absorbent is reversible. However, if this absorbent is then used it will change colour quickly, indicating its exhausted state. Exhausted absorbent should therefore be changed at the end of the day when the colour change is clear.

Absorbents can also release toxic by-products. Dry sodium hydroxide can degrade isoflurane to produce carbon monoxide and can degrade sevoflurane to produce compound A, methanol and formaldehyde. Consequently, it is very important that the absorbent does not dry out. This can be done by ensuring that the fresh gases and inhalational agent are switched off immediately after use to reduce drying by the fresh gases and exposure to the inhalational agent, and that the absorbent is regularly changed

Maintenance of circle systems

Circle systems should be maintained following specific manufacturer's guidelines; however, there are a few basic principles that should always be adhered to.

- Change the CO_2 absorbent frequently, following the absorbent manufacturer's guidelines. It is vital to be aware of the colour change that is present with that particular absorbent (see above).
- Change the CO_2 absorbent in a well ventilated room.
- Wear gloves (most CO_2 absorbents are caustic, especially when damp).
- Wear a face mask to avoid breathing in soda lime dust.
- Empty contents in accordance with local waste disposal regulations, taking care not to breathe in any dust created.
- When the canister is empty, look for any small cracks or signs of damage.
- Check the circle system thoroughly after changing the absorbent:
  1. Once the canister has been refilled, attach it to the anaesthetic machine and attach the Y-piece patient tubing.
  2. Occlude the Y-piece at the patient end.
  3. Close the APL valve.
  4. Fill the circle with O_2 (using either the oxygen flush or flowmeter) until the reservoir bag becomes distended.
  5. Listen and feel for any leaks, watching the reservoir bag for any signs of it deflating.
  6. Open the APL valve to check that it is working and not sticking; this also prevents any accidents caused by inadvertently leaving the valve closed when the circuit is attached to the patient, such as possible barotrauma. Some gas will escape of its own accord and the rest should be removed by squeezing the reservoir bag. By keeping the Y-piece occluded during this process, all gases are removed from the breathing system via the scavenging, preventing environmental contamination from any inhalational agent residue within the system.
  7. Date and initial the canister.

Non-rebreathing systems

Non-rebreathing systems are characterized by the absence of unidirectional valves and CO_2 absorbent. They require higher fresh gas flows than rebreathing systems because the expired CO_2 is removed from the circuit by new fresh gas flushing out the expired gases.

Features of non-rebreathing systems

- High fresh gas flow rates can exacerbate hypothermia – this is particularly problematical in patients of low bodyweight.
- High fresh gas flow rates increase costs associated with both the anaesthetic gases (O_2 and N_2O or medical air) and inhalational agents.
- High fresh gas flow rates lead to greater environmental contamination.
- The patient receives the concentration of volatile agent that is dialled up on the vaporizer with no delay (i.e. next breath). Changes in depth of anaesthesia can be achieved quickly.
- Optimal levels of N_2O can be used safely; total fresh gas flow can be divided in a ratio of 1:2 O_2:N_2O.

- No changes in the fresh gas flow rate are required during the anaesthetic period (unless there are changes to the patient's minute volume due to changes in respiratory rate).
- A circuit factor (Figure 21.49) is required to prevent rebreathing of alveolar gas.

Calculation of fresh gas flow rate

Due to the reliance on the fresh gas flow rate to prevent rebreathing, correct calculation of fresh gas flow rate is essential.

1. Calculate the patient's tidal volume (TV). This is the volume of gas exhaled in one breath and is considered to be between 10 and 15 ml/kg.
   - The size of the patient is the first thing to consider when determining which end of the 10–15 ml/kg range to use. Generally, use the high end of the range (15 ml/kg) for small dogs and cats. For larger patients (e.g. Labrador Retrievers), a tidal volume of 10 ml/kg is appropriate.
   - Consider the body condition of the patient. Only the lean weight, i.e. what the bodyweight would be at a body condition score of 3/5, should be used in the calculation.
   - Consider the shape of the patient's thorax. Deep-chested breeds such as Greyhounds will have a higher tidal volume than would be expected for their bodyweight (12–15 ml/kg).

Tidal volume (ml) = 10–15 x bodyweight (kg)

2. Calculate the patient's minute volume (MV). This is the volume of gas expired by the patient in 1 minute and requires measurement of respiratory rate (breaths per minute). This should be done when the patient has been allowed to acclimatize to its environment. The best way of gathering this information is to observe the patient from a distance when it is in its kennel. If the patient is panting, the respiratory rate should be estimated. Once the patient is anaesthetized the respiratory rate may be different to that used for the MV calculation. It is important to recalculate respiratory rate if it increases, as it will lead to increased MV.

Minute volume (ml/min) = Tidal volume (ml) x Respiratory rate (/min)

3. Multiply the calculated minute volume by the circuit factor of the breathing system being used. The circuit factor varies between different breathing systems (Figure 21.49).

Fresh gas flow rate (ml/min) = Minute volume (ml/min) x Circuit factor

---

Breathing system	Circuit factor
T-piece	2.5–3
Lack and Mini-Lack	1–1.5
Magill	1–1.5
Bain	2.5–3

21.49 Circuit factors for different breathing systems.

T-piece

Many different variations of the T-piece are used within veterinary practice. These differences are centred around the presence or absence of a reservoir bag and APL valve. The Ayre's T-piece (Mapleson E) (Figure 21.50a) has no reservoir bag or valve. An Ayre's T-piece with a Jackson–Rees modification (Mapleson F) (Figure 21.50b) has no valve but an open-ended reservoir bag. A paediatric T-piece (Mapleson D) contains an APL valve and a closed-ended reservoir bag.

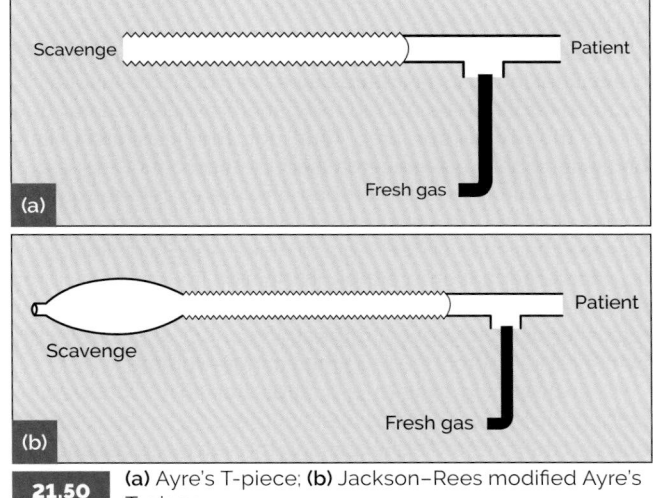

21.50 (a) Ayre's T-piece; (b) Jackson–Rees modified Ayre's T-piece.

Despite these variations, the principle of how a T-piece works is similar. Gases enter the breathing system close to the patient at the 'T' and fill all of the tubing from which the patient inhales. When the patient exhales, the gases move down the expiratory limb (the force of the fresh gas prevents the gases moving towards the anaesthetic machine) where they leave the system: directly into the scavenging system (Ayre's T-piece); through the open-ended reservoir bag and then the scavenging system (Jackson–Rees modification); or out of the APL valve (paediatric system). In the expiratory pause (the gap between breaths) the tubing fills with fresh gas in preparation for the next breath. A high flow rate is required to ensure all of the expired gases are flushed from the system, preventing rebreathing; consequently, a circuit factor of 2.5–3 times minute volume is required (the higher end of the range should be used for smaller patients).

The T-piece is a low-resistance circuit with a small amount of dead space and is the breathing system of choice for small patients (<8 kg). It is not suitable for use in larger patients because the required high flow rates make it uneconomical and the narrow-bore tubing means that resistance will be created for larger patients during inspiration and expiration.

> **WARNING**
>
> Particular care must be taken when using the Ayre's T-piece with the Jackson–Rees modification due to the risk of the scavenging tubing dragging and causing the reservoir bag to twist and become occluded. This is extremely dangerous for the patient (possible pneumothorax, pneumomediastinum and decreased venous return)

T-pieces are suitable for IPPV. This is achieved either by closing the valve, applying positive pressure to the reservoir bag and then opening the valve, or by occluding the base of the reservoir bag as it enters the scavenging and then applying positive pressure. On the Ayres T-piece the end of the breathing tubing is occluded (e.g. with the thumb) creating positive pressure.

Bain

The principle of the Bain circuit (Figure 21.51) is similar to that of the T-piece. Two types of Bain circuit (Mapleson D) are available: coaxial and parallel. The coaxial Bain is more common, the inspiratory limb running inside the expiratory limb. The Bain has an APL valve and reservoir bag, but no unidirectional valves.

The tubing close to the patient is filled with fresh gas. As the patient inhales, gases are taken from both the inspiratory and expiratory limbs. When the patient exhales, gases flow down the expiratory limb (but not the inspiratory limb because of the resistance caused by the continued flow of fresh gas), into the reservoir bag and are expelled from the circuit via the APL valve and scavenging system. A larger reservoir bag than on the T-piece makes the Bain circuit suitable for larger patients, although the high flow rates required make it very uneconomical in patients >15 kg. This high flow rate is required to prevent rebreathing of CO_2 and is reflected by the circuit factor of 2.5–3 times minute volume.

The breathing system is suitable for IPPV, achieved by closing the valve, applying positive pressure to the reservoir bag and then immediately opening the valve. It is essential to open the valve immediately because the high fresh gas flow rates quickly create high pressures within the Bain circuit (often the valve will not need to be completely closed).

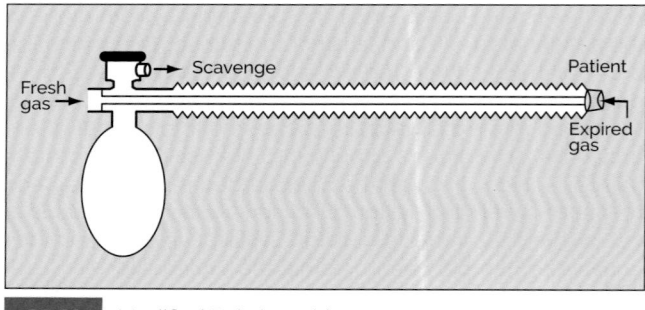

21.51   Modified Bain breathing system.

Lack

The Lack (Mapelson A) can also be either coaxial (Figure 21.52) or parallel (Figure 21.53); the parallel version is the more common. The circuit comprises an APL valve and reservoir bag. The reservoir bag is situated on the inspiratory limb of the system. As the patient inhales, gases are drawn from the inspiratory limb and reservoir bag. When the patient exhales, the first portion of expired gases (dead space gases) enter the inspiratory limb before the rest (alveolar gases) pass down the expiratory limb and out of the APL valve into the scavenging system. The APL valve is situated next to the gas inlet on the anaesthetic breathing system. Rebreathing of the dead space gases in the inspiratory limb at the start of the next breath means that the required fresh gas flow rate is lower than for the T-piece or Bain, and therefore the circuit factor is lower (1–1.5 times minute volume). The circuit is suitable for patients >10 kg.

Lack systems are not ideal for prolonged IPPV as this disrupts the pattern of gas flow within the circuit, resulting in rebreathing. However, if another breathing system that is more appropriate for IPPV is not available, rebreathing can be prevented by increasing the fresh gas flow rate.

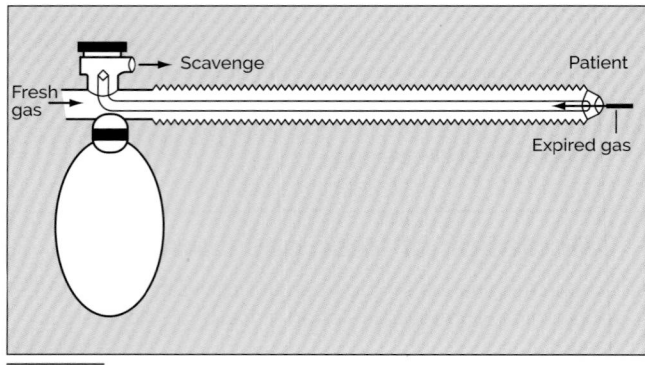

21.52   Coaxial Lack breathing system.

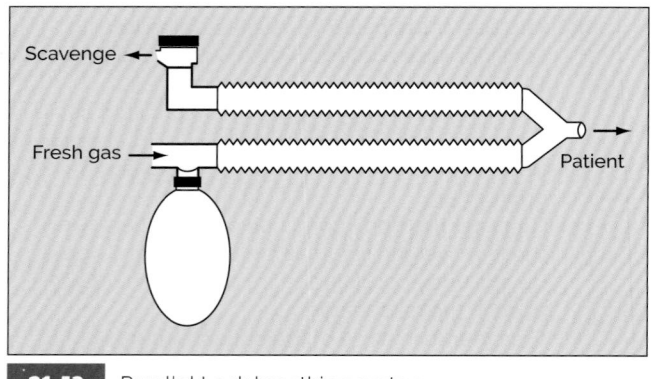

21.53   Parallel Lack breathing system.

Mini-Lack

This system has the same basic design as the conventional Lack, but is suitable for patients <10 kg because it uses narrow low-resistance tubing, with a narrower tubing connector and small reservoir bag. As with the traditional Lack, the design of the mini-Lack enables the use of lower flow rates compared with the T-piece, only requiring 1–1.5 times minute volume. However, this also makes it unsuitable for prolonged IPPV.

Magill

The Magill (Figure 21.54) also has a Mapleson A configuration. It consists of a reservoir bag that is situated by the fresh gas inlet on the breathing system, wide bore tubing, and an APL valve situated next to the patient's head, close to where the breathing system attaches to the ET tube.

When the fresh gases are switched on, the reservoir bag and tubing are filled. As the patient inhales, gases are drawn from the tubing and the reservoir bag. As the patient exhales,

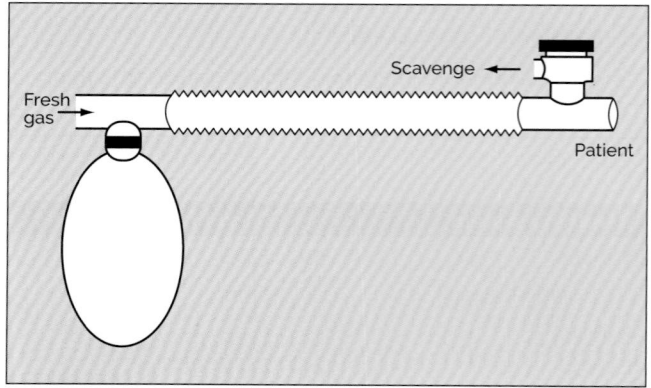

21.54   Magill breathing system.

the first portion of the gas (dead space gas) travels up the tubing before the pressure of new fresh gas entering the system forces the rest of the exhaled gases (alveolar gases) out of the APL valve and into the scavenging system (path of least resistance). This can occur due to the location of the valve next to the patient's head. The system is suitable for patients >10 kg. The circuit factor for the Magill is 1–1.5 times minute volume.

The location of the valve close to the patient's head has some additional disadvantages: it can increase the risk of accidental disconnection from the breathing system and cause accidental extubation; there is an increased risk of the ET tube becoming kinked; and the location of valve makes IPPV difficult and impractical for any surgery around the head and neck due to poor surgical access.

Humphrey ADE and Humphrey ADE–circle system

The Humphrey ADE breathing system (Figure 21.55) was designed to allow three breathing systems in one unit. The Mapelson A circuit is inefficient for controlled ventilation, as is the Mapleson D circuit for spontaneous ventilation. This single circuit can be changed from a Mapleson A system to a Mapleson D by moving a lever on the metallic block that connects the circuit to the fresh gas outlet on the anaesthetic machine. The reservoir bag is situated at the fresh gas inlet end of the circuit and gas is conducted to and from the patient down the inspiratory and expiratory limbs of the circuit.

- When the lever is in the 'up' position (see Figure 21.55) the reservoir bag and respiratory valve are used, creating a Mapleson A type circuit that is ideally suited to spontaneous respiration. It is also suitable for manual ventilation with no change in the fresh gas flow rate, unlike a normal Lack or Magill. The Humphrey ADE–circle system is more efficient than a Magill, therefore average required fresh gas flow rates are 50 ml/kg/min.
- When the lever is in the 'down' position the bag and the valve are bypassed and the ventilator port is opened, creating a Mapelson D (Bain) system for use during IPPV. If no ventilator is attached and the port is left open the system will function like an Ayre's T-piece (Mapleson E).

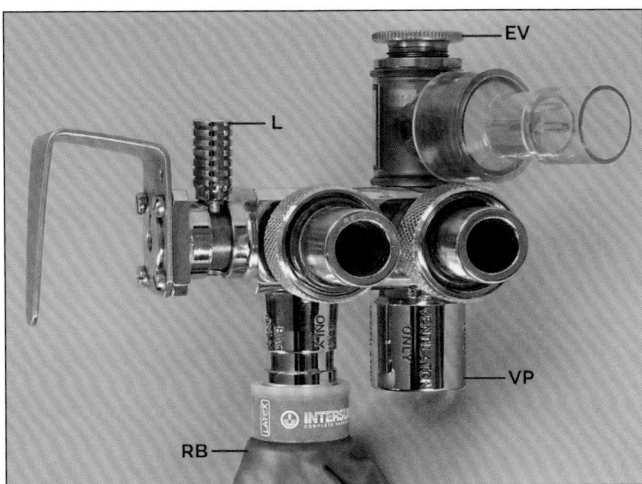

21.55 An ADE circuit. Depending on the position of the control lever (L) at the Humphrey block, gases pass through either the expiratory valve (EV) or the ventilator port (VP). RB = reservoir bag

The three modes centre around the use of the metal block section. The APL valve on this block is especially designed to provide minimal resistance, so the circuit is suitable for use in cats, but also has the benefit of providing 1 cmH_2O positive end-expiratory pressure (PEEP). The Humphrey ADE system uses 15 mm smooth-bore tubing, which encourages laminar flow and has a low resistance and a low volume, making it suitable for small patients when a small reservoir bag is used (e.g. 500 ml or 1 litre).

A later and very useful addition to the Humphrey ADE is that of a removable CO_2 absorber canister, which creates a fourth mode of breathing system: the circle mode (Humphrey ADE–circle system). The canister is easily attached to the main body of the ADE system using two lock nuts on the inspiratory and expiratory limbs. When the CO_2 canister is attached, during induction, when higher fresh gas flow rates are used, the fresh gases automatically pass over and not through the soda lime in the canister; the ADE therefore behaves more like a semi-closed system. Once the fresh gas is reduced, during the maintenance phase of the anaesthetic, the gases pass through the soda lime canister so that the breathing system functions as a circle system. Fresh gas flow rates as low as 1 litre/min can be used.

Before using this system, it is important for the operator to understand fully how it works. Although a basic guide is described here, the authors recommend that the operator's manual is read thoroughly. A number of websites also describe the functioning of the Humphrey ADE/Humphrey ADE–circle systems.

Selection of appropriate circuit and calculation of fresh gas flow rate

Example 1
DSH cat, 4.5 kg, respiratory rate 32 breaths/min

Tidal volume = 4.5 x 15 = 67.5 ml
Minute volume = 67.5 x 32 = 2160 ml

T-piece circuit selected (low resistance, low dead space, low TV).

Fresh gas flow rate = MV x circuit factor = 2160 x 2.5
= 5400 ml (5.4 litres)

The veterinary surgeon requests that nitrous oxide is used.

O_2 flow rate = 5400 ÷ 3 = 1800 ml (c.2 litres)
N_2O flow rate = 1800 x 2 = 3600 ml (c.3.5 litres)

Once the cat is anaesthetized its respiratory rate reduces to 16 breaths/min, allowing recalculation of flow rate. This is not absolutely necessary and maintaining a high flow rate will do no harm, but will increase costs and increase environmental contamination.

Minute volume = 67.5 x 16 = 1080 ml

Fresh gas flow rate
= 1080 x 2.5 = 2700 ml (3 litres – 1 litre of O_2 + 2 litres of N_2O)

Example 2
Labrador, 25 kg, respiratory rate 16 breaths/min

Tidal volume = 25 x 10 = 250 ml
Minute volume = 250 x 16 = 4000 ml →

> **Example 2** *continued*
>
> Lack selected (lower requirement for fresh gas flow compared to a Bain, ease of circuit use compared to a Magill).
>
> Fresh gas flow rate = MV x circuit factor
> = 4000 x 1 = 4000 ml (4 litres)
>
> A circle system could also be used in a semi-closed configuration. This could be achieved by using a fresh gas flow rate of 3 litres/min for the first 20 minutes to ensure denitrogenation and then reducing the fresh gas flow rate to 1 litre/min.

Checking breathing systems

Breathing systems should be checked before every use. The basic principle is the same whatever the breathing system, with small variations towards the end of the check to test individual special features.

Checks to be performed on all breathing systems

1. Visually check for any contamination (e.g. blood) or obvious damage/holes in the tubing or reservoir bag. Dispose of damaged circuits or clean if necessary. Individual parts of systems can often be replaced without the need to replace the whole circuit.
2. Check that the components of the system are in the correct location, e.g. the valve and reservoir bag.
3. Attach the gas inlet on the breathing system to the common gas outlet of the anaesthetic machine.
4. Close the valve or, in the case of the Jackson–Rees modified Ayres T-piece, occlude the neck of the bag where it enters the scavenging system.
5. Occlude the patient attachment end, either with your hand or hold it against your leg (whichever method it is important to create an airtight seal).
6. Fill the system with O^2 (or medical air if available). This can be done either by using the oxygen flush or by the flowmeters. Stop gas flow once the reservoir bag is distended.
7. Listen and feel for any leaks.
8. Open the valve and squeeze the contents out of the reservoir bag to check that the valve opens fully. It is important whilst doing this to keep the patient attachment occluded.

Additional checks should be carried out for coaxial systems, to confirm that there is no damage to the inner limb.

- **Bain:** With the O_2 flowmeter set at 4 litres and the valve closed, use a pen (or disposable Bain breathing systems come with a plastic tool of the correct diameter) to occlude the inner limb. Observe the bobbin within the flowmeter – it will dip if there are no leaks in the system. It should only be transiently occluded as it causes back pressure within the anaesthetic machine, which could be damaging.
- **Lack:** With the O_2 flowmeter set at 4 litres and the valve closed, use a pen of a similar diameter (or disposable Lacks come with a plastic tool of the correct diameter) to occlude the inner limb. Observe the reservoir bag filling and becoming distended.

Scavenging systems

The scavenging of waste anaesthetic gases is controlled by the Control of Substances Hazardous to Health (COSHH) regulations (see Chapter 2). There are two types of scavenging system: active and passive.

Active scavenging

Active scavenging is the preferred technique for removing waste gases as it is the most reliable. It uses an extractor fan to create negative air pressure within the room. Ideally this should be used in combination with a pressure break such as an Anaesthetic Gas Scavenging System (AGSS) receiver unit (Figure 21.56) to prevent excessive negative pressure from being exerted on the patient.

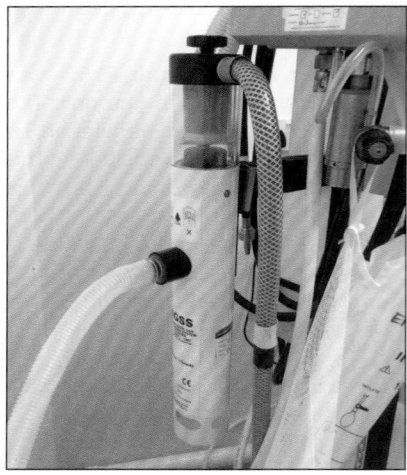

21.56 Anaesthetic gas scavenging system air break.

Passive scavenging

Passive scavenging relies on gases moving either into a system containing activated charcoal or into a tube going outside the building; the latter is not acceptable. Activated charcoal canisters should be weighed regularly to detect when the charcoal is exhausted, following the manufacturer's guidelines. The scavenging tubing should not be too long (ideally no longer than 1.5 m) and it is important that no resistance is created in the tube (e.g. through kinking). Activated charcoal does not absorb N_2O and so should not be used as the scavenging method for this gas.

Other ways of limiting environmental pollution

Along with ensuring that scavenging systems are adequate, other methods are used to decrease environmental contamination by waste anaesthetic gases. These include:

- Checking anaesthetic machines and breathing systems before every use
- Connecting the breathing system to the ET tube and inflating the cuff before switching on the volatile agent or N_2O
- Regularly checking for leaks around the ET tube cuff during anaesthesia
- Maintaining the animal on 100% O_2 for a couple of minutes once the volatile agent has been turned off, to flush anaesthetic gases out of the circuit via the scavenging system. The reservoir bag is disconnected and emptied several times
- Using a rebreathing system wherever possible, to minimize fresh gas flow rates

- Refilling vaporizers at the end of the day using key-fillers (see above). This should not be carried out by the same person every day, but on a rotational basis so as to minimize the individual exposure of staff
- Ensuring that recovery areas are well ventilated, as patients continue to breathe out inhalant agent during the recovery period
- Ensuring regular maintenance of anaesthetic machines
- Monitoring the concentration of inhalant agent in the environment regularly
- Only using inhalational techniques for induction of anaesthesia when absolutely necessary
- Scavenging waste gases from side-stream capnography systems.

Environmental monitoring

Monitoring environmental contamination should be carried out routinely (e.g. every 6 months) using individual dose-meters worn by staff during a normal working day. These are widely available commercially.

Ventilation

The ability to provide patient ventilation manually, through the use of intermittent positive pressure ventilation (IPPV), is an important skill and one that all veterinary nurses should have. The basic technique is given below.

In order to perform IPPV optimally, capnography should ideally be used as it can help to tailor IPPV to the particular patient. For example, a steadily reducing end-tidal carbon dioxide ($ETCO_2$, see below) indicates over-ventilation (hyper-ventilation), due to provision of either a higher respiratory rate than necessary or a larger tidal volume, or both. Conversely, a steadily increasing $ETCO_2$ indicates under-ventilation (hypoventilation) through the provision of an inadequate respiratory rate or tidal volume.

A pulse oximeter is also an important piece of equipment, used to ensure that the IPPV is adequate to maintain the patient's oxygen levels.

IPPV technique

1. Close the valve (or occlude the neck of the reservoir bag as it enters the scavenging system if using an Ayre's T-piece with a Jackson–Rees modification).
2. Squeeze the reservoir bag while watching the patient's chest, to create a normal expansion.
3. Open the valve or stop occluding the reservoir bag.
4. Aim for a 1:2 ratio of inspiration to expiration to minimize the cardiovascular effects of IPPV.

WARNING

If a patient requires prolonged IPPV, this should be performed by a dedicated nurse rather than by the person monitoring the anaesthetic, as it is not possible to concentrate and perform both tasks adequately at the same time.

- The T-piece, Bain and circle circuits are all suitable for prolonged IPPV with no change in fresh gas flow rate
- The Lack and Magill can be used for short periods of IPPV but if prolonged IPPV is necessary the fresh gas flow rate should be increased to prevent rebreathing or, ideally, another breathing system should be used

---

When to ventilate

The correct time to ventilate is ultimately the veterinary surgeon's decision but it is very important for nurses to be aware of the situations when a patient should receive manual IPPV or be placed on to a mechanical ventilator.

Indications for IPPV

- When the patient is unable to breathe adequately and spontaneously and to maintain normal CO_2 and O_2 concentrations in the blood (e.g. due to body position for surgery or obesity).
- Thoracic surgery (including diaphragmatic rupture) that will impair normal respiratory function.
- Pneumothorax.
- Administration of an NMBA that will prevent spontaneous respiration.
- During use of potent opioids that may cause apnoea.
- Spinal cord damage or oedema that hinders respiratory drive or effort.
- Diseases affecting respiratory muscle function (e.g. myasthenia gravis, phrenic nerve paralysis, botulism or tetanus).
- Raised intracranial pressure (due to trauma or other disease processes). Prevention of hypercapnia is important to prevent a further rise in intracranial pressure.
- Severe hypothermia.

Mechanical ventilators

Ventilators are becoming increasingly common in veterinary practice and there are a number of different models available. For the purposes of this chapter, only the basic principles will be explained. Any patient that requires manual IPPV will benefit from being placed on a mechanical ventilator designed for the size of patient. The advantages and disadvantages of using mechanical ventilators are listed in Figure 21.57.

It is recommended that the ventilator parameters are pre-set prior to anaesthesia for cases that are likely to require IPPV in order to expedite a rapid transition to IPPV in an emergency. To test that the parameters are correct, a reservoir bag can be placed where the patient will be attached to the breathing system to act as an artificial lung.

Advantages

- Provide control over respiratory rate and volume
- Constant and regular rhythm help maintain a steady plane of anaesthesia
- No requirement for personnel to provide manual IPPV, allowing them to concentrate on monitoring the patient
- Special features may be used, i.e. PEEP

Disadvantages

- Reduced venous return (especially if there is a long inspiratory time and high airway pressures
- High airway pressures may cause bradycardia
- Mechanical failure or faults may occur
- May cause harm to the patient if used incorrectly
- Expensive to purchase and require regular servicing to ensure safety

---

21.57 Advantages and disadvantages of using mechanical ventilators. IPPV = intermittent positive pressure ventilation; PEEP = positive end-expiratory pressure.

Setting up a ventilator

Important principles to consider when setting up a mechanical ventilator include:

1. Estimate the tidal volume (TV) that the patient will require. For the purposes of setting up a ventilator the TV should always be set on the low end of what is expected for the patient (i.e. 10 ml/kg), as it is safer to increase TV to obtain optimal ventilation than to over-ventilate the patient initially. TV should be reduced if the patient is obese, because obesity decreases lung volume relative to bodyweight due to reduced compliance. This is also the case if there are disease processes present that may affect lung volume (e.g. a lung tumour). Some ventilators do not have a safety feature preventing over-ventilation (pressure cut off); therefore, setting the correct TV is vital.
2. Check that the ventilator and attachments on the ventilator are suitable for the size of the patient (e.g. correct size of bellows).
3. If there is a maximum pressure alarm/limit, set it appropriately. This should be a maximum of 15 cmH$_2$O for most patients.
4. Set the appropriate respiratory rate.
5. If possible set the inspiratory to expiratory ratio. This is the ratio of the time allowed for inspiration and expiration in one breath. Usually this is 1:2 or 1:3. Ensuring that the expiration phase of respiration is 2–3 times longer than the inspiration phase allows adequate time for venous return to the heart, reducing the impact of IPPV on the cardiovascular system.

Placing a patient on a ventilator

1. Ensure the scavenging system is connected correctly – this usually involves taking the scavenging tube off the breathing system and placing it on to an attachment on the ventilator.
2. Switch the ventilator on.
3. Check the pressure gauge to ensure that airway pressure is not excessively low or high. For most patients a pressure of 10–12 cmH$_2$O is appropriate.
4. Observe the patient's chest. Are there suitable chest movements? Change the tidal volume to gain the correct airway pressure and chest movement. Aim to create a breathing pattern that is as natural as possible.
5. Observe the capnogram if available.
6. If the patient is 'bucking' (breathing against) the ventilator, check depth of anaesthesia and increase the respiratory rate. Ventilation can be quite stimulating and the aim is to override the patient's own respiratory drive. It is usually possible to achieve this by increasing the respiratory rate and ensuring an adequate depth of anaesthesia; however, it will sometimes be necessary for the veterinary surgeon to prescribe a drug to facilitate override of spontaneous ventilation (e.g. a potent opioid such as fentanyl or a benzodiazepine such as midazolam).
7. Adjust the rate and volume of respiration in order to maintain optimal ETCO$_2$ (see 'Monitoring the anaesthetized patient', below). The required rate will usually be around 14 breaths/min for cats and small dogs and 6–8 breaths/min for medium to large dogs. These are rough guidelines and it is important to remember that all patients are different.

Weaning a patient off a ventilator

1. Decrease the respiratory rate to increase ETCO$_2$.
2. If the ventilator has an assist mode or pressure trigger (the ventilator detects the patient taking a breath and completes a ventilator breath) switch to this mode first before switching the ventilator off.
3. Switch off the ventilator. If the patient does not start breathing spontaneously, provide occasional manual ventilation while closely observing the patient's O$_2$ saturation using a pulse oximeter.
4. Lighten the plane of anaesthesia.

Monitoring the anaesthetized patient

Monitoring during anaesthesia is one of the most common tasks performed by the veterinary nurse. If done well it can make a significant difference to case outcome; it may make the difference between an animal surviving anaesthesia or not. Anaesthesia has many negative effects on the body, and the aim of diligent monitoring is to identify these effects in order to allow appropriate supportive measures to be put in place, thereby reducing the risk of organ and tissue damage.

Anaesthetic records

Anaesthetic records, such as that shown in Figure 21.58, are legal documents and must give a true account of what occurred throughout the anaesthetic period. However, it is important to remember that monitoring the patient is the most important task to be undertaken and the anaesthetist should not become focused on filling in the record rather than monitoring the patient. Use of an anaesthetic record facilitates the detection of trends that are difficult to see unless parameters are recorded. The recommended format of an anaesthetic record card is graphical, to allow trends to be seen easily and problems to be identified promptly. The patient should be monitored continuously and each parameter recorded approximately every 5–10 minutes, depending on how stable the animal is under anaesthesia. There are many different anaesthetic record designs and choosing or designing a record card can be challenging. With this in mind the Association of Veterinary Anaesthetists have designed two anaesthetic records (low ASA status (Figure 21.58) and high ASA status). The records are free to download from the AVA website (https://ava.eu.com) and the practice logo can be inserted.

Ideally, the following information should be included on an anaesthetic record:

- Date
- Patient name and case number
- Patient species, breed, age, sex, bodyweight
- History of previous anaesthesia
- Details of clinical examination and any problems or concerns
- American Society of Anesthesiologists (ASA) classification
- Drugs used for premedication, along with time, route of administration and effect
- Site of intravenous catheter placement

Anaesthesia record

Name:	
Owner:	
Breed:	
Age:	Sex:
Weight:	
Anaesthetist:	
Clinician:	

Click here to add logo

Date:

ASSOCIATION OF VETERINARY ANAESTHETISTS

History:

Clinical findings/results/medications:

Temperament:

HR: RR:

Pulse quality:

MM: CRT:

Thoracic auscultation:

Temperature: °C

ASA classification

I No organic disease
II Mild systemic disease
III Severe systemic disease (not incapacitating)
IV Severe disease (constant threat to life)
V Moribund (life expectancy < 24 h)
Add 'E' for emergencies

ASA Grade:

Procedure(s):

Anticipated problems:

Pre-GA medication	Dose	Route	Time
....	....	......	......
....	....	......	......
....	....	......	......

Anaesthetic Safety Checklist completed ☐ (see overleaf)

Induction agent(s)	Dose	Route	Time
....	....	......	......
....	....	......	......

☐ IV catheter Position: Size:

ET tube / LMA / Mask | Cuffed / Uncuffed | Size:

Breathing system: | ☐ Eye(s) lubricated

Fluids/Drugs/Monitoring — Time

Notes

220 210 200 190 180 170 160 150 140 130 120 110 100 90 80 70 60 50 40 30 20 10

Patient position	
Patient warming	
Throat pack	Placed ☐ Removed ☐
Swabs	In: Out:
Sharps	In: Out:

Iso / Sevo %
O₂ / N₂O / Air L/min

Symbols
- ● HR
- o RR ø IPPV
- v SAP – MAP ^ DAP
- ⓥ Doppler

SpO₂ %
Jaw tone -/+/++
Palpebral -/+
Eye position ↓ / →

RECOVERY instructions:

IV catheter care: ☐ Remove once recovered ☐ Maintain & flush

	T+0	T+15	T+30	T+45
Time				
Heart rate				
Resp. rate				
MM & CRT				
Temp.				
Pain score				

21.58 An example of an anaesthetic record for low ASA status patients. (© Association of Veterinary Anaesthetists)

- Fluids given and the rate and total volume administered
- Estimation of blood loss
- Breathing system
- ET tube size
- Posture
- Monitors to be used
- Inhalational agent to be used.

Within the graphical section, the following should be included:

- Time of all drug administration and doses given (in mg not ml as drug concentrations can vary and be altered)
- Heart rate
- Respiration rate
- Other monitoring information, e.g. SpO_2 (haemoglobin saturation with oxygen), blood pressure, temperature, $ETCO_2$ (end-tidal carbon dioxide)
- End-tidal inhalational agent concentration or dialled vaporizer setting
- Fresh gas flow rate of the individual gases used.

There must be enough space available to record:

- Extra information, such as the time the patient is moved to theatre and the start of surgery
- Time of disconnection from the anaesthetic machine
- Time of extubation
- Immediate postoperative temperature, pulse and respiration
- Time that the patient lifts its head, moves into sternal recumbency and stands
- Quality of recovery
- General comments about the anaesthetic and the patient.

Anaesthetic records are not only important at the time of the anaesthetic but also afterwards. They can be vital for management of subsequent anaesthesia in the same patient and provide a source of information for both the veterinary surgeon and veterinary nurse to reflect upon in order to improve future case management (not only for that patient but others).

Key times to monitor anaesthesia

The anaesthetic procedure should be monitored throughout; however, there are some key times where monitoring is particularly important.

Premedication

Monitoring during premedication is discussed earlier in the chapter.

Induction

Induction of anaesthesia is a high-risk period. While anaesthesia is being induced the nurse should observe the patient's breathing pattern and mucous membrane colour. If intubation is prolonged the patient will benefit from provision of supplemental oxygen, delivered either by having a break in the attempt to intubate the patient and using a facemask, or by simple flow-by (holding the patient attachment of the breathing system close to the patient's nose).

Once the patient is intubated and the tube has been secured, the patient's pulse should be palpated immediately. Intubation can cause arrhythmias that can result in cardiac arrest (although this is extremely rare) and administration of drugs for induction of anaesthesia can cause marked changes in heart rate. It is also important to check that there are no problems before the introduction of an inhalational agent, i.e. excessive depth of anaesthesia following induction.

Maintenance

It is important to maintain the anaesthesia at an appropriate depth in order to avoid side effects associated with excessively high concentrations of anaesthetic. Although there are many different anaesthetic monitors available, the anaesthetist is the most important monitor and the most reliable. Selection of which parameters are monitored, and use of invasive monitoring techniques such as direct arterial blood pressure measurement, depends on the individual patient and procedure. Minimal monitoring in all patients should include pulse rate, respiratory rate and body temperature.

Monitoring the respiratory system

The rate, depth and characteristics of respiration should all be monitored. Further information on respiratory monitoring is given in the section on capnography.

A respiratory rate higher than expected is described as **tachypnoea** and may be indicative of:

- Inadequate depth of anaesthesia
- Noxious stimulation due to inadequate analgesia
- One lung intubation due to an excessively long ET tube
- Hypercapnia
- Use of an incorrect breathing system for that patient
- Low tidal volume.

A respiratory rate that is lower than expected (<10 breaths/minute) is termed **bradypnoea** and may be indicative of:

- An excessive depth of anaesthesia
- Response to drug administration.

Apnoea – when the patient stops breathing – may be caused by:

- An excessive depth of anaesthesia
- Drugs (e.g. potent opioids)
- Inadequate depth of anaesthesia (breath holding)
- Impending cardiac arrest.

Whilst counting the breathing rate, the characteristics of the breaths should also be observed:

- If the patient has a slow respiratory rate but a large tidal volume (e.g. characteristic of a patient that has received an alpha-2 agonist and an opioid), this is likely to be adequate
- If the patient has a slow respiratory rate and a small tidal volume this is likely to result in hypercapnia and a reduction in O_2 saturation. This type of breathing is described as hypoventilation
- If the patient is breathing rapidly with a normal tidal volume, this is described as hyperventilation and will result in hypocapnia (a reduction in $ETCO_2$).

It is also important to take account of the amount of respiratory effort. If the patient is having difficulty in breathing this is described as dyspnoea and is often characterized by a large abdominal component to the respiratory effort. The size of the thoracic movement should also be compared to the volume of gas movement within the reservoir bag. Dyspnoea represents an emergency and the veterinary surgeon should be informed immediately.

Causes of dyspnoea during anaesthesia include:

- A problem with the breathing system (e.g. a sticking unidirectional valve on a circle circuit)
- A problem with an ET tube (e.g. a very small tube for the size of patient, a plug of secretion, the bevel of the tube resting against the wall of the trachea, or a kink in the tube)
- A concurrent problem (e.g. a pneumothorax).

If the patient appears to be breathing normally but there is no movement of the reservoir bag this could indicate:

- Oesophageal intubation. This can be confirmed with the use of a capnograph: if the oesophagus has been intubated no CO_2 will be detected
- Disconnection of the breathing system
- A fault in the breathing system.

Monitoring the cardiovascular system

Heart rate

Heart rate can be measured by auscultation using either a conventional stethoscope or oesophageal stethoscope and/or by palpation of the apex beat on the left-hand side of the patient's thorax.

A heart rate higher than expected is described as **tachycardia**. Expected heart rate during anaesthesia depends on the drugs that have been used for premedication (e.g. has an alpha-2 agonist been administered in which case heart rate will be lower than after premedication with acepromazine) and the preoperative heart rate measured during the pre-anaesthetic clinical examination. Tachycardia may indicate:

- Inadequate depth of anaesthesia
- Inadequate analgesia
- Result from drug administration (e.g. ketamine)
- Presence of arrhythmias (abnormal heart rhythm on ECG)
- Hypercapnia
- Hypoxaemia
- Hypotension caused by shock and sepsis
- Concurrent disease (e.g. hyperthyroidism (these patients are normally tachycardic before anaesthesia)).

A heart rate lower than expected is described as **bradycardia** and may indicate:

- Excessive depth of anaesthesia
- Result from drug administration (e.g. alpha-2 agonists and opioids)
- Hypothermia
- Hypertension
- Vagal stimulation (stimulation of the vagal nerve caused by pressure or stimulation of the nerve during surgery).

This is common during enuculeation of the eye due to pressure on the eyeball, or during surgical dissection of the neck. If bradycardia occurs, the surgeon should be notified immediately so that they can stop what they are doing; this will normally lead to a rapid correction of the bradycardia. Administration of an anticholinergic (e.g. atropine) may be required to prevent recurrence of the bradycardia as surgery continues

- Hyperkalaemia (high levels of blood potassium)
- Severe acidosis (low blood pH)
- Severe hypoglycaemia (low blood glucose)
- Severe hypoxaemia.

Pulse

Pulse palpation (see also Chapter 14) provides information about the adequacy of cardiac output and the circulation. The most useful information is obtained from peripheral pulses, but if these are not palpable central pulses can be used. In this case, the underlying reason for a failure to palpate a peripheral pulse should be rapidly investigated.

Common sites of peripheral pulse palpation in anaesthetized dogs and cats include:

- Metacarpal artery: Palmar aspect of the forelimb, lateral to the dew claw

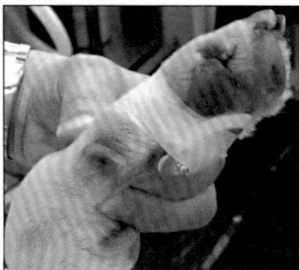

- Dorsal pedal artery: Medial aspect of the metatarsus
- Lingual artery: Midline on the ventral aspect of the tongue

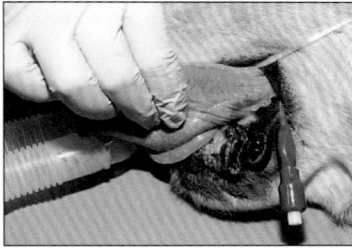

- Labial artery: Inside the upper lip, just behind the level of the canine tooth (the authors find this pulse particularly useful)

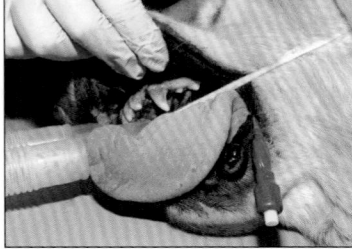

- Coccygeal artery: Ventral aspect of the base of the tail
- Auricular artery: Central ear pinna.

The femoral artery can be palpated but is a central pulse and provides less information than palpation of a peripheral pulse because peripheral pulse quality will be modified first as a result of hypotension or poor peripheral perfusion.

When palpating the pulse, it is important to rest the fingers gently over the pulse point, palpate it and then apply pressure to see how easy it is to occlude. This process is important, as when the pulse is simply palpated, only the difference between systolic and diastolic blood pressure (pulse pressure) is felt. Seeing how easy it is to occlude the pulse provides information about vascular tone and mean arterial blood pressure. A hypotensive patient can have a pulse that is easily palpated but when pressure is applied it can be easily occluded.

It is also important to auscultate the heart and palpate pulses at the same time. If there is not a pulse for every heart sound this is referred to as a pulse deficit. The veterinary surgeon should be told immediately and an ECG obtained as the deficit is likely to indicate a cardiac arrhythmia (see later). The pulse should also be regular; an irregular pulse can indicate an arrhythmia. A commonly seen benign arrhythmia is sinus arrhythmia, characterized by an increase in heart rate on inspiration and decrease in heart rate on expiration. This is especially seen in fit dogs.

Mucous membrane colour and capillary refill time

Mucous membrane colour and capillary refill time (CRT) provide limited information about peripheral perfusion. Normal mucous membranes are described as salmon pink; when blanched (pressure applied), their normal colour returns within 2 seconds (see Chapter 14). Abnormal mucous membrane colours and their causes are shown in Figure 21.59. A prolonged CRT can indicate hypoperfusion, caused by hypovolaemia, hypotension, shock, hypothermia, cardiac failure/depression and vasodilation.

Colour	Possible causes
Pale pink	Vasoconstriction due to: surgical stimulation (e.g. surgeon pulling on a bitch's ovaries); lack of analgesia; haemorrhage or anaemia; drug administration (e.g. alpha-2 agonists); hypoperfusion
Red	Vasodilation, local congestion
Brick red	Severe vasodilation, sepsis, hypercapnia
Blue (cyanosis)	Hypoxia (NB An anaemic patient can be hypoxaemic without the presence of cyanosis due to the reduced oxygen-carrying capacity of the blood)

21.59 Mucous membrane colours during anaesthesia and their clinical interpretation.

Blood loss

Although the surgeon should also be monitoring the amount of blood lost by the patient, the anaesthetist is in the perfect position to monitor the volume of blood loss and provide the patient with necessary intravenous fluid support. Clinically significant blood loss will cause the following signs:

- Tachycardia
- Weak, rapid pulse (often described as thready)
- Hypotension (if using a blood pressure monitor)
- Prolonged CRT
- Pale mucous membranes.

Information on blood loss should be relayed to the veterinary surgeon and the appropriate action taken as prescribed by the veterinary surgeon. Generally, blood loss <10% of circulating blood volume is well tolerated by healthy patients.

Estimating blood loss

1. Collect all used swabs.
2. Count them.
3. Weigh them.
4. Weigh the same number of dry new swabs (if only a couple of swabs have been used weigh 10 swabs and then divide the weight by 10 and multiply by the number used).
5. Subtract the weight of the dry new swabs from the weight of the used, bloody swabs.
6. Calculate the weight of blood contained in the swabs, assuming 1 g equates to 1 ml of fluid/blood.
7. Measure any blood in suction containers and estimate the blood on the floor, drapes and surgeon.
8. Establish the volume of any saline or other fluids used by the surgeon.
9. Add together the volume of blood loss calculated from the swabs, suction, etc., and subtract the volume of any other fluids used by the surgeon to establish the total volume of blood lost.
10. Estimate the patient's blood volume (88 ml x bodyweight (kg) in the dog, 66 ml x bodyweight (kg) in the cat).
11. Divide the estimated blood volume by 100 and multiply by the estimated blood loss (ml).
12. This equates to % blood loss compared to the total blood volume of the patient.

Worked example to estimate blood loss

A 25 kg dog is anaesthetized for ovariohysterectomy. During ligation of the second ovary the ligature around the ovarian pedicle slips and the abdomen starts to fill with blood. The veterinary surgeon gains control of the bleeding after a few minutes but uses a large number of swabs to soak up the haemorrhage. You are concerned about blood loss and wish to calculate the % blood loss in this patient.

1. Ask the surgeon to put the used swabs from the surgical trolley into a container.
2. You count the number of used swabs and find it is 15 small swabs.
3. Weigh a dry swab (6 g) and calculate the weight of the used swabs when dry (6 g x 15 = 90 g).
4. Weigh the used swabs and read off the total weight from the scale. In this case it is 375 g.
5. Calculate the weight of blood in the used swabs (375–90 = 285 g).
6. 1 g of blood is roughly the weight of 1 ml of blood so the total amount of blood lost is 285 ml.
7. The blood volume of a 25 kg dog is 25 x 88 ml = 2,200 ml or 2.2 l.
8. The percentage blood loss in this patient is 285/2,200 x 100% = 12.95%.
9. This percentage blood loss would indicate that fluid therapy with a polyionic solution (containing a number of different ions, e.g. sodium, potassium, chloride, bicarbonate, with an exact composition appropriate for the patient deficits) is indicated to replace blood volume.

Monitoring depth of anaesthesia

Cranial nerve and other reflexes provide information about CNS function and can be used to assess depth of anaesthesia. The deeper the plane of anaesthesia, the greater the depression of the central nervous system. Other information that should be included in the assessment of anaesthetic depth includes heart rate, respiratory rate and blood pressure.

Cranial reflexes commonly used to assess depth of anaesthesia in dogs and cats

- **Palpebral reflex:** Assessed by brushing or lightly touching the medial canthus of the eye or the eyelashes. Brisk or spontaneous movement or blinking indicates a light plane of anaesthesia. As anaesthesia deepens, the palpebral reflex becomes more sluggish and is eventually abolished. A surgical plane of anaesthesia does not require the palpebral reflex to be abolished.
- **Eye position:** If possible, both eyes should be observed as they can be in different positions. A surgical plane of anaesthesia is usually indicated by the eye being in a ventromedial position with mainly the sclera visible. As depth of anaesthesia continues to increase the eye becomes central again. The use of ketamine can interfere with this pattern: the eye remains central regardless of anaesthetic depth.
- **Pupillary diameter:** With increasing depth of anaesthesia the pupil becomes more dilated.
- **Jaw tone:** Jaw tone becomes looser as depth of anaesthesia increases. This is difficult to assess in some breeds of dogs that have a very muscular jaw (e.g. English Bull Terrier). It is important to use a good technique to allow sensitive analysis of this parameter and ensure the safety of the anaesthetist.
- **Pedal reflex:** This is assessed by application of a firm pinch between the patient's toes and observation of a withdrawal response. As depth of anaesthesia increases, the response will reduce until it is abolished.

Other cranial nerve reflexes can be used to indicate depth of anaesthesia; however, they tend to be seen at either inadequate or excessive depth of anaesthesia, thus limiting their routine use:

- **Corneal reflex:** Assessed using a damp cotton-wool bud to touch the cornea gently; the patient should blink in response. This reflex should never be abolished as its absence is an indication of an anaesthetic overdose.
- **Tongue curl:** When a patient is very lightly anaesthetized the tongue will curl when the jaw is opened
- **Lacrimation:** This will reduce as the patient becomes more deeply anaesthetized
- **Salivation:** Excessive salivation may occur with inadequate anaesthesia.

Monitoring body temperature

Anaesthesia inhibits the ability of the patient to thermoregulate. Hypothermia is a major concern with any anaesthetized patient, especially those with the following:

- A high surface area to bodyweight ratio (small patients)
- Neonates because they have an impaired ability to thermoregulate

- Very little body fat
- A thin coat
- A large area of fur clipped
- A large amount of internal tissues exposed.

Hypothermia causes the following physiological changes:

- Reduction in metabolic rate leading to a decreased anaesthetic requirement and increased risk of anaesthetic overdose and prolonged recovery from anaesthesia
- Bradycardia with a potential reduction in cardiac output
- Increased risk of cardiac arrhythmias
- Increased blood loss during surgery due to impaired blood clotting mechanisms
- Shivering during recovery, increases oxygen and glucose demand
- Increased morbidity rate.

Normal body temperature ranges can be found in Chapter 14. To avoid hypothermia, body temperature should be monitored routinely throughout anaesthesia. This can be achieved using a conventional rectal thermometer. A more convenient method is to use a temperature probe that can be placed rectally, nasally or in the oesophagus (the easiest and most convenient location). It also has the advantage of being continuous rather than intermittent, unlike manual measurement of rectal temperature using a conventional thermometer.

Preventing hypothermia

Heat loss from the patient can be minimized by:

- Reducing the preparation and surgery time
- Use of warming devices, starting at premedication
- Minimizing how wet the patient becomes during preparation of the surgical site
- Maintaining a high ambient temperature around the patient
- Use of heat and moisture exchangers
- Use of appropriate flow rates when using non-rebreathing systems
- Use of rebreathing systems when possible
- Providing the surgeon with warmed fluids to use during surgery (e.g. soaking swabs and lavage).

Methods for warming patients during anaesthesia

- Electric heat mats: These can be placed beneath the patient both perioperatively and postoperatively. They should not be left unattended with conscious patients due to the risk of the patient biting the mat and being electrocuted. The use of thermostatically controlled mats is recommended.
- Hot hands: These are examination gloves filled with hot water. Care should be taken when using these because of the risk of their bursting and getting the patient wet, accentuating any hypothermia, or causing scalding if the water is very hot. They also cool down very quickly and need to be replaced regularly; otherwise they will cool the patient.
- Hot air blankets: These are very safe to use. They work by blowing hot air into a disposable blanket that is placed around, under or on top of the patient. Eye lubrication is important to prevent the hot air from drying the cornea and causing a corneal ulcer.
- Microwaveable warming aids: It is particularly easy to overheat these, leading to thermal burns.

It is important to remember that an anaesthetized patient cannot move away from a heat source; measures must therefore be taken to ensure that the patient is not injured. For example, heat mats, hot hands and microwavable aids should be covered with fabric towelling so that they are not placed directly against the skin of an anaesthetized patient.

Aids to patient monitoring

Monitors, particularly multi-parameter monitors, are becoming more common in modern veterinary practice, so it is vital for nurses to be able to use and interpret the information that they provide. It is not appropriate for every monitoring aid to be used on every patient; a cost/benefit analysis should be completed, particularly when using invasive monitoring techniques.

> **WARNING**
>
> The purpose of monitoring aids is to provide additional information about the physiological status of the patient. They should not replace the basic hands-on monitoring described above. Monitors can, and do, go wrong

Cardiovascular system monitoring

Pulse oximetry

Pulse oximeters are probably the most commonly used monitors in veterinary anaesthesia. They provide a non-invasive method of measuring the percentage of oxygen bound to haemoglobin within arterial blood. It is important to monitor oxygen saturation as this will detect tissue hypoxia, which is a common endpoint for many physiological disturbances (see later).

Pulse oximeters have a probe that emits red and infrared light at different wavelengths combined with a photo-detector. Haemoglobin absorbs different wavelengths of the red and infrared light, depending on whether it is bound to oxygen. The amount of red and infrared light absorbed at each wavelength is measured by the photodetector and expressed by the pulse oximeter as a percentage of saturated haemoglobin (SpO_2). This process only takes place for pulsatile blood flow, so only arterial blood is analysed. Pulse oximeters are usually placed on the tongue

(Figure 21.60) but can also be placed on other areas of non-pigmented skin (e.g. prepuce, vulva, between toes, ear pinnae); these are particularly useful if the tongue is not available as a placement site. Some probes cause trauma due to the strength of the spring that closes them. Damage can be avoided by moving the site of the probe frequently. A size of probe should be chosen that is appropriate to the size of the patient and to the area to which the probe will be attached.

All patients should have SpO_2 >90%, as the amount of oxygen contained within arterial blood dramatically decreases when saturation falls below this value. This is expressed in a graphical format by the oxygen dissociation curve (Figure 21.61). The aim during anaesthesia should be to maintain SpO_2 above 95%, to allow a safety margin. If N_2O is being used and SpO_2 drops below 95% use of N_2O should be terminated and the reason for the reduction in O_2 saturation investigated.

Pulse oximeters often give anomalous results, however, so if SpO_2 drops it is also important to look at the patient for signs of cyanosis to confirm the reading, as well as check whether the heart rate given by the pulse oximeter correlates with a manual heart rate; if they do not match it is likely that the reading cannot be trusted. Once checked, the probe should be repositioned. If persistently low readings are obtained the veterinary surgeon should be notified and IPPV performed until the cause is established. Anomalous results can be caused by:

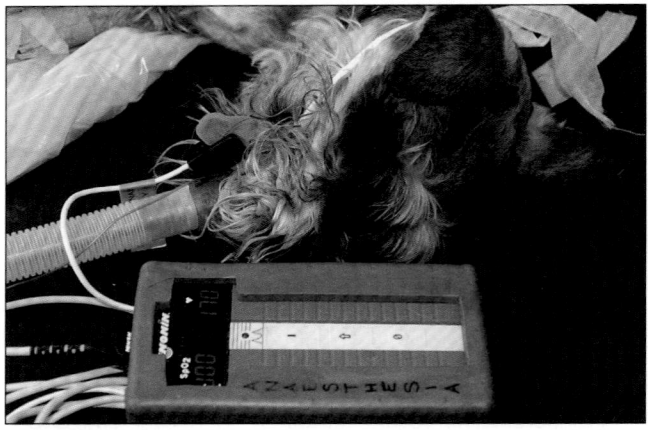

21.60 Pulse oximeter with the probe placed on the tongue.

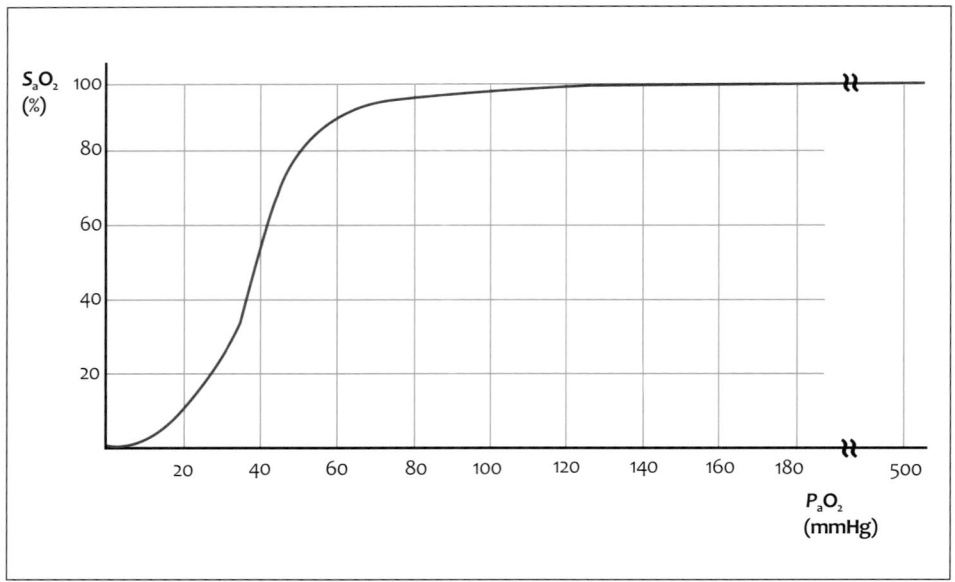

21.61 Oxyhaemoglobin dissociation curve. PaO_2 = arterial oxygen tension; SaO_2 = arterial haemoglobin saturation with oxygen.

- The probe squashing the tissue and preventing pulsatile blood flow
- Abnormal haemoglobin, i.e. carboxyhaemoglobin or methaemoglobin
- Intravenous dyes
- Patient movement (shivering)
- Vasoconstriction (e.g. when using alpha-2 agonists (this is a very common problem, which can often be rectified by doubling/folding the tongue))
- Interference from ambient light
- Skin pigmentation
- Electrosurgical equipment (e.g. diathermy).

Pulse oximeters usually display a pulse rate; the accuracy of this should always be confirmed by pulse palpation. Some oximeters also provide photoplethysmography; the presence of a normal waveform helps to confirm that the reading is correct. The waveform should look like a direct blood pressure trace, as shown in Figure 21.62.

The specifications of pulse oximeters should be read carefully before they are purchased, to ensure that the model selected has the capability to provide accurate readings in a wide range of species.

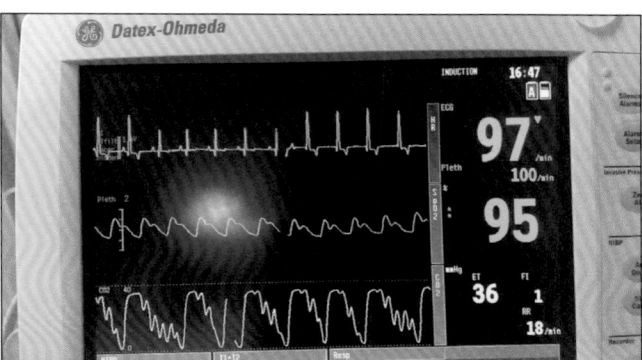

21.62 A screen shot from a multi-parameter monitor. The top line shows the ECG trace (in green) while the middle line shows the plethysmograph trace (in blue). The heart rate and SpO_2 are shown to the right of the screen in green and blue respectively. The heart rate counted from the ECG is 97 beats / minute, while the heart rate counted from the plethysmograph trace is also shown in blue and counted at 100 beats/minute. This slight discrepancy is due to differences in the time period over which the different traces are averaged to calculate heart rate. The lower trace (shown in white) is the capnograph, with the end tidal CO_2 displayed as 36 mmHg and the respiratory rate as 18 breaths/minute.

Blood pressure measurement

Blood pressure measurement provides information about cardiovascular function and is an indirect measure of cardiac output and tissue blood flow.

Blood pressure = cardiac output x total peripheral resistance

It is important to avoid hypotension (mean blood pressure <60 mmHg) as it can have both short-term and long-term physiological effects (Figure 21.63).

Two different techniques are used to measure arterial blood pressure: direct (invasive) (Figure 21.64) and indirect (non-invasive) (Figure 21.65). The relative advantages and disadvantages of direct and indirect blood pressure monitoring are listed in Figure 21.66. In cats and dogs, the decision to use a direct or indirect technique depends on the equipment available, the health status of the patient and the reason for

anaesthesia. For indirect techniques, selection of cuff size is important. The cuff width should be approximately 40% of the circumference of the limb (Figure 21.65c). A cuff that is too wide will artificially lower blood pressure; a cuff that is too narrow will artificially raise blood pressure.

Short-term effects

- Accumulation of lactic acid, leading to metabolic acidosis
- Increased oxygen demand
- Increased glucose demand
- Increased cardiac work

Long-term effects

- Ischaemic tissue damage, leading to organ damage (e.g. renal failure)

21.63 Short- and long-term effects of hypotension.

Blood pressure terminology

- Peripheral vascular resistance – the resistance to blood flow created by the systemic vasculature. This increases in vasoconstriction (e.g. after an alpha-2-agonist has been administered) and decreases during vasodilation (e.g. shock and drugs (e.g. volatile agents) used during anaesthesia)
- Systolic blood pressure is the peak pressure within the arteries that occurs towards the end of the cardiac cycle, when the ventricles are contracting. It is determined by a combination of peripheral vascular resistance, stroke volume and intravascular volume. The normal range for cats and dogs is 90–120 mmHg
- Diastolic blood pressure is the minimum pressure within the arteries that occurs towards the beginning of the cardiac cycle. This is when the ventricles are filled with blood and is predominantly determined by the peripheral vascular resistance. The normal range for cats and dogs is 55–90 mmHg
- Mean blood pressure is the average arterial blood pressure during a cardiac cycle. This provides information about tissue perfusion. The normal range for cats and dogs is 60–85 mmHg. It is important to maintain a mean blood pressure >60 mmHg to ensure adequate organ perfusion

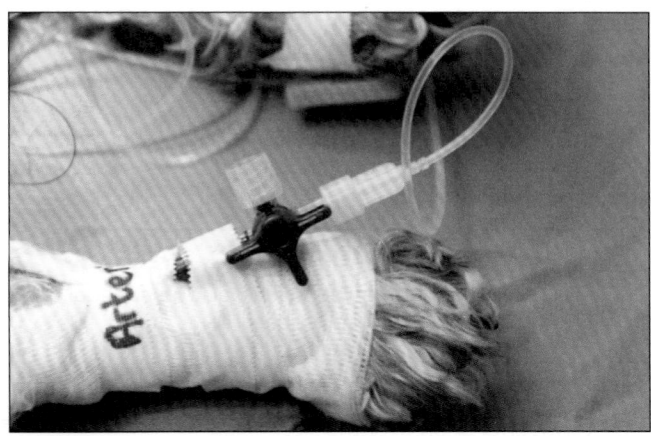

21.64 Arterial catheter placed in the dorsal pedal artery and attached to non-compliant tubing and a blood pressure transducer.

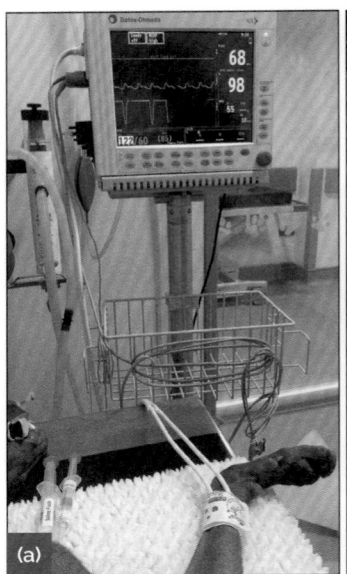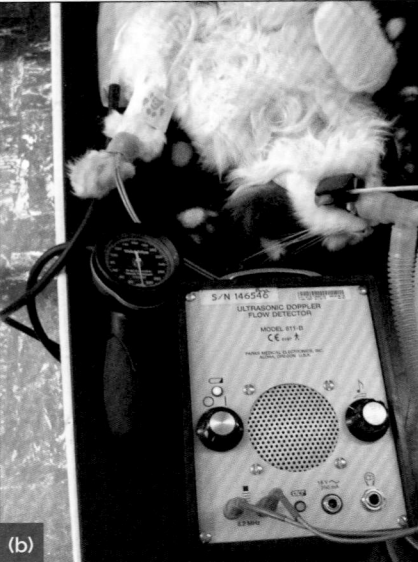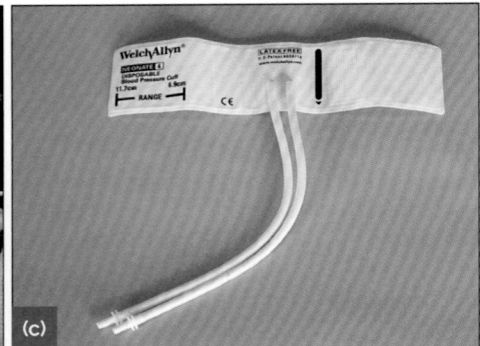

21.65 Indirect blood pressure monitoring techniques. **(a)** Oscillometric measurement in an anaesthetised dog. Cuff placed on forelimb just proximal to the carpus. Cuff attached to multiparameter monitor also performing capnography and pulse oximetry. **(b)** Doppler blood pressure monitor attached to an anaesthetised cat connected to a T-piece and pulse oximetry. Doppler probe is taped in place to aid repeat measurement. **(c)** The width of the cuff for oscillometric and Doppler measurement should be 40% of the circumference of the limb at the site of cuff placement. This cuff is for use with an oscillometric machine. The bold black line across the width is placed over the artery.

Technique	Notes	Advantages	Disadvantages
Direct arterial blood pressure measurement (Figure 21.64)	Electronic transducer converts signal into waveform and blood pressure. Transducer must be placed at level of right atrium and zeroed relative to atmospheric air before use	Gold standard method; most accurate. Gives beat-to-beat assessment. Useful for assessing cardiovascular consequences of a cardiac arrhythmia	Technically demanding: requires placement of arterial catheter (most commonly in dorsal pedal artery). Failure to place catheter correctly can result in haematoma. Risk of sepsis or infection if not placed aseptically
Indirect arterial blood pressure measurement: oscillometric technique (Figure 21.65a)	Uses same principle as Doppler technique but cuff is automatically inflated and deflated by the machine. Presence of pulsatile changes within cuff signals blood pressure	Non-invasive. Very simple to use. Automated and can be set to measure blood pressure every 3–5 min. Systolic, diastolic and mean blood pressure readings are measured or calculated	Less accurate than Doppler in small patients. Difficult to identify whether reading is accurate because process is automated
Indirect arterial blood pressure measurement: Doppler technique (Figure 21.65b)	Cuff placed around distal limb or tail and manually inflated to occlude blood flow. Pressure in cuff released until blood flow can just be detected by Doppler probe over peripheral artery. This is systolic blood pressure, read from a pressure manometer that measures the pressure in the cuff	Non-invasive. More accurate than oscillometric technique in smaller patients. Can be useful for monitoring blood flow in other situations, e.g. during CPR	Less accurate than direct measurement. Does not give continuous reading. Must be measured manually. Most accurate measurement is systolic blood pressure; diastolic pressure not reliable

21.66 Advantages and disadvantages of direct and indirect blood pressure monitoring.

Doppler ultrasonic probes can also be useful to provide an auditory monitor of heart rate and pulse quality in species where feeling pulse quality can be difficult, such as reptiles. The Doppler probe can be placed and secured over a peripheral artery.

Doppler technique

- Palpate the peripheral pulse (carpal, dorsal pedal or coccygeal) as distal as possible
- Clip the hair over the pulse
- Apply ultrasound coupling gel over the pulse and place the Doppler probe with the sound turned down and/or off over the site
- Switch the volume to appropriate level and locate the pulse →

Doppler technique *continued*

- Tape the probe in place
- Apply an appropriately sized cuff and sphygmomanometer
- Inflate the cuff until the pulse is no longer audible, then slowly deflate the cuff until the pulse becomes audible and then obtain a reading
- Deflate the cuff completely
- Repeat reading five times and calculate an average

The Doppler reading obtained equates to the systolic blood pressure in dogs but underestimates the systolic pressure in cats.

Oscillometric technique

This method involves using a monitor to inflate and deflate a blood pressure cuff, as well as detecting the pulsatile movement. The correct placement of the cuff is essential: if a system with a double lumen cuff is being used, then the cuff needs to be positioned with the pulse situated between the two limbs. If a single lumen cuff is being used, then the pulse should be situated directly beneath where the tube enters the cuff. It is also important that the cable connecting the patient to the monitor is resting upon a solid surface and not swinging in the air, as this will cause changes in pressure within the tubing and make it more difficult for the monitor to detect pulsatile movement. This technique provides a systolic, diastolic and mean blood pressure reading (see Figure 21.65a).

High definition oscillometry

High definition oscillometry (HDO) is the next generation of oscillometric blood pressure measurement. It differs from standard oscillometry by providing more rapid and sensitive measurements. HDO measures arterial wall oscillations produced by blood flow entering an artery. When fully inflated, the cuff totally occludes the artery, halting all arterial blood flow. A custom electronic valve under computer control provides for linear cuff deflation over a range of 5–300 mmHg. As the cuff pressure is decreased, blood re-enters the artery and induces characteristic flow-dependent arterial wall oscillations, which are detected by the cuff pressure transducer over a 20–30 second acquisition period.

The software HDO algorithm accurately discriminates between pressure waveform changes that are characteristic of systolic, diastolic and mean arterial pressures. Systole is defined by a unique waveform deflection that accompanies the onset of blood flow. Mean arterial pressure is measured directly and is defined as the period during programmed cuff deflation when individual pulse amplitudes plateau. End-diastole is detected as a characteristic change in the pulsatile blood flow signal. The machine can also be connected to a computer to provide a visual analysis of arterial compliance and/or elasticity and heart rhythm.

Electrocardiography

This is a non-invasive technique that provides information about the electrical activity of the heart (see also Chapter 18). It does not provide information about cardiac output (how well the heart is pumping) but does allow identification of arrhythmias and changes in heart electrical activity associated with other physiological abnormalities such as hypoxia, acid–base balance and electrolyte disturbances (see 'Anaesthetic emergencies', later). The clinical significance of an arrhythmia can be assessed by concurrent pulse palpation or blood pressure measurement, in order to investigate the effect of the rhythm disturbance on cardiac output. A normal electrocardiogram (ECG) trace recorded during anaesthesia in a dog is shown in Figure 21.62

ECG monitoring during anaesthesia uses three electrodes, of which there are two types:

- Crocodile clips that are directly clipped to skin and then sprayed with surgical spirit
- Electrode pads that are stuck to the patient's paws (preferred technique). The gel pad of the electrode should be placed on the footpad of the patient to ensure good contact between the electrode and the patient and reduce noise on the ECG.

Electrode connections in dogs and cats:

- Red: Right forelimb
- Yellow: Left forelimb
- Green: Left hindlimb.

Central venous pressure

Central venous pressure (CVP) measurement provides information about both the volume status of the patient and the ability of the right side of the heart to pump blood to the lungs. Monitoring of CVP is invasive, and placement of the jugular catheter requires skill. A long catheter is placed in the jugular vein so that its tip lies in the cranial vena cava (just past the level of the thoracic inlet). Several types of catheter are suitable, including Seldinger (Figure 21.67), peel-away and basic over-the-needle. If necessary, standard 20 G or 18 G catheters, as used for medium and large-breed dogs, can be used as jugular catheters in cats and small dogs. It is important that the site is prepared aseptically and the catheter placed using surgical gloves and a fenestrated drape. A large window should be clipped around the jugular vein extending cranial-caudally from the caudal edge of the mandible to the point of the shoulder and dorsoventrally from the midline to the 4–5 inches above the jugular groove. In most dogs it is usually easiest to position the animal in lateral recumbency with the neck slightly stretched. In cats and very small dogs either dorsal or lateral recumbency is acceptable depending on the preferences of the person placing the jugular catheter.

> **WARNING**
>
> Contraindications to placement of a jugular catheter include:
> - Sepsis
> - Blood clotting abnormalities

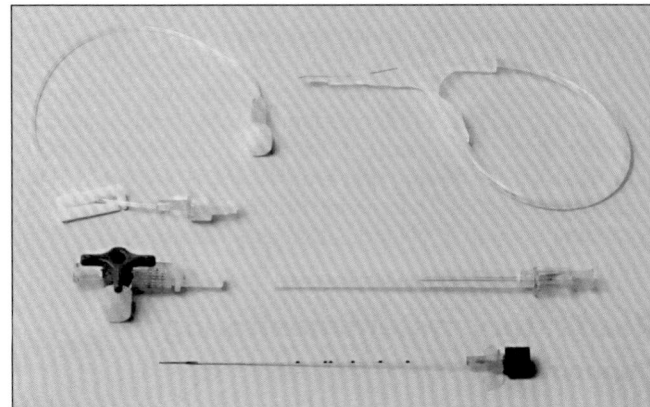

21.67 Central venous Seldinger catheter set, of suitable size for placement in a cat. The needle for jugular venous access has a green hub (middle right). The guidewire is coiled within the introducer device (top right). The catheter (bottom), three-way tap (middle left) and extension set (top left) are also shown.

- The catheter should be measured up against the neck of the patient to ensure it is an appropriate length, with the tip extending just past the point of the thoracic inlet.
- A sandbag can be placed under the point of the shoulder or neck to aid visualization of the jugular vein and to help prevent development of an air embolus.
- Attach the patient to an ECG machine, to monitor for possible electrical disturbances caused by either the guidewire or catheter irritating the myocardium. If an arrhythmia does occur, the catheter or guidewire should be withdrawn slightly.
- Using a Seldinger technique, a needle is used to gain access to the jugular vein. Once the needle is successfully in the vein, a guidewire is placed through the needle to a suitable depth to allow the jugular catheter to be threaded over the guidewire to the correct depth. The tip of the jugular catheter should be placed at a depth to ensure that it lies within the thoracic inlet. The proximal end of the guidewire is normally curved, with a J-tip, to prevent the sharp end of the wire from penetrating the wall of the jugular vein (see Chapter 20).
- Keeping the jugular catheter raised after placement until a bung has been inserted can reduce the risk of air embolus.
- The end of the catheter is attached either to a pressure transducer, which shows continuous readings, or to a water manometer or fluid column, which has to be read every few minutes. Measurement of CVP using a fluid column is relatively easy to perform using readily available equipment (Figure 21.68); this includes a bag of intravenous fluids (saline or Hartmann's solution), a giving set, a three-way-tap, open-ended tubing and a ruler. Manometer kits containing these components can be purchased relatively cheaply.

CVP can be measured in both awake and anaesthetized patients, although placement of a jugular catheter can be problematic in awake, unsedated animals. CVP measurement should be reserved for patients that will benefit:

- Patients that require aggressive fluid therapy – CVP can be used to guide fluid administration to maintain normovolaemia and ward off fluid overload
- Patients in which surgery is likely to cause marked blood loss and fluid replacement
- Patients with cardiovascular dysfunction that are at risk of fluid overload and pulmonary oedema.

The normal range for CVP in the cat and dog is 0–7 cmH_2O. If there is a sudden reduction in CVP this may indicate reduced cardiac output, reflecting decreased venous return to the right atrium. However, a low CVP is more usually indicative of reduced circulating blood volume due to hypovolaemia. A high CVP indicates either fluid overload or cardiac dysfunction.

Respiratory system monitoring

Capnometry

Capnometry involves the measurement of CO_2 concentration in inspired and expired gases and provides the anaesthetist with information about cardiovascular and respiratory function. To understand how this information is obtained it is important to understand the physiology of CO_2 transport in the body. Cells require oxygen and glucose for cell metabolism.

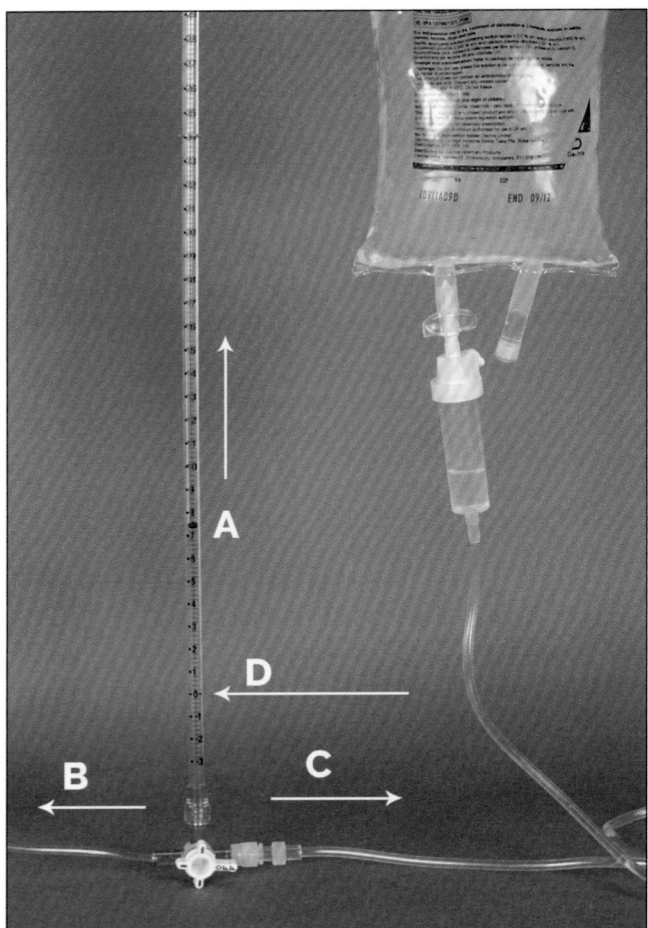

21.68 Measuring CVP using a fluid column. An open-ended section of drip line tubing is fixed in a straight vertical position (A). The red bobbin indicates the height of the water column above 0 cm (D, arrowed). A three-way tap is connected to the bottom of the tubing and also to the jugular catheter (B) and bag of fluid (C). The open-ended drip line is then positioned so that D is level with the animal's heart; this can be achieved by taping the tube to the wall of the kennel. Before measurement, the tubing is filled with fluid from C to a height of approximately 20 cm, using the three-way tap. The tap is then adjusted to the position shown. The height of the fluid column will fall until it is equivalent to the CVP of the animal. In this case CVP = +7.5 cmH_2O.

These are delivered to cells by arterial blood and require adequate tissue perfusion. Cell metabolism uses the oxygen and glucose to create energy, forming CO_2 as a by-product. The CO_2 is transported from the peripheral tissues to the lungs by the venous circulation; this process requires adequate venous return. In the lungs, gaseous exchange takes place and the patient breathes out the CO_2; this process requires adequate ventilation.

A typical capnograph is rectangular in shape, indicating a rapid increase in end-tidal CO_2 concentration ($ETCO_2$) as expired gases are breathed out, a plateau as alveolar gases are breathed out, and then a rapid decline indicating inspiration. $ETCO_2$ is the peak concentration measured by the monitor during expiration. It is typically the concentration measured at the end of the alveolar plateau. In a normal patient this should range between 35 and 45 mmHg (4.6–6 kPa or 5–6% depending on the units used by the monitor) (Figure 21.69a). Between breaths, CO_2 levels should be zero; however this does not occur if the patient is rebreathing (see above).

If the patient has an ETCO$_2$ greater than the reference range, it is described as being **hypercapnic**. This can indicate:

- Increased cardiac output and venous return
- Hypoventilation (Figure 21.69b)
- Increased metabolism (malignant hyperthermia or early sepsis)
- Rebreathing
- Laparoscopy due to absorption of CO$_2$ from the abdomen
- Exhausted CO$_2$ absorbent.

If the patient has an ETCO$_2$ lower than the reference range, it is described as being **hypocapnic**. This can indicate:

- Decreased cardiac output and venous return
- Hyperventilation
- Severe hypothermia
- Rapidly reducing CO$_2$ indicates a failing circulation (impending cardiac arrest)
- Partial airway obstruction (Figure 21.69c).

Absence of CO$_2$ can indicate:

- Apnoea
- Disconnection from the breathing system, with the capnograph attachment being left attached to the breathing system
- Cardiac arrest.

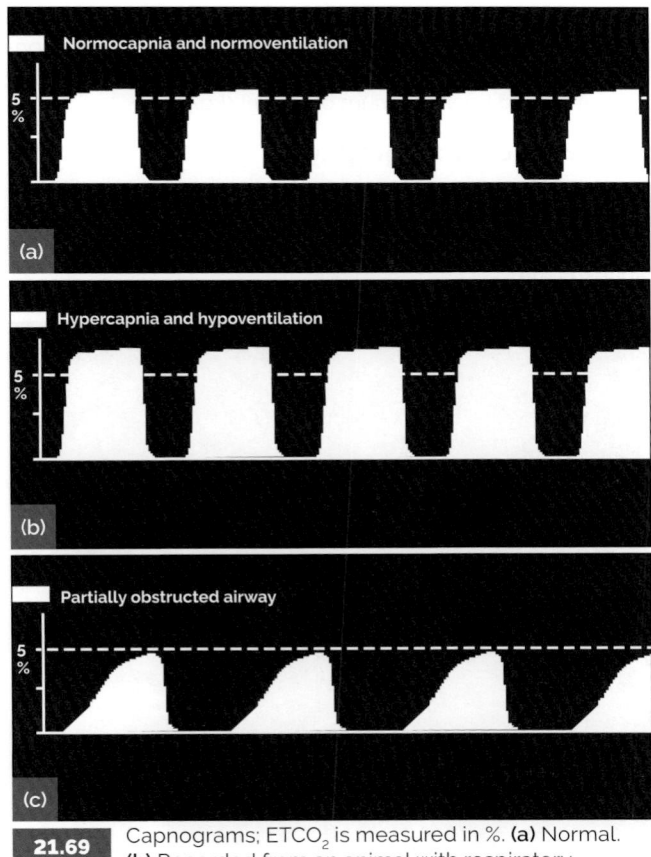

21.69 Capnograms; ETCO$_2$ is measured in %. **(a)** Normal. **(b)** Recorded from an animal with respiratory depression and hypoventilation: ETCO$_2$ is higher than normal. **(c)** Recorded from an animal with a partially obstructed airway. The rise in ETCO$_2$ is delayed due to airway obstruction.

Types of capnometer

- **Mainstream capnometry.** The measurement device is located in a small piece of tubing that connects between the endotracheal tube and the breathing system. This is ideal for measurement in small patients as the increase in dead space is limited and gas sampling is not required. However, the probes are expensive and vulnerable to damage. They can also become contaminated during oral or head and neck surgery. Side stream capnometers may also attach to a side port on heat moisture exchangers (HMEs); see Figure 21.29
- **Sidestream capnometry.** The gases are continually sampled from the respiratory system using a connector that sits between the endotracheal tube and breathing system. The gases are drawn away from the patient via a sample line, and taken to the analyser where measurement occurs. There is less risk of damage to the monitor because it is remote to the patient, but there is a time delay between gas sampling and read-out due to time required for gases to pass along the sampling line to the monitor. The sampling line can also become moist and contaminated with blood, which necessitates replacement of the line

Capnographs also provide additional information about respiration, including:

- Respiration rate
- Apnoea
- Evaluation of respiratory depression
- Inspiratory or expiratory obstruction
- Breathing system leaks.

Variations in the pattern of the capnogram are common during anaesthesia in cats and dogs. Common variations and their causes include:

- Cardiogenic oscillations: Cardiogenic oscillations shown during the expiratory plateau and the descending limb waveform occur as a result of movement of gases in the airway due to cardiac pulsations (Figure 21.70a)
- Lack of relaxation during controlled ventilation: The cleft in the alveolar plateau indicates that the patient is taking a spontaneous breath interspersed between breaths delivered by the ventilator. This pattern can also arise as a result of the surgeon pressing on the chest during expiration, changing the pattern of expired gases (Figure 21.70b)
- Oesophageal intubation: The extremely low ETCO$_2$ concentration at the beginning of the trace suggests that the ET tube has been placed in the oesophagus rather than in the trachea (Figure 21.70c)
- Sudden cessation of measured ETCO$_2$: This may indicate a number of different things in an anaesthetized patient. The most obvious cause is sudden apnoea; however, if the patient is obviously breathing, it is more likely to indicate an equipment fault or disconnection of the breathing circuit with the sampling line connected to the breathing circuit rather than the ET tube (Figure 21.70d).

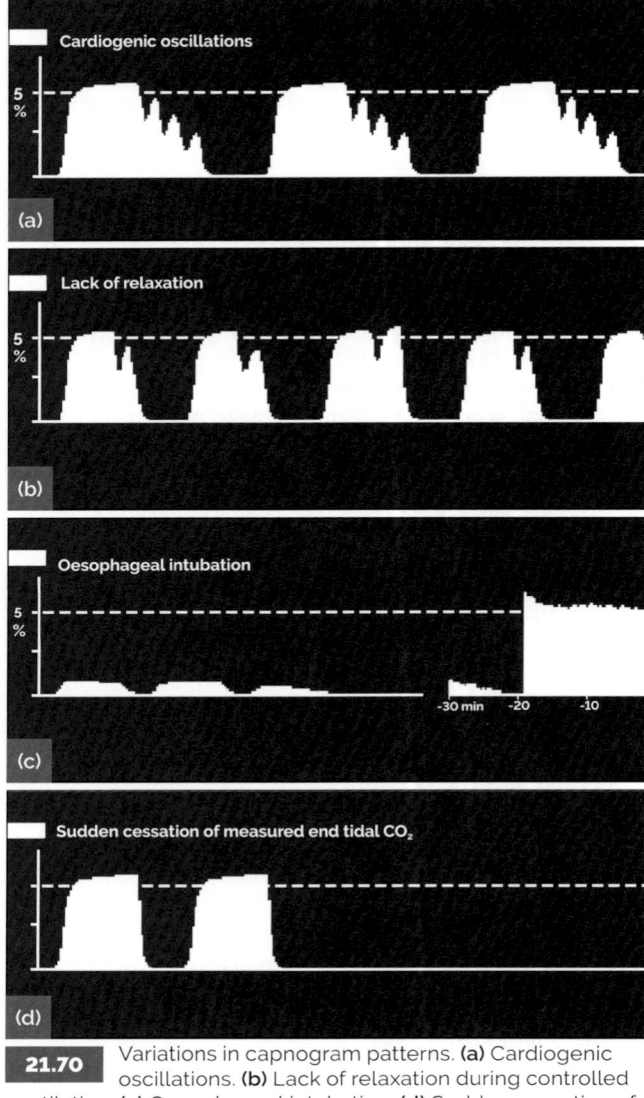

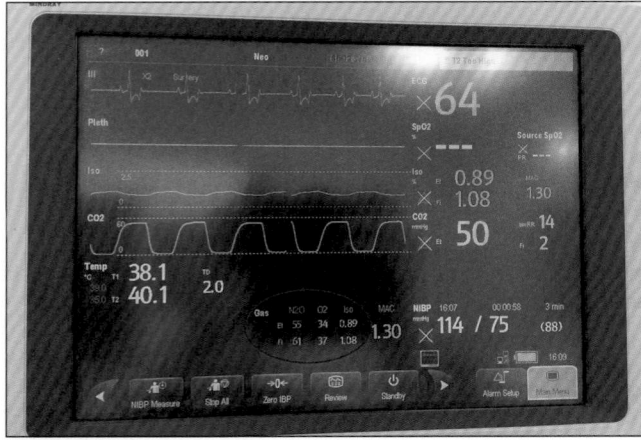

21.71 Multi-parameter monitor showing gas analysis. The expired (Et) and inspired (Fi) concentrations of isoflurane are shown graphically and numerically in pink at 0.89 and 1.08 respectively. The lowest trace is the capnogaph shown in yellow. End tidal (Et) CO_2 is 50 mmHg whilst the inspired CO_2 is 2 mmHg and the respiratory rate is also indicated at 14 breaths / minute. The inspired and expired concentrations of nitrous oxide, oxygen and isoflurane are also shown in the red circle, in this case the patient is breathing a mixture of oxygen and nitrous oxide. This information is useful when using a circle breathing system with nitrous oxide to confirm that you are delivering sufficient oxygen to the patient to prevent hypoxaemia.

21.70 Variations in capnogram patterns. **(a)** Cardiogenic oscillations. **(b)** Lack of relaxation during controlled ventilation. **(c)** Oesophageal intubation. **(d)** Sudden cessation of measured end tidal carbon dioxide.

Urine output

Urine output is easily measured and provides important information about renal function. It can be measured either by manual expression of the bladder, so that urine produced can be collected and the volume measured, or by placement of a urinary catheter connected to a closed collection system (Figure 21.72), so that urine production can be assessed continually and non-invasively in the perioperative period. Urine output should be a minimum of 1–2 ml/kg/h.

Electroencephalography

Electroencephalography (EEG) is not routinely used in clinical practice. It measures the electrical activity of the brain and thus is an alternative method for evaluating depth of anaesthesia.

Airway gas analysers

Airway gas analysers are often found in combination with capnographs. They provide information about the concentrations of different gases in the inhaled and exhaled gas mixture, e.g. O_2 and N_2O concentrations, along with the inhalational agent that is being used (Figure 21.71). End-tidal inhalant concentration, after a period of equilibration, is reflective of the concentration in the brain, and therefore can be useful in the assessment of depth of anaesthesia.

Other monitoring aids

Glucometer

Blood glucose can be monitored easily and cheaply using a hand-held glucometer (specific veterinary monitors are available (see Chapter 17)). Perioperative use can be invaluable. Blood glucose should be routinely monitored in patients at risk of hypoglycaemia; this includes those <3 months old, with hepatic insufficiency or with diabetes mellitus (see later). These patients have a reduced ability to regulate their blood glucose when conscious, and anaesthesia exacerbates this further.

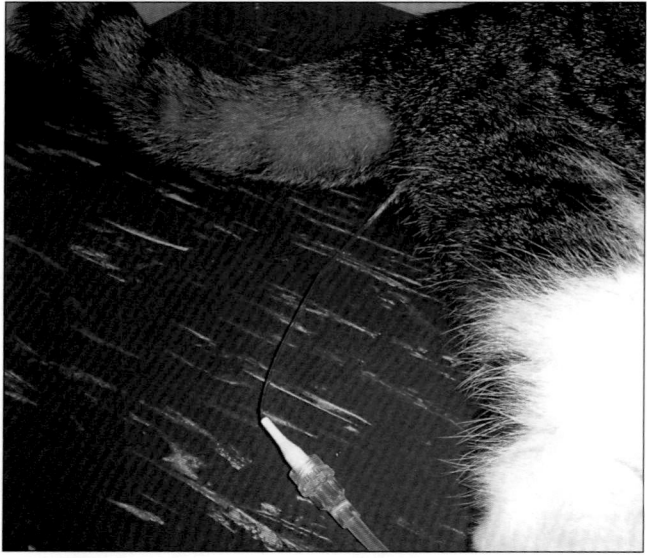

21.72 Closed collection system for monitoring urine output. The tube connects the urinary catheter to a syringe, which is initially air-filled.

Blood gas analysis

A blood gas analyser is used to measure blood pH, partial pressure of oxygen (P_aO_2) and partial pressure of carbon dioxide (P_aCO_2) in arterial (most commonly) or venous (P_vO_2, P_vCO_2) blood samples (Figure 21.73). It can also calculate bicarbonate levels, base excess, and saturation of haemoglobin with oxygen. These parameters provide accurate information about tissue oxygenation and respiratory gas exchange, and metabolic disturbances (e.g. metabolic acidosis). A sample of arterial blood is collected into a heparinized syringe, which can be quite challenging and painful for the patient unless an arterial catheter has been placed. During preparation of the site of arterial puncture using a needle stab, it is important to clip and prepare the site gently to avoid the artery going into spasm. Use of EMLA cream can reduce pain associated with sample collection in conscious animals.

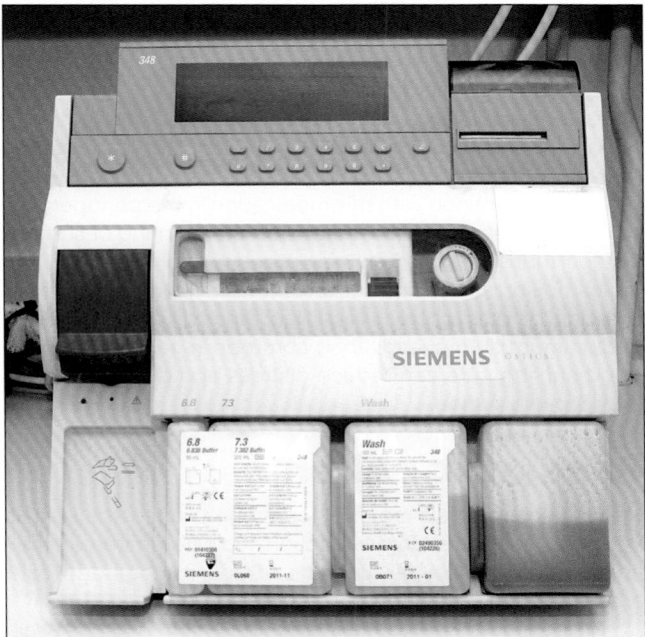

21.73 Blood gas analyser for measurement of blood oxygen and carbon dioxide. The red flap is lifted upwards in order to introduce the sample into the machine.

The anaesthetic recovery period

The recovery period is one of the most high-risk periods of anaesthesia. The Confidential Enquiry into Perioperative Fatalities (CEPSAF) in cats and dogs identified that 60% of anaesthesia-related deaths occurred during the first 3 hours of the recovery period, highlighting the vulnerability of animals during this time. Reasons for this may include:

- Unless a nurse can be dedicated to the recovery area, observation is usually poor
- Monitoring during the recovery period is usually reduced
- Anaesthetic support such as oxygen supplementation is usually withdrawn, whilst the cardiovascular and respiratory depressant effects of the drugs remain
- Body temperature is poorly monitored and heat provision withdrawn.

Extubation

- Dogs: Extubation should take place once the patient has regained the ability to swallow. The ET tube cuff should be kept inflated until just before extubation, as the patient will be unable to protect its own airway until this point. In brachycephalic patients, extubation should be performed as late as possible; this can be facilitated by the use of a role of cohesive bandaging material as a gag (Figure 21.74). Late extubation is also indicated in any patients who have a high risk of the presence of material in the oropharynx, larynx or oesophagus.
- Cats: Extubation should take place before the patient regains the ability to swallow due to the sensitivity of the larynx and the risk of laryngeal spasm. The correct time of extubation is often indicated by increased jaw tone, presence of a brisk palpebral reflex and an ear twitch when the hair is gently touched.

Once extubated, the patient should be assessed to ensure that it can protect its airway adequately. This involves: assessing mucous membrane colour for signs of hypoxaemia; using a pulse oximeter on the tongue (if the patient will tolerate this) or ear fold; monitoring respiratory rate and effort; and looking for signs of paradoxical breathing (asymmetrical chest movements or the chest expanding less rather than more on inspiration).

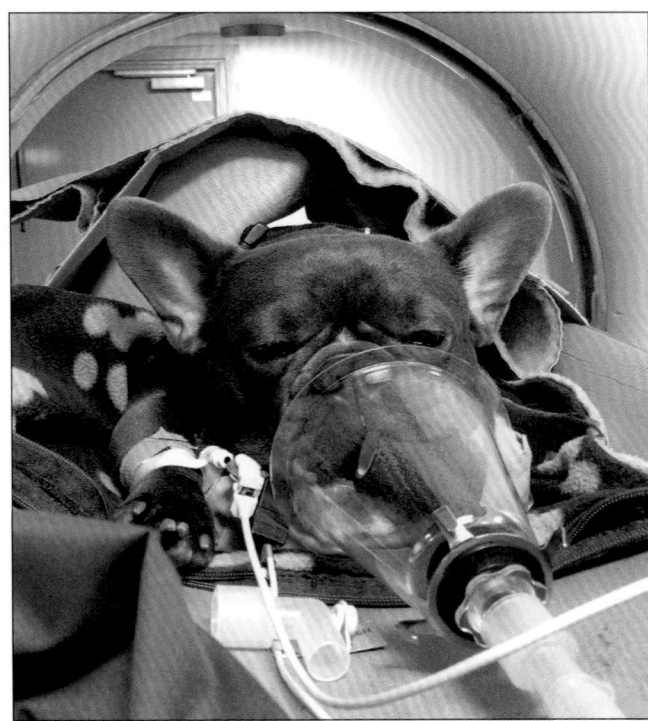

21.74 Use of a cohesive bandage in a sedated brachycephalic patient as a mouth gag. This patient was not intubated but illustrates the use of a cohesive bandage to maintain a patent airway in a patient at risk of respiratory obstruction. The dog was sedated for CT investigation and monitored by pulse oximetry (there are two pulse oximeter probes placed on the tongue in this patient); supplementary oxygen was also being delivered by face mask to prevent hypoxaemia. Note that the head and tongue have been extended and eyes lubricated.

The recovery area

The recovery area for small animals should be:

- Warm (use of a paediatric incubator is ideal)
- Well ventilated (to remove the anaesthetic gases being exhaled by the patient)
- Quiet
- Easily visible from main work area, so that help can be quickly obtained
- Provided with an oxygen supply (either pipeline oxygen from the wall or a dedicated anaesthesia machine with an oxygen cylinder)
- Equipped with accessible power points to allow warming devices and equipment to be plugged in
- Well covered with padded bedding (ideally acrylic fleece bedding so that if the patient urinates it is drawn away from the patient)
- Minimally stressful.

Careful positioning of the patient in the recovery period is important. Generally lateral recumbency is acceptable for most patients unless there is respiratory compromise (e.g. brachycephalic breeds, obese animals or animals with respiratory disease), in which case respiration is usually better supported by placing the patient in sternal recumbency. Make sure that patients in lateral recumbency are placed with their heads facing out of the kennel/cage (legs facing towards the front of the kennel) so that observation of the patient is maximized. Similarly, patients in sternal recumbency should face the front of the kennel/cage. The neck and head should be gently extended and the tongue pulled forward out of the mouth in patients that are still intubated and immobile as this reduces the risk of respiratory obstruction.

The patient's body should also be covered by warm bedding to prevent any further heat loss and to correct any hypothermia. Incubators can be useful for small patients as they provide a warm environment, allow oxygen supplementation and are usually transparent, which enables easy observation of the patient. When patients are placed in an incubator, it is important that their eyes are lubricated frequently with a topical lubricant to prevent corneal drying.

Monitoring during the recovery period

Patients should be closely observed for signs of postoperative complications, such as haemorrhage, with frequent assessment of vital parameters such as temperature, pulse rate and quality, respiratory rate, mucous membrane colour and CRT. Pain should also be assessed frequently. Water can be returned to the patient once it is able to move around the cage in a controlled manner.

The intravenous catheter should be removed once the animal is fully recovered from anaesthesia and there is no further requirement for intravenous fluid therapy. In some cases, it is useful to maintain intravenous access for a longer period; for example:

- In high risk patients for which further intervention might be required (e.g. unexpected fluid support)
- In patients for which intravenous access is required for drug administration, e.g. to allow postoperative analgesia with intravenous opioids, therefore avoiding the need for painful intramuscular injections
- In patients at risk of seizures in recovery
- In patients at risk of airway complications in recovery.

Anaesthesia considerations for specific patient groups

Geriatric patients

It is difficult to define when an animal is geriatric. It depends on the species and breed, and there are no absolute values to define old age. It is more useful to classify animals as old depending on their clinical, rather than their chronological, age.

Geriatric animals do not have normal adult organ reserve function. Therefore, although they may appear to be clinically normal in a resting state prior to anaesthesia, they are less able to regulate organ function to maintain homeostasis in the face of stressors such as anaesthesia. Only drugs with minimal effects on the cardiovascular and respiratory systems should be given, and a balanced anaesthesia protocol should be used. Careful attention should be paid to monitoring during anaesthesia.

Geriatric patients have a high incidence of intercurrent disease. Careful history taking and clinical examination is important, and information must be obtained on current drug therapy. A veterinary surgeon should be consulted about whether to continue with this medication in the perioperative period or whether to stop therapy on the morning of surgery. Osteoarthritis is common, and care is therefore required when moving animals during anaesthesia to prevent an exacerbation of pain on recovery from anaesthesia. Confusion and delirium during recovery is common in geriatric patients; good nursing care can reduce distress and disorientation in the recovery period.

Paediatric patients

Very young animals are not commonly anaesthetized in veterinary practice. Organ function typically matures when animals are around 3–4 months of age in dogs and cats; animals younger than this can be considered paediatric.

Appropriately sized anaesthetic equipment must be available. The large body surface area to volume ratio predisposes young animals to hypothermia. Their body temperature must therefore be monitored and supported during anaesthesia.

Immature liver function results in prolonged metabolism of most anaesthetic agents. Short-acting agents should therefore be used, with a reliance on inhalational anaesthesia to avoid prolonged recovery. Immature renal function means that young animals are less able to regulate their fluid balance. Cardiac output is more dependent on heart rate than in adult animals; young animals therefore have a limited ability to respond to hypotension as they struggle to increase stroke volume. Paediatric patients also have a limited ability to regulate blood glucose concentration, predisposing them to hypoglycaemia during anaesthesia. Blood glucose concentration must therefore be monitored and supplemented intravenously if needed.

Brachycephalic patients

Major considerations relate to maintenance of the airway. The period prior to the induction of anaesthesia and intubation, and the recovery period following extubation (see above) pose the greatest risk. Animals must be closely monitored during these periods so that airway obstruction can be managed promptly.

- Intravenous access must be maintained with an intravenous catheter throughout the perioperative period so that rapid induction of anaesthesia and intubation is possible at all times.
- Pre-oxygenation is strongly advised to reduce the risk of hypoxaemia should the patient become apnoeic and intubation prove difficult.
- Animals should be extubated relatively late in the recovery period, when they are sufficiently awake to maintain a patent airway (see Figure 21.74).
- The equipment for intubation must be kept available close to the animal both prior to intubation and following extubation, and should include a short-acting intravenous induction agent (e.g. alfaxalone or propofol), a laryngoscope, and a selection of suitably sized ET tubes. Topical local anaesthetic should be available for brachycephalic cats.
- Excess sedation after premedication can lead to airway obstruction due to the soft tissues surrounding the larynx and soft palate.
- Stress can exacerbate respiratory compromise. Mild sedation while in the hospital environment may therefore be required.
- Hyperthermia is common in brachycephalic dogs, particularly when they are stressed. Management of body temperature may therefore be required.

Obese patients

- Long needles are required for intramuscular injection of drugs, to avoid injection into fat depots and unreliable drug absorption.
- Obese animals should be weighed, but drug dose based on estimated lean bodyweight rather than actual weight. Fat is metabolically relatively inactive and dosing on 'obese weight' can lead to drug overdose.
- Obese patients are at risk of airway compromise due to fatty tissue around the larynx. Ventilation is often compromised, particularly when animals are in dorsal recumbency.

Patients with cardiovascular disease

Cardiovascular disease is relatively common in cats and dogs and is not a contraindication to anaesthesia. However, this patient group requires careful evaluation before anaesthesia in order to obtain information about the severity of the disease. This allows the anaesthetic protocol to be tailored to meet the demands of the individual patient.

- Animals with cardiovascular disease are generally less able to maintain normal cardiac output and blood pressure during anaesthesia. Monitoring of the cardiovascular system is vital to allow appropriate supportive measures to be implemented. Patients must be monitored from the time of premedication through to the postoperative period. Induction of anaesthesia is a particularly critical time; depending on the nature of the underlying disease, ECG monitoring during induction of anaesthesia may be advisable.
- Oxygen supplementation is important for all patients, but will be of particular benefit for patients with cardiovascular disease. Supplemental oxygen should be provided, to pre-oxygenate patients before induction of anaesthesia.

- Exacerbation of stress is particularly problematical as it increases the circulating levels of catecholamines that can promote cardiac arrhythmias (see later); careful handling and judicious use of sedative drugs is required.
- When planning an anaesthesia protocol, it is important to consider the effect of the specific cardiovascular pathology on the function of the cardiovascular system and adjust drug administration accordingly. For example:
  - In dogs with mitral valve disease, bradycardia will increase the regurgitant fraction (into the left atrium) and reduce cardiac output; therefore, it is prudent to avoid the administration of alpha-2 adrenergic agonists in these cases
  - Cats with hypertrophic cardiomyopathy typically have a thickened left ventricular myocardium, which is associated with a reduced filling capacity of the left ventricle and a reduction in cardiac output. Therefore, heart rate is often increased to maintain sufficient systemic perfusion, which further reduces the time for cardiac filling and myocardial perfusion. Left ventricular outflow tract obstruction may also be present. In some cats with hypertrophic cardiomyopathy, premedication with a low dose of an alpha-2 adrenergic agonist may be a good choice; the alpha-2 agonist will reduce heart rate, thereby allowing more time for ventricular filling, and the reduction in heart rate is associated with a reduced myocardial oxygen demand, which is advantageous. A study also demonstrated reduced left ventricular outflow tract obstruction in cats with hypertrophic cardiomyopathy following the administration of medetomidine (Lamont et al., 2002).

Patients with renal disease

Chronic renal failure is common in geriatric cats. This is not a contraindication to anaesthesia but requires careful management of fluid therapy. It is recommended to assess haematology and serum biochemistry prior to anaesthesia to indicate the severity of renal disease and detect concurrent haematological and biochemical abnormalities. Considerations for acute and chronic renal failure are different.

Acute kidney injury

Acute kidney injury is associated with high plasma concentrations of urea and creatinine, which can cause myocardial depression and altered acid–base balance. Plasma potassium concentration is often raised, which has the potential to cause cardiac arrhythmias, particularly during anaesthesia. Stabilization of the patient prior to anaesthesia with appropriate fluid therapy is paramount, particularly with regard to normalization of plasma potassium concentration.

Chronic renal failure

Animals with chronic renal failure maintain their glomerular filtration rate and stable urea and creatinine plasma concentrations by drinking more and urinating more; anaesthesia disrupts this mechanism. Plasma potassium concentration is likely to be low; supplementation of potassium (orally or through fluid therapy) is therefore advisable before anaesthesia. The patient must be checked for normal hydration before induction of anaesthesia; it can be useful to start intravenous fluid therapy before induction of anaesthesia. Fluids should be provided intravenously throughout the perioperative period until the patient is able to regulate its own fluid balance through drinking. Blood pressure must be monitored and mean arterial pressure maintained at >60 mmHg in order to reduce the risk of renal ischaemia and a worsening of renal function postoperatively.

Patients with liver disease

Most anaesthetic drugs are metabolized by the liver; hepatic disease will therefore slow drug metabolism, with the potential for drug accumulation and a prolonged recovery period. In patients with known liver disease appropriate pre-anaesthetic blood samples should be run to detect the magnitude of liver dysfunction. Short-acting agents should be used where possible, with reliance on an inhalational agent for maintenance of anaesthesia. NSAIDs should be used judiciously; they have the potential to accumulate, leading to side effects in animals with reduced liver function, and may cause a further deterioration in liver function.

Patients undergoing Caesarean operation

Anaesthetic considerations for a Caesarean operation must include both the dam and the offspring. The following principles apply for all small mammals.

- Drugs that cross the blood–brain barrier to cause anaesthesia in the dam will also cross the placental barrier and affect the offspring. Premedication with an opioid drug is usually sufficient to provide sedation prior to induction of anaesthesia. Short-acting drugs should be used for induction of anaesthesia and inhalational agents for maintenance. Further administration of opioids should be restricted until the offspring have been removed from the uterus. There are some data that indicate that puppy vitality is improved after induction of anaesthesia with alfaxalone compared with propofol.
- Placing a pregnant dam on her back can compromise venous return to the heart and ventilation. Therefore, it is advisable to clip and prep the dam in lateral recumbency to reduce the duration of this compromise. The cardiovascular and respiratory systems must be monitored carefully; IPPV is likely to be necessary until the offspring are removed.
- Equipment needed for resuscitation of the offspring should be prepared. This should include: suction to clear the airway; towels to rub the offspring, to dry them and stimulate breathing; a warm environment in which to maintain the offspring until the dam is recovered from anaesthesia; and equipment for providing oxygen support (an oxygen tent is ideal).
- Veterinary nurses should be prepared to give the offspring a drop of naloxone under the tongue if they show signs of respiratory depression resulting from administration of opioids to the dam.
- If alpha-2 agonists have been administered to the dam as part of the anaesthetic protocol, the effects of the drug can be reversed in the offspring by administering a drop of atipamezole under the tongue.
- The dam must have sufficiently recovered from anaesthesia before she is placed with the offspring. She must then be monitored carefully so that she does not squash or otherwise injure the neonates if not sufficiently aware.
- Administering a 'line block' along the midline incision by injection of bupivacaine intramuscularly probably reduces postoperative pain, whilst avoiding systemic effects on the offspring.

Patients with raised intracranial pressure

- If possible, raised intracranial pressure (ICP) should be managed, using diuretic agents such as furosemide and mannitol, before induction of anaesthesia. Further exacerbation of raised ICP during anaesthesia can be prevented by ensuring that there is no obstruction to venous drainage from the head (e.g. placement of a jugular catheter should be avoided and the head and neck raised following induction).
- Coughing should be avoided during intubation as this will acutely exacerbate ICP.
- Administration of drugs that may elicit vomiting must be avoided, as vomiting will also raise ICP.
- An elevation in $ETCO_2$ must be prevented as this will promote vasodilation of blood vessels and therefore raise ICP. This usually necessitates IPPV to maintain the $ETCO_2$ around 33–35 mmHg.
- Generally, fluid replacement with 0.9% saline is preferred to other crystalloid solutions during anaesthesia because it is slightly more hypertonic than plasma and administration is therefore less likely to promote further increases in ICP.
- The patient must be closely observed throughout recovery so that seizures can be identified and managed promptly.
- Ventilatory support must not be withdrawn until the patient's breathing is adequate and it is able to maintain normal $ETCO_2$. This can be monitored using capnography prior to extubation. The sampling line of the capnometer can be attached to a catheter and placed up a nostril to continue monitoring CO_2 concentration after extubation.
- Care must be taken to avoid the patient coughing during extubation as this will raise ICP.
- Measures to reduce ICP must be adopted. These include gentle elevation of the head (a triangular cushion can be useful to place under the head and neck). The neck should be stretched, to prevent obstruction of venous drainage from the head and to maintain normal $ETCO_2$.
- Intravenous access must be maintained until approximately 12 hours after the animal is completely recovered from anaesthesia, to ensure that access can be rapidly achieved in the event of seizures.

Patients with diabetes mellitus

Management of blood glucose concentration is the most important consideration when anaesthetizing patients with diabetes mellitus. Low blood glucose will not be signalled by the onset of clinical signs (changes in mentation, loss of consciousness, seizure activity) in anaesthetized patients; detection and prevention of hypoglycaemia is therefore paramount. Hyperglycaemia is also associated with adverse effects in human patients and tight regulation of blood glucose within narrow limits is recommended; however, in veterinary practice, prevention of hyperglycaemia is currently perceived to be less important than prevention of hypoglycaemia.

For stable diabetic patients managed with insulin, the general recommendation is to advise the owner not to feed their pet on the morning of anaesthesia and to give their pet half their normal insulin dose before anaesthesia at the normal time. This is to prevent hypoglycaemia following insulin administration in patients that have been starved. This recommendation is not supported by clinical evidence, however.

- Premedication with alpha-2 adrenergic agents should be avoided as this class of drugs will result in an elevation of blood glucose. Surgery and anaesthesia alone will result in a destabilization of blood glucose concentration, and therefore administration of drugs with a specific effect on blood glucose regulation should be avoided.
- Following premedication, a blood sample should be taken for measurement of a baseline blood glucose concentration. If the patient is already hypoglycaemic (blood glucose <3.3 mmol/l) then intravenous glucose supplementation should be initiated.
- Blood glucose concentration should be monitored throughout anaesthesia and glucose supplementation initiated if required.
- Glucose is irritant when administered in high concentrations intravenously. Glucose solutions should therefore be diluted with saline or water for injection to 10–20% for administration via a peripheral vein. Glucose supplementation is more effective when a loading dose is given followed by a continuous rate infusion; administration of repeated bolus doses is inefficient and leads to peaks and troughs. The dose of the infusion can be adjusted according to the sequential results following monitoring of blood glucose concentration.
- On recovery from anaesthesia, blood glucose concentration usually returns to within normal limits, or hyperglycaemia develops. A small meal should be given as soon as the patient is awake enough to eat and blood glucose should be monitored every 2–6 hours until the following morning to confirm that the patient is normoglycaemic.
- One method of managing insulin administration before surgery is to give no insulin if the blood glucose is below 8 mmol/l, give a half dose of insulin if the blood glucose is between 8 and 15 mmol/l and to give a full dose of insulin if the blood glucose is >15 mmol/l. Returning the patient to its normal insulin and feeding regimen after surgery (e.g. the following day) is a key goal in these patients.

Anaesthetic emergencies

Commonly occurring anaesthetic emergencies usually involve disturbances in respiratory or cardiovascular system function.

Respiratory emergencies

Apnoea

Cessation of respiration (apnoea) is common during anaesthesia and can easily be recognized by an absence of chest movements, cessation of breathing bag movements and an absence of expired CO_2 (if respiratory function is being monitored using capnography). Apnoea will result in a fall in haemoglobin saturation with oxygen, although changes in O_2 saturation are likely to take a few minutes to occur in animals that have previously been breathing 100% O_2. The

consequences of unmanaged apnoea are hypoxaemia and hypercapnia – potentially life-threatening.

Apnoea can be managed easily by instigating manual or automatic IPPV; however, at the same time as treating apnoea it is important to establish and manage the underlying cause. The most common reason for apnoea is an excessive depth of anaesthesia relative to surgical stimulation; therefore, one of the first things to check is depth of anaesthesia. Other common causes of apnoea are given earlier in this chapter – see 'Monitoring of the respiratory system'.

Hypoventilation

Hypoventilation (inadequate ventilation) is very common during anaesthesia but can be difficult to assess by visual appraisal of chest movements alone. It is most easily diagnosed using capnography, where it will cause an elevation of $ETCO_2$. Hypoventilation does not usually result in hypoxaemia (unless very severe), but prolonged elevations in CO_2 can result in disturbances in acid–base balance, leading to respiratory acidosis. A severe acidosis may result in reduced myocardial function, leading to hypotension and reduced enzyme activity. Hypoventilation can be managed by supporting respiratory function by manual or automatic IPPV; however, it is also important to establish and manage the underlying cause. An excessive depth of anaesthesia is probably the most common reason for hypoventilation. Other common causes include body position (e.g. an overweight dog placed in dorsal recumbency) or administration of potent opioid drugs.

Cardiovascular emergencies

Bradycardia

Ultimately, a severe reduction in heart rate (bradycardia) will reduce cardiac output, due to the relation between heart rate, stroke volume and cardiac output. However, deciding the level at which bradycardia becomes clinically significant and requires management can be difficult. It is important to consider the preoperative heart rate, the species and breed, and the rate of reduction in heart rate; sudden changes may be more clinically significant than a gradual decline. Evaluation of blood pressure and the ECG can help in decision-making: hypotension or the presence of a second- or third-degree AV block indicates that the bradycardia should be managed and heart rate increased. A common cause of bradycardia is an excessive depth of anaesthesia; therefore, it is important to check that anaesthesia depth is appropriate for the surgical procedure and to reduce anaesthetic depth by lowering the delivered concentration of inhalant agent if appropriate. Other common causes of bradycardia include the administration of potent opioids (which cause bradycardia by stimulation of the vagal nerve) or direct stimulation of the vagal nerve due to surgery. Anticholinergics can be administered to increase the low heart rate caused by vagal stimulation.

Tachycardia

Inappropriately high heart rates (tachycardia) will ultimately reduce cardiac output due to inadequate time for cardiac filling between each beat, reducing stroke volume. Definition of tachycardia depends on the species, breed and preoperative heart rate but, in dogs, heart rates >180 bpm will usually reduce cardiac output and have the potential to cause hypotension and hypoxia. Before managing a tachycardia, it is important to establish the underlying cause. Inadequate depth of anaesthesia is an important cause of tachycardia; it is therefore important to evaluate depth of anaesthesia relative to level of surgical stimulation. The tachycardia may also be an appropriate compensatory response to hypotension and may be critical to preventing hypoxia and hypotension in the anaesthetized patient, in which case reducing heart rate may be inappropriate. This should be discussed with the veterinary surgeon in order to establish whether management of the tachycardia is appropriate for the particular patient. There is also a danger that tachycardia can promote cardiac arrhythmias due to myocardial hypoxia or the running of one ECG PQRS complex on to the next, in which case treatment to reduce heart rate is indicated. Pharmacological strategies to reduce heart rate include increasing depth of anaesthesia by the provision of analgesia or hypnosis, or administration of potent opioids specifically to cause vagal stimulation. Short-term specific antagonists of cardiac beta-1 receptors, such as esmolol, can also be given intravenously in an emergency.

Cardiac arrhythmias

These are not uncommon during anaesthesia and can result from a multitude of reasons. Arrhythmias are usually classified as either atrial or ventricular in origin. Ventricular arrhythmias are usually more insidious and include ventricular tachycardia or ventricular extra systoles. Although abnormalities in the electrical activity of the heart may be detected by feeling for changes in the pulse rate or rhythm, the precise nature of the electrical disturbance can only be diagnosed by analysing an ECG trace.

Ventricular tachycardia

Ventricular tachycardia can be recognized by the presence of an increased heart rate or pulse rate and, on the ECG, QRS complexes at a higher than normal rate, without an associated P wave. In order to assess the clinical significance and determine whether treatment is required, the following must be evaluated:

- Pulse rate or heart rate: More severe tachycardias will have a greater effect on cardiac output due to the reduction in time for ventricular filling, thereby reducing stroke volume. Higher ventricular rates are also more likely to result in one QRS complex running into the next, which can promote ventricular fibrillation
- QRS complexes: Ventricular arrhythmias can be defined as unifocal (a single source of abnormal electrical activity) or multifocal (multiple sources of abnormal electrical activity driving the tachycardia). With unifocal abnormalities all QRS complexes look similar, whereas with multifocal abnormalities the QRS complexes look different. Multifocal abnormalities are generally considered to be more insidious due to the increased risk of ventricular fibrillation developing
- Effect on cardiac output or pulse quality: Some ventricular tachycardias are relatively benign, having minimal effects on cardiac output and blood pressure. It is important to assess whether there is a pulse deficit (i.e. whether there is a pulse beat for every QRS complex) and to assess pulse quality. The presence of a pulse deficit or poor pulse quality indicates that the cardiovascular consequences of the arrhythmia are marked, warranting prompt treatment. The effect of a ventricular tachycardia can be more readily assessed if blood pressure is measured using a direct technique.

Direct arterial blood pressure monitoring allows blood pressure to be measured more accurately than an indirect technique or tactile assessment of pulse quality.

Treatment depends on the underlying cause, although this can be difficult to establish as ventricular tachycardia is commonly caused by myocardial hypoxia, which can develop for multiple reasons. Other common causes of ventricular tachycardia include splenic pathology (e.g. tumours of the spleen necessitating removal of the spleen) and gastric dilatation–volvulus syndrome (GDV). Ventricular tachycardia can be managed pharmacologically by the intravenous administration of lidocaine, which decreases automaticity in ventricular muscle.

Ventricular extra systoles

These can be recognized on an ECG by the presence of intermittent QRS complexes without an associated P wave, indicating that the contraction of the myocardium resulting in a heart beat is initiated and generated by contraction of the ventricle only. A P wave may be seen on the ECG but it is usually dissociated from the QRS complex. The clinical significance of ventricular extra systoles depends on their effect on cardiac output and whether the QRS complex generates ventricular contraction adequate to cause a pulse. Other factors to consider are: frequency, presence of a pulse deficit, hypotension and whether the extra systoles are multifocal or unifocal.

Common causes of ventricular extra systoles include myocardial hypoxia and severe bradycardia. Ventricular extra systoles represent escape beats where the intrinsic rate of electrical activity of the ventricles is faster than the intrinsic rate of electrical activity of the sinoatrial node. They can occasionally occur due to a severe bradycardia induced by the administration of an alpha-2 agonist. Management depends on the underlying cause. If the extra systoles result from a severe bradycardia, then management to increase heart rate is appropriate. Measures to improve myocardial oxygenation are required to correct myocardial hypoxia.

Atrial arrhythmias

The most common atrial arrhythmias are bradycardia and tachycardia, which are described earlier. Other common atrial arrhythmias are second- or third-degree AV blocks. This occurs when conduction of electrical activity through the atrioventricular (AV) node is slowed so that each P wave is not followed by a QRS complex. With a second-degree AV block there are some normal PQRS complexes and some P waves that are not conducted through the AV node. The pulse rate will feel irregular, as P waves alone will not result in ventricular activity and generation of a heart beat. A third-degree AV block occurs when no P waves are conducted through the AV node and there is complete dissociation between P waves and QRS complexes. Since no P waves are conducted through to the ventricle the intrinsic electrical activity of the ventricle takes over, generating QRS complexes that can be described as ventricular extra systoles or an escape rhythm. Usually each QRS complex is associated with a heart beat as they result in ventricular contraction. The pulse rate will feel irregular and pulse quality may be reduced.

Common causes of a second- or third-degree AV block include high vagal tone (which slows conduction through the AV node). This may be caused by drug administration (e.g. potent opioids or alpha-2 agonists) or by stimulation of the vagal nerve. Other causes of a severe bradycardia may also result in second- or third-degree AV block. Pharmacological management of an AV block involves administration of an anticholinergic such as atropine.

Hypotension

A low blood pressure is extremely common during anaesthesia due to the effects of anaesthetic drugs on the cardiovascular system to decrease cardiac output and cause vasodilation, combined with the potential for blood and other fluid losses. Although hypotension may be suspected from poor palpable pulse quality and the presence of an increased heart rate (as a compensatory response), it can only be identified definitively by measurement of blood pressure. Common causes of hypotension include excessive depth of anaesthesia, marked blood loss and inappropriate tachycardia or bradycardia.

Management of hypotension depends on the underlying cause. It is important first to check the depth of anaesthesia and adjust if appropriate. If the depth of anaesthesia seems correct for the surgical procedure, yet the patient requires a high concentration of inhalant agent to maintain anaesthesia, it is prudent to switch to a more balanced anaesthesia technique in order to reduce the concentration of inhalant required. Once the depth of anaesthesia has been managed appropriately, there are a number of pharmacological options to manage the hypotension.

A fluid bolus (5–10 ml /kg of a polyionic (containing a number of different ions, e.g. sodium, potassium, chloride, bicarbonate) crystalloid solution such as Hartmann's solution) can be an effective treatment for hypotension in patients that are hypovolaemic (e.g. due to blood loss during surgery). Care should be exercised in patients with concurrent cardiovascular disease to prevent the risk of fluid overload. Other drug options include the administration of ephedrine intravenously as a bolus. Ephedrine is an alpha- and beta-adrenergic agonist that also enhances the release of noradrenaline (norepinephrine) from the sympathetic nerve terminals and, therefore, serves to increase cardiac inotropy and heart rate, as well as provide vasoconstriction. It is a good first-line pharmacological treatment for hypotension in cats and dogs when using non-invasive blood pressure monitoring, particularly if the precise aetiology of the hypotension is unknown.

Other pharmacological options include the administration of vasopressors (e.g. in patients that have inappropriate vasodilation, such as in septic shock) or positive inotropes to increase myocardial contractility (e.g. in patients with poor systolic function). Vasopressors and positive inotropes are potent drugs that are given by continuous rate infusion and should, ideally, be reserved for patients where direct monitoring of arterial blood pressure is in place.

Hypoxia or hypoxaemia

Hypoxia is a failure of normal tissue oxygenation and hypoxaemia is a failure of normal blood oxygenation. Tissue or myocardial hypoxia is a common endpoint pathology, resulting from a multitude of derangements. It is a life-threatening condition and has the potential to cause cardiac arrhythmias or permanent damage to vital organs, resulting in a reduction in organ function on recovery from anaesthesia. However, it is difficult to detect clinically. A pulse oximeter will detect hypoxaemia, and should result in prompt action because hypoxaemia commonly leads to tissue or myocardial hypoxia.

When hypoxaemia is noted it is important to think about the multiple processes that could cause it. It is also important to quickly check that the pulse oximeter is reading accurately (see 'Pulse oximetry', above).

Actions to consider when hypoxaemia occurs

- Check that oxygen delivery via the anaesthetic breathing system is adequate. If <100% O_2 is being delivered, then switch to 100% O_2 administration
- Confirm that the oxygen being delivered to the patient by the breathing system is reaching the patient: Is the breathing system connected? Is the endotracheal tube blocked or kinked?
- Check that the patient is ventilating adequately: Is the patient apnoeic?
- Is the oxygen that is delivered to the lungs being delivered to the central organs and peripheral tissues: Is the animal hypotensive? Is cardiac output adequate?

Cardiopulmonary arrest

Cardiopulmonary arrest is relatively uncommon in anaesthetized patients in general veterinary practice; therefore, when it does occur it can be difficult to respond appropriately and rapidly due to lack of practice.

The techniques used in cardiopulmonary resuscitation (CPR) are described in Chapter 19 and CPR technique should be practised using a critical care model (Figure 21.75). It can be helpful to create arrest scenarios and practise how to manage them. Careful monitoring of the patient during anaesthesia will facilitate the detection of problems early and hopefully allow measures to be put in place to prevent a cardiopulmonary arrest from occurring.

The basic life support techniques described in Chapter 19 are generally applicable to anaesthetized patients. The Reassessment Campaign on Veterinary Resuscitation (RECOVER) (https://recoverinitiative.org) has produced algorithms for CPR and drug administration (Figures 21.76 and 21.77), which may be useful to have printed out in your practice for use in an emergency. The reader is referred to the RECOVER clinical guidelines for a useful summary of their recommendations (Fletcher *et al.*, 2012).

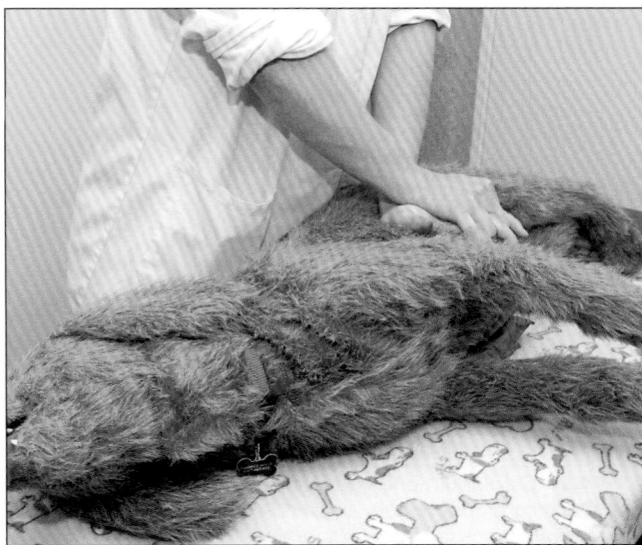

21.75 A critical care model that can be used for CPR training. This person is practicing cardiac massage using the thoracic pump technique.

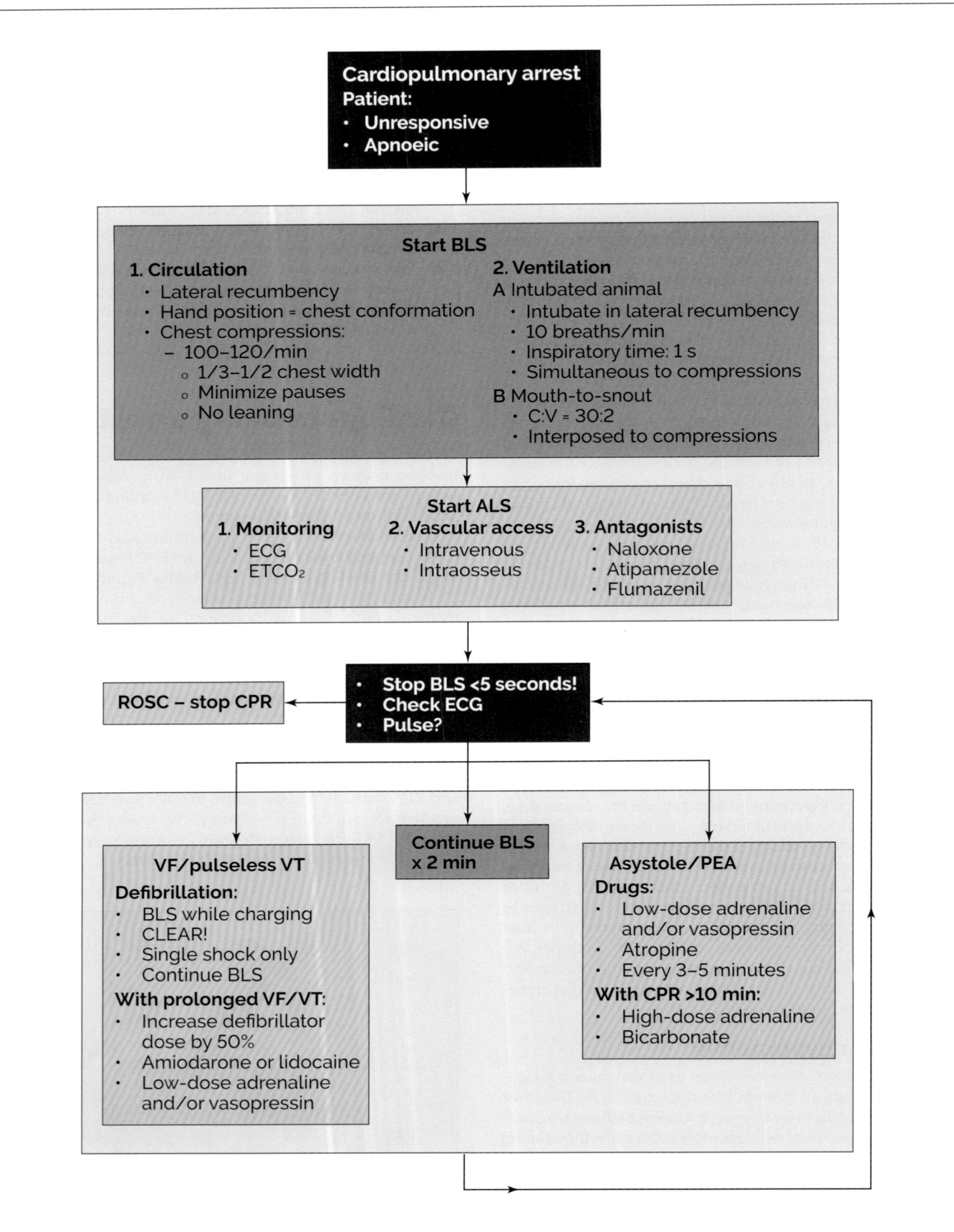

21.76 Cardiopulmonary resuscitation (CPR) algorithm. Basic life support (BLS) is started immediately after recognition of cardiopulmonary arrest (CPA), continued throughout the resuscitation effort and only interrupted every 2 minutes for short patient evaluations (electrocardiogram (ECG) and pulse). Advanced life support (ALS) measures occur whilst BLS is ongoing. C:V = compression:ventilation; ETCO₂ = end-tidal carbon dioxide; PEA = pulseless electrical activity; ROSC = return of spontaneous circulation; VF = ventricular fibrillation; VT = ventricular tachycardia. (Reproduced from the *BSAVA Manual of Canine and Feline Emergency and Critical Care, 3rd edn*).

		Weight (kg)	2.5	5	10	15	20	25	30	35	40	45	50
		Weight (lb)	5	10	20	30	40	50	60	70	80	90	100
	Drug	Dose	ml	ml	ml	ml	ml	ml	ml	ml	ml	ml	ml
Arrest	Epi Low (1:1000; 1 mg/ml) every other BLS cycle x3	0.01 mg/kg	0.03	0.05	0.1	0.15	0.2	0.25	0.3	0.35	0.4	0.45	0.5
	Epi High (1:1000; 1 mg/ml) for prolonged CPR	0.1 mg/kg	0.25	0.5	1	1.5	2	2.5	3	3.5	4	4.5	5
	Vasopressin (20 IU/ml)	0.8 IU/kg	0.1	0.2	0.4	0.6	0.8	1	1.2	1.4	1.6	1.8	2
	Atropine (0.54 mg/ml)	0.04 mg/kg	0.2	0.4	0.8	1.1	1.5	1.9	2.2	2.6	3	3.3	3.7
Antiarrhythmic	Amiodarone (50 mg/ml)	5 mg/kg	0.25	0.5	1	1.5	2	2.5	3	3.5	4	4.5	5
	Lidocaine (20 mg/ml)	2 mg/kg	0.25	0.5	1	1.5	2	2.5	3	3.5	4	4.5	5
Reversal	Naloxone (0.4 mg/ml)	0.04 mg/kg	0.25	0.5	1	1.5	2	2.5	3	3.5	4	4.5	5
	Flumazenil (0.1 mg/ml)	0.01 mg/kg	0.25	0.5	1	1.5	2	2.5	3	3.5	4	4.5	5
	Atipamezole (5 mg/ml)	100 µg/kg	0.06	0.1	0.2	0.3	0.4	0.5	0.6	0.7	0.8	0.9	1
Electrical defibrillation	External defib	4–6 J/kg	10	20	40	60	80	100	120	140	160	180	200
	Internal defib	0.5–1 J/kg	2	3	5	8	10	15	15	20	20	20	25

21.77 CPR drug dosing chart. Drugs are separated by indication and volumes are provided by bodyweight to reduce calculation errors. Defibrillator dosing is for a monophasic electrical defibrillator. BLS = basic life support; CPR = cardiopulmonary resuscitation; Epi = epinephrine (adrenaline). (Data from Fletcher *et al.*, 2012)

Advanced life support

This involves the administration of resuscitation drugs, the use of open chest massage and electrical defibrillation (if appropriate) as described in Chapter 19. Drugs used in advanced life support should be easily available (as a 'crash box') to all anaesthetists. ECG monitoring early in the resuscitation process will guide drug therapy and the requirement for defibrillation.

Death or euthanasia of anaesthetized patients and implications for carcass disposal

Anaesthetized animals may be euthanased by the veterinary surgeon as long as written consent for euthanasia has been obtained from the owner. It is normally expected that the veterinary surgeon will phone the owner to discuss euthanasia while the animal is still anaesthetized, especially if the recommendation for euthanasia is unexpected.

The most common means of achieving euthanasia under anaesthesia is with an overdose of pentobarbital. This can be administered intravenously to cats and dogs. If the patient is being monitored using ECG it is useful to note that the ECG may continue to appear normal despite the absence of any cardiac activity and the cessation of a peripheral pulse.

The owners of domestic pets (e.g. cats and dogs) are allowed to take their animal home, once euthanased, for burial. Other options for carcass disposal are cremation at registered premises with appropriate licensing. A post mortem, with appropriate consent, may be carried out on animals that die unexpectedly under anaesthesia.

Anaesthesia of small mammals and exotic pets

In general, the principles described above for dogs and cats should be adhered to for the management of anaesthesia in small mammals and exotic pets. The purpose of the following section is to highlight where differences occur from the management of dogs and cats.

Pre-anaesthetic considerations

Fasting prior to induction of anaesthesia

Rabbits

Rabbits do not need to be starved before anaesthesia as they are unable to regurgitate food. However, changes in diet during hospitalization should be avoided; it is therefore advisable to ask the owner to bring some of the animal's normal food to the surgery to ensure that a continued diet can be provided. This helps to reduce the risk of gut stasis and anorexia after anaesthesia and surgery.

Rodents

Rats and mice do not vomit during the induction of anaesthesia, so fasting is unnecessary. These animals also have very high metabolic rates, so unnecessary fasting may lead to a low blood glucose concentration and hypoglycaemia.

Guinea pigs

Guinea pigs do not vomit during induction, but food is very occasionally retained in the pharynx during anaesthesia. Guinea pigs may be starved for approximately 2 hours before induction of anaesthesia; more prolonged fasting carries the disadvantage of an increased likelihood of gastrointestinal disturbances after anaesthesia. A pair of atraumatic forceps and a light source should also be readily available at the time of induction so that any food in the pharynx can be carefully removed.

Birds and reptiles

Fasting of birds and reptiles is recommended before anaesthesia. For birds the period of starvation depends on the size of the animal. In birds less than 100 g bodyweight food should be removed for 30 minutes before anaesthesia to empty the crop; in birds between 100 and 300 g bodyweight food should be removed for 1 hour prior to anaesthesia; and in birds greater than 300 g bodyweight the fasting period should be 8–10 hours. Birds of prey should be fasted for 12 hours. Lizards should be fasted for 24 hours to allow live prey to be fully digested, snakes for 2 days and chelonians for 30 mins to 1 hour prior to the procedure. Birds and reptiles are able to regurgitate/vomit around the time of anaesthesia; intubation may reduce the risk of inhalation should this occur.

Weighing

It is useful to have small scales available in the practice (such as digital kitchen scales) that are suitable for weighing rats and mice and other small animals. This ensures that drugs can be dosed accurately based on bodyweight.

Sites for intravenous catheterization

Rabbits

The auricular vein is large in rabbits and the easiest means to achieve intravenous access in this species (Figure 21.78a). Care should be taken to distinguish between the auricular vein (which runs along the lateral aspect of the ear) and the auricular artery (which runs in the middle of the ear) to avoid inadvertent arterial catheterization (Figure 21.78b). The topical application of EMLA cream can be very useful prior to placement of an intravenous catheter in the marginal ear (auricular) vein. Placing a latex glove over the ear and securing it at the ear base can improve drug absorption and therefore effectiveness.

Small mammals

The lateral tail vein is large in rats and an easy site for placement of an intravenous catheter (Figure 21.79), although placement usually first necessitates induction of anaesthesia so that the rat is immobile.

The cephalic and lateral saphenous veins can be used in ferrets and guinea pigs.

Birds

The brachial vein, which can be found on the medial aspect of the wing, is a useful route for catheterization in birds (Figure 21.80). It is also important to remember that the jugular vein is a potential site for intravenous access, although this can be more difficult in conscious animals. The medial tarsal vein is a useful site for intravenous catheterization in larger birds (e.g. chickens, swans).

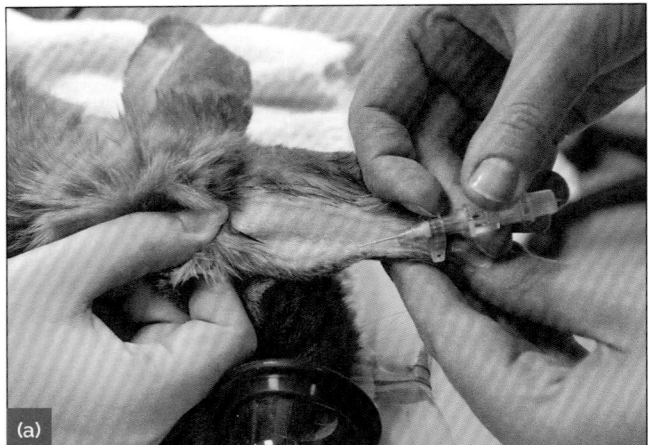
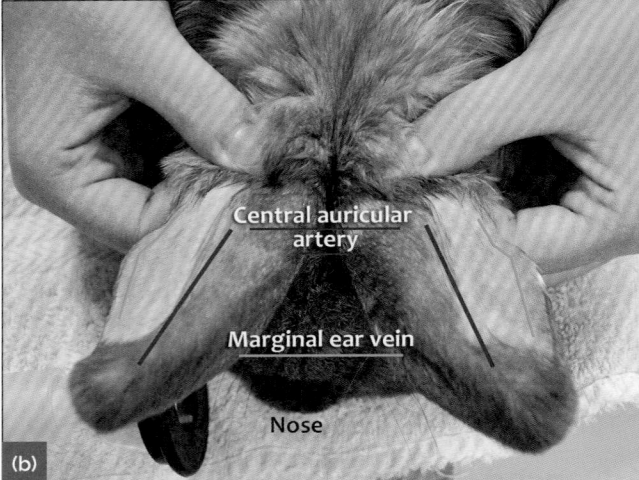

21.78 (a) Intravenous access in a rabbit using the auricular vein, ideally gloves should be worn. (b) Position of the auricular arteries and veins in a rabbit. (Reproduced from *BSAVA Manual of Wildlife Casualities, 2nd edn*)

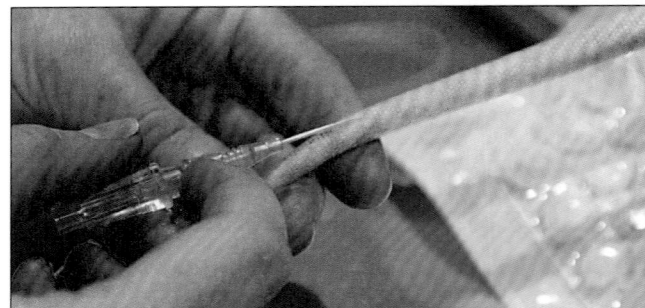

21.79 Catheterization of the lateral tail vein of a rat, ideally gloves should be worn.

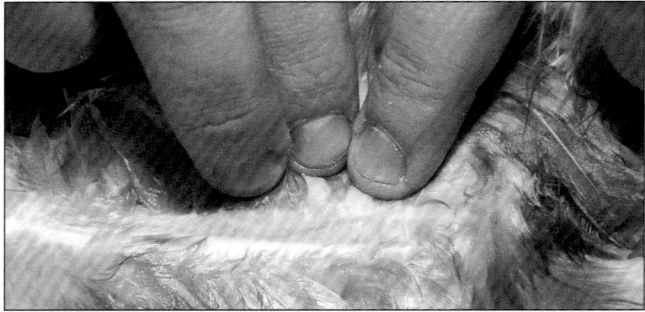

21.80 The brachial vein of a chicken. The medial aspect of the wing is shown, with the feathers dampened by surgical spirit to improve visibility of the vein. The vein is located just ventral to the fingertips.

Reptiles

Veins in reptiles can be difficult to access and are often only used for a bolus of fluids or injectable medication. Sedation or anaesthesia is often frequently for venous catheterisation. The ventral tail vein, palatine vein (in non-venomous species) and jugular veins can be used in snakes. The cephalic vein and jugular vein can be used in lizards. The jugular veins can be used in chelonia.

Assessment of pain

Pain-related behaviour

The effects of the veterinary environment on other pets such as small mammals, birds and reptiles are difficult to evaluate. It should be remembered that many of these animals use sensory systems that are different from those of cats and dogs and therefore they may be distressed by an environment that is appropriate for canine and feline patients. For example, rodents can hear very high frequency noises that humans are unable to detect and may find them distressing. Ideally, exotic species should be isolated from the main cat and dog ward areas and maintained in a quiet environment. Hospitalizing reptiles, rodents and birds in their home cage may reduce stress associated with transfer to a veterinary practice (see Chapter 14).

Rabbits

Rabbits are natural prey species and adept at hiding pain and discomfort. It is essential to remember that they find the veterinary environment particularly stressful and virtually all of the behaviours listed below could be caused by stress. Consequently, the hospitalization environment must be designed specifically to minimize stress, and the importance of this needs to be understood by the whole veterinary team.

A rabbit grimace scale (RbtGS) has been published for use in laboratory rabbits (Figure 21.81) considering orbital tightening, cheek flattening, nostril shape, whisker and ear shape and position, in association with pain. This scale can be useful in pet rabbits, but other changes in behaviour can also be recognized.

Rabbits with foot pain often stretch their legs out behind them; however, this can also be a sign that the rabbit is content and relaxed. This is a good example of how challenging pain assessment in rabbits can be.

Specific behaviours that may be exhibited by rabbits in pain

- Anorexia (potentially leading to gut stasis)
- Reduced drinking
- Hunched up or awkward/abnormal position
- Reduced movement around the cage (almost frozen in position)
- Reduced interaction with environment
- Reluctance to being handled
- Limping or change in gait
- Licking or rubbing at a painful area
- Sudden development of aggression
- Teeth grinding
- Squinting (orbital tightening, see RbtGS)
- Flattening of the cheeks (see RbtGS)
- Wrinkling of the nose (see RbtGS)
- Whiskers pushed away from the face (see RbtGS)
- Flattened and curled ear position (see RbtGS)

Rodents

Facial grimace scales as a means to quantify pain were first developed in mice (Mouse Grimace Scale, MGS; Figure 21.82) and rats (Rat Grimace Scale, RGS; Figure 21.83) and have now been reasonably well validated as a tool to assess pain in these species, as well as in rabbits (see above). The grimace scales consider the variation in facial features associated with pain in these species; closing of the eyes, wrinkling of the nose, bulging of the cheeks and the position of ears and whiskers. These scoring systems can be a very useful aid to quantifying pain in species where behavioural assessment of pain is particularly challenging. These scales are freely available from the NC3R's (National Centre for the Replacement, Refinement and Reduction of Animals in Research) website. A range of other clinical signs of pain, similar to those seen in rabbits (above) can also frequently identified, with careful observation, in pet rodents.

Pain management

Rabbits and rodents

The effects of drugs used in cats and dogs have been evaluated in rabbits, rats and mice, despite difficulties in assessing pain in these species and therefore the outcome of drug administration. It is recognized that opioids provide analgesia in these species, and buprenorphine is reported to be the most widely used opioid analgesic in laboratory small mammals. Buprenorphine has a wide margin of safety in these species, although the associated sedation may be disadvantageous in terms of prolonging recovery from anaesthesia in rabbits. It is therefore recommended to delay repeat doses of buprenorphine until rabbits are fully recovered from anaesthesia and awake. In rats, buprenorphine has been shown to cause pica (an appetite for non-nutritional objects), resulting in animals eating sawdust bedding with the potential to cause gastric obstruction. This can be overcome by using alternative bedding material. Buprenorphine is efficacious when given orally to rats in a 'jelly mixture' and dose rates are published for this technique in the laboratory animal literature.

NSAIDs are also very effective, although it is likely that doses to provide analgesia in rabbits and rodents are higher than in dogs and cats. Injectable carprofen has been shown to be effective given orally in a 'jelly mixture' to rats, avoiding the need for repeated injections. Oral meloxicam has been evaluated in rabbits, but further work is required to establish the optimum dose. Meloxicam is licensed for use in guinea pigs.

Ketamine and alpha-2 agonists are commonly used as part of anaesthetic protocols for rabbits and rodents, although their specific actions as analgesic agents rather than anaesthetic agents have not been evaluated.

Birds

The most challenging part of the provision of effective analgesia is the ability to recognize pain in this diverse group of animals. However, adoption of a precautionary approach is recommended so that analgesia is always provided after carrying out procedures that are likely to be painful in other species, or when birds are presented with pre-existing tissue trauma or injury.

Opioids are frequently used in birds but unfortunately inconsistent experiences and species-specific differences in studies have led to controversial opinions about their use,

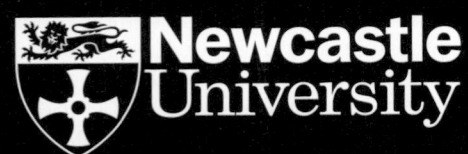

The Rabbit Grimace Scale

Research has demonstrated that changes in facial expression provide a means of assessing pain in rabbits.

The specific facial action units shown below comprise the Rabbit Grimace Scale. These action units increase in intensity in response to post-procedural pain and can form part of a clinical assessment alongside other validated indices of pain.

The action units should only be used in awake animals. Each animal should be observed for a short period of time to avoid scoring brief changes in facial expression that are unrelated to the animal's welfare.

	Action units		
	Not present "0"	Moderately present "1"	Obviously present "2"
Orbital tightening • Closing of the eyelid (narrowing of orbital area) • A wrinkle may be visible around the eye			
Cheek flattening • Flattening of the cheeks. When 'obviously present', cheeks have a sunken look. • The face becomes more angular and less rounded			
Nostril shape • Nostrils (nares) are drawn vertically forming a 'V' rather than 'U' shape • Nose tip is moved down towards the chin			
Whisker shape and position • Whiskers are pushed away from the face to 'stand on end' • Whiskers stiffen and lose their natural, downward curve • Whiskers increasingly point in the same direction. When 'obviously present', whiskers move downwards			
Ear shape and position • Ears become more tightly folded / curled (more cylindrical) in shape • Ears rotate from facing towards the source of sound to facing towards the hindquarters • Ears may be held closer to the back or sides of the body			

21.81 The Rabbit Grimace Scale. (Reproduced with permission of the NC3Rs; www.nc3rs.org.uk/grimacescales: Keating *et al.*, 2012; images provided by Dr Matthew Leach, Newcastle University)

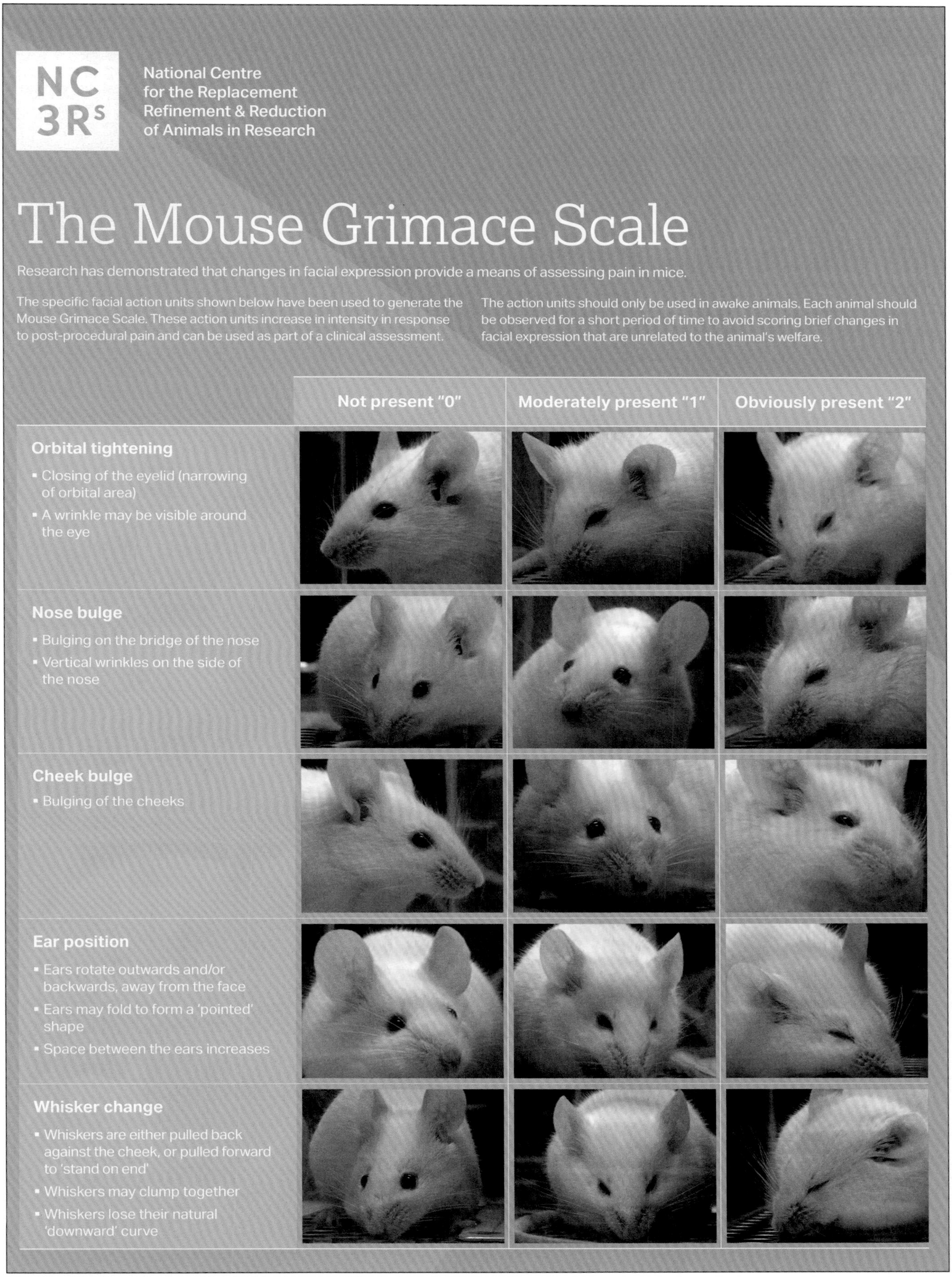

NC 3R^s

National Centre
for the Replacement
Refinement & Reduction
of Animals in Research

The Mouse Grimace Scale

Research has demonstrated that changes in facial expression provide a means of assessing pain in mice.

The specific facial action units shown below have been used to generate the Mouse Grimace Scale. These action units increase in intensity in response to post-procedural pain and can be used as part of a clinical assessment.

The action units should only be used in awake animals. Each animal should be observed for a short period of time to avoid scoring brief changes in facial expression that are unrelated to the animal's welfare.

	Not present "0"	Moderately present "1"	Obviously present "2"
Orbital tightening • Closing of the eyelid (narrowing of orbital area) • A wrinkle may be visible around the eye			
Nose bulge • Bulging on the bridge of the nose • Vertical wrinkles on the side of the nose			
Cheek bulge • Bulging of the cheeks			
Ear position • Ears rotate outwards and/or backwards, away from the face • Ears may fold to form a 'pointed' shape • Space between the ears increases			
Whisker change • Whiskers are either pulled back against the cheek, or pulled forward to 'stand on end' • Whiskers may clump together • Whiskers lose their natural 'downward' curve			

21.82 The Mouse Grimace Scale. (Reproduced with permission of the NC3Rs; www. nc3rs.org.uk/grimacescales: Sotocinal *et al.,* 2011; images provided by Dr Jeffrey Mogill, McGill University)

National Centre
for the Replacement
Refinement & Reduction
of Animals in Research

The Rat Grimace Scale

Research has demonstrated that changes in facial expression provide a means of assessing pain in rats.

The specific facial action units shown below have been used to generate the Rat Grimace Scale. These action units increase in intensity in response to post-procedural pain and can be used as part of a clinical assessment.

The action units should only be used in awake animals. Each animal should be observed for a short period of time to avoid scoring brief changes in facial expression that are unrelated to the animal's welfare.

	Not present "0"	Moderately present "1"	Obviously present "2"
Orbital tightening • Closing of the eyelid (narrowing of orbital area) • A wrinkle may be visible around the eye			
Nose/cheek flattening • Flattening and elongation of the bridge of the nose • Flattening of the cheeks (potentially sunken look)			
Ear changes • Ears curl inwards and are angled forward to form a 'pointed' shape • Space between the ears increases			
Whisker change • Whiskers stiffen and angle along the face • Whiskers may 'clump' together • Whiskers lose their natural 'downward' curve			

21.83 The Rat Grimace Scale. (Reproduced with permission of the NC3Rs; www.nc3rs.org.uk/grimacescales: Langford *et al.*, 2010; images provided by Dr Jeffrey Mogill, McGill University)

effects and doses. It has been suggested that in birds, the kappa opioid receptor is more important in providing analgesia, in contrast to mammals where the mu opioid receptor is predominantly associated with analgesia and the kappa opioid receptor plays a less significant role. The clinical significance of this is that butorphanol (predominantly a kappa agonist) might be more effective in birds than drugs that have a primary action at mu opioid receptors. Generally, butorphanol and buprenorphine are the most widely used opioids in birds; before using them for a particular clinical case it is important to research the literature regarding information for the particular bird species that requires analgesia.

NSAIDs have been widely used in birds but it is important to remember that doses for mammals may not be applicable to birds and side effects such as nephrotoxicity and gastric ulceration are common. This is unlikely to be a problem following administration of a single dose of a NSAID but should be considered for repeated administration.

Reptiles

Recognition of behaviours associated with pain is very difficult in reptiles, although a precautionary principle to the provision of analgesia should again be adopted. Opioids receptors are variable between these species and choice of drug should be made with reference to an appropriate text (e.g. Girling and Raiti, 2018) or exotics formulary (e.g. Meredith, 2015).

Induction of anaesthesia

Chamber induction technique

This technique is particularly useful for small mammals such as rats and mice (see Figure 21.21). Chamber induction should not be adopted for rabbits because they hold their breath when exposed to inhalant agents when conscious and this can lead to hypoxaemia. Chamber induction is also unsuitable for most birds, as flapping can lead to wing trauma; mask induction is preferable if gaseous agents are used. Chamber induction in reptiles is usually unsuccessful as a result of breath-holding. Sevoflurane is preferred over isoflurane for mask inductions in all species, because it is less noxious due to its sweet-smelling odour. Mask induction is also quicker with sevoflurane than isoflurane because it is less soluble in blood.

Mask induction technique

Clear face masks with a diaphragm can be used for the induction of anaesthesia in small animals and exotic pets that can easily be restrained, such as some birds and reptiles. The exception to this rule is ferrets. In the authors' experience, ferrets tend to prefer a black rubber face mask: they will often place their face within the mask of their own accord, due to it being dark. Once the ferret has positioned its face within the mask, it can be easily restrained for anaesthesia. Similarly to chamber induction, sevoflurane is preferred over isoflurane for induction of anaesthesia with a face mask. Reptiles have a strong capacity to breath-hold and mask or chamber inductions may be completely unsuccessful depending on the species. Many snakes and lizards can, however, be intubated conscious and IPPV then used for the induction of anaesthesia.

Intravenous induction

Intravenous induction of anaesthesia should ideally follow premedication with agents suitable for the species.

Premedication will reduce the dose of hypnotic agent required for the induction of anaesthesia and contribute to a balanced anaesthesia technique. Propofol and alfaxalone are suitable for the intravenous induction of anaesthesia in rabbits and ferrets, where intravenous catheterization following premedication is possible. It should be noted that alfaxalone is now licensed for induction of anaesthesia in rabbits. Propofol and alfaxalone can also be used intravenously for induction in reptiles and birds.

Intramuscular drugs for induction

Where intravenous access is difficult in exotic species drugs such as alfaxalone, or combinations of drugs such as medetomidine and ketamine, can be used via the intramuscular route at doses that produce anaesthesia (see 'Total injectable techniques', below). Additional anaesthetic drugs may also be used following deep sedation with intramuscular drugs. Where possible intravenous access should be achieved once the animal is sedated.

Maintenance of anaesthesia

Physiological considerations

Birds

Birds do not have a diaphragm, instead movements of the keel produce respiratory activity. Unidirectional flow of air through the lungs is achieved by the use of air sacs that act as a bellows. The air sacs provide a tidal flow of air to the avian lung but do not contribute significantly to gas exchange. Some bones are also connected to the airways, for example the humerus in most species (see Chapter 3). Due to the long neck of many birds the tracheal dead space is larger than it is in most mammals and can contribute to respiratory depression during anaesthesia. It is also worth noting that mucous production in the trachea can be copious and this can lead to obstruction of the trachea during intubation. This can be detected by a change in the pattern of ventilation with a delay in expiration. Tracheal anatomy can also vary widely between different bird species (e.g. penguins have double tracheas). It is important to be aware of the tracheal anatomy in the species of bird that you are anaesthetizing so that implications for anaesthesia can be appropriately managed. Both inspiration and expiration in birds require muscular activity so respiratory depression during anaesthesia is common necessitating IPPV. Body position during anaesthesia can also significantly affect ventilation. In dorsal recumbency the weight of the abdominal viscera will compress the abdominal air sacs reducing their volume and therefore reducing effective ventilation. Lateral recumbency during anaesthesia is preferred to support effective ventilation.

Reptiles

Reptiles are poikilothermic, i.e. their body temperature is directly dependent on environmental temperature. Changes in body temperature directly influence metabolic rate and many physiological processes. Consequently, it is important to maintain the reptile patient at its preferred optimal body temperature zone in order to be able to better predict the physiological effects of anaesthetic drugs and ensure proper drug metabolism and excretion. The cardiovascular system of reptiles is unique. In chelonians, lizards and snakes the heart has three chambers, comprised of two atria and a single ventricle (see Chapter 3). The atria are completely separate, but the ventricle is partially separated by an incomplete septum. This incomplete septum allows mixing of oxygenated and deoxygenated blood, which may be a mechanism to preserve adequate oxygenation during periods of apnoea (e.g. during diving). Another unique feature of the reptile cardiovascular system is the renal portal system. Valves are located within veins to regulate venous blood through or around the kidney. It is therefore recommended to avoid administration of drugs into the caudal half of the body because of a more rapid clearance and lower plasma levels compared with administration into the cranial half of the body. The reptile lung is generally composed of a simple endothelial lined sac in most species and reptiles (except crocodilians) lack a muscular diaphragm and instead use a variety of skeletal and smooth muscle activity to facilitate respiration. Most reptiles will not breathe for themselves during general anaesthesia, so IPPV is needed throughout the procedure. Chelonians have complete tracheal rings and a very short trachea, therefore an uncuffed ET tube should be used and care should be taken during placement to ensure that one bronchus intubation is avoided. Reptiles have a lower metabolic rate than mammals so that they will tolerate hypoxic conditions better than most mammals.

Endotracheal intubation

Rabbits

Intubation of rabbits may be achieved using either a 'blind' technique or using visualization with either an otoscope, a laryngoscope with a narrow blade or a rigid endoscope. In both cases it is imperative that the rabbit is already at an adequate depth of anaesthesia if intubation is to be successful. The internal diameter of ET tube appropriate for rabbits of 2.5–4 kg bodyweight is between 2.5 and 3.5 mm. Using an uncuffed ET tube will maximize the luminal diameter of the tube that can be placed, which is advantageous.

Blind technique

1. Position the rabbit in sternal recumbency.
2. Use one hand to hold the rabbit's head so that the neck is straight and extended (this often requires the patient to be lifted up off its sternum, so the front legs are hanging).
3. Introduce the tube into the mouth using your other hand.
4. Whilst doing this, position your face (cheek and ear) close to the patient's face and ET tube connector, looking towards the chest of the rabbit so you can see it breathing.
5. In time with inspiration, advance the tube gently but positively, listening for breath sounds.
6. If the tube enters the trachea the patient will often cough; consequently, it is very important to keep a firm grip of the tube. You will also be able to hear and feel the passage of air in the tube. If the tube enters the oesophagus, no passage of air will be present.

Visualization technique

1. Thread a dog urinary catheter down the centre of the ET tube to act as a stylet, so that the urinary catheter protrudes from the end of the ET tube.
2. Ask an assistant to position the rabbit in sternal recumbency and to extend the rabbit's head and neck.
3. Position the endoscope in the rabbit's mouth (a pair of atraumatic forceps can be very useful to pull the rabbit's tongue forward and out of the side of the mouth).
4. Once the larynx is visualized, pass the urinary catheter through the larynx and advance the ET tube down over the catheter.
5. If the tube enters the trachea the patient will usually cough.

The position of the tube can be checked by either feeling or looking for the passage of air:

- Attach the ET tube to the breathing system and watch for movement of the reservoir bag
- Give the rabbit a manual breath and watch for chest movement
- The preferred method is to attach a capnograph to the ET tube: if the tube is in the trachea CO_2 will be present when the patient exhales (or a breath is administered); if the tube is in the oesophagus no CO_2 will be present.

Rodents

Intubation of rats, mice and guinea pigs is a specialized technique and should not be undertaken without training and availability of appropriate equipment.

Birds

Intubation of birds can be relatively simple due to easy visualization of the trachea and glottis; however, use of a laryngoscope is still helpful to aid visualization and prevent trauma. Birds have complete tracheal rings, making the diameter of the trachea very inflexible and increasing the risk of tracheal necrosis if a tube of too large a diameter is placed. Use of cuffed tubes is not recommended in birds.

Reptiles

Intubation is relatively straightforward in most reptiles because they do not have an epiglottis, making visualization of the larynx easy. The glottal folds are maintained in a closed position and only open during inspiration, therefore application of lidocaine on the glottis to facilitate relaxation can be useful in conscious or sedated reptiles prior to intubation. Intubation can then be carried out in conscious in may snakes and lizards. The glottis is at the base of the tongue in chelonians; some chelonians have a fleshy muscular tongue and this can make intubation more challenging unless a laryngoscope is used.

Inhalational agents

Where intubation is possible, maintenance of anaesthesia with inhalational agents is preferred. Inhalational anaesthesia allows the depth of anaesthesia to be rapidly adjusted according to required need. In addition, the time to recovery is not influenced by the duration of the anaesthesia. Maintaining anaesthesia with an inhalant agent using a face mask to deliver the anaesthetic gases to the patient is also possible, but has the major disadvantage that scavenging from the face mask is problematic and, therefore, environmental contamination with the inhalant is inevitable. A suitable sized breathing circuit should be chosen for the patient based on bodyweight; for most species of small mammals and exotic pets a T-piece with a Jackson–Rees modification is appropriate. Ventilatory support, through IPPV or use of an exotic animal ventilator, is likely to be necessary in most reptiles and birds because of their unique respiratory physiology and the adverse impact of anaesthesia on their respiration.

Total injectable techniques

Total injectable techniques to induce and maintain anaesthesia are well described in the literature for rats and mice, and usually involve a combination of medetomidine/dexmedetomidine and ketamine. This approach has the advantage that intubation is not necessary, thus there are no risks associated with the administration of an inhalant and inadequate scavenging. However, the repeated administration of injectable agents to maintain anaesthesia can lead to a prolonged recovery, which is disadvantageous. Weighing the patient to ensure accurate drug dosing is essential. However, it should be remembered that published drug protocols are based on doses required for healthy laboratory animals (rats, mice, rabbits), rather than pet patients that may have a high incidence of subclinical disease. Alfaxalone, or medetomidine and ketamine in combination, can be used for anaesthesia in reptiles. The administration of oxygen via face mask is also important in small mammals maintained with injectable protocols. In reptiles, intubation and IPPV is required.

Monitoring during anaesthesia

As with cats and dogs, monitoring of small mammals and exotic pets during anaesthesia is important to detect changes in physiological parameters promptly and allow action to be taken to correct them.

Depth of anaesthesia

Rabbits

Monitoring depth of anaesthesia in rabbits is very similar to the practice in cats and dogs, although the palpebral reflex is an unreliable guide. Absence of the corneal reflex is always a sign that depth of anaesthesia is excessive and should be lightened immediately. The hindlimb withdrawal reflex can be helpful; absence of a withdrawal reflex usually indicates a depth of anaesthesia suitable for surgery. Changes in respiratory and heart rate with depth of anaesthesia are similar to those in dogs and cats.

Rodents

Slowing of the respiratory rate can easily be assessed visually and will occur as anaesthesia deepens. Palpebral and corneal reflexes are difficult to assess in small rodents. As depth of anaesthesia increases following induction of anaesthesia there is loss of the righting reflex and of spontaneous movement. Presence or absence of a pedal withdrawal reflex to toe pinching is useful during the maintenance phase; at an anaesthetic depth suitable for surgery the pedal withdrawal reflex is abolished.

Birds

Monitoring depth of anaesthesia involves evaluation of muscle tone and various reflexes, including palpebral, corneal and pedal reflexes. At a depth of anaesthesia adequate for surgery, corneal and pedal reflexes will be present but very slow; the palpebral reflex will be absent. Changes in respiratory and heart rate with depth of anaesthesia are similar to those in dogs and cats.

Reptiles

Reptiles relax during anaesthesia from cranial to caudal; motor function returns in the opposite direction during recovery. The righting reflex is lost at light planes of surgical anaesthesia and is useful for monitoring during recovery. The palpebral reflex is generally lost at light planes of anaesthesia, but the corneal reflex persists; loss of the corneal reflex usually indicates excessive anaesthetic depth. At a surgical plane of anaesthesia, the toe pinch or tail pinch withdrawal reflex should be abolished.

Cardiovascular monitoring

Pulse oximetry

It is important to remember that some pulse oximeters are not effective at detecting the high heart rates that occur in rabbits, small rodents and birds, which also limits their ability to measure haemoglobin saturation with oxygen. The specifications of the device should be checked with the manufacturer before purchase. The probe can be put on the tail or ear of rodents and small mammals and across the toe of most birds as long as the skin is unpigmented. Remember that pulse oximeters are calibrated based on the mammalian oxygen-haemoglobin saturation, which may not be applicable to most reptiles, therefore data generated from pulse oximeters in reptiles should be interpreted with caution.

Blood pressure measurement

Use of a Doppler probe is helpful to measure heart rate in most reptiles. In snakes, the Doppler probe can be secured over the heart to give an audible indication of heart rate during anaesthesia. In most snakes the heart is located one-third to one-fourth of its length caudal to the head. In most lizards the heart is located cranially between the forelimbs, so the probe can be positioned ventrally on the chest or in the axillary region. In chelonians placing a flat Doppler probe on the side of the neck within the thoracic inlet can be used to detect the carotid pulse and give an audible signal of pulse rate. Doppler probes are difficult to use to measure blood pressure in most rodents and small birds (<100 g) because of the difficulty of locating a peripheral pulse and finding a cuff small enough to fit around the limb or tail. In rabbits the fore or hind limb can be used for Doppler blood pressure measurement using similar sites to those used in dogs and cats. Alternatively, oscillometric techniques are also suitable for rabbits using the same principles as apply to dogs and cats.

ECG

As in cats and dogs, an ECG is vital for detecting arrhythmias in rabbits and other exotic animals. In rodents and rabbits the same limb configuration can be used that is used in dogs and cats. In birds, the left and right forelimb leads can be placed at the base of the left and right wings, respectively, and the hindlimb lead placed on the left foot to give an ECG trace. In chelonians and lizards, the ECG pads should be placed with the cranial leads in the cervical region (e.g. left and right neck) and with the hind limb lead attached to the left hind limb. In snakes, a two lead ECG is typically measured, with the electrodes placed two heart lengths cranial and caudal to the heart. It is important to adjust the ECG lead (e.g. lead I, II or III) that is being measured to ensure that an ECG trace is obtained with the two leads that are being used.

Respiratory system monitoring

Capnometry

In very small patients (e.g. rodents) the rate of gas sampling is not matched to the respiratory rate and use in these patients is problematic. However, in rabbits, most birds and reptiles capnometry is a useful tool to measure respiratory function. The normal range for expired CO_2 concentration is the same as in cats and dogs (35–45 mmHg). Arterial blood gas analysis to measure arterial concentrations of carbon dioxide and oxygen is an option in patients with a palpable peripheral artery that is amenable to sampling (e.g. the auricular artery in rabbits). After taking an arterial sample it is important to provide firm haemostasis for at least 5 minutes over the vessel to prevent haematoma formation.

Body temperature

Many exotic pet species are particularly prone to hypothermia due to their large body surface area to volume ratio and heat provision should be made for all these species before, during and after anaesthesia. The principles of preventing hypothermia in small mammals and birds are similar to those for cats and dogs. Reptiles are exothermic and derive nearly all their body heat from the external environment. Most reptiles have a Preferred Optimal Temperature Zone (POTZ) that is associated with optimal metabolic function. During anaesthesia, reptiles should be maintained at a body temperature that is at the upper end of the POTZ for that species.

Considerations for recovery

Extubation

- Rabbits and small rodents: Extubation should take place once the patient starts to swallow or regain motor control.
- Birds: Extubation should occur when the patient is fully awake, breathing well and able to swallow.
- Reptiles: Similar to other species, extubation of reptiles should occur when pharyngeal reflexes have returned and the patient is breathing spontaneously.

Rabbits and rodents

It should be remembered that cats and dogs are predators of rabbits and small rodents; allowing these species to recover in the same room as cats or dogs can therefore be extremely stressful for them. Recovery facilities should ideally be provided in an observed area away from noise. Achieving and maintaining normothermia is very important in rabbits and small rodents in order to prevent a prolongation of the recovery period. Monitoring body temperature as the animal awakens from anaesthesia is very difficult in rats and mice; a warm environment should therefore be maintained until normal activity resumes.

> **WARNING**
>
> - Never leave rabbits or rodents unattended with electrical cables or water-filled warming devices, as they are very likely to chew through any unattended cables or rubbery materials
> - Do not allow rabbits and rodents to recover on straw or wood shavings as these materials can easily damage the eyes when the animals are recumbent

It is important to encourage eating and drinking as soon as possible after anaesthesia in order to reduce the risk of anorexia and gut stasis. Water and palatable food should be offered, and intake monitored, as soon as the animal is returned to the recovery environment.

Birds

Wing flapping and emergence delirium is common in birds, particularly after injectable anaesthesia techniques;

preventing self-trauma during the recovery period is therefore vital. Wrapping the animal in a towel so that its wings are constrained is a useful way to control birds during the recovery period. As with other species, achieving and maintaining normothermia is important to hasten recovery. Food and water should be offered as soon as the bird is awake enough to be able to perch.

Reptiles

Prolonged recovery from anaesthesia is not uncommon in reptiles due to their low metabolic rate. In order to hasten recovery, it is usually recommended to terminate delivery of inhalant agents 15–20 minutes before the end of anaesthesia. Reptiles should be maintained in a quiet environment during recovery, at a temperature in the upper end of their POTZ. Aquatic reptiles should not be allowed access to water until they have fully recovered from anaesthesia and are able to swim.

Acknowledgement

The authors would like to acknowledge the help and expertise of Tracey Dewey (Head of Photography, School of Veterinary Science, University of Bristol) for taking some of the photographs used in this chapter.

References and further reading

Aspinall V (2019) *Clinical Procedures in Veterinary Nursing, 4th edn.* Elsevier, Philadelphia

Brodbelt D (2009) Perioperative mortality in small animal anaesthesia. *Veterinary Journal* **182**, 152–161

Challis K and Seymour C (2008) Advanced anaesthesia and analgesia. In: *BSAVA Manual of Canine and Feline Advanced Veterinary Nursing, 2nd edn*, ed. A Hotston Moore and S Rudd, pp. 128–144. BSAVA Publications, Gloucester

Clarke KW, Trim CM and Hall LW (2014) *Veterinary Anaesthesia, 11th edn.* Elsevier, Philadelphia

Clutton E (2007) Surgical muscle relaxation and neuromuscular blockade. *In Practice* **29**, 574–583

Dugdale A (2010) *Veterinary Anaesthesia.* Blackwell, Oxford

Flecknell PA, Orr HE, Roughan JV and Stewart R (1999) Comparison of the effects of oral or subcutaneous carprofen or ketoprofen in rats undergoing laparotomy. *Veterinary Record* **144**, 65–67

Flecknell PA, Roughan JV and Stewart R (1999) Use of oral buprenorphine ('buprenorphine jello') for postoperative analgesia in rats – a clinical trial. *Laboratory Animals* **33**, 169–174

Fletcher DJ, Boller M, Brainard BM *et al.* (2012) RECOVER evidence and knowledge gap analysis on veterinary CPR. Part 7: Clinical guidelines. *Journal of Veterinary Emergency and Critical Care* **22**, S102–S131

Girling S J and Raiti P (2019) *BSAVA Manual of Reptiles, 3rd edn.* BSAVA publications, Gloucester

Harcourt-Brown F and Chitty J (2013) *BSAVA Manual of Rabbit Surgery, Dentistry and Imaging.* BSAVA publications, Gloucester

Hunt JR, Attenburrow PM, Slingsby LS and Murrell JC (2013) Comparison of premedication with buprenorphine or methadone with meloxicam for postoperative analgesia in dogs undergoing orthopaedic surgery. *Journal of Small Animal Practice* **54**, 418–424

Kaka U, Rahman NA, Abubakar AA *et al.* (2018) Pre-emptive multimodal analgesia with tramadol and ketamine-lidocaine infusion for suppression of central sensitisation in a dog model of ovariohysterectomy. *Journal of Pain Research* **11**, 743–752

Keating SCJ, Thomas AA, Flecknell PA and Leach MC (2012) Evaluation of EMLA cream for preventing pain during tattooing of rabbits: changes in physiological, behavioural and facial expression responses. *PLOS ONE* **7**: e44437

King LG and Boag A (2018) *BSAVA Manual of Canine and Feline Emergency and Critical Care, 3rd edn.* BSAVA Publications, Gloucester

Lamont LA, Bulmer BJ, Sison DD, Grimm KA and Tranquilli WJ (2002) Doppler echocardiographic effects of medetomidine on dynamic left ventricular outflow tract obstruction in cats. *Journal of the American Veterinary Medical Association* **221**, 1276–1281

Langford DJ, Bailey AL, Chanda ML *et al.* (2010) Coding of facial expressions of pain in the laboratory mouse. *Nature Methods* **7**, 447–449

Lascelles BD, Cripps PJ, Jones A and Waterman AE (1997) Post-operative central hypersensitivity and pain: the pre-emptive value of pethidine for ovariohysterectomy. *Pain* **73**, 461–471

Lierz M and Korbel R (2012) Anaesthesia and analgesia in birds. *Journal of Exotic Pet Medicine* **21**, 44–58

Meredith A (2015) *BSAVA Formulary 9th Edn, Part B: Exotic Pets.* BSAVA Publications, Gloucester

Meredith A and Johnson Delaney C (2010) *BSAVA Manual of Exotic Pets, 5th edn.* BSAVA Publications, Gloucester

Mullineaux E and Keeble E (2016) *BSAVA Manual of Wildlife Casualties, 2nd edn.* BSAVA Publications, Gloucester

Perpinan D (2018) Reptile anaesthesia and analgesia. *Companion Animal* **23**, 236–243

Seymour C, Duke-Novakovski T and de Vries M (2016) *BSAVA Manual of Canine and Feline Anaesthesia and Analgesia, 3rd edn.* BSAVA Publications, Gloucester

Raftery A (2013) Avian Anaesthesia. *In Practice* **35**, 272–278

Shah MD, Yates D, Hunt J and Murrell JC (2018) A comparison between methadone and buprenorphine for perioperative analgesia in dogs undergoing ovariohysterectomy. *Journal of Small Animal Practice* **59**, 539–546

Sotocinal SG, Sorge RE, Zaloum *et al.* (2011) The Rat Grimace Scale: a partially automated method for quantifying pain in the laboratory rat via facial expressions. *Molecular Pain* **7**, 55

Stanway G and Magee A (2007) Anaesthesia and analgesia. In: *BSAVA Manual of Practical Veterinary Nursing*, ed. E Mullineaux and M Jones, pp. 268–314. BSAVA Publications, Gloucester

Varga M, Lumbis R and Gott L (2012) *BSAVA Manual of Exotic Pet and Wildlife Nursing.* BSAVA publications, Gloucester

Welch E (2009) *Anaesthesia for Veterinary Nurses, 2nd edn.* Blackwell, Oxfordshire

Useful websites

American Society of Anesthesiologists (ASA) – ASA physical status classificaiton system
www.asahq.org/standards-and-guidelines/asa-physical-status-classification-system

Association of Veterinary Anaesthetists (AVA) – Anaesthetic records and patient safety checklists:
https://ava.eu.com

National Centre for the Replacement, Refinement and Reduction of Animals in Research (NC3Rs) – Rabbit, mouse and rat grimace scales:
www.nc3rs.org.uk/grimacescales

Reassessment Campaign on Veterinary Resuscitation (RECOVER):
www.acvecc-recover.org

UNESP-Botucatu Multidimensional Composite Pain Scale for Cats:
www.animalpain.com.br/assets/upload/escala-en-us.pdf

University of Glasgow – Glasgow Composite Pain Scales:
www.newmetrica.com/acute-pain-measurement/

Self-assessment questions

1. What are the six aims of premedication?
2. What is multimodal analgesia?
3. Identify two advantages and disadvantages of total injectable and total inhalational anaesthetic techniques?
4. What are the essential characteristics of red rubber and silicone tubes used for endotracheal intubation in cats and dogs?
5. Compare and contrast rebreathing and non-rebreathing anaesthetic circuits.
6. Calculate the fresh gas flow rate required for maintenance of anaesthesia of an 18 kg dog with a respiratory rate of 13 breaths per minute, maintained on a Lack circuit.
7. How can the respiratory and cardiovascular systems be monitored during anaesthesia?
8. What are the consequences of hypothermia during anaesthesia?
9. What are the main considerations when anaesthetizing a brachycephalic patient?
10. State the routes by which resuscitation drugs can be given during advanced life support.

Chapter 22

Theatre practice

Alison Young and Julie Gerrish

Learning objectives

After studying this chapter, readers will have the knowledge to :

- Explain the principles of surgical asepsis and procedures to minimize the risk of infection in the operating theatre
- Recognize a range of surgical instruments used in all types of veterinary surgery
- Describe the care and maintenance of surgical instruments/packs and equipment
- Describe the different methods of sterilization available and discuss their suitability and use for a range of surgical instruments and equipment used in veterinary surgery
- Describe the preparation of a patient for surgery and the intraoperative and immediate postoperative care of a patient
- Explain the roles of a veterinary nurse in the operating theatre as both a scrubbed and a circulating nurse
- Describe the ideal properties of suture materials and discuss the advantages and disadvantages of different types
- Recognize different suture patterns commonly used in veterinary surgery

---

Introduction

The veterinary nurse is usually given the responsibility of running the operating theatre. This typically involves: maintenance of hygiene in the theatre; care and maintenance of instruments and equipment; preparation of theatre, the patient and the surgical team; and providing assistance as both a scrubbed and circulating nurse.

The most important factor in successful theatre practice is the establishment and maintenance of a good aseptic technique, i.e. all the steps taken to prevent contact with microorganisms (see also Chapter 7). Figure 22.1 gives definitions of commonly used terms in theatre practice.

Factors influencing the development of infection

Infection of a clean surgical wound is always a matter of great concern. It is far better to prevent infection than to try and treat it. With the present day issues of antibiotic resistance, the use of antibiotics should not be relied upon to protect patients from the consequences of poor asepsis (see Chapter 8).

It has been established that most surgical wound infections occur at the time of surgery, not during the postoperative

Term	Definition
Sepsis	The presence of pathogens or their toxic products in the blood or tissues of the patient; more commonly known as infection
Asepsis	Freedom from infection, i.e. exclusion of microorganisms and spores
Antisepsis	Prevention of sepsis by destruction or inhibition of microorganisms using an agent that may be safely applied to living tissue
Sterilization	The complete elimination of all microorganisms, including spores
Disinfection	The removal of microorganisms (but not necessarily spores)
Disinfectant	An agent that destroys microorganisms – generally chemical agents applied to inanimate objects (see Chapters 7 and 14)

22.1 Definitions of commonly used terms in theatre practice .

 BSAVA Textbook of Veterinary Nursing, sixth edition. Edited by Barbara Cooper, Elizabeth Mullineaux and Lynn Turner. ©BSAVA 2020

period (Chemaly *et al.*, 2014). Poor aseptic technique will undoubtedly affect the success of any surgery and, in the long term, the success and reputation of the practice. Strict theatre discipline is essential if high standards are to be maintained. A specific protocol must exist, which should be respected and rigidly adhered to by everyone involved with surgery. The protocol should include:

- Correct theatre attire
- Scrubbing-up procedures
- Patient preparation procedures
- Draping techniques
- Sterilization information and procedures
- Organization of surgical lists, cleaning protocol and conduct during surgery.

Sources of contamination in the operating theatre include the operating room, equipment, personnel and the patient.

General rules for maintenance of asepsis in theatre

- Correct theatre attire should be worn at all times
- There should be the minimum number of people required present within the operating theatre; movement should be kept to a minimum and all doors closed, decreasing the need for people to enter and leave the theatre during surgery
- There should be a new set of sterile instruments for each operation, even when dealing with a contaminated site. More than one set may be required to prevent tumour seeding or contamination
- There should be a plan to perform 'clean' operations first in the day, i.e. orthopaedic operations (especially when implants are used), and to carry out contaminated surgery last (e.g. aural and oral)
- Wherever possible there should be separate rooms for 'dirty' and 'clean' procedures
- An efficient sterilization programme should be adopted
- The theatre should be maintained at an ambient temperature (18–21°C) and the ventilation must be good (a minimum of 20 air changes per hour). Hot, humid conditions encourage the growth of pathogens, in particular *Pseudomonas* spp.
- Patients should be clipped and have an initial skin preparation performed before they are taken to theatre
- The surgical team must ensure that they do not touch any non-sterile surfaces during surgery. Any break in asepsis must be reported and rectified
- No contaminated instruments or equipment should be returned to the sterile trolley
- Good hand hygiene is required before touching a patient, before a clean or aseptic procedure, after touching a patient, after handling bodily fluids and after touching the patient's surroundings
- Sterile gloves should be worn for all aseptic procedures
- A record of all surgical procedures should be kept, so that if any sepsis problems arise the cause can be detected
- A strict cleaning protocol must be maintained
- Dedicated equipment should be available for surgical procedures, which is appropriately maintained and sterilized

---

Operating room and environment

Many microorganisms are airborne and any movement within the operating theatre will disperse them. Good ventilation (20 air changes per hour) is necessary, as is maintaining the theatre at a relative humidity of 50–60% because hot, humid conditions are a threat to asepsis (Dharan and Pittet, 2002). Clean procedures should be performed first on the operating list because microorganisms from contaminated sites will remain in the air. The operating room itself must be easily cleaned and should contain minimal furniture.

Equipment and instruments

All equipment and instruments used in the operative site must be sterile. There must be a fresh sterile set of instruments and spares for each operation.

Personnel

The more people present in theatre, the greater is the likelihood of infection. All theatre personnel should wear theatre clothing: caps, masks, scrub suits and antistatic footwear (Figure 22.2). These should only be worn in the designated theatre area. In addition, those who are in the surgical team should prepare their hands aseptically and wear sterile gowns and gloves.

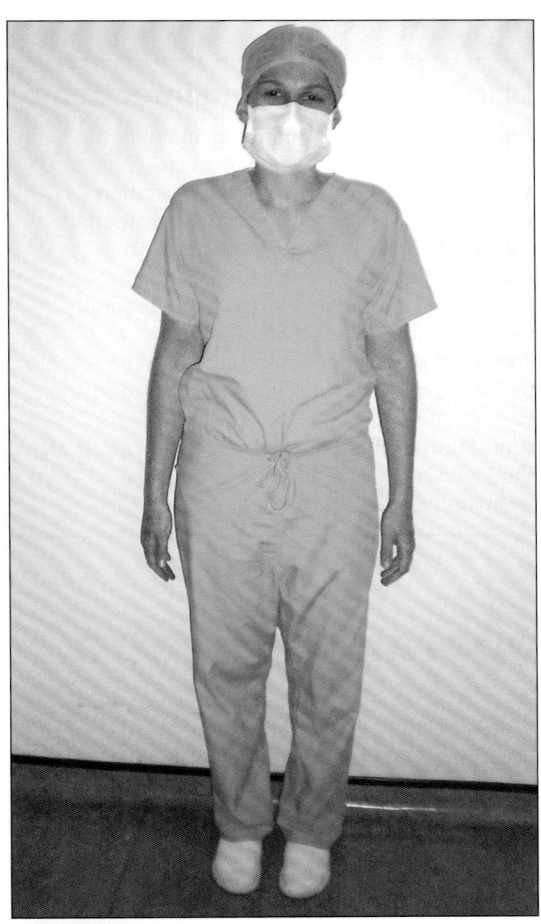

22.2 Correct attire for the operating theatre.

General hand hygiene

The hands can be a portal and transmitter of infection. Risk factors for nosocomial infections include the behaviour of personnel regarding decontamination practices, hand hygiene, antisepsis and compliance with practice theatre protocols. For routine decontamination of hands in the clinical setting, an alcohol-based waterless antiseptic can be used. Hand washing with soap and water (see Chapter 7) is still required if contact with spores (e.g. *Bacillus* spp.) is anticipated. The physical action of washing and rinsing hands under such circumstances is recommended because alcohols, chlorhexidine, idophors and other antiseptic agents have poor activity against spores.

The patient

The patient is the main source of contamination, especially as most animals are covered in hair or feathers. The source of microorganisms may be endogenous or exogenous:

- **Endogenous** – originate from within the body of the patient
- **Exogenous** – found on the outside of the animal, i.e. the skin and coat. This term is also used with reference to environmental sources of microorganisms (e.g. air, equipment).

It does not necessarily follow that the introduction of microorganisms will result in an infected wound. Microorganisms can and will enter any wound that has been exposed to air, but whether infection follows depends on several variable factors.

Factors influencing wound infection

- **Virulence** – the disease-producing ability of the organism and resistance of the patient (see Chapter 7)
- **Duration of surgery** – bacterial contamination increases the longer the wound is open (infection rate doubles for every hour of operative time)
- **Surgical technique** – excessive handling and trauma to tissues and damage to vascular supply may increase the likelihood of infection
- **Impaired host resistance** – may increase the risk of infection if it is due to drugs, nutrition or underlying disease
- **Contamination of the wound** – surgical wounds are classified with respect to their potential for contamination and infection (see Chapter 23)

The operating theatre suite

The design and layout of the operating theatre will rarely be within the control of the veterinary nurse. It is important, however, to have some knowledge of ideal requirements and desirable features in order to appreciate differing standards and to try to make the best of existing facilities. The layout of rooms within the theatre suite is important for the sake of asepsis. The theatre rooms should not be used as a thoroughfare to elsewhere in the building. There

should be a clear separation between the areas where correct theatre attire is worn and the rest of the practice. Clean and used instruments and equipment should not be stored together.

The theatre suite components

- Operating theatre
- Anaesthetic and preparation area
- Area for washing and sterilizing equipment
- Sterile storage area
- Scrubbing-up area
- Changing rooms
- Recovery room

The operating theatre

Many practices have just one operating theatre, which is used for all surgery. Larger veterinary practices may have theatres that are used specifically for particular types of surgery, such as orthopaedic work, general surgery and 'dirty' surgery (e.g. dental work).

The size of the theatre will depend on the purpose for which it is intended. If it is to be used for simple routine surgery, it can be quite compact; if it is to be used for orthopaedic surgery, a large amount of surgical equipment may be needed. If the theatre is too small, working conditions will be compromised and it may be difficult to maintain a high standard of asepsis. It has to be large enough to accommodate the patient, anaesthetic equipment, surgical instrument trolley, other equipment and personnel.

There are several other requirements that are essential, or at least desirable, as follows.

Basic design and materials

The operating theatre should be an end room, not a thoroughfare to other rooms (Figure 22.3).

It must be easy to clean. Walls and floors must be made of impervious non-staining materials; floors should be non-slip and hard-wearing. Walls and ceiling should be painted with a light-coloured 'waterproof' paint. The corners and edges of all walls should be coved to facilitate cleaning.

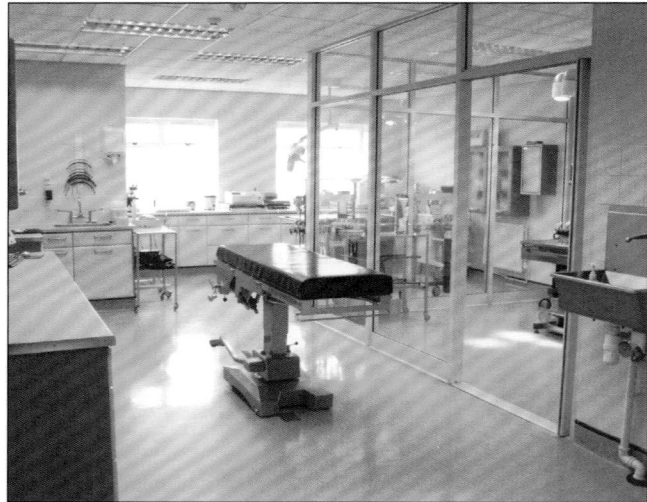

22.3 A theatre has been formed using glass partitioning to leave an L-shaped preparation room, with good visibility throughout the area. (Reproduced from the *BSAVA Manual of Small Animal Practice Management and Development*)

Ceramic tiles are occasionally used on walls in operating theatres. These are hard-wearing, but crevices between the tiles are difficult to keep clean, and harbour dust and bacteria. The use of drains should be avoided within the operating theatre itself, but may be useful in minor and 'dirty' operation areas.

Lighting and electricity

Good lighting is essential. Advantage should be taken of natural daylight. Ideally, lighting should be concealed within the ceiling, with additional side lights on the wall and an overhead theatre light.

There should be a good supply of electrical sockets (in waterproof casing), preferably recessed into the wall.

Heating and air-conditioning

Heating is an important consideration, since anaesthetized animals are unable to control their own body temperature. The ambient temperature should be between 15 and 20°C. Fan heaters cause air and dust movement and should be avoided. Modern wall-mounted radiators are widely available and a common choice for heating. They are, however, difficult to keep clean and will easily trap and harbour dust and dirt behind them. To avoid this, radiators should be included in the cleaning regime. Panel heating within the walls is ideal, but expensive.

A system of air-conditioning and ventilation is necessary. It is recommended that a positive ventilation system is used that can provide a minimum of 20 air changes per hour to ensure that a continuous fresh supply of air is provided to the theatre suite.

Doors and windows

Ideally the room should have double swing doors, which should normally be kept closed.

There should be no clear glass windows to the outside where members of the public could see into the theatres (as per the Royal College of Veterinary Surgeons (RCVS) Practice Standards Scheme requirements).

Operating table

The operating table should be adjustable to facilitate positioning of the patient and to suit the height of the surgeon. The base of the table may be static or maintained on wheels for easy moving. The table should be able to be raised and lowered and tilted as necessary. There is usually a hydraulically operated pump to adjust the height, and some electrically operated pumps are also available. Between cases, the table and instrument surfaces should be cleaned and disinfected.

Other equipment

There should be no shelving and minimal furniture in the theatre as these will harbour dust. All equipment, including the operating table, must be easy to clean.

If required, the radiograph viewer should preferably be flush with the wall. A method of displaying digital images may require a screen or computer to be brought into the theatre. This should not be used outside of the theatre area. It must be kept clean, as it will be a high touch area; washable components such as keyboards are available.

An air supply for power tools may be needed. This should ideally be piped into the theatre from cylinders housed outside it. Anaesthetic gases can be delivered in the same way. A scavenging system for anaesthetic waste gases will also be necessary (see Chapters 2 and 21). A wall clock is required to aid anaesthetic monitoring and timing of surgery.

A dry-wipe board is useful for recording details such as swab numbers, suture details and blood loss. It is standard practice to count supplies (e.g. instruments, needles and sponges) before beginning a case, before final closure and on completing a surgical procedure.

Anaesthetic preparation area

There should be a separate area where the induction of anaesthesia (see Chapter 21) and other preoperative procedures (e.g. clipping, catheterization of the bladder and preparation of the surgical site) can be carried out (Figure 22.4). It should lead directly into the operating theatre.

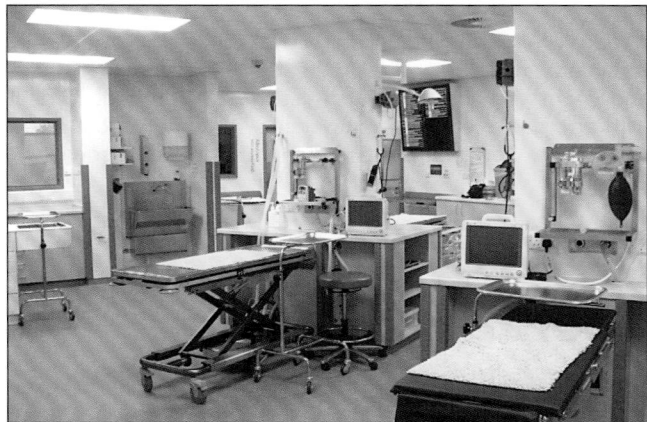

22.4 Preparation room layout will be determined by the space available and the number of stations required. This large preparation area has tables arranged for easy access to theatre and for staff, with wall-mounted anaesthetic machines and clippers. (Reproduced from the *BSAVA Manual of Small Animal Practice Management and Development*)

Areas for washing and sterilizing equipment

There needs to be a separate room or area where dirty instruments are washed and another separate area where clean instrument kits and other equipment can be packed and sterilized. These areas should be situated close to the operating theatre but away from the sterile storage area. They should include sterilization facilities such as an ultrasonic instrument cleaner and an autoclave. A washing machine and tumble drier will be required to facilitate specific cleaning of theatre scrub suits, gowns and drapes. Ideally this should be in another closed room, but situated furthest away from the operating theatres and the clean instrument packing area to confine the dust created when laundering such items.

Sterile storage area

Sterile supplies should be stored in closed cupboards away from the instrument washing area, but adjacent to theatre. Instrument trolleys can have their packed equipment and instruments loaded prior to surgery, to ensure all items are present and available and provide maximum efficiency during the surgery by having all items close by.

Scrubbing-up area

There should be a separate scrub room within the theatre suite, but outside the theatre itself. This should lead directly into the sterile preparation area and theatre. Swing doors, which can be foot operated, should separate the rooms.

Changing rooms

Changing rooms for personnel should be situated at the entrance to theatre. It is useful to have a red line delineating the sterile area and appropriate notices displayed to indicate these areas. Footwear for use in theatre should be placed at the entrance to theatre beyond the red line. This barrier should be adhered to at all times to ensure a high level of asepsis.

Recovery room

A room where the patient can recover following surgery may be situated near the operating theatre suite. It should be quiet and warm and should contain essential equipment to deal with any postoperative emergencies that might occur (see Chapter 21). Good observation of this area is also essential.

Hazards in the operating theatre

The avoidance of accidents to patients and staff in the operating theatre is of the utmost importance. The Health and Safety at Work etc. Act 1974 and the Control of Substances Hazardous to Health (COSHH) Regulations 2002 (see Chapter 2) are designed to ensure safety in the workplace, including the operating theatre. Appropriate risk assessments for the preparation and theatre areas, the activities taking place in them, and the equipment used must be in place (see Chapter 2).

With the increasing use of new and sophisticated equipment, the risk of accidents has also increased. It is very important that all nursing staff are instructed in the use and maintenance of all new equipment. It is also important that all equipment is serviced regularly and tested for electrical safety to minimize risks.

All staff should be aware of the dangers associated with inhaling anaesthetic gases. An anaesthetic gas-scavenging system must be fitted, or absorptive filters used to minimize exposure to gases (see Chapter 21). In the operating theatre, nursing staff will be exposed to various chemicals. Appropriate protective clothing, masks and gloves should be worn.

Maintenance and cleaning of the operating theatre

A routine cleaning programme is essential for a high standard of asepsis to be maintained. Cleaning protocols should be adopted and strictly followed. These protocols should include details of all the daily, weekly and monthly tasks to be completed. Disinfectant agents are discussed in Chapter 14.

Records of cleaning and maintenance tasks conducted at weekly and monthly intervals should be logged and filed as evidence that cleaning protocols are followed. Record keeping allows for clinical audits to be performed at regular intervals to review protocols and ensure they are being adhered to. It will also highlight areas which may require a more vigorous cleaning process or more attention.

Cleaning checks

As well as visual checks of the area to monitor cleanliness, some practices may use bacterial cultures as a monitoring tool. A selection of swab samples for bacterial culture can be taken from a variety of sites in the operating theatre from time to time to ensure efficacy of the cleaning regime and to alert staff to any potential problems. There should be no growth of bacteria from sterilized equipment and most other sites (e.g. sinks, operating tables, trolleys, drains, positioning aids, surfaces, and lights).

Cleaning equipment

Cleaning utensils should be designated specifically for use in the theatre suite only. They should be rinsed and allowed to dry after use. Buckets should always be emptied and rinsed out. All utensils should be stored in a separate cupboard or confined room away from the sterile area.

Cleaning equipment such as cloths and mop heads should be washed daily in a washing machine, but not in the same machine as is used to wash scrub suits and drapes. Cloths should be discarded after a short time and replaced with new ones. Autoclavable mop heads are also available.

Routine cleaning of the operating theatre

- **At the beginning of each day:**
  - All the surfaces, furniture and equipment in the theatre suite should be damp-dusted, using a dilute solution of disinfectant (a dry duster would simply move dust around the room). Damp-dusting is performed to remove any traces of dust particles that may have settled overnight on the surfaces and equipment within the theatre. Starting at the top and working downwards helps ensure all dust is removed.
- **Between cases:**
  - The operating table, stands, instrument trolleys, kick buckets, monitoring equipment and leads should be wiped clean using an appropriate disinfectant
  - The floors should be mopped clean. The operating table should be moved to allow cleaning if the floor has become contaminated with any fluid during a procedure
  - The scrub sink area, including the adjacent wall, should be cleaned
  - All waste material should be removed and disposed of appropriately.
- **At the end of the day:**
  - The floors in all rooms of the theatre suite should be vacuumed or swept to remove debris and loose hair. The vacuum and hose should be emptied and thoroughly cleaned ➜

Routine cleaning of the operating theatre *continued*

- The floors should then be either wet-vacuumed or washed using disinfectant
- All waste material should be removed and disposed of
- Surfaces, equipment, operating tables, lights and scrub sinks should all be thoroughly washed down with disinfectant.
- **Once a week:**
  - There should be a more thorough deep cleaning session of the operating theatres
  - All equipment should be removed from the room and the floors and walls should then be scrubbed
  - A disinfectant with detergent properties that will remove organic matter and that is active against a wide range of bacteria, including *Pseudomonas* spp., should be used
  - After removing any excess solution, the disinfectant should be allowed to dry on the surface rather than being rinsed off, for longer residual activity
  - All equipment should be meticulously wiped over with disinfectant.
- **Once a month:**
  - Vacuum and clean thoroughly all air vents to remove any dust build-up.

Admission of the patient

All relevant details must be recorded on the case records (see also Chapters 1, 9, 14):

- Check the reason for admission and that the correct information is detailed on the consent form
- Where relevant, identify the site (draw or annotate a diagram if necessary)
- Ensure that the owner understands what is to be done, the restrictions of activity postoperatively if relevant and how the patient will look when discharged (e.g. it will have a clipped area and may be wearing a bandage, cast, Elizabethan collar)
- Identify if there are any known allergies or previous drug reactions
- Check any concurrent medication the patient is receiving and a record of the last dose received
- Ensure that the patient is in good general health or that clinical signs have not changed since they were last seen by a veterinary surgeon
- Ensure that there is a contact telephone number and that an anaesthetic consent form has been read, understood and signed
- Weigh the patient
- Fit a plastic identification collar containing the patient's name/number, weight and reason for admission, to minimize the risk of mistakes occurring.

The surgical patient

Surgical cases may be categorized as follows:

- **Elective and non-urgent** – the patient is usually healthy and often young (e.g. ovariohysterectomy, castration, corrective osteotomy)
- **Necessary or urgent** – not immediately life-threatening but requiring prompt attention (e.g. fracture repair, gastrointestinal surgery)
- **Emergency surgery** – life-threatening conditions (e.g. abdominal crisis), often traumatic (e.g. chest injury).

The time between admission and surgery will depend on various factors. In the simplest elective procedures, the patient is admitted on the morning of surgery and returns home later that day. Preoperative preparations in these cases are minimal. In others there may be a delay before surgery is performed. Reasons for this may include:

- **Investigative procedures**, such as diagnostic tests, radiographic and ultrasonographic studies
- **Fluid therapy or transfusion** to improve the patient's physiological status before surgery
- **Presence of other injuries** that require treatment before surgery may be undertaken (e.g. thoracic trauma associated with a limb fracture)
- To allow **reduction of swelling/debridement** of wounds – bandaging of fracture site, application of wound dressings, etc.
- **Stabilization** of patient with concurrent metabolic disturbance (e.g. diabetes mellitus, renal disease, hyperadrenocorticism).

Preoperative preparation of the patient

Withholding food and water

Water should be available at all times up until the time of premedication, when the water bowl can be removed from the patient's kennel. Food is usually withheld for 6–12 hours prior to surgery in dogs and cats. This is primarily to prevent regurgitation of food under general anaesthesia or during recovery. Recent feeding could also interfere with the surgical procedure in very young animals, very old animals and those with metabolic disorders. Prolonged withholding of food may be contraindicated because extending the duration of preoperative fasting has been associated with increased gastric acidity and an increased occurrence of reflux (O'Dwyer, 2016). It is preferable for such cases to be placed as early as possible on the surgical list and then fed promptly afterwards to minimize metabolic disturbances and potential problems in the postoperative period.

Bathing and grooming

Ideally all patients should be bathed before surgery to remove any gross contamination from the fur and skin. This decreases the risk of contamination and thereby reduces the risk of postoperative surgical site infection, but this is not always feasible. It should be considered in elective orthopaedic procedures such as total hip replacement.

Clipping the surgical site is necessary for most procedures (except intraoral and some ophthalmic surgeries). It may be carried out before or during anaesthesia (Figure 22.5),

Timing	Advantages	Disadvantages
Pre-anaesthesia	■ Shorter anaesthetic time ■ Improves asepsis: loose hairs generally shed before surgery ■ Can give initial skin preparation ■ Improves operating theatre efficiency	■ Patient may be uncooperative ■ Requires two or more people ■ Trauma to the skin may cause more irritation/site of infection ■ Clipping more than 12 hours before surgery may increase skin bacteria
During general anaesthesia	■ Often takes less time ■ Fewer people required to restrain animal ■ Desirable with fractious animals or painful/inaccessible sites	■ Decreases asepsis: small loose hairs are extremely difficult to remove, even with a vacuum cleaner ■ Increases anaesthetic time

22.5 Advantages and disadvantages of clipping pre-anaesthesia and during general anaesthesia.

depending on patient cooperation, but should not be done more than 24 hours before the scheduled procedure to avoid bacterial build-up on the patient's skin. Clipping is more commonly performed immediately prior to surgery under general anaesthesia.

Considerations for preoperative clipping

■ Clipping should be performed away from the operating theatre in a separate preparation area or room to minimize contamination by hair
■ Ensure that clipper blades are in good working order and are clean. Tears made in the skin will cause irritation, which may encourage postoperative licking and scratching and will predispose the site to infection
■ Clip a large area around the surgical site. Ensure that the clipping is neat (this is what the owner will notice)
■ When clipping around a wound, a water-soluble sterile gel should be placed in the wound and on the coat at the edges of the wound to help prevent hair entering the wound. Individual sterile sachets of gel should be used for this, rather than multiuse tubes, to prevent contamination from, or of, the wound
■ Clean the clipper blades between patients using a bactericidal disinfectant. It may be necessary to sterilize the blades after clipping contaminated sites (e.g. abscesses)
■ Do not allow clipper blades to become too hot during use, as this may cause inflammation or excoriation that will not be apparent until the postoperative period. Have a second pair of blades ready so that they can be swapped during procedures
■ Shaving the skin after clipping should be avoided as it can lead to severe excoriation, which encourages postoperative licking, scratching and soreness. Well maintained clippers should provide a close-enough clip to remove the hair adequately

Administration of an enema

For some surgeries (e.g. rectal/colonic) it may be desirable to give an evacuant enema prior to surgery. A soap-and-water enema is simplest. The patient may need bathing afterwards to remove faecal contaminants from the skin. However, for some surgical procedures it may not be a sensible option as liquid faeces are more difficult to contain if the area is within or near the sterile field. In these cases, manual evacuation of the rectum and a purse-string suture may be a better option. See Chapter 15 for more information on enemas.

Other possible preoperative procedures

■ Prior to anaesthesia:
  • Placement of intravenous catheters (see Chapter 20)
  • Administration of a premedicant drug, 15 minutes to 1 hour before induction of anaesthesia (see Chapter 21)
  • Covering of any wounds not associated with the surgery, to prevent contamination
  • Application of a foot/tail bandage to cover any unclipped areas where surgery involves a limb or the perineal area (see Chapter 15)
  • Prophylactic antimicrobial use may be considered appropriate in the preoperative period, although it should not be a substitute for good asepsis. Where the risk of infection is low, inappropriate antibacterial use should be avoided so that there are not unnecessary costs for the owner and to avoid increasing the risk of antibacterial resistance and super-infection.
■ Once anaesthetized:
  • Placement of additional venous catheters (e.g. jugular) or of arterial catheters (for anaesthetic monitoring) (see Chapter 20)
  • Catheterization of the bladder (see Chapter 15) may be required to:
    – Monitor urine output during and after surgery
    – Minimize risk of soiling during surgery
    – Facilitate access to abdominal organs
    – Prevent risk of bladder perforation or rupture during surgery
  • Eye lubrication is necessary for all anaesthetized patients to prevent corneal drying during a procedure. A small amount of eye lubricant should be placed into each eye prior to the surgery; depending on the length of the procedure, it may be necessary to reapply during surgery
  • For perianal surgery, application of a purse-string suture around the anus to prevent contamination by faecal material. The nurse should ensure that this is removed at the end of surgery, and a label placed on the head of the dog will be a good reminder
  • For surgery on distal limbs, application of an Esmarch's rubber bandage and tourniquet to give a bloodless operating field. The time of application must be recorded to ensure that the bandage is not left in place for >45 minutes to avoid ischaemic injury to the limb
  • For oral or nasal surgery, introduction of a throat pack (dampened conforming bandage) to prevent aspiration of blood, mucus, etc. should be considered. It is important to remove this following surgery
  • For some ophthalmic surgery, the application of eye drops prior to the surgery may be required.

Aseptic preparation of the skin

The skin and coat are two of the greatest sources of wound contamination, as it is not possible to remove all bacteria. The aim is to reduce significantly the number present without damaging the skin itself. Skin bacteria include species of *Staphylococcus*, *Bacillus* and, occasionally, *Streptococcus*.

As antiseptic and detergent properties are required in skin-cleansing agents, surgical scrub solutions such as chlorhexidine and povidone–iodine are ideal. An antiseptic solution (which may be water- or alcohol-based) is then usually applied to give residual bactericidal activity. Initial skin preparation should be done in the preparation room.

Surgical scrub solutions

The ideal properties of a surgical scrub solution are:

- Wide spectrum of antimicrobial activity
- Ability to decrease microbial count quickly
- Quick application
- Long residual lethal effect against microorganisms (i.e. an agent offering persistent activity, which will keep the bacterial count low under the gloves). Studies have shown that the rate of glove failures (non-visible holes) increases with the duration of surgery. Studies have also shown that bacteria grow faster under gloved than ungloved hands (Hübner *et al.*, 2010)
- Remains active and effective in the presence of organic matter
- Safe to use without skin irritation or sensitization
- No appreciable ocular or ototoxicity
- Economical
- Practical for veterinary use.

Examples of commonly used agents are given in Figure 22.6.

There are several different techniques that are commonly used; however, there is very little evidence to show which method is preferable. The evidence that is available is based on human patients and has small test group sizes. The evidence that is available pertains to the surgical scrub solution

Agent	Properties
Povidone–iodine	■ Iodine combined with a detergent ■ Broad-spectrum antimicrobial activity (bactericidal, viricidal and fungicidal) ■ May cause severe skin reactions and irritation in some individuals ■ Efficacy impaired by organic matter
Chlorhexidine	■ Effective against many bacteria (including *Escherichia coli* and *Pseudomonas* spp.) ■ Viricidal, fungicidal and sporicidal properties ■ Effective level of activity in presence of organic material ■ Longer residual activity than povidone-iodine ■ Relatively low toxicity to tissue
Triclosan	■ Newer agent, claimed to be antibacterial against both Gram-positive and Gram-negative bacteria

22.6 Commonly used surgical scrub solutions.

used, concentration and contact time (World Health Organization, 2009). These are the most important things that the veterinary nurse must ensure are correct for a suitable surgical skin preparation.

Skin preparation technique

1. Put on surgical gloves to prevent contamination of the patient's skin from the hands. It is not necessary, however, for the gloves to be sterile during the initial preparation, although good hand hygiene should be adopted (see above).
2. Using lint-free swabs and a dilute surgical scrub solution (chlorhexidine gluconate diluted 50:50 in water), clean the site. Lint-free swabs should always be used, never cotton wool, to prevent any residue being left on the skin. A reasonable amount of friction is required for the mechanical element of the scrub to be effective. The site should be cleaned from the expected line of surgical incision out to the edge of the clipped area; once the edges of the clipped area are reached, without the surrounding fur being included, the swab should be discarded and a new one used.
3. Continue this procedure until the area is clean, i.e. there is no discoloration or dirt visible on a white swab.

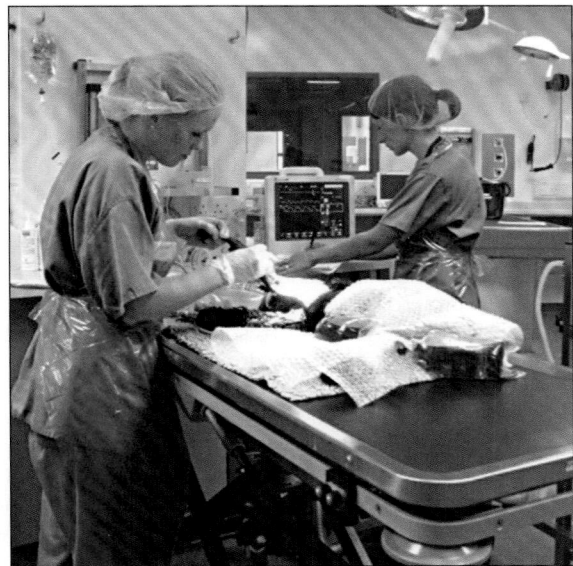

4. Avoid over-wetting the patient. For limb surgery that does not involve the foot, it should be wrapped in a non-sterile cohesive bandage to allow for draping once transferred into the operating theatre. Care should be taken to avoid soaking the coat, as this will increase the risk of 'strike-through' from the drapes, should material drapes be used, and may make the patient hypothermic, especially in the case of small pets.
5. Cover the area with a clean sheet (kennel liners work well). Move the patient into the theatre and position for surgery. For limb surgery, a limb tie or tape is applied over the bandaged foot and attached to a transfusion stand (see Figure 22.12). This allows preparation around all sides of the limb as the limb is suspended. →

Skin preparation technique *continued*

6. If the surgical site was contaminated in the transition to the theatre, clean the skin again in the manner previously described.
7. The final stage of preparation involves the wearing of sterile gloves and the application of an antiseptic skin solution. There are commercially available applicators containing chlorhexidine and isopropyl alcohol at the correct ratio. The manufacturers' guidelines state that these products are applied to the skin in a back and forth method. Products that are sprayed over the surgical site and allowed to dry on to the skin (e.g. chlorhexidine isopropyl), do not provide any mechanical element of cleaning. In addition, they often come in multiuse containers, which raises some concerns about colonization of these items with bacteria that may be detrimental to the goal of skin preparation and the outcome for the patient. Again, there is limited evidence available for all of these methods in the veterinary patient.

Preparation of eyes and mucous membranes

The solutions commonly used for preparation of the skin are likely to be toxic and cause damage to mucous membranes and, in particular, the eye. Dilute povidone–iodine antiseptic solution is commonly used to irrigate the eye and may also be used on oral and other mucous membranes. It is important to ensure the correct antiseptic solution is used; lathering scrub solutions must not be used as these will cause irritation.

- Corneal surfaces: 1:50 dilution (10 ml of povidone–iodine aqueous 10% solution w/w in 500 ml of sterile saline) to give a 0.2% povidone–iodine solution.
- Lids and surrounding skin: 1:10 dilution (50 ml of povidone–iodine aqueous 10% solution w/w in 500 ml of sterile saline) to give a 1% povidone–iodine solution.

The povidone–iodine antiseptic solution should be mixed with sterile saline, although compound sodium lactate or distilled water can be used. Tap water should not be used as it contains compounds that may react and reduce efficacy. Once made up the bottle should be labelled and dated. Although there is no evidence to support how long these preparations can be kept for, it would seem sensible for them to be replaced weekly. This includes discarding the bottle and making a fresh solution in a new bottle, to prevent colonization of the bottle.

Povidone–iodine is not effective in the presence of organic material, and so any debris or ocular discharge must be removed prior to preparing for surgery.

Care must be taken if there is a risk of the eye being perforated, for example, due to a deep ulcer, corneal foreign body or corneal laceration. For these cases, only saline or a balanced salt solution should be used to prevent the povidone–iodine entering the structures of the eye and causing damage.

Chlorhexidine solutions have been shown to be more irritant to the surface of the cornea. Alcohol-based solutions should not be used on this sensitive tissue.

Some surgeons do not advocate clipping around the eye for intraocular surgery but instead use adhesive drapes to protect the eye from the hair and skin. Others prefer to clip a minimal amount of hair around the eye. A water-soluble gel can be applied to the hair and into the eye prior to clipping. Using clippers with a narrow fine blade will help to prevent hair being introduced into the eye. The skin around the eye is extremely thin and sensitive, and so it is important that the clippers are in good order and great care is taken when clipping.

The eye should then be irrigated several times with saline to wash away any loose hair and remaining lubricant before irrigating with a dilute povidone–iodine antiseptic solution. Sterile cotton buds soaked in dilute povidone–iodine can be used very gently to clean inside the eyelids, taking great care not to rub these on the corneal surface. The skin surrounding the eye should also be prepared with dilute povidone–iodine.

For bilateral procedures each eye must be prepared just prior to the surgery, as the ongoing activity is short. Water-soluble lubricating gel should be placed on the other eye to prevent it drying out; this should be removed prior to preparing the second eye for surgery.

Positioning the patient for surgery

Patients should ideally be moved into the theatre on a stretcher or trolley ready to be safely positioned on the theatre table (see also Chapters 2, 21 and 23). It is important to adopt the correct manual handling techniques when moving patients to prevent injury to both the patient and the handler.

Most surgeons have individual preferences with regard to positioning of the patient for surgery, but there are some standard positions for specific operations. The veterinary nurse should be familiar with positioning for different surgical techniques and individual variations. When there is any doubt, the nurse should check well in advance of surgery.

Some operating tables have adjustable sides and tilting facilities that assist in positioning the patient. If not, the use of additional restraining aids such as troughs, sandbags and tapes will be necessary. Care should be taken to avoid placing heavy sandbags over the limbs or tying tapes tightly, as this could occlude blood supply to the area or result in peripheral nerve damage. Raising the limb and securing it with a tie on a fluid stand for a period of time before surgery (see Figure 22.12), for example during the preparation process, may be useful for patients with fractures. This will help with muscle contracture and may help the surgeon to reduce the fracture more easily.

Preparation of the surgical team
Theatre attire

To maintain asepsis, all those involved in the surgery should change from their ordinary clothes into correct theatre attire before entering the operating theatre suite (see Figure 22.2).

- Theatre wear, which should be worn only within the theatre suite, usually consists of a simple two-piece **scrub suit**. A clean laundered suit should be worn each day, and theatre clothing should be changed more frequently if it becomes contaminated. Scrub suits are worn to decrease the shedding of bacteria into the operating room environment.

- Theatre **footwear** should be antistatic and has traditionally consisted of white clogs. These have the advantage of being easy to clean. All footwear should be wiped over with a disinfectant at the end of the day; plastic or rubber footwear can be more thoroughly cleaned in a washing machine and some theatre shoes may be autoclaved. Plastic overshoes are available that fit over normal shoes, but they are not recommended since they wear through in a very short time and the bacterial load on the hands of the person wearing overshoes is higher as they repeatedly take them on and off.
- All personnel should wear a **theatre cap** before entering the theatre suite. All hair should be neatly tucked away inside the hat. To accommodate longer hairstyles and beards, various styles of **headwear** are available. These are usually disposable and paper-based.
- The purpose of **masks** is, in theory, to filter expired air from the nose and stop droplet shedding in order to prevent the transmission of microorganisms from the surgical team to the patient. There is no evidence to show they are effective filters; however, they do provide a barrier for things leaving the nose and mouth and entering the surgical wound (Lipp and Edwards, 2014). Masks should be changed between surgical cases. Conversation should be kept to a minimum to avoid moisture, which can lead to a decrease in mask efficacy.

Scrubbing up

Preoperative scrubbing up is a systematic washing and scrubbing of the hands and arms, which is performed by all members of the surgical team before each operation. As it is not possible to sterilize the skin, the aim of the scrubbing-up routine is to destroy as many microorganisms on the surface of the arms and hands as possible, prior to donning a sterile surgical gown and gloves.

Many different scrub routines have been described and no single technique is necessarily better than another. It is recommended that one of the tried and tested regimes is adopted and adhered to strictly.

The scrubbing procedure should take between 5 and 10 minutes: the clock should be checked at the start of the first stage and again at the start of the final stage, to ensure that the procedure has not been rushed and sufficient contact time with the surgical scrub solution has been allowed.

Before scrubbing up, fingernails should be cut short and any nail varnish removed.

Putting on a surgical gown

There are two different types of gown: back-tie and side-tie. The technique for putting on the gown is similar for both, with slight variations (Figure 22.7).

Example of a scrub routine

1. Remove watch and jewellery.
2. Adjust the water supply (which should be elbow- or foot-operated) to a suitable temperature and flow.
3. Wash the hands thoroughly using an antimicrobial soap, adopting a good hand washing technique (see Chapter 7). At this stage, clean the nails using a nail pick.
4. Once the hands have been washed, wash the arms up to the elbows. Always keep the hands higher than the elbows so that water drains down towards the unscrubbed upper arms. The purpose of this stage of the procedure is to remove organic matter and grease from the skin.
5. Rinse the hands and then the lower arms, allowing water to wash away the soap from the hands towards the elbows.
6. Using a surgical scrub solution begin the surgical scrub. Use only sufficient water to produce a lather, as bactericidal properties of the scrub solution are dependent on contact time with the skin. Excessive amounts of water will rinse away the scrub solution before it has achieved its aim.
7. Lather the surgical scrub solution over the arms before scrubbing the hands. Take a sterile scrubbing brush and systematically scrub the hands. Scrub the palms of the hand, wrist and four surfaces of each finger and thumb (back, front and both sides) and the nails. Either rinse the brush and use it on the other hand or discard it and take a second brush. It is not recommended that the backs of the hands and arms are scrubbed as this may lead to excoriation, which predisposes to infection.
8. When both hands have been scrubbed for the correct contact time, drop the brush into the sink. Begin to rinse the hands and arms as before, ensuring that the hands are constantly kept above the elbows to allow the water to drain away from the hands and off the elbows.
9. The final stage is to wash the hands and wrists in surgical scrub solution. This time the scrubbing process is not extended to the elbow, so that there is no danger that a previously unscrubbed area is touched.
10. Rinse the hands and arms as before.
11. Take a sterile hand towel, holding it at arm's length. Use a different quarter to dry each hand and each arm. Then discard the hand towel.

IMPORTANT NOTE
Once the scrubbing up routine has started, the hands must not touch the taps, sink or scrub dispenser. If these are inadvertently touched, the process must start again at Step 3.

A waterless surgical hand preparation, which involves the use of an alcohol-based solution, is an alternative to chlorhexidine scrub solutions. These solutions are applied using a hand rubbing technique and do not require a scrub brush or water. The recommended protocol may vary according to manufacturer's guidelines, but the majority will provide surgical hand preparation within 1.5–2 minutes, allowing a much faster preparation time compared with the more traditional scrubbing method.

→

Example of a scrub routine *continued*

Scrub routine for alcohol hand solution:

1. Wash hands with a pH neutral detergent to remove gross contamination (see Chapter 7). Dry thoroughly with paper towels (non-sterile).
2. Apply the alcohol-based solution to the hands and arms, up to the elbow. Use enough for good coverage of the whole area.
3. For the first 30 seconds, the alcohol solution is applied up to the elbows; it is important that the areas remain wet with solution. For the second 30 seconds application is only up to the wrists, and for the final 30 seconds the solution is only rubbed into the hands. Care needs to be taken to include the nail beds.
4. Rub the solution into the hands until they are dry. Do not remove any of the solution with a towel or place a gown whilst the hands are still damp.

This method is not a substitute for good hand hygiene, and some basic rules must be followed in order for it to work correctly. Gross contamination must be removed from the hands prior to scrubbing, preferably with a pH neutral soap. Many people find the health of the skin of their hands improves when using this method.

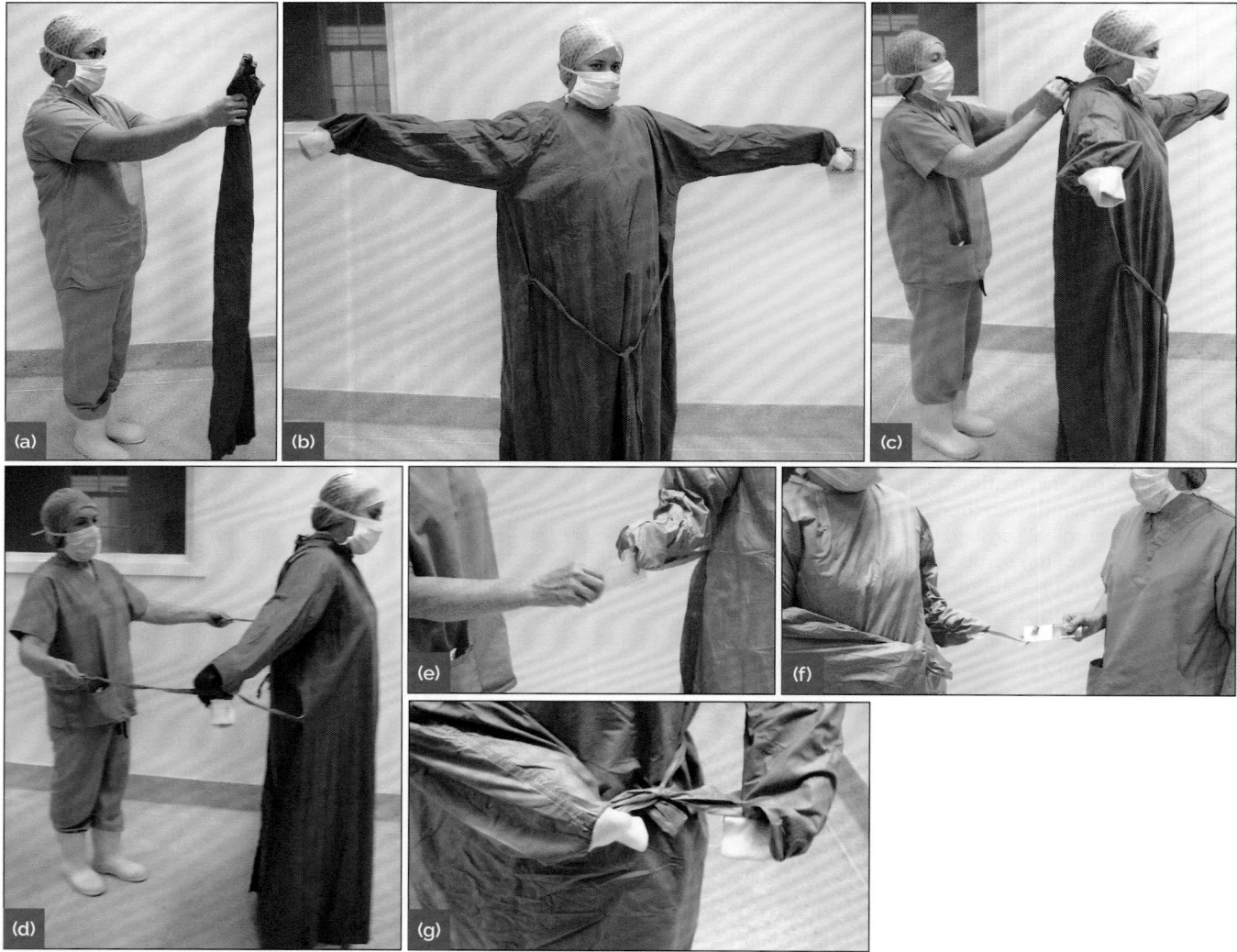

22.7 Putting on a sterile gown. **(a)** The sterile gown (folded inside out) is taken from its sterile pack, held at the shoulders and allowed to fall open. **(b)** One hand is slipped into each sleeve. No attempt should be made to try to pull the sleeves over the shoulder or to readjust the gown, as this will lead to contamination of the hands or outside of the gown. **(c)** An unscrubbed assistant should pull the back of the gown over the shoulders (touching only the inside surface of the gown) and secure the ties at the back. **(d)** With the hands retained within the sleeves, the waist ties should be picked up and held out to the sides. In the case of a **back-tying gown**, the unscrubbed assistant will then take the ends of the waist ties and secure them at the back. The back of the gown is now no longer sterile and must not come into contact with sterile equipment, drapes and gowns. **(e)** In the case of a **side-tying gown**, the unscrubbed assistant takes hold of the paper tape on the longer waist tape and takes the tie around the back to the opposite side. **(f)** The scrubbed person then pulls the tape, so that the paper tape comes away. **(g)** The gown is tied at the waist by the scrubbed person. This type of gown provides an all-round sterile field.

Putting on surgical gloves

Two methods are available: closed gloving and open gloving.

Closed gloving

The hands are kept inside the sleeves of the gown while gloving takes place. The outside of the gown never comes into contact with the hands. This technique has the advantage that it minimizes the chances of contaminating the gloves, since the outside of the gloves do not contact the skin. This method of gloving should be used for all surgical operations, to ensure a high level of asepsis is maintained throughout.

Closed gloving procedure

1. Hands remain within the sleeves of the gown. The glove packet is turned so that the fingers point towards the body. (The right glove will now be on the left and *vice versa*.)
2. The glove is picked up at the rim of the cuff of the glove.
3. The hand is turned over so that the glove lies on the palm surface with fingers of the glove still pointing towards the body.
4. The rim is picked up with the opposite hand.
5. It is then pulled over the fingers and over the dorsal surface of the wrist.
6. The glove is then pulled on as the fingers are pushed forwards.

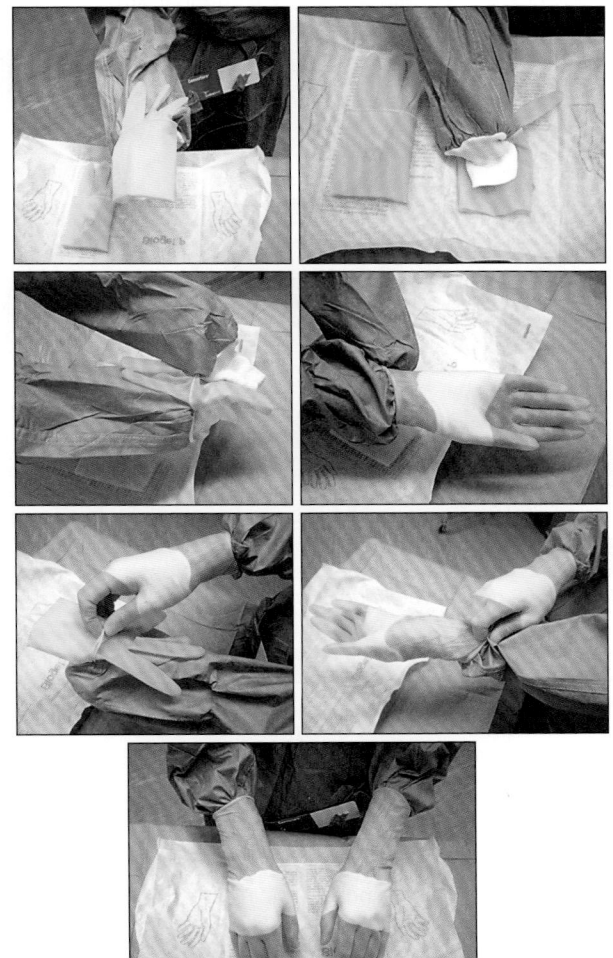

Open gloving

This method of gloving is used when only the hands need to be covered and is not routinely used for gloving and gowning. The technique has the disadvantage that the gloves are relatively easily contaminated by skin contact.

Open gloving is used for the following procedures:

- Jugular catheter placement
- Urinary catheter placement
- Administration of local blocks and epidurals
- Oesophagostomy and pharyngostomy feeding tube placement
- Draining any thoracic, abdominal or wound drains.

Open gloving procedure

1. The glove pack is opened by an assistant.
2. With the left hand, the right glove is picked up by the turned-down cuff, holding only the inner surface of the glove.
3. The glove is pulled on to the right hand. Do not unfold the cuff at this stage.
4. The gloved fingers of the right hand are placed under the cuff of the left glove and pulled on to the left hand, holding only the outer surface of this glove.
5. The rim of the left glove is hooked over the thumb whilst the cuff of the gown (if worn) is adjusted.
6. The cuff of the left glove is pulled over the cuff of the gown (if worn) using the fingers of the right hand.
7. The final steps are then repeated for the right hand.

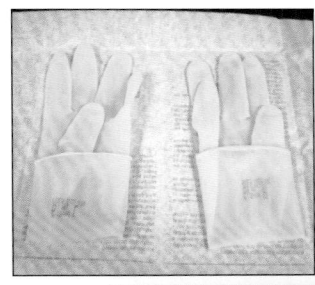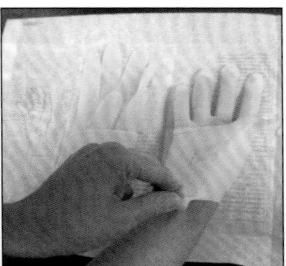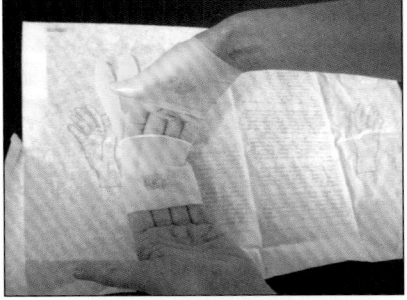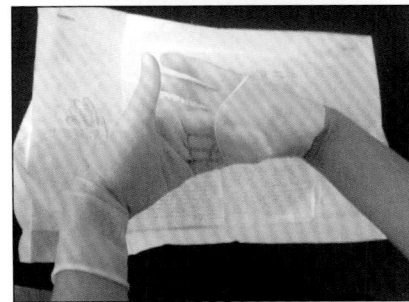

Draping the patient

Draping the patient aims to maintain asepsis by preventing contamination of the surgical site from the hair and the immediate environment. Drapes must therefore cover the entire patient and operating table, leaving only the surgical site exposed.

Types of drape

Drapes may be disposable or reusable. Ideally, disposable drapes should be used in preference to reusable material drapes as they have many advantages. The relative advantages of each type are shown in Figure 22.8.

Disposable drapes

There are many different varieties available. Disposable drapes are usually paper-based and water-repellent and can be purchased pre-sterilized. Cheaper varieties tend to be non-conforming and may tear easily. Many commercial brands are of high quality, and are affordable. Their use is highly recommended for all surgical procedures. Adhesive edges are useful for draping difficult areas. Good disposable drapes tend to be more conformable than cotton drapes and the high water resistance prevents bacterial strike-through. They also help maintain body temperature during surgery.

Reusable drapes

These are usually made from linen or cotton/polyester mixes. They may be custom-made to suit practice needs. Their main disadvantage is the higher risk of strike-through when wet and thus increased risk of break in aseptic technique. This type of drape may appear to be more cost effective than disposables, but the initial cost and the expense of laundering and re-sterilizing after each use needs to be taken into consideration. Each drape is designed to be used a limited number of times, and some manufacturers print a grid in the corner of an item to record when it is used and indicate when it should be discarded. Laundering of reusable items with washing detergents also reduces the function of the drape to prevent penetration of bacteria. In veterinary medicine these items are often reused too many times.

Draping the surgical site

Plain drapes

Four rectangular drapes are used to create a 'window' (fenestration) for the surgical site (Figure 22.9). The fenestration created can be of any size. The first drape should be placed

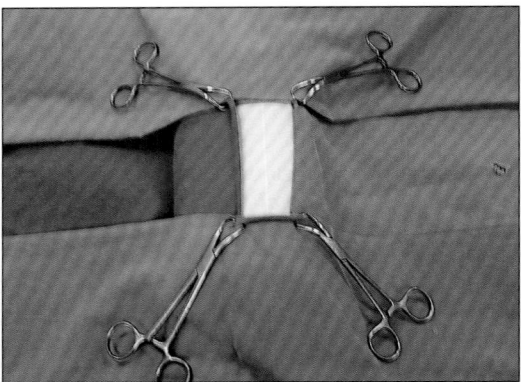

22.9 Draping the surgical site. Plain drapes are first placed longitudinally on both sides of the operating table. More drapes are then placed over each end and secured by towel clips.

between the surgeon and the near side of the table. A drape is then placed over the opposite side of the patient (i.e. away from the surgeon). Drapes are subsequently placed over both ends. They are then secured in place using towel clips.

Fenestrated drapes

Fenestrated drapes achieve the same effect as the plain drapes in leaving a surgery window, but the window is already formed in a single ready-made drape (Figure 22.10). Fenestrated drapes can be large enough to cover the entire animal and table top. A selection of different-sized fenestrations is needed to cater for different surgical sites.

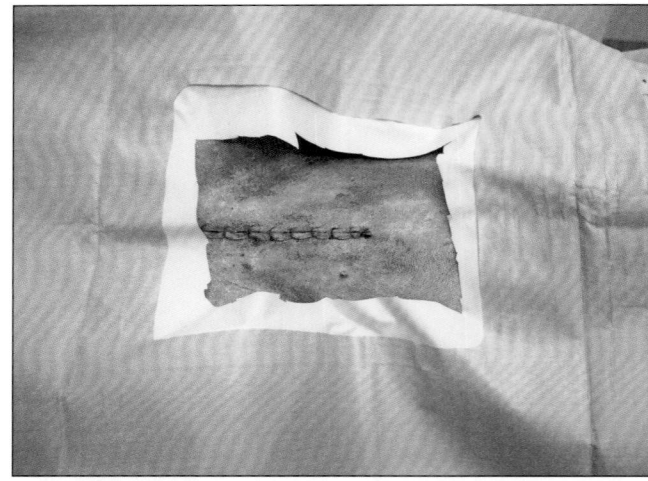

22.10 A patient draped with a disposable adhesive fenestrated drape. (Reproduced from the *BSAVA Manual of Practical Veterinary Nursing*)

Type of drape	Advantages	Disadvantages
Disposable	■ Labour-saving ■ Less laundry ■ Pre-sterilized ■ Usually very water-repellent ■ Always in perfect condition ■ Cost of drape charged to client	■ Initial outlay more expensive ■ Cheaper brands can be less conforming ■ Large stock needed
Reusable drapes	■ Cheaper, although cost of laundering needs to be considered	■ Porous; all fluids leak through, leading to a break in asepsis ■ Time-consuming; washing and folding ■ Danger of threads detaching and gaining access to wounds ■ After repeated use quality becomes poor

22.8 Advantages and disadvantages of disposable and reusable drapes.

Adhesive 'barrier' drapes

Sterile, clear, adhesive plastic sheets are sometimes placed over the surgical site (Figure 22.11). Standard drapes are applied in the usual way, and the adhesive drape is then placed over the skin and the entire draped fenestration. The skin incision is made through the adhesive material. These are particularly useful as they ensure a high level of aseptic technique is maintained, as the patient's skin is completely covered by the drape and is therefore not touched by the surgical team. This type of drape is also completely water-resistant and helps to keep the patient dry during the surgical procedure. This is particularly useful when large volumes of fluid are required for lavage.

Draping limbs

There are various ways of draping a limb for surgery, one of which is shown in Figure 22.12.

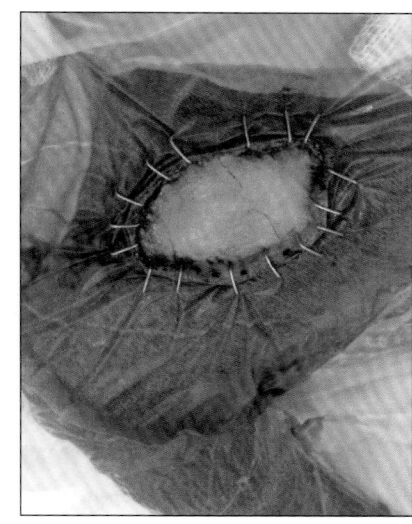

22.11 An adhesive drape can be further secured to the skin using either skin staples or monofilament suture material to prevent inadvertent lifting of the drape and exposure of the adjacent skin. (Reproduced from the *BSAVA Manual of Canine and Feline Musculoskeletal Disorders, 2nd edn*)

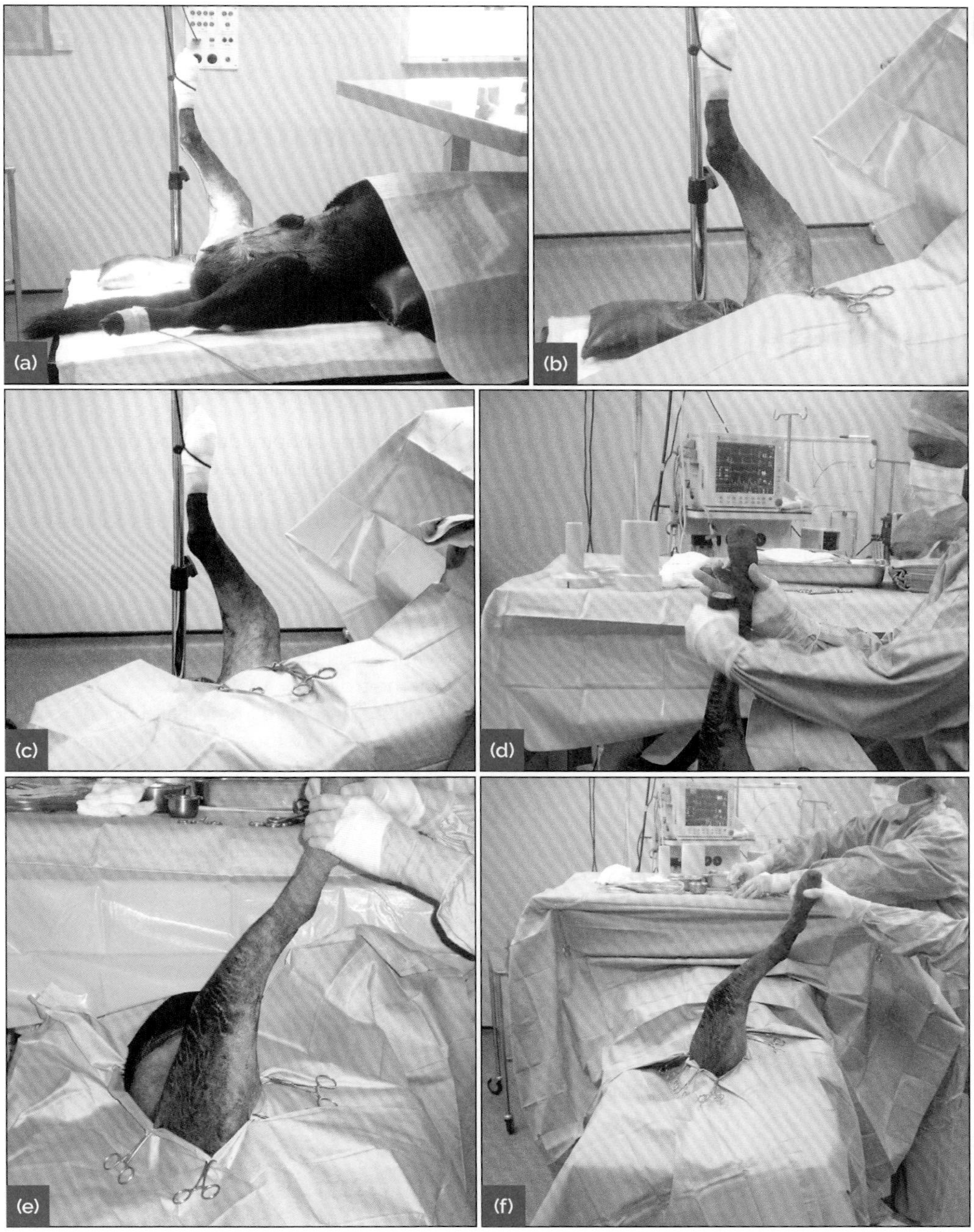

22.12 Draping a limb for surgery. **(a)** The patient lies on the operating table with the limb suspended using a tie and transfusion stand. The patient is then prepared for surgery. **(b)** The instrument trolley is covered and the first drape is placed between the surgeon and the operating table. **(c)** A second drape is placed over the end of the table. **(d)** The surgeon then wraps the foot with sterile cohesive bandage. **(e)** The scrubbed assistant then continues to suspend the limb by holding the foot on the draped side of the table. A third drape is placed on the far side of the table. **(f)** The final drape is placed between the limb and the instrument trolley.

Sub-draping

Additional towels are sometimes used to protect the incision site from contamination. They are applied to each side of the incision by towel clips. The towel is then folded back over the towel clips.

Surgical assistance

The theatre nurse has two main roles: as a circulating nurse and as a scrubbed nurse.

- A **circulating nurse** has not scrubbed up with the surgical team.
- A **scrubbed nurse** has scrubbed up for surgery and wears sterile theatre clothing so that they can work within the operative field and assist the veterinary surgeon.

Duties of a circulating nurse

- Helping to prepare theatre, instruments and equipment for surgery
- Helping to position the patient on the table
- Preparation of the surgical site
- Tying the surgical team into gowns
- Connecting the apparatus (diathermy, suction, airlines, etc.)
- Opening packs of sutures, instruments, etc.
- Counting swabs, sutures, etc. with the scrubbed nurse
- Noting the time of critical surgical activities (e.g. noting that a tourniquet was applied and should be removed)
- Being in theatre at all times when surgery is in progress
- Assisting the anaesthetist
- Preparing postoperative dressings
- Helping to move the patient to recovery
- Helping to clear theatre at the end of surgery
- Recording counts and maintaining patient records during surgery

---

Scrubbed nurse

The role of the scrubbed nurse is an extremely important one and requires rigid adherence to a set of rules. It is very easy to make mistakes if corners are cut or changes made. It is important that the nurse possesses knowledge of the surgical procedure that is to be performed, so that the needs of the surgeon can be anticipated.

- It is essential to know exactly what instruments and equipment are on the trolley at the start and throughout surgery.
- All swabs, sutures, needles, etc., must be counted before surgery begins and again before the wound is closed, to prevent any items being accidentally left within a wound cavity.
- The nurse should watch the operation carefully in order to anticipate the surgeon's needs.
- Instruments should be passed to the surgeon so that they are ready to be used, i.e. not upside down.

- Instruments should be returned to the same place on the trolley each time so that the nurse knows exactly where they are. They should not be left around the surgical site, because they are likely to fall on the floor and because they will not be immediately to hand when needed.
- Instruments should be wiped over with a swab when they are returned to the trolley.
- Only one swab should be given to the surgeon at any time and the nurse must keep a constant check on the number of swabs used.
- Swabs should be applied firmly to a bleeding site, without wiping across the tissue, which may both damage the tissue and disturb a clot.
- All tissues should be handled gently to avoid trauma. Viscera in particular should be handled very carefully.
- One of the nurse's roles may be to irrigate the tissues with warmed sterile saline to prevent desiccation, particularly during long operations.
- For long surgical procedures surgical gloves may need to be replaced.
- On completion of surgery, the nurse should ensure that all instruments, needles and swabs are returned to the trolley and that needles, blades and glassware are disposed of safely.

Preparing an instrument trolley

An instrument trolley is made from stainless steel and is used as either a dressing or surgical instrument trolley. The Mayo trolley is a type of instrument trolley with a tray that is removable for cleaning, is height adjustable and pivots. The framework of this trolley is normally mounted on four swivel brake castors.

Surgical instruments may be laid out on instrument trolleys, for use during surgery (Figure 22.13). A disposable water-resilient plastic drape should ideally be used to cover the trolley first; these can be purchased relatively cheaply and are available pre-sterilized. Should pre-packed plastic trolley drapes not be available, reusable drapes can be used but, due to the higher risk of bacterial strikethrough, the top of the metal instrument trolley must first be covered with a waterproof sterile drape. Instrument sets may be packed in trays, complete with drapes, swabs, blades, etc.; in these cases, the outer wrappings of the set can be unfolded to cover the surface of the trolley.

The trolley should be prepared immediately prior to use. The longer the instruments are exposed to air, the greater the chance of contamination from the environment or personnel.

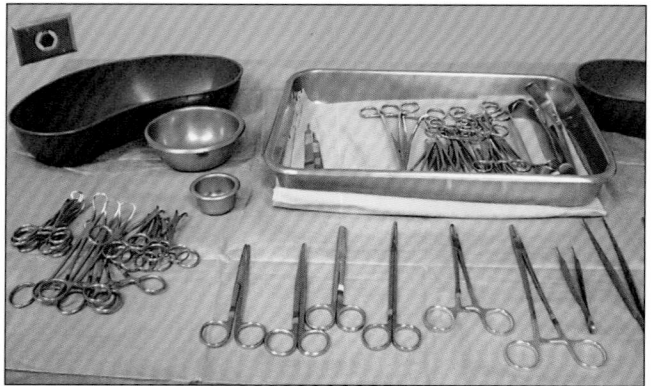

22.13 Instruments laid out on an instrument trolley, ready for use.

If there is a delay once the trolley has been laid out, a sterile drape should be placed over the top.

- Trolleys can be prepared by a scrubbed nurse at the beginning of a procedure, allowing the surgeon to scrub and gown, and drape the patient in the meantime.
- Alternatively, a circulating nurse can lay out the instruments on the trolley using sterile Cheatle forceps. This is not the preferred method, however, as there is greater risk of the trolley becoming contaminated, as the circulating nurse is not sterile and would be leaning over the sterile draped surface to open instruments.

Surgical safety checklist

The surgical safety checklist has been incorporated in many veterinary operating theatres. Guidelines from the World Health Organization (WHO) provide examples and can be used to create a checklist relevant to the practice (www.who.int/patientsafety/safesurgery/checklist/en/; Figure 22.14; see also Chapter 21). The checklists are split into preoperative and postoperative sections and are used to introduce the team, record items opened on to the instrument trolley to ensure the correct numbers are there at the end of the procedure, record any anticipated critical events and discuss any concerns relating to the patient. For some practices, where the team numbers are minimal, it may seem not of value, but the philosophy is to carry out the same procedure every time to ensure that the time you do need the information it is available.

The preoperative checklist is read out and completed by the circulating nurse, after draping but prior to the first incision. It is important that all members of the team stop completely for this brief period of time for full concentration. Any anticipated critical events can be discussed and a plan made for what to do in these situations.

Care of the patient during surgery

It is important to remember that underneath the drapes there is a live patient. Care must be taken by the surgical team to avoid leaning on the animal's chest, which may compromise breathing in a small patient. Careful positioning of towel clips is important to avoid delicate structures such as the eye, which cannot be seen once drapes have been placed.

Attention should be paid to the conservation of heat, especially in the small or very young. Warming devices should ideally be used in all anaesthetized patients (see Chapter 21); 'Bair Hugger' (3M™) warming units work well by circulating warm air close to the patient via a blanket (Figure 22.15). Insulation (e.g. bubble wrap) is useful, particularly around peripheral limbs and the tail, and warmed intravenous and irrigation fluids should be encouraged. Direct

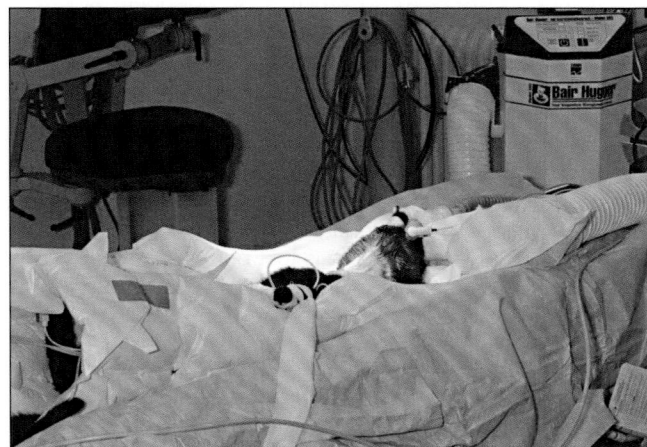

22.15 Warm air units, such as this Bair Hugger (3M™), may be used to keep the patient warm during surgery.

Before anaesthesia	**Before surgical incision**	**Before leaving theatre**
(at least nurse)	*(all theatre staff)*	*(at least surgeon and nurse)*
Confirm: ❑ Patient identity ❑ Procedure ❑ Consent form signed **Check:** ❑ Medications given ❑ Anaesthetic machine ❑ Axillary surgical equipment ❑ Instruments sterilized	❑ **Team have introduced themselves** **Confirm:** ❑ Patient identity ❑ Procedure ❑ Suitability of clip ❑ Bladder empty (abdominal operations) ❑ Specific preoperative preparations ❑ Antibiosis if required ❑ Other perioperative medication **Anticipated critical steps** **Surgeon:** ❑ What are the critical steps? ❑ Anticipated time to completion **Anaesthetist/nurse:** ❑ Anaesthetic specific concerns **Nurse/surgical assistant:** ❑ Sterility of instruments ❑ Any equipment concerns ❑ Essential radiographs displayed	**Nurse verbally confirms:** ❑ Swab count ❑ Sharps accounted for ❑ Specimen labelling *(read aloud)* ❑ Any equipment issues to be addressed **What are the key concerns for recovery and postoperative management?** **Specific medication and care** **Notes:** *(turn over if needed)*
Date: Signed:		

22.14 Veterinary surgery safety checklist, modified form the World Health Organization (WHO) surgical safety checklist. (© Romain Pizzi, Zoological Medicine Ltd)

heat (e.g. hot water bottles) should be avoided during both surgery and recovery periods, as the unconscious animal cannot move away if this is too hot. Serious burns can occur, which will not become apparent until the postoperative period.

Careful positioning of the animal on the table (see above) is also important, to avoid postoperative complications. The patient's core temperature should also be monitored throughout the surgical procedure (see Chapter 21). Other intraoperative care is described in Chapter 23.

Care of the postoperative patient

The patient should not be left unattended until it is conscious. The endotracheal tube is usually removed just before the cough reflex returns (see Chapter 21). The animal should be watched closely to ensure that an adequate airway is maintained once the tube has been removed, especially in brachycephalic breeds or following airway surgery. Cats should be observed closely for any signs of laryngospasm following endotracheal tube removal. A source of oxygen and a means of ventilation should be available during this time in case of any problems. Colour of the mucous membranes and the presence or absence of respiratory noise and effort will be indicators of effective ventilation by the animal. The ability to maintain body temperature is lost under anaesthesia and so steps should be taken to prevent or reverse hypothermia.

The use of checklists improves the management of postoperative complications by providing a standardized, evidence-based approach to various clinical scenarios. They also improve communication and teamwork within the multidisciplinary team.

As these improvements were observed in a simulated environment, clinical implementation studies are required to validate the results.

Haemorrhage

During recovery, the patient should be observed for signs of external haemorrhage (which is usually obvious) or internal haemorrhage (signs of shock).

Recognition of pain

It is important to be able to recognize when an animal is in pain (see Chapter 21). The nurse should obtain instructions from the veterinary surgeon regarding postoperative analgesia.

Application of dressings or casts

Many surgical procedures require a dressing to be placed postoperatively to prevent self-trauma and contamination of the wound to or from the local environment. Wounds should be cleaned with sterile swabs and saline by a member of the team with clean gloves. Any chest drains, feeding tubes or catheters should be dressed and bandaged before the patient is recovered (see Chapters 13, 15 and 20).

Many orthopaedic and some soft tissue cases require postoperative bandages or casts (see Chapter 15). Bandages should be applied before the animal regains consciousness; however, casts are not usually applied until 24–48 hours after surgery. A bandage is placed for this time to allow postoperative swelling to reduce. Due to the restrictive nature of the cast when the limb swells in the initial postoperative period,

if the cast is placed immediately pressure necrosis could occur. Care should be taken not to apply bandages too tightly (especially head and ear dressings). Bandages should be checked again once the patient is awake and in a normal upright position, as a change in position may make the bandage too tight or too loose.

Comfort

- Make sure that the animal has comfortable bedding (see Chapter 14), especially orthopaedic patients.
- Turn the animal regularly if it is disinclined or unable to turn over by itself.
- Give opportunities for the animal to urinate, or empty the bladder manually if necessary.
- Do not forget to offer food and drink if this is allowed, especially in young and old patients and those that are unable to move easily around the kennel.
- Make sure the area is quiet and warm but that the animal is well observed to monitor for signs of pain, shock, respiratory distress, etc.

See also Chapter 14 for information on general patient care.

Instrumentation

The cost of good quality surgical instruments is extremely high, but they will last for years if handled correctly, whereas cheaper instruments of poor quality will require early replacement.

- **Stainless steel** is the material of choice for most surgical instruments. It combines high resistance to corrosion with great strength and it has an attractive surface finish.
- **Tungsten carbide** inserts are often added to the tips of stainless steel instruments that are used for cutting or gripping, such as scissors and needle-holders. They are very hard and resistant to wear but tend to be expensive. Instruments with tungsten carbide inserts are often identified by their gold-coloured handles.
- **Chromium-plated carbon steel** surgical instruments are commonly used in veterinary practice because they are lower in price. However, they will rust, pit and blister when in contact with chemicals and saline and they tend to blunt quickly.
- **Titanium** is used in instruments for ophthalmic surgery. These instruments need to be handled delicately around the eye and are therefore much lighter in weight. Some ophthalmic surgery requires the use of an operating microscope; titanium instruments reduce the glare produced from the microscope light, allowing the surgeon to have increased visibility during the procedure.

Instrument sets

Instrument sets are made up to suit individual requirements and they vary from one veterinary practice to another. Some practices have sets for specific procedures (e.g. bitch spay set). Others have a standard instrument set that is used for all operations, to which other instruments will be added depending on the procedure. Often a smaller set will be available for minor procedures such as a cat spay.

It is important that each of the standard instrument sets contains the same number and type of instruments so that the surgical team always knows what instruments they will have and so that it is easy to check that all are present at the end of the procedure. Instrument sets can be colour-coded by application of a piece of instrument identification adhesive tape. Figures 22.16 to 22.19 list suggested contents for various instrument sets required for soft tissue, orthopaedic and ophthalmic surgery, but these are only guidelines. Dental instruments are described in Chapter 25.

Instrument/equipment	Quantity
Scalpel handle No. 3	1
Dissecting forceps: ■ Rat-toothed fine (Adson) ■ Rat-toothed heavy ■ Dressing forceps (Debakey)	 1 1 1
Mayo scissors – straight or curved	1
Metzenbaum scissors	1
Artery forceps	10
Mosquito forceps	5
Allis tissue forceps	4
Suture scissors	1
Needle holders	1
Langenbeck retractors	2
Gelpi retractors	2
Backhaus towel-holding forceps	10
Poole suction tip	1
Gallipot	1
Kidney bowl	2
Swabs (radiopaque) 10 cm x 10 cm	10
Additional instruments and equipment that may be required for general surgery	
Monopolar electrocautery handpiece	1
Scalpel blades No. 10 and/or No. 15	1 of each
Suction tubing	1

22.16 Standard instrument set.

Abdominal surgery
- Self-retaining retractors
- Doyen's bowel clamps
- Long dissecting forceps
- Long artery forceps (e.g. Roberts)
- Towels to pack abdomen

Thoracic surgery
- Rib cutters
- Finochietto rib retractors
- Periosteal elevator
- Chest drain
- Suture wire
- Oscillating saw if sternotomy approach
- Lobectomy clamps
- Long-handled artery forceps (e.g. Roberts)
- Rib raspatory (e.g. Doyen)

22.17 Additional instruments required for abdominal and thoracic surgery.

Type of equipment	Equipment list
General	Osteotome; Gigli wire and handles; chisel; periosteal elevator; curette; hand drill; mallet; Hohmann retractor; hacksaw; rasp; bone rongeurs; bone holding forceps; Lister's bone cutting forceps
Power tools	Battery drill; air drill; mechanical burr; oscillating saw
Implants	Stainless steel wire; intramedullary pins; Kirschner wires; screws; plates
Bone pinning	Jacobs chuck and key; Steinmann pins; Kirschner wires; pin cutters
Wire fixation	Stainless steel wire (cerclage); wire holding forceps; wire twisters; wire cutters
External fixator	Steinmann pins; ESF connecting bars; ESF clamps; drill or Jacobs chuck; positive profile pins; pin cutters
Bone plating or screw fixation	Bone plates (DCPs/LCPs), cuttable plates, SOP plates); drill bit; air/battery drill; depth gauge; cortical tap; screw driver; plate bender; cortical screws
Association for the Study of Internal Fixation (ASIF) technique	DCPs; LCPs; cortical screws: self-tapping or locking cortical screws; air/battery powered drills; drill bits; drill guides: neutral and loaded; cortical bone tap; tap sleeve and handle; drill insert; depth gauge; countersink; screwdriver; plate bending irons

22.18 Additional instruments required for orthopaedic surgery. DCP = dynamic compression plate; ESF = external skeletal fixation; LCP = locking compression plate; SOP = string-of-pearls.

Equipment
- No. 3 scalpel handle
- Scalpel blade sizes 11, 15 or Beaver handle and blades
- Fine dissecting forceps
- Fine scissors
- Corneal scissors
- Capsule forceps
- Vectis
- Iris repository
- Castroviejo needle-holders
- Eyelid speculum
- Irrigating cannula
- Distichiasis forceps

22.19 Additional instruments required for ophthalmic surgery.

General surgical instruments

There is a wide variety of different surgical instruments available. Veterinary nurses are not expected to be familiar with them all, but a broad knowledge of the names and appearances of the general instruments can be gained by reference to manuals and catalogues.

Scalpel

The scalpel is the best instrument for dividing tissue with minimal trauma. Usually scalpel handles with interchangeable disposable blades are used (Figure 22.20). A size 3 handle is commonly used for small animal surgery with blade sizes 10, 11, 12 and 15. A size 4 handle is used for large animal surgery with blade sizes 20, 21 and 22. The primary

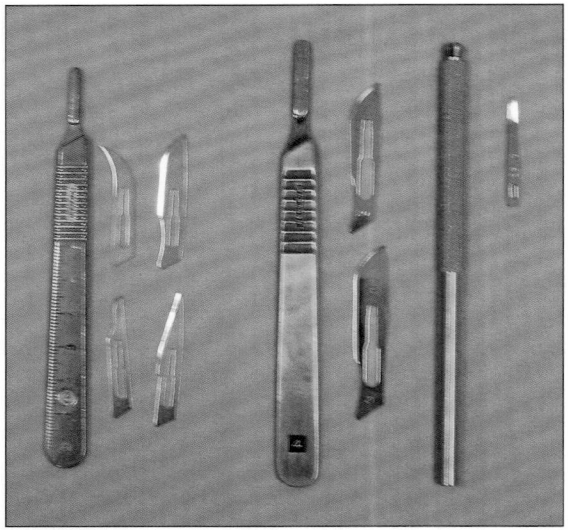

22.20 Scalpel handles and blades. From left to right: size 3 handles and sizes 10, 11, 12 and 15 blades; size 4 handle and sizes 21 and 20 blades; Beaver handle with one blade.

advantage of disposable blades is consistent sharpness. A scalpel with a blade and handle as a disposable package is available, as is a small, rounded (Beaver) handle with smaller disposable blades, which has gained popularity with ophthalmic surgeons.

Dissecting forceps

These are commonly referred to as thumb forceps (Figure 22.21) and are designed to hold tissue. They have a spring action and the jaws are opposed by holding the metal blades together. They may have plain or toothed ends. Generally, forceps with plain ends are used for handling delicate tissues such as viscera, whilst toothed forceps are used for denser tissues. Dissecting forceps should be held like a pencil.

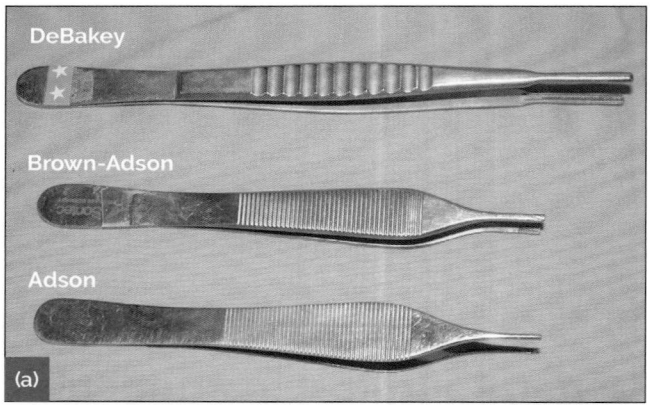

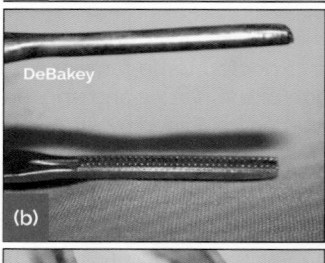

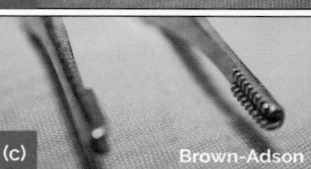

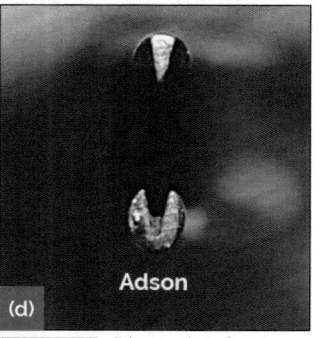

22.21 Dissecting forceps. (a) Thumb forceps. (b–d) Details of tips.

Scissors

Operating scissors are available in various lengths and shapes (Figure 22.22). Mayo dissecting scissors are commonly used for routine surgery; the finer, long-handled Metzenbaum scissors tend to be used for more delicate work. Special suture scissors (e.g. Carless scissors) should be used for cutting sutures to prevent unnecessary blunting of dissecting scissors. For removal of sutures, Payne's scissors are used. These are small and curved with the cutting surface of one blade hollowed out to fit under the suture easily. Scissors should be held with the ring finger and thumb inserted in the ring of the scissor and the index finger placed on the shaft to guide the scissors.

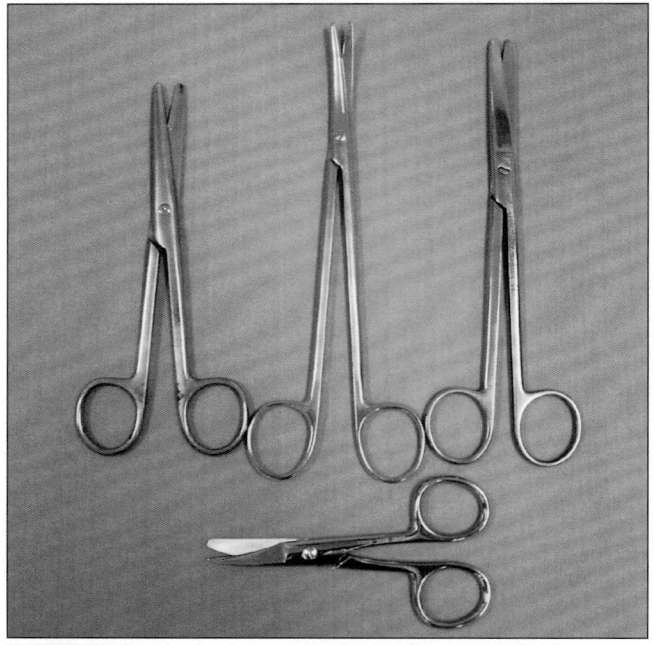

22.22 Surgical scissors. Clockwise from top left: Mayo; Metzenbaum; Carless suture-cutting; Payne's suture removal scissors.

Haemostatic or artery forceps

Artery forceps (Figure 22.23) are designed to clamp blood vessels and thus stop bleeding. They come in several different lengths and shapes. Most have transverse striations to facilitate holding tissue. There are many different patterns of artery forceps. Some of those commonly used include the Spencer Wells, Dunhill, Crile's, Cairn's and Kelly. Mosquito forceps are very small artery forceps for finer blood vessels, the most common type being the Halsted forceps. Like scissors, artery forceps should be held with the ring finger and thumb, using the index finger to steady the forceps. If artery forceps are frequently used to clamp suture material or other items they will become deformed and may not be able to clamp a fine bleeding vessel when required to do so. Care should be taken and separate artery forceps should be used for this purpose.

Bowel clamps

These are designed to clamp bowel in an atraumatic manner. Several different types are available but the most common type used in veterinary surgery is the Doyen's bowel clamp (Figure 22.24).

Sponge-holding forceps

These are designed to hold sponges or swabs for skin preparation prior to surgery (Figure 22.24).

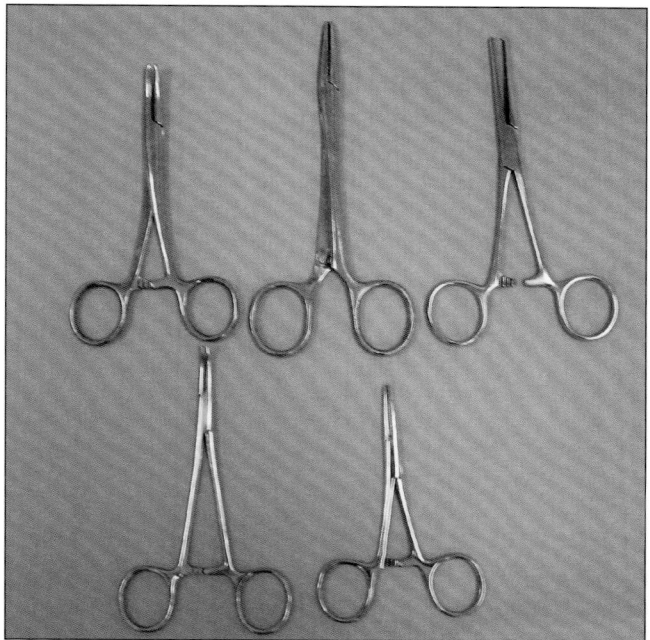

22.23 Artery forceps. Clockwise from top left: Dunhill; Spencer Wells; Kocher's; Criles; Halsted.

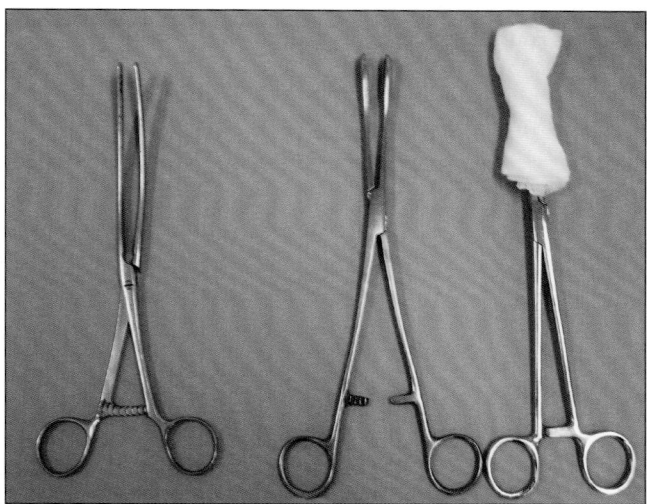

22.24 (Left) Doyen's bowel clamps. (Middle and right) Rampley's sponge-holding forceps.

Tissue forceps

Allis tissue forceps and Babcock's forceps are the most commonly used types of tissue forceps (Figure 22.25). They are designed to grasp tissue with minimal trauma but neither type should be used to grasp and hold viscera, for which more specialized forceps such as Duvall's should be used.

Towel clips

Towel clips (forceps) (Figure 22.26) are used to attach drapes to the patient (see Figure 22.9) and to attach instruments to the operating site. Backhaus and Mayo forceps have a ringed handle and curved, pointed, tongue-like tips. Gray's cross-action forceps, commonly used in veterinary surgery, have a strong spring-clip attachment.

Needle-holders

Needle-holders (Figure 22.27) are forceps that are specifi-cally designed for holding suture needles during suturing and for knot tying.

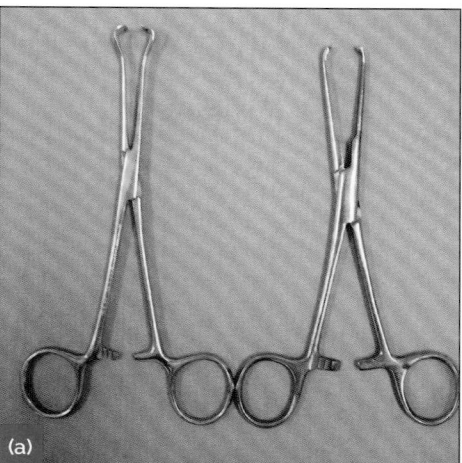

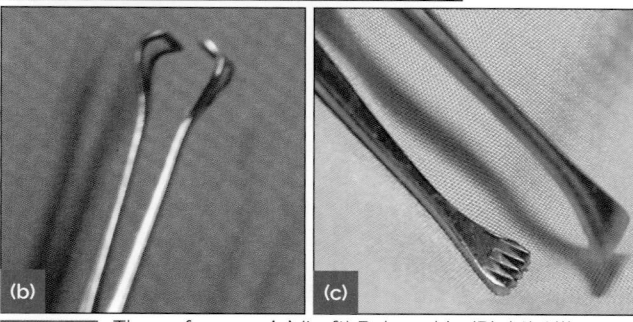

22.25 Tissue forceps. **(a)** (Left) Babcock's. (Right) Allis. **(b)** Close-up of Babcock tip. **(c)** Close-up of Allis tip.

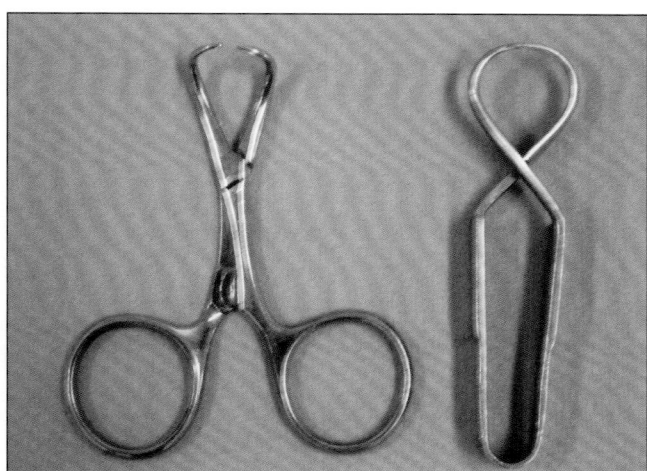

22.26 Towel clips. (Left) Backhaus. (Right) Gray's.

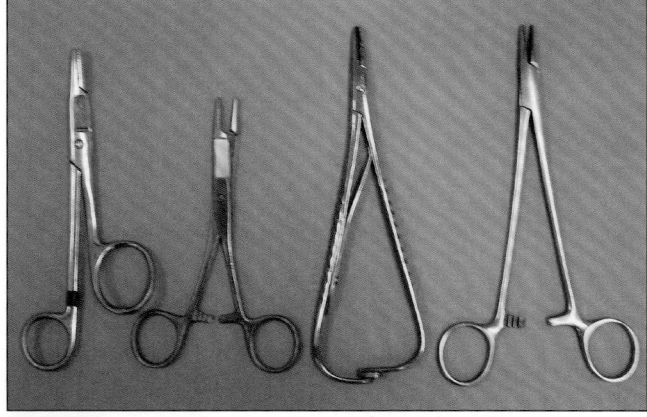

22.27 Needle-holders. From left to right: Gillies; Olsen–Hegar; McPhail's; Mayo–Hegar.

- **Gillies** needle-holders have a scissor action as well, for cutting the suture ends. Their major disadvantage is that they have no ratchet, and so the needle has to be held in place by gripping the blades tightly.
- **Olsen–Hegar** needle-holders also have a cutting edge but have the advantage of a ratchet to hold the needle securely in place. The disadvantage of the scissor edge is that the suture material may be inadvertently cut.
- **McPhail's** needle-holders traditionally have copper inserts in the tips, but those with tungsten carbide inserts are of superior quality. The handles have a spring ratchet so that by squeezing them together the jaws open and release the needle.
- **Mayo–Hegar** needle-holders resemble a pair of long-handled artery forceps. They have a ratchet but no scissor action. This is one of the most popular types of needle-holder.

Retractors

Retractors (Figure 22.28) are used to facilitate exposure of the operating field. They may be hand-held or self-retaining. Hand-held retractors include Langenbeck, Senn and Czerny, Army Navy and malleable. Muscle and joint retractors include Gelpi, West's and Travers. Examples of abdominal wall retractors are Gossett and Balfour; and Finochietto retractors are used for the chest in thoracic surgery.

Orthopaedic instruments

Osteotomes, chisels and gouges

These are used to cut or shape bone or cartilage. They are available in a wide variety of sizes. The cutting edge of the osteotome is tapered on both sides, whereas the chisel is tapered on one side only (Figure 22.29). The gouge has a U-shaped edge to remove larger pieces of cartilage or soft bone.

Curettes

Curettes have an oval-shaped cup (Figure 22.29). They scoop the surface of dense tissue to remove loose or degenerate tissue (e.g. cartilage flaps, necrotic bone). They are also useful for scooping cancellous bone material for a bone graft. The cup has a sharp cutting edge and is available in various sizes.

Periosteal elevators

Periosteal elevators (Figure 22.30) are used to lift periosteum and soft tissue from the surface of bone. The tips require protection and need to be kept very sharp.

Bone-holding forceps

Bone-holding forceps (Figure 22.31) are designed to grip bone fragments during reduction and alignment in fracture repair.

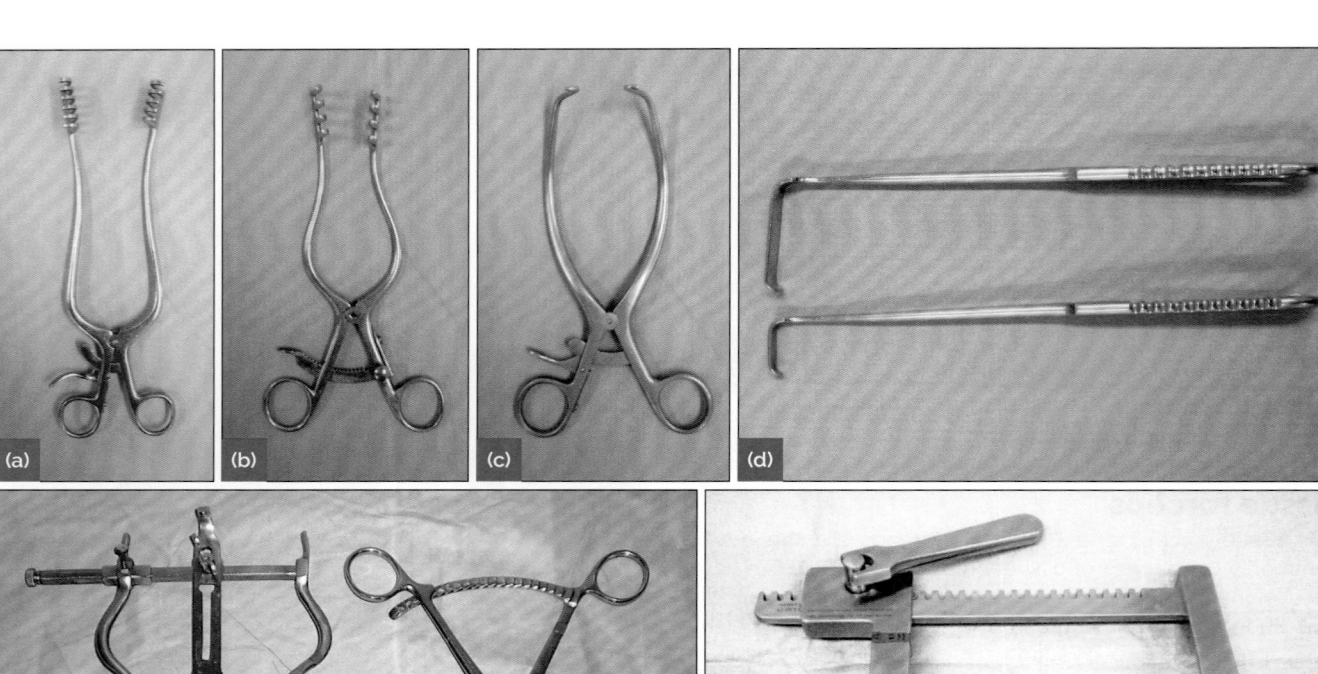

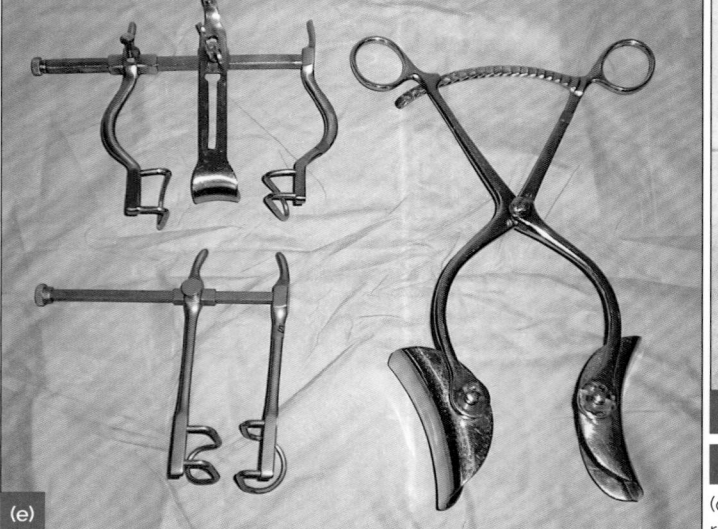

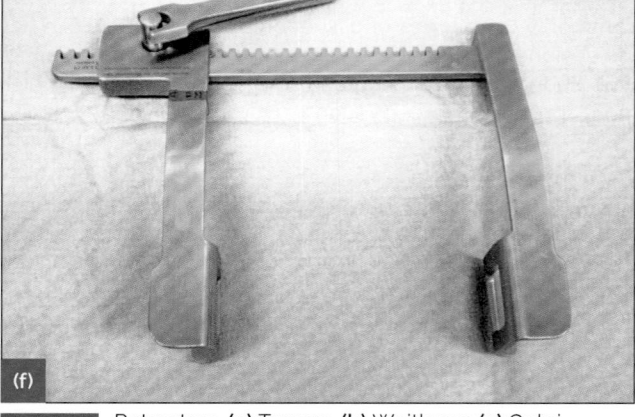

22.28 Retractors. **(a)** Travers. **(b)** Weitlaner. **(c)** Gelpi. **(d)** Langenbeck. **(e)** Abdominal retractors: (clockwise from top left) Balfours, Gosset, Possey. **(f)** Thoracic retractor: Finochietto.

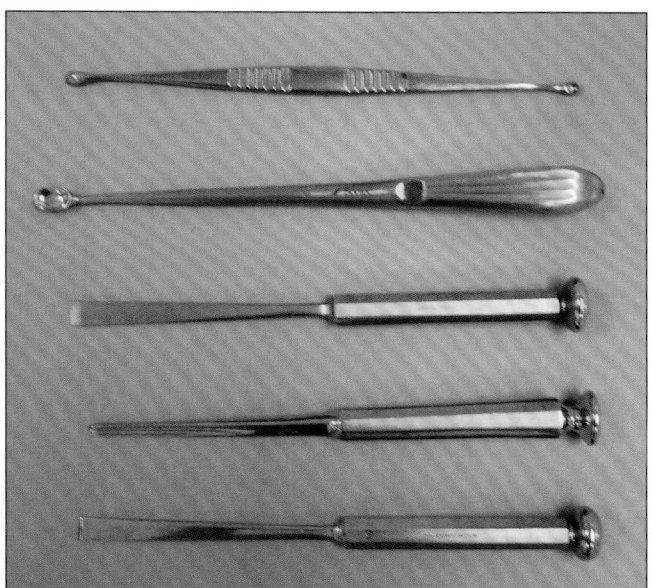

22.29 Some basic orthopaedic instruments. From top to bottom: Volkmann's scoop; curette; chisel; gouge; osteotome.

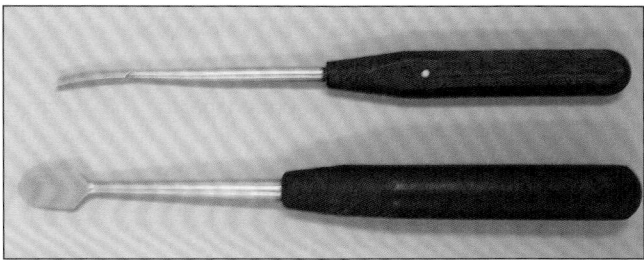

22.30 Small curved and large straight periosteal elevators.

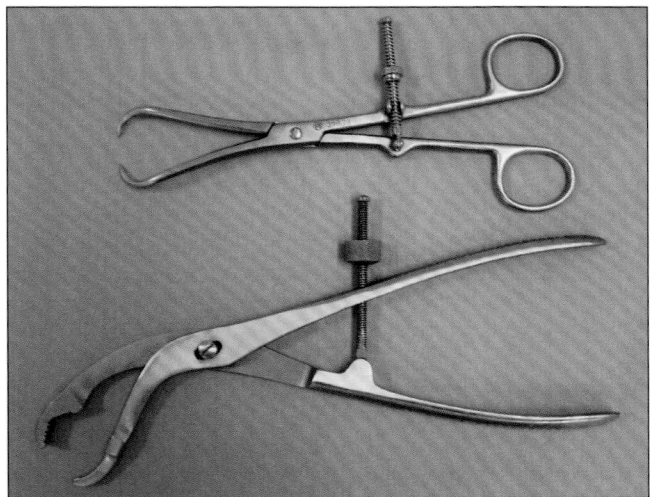

22.31 Bone-holding forceps. Top: Reduction forceps. Bottom: Verbrugge.

Bone cutters and rongeurs

Bone rongeurs (Figure 22.32) are used to cut out or 'nibble' small pieces of dense tissue such as bone or cartilage. Bone cutters (Figure 22.32) are designed to cut larger pieces of bone.

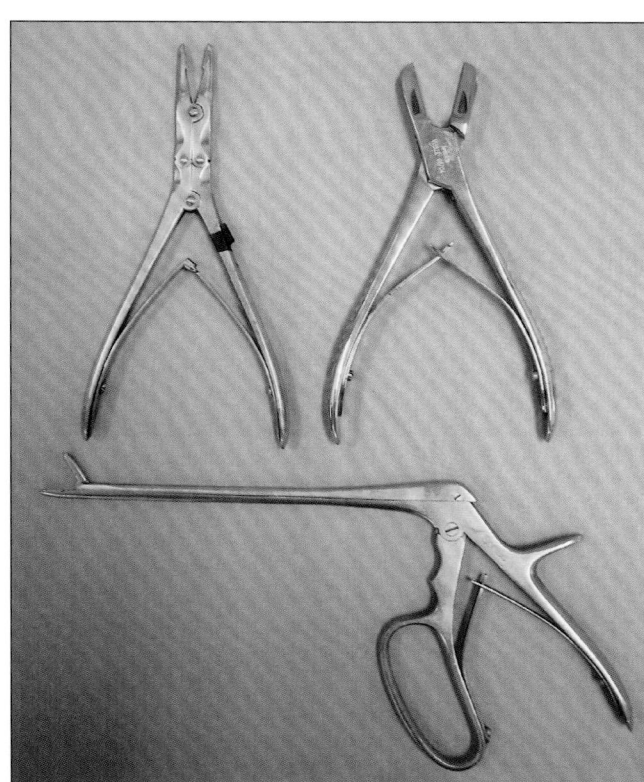

22.32 Clockwise from top left: bone rongeurs; Liston's bone-cutting forceps; arthroscopic rongeurs.

Bone rasps

Bone rasps may be used to remove sharp edges following arthroplasty procedures. They have small teeth that are designed to shape, trim and form bone surfaces.

Retractors

A retractor is used to separate the edges of a surgical incision, or to hold back underlying organs and tissues to allow access to other parts of the body. Standard retractors are commonly used in orthopaedic surgery. In addition, hand-held Hohmann retractors (Figure 22.33) are often used for retracting muscle, tendons and ligaments.

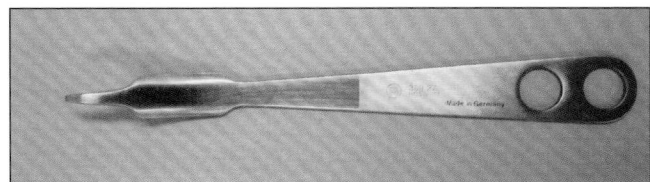

22.33 Hohmann retractor.

Drills, saws and burs

Hand, battery-operated and air drills (Figure 22.34) are commonly used in orthopaedic surgery. Hand drills are useful around delicate structures and when only minimal drilling is required, but for most major surgery a battery-operated or air drill should be a prerequisite. These allow more speed and precision than hand drills. Battery-operated drills are now more common in veterinary medicine and allow the user not to be tethered to an air supply by a hose. There are many extras available for these drills, including chucks and saw attachments. The batteries must be recharged after each use.

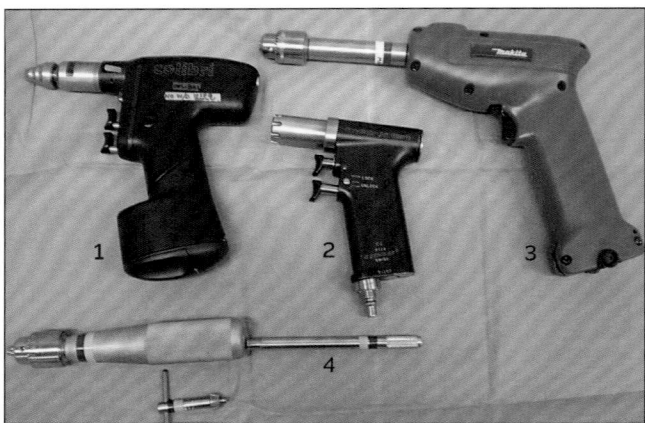

22.34 Orthopaedic drills. **1** = Battery air drill – autoclavable. **2** = Air powered drill. **3** = Battery drill (chuck autoclavable). **4** = Jacobs Chuck and Steinmann pin protector.

Oscillating saws and mechanical burs are either air or electrically driven. Great care should be taken when connecting attachments and during use; there is often a safety switch to prevent accidental activation. The power supply should not be applied until the couplings are assembled.

Wire forceps

Various wire-cutting and twisting forceps are available for applying cerclage wires and for stabilizing bones with wire.

Gigli wire and handles

These are used in osteotomy techniques to saw through bone with a cheese-wire effect.

Instrumentation for fracture repair

The instruments required for fracture repair depend on the technique that is to be used. Materials used to repair fractures internally include Steinmann pins, orthopaedic wire, bone plates, screws and external fixator apparatus (Figures 22.35 and 22.36; see also Chapter 23).

Instruments for laparoscopic surgery

For information on instrumentation for laparoscopic surgery, see Chapter 16.

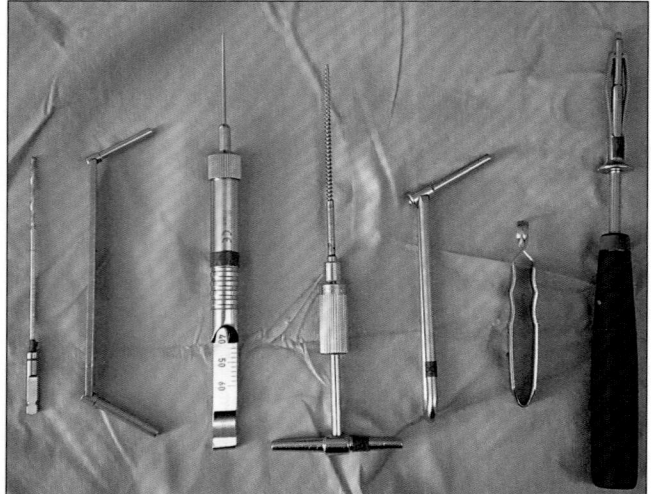

22.35 ASIF (Association for the Study of Internal Fixation) instruments for internal fixation. Instruments in order of use as per ASIF recommendations.

Screw diameter (mm)	Drill – gliding hole (mm)	Drill – pilot hole (mm)	Tap (mm)
5.5	5.5	4.0	5.5
4.5	4.5	3.2	4.5
3.5	3.5	2.5	3.5
2.7	2.7	2.0	2.7
2.0	2.0	1.5	2.0

22.36 Drill and bone tap combinations for ASIF screws commonly used in veterinary surgery.

Care and maintenance of surgical instruments

Surgical instruments should be handled carefully at all times. They should not be dropped into trays and sinks or on to trolleys. Special care should be taken of sharp edges and pointed instruments.

Care of new instruments

Most new instruments are supplied dry without lubrication. Before use, it is therefore recommended that they are washed and dried carefully and their moving parts lubricated with a proprietary instrument lubricant.

Cleaning after use

To comply with health and safety legislation, the veterinary nurse must wear protective clothing (i.e. a plastic apron and gloves) when dealing with surgical instruments.

- Sharp items such as needles, glass vials and scalpel blades should be safely disposed of (see Chapter 2) before removing other disposable items such as suture packets and swabs from the instrument trolley.
- Any specialized or delicate equipment should be separated from the general instruments and cleaned separately.
- Large instruments, such as some orthopaedic instruments, should be washed separately from general instruments as they may cause damage to them or be damaged themselves.

Instruments should be cleaned as soon as possible on completion of surgery to prevent blood, tissue debris or saline drying on them, as this will lead to pitting of the surface and subsequent corrosion. Initial soaking or rinsing in cold water is highly effective for this. Hot water should not be used, as it causes coagulation of proteins (e.g. blood). Alternatively, instruments may be soaked in a chemical cleaning solution specifically manufactured for instrument cleaning.

Where indicated, instruments should be dismantled and ratchets or joints opened before immersion.

Instruments should then be cleaned under cool or warm running water, using a hand brush with fairly stiff bristles. Particular attention should be paid to joints, ratchets, serrations, etc. Abrasive chemical agents should never be used as they may damage the surface of the instrument. Ordinary soap should also be avoided, as it causes an insoluble alkali film to form on the surface, thus trapping bacteria and protecting them from sterilization.

After this initial washing, instruments should be placed in an ultrasonic cleaner (see below). On completion of the ultrasonic cleaning cycle, the instruments are removed from the machine and are rinsed individually under running water – preferably distilled or deionized. After cleaning, each instrument should be inspected for distortion, misalignment, sharpness and incorrect assembly. Pivot movements, joints and ratchets should also be checked for correct function. The instruments are then dried prior to packing and re-sterilization, as water collecting in trapped areas may lead to corrosion.

Ultrasonic cleaners

Bench-top ultrasonic cleaners suitable for veterinary use are readily available and are relatively inexpensive. They are extremely effective at removing debris from areas inaccessible to brushes (e.g. box joints). They work by the production of sinusoidal energy waves with a vibration frequency in excess of 20,000 vibrations per second. This produces minute bubbles within the cleaning solution. These form on the surface of instruments. As the bubbles implode, energy is released and this breaks the bonds that hold debris on the surface.

Instruments are placed in the wire mesh basket of the ultrasonic cleaner and the unit is filled as per manufacturer's recommendation with a specific ultrasonic cleaning detergent. Aqueous cleaning solutions contain detergents, wetting agents and other components, and have a significant influence on the cleaning process. It is generally accepted that cleaning should be at temperatures <45°C to prevent protein coagulation. The basket is placed in the solution, the lid replaced and the unit switched on. Usually a period of approximately 15 minutes is sufficient, although on some machines altering the temperature can reduce this.

Lubrication

Lubrication of instruments on a regular basis is recommended, particularly after using an ultrasonic cleaner. It is important to use lubricants that are recommended by the manufacturer. Mineral oils and grease must be avoided as they leave a film on the surface under which bacterial spores may be trapped, preventing adequate penetration during sterilization. Antimicrobial water-soluble lubricants (instrument milk) are available: instruments are dipped into the solution for a short period and then removed and allowed to dry. They are also available in spray bottles; the spray is applied to the instruments whilst they are laid out with their ratchets and box joints open. They do not need to be rinsed. Instruments that have been washed in a washer/disinfector that uses de-ionized water do not need lubrication.

Sharpening

- Scissors that become blunt should be returned to the manufacturer for sharpening or sent to a company that specifically offers an instrument sharpening service.
- Drill bits may be re-sharpened but replacement will give a more reliable instrument.
- Oscillating saw blades become worn and blunt and will require replacement.

Cleaning compressed air machines

The manufacturer's guidelines must always be followed when equipment is cleaned. Items will come with guidelines; if this is not the case, then the veterinary nurse should contact the supplier. Compressed air machines should never be immersed in water or put in ultrasonic cleaners. The machine should have detachable parts (drills, saw blades, etc.) that can be cleaned in a standard fashion as already described. The main handpiece should be detached from the air hose and cleaned according to the manufacturer's recommendations. Some items can go into a washer/disinfector, but they may need adapters to prevent water from entering the internal mechanisms.

For metal air drills and oscillating saws it is usually possible to wash the outside of the body of the handset. Care must be taken to avoid water getting into the air hose attachment and internal mechanism of the handpiece. With more delicate air- or battery-powered tools, where this is not recommended, cleaning will usually involve wiping over the instrument thoroughly with a disinfectant cleaning solution, paying particular attention to triggers and couplings. Use of a small brush such as a nailbrush may be necessary to remove debris. The air hose should be wiped over using a damp cloth with disinfectant in a similar fashion, and at the same time inspected to check that there is no damage to the outer sheath. The hand piece and hose attachments should be lubricated according to manufacturer's instructions. The machine should then be reassembled, attached to the air supply and run for approximately 30 seconds to allow oil to circulate and ensure patency of the equipment prior to packing and re-sterilization.

Surgical equipment

Suction apparatus

A suction unit in the operating theatre is important for several reasons. It may be used for: aspiration of the oropharynx and nasopharynx during or after surgery; thoracocentesis following surgery; suction of fluids and blood during the surgical procedure. Various suction machines are available and a size suitable for individual requirements should be chosen. It is sensible to choose a unit with two bottles (Figure 22.37) so that there is always a spare when one bottle becomes full. Fluid accumulated in a suction container should be disposed of in a sluice sink if possible to prevent the blocking and contamination of normal sinks. Some units come with disposable liners to prevent any contamination to the environment.

Diathermy

Diathermy is a useful method for coagulation of blood vessels or cutting of tissue during surgery by means of high-frequency alternating electrical current, which produces heat within the tissue at the point of application.

The advantages of diathermy are that it:

- Allows rapid control of haemorrhage and minimizes blood loss (particularly important in very small patients, where even small amounts of blood loss may be life-threatening)

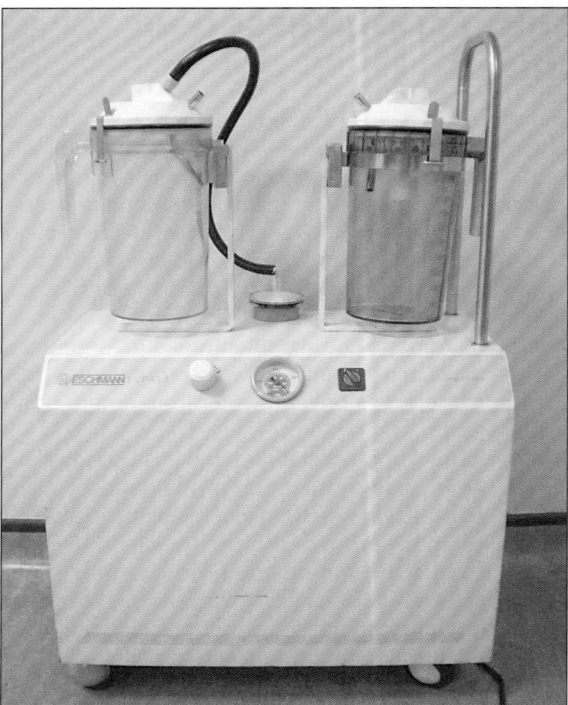

22.37 Suction apparatus with two bottles.

- Allows clear visualization of the surgical field
- Helps to minimize surgery time
- Reduces the amount of foreign material in the form of ligatures that need to be left in the surgical site.

The nature of the waveform of the applied current used in diathermy can vary the effect from cutting to coagulation:

- Continuous waveforms are employed for cutting tissue
- Interrupted waveforms are used for coagulation.

Diathermy unit

There are several different types of diathermy machine available for surgical use. There are two common types of diathermy: monopolar and bipolar (Figure 22.38).

Monopolar diathermy usually involves a finger switch pencil used for cutting and coagulation. This type of diathermy requires the patient to be 'earthed' or 'grounded'. A ground or earth wire transfers the electrical current to a harmless place such as the ground. This 'earth' wire usually takes the form of a plate that is placed under the patient and is connected to the diathermy unit by a cable. If the patient is not sufficiently earthed, the electricity will pass along the line of least resistance, which may be the patient or the surgeon. This may lead to serious burning or electric shock to the patient or surgeon. The earth plate may be disposable or reusable. There must be good contact between the plate and the patient, and coupling gel may be necessary in animals.

With bipolar diathermy the current passes through the tips of the forceps across the tissue. This means a ground/earth plate is not required. The current is usually activated by depression of a foot pedal connected to the machine. Coagulation is achieved by applying the probe or forceps directly to the bleeding vessel or by touching the artery forceps clamping the vessel. Alcohol and other flammable materials should not be used with diathermy, because of the risk of fire.

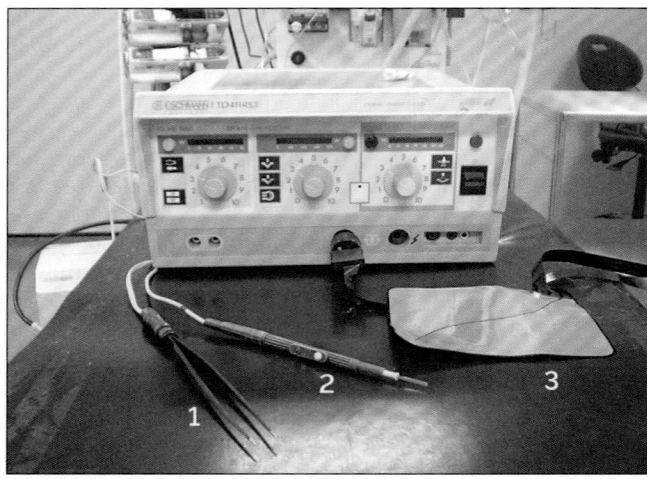

22.38 Diathermy machine. **1** = Bipolar forceps. **2** = Monopolar fingerswitch pencil. **3** = Earth/ground plate.

Care of the diathermy unit

After use, the diathermy earth plate (if of the reusable type) should be disinfected. The cable and lead should be washed, inspected for patency and re-sterilized. The unit should be serviced and maintained by a qualified engineer.

Cryosurgery

Cryosurgery is a technique used to destroy living tissue by the controlled application of extreme cold. The aim is to kill cells in a diseased target while producing minimal damage to normal surrounding tissue.

By the application of a refrigerant (usually liquid nitrogen) to the tissues, the temperature is reduced so that intracellular and extracellular water begins to freeze, with the formation of ice crystals. This leads to cell denaturation and death. A rapid freeze followed by a slow thaw is recommended and usually 2–3 freeze–thaw cycles are necessary to achieve maximal effect. It is usually possible to approach a local hospital or research facility to obtain small amounts of the refrigerant as required.

Alternatively, cryosurgery can be performed using a machine and nitrous oxide cylinder, and there are now products available for this application in an aerosol can.

Precautions

Liquid nitrogen is a harmful substance. To comply with COSHH regulations (see Chapter 2), a standard operating procedure (SOP) should be employed to prevent possible accidents when handling the substance. All persons involved in using liquid nitrogen should be trained and familiar with the SOP.

- Liquid nitrogen should be transported only in containers provided by the supplier of the liquid nitrogen or manufacturer of the cryosurgical equipment. These are insulated metal vessels of varying sizes.
- Protective eye goggles, an apron and insulated gloves must be worn when handling the refrigerant and equipment.
- The splashing of liquid nitrogen on to clothes, floors and equipment must be avoided, as it will disperse over a wide area.
- Skin contact with the refrigerant and probes must be avoided whilst in use.

- Care must be taken when filling the cryosurgical unit. A metal funnel should be used to pour liquid nitrogen from the reservoir vessel into the unit.

Cryosurgical units

In veterinary practice small flask-sized units are normally used. These are easy to handle and manipulate. The liquid nitrogen may be applied via a probe that adheres to the tissue surface or from a more diffuse pulsating spray.

Postoperative care following cryosurgery

Initially there may be erythema and oedema, which should be monitored carefully in the immediate postoperative period. A slough will then follow, which may be moist. This should be cleaned once or twice a day. If there is any discharge, it is a good idea to apply petroleum jelly to the skin around the lesion to prevent excoriation.

Owners should be warned beforehand that following cryosurgery the affected area may be unsightly and there may be a copious foul-smelling discharge. They should also be told that the skin may become unpigmented, resulting in growth of white hair.

Suture materials

The ideal suture material should:

- Be suitable for use in any situation
- Be readily available and inexpensive
- Have a long shelf life and be easily sterilized if necessary
- Show high initial tensile strength, combined with a small diameter
- Have a good knot security (it should tie easily, with no tendency to slip or loosen, and the knot should hold securely without fraying)
- Produce minimal tissue reaction – it should be inert (i.e. not cause pain or swelling or delay healing), non-allergenic, non-carcinogenic and non-electrolytic
- Show good handling characteristics (it should be easy to handle when wet or dry and pass through tissue without friction or cutting)
- Not create an environment for bacterial growth, i.e. not show capillarity or wicking of fluids (ideally monofilament)
- Be absorbed after its function has been served.

No single suture material in the wide range available possesses all of these ideal characteristics. Selection tends to depend on the surgeon's training and preferences. Figure 22.39 explains the terms used to describe the characteristics of suture materials.

Suture material that is presented in a cassette reel should be avoided as sterility cannot be guaranteed. Suture material is the most commonly implanted foreign material into patients and should be thought of in such a way. The smallest size suture material suitable should be selected and as little as possible placed in the animal to try and minimize reaction.

Term	Meaning
Tensile strength	The breaking strength per unit area of tissue
Knot security	Related to the surface frictional characteristics of the material. Every suture is weakest where it is tied. Often the strongest sutures have the poorest knot security
Tissue reaction	The response of the tissue to the suture material involved
Tissue drag	The degree of frictional force developed as the material is pulled through the tissue
Capillarity	The extent to which tissue fluid is attracted along the suture material. Materials with high capillarity act as a wick and encourage fluids to move along them. Such materials should not be used in the presence of sepsis
Memory	The tendency of the material to return to its original shape. A material with high memory tends to unkink during knot tying, i.e. knot security is poor with materials possessing high memory
Chatter	The lack of smoothness as a throw of a knot is tightened down
Stiffness and elongation	The less force required to stretch a suture, the more it will elongate before it ruptures
Sterilization characteristics	The ability of the material to undergo sterilization without deteriorating. Autoclaving is satisfactory for the nylon materials. Repeated autoclaving will, however, weaken them. The natural products and synthetic absorbable materials should not be steam-sterilized. Ethylene oxide sterilization is safe for all sutures provided the packs are sufficiently aerated

22.39 Characteristics of suture materials.

Classification of sutures

Suture materials are either absorbable or non-absorbable. They may be further classified as natural or synthetic, and as monofilament or multifilament (Figure 22.40; see also Chapter 23).

Absorbable sutures

These materials are degraded within the tissues and lose their tensile strength by 60 days. Natural fibres (catgut) are removed by phagocytosis, which tends to produce some degree of tissue reaction. The synthetic absorbable materials are hydrolysed (broken down in the presence of water) and tend to produce minimal tissue reaction. In general, absorbable suture materials are used when closing internal tissue layers or organs that do not require long-term support.

Catgut

For many years, chromic and plain catgut have been used in both human and veterinary surgery. Catgut was made from the submucosa of sheep small intestine or the serosa of cattle intestines. 'Plain catgut' is untreated; 'chromic catgut' is tanned with chromic salts to slow its absorption, increase its strength and decrease the tissue reaction. Both still have

Natural fibres	Synthetic
Absorbable	
Multifilament: Catgut (plain/ chromic)	**Monofilament:** ■ Polydioxanone (e.g. PDS® II) ■ Polyglyconate (e.g. Maxon®) ■ Poliglecaprone 25 (e.g. Monocryl®)
	Multifilament: ■ Polyglactin 910 (e.g. Vicryl®) ■ Polyglycolic acid (e.g. Dexon®)
Non-absorbable	
Multifilament: Silk Linen (e.g. Supramid®)	**Monofilament:** ■ Polyamide (e.g. Ethilon®) ■ Polypropylene (e.g. Prolene®) ■ Polybutylester (e.g. Novafil®) ■ Polyethylene (e.g. Dermalene) ■ Stainless steel (e.g. Flexon®)
	Multifilament: ■ Braided polyamide (e.g. Nurolon®) ■ Polyester (e.g. Mersilene®) ■ Coated polyester (e.g. Ethibond®)

22.40 Examples of absorbable and non-absorbable suture materials.

more disadvantages than advantages, including tissue reaction, poor tensile strength, poor knot security when wet and being prone to wicking. For these reasons synthetic suture materials are preferred. Following an EU ruling they have been withdrawn from manufacture and sale in the United Kingdom for use in human hospitals but are still used in veterinary practice (Field *et al.*, 2016).

Polyglactin 910

This material is a copolymer of lactide and glycolide and is absorbed by hydrolysis. It is available in dyed and undyed preparations, the latter causing less tissue reaction. It is coated to improve its handling characteristics and it is braided.

■ Polyglactin 910 has a higher initial tensile strength than catgut.
■ It loses 50% of its strength in 14 days and is totally absorbed in 60–90 days.
■ There is considerable tissue drag and careful placement of knots is necessary.
■ It is commonly used for subcutaneous, intradermal and muscle layer closure as well as mucous membranes.

Polyglycolic acid

This is an inert, non-antigenic, non-pyrogenic polyester made from hydroxyacetic acid and it is braided. It is absorbed by hydrolysis; the hydrolysed breakdown products have been found to be bacteriostatic experimentally, so its use has been advocated in infected sites.

■ Polyglycolic acid loses approximately 30% of its strength in 7 days and 80% in 14 days.
■ Tissue drag is considerable even in the coated formulation and can cut through friable tissue.
■ It has relatively poor knot security.

Polydioxanone

This is a monofilament absorbable suture that is absorbed by hydrolysis.

■ Polydioxanone loses only 30% of its strength in 2 weeks and is minimally absorbed at 90 days.

■ Tissue reaction is minimal.
■ As it is monofilament, tissue drag is reduced.
■ It is ideal in infected sites and where an absorbable material is required for a long period of time.
■ Its main disadvantage is its springiness.
■ It is commonly used for mucous membranes, subcutaneous, intradermal and muscle layer closure. It is used for closure of the linea alba after laparotomy/ coeliotomy as it maintains its strength for a long period of time.

Polyglyconate

This synthetic monofilament absorbable suture is very similar to polydioxanone. It is slightly less springy and therefore easier to handle than polydioxanone.

Poliglecaprone 25

This new synthetic monofilament absorbable suture is similar to both polydioxanone and polyglyconate, but duration of tensile strength is shorter. It is broken down by hydrolysis.

■ Poliglecaprone 25 is less springy than polydioxanone and polyglyconate.
■ Tissue reaction is minimal.
■ Tissue drag is minimal.
■ Its main disadvantage is that although it has the highest tensile strength, by 14 days only 30% original strength is maintained.
■ It is commonly used for subcutaneous and intradermal closure.

Non-absorbable sutures

These maintain their strength for longer than 60 days. The material is neither hydrolysed nor phagocytosed: it becomes encapsulated within fibrous tissue. Non-absorbable sutures are used where prolonged mechanical support is required. The main indications for use are:

■ In skin closure, where sutures are generally removed after 10 days
■ Within slow-healing tissues
■ When the ligation required is permanent (e.g. patent ductus arteriosus ligation).

Silk

This is available as braided or twisted strands. It is obtained from threads spun by the silkworm larvae. It may be coated with silicone or wax to minimize the capillarity, which may promote infection.

Silk has good handling characteristics, excellent knot security and good tensile strength. It is relatively inexpensive. Its main uses include cardiovascular and thoracic surgery and it can be used on genital mucosa and adjacent to eyes as it is soft and causes less irritation to the surrounding tissue. It should not be used in infected sites, oral mucosa or hollow organs, where it may act as a focus for infection.

Linen

This is twisted from long strands of flax. It is easily sterilized, handles well and has excellent knot security. It does show capillary properties, however, and has been shown to contribute to sinus formation. It is now rarely used, if at all, as it has been largely superseded since the advent of the synthetic non-absorbable materials.

Polypropylene

This is an inert, non-absorbable monofilament material. It has high tensile strength but tends to stretch and is damaged if crushed by needle-holders. The suture material should only be grasped at the ends to prevent this. If it does require clamping, then plastic tips ('shods') should be placed on the end of artery forceps to protect the suture material. The knot security is variable and a bulky knot may be formed. The strands flatten where they cross each other and this increases knot security. It is very springy but shows little tissue drag. It becomes encapsulated in a thin fibrous covering. It is the least thrombogenic suture material and is commonly used in vascular surgery.

Polyamide

This may be either monofilament or braided. The monofilament form causes little tissue reaction, has little tissue drag and is non-capillary. Its handling characteristics are not good and knot security can be poor. It loses approximately 15% of its tensile strength each year. It can be used on fascia and muscle, but the buried ends can be irritant in serous or synovial cavities. The braided form is usually sheathed in an attempt to decrease capillarity, but its use as a buried suture is not recommended. It shows more tissue drag than the monofilament variety, although it handles better.

Polyesters

Various braided polyesters are available. They are easy to handle and retain their tensile strength well. Some are coated with silicone, Teflon® or polybutylate to reduce tissue drag. They tend to have poor knot-tying quality and some have shown signs of capillarity.

Stainless steel

This is available in monofilament or braided varieties. It is very strong, inert and non-capillary. It is relatively difficult to handle as the wire lacks elasticity and knots may be difficult to tie, but knot security is good. It is useful in slow-healing tissues such as bone, tendon and joint capsules, and in contaminated sites. It has become less popular in recent years as newer materials have become available; however, it is commonly used for the thoracic closure of median sternotomy wounds.

Alternatives to sutures

Staples

Metal clips or staples for use in skin and other tissues have gained popularity in veterinary surgery over the last few years. Staples designed for skin closure are packed in a gun-like applicator for rapid insertion. These instruments are intended to be disposable, but they may be safely re-sterilized.

The main advantage of staples is speed of insertion. They are inert and well tolerated. Reusable staple-removing forceps are available to remove metal skin staples.

Stapling instruments have also been designed for a number of soft tissue surgeries, including gastrointestinal anastomosis, splenectomy and lung lobectomy. Although designed for the human market, they are suitable for veterinary applications and are gaining popularity. Their major disadvantage is cost, but as their use can drastically reduce the overall surgery time/fee, often the cost difference is negligible. There may be indications for use in patients with high anaesthetic risks as they can significantly shorten surgery time.

Metal clips are also available for use as ligatures. They come in various sizes with reusable applicators. They are simple and quick to use.

Tissue adhesive

Tissue adhesives are made from cyanomethacrylate monomers that polymerize on contact with moisture in the wound. They are especially useful in small animals, such as guinea pigs and rabbits, and can be used for wounds on pads, for holding catheters in position and in areas where there is limited room for suturing.

Adhesive tapes

Designed for use in humans, these have been of limited use in animals as they do not adhere well to moist skin.

Suture selection

The veterinary surgeon will normally select the suture material (see Chapter 23) but the veterinary nurse should be aware of which materials may be used in different tissues (Figure 22.41) and the sizes (Figure 22.42) that will be required.

Tissue	Suture materials
Skin	Monofilament nylon or polypropylene Metal staples Avoid materials with capillary action
Subcutis	Fine synthetic absorbable material with minimal tissue reaction (e.g. polydioxanone, polyglactin, polyglycolic acid)
Muscle	Synthetic absorbable, non-absorbable (e.g. nylon)
Fascia	Synthetic non-absorbable if prolonged suture strength required
Hollow viscus	Synthetic absorbable or polypropylene In bladder: monofilament synthetic
Tendon	Nylon, polypropylene, stainless steel
Blood vessels	Polypropylene: least thrombogenic is silk
Eyes	Synthetic absorbable (e.g. polyglactin, polydioxanone)
Nerves	Nylon or polypropylene: minimal tissue reaction

22.41 Suture materials suitable for different tissues.

Metric	USP
0.2	10/0
0.3	9/0
0.4	8/0
0.5	7/0
0.7	6/0
1	5/0
1.5	4/0
2	3/0
3	2/0
3.5	0
4	1
5	2
6	3 and 4
7	5
8	6

22.42 Sizes of suture materials. In the metric system, each metric unit represents 0.1 mm.

Packaging of suture materials

Most suture materials are purchased in pre-sterilized individual packets. This guarantees a sterile suture (unless the packet is damaged) and a needle in perfect condition where one is attached. The only potential disadvantage is that of cost. Synthetic absorbable suture materials are only available packaged in this way.

Some suture materials are provided on a reel in surgical spirit, where the suture material is pulled off and a length cut as needed. This is a much less reliable way of storing suture materials and should be avoided.

Suture materials can also be purchased as lengths, which are then threaded on to re-sterilizable needles (see 'Suture needles', below). This causes more tissue trauma, due to drag through the tissues where the suture material is doubled over through the eye of the needle. The needle is also more likely to become blunt.

Multiuse cassettes are still used in veterinary practice for packaging catgut (not UK), nylon and stainless steel sutures. The disadvantage of these is the likelihood of contamination of cassettes during use – they often become damaged. It is also easy to contaminate the material as it is cut from the reel and transferred to the instrument trolley. Their use is to be discouraged.

Suture needles

Suture needles are designed to pass through tissue easily. They must be sharp enough to penetrate tissues with minimal resistance, rigid enough to prevent excessive bending and yet flexible enough to bend before breaking. They should be made from corrosion-resistant stain-less steel.

Swaged needles

Swaged or atraumatic needles are attached to the suture material, i.e. they do not require threading. The advantage of this is that a needle in perfect condition is available with each strand and tissue trauma is minimized by the passage of material and needle of a comparative size. All of the prepacked suture materials are available with a variety of different needle shapes and sizes.

Eyed needles

This type of needle requires threading. The primary indication for its use is economy of suitable material or use of special needles (e.g. for large-animal work). The disadvantages are increased tissue trauma due to the eye size, loss of sharpness of the needle tip, and bending and corrosion following repeated use.

Longitudinal shape

Of the great variety of different sizes and shapes of needle that are available, some of those used in veterinary surgery are shown in Figure 22.43.

Cross-sectional shape

Round-bodied

These are designed to separate tissue fibres rather than cut them, and are used for soft tissue or in situations where easy splitting of tissue fibres is possible.

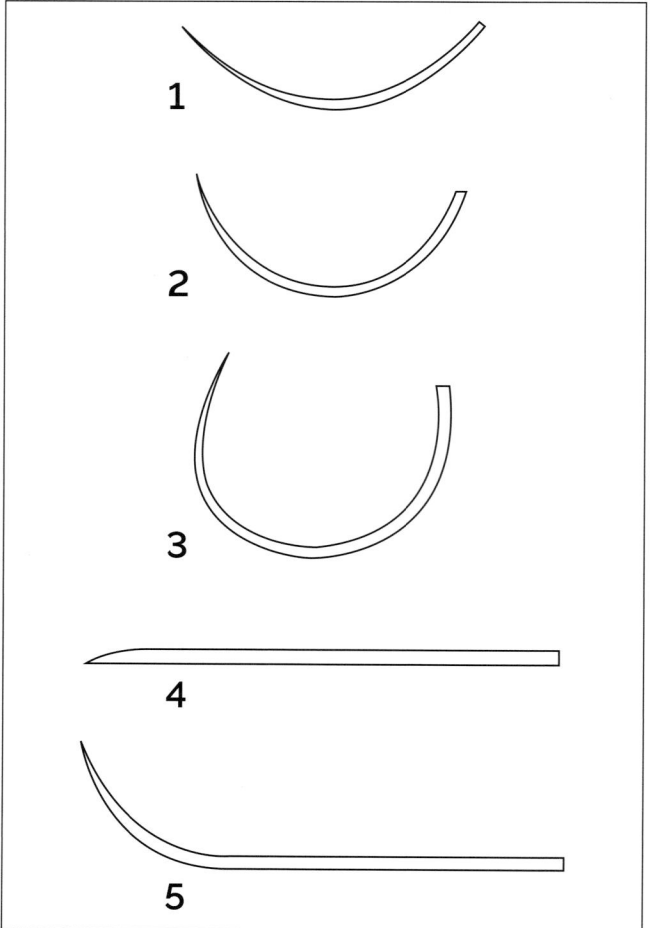

22.43 Suture needle shapes: **1** = ⅜ circle; **2** = ½ circle; **3** = ⅝ circle; **4** = straight; **5** = ½ curved.

Modified point

- The taper-cut needle has a cutting tip on the point of the needle and a round body. This provides increased penetration of the needle without increased tissue trauma.
- The trocar-point needle has a strong cutting head and a robust round body. This is useful in dense tissue.

Cutting needles

These are required wherever dense or tough tissue needs to be sutured. The cross-sectional appearance of the needle is usually a triangular cutting edge, which extends at least half way along the shaft. The reverse cutting needle has the cutting edge on the outside of the needle curvature to improve strength and resistance to bending.

Micropoint needles

These are very fine needles with a sharp cutting edge. They are designed for ophthalmic surgery and microsurgery.

Selection of needles

The use of swaged needles is to be encouraged – their advantages far outweigh those of eyed needles. Other needles should be as close as possible in diameter to that of the suture. A large needle tract invites bacteria and foreign substances to enter the wound, thus delaying healing. The needle should be of the appropriate shape and size to enable the veterinary surgeon to close the wound accurately and precisely.

The smaller and deeper the wound, the greater the curve should be. Straight needles are designed to be handheld and tend to be used in the skin. Half-curved cutting needles have been commonly used in veterinary surgery but have little to recommend their use.

The tissue type will determine the necessary point of the needle. Generally speaking:

- Round-bodied needles are used for viscera, subcutaneous and friable tissue
- Taper-tip needles are used for easily penetrated tissue, i.e. for denser tissue
- Cutting needles are generally used in the skin.

Suture patterns

Veterinary nurses maintained on the Register held by the RCVS are legally allowed to perform minor acts of surgery, including the suturing of wounds, under the direction and supervision of a veterinary surgeon. It is important, therefore, that veterinary nurses are familiar with basic suturing techniques. The veterinary surgeon should give practical instruction and reference should be made to surgical technique textbooks.

Suture patterns may be interrupted or continuous, and may be further classified as apposing, everting or inverting.

- Apposing sutures bring the tissues in direct apposition.
- Everting sutures tend to turn the edges of the wound outwards.
- Inverting sutures turn the tissue inwards (e.g. towards the lumen of a viscus).

A veterinary nurse, however, would only usually perform apposing sutures, as this is the common pattern for wound closure. The other patterns are more commonly used during intestinal surgery.

Surgical knots

A surgical knot has three main components:

- The loop is the part of the suture material within the apposed or ligated tissue
- The knot is composed of a number of throws, each throw linking the two strands of tissue around each other
- The ears are the cut ends of the suture that prevent the knot coming untied.

Knots can be tied by hand or by an instrument. Hand ties may be single or two-handed.

The basic surgical knot is the **reef knot** or **square knot**. A surgeon's knot has an initial double throw instead of a single throw. This reduces the risk of the first throw loosening before the second throw is placed but is usually only required for a wound under tension, which in itself is far from ideal.

Hand-tying helps to prevent slippage of the first throw, since tension can be kept on both ends of the suture throughout the procedure. However, it tends to be wasteful on suture material.

The knots of skin sutures should be pulled to one side of the incision and the suture loop should be loose. During the postoperative period the wound will swell and so sutures should be loose in anticipation of this. Sutures that are too tight compromise the vascular supply, promote infection and delay healing. They are also uncomfortable and encourage the patient to interfere with the wound.

Suture material should not be crushed in the jaws of needle-holders. When tying knots, only the end of the suture material should be grasped. Needle-holders should not be clamped on to the eye of swaged needles, as this will cause damage or breakage of the needle.

Interrupted sutures

The main advantage of the interrupted suture is its ability to maintain strength and tissue apposition if part of the suture line fails. Each suture is individually tied and cut distal to the knot. Its main disadvantage is the amount of suture material used and left within the tissue and the time required to suture.

Continuous sutures

These are neither knotted nor cut, except at each end of the suture line. The advantages of the continuous suture line are ease of application and minimal use of suture material. The main disadvantage is that slippage of either the beginning or end knot is likely to cause failure of the entire suture line, but as long as some basic rules are followed there should be little failure. At the start and end of a continuous suture line there should be a minimum of seven throws on the knot. Continuous suture patterns used in the skin are not ideal; when they are removed all of the suture material that has been on the outside of the patient, and therefore exposed to potential contamination, is pulled through the surgical wound increasing the risk of infection.

Common suture patterns

Common suture patterns used in the skin, in muscle and fascia, and in hollow organ closure are listed in Figure 22.44. Skin sutures (Figure 22.45) should be placed at least 5 mm from the skin edge and be placed squarely across the wound. The skin should be handled gently with fine rat-toothed forceps. The wound edges should be apposed or slightly everted with no gaping or overlapping.

In skin
- Simple interrupted
- Simple continuous
- Ford interlocking
- Interrupted vertical mattress
- Interrupted horizontal mattress
- Cruciate mattress

In muscle and fascia
- Simple interrupted
- Simple continuous
- Ford interlocking
- Cruciate mattress
- Horizontal mattress
- Vertical mattress
- Mayo mattress

In hollow organ closure
- Simple interrupted
- Parker-Kerr
- Purse-string
- Connell
- Cushing
- Lembert
- Gambee
- Halsted

22.44 Common suture patterns.

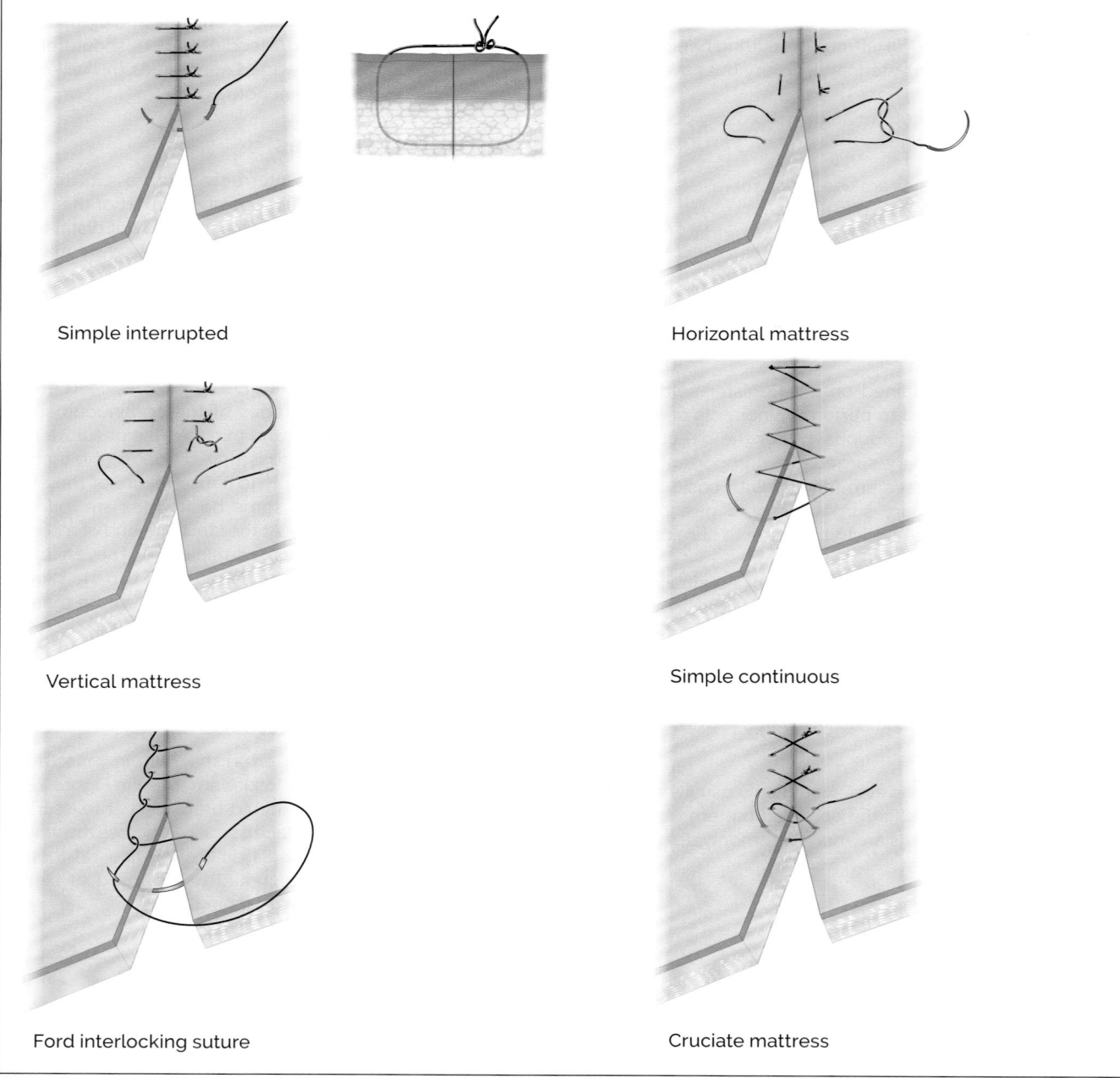

Simple interrupted

Horizontal mattress

Vertical mattress

Simple continuous

Ford interlocking suture

Cruciate mattress

22.45 Common suture patterns used in the skin.

Sterilization of surgical equipment

Sterilization can be divided into heat sterilization and cold sterilization (Figure 22.46).

Heat sterilization

Steam under pressure (autoclave systems)

Steam under pressure is the most widely used and efficient method of sterilization. It is also the most economical, although the initial outlay may be large. Items that may be sterilized in the autoclave include:

Heat sterilization
■ Autoclave (steam under pressure)
• Vertical
• Horizontal
• Vacuum-assisted
■ Dry heat:
• Hot-air oven
• High-vacuum oven
• Convection oven

Cold sterilization
■ Ethylene oxide
■ Commercial solution:
• Chemical
• Alcohol-based
■ Gamma irradiation

22.46 Heat and cold sterilization.

- Instruments
- Drapes
- Gowns
- Swabs
- Most rubber articles
- Glassware
- Some plastic goods.

Heat-sensitive items that may be damaged in the autoclave include fibreoptic equipment, lenses and plastics (especially those designed to be disposable, such as catheters).

The three main types of autoclave are the vertical pressure cooker, the horizontal or vertical downward displacement autoclave and the vacuum-assisted autoclave.

Vertical pressure cooker

This very simple machine operates by boiling water in a closed container, like a household pressure cooker. It usually has an air vent at the top, which is closed once the air has been evacuated and pressure (15 psi) is allowed to build up. As the air vent is at the top, the main disadvantage of this type of autoclave is the danger that some air will be trapped underneath the steam. The temperature in this area will be lower and sterility cannot be guaranteed. It is also manually operated and there is room for human error in the sterilizing cycle.

Horizontal or vertical downward displacement autoclave

This type is larger and usually fully automatic. It uses an electrically operated boiler that is incorporated in the autoclave as a source of steam. Air is driven out more efficiently by downward displacement. There is an air outlet at the bottom and a steam outlet at the top.

Most of these machines are designed for loose instrument sterilization only, rather than packs, as they have insufficient penetrating ability and drying cycles: packs may seem to be dry but they remain damp, allowing entry of microorganisms during the storage period.

There is usually a choice of programmes on this type of autoclave, with temperatures of 112, 121, 126 or 134°C.

Vacuum-assisted autoclave (porous load)

This type of autoclave works on the same principle as the other two but uses a high-vacuum pump to evacuate air rapidly from the chamber at the beginning of the cycle. Steam penetration after evacuation is almost instantaneous and sterilization occurs very quickly. A second vacuum cycle rapidly withdraws moisture after sterilization and dries the load. It is suitable for all types of instruments, drapes and equipment and there is a choice of cycles using different temperatures and pressures.

Vacuum-assisted autoclaves are fully automatic, with failsafe mechanisms (usually warning lights and alarms) that indicate whether the load is non-sterile or has been sterilized effectively. They are generally much larger and more sophisticated than other types and are invariably connected to a central boiler to supply steam. The cost of purchase and maintenance are higher, but the machine's efficiency and reliability in sterilization far outweigh those of the smaller types.

Principles of sterilization using steam under pressure

Although autoclaves vary in size and type, the basic principle of function remains the same. When water boils at 100°C

some bacteria, spores and viruses are resistant to heat, and remain unchanged, even if exposed to such a temperature for a long time. By increasing the pressure, the temperature of the steam is raised and resistant microorganisms and spores will be killed by coagulation of cell proteins. It is the increased temperature, not the increased pressure that leads to this destruction of microorganisms. The higher the temperature, the shorter the time that is needed to achieve sterilization (Figure 22.47).

Temperature (°C)	Pressure (psi)	Pressure (kg/cm²)	Time (minutes)
121	15	1.2	15
126	20	1.4	10
134	30	2	3½

22.47 Autoclave temperature, pressure and time combinations.

The autoclaving proces

The central sterilizing chamber of the autoclave is surrounded by a steam jacket. The pressure in the jacket is raised (depending on the cycle). Steam then enters the chamber and, as it does so, air is displaced downwards, because steam is lighter. When all the air is evacuated, exhaust vents are closed and steam continues to enter until the desired pressure is reached. The more sophisticated types of autoclave have a vacuum prior to introduction of steam to displace air from materials to be sterilized. If any air remains in the chamber, the temperature will be lower than steam at that pressure and sterility cannot be guaranteed.

Once the air has been evacuated, steam that has entered the chamber begins to condense on the colder surfaces in the chamber (e.g. instruments). The steam produces heat, which penetrates to the innermost layer of the pack. The moisture increases the penetrability of the heat. After the given amount of time the steam is exhausted. As the temperature drops, the pressure returns to normal. In vacuum-assisted autoclaves the instruments are then heat dried, with filtered air replacing the exhausted steam. On modern machines the door cannot be opened until the end of this stage.

Effective sterilization also depends on correct loading of packs into the autoclave. There should be adequate space between them to allow steam to circulate freely. Care should be taken to avoid overloading and blocking of the inlet and exhaust valves. Before packing for sterilization, instruments must be free of grease and protein material to allow effective penetration of steam.

Maintenance of the autoclave

All types of autoclave should be serviced by a qualified engineer to ensure that they remain in good working order and remain electrically safe. Vacuum-assisted autoclaves with a separate boiler should be serviced every 3 months to comply with health and safety regulations. Thermocouple testing is recommended at least annually to ensure that effective sterilization is taking place.

Monitoring efficacy of sterilization in the autoclave

External sterility indicators should be used in all cases when sterilizing equipment; however, internal indicators must also be used when sterilizing bulky items so that penetration of heat/steam/chemical can be checked.

- **Chemical indicator strips** (e.g. TST Strips) show colour changes when the correct temperature, pressure and time have been reached. A strip is placed inside each pack (Figure 22.48a). It is important that the appropriate strip is used for each different pressure/time/temperature cycle, otherwise a false result may be given.
- **Browne's tubes** work on the same principle (colour change). Small glass tubes are partly filled with an orange-brown liquid that changes to green when certain temperatures have been maintained for a required period of time (Figure 22.48b). Tubes are available that change at 121, 126 or 134°C. It is essential to ensure that the correct type of tube is selected for any particular temperature cycle. Browne's tubes are also available for hot-air ovens.
- **Bowie–Dick indicator tape** is commonly used to seal instrument and drape packs. It is a beige-coloured tape impregnated with chemical stripes that change to dark brown when a certain temperature is reached (121°C) (Figure 22.48c). As with ethylene oxide indicator tape, it is not reliable as an indicator of sterility as it does not ensure that the temperature was maintained for the required time.
- **Spore tests** are strips of paper impregnated with dried spores (usually *Bacillus stearothermophilus*). A strip is included in the load; on completion of the cycle it is placed in the culture medium provided and incubated at the appropriate temperature for up to 72 hours. If the sterilization process has been successful, the spores will have been killed and there will be no growth.

Spore systems are more accurate than chemical indicators but the delay in obtaining results is a major disadvantage. A combination of both systems is recommended: chemical indicators should be included in each pack and spore strips should be used at regular intervals.

Vacuum-assisted autoclaves will usually have visible temperature and pressure gauges on the front. Some systems have a paper recording chart that indicates the efficiency of sterilization.

Thermocouples (electrical leads with temperature-sensitive tips) are placed in various parts of the sterilizing chamber with the leads passed out through an aperture to a recording device outside. The temperature within the chamber can be constantly recorded throughout a cycle to check that required temperatures are achieved and held for the specified time.

Dry heat

Dry heat kills microorganisms by causing oxidative destruction of bacterial protoplasm. Microorganisms are much more resistant to dry heat than when heated in the presence of moisture and so higher temperatures are required (150–180°C). Dry heat below 140°C cannot destroy bacterial spores in <4–5 hours.

The range of equipment sterilized in this way is restricted: fabrics, rubber goods and plastic cannot withstand these high, dry temperatures and are easily damaged.

There are certain items for which dry heat sterilization is the method of choice. These include glass syringes, cutting instruments, ophthalmic instruments, drill bits, glassware, powders and oils.

Hot-air ovens

These are heated by electrical elements (Figure 22.49). They are usually small but are economical in terms of purchase

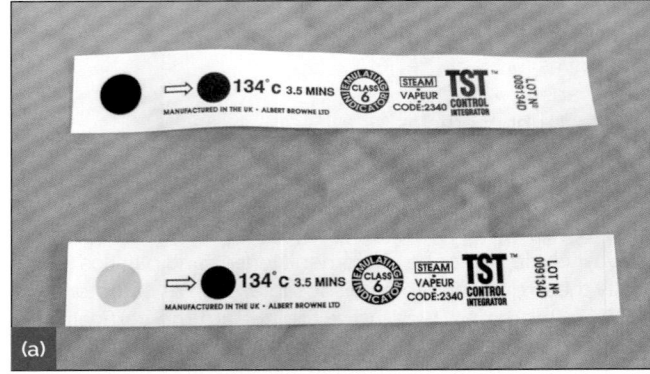

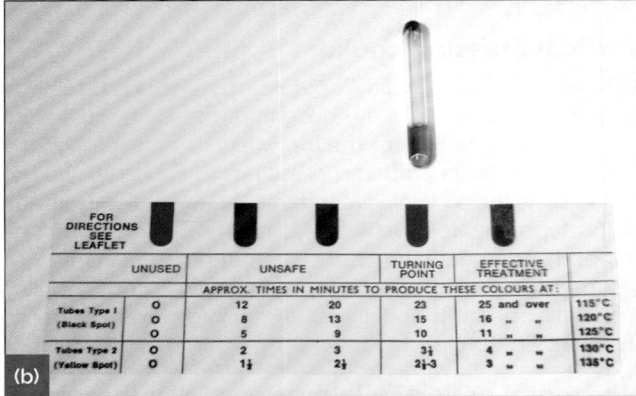

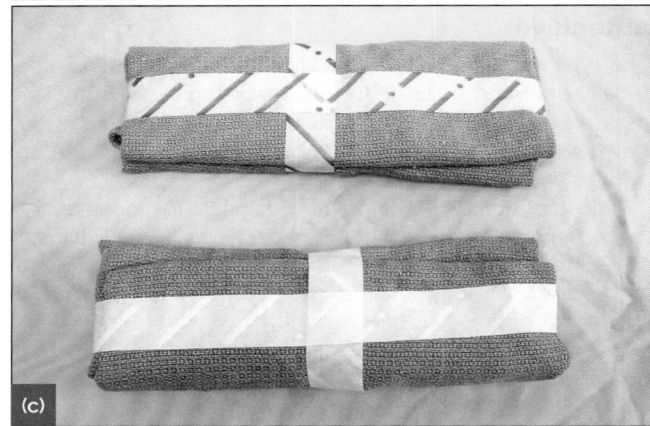

22.48 Indicators of sterilization in common use. **(a)** Chemical indicator strip for steam autoclave (TST strip). Blue = sterile; yellow = not sterile. **(b)** Browne's tube. **(c)** Autoclave (Bowie–Dick) tape after (top) and before (bottom) exposure to steam. (Reproduced from the *BSAVA Manual of Practical Veterinary Nursing*)

Item	Temperature (°C)	Time (min)
Glassware	180	60
Non-cutting instruments Powders, oils	160	120
Sharp-cutting instruments	150	180

22.49 Temperature and time ratios recommended for hot-air ovens.

and running costs. They have been largely superseded by the autoclave, which is more efficient and suitable for most types of material. They are useful for sterilizing glassware, powders, materials that contain oils, and sharp equipment such as scalpels and scissors that may become blunt with repeated moist sterilization.

A long cooling period is needed before the items may be used. The door should be fitted with a safety device to prevent it being opened before the oven is cool. It is important to ensure that the oven is not overloaded and that items are placed so that air can flow freely.

Spore strip tests and Browne's tubes are available that are designed specifically for testing sterility in hot-air ovens.

Moist heat (boiling)

Boiling is no longer considered as a method of sterilization. It cannot be guaranteed to kill all microorganisms and spores, because the maximum temperature of 100°C is insufficient to kill resistant spores.

Cold sterilization

Ethylene oxide

Ethylene oxide is a highly penetrative and effective method of sterilization that can be used on items that would otherwise be damaged by sterilization using heat. However, concerns have been expressed about its use in veterinary practice as it is toxic, irritant to tissue and a very inflammable gas. Its use is currently permitted and the danger to operators should be negligible as long as the manufacturer's recommendations are followed. COSHH Regulations may make its use impractical in some veterinary practices.

Ethylene oxide inactivates the DNA of cells, thereby preventing cell reproduction. The technique is effective against vegetative bacteria, fungi, viruses and spores. Several factors influence the ability of ethylene oxide to destroy microorganisms, including temperature, pressure, concentration, humidity and time of exposure. As the temperature increases, the ability of ethylene oxide to penetrate increases and the duration of the cycle shortens. The only system available in the UK operates at room temperature for a period of 12–24 hours.

Use of the ethylene oxide sterilizer

The sterilizer consists of a plastic container fitted with a ventilation system to prevent gas entering the work area. It should be located in a clean, well ventilated area (e.g. fume cupboard) away from work areas. The temperature of the room must be at least 20°C during the cycle.

Individually packed items to be sterilized are placed in a polythene liner bag. The plastic bag is a gas diffusion membrane of known permeability, the function of which is to contain the gas given off by the ampoule and to release it at a controlled rate during the sterilization cycle. A gas ampoule containing the ethylene oxide liquid surrounded by a plastic shield is placed within the liner bag. Excess air is then pressed out before the mouth of the bag is closed. A flexible plastic purge tube protrudes into the sterilization unit. The end of this purge tube is placed in the mouth of the liner bag and, using a plastic locking bag tie, the neck of the liner bag is sealed around the purge tube. The top of the glass vial is snapped from outside the liner bag to release the sterilant gas. The door to the sterilizer unit is closed and locked, the ventilator switch is turned on and the items are left for 12–24 hours (the sterilization process is frequently performed overnight). At the end of the sterilization period, the unit is unlocked, the liner bag is untied and a purge pump is switched on to aerate the chamber. The door may be opened after 2 hours and the load removed.

The latest model of the Anprolene ethylene oxide sterilizer has a 'cycle start' button, which is pressed when the glass vial is snapped. This then automatically begins a 2-hour purge at the end of sterilization. A green light indicates the end of that period and when the unit may be opened. Items that have been sterilized using ethylene oxide require 24 hours 'airing' time before they can be used.

Preparation of materials for sterilization

Ethylene oxide is effective for the sterilization of many different types of equipment but its use is limited by the size of the container, the duration of the cycle and concerns about toxicity. Its use therefore tends to be restricted to items that are damaged by heat:

- Fibreoptic equipment
- Plastic catheters, trays, etc.
- Bandages for perioperative use
- Anaesthetic tubing, etc.
- Battery-operated drills.

Some commercially available products are sterilized by this method, e.g. syringes, synthetic absorbable suture materials and catheters, although most use gamma-irradiation. Equipment made of polyvinylchloride (PVC) should not be sterilized by this method as the material may react with the gas. Items that have previously been sterilized using gamma-irradiation should not then be re-sterilized.

Materials to be sterilized by ethylene oxide must be cleaned and dried. Water on instruments at the time of exposure may react with the gas and reduce its effectiveness.

Occlusive bungs, caps or stylets must be removed from instruments so that gas can penetrate freely. Syringes should be packaged disassembled.

Ethylene oxide penetrates materials more readily than steam and so a wider variety of packaging materials may be used when preparing items for sterilization and storage. However, nylon film designed for autoclaving should not be used, as it has been shown that there is poor penetration by ethylene oxide.

Testing efficiency of sterilization

- To indicate exposure to ethylene oxide, blue/green **indicator tape** (resembling Bowie–Dick tape in design) with yellow stripes that turn red following prolonged exposure to the gas may be used. It does not guarantee sterility as it gives no indication that exposure was for the correct length of time. In fact, the colour change will occur after a fairly short period of time.
- **Indicator stickers** provided by the manufacturer have a yellow dot/stripes that turns blue following prolonged exposure to ethylene oxide (Figure 22.50). These are useful but not 100% reliable as sterility indicators, as the colour change will also occur following prolonged exposure to light. It is recommended that the box containing the roll of stickers is kept in a drawer or cupboard to prevent this change occurring before use.
- **Dosemeter strips** that undergo a colour change when exposed to ethylene oxide for the correct time may be placed in the centre of a pack or load to test the penetration efficiency.
- **Spore strips** placed into a load are added to a culture medium on completion of the cycle and are incubated for 72 hours. This is a useful test of the efficiency of the system but is obviously not suitable as an immediate indicator of sterility.

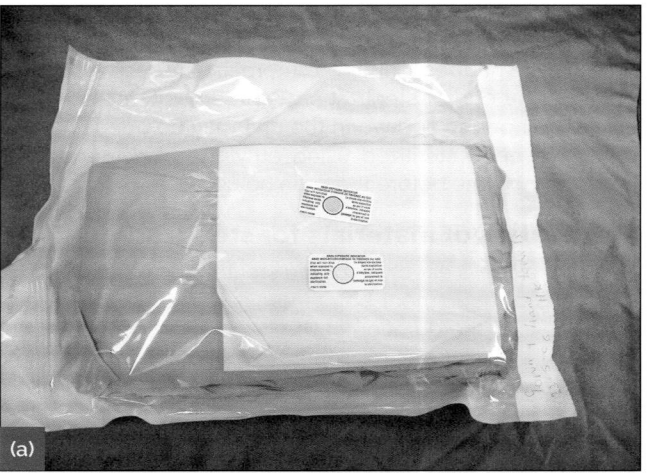

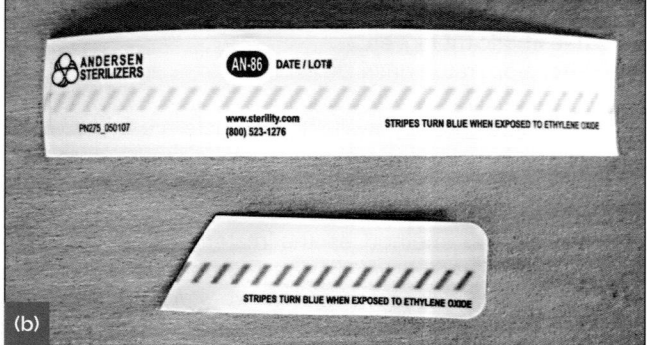

22.50 Ethylene oxide sterilization. The yellow **(a)** dot and **(b)** stripes turn blue when exposed to ethylene oxide. (**a**, Reproduced from the *BSAVA Manual of Practical Veterinary Nursing*; **b**, *BSAVA Manual of Canine and Feline Surgical Principles*)

Hydrogen peroxide sterilizer

This system uses hydrogen peroxide gas plasma at low temperatures. It has a very short cycle time (between 28 and 60 minutes), allowing instruments and equipment to be sterilized and returned to use quickly. It does not require high temperatures and so is suitable for most items that previously used ethylene oxide. Another major advantage is that the only byproducts of the process are water vapour and oxygen. The system can be used for sterilizing endoscopes, arthroscopes and light cables, any plastic goods, batteries and power drills. It cannot be used to sterilize paper or wood products due to absorption. Items with a long lumen will not be fully penetrated by the hydrogen peroxide, and so manufacturers' guidelines must be followed to ensure all items fall within the size limitations.

Chemical disinfectant solutions

A number of chemical disinfectant solutions are produced commercially. Some are ready for use; others require dilution (usually with purified water) prior to use.

Until recently a solution containing glutaraldehyde was the most widely used product for chemical disinfection. Although it is still readily available, COSHH regulations may prevent its use in veterinary (and medical) practice.

The use of chemical solutions should really only be considered as a means of disinfection, although some manufacturers guarantee sterilization following prolonged immersion (usually 24 hours). It remains a useful method for surgical equipment that may not be sterilized by any other means. It

has gained particular popularity for the disinfection of endoscopic equipment. There are several proprietary brands available.

Care should be taken to use the specific concentrations and immersion time stipulated by the manufacturer. Before immersion, a check should be made with the manufacturer that the equipment will not be damaged by wet disinfection. The chemical solution and the article to be disinfected should be placed in a tray or bowl, preferably with a lid to prevent evaporation and contamination by airborne micro-organisms. Following immersion in chemical solutions, instruments should be rinsed in sterile water and dried before use. Chemical solutions should be discarded after use and a fresh solution made up each time.

Alcohol-based solutions

A variety of these have been used, such as ethyl alcohol and isopropyl alcohol. They work by denaturation and coagulation of proteins.

Irradiation

This type of sterilization uses a form of gamma irradiation and can only be carried out under controlled conditions on a large scale in an industrial environment. Many pre-packaged items are sterilized by this method, including suture materials and surgical gloves (Figure 22.51). Items that have previously been sterilized using gamma irradiation should not then be re-sterilized using ethylene oxide because of a contraindicated chemical reaction between the two methods that would affect the patient.

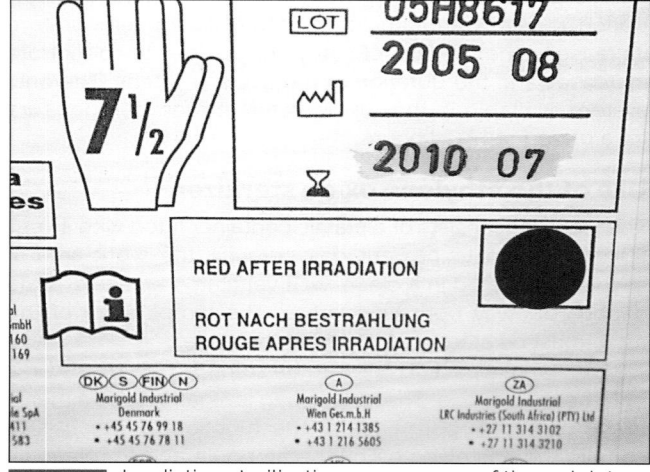

22.51 Irradiation sterilization: appearance of the red dot shows that the package has been subjected to effective sterilization by gamma radiation. (Reproduced from the *BSAVA Manual of Canine and Feline Surgical Principles*)

Packing supplies for sterilization

Various materials and containers are available for packing supplies for sterilization, each having advantages and disadvantages. Choice will depend on several factors:

- The packaging material must be resistant to damage when handled and not damage the equipment to be sterilized

- Steam or gas must be able to penetrate the wrapping for sterilization to occur and must be easily exhausted from the pack once sterilization is complete
- Microorganisms must not be able to penetrate from the outer surface of the wrap to the inner.

Other factors include:

- Size of autoclave/gas sterilizer
- Cost
- Personal preference
- Time taken to achieve sterility.

Materials and containers

Nylon film

Nylon film designed specifically for use in the autoclave is available in a variety of sizes. It has the advantages of being reusable and transparent so that items can be easily seen. Its main disadvantage is that it becomes brittle after use, and this disadvantage may outweigh the advantages. Being brittle results in the development of tiny unseen holes and therefore contamination of the pack. A method of recording the number of uses and discarding it after an agreed number may help resolve this situation. It is also difficult to remove sterile items from packs without contaminating them on the edges of the bag. The packs are often sealed using Bowie–Dick tape.

Seal-and-peel pouches

Disposable bags, consisting of a paper back and clear plasticized front with a fold-over seal, are available in a wide variety of sizes (Figure 22.52). They may be used with ethylene oxide or in the autoclave and there are also seal-and-peel bags made especially for hydrogen peroxide sterilization. The risk of contamination during opening is small. Double wrapping decreases the risk of damage to the instruments during storage or when opening the pack. They are most suitable for individual instruments, although large bags are available for small kits.

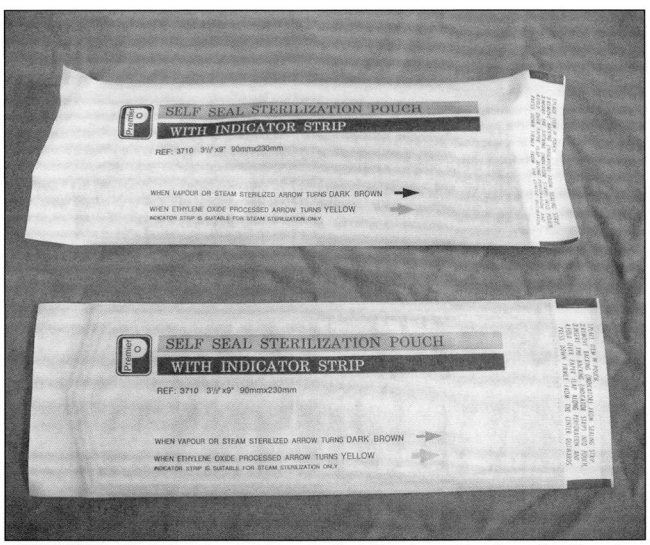

22.52 Peel-and-seal bags after (top) and before (bottom) exposure to steam. (Reproduced from the *BSAVA Manual of Practical Veterinary Nursing*)

Paper

Paper-based sheets are used for packing instruments. The most suitable type consists of a crepe-like paper that is slightly elastic, conforming and water-repellent. It is therefore ideal as an outer dust layer for packs with a drape inner layer although it is acceptable to use these sheets for both inner and outer layers. It is intended to be disposable and should not be reused even if opened carefully, as microholes and damage would not be seen by the naked eye. It is available in different sized sheets that can be cut to the appropriate size.

Textile

Textile (drape) sheets, usually linen or a cotton/polyester combination, are used to wrap surgical equipment for sterilization. They are conforming, strong and reusable but have the major disadvantage of being permeable to moisture. Usually a double layer of linen is covered by a waterproof paper-based wrap for surgical packs. The same concerns with reusing gowns also applies to drapes. The weave of the fabric stretches and, in addition to the damage caused by washing powders, may not be fit for use after a period of time. A grid system should be used to monitor the number of times the item is used.

Drums

Metal drums with steam vents in the side, which are closed after sterilization, can be used for instruments, gowns and drapes. Their main disadvantage is that they are frequently multiuse and so there is a degree of environmental contamination each time the lid is opened. There is also a risk of contamination of items touching the edge or outside of the drum when they are removed. Initial outlay is relatively high but they will last for years.

Boxes and cartons

A variety of boxes and cartons are available for use in the autoclave. They are manufactured from non-toxic ethylene/propylene anti-static material to prevent dust attraction. They are designed for sterilization up to 137°C and for irradiation processes. They are useful for gown or drape packs and for specialized kits (e.g. orthopaedic kits). They are relatively inexpensive and may be reused many times.

Care and sterilization of equipment

Gowns and drapes

After use, reusable surgical gowns and drapes should be washed, dried and inspected for damage. Gowns should then be folded correctly so that the outside surface of the gown is on the inside (Figure 22.53). This is so that the surgical team can put on gowns in an aseptic fashion (see Figure 22.7). Plain drapes may be folded concertina style (Figure 22.54) or so that two corners are on the top surface (Figure 22.55). Fenestrated drapes are usually folded concertina style.

Both gowns and drapes may be sterilized by ethylene oxide but this method is often uneconomical in a large practice, owing to the small size of the sterilizer, duration of the cycle (12 hours) and the airing time (24 hours). Autoclaving is a quicker, more efficient method but it is essential that the machine has a porous load cycle to ensure complete penetration and drying of the load. A hot-air oven is unsuitable as it will lead to charring of the material.

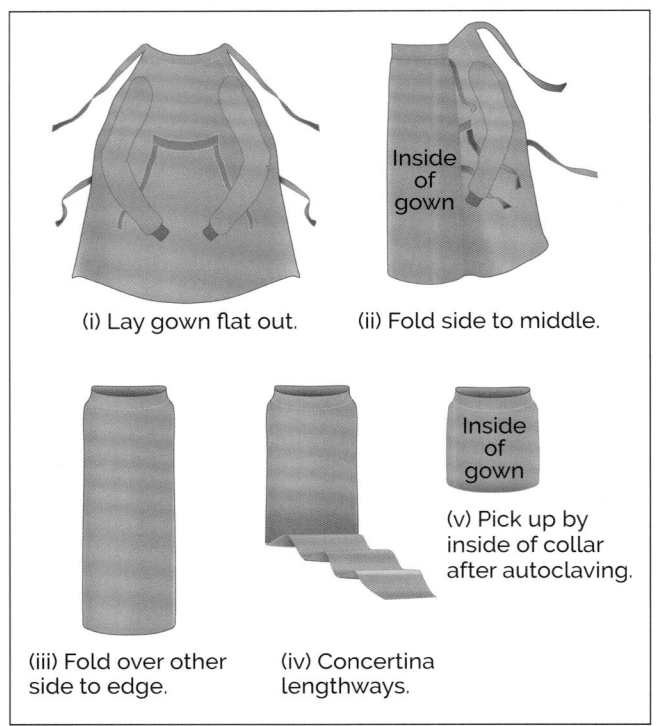

(i) Lay gown flat out.

(ii) Fold side to middle.

Inside of gown

(v) Pick up by inside of collar after autoclaving.

Inside of gown

(iii) Fold over other side to edge.

(iv) Concertina lengthways.

22.53 Folding a gown.

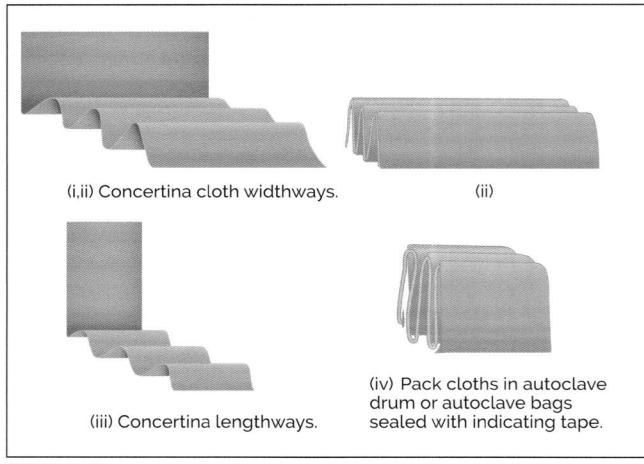

(i,ii) Concertina cloth widthways.

(ii)

(iii) Concertina lengthways.

(iv) Pack cloths in autoclave drum or autoclave bags sealed with indicating tape.

22.54 Folding surgical drapes.

Gowns and drapes may be sterilized in drums, boxes, bags or packs. A hand towel is usually placed with the gown when packing for sterilization. Drapes are sometimes incorporated into the instrument pack.

Disposable sterile gowns and drapes are now widely used and are to be recommended (see above).

Swabs

Swabs may be purchased sterile or non-sterile. Each pack should have a consistent number known to all surgery staff (usually multiples of two or five). Swabs may be incorporated into the instrument pack, supplied in drums or packed individually.

Swabs should be sterilized in the same way as gowns and drapes.

Urinary catheters

Urinary catheters should not be reused as it would be impossible to ensure they are free from any debris. They may be

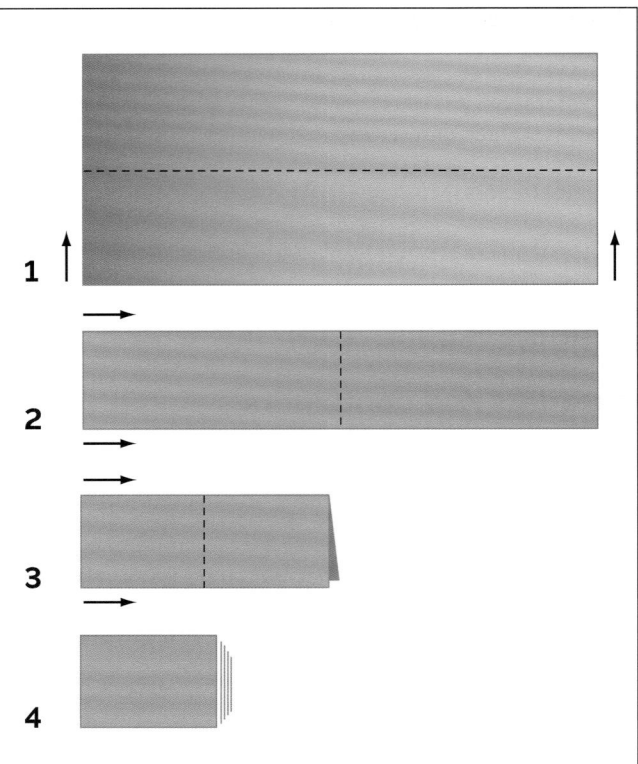

22.55 Folding a plain drape, corner to corner. **1** = The drape is folded in half widthways. **2–4** = it is then folded in half lengthways three times, so that there are two corners at the top.

re-sterilized if opened in error but not used. They should be packed, without coiling if possible, in appropriate bags. Many brands of catheter may be sterilized by autoclaving but some will be damaged by heat. Ethylene oxide can be successfully used for all types of catheter. It is essential to ensure that they are aired for the recommended time before use.

Syringes

Plastic syringes are designed to be disposable and it is not advisable for them to be re-sterilized. Although some practices may do this to save money, it does not work out to be an economical process. Glass syringes may be sterilized using a hot-air oven, autoclave or ethylene oxide.

Liquids

It is usual to purchase liquids pre-sterilized, though more sophisticated autoclaves have a cycle for the sterilization of fluids. The risk of breakage of glass bottles is high and it is probably more economical to purchase fluids that have been commercially prepared.

Power tools

Air drills, saws and mechanical burs are usually autoclavable but individual manufacturer's instructions should always be followed. Autoclaving can, in some cases, lead to jamming of the motor. Ethylene oxide can be used for all air-driven tools. Battery drills used to have a plastic casing that would melt in an autoclave, but they could be sterilized using ethylene oxide or hydrogen peroxide gas plasma. Nowadays most items purchased for veterinary use can be sterilized in autoclaves.

Packing a surgical set

Instrument sets are often packed together with swabs, and sometimes drapes. They are usually wrapped so that, when unfolded, the layers of wrapping will cover the surface of the instrument trolley (see above).

A metal or plastic tray is first lined with a towel or linen drape sheet. The instruments should then be laid out in a specific order on the towel/sheet on the tray. This is generally the order in which they are likely to be used (see Figure 22.13). Swabs, drapes, etc. are then added. A water-resistant paper wrap is laid over the top of an instrument trolley, followed by two layers of linen sheet. The tray is placed on this and the pack is then wrapped, by folding the water-resistant paper wrap and two layers of linen sheet, as well as the towel lining the tray, up and around the instruments (Figure 22.56). The set is secured with Bowie–Dick tape. It should be labelled and dated prior to sterilization. Sharp or pointed instruments can be protected by application of autoclavable plastic tips.

22.56 Instrument set wrapped in crêpe paper. The outer wrappings may be unfolded to cover the base of the trolley. The set has been labelled and dated.

Packing and sterilization of orthopaedic implants

Orthopaedic implants made of stainless steel or titanium are usually sterilized by autoclaving. They may be packed and stored in various ways, from individual packs for each plate, pin, screw or wire to complete sets. Choice will depend on individual preference, facilities and throughput of cases. The ends of Steinmann pins and Kirschner wires (K-wires) should be protected by plastic instrument tips or folded swabs secured with Bowie–Dick tape. All packs or items should be labelled clearly with name, size, length, diameter, etc. as relevant.

Storage after sterilization

There should be a separate area for storage of sterile packs. It should be dust-free, dry and well ventilated. Ideally all packs should be kept in closed cupboards. They should be handled as little as possible to minimize risk of damage, and packed loosely on shelves so that bags are not damaged. The length of time for which packs may be safely stored after sterilization

is the subject of much debate, with recommendations varying from a few weeks to 12 months. A sealed pack should remain sterile for a limitless period but it may become contaminated by excessive handling (resulting in damage to the pack) or moisture. NHS guidelines therefore recommend that unused autoclave packs should be repacked and re-sterilized after 1 year and items sterilized by ethylene oxide in seal-and-peel bags re-sterilized after 6 months.

References and further reading

Arthurs G, Brown G and Pettitt R (2018) *BSAVA Manual of Canine and Feline Musculoskeletal Disorders, 2nd edn.* BSAVA Publications, Gloucester

Baines S, Lipscomb V and Hutchinson T (2012) *BSAVA Manual of Canine and Feline Surgical Principles: A Foundation Manual.* BSAVA Publications, Gloucester

Chemaly RF, Simmons S, Dale C Jr *et al.* (2014) The role of the healthcare environment in the spread of multidrug-resistant organisms: update on current best practices for containment. *Therapeutic Advances in Infectious Diseases* **2**, 79–90

Clarke CJ and Chapman M (2012) *BSAVA Manual of Small Animal Practice Management and Development.* BSAVA Publications, Gloucester

College of Animal Welfare (1997) *Veterinary Surgical Instruments.* Butterworth-Heinemann, Oxford

Dharan S and Pittet D (2002) Environmental controls in operating theatres. *The Journal of Hospital Infection* **51**, 79–84

Field EJ, Hebert S, Friend EJ and Parsons KJ (2016) A survey of current practices and influences on the choice of suture material, pattern and size used in commonly performed procedures in UK small animal veterinary practice. *Vet Record Open* **4**. Available at: https://vetrecordopen.bmj.com/content/4/1/e000189

Hübner NO, Goerdt AM, Stanislawski N *et al.* (2010) Bacterial migration through punctured surgical gloves under real surgical conditions. *BMC Infectious Diseases* **10**, 192

Knecht CD, Allen AR, Williams DJ and Johnson JH (1987) *Fundamental Techniques in Veterinary Surgery, 3rd edn.* WB Saunders, Philadelphia

Lipp A and Edwards P (2014) Disposable surgical masks for preventing infection in clean surgery. *Cochrane Database of Systematic Reviews* **2**, CD002929

McCurnin DM (1990) *Clinical Textbook for Veterinary Technicians, 2nd edn.* WB Saunders, Philadelphia

Mullineaux E and Jones M (2007) *BSAVA Manual of Practical Veterinary Nursing.* BSAVA Publications, Gloucester

O'Dwyer L (2016) Nursing notes: pre-surgery fasting and anaesthesia. *Vet Times* **12** (Available at: www.vettimes.co.uk/app/uploads/wp-post-to-pdf-enhanced-cache/1/nursing-notes-pre-surgery-fasting-and-anaesthesia.pdf)

Savvas I, Rallis T and Raptopoulous D (2009) The effect of pre-anaesthetic fasting time and type of food on gastric content volume and acidity in dogs. *Veterinary Anaesthesia and Analgesia* **36**, 539–546

Scott K and Hotston-Moore A (2007) Surgical nursing. In: *BSAVA Manual of Practical Veterinary Nursing*, ed. E. Mullineaux and M. Jones, pp. 315–370. BSAVA Publications, Gloucester

Slatter D (2003) *Textbook of Small Animal Surgery, 3rd edn.* WB Saunders, Philadelphia

Tracey D (2000) *Small Animal Surgical Nursing.* Mosby, St Louis

Williams D and Niles J (2015) *BSAVA Manual of Canine and Feline Abdominal Surgery, 2nd edn.* BSAVA Publications, Gloucester

Williams J and Moores A (2007) *BSAVA Manual of Canine and Feline Wound Management and Reconstruction, 2nd edn.* BSAVA Publications, Gloucester

World Health Organization (2009) WHO Guidelines on Hand Hygiene in Health Care: First Global Patient Safety Challenge Clean Care is Safer Care. Available at: www.ncbi.nlm.nih.gov/books/NBK144036/#parti_ch13.s3.

Self-assessment questions

1. What five factors can influence the development of wound infection?
2. Identify 10 procedures that may be carried out on a patient prior to surgery.
3. How does the role of the circulating nurse differ from that of the scrubbed nurse?
4. Identify three properties of the following suture materials:
    - Polyglycolic acid
    - Silk
    - Catgut.
5. What are the following surgical instruments used for?:
    - Osteotome
    - Rongeurs
    - Gigli wire and handles.
6. What are the benefits of tissue glue?
7. How should metal surgical instruments be sterilized?
8. How long do instruments remain sterile following sterilization in an autoclave?
9. Describe how an arthroscope should be sterilized.
10. List the different characteristics of two products used for surgical scrub.
11. Describe correct surgical scrub technique.

Chapter 23

Small animal surgical nursing

Davina Anderson and Jenny Smith

Learning objectives

After studying this chapter, readers will have the knowledge to:

- List the common surgical conditions encountered in the dog and cat
- Describe the common terms used to describe surgical conditions
- Describe the basic physiology and treatments of surgical diseases
- Describe the physical signs of normal and delayed healing of tissues and wounds
- Monitor, manage and report the status of wounds
- Discuss the common complications and nursing requirements of surgical diseases
- Provide information to the owner on the postoperative nursing care required for surgical diseases

---

Introduction

This chapter discusses the recognition of surgical diseases, surgical procedures, management and nursing of the post-operative patient, and the stages of normal and abnormal healing (for information on auditing treatment outcomes and surgical procedures see Chapter 9). The chapter relates predominantly to surgical conditions in dogs, cats and some exotic pets; however, the terminology used and many of the basic principles described may be extrapolated to other species. In order to understand this subject a basic knowledge of terminology is required; accurate communication between nursing staff and veterinary surgeons, and reliable record-keeping, can only be accomplished if correct terminology is used (Figure 23.1). Many terms used in the description of surgical diseases or procedures are created by the combination of two or more components. Knowledge of how these terms are created allows a new term to be understood without extensive learning by rote. The first part of the word usually describes the relevant anatomical area or structure whilst the suffix describes the nature of the procedure. For example, cystotomy, cystostomy and cystectomy all describe surgical procedures on the bladder.

Terminology	Meaning
General terms	
Prognosis	The prognosis is an indication of whether the animal is likely to survive the procedure – or at least how long the disease is likely to be controlled. For example a poor prognosis suggests that the animal will die fairly soon despite treatment, whereas an excellent prognosis suggests that the disease may be cured
Postoperative morbidity	This refers to the degree of complications that the animal may be expected to suffer after the surgery. High morbidity would suggest that an animal will need a lot of nursing care (e.g. paraplegics), whereas low morbidity suggests that the animal is expected to make a rapid and full recovery
Emergency surgery	Surgery that is performed immediately as a life-saving procedure despite increased anaesthetic and recovery risks in the ill patient
Elective surgery	Surgery that is planned and can be performed at a time convenient to the veterinary surgeon or owner
Stay sutures	These are long lengths of suture material temporarily placed in tissue so as to hold the tissue without causing bruising during surgery. Usually, the ends are held together with artery forceps, which are used as 'handles' to manipulate the tissue

23.1 Surgical terminology.

continues ▶

Terminology	Meaning
Temporary openings	The suffix **-otomy** denotes a procedure for cutting open or dividing tissue during surgery. The tissue is then repaired to allow it to heal normally
Laparotomy or coeliotomy	A temporary opening into the abdomen. These are the standard terms of abdominal surgery. These terms can be further defined by identifying the site of the incision: ■ Midline (linea alba) ■ Paramedian (slightly to one side of the midline) ■ Parapreputial (to one side of the prepuce) ■ Paracostal (caudal and parallel to the last rib)
Rhinotomy	A temporary opening into the nasal cavity
Tracheotomy	A temporary opening into the trachea
Thoracotomy	A temporary opening into the thorax
Gastrotomy	A temporary opening into the stomach
Enterotomy	A temporary opening into the intestine
Nephrotomy	A temporary opening into the kidney
Urethrotomy	A temporary opening into the urethra
Cystotomy	A temporary opening into the bladder
Hysterotomy	A temporary opening into the uterus (e.g. a caesarean)
Arthrotomy	A temporary opening into a joint space
Osteotomy	A temporary division of a bone
Myotomy	A temporary division of a muscle
Tenotomy	A temporary division of a tendon
Maintained openings	The suffix **-ostomy** denotes the creation of an opening or stoma ('mouth') which communicates with the outside through the skin. Usually a device is used to keep the stoma open, and then this is removed when the opening is allowed to close. Permanent stoma are sutured to the skin and allowed to heal open
Pharyngostomy	An opening in the pharynx, to allow feeding via a tube, or placement of an endotracheal tube bypassing the mouth
Tracheostomy	An opening in the trachea, to allow the animal to breathe when there is an obstruction in the larynx or pharynx, or when it is important not to have the endotracheal tube in the mouth during surgery. The opening may be maintained temporarily via a special tracheostomy tube, or it can be a permanent airway
Gastrostomy	An opening in the stomach to allow decompression or feeding bypassing the oesophagus, via a tube
Jejunostomy	An opening in the jejunum, to allow feeding bypassing the stomach and duodenum via a special feeding tube
Urethrostomy	A permanent opening in the urethra, to allow urination when there is an obstruction or stricture in the urethra distally
Cystostomy	An opening in the bladder, to divert urine from the urethra, via a drain
Removal of structures	The suffix **-ectomy** denotes the surgical removal of all or part of a structure. Where part of a structure is removed, the remaining part must be sutured back together. The point at which the tissue is rejoined is called the anastomosis
Tonsillectomy	Removal of the tonsils
Lung lobectomy	Removal of a lung lobe
Gastrectomy	Removal of part of the stomach
Pancreatectomy	Removal of part of the pancreas
Cholecystectomy	Removal of the gallbladder
Enterectomy	Removal of a length of intestine
Colectomy	Removal of part or all of the colon
Nephrectomy	Removal of a kidney
Cystectomy	Removal of part of the bladder wall
Mastectomy	Removal of some or all of the mammary glands
Orchidectomy	Removal of the testes
Ovariohysterectomy	Removel of the ovaries and uterus (spay)
Splenectomy	Removal of part or all of the spleen
Ostectomy	Removal of a section of bone

23.1 *continued* Surgical terminology.

Physiology of surgical nursing

Inflammation

Inflammation may be a normal physiological response to an injury or irritant, or part of a pathological process causing disease. An inflammatory response will be present as part of the healing process; it then persists for longer if disease develops. For example, the redness and swelling of the inflammation seen along the line of a surgical incision over the first 2–3 days after surgery are normal. If the animal licks the sutures or the surgical incision becomes infected, the inflammation will persist and then would be considered part of a pathological response to the continued injury.

The classical signs of inflammation are:

■ Redness
■ Swelling
■ Heat
■ Pain (see Chapter 21)
■ Loss of normal function of the tissue.

The redness, heat and swelling are due to an increase in the blood flow to the tissue. Swelling occurs as white blood cells and protein-rich fluid leave the blood vessels and accumulate in the tissue. Pain is due to stimulation of the nerve endings in the tissue as a response to the increased pressure due to the swelling, as well as inflammatory mediators and toxins released by the cells in the area. This fluid is known as inflammatory exudate and is an important part of the inflammatory process.

Inflammatory exudate serves a number of functions:

- Dilution of irritant substances in the tissues
- Delivery of immune cells to the tissues
- Delivery of immunoglobulins and other immune response substances
- Delivery of fibrinogen into the area to help with 'walling off' of the inflamed site
- Initiation of the response to injury and start of the healing process.

However, the inflammatory response can also lead to loss of function either due to destruction of the tissue (e.g. destruction of cartilage in erosive arthritis) or due to muscle spasm and pain.

Acute inflammation

Acute inflammation is the immediate and rapid response to injury (Figure 23.2). In ideal circumstances where the injury is self-limiting, the inflammation should settle down very quickly, i.e. within 2–3 days.

There can be systemic signs of acute inflammation, including:

- Fever
- Increased pulse rate
- Increased circulating white blood cells, particularly polymorphonuclear leucocytes (PMNs).

In most circumstances, the acute inflammation resolves quickly once the injury is repaired or the initiating factor is eliminated. Where inflammation persists, it may become chronic and pathological (Figure 23.3). The acute inflammation seen in response to injury is a key stage in the development of normal healing.

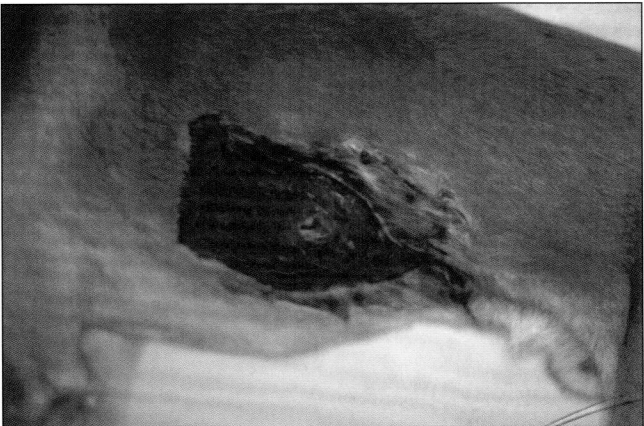

Outcome	Notes
Resolution	No significant tissue injury
Healing	Tissues are slowly regenerated or repaired
Abscessation	An accumulation of pus that persists in a walled-off cavity
Degeneration	Damaged cells degenerate and are not repaired
Mineralization	Calcified deposits are laid down in soft tissues in response to chronic inflammation
Necrosis	Cell death occurs and the affected tissue is sloughed. Particularly seen in the skin or intestinal epithelium in response to severe inflammation
Gangrene	Cell death is associated with loss of the local blood supply and putrefaction of the tissues by anaerobic bacteria

23.3 Outcome of inflammation in tissues.

Chronic inflammation

Chronic inflammation occurs when the inflammatory response has gone on for longer than expected, possibly weeks or months. These changes in the tissue may become irreversible and affect the normal function of the tissue permanently. The main difference in the tissue is that, instead of PMNs, a mononuclear cell population is seen together with proliferation of fibroblasts. There are four common situations where the inflammation persists and chronic inflammation results:

- Persistent low-grade infections (e.g. intracellular organisms or fungi)
- Prolonged exposure to foreign material (e.g. suture material or a grass seed)
- Recurrent local trauma to tissue
- Autoimmune diseases (the inciting cause is the animal's own tissues and treatment aims to reduce the inflammatory response rather than remove the cause).

Inflammation of specific tissues

In different tissues the same basic processes occur, with production of fluid, swelling, oedema, increased blood supply and sometimes increased pain. For example, inflammation of the pancreas (pancreatitis) results in oedema and reddening of the pancreas with severe cranial abdominal pain. Peritonitis has been likened to an 'internal burn' as the peritoneum may become bright red, and produce large amounts of abdominal fluid.

23.2 An acute avulsion of the skin on the flank of a Lurcher. The skin edges are painful and inflamed and there is serous ooze wetting the fur at the edges of the wound. This is a classic example of the very acute inflammatory phase of a wound.

Definitions: Inflammation of tissues

The suffix -itis indicates inflammation and/or infection of that tissue. This may be chronic (long term) or acute (sudden in onset)

- Adenitis – Inflammation of a gland
- Arthritis – Inflammation of a joint
- Colitis – Inflammation of the colon
- Conjunctivitis – Inflammation of the conjunctiva of the eye
- Cystitis – Inflammation of the bladder   →

Definitions: Inflammation of tissues *continued*

- Dermatitis – Inflammation of the skin. Specific terms may be used to describe the nature of the inflammation, e.g. pyoderma – an infected inflammation of the skin
- Enteritis – Inflammation of the small intestines
- Gastritis – Inflammation of the stomach
- Gingivitis – Inflammation of the oral gingiva
- Hepatitis – Inflammation of the liver
- Metritis – Inflammation of the uterine lining Pyometra denotes a concurrent infection of the inflamed uterus
- Nephritis – Inflammation of the kidney, often called pyelonephritis to denote infection in the kidney
- Neuritis – Inflammation of a nerve or nerve roots
- Orchitis – Inflammation of the testes
- Otitis – Inflammation of the ear. This may be the external ear canal (otitis externa) or the middle (otitis media) or inner ear (otitis interna)
- Pancreatitis – Inflammation of the pancreas
- Peritonitis – Inflammation of the abdominal lining
- Pleuritis – Inflammation of the thoracic lining
- Pneumonia – Inflammation of the lungs
- Rhinitis – Inflammation of the nasal cavity
- Tracheitis – Inflammation of the trachea
- Urethritis – Inflammation of the urethra
- Uveitis – Inflammation of the iris of the eye
- Vaginitis – Inflammation of the vagina

Body fluid accumulations

- Exudate is the term used to describe inflammatory fluid that contains white blood cells and proteinaceous debris
- Blood may accumulate in body cavities or between tissues following haemorrhage
- Serosanguineous exudate is fluid that has the appearance of blood, but on analysis has a lower packed cell volume (PCV) than blood, and other inflammatory cells predominate
- Transudate is fluid that has shifted across semi-permeable membranes and is largely acellular. It may accumulate due to loss of osmotic pressure (proteins in the circulating blood) or increased venous pressure (e.g. in heart failure)
- Modified transudate. When a transudate has been in the body cavity for a while, it causes irritation in its own right and some cells start to move into the transudate as part of the inflammatory response
- Physiological fluid in an inappropriate space (e.g. urine, bile, chyle, saliva). The body produces some fluids that should always travel out through lined ducts. If there is a leak in the system, large volumes of these fluids may be identified in inappropriate spaces, such as free urine or bile in the abdomen

Treatment of acute inflammation

The aims of treatment of inflammation are to remove the inciting cause and to prevent the development of chronic inflammation or long-term disease.

Removal of the inciting cause may be as simple as lavage (washing away) of debris or chemicals, or treatment of a bacterial infection with antibiotics. In the early stages, inflammation can sometimes be reduced by using cold compresses to reduce blood flow and thereby reduce swelling. Rapid treatment of burns (within 20 minutes) with cold water can reduce the extent of the injury by dissipating the heat and reducing the inflammatory response around the edge of the burn.

Sometimes it is necessary to limit the inflammatory response with medication. Drugs can reduce inflammation and often have a secondary analgesic effect due to reduced stimulation of nerve endings and reduction of swelling. The commonly used drugs are corticosteroids and non-steroidal anti-inflammatory drugs (NSAIDs). These two groups of drugs have potential side effects; they should never be used together and are only used under the direction of a veterinary surgeon. If ongoing inflammation is caused by infection, topical antiseptics or systemic antibiotics may be used (see Chapter 8).

Fluid accumulation

Fluid can accumulate in tissues or in body spaces as part of a pathological process or as a response to injury and often is part of the inflammatory response. Analysis of the fluid is necessary in order to make a diagnosis of the disease process causing the fluid to accumulate.

Fluid-filled masses

Fluid-filled masses are often identified as part of investigation of disease, and they are differentiated according to the type of fluid within.

Seroma

Seromas are probably the commonest type of fluid-filled mass encountered in surgical nursing. A seroma is usually an accumulation of inflammatory exudate within the tissue underneath a surgical site. Some surgical procedures result in loss of normal tissue structure (dead space) and the spaces fill with fluid rapidly after the surgery. If measures are not taken to prevent this, the fluid may take a long time to resolve or may even need drainage.

Haematoma

This is the term used for a 'blood blister', where a blood vessel bursts due to trauma or surgery and blood accumulates in the surrounding tissues (see Figure 23.26). It is important to differentiate between a haematoma due to direct trauma (or surgery) and a haematoma due to a clotting defect or vessel wall abnormality.

Abscess

An abscess is an accumulation of inflammatory exudate that contains dead and dying white cells (pus) in response to severe irritation or infection. It is usually walled off with a fibrous reaction (see below).

Physiological fluid leak

Sometimes normal body fluids can leak into tissue planes and become walled off by the inflammatory response to form a persistent fluid-filled mass. A good example of this is the salivary mucocele, where saliva leaks from the salivary duct and forms a fluctuant subcutaneous mass.

Abscesses and cellulitis

Abscesses and cellulitis are common presentations of acute inflammatory disease in veterinary practice and are usually very painful. When pyogenic organisms locate in a solid tissue, they cause cell death and a strong inflammatory response. This leads to the formation of pus. If this is not localized, it may distribute diffusely throughout the tissue and is then known as cellulitis.

Abscesses are nearly always secondary to bacterial infection, and the pus is full of bacteria and dead bacteria inside white blood cells. An abscess can also be sterile when there are no bacteria involved but there is an accumulation of dead and dying cells and tissues within a fibrous capsule.

Within an abscess there are often several stages of inflammation going on at the same time, with pus in the centre, an acute inflammatory response around this with PMNs reacting to the toxins produced in the pus and, on the outside, a chronic inflammatory response with mononuclear cells and fibroblasts laying down a fibrous capsule. Sometimes the toxins produced by the abscess are not contained and they cause a toxaemia, which makes the animal systemically ill. The toxaemia can be life-threatening, causing pain, fever, vomiting, shock or even heart or kidney failure. Once the pus is discharged from the abscess, the systemic signs resolve and recovery is usually very rapid.

Abscesses that occur superficially (e.g. cat-bite abscess in the skin, Figure 23.4) often rupture spontaneously, releasing the pus through a break in the overlying skin. Some abscesses occur internally (e.g. prostate, liver or peritoneum). If these abscesses rupture and release pus, the consequences can be fatal.

Treatment

Cellulitis is too diffuse to be drained and is treated with systemic antibiotics, analgesics and anti-inflammatories. Abscesses can often be drained and this provides immediate relief from the clinical signs. Once the abscess is drained, the cavity collapses and the fibrous tissue granulates in and the opening heals over rapidly. If the diagnosis is not certain, a small needle and syringe can be used to aspirate some fluid from the abscess for analysis prior to treatment. Treatment is usually carried out under general anaesthetic, but at the very least, sedation and analgesics should be administered prior to treatment, as abscesses can be extremely painful.

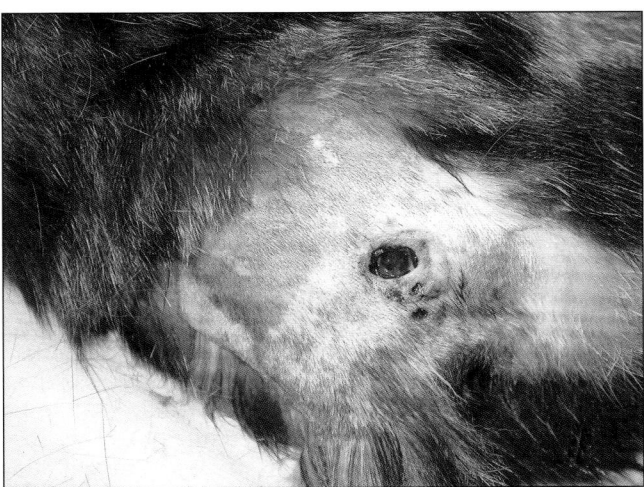

23.4 Cat-bite abscess. This abscess over the gluteal region has ruptured, releasing the pus. It has been clipped and cleaned and will now heal by second intention.

- Hot compresses can be applied to very superficial abscesses. The principle is to soften the overlying skin and encourage rupture of the abscess through the surface. The use of poultices containing boric acid is not to be recommended, as they irritate the surrounding skin.
- Surgical drainage is a much quicker and more reliable way of treating abscesses. An incision is made in the skin at the most superficial point of the abscess, using a scalpel blade. The pus is allowed to drain and the cavity is lavaged with sterile fluids. The incision should be encouraged to stay open for a few days, either by using a drain (see later) or by daily bathing with lavage of the cavity.
- Resection of abscesses. Deep abscesses or internal abscesses are not suitable for treatment by simple lancing. Deep abscesses may be dissected out around the fibrous capsule and removed in one piece. Internal abscesses may be either resected (e.g. a lung lobe abscess) or suctioned out under sterile conditions and the omentum used as a natural drain (e.g. prostatic abscesses).
- Rabbits can develop recurrent abscesses in the submandibular and cheek area. These are filled with a particularly thick type of pus that is very difficult to drain. Rabbit abscesses are very different to those seen in the dog and the cat and rarely respond to simple lancing and drainage (see the *BSAVA Manual of Rabbit Surgery, Dentistry and Imaging*). Where possible they should be removed surgically to access the source of infection (often a tooth root or middle ear). It is important to open up the abscess adequately in order to allow treatments for some days afterwards. Compounds that debride the inside of the cavity, such as hydrogels or debriding solutions, are often used to continue the cleaning process inside the cavity while it granulates. Sometimes the abscess is related to tooth root disease and this must be treated in order to prevent recurrence. In some cases, there are multiple abscesses and it may be necessary to resect all of them.

Wound healing

Generally, acute inflammation of tissue is followed by healing. There are some basic processes that are common to all tissues:

- Removal of dead and foreign material
- Clearance of the inflammatory response
- Regeneration of lost tissue components if possible
- Replacement of lost tissue components by connective tissue.

The different outcomes of the healing process depend on the type of tissue and the degree of damage. There may be resolution, regeneration or organization.

Resolution

Where there is no tissue destruction and the inflammatory process is very mild (e.g. a superficial graze), the tissue can return to its original state prior to the injury.

Regeneration

The damaged tissue is completely replaced by proliferation of the remaining cells. This depends on the type of tissue, as regeneration can only occur if the lost cells can be replaced and if the connective tissue and vascular supply are still intact. In this context, cells are classified into three basic groups:

- Labile cells can divide and proliferate throughout life. They are highly capable of regeneration (e.g. epithelial cells, blood cells and lymphoid tissue)

- Stable cells do not normally divide, but can do so in response to certain stimuli, and may divide following injury to the tissue (e.g. cells in the liver, kidney, endocrine glands, bone and fibrous tissue)
- Permanent cells only divide during fetal growth and are incapable of regeneration (e.g. neurons, cardiac muscle cells and, to some extent, skeletal muscle cells).

Organization

Where the cells cannot repair the damage by regeneration, the tissue heals by the formation of scar tissue, which is organized fibrous tissue with a large number of collagen fibres. Often this means that the tissue will lose its normal function, or be more susceptible to recurrent damage (e.g. scar tissue in skin) (see later).

Most tissues heal by a combination of these processes, with some parts capable of regeneration and others forming scar tissue. Skin is a good example of tissue that heals in the dermis by the formation of scar tissue (organization) and by regeneration in the epidermis.

Normal wound healing in skin

The normal process of healing follows a predictable pattern that can be used to determine the progress of any healing tissue. There is always overlap between the phases as they progress from one predominant cell type to another, and they are not distinct.

Inflammatory phase

After injury, there is an initial inflammatory phase triggered by activation of the platelets and fibrin in the blood clot, which in turn attracts neutrophils to the damaged tissue. The neutrophils will clear up bacteria, necrotic tissue and foreign material. They also release inflammatory mediators that attract macrophages into the tissue. Once the macrophages arrive, the final debridement process begins and the tissue starts to proliferate to repair the damage. The wound will look exudative, swollen and red during this phase (Figure 23.5).

Proliferative phase

The proliferative phase is triggered by the macrophages and involves fibroblasts that lay down the matrix of the tissue, endothelial cells that lay down new blood vessels,

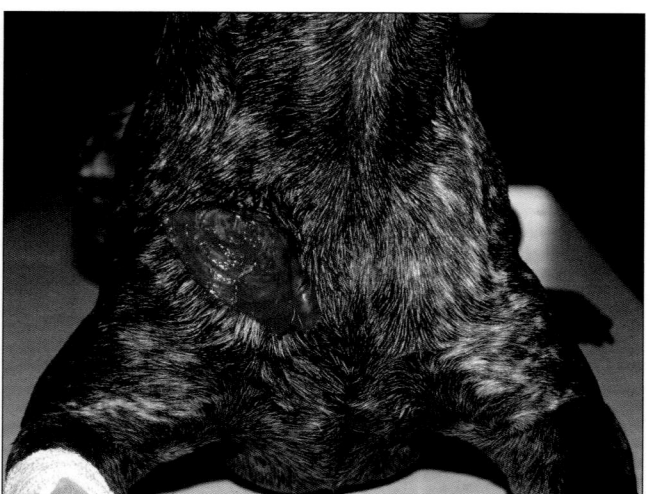

23.5 Gunshot wound across a dog's shoulder. The wound is peracute; there is tissue loss and inflammation and healing processes have not yet started.

and epithelial cells that migrate over the top of the wound to reconstitute the epidermis (epithelialization). This phase is the most crucial part of wound healing, as it demonstrates that it is progressing normally. The classic appearance of this phase is the development of granulation tissue (Figure 23.6). Granulation tissue is bright red, very vascular and has a granular surface due to the capillary loops growing into the tissue. It is highly resistant to infection and is a sign that the wound is clear of both bacterial infection and foreign material. It is important to be able to recognize granulation tissue, as it indicates that the wound is healing. During the formation of granulation tissue, the wound starts to contract and this process alone can close a wound by up to 30% of its area. Gradually, the granulation tissue is replaced by collagen fibres and scar tissue is laid down.

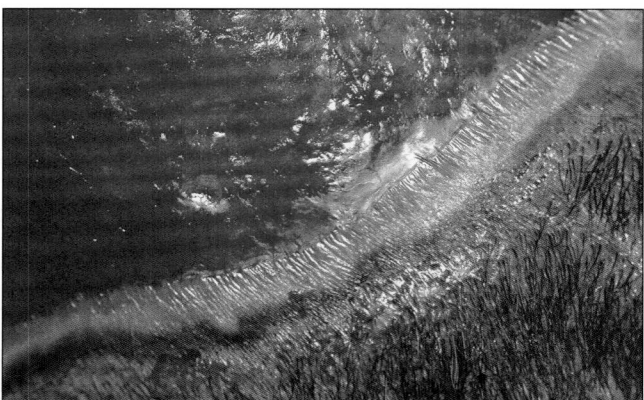

23.6 Close-up of a wound edge, showing healthy granulation tissue with an advancing epithelial edge.

Remodelling phase

Once the proliferation and repair of the tissue is complete, the scar will remodel and strengthen over a period of days to weeks as the hair regrows and the fibroblasts rearrange the matrix of the tissue according to the tensions during normal function.

In a clean surgical wound in skin, the inflammatory phase should last 24–48 hours; then a thin layer of granulation tissue develops between the edges of the surgical wound. By the time the sutures are removed at 7–10 days, the remodelling phase is well under way.

In larger skin wounds, the inflammatory phase may last longer due to infection or foreign material, and the granulation tissue may not start to develop until at least 3–5 days. Depending on how large the wound is, the proliferative phase (granulation, contraction and re-epithelialization) may take days to weeks to be completed.

Normal wound healing in other tissues

All tissues follow the same basic healing pattern as skin, with inflammatory, proliferative and remodelling phases.

Tendon and muscle injuries are often associated with trauma and other tissues may be simultaneously damaged, prolonging the healing process. The basic pattern is as for skin, but the remodelling phase is much more important as tendons and muscles have to regain function as well as strength. Muscle should heal quickly but may have to be immobilized to allow development of strength in the scar. Tendons take a very long time to develop strength; they have to be supported for several weeks and only gradually reintroduced to weight bearing, otherwise they may stretch or rupture.

The gastrointestinal (GI), urinary and reproductive tract tissues heal more rapidly than skin, with the fibrin clot helping to seal the wound initially, and the main support coming from the sutures for the first 3 days. The epithelium can regenerate and starts to close the wound almost immediately, with fibroblast proliferation giving the wound strength by 3–4 days after wounding. The urinary bladder heals the fastest and the colon the slowest. Normal healing in the intestine depends on good nutrition and a good blood supply. Feeding the patient as soon as possible after intestinal surgery will stimulate blood supply to the intestine, provide luminal nutrition and accelerate healing. This simple concept demonstrates the importance of nursing and feeding patients after surgery.

Factors that affect normal wound healing

Normal wound healing in companion animals is reasonably efficient. Most wounds are delayed in healing either because the animal has another undiagnosed disease or because the management of the patient is poor (Figure 23.7). Sometimes treatments affect the rate of healing and these may have to be modified until the wound is healed.

Factors affecting healing	Clinical examples
Systemic diseases	Hypothyroidism, hyperadrenocorticism (Cushing's disease), protein-losing disease, renal or hepatic disease, diabetes mellitus, malnutrition, cachexia, cancer, severe cardiovascular disease
Wound management	Choice of wound dressing (primary layer), bandage technique, inadequate bandage protection, infrequent dressing changes, patient interference with the wound
Surgical factors	Prolonged anaesthetic time, wound infection, overly tight sutures, tension on the suture line, choice of suture material, poor surgical techniques, contamination of instrumentation or surgical site during surgery, inadequate closure or drainage of dead space. Foreign material left in the wound, including suture material, may delay healing by increasing the inflammatory response
Therapy	Corticosteroids, antimetabolite chemotherapeutic drugs, radiotherapy

23.7   Causes of delayed wound healing.

Inflammation: a summary

- Inflammatory processes may be a normal part of the healing process but they can also be part of the pathology
- Prolonged inflammation is usually a sign that the healing process is delayed
- Responses to inflammation can aid in the diagnosis of the disease process
- Some tissues can heal by regeneration, but others may have to heal by the formation of scar tissue

Wounds
Classification of wounds

Wounds may be classified and described according to aetiology (cause), depth of skin loss, contamination or infection, extent of soft tissue or bony involvement, duration since wounding, and site. Accurate descriptions relay information to other nurses and veterinary surgeons about what to expect. For example: 'An abrasive, full-thickness, infected injury to the distal hindlimb with shear and fracture of the lateral metatarsal bone and loss of ligaments' (Figure 23.8). It is important to know how the wound was incurred in order to determine the extent of the injuries and the expected progression of the wound. Some types of injury affect the way in which the tissues heal and their susceptibility to infection.

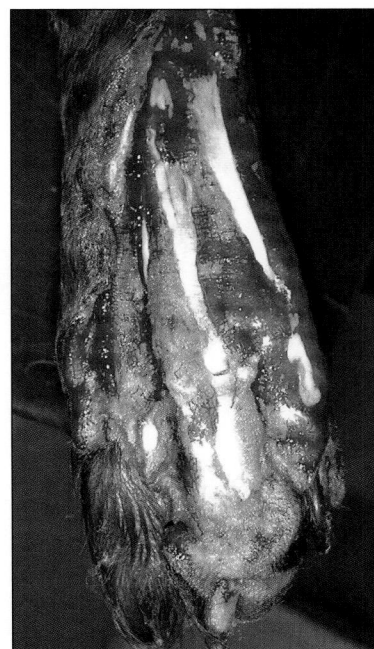

23.8   Traumatic wound on the distal limb as a result of a road traffic accident. The foot has been sheared, losing the skin and some soft tissue and damaging the collateral ligaments and metatarsal bones. This wound is beginning to granulate and has been cleaned of contaminating foreign material. (Courtesy of John Houlton).

Aetiology

There are 11 basic groups of wounds, classified by cause:

- Surgical (incisional)
- Surgical wound dehiscence
- Laceration
- Puncture
- Abrasion/shear
- Degloving/ischaemic/skin slough (avulsion)
- Burns – chemical, cold and heat, electrical
- Ballistic/gunshot
- Crush injury
- Chronic fistulae/sinuses
- Inflammatory (e.g. vasculitis, immune-mediated).

These general groups are distinguished by the degree of tissue trauma, contamination and associated injuries. Identifying the cause of injury helps in determining appropriate wound management and also the expected healing time. Wounds that are heavily contaminated or have large amounts of tissue loss will have longer inflammatory phases and longer healing times. The category also helps to indicate the type and degree of contamination of the wound.

Species differences

There is a different pattern of wound presentations in different species and even in age groups. For example, heat lamp burns are more common in reptiles or neonatal patients. Outdoor, young active dogs or cats are more likely to suffer traumatic injuries and airgun pellet injuries are seen most commonly in cats.

There are also species differences in the timing of the phases of healing as well as the appearance of normal healing wounds. For example, in cats, granulation tissue is slow to appear, is paler, more fragile and appears at the edges of the wounds and is slow to fill an open wound. The inflammatory phase is longer in the cat, but feline wounds also exude less than canine wounds and need to be kept moist.

Degree of contamination

The only truly clean wound is a surgical wound; all other types of wound can be considered contaminated or infected. The optimal time for treatment of an open wound is within the first 6 hours. This is known as the 'golden period' and the wound is considered as contaminated, but not infected:

- 0–6 hours – little bacterial multiplication: contaminated
- 6–12 hours – bacteria beginning to divide: early infection
- Over 12 hours – bacterial invasion of tissues: infection established.

Surgical procedures are also classified according to infection and contamination (see later).

Viability and vascular supply to the tissue

Wounds may also be more susceptible to infection if there is associated tissue damage. Tissue that is devitalized (or necrotic) due to laceration or compression of blood vessels is more likely to become infected. Surgical wounds are more at risk of infection if a tourniquet has been applied, and cardio-vascular disease may also delay healing due to poor blood supply to the limbs. Shock can result in vasoconstriction and if the circulation is not regained there may be reduced blood supply (and therefore increased risk of delayed healing or infection) to wounds in any area of the body.

Different types of tissue have a greater or lesser ability to resist infection. Well vascularized areas of skin have good bacterial defences; they should heal well and resist infection. Tissue may become devitalized due to poor surgical technique or desiccation during surgical debridement, which then increases the risk of infection or delayed healing.

Foreign material

Foreign material has to be removed before the wound is able to heal, with the exception of surgical implants or suture material that has been used to repair damaged structures. It should be noted that the presence of foreign material will slow wound healing. Wound healing can also be affected by the presence of necrotic body tissue underneath the wound such as a bone fragment (sequestrum), tooth root or ingrowing hairs.

Healing of wounds (closure)

Primary closure (first intention healing)

Wounds that are closed surgically heal rapidly with a very short healing phase, because there is little foreign material or bacteria.

Delayed primary closure

Some wounds that are contaminated with foreign material (debris) are better cleaned and managed as open wounds for 1–3 days in order to ensure that there is no residual infection. These wounds are then closed surgically once the earliest signs of granulation tissue formation are seen.

Secondary closure

A wound that is heavily contaminated, or where the surrounding skin is damaged, may be managed as an open wound for several days until it is possible to close the wound surgically. Such wounds will have well established granulation tissue by at the time it is ready for of surgical closure, and it may be necessary to excise some of this in order to close the wound.

Second intention healing

In some instances, it is not possible, or it is unnecessary, to close a wound surgically and it is dressed and bandaged until it heals. In these cases, the wound heals by granulation (Figure 23.9), epithelialization and contraction. Large wounds may take weeks or months to close in this way and during this time the wound has to be regularly re-bandaged. It may be better for the patient and more cost-effective to attempt secondary closure using a reconstructive technique than to continue with second intention healing. The temperament of the patient may also play a part in the decision-making process, depending on whether bandage changes can be easily done without sedation.

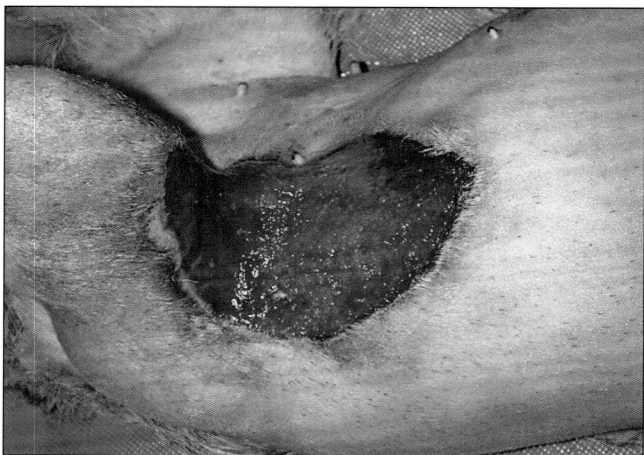

23.9 Large burn wound in the flank fold of a dog. The wound is healing by second intention and has filled in with granulation tissue. The edges of the wound are beginning to epithelialize but there is little evidence yet of contraction.

Management of primary closure wounds

This group of wounds covers all surgical incisions that are sutured, and will be the commonest wound management area that veterinary nurses have to provide advice on. Prevention of complications associated with surgical wounds relies on meticulous management in four main areas:

- Preoperative preparation of the patient (see Chapter 22)
- Systemic or local wound factors that may affect wound healing (see above)
- Surgical technique and wound closure (see later)
- Postoperative management.

Preoperative management of the patient

Preoperative patient management includes:

- Checking the consent form has been signed and the owner understands what procedure is being carried out
- Checking with the owner that food has been withheld according to the instructions provided by the practice and that the animal has not developed any other problems
- Checking that the necessary equipment, results or images, and personnel are available
- Completing a clinical examination and ensuring that the patient is fit for the planned procedure (very important for elective procedures)
- Preparing the skin for surgery (i.e. removal of dirt, hair clipping and cleaning of the skin; see Chapter 22).

Postoperative management of surgical wounds

The patient's wound should be carefully checked prior to discharge from the hospital. Signs of bleeding or bruising should be checked for, as well as that the sutures are intact and have not been interfered with. Abdominal wounds should be checked to ensure they have not been contaminated with urine or faeces while in the hospital. When an animal is discharged, the owner should be given written instructions for wound care, potential problems and when to seek advice. It is a good idea to explain the procedure that has been performed and to show the owner the wound before the animal goes home. Some practices will give specific instructions such as limited exercise, special diet, care of a bandage or physiotherapy. It is advisable that the owner is given written instructions on postoperative care so that there can be no misunderstanding at a later date if there is a complication associated with poor homecare. They should also be very clear on when the next check-up will be and you should ensure that they have made the appointment before leaving.

Immediate perioperative care

At the end of the surgery, blood stains and clots should be gently wiped away using sterile fluid such as saline. Care should be taken not to cause abrasion of the skin. Wetting of the surgical incision should be avoided if possible. Agents such as hydrogen peroxide solutions may be used to help to clean the haircoat, but should not be used on the perisurgical skin as it may cause dermatitis.

The main principles of managing a clean surgical wound are:

- Dressing the wound
- Observation of the wound and patient
- Prevention of self-mutilation
- Suture removal.

Dressing surgical wounds

Surgical wounds (Figure 23.10) are dressed, if required, for various reasons:

- To protect the wound from contamination or trauma
- To protect the wound from self-mutilation by the patient
- To absorb exudate from the wound
- To limit movement of the wound, to reduce pain or tension on the sutures
- To limit swelling of the surgical site.

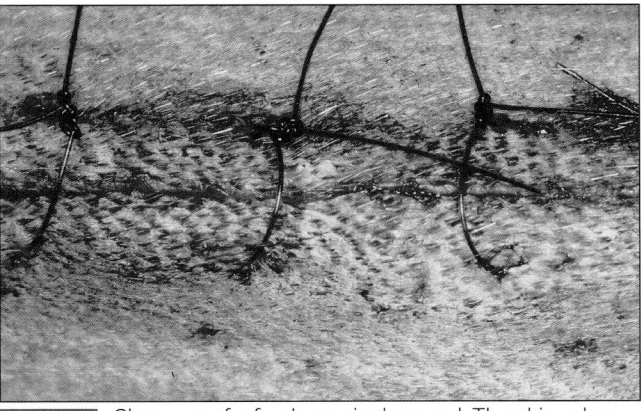

23.10 Close-up of a fresh surgical wound. The skin edges are gently apposed by the sutures and a thin line of blood clot is just visible. The edges of the wound are slightly swollen by the early inflammatory response. The swelling should be resolved by 2 days post-surgery if the wound is healing well.

Some surgical wounds do not require a dressing. Simple dressings consist of a non-adherent primary layer with a thin absorbent pad held in place by an adhesive tape. After 24 hours, this dressing can be removed as the wound will have formed a fibrin seal that is resistant to bacterial contamination. A commercial example of this kind of dressing is Primapore® (Smith & Nephew), which has a strip of non-adherent dressing with an adhesive edge to hold it to the skin. Spray-on dressings can also be used to seal the wound in the first 24 hours with a waterproof and gas-permeable polymer layer.

In some cases, additional padding is required and a thick cover of absorbent material such as cotton wool or gamgee may be used, which is held in place by tertiary dressings. Pressure bandages (e.g. Robert Jones) should always have substantial padding to prevent focal pressure points. All bandages should be replaced 24 hours after surgery to prevent the development of pressure injuries secondary to swelling under the dressing (see Chapter 15).

Wounds that are expected to exude heavily may need to be dressed more than once daily in order to ensure that the absorptive capacity of the dressing is not exceeded and the healthy tissues are kept dry and clean.

Monitoring of postsurgical wounds

Veterinary nurses are well placed to detect early signs of wound complications by careful observation of the surgical wound. If a dressing has been placed on the wound it may not be possible to observe the wound directly, but the skin surrounding the wound and the dressing itself can be observed.

The factors to pay particular attention to are:

- Exudate – note the amount, colour and type (serous or purulent). If exudate continues to leak through a dressing, the dressing must be changed to observe the wound
- Erythema (reddening) – note whether this is limited to the vicinity of the sutures or whether it extends further. Note whether the erythematous area has increased or decreased in size since the surgery
- Oedema – note how severe the oedema is and whether it is increasing or reducing
- Haematoma – note how severe the haematoma is and whether it is increasing or reducing. It is sometimes helpful to draw on the skin with a soft permanent marker

pen around a bruise; this may help to determine whether it changes in size over the following hours. Alterations in the size of a bruise could be an indication of a coagulopathy or postoperative bleeding
- Pain – note the severity of the pain (see Chapters 15 and 21) and whether the pain is continuous, intermittent, only present when the wound is handled, or if there is no pain
- Odour – note if there is a foul odour from the wound.

In addition to monitoring the wound, good post-surgical wound care also involves monitoring the patient for any signs of systemic illness that may be associated with wound complications. Both subjective and objective assessments should be performed:

- Subjective assessment – note whether the animal is bright, alert and responsive or whether there has been a change in demeanour since the surgery. Also note progressive changes in demeanour throughout the postoperative recovery phase. Subtle changes in alertness can be picked up early by an observant veterinary nurse
- Objective assessment – daily monitoring of temperature, pulse and respiration rates, food and water intake, defecation and urination and recording of clinical signs and treatments should constitute the minimum daily assessment of hospitalized patients in the postoperative phase. In some cases, a more detailed clinical examination including other factors such as water intake, neurological reflexes or blood tests may be necessary.

Prevention of self-mutilation

Self-mutilation at the surgical incision often leads to wound dehiscence. Some tendency to lick the wound postoperatively is seen in almost all animals, but persistent licking or chewing at the wound may be an indicator of wound complications. Animals may also lick or chew at the wound because of concern regarding the foreign material on the skin (the sutures) or due to generalized skin disease causing pruritus. Patients can sometimes develop dermatitis following clipping and skin preparation; this can be very painful and cause frantic chewing and licking at the surgical area, causing extensive damage and delayed healing.

Dressings will help to reduce self-mutilation, but a determined animal will soon destroy most bandages. Bitter sprays are available to protect either the bandage or the surgical site, but they are not as effective as preventing access to the wound altogether. The Elizabethan collar (see Chapter 15) is one of the most useful and commonly employed devices. These aids are available in opaque or clear plastic and are placed around the neck secured by a collar or harness. They must be large enough to prevent the nose from reaching over the edge of the collar and accessing the wound. Scratching with the hindfeet can be prevented using well padded bandages on the feet. Other devices available include neck braces or body braces that prevent the animal turning round to reach the wound. Basket muzzles are helpful in preventing animals from destroying bandages, but they must be carefully fitted to ensure that the animal can pant and drink water through the muzzle. Owners should be warned that other pets may interfere with the wound by grooming or playing.

Exotic species may require some ingenuity to prevent them interfering with sutures. The use of subcuticular sutures may be employed so that there are no skin sutures to irritate the fine skin. Elizabethan collars may be made out of light card or plastic, and splints can be made out of syringe cases or ice-lolly sticks. Care should be taken to ensure that the collar does not irritate the skin around the neck. Some species (e.g. rabbits) may 'freeze' on application of an Elizabethan collar and refuse to eat or drink. As it is important that herbivores eat as soon as possible after surgery, an 'anti-scratch' collar may be more appropriate in these situations.

It may be difficult to protect a laparotomy wound in rodents where the surgical site is in constant contact with the floor. These animals should be housed separately until the wound is healed and the bedding changed to a non-powdery form, such as shredded paper. The bedding must be completely changed daily to ensure minimal contamination of the wound with urine or faeces.

Removal of sutures

Sutures approximate the wound edges and this allows rapid first intention healing with minimal scarring. Sutures are removed as soon as the skin is healed and in most cases this will be in 7–10 days. Healing may be quicker in some young animals, whereas in older animals the sutures may be left in for a few extra days. Subcuticular sutures may be used to appose the skin edges using absorbable suture material. In these cases, the wound should still be checked 7–10 days later to ensure that the wound has healed normally.

If the wound has healed, the sutures should be easy to remove and this should not be a painful procedure. As the swelling resolves, the sutures become slightly loose and the tag can be lifted up with fingers or forceps, allowing a scissor blade to be slipped underneath, and the length entering the skin is cut, without needing to touch the skin surface. The suture then slides out of the skin. Skin staples require a special device for removal.

Once the sutures have been removed, the underlying wound should be carefully palpated to check that the tissues underneath the skin have properly healed. Removal of skin sutures from abdominal wounds should be followed by a careful check for hernias underneath the skin.

In snakes the sutures may remain in place until the next ecdysis (moult), as then the epidermis is more active and healing may be considered complete. In chelonians skin sutures are left in place for 4–6 weeks before removal.

Complications of surgical wounds

The main complication of surgical wounds is dehiscence (the breakdown of a wound along all or part of its length) (Figure 23.11). Factors that increase the risk of wound dehiscence are:

- Poor postoperative care of the wound
- Infection of the wound
- Seroma formation or haematoma
- Poor preoperative preparation of the patient
- Poor surgical technique
- Poor suture technique or inappropriate suture materials
- Decreased blood supply to the wound
- Poor general health of the patient.

Infection is the most common cause of dehiscence and may be a result of either the poor postoperative care or the surgical preparation and technique. Other complications of wound healing include sinus formation, fistula and incisional hernia.

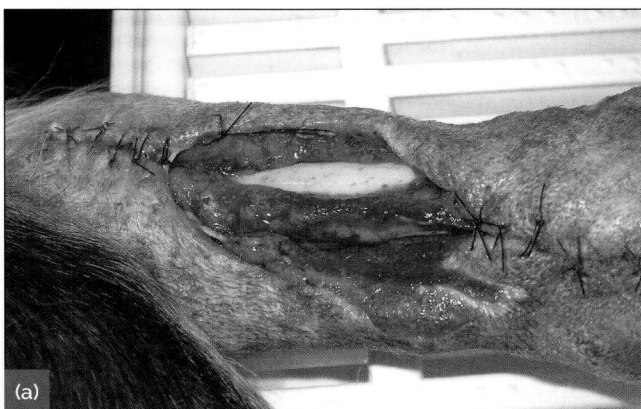

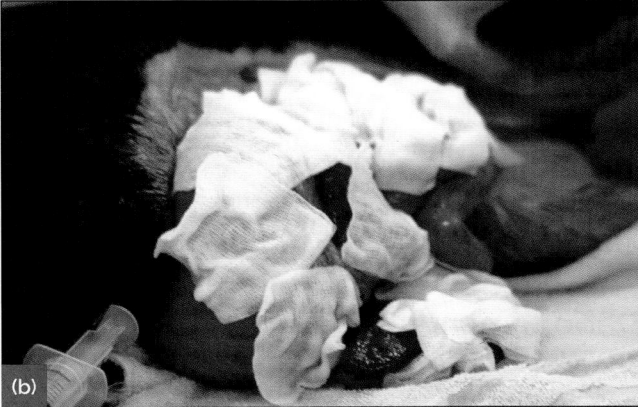

23.11 Surgical wound dehiscence. **(a)** A wound, sutured on the limb of a dog, that has been under too much tension. The central part of the wound has broken open and is now granulating slowly over the exposed bone. The edges of the sutured part are still inflamed. **(b)** A much more serious consequence of wound dehiscence in a bitch spay, where the midline repair has broken down and the abdominal contents (covered here by sterile swabs) have fallen out. This is an acute emergency following dehiscence.

Sinus formation

This is a late infective complication. It is usually a small blind-ending tract lined with granulation tissue leading to an abscess cavity. Sinuses in surgical wounds are often focused around suture material or other foreign material inadvertently left in the wound at the time of surgery. Suture sinuses are often seen surrounding skin sutures if they are left in place for too long. They resolve on removal of the foreign material.

Fistula

This is an abnormal tract that forms between two epithelialized surfaces, or connects an epithelial surface to the skin. It can be a complication of wound healing, for example in anal or oronasal surgery. Occasionally it is seen as a congenital abnormality (e.g. rectovaginal fistula). Fistulae have to be surgically repaired.

Incisional hernia

This is a late complication of abdominal surgery where there is dehiscence of the incision in the muscle layers, while the skin repair remains intact. Abdominal contents may herniate out and lie in the space between the muscles or under the skin. It should be repaired as a matter of urgency in case the skin ruptures and the abdominal contents become contaminated.

Management of contaminated or infected wounds

Initial assessment

First aid measures are important in the initial assessment of the injury:

- Take brief details of the duration and site of the injury
- Assess bleeding and determine whether arterial or venous
- Arrest bleeding using a bandage or tourniquet if necessary
- Cover the wound with a sterile dressing to prevent further contamination in the hospital
- Assess the animal's general state of health; look for signs of shock
- Assess the animal for other life-threatening injuries
- Provide analgesia, as directed by a veterinary surgeon, and treat for shock if necessary
- Antibiotic treatment may be indicated (note, antibiotics are not always indicated until the results of a culture have been received)
- Take a more detailed full history from the owner.

The history helps to determine the origin of the wound and the likely concurrent injuries. It will also determine whether the wound is classified as infected or contaminated.

Note that you should never use your veterinary nurse training to assess or treat a human wound (for example a colleague) unless you have a First Aid qualification and fully understand the differences between species.

Principles of management

The first stage is decontamination as far as possible, given the state of the wound and the condition of the patient. This also means prevention of further contamination in the hospital or by the animal. The second stage is debridement of necrotic or devitalized tissue and removal of any foreign debris. The final result should be control of infection and establishment of a healthy wound bed enabling closure of the skin deficit.

One of the important first steps is to clip and clean the surrounding undamaged skin (Figure 23.12). This not only helps to clean the wound, but also helps to assess the extent of the wound and viability of the skin. Ideally, the wound should be protected from further contamination,

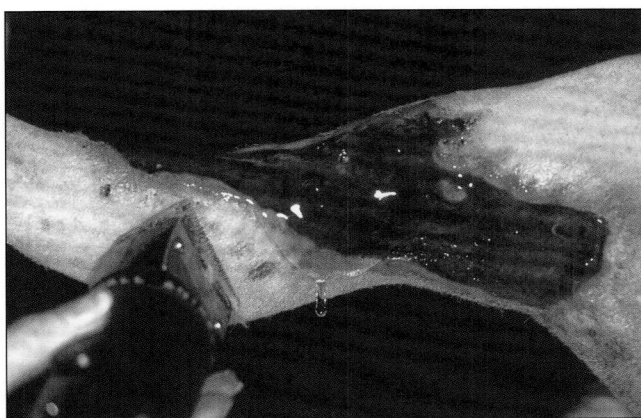

23.12 The skin surrounding a wound should be carefully clipped, using a covering such as K-Y jelly® in the wound to protect it from contamination with hair clippings.

and it may be closed using towel clips or a continuous suture. This is not always possible and so most wounds are packed with sterile swabs or filled with a water-soluble jelly (e.g. K-Y jelly®, Johnson & Johnson) during clipping and cleaning. The jelly can then be washed away with any hair or dirt from the adjacent skin later on. The clipper blades must be properly disinfected and without chips that might cause dermatitis on nearby skin. Hair at the edges may be trimmed with scissors wetted with saline or dipped in mineral oil. Thorough and wide removal of hair is important in keeping the wound clean during the next phases of management.

Lavage of wounds

The aims of wound lavage are to wash debris out of the wound, to dilute the bacteria, and not to cause any further damage. It is therefore important to use large volumes of fluids and not to lavage too vigorously. This may be achieved by using a 20 ml syringe with an 18 G needle or catheter attached to a giving set and bag of sterile isotonic fluid (Figure 23.13). Gross contamination or necrotic tissue may be washed away with gentle tap-water lavage using a hand shower. After this, the wound should be treated in a sterile manner to prevent further contamination.

Not all solutions are suitable for wound lavage; substances added to a lavage solution may damage the host cells and delay healing (Figure 23.14). Although it is tempting

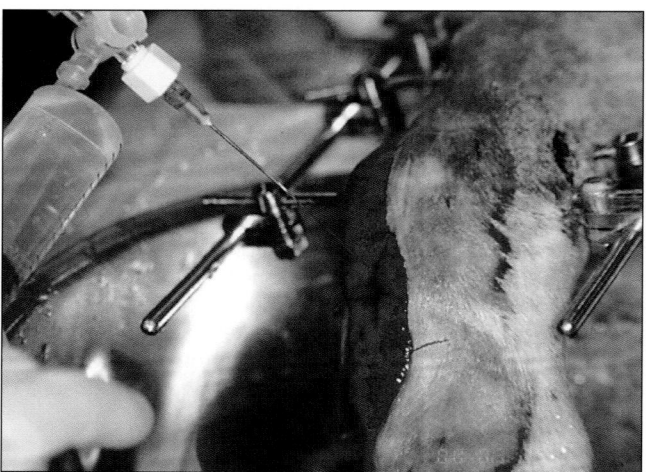

23.13 Once the surrounding skin has been clipped and cleaned, the wound itself can be irrigated or lavaged using sterile isotonic fluids (such as 0.9% saline). A 20 ml syringe is attached to a giving set and a three-way tap is used to fill the syringe with fluids from the fluid bag. The fluid is then sprayed on to the wound using an 18 G needle, as shown here. The procedure is repeated until the wound is completely clean.

to use antiseptic solutions for infected wounds, they do not stay in the wound for long and may delay wound healing. In general, it is better to use large volumes of sterile isotonic fluids to lavage wounds. If antiseptic solutions are used it is important to use the solution at the correct dilution, rather than the surgical scrub, as the latter contains detergents that can irritate an open wound.

Wound lavage procedure

1. Select at least a 1000 ml bag of warmed sterile isotonic fluid.
2. Attach a giving set with a three-way tap on the end.
3. Attach a 20 ml syringe and an 18 G needle or catheter to the three-way tap.
4. Lavage the wound over a bowl or tray to catch the fluid, using the 20 ml syringe to spray the wound surface.
5. Keep refilling the syringe from the fluid bag until all the fluids have been used to clean the wound or the wound fluid runs clear.
6. Carefully dry the healthy skin adjacent to the wound and cover the wound with sterile dressings.

Debridement of wounds

Debridement is the next crucial step in wound management. It involves removal of all infected, necrotic or contaminated tissue from the wound.

Antiseptics or antibiotics should not be a substitute for good surgical debridement. Debridement is the single most important step in the management of a wound and is often performed inadequately.

Surgical debridement

This is the best way to remove grossly contaminated tissue. The wound should be draped and prepared as for surgery and a scalpel used to cut away necrotic or dirty tissue. The instruments, gloves and drapes may be exchanged for sterile ones as the debridement progresses and the wound becomes cleaner. Surgical exploration of the wound also enables visualization of local anatomical structures and determination of the extent of the wound.

Debridement dressings

These are used in the initial stages until it is clear that there is no residual infection or necrotic material. Debridement dressings should not be left on the wound for more than 24 hours and in some instances may need to be changed

Solution	Concentration	Indications
Sterile saline	0.9%	Any wound – no tissue damage; no antibacterial action other than dilution
Lactated Ringer's solution	As supplied	As above
Chlorhexidine	0.5%	Contaminated or infected wounds – *Staphylococcus aureus* often resistant. Toxic to fibroblasts. Residual activity good
Povidone–iodine	1%	Contaminated or infected wounds. Inactivated by debris, pus or blood. Broad spectrum, poor residual activity. Toxic to host cells
Hypochlorite	0.125%	Toxic to cells. Irritant for 4–5 days after use. Not recommended
Hydrogen peroxide	1–3%	No bactericidal activity. Very toxic to all cell types. Not recommended
Cetrimide/chlorhexidine		Very toxic to cells. Irritant. Not recommended

23.14 Suitability of solutions for wound lavage.

Nine Cs of wound assessment (Baranoski *et al.* (2008))

The wound should be carefully assessed at each dressing change. Baranoski *et al* (2008) published a useful framework to guide the assessment process in management of human wounds, the 'Nine Cs of wound assessment':

Consideration	Description
Cause of the wound	Defining the cause of the wound helps with anticipating what tissue loss or factors might affect healing, or whether there might be other injuries
Clear picture of wound appearance	Describe the wound appearance accurately noting the size, location, contamination, granulation tissue, exposure of underlying tissue, epithelialization, etc.
Comprehensive picture of the patient	Note the condition of the patient and whether there are other systemic conditions that might affect outcome (e.g. age, endocrine disease, pyoderma)
Contributing factors	Note any factors that might affect the plan such as patient temperament, financial limitations, concurrent diseases or injuries or species differences in healing. Note the condition of the bandage (e.g. strike through, soiling, poor care) that might contribute to bandage related complications
Communication to other staff in the veterinary practice	Make sure the records are clearly legible and findings shared and discussed with another member of staff when the dressing is changed
Continuity of care	Try and limit the number of people involved so there is some continuity both for clinical decision making and for client communication
Centralized location for wound care information for others in practice to refer to	All records should be kept in one place – ideally on the patient record card or computer file
Components of the wound care plan	Early management strategies will be procedures such as lavage and debridement, and later strategies will include reconstruction or moist open wound healing. Record the plan for the next dressing change
Complications from the wound	Note any consequences of this wound, such as location (e.g. adjacent to vital structures), risk of penetration of a body cavity. Note also complications during ongoing wound management such as bandage related pressure sores, damage to adjacent skin, and keep a record of any suspected complications so that it can be monitored and checked. Photographic records are useful

twice daily. There are three main dressing types available for debridement (see later for details):

- Adherent dressings
- Hydrogels
- Hydrocolloids.

Other techniques

Commercial enzyme preparations can be applied to the wound to break down and allow removal of necrotic debris, but they are stopped once the granulation tissue is established.

Maggots have been used to debride wounds, allowing rapid establishment of healthy granulation tissue. Sterile maggots are produced commercially and are available at the correct larval stage for clinical use. They must be removed from the wound before they start to invade healthy tissue.

Multidrug resistant (MDR) wound contaminants

Meticillin-resistant *Staphylococcus aureus* (MRSA) has been called the hospital 'superbug' by the Press. It is one of many bacterial strains often found in hospital environments that are resistant to a range of commonly used antibiotics (see also Chapter 7). As the bacteria are usually resistant to multiple drugs, it is wise to manage these patients as outpatients where possible. When this is not possible, wounds should be kept covered and patients should be hospitalized in an isolation facility or barrier-nursed. Wearing disposable gloves to handle any patient thought to be at risk, or for changing dressings and cleaning wounds, should be considered standard policy. Multi-resistant wound infections may resolve with adequate debridement, but will persist if there is continued presence of foreign material or necrotic tissue. Commercially available, sterile live maggot dressings are available and have been used to successfully to clear wounds of infection.

Management of secondary closure wounds

Principles of wound dressings

Wound dressings are usually applied to the wound in three layers: the primary, secondary and tertiary layers. The general construction of the dressing depends on the location of the wound and the function of the dressing. Knowledge of the normal process of wound healing enables the veterinary nurse to choose the appropriate dressing at different stages of healing.

Wound dressing functions include:

- Absorption of exudate
- Analgesia
- Protection of the wound
- Prevention of infection
- Promotion of wound healing
- Maintaining a high humidity at the wound dressing interface.

Both the owner and the nursing staff should closely monitor all dressings for signs of complications. Poorly managed dressings will cause delayed wound healing and may cause further damage. Dressings that have been applied too tightly to the limb can cause damage ranging from areas of skin loss to loss of the whole limb or even death.

> ## Reasons to remove the dressing
> - Persistent chewing at the dressing
> - Foul smell from the dressing
> - Soiling or wetting of the dressing with water or urine
> - 'Strike-through' of exudate from the wound to the outside of the dressing
> - Slippage of the dressing from its original placement

Written instructions should always be given to owners if an animal is discharged with a dressing in place, which should include instructions on when to seek urgent veterinary advice.

Primary layer

The primary layer is the material that is placed in contact with the wound itself. The principle behind the primary layer is that it should at least not harm the wound and at best improve the rate of healing of the wound. Current thinking on wound management is that optimal healing occurs in a 'moist' environment. Dressings are therefore designed to provide a controlled environment that is neither too 'wet' nor too 'dry'.

There are numerous products available and it is important to realize that there is no perfect wound dressing. By understanding the way in which the different classes of dressings work, the veterinary nurse should be better equipped to use these dressings appropriately.

The functions of the primary layer will include some or all of the following at different stages:

- Debridement of necrotic tissue (this may require rehydration, lysis of fibrin attachments and physical removal from the wound)
- Absorption of fluid away from wound (if fluid is allowed to remain on the wound surface, it can macerate the tissues or provide a reservoir for infection)
- Stimulation of granulation tissue (some dressings actively promote and speed up the formation of granulation tissue)
- Promotion of epithelialization (epithelialization can only occur across healthy granulation tissue and is faster in a moist warm environment)
- Allowing contraction or controlled contraction of the wound.

Categories of primary layer dressings

Wound dressings can be described according to their basic characteristics. Some dressings may fall into more than one of the following categories, or dressings may be designed so that they have more than one general function:

- Adherent or non-adherent
- Absorbent or non-absorbent
- Passive, interactive or bioactive (passive: having no action on the wound; interactive: responding to the wound environment in some way; bioactive: having a biological effect on the wound)
- Occlusive, semi-occlusive or non-occlusive (this refers to the degree of the dressing's permeability to gas or vapour).

Adherent and non-adherent dressings

Saline-soaked gauze swabs are often used as passive adherent dressings in the early stages of wound management for debridement of necrotic tissue. These are cheap to apply and very effective; however, they may be painful to remove and can damage healthy tissue. They are often referred to as wet-to-dry dressings.

Passive non-adherent dressings are typically used over surgical wounds, skin grafts or granulation tissue. Perforated polyurethane membrane and paraffin gauze are common examples. These do not interact with the wound in any way, but prevent the secondary layers from sticking to the wound.

Absorbent dressing

Sometimes the secondary layer of the dressing is used to absorb exudate, but some primary layer dressings are specifically designed to absorb fluid and prevent it accumulating at the wound surface, causing maceration of the tissues.

Foam dressings (e.g. Allevyn™, Smith and Nephew) usually have a semi-permeable membrane backing that allows absorption of fluid and some controlled evaporation, so that the wound environment remains moist without being too wet. These passive dressings can be useful for exudative granulating wounds, as they allow epithelialization in a moist environment.

Wounds that are producing copious amounts of fluid can be dressed with ordinary disposable baby nappies. These can be weighed to calculate how much fluid the animal is losing and to document improvement as the fluid exudate decreases.

Complex dressings

Alginate dressings are bioactive and interactive. They are sheets of a protein derived from seaweed and release sodium or calcium when in contact with body fluids. This results in the stimulation of haemostasis and inflammation. They are used to stimulate the formation of granulation tissue and for haemostasis in low-level bleeding. Once they are wet, they form a gel that keeps the surface of the wound moist. The disadvantage is that sometimes they cause the formation of excessive granulation tissue.

Hydrogel dressings are interactive, consisting of insoluble hydrophilic polymers. They are provided either as a sheet with a semi-permeable backing or as a gel. The hydrogel can rehydrate necrotic tissue, absorb exudate and reduce oedema. Where it is in gel form, a second primary layer must be put over the gel to prevent it from drying out and often the foam dressings are used for this purpose. It is useful where parts of the wound are granulating well and other parts require further debridement, as the gel will not harm healthy granulation tissue. The disadvantages are that the debridement process is very slow, and the combination of dressings may be expensive.

Hydrocolloids (dressings containing gel-forming agents such as sodium carboxymethylcellulose (NaCMC) and gelatine) are bioactive and interactive suspensions of polymers in an adhesive matrix. They are usually provided as a sheet with an occlusive backing that prevents dehydration of the wound. They can both rehydrate and debride necrotic wounds and will stimulate the formation of granulation tissue. Because they are adhesive, they may prevent contraction of the granulating wound by sticking to the edges and sometimes cause exuberant granulation tissue. They should not be used for infected wounds and they need to be changed regularly so may be expensive.

Topical wound treatments

- Aloe vera ointment actively stimulates the development of granulation tissue but only if very pure products are used.
- Silver sulfadiazine ointment (Flamazine™, Smith & Nephew) is a topical broad-spectrum antibiotic with prolonged activity and is the agent of choice for prevention of sepsis from burns.
- Zinc bacitracin ointments may enhance epithelialization.
- Malic, benzoic and salicylic acid solution (Dermisol™, Zoetis) has a very low pH and is a debriding agent; it is toxic to granulation tissue and should not be left in the wound.
- Nanocrystalline silver can be used for infected wounds, but it is expensive and there are some reports that there is no decrease in infections.

Secondary bandage layer

The secondary layer of a dressing is used either to hold the primary layer in place, to provide padding to the wound underneath, to absorb exudate or to distribute the pressure of the bandage evenly. The secondary layer is most commonly an orthopaedic wool, which is available as rolls of viscose or polyester fleece in different widths. The bandage is applied evenly in a spiral with overlapping layers of 50% of the width of the material. If the bandage is required to distribute pressure (e.g. Robert Jones bandage, see Chapter 15), more substantial materials such as rolls of cotton wool are used. For heavy levels of exudate, cotton wadding such as gamgee may be incorporated into the secondary layer. The secondary layer is then stabilized using a conforming stretch bandage. This layer is again applied evenly with 50% overlap of width, only slightly compressing the wool layer underneath. It is important not to overstretch the bandage during application, particularly over narrow points in the limb, to prevent pressure sores.

Tertiary bandage layer

The tertiary layer is primarily to protect the main functional layers of the bandage from soiling or mutilation by the animal. This outer layer is usually an elastic cohesive or adhesive bandage, applied in a spiral with 50% overlap of width. It is important that this layer is applied with even pressure, as the layers cannot slide over one another to relieve pressure points when the animal moves around in the bandage. At the top of the bandage, this layer must not extend over the top of the secondary layer padding as it will cause chafing of the skin. Finally, adhesive bandages should not be used to stick the bandage to the bare skin or haircoat as an attempt to help keep the bandage in place. The bottom of the bandage may be covered with an elastic adhesive bandage to increase wear. In order to keep the bottom of the bandage dry empty intravenous fluid bags or commercially available canvas boots may be used to protect a foot temporarily, but they should not be left on permanently.

Reconstructive surgery

General principles

Major reconstructive procedures are used when there is inadequate skin or other tissue available to close a deficit created by the surgery or trauma. Usually the surgical procedure is planned in advance so that the patient can be prepared and positioned appropriately. The general principles behind reconstructive surgery include the following:

- The patient should be haemodynamically stable prior to surgery
- The patient should be prepared for a long period of anaesthesia
- A very wide area of skin should be clipped and surgically prepared to allow for moving skin around into the wound
- The skin must be handled gently to prevent bruising that might damage its blood supply.

Reconstructive procedures require good wound management in advance of the surgical procedure. Often the success of the surgery relies on the elimination of infection and foreign or necrotic material prior to surgery.

When an incision is made in the skin, or a skin deficit occurs after trauma, the elastic recoil of the skin makes the edges gape apart. When the skin edges are advanced to close the large wound, there may be too much tension on the edges, causing delayed healing or dehiscence. The skin of the dog and cat generally is extremely mobile and can be manipulated to close skin deficits, but by taking into consideration the tension lines prior to surgery, sometimes the problems associated with the recoil of the skin edges can be avoided.

Suturing skin

Sutures are used to bring the tissues together so that they heal more quickly. Sutures in the skin should appose the tissues and not cause eversion or inversion of the skin edges. Generally:

- Absorbable sutures are used in deep tissues where they are not accessible for removal
- Non-absorbable sutures, which cause less tissue reaction, are used in the skin and then removed about 7–10 days after the surgery.

Sutures should not be placed too tightly, particularly in the skin, which swells slightly in the first 2–3 days after surgery. Tight sutures may either tear out as the skin swells, or cause itchiness, which encourages the animal to interfere with them. Finally, sutures that are placed too tightly may also constrict the vessels at the wound edge and delay wound healing.

Strategies to combat tension may be employed in most simple wounds either as a single procedure or in combination:

- Subcuticular sutures are used to hold the dermis together so that the skin sutures do not have to be too tight
- Walking sutures can advance skin towards the centre of the wound taking the tension off the main incision line
- Vertical mattress sutures can also be used as tension-relieving sutures to take the pressure off the incision line for a few days and then they are removed before the incision sutures.

Many different types of suture material are available and the choice depends on the tissue, technique being used and the procedure. This is covered in more detail in Chapter 22.

Primary closure of large skin deficits

Large skin defects may not be amenable to simple closure and special reconstructive surgical techniques have to be used. These often involve moving flaps of skin around and it is important that the blood vessels supplying the flap are carefully protected from damage during the surgery. Very fine rat-toothed forceps, stay sutures or specialist skin hooks may be used to handle the skin. The blood vessels should also be prevented from going into spasm during the surgery; hypotension, hypothermia, shock, dehydration and pain will all decrease blood flow to the skin and risk damage to the skin flap. These cases need very careful peri- and post-operative nursing:

■ Clip and prepare very wide areas of skin surrounding the surgical site
■ Protect the drapes from 'strike-through' that might compromise aseptic technique
■ Monitor the patient for hypothermia and dehydration during surgery
■ Count the swabs and estimate blood loss
■ Provide soft bedding, good postoperative analgesia and close observation.

Some oncological surgeries will entail removal of part of the abdominal or thoracic wall. In these cases, a synthetic mesh made of absorbable or non-absorbable material may be used to close the defect. These meshes are expensive and can result in the development of sinus tracts if aseptic technique is inadequate.

Subdermal plexus skin flaps

Incisions are made, running away from the skin defect, to create a flap of skin that is then undermined so that it can be advanced to cover the defect. These flaps rely on the network of blood vessels in the dermis to supply the skin edges at the end of the flap. They have to have a wide base to ensure that enough vessels run into the flap to keep it alive and can only be moved into adjacent areas as far as the tension will allow.

Axial pattern skin flaps

These are advanced skin flaps that are defined and named by the specific artery and vein supplying that area of skin. The skin is elevated according to anatomical landmarks and the artery and vein are identified underneath. The flap of skin can then be moved as far as the vessels will allow. This kind of flap is very reliable as it has a well defined blood supply and can be used over wounds that have poor blood supply. They are more mobile than subdermal skin flaps, but surgery is more complex.

Free skin grafts

Free skin grafts are pieces of skin removed from a donor site and then sutured in place on to a wound (Figure 23.15). They are usually used for wounds on the limbs that are difficult to repair using skin flaps. The skin graft is very susceptible to failure, as it has to rely on the wound bed for nutrition from the first day and has no independent blood supply. If the blood supply fails to grow into the skin graft within 3–4 days, the graft will fail.

Skin grafts may be harvested as split-thickness grafts, which include only the epidermis and superficial dermis, or

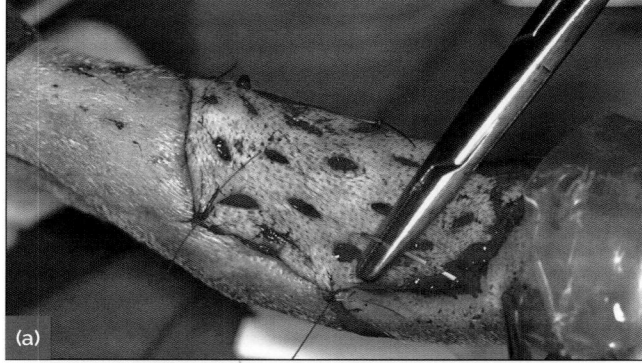
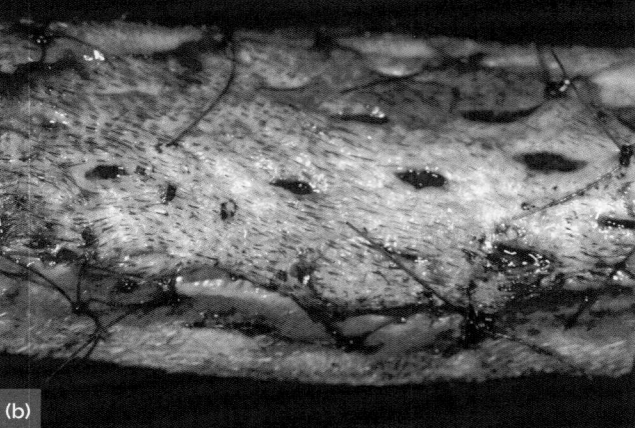

23.15 A free full-thickness skin graft. **(a)** Graft in the process of being applied to the wound; sutures are being placed to secure it. The graft has been punctured with stab incisions so that fluid cannot accumulate under it during healing. **(b)** The same graft 7 days later; the hair is just beginning to grow, the stab incisions have almost healed over and the graft has healed on to the wound bed.

as full-thickness skin grafts (FTSGs), which include the whole of the epidermis and dermis. In animals, full-thickness pieces of skin are usually used, as this also transfers the hair follicles and so the final result is more cosmetic and hard wearing.

If it is difficult to harvest a large piece of skin from the flank, punch grafts or stamp or strip grafts may be taken and embedded into the wound, allowing the surface to re-epithelialize by growing out from the islands of little skin grafts.

■ Punch grafts are usually taken with a skin biopsy punch and pushed into little holes in the granulation tissue.
■ Stamp or strip grafts are small squares or strips of skin laid on to the granulation tissue with gaps between the grafts. These tend to have very sparse hair regrowth between the grafts and are quite fragile.

Usually FTSGs are meshed by making little stab incisions in the skin (see Figure 23.15) to allow them to conform better to the surface of the wound and also to allow drainage of fluid out from underneath the graft.

Management of free skin grafts

■ A well padded bandage (Robert Jones) must be kept on for the first 5–7 days to immobilize the limb.
■ Bandage changes must be carried out carefully in order that the graft does not move.
■ Aseptic wound management is required to prevent infection.
■ A non-adherent primary dressing layer is essential.

Postoperatively grafts are dressed with a non-adherent dressing such as paraffin gauze or silicone mesh and heavily bandaged (e.g. with a Robert Jones bandage) to prevent movement of the graft site. The dressing is changed as infrequently as possible, in order to minimize disruption of the fragile process of graft healing over the first 7 days.

Free skin grafts may fail due to inadequate preparation of the wound bed (e.g. chronic avascular granulation tissue), infection of the graft, failure to immobilize the graft or adherence of the primary dressing to the graft. They may also fail if serum or haemorrhage accumulates underneath the graft and lifts it off the wound surface so that the blood vessels cannot grow into the graft quickly enough.

Complications associated with reconstructive surgery

Many reconstructive procedures are long surgeries with large areas of tissue exposed for some time. Patients may dehydrate and also become hypothermic resulting in longer recovery times and poor skin circulation. If the surgical technique is poor these skin flaps have a high risk of failure. If the circulation fails in the skin flap it rapidly becomes ischaemic and over the first 3–4 days is cold to the touch, finally becoming hard and blackened as the skin dies.

Drains

Drains are used where there is a need to perform repeated lavage of a space, where there is a need for repeated aspiration of fluid (or air) from a space, or where the surgeon wants to prevent the accumulation of fluid in a space (e.g. seroma).

Passive *versus* active drains

Passive drains rely on gravity and capillary action, whereas active drains have a suction apparatus on one end – either intermittent or continuous.

Passive drains

The commonest passive drain is the Penrose drain, which is a soft latex tube (Figure 23.16) usually placed in the dead space created at surgery to allow drainage of fluid after surgery. One end of the drain is anchored in the wound with an absorbable suture and the other is anchored at the skin. The end of the drain should always exit through a separate skin incision site to the surgical incision so that it does not interfere with wound healing. As it relies on gravity, the drain should exit at the lowest possible point. To increase drainage, a larger drain or several drains may be placed (drainage volume depends on the surface area for the capillary action).

Active drains

Active drains usually have rigid walls and may have a radiopaque marker down the side so that their position can be checked (Figure 23.16). The most common is the thoracic drain, where a drain is placed through the skin, under a skin tunnel and then between the ribs into the thorax. The end of the drain is closed securely with clamps and bungs. The drain may be used to aspirate air or fluid out of the chest or to introduce treatment into the chest cavity (e.g. in pyothorax). The drain can be attached to a syringe for intermittent suction or to a suction device that continuously drains the chest. These drains have to be very carefully bandaged in as

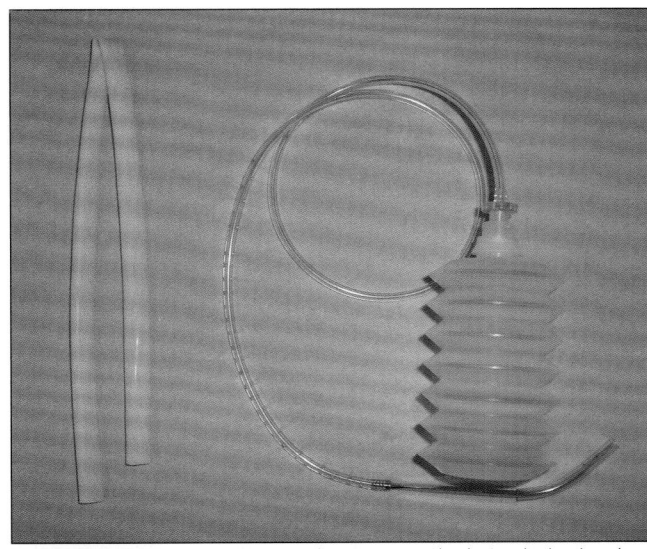

23.16 Drains can be used postoperatively to drain dead space and prevent seroma formation after reconstruction. Penrose drains (left) are soft latex tubes that allow fluid to drain out of the space along the surface of the drain (passive drainage). A dressing should be applied to protect the drain from contamination and to collect the fluid. An active drain (right) is a rigid tube in the wound with a device that exerts constant gentle negative pressure (suction). Active drains often have a sharp curved needle-like device on the end of the tube in order to place the drain through the skin. This 'needle' is then cut off and disposed of.

the animal could die if it chewed the end of the tube and the chest communicated directly with the outside.

Active drains are also used underneath surgical wounds, attached to suction devices that collect the drained fluid. The continuous gentle suction applied to the dead space is a very effective way of preventing the formation of a seroma.

Closed *versus* open drains

The thoracic drain is always a closed drain and the system is sealed from the outside.

- Active drains are closed, as they collect the fluid in a reservoir bottle or tube.
- Passive drains will always be open, as they allow the fluids to drip out on to the patient, dressing or the floor.

When a passive drain is used, there is a potential risk of bacterial contamination of the wound as bacteria may migrate up the sides and lumen of the tube. In addition, there is increased nursing involved in keeping the skin clean and dry underneath the wound and preventing the haircoat from becoming wet. The skin may be protected by using either a thin layer of barrier cream under the end of the drain or a commercial synthetic spray or cream that makes a breathable but waterproof barrier on the skin to help to prevent maceration, e.g. Cavilon™ (3M). Where possible the drain should be bandaged in place with a sterile dressing to absorb the fluid from the end of the drain. This has to be changed regularly to ensure that the skin does not become macerated.

Active drains still have some risk of bacterial contamination as there will be some migration of bacteria up the sides of the tube, but the risk is smaller, particularly as they can often be bandaged into place using antiseptic ointments and sterile dressings.

Care and management of drains

All drains should be handled in an aseptic manner. Antibiotics may be indicated after culture and sensitivity results confirm there is an infection. The animal must be prevented from interfering with the drain and the drain must be protected from the animal's urine or faeces. For removal, the skin suture is cut and the drain is then pulled out quickly with light pressure over the hole to help it to seal. Thoracic drains should have a purse-string suture pre-placed in the skin ready to close the skin on removal. With most other drains, the hole is allowed to granulate over after removal.

Wounds: a summary

- Wounds heal in a predictable manner, which can be manipulated by the veterinary surgeon or veterinary nurse to accelerate or delay the recovery of the animal
- Classification of wounds is important in order to make a rational plan of approach to management of a case
- Wounds allowed to heal by second intention should be assessed closely at each bandage change in order to determine what stage of healing the tissues have reached and to apply the appropriate dressing
- Reconstructive surgery is the technique of choice where possible

---

Fracture management

A fracture is a complete or incomplete break of bone continuity, with or without displacement of the resulting fragments.

Initial assessment and management

It is essential that the patient is adequately restrained before being examined or given first aid. However placid an animal is under normal circumstances it will often attempt to bite when in pain. A muzzle is often required.

Fractures may be accompanied by other injuries and some of these can be life-threatening. The fracture is of less priority and its repair (depending on its nature) can be left for several days until the patient is in a stable condition. It is important to prioritize these injuries and deal with the most life-threatening first (see Chapter 19). A full and careful examination can be carried out by the veterinary surgeon, analgesics administered and the limb temporarily supported with splints and bandages (see Chapter 15). When a fracture is suspected, two orthogonal radiographic views must be taken in order to make a specific diagnosis.

Fracture healing

Indirect fracture healing

This process was previously called secondary healing. Local events immediately after fracture are the same as in other tissues: haemorrhage, formation of a clot, and acute inflammation. The clot is gradually replaced by granulation tissue and blood vessels grow into the organizing clot from periosteal blood vessels and blood vessels in the medullary canal of the bone. Fibrous tissue is produced by fibroblasts in the organizing clot around the fracture and forms a cuff around the bone ends. This fibrous tissue is important: it stabilizes the fracture and allows cartilage to develop. This large cuff of stabilizing tissue is known as callus and is composed of fibrous tissue, cartilage and immature bone; this envelops the ends of the bone.

The cartilage is slowly replaced by bone in endochondral fashion. Cells called chondroclasts resorb cartilage and new bone is formed when osteoblasts line the surfaces and secrete a mineralized matrix. As this process progresses, the callus gradually contains more cartilage and bone and less fibrous tissue. The fracture becomes more stable until eventually the callus rigidly unites the bone ends and this is the point of clinical union. Callus is not always helpful; sometimes the callus formed may be disorganized and excessive and can interfere with the normal movements of muscle and tendons.

There is a long remodelling phase where the callus is replaced by mature bone. Osteoclasts are responsible for bone resorption in the remodelling phase; they remove the mineral part of the callus and degrade the collagenous and non-collagenous proteins. Simultaneously, mature bone is laid down by osteoblasts, thus recreating the original bony structure.

Haversian remodelling is a process of bone resorption and formation within the cortex and is the final step in restoration of the normal compact bone structure. The surface of the cortices becomes smooth and the bone's strength is restored in response to normal weight bearing.

Direct fracture healing

Direct fracture healing (previously called primary healing) occurs when the bone edges are so close together that callus formation does not occur and the bone forms without the interim stage of fibrous tissue and cartilage. In cases where callus formation is detrimental to the return of function (e.g. joint surfaces), direct fracture healing is preferable and this usually requires surgical intervention as soon as possible after the trauma. The fragments must be held in rigid anatomical alignment (i.e. with plates, screws or wires, or a combination), and this allows Haversian systems to cross a minute fracture gap and repair the cortical bone directly with little or no callus formation.

Rate of fracture healing

Provided there are no complications, clinical union is usually achieved in 12–16 weeks in adult dogs and cats. Remodelling may continue for many months, or even years, after clinical union has occurred. The rate of fracture healing is assessed by clinical examination to detect the increase in rigidity and the firm swelling associated with union by callus formation. Radiographs are taken to assess the degree of callus formation and the extent of mineralization within the callus. Many factors influence the rate at which fractures heal and it is important to be aware of these when contemplating fracture repair.

- Fractures in immature animals heal more quickly than in adult animals.
- Fractures in geriatric animals heal more slowly.
- Fractures in debilitated animals heal more slowly. Debilitation may be due to poor nutrition or systemic illness such as hormonal disorder or kidney failure.
- Osteomyelitis interferes with healing and is one of the most common causes of poor fracture healing after surgical repair. Healing can progress normally once the infection is controlled.

- Fractures of cancellous bone heal more quickly than fractures in cortical bone.
- Fractures in bones that have a good blood supply heal more quickly than those in areas with a poor blood supply. For example, the pelvis and scapula are covered by large muscle masses which have a good blood supply and these bones heal well. The distal one-third of the radius and ulna has little muscle cover and a poor blood supply and fractures at this site heal poorly, especially in very small breeds of dog.
- Oblique fractures heal more quickly than transverse fractures, because there is a larger area of contact to promote tissue regrowth.
- Poor reduction or fixation of a fracture will result in a slow rate of healing.
- Movement of the fracture site delays or prevents healing.

Complications of fracture healing

- Non-union – complete failure of the fractured ends of the bone to unite
- Delayed union – fracture healing progresses slowly. Clinical union is not achieved within the expected time
- Malunion – fracture heals in an abnormal position. Untreated fractures and those not treated effectively often heal in an abnormal position
- Shortened limb – limb shortening occurs if there is healing with inadequate reduction of over-riding fracture fragments. Limb function may be severely compromised
- Osteomyelitis – inflammation of the bone. Bacterial osteomyelitis is commonly caused by inadequate asepsis during surgery or in open fractures. It is more likely to occur if there is also damage to the local blood supply. This is recognized by heat, pain and swelling of the affected part, systemic illness, inappetence and fever
- Fracture disease – a syndrome of muscle wastage and inability to flex joints in a limb after fracture repair. One or more joints in the affected limb may be held rigid due to scar formation within the joints or within muscles surrounding the fracture site. Fracture disease is more common after fixation by external coaptation or when there is inadequate reduction
- Sequestrum – a necrotic piece of bone not incorporated successfully in the fracture repair
- Implant failure – this can occur through poor choice of implants or technique, stress applied through the implant caused by overactive behaviour of the patient, or failure of the implant itself. This will result in a sudden deterioration, with instability and pain returning at the fracture site

Classification of fractures

Modern classification of fractures provides information for both treatment and prognosis: the bone involved, type of displacement, direction of the fracture line and the number and type of fragments.

Closed *versus* open fractures

- A closed fracture describes a fracture with no break in the skin.

- An open fracture has a wound that has penetrated the skin and the fracture ends are open to the outside environment. This type carries a greater risk of infection and is often contaminated (e.g. a road traffic accident where the limb has been dragged along the road).

Anatomical description

- Articular – involving the joint.
- Diaphyseal – a fracture in the midshaft or diaphysis of the bone.
- Metaphyseal – a fracture of the area between the midshaft and the end of a long bone (epiphysis).
- Physeal – a fracture through the growth plate of an immature animal.
- Epiphyseal – a fracture of the epiphysis.
- Condylar – a fracture of the epiphysis when condyles are involved, e.g. the distal humerus or femur.
- Other common sites of fractures include the pelvis, the mandibles and the ribs.

Type of displacement

- Greenstick – an incomplete (i.e. only one cortex) fracture of a bone of an immature animal.
- Fissure – a fine crack, which may displace during surgery or when stressed.
- Depressed – especially fractures of the skull, where fragments may be pushed into the underlying cavity.
- Compression – often refers to fracture of a vertebral body where a compressive force has resulted in the shortening of a vertebra by a crushing effect.
- Impacted – cortical fragments forced into cancellous bone.
- Avulsion – a fracture in which a bony prominence has been torn away from the rest of the bone, usually by the pull of a muscle (e.g. fracture of the olecranon or avulsion of the tibial crest).

Direction of fracture line

- Transverse – fracture line is at 90 degrees to the axis of the bone (Figure 23.17a).
- Oblique – fracture line is at an angle of at least 30 degrees.
- Spiral – fracture line curves around the bone.
- Longitudinal, Y or T – refers to the appearance of the fracture lines on the bone.

Number or types of fracture

- Simple – one fracture line, creating two fragments (Figure 23.17a).
- Comminuted – more than one fracture line, creating more than two fragments (Figure 23.17a).
- Wedge – a multifragmented fracture with some contact between the main fragments after reduction.
- Segmental – one or more large complete fragments of the shaft of a long bone.
- Irregular – a diaphyseal fracture with no specific pattern.
- Multiple – more than one fracture in the same or different bones.

Other classifications

Some fractures are further classified to provide more detail about the appearance. Epiphyseal or growth plate fractures are classified by the Salter–Harris system, ranging from Type

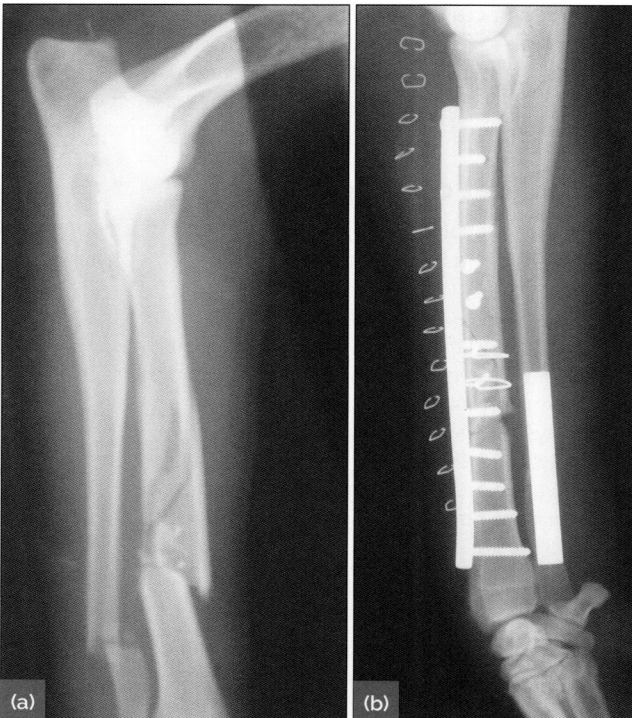

23.17 **(a)** A mid-shaft fracture of the radius and ulna. The ulna has a simple transverse diaphyseal fracture and the radius has a comminuted diaphyseal fracture; **(b)** The radius has been repaired with a 3.5 mm dynamic compression plate (DCP) and 3.5 mm cortical screws. Two lag screws have been placed (screws 5 and 6 from the top) and two cerclage wires have been placed around some of the fragments. The ulna has been repaired with a 2.7 mm DCP. The skin has been closed with skin staples.

I to Type VI. Accessory carpal bone and central tarsal bone fractures are important fractures in racing Greyhounds and are each classified Type I to Type V.

Diagnosis of fractures

Clinical signs

Owners may have witnessed an incident and can give the veterinary surgeon vital information. A good clinical history may then give a good indication of the nature of the injuries.

The first signs, as with any injury, can be attributed to acute inflammation. The major clinical signs seen with fractures are:

- Pain localized to the affected bone
- Local swelling and heat
- Bruising at the fracture site leading to discoloration of the overlying soft tissues
- Marked loss of function (i.e. very lame or non-weight-bearing)
- Visible or palpable deformity of the affected bone
- Abnormal mobility at the fracture site
- Crepitus when the injured part is moved.

Radiography

General anaesthesia is usually necessary to obtain good quality radiographs. At least two views are essential to enable the veterinary surgeon to make a diagnosis and a plan for repair. Radiographs of the normal contralateral limb

are useful in planning reconstruction of a severe fracture, e.g. comminuted or multiple fractures. Although it may be obvious that a limb is fractured, a good-quality radiograph will confirm details such as hairline fractures, small fissures and chips, or alterations in bone density, which could affect the treatment plan (see Chapter 16).

Computed tomography

Computed tomography (CT) scans can be very useful for planning repairs of complex articular fractures or facial and skull fractures. In addition, these scans often reveal information from the 3D reconstruction that would not have been available from conventional radiographs (see Chapter 16).

Principles of fracture repair

The primary aim of fracture fixation (Figure 23.17b) is to restore the functional anatomy of the fractured bone. This is achieved by:

- Restoring the continuity of the bone
- Restoring the length of the bone
- Restoring the functional shape of the bone
- Maintaining essential soft tissue function.

Essential soft tissues include the blood vessels supplying the bone, muscles acting on the bone and the nerves supplying the muscles. Any techniques for fracture repair must be sympathetic to these tissues because without them there is no chance of restoring function to the injured limb. Many techniques exist for successfully restoring bone continuity, length and shape. The same basic principles apply to all the techniques:

- Reduction – the fracture fragments should be brought together in the correct anatomical alignment. This may be carried out 'closed' by traction and manipulation of the limb, or 'open' by performing surgery when the fracture is visualized and the individual fragments are manipulated back into position
- Fixation – the fragments should be immobilized in the correct alignment until clinical union occurs. The fragments may also be compressed together to narrow the fracture gap
- Blood supply – the blood supply to the bone fragments must be preserved. Fractures will heal only if there is an adequate blood supply.

Stabilization of fractures

After reduction of a fracture the bones must be held in position until healing occurs. Indications for immobilization at the fracture site are:

- To relieve pain
- To prevent displacement of the fragment (loss of reduction)
- To prevent movement that might cause delayed union or non-union.

In some cases, such as greenstick fractures and some pelvic fractures, immobilization may be unnecessary and simple restriction of activity will suffice.

Fixation techniques

Fracture fixation techniques are broadly classified into three groups:

- External coaptation, using casts or splints
- Internal fixation, using pins, plates, screws and other devices
- External–internal fixation using 'external fixators'.

There are a number of ways to repair fractures and there are a number of factors to be taken into account before deciding on the technique for repair:

- Classification of the fracture
- Age of the patient
- Size of the patient
- Temperament of patient
- Presence of any underlying disease
- Cost to owner
- Expectations of owner (e.g. working animal *versus* pet).

For example, a young dog's fractures will heal more quickly than an older dog's, and a fracture in a small breed, such as a Chihuahua, presents different problems to those associated with a large breed dog such as a Great Dane with a similar fracture.

External coaptation

The aim of external coaptation is to limit motion at a fracture site by immobilizing the joints above and below the fracture. If the joints above and below the fracture cannot be immobilized, external coaptation is not suitable.

Methods of external coaptation fall into three main groups: casts, splints and extension splints.

External coaptation techniques

Advantages
- Technically simpler than some internal fixation techniques
- Economical
- Non-invasive

Disadvantages
- They have limited applications. For example, casts are most useful for fractures below the stifle in the hindlimb and below the elbow in the forelimb
- They do not provide sufficient stability for many fractures, particularly comminuted or severely oblique fractures
- They are at risk of causing decubital ulcers
- Slower healing of fracture and greater callus formation
- They restrict activity of joints and muscles in the limb and are therefore prone to causing fracture disease

---

Types of fracture suitable for casting

Relatively stable fractures are ideal: greenstick fractures or simple oblique or spiral fractures that are stable after manual reduction. Where one bone is fractured close to an intact bone that provides a splint-like mechanism, a cast can be used (e.g. a fractured radius with an intact ulna). Casts are also used for postoperative support of arthrodeses, internal fixations or tendon repair.

Casting material should:

- Be conformable and easy to apply
- Reach maximum strength quickly.

The ideal finished cast should be:

- Hard wearing
- Radiolucent (to enable monitoring of fracture healing without removal of the cast)
- Strong and lightweight and not bulky
- Easy to remove
- Water resistant and 'breathable'
- Economical.

There are various types of casting materials available:

- Polypropylene impregnated with resin (e.g. Dynacast™, Smith & Nephew) is easy to apply, radiolucent, strong, lightweight and hard wearing
- Fibreglass impregnated with resin (e.g. Vetcast Plus™, 3M) is easy to apply, strong and lightweight. It is porous and allows the skin to breathe, which helps to reduce itching and odour. Softcast™ (3M) is made from knitted fibreglass material and is semi-rigid and flexible
- Thermoplastic polymer mesh (e.g. Vet-Lite™, Runlite SA) is easy to apply, radiolucent (though the mesh creates a distracting pattern on the radiograph), strong and hard wearing. It is unaffected by contact with water, urine or faecal material. It can be reformed or reshaped with hot water
- Plaster of Paris is cheap and conformable but messy to apply. It makes a heavy, bulky and weak cast, is slow to reach maximum strength and loses strength when in contact with water. It is radiopaque and has to be removed to monitor fracture healing.

Application of a cast

The casting material must be applied in close proximity to the bone to be able to give good support to the fracture. There is a fine line between using too much padding and too little. Too much will allow the fractured ends to move within the cast or cause the cast to slip. Too little casting material can lead to decubital ulcers. The cast must contain at least one joint above the fracture and one below, and prevent weight bearing across the fracture.

Applying a cast

The manufacturer's instructions should be followed closely. All the materials needed should be collected before applying the cast.

Equipment
- Gloves
- Stockinette
- Synthetic cast padding, such as Soffban™ (BSN Medical)
- Sufficient rolls of casting material of appropriate size
- A bowl of water at the temperature recommended by the manufacturer →

Applying a cast *continued*

Technique

1. Open or surgical wounds are covered with non-adherent dressing.
2. Stockinette is rolled up the limb, taking care to prevent any creases.
3. Cast padding is carefully and evenly wound on to the limb with 50% overlap at each turn, paying special attention to any bony prominence. These parts should not be overpadded; instead ring 'donuts' are used. Donuts can be made by cutting holes in small pads made out of cast padding; these are usually placed on the accessory carpal bone and olecranon of the forelimb or the calcaneus of the hindlimb. This prevents pressure ulceration on these structures.
4. One roll of casting material is prepared by immersing it in the bowl of water and squeezing several times to allow the water to penetrate into the roll.
5. Excess water is squeezed out and the roll of casting material is applied to the limb in the same manner as the padding but with even tension. The casting material starts to set within minutes (depending on the type used), therefore it is important to work quickly.
6. Each roll is wetted individually just before application. Depending on the type of casting material used and the size of the patient, usually 2–3 layers are applied with 4–6 layers for larger dogs.
7. The pads and nails of the middle two toes are left exposed at the bottom of the cast.
8. A 1–2 cm length of padding is left exposed at the top and bottom of the cast.
9. Once the cast has hardened the stockinette and padding at each end are turned down over the edge of the cast and secured with tape.
10. A cast may be made stronger by applying splints made out of several lengths of casting material laid longitudinally down the compression side of the cast.

Splints

Gutter splints can be used as a fixation technique in some fractures, particularly those occurring below the carpus or hock in cats and small dogs. Splints can also be made from casting material (except plaster of Paris). A cast is applied as before, and then an oscillating saw is used to cut the length of the cast on the medial and lateral sides. The limb is dressed and bandaged appropriately and the two halves of the cast are reapplied to the limb and secured with an adhesive bandage.

Postoperative care of casts and splints

Owners should be given written instructions of how to look after the cast and what to look out for if complications arise.

- When the patient is taken outside, the bottom of the cast should be covered with a plastic bag (old intravenous fluid drip bags are useful for this) and secured with tape – never elastic bands, as these may easily be forgotten and cause problems later on. →

Postoperative care of casts and splints *continued*

- Casts may have to be reapplied if the animal chews extensively or damages the cast. Growing animals will need a new cast every week to allow normal growth of the limb.
- Give medication as prescribed.
- Check cast daily and any of the following signs should be reported to the veterinary surgeon immediately:
  - Swelling of the limb or toes
  - Chafing at the edges of the cast
  - Staining of the cast with a discharge
  - A foul smell coming from the cast
  - Slipping of the cast from its original position
  - Chewing or other signs of discomfort
  - Collapse or bending of the cast (especially plaster of Paris)
  - General illness – depression, lethargy, lack of appetite.

Complications of casts

- Limb swelling – if the cast is too tight it restricts the lymphatic and venous drainage, which results in oedema of the lower limb. This is usually seen within 1 hour of applying the cast and needs urgent attention.
- Decubital ulcers – usually seen if the cast is poorly padded or is slightly loose and sliding on the skin.
- Cast loosening – if the cast was put on when the limb was swollen the cast may loosen once the swelling subsides.
- Prolonged immobilization of the limb may cause any of the following complications:
  - Joint stiffness and fibrosis
  - Cartilage degeneration
  - Muscle atrophy
  - Osteoporosis of disuse.
- Joint laxity – rapidly growing young large-breed dogs are particularly at risk.
- Delayed union, malunion and non-union may be seen with poor case selection, poor cast selection, poor casting technique or frequent reapplication of the cast and movement of the fracture site.
- Refracture on removal of the cast – provided that the limb has good callus formation (clinical union) on the radiograph at the time of cast removal this should not occur.

Removal of the cast

Generally, limbs remain in a cast for 4–6 weeks. Radiographs are taken to establish the degree of healing and callus formation. The patient should be sedated or anaesthetized. An oscillating saw is the most suitable tool for removing casts. Two cuts are made in the cast with the line of cut carefully chosen to avoid bony prominences. The saw should never come into contact with the skin. The saw moves in an arc of 5–6 degrees and only cuts the solid casting material; the padding underneath catches on the blade and is not cut. The oscillating blade can become hot whilst cutting the cast and the saw should be rotated to use a cooler part of the blade. The padding underneath can be removed with scissors. Plaster shears can also be used: they are inserted at the distal end of the cast and the cut is advanced proximally in small regular steps.

Internal fixation

Internal fixation uses pins, plates, screws and wire to repair fractures.

Internal fixation

Advantages
- Suitable for fractures in any bone
- Versatile and can handle the full range of fracture types
- Allows accurate reduction and rigid fixation
- Allows the limb to return to full function early, encouraging fracture healing and minimizing the risk of fracture disease

Disadvantages
- Technique is relatively expensive and time-consuming
- Some internal fixation techniques are technically demanding
- There is capital expenditure on the equipment
- The risks of surgery (wound healing problems, infection) are inherently greater in an open reduction and fixation than in closed reduction and fixation
- Open fractures with extensive soft tissue injury may not be suitable

---

Implants and techniques used in internal fixation

Intramedullary pins

These are called Steinmann pins; they are stainless steel rods with a sharp trocar point at each end, and it is possible to have one end threaded. They come in different widths ranging from 1.6 to 8 mm in diameter and are placed into the medulla of the bone that is fractured. They are inserted with a Jacobs Chuck or power drill.

- Advantages: cheap to purchase, quick to use, require minimal surgical exposure, easier to implant and remove than bone plates.
- Disadvantages: less stable fixation, slower return to function, secondary bone union (i.e. slower healing), greater aftercare required, not suitable for unstable fractures.

Postoperative management of intramedullary pins

- Two radiographic views are required to assess repair
- Provide clients with written instructions outlining convalescent period and dates for follow-up examinations
- Give medication (analgesics and possibly antibiotics) as directed
- Exercise restrictions: lead-exercise only to allow patient to urinate and defecate. Cats should be restricted to a cage or a section of a room
- Avoid stairs and prevent animal jumping on or off furniture
- Sutures are usually removed after 10 days ➜

Postoperative management of intramedullary pins *continued*

- At the first check, evaluate for limb function and assess joints adjacent to the fracture for range of motion. The point where the pin emerges from bone is examined for swelling or evidence of pin migration. There should be regular checks to monitor bone healing and possible pin migration
- The pin is usually removed under anaesthetic once clinical union is achieved

---

Interlocking nail

These are solid rods of 4, 4.7, 6 or 8 mm diameter, with holes through which interlocking nail bolts are inserted. The nails are placed in the medulla and the bolts fix the rod within the bone (Figure 23.18). Diaphyseal fractures are suitable for this method of repair and it gives a more reliable fixation than an intramedullary pin because the rotation and compression forces are resisted. It requires expensive equipment and technical expertise to insert. Equipment and implants are available in the UK but they are mostly used in specialist referral centres.

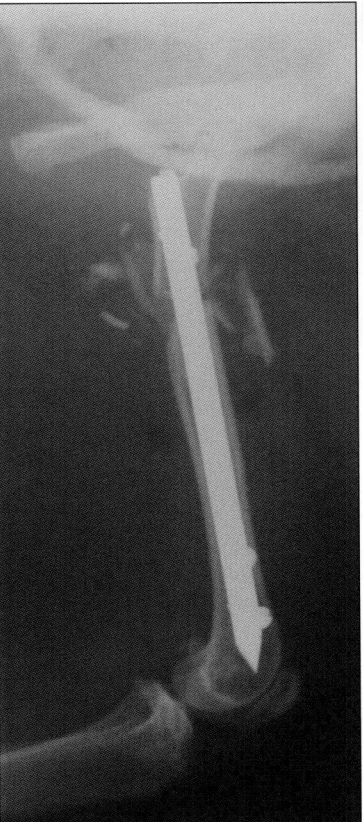

23.18 An interlocking nail has been used to repair this fracture of the femur. Two bolts have been placed in the distal fragment and another two bolts can just be seen in the proximal fragment.

Arthrodesis and Kirschner wire

These are smaller pins with diameters of 0.9 to 2 mm. Arthrodesis wires have trocar points at each end. Kirschner wires (K-wires) have a flattened bayonet point at one end and a trocar point at the other. These pins can be used as intramedullary pins in very small bones, as an aid in stabilizing a fragment while primary fixation is taking place or to create a tension-band wire (see below). They are also used in various types of fractures in small dogs and cats but not for midshaft fractures of long bones.

Cerclage wire

This is malleable monofilament stainless steel wire. It is often used to supplement the use of intramedullary pins, external skeletal fixators and bone plates (see Figure 23.17b). It compresses large fragments by encircling the bone and the fragment and then is twisted with wire twisters, pliers or special tighteners. It is also used to create a tension-band wire (see below).

Tension-band wire

This is used to fix an avulsed fracture. It uses two different directional forces to create compression of the fracture. Two K-wires are placed into the fragment and main bone. A cerclage wire is placed in a figure-of-eight pattern around the end of the pins and anchored through a predrilled hole to a solid part of the bone on the opposite side to the ligament or muscle that pulled off the fragment (Figure 23.19).

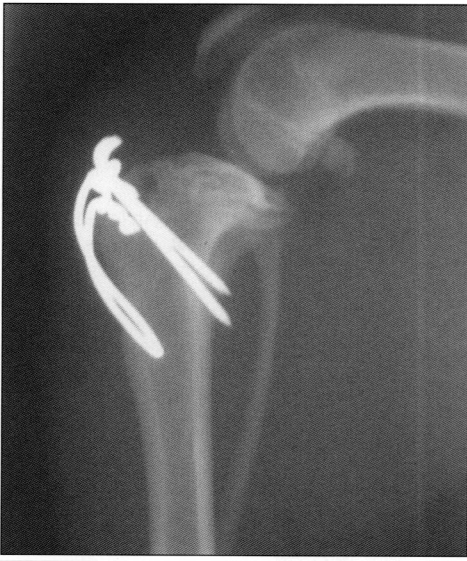

23.19 Two K-wires and a tension-band wire have been used to repair an avulsion fracture of the tibial tuberosity.

ASIF/AO systems

ASIF stands for the Association for the Study of Internal Fixation and is used in North America to name the patent and copyright of the system of orthopaedic equipment used for internal fixation. The European designation for the same equipment is AO, which stands for Arbeitsgemeinschaft für Osteosynthesefragen.

There is a wide variety of different plates and equipment for repairing every conceivable type of fracture. The most commonly used plate in veterinary practice is the dynamic compression plate (DCP; see Figure 23.17b). It is a strong plate with oval holes. These are available in different widths named by the size of screw they take and the length or number of holes. A 2 mm plate takes 2 mm screws; a 2.7 mm plate takes 2.7 mm screws; 3.5 mm and 4.5 mm plates come in narrow or broad widths and take 3.5 and 4.5 mm screws, respectively.

The DCP can serve various functions depending on how it is applied to the fractured bone. It can be used as a compression plate, as a neutralization plate, or as a buttress plate. A compression plate is used in simple transverse diaphyseal fractures to compress the ends of the bone together. A neutralization plate is used in oblique, spiral and comminuted fractures where compression is not possible and the fracture has been reconstructed with wires or screws but the repair needs additional support. A buttress plate is used to help to stabilize the fracture site and to bridge a fracture that is not reconstructable. The defect at the fracture site is usually filled with a cancellous bone graft.

Fracture management systems continue to evolve and specialist orthopaedic surgeons will use a wide variety of implant systems. Newer plates, such as the Locking Compression Plate (LCP), Limited Contact Dynamic Compression Plate (LC-DCP) and String of Pearls plate (SOP) may help to resolve problems that arise in specific situations.

Screws (AO type)

These screws are identified by the hexagonal head, which requires a special type of screwdriver to be able to place them. They are available in different widths and lengths and some larger screws are cortical or cancellous. Figure 23.20 is a guide to the sizes and drill bits to use.

Size of screw (mm)	Drill bit for core (mm)	Drill bit for gliding hole (mm)	Tap (mm)
1.5[a]	1.1	1.5	1.5
2.0[a]	1.5	2.0	2.0
2.4[a]	1.8	2.4	Self-tapping
2.7[a]	2.0	2.7	2.7
3.5[a]	2.5	3.5	3.5
4.0[b]	2.0	4.0	4.0
4.5[a]	3.2	4.5	4.5
6.5[b]	3.2	6.5	6.5

23.20 Sizes of AO-type screws and corresponding drill bits. [a]Cortical; [b]Cancellous.

After the plate has been contoured (bent to fit the shape of the bone), it is held in position with bone-holding forceps. A drill bit is selected to drill a hole the size of the core of the screw to include both near and far cortices; for example, if a 3.5 mm cortical screw is to be used, a 2.5 mm drill bit will be selected. The hole is then measured with the depth gauge and the correct length of screw is selected. The hole is then 'tapped' to create a thread for the screw. A tap is a special device designed to cut the thread in the bone. It is especially important to use the correct tap for the screw being inserted. The tap designed for the 4.0 mm cancellous screw cannot be used for the 3.5 mm cortical screw even though both screws are of similar widths, because the thread has a different pitch. The screw is finally driven into the hole using the hexagonal-head screwdriver.

Self-tapping screws are available in the same widths and lengths, but do not need to be tapped before being inserted into the drilled hole in the bone. Locking screws have a thread cut into the head of the screw, which fits holes in an LCP or LC-DCP and locks the plate to the screw.

Lag screw technique

A lag screw is not a specific type of screw but rather a technique. It is used to stabilize and compress fragments in a fracture (see Figure 23.17b). The fracture is reduced and held in place using bone-holding forceps. A hole the same width as the screw (the gliding hole) is drilled in the fragment, and the far cortex is then drilled with a drill bit the same size as the core of the screw. The far cortex is tapped, but the near cortex (in the fragment) is not. When the screw is driven into the hole it does not grip the fragment but just grips the far cortex; this has the effect of compressing the fragment into place.

Postoperative care after internal fixation

- Two radiographic views are required to assess the repair immediately postoperatively
- Analgesia and nursing are aimed at a smooth and peaceful recovery from the anaesthesia
- Early recovery of appetite and adequate nutrition is important
- Long anaesthetic times and blood loss during reconstruction of the fracture may necessitate continuation of intravenous fluids into the recovery period
- Assisted walking may be necessary to allow the animal an opportunity to urinate and defecate while limiting the use of the fractured limb
- Daily monitoring of temperature, pulse and respiratory rates, food and water intake, urination and defecation and the recording of clinical signs and treatment is required during hospitalization
- Give medication and analgesia as directed in the days following the surgery
- Sutures are usually removed after 10 days
- Clients should be provided with written instructions outlining the convalescent period and dates for follow-up examinations and re-radiography. These should be on a regular basis as directed by the veterinary surgeon. The owners should be instructed on how to recognize possible complications and how to seek veterinary advice if these occur
- Exercise restrictions: cage rest is outdated with modern methods of rigid immobilization. It is considered to be beneficial to fracture healing and to the well being of the patient to give short controlled bouts of lead-exercise: 10–15 minutes (on a lead) a couple of times a day for the first 3–4 weeks is usually sufficient. Hydrotherapy and physiotherapy are also of great benefit once any wounds have healed. This must be controlled in the early stages of healing to prevent overenthusiastic movements

Complications associated with internal fixation

The most common complications are osteomyelitis and infection associated with the implants and implant failure. Both are often due to poor technique or poor choice of implants. In some cases, the postoperative care in the home environment is not sufficiently rigorous to protect the implants from failure. Screw loosening or bone pain associated with implants is sometimes seen some months after surgery; at this point the implants can be removed.

Bone grafts

Bone grafts can be harvested from either cortical or cancellous bone. They are used to supplement fracture repair and accelerate healing across a wide fracture gap during reconstruction. The term autograft refers to bone taken from a site and used elsewhere in the same dog. An allograft refers to bone taken from one patient and transferred into another patient of the same species.

Cortical bone grafts consist of a whole segment of solid bone or chips of cortical bone either in a fracture or taken from a non-essential site. These bone grafts are very robust and can even be taken from a different dog for use in limb salvage although this is a specialized technique. It takes a long time for the cortical graft to become fully incorporated in the repair.

Cancellous bone is harvested from inside the medulla of long bones and the commonest sites used are the proximal humerus or the ilium. A drill is used to make a hole in the cortical bone and the cancellous bone is scraped out from the inside of the bone using a curette. Cancellous bone is very sensitive as it contains live cells. It should be handled in a sterile manner and stored in a blood-soaked swab on the trolley until used. Cancellous bone grafts are an essential part of the repair of complex fractures as they contribute cells and growth factors necessary for bone healing.

External skeletal fixation

External skeletal fixation (ESF) stabilizes fractures using pins that are inserted through a small stab incision in the skin and then into the bone. They usually travel through both cortices and are then fixed on the outside of the limb with bars and clamps (Figure 23.21) or acrylic resin. Different types of frame can be made according to the requirements of the fracture. A simple frame would consist of one bar and three or four pins exiting from the bone. A more complex frame could consist of multiple pins and three or more bars in three different planes.

Pins come in various sizes from 1.1 mm to 4 mm. Pins may be smooth with a trocar end or have threaded ends. End-threaded pins have either a negative thread, where the thread is cut out of the pin and the overall diameter of the pin remains the same, or a positive thread, where a thread is wound on to the pin and the overall diameter of the pin is slightly larger. Pins are also available with a positive thread in the middle of the pin rather than at the end (Figure 23.21). The advantage of a threaded pin is that it is less likely to loosen or be pulled out than a smooth pin. Pins are placed in both cortices of the bone but do not necessarily exit the skin on both sides. The centrally threaded pins are designed to exit both sides of the limb. Various sized clamps (single and double) and bars are available to fit the pins.

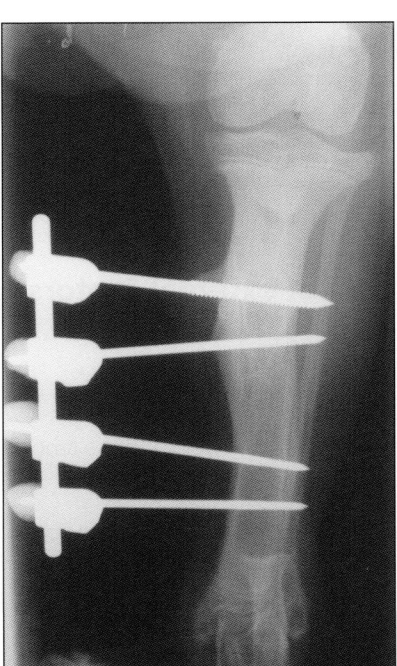

23.21

This radiograph shows an external fixator applied to a fractured tibia using one positively and one negatively threaded pin placed proximally to the fracture, and two negatively threaded pins placed distally. All pins are attached by clamps to a single bar. The tibia is healed and ready for removal of the implant.

Types of fracture suitable for external fixation

- Long bone fractures.
- Comminuted fractures.
- Open and infected fractures.
- Delayed unions and non-union.
- Mandibular fractures.

Acrylic pin external fixator system

The acrylic pin external fixator (APEF) system uses corrugated tubing which is filled with polymethylmethacrylate, a type of bone cement. All the pins are placed in the bone and the corrugated tubing is fixed to the ends of the pins. The cement is mixed and poured into the tubing. The tubing is then held in alignment until the cement has hardened. The hardening process is a chemical reaction between the liquid and powder components and intense heat is generated. It is important to protect the soft tissues (and fingers) from this heat. Heat can also be conducted down the pins and cause necrosis of the bone. Sterile swabs soaked in cool sterile saline can be placed on the tissues to help to protect them; saline can also be dribbled from a syringe on to the pins. The cement takes up to 10 minutes to set. Mandibular fractures are particularly suitable for this system; the acrylic can be formed around the pins and the shape of the jaw into a 'bumper bar'.

Complications of external fixation

- Swelling of the soft tissues impinging on the clamps or acrylic bars.
- Excessive exudate from the pin site caused by movement of the skin and soft tissues.
- Loosening of pins (in some cases individual pins can be removed without losing the stability of the frame).

Luxations and subluxations

A luxation (also called a dislocation) is a displacement of articular surfaces from the normal position within a joint. The joint surfaces no longer touch each other. A subluxation is a partial dislocation of the joint surfaces.

Luxations and subluxations may be classified into two types: congenital and acquired.

- Congenital luxations or subluxations are anatomical abnormalities present at birth, which may or may not be inherited. The most common congenital luxation is that of the patella. In most cases a surgical procedure can replace the patella in its normal position. Some congenital luxations are so severe that they cannot be corrected. Some small dogs and cats may be able to cope with the permanently luxated joint, but in larger breeds severe congenital luxation may cause great disability.
- Acquired luxations and subluxations result from some form of trauma such as a road traffic accident. The ligaments keeping the joint in its normal position are damaged and the joint is forced out of alignment. Acquired luxations most commonly occur in the hip and elbow joints. The phalangeal joints, the hock and shoulder joints are also, less commonly, affected.

First aid treatment for dislocations should follow that for fractures as presenting signs and trauma are often similar.

Clinical signs and diagnosis

The signs shown by the patient can mimic those of a fracture and it can be difficult to differentiate between them. Pain, deformity, loss of motion, non-weight bearing and crepitus are common signs to both. Sometimes typical stance positions are characteristic of an animal with a dislocation. Radiography is essential to confirm the diagnosis and also the presence or absence of other conditions, e.g. small fractures.

Treatment

Treatment of luxations requires the return of the joint to its normal anatomical position and repair of the damaged ligaments. Like fracture reduction, reduction of luxations may be achieved in several ways.

- Closed reduction is reduction of the joint by manipulation of the limb. This is the method that should be attempted first. Closed reduction should be attempted as soon as possible after injury as the longer the delay the less chance there is of successful reduction of the joint. Most joints are impossible to reduce under sedation, causing unnecessary pain and suffering to the patient, and reduction should be carried out under general anaesthetic. The joint should be re-radiographed afterwards to check that the reduction has been successful.
- Open reduction involves a surgical approach to the joint: the luxated bones are visualized and manipulated back into the joint. Some form of stabilization technique is usually required.

Postoperative care

Postoperative care is similar after both open and closed reductions, except that open luxations require the added precautions taken following surgery. The main postoperative aim is to avoid forces that could cause a recurrence of the luxation.

Once the joint is reduced, it must be immobilized. After a hip dislocation the hindlimb is supported in an Ehmer sling (see Chapter 15). After a shoulder dislocation the forelimb can be supported in a Velpeau sling (see Chapter 15). The slings are kept on for 5–7 days. Exercise should be restricted for 3–4 weeks and then slowly increased.

Complications

- Re-luxation is the most common complication especially if activity is not sufficiently restricted or if there is other pathology in the joint such as a fracture.
- Joint infection is a risk especially if an open reduction has been performed.
- There may be injury to surrounding soft tissues associated either with the original trauma or with the reduction of the joint. These injuries may not be obvious at first. They include damage to nerves in the region of the joint.

Oncological surgery

Oncology is the study of cancer and its related diseases. A neoplasm, or tumour, is an abnormal uncontrolled growth of cells that develop faster than the surrounding normal tissues. Most tumours arise as the animal ages and typically they are found in dogs or cats over 8–10 years of age. However, there are some very aggressive tumours that occur in dogs or cats as young as a few months old. Some breeds are specifically susceptible to certain tumours and may develop more than one tumour at the same time (e.g. Boxers, mast cell tumours; Flat-coated Retrievers, sarcomas). Many owners will be very concerned about the possibility that their animal has cancer, and they must be reassured that many tumours are benign and, if removed completely, will not grow again.

Neoplasia

Neoplasia is extremely common in small animal practice and all unexplained lumps on an animal should be investigated with the possibility of neoplasia in mind.

Tumours cause problems in a number of ways:

- The physical mass of the tumour presses on other structures and causes pain or loss of function (e.g. pressing on the pharynx and preventing swallowing)
- A rapidly growing tumour may use up energy resources and cause the animal to feel unwell and depressed
- Cytokines released by the tumour can cause distant physiological effects (see 'Paraneoplastic syndromes', below)
- The tumour may spread to other vital organs (e.g. heart, kidney, liver, lungs) and invade the tissues, causing loss of function and resulting in clinical signs.

Tumours may arise from any body tissue and the name of the neoplasm is derived from its tissue of origin. Very aggressive tumours may lose all their identifying characteristics because they are growing so fast, in these cases it may not be possible for the pathologist to identify the tissue of origin. It is important to know the tissue of origin as this enables the veterinary surgeon to predict how the tumour will behave and also to decide what treatment is most appropriate.

The terminology used in oncology is very specific and often describes both the type of tumour and how it behaves. Neoplasms may be benign or malignant and this description indicates whether or not the tumour is likely to spread to other organs or tissues in the animal and result in its death.

Benign tumours

Benign tumours usually grow quite slowly and are discrete and encapsulated. They are often freely mobile relative to neighbouring tissues. Common examples include:

- Lipoma – a benign tumour of adipose (fat) cells, very common in the subcutaneous tissues of older overweight animals
- Papilloma – a benign wart-like tumour of epithelial cells, most often seen on the skin of cats and dogs (e.g. at the lip margins, eyelid and ear) but they also occur in the bladder and rectum
- Melanoma – a benign pigmented skin tumour of melanocytes; some melanomas, however, are highly malignant, particularly if they arise in the mucous membranes of the mouth
- Fibroma – a benign tumour of fibrous tissue present as firm superficial tumours of the skin, they may be difficult to differentiate from other more malignant skin tumours
- Adenoma – a benign tumour of glandular tissue, it is quite common in older dogs (e.g. peri-anal adenoma).

Malignant tumours

Malignant tumours may grow quickly or slowly. They may not have a definite capsule and may be closely attached to neighbouring tissue. Some malignant tumours will spread (metastasize) very readily to other organs such as the lungs, liver, spleen and bones. Metastasis may occur via various routes:

- In the circulation after invasion of blood vessels
- In the lymphatic system to the draining lymph node and beyond

- By direct contact of tumour cells with neighbouring organs by direct invasion (extension) or by exfoliation of tumour cells into a cavity such as the abdomen (transplantation).

Malignant tumours are also classified according to the tissue from which they arise. Common examples include:

- Carcinoma is a malignant tumour arising from epithelial cells:
  - Squamous cell carcinoma arises from squamous epithelium such as the oral cavity
  - Transitional cell carcinoma arises from the transitional epithelium characteristic of the bladder epithelium
- Adenocarcinoma is a malignant tumour of glandular tissue such as the epithelium of the anal sac
- Sarcoma is a tumour arising from mesenchymal tissues (mainly connective tissues):
  - Lymphosarcoma is a tumour of the lymphoid tissues, common in dogs and may be seen in association with feline leukaemia virus in cats
  - Fibrosarcoma arises from fibroblasts and may be found in any connective tissue
  - Osteosarcoma is a malignant tumour of osteoblasts and is usually in the limb bones. In the dog, these tumours are commonly found in the distal radius or ulna, proximal humerus, distal femur or proximal tibia.

When the tumour is examined histopathologically, it can be further graded to determine its degree of malignancy by assessing its rate of proliferation and degree of differentiation of the cells.

Preparation for oncological surgery

Many forms of neoplasia are amenable to surgery. In order to plan treatment and advise the owner, a specific diagnosis of the type of tumour is necessary. This entails taking a sample from the tumour (biopsy) and submitting it for histopathology or cytology. Benign tumours may be completely cured by excisional surgery and a number of treatments are available for malignant tumours that will extend the lifespan of the animal while maintaining its quality of life.

Tumour staging

All animals with malignant neoplasia should be staged before surgery. Staging is the process used to determine whether the tumour has spread to a distant site such as the lymph nodes, lungs, liver, spleen or bones. Radiographs or a CT scan of the chest are used to assess the lungs, whilst CT or ultrasonography may be used to evaluate the abdomen (see Chapter 16). Lymph nodes local to the tumour can be aspirated for cytological analysis and checked for evidence of tumour cells.

Many animals are older and screening for evidence of other diseases may be necessary before the surgery is carried out. Paraneoplastic disease can cause cachexia, poor body condition or other abnormalities that could increase the risks associated with anaesthesia and surgery. Attention to nutrition and planned postsurgical care and nursing are important for successful oncological surgery.

Paraneoplastic disease

Tumours can cause other signs of illness apart from the physical effects of the mass itself. Some tumours secrete biologically active hormones that may cause generalized non-specific ill health or they may cause well defined disease syndromes. Sometimes the paraneoplastic syndrome is more acutely life-threatening than the tumour itself. For example:

- Anal adenocarcinoma and lymphosarcoma can cause hypercalcaemia, giving rise to polydypsia, polyuria and renal failure
- Insulinomas secrete active insulin which causes episodes of acute hypoglycaemia and collapse or seizures
- Mast-cell tumours can secrete histamine causing generalized or local acute inflammatory responses
- Thyroid adenomas secrete excess thyroid hormone, causing tachycardia, weight loss and hyperactivity.

Tumours can also cause pyrexia, cachexia and generalized poor nutrition due to other substances released into the circulation.

Biopsy
Fine-needle aspiration

This is the commonest and most useful method of obtaining tissue for diagnosis of tumours. It is also used to assess draining lymph nodes for evidence of metastasis (for tumour staging). A fine-gauge hypodermic needle is inserted into the tumour or lymph node to aspirate a few cells for cytological analysis (see Chapter 17). Sometimes ultrasound or CT guidance is used to direct needles into intra-abdominal or intrathoracic tumours.

Bone marrow biopsy

Collection of bone marrow is indicated to evaluate neoplastic or immune mediated disease of circulating white or red cells. It is important to make sure the sample is not contaminated with peripheral blood. The commonest site in the dog and cat is the iliac crest, but occasionally samples are taken from the proximal femur via the trochanteric fossa.

Aspiration is also used to sample bone marrow using a special bone marrow biopsy needle. Usually the sample is taken from the wing of the ilium, under sedation with local anaesthesia or under general anaesthesia. The overlying skin is prepared as for surgery and a small skin incision is made over the bone. The bone marrow biopsy needle is driven through the cortex of the bone with the stylet in place. Once in the medullary cavity the stylet is removed and a syringe is used to aspirate bone marrow. The samples are dripped on to slides tilted at 60 degrees to the vertical so that they run down the slide forming a smear. These are air-dried and submitted for cytology.

Needle core biopsy

A small cylinder of tissue is obtained using a specialized instrument such as a Tru-Cut® needle. There is a central notched obturator with an outer sleeve or cannula with an attached handle. General anaesthesia, or local anaesthesia of the overlying skin, is necessary. A stab incision is made in the skin to allow the loaded instrument to be introduced through the soft tissues, and ultrasound guidance may be used to direct the instrument into the centre of the tumour. Once the obturator is in the tumour the sleeve is pushed sharply over the notch in the obturator cutting out a tiny cylinder of tissue. The closed instrument is withdrawn and a hypodermic needle is used gently to dislodge the sample from the opened obturator into a sample pot and submitted for histopathology.

Other biopsy methods

- Punch biopsy samples are taken from superficial lesions in the skin, using small circular cutters. The biopsy site may be closed using a single interrupted suture.
- Trephine biopsy samples are taken from bony tumours using a trephine or a Jamshidi needle. A core of bone/tumour a few millimetres in diameter is obtained and pushed out of the trephine or needle using a stylet.
- Incisional biopsy is used for tumours that are big enough to remove a piece of tissue from without affecting the ultimate surgical treatment. Usually a wedge of tissue is taken from a part of the tumour that appears to be actively growing and then the wedge is repaired with sutures. This is the most reliable way to obtain a diagnosis.
- Excisional biopsy is usually used for small tumours that are easy to remove with a margin of normal tissue particularly if they are suspected to be benign. It involves the complete removal of the tumour at the first surgery. For further information on biopsies see Chapter 17.

Principles of oncological surgery

The mainstay of any cancer therapy is to maintain the animal's quality of life. Side effects of treatment must be balanced by the clinical improvement – or cure. Most tumours are treated with surgical excision and usually the aim is to remove the entire tumour. Sometimes it is the mass of the tumour that is causing the animal discomfort and in these cases debulking surgery may be used to remove as much of the tumour as possible in order to improve the animal's quality of life until the mass regrows.

Well encapsulated benign tumours may be cured by simple excision of the tumour. However, many tumours require a surgical margin around the tumour in order to ensure that the tumour is entirely removed (Figure 23.22).

Fibrosarcomas are a good example of tumours that are very invasive and require very wide margins of excision in order to attempt to effect a cure. This may in turn require complex reconstructive surgery to repair the defect made where the tumour was removed. Intraoperative techniques may be used to reduce the risk of spreading the tumour into normal tissues; for example, the surgeon may change gloves, instruments or drapes prior to closure.

In some areas, a 'clean' surgical margin may not be possible and further types of therapy for the cancer may be indicated after the surgery. Some tumours are so malignant that postoperative chemotherapy or radiotherapy may be suggested even if the tumour appears to have been completely removed.

Palliative surgery may be used to remove a tumour to improve the animal's quality of life even though it does not alter the prognosis.

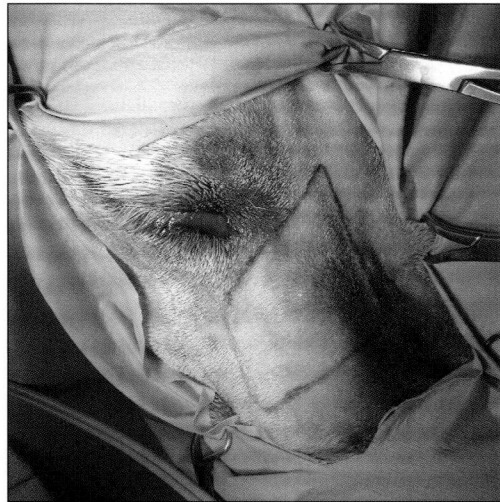

23.22 Skin tumours need to be removed with a margin of unaffected tissue, to ensure that the whole tumour is removed. Here a small mast cell tumour is to be removed with a margin of 2–3 cm. The surgeon has drawn the lines of incision on the skin with a sterile marker.

Submission of tissue for histopathology

All tissue removed from an animal should be submitted for histopathology or stored in formalin in case of recurrence.

Ideally all tissue removed from the animal should be submitted to the pathologist with a detailed history in order to maximize the information available with which to analyse the tumour. Large tumours may be difficult to submit by post, and representative samples may have to be taken from the mass; the main bulk of the tumour should be kept until the pathologist's report is complete in case more tissue is requested. Very bony samples have to be decalcified prior to cutting and this may result in a delay of up to 3 weeks before the report is received by the veterinary practice.

Where the tumour is malignant or locally invasive, the pathologist should be requested to assess the margins of the tumour in order to determine whether excision has been complete. Sometimes the surgeon may orientate the tumour by placing a marker suture at the cranial/caudal ends, or the edges of the mass can be painted with different colours of Indian ink, which are allowed to dry before fixation.

It is important that a clinical history is submitted with the sample in order for the pathologist to be able to provide accurate interpretation of the microscopic findings. In some cases, the pathologist may recommend immunostaining to further characterize the tumour for prognostic purposes. Mast cell tumours (a skin tumour) are a good example of where immunostaining can provide further information on the likely long-term prognosis following removal of the tumour.

Fixation

Tissue should be fixed in 10% neutral buffered formalin in a volume ratio of 1-part specimen to 10-parts of formalin solution. Tissue >1 cm thick may need to be incised to allow more rapid access of the formalin to the deeper parts of the tissue so that adequate fixation occurs. Once the tissue has been fixed for 2–3 days, it can be posted with a 1:1 ratio of tissue to formalin. Formalin is carcinogenic and health and safety regulations must be observed during handling of the solution and preparing packages for posting (see Chapter 17).

Other treatments

- Cryosugery is where tumour tissue is destroyed by freeze–thaw cycles that cause the cells to rupture due to ice crystal formation. This is not very selective and normal cells are also killed.
- Chemotherapy is the use of cytotoxic drugs to kill tumour cells selectively; drugs are selected for specific tumour types.
- Radiotherapy is used in specialist centres to kill dividing tumour cells.
- Hyperthermia is a specialist technique that uses local application of heat via needles introduced into the tumour to try to kill the dividing tumour cells.
- Photodynamic therapy is a specialist technique using photosensitizing chemicals and light to kill superficial tumour cells.

Often treatments may be combined with surgery. Adjunctive therapy in the form of analgesics, antibiotics, anti-inflammatories, specialist nutritional requirements and nursing care may be an important part of managing these patients.

Postoperative management and advice

Ongoing nursing and monitoring of cancer patients is often necessary (see *BSAVA Manual of Canine and Feline Rehabilitation, Supportive and Palliative Care*). Thoracic radiographs (for tumour staging) may be repeated at 4–6-month intervals to check for the development of metastases.

Oncological surgery carries with it the stigma of the dreaded word 'cancer' and many owners will continue to be concerned about the outcome long after the surgical wound has healed. Some animals have a very good quality of life for a considerable period of time even if the treatment has not been curative; owners may need reassurance that the animal is not suffering and how to recognize if they are in pain. Some tumours carry a poor prognosis, despite surgery, and owners may need extra time and advice on how to observe their animal for recurrence and quality of life. It can be very distressing for owners to think that their pet will die from the condition and be waiting for it to happen, and all staff should be made aware of the condition. Discussion about what to look for and how they might want to manage the euthanasia may be best carried out before the animal is terminally ill giving the owners time to come to terms with the inevitable. Many animals have 'good days' and 'bad days' towards the end and it is hard for the owner to understand that 'good days' do not necessarily mean that their pet is having a miraculous recovery.

Surgery and diseases of body systems

This section covers the main surgical diseases in the different body systems, and outlines the surgery and nursing implications of disease or potential surgical complications.

Nearly all surgical procedures are carried out under general anaesthesia and much of the postoperative nursing involves monitoring of the recovery from anaesthesia, and assessment and provision of analgesia (see Chapter 21).

However, some surgical procedures also require postoperative monitoring for specific complications such as haemorrhage, infection, suture dehiscence or respiratory difficulties.

Surgical intervention in different areas of the body can be classified in terms of their potential for infection (Figure 23.23). Areas that can be prepared for aseptic surgery pose a different risk from those that are clearly infected and impossible to make aseptic.

These classifications of surgical procedures enable the surgical team to assess the risk of postoperative infection and treat appropriately. For example, category I does not require postoperative antibiotics and category IV may be treated with antibiotics before, during and after surgery. The most effective way to use antibiotics during surgery is to give an intravenous preparation before the first incision. Antibiotics given after the surgery has been completed will make no difference to the incidence of infection.

Reducing risk of infection

During surgery, the risks of infection can also be reduced by other means:

- Thorough lavage of contaminated tissue using sterile isotonic fluids
- Surgeon changing gloves or re-scrubbing after handling infected or contaminated tissue, prior to closing the unaffected tissue
- Changing instruments that have been used for contaminated or infected tissues prior to closure
- Discarding suture material if used in contaminated areas and supplying new material for closure of clean areas
- Covering drapes with new sterile drapes prior to closure.

These techniques are commonly used after surgery on the GI tract but the surgeon may also change gloves and instruments if concerned that they have been contaminated with tumour tissue, in order to reduce the risk of inadvertently spreading the tumour.

The eye

Ophthalmic surgery is one of the most meticulous areas of small animal surgery, where preparation, technique and postoperative care can have an enormous impact on outcome. General anaesthesia is required for all but the most minor procedures. Specialized instruments, theatre equipment and facilities for magnification (an operating microscope) may be necessary for some ophthalmic surgery.

General principles and preparation for eye surgery

The conjunctival sac is filled with a gel or lubricant and the hair coat is clipped very carefully from a small area surrounding the eye. The first stage is to clean any gross contamination or exudate off the eye and eyelids, using gauze swabs soaked in sterile saline. Skin preparation is completed using diluted povidone–iodine solution in preference to chlorhexidine solutions (note that surgical scrub solutions are not used in eye preparation). The corneal and conjunctival surfaces should then be irrigated with sterile balanced salt solutions or saline and a drop of broad-spectrum antibiotic solution may be instilled on to the surface prior to surgery. Alcohol solutions should not be used near the eye surface. During surgery, ocular lubricants may be used to keep the eye lubricated while the eyelids are held open.

Category	Classification	Definition	Examples of surgical procedures
I	Clean surgery	A surgical wound made under aseptic conditions that does not enter any contaminated viscus, and where there is no break in sterile technique	Neutering. Uncomplicated hernias
II	Clean–contaminated surgery	A surgical wound made under aseptic conditions that enters the oropharynx, respiratory, alimentary or urogenital tracts, but where there is no other source of contamination	Lung lobectomy. Gastrotomy. Tracheotomy
III	Contaminated surgery	There is a major spill of contaminated material at surgery, or a break in sterile technique, or entry into a viscus with a high bacterial load (e.g. colon or rectum)	Abdominal surgery where gut contents spilled accidentally. Oral surgery. Wounds <4 hours old. Lower bowel surgery
IV	Infected surgery	The surgical site is known to be already infected	Aural surgery. Abscesses. Old wounds. Removal of necrotic tissue

23.23 Surgical classifications in terms of infection risk.

Postoperatively, the eye is usually protected using an Elizabethan collar, and sometimes it is necessary to bandage the front paws. Bandages are difficult to keep secure over the eye and they limit postoperative monitoring and treatments.

Inflammation of the eye in the postoperative phase is often detrimental, particularly where specialist surgery has been performed on structures within the eye. In this regard ocular surgery is unusual, as corticosteroids may be used in the postoperative phase to reduce inflammation despite potential steroid-induced delay in wound healing. Postoperative treatments may include topical ointments or drops for administration of antibiotics, steroids or cycloplegics (to reduce pupil spasm). In general, ointments can be applied less frequently than drops and may be easier for the owner to administer.

Analgesia is important and will make administration of treatments easier. Owners may need special advice and instruction on how to administer treatments safely.

Surgical conditions of the cornea and conjunctiva

Conjunctivitis

This is inflammation of the conjunctival membrane and is characterized by reddening of the conjunctiva. Usually the animal also shows increased tear production and overflow (epiphora). If the eye is very sore, the animal may hold the eyelids closed and be very reluctant to allow examination of the eye (blepharospasm). Conjunctivitis is not a surgical disease in its own right, but is often a sign of other conditions in the eye. In cats and rabbits, it can be caused by a primary infection.

Keratitis and ulceration

Keratitis is inflammation of the cornea, which may be accompanied by ulceration. The inflamed cornea has a cloudy appearance due to the oedema. Using the dye fluorescein in the eye allows ulceration to be visualized, and this is important both for diagnosis and in monitoring healing of the ulcer. The eye should be thoroughly flushed to remove any discharge or mucus before the dye is applied to the eye. After a few minutes, the dye will stain the cornea where it is exposed in the presence of an ulcer. Where ointments containing corticosteroids are to be used to treat keratitis, it is extremely important to ensure that no ulceration is present as the corticosteroid would prevent the ulcer from healing.

Ulcers may be secondary to penetration of the conjunctiva by a foreign body or due to keratitis or exposure of the surface of the eye and drying out of the conjunctiva. Severe ulcers may cause erosion of the cornea and ultimately result in rupture of the eye.

Ulcers are treated using techniques to protect the surface of the eye while the ulcer heals by second intention. Small ulcers may be treated with removal of the initiating cause and antibiotic ointment. Large ulcers may require surgical treatment. Traditionally, the third eyelid used to be sutured across the front of the eye to cover the ulcer. However, newer techniques such as con-junctival flaps and corneal contact lenses provide better visualization of the ulcer to monitor healing and make it easier to apply treatments.

Keratitis can also be caused by the instillation of irritant chemicals on to the surface of the eye. This may be accidental, malicious or iatrogenic, and requires emergency treatment to prevent permanent scarring to the cornea. The eye should be irrigated with copious amounts of water or sterile saline to wash out as much of the chemical as possible. The eye should then be closely monitored for ulceration and treated appropriately.

Foreign bodies

Presentation with acute severe conjunctivitis may indicate the presence of a foreign body such as a grass seed trapped behind the eyelids. Careful examination of the inner surfaces of both eyelids and the third eyelid is necessary to identify and remove the foreign material. In calm animals, it may be possible to do this after application of local anaesthetic drops, but many animals will require sedation or general anaesthesia, as it can be very painful. After removal, the eye should be checked for ulceration.

Surgical conditions of the eyelids

Entropion

This is inversion of the eyelid margin such that the eyelashes rub on the cornea (Figure 23.24). There is often secondary conjunctivitis and keratitis or ulceration. Entropion is treated by surgery to return the eyelid margin to its normal position.

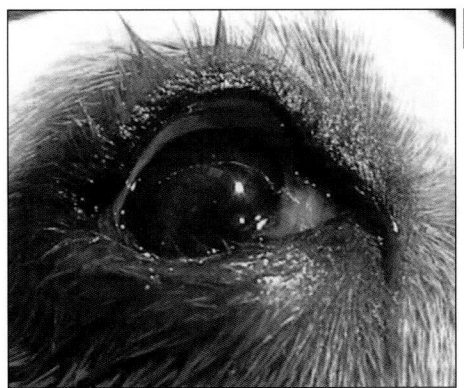

23.24

Entropion (shown here on the lower eyelid) is seen when the eyelid turns inwards and the eyelashes contact the conjunctival surface of the cornea causing constant irritation. (Courtesy of David Williams)

Ectropion

This is eversion of the eyelid margin. In most cases ectropion does not require surgical intervention, but in some dogs it prevents normal lubrication of the eye and gives rise to a chronic exposure keratitis. Certain breeds of dog may have both ectropion and entropion at different points along the eyelid margin.

Distichiasis

This is the most common of a group of disorders characterized by abnormal growth of hairs at the eyelid margin so that the hairs rub the surface of the cornea. In many cases the hairs do not cause a clinical problem but in some cases they cause a chronic keratitis requiring treatment. There are several surgical treatments described to remove the offending hairs and the follicle permanently.

Tumours

Tumours on the margin of the eyelid are very common in older dogs. They cause irritation by rubbing on the surface of the cornea and some are malignant. They are treated by excising a wedge of the eyelid margin containing the tumour.

Surgical conditions of the globe
Eyeball prolapse

Complete prolapse of the eyeball out of its socket (proptosis of the globe) can occur, particularly in brachycephalic dogs or following head trauma. First aid treatment is important if there is to be any chance of saving the eye. The eye must be kept moist using K-Y jelly® (Johnson & Johnson) or Lacri-Lube® (Allergan), supported by sterile saline-soaked swabs. Definitive surgery to replace the eye in the socket must be carried out as soon as possible.

Lens luxation

The lens is usually held in place by ligaments behind the pupil. If these fail, it can luxate either into the anterior chamber of the eye or caudally. This is usually a spontaneous event, often in terrier breeds, but can also be seen as a result of trauma. It requires emergency treatment to remove the lens, as the condition will lead to the development of glaucoma and blindness.

Glaucoma

This is an acute elevation in the pressure within the eye, which can result in permanent blindness within 24 hours if not treated. There are several causes of glaucoma, but the commonest are anterior uveitis and lens luxation. The eye is extremely painful, the sclera engorged and the pupil is usually dilated. Emergency medical treatment includes analgesia and intravenous hypertonic fluids (mannitol) to try to draw fluid out of the eye. Surgical treatments are available in specialist centres.

Cataracts

A cataract is the opacification of the fibres or capsule of the lens of the eye, ultimately resulting in blindness. It should be distinguished from ageing changes in the lens that result in an apparent blue colour of the lens, but through which the animal can still see. Cataracts may be a primary disease or can be secondary to other conditions such as diabetes mellitus. They may be left untreated or can be surgically removed by specialist ophthalmic surgeons. Removal of the lens enables the animal to recognize objects and people as the lens is not as important in focusing as it is in humans. This restores quality of life to the older animal.

Ocular trauma

The eye may be penetrated by foreign bodies or lacerated by claws or teeth during fights with other animals. All these conditions may potentially result in loss of the eye and should be examined and treated as an emergency. Often animals benefit from referral to a specialist ophthalmic surgeon as they are more likely to have the skill to save the eye.

Retina

Most retinal diseases are not amenable to surgery in veterinary medicine, but the retina is an important site of disease in the eye. Of particular importance is a group of inherited diseases of the retina known as progressive retinal atrophy which are known to occur in certain breeds (see Chapter 18).

Skin
Skin biopsy

Skin biopsy is indicated for diagnosis of skin disease. Minimal preparation of the skin surface should be performed in order not to disrupt the surface cells that may aid the pathologist in making a diagnosis. The sample is taken using either a skin biopsy punch or just with a scalpel blade. Several samples should be taken from representative sites and the incisions closed with simple interrupted sutures. In severely diseased skin, there may be delayed wound healing.

Skin tumours

Skin masses should ideally be identified histologically prior to removal. The best way to identify the tumour is using fine-needle aspiration biopsy (see above). Surgery should be performed in the normal aseptic way and the skin closed with sutures. It is important to be aware that some small skin tumours may require tissue margins in three dimensions and therefore some fat and muscle may need to be removed along with the overlying skin.

Surgical management of local pyoderma

Some chronic local skin infections are related to long-term skin disease such as atopy (allergic skin disease) and are then exacerbated by the animal's anatomical skin folds. If the skin folds are not due to obesity, then it may be appropriate to resect the skin folds in order to prevent the recurrence of painful pyoderma. The common examples are vulval folds, screwtail folds and lip folds. Certain breeds, such as the brachycephalics and spaniels, are more likely to suffer from these conditions. Patients with allergic skin disease are most likely to interfere with their sutures as they are always itchy.

Urine/faecal scalding and decubital ulcers

Recumbent or incontinent patients are prone to soiling with urine or faeces and it is a failure of nursing management which then results in the development of decubital ulcers (pressure sores) or 'scald' (dermatitis). The skin and haircoat must be kept clean and dry at all times. In some cases, this may involve several baths per day or clipping away haircoat to enable exposure of the skin so that it can be checked easily. Traditional treatments are to protect the skin with a thin layer of Vaseline® or similar oil-based cream, so that the urine does not irritate the skin surface. However, this does not allow the skin to breathe and although the creams will prevent the skin from becoming worse, they will not help to treat any dermatitis. Commercial spray-on products are available (e.g. Cavilon™ (3M)) that provide a semi-permeable membrane under which the skin can heal while it is protected from the urine/faeces. The skin can also be covered with self-adhesive semi-permeable membranes.

Decubital ulcers (Figure 23.25) are much easier to avoid than to cure and this is an area where intensive nursing can really make the difference between survival and euthanasia. Padded bedding will help to prevent the development of pressure points in recumbent, obese or bony patients, and the use of material such as synthetic fleece bedding or incontinence pads will help to keep the skin dry by wicking moisture away from the surface. Paralysed patients should be turned every 2–4 hours and all pressure points protected. Physiotherapy will encourage the blood supply to the skin and reduce the risk of necrosis (see Chapter 15).

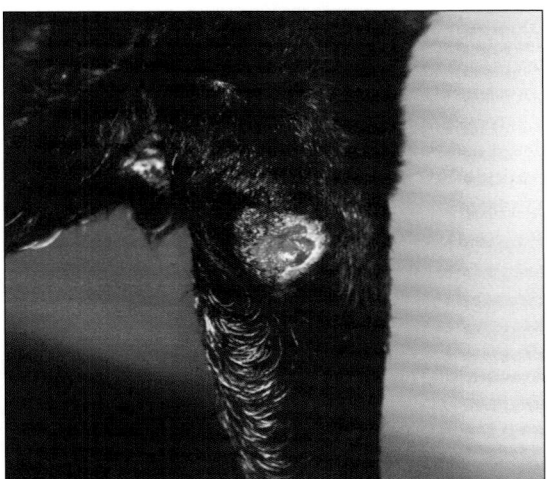

23.25 Decubital ulcers are commonly a sign of poor patient care, but occasionally they are seen in dogs that are predisposed to them due to medical conditions. They are usually on pressure points where the bone is near the surface, such as the elbows or iliac crests. They often appear very round and have a variable depth of tissue loss. Sometimes they are so deep that the underlying bone becomes infected.

Anal sacs

The anal sacs are situated on either side of the anus and contain anal glands, which produce a creamy coloured pungent exudate. The exudate is normally emptied on top of the faeces each time the animal defecates and the sacs should not swell up or cause irritation. If anal sacs become impacted they fill with fluid, which may then become secondarily infected, or they can eventually rupture and spill irritant infected contents into the tissues around the anus. This is often the case with animals that have chronic anal furunculosis, which is a deep-seated infection with sinus tracts in the skin around the anus and under the tail. It is very painful and usually associated with colitis, dietary intolerance and autoimmune disease.

The classic clinical sign of anal sac irritation is persistent chewing at the rump or tail and rubbing the perineum on the ground, particularly after defecation. Anal sac disease may be secondary to a number of non-surgical diseases such as obesity or diarrhoea. In some cases, it is necessary to remove chronically diseased anal sacs to prevent recurrence of infection. When the anal sacs are emptied they should be palpated carefully to screen for anal sac neoplasia.

Anal sac adenocarcinoma is a malignant neoplasm, often seen in middle to older aged dogs, especially Cocker Spaniels. The tumour can cause hypercalcaemia (paraneoplastic disease) as well as spread to the sublumbar lymph nodes. The primary tumour may be tiny, even when the lymph nodes are very large. The treatment consists of removal of the primary tumour and these lymph nodes, and postoperative chemotherapy and remission of up to 3 years has been reported in some cases.

Interdigital disease

Interdigital disease may be part of generalized skin disease, although some breeds are particularly predisposed to the development of interdigital cysts or interdigital foreign bodies such as grass seeds. Dogs with long hair between the toes are particularly at risk of grass seeds becoming embedded in the thin interdigital skin. This causes painful swellings or abscesses. Sometimes it is possible to identify the end of the grass seed in the swelling and it is removed with forceps. If the seed has migrated into the leg, the sinus tract must be surgically explored. During the summer and autumn months, owners should be advised to check between and under the toes daily and keep the hair trimmed very short. Dogs with generalized skin disease (e.g. atopy) may lick their feet a lot, and this drives broken hair shafts under the skin causing painful swellings (trichogranulomas) between the toes.

Abscesses

Long-haired breeds are particularly prone to migration of foreign bodies such as grass seeds and may then present with a painful swelling under the skin. The abscess may burst spontaneously but sometimes the grass seed continues to migrate and spreads the infection deep into the abdomen or chest. In these cases, advanced imaging such as magnetic resonance imaging (MRI) or CT may be necessary to locate the foreign body prior to surgical removal.

Aural surgery

The most common conditions of the ear are usually related to generalized skin disease. Recurrent shaking of the head and scratching at the ears can result in an aural haematoma, and persistent dermatitis may result in otitis externa.

Aural haematoma

This is the most common injury of the pinna. It is secondary to self-induced trauma and there is nearly always underlying otitis externa. A blood vessel bursts, usually on the underside of the pinna, and forms a large haematoma (Figure 23.26). This is painful and, if not treated, will cause the pinna to scar in a deformed shrivelled shape. Generally, a haematoma is treated surgically. The haematoma is drained and cleaned allowing the skin to flatten again against the cartilage. Recurrence is prevented by suturing the skin to the cartilage to close the dead space with the knots tied on the outer surface of the pinna. Buttons, quills or X-ray film have all been used to help to flatten the skin and prevent the sutures from pulling out.

Postoperatively it is important to treat any underlying skin or ear disease and to prevent the patient from scratching at the ear again. This is achieved either with an Elizabethan collar or with a figure-of-eight head bandage (see Chapter 15).

Otitis externa

Otitis externa (Figure 23.27) is very common in both dogs and cats. There are many causes and these have to be investigated prior to treatment (see Chapter 18). Most cases of otitis are treated medically, but surgery may be indicated if there

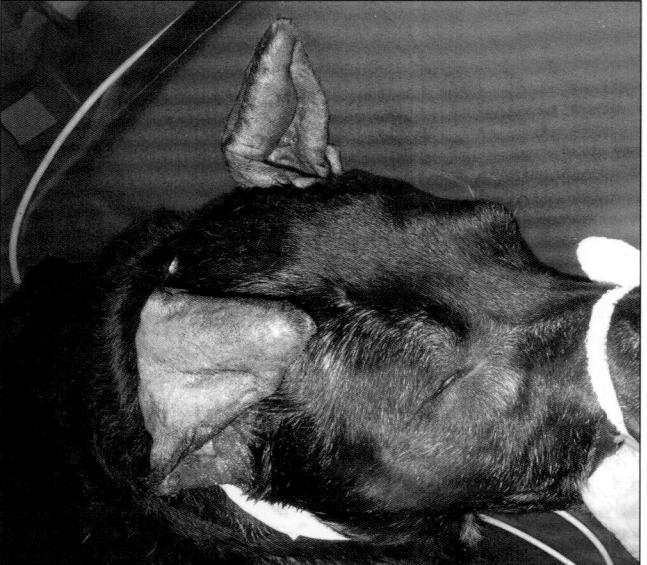

23.26 An aural haematoma forms when a blood vessel bursts and bleeds into the subcutaneous space between the skin and cartilage of the underside of the pinna. Often the pinna is heavy and painful, and drainage of the haematoma provides considerable relief. It is important to treat the underlying ear disease. This dog has been prepared for surgical drainage of bilateral aural haematomas, and the pinnae have been clipped.

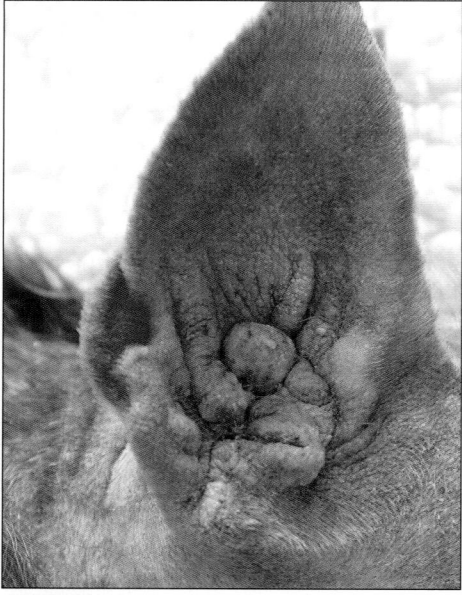

23.27 Chronic otitis externa. The external ear canal is completely obliterated with chronic greyish proliferative tissue. At this stage, it is not possible to salvage the ear by controlling the underlying skin disease and surgery would be recommended.

is a tumour, polyp or irreversible changes in the external ear canal. Where infection has extended into the middle ear, it is harder to resolve the otitis and surgery may be indicated.

There are four surgical options in dogs and cats:

- Lateral wall resection: the lateral wall of the vertical canal is removed so as to open up the ear to the air and allow better drainage and access for cleaning. This is only suitable for ears that have no disease on the medial wall of the vertical canal or in the horizontal canal

- Vertical canal ablation: the vertical canal is completely removed and the horizontal canal opening is sutured to the skin. This is only for ears where the disease is confined to the vertical canal (e.g. neoplasia)
- Total ear canal ablation (TECA): this procedure is most commonly used and is usually for severe long-term otitis externa. Often the infection has ruptured the tympanic membrane and there is also otitis media or severe chronic changes. The middle ear (tympanic bulla) is accessed at the time of surgery by enlarging the bony opening (bulla osteotomy) and the middle ear is scraped and lavaged clean. The whole of the vertical and horizontal ear canal are removed and the tissue and skin sutured closed over the top. This procedure is more challenging than the others but often is the only solution as it removes all the diseased tissue.

Ear surgery is regarded as infected and antibiotics are usually given both before, during and after the surgery. Ear infections are often longstanding, and opportunistic pathogens such as *Pseudomonas* or *Proteus* establish. They are difficult to treat as they are often resistant to most of the antibiotics commonly used. A foul-smelling greenish discharge may be an indication of these pathogens and a swab should be submitted for culture and sensitivity testing.

Postoperatively, the patients require analgesia and the ear must be protected from self-inflicted injury. An Elizabethan collar may be used, or a head bandage, or the pinnae may be bandaged together to stop them flapping against the wound. There is often a discharge of blood or exudate from the wound for several days and this must be gently cleaned away using sterile saline. The sutures may have to stay in slightly longer than usual, but small areas of dehiscence are allowed to heal by second intention.

Otitis media

In the dog this is usually an extension of otitis externa, but in the cat it may occur as a primary disease as an ascending infection via the eustachian tube. Access to the middle ear is either via a total ear canal ablation as described above if there is external disease or via a ventral approach (ventral bulla osteotomy). The animal is placed in dorsal recumbency and the dissection made directly over the tympanic bulla. A small drill is then used to make a hole in the bulla to allow drainage and lavage. Damage to the nerves in the middle ear can occur during this procedure and Horner's syndrome may be seen (see Chapter 18).

Otitis interna

Inflammation of the inner ear structures causes loss of balance, vomiting, head tilt, nystagmus and disorientation (vestibular syndrome) (see Chapter 18). If this is secondary to severe middle ear disease, surgical management of the middle ear disease may be necessary to resolve the otitis interna.

Mammary tumours

Mammary neoplasia is the commonest tumour in the bitch, and the second most common tumour in all dogs. It is less common in the cat but it is seen in breeding queens (particularly Siamese) or cats that have been treated for oestrus suppression or skin disease using megoestrol acetate.

In bitches the most commonly affected glands are the two caudal pairs, while in queens the cranial glands are most often affected. About 50% of mammary tumours in the bitch are benign but in cases with multiple masses they may all be different tumour types (Figure 23.28). In cats, over 80% of

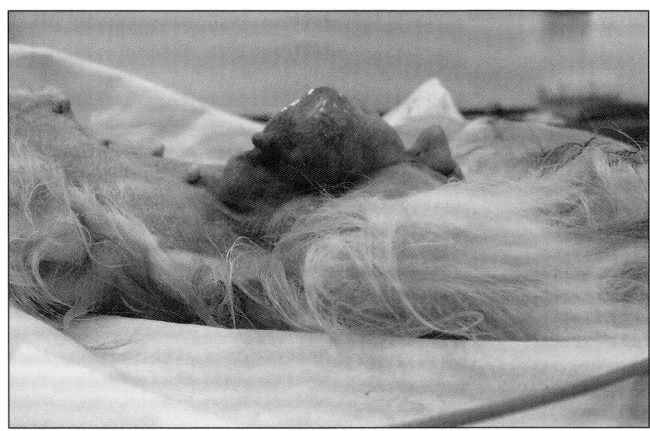

23.28 Mammary tumours in dogs may be benign or malignant and can grow to considerable size by the time the owner presents the animal for treatment. (Courtesy of Pierre Barreau).

mammary masses are malignant and carcinomas tend to be particularly aggressive, most having metastasized by the time of presentation.

Fine-needle aspiration biopsy is rarely helpful except to differentiate mammary tumours from mastitis, hypertrophy or other tumours. The type of tumour is rarely confirmed prior to surgery as it does not change the management of the disease.

Surgery is the treatment of choice for mammary tumours. In the bitch the type of surgery has little effect on the survival time, and radical surgery is generally unnecessary, as many tumours are benign. Surgery involves removing either just the affected gland (mammectomy) or that gland and an adjacent gland (local mastectomy) or all the glands on the affected side (radical mastectomy or 'mammary strip'). In the cat, the tumours are usually aggressive and radical mastectomy, often including part of the body wall, is always recommended.

All mammary gland surgery is prone to dehiscence and ideally a drain should be used. To reduce the risk of wound complications surgery on both sides simultaneously is usually avoided.

Although in humans there are many other treatments used alongside surgery for mammary tumours, in dogs and cats there are currently no other treatments that are known to make a difference to survival after removal of malignant mammary tumours.

Digestive tract

Many diseases affecting the digestive tract have serious adverse effects on the fluid and electrolyte status of the patient. These deficits should be identified and stabilized prior to anaesthesia and surgery (see Chapter 20). Long periods of anorexia or vomiting and diarrhoea will cause the animal to be dehydrated and in a negative energy balance and, therefore, a poor candidate for anaesthesia. Steps must be taken to replenish nutritional deficits and to maintain nutrition to minimize the effects of surgery on the patient. This may mean placement of feeding tubes prior to or during the surgical procedure to help with nursing the patient postoperatively. For example, an anorexic cat is likely to recover much more quickly if feeding tubes are placed at the time of surgery than if hand feeding or 'tempting' food is relied upon in the early postoperative stages.

Oral surgery
Oral tumours

These are generally seen in older dogs and cats. Tumours may arise on any structure of the oropharynx (tongue, gingiva, lips, palate, tonsils, etc.), and the prognosis depends very much upon both the site of the tumour and the type of tumour. As owners generally do not inspect their pet's mouth regularly these tumours may be large before they are presented for treatment. The first sign of a tumour may be halitosis, loss or displacement of teeth or facial swelling, and the tumour may only be identified at the time of dental examination by the veterinary surgeon.

Surgical resection carries the best prognosis for all oral tumours in the dog and cat. Where tumours are on the mandible or maxilla (Figure 23.29), bone and teeth may have to be removed along with the tumour in order to obtain adequate margins. The defect is then closed using flaps of mucosa from the lips and sutured with absorbable suture material. Postoperative nursing focuses on analgesia and ensuring that the patient can eat and drink easily. Food should be soft and formed not dry or abrasive (which might tear the sutures) or too sloppy (which might seep between the sutures). Tumours of the tonsils or palate often carry a worse prognosis particularly in cats.

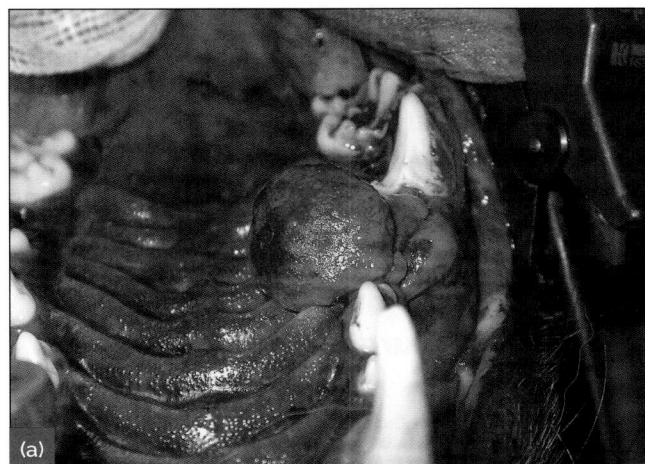

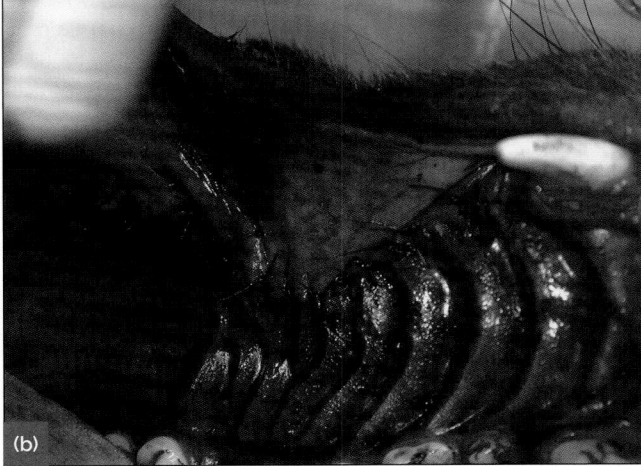

23.29 Maxillary tumours are usually seen in middle-aged to older dogs. **(a)** This dog has a tumour centred between premolar 3 and the carnassial tooth. The tumour must be removed with a margin of at least one uninvolved tooth on each side as well as the oral mucosa and underlying bone. **(b)** The maxilla after the tumour has been removed along with all of the dental arcade up to the incisor. The defect has been repaired with a flap of mucosa from the lip.

Oronasal fistulae

These may be secondary to trauma, dental extraction or tumour resection. All fistulae should be repaired surgically to prevent food material impacting in the nasal cavity and causing a rhinitis. Preoperative preparation involves the use of saline and then dilute chlorhexidine or povidone–iodine solution to flush out debris accumulated in the cavity and nasal passages. Postoperatively, the defect should heal rapidly and may be kept clean with gentle oral lavage using chlorhexidine solutions.

Cleft palate

Puppies should always be checked for cleft palate at the time of birth, but it can also be traumatic in origin. Some clefts are repaired using simple advancement flaps; others require more advanced techniques, depending on the degree of involvement of the soft and hard palate. Protection of the suture line in the mouth is difficult and restriction of food intake or use of feeding tubes is counterproductive. The animal should be given soft formed food that will not get stuck in the suture line and is easy to swallow.

Foreign bodies and penetrating injuries

Foreign bodies such as sticks, bones, fish hooks, blades of grass or grass seeds may lodge in the soft tissues of the mouth and pharynx. All cause pain associated with the mouth, difficulty in swallowing and drooling.

The mouth can be opened in the conscious animal by using ropes behind the canine teeth of the upper and lower jaws, but the examination will be more effective and less stressful under general anaesthesia. Penetrating injuries of the oesophagus and pharynx caused by sticks thrown for dogs by the owners can be potentially life-threatening and should be surgically explored as an emergency. Referral may be required to surgically explore the injury and repair the pharyngeal tear.

Oesophageal surgery
Foreign bodies

Partial obstruction of the oesophagus with bones is common in terrier breeds and results in regurgitation of food and sometimes fluids. In cases where there is complete obstruction, dehydration is extremely rapid and hypovolaemia may be life-threatening. These cases are always emergencies. The foreign body is usually retrieved by extraction via the mouth through a rigid endoscope. Occasionally bones may have to be pushed down into the stomach. Digestible foreign bodies (such as bones) are not removed from the stomach but plastic toys or balls have to be removed via a gastrotomy. Postoperatively, the patient is treated with drugs to reduce gastric acidity in case of gastric reflux, which will exacerbate oesophagitis. The oesophagus is also assessed for tears and inflammation, using the endoscope. Small tears or bruising may be treated with nil by mouth and food and water via a gastrostomy tube for 3–5 days. Severe full-thickness tears may have to be explored via a thoracotomy to prevent development of sepsis, and the prognosis may be poor.

Oesophageal stricture

This condition may arise as a result of trauma secondary to an oesophageal foreign body but is also known to arise as a consequence of general anaesthesia. The animal presents 2–4 weeks after having an anaesthetic or an episode of reflux or vomiting, with a history of regurgitating all solid food. It is difficult to treat successfully. Therapy relies on stretching the stricture using expanding balloons positioned using an endoscope, and steroid therapy to reduce the rate of recurrence of scar tissue. Animals may manage on a liquidized diet.

Gastric surgery
Foreign bodies

The cardinal sign of a gastric foreign body is persistent or intermittent vomiting. Diagnosis may be confirmed by radiography, contrast radiography, ultrasonography or gastroscopy. Some foreign bodies may be retrieved endoscopically but many will require surgical removal. The stomach is accessed via a cranial midline laparotomy and pulled out of the abdomen as far as possible. Stay sutures are used in the stomach wall to prevent it falling back into the abdomen and the gastric contents spilling into the abdomen. The rest of the abdominal organs are packed off with sterile moist towels or swabs to protect them from contamination. The incision is usually made in an avascular area of the body of the stomach. The whole stomach and small intestine should be inspected for other foreign bodies and mucosal damage prior to closure with a synthetic absorbable suture material.

Pyloric obstruction

This can be caused by a foreign body but more often it is because of pyloric thickening, due either to hypertrophy of the muscle or to neoplasia. These diseases are often known as gastric outflow diseases and congenital forms are more common in specific breeds such as brachycephalic dogs or Siamese cats. Once the diagnosis is confirmed, surgery is performed either to widen the pylorus (pyloroplasty) or to remove the pylorus altogether (pyloric resection).

Immediately postoperatively, small amounts of water are made available to the patient and then small quantities of a liquidized low-fat diet are offered 24 hours later. It is important to stimulate normal gastric motility without inducing vomiting, and some cases may have a gastrostomy tube placed at the time of surgery to help to decompress the stomach postoperatively for a few days.

Gastric dilatation–volvulus

This is a peracute rapidly fatal syndrome resulting from accumulation of food and gas in the stomach. The stomach dilates initially and this precipitates rotation of the stomach around its axis, resulting in occlusion of the oesophagus and the venous drainage. Severe hypovolaemic and toxic shock starts during the dilatation phase and escalates once rotation occurs. If not treated promptly, death results from the shock, gastric wall necrosis, ventricular dysrhythmias and disseminated intravascular coagulation (DIC). The specific aetiology is poorly understood, but usually the dogs are deep chested, often middle to older aged, and the condition may be associated with a nervous temperament. Preoperatively, nursing involves aggressive management of the shock and attempts to deflate the stomach either by passage of a stomach tube or by percutaneous needle gastrostomy (see Chapter 19).

Confirmation of rotation of the stomach is obtained with a right lateral abdominal radiograph (Figure 23.30) and indicates that surgery is necessary.

Usually a gastrostomy tube is placed at the time of surgery to allow decompression of the stomach if there is reduced gastric motility postoperatively, and the tube may also be used for feeding if the animal is moribund. In order to prevent recurrence of the rotation, a gastropexy may be carried out where the pylorus is anchored to the right body wall with sutures, but this does not prevent the recurrence of

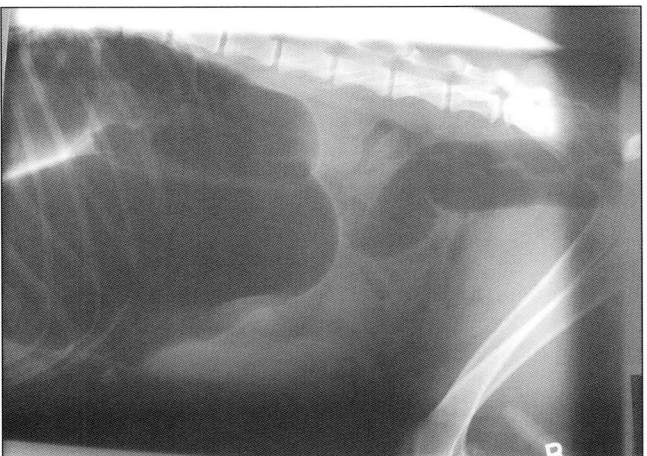

23.30 Right lateral abdominal radiograph of a dog with gastric dilatation–volvulus. The stomach can be seen hugely dilated with air and there is a characteristic fold of tissue crossing the dilated stomach, which indicates torsion.

Gastric dilatation–volvulus: treatment

1. Treat for shock with rapid administration of large volumes of intravenous fluids.
2. Blood tests for haematology, biochemistry and blood gas analysis including lactate.
3. Decompression of the stomach via passage of a stomach tube.
4. Right lateral radiograph to confirm volvulus (twist).
5. Electrocardiography (ECG) – treat if necessary for ventricular dysrhythmias.
6. Surgery for decompression, derotation and assessment of stomach wall viability.

---

dilatation. Postoperative nursing continues treatment of fluid and electrolyte losses and in particular monitoring and treating ventricular arrhythmias.

Gastric neoplasia

Gastric neoplasms are often aggressive and may be very advanced before diagnosis. Clinical signs include haematemesis, weight loss and gastric pain. Some neoplasms can be resected if they are on the greater curvature of the stomach.

Tube gastrostomy

This is a useful tool for nutritional support (see Chapter 13) or decompression of the stomach. The tube is anchored in the stomach and exits through the body wall, where it is sutured to the skin and bandaged in place. The tube can be placed without surgery, using an endoscope to push the end of the tube through the skin (percutaneous endoscopic gastrostomy tube or 'PEG' tube) or it is placed surgically via a laparotomy. A mushroom-tipped catheter is usually used, although a Foley catheter may be substituted (Figure 23.31). It is important to protect the tube from mutilation by the animal, particularly if the tube was placed endoscopically, as it is less secure in the stomach wall than if placed surgically. Mushroom-tipped tubes are removed by pushing a probe into the end of the mushroom tip to straighten it out and allow the tube to be pulled through the abdominal wall. Other tubes can be cut short and allowed to pass through the intestinal tract, or removed endoscopically. Tubes should

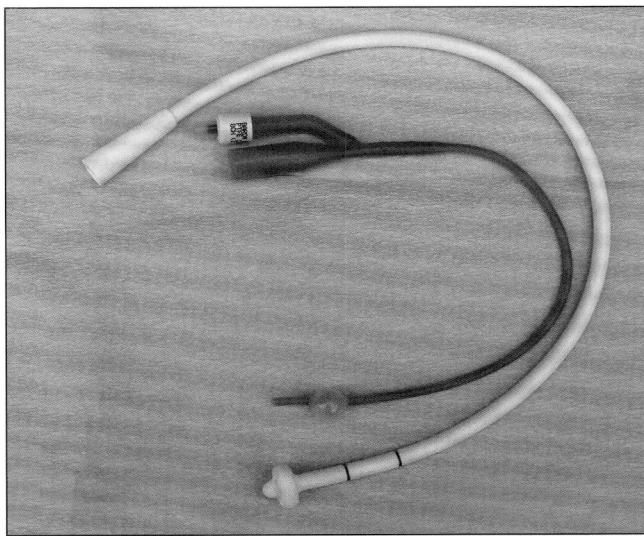

23.31 Depezzer (mushroom-tipped) and Foley catheters. These catheters can be used in situations where they need to be self-retaining (e.g. as a tube gastronomy). To remove it, the Depezzer has to have the tip cut off, or straightened out. The Foley is removed by drawing the fluid out of the bulb.

not be removed too early (<3 days) before a seal has formed around the hole in the gastric wall. The resultant wound in the body wall may leak gastric contents for 1–2 days, but is kept clean with skin antiseptics and allowed to granulate closed.

Small intestine

Surgery on the small intestine (duodenum, jejunum and ileum) is common in small animal practice. The intestines are lifted out of the abdomen during surgery so that other organs are not contaminated if gut contents spill (Figure 23.32). They should be kept moist using sterile saline-soaked swabs or towels but this will mean that waterproof surgical drapes are necessary. Heat loss is rapid when the intestines are removed from the abdomen and it is necessary to provide a heating pad or warmed fluids. Postoperative nursing is important to ensure that the animal eats and drinks soon after surgery. Observation for regurgitation, nausea or other signs of ileus (lack of peristalsis) is important to enable prompt treatment of any postoperative complications.

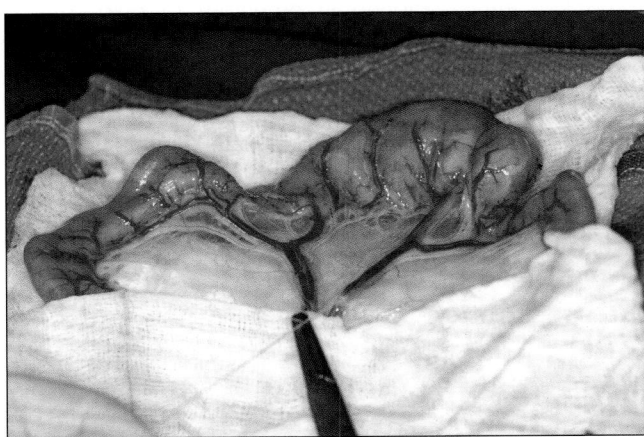

23.32 Intestinal surgery in a cat to remove a tumour in the small intestine (enterectomy). Note how the affected segment of intestine has been exteriorised from the abdomen and packed off with sterile swabs. The drapes underneath are also waterproof.

Biopsy

Intestinal biopsy is usually indicated when investigations of GI signs such as persistent or recurrent vomiting or diarrhoea have been unrewarding. It is not possible to sample the jejunum or ileum via endoscopy and these have to be accessed via a laparotomy. Animals presented for intestinal biopsy may be poor candidates for surgery. Healing may be delayed due to hypoproteinaemia or cachexia. Small samples of intestine are taken from several sites all the way down the GI tract and submitted in separate containers each labelled with the site of the sample. All the biopsy sites are sutured closed and wrapped with omentum.

Postoperatively, the animal is encouraged to eat and drink as soon as possible in order to encourage rapid healing of the biopsy sites.

Enterotomy: foreign body removal

Foreign bodies in the cat small intestine are often linear, e.g. string, wool, thread and needle. The material may be lodged behind the back of the tongue or trapped at the pylorus and travel all the way into the small intestine. Smooth muscle contraction of the gut wall then 'concertinas' the gut up the linear material and eventually either blocks the lumen or cuts through the wall of the intestine. Dogs more commonly ingest balls or plastic toys, which pass to a point along the jejunum and then become lodged.

Sometimes the foreign body can be palpated through the abdominal wall but often radiography or ultrasonography is necessary to make the diagnosis. The animal is stabilized and the foreign body removed via a laparotomy.

Usually the foreign body can be removed via a scalpel incision in the intestinal wall and then the hole is closed with synthetic absorbable sutures. Sometimes the intestine is very inflamed and appears necrotic, in which case an enterectomy may be necessary.

Enterectomy

Enterectomy is indicated where the intestine is necrotic or there is a tumour in the wall. A section of the intestine is removed and then the ends are sutured together to form an anastomosis. The affected section of intestine is separated off, using Doyen bowel clamps or just an assistant's fingers to prevent leakage from the remaining bowel, and then cut with a scalpel to remove it. Once it is removed, the cut ends are held close together while the surgeon sutures the edges using synthetic absorbable suture material. Often the anastomosis is then wrapped in omentum to help to seal the surgical site. Postoperatively, healing is enhanced if the animal is encouraged to eat as soon as possible.

In some cases, it may be necessary to remove a large proportion of the small intestine. This can result in a condition known as 'short bowel syndrome', which is characterized by persistent diarrhoea and poor body condition due to inadequate nutrition from the shortened bowel. Some animals will recover and regain more normal function, but this may take many months.

Intussusception

In this condition the small intestine invaginates into itself (like a telescope closing up). It is very rare in the cat and usually seen in young dogs often secondary to an episode of diarrhoea. The invaginated portion of intestine is called the intussusceptum and the outer part is the intussuscipiens. The blood supply to the intussusceptum is compromised and it often becomes necrotic. Clinical signs are similar to those for intestinal obstruction and the diagnosis is usually made

by radiography or ultrasonography. Surgery to reduce the intussusception is necessary and if the intussusceptum is necrotic it is resected. Sometimes the disease recurs and the intestines may be sutured to each other (enteropexy) to prevent this. Resolution of the underlying disease is important to prevent recurrence.

Volvulus

Mesenteric volvulus is rarely reported in the dog or cat. In this condition, all of the small intestine twists on itself and this obstructs the blood supply. In all species it is rapidly fatal due to endotoxic and hypovolaemic shock secondary to death of most of the small intestine.

Large intestine

Surgery of the large intestine carries greater risk than surgery of the small intestine or stomach as there is an increased bacterial load and a slower rate of healing. Enemas near the time of surgery are detrimental to surgical asepsis as the slurry is more likely to spill and contaminate the abdomen. Preoperative oral antibiotics with anaerobic activity may help to reduce the bacterial load but perioperative antibiotics are essential and should be continued postoperatively. Hospital feeding should be careful not to induce a dietary enteritis, i.e. easily digested protein sources may be better than high-protein diets which may cause a nutritional diarrhoea. Often constipation or tenesmus is a sign of the disease and dietary fibre supplements and faecal modifiers such as ispaghula or sterculia are used to increase faecal mass and increase peristalsis. Paraffin pastes or liquids are less suitable as they only lubricate the faeces and do not alter the water content or soften impacted faeces.

Biopsy

Biopsy samples of the rectum and distal colon can be taken using rigid proctoscopy, but these are only of partial thickness. Full-thickness samples are taken via laparotomy, and carry an increased risk compared with small intestinal biopsy. Strict aseptic technique, packing off the uncontaminated viscera and thorough lavage of the abdomen at the end of the procedure are important.

Colectomy

Removal of the colon is most often indicated for the treatment of chronic constipation in cats. Cats present with multiple episodes of complete obstipation requiring enemas and evacuation each time. Eventually the episodes become more frequent and the colon loses all function. It is important to check that the cat does not have an obstruction to defecation in the pelvic canal by rectal examination and radiography of the pelvis. Surgery involves careful identification and ligation of the vessels supplying the colon, and resection and re-anastomosis of the colon ends. In animals that are severely affected the ileocaecocolic valve may need to be removed as well. The animal is prepared for surgery with antibiotics but an enema is not performed as it is easier to prevent contamination of the abdomen during surgery if the faeces are dry and hard and can be removed within the colon.

These animals are often inappetent postoperatively and early nutritional support is important to healing in the colon. Dehiscence of the anastomosis is often fatal.

Rectal polyps/tumours

Rectal polyps (papillomas) cause faecal tenesmus, bleeding and discomfort and are often treated initially as colitis. Removal of the polyps is indicated because they are a pre-malignant change of the rectal mucosa. They can be removed by using a 'pull out' technique where the rectum is everted through the anus to allow removal of the polyp (Figure 23.33). The defect should be sutured using monofilament absorbable material and postoperative care is directed at reducing postoperative straining using analgesics, anti-inflammatories, local anaesthetic gel and dietary fibre. Where the tumour is identified as malignant or has invasive characteristics, a wider excision is carried out to remove the full thickness of the rectal wall.

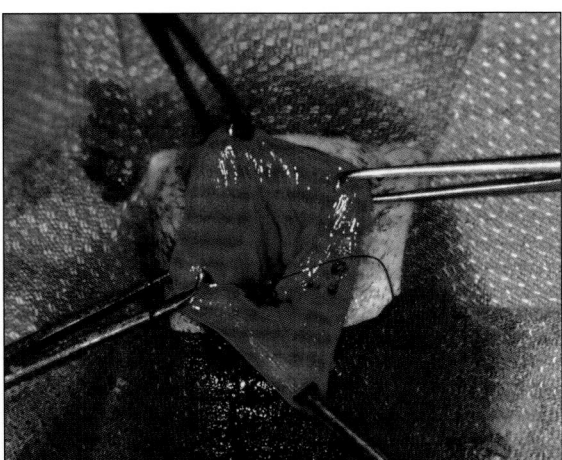

23.33 An intraoperative view of a rectal pull-out procedure to remove a rectal polyp. The everted rectal mucosa is stabilized using Allis tissue forceps.

Rectal prolapse

This is eversion of the wall of the rectum through the anus. It is usually secondary to chronic straining and may be associated with a rectal tumour or chronic colitis. Successful management requires treatment of the primary disease as well as reduction of the prolapse itself. The prolapse should be protected from self-mutilation and kept moist and lubricated, using lidocaine gel. Once the rectum is reduced it is maintained using a loose temporary purse-string suture around the anus. This may have to be loosened intermittently to allow defecation. Dietary faecal modifiers should be given to make the faeces soft and bulky. If the prolapse does not resolve, then surgery can be carried out to suture the distal rectum and colon to the body wall via a laparotomy.

Imperforate anus

This is a congenital condition where the anus fails to unite with the rectum, thus creating complete obstruction to the normal passage of faeces from the moment of birth. Sometimes it is possible to correct this condition surgically.

Peritoneum

The peritoneum is the lining of the abdominal cavity and functions to help with healing of the intestinal tract and to protect it from infection if it becomes contaminated. Peritonitis occurs if there is contamination or irritation that results in an inflammatory response. Peritonitis can be due to surgical contamination, urine leakage from the bladder, intestinal content leakage due to perforation of any part of the GI tract, penetrating abdominal injury or leakage from the biliary or pancreatic systems. Initially, if there is no infection, peritonitis develops in response to the irritant nature of the fluid (e.g. urine or bile) and clinical signs may take a few days to

develop. However, if the fluid is septic, or where there is leakage from the GI tract, the peritoneum becomes infected and this rapidly leads to severe illness, with septicaemia, shock and cardiovascular collapse within a few hours.

It is important for nurses to recognize peritonitis as part of postoperative monitoring of a patient, particularly after surgery on the GI tract. An animal may show some, or all, of the following clinical signs:

- Pyrexia
- Anorexia
- Depression
- Tachycardia
- Vomiting
- Ascites
- Abdominal pain.

The mainstay of treatment is to explore the abdomen surgically and find the source of contamination. In mild cases, or where there is no infection, thorough lavage of the abdomen may be sufficient. Where there is severe infection that cannot be resolved with surgery, the abdomen is best treated with open peritoneal drainage.

Abdominal lavage

Abdominal lavage involves pouring large volumes of warmed sterile isotonic fluids into the abdomen via a laparotomy and using suction to remove them until they come out clear. It is important to remove all the contaminated fluid to be effective and waterproof surgical drapes should be used.

Abdominal lavage technique

1. Take a sample of the abdominal fluid for culture and sensitivity at the start of the surgery.
2. Use sterile isotonic fluids (Hartmann's (lactated Ringer's) or saline) at body temperature.
3. Repeat lavage until the fluids come out clear.
4. All lavage fluid must be removed from the abdomen, as remaining fluid reduces the ability of the immune system to clear remaining bacteria.
5. Use omentum to cover any potential sites of leakage.
6. Change the surgeon's gloves and instruments. Re-drape with sterile drapes over the top of the contaminated drapes (preferably with waterproof drapes).
7. Topical antibiotics and antiseptics should not be used in the abdomen. Broad-spectrum bactericidal antibiotics are given intravenously pending the results of culture and sensitivity on a sample of abdominal fluid.

Open peritoneal drainage

Open peritoneal drainage is a technique whereby the abdomen is not fully closed after the lavage and is dressed with sterile dressings and a thick absorbent bandage (or disposable nappies). This dressing is changed using sterile technique 2–3 times per day while the infection drains from the abdomen. At each dressing change, the abdomen may be lavaged again through the open wound. Nursing of these patients is very complex and involves close monitoring of blood albumin and electrolyte levels, hydration, assisted feeding and care of the bandage.

Respiratory tract

Respiratory distress is potentially life-threatening in any species and the veterinary nurse must be able to recognize respiratory difficulties quickly in order to respond with potentially life-saving first aid (see Chapter 19).

Respiratory difficulty arises from inadequate oxygen delivery to the tissues which causes hypoxia. There are a number of ways this can come about and further details can be found in Chapters 18 and 19. First aid treatment is essential even for only mildly affected patients. Animals that show any signs of respiratory difficulty may suddenly decompensate when they are stressed during examination and become profoundly hypoxic. Most respiratory tract diseases that require surgery relate to obstruction of the free flow of air through the nose, the larynx, the trachea or into the lungs.

Nasal disease

The dog and cat have different patterns of nasal disease, with the cat being predominantly affected by infectious agents causing acute or chronic rhinitis. Diagnosis of nasal disease can be very challenging and relies mainly on radiography, rhinoscopy, biopsy and in some cases MRI or CT scanning. Rhinoscopy is used to visualize the nasal turbinates and to examine the nasopharynx above the soft palate. Biopsy samples may be taken to confirm the diagnosis. There are a few conditions that are treated surgically.

Rhinotomy

Occasionally it is necessary to open the nasal cavity to take biopsy samples, remove foreign bodies or remove a benign tumour or fungal plaque. This is done via an incision on the bridge of the nose and the nasal cavity is accessed using a burr or oscillating saw to create a passage through the nasal bones. Postoperative complications can include emphysema of the head and neck due to air leaking out through the rhinotomy incision. The turbinates often bleed profusely when biopsied.

Nasal aspergillosis

This is a fungal infection of the nasal cavity usually seen in younger dolichocephalic breeds of dog. It causes a purulent nasal discharge and often causes epistaxis, which can be very severe. Diagnosis is made sometimes on biopsy or rhinoscopy but it is more usually diagnosed by a blood test for Aspergillus antibodies. Treatment usually involves treating the nasal cavity with an antifungal agent via tubes implanted through the frontal sinus. This may be done under anaesthetic, leaving the antifungal agent to soak in the nasal cavity for an hour, or the flushing may be carried out daily in the conscious animal for 5 days. The success rate of these techniques is about 70–80% but some dogs will need more than one treatment.

Nasal neoplasia

Nasal tumours tend to affect older dolichocephalic dogs and are most often carcinomas. In cats adenocarcinoma is the most common diagnosis but lymphoma is also seen. The Siamese may be more at risk. The diagnosis is made by radiography and biopsy of the abnormal region seen on the radiograph. Surgical treatment is not usually an option and nasal tumours are treated with a course of radiotherapy.

Stenotic nares

Brachycephalic obstructive airway syndrome (BOAS) affects brachycephalic breeds with deformed airways, resulting in difficulty with breathing. The commonest breeds affected are the English Bulldog, Pekingese, French Bulldog and Pug; occasionally Persian cats may be affected. The animal presents with noisy breathing, snoring when asleep and exercise intolerance, which results from a combination of obstructions to the upper airway:

- Stenotic nares
- Overlong soft palate
- Tonsillar hypertrophy
- Pharyngeal hypertrophy
- Laryngeal collapse.

Many brachycephalic breeds also have problems with regurgitation of food and/or saliva. Some dogs may have a collapsed larynx and a narrow trachea. Laryngeal collapse occurs secondary to the upper airway obstruction. It may be managed with weight loss and surgery of the upper airways, but if there is insufficient improvement, a permanent tracheostomy or laryngeal surgery can be considered. The overall prognosis is guarded.

Severely affected animals may have exercise intolerance and episodes of cyanosis and syncope. Animals may present as an emergency in hot weather when they may be suffering from heat stroke, dehydration, cyanosis and severe stress. Nursing requires oxygen supplementation, cooling, sedation and if necessary an emergency tracheostomy.

Surgical treatment depends on the most severely affected part of the airway: the stenotic nares can be widened and the tonsils and part of the soft palate resected to improve upper airway flow. Laryngeal collapse should not be confused with laryngeal paralysis (see below).

Laryngeal surgery

Surgery on the larynx is a complex procedure and can potentially result in severe difficulty during recovery due to mucosal swelling. The animal must be closely observed for signs of respiratory distress and facilities should be available for oxygen supplementation or emergency tracheostomy if necessary.

Laryngeal paralysis

This typically occurs in the older medium-sized breeds of dog. It is occasionally seen in the cat. The disease results from paralysis of the recurrent laryngeal nerve, which means that the dog cannot abduct the arytenoid cartilages to open the airway on inspiration. The clinical signs range from increased noise on breathing when excited, panting on exercising, to cyanosis and collapse. These dogs often present in the summer when they are panting more to lose heat and the paralysed larynx becomes oedematous and swollen thereby further reducing airflow. They may collapse and be brought into the practice cyanotic and struggling to breathe. In hot weather they may also have heat stroke.

In an acute situation the animal may have to be anaesthetized so that the airway can be intubated and oxygen administered. Prior to recovery, the appropriate surgery is to 'tie back' the arytenoid cartilage so that it no longer obstructs the airway. This procedure is carried out through an incision over the larynx in the side of the neck. If this is not possible, then it would be necessary to place a tracheostomy tube to bypass the larynx and allow the dog to breathe until surgery is possible. This is not an easy procedure and is often carried out in referral centres. Laryngeal paralysis should be distinguished from laryngeal collapse, which is usually seen in small-breed dogs.

Laryngeal tumours

These are rare, but also cause respiratory obstruction. Small tumours on the arytenoid cartilages can be treated with partial resection of the cartilage. Complete resection of the larynx is not very successful and there is little treatment possible, unless the tumour is sensitive to chemotherapy (e.g. lymphoma).

Trachea

The trachea is a rigid cartilaginous structure that prevents collapse of the airway when the animal creates negative pressure on inspiration.

Collapsing trachea

This is most often seen in toy or miniature breeds of dog, most notably the Yorkshire Terrier. The tracheal rings are not rigid, and when the dog is excited, or exercising, the trachea flattens and causes a harsh honking cough. Severely affected dogs may become cyanotic during coughing episodes, or even syncopal. Some dogs respond to medical management of weight loss, anti-inflammatories, antitussives (see Chapter 8), anti-cholinergics and use of a harness rather than a collar. Dogs that are severely affected may require placement of a stent along the inside of the trachea, which holds it open, and this has been very successful. Measurement and placement of the stent is complex and is usually done in referral centres.

Avulsion of the trachea

Typically, this is seen in the cat after a road traffic accident. The trachea is torn apart usually quite distal within the thorax. The cat may initially appear normal, but becomes tachypnoeic over the first few days after the accident and may develop emphysema over the neck and shoulders. Surgical repair is urgent and involves a thoracotomy to re-anastomose the ends of the trachea. The surgery is technically difficult and the anaesthetic complicated by the fact that the cat requires intermittent positive pressure ventilation (IPPV) during the surgery through a sterile endotracheal tube placed by the surgeon through the thoracotomy incision into the distal trachea. Postoperatively, a chest drain is placed to monitor for pneumothorax and the cat is closely monitored for signs of leakage from the anastomosis.

Ruptured trachea

Ruptured trachea can occur secondary to traumatic events such as road accidents or bite wounds; however, it is also reported subsequent to endotracheal intubation. In one study of iatrogenic tracheal rupture in cats, it was noted that it was more common after anaesthesia for routine dentistry. Inflation of the cuff and twisting of the head and neck during anaesthesia may be contributory factors. The cat presents either with subcutaneous emphysema 24 hours after the injury or with progressive dyspnoea 4–5 days later as the ends of the trachea scar and become narrow. Surgical repair is sometimes necessary.

Tracheostomy

This may be temporary or permanent. It may be used for administration of anaesthetic gases during oral surgery or as a means of bypassing an obstructed upper airway. Most often it is used as a life-saving procedure in an emergency situation to bypass an obstructed upper airway.

Usually the airway is not completely blocked and administration of oxygen with a face mask provides some relief while the animal is prepared for tracheostomy. However, where the animal is unconscious or severely cyanotic, the veterinary nurse should prepare for the veterinary surgeon to perform the tracheostomy using only local anaesthetic or no anaesthetic and no surgical preparation if the animal is likely to die with any delay. If airway obstruction is anticipated (e.g. after surgery on the upper airway), the ventral aspect of the neck may be prepared in readiness for an emergency tracheostomy. Tracheostomy tubes are illustrated in Figure 23.34.

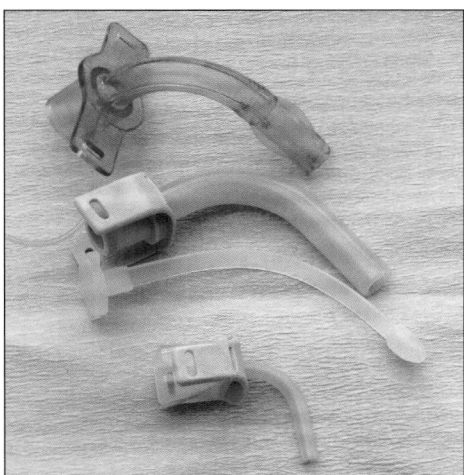

23.34 These are different types of tracheostomy tubes but all have a curved tube that enters through the skin into the trachea. The middle tube shown here also has a trochar that fits inside the tube. They are available in different sizes to accommodate different sizes of animal.

Emergency tracheostomy

- Make sure that the oxygen delivery tube will fit the tracheostomy tube
- Clip and surgically prepare the ventral aspect of the neck
- Have a sterile surgical kit ready, together with the appropriate-sized tracheostomy tube and suture material to open up the tracheal incision
- Suction may be necessary for the lower airway
- Prepare for continuous postoperative monitoring

Management of a tracheostomy tube

- Constant one-to-one monitoring for at least the first 12–24 hours
- Regular suction of the tracheostomy tube every hour
- Humidification of the trachea by instilling 2–10 ml sterile saline into the tube every hour, or use of a nebulizer
- Changing the tracheostomy tube for a new sterile one every 2–6 hours, depending on the quantity of exudate

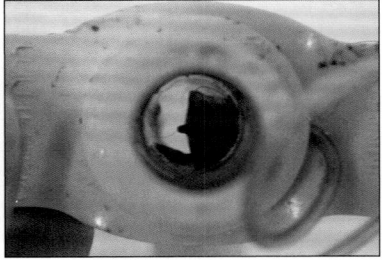

Tracheostomy tubes can block quickly with dried secretions and blood. Meticulous care is necessary to prevent sudden death.

Emergency airway

If an animal is very close to death and the materials are not immediately available, oxygen can be administered via a wide-gauge hypodermic needle or intravenous cannula pushed quickly through the ventral midline of the neck between the tracheal rings. This can then be used to administer oxygen via a narrow tube or urinary catheter

Tracheal foreign bodies or neoplasia

Rarely an animal presents with obstruction of the trachea. If this is a foreign body it may be removed under anaesthesia using endoscopic forceps. Small tumours can be removed by resection of some of the tracheal rings and re-anastomosing the trachea.

Lungs

Principles of thoracotomy

The thorax can be approached either by entering the cavity between the ribs (lateral or intercostal thoracotomy) or by splitting the sternum and approaching the thorax from the ventral aspect (sternal thoracotomy or sternotomy). If more access is required, a rib can be resected.

Intercostal thoracotomy is the commonest approach and allows the surgeon access to the lungs, heart, oesophagus and pleural cavity on one side only. The advantage of sternotomy is that both sides of the chest can be explored at the same procedure. Sternotomy in large dogs requires the facilities to saw through the sternum. During the thoracotomy, the animal must be on IPPV continuously, and it should be monitored for heat loss, hypotension and dehydration.

Following thoracotomy, great care is taken to close the incision with an airtight seal. A chest drain is used to remove the pleural air during closure and also postoperatively to monitor air or fluid leaks within the chest (Figure 23.35). A sterile drain is placed through a skin tunnel between the ribs and the other end is linked to a water seal which allows continual aspiration of air, or it may be occluded and drained intermittently (see 'Drains', above).

Analgesia is very important after thoracotomy. It is also important to get large dogs up and moving around as soon as possible to reduce the risk of thromboembolism (obstruction of a blood vessel by a blood clot that has become dislodged from another site).

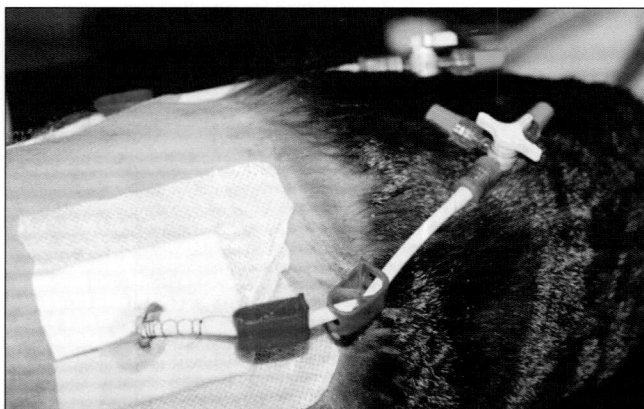

23.35 Chest drains placed in a cat for the treatment of pneumothorax. The drains are secured to the skin with a finger-trap suture. The drains should be further stabilized by a dressing and monitored continuously, as interference could be fatal. (Courtesy of C. Sturgeon).

Lung lobectomy

Lung lobes are removed via an intercostal thoracotomy as this gives the best access to the arteries, veins and bronchus. The vessels and bronchus may be ligated and oversewn manually or a lung lobectomy stapling device can be used to perform the procedure in one step. After the lung lobe has been removed, the bronchus is checked for air leaks by filling the chest with warm sterile saline, inflating the lungs, and looking for bubbles.

Pyothorax

This is an infection of the pleura in the thoracic cavity. It is commonly seen in cats probably secondary to cat bites and in dogs probably due to migrating grass seeds. The animal presents with difficulty in breathing, due to large volumes of pus in the thoracic cavity. Mostly these cases are treated by placing thoracic drains in both sides of the chest and draining and lavaging the chest twice daily with sterile fluids and anti-biotics. Persistent cases may require a thoracotomy to open up the chest cavity and debride infected tissue or look for the foreign body.

Cardiovascular system

Heart

Persistent ductus arteriosus

Persistent ductus arteriosus (PDA) occurs when the ductus arteriosus fails to close at birth, and blood bypasses the lungs and left side of the heart, travelling from the pulmonary artery directly into the aorta. It creates a characteristic heart murmur that should be easily detected at the first vaccination check. If the condition is left untreated, the dog will eventually die from heart failure. Surgical treatment can be performed in patients weighing less than about 10 kg; the PDA is accessed via a left lateral thoracotomy and ligated. In larger patients, interventional radiology is required to place coils via the femoral artery to occlude the PDA.

Vascular ring anomaly

Congenital defects of the heart and great vessels sometimes occur and result in entrapment of the oesophagus between the ligamentum arteriosum (the remnants of the closed ductus arteriosum) and the other vessels. The commonest is a persistent right aortic arch (PRAA) when the aorta is found on the right side instead of the left and the ductus crosses the oesophagus and makes a constriction that prevents the normal passage of food on swallowing. The treatment is ligation and separation of the ductus from the surface of the oesophagus via a left-sided thoracotomy.

Arteries and veins

Vascular access: 'cut-down'

Intravenous treatments are usually given via an intravenous catheter placed in the cephalic vein. In patients that are collapsed, dehydrated or in severe shock it can be very difficult to identify the superficial veins in order to place the catheter. If it is not possible to place a jugular catheter, a 'cut-down' technique may be used instead to access a vein. The area over the vein is clipped and prepared surgically and a tourniquet is placed above the vein to increase visibility. An incision is made directly over the vein, and careful dissection down through the tissue planes is used to identify the vessel. The catheter is then placed routinely, flushed with heparin–saline and usually sutured in place. The skin is sutured over the surgical site and the wound is dressed.

Aortic thromboembolism

This is a serious emergency condition, usually seen in the cat, when a blood clot (embolism) breaks off and travels down the aorta to block the iliac arteries at the end of the aorta. This completely blocks the blood flow to one or both hindlimbs. The hindlimbs are cold, stiff and very painful and there is no palpable femoral pulse. Occasionally the condition is responsive to medical management; and surgical removal of the thromboembolism has been reported, but is only rarely successful. The condition is usually secondary to heart disease and the prognosis is poor.

Emergency vessel occlusion

Vessels may be lacerated or ruptured during the course of surgery or as a result of severe trauma. If the event occurs during surgery, small arteries (<2 mm) and veins (<4 mm) can be sealed using electrodiathermy, or may stop bleeding after a few minutes of direct pressure. Large vessels are ligated or double ligated, using absorbable synthetic suture material with good knot security. There are also commercial staples available to seal arteries and veins during surgery.

Traumatic haemorrhage may have to be stemmed prior to identifying the specific vessel. If the bleeding is clearly arterial (pumping), surgical exploration and ligation of the artery is a priority. However, the bleeding may be profuse and non-specific. Initially direct hand-held pressure on the wound using a sterile pack of absorbent material may be sufficient to slow the bleeding. If the bleeding continues to be profuse, other options are a tourniquet above the site of bleeding on a limb, application of a very heavily padded bandage or immediate surgical exploration under anaesthesia. It is very important to time the duration of a tourniquet to prevent ischaemic necrosis. It is also important to remove the bandage as soon as possible, otherwise high pressure underneath the bandage may result in the same effect. Weighing the material used to absorb the blood before and after use will help in estimating blood loss.

Major arteries may be repaired if necessary and blood flow can be temporarily stopped during the repair using bulldog clips or a Rommel tourniquet. Very fine-gauge polypropylene suture material is usually used to repair arteries or veins, as it causes very little tissue reaction.

Endocrine system

Thyroid gland

Thyroidectomy (dog)

In the dog, thyroidectomy is usually carried out as treatment for thyroid carcinoma. Small tumours may be easy to remove, but they can be very vascular and may be attached to vital structures in the neck. In some cases, they are treated with radiotherapy or chemotherapy if they are deemed inoperable.

Thyroidectomy (cat)

Hyperthyroidism is a common condition in the older cat. The majority of cases are due to a thyroid adenoma (a benign tumour) of one, or more usually both, thyroid lobes, which secretes excess thyroid hormone. It results typically in hyperactivity and restlessness, weight loss, polyphagia, polyuria/polydipsia, diarrhoea and tachycardia. Some cats may also have concurrent kidney disease and heart failure. The enlarged thyroid gland may be palpated in the neck, or the condition may be diagnosed from a blood sample (see Chapter 18).

Initially, the cat is usually stabilized using an orally administered drug that controls the thyroid hormone levels, e.g. methimazole and carbimazole, but this would have to be continued for life unless a definitive treatment is employed. Surgical removal of the thyroid gland is one option, but there is a risk of recurrence if the thyroid tumour is not completely removed. The main perioperative risk associated with surgery is damage to the parathyroid glands, which are closely attached to the thyroid gland. This results in loss of control of calcium metabolism, and hypocalcaemia develops in the first 2–3 days after surgery. Thus, cats should be frequently tested and closely observed for signs of hypocalcaemia in the first 2–3 days postoperatively. If the damage is severe, the cat may need calcium supplementation intravenously and then orally for 8–12 weeks until the parathyroid glands recover. The gold standard treatment is injection with a radioactive isotope of iodine, which has a 95% success rate and few complications.

Adrenal glands

The adrenal glands in the dog and cat are sometimes removed as a treatment for hyperadrenocorticism (Cushing's disease) or phaeochromocytoma, where the adrenal gland is the primary source of the condition. Surgery involves deep dissection in the region of the dorsal abdominal vena cava and there can be severe haemorrhage. The patient may have delayed wound healing due to the medical condition and should be closely monitored for wound dehiscence. Sudden hormonal changes in the postoperative period can also destabilize a patient and they should be closely monitored for electrolyte abnormalities, hypotension and vomiting/diarrhoea. Adrenal tumours are common in ferrets and are often removed successfully.

Pancreas

The pancreas is a lobulated gland that is closely associated with the stomach and duodenum. The commonest disease is a sterile inflammation (pancreatitis), which causes severe abdominal pain and vomiting. This is not a surgical disease and surgical exploration will make the clinical signs worse. Other conditions include pancreatic abscesses, damage due to abdominal trauma and pancreatic tumours.

Pancreatectomy

Abscesses and tumours may be removed by a partial pancreatectomy. If the lesion is in the body of the pancreas or involves the blood supply to the duodenum it is generally considered inoperable.

The most common tumour of the pancreas is an insulinoma. This is a tumour that secretes excess insulin and causes hypoglycaemia. After surgery the animal has to be carefully managed to ensure that acute pancreatitis does not occur; pain monitoring and management is also important. Pancreatic surgery may cause nausea, vomiting or swelling and obstruction of the common bile duct. Monitoring of the glucose levels is critical in postoperative management of insulinoma patients and they may need either glucose or insulin therapy. When the animal is fed it should initially be given small quantities of a low-fat diet.

Pancreatic biopsy

In some patients with chronic low-grade pancreatitis, it is difficult to diagnose the disease without biopsy. Ideally, this is performed via laparoscopy to reduce the risk of a flare-up of the disease. Otherwise, a small piece of pancreas is removed via laparotomy and the patient is managed as for pancreatectomy.

Liver and gallbladder

Liver disease can potentially result in a number of medical conditions that would adversely affect the success of surgery. Many patients may have low levels of albumin and vitamin K and increased susceptibility to sedatives or anaesthetic agents. Animals with suspected liver disease should always have blood-clotting times tested prior to surgery and they may require a transfusion of plasma. The liver has remarkable powers of regeneration and can compensate for removal or damage to liver lobes.

Biopsy

The purpose of performing a liver biopsy is to achieve a specific diagnosis. Samples can be obtained either by laparoscopy or via a laparotomy incision. Usually just a small piece of the edge of a liver lobe is removed and normal clotting stops the bleeding spontaneously. Occasionally a core needle biopsy (e.g. using a Tru-Cut® needle) may be used with ultrasound guidance to obtain the sample.

Lobectomy

A whole liver lobe may need to be removed if it is diseased or damaged. The blood supply to the liver may be temporarily shut off using a small tourniquet during the surgery. Postoperatively, the animal must be monitored closely for haemorrhage into the abdominal cavity as this is the most common complication of the surgery.

Portosystemic shunts

A portosystemic shunt (PSS) is a congenital or acquired vascular anomaly that redirects blood flow in the portal vein so that it bypasses the liver. The clinical signs include poor growth, abnormal behaviour a few hours after feeding, seizures, urate calculi in the urinary tract and hypoglycaemia. The disease is usually diagnosed with blood tests and ultrasound scans of the liver. More detailed investigations such as a portovenogram (contrast material injected into a mesenteric vein), CT angiogram or contrast fluoroscopy may be necessary.

- Small breeds of dog are most commonly affected with congenital shunts; these are usually single large vessels draining into the abdominal vena cava (extrahepatic shunts).
- Large breeds of dog are usually affected with intrahepatic shunts.
- Acquired shunts are seen in older dogs or cats and are related to the development of veins that bypass the liver secondary to chronic liver disease that obstructs the normal flow of blood in the portal vein.

Only congenital PSS is treated surgically. The patient is usually stabilized with medical management first and then the shunt is partially ligated via a laparotomy in one or more surgical procedures. Some referral centres use constrictor devices or cellophane around the shunt to occlude the vessel slowly, allowing the liver more time to adapt to the increased blood flow. Interventional radiology techniques can be used to occlude intra hepatic shunts. Postoperative complications include abdominal pain, hypoglycaemia, diarrhoea, vomiting, hypotension, hypothermia, prolonged recovery time due to poor metabolism of anaesthetic drugs, seizures text and shock. Seizures can occur up to 5 days after surgery and are associated with a guarded prognosis for recovery; sometimes anaesthesia for several days and long-term hospitalization are required.

Cholecystectomy

Cholangitis or cholecystitis (infection or inflammation of the biliary ducts and gallbladder) and cholelithiasis (stones in the gallbladder) may be treated by removal of the gallbladder. The most common indication for cholecystectomy is gallbladder mucocoele. The gallbladder fills with thick jelly-like bile which may be infected. It is often seen in Border Terriers. The surgery is carried out through a cranial midline laparotomy and the gallbladder is ligated and removed. The bile continues to drain from the liver into the duodenum through the common bile duct, the only difference being that it does not collect in the gallbladder between meals. Postoperatively, the animal should be treated with antibiotics and monitored for pancreatitis or bile leakage.

Spleen

The spleen is a large vascular organ in the abdomen on the left side next to the stomach. Although removal of the spleen in humans can result in the development of septicaemia, this has not been reported in dogs and cats and total splenectomy is not usually associated with any long-term problems.

Splenectomy

Indications for removal of the spleen include neoplasia, splenic torsion, trauma and haemorrhage. Haemangiosarcoma is the most common primary tumour of the spleen, and some tumours will be metastases from elsewhere. Up to half of splenic tumours may be benign or even just haematomas, and splenectomy can carry a good prognosis.

Sometimes patients present with acute haemorrhage from the spleen, and splenectomy is performed as an emergency procedure. More often, the bleeding is intermittent and the spleen is removed as an elective procedure to prevent a haemorrhagic crisis. If the haemorrhage has been severe, the animal may require a blood transfusion prior to surgery; if the haemorrhage is due to trauma and not neoplasia, an autotransfusion of blood can be carried out. At the time of the laparotomy the blood is suctioned via sterile apparatus out of the abdomen, mixed with the appropriate volume of anticoagulant, filtered and transfused into a peripheral vein. If there is any likelihood of neoplastic disease, autotransfusion should not be carried out.

Splenectomy may be performed using conventional surgical instruments and technique, using a stapler or using a harmonic scalpel (Figure 23.36).

The most common postoperative complication is haemorrhage as a result of displacement of a ligature in the abdomen. The patient needs to be closely monitored for signs of intra-abdominal bleeding.

Urinary tract

All surgery of the urinary tract runs the potential risk of acute kidney injury if kidney function is affected and urine production stops postoperatively. Urine production should be maintained at a minimum of 2 ml/kg/h using intravenous fluid therapy as required during the postoperative period. Urine needs to be collected and measured in order to monitor output. Diuretics or other treatments may be given if urine output is inadequate. Blood samples can also be analysed for urea, creatinine and electrolyte (potassium) levels, which also indicate renal function.

Kidney

The kidneys are retroperitoneal, which means that they lie outside the peritoneal cavity of the abdomen. They receive

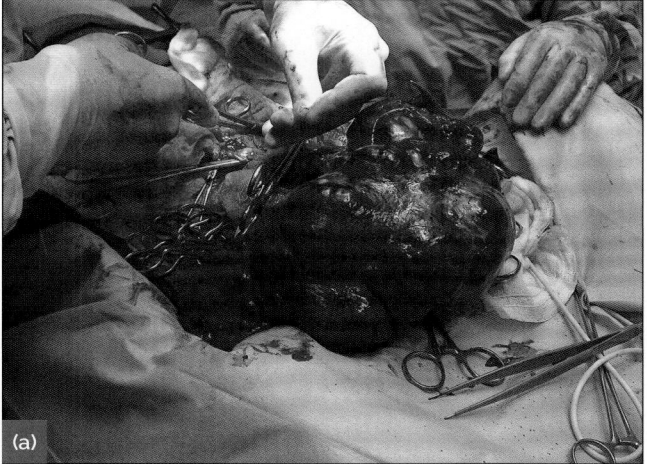

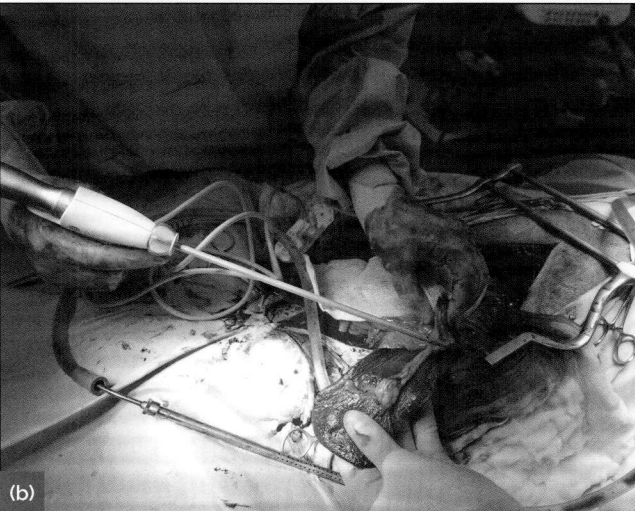

23.36 Splenectomy. **(a)** A splenectomy being carried out using conventional surgical technique, with hand-tied sutures and artery forceps for haemostasis. **(b)** A splenectomy being carried out using a harmonic scalpel.

25% of the total cardiac output and are one of the vital organs of the body. Surgical handling or trauma that might disrupt the blood supply or cause the artery to spasm could be potentially life-threatening.

Ureteronephrectomy

A kidney may be removed if there is severe trauma, neoplasia, hydronephrosis (enlargement of the kidney secondary to back pressure from the bladder), or severe pyelonephritis (infection). It is essential to be sure that the other kidney is functioning normally prior to this procedure otherwise the animal may go into postoperative renal failure. The kidney is removed together with its ureter, which is traced all the way down to the bladder and the arteries and veins are ligated. Postoperatively, intravenous fluids should be given until normal urine flow has been monitored and recorded.

Nephrotomy

Calculi can occasionally form in the kidney. These are very painful and may result in severe secondary infections of the kidney, which may cause permanent damage. They are removed by a nephrotomy into the renal pelvis, when the calculus is removed and the incision repaired. However, it should be noted that any incision will compromise the function of the kidney for days or even weeks postoperatively, and renal function needs to be carefully monitored in the

postoperative period. Postoperative intravenous fluid therapy is important to ensure good urine production, along with close monitoring of blood urea and creatinine to check for evidence of urine leakage.

Renal biopsy

Biopsy of the kidney can be performed, but this is only done after extensive investigation of the renal disease as it carries considerable risks of haemorrhage and damage to renal function. Ideally, the sample is taken through a surgical incision, but sometimes it is carried out percutaneously using a core needle (e.g. Tru-Cut® needle) with ultrasound guidance. Postoperatively, pressure is used to stop bleeding and urine output is monitored and the urine analysed.

Ureters

The ureters travel in the retroperitoneal space from the kidney to the bladder. They can be imaged using intravenous excretory urography or ultrasound examination. They are not seen on plain radiographs.

Avulsion of the ureter

Rarely, the ureter may be torn secondary to abdominal trauma. This causes urine leakage into the retroperitoneal space, causing cellulitis with electrolyte abnormalities and azotaemia. In some cases, the damage can be repaired surgically, but often ureteronephrectomy is necessary. It is important to stabilize the animal with respect to renal and electrolyte parameters prior to anaesthesia.

Ectopic ureters

This is a congenital condition where one or both ureters implant distal to the bladder, so that urine flows directly into the urethra. This results in a constant urinary incontinence, usually in a young dog. Golden Retrievers, Poodles and Labrador Retrievers are most commonly affected. The condition is diagnosed using excretory urography and ultrasonography. The ureters are often enlarged and abnormal due to ascending infections. In some cases, the ascending infection results in severe pyelonephritis and a ureteronephrectomy is carried out. Where the ureter and kidney are healthy it is possible to reimplant the ureter surgically into the bladder, or using endoscopy an incision is made to adjust the level of the opening. Surgery on the ureter can result in spasm that causes the kidney to stop producing urine on that side for up to 48 hours. Therefore, ideally, if both ureters require surgery, one side should be done at a time. As in renal surgery, urine production is carefully monitored postoperatively. In some cases, the incontinence may persist due to other bladder abnormalities.

Ureteric entrapment

The ureters run down to the bladder and in the female pass the uterine body and cervix. At this position they are at risk of entrapment in the ligature during routine ovariohysterectomy. This is life-threatening, particularly if both ureters are involved. If the ligature is removed within 7 days, little damage is done to the kidney and it should completely recover, thus postoperative nursing observations are important in routine neutering procedures to pick up these complications.

Ureteral obstruction

Urolithiasis can result in stones that dislodge from the kidney and pass into the ureter causing obstruction. This is most commonly seen in cats with calcium oxalate uroliths. The ureteric obstruction causes pain and requires urgent referral for specialist treatment. Sometimes small uroliths can be flushed to the bladder with intravenous fluids, but usually a bypass device is required to divert urine from the kidney to the bladder. The subcutaneous ureteric bypass (SUB) requires long-term management to ensure that it does not obstruct again.

Urinary bladder

Surgery on the bladder is common in veterinary practice. The bladder lies in the caudal abdomen and can be accessed via a midline laparotomy. The bladder should be emptied prior to surgery, either using a catheter via the urethra or by cystocentesis using a small-gauge needle and syringe at surgery. The bladder wall is delicate and prone to oedema and bruising with rough handling, so it is usually held during surgery using stay sutures or fine forceps. Urine continues to collect in the bladder during surgery so it is important to protect the other abdominal organs from contamination with the urine during cystotomy.

Cystotomy and cystectomy

The most common indications for cystotomy are to remove calculi (stones) or tumours. Usually the incision in the bladder wall is made in the ventral aspect and more stay sutures may be placed lateral to the incision to assist opening the bladder for inspection. Sometimes the calculi are located far down the bladder neck and it may be necessary to place a urethral catheter and flush them into the bladder with sterile saline. For removal of neoplasms, the full thickness of the bladder wall is removed with a margin around the tumour and the bladder reconstructed. The incision is closed in two layers using a synthetic absorbable suture material. Postoperatively, the animal should be given the opportunity to empty the bladder as frequently as possible and monitored for normal urination and evidence of urine leakage (uraemia, hypothermia, abdominal pain) for 3–4 days.

Bladder rupture

This occurs either secondary to blunt abdominal trauma or due to prolonged urethral obstruction causing severe back pressure and accumulation of urine. Occasionally, bladder rupture occurs when attempts are made to express the bladder manually in paralysed patients. The condition may be diagnosed from the history, an absence of urine in the bladder or using diagnostic imaging. The immediate concern is the uroperitoneum and the metabolic consequences of the absorption of urine from the peritoneum. There may be azotaemia, electrolyte imbalances, dehydration and shock, which may have to be treated prior to surgery. At surgery, the abdomen should be lavaged with sterile saline to remove urine and contaminants, and the bladder is repaired. Postoperatively, blood urea levels and urine production should be closely monitored.

Tube cystostomy (urinary diversion)

This is the placement of a drain through the abdominal wall in order to drain the bladder, bypassing the urethra. This may be used as a temporary measure prior to urethral surgery or after bladder or urethral surgery to divert urine flow. It can also be used for diversion of urine in patients with urethral obstruction due to tumours or paralysis of the bladder. A Foley catheter is drawn into the abdomen through a stab incision lateral to the midline (Figure 23.37). The tip is placed into the bladder, the balloon inflated with sterile saline and the catheter secured with sutures and omentum. The catheter is then secured to the outside of the body wall with sutures or zinc

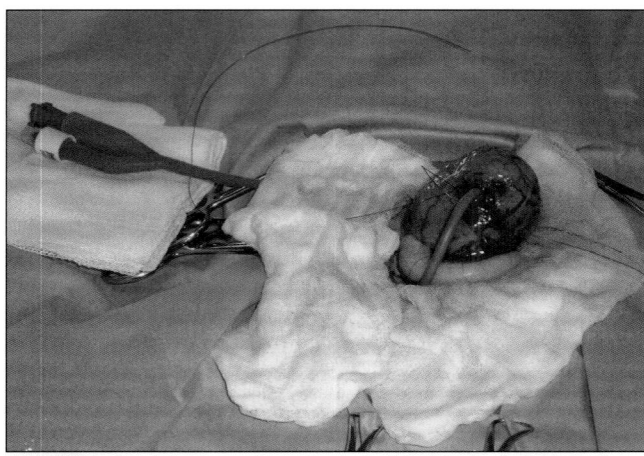

23.37 An intraoperative view of a bladder exteriorised for placement of a cystostomy tube using a Foley catheter.

oxide butterfly tapes. In the hospital, this should be attached to a closed urine collection system to prevent the risk of ascending infections. In the longer term, the bladder is emptied at least four times daily by removing a bung from the end and attaching a syringe. When the drain is removed, the tip should be submitted for culture and then appropriate antibiotics used to treat any associated infection. Use of antibiotics while the drain is in place will not prevent infection and will only increase the likelihood of resistant strains developing. Owners should be shown how to use the tube by a veterinary nurse when the patient is discharged, and regular contact maintained with the owner to ensure sure that they are using it properly and managing the tube in a sterile manner.

Percutaneous cystostomy tube placement is also possible. In this technique a 'locking loop' catheter is used to puncture a full bladder through the skin under ultrasound guidance. Once the sharp stylet has been removed, the tip of the catheter is curled into a 'pigtail' shape to keep it within the bladder wall. This catheter can be used to temporarily keep the bladder empty pending further treatment or stabilization of post-renal azotaemia.

Urethra

Surgery on the urethra is most often carried out following damage caused by calculi. Preoperatively, the systemic consequences of urethral obstruction may need to be addressed prior to anaesthesia, and often a urinary catheter is passed before surgery to make identification of the urethra easier.

Urethral obstruction

Blockage of the urethra in any species results in accumulation of urine in the bladder, which, if not relieved, causes back pressure on the kidneys and then bladder rupture. The urine spills into the abdomen and causes azotaemia and death. The clinical signs may be severe abdominal pain with persistent straining to urinate.

Animals straining to urinate should be checked as an emergency to assess the bladder.

Cats are usually more severely affected than dogs, which may have only partial obstruction.

The urethra in the female is short and wide and unlikely to obstruct except secondary to neoplastic growth. In the male dog and cat the urethra is narrower, particularly at the tip in the male cat and at the level of the os penis in the male dog. This anatomical characteristic makes it prone to obstruction by urinary calculi. The type of stone that blocks the urethra depends on the disease and it should always be submitted for analysis in order to determine the most appropriate prophylactic treatment for the future.

Male cats also develop obstruction of the urethra secondary to feline lower urinary tract disease (FLUTD) and, in these cases, the obstruction is not always due to a calculus, but can be caused by a mucoid plug or spasm of the urethra in response to inflammation.

The priority is to stabilize the animal with intravenous fluids and decompress the bladder. If a urinary catheter cannot be passed, then it may be necessary to empty the bladder by cystocentesis. Once the pressure is reduced, it may then be possible to pass a catheter or to flush the urolith or plug back into the bladder with sterile saline (retropulsion). If it is not possible to remove the calculus in this way, urethrotomy is necessary.

Cystocentesis

1. Sedation is only necessary in fractious animals but analgesia should always be provided.
2. The distended bladder is identified as a hard mass in the caudal abdomen.
3. A small area of skin on the ventrolateral abdomen directly over the bladder is clipped and surgically prepared.
4. A 20 G needle of the appropriate length for the size of animal is selected and attached to a 20 ml syringe via a three-way tap.
5. Sterile gloves are used or a hand scrub is performed.
6. The bladder is gently held still with one hand and the needle is introduced into the bladder through the prepared area of skin.
7. The urine is drawn off and the three-way tap is used to expel the urine into a bowl. This is repeated until the bladder feels empty.
8. The volume of urine is recorded.

Urethrostomy

In some circumstances, either the cause of the urethral obstruction cannot be treated (e.g. calcium oxalate crystals) or the tip of the urethra is so damaged that it is prone to recurrent obstruction. In these cases, it may be necessary to create a new opening for urination through a wider part of the urethra. In the dog this is done at the level of the scrotum. In an intact male dog, castration and scrotal ablation are performed and then an incision into the urethra at that level is sutured to the skin edges (scrotal urethrostomy). In the male cat, the penis is amputated and the urethra is opened out and sutured to the skin edges (perineal urethrostomy). A urinary catheter should not be placed after surgery, and it is extremely important that the animal does not lick at the site at any stage during the healing process. Initially, there may be considerable bleeding associated with urination and it may be advisable to hospitalize the patient until this has reduced. Nursing involves keeping the site clean and free of urine or blood and preventing urine scald until the animal learns how to reposition during urination.

Urethral rupture

The urethra is exposed to damage in the male dog as it runs down the perineum and inguinal area and in all animals as it runs through the pelvic canal. The most common cause of rupture is trauma to the pelvic area and it is often seen secondary to pelvic fractures. The urine leaks out of the urethra and can cause severe inflammation of the pelvic tissues. Re-absorption of the urine then causes changes in the blood biochemistry such as azotaemia and hyperkalaemia, which cause systemic illness. If the tear is small, the urethra may be treated with placement of a soft silicone indwelling urinary catheter, allowing it to heal by second intention. Larger tears or complete ruptures (avulsion) should be repaired surgically once the animal has been stabilized for the anaesthetic. Urine is then diverted through a cystostomy tube until the site is healed.

Urethral neoplasia

This is more common in the bitch than the dog and is occasionally seen in the cat. It usually presents with acute obstruction to urination although there may be a history of cystitis. Surgery can be performed to remove the urethra and reconstruct it using part of the vagina; however, the prognosis is very poor. It is important that a biopsy is done to confirm the diagnosis, as granulomatous urethritis can look very similar to neoplasia but can be treated successfully with steroids.

Urinary incontinence

Incontinence is most common in the bitch. It has to be investigated in order to determine the primary cause or causes:

- Ectopic ureter
- Pelvic bladder
- Short bladder neck
- Urinary tract infection
- Urinary sphincter mechanism incompetence (USMI).

The only condition that has to be treated surgically is ectopic ureter (see above). The other conditions often present in a slightly older bitch or in the young bitch after spaying. They usually respond to medical management, but occasionally surgery is necessary to reposition the bladder neck and increase the pressure around the sphincter; this increases the holding capacity of the bladder and reduces incontinence. This surgery is usually carried out in specialist referral centres. Different techniques may be employed depending on the exact anatomical cause of the urinary incontinence, e.g. collagen injections into the urethral wall, urethropexy, colposuspension or placement of an artificial urethral sphincter. Postoperative care involves carefully monitoring for urinary tract infections and ensuring that there is no retention of urine.

Incontinence in the male dog is usually secondary to prostatic disease. Castration may make the incontinence worse; it is very difficult to treat successfully with drugs, but artificial urethral sphincters have been used successfully.

Reproductive system

Conditions are discussed in detail in Chapter 24.

Testes

The testes are the reproductive organ producing spermatozoa in male animals. They should normally descend after birth into the scrotum and remain externally located.

Elective castration (orchidectomy)

Castration may be carried out for therapeutic reasons (treatment of orchitis, perineal hernia, anal adenoma, testicular tumours or prostatitis), social reasons or as part of a neutering programme. Occasionally, castration is recommended to control behavioural abnormalities or difficulties such as roaming, excessive libido or aggression. Castration in the tomcat is usually carried out to prevent territorial spraying. Castration of the male dog at less than 6 months of age is associated with a decreased risk of prostatic neoplasia.

Castration in the cat is usually carried out via an incision in the scrotum; the testis is pulled out gently and then either it is ligated with suture material or the vas deferens and vascular bundle are tied in a knot to secure haemostasis. The vascular bundle is released into the scrotum and the procedure repeated on the other side. The cat is observed postoperatively for signs of haemorrhage, and then discharged with instructions for a litter tray to be used with shredded newspaper for 2–3 days. The wounds in the scrotum are not sutured, but allowed to heal by second intention.

Castration in the dog can be carried out either through a prescrotal midline incision or via scrotal ablation. Prescrotal castration involves pushing the testes forwards into the single incision and then the arteries and veins are ligated before removal of each testis. The skin incision is sutured closed, and the scrotum is left in place. Scrotal ablation involves removal of the scrotum and then the testes are removed with ligation as described above directly through the scrotal area. The skin is sutured closed. Prescrotal castration is quicker but leaves an unsightly scrotal sac behind and risks seroma or haematoma formation in the scrotum. Scrotal ablation takes longer, but has fewer complications associated with the healing of the surgical site.

Postoperatively, it is important that the owner is warned not to let the dog lick the sutures and that the dog is monitored for signs of ventral abdominal or scrotal swelling or bruising that might indicate ligature slippage.

Castration of rabbits may be carried out to reduce aggression and improve their behaviour as pets or in groups. Incisions may be made in a prescrotal or scrotal position and usually subcuticular sutures are used to close the incision. There is a theoretical risk of herniation through the inguinal canal and some surgeons will close the canal with one or two sutures before skin closure.

Retained testes (cryptorchidism)

Failure of one or both testes to descend is an inherited condition (see Chapter 24). It is more common in small-breed dogs, and is very rare in the cat. The retained testicle has an increased risk of developing neoplasia and should be removed. Owners should be encouraged not to breed from affected animals and ideally both testicles should be removed in affected males.

The retained testis may be found at any point from the kidney down through the inguinal canal to just above the scrotal sac. The path is carefully explored surgically to locate the testicle, which is then removed in the standard way. The removed testis should be submitted for analysis to confirm that the correct tissue was removed.

Testicular neoplasia

These tumours are relatively common and are usually seen in older dogs. There are three main tumour types:

- Sertoli cell tumour (SCT)
- Seminoma (SEM)
- Interstitial cell tumour (ICT).

Sertoli cell tumours are more likely to metastasize than the other types to the lymph nodes, lung or liver. Sometimes SCTs or SEMs can cause a paraneoplastic syndrome

associated with the production of hormones. Usually a feminization syndrome is seen that causes hair loss, gynaecomastia (enlarged mammary glands), prostatitis, atrophy of the unaffected testis and a pendulous prepuce, and the dog may become attractive to other male dogs. More severely affected dogs may also have bone marrow suppression, causing changes such as anaemia. Treatment with castration should carry a good prognosis.

Prostate

The prostate gland completely regresses after castration and should not develop disease later in life. Uncastrated dogs may develop prostatic disease secondary to the influence of the hormone testosterone. Clinical signs may include infertility, impotence, incontinence, dysuria, haematuria, caudal abdominal pain and faecal tenesmus. The prostate can be examined by caudal palpation of the abdomen or rectal examination. Ultrasonography and radiography are also useful. Samples of the prostate gland can be taken by needle aspirates through the abdomen, alongside the rectum or via a urinary catheter. Ejaculation samples will also give some information about the fluid that the prostate is secreting.

Benign prostatic hyperplasia

Benign prostatic hyperplasia (BPH) occurs in the older male dog, when the prostate becomes acutely enlarged and very painful and secondary infection may occur. Castration may be indicated to prevent recurrence but in some cases may cause urinary incontinence. BPH may also be treated medically with drugs that inhibit the effect of testosterone, e.g. deslorelin by implant, delamadinone acetate by injection, osaterone orally or other licensed products (see Chapter 24).

Prostatic cysts and abscesses

If BPH persists the prostate may develop cysts or abscesses, which can become enormous. Prostatic abscesses may be life-threatening, presenting with toxaemia and systemic disease similar to pyometra in the bitch. Cysts and abscesses should be operated on before they rupture and cause peritonitis. The approach is through a midline laparotomy; the abscess or cyst is drained and lavaged with sterile fluids until clean, and then packed with omentum before routine closure. Castration is recommended at the same time and a biopsy sample of the prostate is taken to screen for underlying neoplastic disease.

Prostatic neoplasia

Cancer can develop in the prostate gland of older dogs, and is more common in neutered males. Prostatic neoplasia is often very painful and has similar presenting signs to other prostatic diseases. Prostatic carcinoma rapidly spreads to the adjacent lymph nodes and sometimes the vertebral bodies. The prognosis is poor. Prostatectomy combined with postoperative chemotherapy may improve quality of life for a few months, but is rarely successful at achieving a cure and can result in urinary incontinence.

Penis
Amputation

Penile amputation is indicated where there is severe trauma to the penis or if there is neoplastic disease. The penis is extremely vascular and the procedure should be done under a tourniquet. Usually the whole of the os penis is removed and the urethra is reconstructed at the end of the inguinal part of the penis.

Mucosal eversion

Occasionally, hypersexed dogs may present with mucosal eversion of the tip of the urethra on the end of the penis. The mucosa is very vascular and bleeds because of the trauma. Castration may help, but usually the mucosa has also to be resected from the end of the penis. Again it helps to use a tourniquet during surgery and then absorbable fine-gauge suture material is used to resuture the mucosa at the end of the urethra. Postoperatively there may be some bleeding, and wadding may be used inside the prepuce to help to provide gentle pressure to stop this. The dog's behaviour has to be stopped and sometimes cold-packing the swollen mucosa helps.

Ovaries and uterus

Elective ovariohysterectomy (spay)

In the UK, female companion animals are usually neutered (removal of the uterus and ovaries) to prevent unwanted litters and to prevent oestrous activity (see Chapter 24). Bitches are also neutered to decrease the risk of development of mammary tumours; the best effect of this is seen if the bitch is neutered before the first season. Bitches and queens are also neutered to prevent the development of pyometra (uterine infection) later in life. Female rabbits are neutered to prevent uterine neoplasia.

The ovaries are identified and the arteries tied off before cutting the ovarian ligament. A ligature is then placed around the uterine stump as close to the cervix as possible, to tie off the uterine arteries, before removal of the whole of the genital tract. The most important part of the procedure is to ensure that the ovaries are removed intact and no remnants are left behind that might secrete hormones. Whilst in the UK ovariohysterectomy is routinely performed, in a healthy bitch or queen, it is only necessary to only remove the ovaries (ovariectomy); this is a shorter procedure and there is no documented increased risk of uterine disease. Laparoscopic techniques (see later) are increasingly used to perform ovariectomy, which result in much shorter recovery times and postoperative restriction. Bitches and many pedigree cats are usually operated from the midline and the majority of cats are operated on via a left flank approach with the patient lying in lateral recumbency. Neutering increases the likelihood of urinary incontinence in some at-risk breeds of dog (medium to large breeds), but it is also likely that there is already an underlying bladder abnormality that is exacerbated by the loss of hormonal influence. The risk of urinary incontinence is outweighed by the life-threatening nature of pyometra or mammary neoplasia.

Postoperative analgesia and observation are important. The wound should be observed for signs of bleeding or bruising and the recovery monitored. Any postoperative spay patient that has a prolonged recovery from anaesthesia should be assessed for the possibility of intra-abdominal haemorrhage. Pale mucous membranes, generalized weakness, a rapid thready pulse, hypothermia, or bleeding from the laparotomy wound or vagina are all clinical signs that should be investigated. Postoperative instructions relate to wound care and restricted activity to prevent dehiscence of the abdominal repair.

Pyometra

This is the accumulation of pus in the uterus (Figure 23.38), which may be infected or sterile. It occasionally occurs in the uterine remains in spayed females, if there are ovarian remnants. It occurs most commonly in middle to older aged

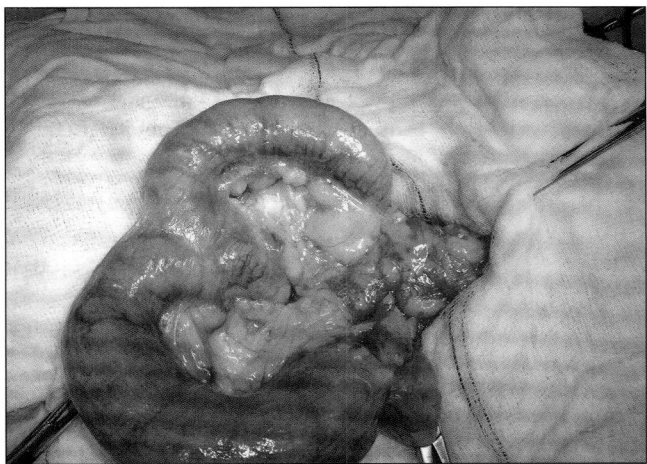

23.38 Intraoperative view of a pyometra. The uterus is grossly swollen and very vascular.

entire bitches. It is potentially life-threatening and often presents as an emergency. Disease occurs during metoestrus and the bitch may have a history of irregular oestrous patterns or of receiving oestrogens and progestogen medications. Clinical signs include depression, lethargy, anorexia, polydipsia and polyuria, vomiting and diarrhoea, and pyrexia. If the cervix is open (open pyometra), there is a vaginal discharge and the patient may be less ill than when the cervix is closed (closed pyometra) and all the pus is retained in the uterus.

The bitch may be in severe toxaemic shock and will often require intensive fluid therapy before being fit for anaesthesia. Ovariohysterectomy is required as a life-saving procedure as soon as the animal is stable enough for surgery. Intensive nursing is required in the postoperative phase to monitor recovery with regard to blood pressure, analgesia, shock, dehydration and infection. Fluid therapy should continue until renal function and urine output are normal.

Caesarean operation

This is removal of fetuses by hysterotomy. It may be necessary when a bitch or queen presents with dystocia (see Chapter 24).

Usually the Caesarean operation is carried out under general anaesthetic, but epidural anaesthesia is the technique of choice where the facilities are available. Preparation for the Caesarean operation focuses around the provision of enough personnel to resuscitate the puppies or kittens (see Chapter 24). Most veterinary surgeons use a midline approach to the abdomen, despite the possibility of subsequent interference with the sutures by the young. Preparation of the abdomen for aseptic surgery must be thorough, but the use of antiseptics that might cause dermatitis around the mammary glands should be avoided. The incision is closed routinely, though some surgeons may use a subcuticular closure in order that there are no skin sutures in the region where the offspring will be suckling.

Postoperative care involves close monitoring of the recovery from anaesthesia, and prevention of hypothermia. Regular postoperative checks are necessary to ensure that the dam is feeding and caring for the litter, despite the stress of hospitalization and surgery. Many cases will be discharged to their home environment as soon as possible after recovery and monitored with home visits. It is particularly important that the owner is given advice on postoperative nutrition of the dam and that frequent small meals are offered in the early stages postoperatively. Often these patients will develop transient diarrhoea due to hormonal influences. The litter and bedding must be kept as clean as possible to prevent postoperative sepsis.

In some circumstances an ovariohysterectomy will be performed at the same time as the Caesarean operation. This is not ideal but is sometimes indicated where there is uterine rupture or risk of recurrent unwanted pregnancy (e.g. in 'stray' animals).

Neoplasia

Older animals may develop tumours of the ovaries or uterus. These can be very aggressive, but some are benign. Ovario-hysterectomy is indicated.

Vagina

The vagina is usually only affected by disease in the entire bitch or queen. It rarely causes problems after neutering. See Chapter 24.

Neoplasia

Neoplasia of the vulva and vagina is seen occasionally. Most large fibrous tumours identified in the wall of the vagina are leiomyomas (benign) or leiomyosarcomas, and are infiltrative hard nodules usually in the dorsal vaginal wall. The tumours are removed using an episiotomy to access the vaginal lumen from the perineum, and the bitch is also neutered. The urethra should be catheterized during surgery, so that the urethral orifice can be identified during the resection. Neoplasms of the vulva tend to be more aggressive carcinomas or mast cell tumours and require complex surgery for removal and reconstruction.

Hernias and ruptures

- A hernia is an abnormal protrusion of an organ or organs through a physiological opening in the lining of the cavity in which it is normally enclosed.
- A rupture is a pathological tear in the lining of the cavity through which enclosed organs may protrude.

Most hernias and ruptures affect the abdominal cavity, but a few occur elsewhere. An example outside the abdomen includes herniation of the occipital or temporal lobes of the brain under the bony tentorium cerebelli as a complication of space-occupying lesions of the cranium.

The openings through which a hernia may occur are either a normal opening that has enlarged to allow organs through (e.g. inguinal canal), or an opening that should have closed during normal development (e.g. umbilicus). Hernias and ruptures share some characteristics in terms of the risks associated with the protrusion of viscera; however, as hernias are physiological, they are usually lined by an outpouching of the cavity lining (e.g. the peritoneum). Ruptures are not lined and the cavity lining is ruptured along with the body wall.

Hernias and ruptures are further described by the following terms:

- Reducible – the contents of the hernia or rupture can be replaced in the original anatomical location by gentle pressure on the swelling to push the viscera back through the defect itself
- Irreducible or incarcerated – the contents of the hernia or rupture cannot be replaced, usually because of the formation of adhesions in chronic cases
- Strangulated – the contents of a hernia or rupture can become devitalized due to entrapment of the blood vessels passing through the defect. Strangulation is life-threatening and a serious emergency.

Umbilical hernia

This is a congenital condition where the umbilicus fails to close over and fat and abdominal contents protrude through under the skin. Small hernias are of no consequence as they usually do not increase in size as the animal grows. Large hernias should be repaired due to the risk of incarceration of small intestine or other abdominal organs.

Inguinal hernia

Herniation occurs through the inguinal canal, which is a physiological opening in the muscle of the caudal abdominal wall. It is more common in females than males, particularly in elderly overweight small-breed dogs. In the bitch a swelling may be seen in the groin extending towards the vulva. The hernia may contain fat in the broad ligament, uterus, intestines or bladder. If the bitch is pregnant, the gravid uterus can become strangulated. In male dogs, fat or intestine may herniate into the scrotal sac and can become strangulated because of the small opening.

Ultrasonography or radiography may be used to determine what structures the hernia contains. The owner should be warned about the possibility of strangulation. All hernias should be surgically repaired and the inguinal canal narrowed to prevent recurrence. Ideally the animal should also be neutered as hernias are heritable.

Perineal hernia

Perineal hernia occurs almost exclusively in older male dogs. It is associated with degeneration of the muscles of the pelvic diaphragm (coccygeus and levator ani). Affected dogs have difficulty defecating and have an obvious swelling on one or both sides of the anus (Figure 23.39). The swelling is associated with impaction of faeces in the rectum as well as herniated abdominal contents. An important complication of perineal hernia is retroflexion and incarceration of the bladder and prostate. This can result in acute urethral obstruction and is an emergency.

There are a number of surgical techniques described for hernia repair that involve apposing the remains of the atrophied muscles using a monofilament long-lasting suture material (e.g. polydioxanone or polypropylene). More often than not, the remaining muscles are not adequate and muscle flaps are required to help support the hernia repair, making the repair more successful. All dogs are castrated to help to prevent recurrence.

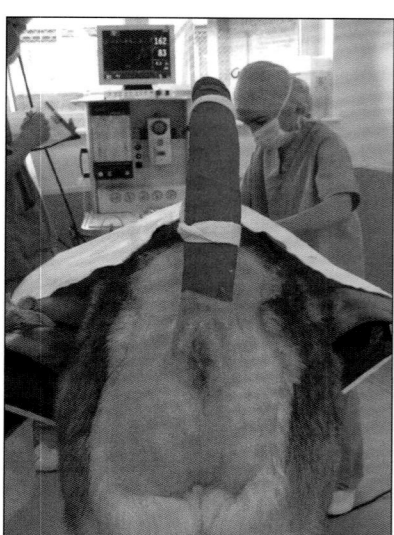

23.39 A bilateral perineal hernia. The perineal area is swollen with herniated contents of the caudal abdomen. Faeces are sometimes impacted in the caudal rectum, contributing to the perineal swelling. Rectal examination confirms the absence of the pelvic diaphragm.

Pre- and postoperative nursing

Preoperatively, the animal should be assessed for bladder position and the possibility that the bladder could be retro-flexed into the hernia, obstructing the urethra. If there is doubt, the hernia may be radiographed or the urethra catheterized in order to empty the bladder. Sometimes the bladder has to be emptied by cystocentesis before it can be catheterized or reduced. The surgical site is considered contaminated and peri- and postoperative antibiotic cover is required. Before the surgical preparation, the rectal sac-culation is manually emptied of faeces and a purse-string suture is placed to prevent faecal material contaminating the surgical site during surgery. Enemas are not used as they may result in loose slurry that could easily spill into the surgical site. Postoperatively, the purse-string is removed and faecal modifiers (ispaghula, sterculia) are given in the food to prevent straining against the hernia repair and also to improve rectal function. Bilateral hernia repairs some-times develop rectal prolapse which requires a loose purse-string suture around the anus for a few days until the anus regains normal tone.

Diaphragmatic hernias and ruptures

Diaphragmatic rupture is most commonly associated with trauma such as a road traffic accident, causing a sudden increase in abdominal pressure when the glottis is closed. The diaphragm tears either around the edge (circumferen-tial) or across from the centre to the edge (radial). The loss of a functional diaphragm makes breathing difficult and this is coupled with herniation of abdominal contents such as intestine, liver, spleen or stomach into the pleural space. The trauma may also cause pulmonary contusion (bruising of the lungs), which adds to the animal's respiratory distress. Some cases are undiagnosed at the time of the original trauma and can present months later with dyspnoea when more abdominal contents herniate.

Congenital defects in the diaphragm are also seen, the most common of which is the pericardial–peritoneal dia-phragmatic hernia. In this condition, the ventral portion of the diaphragm is absent and abdominal contents herniate into the mediastinum (not the pleural space). Often the animal also has a large umbilical hernia.

All diaphragmatic hernias are repaired surgically. Congenital defects are repaired as elective procedures, but ruptures may need to be repaired as an emergency if the stomach is in the chest and it begins to dilate. Ideally, the animal should be stabilized after the accident to improve the anaesthetic risk, but in some cases the dyspnoea is so severe that immediate surgery is necessary. The tear is sutured closed using long-lasting absorbable suture material. Chronic cases may be difficult to reduce due to adhesions to the pleura. Due to contraction of the abdominal muscles, the abdomen may be difficult to close once all the abdominal contents are returned. A chest drain may be necessary, particularly in chronic cases where there may be a pleural effusion.

Pre- and postoperative nursing

Preoperative nursing focuses on provision of supplementary oxygen, reducing stress on handling, analgesia and treat-ment of shock. The nurse should be prepared to provide IPPV during the anaesthesia (see Chapter 21) and to monitor for sudden changes in blood pressure when the abdominal viscera are moved back into the abdomen. A catheter may be used to aspirate air from the thorax as the rupture is closed or a chest drain may be used. Postoperatively, the animal should be watched carefully for signs of discomfort associated with increased abdominal pressure and evidence of continuing difficulty with breathing due to pulmonary contusions. Some cats may be inappetent after surgery, due to liver damage.

Prepubic tendon or abdominal wall rupture

This condition is usually seen as a consequence of abdomi-nal wall trauma, most commonly a road accident, but also due to a blunt blow such as a kick. There may be other injuries associated with the trauma. Usually there is an exten-sive area of severe bruising over the rupture and the asso-ciated subcutaneous swelling.

The rupture is repaired surgically using long-lasting absorbable materials such as PDS® (Ethicon). Macerated muscle tissue may not repair easily, and a synthetic mesh might be necessary to replace devitalized muscle. Where the prepubic attachment is ruptured, wire sutures may be used to reattach the ventral abdominal wall to the pubic bone.

Pre- and postoperative nursing

The animal should be stabilized and given analgesia prior to surgical repair. If the bladder is in the rupture, urine produc-tion should be closely monitored or the animal catheterized to ensure that the bladder neck is not entrapped. Analgesia is important as the abdominal wall is often bruised. Anti-inflammatories may help with resolution of bruising in addition to padded bedding and cage rest. Faecal modifiers should be given to assist with defecation so that the animal does not strain and put pressure on the abdominal repair. Animals that require a mesh implant should be closely monitored for signs of infection or sinus tracts associated with the implant. Postoperative exercise is restricted and the animal should be prevented from jumping up or stretching the abdomen.

Musculoskeletal system

Tendon and muscle repair

Tendon and muscle damage are usually secondary to trauma, unless a myotomy or tenotomy has been performed as part of a surgical approach to a joint.

Muscle damage is usually repaired as soon as possible after injury, using absorbable monofilament material. Trauma to muscle often results in macerated fragile tissue and it can be difficult to reappose successfully. Normal healthy muscle heals quickly after a myotomy as it has a good blood supply.

Tendons heal very slowly and have to be supported to ensure that they do not stretch and lose function. Ortho-paedic implants, a cast or a supportive bandage may be used to protect the tendon until it has fully repaired and remodelled. Postoperative care with controlled exercise for at least 6–8 weeks is also important, and physiotherapy may be useful to improve gradual regain of tendon strength.

Limb amputation

Amputation is an unfortunate but not infrequent surgical pro-cedure in all companion animals. It is a very difficult concept for many owners to come to terms with and they may need counselling and advice. Most animals cope with amputation much better than the owner expects (Figure 23.40) and some may even be walking within hours of anaesthetic recovery.

Amputation may be recommended for the following reasons:

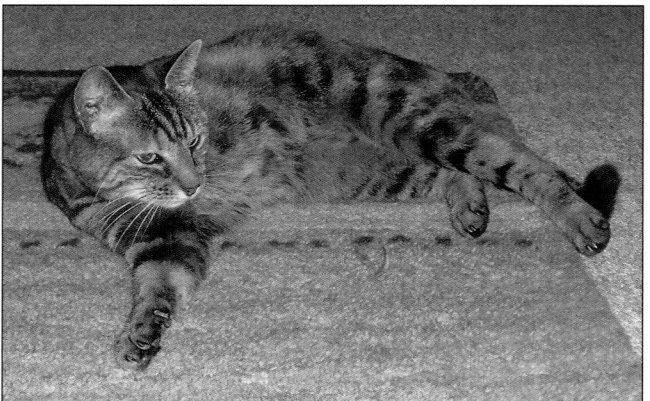

23.40 Animals frequently tolerate limb amputation remarkably well, as long as the remaining three limbs are free of any other orthopaedic or neurological disease. This cat has had her left forelimb amputated yet lives a full and normal life.

- Curative removal of a benign tumour (e.g. haemangiopericytoma)
- Palliative removal of a malignant but very painful tumour (e.g. osteosarcoma)
- Injury to the distal limb that is beyond repair (e.g. shear injury)
- Nerve root avulsion resulting in permanent paralysis of the limb
- Economic reasons, if the complex fracture or soft tissue injury is too expensive for repair.

The most important aspect of assessment of a patient for amputation is establishing that the other three limbs are fit and free of disease, and there is no disc disease that may get worse after amputation. On admission it is important to check and state on the consent form which limb is to be amputated. Obese patients or very large breeds may not be suitable candidates for amputation as they will have difficulty shifting the centre of gravity over to the remaining legs and may be less agile. Cats often do very well after amputation and remain very agile.

Postoperative nursing

Surgery may be prolonged and there can be considerable blood loss from the cut muscle ends if diathermy is not available, so intravenous fluids are important to ensure a rapid recovery. Prevention of seroma formation at the site of the amputation can be achieved by bandaging or use of a drain. Postoperative nursing is important to help these patients to their feet as soon as possible in order that they can quickly adapt to a new gait. Walking must be assisted if the floor is slippery or rubber mats may be placed to give the animal confidence. Postoperative physiotherapy may help the animal adjust their gait.

Arthrotomy

Some surgical conditions of the joints require surgery inside the joint itself (arthrotomy). The most common indications for joint surgery in the dog and cat are dislocations, ligamentous injuries (in particular, cruciate ligament rupture), osteochondrosis (abnormal development of cartilage in the joint), penetrating wounds of the joint and fractures involving the joint surface. The elbow, stifle and hip are the most commonly affected joints.

Strict asepsis is extremely important as postoperative infection in the joint is devastating. Equally important are haemostasis and meticulous repair of the surgical approach through the joint capsule. The joint is usually flushed with sterile saline at the end of the surgery, and the repair made using monofilament suture materials. Joint surgery can be very painful and good analgesia is important; some surgeons may use local anaesthetic into the joint. Seroma formation is a common postoperative complication and some veterinary surgeons will use a pressure bandage on the joint to prevent this and to immobilize the joint for a few days. However, it is difficult to immobilize the elbow and stifle and often bandages are ineffective. Exercise is usually limited to a strict regime and it is important that the owner is given clear written instructions.

In some specialist centres, joint surgery may be carried out using arthroscopy. This enables access to the joint without the disadvantages and postoperative complications of a surgical approach. The arthroscope must be sterile, and specialist instruments are used that are introduced into the joint via a separate opening. The joint is subject to a continuous high-pressure sterile fluid lavage during surgery. A sterile sleeve is used to cover the cable from the arthroscope to the viewing screen. In dogs, only the stifle, elbow and shoulder are routinely investigated with arthroscopy and occasionally in larger breeds it is possible to scope the other joints. It is possible to remove fragments of cartilage or bone without opening the joint by using special instruments alongside the camera inside the joint.

Cruciate disease

The cruciate ligaments are two crossed ligaments within the stifle joint that stabilize the joint within its range of movement. There are also two C-shaped menisci that serve as 'shock absorbers' in the stifle. Disease of this complex joint is very common. It is often the cranial cruciate ligament that ruptures and the medial meniscus that is damaged. The instability results in the femur slipping on the tibia as the dog bears weight. The patient may be presented acutely lame, following trauma during exercise or with a low-grade, slowly progressing lameness of the affected hindlimb.

Some breeds with upright conformation are prone to cruciate degeneration and may present with both hindlimbs affected. In dogs less than 15 kg bodyweight, the joint will eventually stabilize with rest and physiotherapy, but may remain painful without surgery. In larger breeds, there is a better result if the joint is stabilized surgically. There are a number of surgical techniques that have been described and new methods continue to be developed. In all cases, the joint should be examined (sometimes using arthroscopy) to remove damaged meniscus prior to treatment for the instability. Veterinary nurses may encounter a number of surgical techniques, the most popular of which are listed below.

- Extracapsular techniques: These techniques use a lateral retinacular suture, where non-absorbable suture material is placed around the lateral fabella and through a hole drilled in the tibial crest, and then secured with metal crimps or a locking knot.
- Intracapsular technique: This is where a strip of patellar ligament and fascia is pulled through to the inside of the joint and secured with sutures.
- Tibial Plateau Levelling Osteotomy (TPLO): This procedure aims to make the stifle joint stable during weight bearing by changing the angle of the tibial plateau, allowing the dog to move without pain – although the ruptured ligament has not been 'repaired'. A curved cut is made with a saw and special radial blade

in the proximal tibia. The tibia is then rotated through the appropriate number of degrees as measured from the radiograph taken prior to surgery. The bone is stabilized with a specially designed TPLO plate and screws to keep the tibial plateau in its new position.

- Cranial Closing Tibial Wedge Osteotomy (CCTWO): This procedure is similar to TPLO except that a wedge of bone is removed from the proximal tibia and a plate similar to a T plate is screwed into place over the cut.
- Tibial Tuberosity Advancement (TTA): This technique also aims to change the forces on weight bearing in the stifle. This is a simpler procedure than TPLO, but still requires special equipment, plates and screws and is not suitable for large breed dogs.

Postoperative care after cruciate surgery depends on which technique has been used; however, there is usually a strict regime of rest followed by carefully controlled return to activity and fitness. Postoperative physiotherapy (see Chapter 15) has an important role to play in recovery. The last three techniques (TPLO, CCTWO and TTA) require special training and should only be carried out by orthopaedic surgeons. The postoperative instructions must be carefully followed as the bone has been cut (fractured) and repositioned and there is a risk of severe complications if there is infection or overactivity postoperatively. All cruciate surgery is painful postoperatively and multimodal analgesia is an important part of nursing these patients.

Joint replacement

Dogs with chronically painful hips or elbows due to osteoarthritis may be candidates to have these joints replaced with artificial joints (prostheses). These are expensive procedures, but the success rate in experienced hands is as high as 90% for hip replacement and 80% for elbow replacement. When there are complications, they are major and may result in loss of the joint function completely. These procedures are only carried out by specialist orthopaedic surgeons.

- Total Hip Replacement (THR): The diseased femoral head is removed and replaced with a metal femoral stem prosthesis, which is anchored into the femur (some systems use a special bone cement for this). The acetabulum is reamed out and a high-density polyethylene cup is anchored in position (again, with or without cement). A metal femoral head is then placed on to the femoral stem and this sits in the acetabular cup.
- Total Elbow Replacement (TER): This procedure is currently carried out at a few centres in the UK. The humeral joint surface is replaced with a metal component and the radius and ulna joint surfaces are replaced with high-density polyethylene component. This technique is still being developed.
- Total Knee Replacement (TKR): This procedure is beginning to be performed in the UK in a few specialist centres, but there are few long-term data on their success.

Arthrodesis

Arthrodesis is the surgical fusion of a joint to prevent its movement, and is used when there is intractable joint pain, chronic instability of the joint or an irreparable joint fracture. The principle is that the joint surfaces are obliterated using curettes or power-driven burrs or saws, and then the joint is fused in a normal standing position, using plates or screws to compress the surfaces together. The joint is often supported with a cast postoperatively until the arthrodesis has fully healed and can support the animal's weight. Strict asepsis is essential to the success of the procedure. Sometimes the surgery is carried out using a tourniquet (e.g. carpal arthrodesis) to reduce blood loss and improve visibility during surgery.

Fractures

Fractures are usually the result of traumatic incidents. In small-breed dogs they can occur if the dog jumps down from a height (e.g. out of the owner's arms or off the sofa), or some dogs have a predisposition to certain spontaneous fractures (e.g. Springer Spaniels with fractures of the distal humerus). Some fractures are pathological and are associated with bone disease or neoplasia.

In most instances, fractures are repaired surgically, though this depends on the type of fracture (see earlier). It is important that two good quality orthogonal radiographs are obtained of the fracture prior to surgery, in order to plan the repair. Immediately postoperatively, two views are taken to assess the success of the repair and to determine the position of any implants. The healing is then followed up with regular radiographs in the weeks following surgery until evidence of union is seen.

Nursing the fracture patient

- Assessment and treatment of concurrent injuries
- Provision of analgesia
- Assisted walking to ensure that the animal does not slip when taken out
- Provision of adequate dry bedding so that the animal remains dry and clean
- Monitoring for decubital ulcers
- Monitoring the temperature, pulse and respiration rate as indicators of pain, infection or distress
- Observation of the surgical wound for signs of postoperative infection
- Detailed communication with the owner over the exercise regime and prevention of excessive use of the limb during the healing process
- Regular radiography of the repaired fracture to monitor healing

Physiotherapy by a qualified physiotherapist is sometimes used for fracture patients, but the programme must be assigned on an individual basis by a veterinary surgeon, as inappropriate manipulation may cause more harm.

Specialist orthopaedic surgery

Some orthopaedic surgery is only carried out in referral centres, such as angular limb correction, joint replacement or very complex fractures. These procedures require detailed assessment of the animal and the surgery is performed under strict aseptic conditions. The equipment is expensive and the nursing staff must be experienced in the use and care of these instruments.

For example, when a total hip replacement is carried out, the animal is assessed for skin disease that may increase the risk of bacterial contamination at the time of surgery, obesity, and GI disease that might cause diarrhoea during hospitalization, as well as its orthopaedic disease.

During surgery, the surgeons may wear two pairs of gloves. Adhesive waterproof disposable drapes are used and personnel in theatre are limited to reduce aerosol contamination. Often a culture swab is taken from the surgical wound just before closure to check for any contamination in the surgical wound during surgery.

Spinal surgery

Neurosurgical procedures require certain specialized equipment and skills and are usually carried out in referral centres. Diagnoses of spinal injuries or diseases are carried out using a combination of clinical examination and neurological tests and radiographs, contrast radiography (myelography) and advanced imaging techniques (e.g. MRI or CT). Samples of spinal fluid may be taken for analysis either from between the skull and first cervical vertebra (cisternal puncture) or from between the lumbar vertebrae (lumbar puncture).

Spinal cord injury arises from any pressure on the cord within the vertebral canal. The resulting inflammatory response can result in continued injury to the nerves even after the cause of the pressure has been relieved. Recovery from spinal injuries can be very slow and requires committed and caring nursing staff. Spinal patients are at risk from:

- Pneumonia
- Decubital ulcers
- Dermatitis due to urine or faecal skin soiling
- Limb oedema
- Muscle wasting
- Urinary tract infection.

Nursing spinal injuries

Recumbent animals are at high risk of a number of complications that can be alleviated or prevented by good nursing (see Chapter 15):

- Analgesia/pain management
- Wound management/assessment
- Ensuring that the bladder is emptied regularly
- Checking for decubital ulcers three times daily
- Turning the patient regularly – at last every 2 hours
- Monitoring conscious or unconscious defecation and urination
- Monitoring neurological reflexes and recording improvements
- Maintaining adequate nutrition
- Administering physiotherapy to all joints to prevent stiffness and cartilage degeneration – hydrotherapy can be very useful in this regard
- Keeping the skin clean and dry
- Providing regular assisted walks and attention
- Moving the patient into a place where it can watch general activity, and improve its mental wellbeing.

Most dedicated owners can manage small to medium-sized recumbent patients at home once the animal is urinary continent, but will need detailed written guidelines on nursing care. Regular visits help to monitor the animal's progress and to provide support to the owners that they are doing everything correctly.

Spinal fractures

Spinal fractures are usually the result of trauma, and the radiograph may not accurately reflect the degree of spinal cord damage inflicted at the time of impact if the spinal muscles have pulled the bones back into alignment. If a spinal fracture is suspected, the patient should not be sedated or anaesthetized for radiography, as the muscles may be holding the bones in place and preventing further spinal cord damage. A conscious CT scan is much safer and will provide more accurate information. Some fractures are managed with cage rest if the spinal cord injury is not severe. In other cases, the vertebrae have to be stabilized using pins, plates or external fixation.

Disc disease

The intervertebral discs can cause severe spinal cord injury if they dislodge and erupt into the spinal canal, contacting the ventral aspect of the spinal cord. This classically occurs in the small-breed dogs such as Dachshunds, Pekingese and Jack Russell Terriers, which have a defect in the cartilage component of the disc (Type 1). These disc protrusions can occur very suddenly and result in acute paralysis of the patient. Another disc disease syndrome is seen in ageing larger-breed dogs, which causes slow compression of the spinal cord and results in chronic nerve pain (Type 2).

Both types of disc disease are alleviated by surgery to open up the spinal canal (laminectomy) and to remove the fragments of disc pressing on the spinal cord. This is specialized surgery and careful assessment of the patient is necessary to determine which part of the spinal canal is affected. Diagnostic imaging with CT or MRI is necessary to determine where the approach to the spinal canal should be made. Postoperatively, the patient may be slightly worse before the neurological signs improve. They will require prolonged nursing care. Acute cases of paraplegia should be operated on as soon as possible to minimize the damage to the spinal cord and maximize the chances of a full recovery to normal function. However, even if surgery is successful, there is a risk that another disc could protrude at a later date.

Neoplasia

Tumours are occasionally diagnosed causing neurological signs secondary to slow compression of the spinal cord as they grow within the confined space of the spinal canal. Surgical removal of benign tumours of the meninges via a laminectomy can be successful, but tumours arising from the vertebrae themselves are usually inoperable.

Minimally invasive surgery

Therapeutic techniques are constantly evolving and recent developments in veterinary surgery include the use of minimally invasive techniques (MIS).

Rigid endoscopes can be used to enter cavities such as the abdomen, thorax or joint space to visualize structures (see also Chapter 16) and to undertake diagnostic or therapeutic procedures. This enables procedures to be carried out using two or three small holes instead of large incisions (so-called 'key hole' surgery). Laparoscopy relates to entering the abdomen and thoracoscopy is related to the thorax. In dogs and cats, minor procedures such as pancreatic, hepatic and lung biopsy, ovariectomy and gastropexy have been described, but in experienced hands it is also possible to carry out splenectomy, lung/liver lobectomy and pericardectomy.

These are difficult techniques to master and are generally carried out by surgeons who are in referral centres and are carrying out these techniques regularly. As with all surgery, there has to be a 'Plan B'. If the arthroscopy/laparoscopy/

thoracoscopy does not go as planned, or it is not possible to complete the procedure using MIS, the surgeon has to have the skill and equipment to convert to a conventional surgical approach.

The surgical technique is based on the principle of triangulation. The telescope and instruments are introduced into the abdomen through trocars (cannulae) and form a triangle. At the base of the triangle, the surgeon and assistant manipulate the telescope (attached to the camera so the image is viewed on a screen) and an instrument, which meet at the tip of the triangle within the abdomen (Figure 23.41). Distension of the cavity with gas makes a space so that the surgeon can see the tips of the instruments and organs on the monitor.

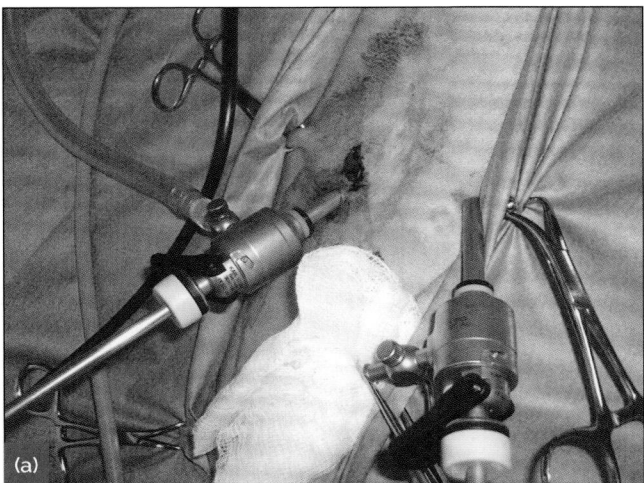

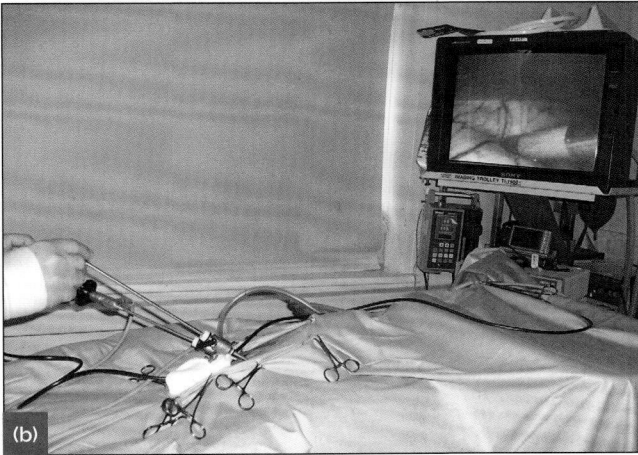

23.41 (a) Laparoscopy of an abdomen. Small incisions are made through which the laparoscope is inserted. Fine instruments are introduced through a trochar in another incision. **(b)** A light source and a camera are attached to the laparoscope and images appear on the monitor. Organs and abdominal contents can be inspected and the procedures being performed with the instruments through the other ports can be viewed in real time. (Courtesy of T. Charlesworth).

Equipment

- Light source – The type of light source and the strength is important in the quality of the image obtained.
- Camera – This is attached to the end of the endoscope so that the surgeon can view the image on a screen.
- Trocars – These are used to make entry holes (portals) through which the instruments and endoscope can be introduced. Generally, three portals are made; one for the camera and two for the instruments.

- Insufflator – This gently pumps carbon dioxide into the cavity (abdomen or thorax), which separates the organs so that the surgeon can see each one individually.
- Fluid pump – In arthroscopy, the joint space is separated for the camera by sterile saline (rather than carbon dioxide).
- Veress needle – This is a needle with a spring-loaded insert that slips out and covers the sharp tip after introduction into a cavity. This then enables the carbon dioxide to be introduced to make space in the cavity so that the other portals can be made safely (without the trocars damaging an organ). Not all surgeons use the Veress needle to enter the abdomen and sometimes make a mini surgical approach to place the first trocar.
- Endoscopes – These come in different sizes depending on the size of the patient and the cavity to be inspected. For example, the laparoscope used for an equine liver biopsy would be 10 mm, and for a Labrador ovariectomy would be 5 mm. Arthroscopes are usually between 2 and 4 mm in diameter. The endoscopes are also designed to have the view end-on or at an angle (10–40 degrees), which can make it easier to look around.

Surgical instruments

Special surgical instruments are used for MIS. These very fine, long-handled instruments fit down the trocars and are designed for specific purposes:

- Some can be attached to the diathermy unit so that they seal and cut at the same time
- Some are just for holding tissue
- Some are blunt ended and are used for moving tissue, as well as for other specialist applications.

Special diathermy units are used for MIS, as the power must be higher than in conventional surgery. A special unit called a LigaSure™ may be used to cut tissue by heat sealing. This unit can also be used to ligate vessels up to 7 mm in diameter. Another option is the harmonic scalpel, which seals and cuts vessels using high frequency ultrasound waves.

MIS is a very advanced technique in human surgery but is in its infancy in veterinary surgery. There are specialist instruments for a variety of techniques; for example, special bags are used to hold removed organs, before they are pulled out through a small hole in the body wall.

MIS involves expensive equipment and considerable experience. There is a risk of damage to organs or vessels when the sharp trocars are introduced. There are also reported risks associated with the insufflation of the cavity with CO_2, such as air embolism, hypercapnia, emphysema and peritoneal irritation. However, recovery from the procedure is quick and healing of the access incisions is very rapid.

References and further reading

Aspinall V (2014) *Clinical Procedures in Veterinary Nursing, 3rd edn.* Butterworth-Heinemann, Oxford

Baines S, Lipscomb V and Hutchinson T (2012) *BSAVA Manual of Canine and Feline Surgical Principles*. BSAVA Publications, Gloucester

Baranoski S, Ayello EA and Langemo DK (2008) Wound Assessment. In: *Wound Care Essentials: Practice Principles*, ed. S Baranoski and EA Ayello, pp. 77–92. Lippincott, Williams and Wilkins, Pennsylvania

Cian F and Freeman K (2017) *Veterinary Cytology: Dog, Cat, Horse and Cow: Self-Assessment Color Review, 2nd edn.* CRC Press, Florida

DeCamp CE (2015) *Brinker, Piermattei and Flo's Handbook of Small Animal Orthopaedic and Fracture Repair, 5th edn.* W B Saunders, Philadelphia

Gemmill T and Clements D (2016) *BSAVA Manual of Canine and Feline Fracture Repair and Management, 2nd edn.* BSAVA Publications, Gloucester

Griffon D and Hamaide A (2016) *Complications in Small Animal Surgery.* Wiley Blackwell, Oxford

Harcourt-Brown F and Chitty J (2013) *BSAVA Manual of Rabbit Surgery, Dentistry and Imaging.* BSAVA Publications, Gloucester

Lhermette P and Sobel D (2008) *BSAVA Manual of Canine and Feline Endoscopy and Endosurgery.* BSAVA Publications, Gloucester

Lindley S and Watson P (2010) *BSAVA Manual of Canine and Feline Rehabilitation, Supportive and Palliative Care.* BSAVA Publications, Gloucester

Moore AH and Rudd S (2008) *BSAVA Manual of Canine and Feline Advanced Veterinary Nursing, 2nd edn.* BSAVA Publications, Gloucester

Morgan DA (2000) *Guides for Health Care Staff, 9th edn.* Euromed Communications Ltd, Surrey

Pavletic M (2010) *Atlas of Small Animal Wound Management and Reconstructive Surgery.* Wiley Blackwell, Oxford

Risselada M (2017) Wound Management. *Veterinary Clinics of North America: Small Animal Practice* **47**, pp. 1123–1262

Williams J and Niles JD (2015) *BSAVA Manual of Canine and Feline Abdominal Surgery, 2nd edn.* BSAVA Publications, Gloucester

Self-assessment questions

1. What does the term pleuritis indicate?
2. What is the difference between a tracheotomy and a tracheostomy?
3. What is the difference between an enterotomy and an enterectomy?
4. What does the presence of bright red granulation tissue indicate?
5. How many days post surgery are skin sutures usually removed?
6. What are the signs of pancreatitis following abdominal surgery?
7. List three signs of wound complications.
8. Which type of drain requires suction?
9. What is the difference between a sequestrum and a sinus?
10. What is one of the most common causes of poor fracture healing after surgical repair?
11. Is a fibrosarcoma a benign or malignant tumour?
12. List three common locations for metastasis.
13. Identify three preventative postoperative nursing considerations in a spinal patient.

Chapter 24

Reproduction, obstetric, neonatal and paediatric nursing

Gary England and Wendy Adams with exotic pets by Simon Girling

Learning objectives

After studying this chapter, readers will have the knowledge to:

- Recognize typical behaviour and function of the reproductive system
- Understand the basic endocrine control of reproduction
- Be aware of the procedures involved in performing a clinical examination of the reproductive tract in males and females to enable detection of normal and abnormal function
- Appreciate which abnormalities are common, especially with respect to parturition
- Describe the unique physiology of neonatal animals
- Describe how to optimize care of the dam and neonate at normal parturition and after assisted delivery
- Understand the requirements of puppies and kittens in their first few weeks of life during the neonatal period

Breeding domestic pets

Breeding of domestic pets may occur as a planned event by the experienced breeder or novice but enthusiastic owner. Commonly, however, pet animals also become pregnant as a result of an unintentional mating. The latter situation occurs most frequently because of a lack of education on the part of the owner. This situation is lamentable, especially considering the thousands of unwanted pets that are destroyed by humane societies every year. It is the responsibility of the veterinary profession to educate owners of new pets so that they are fully aware of the reproductive physiology and the risks of pregnancy. In the majority of cases neutering of the pet is recommended.

Assessment of animals for breeding

Breeding should not be undertaken lightly. Potential breeders should take advice from many sources before breeding from any animal. The male and female should be carefully assessed before making the decision to breed. Both potential parents should:

- Be clinically sound (in good general health and well being)
- Be of a suitable age for reproduction (females should be skeletally mature, and both males and females should

be of an age at which their temperamental and conformational qualities can be properly assessed)
- Be free from hereditary diseases (all the necessary checks for the particular breed should have been undertaken)
- Have excellent temperaments
- Be free from infectious disease (in the UK (but not other countries), there are currently no bacterial venereal pathogens in dogs and therefore routine bacteriological swabbing of the prepuce or vagina is not necessary. In the cat, however, it is important to screen for feline leukaemia virus before embarking upon breeding).

Many animals used for breeding do not meet these criteria, and it is the responsibility of the veterinary profession to make sure that owners are aware when their potential breeding animals fall short of the required characteristics. Before breeding from a pet, the owner should give careful consideration to the quality of their animal, the availability of homes for the potential offspring, available facilities and equipment required to whelp and rear a litter (especially if it is a large litter) and the potential costs involved, which may include a Caesarean operation if the female has difficulties during parturition. Thought should also be given to how the litter will be reared should something happen to the mother and whether or not the breeder would have the facilities to rear and care for any offspring should they be returned to the breeder following sale. In England and Wales the conditions for the housing and rearing of dogs should comply with guidance provided by the Animal Welfare Act (2006).

There are moral and legal responsibilities (under the Sale of Goods Act) for breeders of animals to ensure that the off-spring are clinically healthy and have a sound temperament. There are many hereditary defects that should preclude animals from breeding and these are discussed in detail in other chapters. In the case of cryptorchidism, for example, the affected male and both parents should be considered to be carriers and should not be used for breeding. The Department of Veterinary Medicine at Cambridge University hosts a website termed the Inherited Diseases in Dogs Database (www.vet.cam.ac.uk/idid), and this is a useful resource for veterinary professionals and breeders.

Dogs

Control of hereditary disease

Four schemes created in collaboration with the Kennel Club (KC) and the British Veterinary Association (BVA) aim to control the incidence of hereditary diseases in pedigree dogs. These are the BVA/KC Elbow Dysplasia Scheme, the BVA/KC Hip Dysplasia Scheme, the BVA Chiari Malformation/Syringomyelia Scheme and the BVA/KC/ISDS (International Sheep Dog Society) Eye Scheme (see Chapter 4). There are also several health schemes that include DNA testing (see Chapter 4). Where they exist, it is strongly recommended that both potential parents are screened before breeding is undertaken. Other schemes have been adopted by certain breed societies to monitor the level of specific diseases.

There are a number of laboratories that provide a wide range of genetic screening tests for breeding animals and domestic pets. Breeders should be encouraged to review what hereditary diseases occur within their breed and what genetic tests are available for their particular breed. They should be prepared to undertake any genetic testing that has been recommended for that breed as advised by the Kennel Club.

Certain breed societies have established codes of conduct that aim to control the number of litters bred per bitch and the age of first mating. The Kennel Club may NOT register a litter of puppies born to a bitch if:

- The dam has already whelped 4 litters
- The dam has already reached the age of 8 years at the date of whelping. (Relief from this restriction may be considered provided an application is made prior to the mating, the proposed dam has previously whelped at least one other registered litter, and the application is supported by veterinary evidence as to the suitability of the bitch involved in the proposed whelping)
- The dam was less than 1-year-old at the time of mating
- The offspring are the result of any mating between father and daughter, mother and son, or brother and sister, save in exceptional circumstances or for scientifically proven welfare reasons
- The dam has already had two litters delivered by Caesarean section, save for scientifically proven welfare reasons and only normally provided the application is made prior to the mating (introduced from the 1st January 2012)
- The dam was not resident at a UK address at the date of whelping.

Breeders must also agree to adhere to a code of ethics set by the Kennel Club if they wish to register puppies.

Breeder licences

A breeder must obtain a breeder licence from their local authority if:

- They breed three or more litters and sell at least one puppy in a 12 month period (note this is a reduction from the previous five or more litters)
- They breed one or two litters in a 12 month period and are deemed to be 'breeding dogs and advertising a business of selling dogs'
- They are deemed to need a licence by virtue of the number of animals sold. Note: a breeder can breed as many puppies as they wish without a licence 'if the person carrying out the activity (breeding) provides documentary evidence that none of them have been sold (whether as puppies or as adult dogs)'.

Under this licence, breeders must not whelp two litters from the same bitch within a 12-month period.

Further details about breeder schemes, health schemes and licensing can be found on the Kennel Club website (www.thekennelclub.org.uk).

Microchipping legislation

All puppies must have a microchip implanted before 8 weeks of age. The breeder is considered the first keeper of their litter of puppies and it is their legal responsibility to get their puppies microchipped and recorded on a database compliant with the new regulations. The breeder may not record the new owner as the first keeper of a puppy instead of themselves; it is an offence if they are not listed as the first keeper of their puppies on a microchipping database compliant with the regulations. A puppy may only be passed to its new keeper once it has been microchipped.

No minimum age for microchipping is currently specified; however, it is advised that microchipping does not take place before the puppy is 6 weeks old, but 8 weeks of age is the legal maximum unless an exemption applies. There are two exemptions to the microchipping regulations:

- A veterinary surgeon has certified the dog as a working dog and docked its tail in accordance with the Animal Welfare Act 2006. In such cases, the time limit for the dog to be microchipped and details recorded with a database is extended to 12 weeks. This exemption is applicable in England and Wales only. Exemptions exist in Northern Ireland where some working breeds can be legally docked and have to be microchipped by 8 weeks of age. Scotland has no such exemptions
- A veterinary surgeon certifies that a dog should not be microchipped because it could adversely affect its health. In such cases a veterinary surgeon would have to certify that this was the case and state when the exemption expired. The dog would then need to be microchipped on the expiry of that time limited certificate unless a veterinary surgeon issued a further exemption certificate because of ongoing concerns with the dog's health. In this case the decision to exempt a dog from being microchipped would be made by the veterinary surgeon. In such a case, a breeder may pass the puppy on with a copy of the veterinary exemption certificate and any time limit for microchipping, although it would be for the puppy buyer to decide whether to take the dog given this information.

Artificial insemination

There are regulations concerning artificial insemination (AI) in dogs. For the Kennel Club, prior approval is not necessary to register a litter produced by AI provided that the AI involves non-surgical insemination and that all of the following apply:

- All litters produced by AI are subject to existing Kennel Club registration regulations
- The Kennel Club will accept an application to register a litter produced by AI from either overseas dogs or those domicile in the UK, but the AI must be declared on the litter application form
- Litters produced by AI from maiden dogs or bitches will be accepted, but their progeny should produce a natural litter before they themselves are involved in an AI breeding. If the sire or dam subsequently produces a litter naturally the restriction on AI for the progeny no longer applies.

The Royal College of Veterinary Surgeons (RCVS) confirmed in 2019 that canine surgical AI is prohibited by animal welfare legislation (see 'Useful websites', below).

Cats

The Governing Council of the Cat Fancy (GCCF) provides for the registration of cats and the production of certificates. In addition, it classifies breeds, licenses shows and publishes rules that control these functions. Whilst the GCCF publishes leaflets of general advice, it issues no specific guidelines regarding hereditary disease. Further information can be found on their website (www.gccfcats.org/).

Exotic pets

There are several organizations that offer advice to those breeding and showing exotics pets. These include the British Rabbit Council, Rabbit Welfare Association and Fund, British Cavy Council, British Herpetological Society and British Bird Council. Such organizations promote breed standards and offer advice on breeding, with increasing emphasis on the issues of in-breeding and welfare.

Breeding dogs and cats

The male dog and tomcat

Male dogs and tomcats are sexually active throughout the year, although a minor seasonal effect may be noted in some countries. In the cat, the testes are descended into the scrotum at birth; in the dog, they descend into the scrotum by 10 days after birth. Puppies and kittens may show sexual activity from several weeks of age, but puberty does not occur until 6–12 months in the dog and 8–12 months in the cat. For both species, spermatogenesis (the production of spermatozoa) commences at approximately 5 months of age.

It is preferable not to use a male at stud until he is at least 12 months of age as it is not possible to evaluate his qualities fully until this time, and even then the occurrence of certain hereditary diseases may not be apparent. It is advisable that the first mating attempts should be with an experienced female.

The fertile lifespan of a male varies considerably and is probably related to the longevity of the breed. It is certain that average seminal quality of male stud dogs is reduced from 7 years of age onwards. This may result in small litters or fewer bitches becoming pregnant.

Endocrinology

The production of hormones from the testes is under the control of the hypothalamic–pituitary–gonadal axis. The interstitial (Leydig) cells are the source of testosterone production from the testes. Luteinizing hormone (LH), a gonadotrophin hormone released from the pituitary gland, stimulates the production of testosterone. A second pituitary gonadotrophin called follicle-stimulating hormone (FSH) appears to increase the process of spermatogenesis directly via the Sertoli cells. Testosterone has a negative feedback effect upon the release of FSH and LH, which is mediated by gonadotrophin-releasing hormone (GnRH) (Figure 24.1).

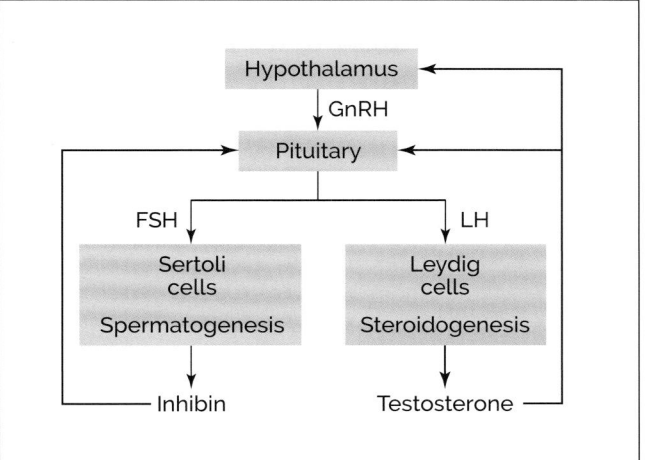

24.1 Schematic representation of the endocrine control of testicular function in the male. Testosterone and inhibin have negative feedback roles. FSH = follicle-stimulating hormone; GnRH = gonadotrophin-releasing hormone; LH = luteinizing hormone.

Antisocial behaviour

In many cases, behaviour that may be normal for a male animal is considered to be antisocial by humans. These problems include territory marking, mounting inappropriate objects and aggression towards other males. These problems often necessitate treatment, which may include behavioural modification therapy in conjunction with drugs that inhibit male hormone production, such as gonadotrophin-releasing hormone agonists (e.g. deslorelin) and progestogens. Castration may be required in certain cases.

Diseases of the reproductive tract

There are a variety of conditions that may affect the reproductive organs of both the tomcat and the male dog.

Endocrinological abnormalities

Primary abnormalities in the secretion of pituitary hormones may result in poor development of gonadal tissue, a condition called hypogonadism. This is rare but has been reported in both species.

Diseases of the testes

Cryptorchidism

An absence of the testes (anorchia) is very rare; in most cases the testes are retained within the abdomen. These undescended testes belong to the condition known as cryptorchidism (literally, 'hidden testicle'). Often the condition is unilateral, with one testicle present within the scrotum and the other retained within the abdomen. These cases are often wrongly called monorchids; monorchidism actually refers to an animal with a single testicle. Some cryptorchid animals are bilaterally affected and no testes are seen within the scrotum. The treatment for all cryptorchids is removal of both testes, because of the high incidence of neoplasia in abdominal testicles, and because the condition is likely to be inherited.

Orchitis

This is inflammation of the testes; it is rare but may follow trauma (particularly in the tomcat) or ascending bacterial infection. In some countries (but not the UK), orchitis may be caused by the bacterium *Brucella canis*, which is a venereal pathogen transmitted during mating.

Testicular tumours

Testicular tumours are the second most common tumour affecting the male dog but are rare in the tomcat. There are three common tumour types: those affecting the Leydig cells (Leydig cell tumour); those affecting the Sertoli cells (Sertoli cell tumour); and those affecting the germ cells (seminoma). Some of these tumours may be endocrinologically active and secrete female hormones (oestrogens), which produce signs of feminization.

Diseases of the accessory glands

The prostate gland in the male dog is the only accessory sex gland. The tomcat has both prostate and bulbourethral glands, but disease of either is rare. Prostate abnormalities in the dog are common and include benign enlargement (hyperplasia), bacterial prostatitis, prostatic cysts and prostatic tumours. The clinical signs of these diseases may be similar and include difficulty urinating and defecating and the presence of blood within the urine or semen.

Diseases of the penis and prepuce

It is common for there to be a creamy discharge from the prepuce of the male dog and this should be considered normal unless it is excessive. It is not seen in the tomcat.

Lymphoid hyperplasia

This is a relatively common condition in the male dog, where the bulbus glandis is covered with multiple nodules 2–3 mm in diameter. These are usually smooth and do not cause any significant disease, but they may be traumatized at the time of mating or semen collection. Lymphoid hyperplasia may be present where there is excessive preputial discharge.

Phimosis

This is the inability to extrude the penis due to an abnormally small preputial orifice. It may occur either congenitally or as a result of trauma or inflammation and may result in pain during erection.

Paraphimosis

This is failure to retract the penis into the prepuce and may also be due to a small preputial orifice. The penis becomes dry and necrotic and urethral obstruction may result.

Priapism

This refers to the persistent enlargement of the penis in the absence of sexual excitement.

Assessment of fertility

Male fertility may be assessed by the evaluation of semen quality. Semen may be collected by stimulating the male dog to ejaculate by hand (Figure 24.2) (artificial vaginas are no longer used for this purpose). Semen collection is more difficult in the tomcat and may require general anaesthesia and electroejaculation. A special artificial vagina may be used to collect semen from trained tomcats. Collection equipment should be warmed before use.

Once collected, semen should be placed into a water bath at body temperature to prevent damage to the sperm. The second fraction of the dog ejaculate and the entire cat ejaculate should be used for evaluation (Figure 24.3).

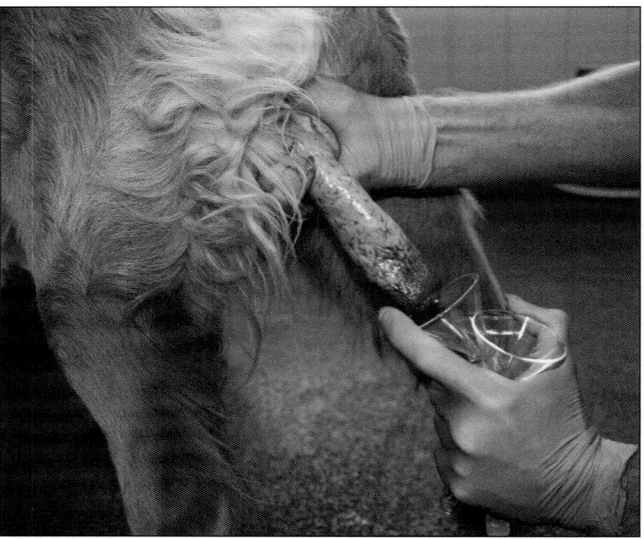

24.2   Semen collection from the male dog.

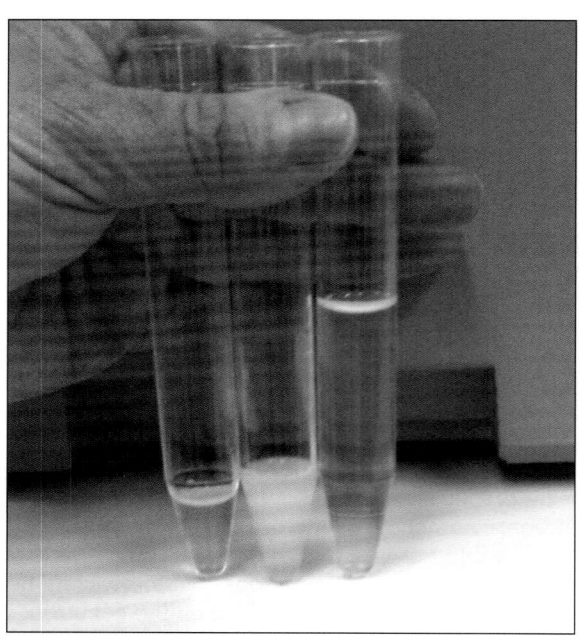

24.3   Dog ejaculate (from left to right): 1st fraction, prostatic fluid; 2nd fraction, semen-rich; 3rd fraction, prostatic fluid.

Examination of canine ejaculate

1. The volume should be measured and the colour recorded. Normal semen is white and milky. Second fraction volume is up to 2 ml for the dog and ejaculate volume is 0.1–0.5 ml in the tomcat.
2. After gently mixing the sample, a drop should be placed upon a warmed microscope slide and a subjective assessment made of the percentage of sperm with vigorous forward progression.
3. A small portion of the sample should be diluted with water to kill the sperm and therefore stop their movement. The spermatozoal concentration can then be measured using a haemocytometer.
4. The total sperm output should be calculated by multiplying this value by the volume of the sample.
5. A portion of the sample should be stained to allow differentiation of live and dead sperm and the assessment of spermatozoal morphology. A combination of the two stains nigrosin and eosin is suitable for this purpose. Normally four-parts stain are mixed with one-part semen, and then a smear is immediately made on to a glass microscope slide. When examined under high magnification, nigrosin appears as a background stain. The eosin is a vital stain – it stains only sperm with a damaged membrane, i.e. dead sperm (Figure 24.4). When using nigrosin and eosin, sperm are either stained pink (dead) or are unstained (live).

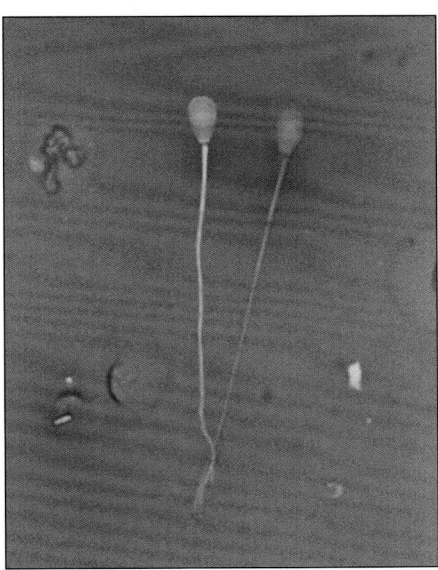

24.4 Photomicrograph of dog sperm: live (left) and dead (right) sperm with lost acrosome.

The semen characteristics of fertile dogs are given in Figure 24.5.

The bitch and queen

The oestrous cycle

The domestic bitch

In the bitch, the onset of cyclical activity (puberty) normally occurs between 6 and 23 months of age, with most bitches having their first oestrus by the age of 12–14 months. Bitches that do not exhibit oestrous behaviour by the anticipated age are considered to have delayed puberty; however, it should be remembered that many normal bitches will not cycle until they are 2 years old. The majority of bitches start to cycle about 6 months after they have reached adult height and weight, which may explain some of the variations exhibited between breeds. The bitch is polytocous (produces numerous offspring in each litter) and the oestrous periods are non-seasonal.

Bitches generally have one or two oestrous cycles per year. The interval between each oestrous cycle can vary between 5 and 13 months, but the average is 7 months. For individual bitches, cyclicity may range from being highly variable to almost regular. The stages of the oestrous cycle in the bitch are **pro-oestrus** (7–10 days), **oestrus** (7–10 days), the **luteal phase** or **metoestrus** (**dioestrus**) (2 months), during which the bitch may be pregnant or not pregnant, and **anoestrus** (4.5 months) (Figure 24.6).

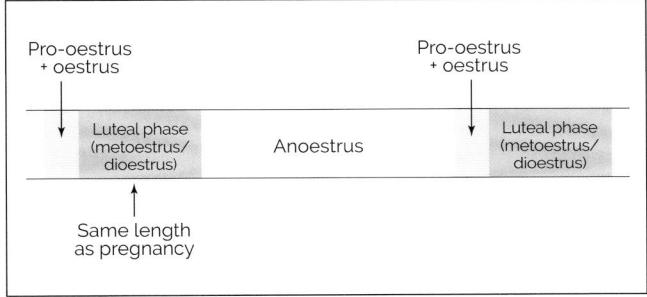

24.6 Sequence and length of various stages of the oestrus cycle of the bitch.

- The beginning of each oestrous cycle is signified by the presence of the 'season', the onset of which is signalled by a bloody vulval discharge. The term 'season' refers to the period of pro-oestrus and oestrus.
- Oestrus ends with spontaneous ovulation (i.e. ovulation occurs automatically and does not have to be 'induced' by mating). The terms 'in season' or 'in heat' are both used to refer to this stage of the oestrous cycle when the bitch is receptive to the male dog.
- Each 'season' (pro-oestrus and oestrus) will normally last an average of 3 weeks in the domestic bitch, but can be shorter in length or can extend to 4 weeks or more in some cases. The 'season' length can vary between bitches and from 'season' to 'season'. The bitch is said to be 'out of season' once the vulval discharge has stopped.

Parameter	Normal progressive motility (%)	Volume (ml)	Concentration (x 10⁶/ml)	Total sperm output (x 10⁶)
Mean	85.2	1.3	310.5	403.4
Standard deviation	6.2	0.4	82	120
Range	42–92	0.4–3.4	50–560	36–620

24.5 Characteristics of the second fraction of the ejaculate from 53 fertile dogs.

- Oestrus is followed by the luteal phase or metoestrus (dioestrus). This phase lasts the same length of time, regardless of whether the bitch is pregnant or not.
- A variable period of acyclicity (anoestrus) follows the luteal phase.

Late anoestrus

During late anoestrus two hormones are released from the pituitary gland: follicle-stimulating hormone (FSH) and luteinizing hormone (LH). These initiate the growth of follicles within the ovaries and cause the follicles to produce the hormone oestrogen.

Pro-oestrus

During pro-oestrus the bitch will not allow mating but may show increased receptivity to the male. Pro-oestrus is characterized by increased plasma concentrations of oestrogen, causing swelling of the vulva and the development of a serosangineous (bloody) vulval discharge. Oestrogen also induces the release of specific pheromones that are responsible for attracting male dogs. This period lasts for approximately 7–10 days. Oestrogens also cause thickening of the vaginal wall and an increase in the number of epithelial cell layers. During pro-oestrus the elevated concentrations of oestrogen have a negative feedback effect upon the release of the gonadotrophin hormones from the pituitary gland, and the concentrations of FSH and LH are reduced compared with late anoestrus.

Oestrus

During oestrus the bitch demonstrates characteristic behaviour towards the male dog, including deviation of the tail and presentation of the vulva and perineum. The bitch will stand to be mated (standing oestrus). This period lasts for approximately 7–10 days. The onset of oestrus is related to a decline in the concentration of plasma oestrogen and at the same time the production of the hormone progesterone. The bitch is unusual in that progesterone is produced in low concentrations by luteinization of the follicle, a process that occurs before ovulation (in many species progesterone is only produced after ovulation). It is this decline in the concentration of oestrogen and the slight increase in the concentration of progesterone that is responsible for stimulating a surge of both FSH and LH. This surge is the trigger for the release of eggs from the ovaries (ovulation) which occurs spontaneously

approximately 2 days later, towards the end of oestrus. The bitch is said to be a spontaneous ovulator. It can therefore be seen that the hormonal stimulus for ovulation occurs during standing oestrus and that the release of eggs also occurs during this period. Each egg is contained within a fluid-filled structure called a follicle. After ovulation the follicle develops into a solid structure called a corpus luteum. One corpus luteum forms from each follicle that has ovulated and the corpus luteum produces progesterone. The end of standing oestrus is associated with relatively high concentrations of progesterone in the blood.

Metoestrus (also called dioestrus)

In many species the period of progesterone production (the luteal phase) is divided into two phases. The early luteal phase is termed metoestrus and the mature luteal phase is termed dioestrus. In the bitch, however, the early luteal phase occurs during standing oestrus, making this terminology difficult to adopt (since metoestrus would then be occurring during oestrus). In the bitch, the terms metoestrus and dioestrus are therefore often used interchangeably to reflect the luteal phase of the cycle after the end of standing oestrus. This phase is characterized by the presence of the corpora lutea within the ovaries and the presence of the hormone progesterone in the blood.

The period of metoestrus lasts whilst the corpora lutea continue to produce progesterone and it is approximately 2 months in length. In the pregnant bitch, the period of metoestrus is synonymous with pregnancy. The bitch is unusual, compared with other species, in that the duration of metoestrus is similar whether the bitch is pregnant or not (Figure 24.7). The birth of puppies occurs when progesterone secretion is terminated. In the non-pregnant bitch, the corpora lutea persist for a similar period of time.

From the middle of metoestrus another hormone, called prolactin, is released from the pituitary gland. This is responsible for the development of mammary tissue and the onset of lactation. Prolactin is produced in both the pregnant and the non-pregnant bitch and is the reason why false or pseudopregnancy is a common event in the bitch (see 'Pseudopregnancy', below). Prolactin also has another role in supporting the production of progesterone from the corpus luteum (prolactin is said to be 'luteotrophic').

The hormonal changes of the oestrous cycle are summarized in Figure 24.8.

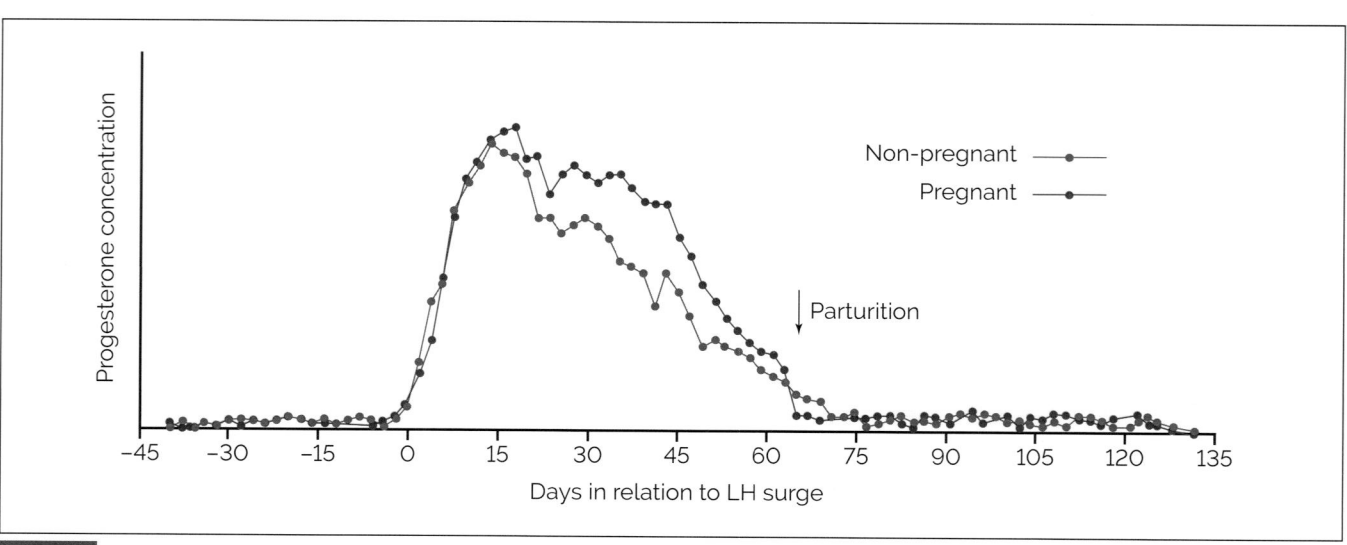

24.7 Changes in plasma progesterone concentration in the pregnant and non-pregnant bitch.

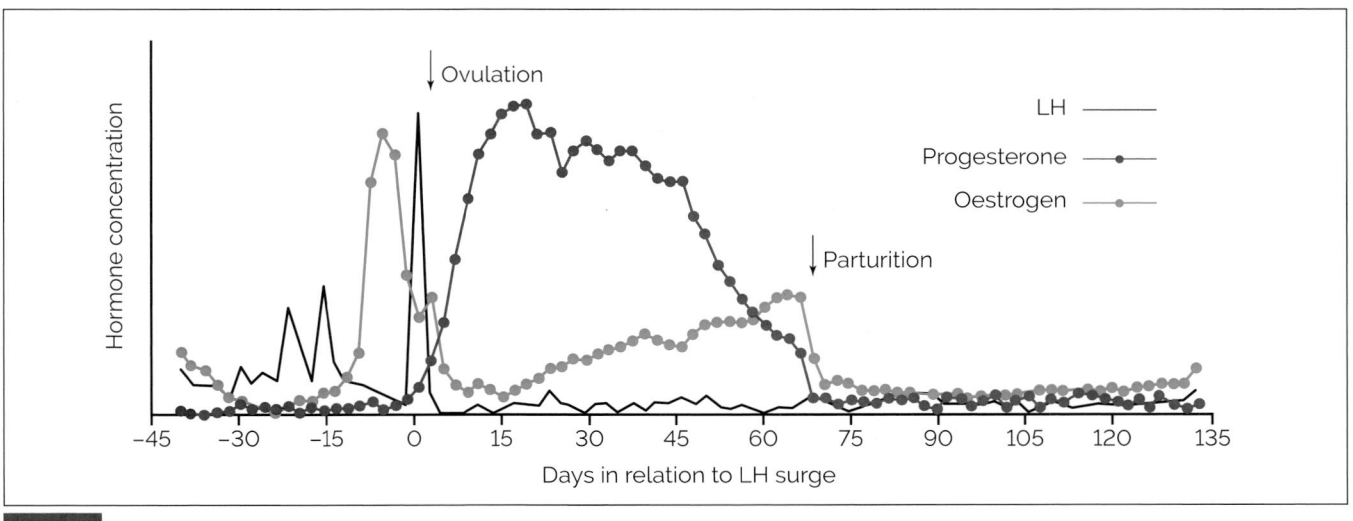

24.8 Changes in plasma hormones during the oestrus cycle of the pregnant bitch.

Anoestrus

Metoestrus is followed by a period of quiescence, during which time there is effectively no hormonal activity. In the non-pregnant bitch there is no sudden decline in the concentration of progesterone but values gradually reduce and the transition to anoestrus is smooth. The situation is slightly different during pregnancy because progesterone concentrations rapidly decline, and it is this event that stimulates the onset of parturition. The length of anoestrus varies considerably between bitches, but on average it is 5 months.

The domestic queen

Female cats generally exhibit their first oestrus at 6–9 months of age, but this is dependent upon photoperiod. Those that are born in the summer frequently commence cycling at the first spring; those that are born in the winter may not cycle until they are least 12 months of age.

Queens have multiple oestrous cycles each year. They typically cycle from February to September and are seasonally polyoestrous. Ovulation is not spontaneous as for the bitch but is induced by mating. Queens are said to be induced ovulators. The interval between each oestrous cycle varies depending upon whether the queen has ovulated, or fails to ovulate either because she is not mated or because there is insufficient hormone release at mating. Unmated queens return to oestrus at intervals of 14–21 days. Queens that ovulate but do not become pregnant generally return to oestrus after approximately 45 days. Pregnancy is approximately 64–68 days in duration, and queens do not return to cyclicity immediately after parturition as this is inhibited during early lactation.

The stages of the oestrous cycle in the queen are anoestrus, pro-oestrus, oestrus and interoestrus (Figure 24.9). The terms 'in season' or 'in heat' are used to indicate the stage of the cycle when the queen is receptive to the male, i.e. oestrus. During winter there is essentially no hormone activity; the queen is in anoestrus. This is a seasonal anoestrus, unlike in the bitch. In springtime, cyclical activity commences and, in the unmated queen, periods of sexual activity (pro-oestrus and oestrus) are interrupted by periods of non-receptivity (interoestrus). If the queen is mated and ovulation is induced, she enters metoestrus or pregnancy.

Pregnancy follows a fertile mating; metoestrus (also called pseudopregnancy) follows a sterile mating. The duration of

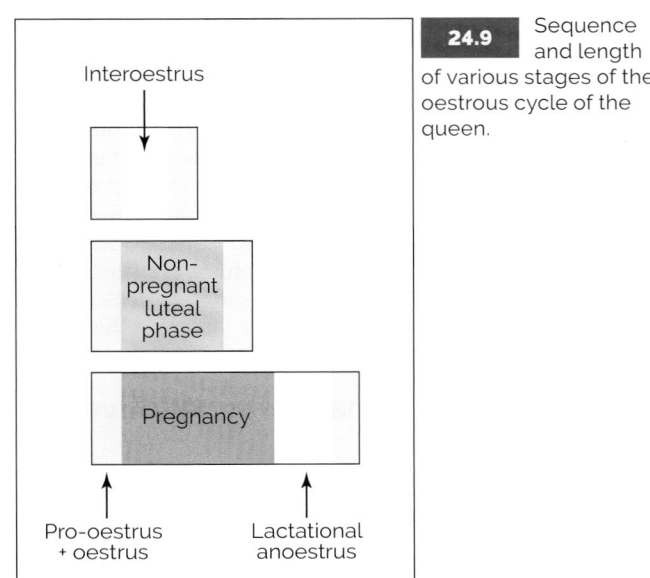

24.9 Sequence and length of various stages of the oestrous cycle of the queen.

pseudopregnancy in the queen is shorter than that of pregnancy, unlike the situation in the bitch.

Pro-oestrus

Follicular development occurs during this phase due to the release of LH and FSH. This causes the secretion of oestrogen that is responsible for the development of the signs of pro-oestrus, including attraction of the male and the changes in the vaginal epithelium similar to those seen in the bitch. Pro-oestrus in the queen is often poorly recognized unless a male is present, but during this stage the queen will not accept mating. Pro-oestrus lasts for 2–3 days.

Oestrus

The exact hormonal changes that cause the onset of standing oestrus are uncertain, but may be associated with increasing concentrations of oestrogen. The clinical signs of oestrus (also termed calling) include persistent vocalization, and rolling and rubbing against inanimate objects. In the presence of the male the queen may show persistent treading of the hind feet, lateral deviation of the tail and lordosis of the spine. Oestrus lasts between 2 and 10 days.

Interoestrus

In the absence of mating, or when mating does not result in ovulation, the signs of oestrus gradually subside and the queen enters a stage of non-receptivity. This period may last for between 3 and 14 days. After this time the queen returns to pro-oestrus and oestrus.

Pregnancy

Ovulation in the queen is caused by the release of LH, which is stimulated by mating. Each mating results in a surge of LH, however, there appears to be a threshold value below which ovulation will not be induced. Multiple matings are therefore more likely to result in ovulation than are single matings.

Ovulation is followed by an increase in the plasma concentration of progesterone released from the newly formed corpora lutea. Peak progesterone concentrations are reached approximately 1 month after mating and are maintained for the duration of the pregnancy, which varies between 64 and 68 days. Queens do not return to cyclical activity immediately after parturition, as this is inhibited in early lactation, and it is not uncommon for queens to have an absence of cyclical activity during lactation. This has been called lactational anoestrus.

Metoestrus (pseudopregnancy)

Non-fertile matings result in ovulation without conception. Ovulation may also occur following stimulation of the vagina (e.g. following collection of a vaginal smear), stimulation of the perineum (which may be self-induced) or spontaneously in some queens. Ovulation results in the formation of corpora lutea and the production of progesterone in a similar manner to early pregnancy. After approximately 40 days, progesterone concentrations decline, and the queen returns to cyclical activity approximately 45 days after the previous oestrus. Should pseudopregnancy occur late in the year (autumn), the queen may not return to cyclical activity but may enter anoestrus.

Diseases of the female reproductive tract

The domestic bitch

There are several abnormalities of the reproductive tract in the domestic bitch. These may be considered under general headings of endocrinological, ovarian, uterine and external genital abnormalities.

Endocrinological abnormalities

The common endocrinological abnormalities of the bitch include:

- Delayed onset of puberty – cyclical activity is not present at 24 months of age
- Prolonged anoestrus – failure of return to cyclical activity, resulting in a prolonged interoestrus interval
- Silent oestrous cycles – normal cyclical activity, including ovulation, but without the external signs of oestrus
- Split oestrus – signs of pro-oestrus but this does not terminate in ovulation and is followed 2–12 weeks later by a normal cycle. This is also called ovulation failure.

Pseudopregnancy

One specific endocrinological condition frequently seen in the bitch is pseudopregnancy (also called false pregnancy, phantom pregnancy or pseudocyesis). The signs of the condition may include anorexia, abdominal enlargement, nest making, nursing of inanimate objects, mammary development and lactation. False pregnancy should be considered normal in the bitch, because the changes in plasma hormones are similar in both pregnant and non-pregnant individuals. It

has been wrongly thought that pseudopregnancy is produced by either an overproduction of progesterone or abnormal persistence of the corpus luteum. The actual mechanism is related to the decline in plasma progesterone concentration during late metoestrus, which is associated with an increase in plasma concentrations of prolactin. It is prolactin that causes lactation and the behavioural changes.

In many cases treatment is not required, because the signs will gradually decline. Often, removal of the bedding material that the bitch is using to make a nest or removal of the toys that she is nursing will be enough to help the bitch to overcome a false pregnancy. In certain cases, it may be necessary to use hormonal therapy to reduce the plasma concentrations of prolactin. Most commonly, this is achieved using the prolactin inhibitor cabergoline.

Diseases of the ovary

There are few abnormalities of the ovary. An absence of ovarian development (agenesis) may occur; this usually affects one side only and may not affect fertility, only litter size. Ovarian cysts are rare and may be associated with signs of persistent oestrus, but most cysts originate from the ovarian bursa and are not endocrinologically active. Ovarian tumours are also rare.

Occasionally, bitches with mixed ovarian and testicular tissue are seen. These animals are termed 'intersex' and are often recognized because of the appearance of their external genitalia. The vulva may be cranially positioned and an os clitoris may develop. The gonads may be found in a normal ovarian position or within the scrotum. These animals are usually sterile.

Diseases of the uterus

Developmental problems of the uterus include aplasia (abnormal development) or agenesis (failure of development); in these cases, reproductive cyclicity will be normal but the bitch may fail to become pregnant. Intersex animals may have the presence of both uterine tissue and male internal genitalia (e.g. the vasa deferentia).

The most common uterine disease of the bitch is **cystic endometrial hyperplasia** (CEH), which may develop into **pyometra**. Hyperplasia of the endometrium occurs in response to progesterone during normal metoestrus. In young animals the hyperplasia resolves at the end of the luteal phase. This is not the case in older bitches and small cystic regions develop within the glandular tissue. The uterus in this state is probably more prone to infection than the normal uterus, and should bacteria enter during oestrus (when the cervix is open) they may proliferate. The accumulation of pus within the uterus (pyometra) leads to the bitch becoming unwell. This nearly always occurs from 3 weeks after oestrus onwards.

Clinical signs may include the presence of a malodorous, creamy yellow to blood-stained vulval discharge (pus) (Figure 24.10), lethargy, inappetence, pyrexia, vomiting, polydipsia and polyuria. In some cases, the cervix is not open and a vulval discharge is absent; these cases are called closed pyometra.

In all cases of pyometra the treatment of choice is ovariohysterectomy following stabilization of the patient using appropriate fluid therapy. Medical treatment (with combinations of prolactin inhibitors and prostaglandins or with progesterone receptor antagonists) has been advocated and success rates can be up to 80% for resolving the acute problem, although in up to 50% of cases pyometra returns after the next oestrus. In most cases the best option is surgery.

Treatment of bitches with progestogens for the prevention or suppression of oestrus, or with oestrogens for the treatment of unwanted matings, may predispose to the development of pyometra.

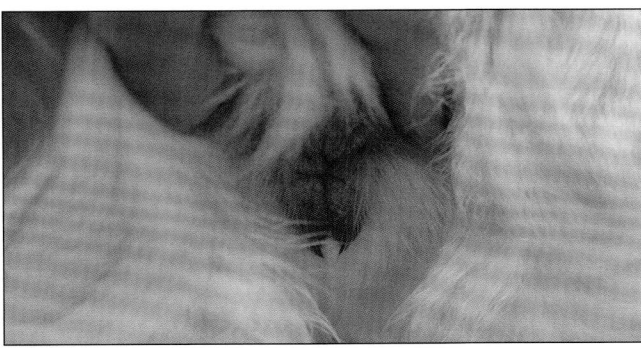

24.10   Pyometra discharge in the bitch.

Diseases of the vagina and vestibule

Congenital abnormalities of the caudal reproductive tract include hymenal or vestibular constrictions and are relatively common. These constrictions frequently occur just cranial to the external urethral orifice and can be associated with pain at attempted mating.

Vaginitis (inflammation of the vagina) is sometimes seen in prepubertal bitches and usually resolves after the first oestrus. Specific infectious causes of vaginitis include *Brucella canis* (not currently present and transmitted in the UK, although imported cases are occasionally seen) and canine herpesvirus. Many bacteria are found within the vagina as normal commensal organisms (including beta-haemolytic streptococci), which many dog breeders wrongly consider to be venereal pathogens. There is little value in routine bacteriological swabbing of the vagina before breeding, since usually only these commensal bacteria are isolated.

During normal proestrus and oestrus there is thickening (hyperplasia) of the vaginal wall, which is a normal mechanism to prevent the vagina from being damaged at the time of mating. In some bitches for an unknown reason the hyperplasia of the ventral vaginal wall just cranial to the urethra is excessive, leading to a tongue-shaped mass that protrudes into the vaginal cavity. This mass may make breeding difficult. In some cases, the hyperplastic tissue is so large that it protrudes from the vulva.

Diseases of the external genitalia

Congenital abnormalities such as vulval atresia (abnormal narrowing) and agenesis (failure of development – may be completely absent) are rare. Clitoral hypertrophy may occur associated with intersexuality.

The domestic queen
Endocrinological abnormalities

Delayed puberty may be difficult to assess in the queen, since the onset of cyclical activity is related to the season of the year at birth (see above). Delayed puberty and prolonged anoestrus have been seen but they are rare.

The most common abnormality is ovulation failure, which often results from insufficient reflex release of LH at mating. Frequently, the owner does not allow the queen to be mated a sufficient number of times to induce ovulation. The majority of queens will ovulate if 4–12 matings are allowed in a 4-hour period.

Pseudopregnancy also occurs in the queen. This condition is dissimilar to that seen in the bitch and usually follows a sterile mating (or occasionally following spontaneous ovulation). After ovulation there is an increase in plasma progesterone (Figure 24.11) (which does not occur in the absence of mating) and no return to oestrus for a further 40–45 days. The clinical sign is an absence of oestrus; treatment is not required.

Diseases of the ovary

Congenital diseases of the ovary such as ovarian agenesis and ovarian hypoplasia are rare. Ovarian cysts and neoplasms may develop similar to those seen in the bitch but are also rare.

Premature ovarian failure may be seen in queens aged 8 years and above; these animals stop cycling for an unknown reason.

Diseases of the uterus

The range of uterine abnormalities seen in the cat is similar to that seen in the bitch. Pyometra may be less common, because in the absence of mating ovulation does not occur and the luteal phase is therefore absent. Spontaneous ovulations or the common use of progestogens (to prevent oestrus) may cause the development of CEH and pyometra.

Diseases of the vagina, vestibule and external genitalia

Congenital abnormalities of the vagina, vestibule and external genitalia are rare but include vaginal and vulval aplasia and defects associated with intersexuality. Vaginitis is uncommon.

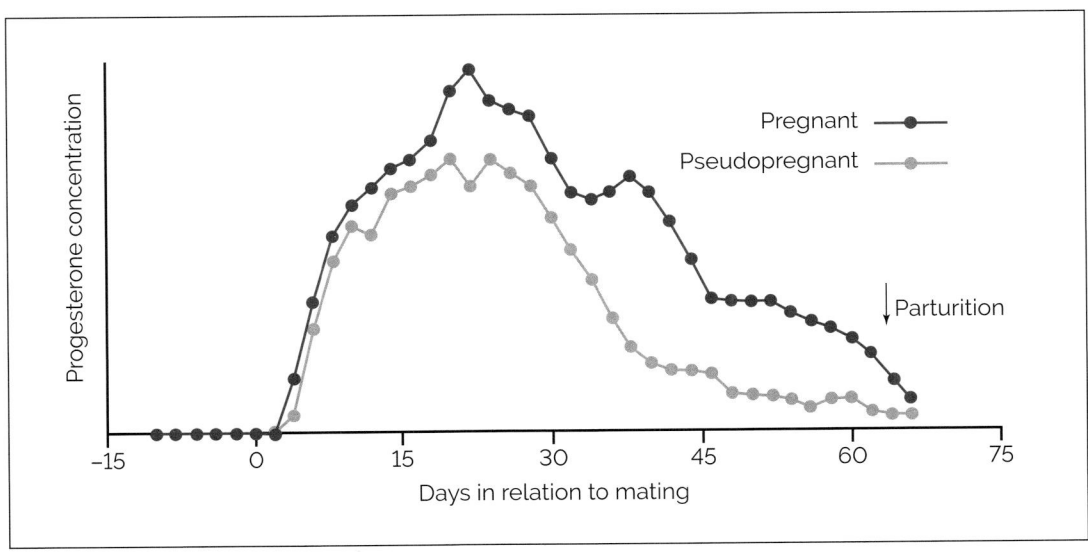

24.11 Progesterone profiles in the pregnant and pseudopregnant queen.

Control of reproduction

The male dog and tomcat

The majority of male dogs do not cause problems if they remain entire, but there are situations where control of 'anti-social' behaviour may be necessary. The situation in the entire tomcat is rather different, because the problems of territory marking, roaming and aggression are greater than in the dog.

Exogenous hormones

Hormonal control of reproductive function can be achieved in both dogs and cats on a short-term basis with hormones that suppress the normal release of testosterone. A GnRH agonist drug, deslorelin, causes an initial stimulation of the pituitary–gonadal axis and then a long duration (for as long as the product is active) of down-regulation. Deslorelin is available as an implant (Suprelorin®), and is licensed for the induction of temporary infertility in male dogs. Approximately 6 weeks after placing the implant the dog becomes infertile, and this situation is maintained for at least 6 months after the initial treatment. This drug may be useful for medium duration suppression of reproductive function (as well as the treatment of male reproductive diseases stimulated by testosterone, such as prostatic disease and anal adenoma). Furthermore, this product is also effective but not licensed for tomcats (and for females).

The other commonly used drugs include the progestogens (progestagens; drugs with progesterone-like activity), which may be administered daily orally (e.g. megestrol or osaterone) or as a depot injection (e.g. proligestone or delmadinone acetate). These drugs do not produce infertility, only poor semen quality and reduced libido.

Surgical neutering

The most common method of regulating sexual activity is castration, which is not reversible.

- Castration of the domestic dog is generally carried out at 8–12 months of age, after the dog has reached puberty. Castration before puberty may result in failure of development of the secondary sexual characteristics. It may also delay growth plate closure, resulting in increased length of the long bones, leading to the male being taller. In some males a change in metabolic rate may result in increased bodyweight. Castration after puberty and correct dietary control eliminate the majority of problems associated with castration.
- Castration of the tomcat is normally performed at approximately 5–6 months of age just prior to puberty, although in some centres, castration is undertaken as early at 8 weeks of age.

Vasectomy is rarely performed in the dog or tomcat. It involves removal of part of the vas deferens, thus preventing ejaculation of sperm. The procedure does not interfere with sexual behaviour. Since in many cases the latter is the primary aim, vasectomy has no advantages over castration.

Intra-testicular administration of a variety of noxious substances (e.g. hypertonic saline/zinc gluconate based solutions) has been used in some countries as a relatively simple method of inducing testicular degeneration and preventing breeding. It has not reached wide acceptability in the UK.

Vaccination

As technology advances it is becoming more likely that vaccines will be developed against components of the reproductive system. Currently, whilst some experimental vaccines are available for use in females in other species (directed against the zona pellucida), there are none available for use in the male dog or cat.

The domestic bitch

Many methods have been employed to control the reproductive cycle of the bitch and queen. These include surgical methods and medical control of cyclical activity. More recently advances have been made in the induction of oestrus and in the termination of pregnancy.

Surgical neutering

Ovariohysterectomy is the removal of both ovaries and the uterus to the level of the cervix. The term 'spaying' is commonly used to describe this procedure. In some countries it is more common to remove only the ovaries (ovariectomy). Either technique should be considered in any bitch not required for breeding. Both have several advantages, including a reduction in the incidence of mammary tumours and elimination of the problems of false pregnancy and of pyometra, as well the obvious advantages of absence of oestrous behaviour and inability to produce offspring. BSAVA have a position statement on neutering (www.bsava.com/Resources/Veterinary-resources/Position-statements/Neutering).

There are several adverse effects, including an increased incidence of incontinence, changes in coat texture and a tendency to gain weight. Whilst little can be done regarding the former two conditions, the latter may easily be controlled by correct dietary management. Recent information shows an increase in the occurrence of some cancers in dogs that have been spayed. As a result of the risk of non-reproductive neoplasia, some veterinary surgeons are currently advocating removal of the uterus and leaving the ovaries in place (hysterectomy; also colloquially called 'ovary-sparing spay'). The real benefits of this technique have not yet been evaluated. One of the largest changes to neutering practices has been the introduction of laparoscopic surgery. This can have a number of advantages specifically relating to recovery from surgery and is most suitable for young animals. For older animals with uterine disease, it is often preferable to perform ovariohysterectomy via laparotomy.

Age for neutering

There is considerable discussion concerning the correct time to perform the procedure on a bitch. The BSAVA position statement does not give any guidance on this. Some veterinary surgeons prefer to perform the procedure before puberty when there is no doubt that the surgery is technically easier and recovery is more rapid than in older animals; some veterinary surgeons perform the surgery as early as 4 months of age. However, it has been suggested that when such surgery is performed before puberty (the first oestrus) there is an increased chance that the external genitalia will be underdeveloped (for example, resulting in a recessed vulva) and there may also be effects on the closure time of the animal's growth plates (resulting in the animals having long limbs). However, it is important to note that prepubertal neutering does significantly protect the female against the development of mammary tumours later in life. Other veterinary surgeons prefer to wait until after the first oestrus to avoid some of these possible adverse effects; however, waiting increases the risk of pregnancy and false pregnancy.

Advice from veterinary practices on the best time to neuter a bitch is, therefore, variable and based on personal experience. Whilst some practices recommend that the bitch should have her first 'season' before being neutered, many practices advise that a larger breed bitch that is not required for breeding should be neutered at approximately 6 months of age, which would normally be before the first oestrus. In smaller breeds, the advice is usually to wait until after the first oestrus, as smaller breeds tend to have their first oestrus at a younger age, normally around 6 months old. The advice should also take into account that there are some specific reasons not to perform surgical neutering before puberty, including bitches with prepubertal vaginitis, bitches with urinary incontinence and bitches of certain breeds where changes in coat colour after neutering are common (e.g. red-coated breeds).

Medical inhibition of cyclical activity

A variety of compounds may be used to inhibit cyclical activity, including progesterone or progesterone-like compounds (progestogens), testosterone or other male hormones (androgens) and depot GnRH agonists. Drugs may either be administered during anoestrus to prevent the occurrence of an oestrus (the term prevention is used), or be given during pro-oestrus or oestrus to abolish the signs of that particular oestrus (the term suppression is used).

The most commonly used compounds are the progestogens, which are formulated as depot injections or as oral tablets. Depot injections (e.g. proligestone) may be used during anoestrus to prevent the occurrence of the next anticipated oestrus. Oral tablets (e.g. megestrol acetate) may be used either during anoestrus for oestrus prevention, or during pro-oestrus to suppress the signs of that oestrus.

These drugs are not recommended for use before the first oestrus or in an animal that is required for breeding. The side effects of these drugs may include increased appetite, weight gain, lethargy, mammary enlargement, coat and temperament changes and the risk of inducing pyometra. All progestogens have the potential to induce a reversible diabetes and acromegaly.

Termination of pregnancy

Unwanted matings are commonly seen in general practice. The term 'misalliance' is often used to describe such cases. There are several treatment options should pregnancy termination be necessary. If the bitch is not required for breeding, an ovariohysterectomy may be performed early in metoestrus, approximately 2–4 weeks after the end of oestrus. Medical therapy is usually successful in preventing conception; until recently this was done using oestrogens on several occasions after mating and now has been largely superseded by use of progesterone receptor antagonists (e.g. aglepristone). In later pregnancy it is possible to use various drugs (e.g. progesterone receptor antagonists or prolactin inhibitors (cabergoline) and/or prostaglandins (cloprostenol)) that lower the concentration of progesterone in the blood or block its actions and therefore induce resorption or abortion.

Induction of oestrus

With the development of new drugs and new drug regimes, it has become possible to induce an oestrous cycle in the bitch. The best success rates occur with prolactin inhibitors such as cabergoline. These methods may be useful in bitches that have longer than average interoestrus intervals, those that are slow to reach puberty and those that do not exhibit behavioural signs of oestrus.

The domestic queen
Surgical neutering

There is little data on the adverse effects of surgical neutering in the cat but they are assumed to be similar to those in the bitch. The procedure is usually performed when the queen is 5–6 months of age, regardless of the onset of puberty; poor development of the external genitalia does not cause problems. In the UK the surgical procedure is frequently performed through a flank incision, but this approach is best avoided in oriental breeds where coat colour is temperature-dependent and clipping of the coat may result in the regrowth of dark-coloured hairs.

Medical inhibition of cyclical activity

The drugs available for use in the queen are similar to those described for the domestic bitch. Long-term drug therapy is less commonly used, because queens that are not wanted for breeding are usually surgically neutered.

Termination of pregnancy

Treatment of an unwanted mating can be achieved by the administration of progestogens if the queen is still in oestrus, or progesterone receptor antagonists (aglepristone) if she has ovulated. In many cases pregnancy termination is performed 1 month after mating, using similar drug regimes to those described for the bitch.

Induction of oestrus

Various drugs may be used for the induction of oestrus and ovulation. In most cases it is important to remember that the queen is a seasonal breeder, and that her cyclicity is governed by photoperiod.

Mating
Optimum time
The domestic bitch

Determination of the time of ovulation in the bitch is important since the bitch is monoestrous (has one oestrous cycle followed by an obligatory period of anoestrus). The clinical signs of oestrus are not always reliable indicators of the time of ovulation; in many bitches the behavioural signs do not correlate well with the changes in hormone concentration.

There are two factors that increase the likelihood of conception: the relatively long fertile period of the eggs and the relatively long survival of spermatozoa within the female reproductive tract.

There are several methods by which the optimum time for mating can be detected, including clinical assessments, measurement of plasma hormone concentration and vaginal cytology.

Clinical assessments

The clinical signs of oestrus do not correlate well with the underlying hormonal events. The 'average bitch' ovulates

12 days after the onset of pro-oestrus and should be mated from day 14 onwards, when oocytes have matured. In some bitches, ovulation may occur as early as day 5 or as late as day 32 after the onset of pro-oestrus, and these bitches would be unlikely to become pregnant if mated on the 12th and 14th day, which is common breeding practice.

Studies on laboratory dogs have shown that the LH surge often occurs around the same time as the onset of standing oestrus. Although there is some variation of this event, commencing mating 4 days after the onset of standing oestrus may be a suitable time in many bitches.

One clinical assessment that may be useful in the bitch is the timing of vulval softening (Figure 24.12). This often occurs during the LH surge when there is a switch from oestrogen dominance to progesterone dominance of the reproductive tract.

If only clinical assessments are available, the combination of the onset of standing oestrus (noted as the first day that the bitch will accept mating) and the timing of distinct vulval softening may be useful in the prediction of the best mating time, since each event occurs on average 2 days before ovulation.

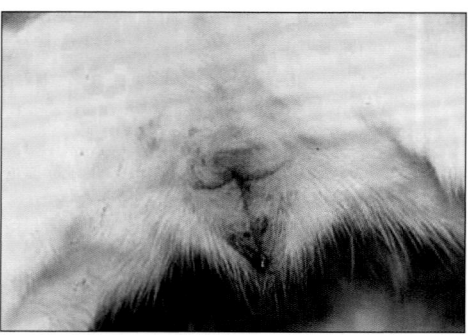

24.12

Bitch's softened vulva, just after the LH surge.

Measurement of plasma hormone concentration

The three relevant plasma hormones are LH, oestrogen and progesterone.

- Plasma concentrations of LH indicate impending ovulation; the fertile period is between 4 and 8 days after the LH surge. Unfortunately, there is no simple method by which plasma LH concentrations can be readily measured.
- There is little value in the measurement of plasma oestrogen concentrations because the oestrogen plateau is not predictive of the timing of ovulation.
- Plasma progesterone concentrations are very useful, since this hormone is absent during pro-oestrus and begins to increase at the same time as the plasma surge of LH. Thus detecting a rise in the concentration of plasma progesterone is predictive of ovulation.

Progesterone can be easily measured in the practice laboratory within 30 minutes of sample collection, using a commercial enzyme-linked immunosorbent assay (ELISA) test kit. This method simply involves comparison of a colour change in the sample with the colour change in low- and high-concentration progesterone controls. Many commercial laboratories also offer a rapid turnaround measurement of progesterone using either chemoluminescence or a radio-immunoassay.

Vaginal cytology

The concentration of plasma hormones has a marked effect upon the vaginal mucosa. When the bitch is in anoestrus,

there are approximately two or three layers of cells lining the vagina. During pro-oestrus, the vagina develops many cell layers in order to protect itself during mating. The cells within these layers differ from each other in their shape and size. When cells are collected from the vagina (the technique called a vaginal smear), only the cells on the surface of the vagina are removed. Different cell types are therefore collected at the various stages of the reproductive cycle. Staining of these cells and subsequent microscopic examination allows an assessment of the underlying hormone changes to be made. Cells can be collected either by aspirating vaginal fluid using a pipette, or using a cotton swab. Once collected, cells are placed on a glass microscope slide, spread into a thin film and stained so that they can be individually examined.

- During anoestrus (Figure 24.13a) the vaginal wall is only a few cells in thickness and these cells are small and spherical in shape. Because they are positioned close to the basement membrane they are called parabasal cells. The anoestrus vaginal smear is characterized by the presence of these cells. There are also normally a few white blood cells (neutrophils), which remove cell debris and bacteria.
- During pro-oestrus (Figure 24.13b) the vaginal mucosa increases in thickness under the influence of oestrogen. The mucosa may be up to five or six cells thick. The cells further away from the basement membrane are larger in diameter than those nearer to the membrane. These cells have a large area of cytoplasm surrounding the cell nucleus and are called small intermediate cells. When the surface cells are collected during pro-oestrus they are therefore predominantly these small intermediate cells, although there will also be a small number of the parabasal cells present. White blood cells are also present during pro-oestrus, but numbers are reduced compared with anoestrus. This is because the increased thickness of the vaginal mucosa prevents movement of the white blood cells into the lumen of the vagina. Red blood cells are also present in the vaginal smear during pro-oestrus. These cells originate from the uterus and pass into the vagina via the cervix.
- During oestrus (Figure 24.13c) the vaginal mucosa continues to thicken and the number of cell layers increases. There may be up to 12 cell layers during oestrus. Surface cells are large and irregular in shape and are called large intermediate cells. Cells of this size may accumulate the material keratin and are then termed keratinized. The nucleus of these large keratinized cells often disappears. The cells are then called anuclear because of the absence of the nucleus. White blood cells are not found in the vaginal smear during oestrus because the thick vaginal wall does not allow them to penetrate. Red blood cells are present in large numbers during oestrus.
- During metoestrus (Figure 24.13d) there is sloughing of much of the vaginal mucosal epithelium. This is caused by the increasing concentrations of the hormone progesterone. The number of cell layers is reduced and the surface cells are again the small intermediate epithelial cells or parabasal cells. Several of the epithelial cells may have vacuoles within the cytoplasm, giving the cell a 'foamy' appearance. Foam cells and epithelial cells with cytoplasmic inclusion bodies are characteristic of metoestrus. Because of the large amount of degenerate cellular material within the vaginal lumen, there is a rapid influx of white blood

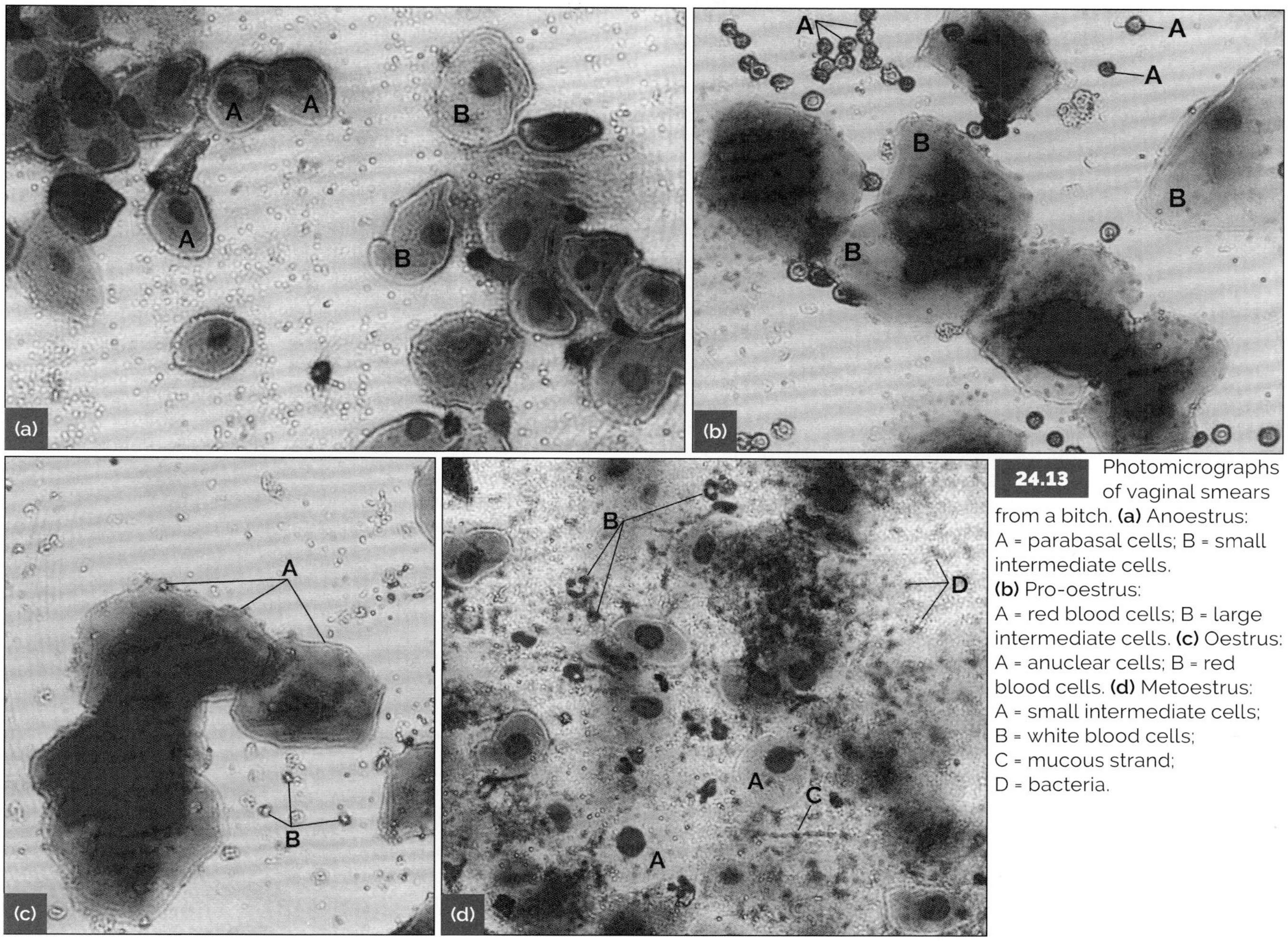

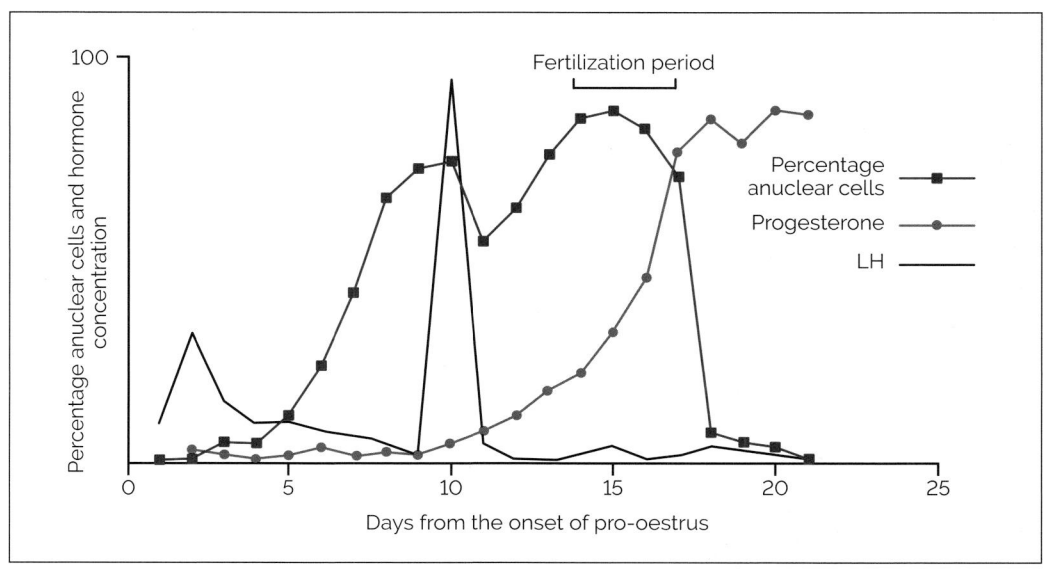

24.13 Photomicrographs of vaginal smears from a bitch. **(a)** Anoestrus: A = parabasal cells; B = small intermediate cells. **(b)** Pro-oestrus: A = red blood cells; B = large intermediate cells. **(c)** Oestrus: A = anuclear cells; B = red blood cells. **(d)** Metoestrus: A = small intermediate cells; B = white blood cells; C = mucous strand; D = bacteria.

cells as soon as the mucosa is thin enough to allow their penetration. Large numbers of white blood cells are therefore found in the metoestrus vaginal smear. Few red blood cells are present during metoestrus.

The bitch should first be mated when the percentage of anuclear cells is maximal (usually 80% or above) (Figure 24.14). There are variations from the normal: some bitches may have two peaks of anuclear cells and some have a low percentage of anuclear cells during the fertile period.

Other tests

A number of other tests have been evaluated in the past, including the measurement of electrical resistance, pH and glucose concentration in the vagina. None of these methods are reliable.

Examination of the vaginal wall using an endoscope (vaginoscopy) may be valuable for identifying the optimal time for breeding, as the vaginal wall undergoes specific changes around the time of ovulation.

24.14 Changes in percentage of anuclear cells during oestrus in the bitch.

The domestic queen

Unlike the bitch, ovulation in the queen is induced by coitus. After mating, assuming that a sufficient release of LH has occurred, follicles increase in size and ovulation follows 24–36 hours later. Mating is best planned during the peak of oestrus, and vaginal cytology may be used to assess this time, but collection of the smear may itself induce ovulation. Multiple copulations should be permitted to ensure an adequate release of LH and therefore ovulation.

Normal mating behaviour

It is important that the events of natural mating are understood so that abnormalities can be recognized, whilst remembering that the mating environment is often artificial. On the day of mating, bitches and queens are frequently transported large distances, are introduced to the male briefly and then expected to mate immediately. This situation eliminates the normal courtship phase associated with pro-oestrous behaviour and may result in mating problems. In addition, many females are presented to males at inappropriate times, either because this is convenient for the owner or because of inexact assessment of the stage of the oestrous cycle. On such occasions sexual behaviour of both males and females may not be optimal.

Dogs

The dog and bitch will normally exhibit play behaviour when they are first introduced to each other. Generally, the bitch should be taken to the designated area first. The dog can then be introduced. He should be restrained on a lead to ensure that the bitch is comfortable with the dog being near her and is receptive to him. Once this has been established the dog can be allowed off his lead. The dog and bitch will normally play for a few minutes (Figure 24.15a). Very experienced studs may forego this playtime and mount the bitch straight away, so it is important to establish the willingness of the bitch to be mated in the first instance. The bitch will normally settle and stand with her tail deviated to one side in order to allow mating to take place. This tail deviation is known as 'flagging'.

The dog may ejaculate a small volume of clear fluid either before mounting the bitch or whilst he is trying to gain intromission into the bitch. This fluid is the first fraction of the ejaculate and does not contain sperm. It originates from the prostate gland and its function is to flush any urine or cellular debris from the urethra. The dog will continue to mount, thrust and dismount until his position allows the tip of the penis to enter the bitch's vagina. This is known as intromission (Figure 24.15b). The dog will now achieve a full erection. The dog appears to move much closer to the bitch and the thrusting movements increase rapidly. He will now ejaculate the second fraction of the ejaculate, which is sperm rich. Once thrusting has subsided the dog will turn through 180 degrees and dismount the bitch whilst his penis remains within the vagina. The dog and bitch will now stand tail-to-tail and this is called the tie (Figure 24.15c). The tie is associated with the dog ejaculating the third fraction of the ejaculate. This is again clear fluid and prostatic in origin and its purpose is to flush the sperm forwards through the cervix into the uterus. The tie will last on average for 20 minutes but varies considerably between dogs and can be as short as 5 minutes or over an hour in length.

Once the swelling of the bulbous gland subsides, the dog and bitch will separate and the mating is finished (Figure 24.15d). The bitch should be checked for any bleeding. There is normally a small amount of fluid that comes away when the tie ends; this is just the last portion of prostatic fluid and is normal. The fluid can sometimes be bloodstained, depending on the bitch's discharge. Bitches with a coloured discharge tend to have a heavier staining of this fluid. If this fluid is very heavily bloodstained, the bitch and the dog should be checked thoroughly.

If all is normal, the bitch is taken away from the area first. The dog will usually lick at himself to help the penis re-enter its sheath. At this time the dog should be checked to ensure that his penis has returned to its sheath correctly. Occasionally, during the mating process, small blood vessels in the dog's penis will burst, resulting in a small amount of bloody discharge. This should subside quickly.

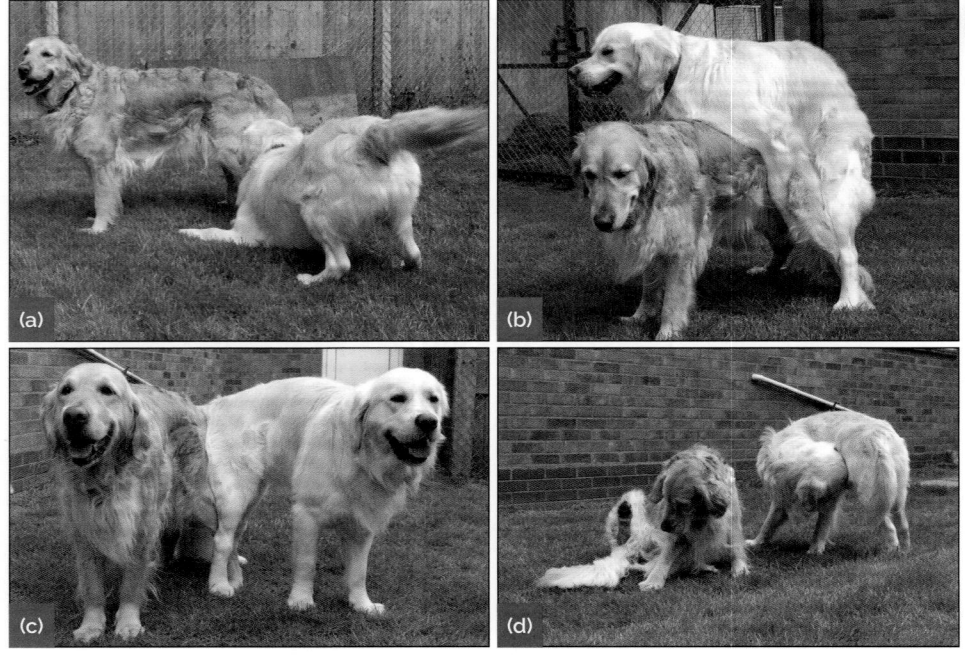

24.15 Normal mating behaviour in the dog: **(a)** playing prior to mating; **(b)** intromission; **(c)** the 'tie'; **(d)** separation after mating.

Cats

The period of sexual introduction and play is variable in the cat, depending upon the experience and aggression of the male. The normal sequence of events occurs rapidly compared with the dog. The male usually approaches the female from the side or back and grasps her neck in his mouth. Whilst maintaining this grasp he mounts the female and positions himself to align the genital regions. The queen normally lowers her chest and elevates the pelvic region whilst deviating her tail. Pelvic thrusting and ejaculation occur rapidly. During intromission the queen often emits a cry and attempts to end mating by rolling, turning and striking at the male. The female then exhibits a marked postcoital reaction consisting of violent rolling and excessive licking. She will not allow further mating at this time.

Problems in mating

Dogs

The mating of dogs and bitches always seems a straightforward process, but there can often be problems. The most common difficulty is that the dog does not tie with the bitch. This is not considered a satisfactory outcome, although it is quite possible that such matings will still result in the bitch conceiving if the dog has ejaculated. The most common reason for a mating with no tie is that there is a height difference between the dog and the bitch. The dog must be able to enter the bitch as straight as possible and this could be difficult if he is too short or too tall. If the dog is too short, a step should be used to make him 'taller'; a step can be used by the bitch if the stud is too tall. Sometimes the dog will not tie because he has had an unpleasant past experience that has resulted in a loss of confidence, often causing a failure to achieve a full erection. In these instances, holding the dog and bitch together as soon as the dog's thrusting has stopped may be helpful. This is known as a held tie, but this in itself can be very difficult to achieve. The dog should not be allowed to mate the bitch too many times without achieving a tie. It is better to try a few times and then rest the dog until the next day.

Often the bitch's position can be a problem: she may not elevate her vulva correctly, she may not deviate her tail very well, or she may keep moving her tail from side to side. In these instances, elevating the bitch's vulva to the correct position or holding her tail out of the way can help the dog. These problems are commonly associated with inexperienced bitches. Maiden bitches (bitches that have not been mated before) can be a little overwhelmed by the whole process and require much more support than an experienced bitch. Inexperienced bitches will often stand at first but then appear to change their minds. In these cases, the owner must be patient. Often the bitch just requires a little more time to get used to the stud and the idea of being mated. These matings can sometimes take several hours to achieve, but the bitch should not be rushed and must not be forced to stand. This can result in her not standing to be mated at all.

Some bitches can be difficult if the stud dog is playing too much and leaping on the bitch. The more inexperienced stud will exhibit this type of behaviour. The problem is rectified by gentle restraint of the bitch, ensuring that the human presence does not upset the stud. Whenever possible a new stud dog should be put with an experienced bitch, and a new bitch with an experienced stud.

Cats

In the cat, it is frequently very difficult to be present during a mating since this puts off all but experienced males; in most cases, it is necessary to observe from a distance. It is always better to have an experienced partner when a queen or tomcat is mated for the first time.

Assisted reproduction

Dogs

There are several techniques that may be used to assist reproduction in the bitch. These include the induction of oestrus (see 'Induction of oestrus' above) and artificial insemination.

Artificial insemination

Artificial insemination (AI) is the technique of placing semen collected from a male into the reproductive tract of the female. It may involve the use of freshly collected semen, semen that has been diluted and chilled, or semen that has been frozen and then thawed. AI has several advantages over natural mating:

- It reduces the requirement to transport animals
- It is an acceptable way of overcoming, to some extent, the quarantine restrictions that prevent the movement of animals from one country to another
- It increases the genetic pool available to an individual breed within a country
- It reduces the disease risk that is always present when unknown animals enter a kennel for mating. (In some countries the use of AI may reduce the spread of infectious diseases)
- It may be useful when natural mating is difficult (for example, bitches that ovulate when they are not in standing oestrus or bitches that have hyperplasia of the vaginal floor)
- Semen can be collected from male animals that, due to age, debility, back pain or premature ejaculation, are unable to achieve a natural mating.

The greatest area of interest is probably in the storage of genetic material by freezing semen for insemination at a future date. This may be necessary in male animals that are likely to become infertile due to castration or to medical treatments with certain hormones. The more common reason is the preservation of semen from superior animals for use in future generations.

Collected semen may be deposited easily into the vagina of the bitch using a long inseminating pipette (Figure 24.16) that is gently introduced near to the cervix. When semen is placed in this position, spermatozoa must swim through the cervix, into the uterus and up the uterine horns. During a

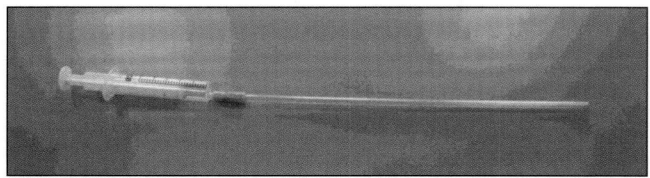

24.16   Inseminating pipette.

natural mating, contractions of the vagina and uterus help in transporting semen. These contractions generally do not occur during insemination, though some may be produced by stimulating the vagina. Vaginal insemination is therefore not ideal, but usually when fresh or chilled semen is used the spermatozoa will live long enough to fertilize the eggs. In the case of frozen semen, the spermatozoa do not live for long after thawing and so vaginal inseminations are not very satisfactory.

The chance of pregnancy can be improved if the semen is placed directly into the uterus rather than into the vagina. It is very difficult to place a catheter through the bitch's cervix into the uterus (a technique that is simple in many other animals) because the vagina is long and narrow and because the cervical opening is small and at an angle to the vagina. A special insemination pipette has been developed for this purpose. Some veterinary surgeons are able to catheterize the cervix using an endoscope, although this requires training and experience. In several countries the commonest way of performing uterine insemination is surgically via a laparotomy. In the UK the RCVS confirmed in 2019 that surgical insemination in dogs is prohibited by animal welfare legislation.

Because of the short lifespan of the preserved sperm, it is most important that inseminations are accurately timed in relation to ovulation. The ideal time is 2–5 days after ovulation, and this is best assessed by using the measurement of plasma progesterone concentration and the study of vaginal cytology (see 'Optimum time' above).

In the UK, puppies that are the result of artificial insemination can be registered with the Kennel Club without prior permission, providing certain requirements are met (see above). The permission of the Kennel Club is not required before semen is imported or exported. There are specific regulations set by the Department for Environment, Food and Rural Affairs (Defra) in the UK and by similar organizations in other countries, which aim to prevent the introduction of infectious diseases. Import regulations vary between countries but are particularly stringent for the UK. Import permit requirements usually include: health certification before, and a set time period after, semen collection, quarantine of semen until the second health examination, and various serological tests.

Cats

Whilst artificial insemination has been widely practised in the domestic cat as a research model for wild cats, the technique is not commonly used in the UK. Techniques used in the cat are further advanced than those in the dog and include the induction of ovulation, *in vitro* fertilization and embryo transfer.

Embryological development

Fertilization

The egg (ovum) which is released at ovulation from the follicle is surrounded by a thick protective coat. The inner layer comprises glycoprotein and is called the zona pellucida, whilst the outer layer is made up of small follicular cells and is called the corona radiata (Figure 24.17).

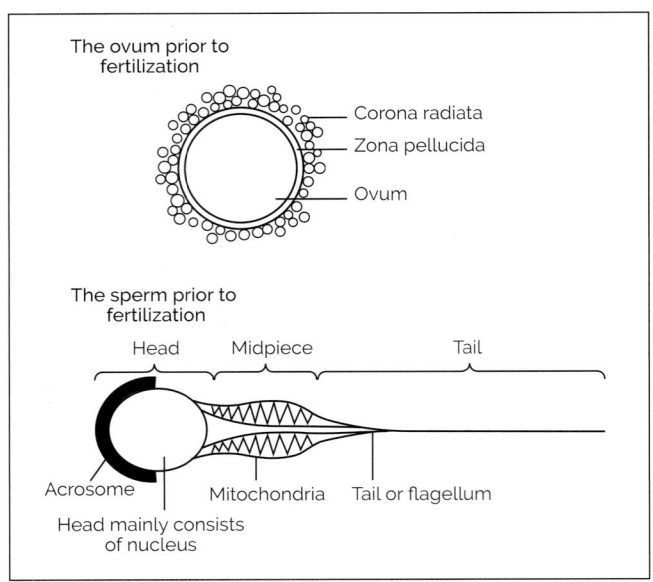

24.17 Structure of ovum and sperm. (Not to same scale.)

The egg is fertilized during its passage through the uterine tube. Just before fertilization, sperm change their type of motility so that they are able to burrow through the cells surrounding the egg. During this process a reaction occurs in the head region of the sperm, resulting in the release of an enzyme that starts to digest the zona pellucida. These sperm are said to be acrosome-reacted. The sperm is then able to penetrate into the egg (the process called fertilization).

The fertilized egg is frequently called a zygote or conceptus (it is sometimes also called an embryo, but this term needs to be differentiated from the embryo proper, which is the mass of cells that form the true body of the developing animal – see below).

The conceptus

After fertilization the conceptus continues to travel down the uterine tube towards the uterus and generally reaches the uterus by day 7 after ovulation. During its journey, the cells of the conceptus begin to divide (Figure 24.18). By doubling at each division the conceptus has two, then four and then eight cells, before forming a solid ball of cells called a morula.

The spherical morula develops a central fluid-filled cavity. The cells lining the cavity are called the trophoblast. Cells tend to accumulate at one end of the conceptus and are called the inner cell mass. This gathering of cells will eventually form the embryo proper. Three separate layers then develop and these will finally form specific recognizable areas of the body.

- The outer layer of the inner cell mass is called the ectoderm – this will form the skin and the nervous system.
- The middle layer of the inner cell mass is called the mesoderm – this will form several organ systems and the musculoskeletal system.
- The inner layer of the inner cell mass is called the endoderm – this will form the lining of the gastrointestinal tract and of other visceral organs.

Two long blocks of mesoderm develop. Underneath these, the endodermal cells spread out and form a lining to the trophoblast which is called the yolk sac. In birds (and

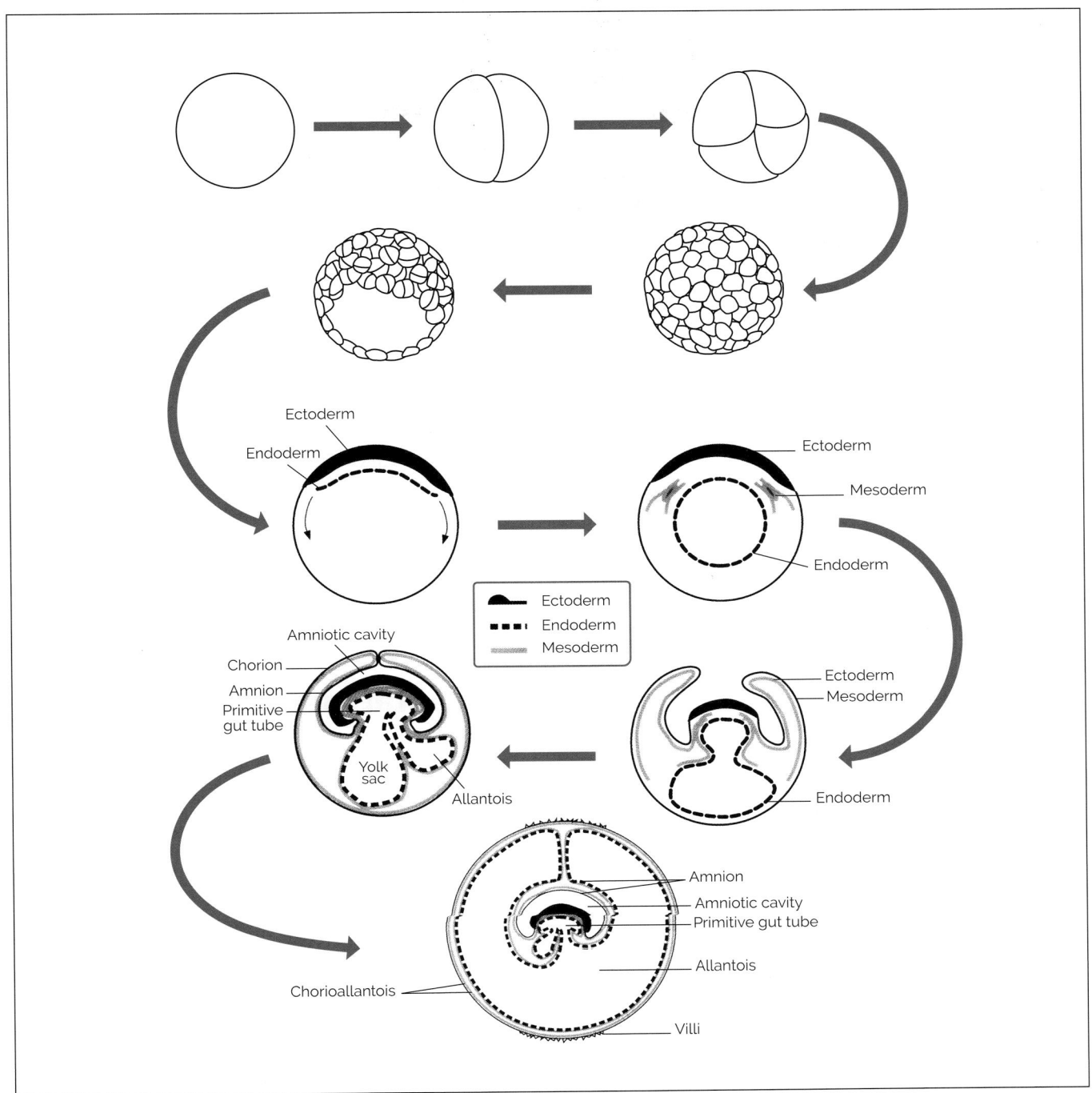

24.18 Early embryonic development.

reptiles) this contains a true yolk, which provides nourishment, but in mammals it is a fluid-filled sac for nutrient transfer. The two blocks of mesoderm then align themselves, one next to the ectoderm and one next to the endoderm. A cavity forms between these two layers of the mesoderm. The inner cell mass curls around and encloses the mesoderm and endoderm layers, which will then form the internal organs of the embryo. The yolk sac and the trophoblast form the placental membranes.

Implantation

During the period of maturation of the conceptus it has been slowly moving down the uterine tube and has entered the uterus. Usually there are multiple conceptuses, which tend to move around within the uterus and become relatively evenly spaced apart. The conceptuses lie close to the wall of the uterus and the process of implantation starts at approximately day 14 in the bitch and day 11 in the queen. During implantation the conceptus partly destroys an area of the uterine wall (the endometrium) and becomes firmly attached.

The placental membranes

The placental membranes form around the embryo and are therefore called the extra-embryonic membranes. There are four basic components to the extra-embryonic membranes: the yolk sac, the chorion, the amnion and the allantois.

As the gut starts to develop (from the endoderm), a specific part of this forms the allantois. The allantois receives urine from the kidneys via a special tube (the urachus) present only in the embryo and fetus (it regresses in the adult).

Whilst the allantois is developing, the trophoblast continues to expand and it spreads around the embryo as a double sheet. The outer membrane is called the chorion and the inner layer is called the amnion. Throughout the period of this development the allantois continues to be filled with fetal urine and ultimately the allantois comes into contact and then fuses with the chorion. This combined structure is called the chorioallantois.

The placenta is the thickened area of the extra-embryonic membranes that attaches the fetus to the endometrium. The placenta is an interface between the fetus and the mother that allows transmission of oxygen and nutrients to the fetus whilst ensuring the elimination of waste products. To do this the fetus develops a blood supply to the placenta (actually within the chorioallantois), which has a large surface area of contact with the maternal tissue.

In the bitch the placenta is described as having a zonary nature, because it forms as a broad belt around the fetus (Figure 24.19). At the edge of the placenta is the marginal haematoma. This is a region where there is degeneration of the maternal endothelium with a resultant bleeding into the spaces formed by the degeneration. Substances secreted by the chorion prevent the blood from clotting, and it is thought that this blood may form a source of iron for the fetus. The fluid in the marginal haematoma is green in bitches and brownish in queens. These are the colours that are noted at the time of placental separation in these species.

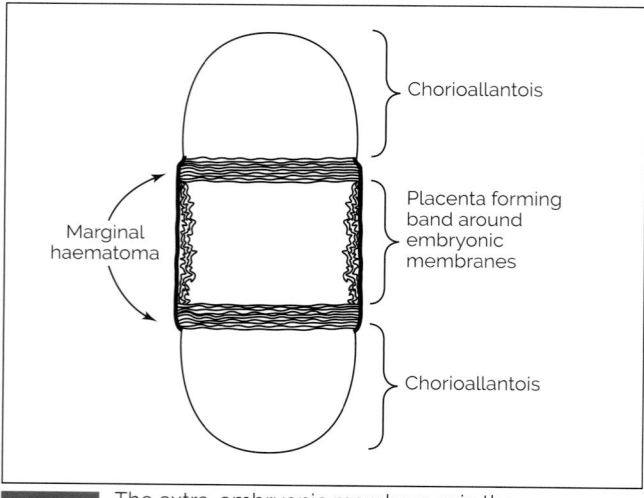

24.19 The extra-embryonic membranes in the zonary placenta of the bitch.

Development of the embryo

As the cells of the inner cell mass multiply and then start to curve underneath themselves, they form the head and trunk of the embryo. Within the embryo an inner cavity forms which is called the coelom (the main body cavity). The coelom is divided into two separate zones by the diaphragm. The cranial zone is the thorax and the caudal zone is the abdomen.

- Generally, by 3 weeks after ovulation the amnion and the allantois have formed and the embryo (in the dog) is approximately 5 mm in length. Normally the uterus itself is now slightly enlarged at the site of the placental attachment.

- By 4 weeks of age it is possible to identify the forming vertebrae and limb buds and the embryo is approaching 20 mm in length. Usually at this stage there is the first evidence of ossification (though this is not yet visible on a radiograph).
- By 5 weeks of age the eyelids, internal ears and canine teeth have started to form, and the embryo is approximately 35 mm in length.

Development of the fetus

From approximately day 35 the external features of the developing canine embryo allow it to be recognized as a dog and from this time onwards it is referred to as a fetus. By this time all the major internal organs have formed, and further development is characterized by an increase in size, especially elongation of the trunk and an increase in diameter of the head.

- By 6 weeks the digits and the external genitalia are well developed and the fetus is approximately 60 mm in length.
- By 7 weeks the fetus is approximately 100 mm in length and there is significant ossification of the vertebral bodies and some of the long bones.
- At 8 weeks the fetus is approximately 150 mm in length and has hair and pads. Fetuses are normally delivered at approximately 9 weeks (65 ± 1 days after ovulation).

Placental membranes at birth

During birth the chorioallantois is recognized as the outer fetal sac (often called the 'water bag') which ruptures as the fetus moves into the birth canal. The amnion, which is the inner fetal sac, is designed also to rupture and provide additional lubrication, but it does not always rupture and in some cases the fetus may be delivered within the amnion.

Pregnancy
The domestic bitch

The length of pregnancy in the bitch is relatively consistent, at 64, 65 or 66 days from the pre-ovulatory LH surge. However, the apparent length of pregnancy, assessed from the time of mating, may vary between 56 and 72 days, since both early and late matings may be fertile.

- Early matings require sperm survival within the female reproductive tract until ovulation and egg maturation; such matings produce an apparently long pregnancy.
- Late matings occur when eggs are waiting to be fertilized for some time after ovulation; such matings produce an apparently shorter pregnancy.

The clinical signs of pregnancy may include:

- Increased bodyweight and abdominal enlargement (these signs may not be obvious if the number of puppies is small)
- A reduced food intake and a vulval discharge, these are common approximately 1 month into the pregnancy

- Enlargement and reddening of the mammary glands – may be noted especially from 40 days after mating (but may also be present in bitches with pseudopregnancy)
- Production of milk – a variable finding (some bitches produce serous fluid from day 40 and milk from day 55 onwards, whilst in others this may not occur until just before parturition).

Certain physiological changes also occur during pregnancy and include the development of a normochromic, normocytic anaemia and a reduction of the packed cell volume; these changes are normal.

Uterine changes during pregnancy

Under the influence of progesterone, the uterus becomes prepared to accept and nourish a pregnancy. This occurs in both pregnant and non-pregnant bitches, since both have elevated concentrations of progesterone. The specific change that occurs is an increased thickness of the uterine wall (the endometrium) associated with enlargement of specific glandular regions.

Overall, the uterus increases in diameter only slightly under the influence of progesterone and it is not until approximately 21 days that there is any enlargement related to the presence of a pregnancy. At this time there is slight swelling at the site of each pregnancy. By approximately 4 weeks the uterine swellings are significant in size and can be readily detected by palpation: the swellings are approximately 4 cm x 7 cm in size at 5 weeks and 5 cm x 8 cm at 6 weeks. Normally by 7 weeks the uterus has enlarged to such a degree that the individual swellings are no longer apparent and the adjacent fetuses are in contact with one another. From here onwards the uterus is very large and the fetuses can move freely within the allantoic fluid.

Pregnancy diagnosis

As well as observation of the clinical signs described above (noting that mammary gland development, increased weight and abdominal enlargement may be present in pseudopregnancy as well as in pregnancy), there are several methods for pregnancy diagnosis in the bitch.

Abdominal palpation

This is best performed approximately 1 month after mating, when the conceptual swellings are approximately 2 cm in diameter. The technique can be highly accurate but may be difficult in obese or nervous animals, and may be inaccurate if the bitch was mated early such that pregnancy is not as advanced as anticipated. After day 35 individual conceptuses cannot easily be palpated and diagnosis becomes more difficult.

Ultrasonography

Diagnostic B-mode ultrasonography is now commonly used for pregnancy diagnosis (Figure 24.20). The technique is non-invasive and without risk to the puppies, dam or veterinary surgeon. The bitch can be examined in the standing position with minimal restraint.

Using ultrasonography, it is possible to diagnose pregnancy as early as 16 days after ovulation, but in most cases this time is not known and so it is prudent to wait until 28 days after mating. At that time the fluid-filled conceptuses can be easily imaged and embryonic tissue can be identified. It is possible to assess the number of conceptuses, though this can be inaccurate, especially when the litter size is large.

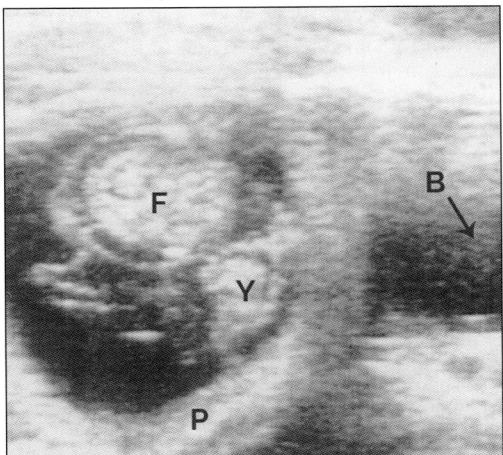

24.20 Ultrasonogram of a pregnant bitch. B = urinary bladder; F = fetus; P = placenta; Y = yolk sac.

Movement of the fetal heart can be seen and this confirms fetal viability. It is possible to examine the bitch at any time after day 28 to diagnose pregnancy and to confirm fetal viability and growth. With later examinations it is less easy to estimate the number of puppies.

Radiography

From day 30 it is possible to detect uterine enlargement with good-quality radiographs. This is not actually diagnostic of pregnancy, since pyometra may have a similar appearance. Pregnancy diagnosis is not possible until after day 45, when mineralization of the fetal skeleton is detectable radiographically. At this stage it is unlikely that there will be radiation damage to the fetus, but sedation or anaesthesia of the dam may be required and is a potential risk. In late pregnancy the number of puppies can be reliably estimated by counting the number of fetal skulls.

Identification of fetal heart beats

In late pregnancy it is possible to auscultate the fetal heart beats using a stethoscope, or to record a fetal ECG. Both of these methods are diagnostic of pregnancy; fetal heart rate is more rapid than that of the dam (usually more than twice the maternal heart rate).

Hormone tests

Plasma concentrations of progesterone are not useful for the detection of pregnancy in the bitch. Measurement of the hormone relaxin is diagnostic of pregnancy, and there is a rapid ELISA test kit that can be run within the practice laboratory to measure this hormone. Alternatively, a blood sample can be sent away to a commercial laboratory.

Acute-phase proteins

The rise in the concentration of acute-phase proteins has been used as the basis of a commercial pregnancy test in the bitch. Concentrations of these proteins (including fibrinogen and C-reactive protein) increase from approximately 25 days onwards. The test is reliable although these proteins are also released in inflammatory conditions such as pyometra.

Care of the bitch during pregnancy

Food intake does not increase during the first 30 days of pregnancy. After this time the absolute requirement for carbohydrate and protein increases. During the last half of pregnancy, food consumption may be doubled. Provided that the diet is well balanced and contains suitable amounts of vitamins and minerals it is not necessary to provide extra supplementation, but it may be necessary to divide the food into two or three meals during the day. Supplementation with calcium and vitamin D should be avoided, since this does not prevent eclampsia and can be dangerous. Supplementation with folic acid prior to mating is widely practiced in breeds and lines with a history of cleft palate.

Regular exercise should be provided throughout pregnancy, limited by the amount the bitch is willing to undertake.

For the control of ascarid infections (*Toxocara*; see Chapter 6) it is necessary to administer medication during pregnancy to reduce or prevent perinatal transmission. Various drugs (benzimidazoles, milbemycin) and treatment regimes have been advocated for the treatment of pregnant bitches. Many veterinary practices would advise that ascarid control should be undertaken prior to mating and after parturition, normally carried out at the same time that the puppies are treated. If it does become necessary to treat the dam, then this can be done during pregnancy.

It is advisable to ensure that routine vaccination has been performed before mating. Vaccination during pregnancy is unlikely to be damaging to the fetus and therefore may be undertaken if necessary, but no live vaccine is licensed for this purpose.

The domestic queen

The average length of pregnancy in the queen is 65 days, with a range of 64–68 days. The clinical signs of pregnancy include increased bodyweight and abdominal enlargement (these signs are often apparent in all but young queens) and mammary development, which is obvious from approximately day 40. These changes are usually diagnostic for pregnancy, since pseudopregnancy is not common and is not usually associated with clinical signs.

Pregnancy diagnosis

Abdominal palpation

Conceptual swellings can be palpated from approximately 21 days after mating. These are discrete until 30 days after mating but become more difficult to palpate from this time onwards.

Ultrasonography

Diagnostic B-mode ultrasonography may be used for pregnancy diagnosis in the cat. The pregnancy length can be assessed from mating time, unlike in the bitch. Conceptuses can be imaged from 12 days after mating and embryonic tissue can usually be seen from day 14. From this time onwards it is possible to identify pregnancy, confirm fetal viability and assess fetal growth. It is more difficult to assess the number of kittens in later pregnancy.

Radiography

From day 30 it is possible to detect uterine enlargement with good-quality radiographs. Mineralization of the fetal skeleton is detectable radiographically from 40 days after mating.

Identification of fetal heartbeats

In late pregnancy the fetal heartbeats may be auscultated using a stethoscope. At this time, it is also usually possible to palpate the fetus in all but the most obese cats.

Hormone tests

Plasma concentrations of progesterone are elevated in both pregnancy and pseudopregnancy, therefore measurement of this hormone is not diagnostic. Plasma relaxin concentrations are elevated from day 25; this hormone is diagnostic of pregnancy and can be measured as described for the bitch.

Care of the queen during pregnancy

During the second half of pregnancy there is an increase in food intake and in the requirement for both carbohydrate and protein. Provided that diet is well balanced and contains suitable amounts of vitamins and minerals, it is not necessary to provide extra supplementation.

Many queens continue to be active during pregnancy and the amount of exercise is best limited by the individual cat.

It is advisable to ensure that routine vaccination has been performed prior to mating.

Abnormalities of pregnancy

Resorption and abortion

A great concern for owners is the risk of resorption or abortion during pregnancy. To understand the differences in these processes, it is necessary to define the stages of development. In general, the term 'embryo' is used when the characteristics of the species are not discernible (see 'Embryonic development' above). From approximately 35 days after ovulation the characteristics of a puppy or kitten become obvious and the term 'fetus' is used.

- **Resorption** refers to the resorption of the entire conceptus and occurs during the embryonic stage of development.
- **Abortion** refers to the expulsion of the fetus and the fetal membranes before term (i.e. before 58 days after ovulation).
- A **stillbirth** is the expulsion of the fetus and fetal membranes after day 58 (i.e. close to term).

The incidence of resorption or abortion of the entire litter is not known, but it is certain that up to 5% of bitches and queens suffer isolated resorption of one or two conceptuses, with continuation of the remaining pregnancy.

There are many potential causes of resorption and abortion, including infectious agents, trauma, fetal defects and maternal environment.

- In the dog, the infectious agents *Brucella canis* (not currently present in the UK), canine distemper virus, canine herpesvirus and *Toxoplasma gondii* have all been implicated as causes of abortion and resorption. It is possible to vaccinate the bitch against canine herpesvirus; the vaccine is given on two occasions during pregnancy and is very effective in reducing subsequent pregnancy loss, stillbirths and fading pups.
- In the cat, feline herpesvirus-1, feline panleucopenia virus, feline leukaemia virus, feline infectious peritonitis virus and *Toxoplasma gondii* infection may produce abortion, resorption or stillbirths.

In many cases embryonic death and pregnancy loss are best assessed using real-time diagnostic B-mode ultrasonography. Resorptions may not be recognized by the owner unless associated with a period of illness. Abortion of fetal tissue may be obvious, but may not be noticed should the dam eat the aborted material. In the face of an abortion, there is little that can be administered to the patient except supportive therapy.

Hypoglycaemia

Pregnancy hypoglycaemia has been reported in the bitch and is associated with reduced blood glucose concentrations during late pregnancy. The clinical signs include weakness that may progress to coma. The condition may be confused with hypocalcaemia, which can occur at a similar time (see 'Hypocalaemia', below).

Parturition
Preparation for parturition in the bitch

In the last few weeks of pregnancy, attempts should be made to encourage the bitch to accept a nest in a suitable place for parturition and rearing. Ideally, this should be a warm, clean, draught and damp-proof room that can be heated. The room is best isolated from the main thoroughfare of the household, where the bitch can rest quietly, but it is beneficial for socializing the litter if noises from washing machines, radios and people talking can be heard. The room should be of a sufficient size to allow the growing litter to play and, where possible, for puppies to have access to an outside area (should the weather permit).

The room should contain a whelping bed. The bed should be large enough to allow the dam to stretch and have sufficient room for a large litter. The sides should be high enough to prevent the puppies escaping until they are approximately 4 weeks old.

In some cases, particularly in a bitch with a long or thick hair coat, it might be useful to remove some of the coat from around the perineum and ventral abdomen, prior to the whelping. This will help the puppies gain access to the nipples and allows cleaning of the dam after parturition.

Heating

Hypothermia is a major cause of neonatal mortality and so the environmental temperature is critical. Neonates are unable to regulate their own temperature for the first week of life and rely on the dam and other neonates to keep warm. A chilled neonate will not respond normally, move properly or be able to suck, and this may result in it being neglected by the dam. It is therefore recommended that the room must be able to be heated to 25–30°C for the first few days of the neonates' life. This temperature is often unbearable for the dam and so can be safely reduced to approximately 22°C after this time. It is most important that the litter is kept well away from any draughts that might chill them.

The room can easily be heated using a thermostatically controlled heater. A heat lamp can be suspended over the bed, but care must be taken to ensure that the neonates do not overheat. It is recommended that perhaps only half of the bed or box is heated, so that the dam can move out of the heat if she wishes. A well protected hot-water bottle provides a good alternative.

Useful equipment

A plentiful supply of newspaper is necessary for the area. Plenty of bedding that can easily be removed when soiled should be available. Shredded paper can be used but with care, since very small neonates may get caught up in it. If using a fabric bedding material, then at least three or four of these will be needed. A supply of blankets will suffice.

A pair of weighing scales, clock and notepad are useful, to enable a record to be kept of the times of birth and weights of neonates. A thermometer should be kept in order to record the dam's rectal temperature prior to parturition.

Sometimes dams can be clumsy at the time of parturition. If there is a large litter, it may be useful to put some of the neonates out of harm's way in a small box within the nesting bed. It is important to ensure that the neonates are kept warm whilst away from their mother. This can be achieved by wrapping a hot-water bottle in some towels and placing it in the bottom of the box.

A supply of milk substitute can be offered to the dam during parturition. No food should be offered at this time, in the event that the dam gets into difficulty and requires veterinary intervention.

There should be suitable equipment to facilitate the artificial rearing of the neonates should this be required. This should include small syringes, feeding bottles and teats and substitute milk for feeding the neonates, along with cotton wool for cleaning any spilt milk off them and to aid urination and defecation if the dam is unable to care for them at all.

Stages of parturition

In the last week of pregnancy, it is prudent to record the dam's rectal temperature at least twice daily. This is to detect the prepartum drop in temperature that precedes the onset of parturition by 24–36 hours. This decline in body temperature is mediated by a sudden reduction in the plasma concentration of progesterone. The rectal temperature usually changes from approximately 39°C to below 37°C.

There are five stages of parturition:

1. Preparation.
2. First stage (onset of uterine contractions).
3. Second stage (propulsion of fetus).
4. Third stage (passage of placenta).
5. Puerperium (after parturition).

Preparation stage

The preparation stage is associated with the decline in plasma progesterone concentration and hence the decrease in rectal temperature. At this time the vaginal and perineal tissue will relax and the dam may show some signs of impending parturition.

She may start to prepare her nest by shredding and ripping up the bedding and may be more restless than usual. She may also show an increased mucus discharge from her vulva, which will probably be slightly more swollen. It is important to remember that some bitches may show no signs of preparation at all.

Some bitches may seek the company of others, while some will try to find solace in a quiet place on their own. Few bitches will be happy with an audience for whelping and so it is best if just one person can stay with the bitch for the birth.

Many queens will seek seclusion to give birth to their kittens, preferring not to have people around them at this time.

First stage of parturition

The first stage of parturition commences with the onset of uterine contractions and can be 1–12 hours in duration, but this is very variable. By this time, milk is usually present within the mammary glands or should appear at this stage.

With the onset of contractions, the bitch might become increasingly restless, pant and/or shiver and her nesting behaviour might become more frantic. Some bitches will refuse food at this time or may vomit their last meal. Most cats will seek seclusion at this time.

The uterine contractions will push the fetus against the cervix, which has begun to dilate. This may result in the rupture of the allantochorion and so allantoic fluid may then be produced from the vulva.

Second stage of parturition

The second stage is characterized by an increase in uterine contractions and propulsion of the fetus through the cervix into the vagina. These will begin when the first fetus enters the pelvic canal. Abdominal contractions then start and are normally quite noticeable. The bitch will appear to squeeze from her ribs towards the perineal area and then relax.

The time of the first abdominal contractions should be recorded, in case there is any delay in the whelping. The time between the onset of straining and the birth of the first fetus is variable. It can be as short as 10 minutes or up to 30 minutes or longer, particularly in maiden bitches. If the bitch continues to have contractions as described earlier, for more than 1 hour without producing a puppy, or if her waters have broken and a puppy has not been produced, the veterinary surgeon should be contacted. It may be necessary for the veterinary surgeon to attend the bitch to assess whether the she is suffering from dystocia and whether assistance is required for the delivery.

Most bitches will be in lateral recumbency during whelping, but some prefer to stand. Delivery of the head is often the most difficult part of the birth and may be associated with some pain, but once this is delivered the rest of the fetus is usually expelled rapidly.

A membrane, the amnion, surrounds the fetus and is often seen at the vulva during straining. It may appear and then disappear with the contractions, and it may rupture spontaneously or be broken by the dam. The puppy may also be born within it.

After delivery, the dam will normally commence vigorous licking, removing the membranes and clearing fluid from around the neonate's face. If the dam fails to remove the membranes immediately after the birth, it must be done for her swiftly. Occasionally young or inexperienced bitches may need help and encouragement with the immediate licking and cleaning. This can be achieved using a clean soft towel. The neonate should be given a vigorous rub with a towel to stimulate it, to help to clear the airways of any fluid and to dry it so as to avoid chilling. When rubbing a neonate, it is recommended that the animal is held with its head lower than its bottom (to aid the drainage of fluid from its lungs).

The birth of the fetus is usually followed by the passage of the allantochorion placenta (afterbirth). Normally a dam separates the neonate from the placenta by chewing through the cord and then eating the placenta when it is expelled. It is important to ensure that the dam does not chew the umbilicus excessively, as this can cause damage to the neonate. If the dam does not sever the umbilicus, the placenta can be separated by tearing or cutting the cord using scissors. Care must be taken if the cord is to be torn. The procedure can be

achieved by holding the cord an inch or so away from the neonate's abdomen and tearing the cord with the other hand. The dam should be given every opportunity to clean and fuss over the neonate before it is removed for weighing and clinical examination.

Once all the procedures have been carried out, the neonate can be returned to the dam. The neonates are best left with their mother during the remainder of the delivery, as removing them might cause distress to the dam, inhibiting further straining. If the dam is young, inexperienced or particularly clumsy, it can be a good idea to put a few of the neonates in a warm box, once the dam has attended to them. This will keep them safer whilst the dam continues giving birth.

Third stage of parturition

The third stage is the passage of the placenta. In the bitch and the queen, the passage of the placenta occurs usually during the second stage of parturition, but occasionally one or more fetuses are delivered without their placentae, which are expelled at a later stage or delivered with subsequent fetuses. It is useful to count the number of placentas passed, as a larger number of fetuses compared with the number of placentas may indicate that the dam has retained one or more.

After a bitch has finished whelping, there is normally a dark-coloured vulval discharge. This contains a green pigment that originates from the placenta. This discharge should normally decline after about a week.

Puerperium

The puerperium is the period after parturition during which the reproductive tract returns to its normal non-pregnant state. During this time the uterus starts its involution and it is common to see a mucoid vulval discharge that may last for up to 6 weeks.

Dystocia

The term dystocia literally means difficult birth; it is used to indicate any problem that interferes with normal birth. Dystocia is rare in the queen but problems are not uncommon in the bitch, especially in brachycephalic breeds such as the Bulldog and Boston Terrier. The two main causes of dystocia are maternal factors and fetal factors.

Maternal dystocia

Maternal dystocia may be divided into two categories: poor straining efforts by the dam and obstruction of the birth canal.

Poor straining efforts of the dam

Poor straining may be the result of nervousness or pain that inhibits normal parturition, but it is more commonly the result of poor myometrial contractions, a condition that has been termed uterine inertia. Inertia may be primary, in which case parturition does not commence, or may be secondary to some other factor occurring during parturition.

Primary uterine inertia

This rarely occurs in the queen, but is a common cause of dystocia in the bitch. It is frequently seen in young bitches with only one or two puppies, or in older overweight bitches with large litters. The cause of the condition is unknown, but it may relate to poor condition of the uterine musculature in overweight or debilitated animals, overstretching of the uterus when the litter size is large, poor stimulus for parturition when there are only a few fetuses or low plasma calcium concentrations.

The endocrinological events of parturition are usually normal, but subsequent uterine contractions are not fully initiated and parturition does not follow. A green vulval discharge, which indicates placental separation, may be seen some days after the expected date of parturition. In some cases, the owner may have observed initial weak uterine contractions or have noted the decline in body temperature. At this stage the administration of the hormone oxytocin may stimulate uterine contractions. Some cases may respond to the intravenous administration of calcium borogluconate. Repeated doses of oxytocin may be necessary but oxytocin should only be given when it is certain that there is no obstruction to the birth canal. It is not possible in the bitch to assess the patency of the cervix by digital palpation (the vagina of an average 20 kg bitch is 20 cm long). In certain cases, a Caesarean operation may be necessary.

Primary uterine inertia may be anticipated in some bitches because of a previous history of this problem or because of their age, physical condition or the number of puppies. The best assessment of the bitch is to monitor the rectal temperature twice daily during the last 7–10 days of pregnancy.

Secondary uterine inertia

This is the cessation of uterine contractions after they have started. Most commonly it is the result of uterine exhaustion following obstructive dystocia, but it may occur spontaneously during the second stage of parturition, presumably because of factors similar to those seen with primary uterine inertia. If the cause of the dystocia can be relieved, the administration of oxytocin and calcium may be suitable treatments. In some cases, Caesarean operation may be necessary.

Obstruction of the birth canal

Obstruction may be the result of abnormalities of the birth canal, such as:

- Deformity of the pelvic bones – these may be congenital malformations, developmental abnormalities or the result of previous trauma, commonly following a road accident
- Soft tissue abnormalities within the pelvis which press against the reproductive tract – they might include pelvic neoplasms, though these are rare in animals of breeding age
- Abnormality of the reproductive tract itself – for example, torsion of the uterus or congenital vaginal or uterine constrictions.

Fetal dystocia

Fetal oversize

Oversize of the fetus relative to the birth canal may be the result of:

- Breed conformation – dystocia may be considered almost normal for certain breeds with exaggerated physical characteristics such as a large head size
- Actual fetal oversize – when the litter size is small and large fetuses develop within the uterus
- Fetal abnormalities – including fetal 'monsters', resulting in relative oversize and dystocia.

In the majority of these cases a Caesarean operation is necessary for the delivery of the fetuses, whether normal or abnormal.

Abnormalities of fetal alignment

Variation from the normal presentation, position and posture of the fetus during delivery may result in dystocia. This may be corrected in certain cases by manipulation per vaginum; however, a Caesarean operation may be necessary.

- The presentation of a fetus is a description of the direction of its long axis in relation to the long axis of the dam (Figure 24.21). Puppies and kittens can only be delivered in longitudinal presentation (i.e. the long axis of the fetus is parallel to the long axis of the dam) but may have either anterior (fetal head delivered first) or posterior (fetus delivered backwards) presentation.
- The position of a fetus is a description of its dorsal axis with respect to the dorsum of the dam; this describes the degree of rotation of the fetus. Most species are normally born in dorsal position; i.e. the back of the fetus is uppermost in the same orientation as the dam.
- The posture of a fetus is a description of the orientation of the head and legs, which may be extended or flexed. For anterior presentation the head must be extended, and this occurs naturally during a posterior presentation.

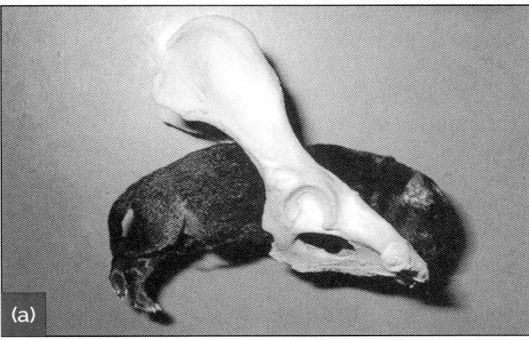

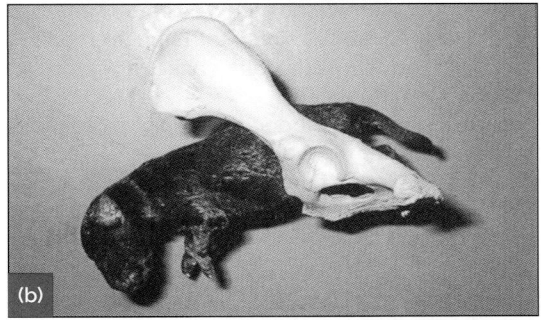

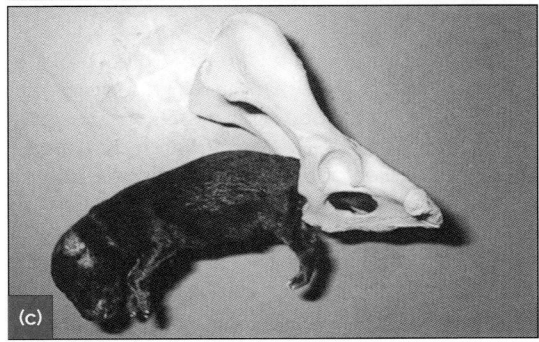

24.21 Presentation of a fetus: **(a)** normal anterior presentation; **(b)** normal posterior presentation; **(c)** breech presentation.

A breech birth refers to a fetus delivered in posterior longitudinal presentation, usually in dorsal position with the hindlimbs flexed. This means that the fetus is presented 'bottom first' with its hindlimbs directed towards the dam's head. A fetus delivered in posterior presentation with the legs extended is not a breech presentation.

Recognition of dystocia

The normal events of parturition should be clearly understood so that recognition of dystocia can be achieved rapidly, thus allowing prompt intervention.

Collection of a relevant history is essential in the evaluation of a potential case of dystocia. This includes the estimation of the stage of pregnancy. Determining the mating time is most helpful for establishing the stage of pregnancy in queens but this is not very useful in bitches, where apparent pregnancy length can vary between 56 and 72 days from mating (see above). Regular monitoring of rectal temperature is therefore essential in the bitch. It should be established whether this has been done by the owner, and, if so, what changes were observed.

Of particular importance is the time-course of events from the onset of parturition, e.g. the onset of behavioural changes such as restlessness, nest making and panting. The time when straining first occurred and the character of the straining efforts may also be useful as an indicator of dystocia, as will the times that any fetuses were produced.

It is not possible to give definite guidelines regarding potential cases of dystocia but examination of the patient is warranted in certain situations:

- A bitch that has exceeded 70 days from the last mating and has no signs of impending parturition
- A queen that has exceeded 65 days from the last mating and has no signs of impending parturition
- The dam is unsettled and strains forcefully but infrequently
- There are signs of straining which then cease
- There is a black/green vulval discharge with no signs of parturition
- There has been a decline in rectal temperature and parturition has not commenced within 24 hours
- There has been ineffectual straining for 1 hour or more, i.e. the bitch has been having regular contractions, but a puppy has not been produced
- Several fetuses have been produced, the last more than 2 hours ago and the dam is restless
- Several fetuses have been produced, the last more than 2 hours ago and a larger litter is expected (may not be known by the owner).

Investigation of potential cases of dystocia

In most cases it is necessary to ensure that the animal is pregnant and/or that viable fetuses remain within the uterus. This can be achieved by transabdominal palpation, auscultation of fetal heartbeats, real-time ultrasonography and radiography, as described earlier for pregnancy diagnosis.

Further investigation involves digital examination of the vagina to assess whether a fetus is present and to establish fetal alignment. This should only be performed after cleaning the vulval area thoroughly with an antiseptic solution and scrubbing the hands or wearing surgical gloves. A water-soluble lubricant should be applied to the fingers and the vestibule and vagina should be carefully examined. The presence of bone or soft-tissue abnormalities of the pelvis should be noted. The presentation, position and posture of the fetus should be established before any further intervention is contemplated.

For normal presentations delivery can be assisted using the thumb and forefinger placed in a cradle manner around the fetal head (anterior presentation) or pelvis (posterior presentation). Traction should only be applied during the straining effort of the bitch, but pressure on the roof of the vagina may be applied with the finger to stimulate straining. Sterile gauze or similar fabric may help to grip the puppy or kitten when assisting delivery. Undue force should never be applied to the feet, as these are easily damaged or deformed.

Caesarean operation

There are a number of reasons for performing a Caesarean operation. In many cases this may be for the relief of dystocia, whilst occasionally it may be an elective procedure when there is concern over feto-maternal disproportion.

Anaesthesia

It is important to remember that there are several marked physiological changes during pregnancy that may affect the requirements for anaesthesia. These physiologica changes result in decreased minimum alveolar concentrations of anaesthetic gases, an increased oxygen requirement, and commonly hypoventilation and subsequent hypoxia and hypercarbia. In addition, in cases of dystocia, the animal may be debilitated and may have recently been fed.

The general aims are to:

- Ensure adequate oxygenation (intubation and oxygen administration)
- Maintain blood volume and prevent hypotension (intravenous fluid therapy)
- Minimize depression of the fetus and dam during and after surgery (reduce the dose of anaesthetic agents used).

There are many anaesthetic regimes suitable for this procedure, including the use of volatile agents for induction and maintenance of anaesthesia and the use of rapid-acting intravenous induction agents (such as propofol) followed by maintenance of anaesthesia using a volatile inhalational anaesthetic.

Complications

There are several complications of Caesarean operations seen in both bitches and queens. These include:

- Anaesthetic risks in the dam and the neonate
- Risks during surgery of uterine rupture and haemorrhage resulting in hypovolaemia
- Postoperative risks, including wound infection and wound breakdown
- Interference with the wound by neonates trying to suck
- Problems in the dam of accepting the litter.

Some veterinary surgeons prefer to perform the operation via a flank incision to avoid the problem of wound interference when the neonates try to suck.

The problem of rejection of the litter by a young dam after a Caesarean operation may be overcome by placing the offspring with the dam as soon as possible after surgery. The mother's milk should be squeezed on to the newborn's heads if rejection is a problem. The dam should be carefully observed until she is able to coordinate sufficiently not to damage them and she must not be left unattended until successful sucking has been noted.

Post-parturient care of the dam

Once the dam has finished giving birth she should be cleaned, paying particular attention to her perineum. This will make her feel more comfortable. She should now be given the opportunity to exercise and urinate or defecate. Usually the dam will then settle with her litter during feeding. Soiled bedding should be changed for clean, fresh material.

The dam should now be offered some food. It must be remembered that, depending on the amount of afterbirths she has eaten, if any, she may be prone to gastrointestinal upset. It is therefore recommended that for the first day or so she should be offered something nutritious but 'light'. Chicken, fish, rice and pasta are all suitable. The dam should be offered her diet in five or six small meals. This can be a pre-prepared diet specifically suitable for lactation. The amount she receives should depend on the litter size. A dam with a large litter will need significantly more food than a dam with only a small litter. The dam should remain on five or six small meals per day for the first few weeks. It should also be remembered that the diet should not be altered too quickly, as this may worsen any gastrointestinal upset.

During the first 2 weeks after the birth of the litter, the dam will spend much of her time with the litter and therefore it may be preferable to feed her close to the nest. A readily accessible supply of fresh water should be close by. Once weaning begins the dam should be encouraged to leave the nest for increasingly longer periods.

The dam should be encouraged to exercise during lactation. Where possible, to minimize the risk of infection of the litter, this should be where she will not come into contact with other animals.

Once weaning has begun and is well underway, the demands on the dam start to reduce and therefore her relevant food intake should also gradually begin to lessen. If the dam has lost a great deal of weight through her efforts to feed the litter, then her food intake should remain high so that she can replace some of the lost bodyweight. When she has regained some weight her food intake can be reduced.

Normally a veterinary surgeon should be called to examine the dam when parturition is finished, in order to check her health and that of her newborn litter. Thereafter the dam's general health should also be closely monitored throughout lactation. Common problems to look for are signs of eclampsia (see 'Hypocalcaemia', below), mastitis (see 'Mastitis', below), pyrexia, and a foul-smelling vulval discharge. If any of these are observed, veterinary attention should be sought. The litter should also be closely monitored for fading syndrome (see 'Fading puppy and kitten syndrome', below).

Lactation

The development of the mammary gland after puberty is under hormonal control. Progesterone from the corpus luteum causes the glands to enlarge during pregnancy; this is sometimes seen in false pregnancies. Hormones are responsible for the initiation of milk secretion (see below). They also play a vital role in the maintenance of milk secretion after it has been established. The terminology used to describe the various aspects of lactation is often confused:

- **Milk secretion** refers to the synthesis of milk by the epithelial cells and the passage of milk from the cytoplasm of the cells into the alveolar lumen
- **Milk removal** includes the passive withdrawal of milk from the cisterns and sinuses and the ejection of milk from the alveolar lumina
- **Lactation** refers to the combined processes of milk secretion and removal
- **Lactogenesis** is the initiation of milk secretion
- **Mammogenesis** describes the development of the mammary gland
- **Galactopoiesis** refers to the enhancement of established lactation.

In the bitch, there is a long luteal phase in both pregnancy and non-pregnancy. Progesterone primes the mammary glands; mammary gland secretion and the development of obvious clinical signs of pregnancy (and pseudopregnancy) are associated with a rise in plasma concentration of prolactin, which commences at 30–35 days after ovulation. Prolactin is the principal luteotrophic factor in the bitch. Prolactin concentration continues to increase during late pregnancy to a plateau at approximately day 60. Prolactin concentration surges during the prepartum decline in progesterone, and reaches a peak at, or shortly after, parturition.

Initiation of milk secretion

The hormonal control of the initiation of lactation has not been fully investigated in the bitch and queen. It is likely to be either a rise in the blood concentrations of prolactin and glucocorticoids at the time of parturition, or a decrease in the concentrations of compounds that have an inhibitory effect on the milk secretion process, namely progesterone and transcortin.

Prior to parturition, lipid and protein granules form in the epithelial cells and accumulate in the lumen of the alveolus as colostrum. Colostrum is the first milk produced and is a source of antibodies for the neonate. In the bitch and queen, antibodies are present in the milk for several days after parturition. Antibodies are readily absorbed on the first day after birth, the rate of absorption varies for different antibodies and the intestinal tract ceases to absorb different antibodies at different times. As a general rule, puppies and kittens should have sucked (or be given colostrum) within 8 hours of birth; ideally they should suck within the first few hours of birth.

Oxytocin secreted by the posterior pituitary gland in the few hours around parturition enables the release or 'letdown' of milk in response to sucking by the neonate. Continuation of sucking is necessary to maintain the production of milk.

Milk

Milk is the liquid produced after the colostrum. The composition of milk varies between species: milk produced by the bitch and queen is more concentrated and contains more protein and twice as much fat as cow's milk. The average composition of milk is shown in Figure 24.22. The basic milk sugar is lactose. A variety of milk substitutes are commercially available and these are discussed later.

	Bitch	Queen	Cow	Goat
Protein (g/L)	70	90	32	32
Fat (g/L)	110	130	33	36
Carbohydrate (g/L)	35	36	47	43
Energy (Kcal/L)	1400	1000	670	610

24.22 Composition of the milk of various species. The approximate composition of milk of the bitch and queen is quite different to that of milk from the cow and goat and neither of the latter milk offers a good substitute; a commercial product is more likely to be suitably formulated.

Periparturient abnormalities

There are several conditions that may occur during late pregnancy or soon after parturition in both the domestic bitch and the queen. Some conditions are emergencies and prompt recognition of the clinical signs is essential to allow successful treatment.

Hypocalcaemia (eclampsia, puerperal tetany)

Low plasma concentrations of calcium are related to calcium loss in the milk and poor dietary calcium availability. The condition can be seen during late pregnancy or early lactation but is most common 10–30 days after whelping. It is rare in the queen. The clinical signs include restlessness, panting, increased salivation, tremors and a stiff gait that may progress to muscle fasciculation, pyrexia and tachycardia. If untreated, seizures and death result. The slow administration of calcium borogluconate by intravenous infusion produces a rapid resolution of the clinical signs. During administration, cardiac rate and rhythm should be monitored. Calcium supplementation may then be given orally or by subcutaneous injection to prevent recurrence of the condition. The litter should be hand fed, or older litters weaned.

Placental retention

The retention of placental tissue is uncommon in both the bitch and the queen. Placentas are normally delivered following each puppy or kitten and may be quickly eaten by the dam. If a placenta is retained, the clinical signs are a persistent green vulval discharge. This should be differentiated from the normal haemorrhagic discharge that may persist for 1 week after parturition (a mucoid discharge may be present for up to 6 weeks). If a retained placenta is diagnosed by either ultrasound examination or palpation, the administration of oxytocin will usually allow its delivery.

Postpartum metritis

Infection and inflammation of the uterus may occur following prolonged parturition, abortion, fetal and/or placental retention or obstetrical manipulation. The clinical signs commonly include a persistent purulent vulval discharge, lethargy and pyrexia. Treatment with broad-spectrum antibiotics should be instituted immediately; fluid replacement therapy may be required.

In some cases, the condition may be acutely septic resulting in dehydration and collapse and requires aggressive treatment to prevent mortality.

Postpartum haemorrhage

Excessive blood loss after parturition may indicate uterine or vaginal tearing, or an underlying coagulation disorder. A vaginal tampon can be useful when the lesion is within the wall or the vagina, and oxytocin administration may be useful to promote uterine involution. The dam should be monitored for signs of shock and a blood transfusion may be necessary. In severe cases an exploratory laparotomy may be required.

Subinvolution of placental sites

The persistence of a blood-coloured vulval discharge for more than 6 weeks after parturition should raise suspicion of subinvolution of placental sites. This is where one or more areas of the uterus fails to completely involute and there is continued blood loss often until re-vascularization at the subsequent oestrus. Most cases resolve spontaneously and require no treatment.

Uterine prolapse

Uterine prolapse is a very uncommon complication that occurs within a few hours of delivery of the last neonate. The condition requires urgent treatment, usually via laparotomy, and frequently because of trauma to the uterus an ovariohysterectomy is performed.

Agalactia

Agalactia is the term often used to describe absence of milk after parturition. It is important to differentiate two conditions:

1. Failure of milk production (true agalactia).
2. Failure of milk letdown.

Whilst failure of milk letdown can be treated by the administration of oxytocin, this drug is not effective when there has been failure of milk production. Some success has been reported in treating bitches with failure of milk production using metoclopramide, but careful management of the litter will be required as they will require supplementary feeding with an alternative source of colostrum until lactation commences. Alternatively, the puppies may be fostered, if possible.

Mastitis

Inflammation of the mammary gland is not common in the bitch or queen, but it may have disastrous results should the dam reject the litter because of pain on suckling. It is usually the result of bacterial infection either blood-borne or through the teat. The mammary glands are tender, warm and firm upon palpation and the milk may be contaminated with blood and inflammatory cells so that it becomes yellow, pink or brown. The dam may become lethargic and anorexic if the condition is not treated. Bathing and massaging the gland with warm water and gently removing the infected fluid may be helpful, but antibiotics are usually required. It should be remembered that these agents will be excreted in the milk and ingested by the neonates.

Breeding exotic pets

Many of the reproductive principles described for dogs and cats also apply to many exotic pets, in particular mammalian species. However, each species may differ considerably in other ways. Only basic details of reproduction of the individual exotic species can be covered in this chapter and the reader is referred to other texts such as the *BSAVA Manual of Exotic Pets, 5th edn.*

Small mammals

Descriptions of the basic reproductive parameters for a variety of common small mammals are given in Figure 24.23.

Ferrets

The male ferret (hob) is often twice the size of the female ferret (jill). It is also simple to differentiate the sexes by inspection of the external genitalia; the testes are situated in the perineal region (similar to cats), although the prepuce is found on the ventral caudal abdominal surface.

The size of the testicles of the hob vary during the year and can be very small during the non-breeding season. Surgical neutering of hobs is no longer favoured, as studies have shown that adrenal disease is highly likely to develop around 2.5–3 years post-neutering due to the removal of the negative feedback (testosterone) on luteinizing hormone (LH) release from the pituitary gland and the high numbers of LH receptors on the ferret adrenal glands. Instead, a gonadotrophin-releasing hormone (GnRH) agonist (deslorelin) is licensed in the UK for use in hobs as a form of chemical castration (reversible). The depot preparation is implanted subcutaneously between the shoulder blades and results in a reduction in testicular size, sexual activity and the musky odour of entire hobs within 5–14 weeks of implantation. It should be used only once the hob has reached sexual maturity, and preferably at the beginning of the breeding season (February). Its effects last between 16 months and 4 years, depending on the individual.

Jills are sexually mature in the spring after their birth. The breeding season for ferrets in the UK stretches from February/March to September/October and the jill is in a near-permanent (persistent) state of oestrus, as she is an induced ovulator. Persistent oestrus may result in bone marrow suppression and potentially lethal pancytopenia. Mating with a vasectomized male ferret provides a short-term solution in females that may be required for breeding in the future, as does the use of proligestone. Surgical neutering is no longer recommended as a method of preventing oestrus in jills unless there is evidence of uterine disease, as such neutering has been associated with endocrinopathies. Proligestone injections or GnRH-agonist implants (lasting 18–24 months) are preferred, although the latter is not currently licensed for this use in the UK.

Rabbits

Sexual maturity in rabbits varies between breeds but is typically reached at 4–5 months in females (does) and 5–8 months in males (bucks). Rabbits are seasonally polyoestrus and are induced ovulators. Both males and females may be territorially aggressive during the breeding season and this, as well as unwanted litters, is a major reason for neutering pet animals. Neutering is usually carried out from 5–6 months of age in does, but may be carried out once the testes have descended into the scrotum (12 weeks of age) in bucks. Importantly, early neutering of female rabbits prevents uterine adenocarcinoma, the most common neoplasia in female rabbits, in addition to other uterine and mammary conditions.

Species	Sexual maturity	Oestrus cycle interval	Duration of oestrus	Ovulation	Gestation length	Pseudopregnancy	Litter size
Rat	8–10 weeks	4–5 days Non-seasonally polyoestrus	10-20 hours	Spontaneous	21–23 days	Approximately 14 days after non-fertile mating	8–18
Mouse	6–7 weeks	4–5 days Non-seasonally polyoestrus	10-20 hours	Spontaneous	19–21 days	Approximately 14 days after non-fertile mating	5–12
Syrian hamster	6–12 weeks	4 days	8-26 hours	Spontaneous	15–18 days	Approximately 8–10 days after non-fertile mating	5–10
Gerbil	8–10 weeks	4–7 days	12-18 hours	Spontaneous	23–26 days (42 days if delayed implantation)	Approximately 16 days after non-fertile mating	3–8
Guinea pig	1.5–3 months	15–17 days	6-11 hours	Spontaneous	59–72 days (average 63 days)		1–6 (average 3–4)
Chinchilla	6–9 months	30–50 days Seasonally polyoestrus	40 hours	Spontaneous	111 days	Approximately 16 days after induced ovulation	2
Rabbit	4–8 months	Seasonally polyoestrus	Variable during the breeding season	Induced	29–35 days (average 31 days)	Approximately 42 days after induced ovulation	4–10
Ferret	4–8 months First Spring after birth	Seasonally polyoestrus	7 months. Persistent according to day length	Induced	41–42 days		2–14

24.23 Reproductive parameters for small mammals.

Pregnancy can be detected by palpation or ultrasonography from approximately 10–14 days gestation and by radiography from 11 days. Average gestation is around 31 days (30–32 days). Parturition is called kindling.

Rodents

Sexing

Female rodents have separate external orifices for their urinary and reproductive systems. This can be used for sexing the animals, in conjunction with the spacing of the urinary papilla (the nodule-like lump on the ventrum through which the urinary tract exits in the female rodent) from the anus. In females, the urinary papilla is closer to the anus and, if care is taken, the entrance to the genital tract may be seen between the urinary papilla and the caudally situated anus (Figure 24.24). In males, the prepuce is spaced at a greater distance from the anus. There are also prominent testes in adult males, but these may be retracted into the caudal abdomen. The testes may be encouraged to descend by gently holding the male rodent vertically, with head uppermost and resting its rear on the palm of one hand.

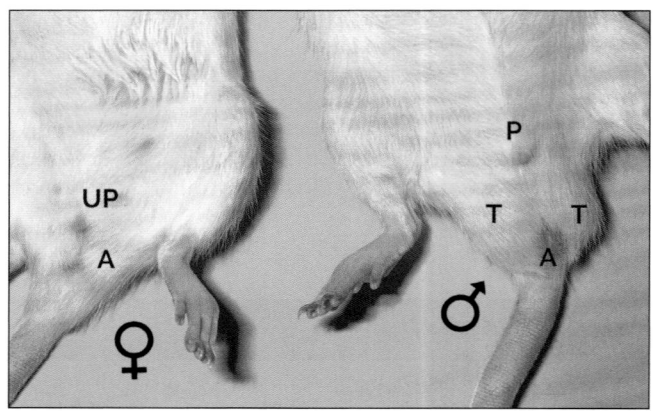

24.24 Differences in anogenital distance in rats: (left) female; (right) male. A = anus; P = prepuce; T = testes; UP = urinary papilla. (Reproduced from *BSAVA Manual of Exotic Pets, 4th edn*).

Guinea pigs

Guinea pig sows have a higher risk of complications during parturition because the piglets are large and fully formed at birth. If a sow is to be bred from, she should have her first litter prior to 8 months of age. Upon reaching adulthood her pelvic symphysis will stiffen (around 1 year of age) and she may not be able to deliver her piglets, resulting in dystocia and a need for a Caesarean operation.

Birds

Many bird species will breed predominantly at one time of the year. Some seasonal breeders are triggered to start breeding by an initial decrease in day length, as is seen over the winter, followed by an increase, as occurs in the spring. This day length variation stimulates the pineal gland, which is connected to the pituitary gland, to alter concentrations of melatonin and GnRH; this can stimulate the reproductive cycle. Other seasonal breeders are stimulated to cycle by other external stimuli, such as rainfall and food availability. Sexual maturity may be reached quickly in smaller species, such as finches, or may take several years, as with many of the larger parrots.

Some bird species are sexually monomorphic, i.e. the two sexes look physically identical (e.g. Amazon parrots, macaws). In other species there is a distinct difference: they are sexually dimorphic. For example, in budgerigars the male has a blue cere (fleshy covering located above the beak) and the female a brown or pinkish one. In many birds of prey, the female is up to twice the size of the male.

Mating involves the male mounting the female and pressing his vent to hers. A few species of birds possess a phallus (for example, some species of ducks and ratites such as the emu and ostrich). Where present, it is purely an organ of intromission to guide semen from the male vent into the female vent; it plays no part in urination. Most species of birds (e.g. parrots) do not possess a phallus and semen transfer from vent to vent is passive and gravity fed. Following mating, the sperm may be stored in the oviduct for a short period. The whole process from shedding of the oocyte to laying of the egg takes approximately 2 days. The number of eggs laid in a 'clutch' varies between species.

Occasionally a female will not pass an egg efficiently, resulting in her becoming egg-bound. The fully formed egg may lodge in the vagina or in the shell gland. The causes of egg-binding can include hypocalcaemia, oversized/malformed eggs and trauma to the pelvis or vent.

Incubation of the eggs may be performed by just the female or just the male or by both parents, depending on the species. Incubation periods vary between species, as do weaning ages (Figure 24.25). Artificial incubation may help increase hatching rates. Parent-reared birds take longer to wean on average than hand-reared ones and are usually less hand-tame.

Reptiles

Reptiles are classified as:

- **Oviparous:** Lay eggs externally
- **Ovoviviparous:** Produce live young instead of laying eggs, but the eggs are produced internally
- **Viviparous:** A form of placenta/thin-walled egg structure is produced in the reproductive system, which allows the fetus to develop and live young are produced.

Reptile eggs are generally soft-shelled and more leathery than birds' eggs, although egg production in lizards is similar to the process in birds. Incubation length depends upon the temperature at which the eggs are kept. Unlike birds' eggs, reptile eggs should not be moved during incubation but kept with the same side up as when they were deposited. Figure 24.26 gives an idea of some common incubation lengths, or, where the species is viviparous, the gestation length.

Chelonians

Male chelonians often have longer tails as the phallus is located on the floor of the cloaca. As in birds, the phallus plays no part in urination but is simply an organ of intromission used to guide semen from the male cloaca into the female (Figure 24.27). In some species the male and female vary significantly in size (e.g. Indian star tortoise, striped mud turtle, red-eared terrapin); in others there are other differing secondary sexual characteristics, such as longer claws in females (e.g. leopard and Indian star tortoises) and differing eye colours (box turtle). Males of many Mediterranean species of tortoise and turtle possess a dished (concave) plastron, to make mounting the female easier, and often

Species	Incubation period (days)	Weaning (days): parent-reared	Weaning (days): hand-reared	Sexual maturity
African Grey parrot	26–28	100–120	75–90	4–6 years
Amazon parrot	26–29	90–120	75–90	4–6 years
Barn owl	30–31	70–75		1 year
Budgerigar	16–18	30–40	30	6–9 months
Canary	12–14	21		<1 year
Cockatiel	18–20	47–52	42–49	6–12 months
Cockatoo: large spp. Cockatoo: medium spp.	23–30 (depending on spp.)	60–80 45–60	95–120 75–100	5–6 years 3–4 years
Harris hawk	32	35–45 (fledging)[a]		>3 years
Lovebird	18–24	45–55	40–45	6–12 months
Macaw: large spp. Macaw: small spp.	26–28 23–26	120–150 90–120	95–120 75–90	5–7 years 4–6 years
Peregrine falcon	29–32	35–42 (fledging)[a]		>3 years
Pheasant	22–24	Precocial[b]		
Pigeon	16–19	35		1 year
Zebra finch	12–16	25–28		9 months

24.25 Reproductive parameters for selected bird species. [a] Fledging refers to a time when bird can first fly. [b] Self-feeding from hatchling.

Species	Method of reproduction	Incubation/ gestation period (days)	Incubation/ temperature ranges (°C)
Boa constrictor	Viviparous	100–120	28–32.5
Burmese python	Oviparous	55–65	28–32
Corn snake	Oviparous	55–70	28–30
Garter snake	Viviparous	90–100	24–29.5
Kingsnake	Oviparous	55–70	28–30
Bearded dragon	Oviparous	65–115	28–32
Green iguana	Oviparous	60–70	25–30
Jackson's chameleon	Ovoviviparous	90–180	27–29
Leopard gecko	Oviparous	150–170	28–32
Hermann's tortoise	Oviparous	85–100	30–33
Leopard tortoise	Oviparous	140–155	28–32
Red-eared terrapin	Oviparous	54–80	28–29
African spurred tortoise	Oviparous	120–170	28–32

24.26 Reproductive parameters for selected reptiles.

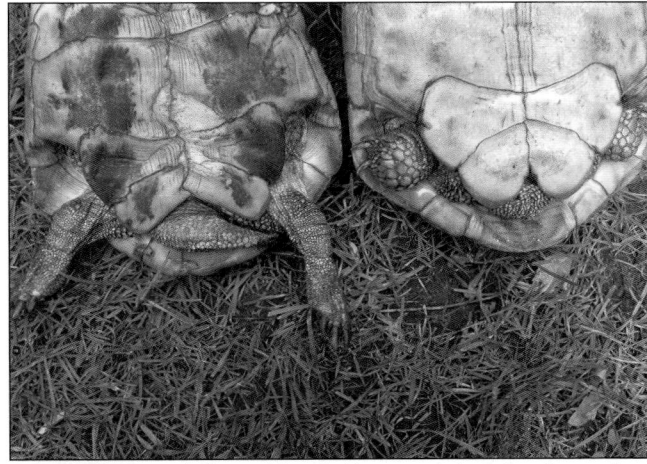

24.27 Sexual dimorphism in Hermann's tortoise: the male (left) has a longer tail and wider anal scutes than the female (right). (Courtesy of Alan Humphreys)

Inability to pass the egg (called 'egg binding') may occur in chelonians, often caused by the development of an abnormally large egg but sometimes due to a damaged pelvis, which results in an inability to pass even normal-sized eggs. Another cause of egg binding is egg retention, which can be related to behavioural stress, often due to an unsuitable habitat or substrate for laying the eggs and/or creating a nest.

Incubation temperature control is important in sex determination. For example, the eggs of the spur-thighed tortoise will produce males if kept at 29.5°C and females if kept at 31.5°C. This principle seems to apply to a large number of tortoise species, with males being predominantly produced at lower temperatures than females. If the temperature range is kept at 28–31°C, a mixture of sexes is likely to be achieved.

Lizards

In most species of lizard there are external physical differences that allow differentiation of the sexes. These include: prominent prefemoral pores in male iguanids and agamids;

have wider anal scutes than the egg-bearing females. Some female Mediterranean species have a hinge to the caudal part of the plastron to allow easier egg-laying.

In the colder northerly climes of the UK the incubation of chelonian eggs in an outside environment is not possible. It is necessary to remove the eggs from wherever they have been laid by the female and to transfer them to a purpose-built incubator for hatching. Incubators may be purchased from many reptile outlets, or from commercial poultry or cage-bird suppliers.

prominent precloacal pores in male geckos; larger scales caudal to the vent in male anoles; wider tail bases in male green iguanas; greater ornamentation such as larger crests in plumed basilisks; horns in Jackson's chameleons; and larger crest spines in male water dragons. In other species, such as the beaded lizard, some monitors and the Gila monster, sexual identification must be performed by surgical probing. This involves inserting a blunt-ended sterile probe carefully into one of two orifices in the base of the tail just caudal to the vent. This is where the hemipenes are located; all lizards have two hemipenes and, as with chelonians, they are organs of intromission and have no urethra, so play no part in urination. When not engorged, they sit in an invagination into which the probe can be passed to a depth of several skin scales (usually greater than five).

Sexual maturity varies according to the species and also according to the husbandry provided, as poor nutrition and poor heat or ultraviolet light provision may lead to delays in maturation.

Lizard eggs may be incubated in vivaria. Incubation periods vary from 45–70 days for smaller lizards to 90–130 days for larger lizards (see Figure 24.26). A few species are parthenogenic, i.e. females give birth to females with no need for male fertilization.

Obstructive (eggs too large) and non-obstructive (insufficient nesting site, digging substrate, poor physical condition, hypocalcaemia or infection of the oviduct) dystocia are common problems in egg-laying lizards.

Sex determination in most lizards is dependent on genetic factors, with the exception of some geckos, for which sex determination is dependent on the temperature at which the egg was incubated.

Snakes

Telling the sexes apart can be difficult in snakes and is best performed by surgical probing. A fine sterile blunt-ended probe is inserted through one of two small orifices just caudal to the vent (on either side of the midline) and advanced in a caudal direction. If the snake is a male, the probe will pass into one of the inverted hemipenes and so will insert to a depth equivalent to 8–16 subcaudal scales. In females there are anal glands in this region and so the probe may be inserted to a depth of only 2–6 subcaudal scales. In some species, such as boas, males possess a paracloacal spur (the remnant of the pelvic limb) on either side of the body ventrally at the level of the cloaca. In very young snakes it may be possible to evert the hemipenes manually, with care, in a technique known as 'popping'. As with lizards and chelonians, the hemipenes are organs of intromission and play no part in urination.

Sex determination in snakes is entirely chromosomally dependent; the process is not influenced by the temperature at which the eggs are hatched.

The average incubation period in snakes is generally 45–70 days, but this varies with species (see Figure 24.26); artificial incubation improves hatching rates. Temperatures for incubation vary from 24 to 32°C; it is important to have a thermometer and humidity gauge within the incubator. When eggs are retrieved from the nest site, particular care should be taken to maintain the same position of the egg in the incubator. The eggs should not be turned or touched during the incubation process, as this can cause significant fetal mortality.

Egg impaction, which is thought to be a result of exhaustion or calcium deficiency, may occur in egg-laying species.

Care and management of the neonate

Dogs and cats

The first essential steps after birth are to:

- Establish a clear airway and stimulate respiration
- Separate the umbilicus from the placenta
- Keep the neonate warm until active
- Encourage the neonate to suck.

It is essential that a clear airway is established as soon as a fetus is born (or delivered via a Caesarean operation). This is usually done by the dam, but if she does not or is unable to, then this can be done by the assistant. It involves removal of the surrounding fetal membranes using a soft dry towel. This will usually stimulate respiration. The mouth and nose can be cleared of fetal fluid by suction. The practice of swinging the neonate in an arc should be avoided because of the risk of cerebral haemorrhage. If vigorous rubbing does not stimulate respiration positive pressure ventilation using a snug fitting mask may be started ensuring that the head and neck are extended.

If the heart is not beating, external cardiac massage combined with artificial respiration may be attempted.

The umbilicus should be clamped and cut approximately 3 cm from the abdomen; excessive bleeding can be prevented by the application of a ligature.

Once regular respiratory efforts are maintained, the neonate may be placed into a pre-warmed box or incubator until it is active, when it may be returned to the dam and encouraged to suck. Sucking normally occurs immediately after birth and at intervals of 2–3 hours for the first few days.

Examination

Once the dam is content for the neonate to be removed, it should be checked for abnormalities.

- The birth weight should be recorded. Normally the neonate will gain between 5% and 10% bodyweight per day; failure to do so may indicate poor health.
- The neonate should be checked for congenital abnormalities, such as cleft palate or harelip.
- The umbilicus should be checked for herniation. It should be clean and show no evidence of further bleeding. If the umbilicus is bleeding, this can be ligated to prevent further blood loss.
- Respiration should be regular and even. The normal respiratory rate for a neonate is 15–40 breaths per minute. There should not be excessive noise. If there is excessive noise, this may indicate that the neonate still has fluid in its lungs and the appropriate action should be taken (see 'Second stage of parturition' above).
- There should be no discharge from the eyes or ears.
- Any other birth defects should also be recorded, as well as the neonate's colour and sex.
- The neonate's rectal temperature could also be taken and recorded at this time, but in reality this is often unnecessary. The normal rectal temperature for the first week after birth should be 32–34°C.

Neonatal characteristics

Neonatal puppies and kittens are unable to stand at birth but should be quite mobile, using their limbs to crawl. Neonates need to be assessed for their general strength. The weakest must be carefully observed, since they do not feed adequately and may fail to thrive. Standing may be seen from 10 days after birth and most neonates should be able to walk at 3 weeks of age.

Puppies and kittens are born with their eyes closed; separation of the upper and lower lids with opening of the eyes should occur by approximately 10–14 days after birth. The cornea at this stage may appear slightly cloudy, but this will disappear over the first 4 weeks. Many kittens are born with strabismus, which persists until they are 8 weeks old.

Care of the litter

During the first few weeks of life the dam will take care of the needs of the litter. However, the litter need to be checked regularly for signs of problems, ensuring that all of them are receiving an adequate supply of milk from the dam and that no individual is missing out on feeding opportunities. There should be a plentiful supply of clean bedding available, so that the dam and her offspring are comfortable and not lying on soiled or wet bedding.

Normally the dam will lick the perineal region in order to stimulate the neonates to defecate or urinate and she continues to do this for the first 2–3 weeks after birth. After this time the neonates will urinate and defecate voluntarily and therefore the amount of soiling in the nest will increase and will require more frequent changing.

The litter should be weighed on a regular basis, usually weekly to ensure that all of them are gaining weight adequately. At 10–14 days, when the eyes of puppies and kittens should open, they will gradually be able to focus on objects. They will become stronger on their legs and begin to crawl around. At this time, it is advisable to ensure that all the puppies are able to use their hindlegs properly; sometimes very large or fat puppies fail to get up on their hindlegs and will haul themselves around on their front legs and bellies. If this becomes apparent, the puppy should be checked to ensure that there is nothing physically wrong with the legs, and then be encouraged to use its hindlegs by placing a hand under its bottom and pushing it on to its hindlegs. This condition rarely persists, due to the increased competition for food, but with a small litter it may become a problem.

Once weaning commences the dam may be less inclined to clean up their mess. The litter should be encouraged to soil away from the nest so that cleaning is more easily facilitated. This may hasten toilet training.

Small mammals

It should be noted that, in pet species other than the dog and cat, there may be a tendency towards cannibalism of the litter by the dam, or at least abandonment or abuse, if she is disturbed with her young in the first few weeks after parturition. For this reason, female rats, mice, hamsters, gerbils and rabbits should be left alone with their litters, except for replenishing food and clearing the worst of any cage soiling. Cannibalism is especially common in the hamster, though the female will also protectively place the young in her cheek pouches to move them, which may appear as her 'eating' the young.

Neonatal characteristics of small mammalian species likely to be seen in small animal practice are described in Figure 24.28. Most small mammal species are altricial at birth (wholly dependent on the mother for nutrition and survival in the first few weeks of life); they are born blind, deaf, hairless and without teeth. Guinea pigs and chinchillas are precocial (relatively mature and mobile) at birth.

Ferrets

The average number of ferret kits in a litter is eight. They are altricial but are born with a prominent fat pad on the dorsum of the neck, which provides some calorific value during the early stages of life. They have a higher caloric requirement than adult ferrets, at 1.5–2 times adult maintenance levels.

Rabbits

Rabbit does will suckle their kits for only 3–5 minutes at a time and only once or twice in a 24-hour period, even though they are totally dependent on her milk up to 21 days postparturition. They will begin to take solid foods from the age of 2–3 weeks and at this time they should be weighed. Solid foods offered will increasingly be consumed and weight losses may be seen during this changeover period. Weaning

Species	Terminology	Precocity	Development			Weaning age
			Eyes open	Ears open	Hair and skin	
Rat	Pups	Altricial	12–15 days	4–5 days	Fur appears at 7–10 days	17–21 days
Mouse	Pups	Altricial	12–14 days	4–5 days	Fur appears at 10 days	21–28 days
Syrian hamster	Pups	Altricial	12–14 days	1.5–3 days	Skin changes from pale pink to darker at 2–3 days	20–28 days
Gerbil	Pups	Altricial	12–14 days	4–5 days	Skin changes from pale pink to darker at 7 days with fur appearing	20–30 days
Guinea pig	Piglets	Precocial	At birth	At birth	Born fully furred	14–28 days (eating solids from day 1)
Chinchilla	Kits	Precocial	At birth	At birth	Born fully furred	36–48 days (eating solids from day 1)
Rabbit	Kits/kittens	Altricial	8–10 days	11–12 days	Fur appears at 5–6 days	6 weeks (eating solids from 2–3 weeks)
Ferret	Kits	Altricial	4–5 weeks	10 days	Fur appears 2 days, pronounced at 3 weeks	6–8 weeks (ideally 8 weeks)

24.28 Neonatal characteristics of small mammals.

occurs at around 6 weeks of age. The growing kits require higher levels of vitamin D3 and calcium than adult rabbits and should be offered a balanced diet, such as a combination of a pelleted growing-rabbit formulated food along with good-quality grass hay and some greens. The pelleted foods should be chosen carefully; many are nutritionally balanced but it is preferable to use a homogeneous pelleted diet, as rabbits are selective eaters of concentrates and will pick and choose if offered a mixed dry food. They should also be given access to unfiltered natural sunlight, even if for only 15–20 minutes a day, to ensure adequate synthesis of vitamin D.

Birds

After hatching, the chick must be supplied with high levels of energy and protein for the growth phase within 3–4 days, but it does not require food in the first 24 hours. This delay is possible due to the remnants of the yolk sac inside the body cavity still providing some nutrition and immunity for the first few hours/days of life. Failure to internalize the yolk sac prior to hatching is sometimes seen and can lead to septicaemia. Surgical removal of the non-internalized yolk sac is possible but the chick will require immediate supplementary nutritional support due to the removal of this energy/nutrient source.

When feathers are produced, a huge demand for protein occurs; there are several feather changes during the first 2 years of life. Young birds also have a large requirement for calcium and vitamin D3 for developing and mineralizing the skeleton.

It has been estimated that minimum energy requirements for small psittacine and passerine birds is five times that of adults, with young chicks nearly doubling their weight over 48 hours, with a protein need of 15–20% compared with an adult protein need of 10–14%. Diets for chicks have therefore concentrated on pre-formulated mashes with this level of protein, or the use of eggs and dairy products, which have a good broad spectrum of amino acid supplementation and 20% protein levels.

However, excessive protein supplementation (>25% of diet) has been shown to lead to behavioural problems and claw, beak and skeletal deformities, particularly if combined with a lack of calcium. Excessive protein levels, poor calcium and vitamin D3 can lead to rapid growth, bowing of the long leg bones due to metabolic bone disease and, in waterfowl in particular, lateral rotation of the carpi when the flight feathers first start to come through due to their weight. This condition is known as 'angel wing'.

Reptiles

Parental neonatal care varies greatly between species, from no care at all, to careful tending of infants in, for example, many crocodilian species. In some herbivorous species, direct neonatal care is absent but proximity to adults is essential for the development of normal gut flora. Temperature, environmental enrichment and single versus group rearing may all affect the behavioural development and survival of reptile neonates. Reptiles survive initially on the nutrients within the yolk sac before progressing to eat adult type diets; however, it should be noted that many species have different diets as young reptiles compared with adult animals. One example is the bearded dragon, which is predominantly insectivorous as a hatchling/juvenile, but becomes more herbivorous as an adult.

Neonatal reptiles may suffer from retained or infected yolk sacs, often as a result of premature birth or hatching in artificial rearing situations or where there is suboptimal maternal nutrition. Surgical intervention is usually required in such cases, with subsequent supportive feeding until normal eating commences.

Diseases of the neonatal period

A number of diseases may affect puppies and kittens early in life. A certain percentage of neonates may die before weaning and it has been suggested that this can be as high as 15–20%. With good management systems (including the avoidance of hypothermia), the number of offspring lost should not be >5%.

Fading puppy and kitten syndrome

The most common problem noted within the neonatal period is that of fading puppies or kittens. Most commonly, neonates die when <1 week of age. There are numerous factors associated with this loss, but usually it is the inherent susceptibility of the newborn that results in its ultimate demise. Neonates have poor mechanisms of thermoregulation, fluid and energy balance; they are immunologically incompetent; and they may have abnormal lung surfactant composition. When combined with poor management regimes and poor mothering behaviour of the dam, the risk of neonatal mortality can be high. Approximately 50% of neonatal deaths can be attributed to infection, maternal and management-related deficiencies, low birth weight or congenital abnormalities.

Neonatal septicaemia

The inherent vulnerability of the neonate puts it at risk of colonization by a number of bacterial agents. This may result in rapid death with very few initial clinical signs. In some circumstances, ill health results in frequent crying, restlessness and hypo-thermia, progressing to clinical signs of diarrhoea and/or dyspnoea with resultant dehydration or cyanosis, and ultimately death. In other instances, neonates are more chronically affected and fail to grow as expected prior to the onset of obvious clinical disease.

The majority of passive immunity follows from the intake of colostrum, and gut transfer occurs only during the first 48 hours of life. It is vital, therefore, to ensure an adequate intake of colostrum at this time to protect against these organisms. It is always sensible to have either frozen colostrum or a commercial preparation available.

Regardless of the cause, rapid and aggressive treatment using intravenous fluid therapy, oral electrolytes, broad-spectrum antimicrobial agents and oxygen administration is essential. Despite such treatment, the mortality rate can be high.

Neonatal viral infection

Viral infections are not common in the neonate, especially when vaccination programmes are practised in the adult.

Maternally derived antibodies (MDA) frequently provide protection for several weeks.

- Canine herpesvirus may result in the birth of congenitally infected puppies that are weak and die soon after birth. Vaccination of the pregnant bitch can reduce neonatal losses.
- Feline immunodeficiency virus and feline leukaemia virus in the queen can infect kittens transplacentally as well as perinatally, and result in neonatal death after a few weeks of age.
- Neonatal deaths and the birth of kittens with cerebellar hypoplasia are not uncommon following infection with feline panleucopenia virus during pregnancy.
- Feline infectious peritonitis virus has also been implicated in cases of upper respiratory tract disease and fading kitten syndrome.

Congenital abnormalities

Congenital abnormalities are those that are present at birth. Common problems include cleft palate, where there is failure of the normal fusion of the palatine arches. The defect may occur anywhere along the length of the hard or soft palate, though most commonly it arises caudal to the incisor ridge. The defect is common in certain breeds and it has been suggested that it is a trait inherited in either a recessive or polygenic manner. In most cases euthanasia of the neonate is advisable, because of the problems with sucking and the aspiration of milk. As noted previously, supplementation of the dam with folic acid may reduce the occurrence of this defect.

There are many other congenital abnormalities that may affect organ systems, such as hernias, fetal 'monsters', hydrocephalus, microphthalmus, flat puppies ('swimmers'), congenital heart disease and atresia of the terminal rectum. A thorough clinical examination of each neonate after birth should allow these abnormalities to be readily detected.

Artificial rearing of neonates

In some circumstances it may be necessary to rear some or all of the litter artificially. These include:

- Death of the dam
- A sick dam
- A dam showing no interest in her litter
- A dam with an inadequate milk supply
- A large litter.

Artificial rearing is best avoided where possible. In some cases, it may be possible to foster the neonates on to another dam. Suitable candidates to foster orphans might include a lactating bitch or queen that has just given birth and lost her litter, one that has been through a pseudopregnancy and is currently lactating, or a dam with a small litter.

In the case of an excessively large litter, it may be possible to rotate some of the neonates between artificial rearing and being reared by the dam. It has been suggested that a small number of neonates should be entirely artificially reared, rather than rotated, but this method is not advocated. The neonates should, where possible, remain in the nest with the dam to ensure normal socialization.

It is essential that all neonates receive colostrum from the dam to ensure an adequate uptake of immunoglobulins. If the dam has died, it may still be possible to express some colostrum from her, as long as it is not contaminated with drugs or toxins.

Equipment

All the equipment for artificial rearing should be readily available and where possible should be included in the equipment needed in preparation for parturition, so it is available if needed.

Milk substitutes

There are several commercially available milk substitutes for artificial rearing of both puppies and kittens. It is important that the neonate receives the right formulation of milk. Cow's and goat's milk are not suitable substitutes, since their composition is very different to that of milk from the bitch or queen. It is possible to make up a milk substitute, but this must have the appropriate lactose, fat and protein content, and achieving this is time-consuming. It is better to make up a pre-prepared milk substitute. The milk should be warmed to body temperature (39°C) and fed according to the manufacturer's instructions, with regard to bodyweight and age.

Feeding bottles

Artificial rearing is both demanding and time-consuming, especially if rearing is done entirely without the dam. The neonates normally feed every 2–4 hours during the first 5 days of life, which then reduces to every 4 hours after day 5.

- Feeding can be achieved using a commercial feeding kit, which contains a bottle and teat. This encourages normal sucking, but can be more time-consuming. The teat aperture should be large enough to prevent the neonate sucking in air but small enough to prevent excessive volumes of milk flowing through it.
- Feeding can also be achieved using a dropper bottle or syringe feeding. A 2 ml syringe should be adequate for the first few days.

When using either of these methods, care must be taken not to rush the neonate, as this may result in inhalation of milk rather than swallowing, which may cause pneumonia.

Orogastric tube feeding

In some cases, it may be beneficial to feed neonates by means of a stomach tube (orogastric tube), especially during the first few days of life, for rapid feeding or for particularly sick neonates. The procedure is relatively simple. A small 2 mm diameter piece of soft polythene tubing should be measured against the neonate's mouth and to the end of the level of the ninth rib. This length should be marked on the tube. The outside of the tube should be lubricated with a small volume of water.

The neonate's head is held in the normal position and the mouth is held just open using a finger and thumb; if the head is extended or flexed, passage of the tube into the trachea is more likely. The tube is directed gently over the tongue into the back of the throat. Swallowing greatly assists passage into the oesophagus, but is not essential. The tube can usually be seen on the left side of the neck as it passes down the oesophagus. There is little resistance as the tube is introduced into the stomach; the length of the tube is the best guide. Once the tube is in position, the syringe can be attached and its contents slowly injected into the stomach. The tube is then gently removed.

General care

Dogs and cats

When artificial rearing has to take place entirely without the dam, the neonate is fully reliant upon its human carer.

Neonates are unable to open their bladder or bowels voluntarily; normally the mother would stimulate urination or defecation by licking the anogenital region after feeding. In the absence of the mother, this stimulation can be carried out manually by using a moistened piece of cotton wool. This should be performed every 2 hours.

Any spilt milk should be cleaned off the neonate immediately, as during the early days of life this might otherwise result in chilling. Once any spilt milk is allowed to dry, it will cause matting of the coat.

The orphaned neonates' only other need is to be kept warm and out of draughts. They should be maintained at an environmental temperature of 25 °C.

Exotic pets

Small mammals

The basic principles of artificial rearing of small mammal neonates are similar to those described above for dogs and cats; they require suitable feeding, a warm environment and stimulation to urinate and defecate. An overview of species specific requirements is given here. More detailed information can be found in appropriate texts, including the *BSAVA Manual of Rabbit Medicine* and the *BSAVA Manual of Rodents and Ferrets*.

Ferrets

Milk replacers for ferret kits have been adapted from puppy or kitten milk replacers, enriched with cream until the fat content reaches 20% (e.g. 3-parts puppy milk replacer to 1-part whipping cream). This can be fed on demand 4–6 times daily and the kits may be weaned on to adult food at 4–5 weeks of age.

Rabbits

Rabbit kits are altricial and also rely upon the doe for the development of intestinal microflora. In hand-reared kits this may not occur properly and subsequent deaths from enterotoxaemia are commonplace. It may be possible to prevent this situation by transfaunation of gut flora from a healthy parasite-free adult rabbit to the kits. For hand-rearing (Figure 24.29), diluted kitten milk replacers or a homemade formula

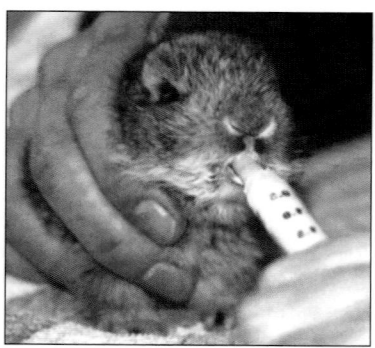

24.29 Hand feeding a rabbit kit. (Reproduced from *BSAVA Manual of Rabbit Medicine and Surgery, 2nd edn*).

of 1-part whole full-fat cow's milk to 3-parts condensed milk, adding 6 g skimmed milk powder per 100 ml of the mixture can be used. Adult foods (including weaning formulated dry foods) should be offered from 2 weeks of age and weaning attempted at 3 weeks, although a naturally reared kit would not be weaned until 6 weeks of age.

Rodents

Hand-rearing of small rodents is challenging and has a high failure rate, owing to the altricial nature of the young of most species (see Figure 24.28).

All of the altricial species show evidence of poor thermoregulation and require environmental temperatures of around 35°C while they are hairless, and around 32°C once they are furred. After their eyes open, the temperature may be reduced by 2.5°C per week and a temperature gradient should be provided.

The first concern when providing supportive feeding for orphaned rodents must be to ensure hydration. Initially, oral rehydration solutions suitable for cats and dogs may be used. Once hydration is established, the orphans may be offered dog or cat milk replacers or homemade diets. The milk replacer may be fed from the tip of a paintbrush, or using kitten feeders for older and larger individuals. Feeding should be once every hour during daylight and once every 2 hours overnight. Up to 35–40% of bodyweight may be fed per day.

Precocial young guinea pigs and chinchillas are able to eat small amounts of solid food within 24 hours of birth, but they are often not hungry for the first 12–24 hours as they are able to make use of brown fat reserves; they should not be force-fed during this period. Thereafter, it is important to ensure that high-fibre foods are offered preferentially (to avoid fussy eating in later life). A hand-rearing formula for guinea pigs might be 1-part condensed milk to 2-parts cooled boiled water, fed every 3–4 hours at a rate of 1–3 ml; this may be adapted for chinchillas with the addition of 6 g skimmed milk powder to 100 ml of the formula to help to increase protein levels. Early weaning on to solid adult food is encouraged for both species, and is advised after 7–10 days. As with rabbits, which are also hindgut fermenters, transfaunation of caecotrophs from healthy adults can be helpful in colonizing the neonatal gut with a healthy flora.

Birds and reptiles

Some information on rearing of birds and reptiles has been given above under 'Care and management of the neonate'. More detailed information can be found in appropriate texts, including the *BSAVA Manual of Exotic Pet and Wildlife Nursing*, the *BSAVA Manual of Reptiles, 3rd edn*, the *BSAVA Manual of Psittacine Birds, 2nd edn* and the *BSAVA Manual of Avian Practice*.

Weaning

Weaning is a gradual process, which normally starts at about 2.5 weeks for puppies and kittens and will be complete by about 5 weeks. The neonates will still suckle from their mother throughout the process, but once weaning has begun the dam will normally spend an increasing amount of time away from her offspring. She should still be allowed frequent access to them during the day and will normally still spend the night with them.

Until the weaning process begins, the neonate is reliant on the dam for all of its nutritional needs, but once weaning has begun each puppy or kitten should be closely monitored for continued weight gain. Signs associated with under-nutrition include crying, inactivity and poor weight gain.

Small quantities of food can be offered to neonates on a finger, allowing them to lick or suck the finger. The range and volume of food can be increased as the neonates get used to feeding. The food offered can be of a proprietary brand specifically designed for weaning. Some animals will wean easily, taking solids and lapping straight away, whilst others may take longer. It is therefore especially important to treat each neonate individually and to be patient.

Neonates that are weaned directly from the dam should gradually increase the amount of solid food they eat, and should be on five or six feeds per day by the age of 5 weeks old. Those neonates being hand-reared should have the volume of milk they receive gradually reduced as the weaning process continues, in a similar manner to being weaned from the dam.

References and further reading

England GCW (2013) *Dog Breeding, Whelping and Puppy Care.* Blackwell Scientific Publications, Oxford

England GCW and von Heimendahl A (2010) *BSAVA Manual of Canine and Feline Reproduction and Neonatology, 2nd edn.* BSAVA Publications, Gloucester

England GCW, Russo M and Freeman SL (2016) Laboratory evaluation of the reproductive system. In: *BSAVA Manual of Canine and Feline Clinical Pathology, 3rd edn*, ed. E Villiers and J Ristic, pp 373–388. BSAVA Publications, Gloucester

Chitty J and Monks D (2018) *BSAVA Manual of Avian Practice: A Foundation Manual.* BSAVA Publications, Gloucester

Girling SJ (2013) *Veterinary Nursing of Exotic Pets.* Wiley-Blackwell, Oxford

Girling SJ and Raiti P (2019) *BSAVA Manual of Reptiles, 3rd edn.* BSAVA Publications, Gloucester

Harcourt-Brown F and Chitty J (2013) *BSAVA Manual of Rabbit Surgery, Dentistry and Imaging.* BSAVA Publications, Gloucester

Harcourt-Brown N and Chitty J (2005) *BSAVA Manual of Psittacine Birds, 2nd edn.* BSAVA Publications, Gloucester

Hoskins JD (2001) *Veterinary Pediatrics: Dogs and Cats from Birth to Six Months, 3rd edn.* WB Saunders, Philadelphia

Keeble E and Meredith A (2009) *BSAVA Manual of Rodents and Ferrets.* BSAVA Publications, Gloucester

Meredith A and Flecknell P (2006) *BSAVA Manual of Rabbit Medicine and Surgery, 2nd edn.* BSAVA Publications, Gloucester

Meredith A and Johnson-Delaney C (2010) *BSAVA Manual of Exotic Pets, 5th edn.* BSAVA Publications, Gloucester

Meredith A and Lord B (2014) *BSAVA Manual of Rabbit Medicine.* BSAVA Publications, Gloucester

Okerman L (1994) Breeding problems. In: *Diseases of Domestic Rabbits, 2nd edn*, ed. L Okerman, pp. 113–120. Blackwell Scientific Publications, Oxford

Reineke E and Lewis D (2018) Reproductive and paediatric emergencies. In: *BSAVA Manual of Canine and Feline Emergency and Critical Care, 3rd edn.* ed. LG King and A Boag, pp. 249–263. BSAVA Publications, Gloucester

Varga M, Lumbis R and Gott L (2012) *BSAVA Manual of Exotic Pet and Wildlife Nursing.* BSAVA Publications, Gloucester

Wright K and Raiti P (2019) Breeding and neonatal care. In: *BSAVA Manual of Reptiles, 3rd edn*, ed. SJ Girling and P Raiti, pp. 70–88. BSAVA Publications, Gloucester

Useful websites

BSAVA position statement on neutering:
www.bsava.com/Resources/Veterinary-resources/Position-statements/Neutering

Inherited Diseases in Dogs Database–Department of Veterinary Medicine at Cambridge University:
www.vet.cam.ac.uk/idid

Governing Council of the Cat Fancy:
www.gccfcats.org/

Guidance on surgical artificial insemination in dogs – RCVS:
www.rcvs.org.uk/setting-standards/advice-and-guidance/code-of-professional-conduct-for-veterinary-surgeons/supporting-guidance/miscellaneous/

The Kennel Club:
www.thekennelclub.org.uk/

Self-assessment questions

1. Name the four stages of the oestrous cycle in the dog.
2. What is the difference between spontaneous and induced ovulation and in which species do these occur?
3. What is the role of prolactin in pregnant and non-pregnant bitches?
4. What is the difference between cryptorchidism and monorchidism?
5. Name the three layers of cells that make up the inner cell mass of a conceptus.
6. What are the membranes called that surround an embryo and what are their four basic components?
7. What are the two main causes of dystocia?
8. What are the clinical signs of eclampsia?
9. What age do puppies open their eyes?
10. What is the gestation length of a guinea pig?
11. What are the three classifications of reptiles in terms of breeding?
12. What are ferret young called?

Chapter 25

Dentistry

Cedric Tutt and Ursula van der Riet

Learning objectives

After studying this chapter, readers will have the knowledge to:

- Define the terms used to describe dental disease
- Complete a dental chart accurately
- Describe how to handle an avulsed tooth
- List and describe the power-driven and hand dental instruments used in dentistry in general small animal practice
- List the surgical equipment required for extractions
- Describe the scale and polish procedure
- List the indications for dental radiography
- Instruct a client in dental homecare
- Describe the common dental conditions in lagomorphs and rodents

Dental disease

Periodontal disease

Periodontal disease is one of the most commonly seen diseases in small animal practice. Approximately 85% of dogs and cats older than 3 years of age show signs of periodontal disease, the term used for plaque-induced diseases of the supporting structures of teeth. The prevention of this disease is discussed later.

The two main forms are:

- Gingivitis, a reversible condition, defined as inflammation of the gingiva
- Periodontitis, an irreversible condition, is a progression from gingivitis affecting the gingiva, alveolar bone, periodontal ligament and cementum of the tooth. Periodontitis is also commonly seen around the apices of teeth that have crown fractures, pulp necrosis or other causes of pulp death. These lesions are seen on dental radiographs of the affected teeth.

For teeth to be firmly held in the mouth the periodontium must be healthy.

Aetiology

Periodontal disease begins when bacteria in the mouth form a substance called plaque that sticks to the surfaces of the teeth. Over 300 species of bacteria can be present in the oral cavity of dogs and cats. These bacteria colonize the surfaces of the teeth and other areas of the mouth, forming biofilms, communities of bacteria that progress to plaque. From the time the teeth erupt into the mouth, plaque begins to accumulate on the tooth surface. Plaque consists of desquamated oral epithelial cells, food particles and bacteria. Initially, Gram-positive aerobic bacteria colonize the tooth surface and this population creates conditions that are optimum for Gram-negative anaerobic organisms to thrive. Bacteria, their by-products and toxins, as well as the host's own defence systems, contribute to the initiation and continuation of periodontal disease and result in damage to the supporting structures of the teeth.

Local secondary factors that predispose the host to the initiation and contribute to the rate of progression of the disease process include calculus, tooth crowding (especially in small breeds), tooth morphology, supernumerary teeth, mouth breathing which dries the mucosal surface and salivary gland dysfunction with subsequent decreased saliva flow (saliva flow aids in the clearance of unattached oral bacteria) as well as the loss of natural antimicrobials, including immunoglobulin A (IgA), found in saliva. Dental calculus is mineralized plaque, and a layer of plaque always covers the calculus. It has been shown that the surface roughness of calculus increases its plaque retentiveness. Supragingival and subgingival plaque can develop into calculus which hosts the plaque organisms, leading to persistent inflammation.

BSAVA Textbook of Veterinary Nursing, sixth edition. Edited by Barbara Cooper, Elizabeth Mullineaux and Lynn Turner. ©BSAVA 2020

Gingivitis

The gingiva is made up of an attached part, tightly adhered to the alveolar bone, and a free part that forms the normal gingival sulcus (a collar surrounding the crown of each tooth). Gingivitis is the earliest sign of periodontal disease. Gingivitis presents as redness, swelling and bleeding of the gums, and is graded depending on its severity:

- Mild gingivitis (G1) – marginal redness of the gums
- Moderate gingivitis (G2) – the gums bleed when the gingival sulcus is probed
- Severe gingivitis (G3) – the gingivae are swollen and bleed spontaneously.

Gingivitis affects only the gingiva; it does not extend beyond to the deeper supporting tissues and is reversible (as there is no loss of periodontal attachment). The severity of gingivitis is scored according to how much bleeding there is on gentle probing of the sulcus (Figure 25.1). In patients with uncomplicated gingivitis there will be normal periodontal sulcus probing depths (<3 mm in dogs and <0.5 mm in cats). Gingivitis is often accompanied by halitosis (oral malodour). However, accompanying complications to gingivitis such as gingival overgrowth may cause additional problems (see below). Gingivitis can occur within days of plaque accumulation but, if treated correctly, is reversible and gingival health can be quickly restored. In some breeds of dog (e.g. Boxers), plaque causes the gingiva to enlarge, termed gingival hyperplasia or gingival overgrowth. In these situations, the probing depth of the sulcus is increased even though there is not sufficient attachment loss to cause a pocket – known as a pseudo-pocket.

Gingival overgrowth

Gingival overgrowth may be the result of plaque-induced inflammation (e.g. gingival hyperplasia); it may be idiopathic or hereditary. Boxers and, to a lesser extent, Border Collies and Labrador Retrievers show a predisposition to the condition.

The significance of gingival overgrowth is the development of a 'pseudo-pocket' due to the altered position of the gingival margin. This 'pseudo-pocket' is formed due to the enlarged gingiva and not because of destruction of the periodontal ligament and alveolar bone. In other words, the free gingiva has become taller, giving the impression that there is a pocket. Intraoral radiography helps to confirm the level of the alveolar margin in these cases. The presence of overgrown gingiva compromises normal tooth cleaning from mastication and therefore predisposes to periodontitis. It can also lead to bleeding as a result of trauma during mastication.

Calculus

Dental calculus is mineralized plaque and in itself does not initiate periodontal disease. However, it does provide a roughened surface for plaque to adhere to, as well as interfere with homecare and plaque removal. Therefore, calculus indirectly contributes to the pathogenic process of periodontal disease. As a result, supragingival and subgingival plaque can develop into calculus that can host the plaque organisms, leading to persistent inflammation.

Once formed, calculus is difficult to remove with conventional home oral hygiene practices (i.e. tooth brushing) and its removal necessitates professional scaling under general anaesthesia.

Periodontitis

Periodontitis *may* develop in an individual with untreated gingivitis. The inflammation seen with periodontitis involves not only the gingiva but also the surrounding periodontal ligament, alveolar bone and cementum (Figure 25.2). The end result of untreated periodontitis is exfoliation of the affected teeth (teeth fall out), due to the destruction of the periodontal ligament and alveolar bone (Figure 25.3). Periodontitis is not site-specific; it may affect one or more sites around one specific tooth or numerous teeth.

Periodontitis is not reversible: once the alveolar bone and periodontal ligament have been destroyed it is impossible to replace them without expensive and complicated periodontal surgery. However, it can be managed with the correct treatment and homecare to prevent disease progression.

Clinical signs of periodontitis include the presence of severe halitosis and large amounts of dental deposits. Oral bacteria, especially anaerobic organisms, produce volatile sulphur compounds that lead to oral malodour.

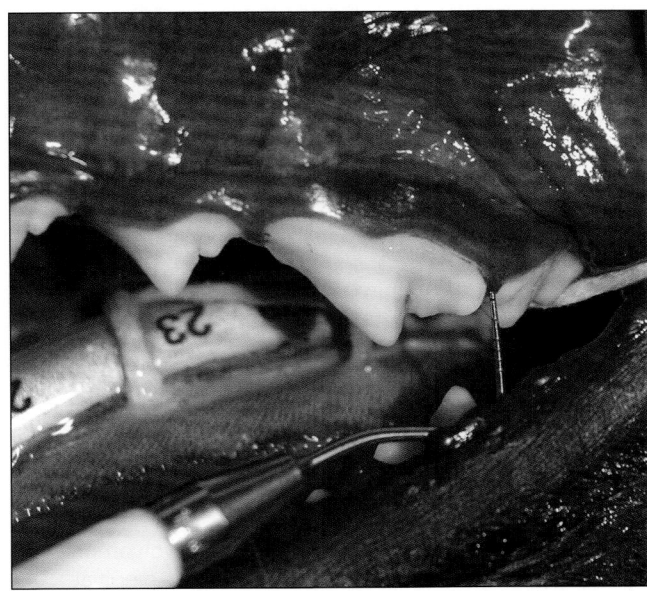

25.1 Gingivitis grade 2 (G2). The gum bleeds when gently probed during the dental examination.

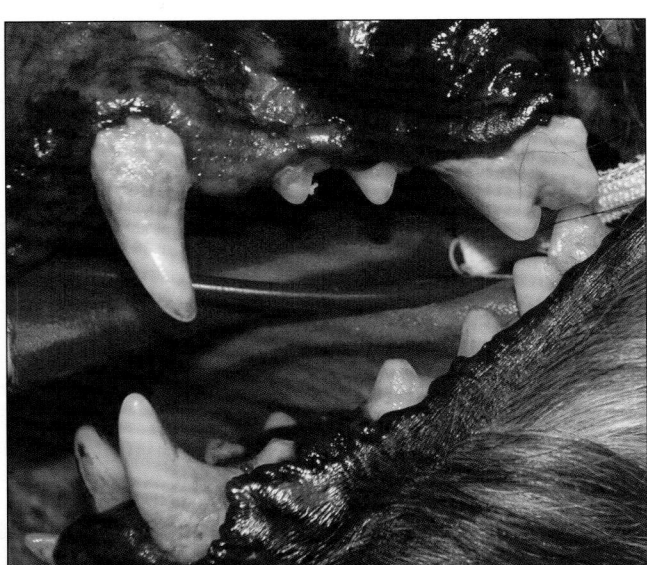

25.2 Periodontal disease in a dog. Note the gingival and bone recession over the canine tooth due to periodontitis. (© Cedric Tutt)

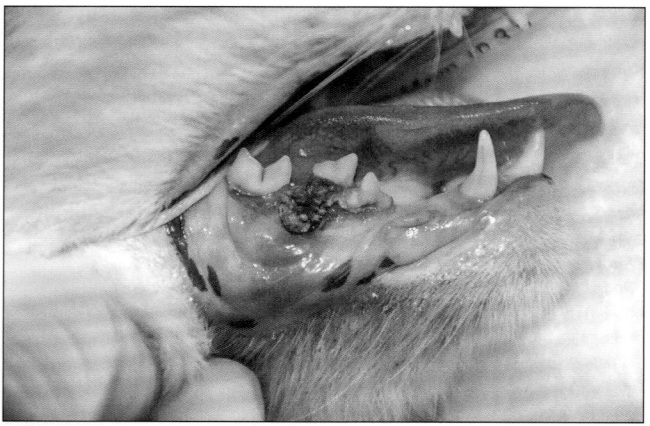

25.3 Severe periodontitis in a cat. The tooth is being shed due to extensive bone loss. (© Cedric Tutt)

Periapical periodontitis is usually associated with an exposed pulp that has become necrotic, resulting in inflammation of the tissues surrounding the apex of the root. This may cause a swelling in the jaw or face, and in some cases a draining sinus tract may connect the periapical lesion with the gingival sulcus. Where this occurs there will be a deep narrow pocket extending all the way to the affected root apex. In other cases, the swelling in the jaw may communicate with the oral mucosa or the skin. Blunt trauma to the crown of the tooth can also result in pulp death and periapical periodontitis, even though the tooth crown is intact and has a healthy appearance. Treatment of these teeth involves endodontic procedures (root canal therapy) or extraction.

There may be associated mucosal and glossal ulcers, gingival recession and furcation lesions (loss of alveolar bone between the roots at the neck of the tooth), bleeding from the mouth and/or loose teeth. Other clinical signs include excessive salivation, dysphagia, pain on chewing and lethargy. However, dogs with periodontal disease often show few or no signs until the disease is well advanced. This may contribute to the late presentation of these dogs to the veterinary practice, making management of their disease more difficult. Patients with severe oral infections may develop transient bacteraemia when they eat and groom themselves. This may be associated with organ disease affecting the heart, liver, lungs and kidneys.

Other terms defining inflammation of oral tissues

Glossitis

Glossitis is defined as inflammation of the tongue and can be associated with plaque and its by-products (Figure 25.4).

Stomatitis

Stomatitis is inflammation of the oral mucosal surfaces and can be further defined as:

- Buccal stomatitis – inflammation of the cheek mucosa
- Palatitis – inflammation of the palatal mucosa
- Caudal oral stomatitis – inflammation of the caudal aspects of the oral cavity, rostral to the oropharynx

---

Stages of periodontal disease:

Periodontal disease is classified in stages and is based on the extent of attachment loss (i.e. loss of periodontal attachment surrounding the tooth) as measured using a periodontal probe and confirmed radiographically. Staging of periodontal disease allows the clinician to determine how far the disease process has progressed for each individual tooth. Any staging refers to the tooth only and not the mouth in general. Assessment of the degree of attachment loss can be estimated with a probe, but must be confirmed radiographically.

- **Stage 0: Normal and healthy periodontium**
  Healthy periodontium, the gingiva should be pink (no gingivitis), except when pigmented, firmly attached to the underlying bone and form a sharp margin where the soft tissues meet the tooth. Radiographs should show good bone height to the cementoenamel junction, no pockets and uninterrupted lamina dura. The periodontal ligament space is seen as a radiographically less dense area surrounding the roots (also known as the lamina lucida). No bleeding evident on probing.
- **Stage 1: Gingivitis**
  Gingivitis only, due to plaque deposition and lack of homecare. Variable amounts of plaque and calculus may be present. Reversible by professional scaling and polishing, followed by diligent homecare practices. There is no attachment loss. Without treatment and with an increase in quantity or virulence of bacteria, this will lead to Stage 2. Sulcus bleeds on probing.
- **Stage 2: Early (mild) periodontitis (early attachment loss)**
  Early disease is defined by attachment loss of up to 25% along with evidence of gingival recession or pocketing, loss of gingival contour and furcation involvement in multirooted teeth. There are early radiographic signs of periodontitis. The loss of periodontal attachment is <25% as measured by probing the clinical attachment or by radiographic determination of the distance of the alveolar margin from the cementoenamel junction relative to the length of the root. Pocket/sulcus bleeds on probing.
- **Stage 3: Moderate periodontitis (moderate attachment loss)**
  Moderate disease is defined by attachment loss of 25–50% as measured by probing and radiographs. Note that gingival recession occurring at the same time as deepening pockets may not increase the probing depth. However, attachment loss is still significant. More noticeable furcation involvement and tooth mobility present. Pocket bleeds on probing.
- **Stage 4: Severe periodontitis (severe attachment loss)**
  Attachment loss is now greater than 50% as measured by probing and radiographs. Significant furcation involvement and more prominent tooth mobility. May be associated with purulent discharge from pockets, spontaneous gingival bleeding and/or possible periodontal abscess formation.

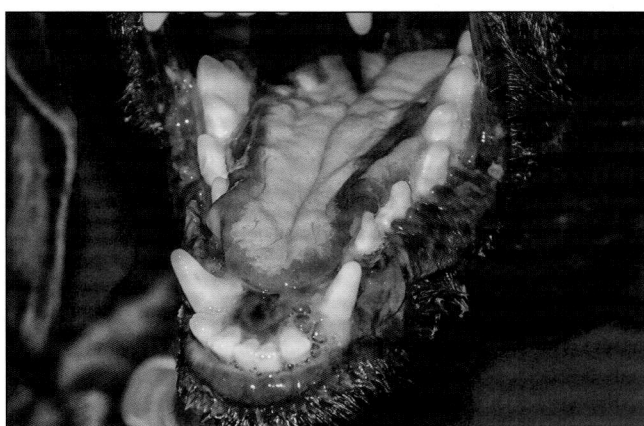

25.4 Gingivostomatitis with periodontitis and marginal glossitis in a dog. (© Cedric Tutt)

- Faucitis – inflammation of the tissues situated medial to the glosso-palatine folds; the area which houses the tonsils in their fossae
- Cheilitis – inflammation of the lips.

The term 'faucitis' is often, incorrectly, used to describe caudal oral inflammation. Caudal oral inflammation describes inflammation of the oral mucosa lateral to the glosso-palatine folds. Generalized gingivitis and stomatitis is common in cats and is being seen more commonly in dogs, especially Maltese and Cocker Spaniels.

Other dental diseases and conditions

Caries

Caries, or dental decay, occurs in dogs, rabbits and chinchillas. In dogs, it usually affects the molars (Figure 25.5), as these teeth have occlusal tables that can trap food that is then fermented by bacteria, forming acids that induce demineralization of the hard tissues of the tooth. Extensive caries can involve tooth dentine and even invade the pulp tissue. Once the dentine has been destroyed the unsupported enamel crown will fracture; in severe cases, the only remaining tooth remnants may be roots protruding through the gingiva.

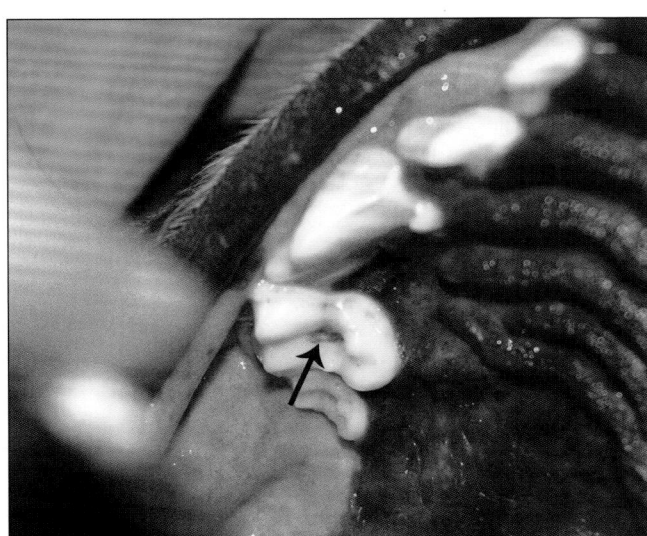

25.5 A typical site for caries in the dog is maxillary molar 1 (tooth 109). There is a discoloured carious lesion on the occlusal surface of tooth 109 (arrowed).

Clinically, caries can usually be seen as craters in the dentine that may be filled with soft brown to grey material (although not all lesions are discoloured). A dental explorer will stick into the tooth surface softened by caries. Teeth with carious lesions should be radiographed to reveal the extent of the disease so that appropriate treatment can be carried out.

Teeth with caries need treatment. If the lesion is extensive, with most of the crown lost, the only treatment option is extraction. It is possible to restore a tooth with a small caries lesion, as long as there is no radiographic evidence of endodontic disease. More severely affected teeth, where the lesion involves the pulp, may need endodontic therapy, but this ideally requires referral to a specialist veterinary dentist. Where parts of the tooth have been destroyed, the only option will be extraction.

Teeth can become stained for a number of reasons and these lesions should not be confused with caries. Stained teeth usually have intact enamel and dentine, and the surface of these lesions will be hard and smooth when examined with a dental explorer. Tooth staining may be intrinsic, where the dentine is discoloured (e.g. antibiotic is incorporated in the tooth substance during tooth development), or extrinsic, where external pigments affect the tooth colour.

Discoloured teeth

Teeth subjected to trauma, whether from a blunt blow (road traffic accident), or as a result of play where teeth have clashed or play with certain toys (tug toys), may become discoloured due to pulp inflammation and bleeding. Blood cells permeate the dentine and initially the tooth may appear pink; thereafter, it will progress through the colour changes experienced in bruised soft tissue, ending up being a dull grey. Discoloured teeth may no longer be vital (living). A vital tooth can be distinguished from a non-vital tooth using a bright light source (e.g. auroscope light source). A non-vital tooth will 'absorb' the light, rather than 'transmitting' it as a vital tooth would. This technique of tooth examination is called transillumination (Figure 25.6). Radiographic examination is required to rule out endodontic disease in these teeth.

Teeth with enamel defects will become discoloured due to pigments in food and also as a result of gingival bleeding. The use of tetracyclines during odontogenesis (development of the tooth – up to about 3 months of age) may cause discoloration of the tooth, as it chelates the calcium laid down in the dental hard tissues and becomes permanently incorporated in the tooth.

Plaque and calculus commonly discolour teeth, but once removed usually a clean crown is revealed. Sometimes calculus formation is associated with demineralization of the crown, leading to discoloration.

Tooth resorption lesions

Tooth resorption lesions (TRs) are common in cats and dogs (Figure 25.7). There are two commonly seen types of tooth resorption, both of which may occur on the same tooth:

- Tooth resorption associated with periodontitis
- Idiopathic tooth resorption with replacement, not associated with inflammation.

Tooth resorption associated with periodontitis is clinically evident (i.e. the resorptive lesion can be seen on the exposed root and crown) and appears as an 'apple-core' lesion on radiographs. With the idiopathic form there is no associated inflammation and most of the lesions are not visible clinically, with the exception of those that have

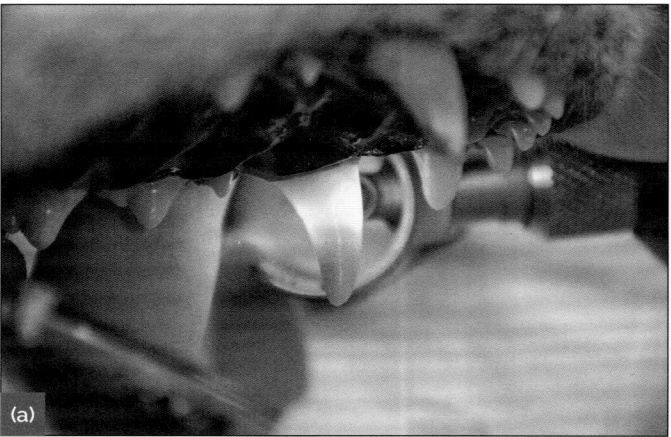
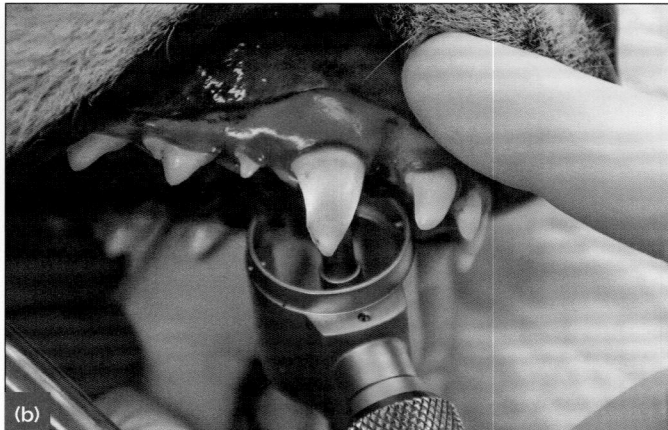

25.6 Transillumination of a canine tooth. (a) Living teeth 'transmit' light and appear 'clear', while (b) 'dead' teeth absorb light and appear dull. (© Cedric Tutt)

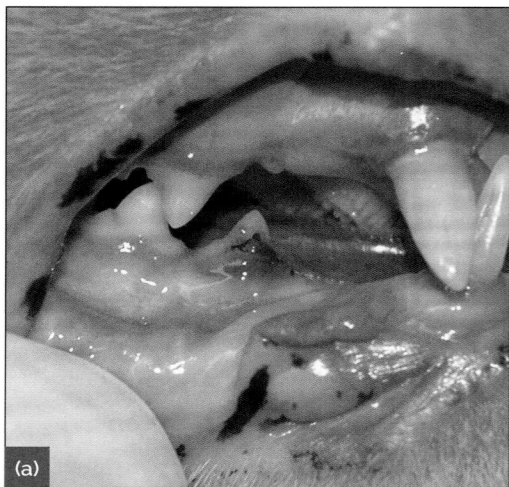

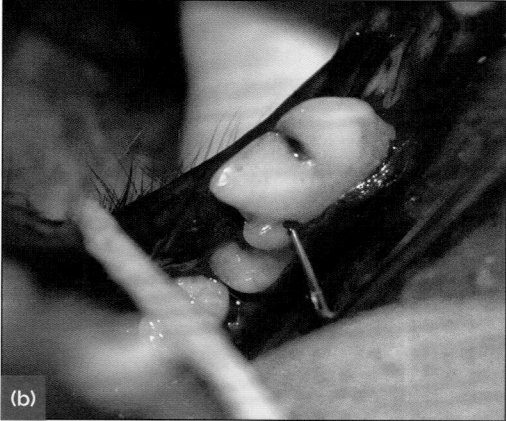

25.7 Tooth resorption lesions (TRs). (a) TR affecting the mandibular right premolar 3 in a cat. (b) TR affecting the mandibular left molar 1 in a dog.

developed up the crown and have associated hyperplastic gingiva. This gingival overgrowth often bleeds when probed with a periodontal probe.

Idiopathic external root resorption begins on the root surface (cementum) and can progress into the root and crown dentine and through the enamel. Often the crowns of affected teeth fracture and remnants may be visible during an oral examination. In these cases, roots undergo replacement resorption where the root substance is resorbed and replaced with bone-like material. Some tooth roots may be partially affected by replacement resorption and may be ankylosed

to the bone; these often fracture during extraction attempts. It is essential to take radiographs of the teeth to be extracted to determine the extent to which the roots are affected by resorption. It does not make sense to try to extract roots that no longer exist. The aetiology of non-inflammatory TRs is unknown.

Enamel hypoplasia/dysplasia

Enamel hypoplasia or dysplasia is incompletely formed or absent enamel on the tooth crown and can be caused by systemic disease, infectious, nutritional, inflammatory, hereditary or traumatic factors. Traumatic injuries to the face and mouth before 3 months of age can damage the enamel organ (enamel-producing and maturing cells), resulting in enamel dysplasia or hypoplasia that is evident when the permanent teeth erupt into the mouth.

Enamel hypoplasia can affect one, several or all of the teeth; it can also affect the primary or secondary teeth depending on when the insult occurred. Clinically, the lesions can affect part of the tooth or the whole tooth, depending on when the developing tooth was affected. The longer the noxious cause is present, the greater the area that will be affected (enamel is not produced over the whole crown at the same time). Distemper virus enters the ameloblasts and destroys them, leading to enamel defects. In addition, Hertwig's root sheath, which is formed by the inner and outer layers of epithelial cells (of the enamel organ), will be affected, disrupting dentine production and root development.

Where enamel production has been deficient, dentine will be exposed and can become infected with plaque bacteria, leading to pulp necrosis and periapical pathology (Figure 25.8) that can lead to abscessation.

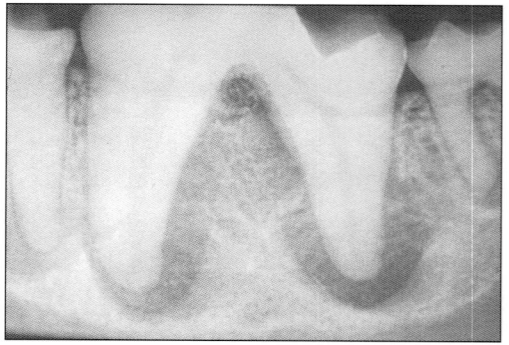

25.8 Radiograph showing periapical pathology due to enamel dysplasia. This resulted in pulpitis and pulp necrosis. (Courtesy of C Gorrel)

Other causes of enamel defects

Fractured deciduous teeth can develop periapical lesions, which can cause enamel defects in the secondary teeth (the inflammatory reaction as a result of pulpitis and pulp necrosis can damage the enamel organ of the developing secondary tooth).

Pyrexia during amelogenesis (development of tooth enamel) causes enamel defects that present as bands of malformed enamel. These teeth may also have an abnormal shape.

Traumatic tooth injuries

Fractured teeth (Figure 25.9) are commonly found on clinical examination and may require referral to a specialist for treatment. Complicated crown fractures, where the pulp is exposed, should be treated either by extraction or by endodontic therapy (root canal therapy). Uncomplicated crown fractures, where the pulp is not exposed, may be treated with a restoration if necessary. Immature teeth (those that have not yet developed a root apex) run the risk of pulpitis when the enamel is damaged exposing the dentine, which has wide tubules at this stage. Dentinal sensitivity often occurs after uncomplicated tooth crown fractures and restoration is required to seal the exposed dentinal tubules, eliminating pain and reducing the likelihood of pulp infection.

Fractures that extend below the gum line compromise the periodontium and therefore should be evaluated by a veterinary surgeon who accepts dentistry referrals to determine whether a restoration can be placed, whether the tooth should be extracted or treated endodontically. Subgingival fractures are more plaque retentive than the normal healthy enamel surface and therefore give plaque a foothold.

Sometimes teeth are luxated or avulsed as a result of trauma. Avulsed teeth (those wrenched from the alveolus) must be handled by the crown, placed in milk at room temperature and sent with the patient to a veterinary surgeon experienced in orthodontics to be replaced in the mouth. This is a dental emergency and the patient must be attended to within hours if the tooth is to be successfully replanted in the alveolus. Replanted teeth inevitably require endodontic treatment because the communication between the pulp and its neurovascular supply has been severed. Luxated teeth (sometimes seen protruding from beneath the lip) also require urgent attention to reduce and stabilize them. Teeth may be traumatically intruded into the jaw, resulting in destruction of the neurovascular supply to the pulp. Endodontic therapy is inevitably required.

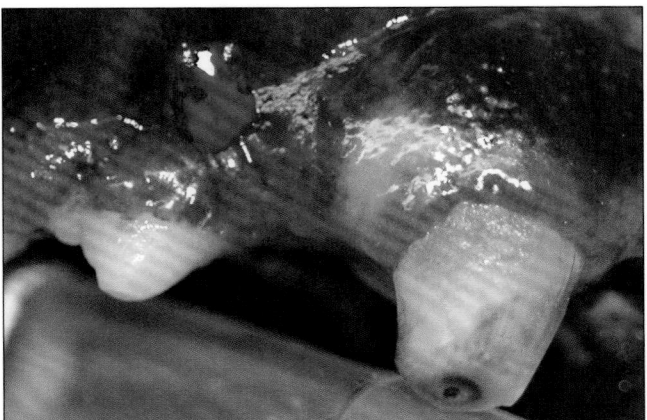

25.9 The pulp in this fractured maxillary right canine tooth has died and caused a root 'abscess' that is draining through the sinus tract at the mucogingival line caudal to the tooth. This dog is also missing maxillary right premolar 1.

Feline oral cavity disease

Chronic gingivostomatitis is commonly seen in cats. These cats are usually in severe pain and need immediate treatment. The aetiology of this disease complex is unknown (probably multifactorial), but affected animals should always be tested for feline leukaemia virus (FeLV), feline immunodeficiency virus (FIV), feline calicivirus (FCV) and feline herpesvirus (FHV). FCV will be isolated from the majority of cats with chronic gingivostomatitis, but the association between this condition and this virus is at present unknown.

Treatment includes antibiotic therapy, professional teeth cleaning, extraction of many or all of the teeth (full-mouth extraction) and dental homecare. Radical extraction is the best long-term option in most cases (about 85% of cats will recover within about 2 years following full-mouth extraction). Full-mouth extraction is a major procedure and it may be advisable to stage the surgery. All affected teeth and any remaining healthy premolars and molars should be extracted during the first procedure; extraction of the canine and incisor teeth should be scheduled later unless it proves necessary to extract them during the initial procedure. It may not be necessary to extract the incisors and canines. Oral rinses or gels containing chlorhexidine gluconate are useful in maintaining oral hygiene postoperatively, as are lactoferrin-containing oral sprays.

The oral examination

Dental formulae

Puppy

2x $\dfrac{\text{i3 c1 pm3}}{\text{i3 c1 pm3}}$ = 28 teeth

Adult dog

2x $\dfrac{\text{I3 C1 PM4 M2}}{\text{I3 C1 PM4 M3}}$ = 42 teeth

Kitten

2x $\dfrac{\text{i3 c1 pm3}}{\text{i3 c1 pm2}}$ = 26 teeth

Adult cat

2x $\dfrac{\text{I3 C1 PM3 M1}}{\text{I3 C1 PM2 M1}}$ = 30 teeth

Where: C = canine; I = incisor; M = molar; PM = premolar. Deciduous teeth are signified by lower case letters.

Dental charting

The oral cavity should be examined thoroughly under general anaesthesia as the conscious examination will reveal only the most superficial and obvious pathology. The animal's head shape (brachycephalic, mesocephalic or dolichocephalic), orientation of canine teeth, occlusion and each individual tooth should be examined and the findings recorded on a dental chart; this is an essential part of the patient's medical records. The lips, cheeks, tongue, hard and soft palates, oropharynx and larynx, tonsils and the oral mucous membranes should also be examined prior to intubation and any abnormalities noted on the chart.

There are many types of dental chart available; examples are shown in Figure 25.10. Each chart has its own system for

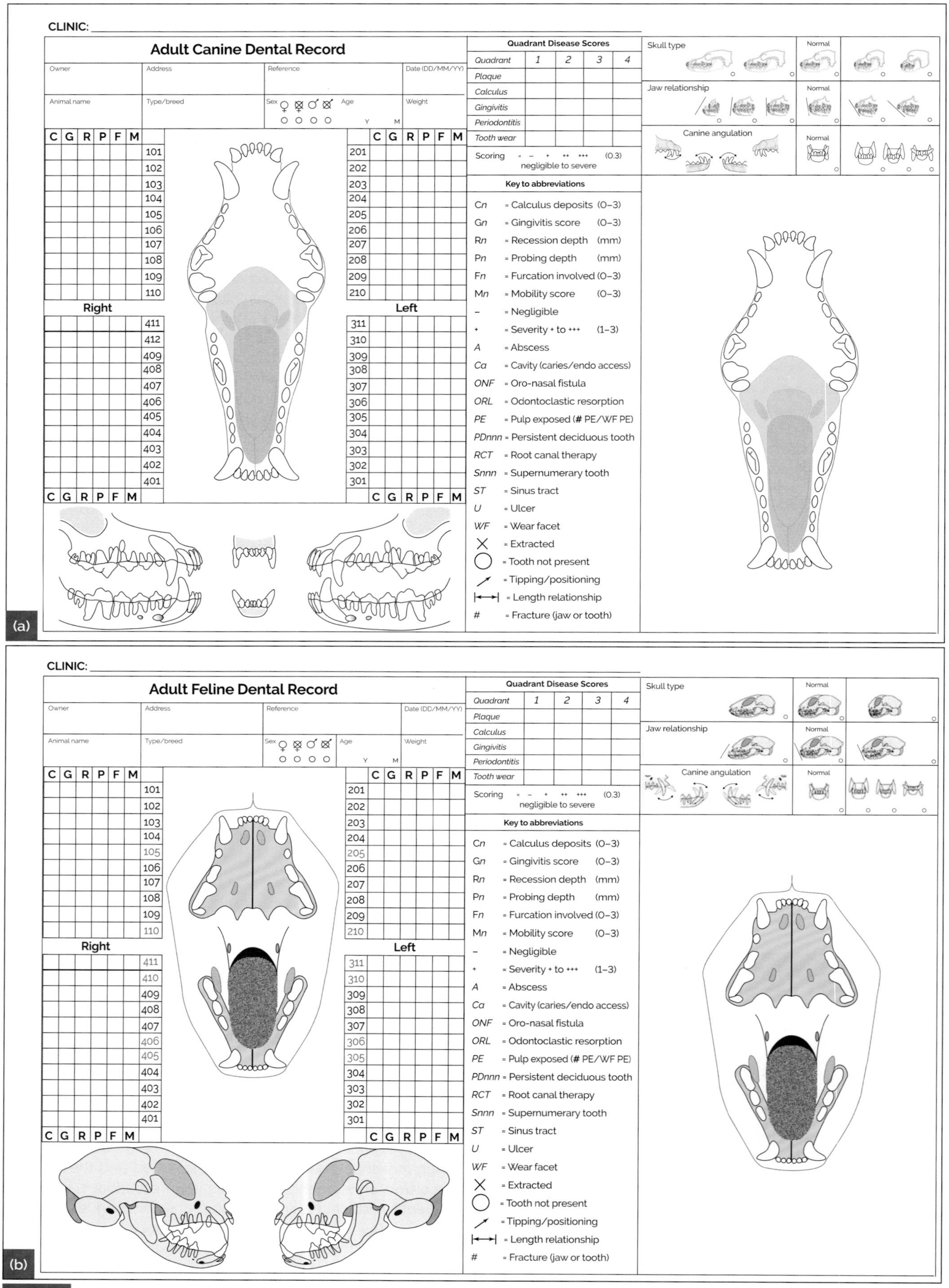

(a)

CLINIC: _____

Adult Canine Dental Record

Owner	Address	Reference	Date (DD/MM/YY)

Animal name	Type/breed	Sex ♀ ⚭ ♂ ⚭ Age	Weight
		○ ○ ○ ○ Y M	

C	G	R	P	F	M		
						101	
						102	
						103	
						104	
						105	
						106	
						107	
						108	
						109	
						110	

Right

C	G	R	P	F	M		
						411	
						412	
						409	
						408	
						407	
						406	
						405	
						404	
						403	
						402	
						401	
C	G	R	P	F	M		

	C	G	R	P	F	M
201						
202						
203						
204						
205						
206						
207						
208						
209						
210						

Left

	C	G	R	P	F	M
311						
310						
309						
308						
307						
306						
305						
304						
303						
302						
301						
	C	G	R	P	F	M

Quadrant Disease Scores

Quadrant	1	2	3	4
Plaque				
Calculus				
Gingivitis				
Periodontitis				
Tooth wear				

Scoring   = − + ++ +++   (0.3)
negligible to severe

Key to abbreviations

Cn = Calculus deposits (0–3)
Gn = Gingivitis score (0–3)
Rn = Recession depth (mm)
Pn = Probing depth (mm)
Fn = Furcation involved (0–3)
Mn = Mobility score (0–3)
− = Negligible
+ = Severity + to +++ (1–3)
A = Abscess
Ca = Cavity (caries/endo access)
ONF = Oro-nasal fistula
ORL = Odontoclastic resorption
PE = Pulp exposed (# PE/WF PE)
PDnnn = Persistent deciduous tooth
RCT = Root canal therapy
Snnn = Supernumerary tooth
ST = Sinus tract
U = Ulcer
WF = Wear facet
✕ = Extracted
○ = Tooth not present
↗ = Tipping/positioning
|↔| = Length relationship
= Fracture (jaw or tooth)

Skull type   Normal

Jaw relationship   Normal

Canine angulation   Normal

(b)

CLINIC: _____

Adult Feline Dental Record

Owner	Address	Reference	Date (DD/MM/YY)

Animal name	Type/breed	Sex ♀ ⚭ ♂ ⚭ Age	Weight
		○ ○ ○ ○ Y M	

C	G	R	P	F	M		
						101	
						102	
						103	
						104	
						105	
						106	
						107	
						108	
						109	
						110	

Right

C	G	R	P	F	M		
						411	
						410	
						409	
						408	
						407	
						406	
						405	
						404	
						403	
						402	
						401	
C	G	R	P	F	M		

	C	G	R	P	F	M
201						
202						
203						
204						
205						
206						
207						
208						
209						
210						

Left

	C	G	R	P	F	M
311						
310						
309						
308						
307						
306						
305						
304						
303						
302						
301						
	C	G	R	P	F	M

Quadrant Disease Scores

Quadrant	1	2	3	4
Plaque				
Calculus				
Gingivitis				
Periodontitis				
Tooth wear				

Scoring   = − + ++ +++   (0.3)
negligible to severe

Key to abbreviations

Cn = Calculus deposits (0–3)
Gn = Gingivitis score (0–3)
Rn = Recession depth (mm)
Pn = Probing depth (mm)
Fn = Furcation involved (0–3)
Mn = Mobility score (0–3)
− = Negligible
+ = Severity + to +++ (1–3)
A = Abscess
Ca = Cavity (caries/endo access)
ONF = Oro-nasal fistula
ORL = Odontoclastic resorption
PE = Pulp exposed (# PE/WF PE)
PDnnn = Persistent deciduous tooth
RCT = Root canal therapy
Snnn = Supernumerary tooth
ST = Sinus tract
U = Ulcer
WF = Wear facet
✕ = Extracted
○ = Tooth not present
↗ = Tipping/positioning
|↔| = Length relationship
= Fracture (jaw or tooth)

Skull type   Normal

Jaw relationship   Normal

Canine angulation   Normal

25.10 Examples of dental recording charts used in **(a)** dogs and **(b)** cats. (© Cedric Tutt and David A Crossley)

recording clinical findings and the choice of charting system is a matter of personal preference. It should be noted that dental charts are viewed as if one is looking at the animal face on, i.e. the right side of the mouth is shown and recorded on the left of the chart, the maxillary crowns face down and the mandibular crowns face up.

Triadan numbering system

On most of the commercially available charts for dogs the teeth are numbered using the three-digit Triadan numbering system. The first numeral denotes which quadrant the tooth is in and whether the tooth is part of the permanent or deciduous dentition:

Quadrant	Deciduous dentition numeral	Secondary dentition numeral
Right maxilla	5	1
Left maxilla	6	2
Left mandible	7	3
Right mandible	8	4

The second and third numbers in this system denote the tooth.

Examples:

- The tooth numbered 104 is the right maxillary canine tooth
- The tooth numbered 208 is the left maxillary fourth premolar tooth
- The tooth numbered 401 is the right mandibular first incisor.

The Triadan system is used for the dog. The cat has fewer teeth and the missing teeth are therefore omitted from the chart, known as the Modified Triadan System of dental nomenclature (e.g. the mandibular first and second premolars and the second and third molars are not present in the cat; see Figure 25.10b).

When completing dental charts, abbreviations are used to record the information.

Commonly used abbreviations

- Ca = Caries lesion
- CCF = Complicated crown fracture (may be recorded as '#PE')
- ED = Enamel defect
- GH = Gingival overgrowth
- GR = Gingival recession
- NAD = No abnormality detected
- ONF = Oronasal fistula
- PE = Pulp exposure
- TD = Tertiary dentine
- TR = Tooth resorptive lesion
- UCF = Uncomplicated crown fracture
- WF = Wear facet
- # = Fracture

Tooth fractures are denoted by a line drawn on the chart showing the location and orientation of the fracture. For example, if the fracture extends below the gingiva the line should be drawn correspondingly on the chart. Missing teeth are circled. Teeth extracted are crossed through. The patient's occlusion (e.g. scissor bite, short mandibles, short maxillae) can also be recorded on some charts.

The examination and recording procedure

The following information should be recorded for each individual tooth on the charts:

- Calculus scores
- Gingivitis scores
- Periodontal probing depth
- Mobility
- Gingival recession
- Gingival overgrowth
- Presence of traumatic injuries
- Exposed pulp
- Enamel defects, abrasion and attrition
- Caries
- Stain
- Supernumerary teeth
- Mixed dentition (simultaneous presence of deciduous and secondary teeth)
- Retained teeth (unerupted teeth)
- Persistent deciduous teeth
- Soft tissue injuries
- Oral masses.

Calculus scores

Gross calculus should be removed prior to examining the teeth and therefore calculus scoring should be carried out first. A slight (CS or 1), moderate (CM or 2) and heavy (CH or 3) scoring method is used. By scoring and recording calculus at the initial consultation, the examiner is able to compare the teeth against these scores at subsequent examinations. This enables the examiner to monitor the effectiveness of dental homecare programmes. If homecare programmes are correctly implemented the amount of calculus seen at subsequent examinations should be significantly decreased.

Some animals may have heavy calculus on the teeth on one side of the mouth and slight to moderate on the other. There is often a reason for this; for example, there may be a fractured tooth preventing chewing on the side with heavy calculus. Heavy calculus deposits on the teeth on one side of the mouth should also alert the examiner to the possibility of occult disease.

Calculus is rough and porous and highly plaque retentive, and although it does not cause periodontitis directly, the fact that it allows the accumulation of plaque often leads to gingivitis.

Gingivitis scores

The modified Löe and Silness gingival index is generally used. It relies on visual inspection and the presence of bleeding on probing of the gingival sulcus (Figure 25.11).

Periodontal probing depth

The periodontal probe (see 'Dental instrumentation and equipment' below) should be inserted gently into the gingival sulcus until resistance is encountered at the sulcus base. The depth from the free gingival margin to the base of the sulcus is measured in millimetres. The normal depth of the gingival sulcus is 1–3 mm in dogs and <0.5 mm in cats. Measurements that exceed these values indicate the presence of pockets or pseudo-pockets. The measurement should be marked on the dental chart as close to its position on the actual tooth as possible.

Grade	Furcation	Mobility	Gingivitis	
0	No furcation involvement	No mobility	Healthy gingiva	
1	Probe dips in at the furcation – little bone loss	Horizontal movement of 1 mm or less in one plane	Marginal redness with slight thickening of marginal gingiva	
2	Probe passes to mid-furcation – significant bone loss	Horizontal movement of 1 mm or more in two planes	Gingival margin thick and red. Bleeds on probing	
3	Probe passes from buccal to lingual/palatal – no furcation bone remaining	Vertical as well as horizontal movement is possible	Gingiva thickened and red (to bluish). Bleeds spontaneously or when touched	

25.11 Grading of gingivitis, tooth mobility and furcation lesions.

Where probing depths are increased, measurements should be recorded at four sites around the tooth. Some examiners prefer to have one recording per tooth; for example, if the probing depths were as follows: mesiopalatal = 3 mm, mesiobuccal = 3 mm, distobuccal = 5 mm, and disto-palatal = 6 mm, they would record a probing depth of 6 mm (i.e. the worse score is recorded) for the tooth. If the tooth has a single root it may be appropriate to use this scoring system but if there are multiple roots, recording four measurements per tooth is more suitable.

Furcation lesions

In patients with periodontitis, the roots of multirooted teeth can become exposed and the furcation between them becomes visible. Furcation exposure is graded from 0 to 3, depending on severity (grade 3 being when the probe passes through the furcation from one side to the other; see Figure 25.11).

Mobility

Tooth mobility can be tested by using the blunt end of a dental instrument (e.g. the handle of the mirror) in an attempt to move the tooth from its normal position. Using fingers can give a false-positive movement due to the give in the finger. The grading of tooth mobility is shown in Figure 25.11.

Gingival recession

Gingival recession is measured using a periodontal probe (Figure 25.12) and is the distance between the clinical gingival margin and an imaginary line drawn across the normal gingival height at the mesial and distal edges of the tooth or mid-buccal surface, depending upon where the defect is. The gingival contour can be drawn on the dental chart, showing the shape of the defect. In some cases, the bone will have receded as well and this should also be noted on the chart.

Gingival overgrowth

Overgrown gingiva forms pseudo-pockets as there is an increased probing depth from the margin of the overgrown tissue to the bottom of the sulcus. In some animals with gingival overgrowth, true pockets may also be present in response to plaque on the tooth surface (i.e. they may have concurrent periodontitis). The term gingival overgrowth should be used where the gingiva is enlarged. Boxers and, to a lesser extent, Border Collies and Labrador Retrievers show a predisposition for the condition. Gingival hyperplasia is a histopathological/laboratory diagnosis.

Presence of traumatic injuries

This includes, for example, fractured teeth, fractured jaws, symphysial separations/fractures, temporomandibular joint (TMJ) dislocations, gingival clefts, traumatic cleft palates and foreign bodies. Foreign bodies may become lodged across the palate between the maxillary carnassial teeth (Figure 25.13) or longitudinally along the cheek teeth, and may cause the jaws to lock closed or prevent the animal from closing its jaws. Patients with oral foreign bodies are often presented with halitosis. This is due to food and other foreign matter around the object becoming necrotic. Some foreign bodies are found during routine oral examinations, without prior clinical signs having been noted. Fractures are denoted on the chart using a #, written adjacent to the affected tooth.

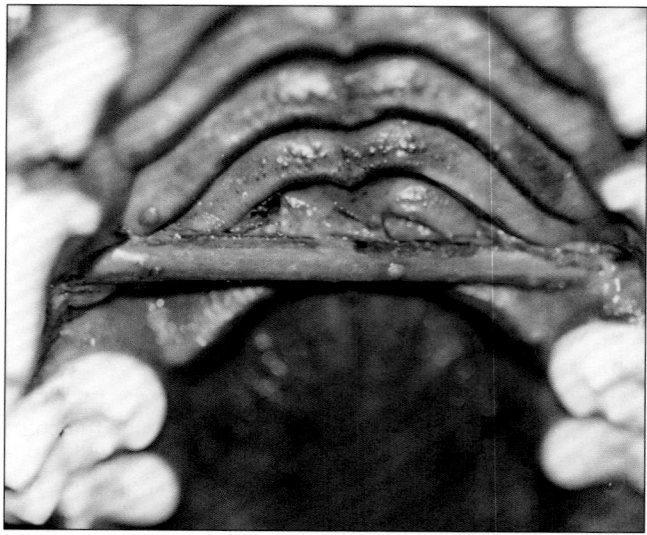

25.12 Gingival recession is measured from the clinical gingival margin to a line joining the normal gingival height mesially and distally on the tooth.

25.13 This foreign body trapped across the palate was an incidental finding in a patient that had a recent history of halitosis.

Exposed pulp

Exposed pulp is denoted on the chart by PE, written adjacent to the affected tooth.

Enamel defects, abrasion and attrition

Enamel defects may be due to trauma or developmental abnormalities.

- Abrasion is the abnormal wear of teeth as a result of the animal's behaviour, e.g. stick or stone chewing, cage biting or playing with a tennis ball (tennis balls are inappropriate toys as they gather sand and grit and abrade the teeth each time they come in contact with them).
- Attrition is abnormal wear due to tooth-to-tooth contact, often seen in dogs with a malocclusion (e.g. brachycephalic dogs with a tight canine–canine–lateral incisor interlock).

Caries

Teeth affected by caries must be differentiated from those that are stained or undergoing resorption. Caries usually present as enamel defects on the tooth surface, into which the dental explorer will stick when gently explored. It is often associated with deep dentine craters and halitosis. Surface caries may be seen on carnassial teeth and appear as black pits in the enamel. Animals suffering from caries are often presented due to halitosis recognized by the owner.

Stain

Teeth that become worn and have exposed secondary or tertiary dentine often become stained. Tertiary dentine is less structured than secondary dentine and becomes stained by food and other pigments. Arrested caries often also become stained due to the increased permeability of the enamel before remineralization occurs. Surface stain may be removed by polishing, but care must be taken not to damage the pulp as a result of the frictional heat of polishing.

Supernumerary teeth

Supernumerary teeth (teeth in addition to the normal number) may be smaller than their normal counterparts. Some are termed peg teeth, due to their conical shape. These teeth should be drawn on the dental chart. These teeth may require extraction, depending on their relationship to the surrounding secondary dentition (Figure 25.14).

Mixed dentition

The patient's dentition is considered mixed if there are deciduous and secondary teeth in the mouth at the same time (Figure 25.15). Deciduous teeth that are still present in the mouth when the secondary teeth have come into occlusion are considered persistent deciduous teeth and should be extracted to prevent compromise of the secondary dentition. Extraction of deciduous teeth should be performed with extreme care as they have long and narrow roots that may be partly resorbed. Radiographs should be taken prior to extraction to help determine which of the teeth are deciduous and if root substance is still present.

Retained teeth

Retained teeth are those that are found by radiographic examination after they were noted to be clinically missing from the mouth. In other words, they have not erupted and

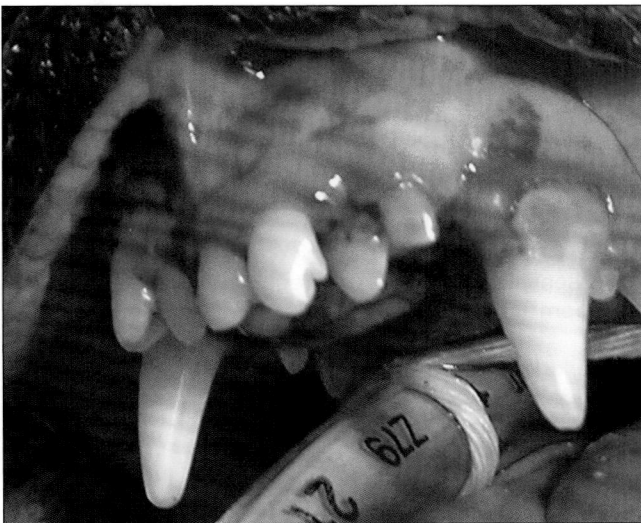

25.14 This dog has supernumerary incisors. The incisor set back in the palate has periodontal disease as a result of trapped food and other debris. There is also bony and gingival recession affecting the canine tooth.

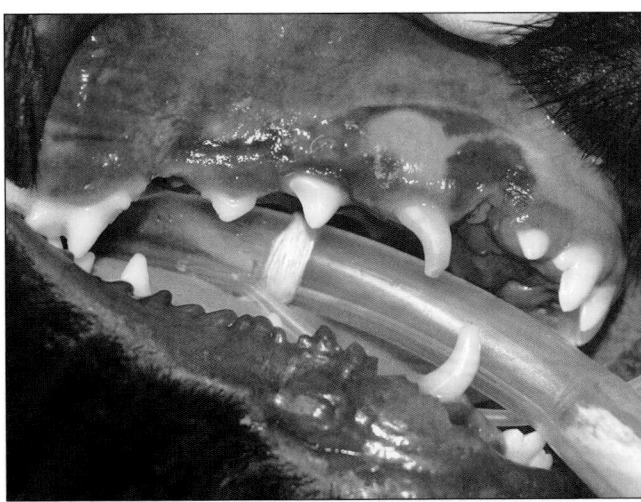

25.15 This puppy has mixed dentition: some secondary teeth have already erupted, while some deciduous teeth are still present. None of the deciduous teeth here would be considered persistent as they do not occupy the same location as a secondary tooth.

remain below the alveolar margin and gingiva. This may be due to impaction where the eruption pathway is obstructed by an adjacent tooth. These teeth may be associated with other pathology (e.g. dentigerous cysts).

Soft tissue injuries

Oral soft tissue injuries should be charted. These include ulcers, lacerations secondary to tooth trauma and degloving injuries.

Oral masses

The presence of oral masses should be noted on the dental chart; a periodontal probe can be used to measure the dimensions. Biopsy of the mass is required for a diagnosis and to establish a prognosis for the patient. It is recommended that a deep incisional biopsy sample be taken and submitted for histopathological evaluation by an experienced oral pathologist.

Dental instrumentation and equipment

It is important that all instruments are clean, sterilized and sharpened (if necessary) before use on each patient. Equipment care and maintenance is of utmost importance. The power equipment should also be regularly maintained and serviced to ensure good working order.

Essential instruments used regularly in the dental operating room are:

- Periodontal probe
- Periodontal (dental) explorer
- Mirror
- Calculus-removing forceps
- Hand scaler and curette
- Ultrasonic and sonic scalers
- Dental unit (power equipment)
- Dental Luxator®
- Dental elevator
- Periosteal elevator
- Extraction forceps
- Surgical kit.

Periodontal probe

This is a blunt-ended graduated instrument used to measure gingival sulcus and periodontal pocket depths. It can also be used to measure gingival recession (see Figure 25.12) and overgrowth and for gingivitis scoring, as it is circumscribed around the tooth in the gingival sulcus. It can be used to grade furcation lesions, and the handle (on single-ended instruments) can be used to grade tooth mobility. The graduations on the periodontal probe should be measured so that pocket depth and other measurements are accurate. A Williams 14 periodontal probe (Figure 25.16) is ideal.

Periodontal (dental) explorer

This is a needle-sharp, straight or curved instrument (see Figure 25.16b) used to explore the tooth surfaces for the presence of caries or other enamel defects (e.g. enamel hypoplasia, fractured teeth and tooth resorptive lesions). It is also possible to explore subgingivally using a dental explorer to examine for residual calculus after the scale and polish

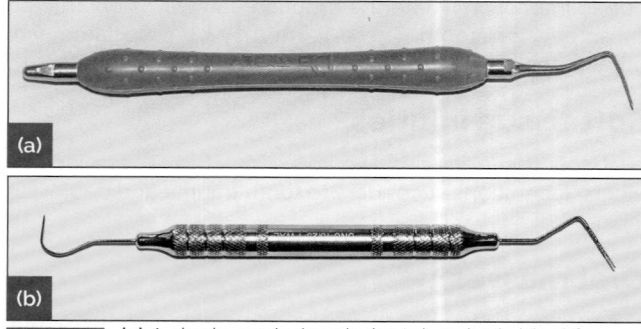

25.16 **(a)** A single-ended periodontal probe is ideal for measuring gingival recession and periodontal pocket depth. The blunt end can be used to grade tooth mobility by gently pressing it against the tooth. **(b)** Periodontal probe (right end) combined with a dental explorer (left end). Some clinicians prefer a double-ended instrument, whilst others prefer individual probes and explorers. (© Cedric Tutt)

procedure. It is important to keep the dental explorer sharp. This instrument should be replaced when damaged, as excessive hand-sharpening produces a roughened tip that is undesirable.

Mirror

A dental mirror is commonly used in human dentistry, less commonly in veterinary dentistry. It can be used to visualize the palatal and lingual surfaces of teeth, as well as the distal surfaces of the caudal teeth. It can also be used to reflect light into poorly lit areas of the mouth and to examine the nasopharynx. Wiping the surface of the mirror against a moist mucosal surface prevents the mirror from fogging.

Calculus-removing forceps

Calculus-removing forceps (Figure 25.17) must be correctly used by placing one beak on the gingival extent of the calculus and the other on the incisal tip of the tooth. This generates a shearing force that dislodges the calculus from the tooth surface. Under no circumstances should the tooth surface be 'pinched' between the beaks of the forceps, or the crown may shatter. Care must also be exercised when placing the forceps at the gingival margin, or the gingiva can be damaged as well.

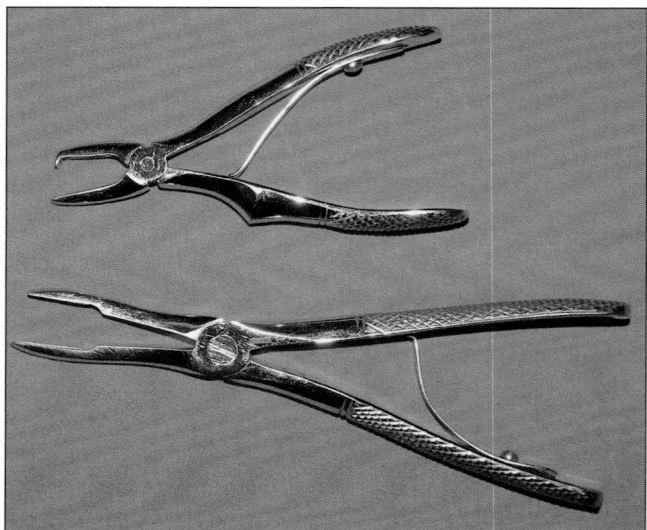

25.17 Calculus-removing forceps are available in numerous patterns. They must be used with care to prevent damage to the tooth and gingiva.

Hand scaler and curette

The dental scale and polish procedure is described in a later section. The scaler and curette (Figure 25.18) are used to remove dental deposits from the tooth surfaces. They consist of a handle, shank and a working tip. The scaler has a sharp, pointed tip that should only be used supragingivally (subgingival use will result in laceration of the gingival tissues). The curette has a blade that ends in a blunt, rounded tip that can be used subgingivally for removal of subgingival deposits and root debridement. Both the scaler and curette should be pulled away from the gingiva towards the tip of the crown of the tooth. It is important to maintain the sharp edges of these instruments for efficient use.

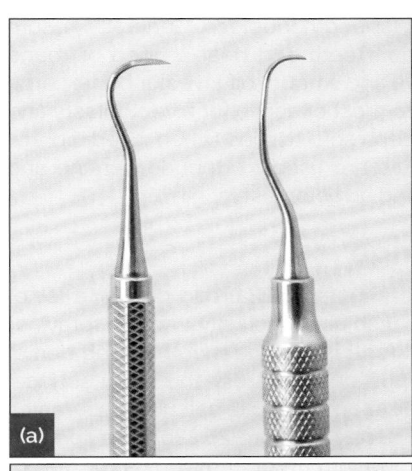

25.18 (a) The hand curette (right) has a blunt end, while the scaler (left) has a sharp tip and is only used above the gum line. (b) The hand scaler (left) and curette (right) as viewed from the working side. (© Cedric Tutt)

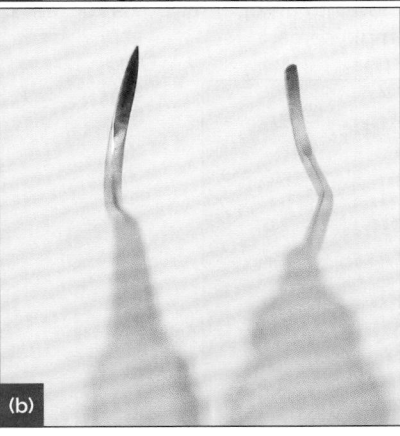

Ultrasonic and sonic scalers

The tip of an ultrasonic scaler oscillates at ultrasonic frequencies and is driven by an electromagnetic or a piezo-electric (Figure 25.19) handpiece. Some ultrasonic tips are manufactured for supragingival or subgingival use. Some subgingival ultrasonic scaler tips are designed to be used on the 'push' rather than 'pull' stroke. Sonic scalers are air-driven and rather than being electrical are mechanical. Sub- and supragingival tips are available for sonic scalers too.

Tip vibration in magnetostrictive scalers is created by an electromagnetic field in the handpiece that surrounds a metal stack or ferrite rod. When an alternating electric current is applied to the handpiece, the insert vibrates. Piezoelectric scaler tips vibrate because of deformation of a crystal in the handpiece when an alternating electric current is applied to it. Sonic scalers are available that are

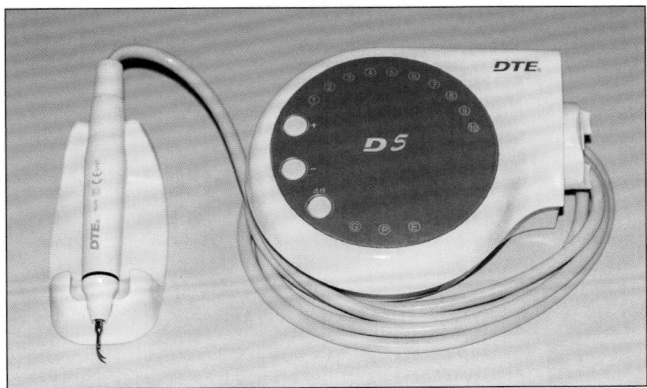

25.19 The piezoelectric ultrasonic scaler unit. (© Cedric Tutt)

driven by compressed air. Tip vibration is caused when air is driven through an eccentric hole in the shaft to which the tip is attached.

All electromechanical scalers have coolant water directed at their tips and this must be adjusted for optimal function. The water is also responsible for the phenomenon known as cavitation, by which very small bubbles that develop within the coolant liquid implode on the calculus, helping to dislodge it. Cavitation has also been shown to cause disruption of the cell walls of some plaque bacteria (spirochaetes).

Scalers must never be used with their tips perpendicular to the tooth surface, as the action of the vibrating tip will damage the tooth surface (gouge the enamel). Ultrasonic instruments were first invented to section (cut) teeth prior to extraction, therefore improper use will damage teeth.

The dental unit (power equipment)

Dental units (Figure 25.20) are available with numerous attachments but the minimum requirements are: high-speed handpiece; low-speed handpiece with contra-angled 'prophy' attachment; (low-speed straight handpiece for rabbit dentistry); three-way air–water syringe; and an ultrasonic scaler. The ultrasonic scaler may be combined into the dental unit or be a stand-alone piece of equipment (see Figure 25.19).

High-speed handpiece

The high-speed handpiece facilitates tooth extractions by allowing the operator to section multirooted teeth prior to extraction. The bur in the handpiece rotates at about 400,000 rpm (revolutions per minute). High-speed handpieces are more efficient at sectioning teeth, but care must be exercised when using them to prevent air emboli and emphysema formation. Some high-speed handpieces have an integrated fibreoptic or LED light that improves visibility in the work field. It is essential that protective eyewear is worn by both the operator and the assistant when this equipment is used.

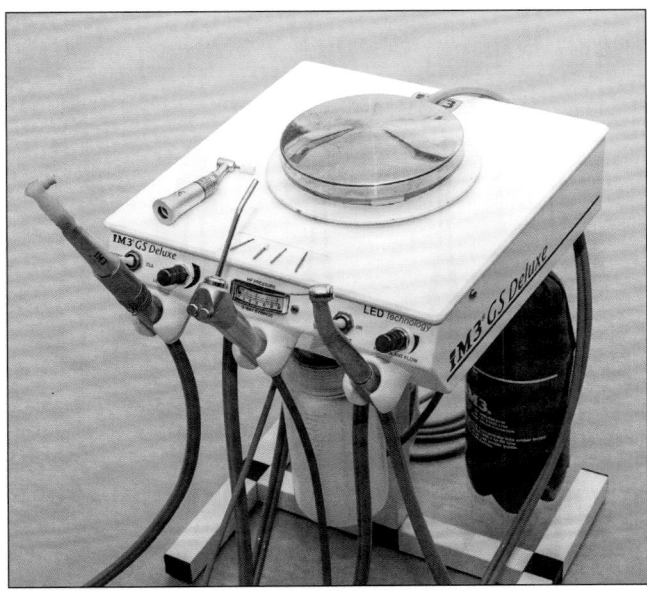

25.20 The dental unit. From the left: low-speed handpiece with reciprocating polishing head; three-way air–water syringe; and high-speed handpiece. This unit has cooling fluid for low- and high-speed handpieces. (© Cedric Tutt)

Low-speed handpiece

The low-speed air motor on the dental unit can accept contra-angle or straight handpieces. It also accepts the contra-angled polishing head. The rotation speed of this air motor is adjustable up to 5500 rpm (but speed-reducing and speed-increasing handpieces may also be used), however polishing is normally performed at less than 3500 rpm. Straight surgical handpieces are available for use with the low-speed air motor. These can be used for removing and shaping alveolar bone. When being used for sectioning teeth (in combination with a speed-increasing handpiece) and alveolotomy (incision into the dental alveolus) or alveoloplasty (surgical shaping of the dental alveolus), the tooth or bone must be kept cool by applying sterile coolant to the bur and tooth or bone. This is most effectively carried out by an assistant squirting a gentle stream of polyionic fluid from a syringe on to the operating site. It should be noted that it is not ideal to use a low-speed handpiece to section teeth; however, they are efficient at removing compromised dentine in carious lesions. Electric motor driven low-speed units are also available and these have a greater torque than the air motor units. Some low-speed air and electric motors have internal cooling, which not only keeps the motor cool, but also supplies coolant to the bur as well.

Burs

Various burs are available for the high- and low-speed handpieces (Figure 25.21). Friction grip (FG) burs fit into the turbine of a high-speed handpiece and right angle (RA) burs fit into the grip/latch of a low-speed handpiece. Generally, fissure burs are used to section teeth and pear-shaped or round burs are used to remove and smooth off alveolar bone. Large round diamond burs are most effective for alveoloplasty and do not damage adjacent soft tissues when used appropriately. Low-speed burs are used to debride dentine and perform alveolotomy and alveoloplasty.

Three-way syringe

The three-way syringe (Figure 25.22a) can deliver a jet of water, or a jet of water with air (effectively a water spray), or just air. It is very useful for flushing the mouth during dental procedures. A gentle puff of air will dry the tooth surface, enabling better visualization; residual calculus resembles chalk on the dry tooth surface (Figure 25.22b). The spray or air should not be directed into an open alveolus for fear of causing air emboli or emphysema.

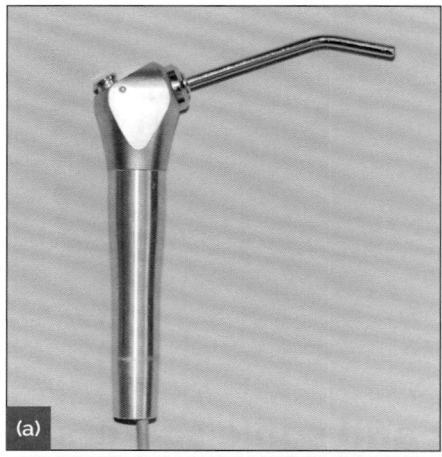

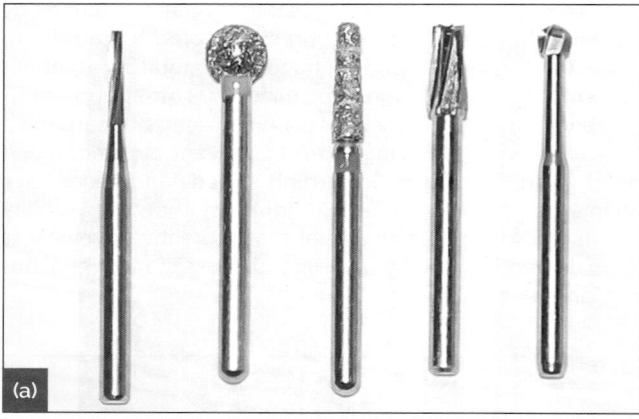

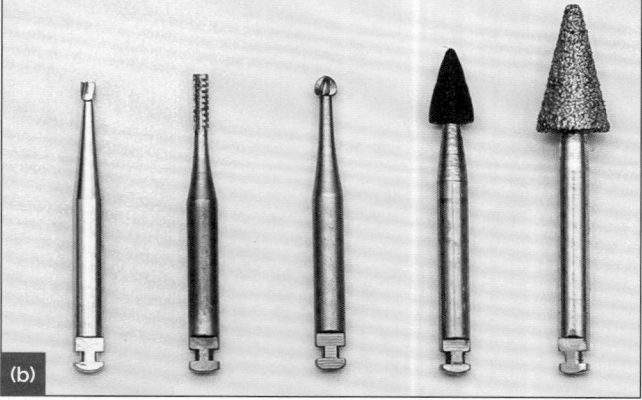

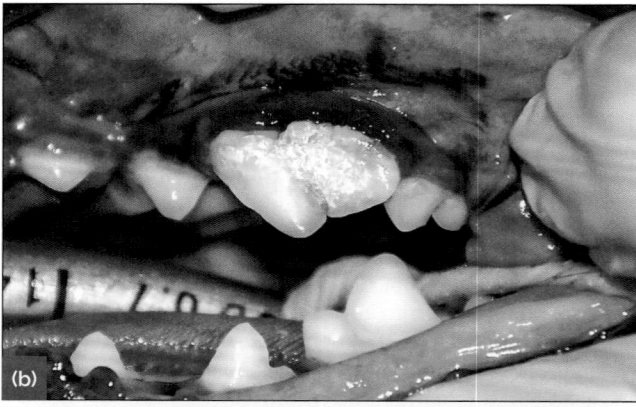

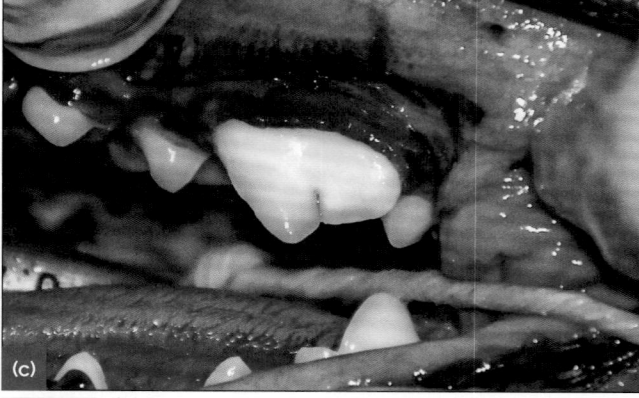

25.21 (a) Friction grip (FG) burs (high-speed burs). From the left: tapered fissure cross-cutting tungsten carbide; round diamond; tapered diamond fissure; tapered fissure cross-cutting tungsten carbide; and round tungsten carbide. (b) Right angle (RA) burs (low-speed burs). From the left: inverted cone tungsten carbide; straight fissure tungsten carbide; round tungsten carbide; flame shape polishing bur; and flame shape diamond bur for odontoplasty/alveoloplasty. (© Cedric Tutt)

25.22 (a) Three-way syringe which delivers air, water or a mist. (b) Dried calculus on the tooth surface and (c) the same tooth after a scale and polish procedure has been performed. (© Cedric Tutt)

Dental Luxator®

The dental Luxator® (Directa Dental AB, Sweden) is used to sever the periodontal ligaments during tooth extraction. It has a fine, sharp tip (Figure 25.23) that is used to cut the epithelial attachment and periodontal ligament, which hold the tooth in the alveolus. An appropriately sized instrument should be used for the root in question (the curvature of the Luxator® blade should approximate that of the root being extracted). When the Luxator® is driven into the periodontal ligament space it causes condensation of the alveolar bone, creating more space that will allow insertion of the dental elevator to further loosen the tooth.

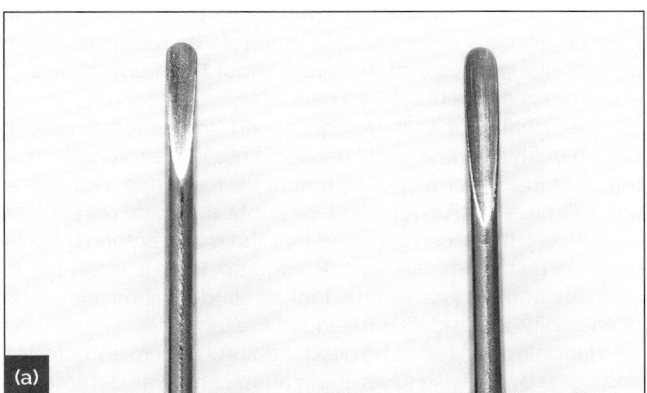

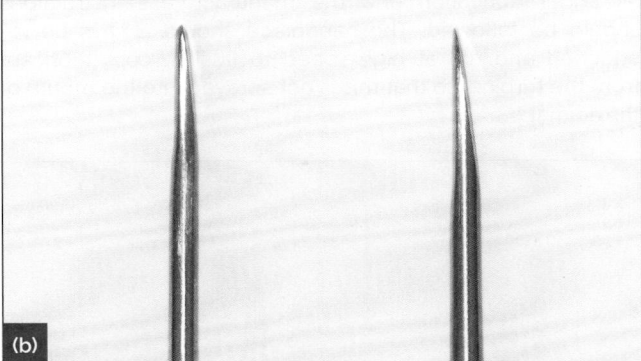

25.23 **(a)** The Luxator Forte® (left) is more robust and is less tapered at the tip, enabling increased rotational leverage. The Luxator® (right) has a fine sharp point that facilitates severing of the periodontal ligament and compression of the alveolar bone, creating space to use the Luxator Forte® (left). **(b)** The Luxator Forte® (left) and Luxator® (right) as viewed from the side. (© Cedric Tutt)

Dental elevator

Once the gingival attachment has been severed and most of the periodontal ligament has been severed and torn and sufficient space has been created by using the Luxator®, the dental elevator (Figure 25.24) can be worked into the alveolus and used to apply rotational leverage on the root, disrupting its attachment further and leading to it being delivered from the alveolus. The Luxator Forte® (see Figure 25.23) can also be used following the Luxator®.

Periosteal elevator

The periosteal elevator (Figure 25.25) is necessary for surgical extraction procedures and other oral surgery. It is used to raise the gingival and mucoperiosteal flap to expose the

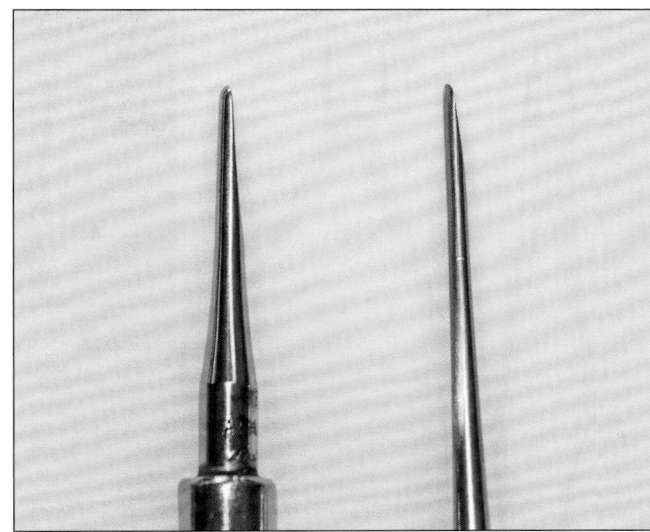

25.24 The Luxator® (right) is sharpened to a fine point, whereas the elevator (left) is sharpened to about 45 degrees. (© Cedric Tutt)

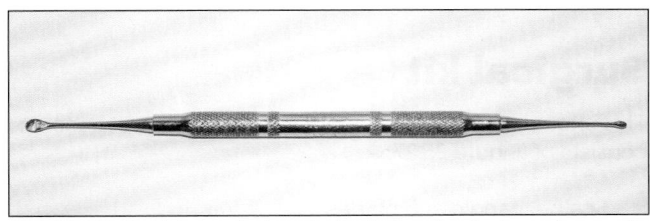

25.25 Double-ended periosteal elevator that can be used in small dogs and cats. (© Cedric Tutt)

alveolar bone. Once the gingival and releasing alveolar mucosal incisions have been made, the periosteal elevator is inserted below the periosteum beneath the alveolar mucosa and worked along the bone surface, raising the periosteum. Once the alveolar mucosal periosteum has been raised from the bone, the instrument is worked along the bone in the direction of the alveolar margin and then under the attached gingiva. If approached via the gingival sulcus there is a risk that the periosteal elevator will puncture the flap at the mucogingival junction.

Extraction forceps

Extraction forceps should not be used by the veterinary surgeon without prior training. Extraction forceps must be used appropriately, as incorrect use could fracture the crown of the tooth. There are numerous extraction forceps beak patterns manufactured to fit human teeth. Most of these are inappropriate for use in veterinary dentistry. The beak size used should approximate to the size of the root to be extracted to ensure an appropriate fit (Figure 25.26).

The tooth crown/root must be firmly grasped using the forceps and an intrusive force applied, followed by clockwise and anticlockwise rotational forces. At the end of each rotation, the intrusional and rotational forces must be maintained for about 10 seconds before rotation in the opposite direction. When the tooth is loose, an extrusional force can be applied to try and deliver the tooth from the alveolus. If this is unsuccessful, additional luxation and elevation techniques must be employed, followed by forceps manipulation.

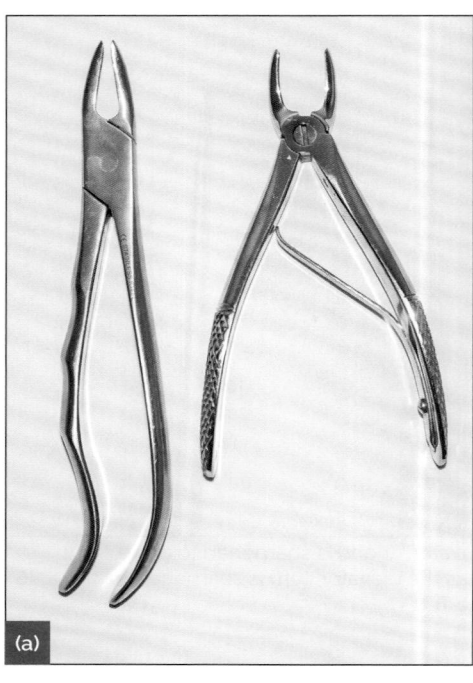

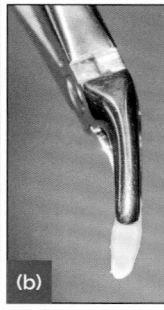

25.26

(a) Extraction forceps. **(b)** Forceps fitting the tooth root surface. (© Cedric Tutt)

Surgical kit

This should be readily available for surgical extractions and consists of (Figure 25.27):

■ Scalpel handle and blades
■ Periosteal elevator

■ Small scissors (sharp–sharp Metzenbaum and iris scissors are ideal)
■ Synthetic, monofilament absorbable suture material, 1 metric (5/0 USP)
■ Fine needle holders
■ Small rat-toothed tissue forceps (Adsons)
■ Suture cutting scissors.

Maintenance of instruments and power equipment

When dropped, dental explorers and periodontal probes inevitably bend. Attempts at straightening them may result in their breakage and they should therefore be replaced. Spare periodontal probes and explorers should be kept in case of emergency and replaced as necessary.

The dental unit, handpieces and instruments require daily, weekly, monthly and annual maintenance to ensure that they continue operating at optimum performance. The dental unit will have instructions and, possibly, a service agreement unique to it. It is recommended that the manufacturer's maintenance guidelines are strictly adhered to. It is essential to drain the compressor storage tank of condensation at the end of each day. This reduces rusting of the tank.

Handpieces need to be oiled regularly prior to autoclaving and again before use. Over-lubrication can be as detrimental as under-lubrication and the manufacturer's instructions should be followed. The handpiece should always be re-attached and run at high-speed to flush excess lubricant from the turbine, so that this is not sprayed into the mouth of the animal.

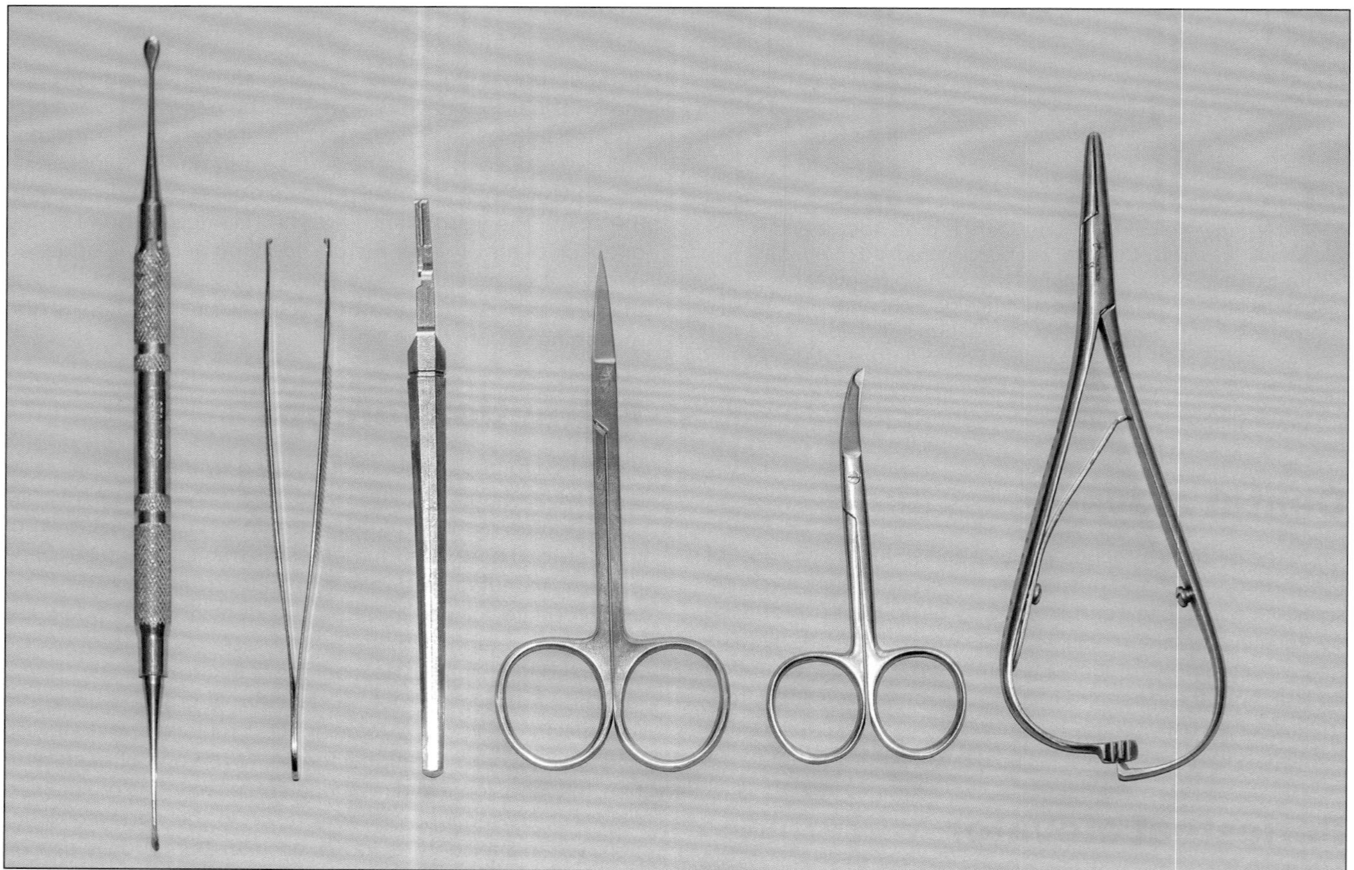

25.27 A surgical kit adequate for raising mucoperiosteal flaps. From the left: periosteal elevator; fine rat-toothed forceps; No. B3 scalpel handle; iris scissors; suture scissors; and comfortable needle holder able to accommodate fine suture material needles. (© Cedric Tutt)

Sharpening instruments

Hand instruments need to be cleaned, sterilized and sharpened. Sharpening these instruments regularly not only increases their useful life but also prevents injuries to the patient and operator due to instrument slippage.

- Hand scalers are sharpened by placing the blade of the scaler on a flat sharpening stone (Figure 25.28a). Using the fourth finger as a guide on the table surface to keep the instrument at the correct angle to the sharpening surface, it is drawn towards the operator in a pull-stroke. Both sides must be sharpened.
- Dental hand curettes are sharpened by holding the instrument in the palm grip with the curette tip projecting from the back of the hand. A sharpening stone is held in the other hand, applied to the curette blade and drawn across it in an arc to accommodate the slight curvature of the cutting edge (Figure 25.28b).
- Luxators are sharpened on the concave surface. The instrument should be placed on a conical or cylindrical sharpening stone that is held firmly on a solid surface and then pushed along the stone (Figure 25.28c). This sharpens the tip without forming a 'bur' on the convex side.
- Dental elevators are sharpened on a flat sharpening stone. The convex side of the instrument is applied to the stone at the correct inclination (Figure 25.28d) and the instrument is sharpened using a back-and-forth wrist motion. Some elevators are sharpened by engaging the cutting surface with a flat sharpening stone and gently applying a push-stroke (Figure 25.28e).

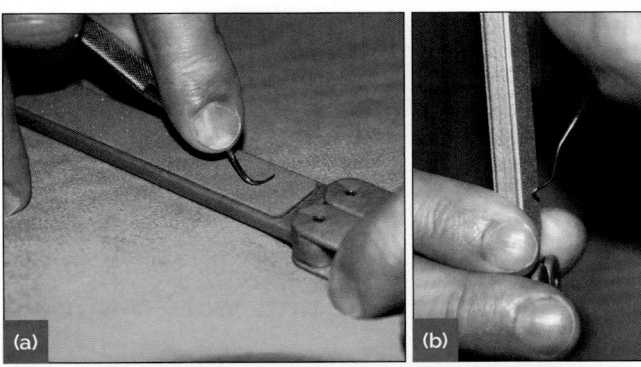
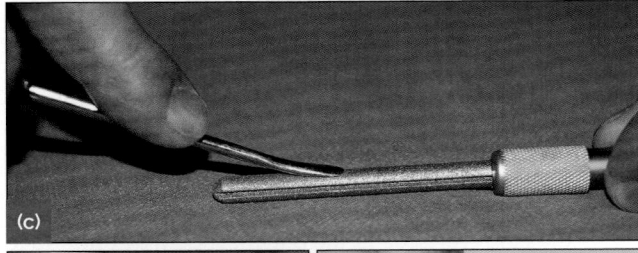
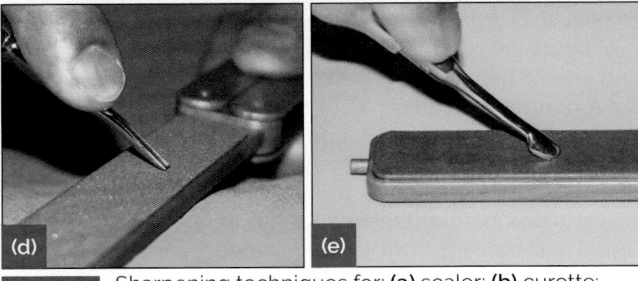

25.28 Sharpening techniques for: **(a)** scaler; **(b)** curette; **(c)** Luxator®; **(d)** elevator and **(e)** winged elevator. (e, © Cedric Tutt)

Health and safety considerations

Dental operating room

The dental operating room should not share airspace with the surgical preparatory room, sterile procedures room or theatres, due to aerosolized plaque and bacteria generated during the dental procedure.

Some dental materials contain solvents and for this reason the dental operating room should be well ventilated. Ideally it should have an air extraction system that discharges the air outside so that it does not re-enter the building via the clean air supply.

There must be sufficient light in the room, which may be supplemented by an additional light source directed on to the work area. The operating light should not be excessively brighter than the room light or a dazzle effect will be experienced.

Operator and assistant

To reduce fatigue, both the operator and the assistant should be seated, with the patient, instruments and anaesthetic equipment all within easy reach during the dental procedures.

Safety spectacles must be worn by the operator and assistant to prevent injury to the eye from flying debris or a fractured high-speed bur. The high-speed bur rotates at approximately 400,000 rpm and will travel at an enormous speed if it fractures. Spectacles also prevent splatter and aerosolized material from landing in the eye. Safety spectacles must be kept on at all times as this will allow them to warm up to body temperature and not to fog.

Integrated face mask/face shield devices may also be used to protect the operator and assistant from aerosols generated during dental procedures. Surgical (not paper) face masks must be worn by the operator and assistant and these should be replaced regularly. Once moisture from expired air has condensed in the mask it is no longer an efficient microbial barrier.

Examination gloves should be worn, as should protective clothing. It is also recommended that the veterinary surgeon and nurse wear head coverings.

Instruments

All instruments must be kept sharp to prevent accidents that may occur when blunt instruments slip off the tooth or alveolar bone. Care must be exercised when sharpening and washing instruments and the manufacturer's instructions must be followed. Instruments should be sterilized between patients; chemical sterilization is adequate for disinfection of dental instruments between patients. Sharps must be disposed of correctly (see Chapter 2).

Handling dental instruments

- Correct handling of dental instruments is essential to prevent repetitive strain injury
- Approximately 300 different types of bacteria can be cultured from the mouths of cats and dogs. Adequate disinfection of instruments must be performed between patients

---

Patient safety

The patient should be placed on a soft surface that will maintain its body heat. Covering the patient with bubble wrap will help maintain body temperature. Adequate provision should be made to remove water delivered from dental equipment in order that the animal does not become wet and cold. The patient's face should be protected from the aerosolized bacteria by a towel or drape. An ocular lubricant should be placed in both eyes to prevent desiccation of the corneas and regularly reapplied throughout the dental procedure.

Scaling and polishing

Tooth scaling and polishing is performed routinely in patients that have slight calculus and mild gingivitis or may be required in the treatment of patients suffering from periodontal disease or in preparation for tooth extraction.

Intubation

Scale-and-polish procedures are performed in animals that are anaesthetized and intubated. The cuff of the endotracheal (ET) tube should be inflated to the correct pressure so as not to cause damage to the trachea or respiratory epithelial lining. Applying a thin layer of sterile water-soluble lubricant will ensure that the ET tube does not adhere to the respiratory epithelium. Inflation of the cuff does not prevent liquid from passing down the trachea and so it is important to keep the mouth lower than the pharynx, enabling liquids to flow from the mouth. It is good practice to place a pharyngeal pack into the pharynx to trap calculus and other debris and prevent blood from accumulating around or passing by the ET tube.

The cuffed ET tube ensures that anaesthetic gases are confined to the anaesthetic circuit and disposed of via the scavenging system. It also prevents the anaesthetized animal from inhaling aerosolized bacteria, plaque and calculus.

Scaling

Prior to scaling the teeth, the oral cavity should be flushed with chlorhexidine, as this has been shown to significantly reduce aerosolized bacteria.

After the mouth has been examined and charted, gross calculus can be removed from the teeth using calculus forceps, as described earlier. The remaining calculus can then be removed using hand or electromechanical scalers. When using electromechanical scalers, the scaler tip must be applied side-on to the crown surface (Figure 25.29). If the calculus is tenacious, the operator should move on to an adjacent tooth before returning to complete scaling on the first tooth. This will prevent iatrogenic damage to the tooth by heating. Electromechanical scalers should be applied to the calculus using a brush-stroke technique without applying downward force against the tooth. If the scaler tip is pushed against the tooth, resulting in less vibration, the efficiency of scaling is decreased. Some scaler tips vibrate in an orbital pattern, whilst others oscillate in a linear manner. Knowledge of the scaler tip oscillation pattern will help the operator to use the instrument effectively.

- The point of the ultrasonic scaler tip should never be used against the tooth, as it will etch (engrave) the tooth surface.
- Plenty of water coolant should be used to keep the scaler and tooth cool and to flush away debris.

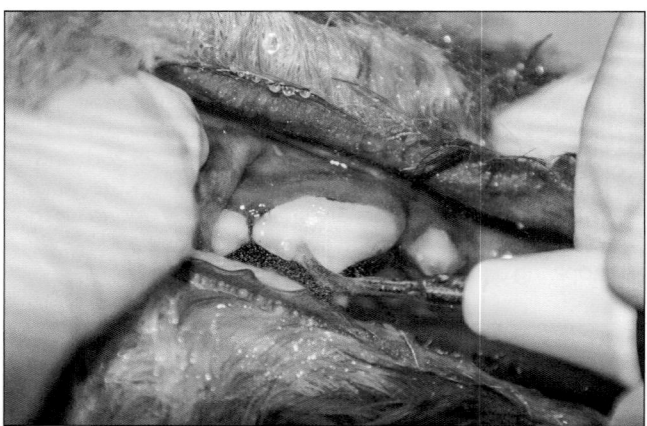

25.29 Piezoelectric scaler being used appropriately with the edge of the scaler tip against the tooth. The scaler should not be in continuous contact with a tooth for >8 seconds to prevent heating of the tooth. (© Cedric Tutt)

Subgingival scaling and root debridement

Short excursions may be made subgingivally to remove calculus; under ideal circumstances a subgingival scaling tip should be used for this to prevent thermal damage to the crown and gingiva. Hand curettes can be used to remove subgingival calculus, and a dental explorer gently circumscribed around the subgingival crown will reveal residual calculus. Where pockets are deep it may be necessary to debride the root surface, using a curette to remove necrotic cementum. In severe cases, the patient should be referred to a specialist veterinary dentist for open root debridement; this procedure involves raising a gingival flap to expose the roots and enable debridement before being sutured back in place.

A curette is used for both subgingival scaling and root debridement. It is inserted into the gingival sulcus; the cutting edge should then be engaged against the tooth surface and the curette pulled in a coronal direction. This should be carried out around the whole circumference of the tooth using overlapping strokes. This procedure also debrides the gingival wall of the pocket. An explorer can then be used to judge the smoothness of the subgingival part of the tooth. Care must be exercised not to denude the root of cementum, as this will expose the dentine and may lead to dentinal hypersensitivity. Cementum is required for re-attachment of the periodontal ligament and must be preserved as far as possible.

Polishing

Polishing removes the remaining plaque that is usually not visible and helps to smooth the roughened tooth surface. If the tooth has been scaled it must be polished, as minor scratches left on the tooth after scaling facilitate plaque retention due to the roughened surface. Polishing does not render the enamel surface completely smooth but does make it less plaque retentive. To minimize the amount of frictional heat generated, the prophylaxis cup or brush, used in a low-speed contra-angle handpiece, should not rotate faster than 1000 rpm. Some prophylaxis cups oscillate (Figure 25.30a) rather than rotate, generating less frictional heat during polishing. In addition, large volumes of prophylaxis paste should be used as it acts as a lubricant during polishing. Using paste and a rubber cup, the tooth surfaces can be polished. When gentle pressure is exerted on the prophylaxis cup against the tooth surface, it flares and can pass under the gingival margin to remove subgingival plaque (Figure 25.30b). 'Prophy' brushes can also be used, although those made of nylon filaments may strip cementum from the root when polishing subgingivally, resulting in dentinal hypersensitivity.

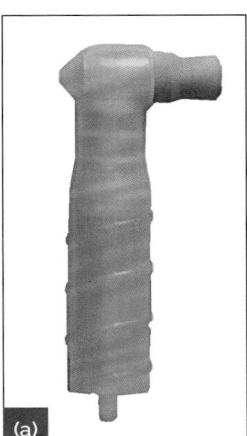 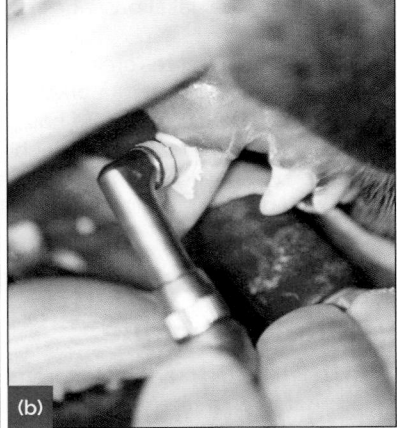

25.30 (a) Reciprocating polisher head. (b) The 'prophy' cup should be gently pressed on to the tooth to flare out and polish the tooth surface, as well as subgingivally. (a, © IM3 Pty Ltd)

Radiography of teeth and supporting structures

It is essential to take radiographs when performing veterinary dentistry, as the extent of pathology cannot be seen without them (see Chapter 16). Whereas the clinical examination enables visualization of the tooth crown, radiography reveals the root, which can make up about 75% of the length of the tooth in deciduous canines. Radiographs also show the extent of bone loss in periodontitis and periapical pathology in teeth with inflamed or necrotic pulps.

Indications for radiography

- Missing teeth
- Retained (subgingival/alveolar) teeth
- Fractured teeth
- Supernumerary teeth (to determine association with adjacent normal teeth)
- Mixed dentition
- Prior to extraction
- Monitoring treatment progress (e.g. when retrieving root remnants)
- Teeth affected by caries
- Differentiating teeth with tertiary dentine from those that may have exposed pulps
- Teeth affected by periodontal disease
- Persistent deciduous teeth
- Discoloured teeth
- Teeth affected by resorption
- Jaw fractures
- Investigation of sinus tracts that may be associated with teeth
- Investigation of nasal discharge
- Investigation of oral masses

Good technique is vital; for the radiograph to be diagnostic it must be an accurate representation of the tooth and associated structures. It is therefore best practice to use intraoral digital dental radiography.

X-ray generators

Medical X-ray machines

Although cumbersome and usually fixed to the wall or floor in one room, medical X-ray machines (described in detail in Chapter 16) can be used to take diagnostic dental radiographs. The focus–film distance should be adjusted to approximately 40 cm, either by lowering the X-ray tube head or by placing the patient on an object on top of the X-ray table. The kV should be set at 70 and the mAs at 15–25, depending upon the size of the patient. If dental X-ray film is not available, mammography film can be used to good effect but superimposition of structures may be problematic. Using mammography film in flexible cassettes will eliminate superimposition. Medical computed radiography (CR) and direct radiography (DR) systems can be used to obtain digital radiographs.

Dental X-ray machines

A dedicated dental-specific X-ray machine has numerous advantages:

- The machine can be installed in the dental operating area (thus the anaesthetized animal does not need to be transported from the dental room to the radiography room each time a radiograph is required)
- The machine can be manoeuvred around the animal
- Cylindrical collimators of a fixed length, reducing scatter radiation (Figure 25.31)
- Using a dedicated dental X-ray machine frees up the radiography room to be used for other patients.

Dental X-ray machines can be attached to a wall (Figure 25.32a), suspended from the ceiling, on castors so they can be wheeled or portable and hand-held (Figure 25.32b). Dental

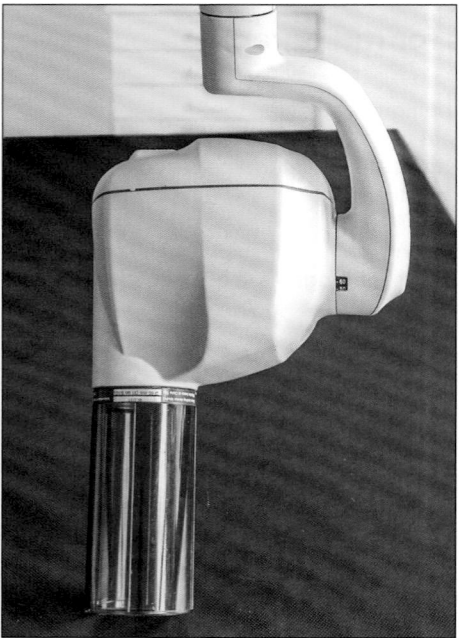

25.31 A cylindrical collimator is the best choice for dental radiography as it can be manoeuvred around the animal and produces less scatter radiation. (© Cedric Tutt)

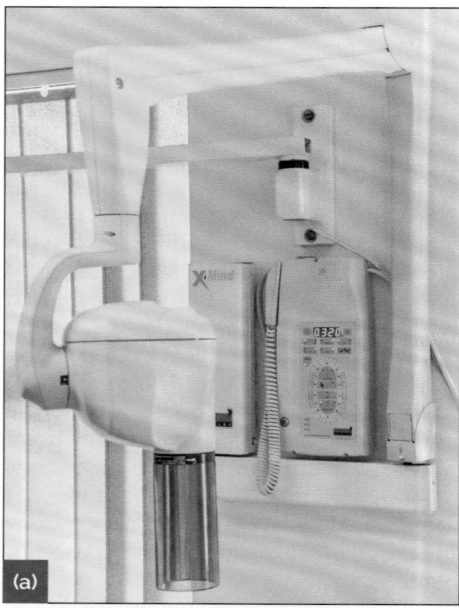

(a)

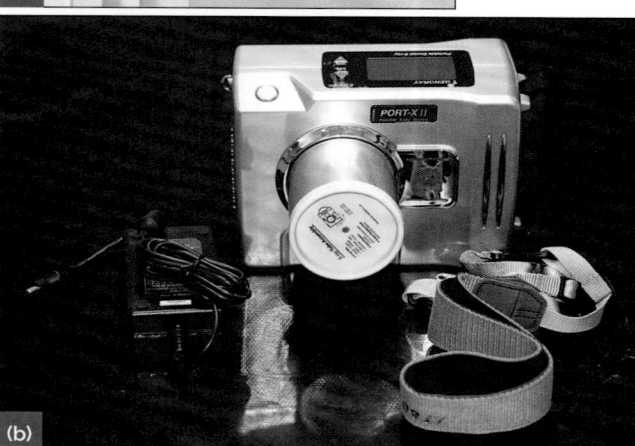

(b)

25.32 (a) Dental X-ray machine mounted to a wall.
(b) Portable dental X-ray machine. (© Cedric Tutt)

X-ray generators usually have a fixed kV and mA, with time being the only adjustable setting on most machines. Modern dental X-ray machines have a fixed kV of 60–80 and mA of 2–8. Time can be adjusted from 0.1 to about 2 seconds. The hand-held portable units have a kV of 60 to 75 and mA of 2.

Dental operating room

The dental room should be planned in such a manner that the X-ray machine can be discharged from outside to improve safety for the operator and assistant. The machine may be discharged from outside by depressing a button mounted on the wall or remotely using an extension cable. The door to the dental operating area should be lead-lined, with a window permitting constant observation of the patient. Radiation safety advice should be sought before investing in a portable machine.

Dental imaging plates and transducers

Dental X-ray CR plates are available in a number of sizes. The most commonly used in veterinary dentistry are:

- Adult periapical film: 3 x 4 cm (#2)
- Occlusal film: 5 x 7 cm (#4)
- Paediatric periapical film: 2 x 3.5 cm (#1)
- Size #0 is useful in small cats
- Sizes #5 and #7 are preferred in large dogs and for examining the nasal passages of large dogs.

The dental CR plates are packed in impervious envelopes that have a clear side and a black back to protect the plate from ambient light. Each plate has a radiolucent triangle (or the letters 'cr') in one corner, which allows the image to be oriented for viewing. Some CR plate manufacturers make plates suitable for intraoral radiography in lagomorphs.

Intraoral techniques

Parallel technique

This is used for the mandibular premolars and molars caudal to premolar 2 in the dog (including this tooth in some animals). The patient is positioned in lateral recumbency and the film is placed adjacent to the tooth or teeth to be radiographed (between the tongue and the mandible) and pushed ventrally so that it becomes palpable beyond the ventral margin of the mandible (Figure 25.33). A piece of scrunched-up paper towel can be used to keep the film in the correct position. The incident beam is then directed at right angles to the long axes of the tooth and film. The tooth and film are parallel to each other and the incident beam is directed perpendicular to both.

Bisecting angle technique

This technique is used when taking radiographs of the maxillary teeth and the incisors, premolars 1 and 2 and canines in the mandible. The film is placed as close as possible to the tooth or teeth to be radiographed. When maxillary teeth are radiographed, the film spans the palate or is placed on the incisal tips of the canines (Figure 25.34). The tooth axis (an imaginary line joining the tip of the crown and the root tip) is determined and the angle formed by this line and the film axis is bisected. The incident beam is directed

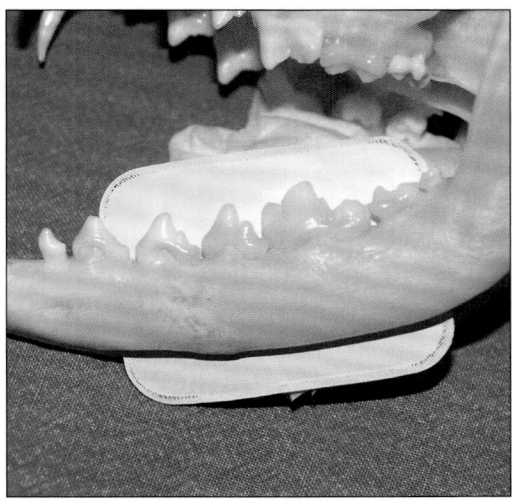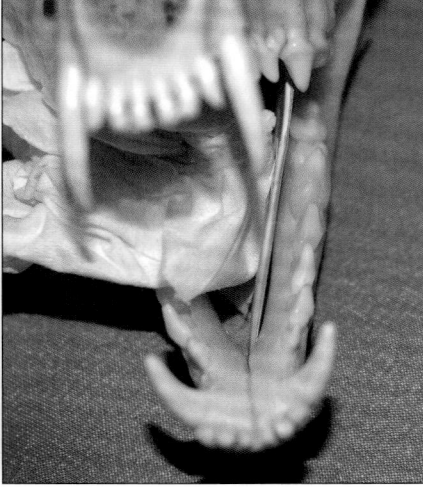

25.33 For the parallel technique, the film is placed between the tongue and teeth/mandible so that the film protrudes past the ventral margin of the mandible. The film should be parallel to the teeth and the incident beam directed perpendicular to the teeth and film.

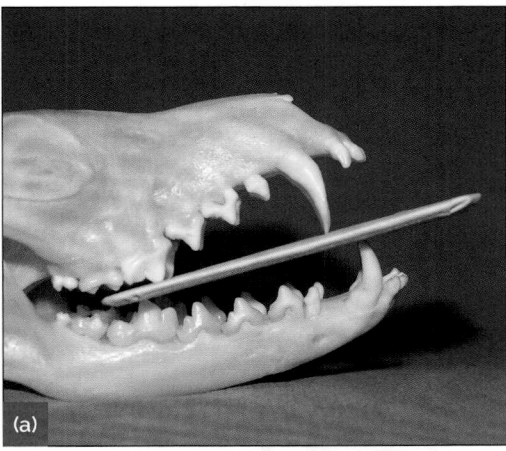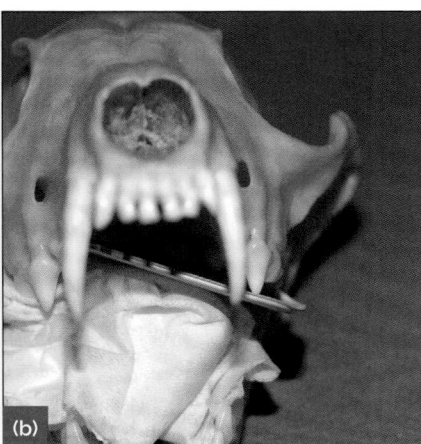

25.34 For the bisecting angle technique, the film is placed as close to the teeth as possible. **(a)** Film positioned for imaging the maxillary incisors including a rostrocaudal view of the maxillary canines. **(b)** Film positioned for imaging maxillary premolars and molars.

perpendicular (at right angles) to the bisecting line, giving a true representation of the tooth on the radiograph. If the incident beam is close to perpendicular to the film axis, the tooth will appear short and the image is termed foreshortened. If the beam is close to perpendicular to the tooth axis, the resultant image will be lengthened and termed elongated.

When radiographing the maxillary carnassial tooth, which has three roots (two mesially (towards the dental arch midline) and one distally), the mesial roots are often superimposed on each other. To separate these roots on the radiograph, the incident beam must be directed from either rostrally or caudally (maintaining the same bisecting angle). On the resultant image the SLOB (Same Lingual Opposite Buccal) rule is used to identify which root is which. Using the SLOB rule, if the incident beam is directed from rostrally the most rostral of the mesial roots will be the palatal root. If the incident beam is directed from caudally, the more caudal of the mesial roots will be the palatal root and the more rostral of the mesial roots will be the buccal root.

Incident beam technique

To overcome the difficulty many people experience with three-dimensional (3D) perception (which makes determining the bisecting line difficult), the incident beam technique can be used to position the X-ray machine and obtain diagnostic radiographs. The CR plate is placed in the mouth, as it

would be for the bisecting angle technique, and the film axis is extrapolated out of the mouth to form an angle with the tooth axis. This angle is divided by the line along which the incident beam is to travel (Figure 25.35).

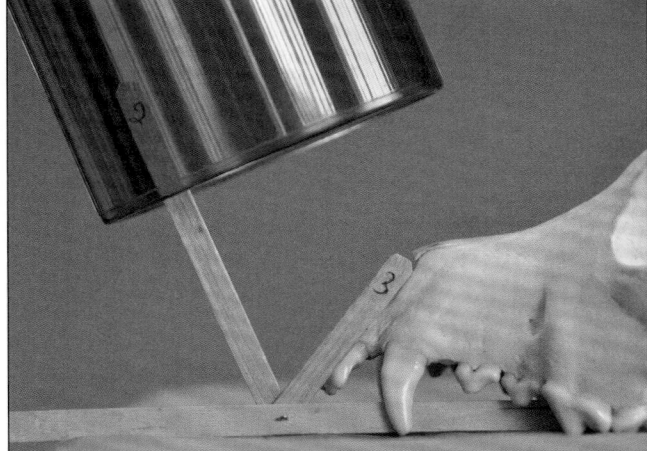

25.35 For the incident beam technique, the film is placed in the mouth as for the bisecting angle technique (see Figure 25.34). The film axis is then extrapolated out of the mouth to form an angle with the tooth axis. The extraoral angle is bisected and this is the line along which the incident beam will travel. (© Cedric Tutt)

Positioning the patient

It may be helpful to position the patient as follows:

- Sternal recumbency for the maxillary incisors
- Lateral or sternal recumbency for the maxillary canines, premolars and molars
- Dorsal recumbency for the mandibular incisors
- Dorsal or lateral recumbency for the mandibular canines
- Lateral recumbency for the mandibular premolars and molars.

When radiographing the maxillary carnassials of a cat, superimposition of the zygomatic arch presents a problem. Lifting the cat's nose or tilting its head in order that the upper dental arch is parallel to the table helps to prevent this superimposition.

Digital dental radiography

Veterinary practices are increasingly investing in digital dental radiographic technology. There are two main digital radiographic systems:

- Direct (direct radiography, DR)
- Indirect (computed radiography, CR).

The direct system uses a digital sensor (Figure 25.36) that is placed in the mouth in the same way as intraoral film. The tooth/teeth are exposed and the image appears on the computer screen within seconds. The sensor may be attached to the computer via a docking station and USB cable, or transmit the captured information via Bluetooth technology. At present, there is a limited selection of transducer sizes, some of which are bulky, making their use in smaller dogs and cats challenging.

Using the indirect system (CR) (Figure 25.37), phospho-stimulable plates (within protective envelopes) are placed in the mouth in the same way as intraoral film and the tooth/teeth exposed in the usual way. The exposed plate is then placed in a laser reader (Figure 25.38), which converts the phosphorescent image into a digital image that is viewed on a computer screen. This system takes slightly longer than the direct system but has a wide range of plate sizes and currently delivers a higher resolution image.

Digital radiographs can be enhanced in a number of ways to help produce a clearer image: brightness, contrast, reverse-image, 3D, measurement and magnification can all be altered. Digital radiographs can be appended to the patient record and also emailed to a colleague for a second opinion.

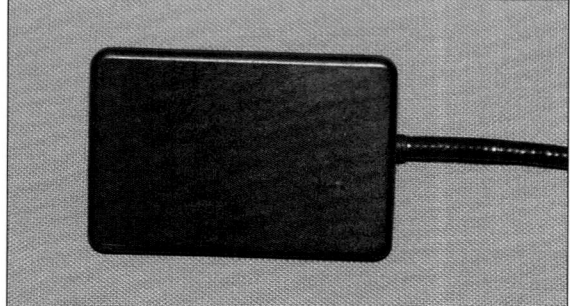

25.36 This transducer is used to take digital dental radiographs using the direct technique. The image is displayed almost immediately on a computer screen.

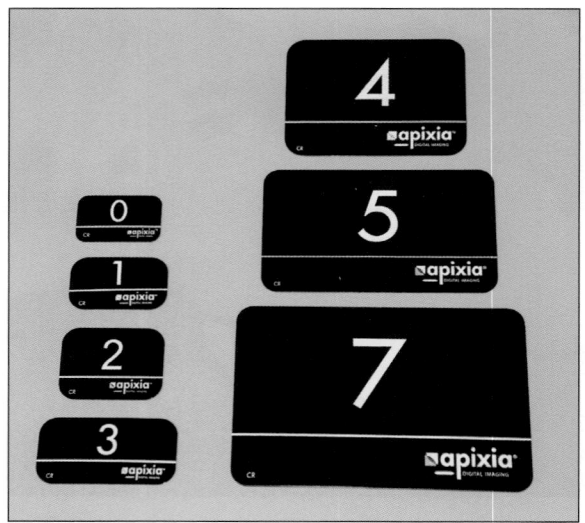

25.37 Examples of high resolution intraoral dental CR plates used in the indirect radiographic system. Sizes shown are: 0, 1, 2, 3, 4, 5 and 7. Each image plate has to be placed in a protective envelope during the exposure. (© Cedric Tutt)

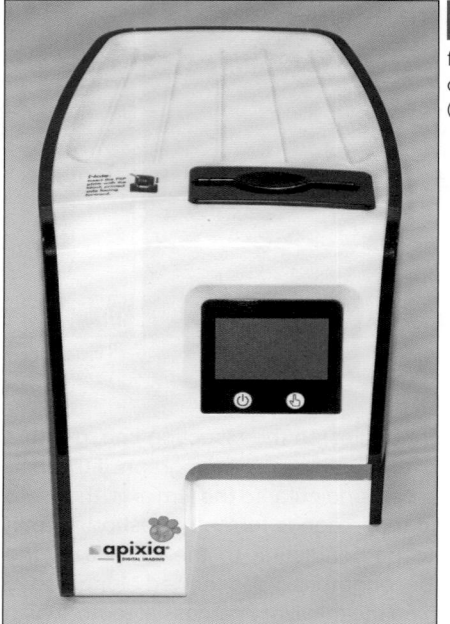

25.38 Plate reader for computed dental radiography. (© Cedric Tutt)

Maintenance of dental health and prevention of dental disease

Disease prevention is vital in the maintenance of dental and oral health. As mentioned above, approximately 85% of dogs and cats >3 years of age suffer from early signs of periodontal disease, probably making dental disease the most common condition seen in general veterinary practice. Periodontitis almost exclusively follows on from gingivitis, a reversible condition; consequently, its control is within reach. Treating gingivitis prevents most cases of periodontitis.

In the minority of cases, as a result of periapical pathology (secondary to necrotic pulp), periodontitis may spread along the root surface in the periodontal space and eventually surface in the gingival sulcus. In these cases gingivitis may be secondary to the periapical lesion, called an endodontic–periodontic lesion.

The causes of gingivitis are discussed above. The treatment is routine dental scale-and-polish followed by thorough dental homecare.

Dental homecare

This consists of daily tooth brushing, feeding an appropriate diet, providing dental chews and encouraging play with tooth-friendly toys. Tooth brushing is the most important of these routines. As veterinary patients cannot be taught to brush their own teeth, owners must be relied upon to institute and continue dental homecare. Thus, an essential part of professional periodontal therapy is client education. Oral antiseptic agents, such as chlorhexidine gluconate, have also been shown to help prevent gingivitis.

Pet owners must be made aware that, whatever professional treatment is performed, it is only part of the ongoing therapy. Plaque begins to accumulate on tooth surfaces within 24 hours of a scale-and-polish procedure. Where homecare is not implemented, gingivitis scores 3 months after professional periodontal therapy (supra- and subgingival scaling and polishing) have been found to be the same as those prior to treatment. The aim of dental homecare is to minimize the accumulation of plaque and therefore reduce the risk of periodontal disease developing or progressing. Continuous monitoring of dental homecare is essential, to keep owners motivated and to check on the adequacy of the oral hygiene carried out. Nurse-led clinics should be instituted during which plaque-disclosing solution may be applied to the pets' teeth and gums to show how effective the dental homecare is.

Tooth brushing

Tooth brushing is the most effective method of removing plaque from the pet tooth surfaces at home. Daily tooth brushing can return the gingivae to health, but this will not be maintained if carried out less than daily. In addition, an animal may require professional periodontal therapy at regular intervals, just as some people need to visit the dentist or dental hygienist on a more regular basis. Some animals are more predisposed to plaque accumulation and hence regular professional treatment may be required despite conscientious thorough dental homecare.

The success of plaque control by tooth brushing depends on the owner's ability and the animal's cooperation. Owners should therefore start brushing their pet's teeth as early in its life as possible. Even the youngest puppies and kittens can have their teeth brushed. The primary dentition will be exfoliated but the animal will have become accustomed to the tooth brushing process by the time the secondary dentition has erupted. It is important to brush kittens' teeth, as it is particularly difficult to introduce adult cats to the process.

Most young animals will tolerate tooth brushing as it is begun when the gingivae are healthy and the procedure is not associated with pain (which can lead to a negative response). Pets that have their teeth brushed regularly enjoy increased intervals between professional dental treatments. Tooth brushing (Figure 25.39) should be introduced as part of the daily routine. A treat or a walk can be the reward at the end of a tooth brushing session. In multi-pet households, the added individual attention appears to appeal to pets and they will queue to have their turn.

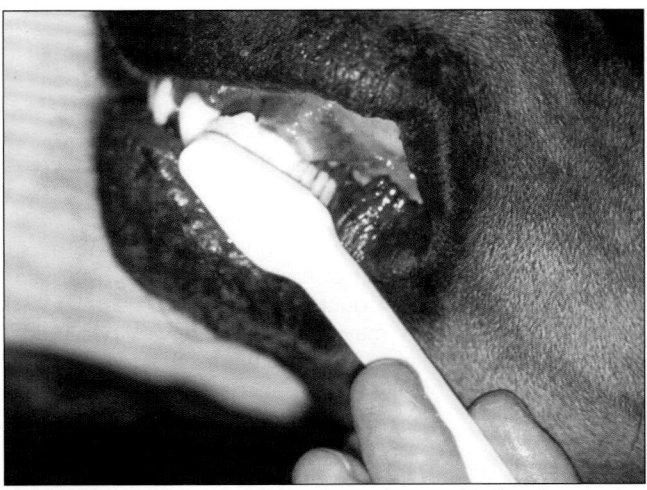

25.39 A medium toothbrush can be used to brush a dog's teeth. Pet toothpaste must be used as human toothpaste contains a foaming agent and fluoride which can cause toxicity.

Tooth brushing procedure

- Put the animal at ease: make sure it is comfortable (sitting on your knees, on the floor, or on a table as it prefers). Stroke it frequently to reassure it. You may prefer a second person to assist you with this
- Apply the toothpaste to the brush, pushing it down into the filaments so that the animal cannot lick it off
- Introduce the brush into the cheek and start brushing the molars and premolars and brush a few teeth each day until eventually all the teeth can be brushed in one session
- Gentle circular motions are used to brush the teeth and gingival margin
- Using a circular movement with the brush at an angle of 45 degrees near the gingival margin, the filaments of the brush can be made to flare slightly into the gingival sulcus, removing subgingival plaque

---

Toothbrushes and toothpaste

A medium texture human toothbrush with rounded filaments can be used (or medium child's toothbrush) in both dogs and cats. Human toothpaste must never be used, due to the high fluoride content, which can cause toxicity when pets swallow it rather than rinsing and spitting. Human toothpastes also usually contain a detergent that causes foaming, a sensation apparently disliked by animals. Pet toothpastes are available in a variety of flavours and, although not essential, help to familiarize the pet with the tooth brushing process.

Initially it is acceptable to concentrate on brushing the buccal surfaces of the maxillary teeth by placing the toothbrush in the animal's cheek, but eventually it is advisable to open the mouth to brush the lingual/palatal surfaces as well. When the mouth is opened slightly, the mandibular carnassial teeth will be exposed and can also be brushed. It may take longer for the animal to become accustomed to this, so incorporating rewards may be beneficial.

In patients with periodontal disease, the gums will bleed when tooth brushing is first instituted. The owners should be informed that this will happen and that they should continue brushing gently. As the gingivae return to health there will be less bleeding, until brushing does not elicit any bleeding at all.

Diet, chews and toys

There are numerous diets formulated to be tooth friendly. Some have a structure that ensures that the food is chewed mechanically cleaning the tooth surface. Other diets contain minerals that prevent mineralization of plaque to calculus by binding with calcium.

Some dental chews contain enzymes that prevent calculus formation with or without a physical cleansing effect (the Veterinary Oral Health Council (www.vohc.org/) maintains a list of accepted products for dogs and cats).

Tooth-friendly toys may have a 'window-wiper blade' effect or have projections that clean the tooth surface. Some also dispense toothpaste as the animal plays with the toy (Figure 25.40).

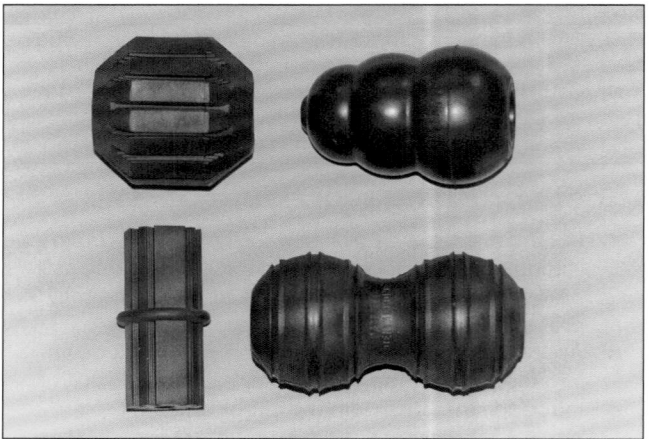

25.40 A selection of rubber toys (Kong®) suitable as tooth-friendly toys. (© Cedric Tutt)

Bones and hooves

Dry bones, hooves and antlers should not be fed as they cause tooth fractures and other trauma to the oral cavity.

Uncooked bones that have a high proportion of spongy bone are fed in some countries without tooth fractures being reported.

Dentistry in rabbits and rodents

Definitions

- **Brachyodont** – short crown:root ratio with a true root. The mature tooth has a closed root apex (e.g. humans, dogs, cats, ferrets and cheek teeth of some rodents
- **Hyposodont** – tooth with a long crown and comparatively short or no true root. The subgingival part is called the reserve crown. The dentition or part thereof may be radicular or aradicular:
  - Radicular hyposodont – true tooth root develops later in the life of the animal (e.g. horses, cattle)
  - Aradicular hyposodont – tooth never forms a true root with an apex, and continues to grow throughout life (e.g. rabbits, hares, guinea pigs, chinchillas and incisors of rats and mice).

Normal dentition

Rodents have aradicular hypsodont incisors and either aradicular hypsodont or brachyodont cheek teeth. Rodents have only one pair of upper and lower incisors. Guinea pigs and chinchillas have aradicular hypsodont dentition, whilst rats and mice have aradicular hypsodont incisors and brachydont cheek teeth.

Lagomorphs (hares and rabbits) have aradicular hypsodont dentition. They have four incisors in the maxillae in two rows, two large central incisors labially and two peg teeth palatally. They have no canine teeth. The incisor teeth grow at a rate of about 2 mm per week.

The teeth of rabbits, hares, chinchillas and guinea pigs grow continuously. An abrasive diet, such as grass supplemented with hay, keeps the teeth worn to a physiological length. Commercial mixes, whilst providing a nutritionally balanced diet, do not provide the wear required for dental health and thus should be fed sparingly.

In lagomorphs, the incisors are in occlusion (touching each other) at rest and the cheek teeth are apart. This is in contrast to rodents, where the cheek teeth are in occlusion at rest and the incisors are apart. Rodents gnaw with their incisors, whereas lagomorphs use their incisors in a sideways cutting action. As with many other species, the jaws of rabbits and rodents are anisognathic (upper and lower jaws of unequal length and width). In rabbits the mandibular arcades are narrower than the maxillary arcades, while in guinea pigs the mandibular arch is wider than the maxillary arch (Figure 25.41).

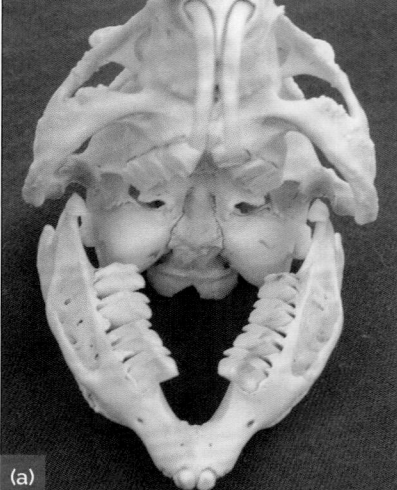

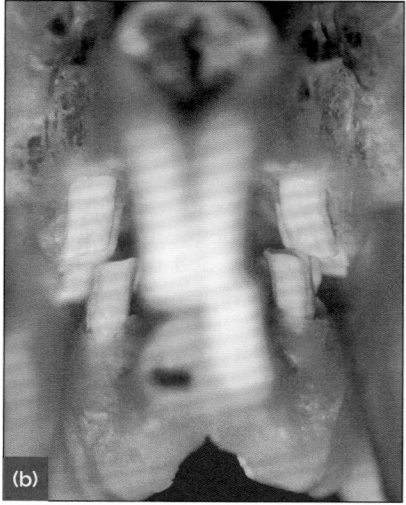

25.41 **(a)** Guinea pig skull, showing mandibular cheek teeth arch set wider apart than maxillary cheek teeth arch. **(b)** Rabbit skull, showing mandibular cheek teeth arch set narrower than maxillary cheek teeth arch.

Malocclusion

This is the most common presentation of dental disease. It may be caused by:

- Incorrect diet leading to lack of wear and tooth overgrowth
- Congenital deformity of the maxillae – seen most commonly in brachycephalic rabbits (e.g. dwarf rabbits)
- Tooth or mandibular trauma
- Tooth apex infection
- Neoplasia.

Incisor malocclusion

Incisor malocclusion may be primary or secondary. In brachycephalic breeds the malocclusion is primary, as a result of the maxillae being short and the mandibular incisors consequently protruding rostrally.

Secondary incisor malocclusion occurs in animals whose diet lacks fibre, resulting in cheek tooth overgrowth. As the cheek teeth do not undergo normal wear, they come into occlusion, and the force of occlusal contact causes the jaws to be pushed apart and the mandibular incisors to lose occlusal contact with the maxillary incisors and protrude rostrally. The maxillary incisors may come to occlude on the lingual surface of the mandibular incisors, causing them to curl back into the mouth and in severe cases they may impinge on or penetrate the palate.

Maloccluding incisors cannot prehend food. Rabbits that chew in one direction (normally they will chew clockwise and anticlockwise alternately) develop an inclination in the occlusal surfaces of the incisor teeth. Clinical signs include anorexia and weight loss, lack of grooming, grinding of the teeth and slobbering (wet chin and neck). Treatment involves tooth trimming or in some cases incisor extraction. When the incisors are completely out of occlusion and protruding from the mouth they should be extracted as they are no longer functional but rather obstruct cheek tooth function.

Cheek teeth malocclusion

This may occur as a result of one of the factors listed above. An important cause of the acquired condition is abnormal tooth wear. Rabbit cheek teeth erupt at about 1 mm per week and if normal wear does not occur the cheek teeth develop sharp spikes. The mandibular cheek teeth form sharp spikes that protrude lingually and can lacerate the tongue, whilst the maxillary cheek teeth develop spikes that protrude buccally often lacerating the cheeks. Spikes can be so long that they entrap the soft tissues.

When the overgrowing cheek teeth come into occlusion, the force exerted by the opposing cheek teeth prevents normal tooth eruption, resulting in retrograde eruption of the teeth into the mandibles and maxillae. This causes periosteal pain. Irreversible changes occur if the growth tip penetrates the jaw and the ventral mandibular margin or the orbit is perforated. Swellings may be palpated on the upper and lower jaws. Retrograde eruption of maxillary cheek and incisor teeth may cause obstruction of the nasolacrimal duct, leading to lacrimation and/or dacryocystitis. This may progress to tooth root-associated abscessation and osteomyelitis.

Selective feeding may be the initial clinical sign, progressing to anorexia, weight loss, excessive salivation and difficulty in eating. Signs of pain include slobbering (wet chin and neck), teeth grinding, aggression and depression. An animal with tooth root abscessation will present with facial swelling, by which time the prognosis is grave. Diagnosis is confirmed by lateral intra- or extraoral radiographs of the patient's jaws, and the condition can be monitored by dental radiography.

Analgesia is essential. If the ventral mandibular margin and the orbit are intact, recreating the normal occlusal surfaces is advised. Following treatment, the normal abrasive diet of fresh grass or hay (less effective than fresh grass) should be fed to help prevent recurrence. Commercial mixes do not provide the tooth wear required.

Regular weighing is an ideal method of monitoring patients that may be affected by this form of dental disease. A 5% reduction in body mass is a good indication of dental disease. Owner education is essential.

Chinchillas are often presented with advanced dental disease and euthanasia may be the only option. Radiographs should be taken to confirm the diagnosis and aid in treatment planning or the decision to euthanase the animal.

Guinea pigs are often presented with cheek teeth overgrowth to the extent that the premolars bridge the tongue, limiting its function. The tongue of a guinea pig has both a movable and an attached part. The jaw configuration of the guinea pig is different to that of the rabbit – the mandibles are at a wider angle than the maxillae and, therefore, the mandibular cheek teeth overlap the maxillary cheek teeth in the normal animal.

Tooth trimming

Teeth should not be clipped, as the uneven pressure applied to the tooth surfaces can cause the tooth to crack or shatter. Clipping can cause damage to the periapical tissues, affecting future tooth growth, or fissures may be produced, leading to periodontal problems and pulp infection. In addition, sharp edges occur, leading to oral discomfort.

The incisors are effectively trimmed using a high-speed dental fissure bur (diamond or tungsten carbide). This can be performed in the conscious animal if it is properly restrained. Care should be exercised to prevent thermal damage to the teeth. While trimming and reshaping is performed, the soft tissues should be protected by placing a tongue depressor or empty syringe case behind the incisors. The cheek teeth can be trimmed using a long-shank fissure bur in a soft tissue protective shroud or using an acrylic trimming bur. Cheek teeth are trimmed when the animal is anaesthetized. Care must be exercised to ensure the soft tissues are kept well away from the rotating instruments or severe, extensive trauma may result.

Extraction of maloccluding incisor teeth should be performed by a veterinary surgeon experienced in the technique.

Lagomorphs and rodents undergoing dental treatment should be treated with analgesics to relieve existing and postoperative pain and discomfort. Gut motility modifiers are useful in animals that have been anorexic and fluid administration is also indicated.

Equipment

Equipment for lagomorph and rodent dentistry includes the following (Figure 25.42):

- High-speed handpiece and fissure burs
- Low-speed straight handpiece with acrylic, diamond or long-shank fissure bur
- Cheek dilator
- Oral speculum
- Cheek protector
- Cheek tooth luxator
- Incisor luxator

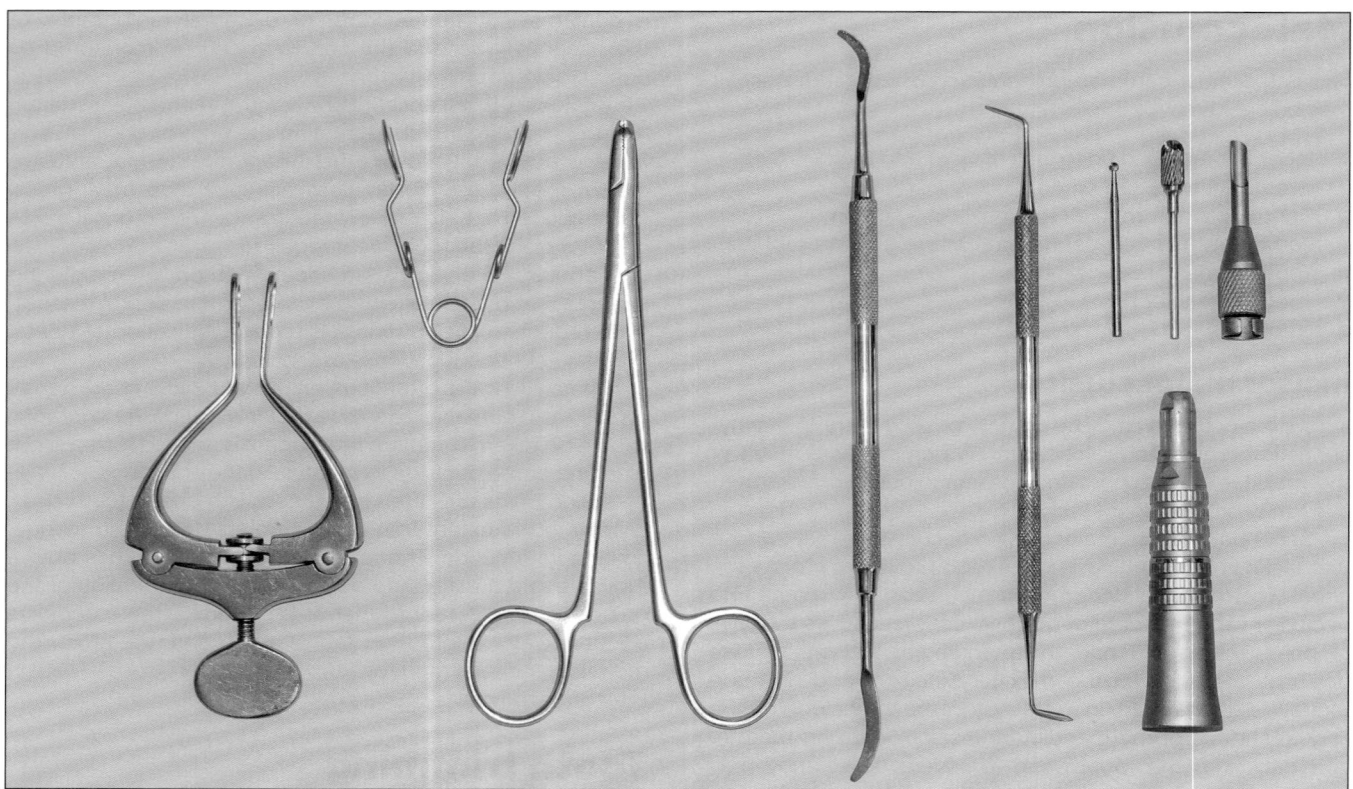

25.42 Rabbit dental kit. From left: mouth opener; cheek dilator; cheek teeth extraction forceps; incisor luxators; cheek tooth luxator; straight surgical round bur; acrylic bur for shortening cheek teeth; soft tissue guard and below straight low-speed handpiece. (© Cedric Tutt)

- Molar extraction forceps
- Good light source
- Cotton buds to remove tooth dust from the mouth.

It should be noted that damage to the temporomandibular joint (TMJ) capsules may occur if the mouth is opened excessively using the oral speculum. Using sprung mouth gags is not recommended as they keep the TMJs under continuous tension.

References and further reading

Capello V (2005) *Rabbit and Rodent Dentistry Handbook.* Zoological Education Network, Florida

Gorrel C, Andersson S and Verhaert L (2013) *Veterinary Dentistry for the General Practitioner, 2nd edn.* Elsevier, St Louis

Harcourt-Brown F and Chitty J (2013) *BSAVA Manual of Rabbit Surgery, Dentistry and Imaging.* BSAVA Publications, Gloucester

Holmstrom S (2018) *Veterinary Dentistry: A Team Approach, 3rd edn.* Elsevier, St Louis

Reiter AM and Gracis M (2018) *BSAVA Manual of Canine and Feline Dentistry and Oral Surgery, 4th edn.* BSAVA Publications, Gloucester

Tutt C (2006) *Small Animal Dentistry: A Manual of Techniques.* Blackwell Publishing, Oxford

Useful websites

British Veterinary Dental Association:
www.bvda.co.uk

Veterinary Oral Health Council:
www.vohc.org/

Self-assessment questions

1. Describe the dental formula of a kitten.
2. Describe the dental formula of an adult dog.
3. Explain the incident beam technique used to radiograph most teeth in dogs.
4. List the abbreviations used during charting.
5. The upper and lower jaws of rabbits and guinea pigs are of unequal size. What term describes this phenomenon and what is the difference between rabbits and guinea pigs?
6. Describe periodontitis. How does it differ from gingivitis?
7. Describe why scaling a tooth with an ultrasonic scaler for more than 8–10 seconds continuously is detrimental to the tooth.
8. Why should the tip of an ultrasonic scaler not be applied at right angles (perpendicular) to the tooth surface?
9. Formulate a dental homecare programme for a 6-week-old Golden Retriever puppy.
10. List the advantages of using a reciprocating polisher head.

Some common breeds

Dogs

The Kennel Club website (www.thekennelclub.org.uk) lists seven Dog Groups. Individual breeds, with their own specified Breed Standards, are placed within these groups. The heights listed below are taken from the Kennel Club Breed Standards.

Gundog group Includes: English Setter, Labrador Retriever, Cocker Spaniel, Weimaraner

Golden Retriever

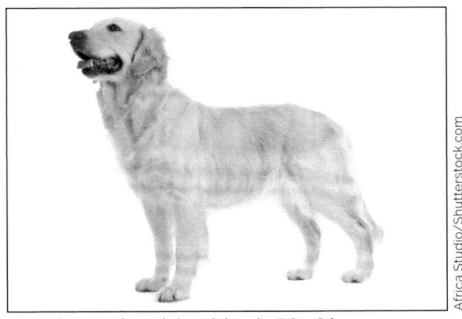

Height at shoulder (dog): 56–61 cm
Height at shoulder (bitch): 51–56 cm

Gordon Setter

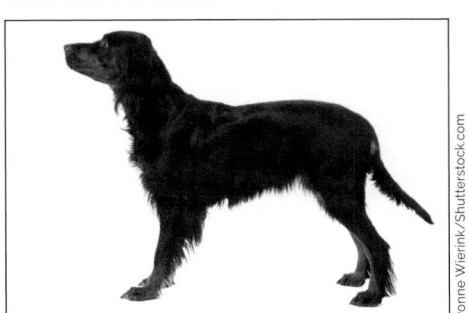

Height at shoulder (dog): 66 cm
Height at shoulder (bitch): 62 cm

Hound group Includes: Afghan Hound, Beagle, Whippet, Wire-haired Dachshund

Finnish Spitz

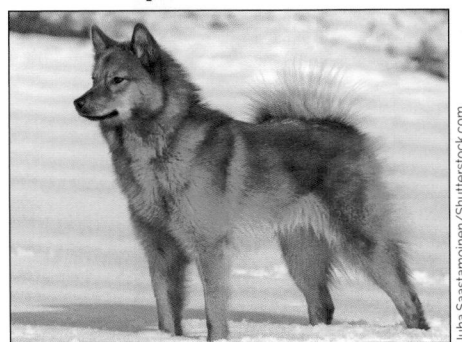

Height at shoulder (dog): 43–50 cm
Height at shoulder (bitch): 39–45 cm

Irish Wolfhound

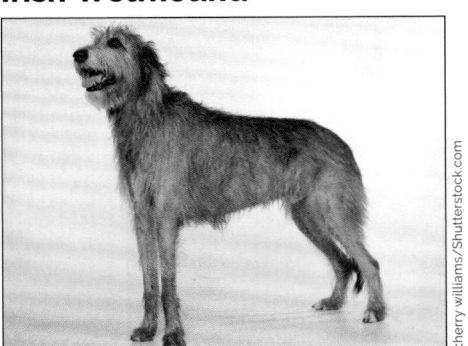

Height at shoulder (dog): ≥79 cm
Height at shoulder (bitch): ≥7 1cm

Pastoral group Includes: Border Collie, Old English Sheepdog, Pembroke Welsh Corgi

Border Collie

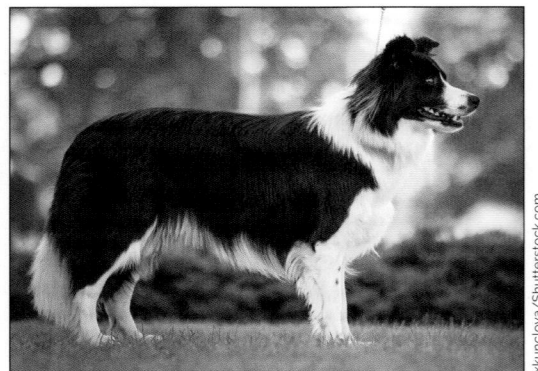

xkunclova/Shutterstock.com

Height at shoulder (dog): 53 cm
Height at shoulder (bitch): slightly less than 53 cm

German Shepherd Dog

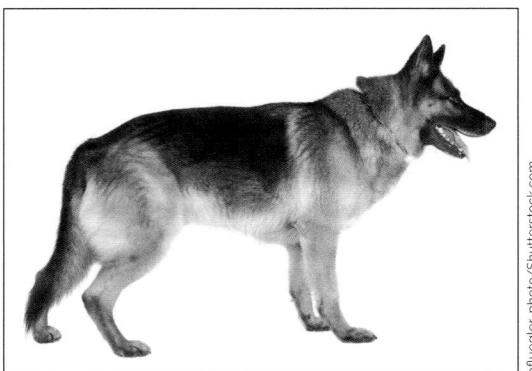

pfluegler-photo/Shutterstock.com

Height at shoulder (dog): 60.5–65.5 cm
Height at shoulder (bitch): 55.5–60.5 cm

Terrier group Includes: Bedlington Terrier, Norfolk Terrier, West Highland White Terrier

Cairn Terrier

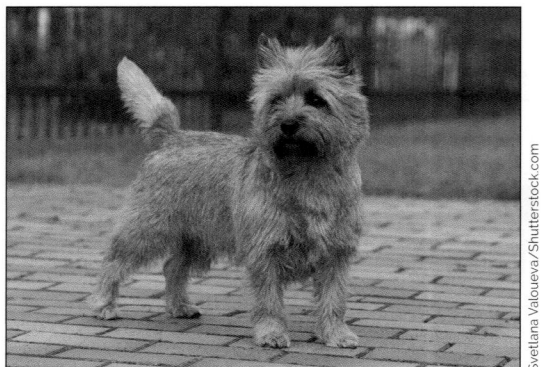

Svetlana Valoueva/Shutterstock.com

Height at shoulder (dog): 28–31 cm
Height at shoulder (bitch): 28–31 cm

West Highland White Terrier

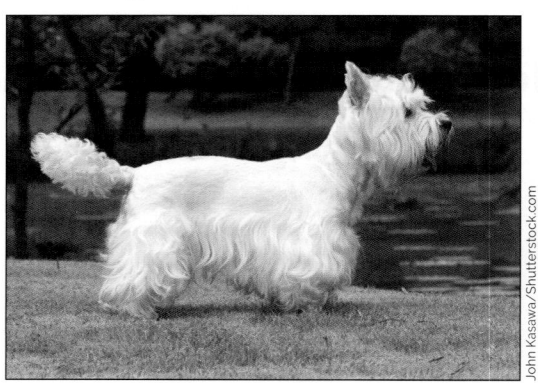

John Kasawa/Shutterstock.com

Height at shoulder (dog): approximately 28 cm
Height at shoulder (bitch): approximately 28 cm

Toy group Includes: Bichon Frise, Cavalier King Charles Spaniel, Yorkshire Terrier

Bichon Frise

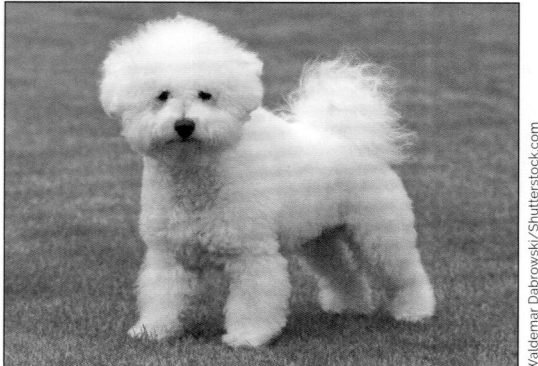

Waldemar Dabrowski/Shutterstock.com

Height at shoulder (dog): 23–28 cm
Height at shoulder (bitch): 23–28 cm

Papillon

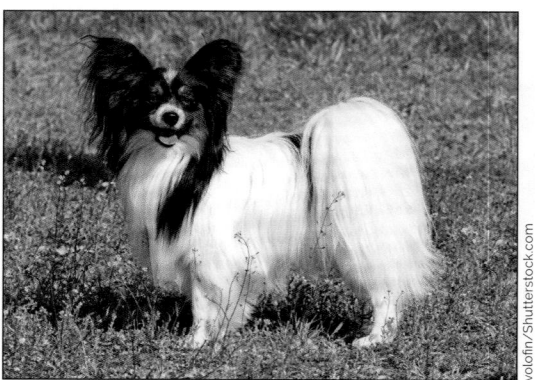

volofin/Shutterstock.com

Height at shoulder (dog): 20–28 cm
Height at shoulder (bitch): 20–28 cm

Utility group Includes: Chow Chow, Dalmatian, Shuh Tzu, Standard Poodle

Dalmation

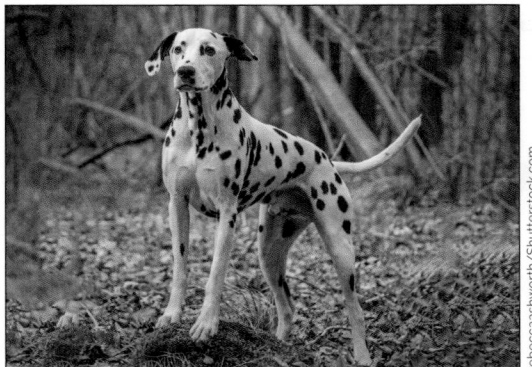

Height at shoulder (dog): 58–61 cm
Height at shoulder (bitch): 56–58 cm

Shar Pei

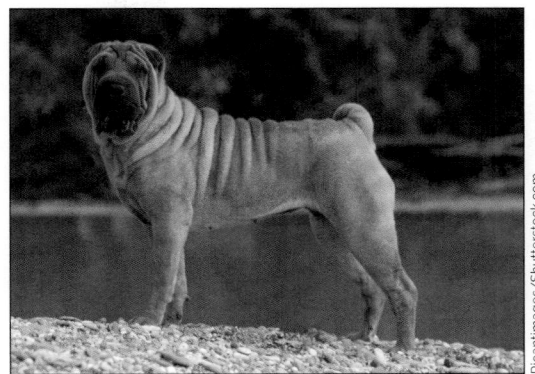

Height at shoulder (dog): 46–51 cm
Height at shoulder (bitch): 46–51 cm

Working group Includes: Boxer, Mastiff, Great Dane, Newfoundland, St Bernard

Alaskan Malamute

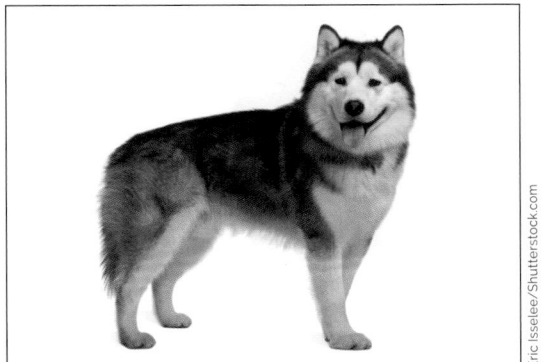

Height at shoulder (dog): 64 cm
Height at shoulder (bitch): 58 cm

Great Dane

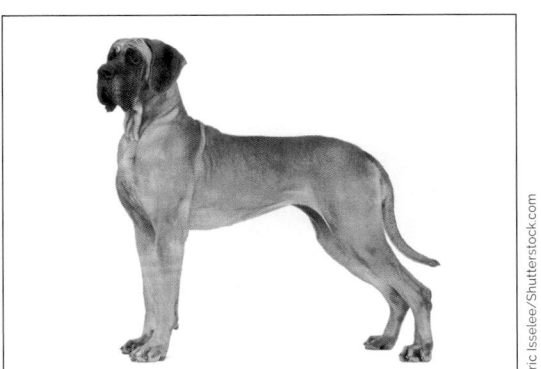

Height at shoulder (dog): ≥76 cm
Height at shoulder (bitch): ≥71 cm

Cats

The weights listed below are taken from the Governing Council of the Cat Fancy website (www.gccfcats.org/Cat-Breeds).

Abyssinian

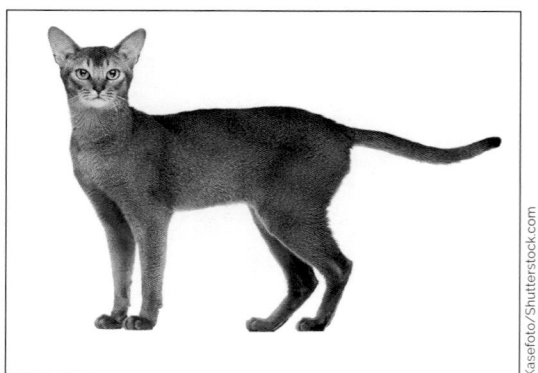

Average weight (male): 4.5 kg
Average weight (female): 4.5 kg

Bengal

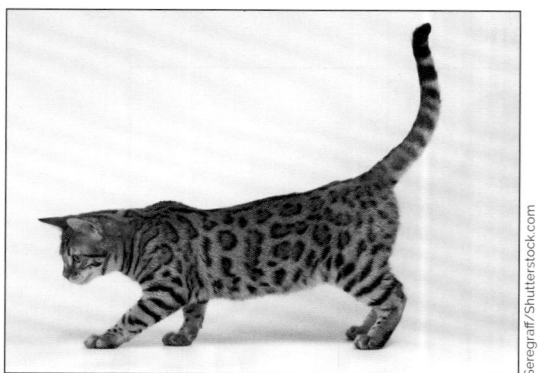

Average weight (male): 4.5–6.8 kg
Average weight (female): 3.6–5.4 kg

Birman

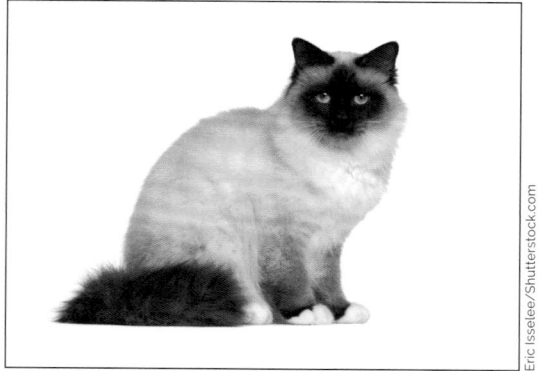

Average weight (male): 4.5–6.8 kg
Average weight (female): 2.7–4.5 kg

British Shorthair

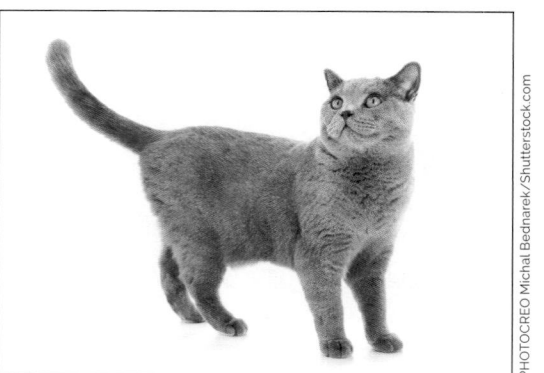

Average weight (male): 4.1–7.7 kg
Average weight (female): 3.2–5.4 kg

Burmese

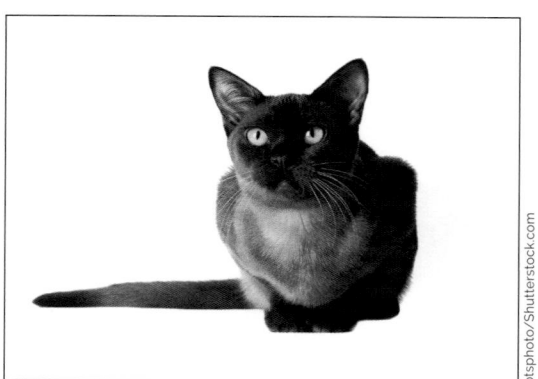

Average weight (male): 5–6.4 kg
Average weight (female): 2.7–4.1 kg

Cornish Rex

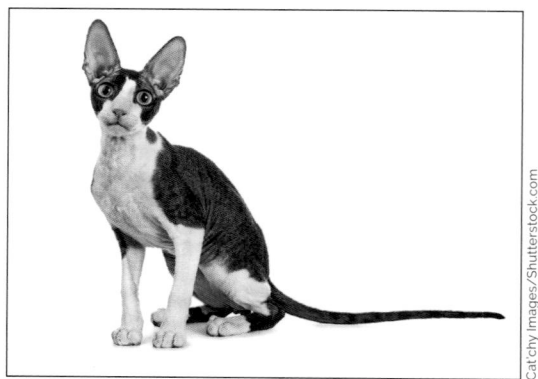

Average weight (male): 3.6–4.5 kg
Average weight (female): 2.3–3.2 kg

Maine Coon

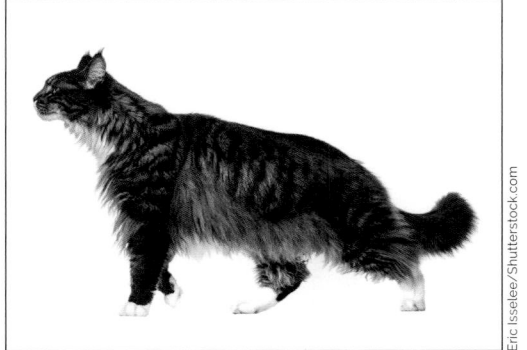

Eric Isselee/Shutterstock.com

Average weight (male): 4.5–8.2 kg
Average weight (female): 3.2–5.4 kg

Siamese

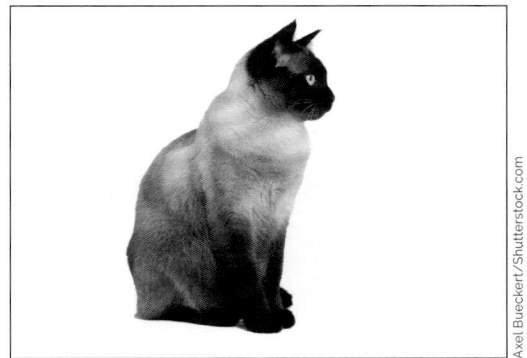

Axel Bueckert/Shutterstock.com

Average weight (male): 4.5–6.8 kg
Average weight (female): 3.6–5.4 kg

Oriental

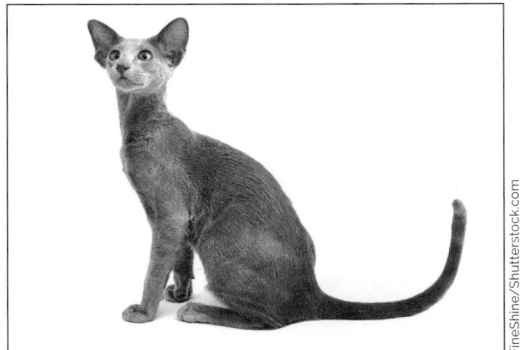

FineShine/Shutterstock.com

Average weight (male): 3.6–6.4 kg
Average weight (female): 3.6–6.4 kg

Sphynx

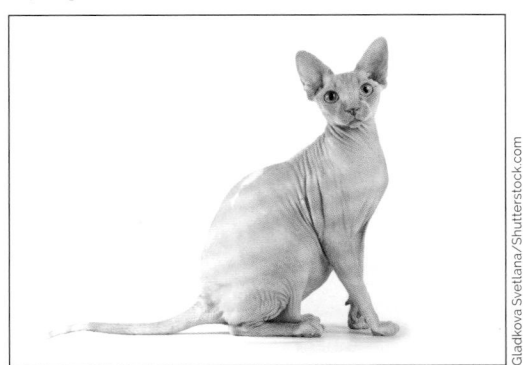

Gladkova Svetlana/Shutterstock.com

Average weight (male): 3.6–5 kg
Average weight (female): 2.7–3.6 kg

Persian

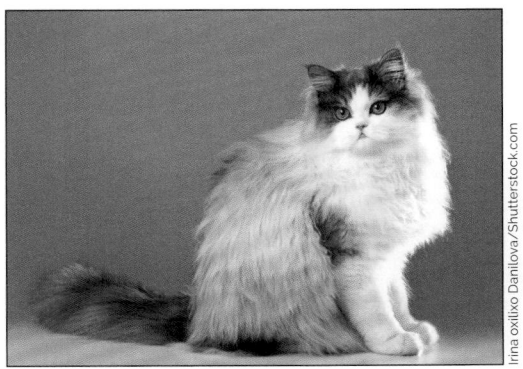

Irina oxilixo Danilova/Shutterstock.com

Average weight (male): ≥5.4 kg
Average weight (female): 2.7–5.4 kg

Turkish Van

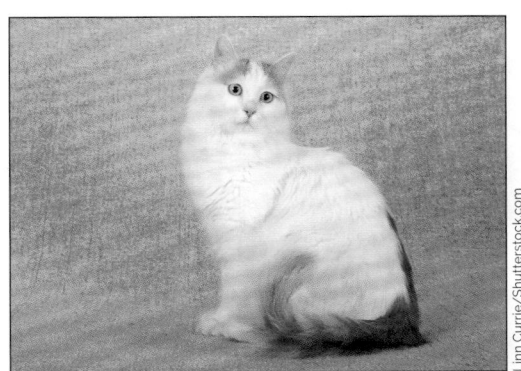

Linn Currie/Shutterstock.com

Average weight (male): 4.5–9 kg
Average weight (female): 3.2–5.4 kg

Rabbits

The weights listed below are taken from the British Rabbit Council Breed standards (www.thebritishrabbitcouncil.org/standards.htm).

Angora

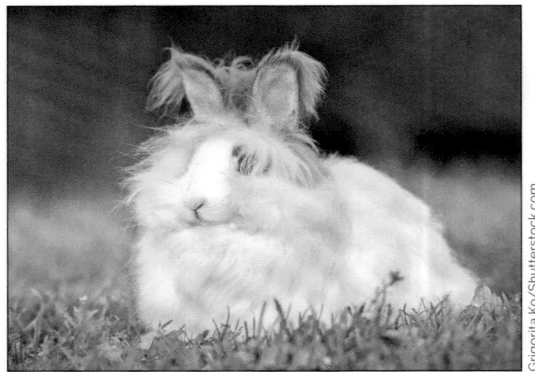

Maximum weight: 3.4 kg

English

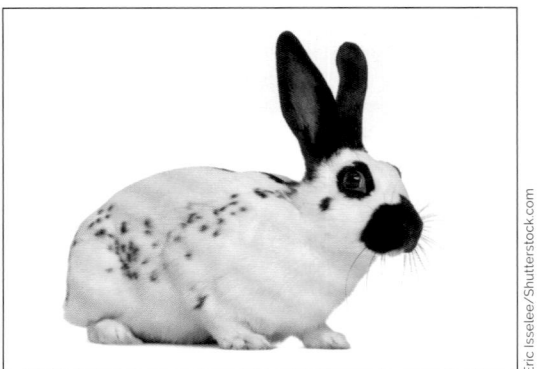

Average weight: 2.72–3.63 kg

Castor Rex

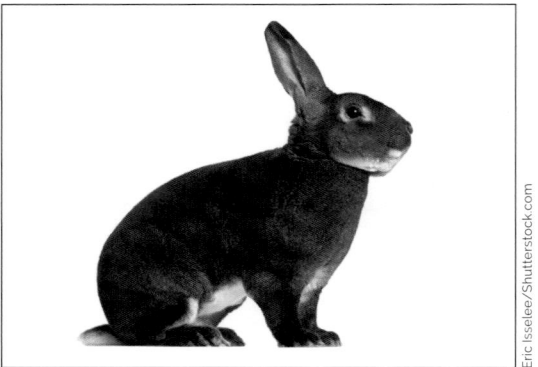

Average weight: 2.72–3.62 kg

Flemish Giant

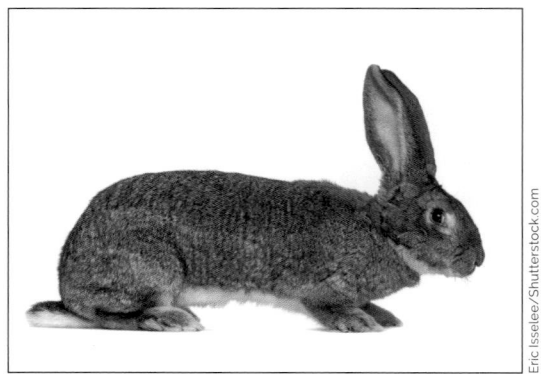

Minimum weight (buck): 4.97 kg
Minimum weight (doe): 5.44 kg

Dutch

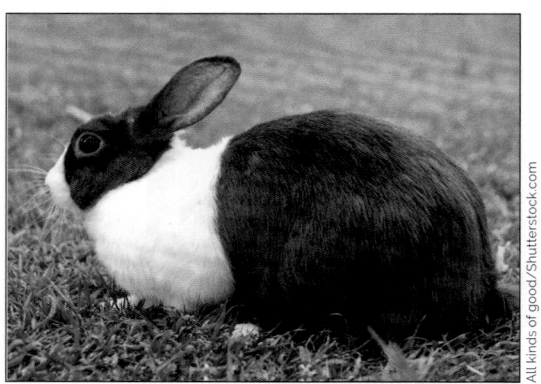

Average weight: 2.04–2.26 kg

French Lop

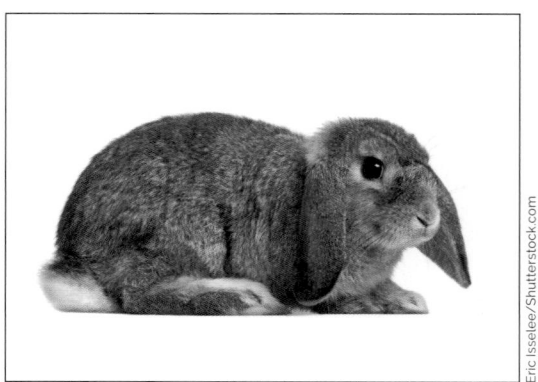

Minimum weight: 4.54 kg

Lionhead

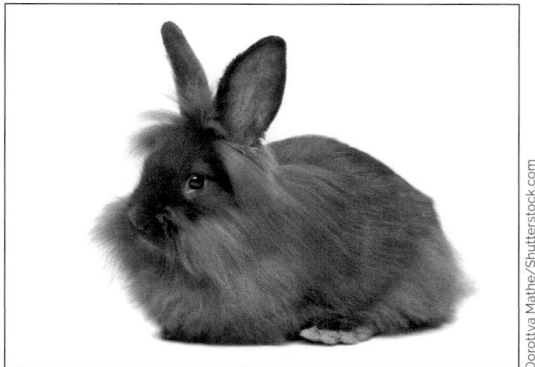

Average weight: 1.36–1.7 kg

New Zealand White

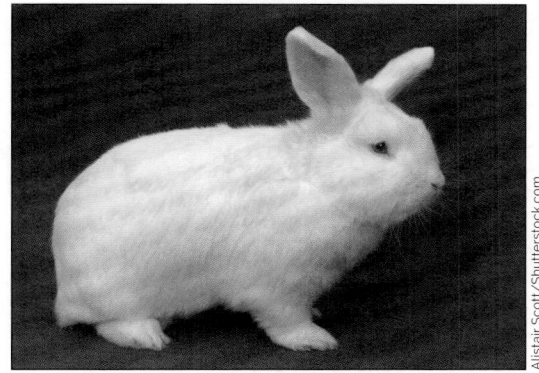

Average weight (buck): 4.08–4.99 kg
Average weight (doe): 4.53–5.44 kg

Miniature Lop

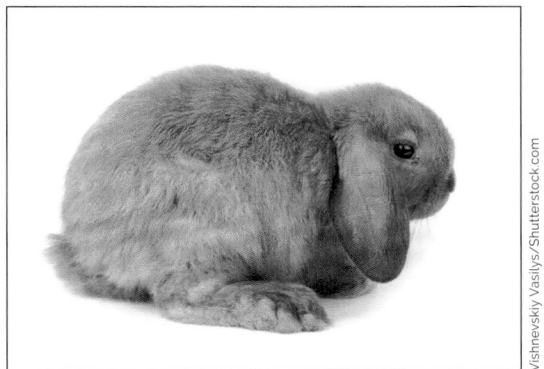

Average weight: 1.5–1.6 kg

Netherland Dwarf

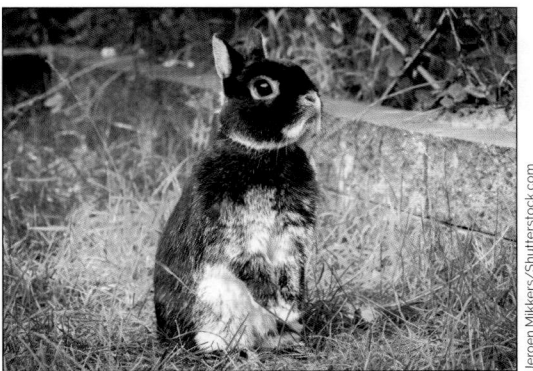

Maximum weight: 1.13 kg

A summary of normal parameters in dogs, cats and rabbits

Parameter	Normal range	Comments	
Dogs			
Body temperature	38.3–39.2°C	Depends on individual physiology and environmental effects	
Pulse/heart rate	70–140 beats/min	Depends on individual physiology and excitement/stress	
Respiration rate	10–30 breaths/min	Depends on individual physiology and excitement/stress	
Water intake	40–60 ml/kg/day	Depends on individual physiology	
Urine production	24–48 ml/kg/day	Depends on intake	
Cats			
Body temperature	38.2–38.6°C	Depends on individual physiology and environmental effects	
Pulse/heart rate	100–200 beats/min	Depends on individual physiology and excitement/stress	
Respiration rate	20–30 breaths/min	Depends on individual physiology and excitement/stress	
Water intake	40–60 ml/kg/day	Depends on individual physiology	
Urine production	24–48 ml/kg/day	Depends on intake	
Rabbits			
Body temperature	38.5–40.0°C	Depends on individual physiology and environmental effects	
Pulse/heart rate	130–325 beats/min	Depends on individual physiology and excitement/stress	
Respiration rate	30–60 breaths/min	Depends on individual physiology and excitement/stress	
Water intake	50–150 ml/kg/day	Very variable	
Urine production	12–48 ml/kg/day	Very variable	

BSAVA Textbook of Veterinary Nursing, sixth edition. Edited by Barbara Cooper, Elizabeth Mullineaux and Lynn Turner. ©BSAVA 2020

Conversion tables

Biochemistry

	SI unit	Conversion	Conventional unit
Alanine aminotransferase	IU / l	x 1	IU / l
Albumin	g / l	x 0.1	g / dl
Alkaline phosphatase	IU / l	x 1	IU / l
Aspartate aminotransferase	IU / l	x 1	IU / l
Bilirubin	µmol / l	x 0.0584	mg / dl
Calcium	mmol / l	x 4	mg / dl
Carbon dioxide (total)	mmol / l	x 1	mEq / l
Chloride	mmol / l	x 1	mEq / l
Cholesterol	mmol / l	x 38.61	mg / dl
Cortisol	nmol / l	x 0.362	ng / ml
Creatine kinase	IU / l	x 1	IU / l
Creatinine	µmol / l	x 0.0113	mg / dl
Glucose	mmol / l	x 18.02	mg / dl
Insulin	pmol / l	x 0.1394	µIU / ml
Iron	µmol / l	x 5.587	µg / dl
Magnesium	mmol / l	x 2	mEq / l
Phosphorus	mmol / l	x 3.1	mg / dl
Potassium	mmol / l	x 1	mEq / l
Sodium	mmol / l	x 1	mEq / l
Total protein	g / l	x 0.1	g / dl
Thyroxine (T4) (free)	pmol / l	x 0.0775	ng / dl
Thyroxine (T4) (total)	nmol / l	x 0.0775	µg / dl
Tri-iodothyronine (T3)	nmol / l	x 65.1	ng / dl
Triglycerides	mmol / l	x 88.5	mg / dl
Urea	mmol / l	x 2.8	mg of urea nitrogen / dl

Temperature

- To convert Fahrenheit to Celsius: subtract 32, multiply by 5 and divide by 9
- To convert Celsius to Fahrenheit: multiply by 9, divide by 5 and add 32

Haematology

	SI unit	Conversion	Conventional unit
Red blood cell count	10^{12} / l	x 1	10^6 / µl
Haemoglobin	g / l	x 0.1	g / dl
MCH	pg / cell	x 1	pg / cell
MCHC	g / l	x 0.1	g / dl
MCV	fl	x 1	µm³
Platelet count	10^9 / l	x 1	10^3 / µl
White blood cell count	10^9 / l	x 1	10^3 / µl

Hypodermic needles

	Metric	Non-metric
Needle gauge (External diameter)	0.8 mm	21 G
	0.6 mm	23 G
	0.5 mm	25 G
	0.4 mm	27 G
Needle length	12 mm	½ inch
	16 mm	⅝ inch
	25 mm	1 inch
	30 mm	1 ¼ inch
	40 mm	1 ½ inch

Suture material sizes

Metric	USP	
0.1	11/0	
0.2	10/0	
0.3	9/0	
0.4	8/0	
0.5	7/0	
0.7	6/0	
1	5/0	
1.5	4/0	
2	3/0	
3	2/0	
3.5	0	
4	1	
5	2	
6	3	

Appendix 4

Common prefixes and suffixes in veterinary terminology

Prefix	Meaning	Example
a-/an-	without	apnoea (absence of breathing)
ante-	before or in front of	antenatal (before birth)
dys-	difficult or bad	dyspnoea (difficult/laboured breathing)
ecto-	outside	ectoparasite (a parasite that lives on the outside of its host)
endo-	inside	endotracheal (inside the trachea)
extra-	outside	extravascular (occurring outside of the vascular system)
haem-	blood	haemolysis (breakdown of blood)
hemi-	half	hemiparesis (weakness in one side of the body)
hyper-	greater	hyperthyroid (with excessive amounts of thyroid hormone)
hypo-	less	hypoglycaemia (low blood sugar levels)
infra-	below	inframaxillary (below the maxilla/upper jaw)
intra-	inside	intravenous (existing or taking place within, or administered into, a vein or veins)
neo-	new or young	neonatal (relating to newborn mammals)
peri-	around	pericardial (around the heart)
poly-	many	polyoestrus (having several oestrus cycles per annum)
post-	after	postpartum (following the birth of young)
pre-	before	preoperative (occurring in the period before a surgical operation)
pro-	forwards	projectile (propelled with force)
pyo-	pus or white blood cells	pyometra (infection of the uterus)
retro-	behind	retrobulbar (situated or occurring behind the eyeball)
sub-	under	subcutaneous (situated or applied under the skin)
super-	over	supernumerary (present in excess of the normal or requisite number)
supra-	above	supragingival (relating to part of the tooth not covered by gingiva)
trans-	across or through	transdermal (route of administration through the skin)
ultra-	Increased or greater than normal	ultrasound (sound waves with frequencies higher than the upper audible limit of human hearing)

Suffix	Meaning	Example
-algia	pain	myalgia (muscle pain)
-centesis	puncture	cystocentesis (needle is placed into the urinary bladder through the abdominal wall of an animal and a sample of urine is removed)
-cyte	cell	leucocyte (white blood cell)
-ectomy	removal of anatomic structure	prostatectomy (surgical removal of the prostate gland)
-emesis	vomiting	hyperemesis (severe or prolonged vomiting)

continues ▶

Suffix	Meaning	Example
-ia	condition	leucopenia (a reduction in the number of white cells in the blood)
-itis	inflammation	urethritis (inflammation of the urethra)
-logy	area of study	nephrology (study of the kidney)
-oma	tumour/mass	haematoma (a solid swelling of clotted blood)
-opsy	examination/inspection	necropsy (a post-mortem examination)
-osis	abnormal condition	proptosis (abnormal protrusion or displacement of an eye or other body part)
-ostomy	to furnish with an opening	pharyngostomy (creation of an opening into the pharynx)
-otomy	surgical incision	cystotomy (a surgical incision into the urinary bladder)
-penia	deficiency	leukopenia (a reduction in the number of white cells in the blood)
-pexy	attach	nephropexy (the surgical fixation of a floating or hypermobile kidney)
-phagia	eating	polyphagia (excessive eating or appetite)
-phobia	dislike or fear	Lipophobia (a chemical property of compounds which means 'fat rejection')
-plasia	formation	neoplasia (presence or formation of new, abnormal growth of tissue)
-rrhoea	flowing	creatorrhea (abnormal excretion of muscle fibre in faeces)

Index

Page numbers in *italics* refer to figures.

Capillaria spp. 166
Capillaries *88*, 89
Capillary refill time (CRT) 359, 645, 720
Capnometry 726–8, 745–6
Capsule history 605
Carbohydrate, dietary 312–13, 318–19, 325
Carbon dioxide absorption, rebreathing systems 709–10
Carcass disposal 45
    anaesthetized patients 737
Carcinoma
    squamous cell 814
    transitional cell 814
Cardiac arrest
    resuscitation 607–9
    signs 607
Cardiac arrhythmias 540–1, 719
    during anaesthesia 734–5
    as emergencies 613–14
    (see also specific arrhythmias)
Cardiac glycosides *208*
Cardiac muscle 75
Cardiac sphincter 101
Cardiac tamponade 538
Cardiogenic shock 611, 646
Cardiomyopathy 538, 540
Cardiopulmonary arrest 607–9, 735–7
Cardiopulmonary resuscitation (CPR) 607–9, *736*, *737*
Cardiovascular system 86–94
    anaesthesia and 670, 672, 702, 719–20, 722–6, 731
    assessment, emergency 602
    disease, nutrition and 326, 328
    drugs 207–8
    emergencies 612–14, 733–5
    opioids and 681
    surgery 828–9
L-Carnitine 318
Carprofen 682, 739
Carpus
    anatomy 68
Carriers of infection 175
Cartilage 60
Cascade, prescribing 217
Castration 833–4, 852
    rabbit, care plan *305–6*
Casts
    for fracture fixation 807–8
    postoperative 764
    in urine sediment 516–17
Cat 'flu 591–2
Cataracts 818
Catgut suture material 773–4
Catheterization
    epidural 689
    intraosseous 652–3
    intravenous
        catheter care 652
        catheter management 424, 606
        complications/contraindications 652
        methods 650–2, 673–4, 738–9, 828
    urinary 396–403
        catheter management 402, 424
        catheter sterilization 784
        catheter types 396–8
        complications 402–3
        equipment for 398–9
        indications 396
        methods 399–402
        for sample collection 512
    wound 690
Catteries 343–5
CEH *see* Cystic endometrial hyperplasia
Cell cycle 125

Cell division
    meiosis 57, 122, 125, 126–7
    mitosis 56–7, 122, 125, 126
Cells
    structure 55–7
    in urine sediment 516
Cellulitis 791
Central nervous system 76–9
    anaesthesia and 672
Central venous pressure (CVP) 645, 725–6
Centrifuges 497–8
Centrosome 56
Cephalic vein injection 198
CEPSAF 729
Cerclage wire 810
Cerebellar hypoplasia 875
Cerebellum 78
Cerebrospinal fluid (CSF) 78–9
    sampling 524
Cerebrum 76
Ceruminous glands 118
Cervix 114
Cestodes 158–62
Chamber induction technique 692
Changing rooms, theatre 752
Chelonians
    anatomy *106*
        intradermal bone 118
        reproductive system 114, 115
    breeding 870–1
    feeding 339
    handling and restraint 286
    injection sites *200*
    parasites *170*
    sexual dimorphism *871*
    venepuncture sites *500*
Chemical disinfectant solutions 782
Chemical indicator strips 780
Chemicals, hazardous 38
Chemosis 654
Chemotherapy 40, 213, 816
Chest
    bandaging 387–8
    drains *828*
    (see also Thorax)
Chews 900
Cheyletiella spp. *153*, 156, *215*
CHF *see* Congestive heart failure
Chiari-like malformation/syringomyelia scheme, BVA/KC 132
Chinchillas
    accommodation 346
    coat care 374
    dental disease 901
    dentition 65, 900
    feeding 336
    handling and restraint 282
    neonatal characteristics *873*
    radiography in 480
    reproductive parameters *869*
Chipmunks
    accommodation 346
    handling and restraint 282
Chiropractics 406–7
Chisels 768, *769*
Chlamydia
    felis 145, *184*, *205*, 591
    psittaci 144–5
Chloramphenicols *203*
Chlorhexidine *755*
Chloride 511
Chocolate agar 526
Cholecystectomy 830
Cholecystokinin 109

Ulcers
  decubital 368, *418*, 421, *422*, 818–19
  eye 817
Ulna 68
Ultrasonography
  equipment 483
  pregnancy diagnosis 861, 862
  principles 482–3
  techniques 483–5
Ultrasound
  dental scalers 889
  examination *see* Ultrasonography
  heart rate/pulse detection 724
  instrument cleaners 771
  therapy 408
Umbilical hernia 836
Umbilicus
  cutting 864, 872
Uncinaria stenocephala 164, *165*
Unconscious patients
  assessment 609–10
Upper airway disease, emergency 614
Upper respiratory tract disease 532–5, *590*, 591–2
Urachus 860
Ureteronephrectomy 831
Ureters
  anatomy 111
  avulsion 831
  ectopic 831
  entrapment 831
  surgery 831–2
Urethra
  anatomy 111
  damage from catheterization *402*
  neoplasia 833
  obstruction 621, 832–3
  rupture 833
  surgery 832–3
Urethritis 790
Urethrography 478
Urethrostomy 833
Uric acid 111
  crystals 517, *518*
Urinalysis *see* Urine
Urinary bladder
  anatomy 111
  manual expression *419*
  radiography 477–8
  rupture 832
  surgery 832
Urinary calculi 560
Urinary catheters *see* Catheterization
Urinary diversion 832
Urinary incontinence *213*, 559, 561, 833
Urinary system
  anatomy and physiology 110–12
  drugs acting on 212–13
  emergencies 621–2
  lower, disease 559–63
  surgery 830–3
Urinary tenesmus 559
Urination
  In critically ill patients 424
  in geriatric patients 412–13
  in neonatal patients 414
  in recumbent patients 419–20
  in soiled patients 417
  in vomiting patients 416
Urine
  analysis
    appearance 362, 514
    chemical tests 515
    microscopic 515–18
    specific gravity 514–15

collection 399, 512–14
formation, physiology of 110–11
output
  monitoring 728
  rates 362, 910
  shock and 612
samples
  collection 512–14
  patient preparation 512
scalding 420, 818–19
Uroabdomen 621
Urodeum 111
Urography 477
Urolithiasis 517, 560
  drugs *213*
  nutrition and 329
Uterus
  anatomy 114
  changes in pregnancy 861
  diseases 850, 851
  inertia 864–5
  prolapse 868
  surgery 835–6
Utilitarianism 15
Uvea 82–3
Uveitis 583, 629–30, 790

Vaccination
  contraception 852
  nursing clinics 256
  principles 182–5
  Schedule 3 5
  vaccines 182–3, 204, *205*
Vacutainers 501, *502*
Vagina
  anatomy 114
  cytology 854–5
  diseases 851
  surgery 836
Vaginitis 790, 851
Vaginoscopy 855
Vaginourethrography 478
Vago-vagal reflex, in lizards 287
Vaporizers 706–7
Vas deferens 113
Vascular access *see* Catheterization, Intravenous injection
Vascular ring anomaly 828
Vasectomy 852
Vasopressin 108, *737*
Vasotocin 109
VDUs *see* Visual display units
Vectors of disease 174–5
Vehicle safety 46
Veins *88*, 89–91
Velpeau sling 390, *391*
Venepuncture sites/techniques 500–1, *664, 665*
Venography, portal 479
Ventilation
  of accommodation 345
  during CPR 608–9
  of patient during anaesthesia 715–16
Ventilators 715–16
Ventricular extra systoles 734
Ventricular system, brain *77*
Ventricular tachycardia *613*, 734
Ventriculus, avian 104
Veress needles 841
Vernier scales 496
Vertebrae 66–7
Vertebral column *see* Spine
Vertebral formulae *67*
Vestibular disease 618–19